Abrams' Angiography

Interventional Radiology

THIRD EDITION

Abrams'
Angiography

Interventional Radiology

THIRD EDITION

Jean-François H. Geschwind, MD

Professor of Radiology, Surgery, and Oncology
Director, Vascular and Interventional Radiology
Johns Hopkins University School of Medicine
Baltimore, Maryland

Michael D. Dake, MD

Thelma and Henry Doelger Professor (III)
Department of Cardiothoracic Surgery
Stanford University School of Medicine
Falk Cardiovascular Research Center
Stanford, California

Wolters Kluwer Health | Lippincott Williams & Wilkins

Philadelphia • Baltimore • New York • London
Buenos Aires • Hong Kong • Sydney • Tokyo

Senior Executive Editor: Jonathan W. Pine, Jr.
Product Development Editor: Amy G. Dinkel
Production Project Manager: David Orzechowski
Senior Manufacturing Coordinator: Beth Welsh
Senior Marketing Manager: Kimberly Schonberger
Senior Design Coordinator: Teresa Mallon
Production Service: S4Carlisle Publishing Services (P) Ltd

Library of Congress Cataloging-in-Publication Data

Abrams' angiography : interventional radiology / editors, Jean-François H. Geschwind,
    Michael D. Dake.—Third edition.
        p. ; cm.
Angiography
Interventional radiology
Preceded by Abrams' angiography / editors, Stanley Baum, Michael J. Pentecost. 2nd ed. c2006.
Includes bibliographical references and index.
ISBN 978-1-60913-792-2 (hardback)
I. Geschwind, Jean-François H., 1963- editor of compilation.   II. Dake, Michael D., editor of
    compilation.   III. Title: Angiography.   IV. Title: Interventional radiology.
[DNLM: 1. Angiography. 2. Radiology, Interventional. WG 500]
RC691.6.A53
616.1'307572—dc23

2013018773

Care has been taken to confirm the accuracy of the information presented and to describe generally accepted practices. However, the authors, editors, and publisher are not responsible for errors or omissions or for any consequences from application of the information in this book and make no warranty, expressed or implied, with respect to the currency, completeness, or accuracy of the contents of the publication. Application of the information in a particular situation remains the professional responsibility of the practitioner.

The authors, editors, and publisher have exerted every effort to ensure that drug selection and dosage set forth in this text are in accordance with current recommendations and practice at the time of publication. However, in view of ongoing research, changes in government regulations, and the constant flow of information relating to drug therapy and drug reactions, the reader is urged to check the package insert for each drug for any change in indications and dosage and for added warnings and precautions. This is particularly important when the recommended agent is a new or infrequently employed drug.

Some drugs and medical devices presented in the publication have Food and Drug Administration (FDA) clearance for limited use in restricted research settings. It is the responsibility of the health care provider to ascertain the FDA status of each drug or device planned for use in their clinical practice.

To purchase additional copies of this book, call our customer service department at (800) 638-3030 or fax orders to (301) 223-2320. International customers should call (301) 223-2300.

Visit Lippincott Williams & Wilkins on the Internet: at LWW.com. Lippincott Williams & Wilkins customer service representatives are available from 8:30 AM to 6 PM, EST.

10 9 8 7 6 5 4 3 2 1

RRS1308

DEDICATION

To my parents for allowing me to fulfill my dream of an academic career in the United States and
to my beloved wife Meg and my two wonderful sons, David and Marc,
who mean everything to me.
—J.F.G.

To Barbara, whose love, support, encouragement and patience have enabled
me to understand what's important.

To the songs of our life, Ben, Ellery, Austen, and Emma, whose passion, enthusiasm
and indomitable spirits have made all the difference.

To my parents, whose wisdom, gentle guidance, and infinite kindness have always inspired me.
—M.D.D.

CONTRIBUTORS

Andreas Adam, MB, BS
Professor of Interval Radiology
Department of Radiology
King's College
Clinical Director
Clinical Imaging and Medical Physics
St. Thomas' Hospital
London, United Kingdom

Joshua D. Adams, MD
Assistant Professor
Department of Surgery and Radiology
Medical University of South Carolina
Charleston, South Carolina

Muneeb Ahmed, MD
Assistant Professor of Radiology
Section of Interventional Radiology
Beth Israel Deaconess Medical Center
Harvard Medical Center
Boston, Massachusetts

Sun Ho Ahn, MD
Assistant Professor
Department of Radiology
Division of Vascular and Interventional
    Radiology
Alpert Medical School of Brown
    University
Providence, Rhode Island

Andrew S. Akman, MD, MBA
Assistant Professor
Department of Radiology
George Washington University School
    of Medicine and Health Sciences
Washington, DC

Ali Albayati, MBChB
Clinical Instructor
Department of Radiology
The George Washington University
    Hospital
Washington, DC

Janivette Alsina, MD, PhD
Fellow, Surgical Oncology
Division of Surgical Oncology, Department
    of Surgery
Johns Hopkins University
Baltimore, Maryland

Hiroshi Anai, MD, PhD
Assistant Professor
Department of Radiology
Nara Medical University
Kashihara, Nara, Japan

R. Torrance Andrews, MD
Clinical Associate Professor
Department of Radiology
University of Washington
Vascular & Interventional Radiology
Swedish Medical Center, First Hill
Seattle, Washington

Daniel Anghelescu, MD
Interventional Radiologist
Radiology
Doctors Hospital
Modesto, California

John F. Angle, MD
Professor of Radiology
Department of Radiology and Medical
    Imaging
University of Virginia Health System
Charlottesville, Virginia

Gary M. Ansel, MD
Associate Director
Ohio Health Research Institute
Director
Center for Critical Limb Care
Riverside Methodist Hospital
Columbus, Ohio

Anjali N. Avadhani, MD
Staff Oncologist
Department of Medical Oncology
Thomas Jefferson University
Jefferson Medical College
Philadelphia, Pennsylvania

Mark Otto Baerlocher, MD
Department of Interventional Radiology
Division of Medical Imaging
Royal Victoria Hospital
Barrie, Ontario, Canada

Joshua A. Beckman, MD, MS
Associate Professor
Department of Medicine
Harvard Medical School
Director, Cardiovascular Fellowship
    Program
Brigham and Women's Hospital
Boston, Massachusetts

James F. Benenati, MD
Clinical Associate Professor
Department of Radiology
University of South Florida College
    of Medicine
Tampa, Florida
Medical Director, Non Invasive Laboratory
Baptist Cardiac and Vascular Institute
Baptist Hospital of Miami
Miami, Florida

Nik Bhagat, MD
Assistant Professor
Departments of Surgery and Radiology
Mayo Clinic College of Medicine
Rochester, Minnesota

Haraldur Bjarnason, MD
Professor
Department of Radiology
Mayo Clinic College of Medicine
Rochester, Minnesota

Chase R. Brown, BS
Medical Student
Department of Vascular Surgery
Cleveland Clinic
Cleveland, Ohio

Brendan Buckley, BSc, MB, BCh, BAO
Interventional Radiologist
Department of Interventional Radiology
Auckland City Hospital
Grafton, Auckland, New Zealand

Matthew R. Callstrom, MD, PhD
Associate Professor
Department of Radiology
Mayo Clinic
Rochester, Minnesota

Rabih A. Chaer, MD
Assistant Professor
Division of Vascular Surgery
UPMC
Pittsburgh, Pennsylvania

Michael A. Choti, MD, MBA
Jacob C. Handelsman Professor of Surgery
Department of Surgery
Johns Hopkins University
Vice Chair
Department of Surgery
Johns Hopkins Hospital
Baltimore, Maryland

Howard B. Chrisman, MD, MBA
Professor
Department of Radiology and Surgery
Northwestern Feinberg School of Medicine
Chicago, Illinois

Brigid N. Connor, MBChB
Interventional Radiologist
Department of Radiology
Auckland City Hospital
Auckland, New Zealand

Francisco J. Contreras, MD
Vascular & Interventional Radiology Fellow
Department of Interventional Radiology
Baptist Cardiac & Vascular Institute
Miami, Florida

David Cosgrove, MB, BCh
Assistant Professor
Department of Medical Oncology
Sidney Kimmel Comprehensive Cancer Center,
    Johns Hopkins University
Baltimore, Maryland

Andrew H. Cragg, MD
Clinical Professor
Department of Radiology
University of Minnesota School of Medicine
Director, Endovascular Research
Minneapolis Heart Institute
Minneapolis, Minnesota

Mark A. Creager, MD
Professor of Medicine
Department of Medicine
Harvard Medical School
Director, Vascular Center
Cardiovascular Division
Brigham and Women's Hospital
Boston, Massachusetts

Michael Darcy, MD
Professor
Department of Radiology
Washington University in St. Louis
Chief of Interventional Radiology
Radiology
Barnes Jewish Hospital
St. Louis, Missouri

Ingemar J. Davidson, MD
Professor
Department of Surgery
UT Southwestern Medical Center
Dallas, Texas

Thierry de Baère, MD
Head of Department
Department of Image Guided Therapy
Institut Gustave Roussy
Villejuif, France

G. Michael Deeb, MD
Herbert Sloan Collegiate Professor
    of Cardiac Surgery
Cardiac Surgery
University of Michigan
Ann Arbor, Michigan

Eric Desruennes, MD
Chief
Central Vascular Access Unit
Gustave Roussy, Cancer Campus Paris
Villejuif, France

Sabeen Dhand, MD
Resident
Department of Radiology
Northwestern University
Chicago, Illinois

Bart L. Dolmatch, MD
Interventional Radiology
The Palo Alto Medical Foundation
Interventional Radiology
El Camino Hospital
Mountain View, California

Bertrand Janne d'Othée, MD, MPH
Associate Professor
Attending Physician
Division of Vascular and Interventional
    Radiology
Department of Diagnostic Radiology and
    Nuclear Medicine
University of Maryland Medical Center
Baltimore, Maryland

Alexander D. Drilon, MD
Thoracic Oncology Fellow
Department of Medicine
Memorial Sloan-Kettering Cancer Center
New York, New York

Jessica H. Duman, PharmD
Oncology Pharmacist
Oregon Health and Sciences University
Portland, Oregon

Khashayar Farsad, MD, PhD
Assistant Professor
Dotter Interventional Institute
Oregon Health and Science University
Portland, Oregon

Andrew S. Ferrell, MD
Assistant Professor
Department of Radiology
University of Tennessee Knoxville Graduate
    School of Medicine
Knoxville, Tennessee

Dominik D. Fleischmann, MD
Professor of Radiology
Department of Radiology
Stanford University School of Medicine
Director of Computed Tomography
Stanford Hospital
Stanford, California

Matthew D. Forrester, MD
Resident
Department of Cardiothoracic Surgery
Stanford University
Stanford, California

Terence P. Gade, MD, PhD
Clinical Fellow
Department of Radiology
Hospital of the University of Pennsylvania
Philadelphia, Pennsylvania

Ripal Gandhi, MD
Baptist Cardiac and Vascular Institute
Miami Vascular Specialists
Associate Clinical Professor
FIU Herbert Wertheim College of Medicine
Assistant Clinical Professor
University of South Florida College
    of Medicine
Miami, Florida

Ricardo D. Garcia-Monaco, MD, PhD
Professor
Department of Radiology
University of Buenos Aires
Head
Vascular and Interventional Radiology
Hospital Italiano
Buenos Aires, Argentina

John R. Gaughen, Jr., MD
Instructor
Department of Radiology and Medical
    Imaging
University of Virginia Health System
Charlottesville, Virginia

Christos Georgiades, MD, PhD
Associate Professor
Radiology & Surgery
Johns Hopkins University
Baltimore, Maryland
Attending Physician
Vascular & Interventional Radiology
American Medical Center
Nicosia, Cyprus

S. Nahum Goldberg, MD
Professor of Radiology
Department of Radiology
Hebrew University
Vice-Chairman for Research
Department of Radiology
Hadassah Hebrew University Medical Center
Jerusalem, Israel

Jafar Golzarian, MD
Interventional Radiologist
University of Minnesota Medical Center,
    Fairview
Minneapolis, Minnesota

William A. Gray, MD
Associate Professor
Department of Medicine
Director of Endovascular Services
Division of Cardiology
Columbia University Medical Center
New York, New York

Roy K. Greenberg, MD
Professor
Director, Endovascular Research
Department of Vascular Surgery, Cardiac
    Surgery, and Biomedical Engineering
Cleveland Clinic
Cleveland, Ohio

Ramona Gupta, MD
Assistant Professor
Department of Radiology
Attending Physician
Section of Interventional Radiology
Northwestern University
Chicago, Illinois

Narendra B. Gutta, MD
Research Fellow
Department of Interventional Radiology
Memorial Sloan Kettering Cancer Center
New York, New York

Klaus D. Hagspiel, MD
Professor
Department of Radiology and Medical
    Imaging
Chief
Division of Noninvasive Cardiovascular
    Imaging
Department of Radiology and Medical
    Imaging
University of Virginia School of Medicine
Charlottesville, Virginia

Richard L. Hallett, MD
Adjunct Clinical Assistant Professor
Department of Radiology
Stanford University School of Medicine
Stanford, California
Chief, Cardiovascular Imaging
Department of Medical Imaging
St. Vincent Hospital - Indianapolis
Indianapolis, Indiana

Ziv J. Haskal, MD
Professor
Department of Diagnostic Radiology and
    Nuclear Medicine
Vice Chair & Chief
Division of Vascular and Interventional
    Radiology
University of Maryland School
    of Medicine
Baltimore, Maryland

Robert J. Herfkens, MD
Professor
Department of Radiology
Stanford University
Stanford, California

Kevin Herman, MD
Department of Vascular and Interventional
    Radiology
Holy Name Medical Center
Teaneck, New Jersey

Ryan M. Hickey, MD
Health Systems Clinician
Department of Radiology
Northwestern Memorial Hospital
Chicago, Illinois

Andrew Holden, MBChB
Associate Professor
Radiology
University of Auckland
Auckland, New Zealand

Kelvin Hong, MD
Assistant Professor
Division of Vascular and Interventional
    Radiology
Johns Hopkins University School
    of Medicine
Baltimore, Maryland

David M. Hovsepian, MD
Professor
Department of Radiology
Stanford University School of Medicine
Attending Physician
Department of Radiology
Stanford Hospitals and Clinics
Stanford, California

Steven L. Hsu, MD, MBA
Assistant Professor
Department of Radiology
University of Texas Southwestern Medical
    Center
Dallas, Texas

Rehan Hussain, MD
Resident
Henry Ford Hospital
Detroit, Michigan

Gloria L. Hwang, MD
Assistant Professor
Department of Radiology
Stanford University School of Medicine
Stanford, California

Augustinus L. Jacob, MD
Professor of Radiology
Swiss Intervention Center for Mikrotherapy
Klinik Hirslanden
Zurich, Switzerland

Michael R. Jaff, DO
Professor in Medicine
Harvard Medical School
Chair
MGH Institute for Heart, Vascular, and Stroke
    Care
Massachusetts General Hospital
Boston, Massachusetts

Priya Jagia, MD, DNB Radiology
Associate Professor
Department of Cardiac Radiology
All India Institute of Medical Sciences (AIIMS)
Delhi, India

Mary E. Jensen, MD
Professor of Radiology and Neurosurgery
Department of Radiology and Medical
    Imaging
University of Virginia Health System
Charlottesville, Virginia

Amardeep Johar, MD
Resident
Department of Radiology
Maricopa Medical Center
Phoenix, Arizona

Matthew S. Johnson, MD
Professor
Radiology
Indiana University School of Medicine
Indianapolis, Indiana

Christian N. Johnson
Graduate Student
Indiana University
Indianapolis, Indiana

Barry T. Katzen, MD
Clinical Professor
Radiology and Surgery
FIU Herbert Wertheim College of Medicine
Founder and Medical Director
Baptist Cardiac and Vascular Institute
Miami, Florida

John A. Kaufman, MD, MS
Professor of Interventional Radiology
Director
Dotter Interventional Institute
Oregon Health & Science University
    Hospital
Portland, Oregon

Moazzem Kazi, MD
Research Fellow
Department of Radiology
Weill Cornell Imaging
New York, New York

Stephen T. Kee, MB, BCh, BaO
Professor
Radiology
Section Chief
Division of Interventional Radiology
UCLA
Los Angeles, California

Frederick S. Keller, MD
Cook Professor
Dotter Interventional Institute
Oregon Health & Sciences University
Portland, OR

Robert K. Kerlan, Jr., MD
Professor of Clinical Radiology and Surgery
Chief of Interventional Radiology
Department of Radiology
University of California
San Francisco, California

Tanaz A. Kermani, MD, MS
Assistant Clinical Professor
Division of Rheumatology
Department of Medicine
University of California Los Angeles
Santa Monica, California

Darren D. Kies, MD
Assistant Professor
Department of Radiology
Emory University School of Medicine
Atlanta, Georgia

Hyun S. Kim, MD
Associate Professor
Director of Interventional Radiology and
    Image-Guided Medicine
Attending Physician
Interventional Radiology and Image-Guided
    Medicine
Department of Radiology and Imaging
    Sciences
Emory University School of Medicine
Atlanta, Georgia

Hiro Kiyosue, MD
Associate Professor
Department of Radiology
Oita University, Faculty of Medicine
Yufu, Oita, Japan

Kenneth J. Kolbeck, MD, PhD
Associate Professor
Dotter Interventional Institute
Oregon Health and Science University
Portland, Oregon

Sebastian Kos, MD, PhD
Deputy Head, Interventional Radiology
Department of Radiology and Nuclear
    Medicine
University of Basel Hospital
Basel, Switzerland

Steven J. Krohmer, MD
Assistant Professor
Department of Radiology
Johns Hopkins Hospital
Baltimore, Maryland

Lee M. Krug, MD
Associate Professor
Department of Medicine
Weill Medical College of Cornell University
Associate Attending Physician
Department of Medicine
Memorial Sloan-Kettering Cancer Center
New York, New York

William T. Kuo, MD
Assistant Professor
Division of Vascular and Interventional
    Radiology
Stanford University School of Medicine
Stanford, California

A. Nicholas Kurup, MD
Assistant Professor
Consultant
Department of Radiology
Mayo Clinic College of Medicine
Rochester, Minnesota

Jeanne M. LaBerge, MD
Professor
Department of Radiology
University of California
San Francisco, California

David Lee, MD
Associate Professor
Medicine
Stanford University
Director
Cardiac Catheterization and Intervention
    Laboratories
Stanford University
Stanford, California

Justin S. Lee, MD
Assistant Professor
Department of Radiology
Georgetown University School of Medicine
Attending Physician
Department of Radiology
Medstar Georgetown University Hospital
Washington, DC

Riccardo Lencioni, MD
Professor
Department of Radiology
University of Pisa School of Medicine
Director
Division of Diagnostic Imaging and
    Intervention
Pisa University Hospital
Pisa, Italy

Leanne Doré Lessley, RT (R) VI
Interventional Radiology Technologist
Fletcher Allen Health Care
Interventional Radiology
Burlington, Vermont

Robert J. Lewandowski, MD
Associate Professor
Department of Radiology
Section of Interventional Radiology
Division of Interventional Oncology
Northwestern University Feinberg School
    of Medicine
Chicago, Illinois

Eleni Liapi, MD
Assistant Professor
The Russell H. Morgan Department of
    Radiology and Radiological Science
Johns Hopkins University School of
    Medicine
Baltimore, Maryland

David M. Liu, MD
Clinical Associate Professor
Department of Radiology
University of British Columbia
Vancouver, British Columbia, Canada
Adjunct Faculty
Department of Radiologic Sciences
University of California Los Angeles David
    Geffen School of Medicine
Los Angeles, California

Shaun Loh, MD
Interventional and Diagnostic
    Radiologist
Department of Radiology
San Rafael Medical Center
San Rafael, California

Robert A. Lookstein, MD
Associate Professor of Radiology
Associate Professor of Surgery
Division of Vascular and Interventional
    Radiology
The Mount Sinai Medical Center
New York, New York

Lindsay Machan, MD
Associate Professor
Department of Radiology
University of British Columbia
Interventional Radiologist
Department of Radiology
Vancouver, Hospital
Vancouver, British Columbia,
    Canada

David C. Madoff, MD
Professor of Radiology
Department of Radiology
Division of Interventional Radiology
Weill Cornell Medical Center
New York, New York

Michel S. Makaroun, MD
Professor and Chair
Division of Vascular Surgery
University of Pittsburgh School
    of Medicine
Co-Director
UPMC Heart and Vascular Institute
UPMC
Pittsburgh, Pennsylvania

Sean M. Marks, MD
Assistant Professor
Medicine Section Palliative Medicine
Medical College of Wisconsin
Milwaukee, Wisconsin

Francis E. Marshalleck, MD
Assistant Professor
Department of Radiology
Indiana University School of Medicine
Indianapolis, Indiana

Louis G. Martin, MD
Professor
Radiology
Emory University School of Medicine
Atlanta, Georgia

Tara M. Mastracci, MD, MSc
Associate Professor
Department of Vascular Surgery
The Cleveland Clinic Foundation
Cleveland, Ohio

Alan H. Matsumoto, MD
Chair & Theodore E. Keats Professor of Radiology
Department of Radiology & Medical Imaging
University of Virginia Health System
Charlottesville, Virginia

Jon S. Matsumura, MD
Professor and Chair
Division of Vascular Surgery
University of Wisconsin School of Medicine
    and Public Health
Madison, Wisconsin

Andrew D. McBride, MD
Attending Physician
Mori, Bean & Brooks, P.A.
Jacksonville, Florida

James C. McEachen, MD, MPH
Fellow
Department of Radiology
Division of Interventional Radiology
Mayo Clinic
Rochester, Minnesota

Khairuddin Memon, MD
Resident
Department of Radiology
Northwestern University Feinberg School
    of Medicine
Chicago, Illinois

Wells A. Messersmith, MD
Professor
Department of Medical Oncology
University of Colorado School of Medicine
Director
Gastrointestinal Medical Oncology Program
University of Colorado Cancer Center
Aurora, Colorado

Andrew Misselt, MD
Assistant Professor of Radiology
Department of Diagnostic Radiology
University of Minnesota
Minneapolis, Minnesota

Sally E. Mitchell, MD
Professor of Radiology, Surgery, and Pediatrics
Division of Interventional Radiology
Johns Hopkins Hospital
Baltimore, Maryland

John M. Moriarty, MD
Assistant Professor
Cardiovascular and Interventional Radiology
David Geffen School of Medicine at UCLA
Los Angeles, California

Mary F. Mulcahy, MD
Associate Professor
Division of Hematology/Oncology
Northwestern University
Chicago, Illinois

Timothy P. Murphy, MD
Professor
Diagnostic Imaging
Alpert Medical School of Brown University
Attending Physician
Interventional Radiology
Rhode Island Hospital
Providence, Rhode Island

Albert A. Nemcek, Jr., MD
Professor of Radiology and Surgery
Feinberg School of Medicine at Northwestern
    University
Northwestern Memorial Hospital
Department of Radiology
Chicago, Illinois

Patrick T. Norton, MD
Assistant Professor
Department of Radiology, Cardiology,
    and Pediatrics
University of Virginia
Charlottesville, Virginia

Cindy L. O'Bryant, PharmD, BCOP
Associate Professor
Department of Clinical Pharmacy
University of Colorado Skaggs School
    of Pharmacy and Pharmaceutical
    Sciences
Aurora, Colorado

Keigo Osuga, MD, PhD
Associate Professor
Department of Diagnostic and Interventional
    Radiology
Osaka University Graduate School
    of Medicine
Osaka, Japan

Siddharth A. Padia, MD
Assistant Professor
Section of Interventional Radiology
University of Washington and Harborview
    Medical Center
Seattle, Washington

Himanshu J. Patel, MD
Associate Professor of Cardiac
    Surgery
Cardiac Surgery
University of Michigan
Ann Arbor, Michigan

Timothy M. Pawlik, MD, PhD
Associate Professor
Surgical Oncology
Johns Hopkins University
Baltimore, Maryland

Peter D. Peng, MD
Staff Surgeon
Kaiser Permanente Oakland Medical
    Center
Oakland, California

Todd S. Perlstein, MD
Staff Cardiologist
Tri-City Cardiology Consultants
Gilbert, Arizona

John A. Phillips, MD
Staff Cardiologist
Ohio Health and Vascular Physicians
Columbus, Ohio

Alex Powell, MD
Baptist Cardiac and Vascular Institute
Miami, Florida

Martin R. Prince, MD, PhD
Professor
Attending Radiologist
Department of Radiology
Weill Cornell Medical College, Columbia
    University College of Physicians and
    Surgeons
New York, New York

Bradley B. Pua, MD
Assistant Professor
Department of Radiology
New York Presbyterian-Weill Cornell Medical
    College
New York, New York

Kathcrinc B. Puttgcn, MD
Assistant Professor
Departments of Dermatology & Pediatrics
Johns Hopkins University
Baltimore, Maryland

Reshma A. Rangwala, MD
Merck & Co., Incorporated
Whitehouse Station, New Jersey

Aljoscha Rastan, MD
Department of Cardiology and Angiology II
Albert-Ludwig-Universitat Freiburg
Senior Physician
Department of Cardiology and Angiology II
Universitats-Herzzentrum Freiburg-Bad
    Krozingen
Bad Krozingen, Germany

Mahmood K. Razavi, MD
Director of Clinical Trial and Research Center
Vascular and Interventional Specialists of
    Orange County, Inc.
Orange, California

Richard J. Redett, MD
Associate Professor
Program Director
Department of Plastic and Reconstructive
    Surgery
Johns Hopkins School of Medicine
Baltimore, Maryland

Ahsun Riaz, MD
Resident
Department of Radiology
Northwestern University Feinberg School
    of Medicine
Chicago, Illinois

William S. Rilling, MD
Professor of Radiology & Surgery
Radiology
Medical College of Wisconsin
Faculty Physician
Radiology
Froedtert Memorial Lutheran Hospital
Milwaukee, Wisconsin

Adnan Z. Rizvi, MD
Attending Vascular Surgeon
Minneapolis Heart Institute
Minneapolis, Minnesota

Anne C. Roberts, MD
Clinical Professor
Division Chief, Vascular/Interventional
    Radiology
University of California, San Diego Health System
San Diego, California

Ronald Rodriguez, MD, PhD
Associate Professor
Department of Urology
Johns Hopkins University School of Medicine
Baltimore, Maryland

Thom W. Rooke, MD
Krehbiel Professor of Vascular Medicine
Vascular Medicine
Mayo Clinic
Rochester, Minnesota

Josef Rösch, MD
Professor
Dotter Interventional Institute
Oregon Health & Science University
Portland, Oregon

Robert E. Roses, MD
Assistant Professor
Division of Endocrine and Oncologic Surgery
Hospital of the University of Pennsylvania
Philadelphia, Pennsylvania

Drew A. Rosielle, MD
Assistant Professor
Department of Medicine
University of Minnesota Medical School
Palliative Medicine Consultant
Fairview Health Services Palliative Care
    Program
University of Minnesota Medical Center
Minneapolis, Minnesota

John H. Rundback, MD
Medical Director
Interventional Institute
Holy Name Medical Center
Teaneck, New Jersey

Robert K. Ryu, MD
Professor of Radiology
Department of Radiology
Northwestern University Feinberg School
    of Medicine
Chicago, Illinois

Wael E. Saad, MB, BCh
Professor of Radiology
Department of Radiology
University of Virginia Health System
Charlottesville, Virginia

Tarun Sabharwal, MD, ChB
Consultant Interventional Radiologist
Department of Interventional Radiology
Guy's and St. Thomas' Hospital
London, United Kingdom

Saher S. Sabri, MD
Assistant Professor
Department of Radiology and Medical Imaging
University of Virginia
Charlottesville, Virginia

Riad Salem, MD
Professor
Radiology, Medicine-Hematology/Oncology
    and Surgery-Organ Transplantation
Northwestern University Feinberg School of
    Medicine
Chicago, Illinois

Naveed U. Saqib, MD
Fellow
Division of Vascular Surgery
UPMC
Pittsburgh, Pennsylvania

Shawn Sarin, MD
Assistant Professor
Department of Radiology
George Washington School of Medicine
    and Health Sciences
Washington, DC

Andrej Schmidt, MD
Center for Vascular Medicine
Angiology, Cardiology and Vascular Surgery
Park-Hospital Leipzig
Leipzig, Germany

Charles P. Semba, MD
Associate Clinical Professor
Department of Interventional Radiology
Stanford University School of Medicine
Stanford, California

Sanjiv Sharma, MD
Professor and Head
Department of Cardiac Radiology
All India Institute of Medical Sciences
Delhi, India

Onur Sildiroglu, MD
Assistant Professor
Department of Radiology
GATA Haydarpasa Teaching Hospital
Istanbul, Turkey

Tony P. Smith, MD
Professor
Radiology
Duke University
Durham, North Carolina

Bob R. Smouse, MD
Associate Professor
Radiology, Surgery
University of Illinois College of Medicine
    at Peoria
Peoria, Illinois

Luigi A. Solbiati, MD
Chairman
Department of Interventional Oncologic Radiology
General Hospital of Busto Arsizio
Busto Arsizio, Italy

Stephen B. Solomon, MD
Professor
Department of Radiology
Weill Cornell Medical College
Attending
Department of Radiology
Memorial Sloan-Kettering Cancer Center
New York, New York

Michael C. Soulen, MD
Professor
Department of Radiology
University of Pennsylvania School of Medicine
Philadelphia, Pennsylvania

James B. Spies, MD, MPH
Professor
Department of Radiology
Georgetown University School of Medicine
Chair
Department of Radiology
Georgetown University Hospital
Washington, DC

James R. Stone, MD
Assistant Professor
Department of Radiology and Medical Imaging
University of Virginia
Staff Physician
Division of Interventional Radiology
University of Virginia
Charlottesville, Virginia

Weijing Sun, MD
Professor of Medicine
Medicine, Hematology and Oncology
University of Pittsburgh
Director of GI Medical Oncology
Co-Director of UPMCGI Cancer Center of
    Excellence
University of Pittsburgh Cancer Institute
Pittsburgh, Pennsylvania

Daniel Y. Sze, MD, PhD
Professor
Division of Interventional Radiology
Stanford University
Stanford, California

Aylin Tekes, MD
Assistant Professor
Department of Radiology
Johns Hopkins Hospital
Baltimore, Maryland

Lisa A. Thompson, PharmD, BCOP
Assistant Professor
Department of Clinical Pharmacy
University of Colorado Skaggs School
 of Pharmacy and Pharmaceutical
 Sciences
Aurora, Colorado

Margaret Clarke Tracci, MD, JD, MBA
Assistant Professor
Division of Vascular and Endovascular
 Surgery
University of Virginia
Charlottesville, Virginia

David W. Trost, MD
Clinical Associate Professor
Attending Physician
Department of Radiology
Weill Cornell Medical Center
New York, New York

Ulku Cenk Turba, MD
Associate Professor
Interventional Radiology
Rush University Medical Center
Chicago, Illinois

Heiko Uthoff, MD
Consultant
Vascular and Interventional Radiology
Baptist Cardiac and Vascular Institute
Miami, Florida
Attending Physician
Angiology
University Hospital Basel
Basel, Switzerland

Karim Valji, MD
Professor and Chief of Interventional
 Radiology
Department of Radiology
University of Washington
Seattle, Washington

Mark G. van Vledder, MD, PhD
Resident
Department of Surgery
Erasmus University Medical Center
Rotterdam, The Netherlands

Jean-Nicolas Vauthey, MD
Professor
Department of Surgical Oncology
MD Anderson Cancer Center
Houston, Texas

Miguel A. Vazquez, MD
Professor
Department of Medicine
University of Texas Southwestern Medical Center
Dallas, Texas

Suresh Vedantham, MD
Professor of Radiology & Surgery
Mallinckrodt Institute of Radiology
Washington University School of Medicine
St. Louis, Missouri

Anthony C. Venbrux, MD
Professor
Radiology and Surgery
Director
Cardiovascular and Interventional Radiology
George Washington University Hospital
Washington, DC

Robert L. Vogelzang, MD
Professor
Department of Radiology
Northwestern Feinberg School of Medicine
Senior Attending Physician
Division of Interventional Radiology
Northwestern Memorial Hospital
Chicago, Illinois

Cynthia E. Wagner, MD
Resident
Cardiothoracic Surgery
University of Virginia
Charlottesville, Virginia

Arthur C. Waltman, MD
Professor in Radiology
Harvard Medical School
Staff Radiologist
Cardiovascular Interventions
Massachusetts General Hospital
Boston, Massachusetts

Kenneth J. Warrington, MD
Associate Professor
Department of Medicine
Mayo Clinic
Rochester, Minnesota

Ido Weinberg, MD, MSc, MHA
Instructor
Medicine
Harvard Medical School
Attending Physician
Cardiology
Massachusetts General Hospital
Boston, Massachusetts

Clifford R. Weiss, MD
Assistant Professor
Interventional Radiology Center/Russell H.
 Morgan Department of Radiology
 and Radiologic Science
Clinical Director
Center for Bioengineering, Innovation and Design
Whiting School of Engineering
Johns Hopkins University School of Medicine
Baltimore, Maryland

Jonathan K. West, MD
Resident Physician
Department of Radiology and Medical
 Imaging
University of Virginia Health
 System
Charlottesville, Virginia

David M. Williams, MD
Professor
Department of Radiology
University of Michigan
Ann Arbor, Michigan

Neil J. Wimmer, MD
Clinical Fellow
Cardiovascular Medicine
Brigham and Women's
 Hospital
Boston, Massachusetts

Kei Yamada, MD
Assistant Professor
Department of Radiology
Emory University School of
 Medicine
Atlanta, Georgia

Dai Yamanouchi, MD, PhD
Assistant Professor
Attending Physician
Department of Surgery
Division of Vascular Surgery
University of Wisconsin School of Medicine
 and Public Health
Madison, Wisconsin

Douglas B. Yim, MD
Assistant Professor of Radiology
Interventional Radiology and Image Guided
 Medicine
Emory University School of
 Medicine
Director
Interventional Radiology Lab
Emory Johns Creek Hospital
Atlanta, Georgia

Phillip M. Young, MD
Associate Professor
Consultant
Department of Radiology
Mayo Clinic College of Medicine
Rochester, Minnesota

Marjorie G. Zauderer, MD, MS
Assistant Attending Physician
Department of Medicine
Memorial Sloan-Kettering Cancer
 Center
New York, New York

Thomas Zeller, MD
Associate Professor
Department of Angiology
Universitäts Herzzentrum Freiburg–Bad
 Krozingen
Bad Krozingen, Germany

PREFACE

Nothing stays the same. Politics, art, science, technology, the environment—if there is one constant in life, it is the inevitability of change.

In the last half century, the speed of that change has increased at a pace unique in human history. We live in an era that has been called "the age of acceleration," in a rapidly evolving world that increasingly delights in pulling the rug out from under us. Just when one starts to feel comfortable with a predictable routine, life imposes a new reality. Change is as inescapable as it is impenitent.

Without a doubt, this shift in momentum has affected the field of medicine. A look at the table of contents from the last edition of Abrams' Angiography, released in 2006, reveals that interventional radiology has kept pace. The hot topics and procedures at the time of publication were on the leading edge of medical innovation. In less than a decade, these advances would be eclipsed by new interventions of startling impact and clinical benefit. The field changed so quickly that many of these image-guided less invasive procedures were completely unanticipated when the last volume of Abrams' was released.

This rapid evolution makes sense. Interventional radiology has always been about what's next, with deep roots in the future. Today, just as when the 1st edition of Abrams' Angiography was introduced in 1961, innovation and interventional radiology remain synonymous. Change through innovation is where the early interventional pioneers planted their flag and that is where the field continues to grow and prosper.

As editors of this new edition of Abrams', we felt compelled to honor this legacy of innovation. Thus, the focus and content of the book have been completely revamped to reflect the fast-moving landscape of the practice of interventional radiology. The organizational format of this volume, including chapter titles and authors, was created from scratch with the goal of providing a fresh take on leading edge subjects by the most knowledgeable current authorities.

Traditionally, one of the goals of a standard reference text is to be a comprehensive compendium of a given field. We took on that challenge in this edition of Abrams', but we also intentionally pruned its scope to 100 chapters—what we consider the most salient top 100 topics that are key to mastering contemporary interventional radiology. Obviously, this means some aspects of the field will receive less emphasis. We acknowledge the arbitrary nature of our chapter selections, but in the end we believe it is important to limit the project to one relevant volume.

One obvious change over the last decade has been a crescendo of interest in the area of interventional oncology. This important aspect of contemporary interventional radiology is a natural extension of the percutaneous and endovascular procedures that were initially applied to hepatic malignancies, but were only briefly described in the last edition.

In this latest edition, we devote about one-third of the content to topics directly associated with interventional oncology. Two-thirds of the text addresses the management of arterial and venous disease. Many of the themes considered in the vascular sections are rooted in the original stock of the initial Abrams' volume. All of the new chapters, however, focus on the current understanding and management of vascular disease.

In regard to authors, we have been blessed with the wisdom and talent of the best and brightest experts in interventional radiology. We take this opportunity to express our deepest appreciation to these friends and colleagues. Their contributions captured the groundbreaking achievements and vibrating excitement of interventional radiology today. It has been an honor and privilege to work with them on this text.

In addition, we must thank our administrative assistants, Monique Chang and Lora Stepan, who helped manage many of the details throughout the course of the book's preparation. We are also grateful for the sage editorial advice and guidance provided by Jonathan Pine, Sarah Granlund, and Amy Dinkel at Wolters Kluwer and the production help provided by David Orzechowski, also of Wolters Kluwer, and Mohamed Hameed of S4Carlisle.

We trust you will find this edition of Abrams' Angiography to be a worthy companion, providing a source of valuable information and guidance that enhances your care of patients. Above all, we hope this state of the art overview inspires the next generation of interventional radiologists, reminding them that the great gift and promise of our field lies in its capacity to change the future through innovation.

Michael D. Dake
Jean-François H. Geschwind

CONTENTS

Evaluation of the Cancer Patient

RESHMA A. RANGWALA, ANJALI N. AVADHANI, and WEIJING SUN

The care of the cancer patient requires a multidisciplinary team approach, involving medical, surgical, radiation, and interventional oncologists as well as social work support and palliative care experts. The goal is to create treatment plans individualized to the patient while supporting his or her psychosocial needs. Such communication among physicians and teams is essential to the patient's overall well-being and success. Interventional oncologists require the ability to accomplish a thorough and comprehensive assessment of patients who have a variety of malignancies and a range of associated medical problems, including comorbidities, previous treatment history, and social status. Their skills are vital because of their ability to perform procedures in patients who have various malignancies with a range of medical problems and types of organ dysfunctions. As such they play an integral role in the management of cancer patients. Evaluation of cancer patients comprises several fundamental principles, including a complete medical history, performance status grading, quality-of-life assessment, physical examination, laboratory and data review, and an in-depth discussion with the patient and family regarding treatment options, choices of plans, rationale and expectation of the outcomes, and potential risks.[1,2]

The physician should first elicit information regarding the patient's symptoms, yielding as much information as possible on the progression of these symptoms, their impedance on the patient's activities of daily living, and the chronicity and tempo of the disease. Other components of the medical history, which are discussed in detail later, include history of present illness, review of systems, pertinent listing of previous medical and surgical details, review of records, hereditary and environmental factors, use of drugs and medications, allergies (both to prescription and over-the-counter drugs), and alternative treatments. Subsequently, the physician performs a relevant physical examination to obtain insight on organ dysfunction. The history and physical examination can be a fluid process, because such findings may prompt the health care provider to obtain additional medical history in a targeted fashion. The history and physical examination should be cohesive and similarly structured[3] to provide a platform on which further diagnostic information from laboratory and ancillary data can build. It also serves as the foundation for information sharing among the many teams involved in an individual patient's care.

MEDICAL HISTORY

A comprehensive and thorough history and physical exam, even in the era of technology-driven medicine, provides the most vital and crucial basis for any resulting diagnosis or treatment plan.

History of Present Illness

The history of present illness (HPI) is the chronologic sequence of symptomatic events and includes detailed descriptions of each associated symptom; it builds around the original "chief complaint," or the major health problem for which the patient is seeking medical attention. The HPI should include information regarding the patient's original cancer diagnosis, such as presenting symptoms, the mode of diagnosis, any radiographic and laboratory data obtained, and any progression in symptoms since the diagnosis. All consultants' notes should be reviewed. Any surgical procedure(s) and complications associated with the patient's primary malignancy or metastatic disease should be viewed in detail, which may influence both the choices and effects of subsequent interventional therapy. In addition, the HPI should cover a comprehensive list of all systemic chemotherapies, including dose, schedule, and number of treatments received as well as any previous radiation, the sites of administration, and the doses administered. For example, particular attention should be given to total lifetime anthracycline dose; this is associated with a dose-dependent cumulative cardiomyopathy[4] and is often used in the setting of chemoembolization (TACE) for hepatocellular carcinoma or liver-limited metastases of malignancies. A detailed review of adverse treatment-relative events and symptomatology, as well as any treatment complications, should be brought forth.[2]

Review of Systems

Review of systems (ROS) is an imperative component of a thorough medical history. All symptoms associated with the primary diagnosis and the secondary effects of the tumor or different previous treatment versus current treatment should be explored in detail. Systemic complaints such as malaise, fatigue, lethargy, anorexia, weight loss, fevers, chills, and drenching night sweats are common. For example, patients with primary hepatocellular carcinoma (HCC) or liver metastases from other cancer may manifest gastrointestinal symptoms, which may range from right upper quadrant pain from capsular stretch to abdominal distention to jaundice secondary to biliary obstruction or severe liver dysfunction. They also may manifest as constipation, diarrhea, melena, early satiety, nausea, vomiting, and/or a change in bowel habits. Neuroendocrine tumors (NET) can cause systemic symptoms based on their point of origin and metastases; flushing and diarrhea are associated with small-bowel carcinoids, whereas shortness of breath, bronchospasm, palpitations, and heart failure can result from nongastrointestinal carcinoids; and hormonal-related symptoms may be the initial symptom of pancreatic islet cell tumors (e.g., insulinoma, gastrinoma). An in-depth knowledge of the respective tumors can allow one to explore with the patients symptoms specific to their disease; a fluid knowledge of the chemothera-peutic options can also allow one to explore symptoms related to the drugs. Other symptoms to review with all cancer patients include oropharyngeal soreness, chest pain, hemoptysis, flank and back pain, hematuria, and enlarged lymph nodes.[5] Skeletal metastases typically lead to severe bony pain, either isolated to the thoracolumbar spine or diffuse in nature (ribs, shoulders, hips). Neurologic symptoms such as bowel or bladder inconti-nence, saddle anesthesia, gait instability, and back pain should raise concern for cord compression, requiring emergent workup and intervention. New-onset headaches, worsening headaches, vision changes, or isolated weakness should also raise concern for metastatic disease to the brain, requiring prompt imaging by magnetic resonance imaging (MRI). Pain is commonly associ-ated with a variety of malignancies, and a verbally administered pain scale of 0 to 10 is a useful, easy way to assess severity and, therefore, to guide treatment, especially in older adults.[6]

Past Medical and Surgical History

Past medical and surgical history (PMH/PSH) includes major current comorbidities, ongoing illness, and all previous surgical procedures. Any coexisting medical problems should be elicited that may impact the primary oncologic diagnosis and specifically may influence choice and impact of certain therapies. Chronic medical problems including but not limited to chronic obstruc-tive pulmonary disease (COPD), emphysema, diabetes mellitus, hypertension, cardiovascular disease including congestive heart failure and coronary artery disease, as well as prior myocardial infarctions, peripheral vascular disease, chronic liver disease, and chronic renal insufficiency should be detailed in this sec-tion. COPD and emphysema are especially pertinent in the care of the patient with lung cancer; chronic liver disease/cirrhosis and hepatitis B and C status are especially pertinent in patients who are being considered for chemoembolization (TACE). Any immunocompromising state, such as HIV, should also be elic-ited because chemo- and radiotherapy including radioisotope-based interventional therapy can lead to marrow suppression and increase the risk for infections. Transfusion history should be obtained to assess risk factors for viral hepatitis and to assess prior transfusion needs. Any previous psychological disorders, including depression and anxiety, should be ascertained in order to facilitate patient discussion in the future, determine cop-ing mechanisms, and determine whether any current or prior antidepressant/anxiolytic medications with significant hepatic metabolism may interact with planned interventional thera-peutics. Surgical history must address the date of resection of the primary cancer, any history of prior liver resections, and placement of hepatic arterial infusion pumps or portal shunt. A complete list of any prior malignancies and their treatment dates should be obtained because this may influence subsequent therapeutic options. Examples of such include use of prior anthracyclines or radiotherapy because lifetime dose limitations may warrant changes in the treatment plan.[4]

Family History, Social History, and Medications

It is essential to have a detailed family history described for most common malignancies. Often, the observation of multiple fam-ily members with similar cancers generates referrals for genetic counseling in order to ascertain risk to unaffected individuals. An example of this includes familial adenomatous polyposis (FAP) or hereditary nonpolyposis colon cancer (HNPCC).[7] This entity affects multiple first-degree family members with early diagnoses of colon cancers or detection of numerous colonic adenomas.

A complete medical evaluation for the cancer patient should include the social history. It yields information regarding any occupational or environmental exposures that may associate with tumorigenesis.[5] This segment of the history should include an in-depth assessment of a patient's alcohol and tobacco use (both current and past use, first-hand versus second-hand expo-sures), illegal/recreational/intravenous drug use, and any pos-sible risk factors for hepatitis including tattoos, incarceration, and blood or blood product transfusion history. Tuberculosis exposure risks should be investigated as well. The social his-tory should also include a broad review of the patient's social support, home environment, and functional status, particu-larly for elderly patients. These details may have a significant impact on the choice of treatment and can affect compliance with therapies, ability to follow up, and capacity to cope and manage the side effects and toxicities of therapy. It is also cru-cial to obtain information on the home environment, ability to work and the nature of the patient's employment, availability and proximity of friends and family, driving capacity, and per-formance of activities of daily living.[8] A detailed list of current medications and doses, including prescription drugs, over-the-counter drugs, and supplements, should be obtained. Because most patients typically use multiple medications that have some element of hepatic metabolism, it is essential to avoid concur-rent use of hepatotoxic drugs. Because many patients may take alternative medicines or therapies without telling physicians or health providers, and these may interfere with the interventional therapies/procedures, investigational efforts should be taken to look into this issue. On the other hand, it is also important to note compliance in drugs and obstacles that prevent the patient from taking the drug(s) as prescribed. Any drug or food aller-gies and their reactions, particularly to antibiotics, should be recorded in detail.[9]

▎ PHYSICAL EXAMINATION

A comprehensive physical examination should be performed on every patient. During the initial office visit, a full-systems approach should be obtained to gather information regarding the general health of the individual, including vital signs: blood pressure, pulse, respiratory rate; weight and height; and pulse oximetry. During subsequent follow-up visits, the physical exam can be more focused for the patient's specific tumor type and extent of disease. For example, HCC or metastatic liver disease not only affects the abdomen (distention, ascites, hepatomegaly, pain) but can also affect the lower extremities (edema), the skin (jaundice), and the eyes (icterus), to name a few organ systems. Following assessment of the vital signs, assessment of the overall health status of the patient should be obtained. This includes an evaluation of the patient's body habitus and assessment of cachexia (bitemporal wasting). An assessment of the patient's fluid status should be performed next. Dry mucous membranes, poor skin turgor, and chapped lips can indicate a hypovolemic state. If these are found, it is useful to also ask about symptoms of orthostasis and to assess orthostatic blood pressures/heart rate evaluation in the prone, sitting, and standing position at the end of the exam. An overall assessment of the skin can be indicative of the general health of the patient as well as point to specific organ dysfunction. For example, general pallor and pale conjunctivae can signify anemia.[5] Jaundice of the skin, sclerae, and mucous membranes is frequently a late-presenting physical exam finding of biliary obstruction, often found in pancreatic or biliary malignancies, or metastatic disease to this site. It is caused by accumulation of the conjugated form of bilirubin,[3] often associated with biliary obstruction or dilatation, and usually observed if the serum bilirubin level is greater than 3 mg/dl.[10] Evaluation of enlarged lymph nodes should be performed, with specific attention to cervical, submandibular, occipital, supraclavicular, axillary, and inguinal regions. Pathologically enlarged lymph nodes are typically detected by palpation when they are located in anatomically superficial areas. Specific attention should be made to the size, texture, and possible impingement on surrounding structures, including the trachea. Lymph nodes that are too deep to palpate may be detected by multiple imaging modalities, including ultrasonography (US), computed tomography (CT), magnetic resonance imaging (MRI), and positron emission tomography (PET).[3] Biopsy of pathologically enlarged lymph nodes may be needed for diagnosis. The general approach to the head and neck exam should include assessment of alopecia because this may be indicative of poor nutritional status or prior chemotherapy. Specific attention should be made to the oropharynx: dentition; peritonsillar masses/erythema, which may be indicative of an abscess; white plaques, especially on the tongue and buccal areas, which may be concerning for thrush; and posterior oropharynx erythema and exudates. Asymmetry in the oropharynx may be indicative of masses and/or cranial nerve deficits.

The general approach to the abdominal examination should include detection of ascites, abdominal masses and/or bruits, abdominal distention, hepatic and/or splenic enlargement, tenderness, and nodules. Patients with liver metastases or hepatocellular carcinoma can often present with a firm, enlarged, and irregular liver on palpation. Palpation of the liver edge within the right upper quadrant usually indicates hepatomegaly. The normal liver may be palpated 4 to 5 cm below the right costal margin but is often not detected within the epigastric area.[10] Presence of cirrhosis is usually manifested by a nodular, small-sized liver. Patients may have complaints of tenderness within the right upper quadrant with abdominal palpation and sometimes with percussion. Occasionally a vascular bruit over the liver caused by increased vascularity from the tumor can be appreciated.[11] A common complication of HCC includes portal vein involvement by tumor. This complication can lead to portal hypertension and effectively decrease blood flow to the liver.[11] Advanced liver disease and cirrhosis can present with massive ascites, gynecomastia, splenomegaly, portal hypertension, testicular atrophy, proximal muscle wasting, palmar erythema, spider angiomas on the anterior chest and trunk, lower extremity edema, and encephalopathy. Splenomegaly is detected by movement during inspiration because enlarged spleens typically are present just beneath the abdominal wall.[3] Lying the patient on the right side, in a supine position with flexion of the left knee, can help in identifying splenomegaly.

A thorough cardiovascular and chest examination should be performed, particularly in those patients receiving any type of anesthesia or intra-arterial therapies. Evaluation of cardiac rate, rhythm, auscultation for murmurs and rubs, and a full assessment of peripheral pulses should be done. For patients with pulmonary involvement of their disease, physical exam findings can include decreased unilateral breath sounds and dullness to percussion caused by pleural effusion and/or lobar collapse and atelectasis. Inspiratory and/or expiratory wheezes may be a sign of intrinsic or extrinsic obstruction of the airways by tumor. Finally, a thorough neurologic exam is warranted. This includes assessment of the cranial nerves, motor strength, sensation, cerebellar function, and gait. Dysfunction in any of these areas may be indicative of metastases to the brain parenchyma, leptomeninges, and/or the spinal cord, requiring emergent imaging and treatment. Spinal cord compression, for example, can present with either unilateral or bilateral weakness, back pain with focal vertebral tenderness, decreased rectal tone, and incontinence.

■ PERFORMANCE STATUS ASSESSMENT

Several parameters have been used to assess performance status (PS) of cancer patients. *Performance status* is defined as the global evaluation of a patient's practical functional level and the patient's ability to care for himself or herself.[12] PS should correlate to the clinical health and overall well-being of the cancer patient. It is a vital tool used to determine whether a patient can withstand the toxicities associated with various modes of treatment. It is similarly used in the surveillance of the cancer patient during a therapy to assess whether the toxicities are becoming too overwhelming to the patient's overall well-being. PS has been used to estimate prognosis, to measure treatment efficacy, and to help in selection of patients for clinical trials. Two of the most commonly used scales for PS assessment include the Karnofsky's Scale of Performance Status (KPS) and the Eastern Cooperative Oncology Group Scale of Performance Status (ECOG PS).[9] KPS, initially used in the 1940s, rates PS from a scale of 0 to 100 in increments of 10 and incorporates information on the ability to perform normal activity versus need for assistance.[12] A score of 100 correlates to completely normal function, whereas a score of 0 signifies death. The ECOG PS emerged in the 1960s and provided an alternative 5-point scale rather than the 100-point Karnofsky scale. An ECOG PS score of 0 correlates to full activity without restriction, whereas a score of 5 indicates death.[13] For example, a ECOG PS of 1, often the limit used in enrollment in phase 1 trials, requires that a patient be only marginally limited and thus should be able to perform all activities of daily living, including grocery shopping and vacuuming. Although both scales are commonly used by medical oncologists, the ECOG scale has shown improved predictive value over the KPS, specifically in terms of patient prognosis.[12] It is important, however, for an interventional radiologist to evaluate and distinguish between suboptimal or poor PS of a particular patient caused by the individual's cancer or cancer-related effects versus comorbidities that are not directly cancer related and, therefore, should not be reflected by the specific PS score. In addition to the assessment of PS, quality of life can be an important indicator of treatment effect and overall impact of disease. Evaluation of quality of life can be particularly relevant for older patients, because this population is typically most concerned about changes in quality of life rather than disease progression and death.[14] Questions pertaining to activities of daily living (ADLs) and instrumental activities of daily living (IADLs) are useful quality of life indices. ADL questions typically refer to basic functioning within the home such as bathing and dressing, whereas IADL assessments focus on community activities including driving, shopping, and handling of finances.[15]

LABORATORY

Routine laboratory evaluation in cancer patients is essential and critical for diagnosis and assessment prior to any treatment and procedure. Basic laboratory tests should include complete blood count (CBC) with white blood cell (WBC) differential, and liver and kidney functions. Prothrombin time (PT) and partial thromboplatin time (PTT) should also be tested, especially in those patients undergoing anticoagulation therapies with either warfarin or low-molecular-weight heparin. Tissue diagnose of malignancy is mandatory before any kind of therapy in most types of cancer. Some serum tests may be valuable as "surrogate markers" in disease diagnosis and estimation results of treatment and ablative procedures, including AFP, CEA (carcinoembryonic antigen), CA19-9 (cancer antigen 19-9), CA 125, and Chromogranin A. These "tumor markers" should be used to evaluate the response to therapy with caution because, due to their short half-lives, they may fluctuate substantially and with widely variant normal ranges based of the specific types of assay performed within an individual laboratory. Trends from serial measurements of these markers are far more useful than a single reading.

IMAGES

Cross-sectional images (CT, MRI) of targeted organs are essential for planning image-guided therapy. Baseline images should be done within 1 month of the procedure for baseline assessment.

The images should be reviewed by the treating physician personally because written reports rarely provide sufficient or accurate information. All of the following elements should be considered when formulating a treatment plan and judging its risks and benefits: size, number, and location of tumors; anatomy and patency of relevant arteries and veins; evidence of organ obstruction; alterations caused by surgery or stenting; critical adjuvant structures; and presence of substantial amounts of disease outside the target organ. Again, post therapy images should be reviewed personally by the physician who performs the procedure because diagnostic radiologists may not be aware of the nature of the therapy, the expected imaging appearance, or how to report the image outcomes appropriately.

Image-guided therapy has an important role in the treatment of many cancers. However, the interventional oncologist's expertise in therapy must be integrated into an overall multidisciplinary care plan for each cancer patient. Other treatment modalities should be disclosed, and expert referrals should be offered when appropriate. Communication between the treating physician and the patient and family should be emphasized as well. The patient and family should be informed so that they understand that most image-guided procedures performed by interventional radiologists are not based on curative intent and must be provided with a comprehensive overview of the disease status and prognosis; the goals of the treatment and achievement; the expected outcome with and without therapy; the pros and cons; the reasonable expectations for risk, tolerability, toxicity, and disruption of quality of life; and any potential alternative options.

In summary, the evaluation of the cancer patient needs to entail a comprehensive systemic workup, which is crucial for interventional oncologists to optimize the assessment and management of patient care.

REFERENCES

1. Schwartz JH, Ellison EC. Focal liver lesions. Evaluation of solid neoplasms. *Postgrad Med* 1994;95(1):157–160, 165–168, 171–174.
2. Tuite CM, Sun W, Soulen MC. General assessment of the patient with cancer for the interventional oncologist. *J Vasc Interv Radiol* 2006;17:753–758.
3. Kaushansky K, Lichtman MA, Beutler, E, et al. Initial approach to the patient: history and physical examination. In: *Williams Hematology* . 8th ed. New York, NY: McGraw-Hill Professional; 2010:3–9.
4. Lefrak EA, Pitha J, Rosenbaum S. A clinicopathologic analysis of adriamycin cardiotoxicity. *Cancer* 1973;32:302–314.
5. Bitran JD. *Establishing a Diagnosis. Expert Guide to Oncology* . Philadelphia, PA: American College of Physicians; 2000:23–38. ACP Expert Guides Series.
6. Herr K. Pain in the older adult: An imperative across all health care settings. *Pain Manag Nurs* 2010;11(suppl 2):S1–10.
7. Pérez Segura P, Guillén Ponce C, Ramón y Cajal T, et al. TTD consensus document on the diagnosis and management of hereditary colorectal cancer. *Clin Transl Oncol* 2010;12(5):356–366.
8. Extermann M, Hurria A. Comprehensive geriatric assessments for older patients with cancer. *J Clin Oncol* 2007; 25(14):1824–1831.
9. Conill C, Verger E, Salamero M. Performance status assessment in cancer patients. *Cancer* 1990;65(8):1864–1866.
10. Bickley LS, Szilagyi PG. *Bates Guide to Physical Examination and History Taking.* 10th ed. Philadelphia, PA: Lippincott Williams & Wilkins; 2008.
11. DiBisceglie AM. Epidemiology and clinical presentations of hepatocellular carcinoma. *J Vasc Interv Radiol* 2002;13:S169–S171.
12. Buccheri G, Ferrigno D, Tamburini, M. Karnofsky and ECOG performance status scoring in lung cancer: A prospective, longitudinal study of 536 patients from a single institution. *Eur J Cancer* 1996;32A:1135–1141.
13. Sorenson JB, Klee M, Palshof T, et al. Performance status assessment in cancer patients: An inter-observer variability study. *Br J Cancer* 1993;67:773–775.
14. Abernethy AP, Wheeler JL, Currow DC. Utility and use of palliative care screening tools in routine oncology practice. *Cancer J* 2010;16(5):444–460.
15. Enelow AJ, Forde DL, Brummel-Smith K. *Interviewing and Patient Care* . 4th ed. New York, NY: Oxford University Press; 1996.

CHAPTER 2

Principles of Chemotherapy

LISA A. THOMPSON, CINDY L. O'BRYANT, JESSICA H. DUMAN, and WELLS A. MESSERSMITH

INTRODUCTION

Chemotherapy is an important component in the treatment of cancer. The term traditionally refers to the use of conventional cytotoxic drugs but also includes hormonal agents and, more recently, targeted anticancer agents. Chemotherapy is most frequently used in the treatment of disseminated or advanced stage cancers and may be used in combined modality programs with surgery and radiation for early stage disease. For the interventional radiologist, the administration of regional chemotherapy is an integral part of clinical practice. It is therefore essential to have an understanding of the general principles of chemotherapy and the chemotherapeutic agents, including associated toxicities, most commonly utilized by the interventional radiologist.

GENERAL PRINCIPLES

Cell Cycle

The cell cycle is the process by which normal and cancer cells replicate and divide. During this process tumor cells are much more likely to experience genetic abnormalities that lead to uncontrolled growth. Chemotherapy drugs interfere with the steps of the cell cycle; thus understanding the cell cycle and the events that occur in each phase is central to understanding the role of these agents in the treatment of cancer.

The cell cycle is made up of five phases: Gap0 (G_0), Gap1 (G_1), synthetic phase (S), Gap2 (G_2), and mitosis (M), as shown in FIGURE 2.1. The majority of cells within the body exist in the resting, nonreplicating G_0 phase but retain the ability to divide

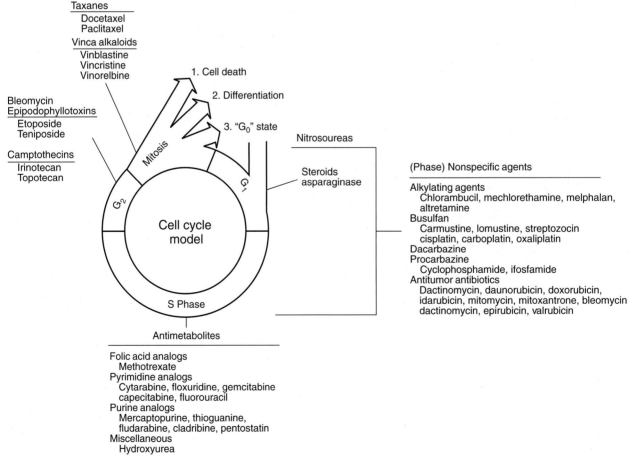

FIGURE 2.1 The cell cycle and effects of cytotoxic chemotherapy.

Reproduced with permission from Koda-Kimble MA, Young LY, Kradjan WA, et al. *Applied Therapeutics: The Clinical Use of Drugs.* 8th ed. Philadelphia, PA: Lippincott Williams & Wilkins, 2005.

again when stimulated by the appropriate growth factor. In this quiescent state, cells are not generally susceptible to the effects of cytotoxic chemotherapy. Once stimulated, a cell will reenter the cell cycle in the G_1 phase where the synthesis of enzymes necessary for DNA replication occurs. Once the cell is stimulated to begin the S phase, it is committed to proceed through the cell cycle. It is in the S phase that DNA synthesis occurs and results in the doubling of the chromosomes. During the G_2 phase, RNA and protein synthesis occurs as well as a "G_2 checkpoint" that assesses the replicated DNA for errors and ensures the cell is prepared to enter the M phase.[1] The mitosis phase is made up of a series of events that result in the separation of chromosomes into two identical sets in two nuclei followed by cytokinesis, the process of dividing the cell into two cells. Once this occurs cell division is complete and the cell can then die, reenter the cell cycle in the G_1 phase, or enter the resting G_0 phase.

Tumor Growth/Chemotherapy Strategy

It is generally believed that cancer develops from a single cell that has undergone a malignant change and continues to grow into a mass. A tumor mass is generally undetectable by physical exam or radiologic studies until it is at least 1 cm in diameter. A tumor this size weighs about 1 gram and is made up of approximately 1 billion (1×10^9) cells. Tumors deep within organs may not be detected until they are even larger. Net tumor growth depends on the rate of cell death and the rate of cell division within the mass. The percentage of actively replicating cells within the tumor is known as the growth fraction. The mitotic index is the percentage of the replicating cells that are in mitosis. Initially, as a tumor grows in size, the growth fraction is high but this decreases as the tumor size increases due to restrictions of space, nutrients, and blood supply. The Gompertzian model of tumor growth represents this growth pattern, as shown in FIGURE 2.2.[2]

As stated previously, chemotherapy works primarily on cells that are actively replicating and, as such, tumors that are small in size and have a high growth fraction and mitotic index are more susceptible to the cytotoxic effects of chemotherapy. To maximize the killing effects of chemotherapy, the use of early intensive chemotherapy is preferred over delayed or low-dose treatment. This signifies the importance behind finding smaller tumors earlier in the disease by utilizing screening methodologies, and the rationale for treating patients with microscopic disease after surgery with multiple cycles of aggressive, high-dose, "adjuvant" chemotherapy.

Drug Selection

When selecting a chemotherapy agent for use against a specific tumor type several factors come into play. First, the drug has to be shown to be effective for the treatment of that cancer type. Next, the optimal dose for maximal cell kill within the toxicity range must be determined. Lastly, the optimal schedule and duration of treatment to improve response, yet keep toxicity to a minimum, should be established. For the interventional radiologist, the selection of chemotherapeutic agents to be used for regional administration is typically limited to agents that are proven effective when given systemically. In some cases, a chemotherapeutic agent may be too toxic to give systemically, and direct administration to a localized area may allow for increased tumor response while minimizing systemic exposure and thus unacceptable toxicity.

Pharmacokinetics/Pharmacodynamics

The study of drugs in humans can be divided into two parts: pharmacokinetics and pharmacodynamics.[3] It is important to understand the pharmacokinetics and pharmacodynamics of a chemotherapy agent to maximize its therapeutic effects. Pharmacokinetic properties including absorption, distribution, metabolism, and excretion provide information regarding the behavior of the drug in the body ("what the body does to the drug"). Using this information, clinical determinants, such as appropriate dose, schedule, and dose adjustments based on organ dysfunction (renal or hepatic), age, albumin status, and absorption issues, can be established. Pharmacodynamics relates the dose and kinetics of the drug to the observed clinical effects, for example, toxicity or response ("what the drug does to the body"). It is important for interventional radiologists to understand the general pharmacokinetic and pharmacodynamic properties of chemotherapeutic agents used in practice to ensure safe and effective use.

Concepts Behind Regional Administration

The rationale for the regional administration of chemotherapy is to deliver a higher concentration of the agent to the tumor present within a particular region of the body, to expose the tumor to active drug for longer periods than safely possible with systemic administration, and to improve clinically relevant concentration-dependent synergy between anticancer agents.[4] Intra-arterial therapies, such as chemoembolization, have become a rational treatment strategy in a number of clinical practice settings. The principles, management, and outcomes of intra-arterial therapies are discussed further in other chapters of this book.

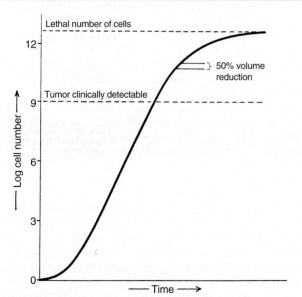

FIGURE 2.2 Gompertzian model of tumor growth.

Reproduced with permission from Casciato DA, Territo MC. *Manual of Clinical Oncology.* 6th ed. Philadelphia, PA: Lippincott Williams & Wilkins, 2009.

Concepts Behind Systemic Administration

With few exceptions, the use of a single chemotherapy agent is not curative in the treatment of cancer. Combination chemotherapy has been shown to be curative in the adjuvant (postsurgical) and neoadjuvant (presurgical) setting.[1] The advantages to combination chemotherapy regimens can be summarized in three basic premises. First, the use of multiple agents will increase the tumor cell kill of a treatment regimen. Second, utilizing agents with different mechanisms of action increases the range of interactions between tumor cells and drug, thus enhancing the synergy of the chemotherapeutic agents and targeting the heterogeneity of a tumor. Third, combination chemotherapy may prevent or slow the development of drug resistance.[5] Drug resistance is, in fact, the most common reason for failure of a chemotherapeutic regimen.[6] When combining chemotherapeutic agents together in a regimen the primary principles are to use (1) agents with different pharmacologic mechanisms of action, (2) agents with different organ toxicities, (3) agents that are active against the tumor and are preferably synergistic when used together, (4) agents at their optimal dose and schedules given at consistent intervals, and (5) agents that do not result in significant drug interactions.[5]

Concepts Behind Radiosensitization with Chemotherapy

Chemotherapeutic drugs that are able to produce significant sensitization of tumor cells to radiation treatment are termed *radiosensitizers*. The combination of radiotherapy and chemotherapy involves the individual cytotoxic actions of each treatment modality as well as the interactions between them and is termed *chemoradiation*.[7]

There are several mechanisms by which the combination of chemotherapy and radiation may increase tumor cell kill. Radiation itself induces many different lesions in the DNA molecule including single- and double-strand breaks, base damage, and inhibition of DNA repair. Chemotherapeutic agents that incorporate into DNA enhance cell killing by making DNA more susceptible to radiation damage. Many agents used in chemoradiation therapy also interfere with cellular repair mechanisms. Nucleoside analogs, such as gemcitabine, potently inhibit repair of genomic damage induced by ionizing radiation. In addition, they are preferentially cytotoxic to proliferative cells, thus slowing cell repopulation following fractionated radiation therapy.[8] Antimitotic agents, such as taxanes, block the transition of cells through mitosis, resulting in an accumulation of cells in the more radiosensitive G_2 and M phases of the cell cycle.[9]

Randomized trials have shown that combination treatment improves patient outcomes compared with radiation alone in the treatment of locally advanced cancers of the head and neck, lung, esophagus, stomach, pancreas, anus, and rectum.[8,10] The most commonly used radiosensitizing chemotherapeutic agents include the fluoropyrimidines (5-fluorouracil, fluorodeoxyuridine), taxanes, platinums, and gemcitabine. Chemoradiation therapy is limited by its narrow therapeutic index and significant potential toxicity to normal tissues during treatment. Efforts are ongoing to develop more selective and effective chemotherapeutic agents as well as agents that protect normal tissues or selectively target molecular processes responsible for tumor radioresistance or chemoresistance.[9]

■ CYTOTOXIC AGENTS

History of Modern Chemotherapy

Alkylating agents are among the oldest antineoplastic drugs that are still in use today. Before their use in the treatment of cancer, alkylating agents were better known for their use as chemical warfare agents ("mustard gas") in World War I. It was not until after an exposure incident occurred during World War II, however, that these poisons were considered by the medical community as potential therapeutic agents in oncologic disorders. The survivors of the exposure event, who had been submerged in nitrogen mustard-rich waters, experienced profound bone marrow suppression and lymph node shrinkage. This effect was later harnessed in an effort to develop similar agents that would be useful for treating cancerous overgrowth of lymphoid tissues.[11] The commencement of clinical studies with these agents launched the era of modern cancer chemotherapy.[12] Select chemotherapy agents that are utilized in the interventional radiology setting, or that patients undergoing interventional radiology procedures may be concomitantly receiving, are briefly described in Table 2.1.

Alkylating Agents

Although there are different classes of alkylating agents, they all share a common mechanism of action. The major cytotoxic effect results from covalent bonding of highly reactive alkyl groups with nucleophilic sites on biologic molecules, such as DNA. Binding of alkyl groups to reactive DNA molecules leads to inhibition of replication and transcription, DNA mispairing, and strand breakage that ultimately results in cell death.[13] Alkylating agents are classified as cell cycle nonspecific agents because they are capable of damaging DNA during any phase of the cell cycle. Despite this classification, their greatest cytotoxic effects are seen in rapidly dividing cells.[14]

Alkylating agents differ in their pharmacokinetics, lipid solubility, chemical reactivity, and properties of membrane transport. Alkylating agents are often used in combination regimens with other chemotherapy agents, especially in the systemic treatment of hematologic malignancies. The dose-limiting toxicity for alkylating agents is generally myelosuppression that manifests as neutropenia. Other common toxicities include nausea and vomiting, alopecia, and infertility; rarely, secondary malignancies, such as leukemia, may occur due to DNA damage inflicted by the antineoplastic drugs themselves. Alkylating agents are not commonly used in interventional radiology procedures at the time of this review.

Platinum Salts

Platinum derivatives were serendipitously discovered in the 1960s when it was observed that bacterial growth was inhibited following electrical current delivery to the media through platinum electrodes. The antiproliferative action was noted to be similar to that produced by alkylating agents and radiation.[13,15]

Cisplatin, carboplatin, and oxaliplatin are "alkylating-like" agents used commonly in clinical practice. Platinum compounds enter the cell predominantly by passive diffusion and bind to DNA, forming intrastrand crosslinks or adducts

Table 2.1			
Select Chemotherapy Agents			
Agent class	**Agent used in IR**	**Clinical application in IR**	**Adverse effects**
Alkylating agents		None common	Myelosuppression, GI symptoms, potential for sterility and carcinogenesis
Platinum derivatives	Cisplatin	TACE—HCC, cholangiocarcinoma, carcinoid, liver metastases (neuroendocrine tumors, sarcoma)	Nausea/vomiting, ototoxicity, nephrotoxicity, myelosuppression, neuropathy
Antimetabolites	Fluorouracil (5-FU)	HAIC—HCC	Mucositis, diarrhea, nausea/vomiting, skin reactions, neuropathy, cardiotoxicity, myelosuppression, alopecia
Topoisomerase inhibitors	Doxorubicin	TACE, DEB—HCC, cholangiocarcinoma, carcinoid, liver metastases (neuroendocrine tumors, sarcoma)	Cardiotoxicity, myelosuppression, alopecia, nausea/vomiting, mucositis, red-tinged urine (not hematuria), palmar-plantar erythrodysesthesia
	Irinotecan	TACE—liver metastases from colorectal cancer	Diarrhea, fever, myelosuppression, nausea/vomiting, pancreatitis, thromboembolism, typhlitic colitis, and toxic megacolon
Other agents	Bleomycin	Pleurodesis of malignant pleural effusion	Fever, local pain
	Mitomycin C	HIAC, TACE—HCC, liver metastases (colorectal, ocular melanoma, neuroendocrine tumors)	Fever, anorexia, nausea/vomiting, myelosuppression, hemolytic uremic syndrome, local hepatic arterial thrombosis
Antimicrotubule agents	None common	None common	Peripheral neuropathy, mucositis, GI symptoms, alopecia
Monoclonal antibodies	Bevacizumab	TACE—liver metastases from colorectal cancer	Hypertension, proteinuria, epistaxis, headache, impaired wound healing, GI perforation, exfoliative dermatitis, taste alteration, lacrimation disorder
	Cetuximab	Not commonly used in regional chemotherapy but used in systemic regimens for CRC, H & NC, and others	Infusion reactions, malaise, acneiform rash, headache, edema, paronychia, hypomagnesemia, anorexia, conjunctivitis, cough, interstitial lung disease
	Panitumumab	Not commonly used in regional chemotherapy but used in systemic regimens for CRC and others	Acneiform rash, fatigue, infusion reactions, paronychia, edema, hypomagnesemia, anorexia, conjunctivitis, cough, interstitial lung disease
	Trastuzumab	Not commonly used in regional chemotherapy but used in systemic regimens for breast, gastric, and other cancers	Impaired cardiac function, asthenia, headache, dizziness, rash, infusion reactions, arthralgias, myalgias, cough, interstitial lung disease, flulike syndrome

(continued)

Table 2.1			
Select Chemotherapy Agents (*Continued*)			
Agent class	Agent used in IR	Clinical application in IR	Adverse effects
Multikinase inhibitors *None commonly used in regional chemotherapy*	Sorafenib	Used in systemic regimens for HCC, RCC, and others	Diarrhea, weight loss, hand-foot skin reaction, hypertension, fatigue, neuropathy, elevated transaminases/lipase/amylase, hypophosphatemia, GI symptoms, myelosuppression, bleeding events
	Sunitinib	Used in systemic regimens for GIST, RCC, and others	Hypertension, fatigue, asthenia, neuropathy, yellow skin discoloration, reversible hair depigmentation, hypothyroidism, diarrhea, nausea, anorexia, elevated transaminases/lipase/amylase, myelosuppression, electrolyte alterations
	Pazopanib	Used in systemic regimens for RCC and others	Hypertension, diarrhea, hair color changes, nausea, anorexia, headache, fatigue, fatal hepatotoxicity, asthenia, elevated transaminases, hypophosphatemia, hypomagnesemia, myelosuppression
	Erlotinib	Used in systemic regimens for NSCLC, pancreatic cancer, and others	Fatigue, acneiform rash, diarrhea, anorexia, elevated transaminases, dyspnea, interstitial lung disease, conjunctivitis

IR, interventional radiology; GI, gastrointestinal; TACE, transarterial chemoembolization; HCC, hepatocellular carcinoma; HAIC, hepatic arterial infusion chemotherapy; HIAC, hepatic intra-arterial chemotherapy; DEB, drug eluting beads; CRC, colorectal cancer; H & NC, head and neck cancer; RCC, renal cell carcinoma; GIST, gastrointestinal stromal tumor; NSCLC, non–small-cell lung cancer.

between adjacent guanines.[16] The intrastrand crosslinks cause cellular damage through bending and distortion of normal DNA conformation, which is thought to trigger an enzymatic cascade that ends in apoptosis.[17] Less frequently, *interstrand* crosslinks are formed, which also contribute to the demise of tumor cells. Platinum compounds cause apoptosis most readily in cells that are actively replicating and are thus relatively cell-phase specific.

Cisplatin is a highly toxic antineoplastic agent that can cause potentially severe adverse events including dose-limiting nausea and vomiting (acute and delayed), nephrotoxicity with electrolyte disturbances, myelosuppression, ototoxicity, and peripheral neuropathies. Other, less toxic platinums have been developed, but all platinum agents are not active in the same cancers. Cisplatin has shown superior efficacy in many tumor types and is, therefore, still considered a valuable platinum agent despite its significant toxicity profile. In addition, most adverse events can now be reasonably controlled with aggressive supportive care including antiemetics and aggressive hydration to prevent nephrotoxicity.[18]

Carboplatin and oxaliplatin are platinum derivatives that were developed in an effort to decrease the severe toxicity encountered with cisplatin. Their potential to cause renal damage, ototoxicity, and nausea or vomiting is much less when compared to that of cisplatin in equivalent doses. In contrast to cisplatin, the dose-limiting toxicities for carboplatin and oxaliplatin are myelosuppression and neuropathies, respectively. Carboplatin is most commonly dosed according to the Calvert formula, a calculation that uses target area under the curve and

renal function parameters to estimate the dose for individual patients.[13] The acute and rapidly reversible neurosensory toxicity that occurs during or shortly after oxaliplatin infusion manifests as paresthesias or dysesthesia in the extremities and is often triggered by exposure to cold. Delayed neurosensory toxicity is cumulative and less readily reversible. It often presents as deep sensory loss, sensory ataxia, or functional impairment.[19]

Platinum compounds are used in a wide variety of systemic chemotherapy regimens in the treatment of lung, testicular, bladder, breast, ovarian, colorectal, head and neck, and gastric carcinomas. Cisplatin is often used in the treatment of liver tumors during transarterial chemoembolization (TACE) procedures.

Antimetabolites

Antimetabolites are structural analogs of naturally occurring physiologic molecules found in the body. These agents exert damage to DNA through competitive enzyme binding or by direct incorporation into DNA or RNA. Macromolecules that are formed following incorporation of antimetabolites are incapable of carrying out their intended physiologic functions, ultimately resulting in apoptotic cell death. Because DNA synthesis occurs during the S phase of the cell cycle, antimetabolites are considered cell cycle-specific agents. Antimetabolites are considered the most versatile drug class in chemotherapy,[20] and they are used to treat multiple tumor types including lymphocytic leukemia, breast cancer, gastrointestinal (GI) adenocarcinoma, squamous cell carcinoma, and hepatocellular carcinoma (HCC).

Fluoropyrimidines have been the mainstay of treatment for several solid tumors, including colorectal, breast, and head and neck cancers, for over 40 years. Fluorouracil (5-FU) is a fluorinated analog of the naturally occurring pyrimidine uracil. It is a prodrug and must be metabolized to the nucleotide form, fluorodeoxyuridine monophosphate (FdUMP), to be active. FdUMP binds tightly to the enzyme thymidylate synthase (TS), which is normally involved in the synthesis of thymidine, an essential building block of DNA. Fluorouracil is usually administered with calcium leucovorin, a reduced folate, to enhance stability of the FdUMP-TS complex and increase cytotoxicity of the drug.[13]

Capecitabine is an orally active prodrug of 5-FU. It is almost 100% bioavailable and is absorbed through the GI tract in an inactive form and subsequently converted to 5-FU in a three-step process that starts in the liver. The process is completed by thymidine phosphorylase, an enzyme found in much higher concentrations in tumor tissue than in normal tissue. Theoretically, tumor "selective" conversion of capecitabine into 5-FU may provide greater targeted antitumor effects while reducing toxicity. Chronic twice-daily dosing of capecitabine produces a similar toxicity pattern to that of infusional 5-FU.[21]

Fluorouracil is the most frequently used chemotherapeutic agent for hepatic arterial infusion chemotherapy (HAIC). In these procedures, it is often used in combination with other drugs, such as cisplatin, which amplify the effects of 5-FU through biochemical modulation and enhancement of antitumor effects.[22] Approximately 95% of a dose of 5-FU is absorbed by an HCC on first pass through the liver, which allows a high intratumoral concentration while maintaining a low systemic toxicity.[23]

Other antimetabolites are not commonly used in locoregional therapy; however, they are discussed briefly for the sake of completeness. Cytarabine and gemcitabine are antimetabolite drugs that are structurally related to one another. They exert antineoplastic effects through competitive inhibition of DNA polymerase following conversion to their active triphosphate nucleotide forms.[13] Purine analogs such as thioguanine (6-TG) and mercaptopurine (6-MP) are structural analogs of guanine, which undergo conversion to substrates that are incorporated into DNA and prevent purine synthesis. Fludarabine is an analog of the purine adenine that works by interfering with DNA polymerase, causing chain termination.[13]

Methotrexate (MTX) is a folate antagonist that prevents the conversion of folic acid to tetrahydrofolate by inhibiting the enzyme dihydrofolate reductase (DHFR). This depletes intracellular pools of reduced folates required as cofactors for DNA synthesis. Because this mechanism of action affects both tumor and normal cells, high-dose therapy with MTX requires neutralization through administration of exogenous reduced folates to overcome the toxic effects of MTX. The reduced folate used in clinical practice to "rescue" normal cells is calcium leucovorin.[13]

Topoisomerase Inhibitors

DNA topoisomerases are enzymes that maintain DNA topologic structure during replication and transcription. They relieve torsional strain during DNA unwinding and allow for necessary strand breaks followed by religation during DNA transcription and replication. Topoisomerase I enzymes produce single-strand breaks and inhibit resealing, whereas topoisomerase II enzymes produce double-strand breaks.[13]

Anthracene derivatives such as doxorubicin induce formation of covalent complexes between topoisomerase II and DNA. Their characteristic four-ring structure binds tightly to DNA by intercalation and results in local uncoiling of the double helix followed by double-stranded DNA breaks. Inhibition of topoisomerase II prevents the normal resealing step after double-strand breakage. Tumor cell death ensues when strand breaks cannot be repaired before cell division is attempted. Anthracyclines also undergo electron reduction, which produces highly reactive free-radical species. Although free-radical production is not a major mechanism for tumor destruction, it is a well-studied cause of anthracycline toxicity and is responsible for cardiac damage as well as extravasation injury.[24]

Doxorubicin is used extensively as a systemic agent in many types of solid tumors and hematologic malignancies. It is also one of the most common agents used by interventional radiologists for TACE or in drug-eluting beads. Intra-arterial administration allows for highly concentrated local drug delivery with relatively less systemic toxicity and is frequently used in the treatment of HCC.[25]

Camptothecin derivatives, such as irinotecan and topotecan, are potent inhibitors of DNA topoisomerase I. Inhibition of this enzyme results in stabilization of cleavable complexes, thus allowing the process of uncoiling to continue while preventing religation of DNA single-strand breaks.[26] Camptothecin derivatives are used in the treatment of GI, cervical, ovarian, and lung cancers. Irinotecan is currently used in interventional radiology procedures as irinotecan-loaded DC beads (PARAGON beads) via Biocompatibles UK Ltd.

Etoposide and teniposide are semisynthetic *podophyllotoxin derivatives* that are synthesized from extracts of the mayapple or mandrake plant. These drugs damage tumor cells by causing DNA strand breakage through inhibition of topoisomerase II.[13] They are effective in the treatment of testicular, ovarian, and small-cell lung cancers as well as several hematologic malignancies. Epipodophyllotoxins are not commonly used in interventional radiology procedures at this time.

Antimicrotubule Agents

Antimicrotubule agents bind to tubulin, the structural protein that polymerizes to form microtubules. Inhibiting the movement of microtubules interferes with the normal balance of tubulin assembly or disassembly during mitosis, ultimately resulting in apoptosis.[13] Antimicrotubule agents are not commonly used in interventional radiology procedures but are summarized briefly. These agents are severe vesicants that may produce epithelial blistering and tissue necrosis if leakage from the IV site occurs.

Vinca alkaloids are natural products derived from the periwinkle plant. They bind to tubulin, inhibiting its polymerization and formation of the mitotic spindle during mitosis.[27] Vinca alkaloids exert most of their action during the M phase of the cell cycle through inhibition of cell division. They also retain some activity during the quiescent portion of the cell cycle because microtubules are involved in intracellular transport processes that occur throughout all phases of cellular development. The dose-limiting toxicity of vincristine is a peripheral neuropathy that is common to all antimicrotubule agents because functional microtubules are required for intracellular axonal transport. The neuropathy usually begins as parasthesias in the hands before progressing to the feet and persists for a variable time period after completion of therapy.[28]

Taxanes, specifically paclitaxel, were initially extracted from the bark of the Pacific Yew tree.[13] The taxanes are similar to vinca alkaloids in that they are active during the M phase of the cell cycle; however, instead of preventing microtubule polymerization, they promote microtubule assembly and prevent depolymerization. This leads to inappropriately stable and nonfunctional microtubules, eventually causing cell death.

Other Agents

Bleomycin is an antineoplastic antibiotic that is a mixture of peptides from fungal *Streptomyces* species. It binds DNA and produces strand breakage through generation of free radicals formed using free iron in the cell nucleus. Bleomycin is used in many systemic combination regimens, where the dose-limiting toxicity is pulmonary toxicity that can ultimately lead to pulmonary fibrosis. It is widely used by interventionalists as a sclerosing agent in the treatment of malignant pleural effusions.[29] Of the intracavitary dose delivered, approximately half enters into the systemic circulation.[30]

Mitomycin C is an antineoplastic antibiotic that has functional similarities to nitrogen mustard compounds and may function as an alkylating agent to inhibit DNA and RNA synthesis. This reaction is best catalyzed in an oxygen-poor environment.[31] The dose-limiting toxicity is delayed myelosuppression that may take 6 to 7 weeks to recover. Mitomycin C is used systemically to treat gastric, pancreatic, breast, and lung cancers. It is also utilized by interventionalists in hepatic intra-arterial chemotherapy and chemoembolization procedures.[32]

▌ TARGETED ANTICANCER THERAPY

Targeted chemotherapy inhibits cancer growth and spread through interference with specific molecular pathways and receptors that are overexpressed by tumors. This differs from traditional cytotoxic chemotherapy and allows the agent to have greater selectivity for cancer cells, typically resulting in less harm to normal tissue. Although this does not mean that these agents are without adverse effects, their use frequently results in a different adverse effect profile than cytotoxic agents.

Monoclonal Antibodies

Monoclonal antibodies bind to receptors preferentially expressed on the cell surface of some cancers. They may be "naked" or bound to a toxin, chemotherapy drug, or radioactive isotope ("conjugated").[33] Once bound, the antibodies exert their antitumor effects by activating the cells of the innate immune system to lyse the marked tumor cells, blocking growth stimuli from the receptor, or delivering the conjugated material to cause cell death. Naked monoclonal antibodies act through the first two mechanisms and are more frequently used in clinical practice.

Naked monoclonal antibodies are used as single agents or in combination with cytotoxic chemotherapy regimens for treatment of malignancies such as non-Hodgkin lymphoma (rituximab), metastatic colorectal cancer (bevacizumab, cetuximab, panitumumab), and metastatic breast cancer (trastuzumab).[34] These monoclonal antibodies target receptors for CD20 (rituximab), vascular endothelial growth factor (VEGF)

(bevacizumab), and HER family receptors (trastuzumab, cetuximab, panitumumab), including multiple endothelial growth factor receptor (EGFR) subtypes. Conjugated monoclonal antibodies are used to treat some lymphomas (e.g., ^{90}Y ibritomomab tiuxetan). Currently, monoclonal antibodies are not typically used in combination with other antibodies outside of clinical trials.

Adverse effects of monoclonal antibodies vary and are often related to the receptor to which it is targeted.[35] For example, bevacizumab inhibits VEGF and as a result of these effects on the vasculature may cause decreased wound healing, GI perforation, hemorrhage, thromboembolic events, hypertension, and proteinuria. The EGFR inhibitors cetuximab and panitumumab cause an acneiform rash due to the effects of EGFR inhibition in the skin. Trastuzumab may cause cardiotoxicity due to its effects on HER receptor subtypes expressed in cardiac tissue.[36]

Because some of these agents retain some characteristics of the animal antibody from which they were derived, hypersensitivity or infusion reactions may occur. Infusion reactions may occur at any point during treatment, although rituximab reactions occur most commonly with the first infusion.[35] The incidence varies with the agent, and patients may experience reactions that range from mild itching or rash to severe anaphylaxis. The more humanized antibodies typically carry a lower chance of these reactions.

Multikinase Inhibitors

Protein kinases are transmembrane proteins that regulate cell signaling pathways involved in cancers, including cellular proliferation, invasion, metastasis, and angiogenesis.[37] In normal tissue, kinases and their respective pathways are inactive unless phosphorylated. A component of the multistep carcinogenic pathway observed in cancers such as colorectal cancer involves a mutation that causes constitutive activation of the kinase so that it is always "on."[38] This results in abnormal cellular proliferation and differentiation. The class of small molecules that inhibit these kinases is known as tyrosine kinase inhibitors (TKIs). The TKIs reversibly inhibit a variety of kinases and molecular pathways; there are many TKIs currently in development. Although the TKIs typically have shorter half-lives than monoclonal antibodies that may affect the same receptor, they are administered orally which many patients may prefer.

Similarly to the monoclonal antibodies, the adverse effect profile of a TKI is frequently related to the agent's mechanism of action. The TKIs that inhibit VEGF (sorafenib, sunitinib, pazopanib) are also associated with hypertension and increased risks of bleeding and clotting; TKIs that inhibit EGFR are also associated with skin rash (erlotinib, gefitinib); TKIs that inhibit HER2 are associated with impaired cardiac function (lapatinib). Additionally, the TKIs are also associated with GI adverse effects, such as diarrhea, as well as nonrelated adverse effects, such as hand-foot syndrome.

One TKI frequently used by patients presenting to interventional radiology (IR) for treatment is sorafenib, an oral multikinase inhibitor of the VEGF receptor and other pro-oncogenic cellular pathways. It is used in the systemic treatment of highly vascular tumors such as HCC and renal cell carcinoma (RCC). A placebo-controlled, multicenter study published in 2008 by Llovet et al. demonstrated a mean 3-month increased survival time and time to radiologic progression in the treatment of

HCC (in Child's A patients),[39] and now it is commonly used for treatment of advanced HCC in addition to localized therapy provided by IR. Other TKIs that may be seen in the IR population include sunitinib (RCC), pazopanib (RCC), and erlotinib (non–small-cell lung cancer [NSCLC]).

Specific Concerns with Angiogenesis Inhibitors

Angiogenesis inhibitors are used to treat multiple cancers, including colorectal cancer, NSCLC, RCC, HCC, ovarian cancer, glioblastoma, and breast cancer. Angiogenesis inhibitors include both monoclonal antibodies (bevacizumab) and small-molecule kinase inhibitors (sorafenib, sunitinib, pazopanib) that inhibit the effects of VEGF by binding the VEGF receptor or inhibiting downstream signaling, respectively. VEGF is overexpressed in many solid tumors, allowing increased inhibitory effects in tumor tissue over regular tissue. VEGF inhibition decreases angiogenesis within the tumor to inhibit cancer growth and spread. Angiogenesis inhibitors also may exert other antitumor effects, most notably enhancing permeation and cytotoxicity of chemotherapy agents through vascular normalization.

Because inhibition of VEGF can also prevent angiogenesis in normal tissue, prior or concomitant treatment with an angiogenesis inhibitor may impact outcomes after portal vein embolization of hepatic colorectal cancer metastases.[40] Some studies have noted lower remnant liver volume in patients receiving bevacizumab; however, other studies have noted no differences between patients receiving chemotherapy alone or in combination with bevacizumab.

The TKIs that inhibit VEGF (sorafenib, sunitinib, pazopanib) may also prevent angiogenesis after procedures, affecting the sequencing of these treatments. This has been hypothesized to improve efficacy by preventing angiogenesis after TACE has been performed, but it may also increase complications during or after TACE and worsen outcomes. Historically, due to concern for increased bleeding risk and changes in tumor vasculature impacting the ability to deliver TACE, treatment of HCC with sorafenib has been reserved until after TACE has been performed. Phase II studies suggest that performing TACE while patients are receiving sorafenib may be safe and effective[41]; however, larger phase III studies evaluating concurrent administration are currently ongoing.[42]

Miscellaneous Targeted Agents

Targeted cancer treatments include a diverse array of other agents, and although they are not commonly used in locoregional therapy, the major classes are discussed briefly for the sake of completeness. *Interferons* are immunomodulators that activate cellular pathways to cause innate immune system upregulation and are used in both hematologic malignances and solid tumors.[43] *Interleukin-2* enhances the activity of cytotoxic and natural killer T cells and is used in the treatment of metastatic RCC and metastatic melanoma.[44] *Histone deacetylase inhibitors* affect DNA packaging proteins used in the transcription process, causing apoptosis and arresting cell growth. These agents are used to treat hematologic malignancies.[45] *Hormonal agents* manipulate the endocrine pathways of susceptible tumor types, such as prostate cancer and hormone receptor-positive breast cancer, and include selective estrogen receptor modulators, aromatase inhibitors, antiandrogens, and GnRH agonists.[46] The *mTOR inhibitors* affect multiple intracellular pathways to decrease cell growth and proliferation and are currently approved for the treatment of RCC and pancreatic neuroendocrine tumors, although they have been studied in other tumor types.[47]

CONCLUSION

The image-guided, regional chemotherapeutic techniques used by interventional radiologists offer high-concentration, directed delivery of agents to local tumor environments. As the model of IR practice continues to involve direct patient management, it has become increasingly important for interventionalists to be familiar with the systemic chemotherapy regimens that their patients are receiving in addition to the agents used in regional chemotherapy. Increasing the knowledge of chemotherapeutic principles, agents, and toxicities will help to optimize outcomes and minimize toxicity in patients receiving multimodality treatment for their cancer.

REFERENCES

1. Lees J, ed. Control of the cell cycle. In: Abeloff M, Armitage J, Niederhuber J, et al., eds. *Abeloff's Clinical Oncology*. 4th ed. Philadelphia, PA: Churchill Livingstone/Elsevier; 2008:50.
2. Norton L. A Gompertzian model of human breast cancer growth. *Cancer Res* 1988;48:7067–7071.
3. Takimoto C, Ng C, eds. Pharmacokinetics and pharmacodynamics. In: DeVita V, Hellman S, Rosenberg S, eds. *Cancer: Principles & Practice of Oncology*. 8th ed. Philadelphia, PA: Lippincott Williams & Wilkins; 2005:392.
4. Markman M, ed. Regional chemotherapy. In: Kufe DW, Pollock RE, Weichselbaum RR, et al., eds. *Holland-Frei Cancer Medicine*. Hamilton (ON): BC Decker; 2003.
5. DeVita V, Chu E, eds. Basic principles. In: DeVita V, Hellman S, Rosenberg S, eds., *Cancer: Principles & Practice of Oncology*. 8th ed. Philadelphia, PA: Lippincott Williams & Wilkins; 2005:337.
6. Kinsella A, Smith D. Tumor resistance to antimetabolites. *Gen Pharmacol* 1998;30:623–626.
7. Pauwels B, Korst AE, Lardon F, et al. Combined modality therapy of gemcitabine and radiation. *Oncologist* 2005;10:34–51.
8. Lawrence TS, Blackstock AW, McGinn C. The mechanism of action of radiosensitization of conventional chemotherapeutic agents. *Semin Radiat Oncol* 2003;13:13–21.
9. Halperin EC, Perez CA, Brady LW. *Perez and Brady's Principles and Practice of Radiation Oncology*. 5th ed. Philadelphia, PA: Wolters Kluwer Health/Lippincott Williams & Wilkins; 2008.
10. Uronis H, Bendell J. Anal cancer: an overview. *The Oncologist* 2007;12:524–534.
11. Hirsch J. An anniversary for cancer chemotherapy. *JAMA* 2006;296:1518–1520.
12. Chabner BA, Ryan DP, Paz-Ares L, et al. Antineoplastic agents. In: Hardman JG, Limbird LE, Gilman AG, eds. *The Pharmacological Basis of Therapeutics*. New York, NY: McGraw-Hill; 2001:1389. Chabner BA, Bertino J, Cleary J, et al. Chapter 61. Cytotoxic Agents. In: Chabner BA, Brunton LL, Knollmann BC, eds. Goodman & Gilman's *The Pharmacological Basis of Therapeutics*. 12th eds. New York, NY: McGraw-Hill; 2011:online edition.
13. Balmer CM VA, Iannucci A. Cancer treatment and chemotherapy. In: Dipiro J, Talbert R, Yee G, et al., eds. *Pharmacotherapy: A Pathophysiologic Approach*. 6th ed. New York, NY: McGraw-Hill; 2005:2279–2328. Medina PJ, Shord SS. Chapter 135. Cancer treatment and chemotherapy. In: Talbert RL, DiPiro JT, Matzke GR, Posey LM, Wells BG, Yee GC, eds. *Pharmacotherapy: A Pathophysiologic Approach*. 8th ed. New York, NY: McGraw-Hill; 2011: online edition.
14. Huitema AD, Smits KD, Mathot RA, et al. The clinical pharmacology of alkylating agents in high-dose chemotherapy. *Anticancer Drugs* 2000;11:515–533.
15. Alama A, Tasso B, Novelli F, et al. Organometallic compounds in oncology: implications of novel organotins as antitumor agents. *Drug Discov Today* 2009;14:500–508.
16. Gately DP, Howell SB. Cellular accumulation of the anticancer agent cisplatin: a review. *Br J Cancer* 1993;67:1171–1176.

17. Johnson S, O'Dwyer P. Cisplatin and its analogues. In: DeVita V, Hellman S, Rosenberg S, eds. *Cancer: Principles & Practice of Oncology*. Philadelphia, PA: Lippincott Williams & Wilkins; 2005:344–358.

18. O'Dwyer PJ, Stevenson JP, Johnson SW. Clinical pharmacokinetics and administration of established platinum drugs. *Drugs* 2000;59(suppl 4):19–27.

19. Pasetto LM, D'Andrea MR, Rossi E, et al. Oxaliplatin-related neurotoxicity: how and why? *Crit Rev Oncol Hematol* 2006;59:159–168.

20. Kummar S, Noronha V, Chu E. Antimetabolites. In: DeVita V, Hellman S, Rosenberg S, eds. *Cancer: Principles & Practice of Oncology*. Philadelphia, PA: Lippincott Williams & Wilkins; 2005:358.

21. Mikhail SE, Sun JF, Marshall JL. Safety of capecitabine: a review. *Expert Opin Drug Saf* 2010;9:831–841.

22. Eun JR, Lee HJ, Moon HJ, et al. Hepatic arterial infusion chemotherapy using high-dose 5-fluorouracil and cisplatin with or without interferon-alpha for the treatment of advanced hepatocellular carcinoma with portal vein tumor thrombosis. *Scand J Gastroenterol* 2009;44:1477–1486.

23. Ray C, Koczwara B. Principles of chemotherapy. In: Ray CE, Hicks ME, Patel NH, eds. *Interventions in Oncology*. Fairfax, VA: Society of Interventional Radiology; 2003:9–15.

24. Simunek T, Sterba M, Popelova O, et al. Anthracycline induced cardiotoxicity: overview of studies examining the roles of oxidative stress and free cellular iron. *Pharmacol Rep* 2009;61:154–171.

25. Liapi E, Geschwind JF. Intra-arterial therapies for hepatocellular carcinoma: where do we stand? *Ann Surg Oncol* 2010;17:1234–1246.

26. Liu EH, Qi LW, Wu Q, et al. Anticancer agents derived from natural products. *Mini Rev Med Chem* 2009;9:1547–1555.

27. Risinger AL, Giles FJ, Mooberry SL. Microtubule dynamics as a target in oncology. *Cancer Treat Rev* 2009;35:255–261.

28. Verstappen CC, Koeppen S, Heimans JJ, et al. Dose-related vincristine-induced peripheral neuropathy with unexpected off-therapy worsening. *Neurology* 2005;64:1076–1077.

29. Zimmer PW, Hill M, Casey K, et al. Prospective randomized trial of talc slurry vs bleomycin in pleurodesis for symptomatic malignant pleural effusions. *Chest* 1997;112:430–434.

30. Copur M, Rose M, Chu E. Miscellaneous chemotherapeutic agents. In: DeVita V, Hellman S, Rosenberg S, eds. *Cancer: Principles & Practice of Oncology*. Philadelphia, PA: Lippincott Williams & Wilkins; 2005:417.

31. Colvin O, Friedman H. Alkylating agents. In: DeVita V, Hellman S, Rosenberg S, eds. *Cancer: Principles & Practice of Oncology*. Philadelphia, PA: Lippincott Williams & Wilkins; 2005:332–344.

32. Herber S, Otto G, Schneider J, et al. Transarterial chemoembolization (TACE) for inoperable intrahepatic cholangiocarcinoma. *Cardiovasc Intervent Radiol* 2007;30:1156–1165.

33. Argyriou A, Kalofonos H. Recent advances relating to the clinical application of naked monoclonal antibodies in solid tumors. *Mol Med* 2009;15:183–191.

34. Cheng J, Adams G, Robinson M, et al. Monoclonal antibodies. In: DeVita V, Hellman S, Rosenberg S, eds. *Cancer: Principles & Practice of Oncology*. Philadelphia, PA: Lippincott Williams & Wilkins; 2005:445–456.

35. Boyiadzis M, Foon K. Approved monoclonal antibodies for cancer therapy. *Expert Opin Biol Ther* 2008;8:1151–1158.

36. Chien K. Herceptin and the heart—a molecular modifier of carciac failure. *N Engl J Med* 2006;354.

37. Giamas G, Man Y, Hirner H, et al. Kinases as targets in the treatment of solid tumors. *Cell Signal* 2010;22:984–1002.

38. Ito Y, Sasaki Y, Horimoto M, et al. Activation of mitogen-activated protein kinases/extracellular signal-regulated kinases in human hepatocellular carcinoma. *Hepatology* (Baltimore MD) 1998;27:951–958.

39. Llovet JM, Ricci S, Mazzaferro V, et al. Sorafenib in advanced hepatocellular carcinoma. *N Engl J Med* 2008;359:378–390.

40. Geva R, Prenen H, Topal B, et al. Biologic modulation of chemotherapy in patients with hepatic colorectal metastases: the role of anti-VEGF and anti-EGFR antibodies. *J Surg Oncol* 2010;102:937–945.

41. Pawlik T, Reyes D, Cosgrove D, et al. Phase II trial of sorafenib combined with concurrent transarterial chemoembolization with drug-eluting beads for hepatocellular carcinoma. *J Clin Oncol* 2011;29:3960–3967.

42. Hoffmann K, Glimm H, Radeleff B, et al. Prospective, randomized, double-blind, multi-center, phase III clinical study on transarterial chemoembolization (TACE) combined with sorafenib versus TACE plus placebo in patients with hepatocellular cancer before liver transplantation - HeiLivCa [ISRCTN24081794]. *BMC Cancer* 2008;8.

43. Sondak V, Redman B. Pharmacology of cancer biotherapeutics. In: DeVita V, Hellman S, Rosenberg S, eds. *Cancer: Principles & Practice of Oncology*. Philadelphia, PA: Lippincott Williams & Wilkins; 2005:423–430.

44. Mier J, Atkins M. Interleukin-2. In: DeVita V, Hellman S, Rosenberg S, eds. *Cancer: Principles & Practice of Oncology*. Philadelphia, PA: Lippincott Williams & Wilkins; 2005:431–438.

45. Marks P, Richon V, Miller T, et al. Histone deacetylase inhibitors: new targeted anticancer drugs. In: DeVita V, Hellman S, Rosenberg S, eds. *Cancer: Principles & Practice of Oncology*. Philadelphia, PA: Lippincott Williams & Wilkins; 2005:439–445.

46. Goetz M, Erlichman C, Loprinzi C. Pharmacology of endocrine manipulation. In: DeVita V, Hellman S, Rosenberg S, eds. *Cancer: Principles & Practice of Oncology*. Philadelphia, PA: Lippincott Williams & Wilkins; 2005:457–469.

47. Di Lorenzo G, Buonerba C, Biglietto M, et al. The therapy of kidney cancer with biomolecular drugs. *Cancer Treat Rev* 2010;36(suppl 3):S16–S20.

Principles of Locoregional Therapy: Intra-Arterial Therapies

ELENI LIAPI and JEAN-FRANÇOIS H. GESCHWIND

INTRODUCTION

Intra-arterial therapies are image-guided locoregional therapies that deliver targeted anticancer therapy via intra-arterially inserted catheters for treatment of various malignancies, mostly for palliation. Intra-arterial therapies are widely employed for patients with unresectable hepatic malignancies with proven prolonged overall survival in selected patient populations.[1] Other sites of application include the lungs, brain, uterus, kidneys, bones, oral cavity, and anterior oropharynx.[2–4] The goal of an intra-arterial therapy is to selectively deliver therapeutic agents to the arterial supply of a tumor. In this way, increased concentration of chemotherapy reaches the tumor, while concurrently systemic toxicity is minimized. In this chapter, we focus on the principles of intra-arterial therapies for hepatic malignancies. Hepatic malignancies that are amenable to intra-arterial therapies include hepatocellular carcinoma (HCC) (and its variant, fibrolamellar), primary intrahepatic cholangiocarcinoma, hepatic neuroendocrine metastases, colorectal, and other metastases to the liver (uveal melanoma, breast cancer, leiomyosarcoma).[5–7] The most commonly performed intra-arterial therapies for hepatic malignancies include transcatheter arterial chemoembolization (TACE) with ethiodized oil, transcatheter arterial chemoembolization with drug-eluting beads (DEB-TACE), and radioembolization. These procedures are further described and discussed in Chapter 7.

The constantly evolving field of interventional oncology can be considered as an integrative part of the complex area of medical and surgical oncology. The medical oncologic component of any intra-arterial therapy relates to the pharmacologic oncologic principles and patient management, whereas the surgical oncologic component relates mostly to the technical procedural details. In this chapter, we focus first on the medical oncologic principles of intra-arterial therapies for hepatic malignancies. These principles are based on the comprehensive evaluation of the clinical setting, the tumor characteristics and the underlying biology, as well as the pharmacologic oncologic background of the agents that are commonly used for intra-arterial therapies. For the surgical oncologic perspective of intra-arterial therapies, important anatomic details, arterial flow dynamics, principles of embolotherapy, as well as technical considerations are covered.

HISTORICAL BACKGROUND

Intra-arterial delivery of chemotherapy for liver cancer was first attempted in the early 1960s in the form of regional arterial infusion chemotherapy with surgically placed catheters.[8] In subsequent years, several techniques for placement of percutaneous catheters were developed for patients with both primary and metastatic tumors.[9] Although the toxicities associated with the various chemotherapeutic agents were documented

as relatively mild, there were significant problems associated with the catheter thrombosis, infection, and leakage or catheter malposition. These issues were noted with both surgically and radiographically placed intra-arterial infusion catheters.[10] Interestingly, thrombosis of the catheter during delivery of intra-arterial chemotherapy was described as beneficial for inducing an improved tumor response.[11,12]

Hepatic arterial ligation with intra-arterial injection of chemotherapy was another initial attempt of targeted chemotherapeutic delivery to hepatic tumors via the hepatic artery.[12,13] Soon, this method was replaced by the purposeful long-term insertion and securement of intra-arterial catheters for the creation of complete or partial thrombosis of the hepatic artery with concurrent administration of chemotherapy.[12] By the early 1970s, intra-arterial embolization had already been developed with the injection of gelfoam particles in the hepatic artery and nonocclusive embolization was thought as beneficial due to the development of only few collaterals to the tumor.[14] At that time, intrahepatic arterial injection of adriamycin, 5-fluorouracil, mitomycin-C, or their combinations was also introduced for treatment of HCC.[15] The technique of chemoembolization with the injection of a combination of ethiodized oil and chemotherapy was developed in Japan a few years later.[13,16,17] Since then, multiple variations on the technique and drug combinations have been developed for intra-arterial delivery, leading to significant tumor necrosis and improved overall survival in selected patients.[5,18–20]

RATIONALE FOR INTRA-ARTERIAL DELIVERY OF THERAPY

The hepatic tumor microenvironment consists of a dynamic infrastructure that includes cancer cells, their surrounding extracellular matrix, cancer-associated fibroblasts, pericytes, multiple immune cells, and vascular and lymphatic endothelial cells. Given the complexity both within and outside the cancer cells, and the interactions between cancer cells and the surrounding stroma, it is not surprising that a single event within a tumor can create a cascade of changes in multiple pathways.[21] This interplay among the elements of the hepatic tumor microenvironment for tumor growth and disease progression has been demonstrated in several studies and has been extensively described in the literature.[21–23] Several elements of structural aberrant architecture of neovessels, such as an increased number of proliferating endothelial cells, a deficiency in pericytes, and an aberrant basement membrane formation, all result in enhanced vascular permeability, facilitating transport of nutrients and oxygen to the tumor microenvironment.[23] Although tumor vessel development and function has become a therapeutic target for which there are agents that have shown therapeutic efficacy and impact in survival, tumor vessels are also the avenues for cytotoxic chemotherapy to directly reach the tumor.

The rationale for delivering chemotherapy to hepatic tumors via the arteries is based on the established knowledge that both primary and secondary liver tumors derive their blood supply from the hepatic artery, whereas approximately 50% of the oxygen supply to normal liver comes from the portal system.[24–26] A hepatic tumor may receive twice as much blood flow from the hepatic artery compared to the flow received from the portal vein.[27] Initial experiments with intraoperative intra-arterial injection of chemotherapy showed a 10 times higher intratumoral concentration of chemotherapy administered via the hepatic artery compared to chemotherapy delivered via the portal vein.[28] Drugs with a high first-pass metabolism, and therefore high extraction rates, result in high local concentrations with minimal systemic drug exposure. Moreover, drugs with a steep dose-response curve are more appropriate for intra-arterial delivery.[29] Thus, regional chemotherapy administered into the hepatic artery may expose tumor cells to high-dose chemotherapy while sparing the normal liver and minimizing systemic toxicities. This makes any intra-arterial therapy particularly attractive from both the delivery and safety points of view.

Similarly, the rationale for delivering embolic particles via the hepatic artery (embolization) lies in the preferential blood supply of tumors by the hepatic artery. Embolization may be part of the chemoembolization procedure or may stand alone as a palliative treatment option for hepatic malignancies.[30–32] Several embolic particles have been employed over the past three decades for transcatheter intra-arterial delivery and treatment of hepatic tumors.[33–36] These particles may produce different effects on vasculature, resulting in permanent or transient obstruction, by acting at different levels in the arterial system.[37]

Early studies have shown that proximal embolization of tumor-feeding arteries in hepatic metastases with large particles or coils may lead to immediate peripheral hepatic circulation reconstitution through collateral vessels.[38] It seems that the earlier the revascularization of the tumor occurs, the more incomplete the necrosis will be. An occlusion of more peripheral vessels generates a nearly complete tumor necrosis and current trends in oncology embolotherapy seem to favor for distal occlusion.[39,40]

Radioembolization should be distinguished from bland embolization or chemoembolization because it is rather a microembolic procedure and will not result in complete arterial occlusion.[41] Because the liver is sensitive to external beam radiation doses exceeding 35 Gy, with subsequent radiation-induced liver disease occurring weeks to months after therapy, radioembolization achieves the delivery of high radiation dose to tumors with minimal hepatic parenchymal damage.[41]

PHARMACOLOGIC ASPECTS OF COMMON INTRA-ARTERIALLY INJECTED DRUGS

In a recent review of the literature on the most commonly injected intra-arterial agents, single-drug injection was performed in 75% of referenced studies, whereas double-drug therapy was cited in 15% of studies and triple-drug therapy in 6% of studies.[42] Doxorubicin was used in 36% of studies, cisplatin in 31%, epirubicin in 12%, mitoxantrone in 8%, mitomycin C in 8%, and zinostatin stimalamer (SMANCS) in 5% of referenced studies.[42] In Japan, epirubicin (74%) is the most commonly used drug, followed by doxorubicin (9%), mitomycin C (9%),

cisplatin (4%), and SMANCS (4%). The increased use of epirubicin is explained by the fact that epirubicin (and not doxorubicin) is covered by the National Insurance System. A short review of the most commonly used chemotherapeutic drugs for intra-arterial injections will aid in appreciating the existing level of clinical evidence for their use as well as identifying opportunities for therapeutic advances.

Doxorubicin is an anthracycline, DNA-binding, topoisomerase II inhibitor, which is among the most effective chemotherapy drugs in cancer treatment.[43–45] Doxorubicin was first isolated from the pigment-producing *Streptomyces peucetius* early in the 1960s. Doxorubicin is metabolized predominantly by the liver to the major metabolite, doxorubicinol, and several cytotoxic aglycone metabolites.[46] Interestingly, doxorubicin is a drug with low first-pass liver metabolism. Doxorubicin is the most commonly injected single chemotherapeutic drug during TACE worldwide (36%).[22] Intrinsic or acquired resistance to doxorubicin in HCC is common, resulting in treatment failure and disease progression.[47] Multiple mechanisms for doxorubicin resistance have been identified in vitro, such as the increased expression of drug transporters, alterations in doxorubicin metabolism or localization, and defects in the drug's ability to induce apoptosis.[47] Reported dosages of doxorubicin intra-arterially injected range between 50 and 150 mg per procedure.[48] Doxorubicin has been successfully tested in combination with several antiangiogenic agents over the past 7 years.[49,50] Interestingly, the combination of sorafenib and doxorubicin has been shown to increase doxorubicin's area under the concentration curve (AUC) by almost 20%.[50] There are several hypotheses that may support a possible synergism between sorafenib and doxorubicin. Inhibition of the Ras/Raf/MEK/ERK pathway may prevent activation of the multidrug resistance pathway.[51] Moreover, anthracyclines have also been described as modulators of angiogenesis.[52] The last three decades have witnessed numerous attempts to identify novel anthracyclines with improved antitumor activity and reduced cardiotoxicity. Not surprisingly, more than 200 analogs have been developed; yet only few of them have reached the stage of clinical development and approval. Among them, epirubicin and idarubicin have been recently introduced as viable and potent alternatives to doxorubicin or daunorubicin, respectively.

Epirubicin is a semisynthetic derivative of doxorubicin obtained by an axial-to-equatorial epimerization of the hydroxyl group at C-4' in daunosamine.[53] This positional change has little effect on the mode of action and spectrum of activity of epirubicin compared with doxorubicin, but it introduces pharmacokinetic and metabolic changes like increased volume of distribution, 4-O-glucuronidation, with subsequent enhanced total body clearance and shorter terminal half-life. It is because of these kinetic and metabolic changes that epirubicin can be used at cumulative doses almost double those of doxorubicin, resulting in equal activity but not in increased cardiotoxicity.[54]

Idarubicin is another anthracycline, commonly used to treat leukemias, that has been recently tested for its in vitro and in vivo cytotoxicity against HCC.[55,56] Idarubicin seems a viable alternative to doxorubicin with high cytotoxicity and ability to overcome multidrug resistance. Furthermore, idarubicin is much more lipophilic than doxorubicin, leading to higher penetration through the lipidic double layer of tumor cell membranes and thus has better efficacy.

The second most common single drug used during TACE is cisplatin.[42] Cisplatin was discovered in 1965 and was first introduced into clinical trials in the early 1970s.[57,58] The mechanism of action of cisplatin is briefly described here. After entering the target cells, cisplatin binds to the cellular DNA and causes reversible alkylation of guanine and adenine by forming intra- and interstrand cross-links in the DNA, thereby inhibiting DNA elongation and resulting in cellular conformation changes.[57] These changes induce apoptosis and necrosis of the cancer cells and underlie the antitumor effect of cisplatin, which is based on both concentration-dependent and time-dependent features. The proportion of cisplatin into the hepatic tumor by first-pass kinetics has been reported to be less than 5% after intravenous administration, but that of intra-arterial infusion was reported to be 48.4% (34% to 55%).[59] Combined with lipiodol, cisplatin has been reported to yield response rates of 15% to 57%, whereas corresponding rates of 45% to 73% have been reported for the treatment combined with embolization using gelatin sponge particles.[60] In one of the two RCTs testing chemoembolization against best supportive care, Lo et al.[20] reported a significantly better overall survival with a relatively low dose of cisplatin (median 10 mg/20 mL). Cisplatin dosages reported in the literature range between 10 and 100 mg.[42,61] Interestingly, the lipiodol suspension is thought to prevent cisplatin inactivation by protein binding, allowing a higher concentration of the drug to be maintained inside the tumor.

Miriplatin is a new third-generation platinum derivative and has been recently tested for intra-arterial treatment of HCC.[62] Unlike other hydrophilic anticancer agents, miriplatin contains myristates as lipophilic side chains, making the drug easily dissolved in ethiodized oil without the need for emulsification. Following intra-arterial administration, the miriplatin-iodized oil suspension accumulates in the target tumor, and continuous antitumor effects caused by gradual release of active platinum compounds are expected.[62] Initial clinical studies suggest that miriplatin may be successfully used as an alternative to conventional hydrophilic chemotherapeutic agents, such as cisplatin or doxorubicin, for treating unresectable HCC. Miriplatin has been recently approved for clinical use and covered by public health insurance in Japan.[63]

Mitomycin C is an alkylating agent used for intra-arterial hepatic administration since the 1980s.[64,65] Reactive metabolites of mitomycin C can cross-link DNA, and its cytotoxicity has been attributed in part to the capacity of guanine residues. Its pharmacologic activity is increased under conditions of cellular hypoxia.[66] Mitomycin C has been shown to induce vascular injury, including alterations to endothelial cells.[67] Mitomycin C has been tested for intra-arterial injection in doses ranging between 2 and 30 mg.[42,61,68]

▌ PRINCIPLES OF DRUG DELIVERY SYSTEMS

Drug delivery systems may provide with reliable and controlled drug release to tumors. Ideally, a drug delivery system that can be injected intra-arterially should target cancer effectively, promote drug absorption, control and sustain drug release, increase exposure time of tumor to chemotherapy, and reduce systemic drug levels and subsequent undesirable side effects and toxicity to normal tissue.[69] Several materials have been tested for effective drug loading and drug release. Currently, the most popular materials used for intra-arterial drug delivery include polyvinyl alcohol (PVA) hydrogels and acrylic copolymers.[48]

PVA hydrogels are nonbiodegradable and biocompatible materials that can be easily and reliably fabricated with high stability under a range of temperature and pH conditions.[70] Moreover, they have been shown to provoke a limited inflammatory response.[71] Because of their amphiphilic nature and microporous architecture, drugs can be incorporated in hydrogel coatings and can be typically released within hours to weeks.[71] The release of the loaded drugs in acidic environment represents another important property of these polymers.

Doxorubicin-eluting beads (DC Bead for loading by the physician and PRECISION Bead preloaded with doxorubicin, Biocompatibles UK Ltd., Surrey, UK) are PVA hydrogel-based microspheres designed for intra-arterial therapy and selective tumor targeting.[72] They can be formulated in different ranges of sizes (from 75 to 900 µm). DC Bead microspheres actively sequester oppositely charged drugs through an ion-exchange mechanism. Initial in vitro studies showed that doxorubicin can be efficiently sequestered by the DC Beads to a maximum loading of approximately 45 mg/mL of hydrated beads, irrespective of the size range of beads used.[40] The rate at which the beads sequester the doxorubicin depends on bead size, drug concentration, and salt loading solution concentration. Larger-sized (700 to 900 µm) beads show an approximately 35% decrease in average diameter when loaded with the maximum dose of drug, whereas smaller-sized microspheres (100 to 300 µm) shrink less after drug loading. Moreover, larger-sized beads (700 to 900 µm) release the drug more slowly than the smaller 100- to 300-µm beads.[40] DC Bead microspheres can load a maximum of around 45 mg doxorubicin/mL with greater than 99% of drug being sequestered from the doxorubicin solution.[39] Loading with 37.5 mg doxorubicin/mL beads is currently recommended, combining a practical therapeutic dose and optimum handling characteristics.

Paragon Bead microspheres (Biocompatibles, UK) are irinotecan-loaded drug-eluting microspheres for palliation of hepatic colorectal metastases. Initial in vitro experiments of irinotecan drug-eluting beads, prepared by combining embolization beads (DC Bead, Biocompatibles, UK) with irinotecan hydrochloride solution, showed that the rate of drug uptake was seen to be bead size dependent, the smaller beads loading more quickly due to increased surface area to volume ratio. The maximum loading of bound drug was shown to be around 50 to 60 mg irinotecan/mL beads for all sizes.[67] The time required to reach suspension in contrast agent/saline mixture was both bead-size and drug-dose dependent, ranging between 1 and 12 minutes. In another study, irinotecan-loaded beads were shown to decrease in size (by a maximum 25% to 30%) with a concomitant increase in their modulus of compression and drug loading.[68]

Superabsorbent polymer (SAP) QuadraSphere (HepaSphere for Europe) microspheres (Merit Medical Systems, Inc. South Jordan, UT) are biocompatible, hydrophilic (absorbent), nonresorbable, acrylic copolymer microspheres, designed for hepatic arterial embolization with an ability to absorb fluids up to 64 times their dry state volume. The expansion rate depends on ionic concentration of their surrounding media. The size of dry particles ranges between 50 and 200 µm, corresponding to an expanded size range of 200 and 800 µm. The SAP microspheres can be loaded with doxorubicin or cisplatin for drug delivery during TACE.[18] Initial in vitro and in vivo studies showed encouraging results, and these microspheres now have CE mark approval for TACE of unresectable HCC in combination with doxorubicin. An in vitro study tested the reservoir capacity of SAP, using two different contrast media and optimal loading doses of cisplatin powder into SAP for hepatic arterial embolization. Interestingly, 100 mg of SAP, when mixed with iohexol, could carry 10 times larger dose of cisplatin than when mixed with ioxaglic acid. Moreover, cisplatin-loaded SAP with ioxaglic acid were double in size than those loaded with iohexol, suggesting that they may occlude vessels at a more proximal level than required.

MULTIDISCIPLINARY CLINICAL APPROACH

A multidisciplinary team approach is essential for the management of all patients that are candidates for intra-arterial therapies.[73,74] Multidisciplinary tumor boards may discuss available treatment options and recommend in consensus individually tailored therapeutic strategies. Diagnostic radiologists and/or body imaging specialists may assess baseline patient and tumor staging and characterize tumor response to intra-arterial therapy. Medical oncologists may provide their expertise on the available chemotherapeutic, targeted molecular, or combination regimens. Radiation oncologists may provide expertise on radiologic oncologic therapeutic options. Liver pathologists may provide expertise on tumor histologic morphology, variants, and underlying cirrhosis.[75] Gastroenterologists and hepatologists may provide insight on the management of underlying liver cirrhosis. Surgical oncologists and transplant surgeons may identify patients who are eligible for surgery or transplantation. Physician assistants and oncology nursing staff members are a critical component of patient care because these providers may coordinate patient care and help to ensure patient compliance to treatment.

TUMOR STAGING SYSTEMS

Tumor size, number of tumors, and location are all tumor morphologic characteristics that are important for characterizing tumor burden at presentation. For patients with HCC, tumor size and number of tumors are important markers of resectability and eligibility for transplantation. The Milan Criteria (a single tumor ≤5 cm in diameter or three or fewer nodules ≤3 cm in diameter) have been recommended as the major reference system for liver transplantation in patients with HCC.[76] Most patients who are eligible for intra-arterial therapy do not fulfill these criteria. Selected transplant candidates, however, may receive an intra-arterial therapy as a bridge to transplantation or as treatment of intrahepatic recurrence following transplantation. Moreover, few patients within the Milan Criteria are deemed inoperable due to other comorbidities and may, therefore, be eligible for intra-arterial therapies. For patients with small tumor burden who are otherwise eligible for surgery, however, it is not clear whether there is a clinical benefit of receiving intra-arterial treatment. Although there is certainly no clear limitation up to which tumor size are intra-arterial therapies effective, there is evidence that multiple treatment sessions are more beneficial than single ones. There is also no clearly defined upper limit of total tumor volume that can be treated via the intra-arterial route. Tumor volume greater than 50% of liver parenchyma is a predictor of poor outcome, however. Moreover, multinodular and infiltrative lesions may not respond as favorably to intra-arterial therapies.

Contrary to other malignancies, long-term survival in patients with HCC depends on both pathologic stage of the disease as well as severity of underlying liver dysfunction. Several tumor staging systems have been developed for HCC, yet none has been universally adopted, primarily due to the lack of a multidimensional comprehensive representation of all factors influencing patient survival.[77] Most systems variably incorporate four features that have been recognized as important determinants of survival: the severity of underlying liver disease, tumor size, extension of the tumor into adjacent structures, and the presence of metastases.[78] In general, pathologic staging systems, such as the American Joint Committee on Cancer (AJCC) tumor-node-metastasis (TNM) staging system, are suitable for assessing the outcomes of resection or liver transplantation.[79] For patients with unresectable HCC, several clinical staging systems have been proposed. The most commonly used systems for patients with unresectable HCC are the Okuda and Barcelona Clinic Liver Cancer (BCLC) systems and the Cancer of the Liver Italian Program (CLIP) Investigators score (Table 3.1).

The BCLC staging system, which was devised from the results of cohort studies and randomized controlled trials (RCTs), is widely recognized and endorsed.[80,81] It includes variables related to tumor stage and function, physical status, and cancer-related symptoms, and it combines each stage with a treatment algorithm. This system has been criticized because of its algorithmic, rather than patient-centered, approach. Patients classified as having early-stage HCC (stage A), with either a single nodule or three nodules less than 3 cm in diameter and a performance status (PS) score of 0, are suitable for treatment with potentially curative therapies (resection, transplantation, or ablation). Patients with intermediate-stage HCC (stage B) are asymptomatic (PS score, 0) with multinodular tumors but without vascular invasion or extrahepatic spread, and are eligible for locoregional therapy (TACE). Those with advanced-stage HCC (stage C) are either symptomatic (PS score, 1–2) or have evidence of vascular invasion or extrahepatic spread; these patients are eligible for sorafenib. Finally, patients with terminal-stage HCC (stage D) have either severe cancer symptoms (PS score, 3–4) or severely decompensated cirrhosis (Child-Pugh class C) and should receive symptomatic treatment only. Unlike many of the proposed staging systems, the BCLC system has been externally validated and is endorsed by both the American Association for the Study of Liver Diseases (AASLD) and the European Association for the Study of the Liver (EASL).

The oldest prognostic scoring system was proposed by Okuda back in 1985 and includes tumor size and three measures of the severity of cirrhosis (the amount of ascites, serum albumin, and total bilirubin levels).[82] The Okuda system does not classify patients by vascular invasion or the presence or absence of nodal metastases. The CLIP staging system was created in 1998 and incorporates hepatic cirrhosis (Child-Pugh Turcotte score), tumor morphology, alpha fetoprotein (AFP) levels, and the presence of portal vein thrombosis (PVT), with an index of the severity of cirrhosis to determine a prognostic score ranging from 0 to 6.[83] A modified version of the score (incorporating the Model for End-Stage Liver Disease [MELD] score) has also been proposed.[84] Some groups are investigating whether prognostication with the CLIP score can be improved by the addition of serum factors, such as vascular endothelial growth factor (VEGF) and insulin-like growth factor-I (IGF-1).[85,86] The Japan Integrated Staging Score from the Cancer Study Group of Japan combines Child

Table 3.1

Most Commonly Used Staging Systems for Hepatocellular Carcinoma with Parameters Included in the Staging Systems

Staging system	Grades	Tumor assessment	Liver function assessment	Clinical performance
Child-Pugh	A–C 1–15	N/A	Bilirubin Albumin PT or INR Ascites Hepatic encephalopathy	N/A
TNM (AJCC 2010)	0–IVB	Number and size of tumor(s) (Tx-T4) Vascular invasion Regional lymph nodes (Nx-N1) Distant metastasis (M0-M1)	N/A	N/A
Okuda	I–III	Tumor load ≤ or >50%	Bilirubin Albumin Ascites	—
CLIP	0–6	Tumor extension ≤ or >50% Single or multiple nodes AFP Portal vein thrombosis	Child-Pugh score	—
BCLC		Tumor extension Metastasis Portal vein thrombosis Okuda score	Child-Pugh score Portal hypertension Bilirubin	ECOG PS
GRETCH		AFP Portal vein thrombosis	Bilirubin Alkaline phosphatase	Karnofsky PS
JIS		TNM-Classification of the LCSGJ (singular, <2 cm, vascular invasion, lymph node metastasis)	Child-Pugh score	—

PT, prothrombin time; INR, international normalized ratio; TNM, tumor-node-metastasis; AJCC, American Joint Committee on Cancer; CLIP, Cancer of the Liver Italian Program; AFP, alpha fetoprotein; ECOG, Eastern Cooperative Oncology Group; GRETCH, Groupe d'Etude et de Traitement du Carcinome Hepatocellulaire; JIS, Japan Integrated Stage; LCSGJ, Liver Cancer Study Group of Japan; PS, performance status.

staging with a modified TNM staging and incorporates measures of functional status as well.[87] The French Groupe d'Etude et de Traitement du Carcinome Hepatocellulaire (GRETCH) developed a prognostic classification system based on a multivariate analysis of prognostic factors in 761 patients from 34 countries who were diagnosed and treated over a 30-month period.[88] They identified five prognostic factors: (a) Karnofsky PS, (b) serum bilirubin greater than 50 micromol/L (>2.9 mg/dL), (c) serum alkaline phosphatase at least twice the upper limit of normal, (d) serum AFP greater than 35 ng/mL, and (e) ultrasonographic portal obstruction. Other classifications include the Chinese University Prognostic Index (CUPI) and simplified Vauthey staging system.[89,90] The consensus of the American Hepato Pancreato Biliary Association (updated in 2010) reasserts the need to use different systems in different patients. Its consensus

statement recommends the use of the TNM system to predict outcome following resection or liver transplantation and the BCLC scheme for patients with advanced HCC who are not candidates for surgery.[91]

▌ EVALUATION OF LIVER FUNCTION

The most common way to stratify patients according to hepatic reserve is the Child-Turcotte-Pugh (CTP) classification. The CTP classification, in combination with clinical assessment, provides a simple and reliable method to identify patients with unresectable liver cancer at risk for liver insufficiency. It was initially developed by Child and Turcotte in 1964 and modified by Pugh in 1972.[92] The current CTP scoring system is based on five parameters: serum bilirubin, serum albumin, prothrombin

Table 3.2

Modified Child-Pugh Classification of Severity of Liver Disease

Parameter	Points assigned		
	1	*2*	*3*
Ascites	Absent	Slight	Moderate
Bilirubin (mg/dL)	<2	2–3	>3
Albumin (g/dL)	>3.5	2.8–3.5	<2.8
Prothrombin time			
Seconds over control	1–3	4–6	>6
International normalized ratio	<1.7	1.8–2.3	>2.3
Encephalopathy	None	Grade 1–2	Grade 3–4

Modified Child-Pugh classification of the severity of liver disease according to the degree of ascites, the plasma concentrations of bilirubin and albumin, the prothrombin time, and the degree of encephalopathy. A total score of 5 to 6 is considered grade A (well-compensated disease); 7 to 9 is grade B (significant functional compromise); and 10 to 15 is grade C (decompensated disease). These grades correlate with 1- and 2-year survival: Grade A, 100% and 65%; Grade B, 80% and 60%; and Grade C, 45% and 35%.

time, ascites, and encephalopathy. The sum of the points for each of these five parameters gives the total score and patients with chronic liver disease are placed into one of three CTP classes (A, B, or C) (Table 3.2).

Severe hepatic dysfunction, as quantified with the Child-Pugh score, has long been considered to be a contraindication to the intra-arterial approach, not only because of the possibility of severe complications following the procedure but also due to the poor prognosis despite treatment in patients with CTP class C disease. In patients with advanced HCC, but with CTP class A or B cirrhosis, immediate hepatic dysfunction after TACE gradually improves in about 4 weeks, which is the time necessary for liver regeneration. Surprisingly, the effect of intra-arterial therapies to the cirrhotic liver has not been reported very extensively. In the case of TACE in patients with cirrhosis, few authors have reported extensively on the effect of the procedure on liver function and the damage caused by TACE to nontumorous liver tissue.[93]

Another commonly used prognostic system for the evaluation of the hepatic reserve is the MELD scoring system. MELD is a prospectively validated chronic liver disease severity scoring system that uses a patient's laboratory values for serum bilirubin, serum creatinine, and the international normalized ratio for prothrombin time (INR) to predict survival. The MELD scoring system was developed initially by using data from patients with cirrhosis treated with transjugular intrahepatic portosystemic shunt (TIPS).[94] An increasing MELD score in patients with chronic liver disease is associated with increasing severity of hepatic dysfunction and 3-month mortality risk.

The formula used for calculation of the MELD score is:

$$3.8[\text{Ln serum bilirubin (mg/dL)}] + 11.2[\text{Ln INR}] + 9.6[\text{Ln serum creatinine (mg/dL)}] + 6.4[\text{etiology: 0 if cholestatic or alcoholic, 1 if other etiologies}]$$

Patients with cirrhosis secondary to either alcoholic or cholestatic liver disease demonstrated slightly better survival compared with patients with viral or "other" disease etiologies. As a result, the MELD score was initially designed to reflect this mortality difference. The Child-Pugh score has been tested against the MELD score for patients treated with TACE and has been shown to correlate better than the MELD score to overall patient survival. Of the components of the Child-Pugh and MELD systems, albumin level is the most useful predictor of survival.[95]

■ TECHNICAL CONSIDERATIONS

A thorough understanding of the tumor flow dynamics, the embolization effect, as well as the hepatic arterial anatomy are essential to ensure reliable results for all intra-arterial therapies. Knowledge of hemodynamic parameters of tumor vascularity is essential for a successful embolization. Inadequate embolization can lead to subsequent quick tumor regrowth. Overembolization, on the other hand, may lead to nontargeted embolization and can accelerate the onset of liver failure.

Anatomic variations of the hepatic arteries and celiac trunk are of considerable importance in intra-arterial therapies. A thorough understanding of the anatomic variants and hemodynamic features of the hepatic arteries, tumor-feeding arteries, and portal vein is the first step in performing an effective and safe intra-arterial therapy. Differences arising during several developmental stages in the embryonal process lead to a range of variations in vascular structures supplying the gastrointestinal tract. According to the Michels[96] classification of the hepatic arterial system, 10 variant subtypes have been identified. The most common variants of the hepatic artery are the replaced left hepatic artery (LHA) from the left gastric artery (LGA) and the replaced right hepatic artery (RHA) from the superior mesenteric artery (SMA).[96] A replaced or accessory RHA can also originate early from the celiac trunk, or it can originate directly from the aorta, hepaticomesenteric trunk, or celiacomesenteric trunk.[97] Other variants include the common hepatic artery (CHA) arising off the SMA, whereas the rarest variant of the CHA is the replaced CHA from the LGA[98] (FIGURE 3.1A–C).

Extrahepatic tumor collaterals can develop either due to repeated intra-arterial treatments or to exophytic tumor growth. There is also a predilection for tumor size with more than 50% of large tumors (>6 cm) demonstrating collateral blood supply, in contrast to only 3% of small tumors (<4 cm).[99] Intra-arterial therapy via the extrahepatic collateral routes has been well described and with survival rates that are comparable to those for patients treated via the hepatic artery. There are numerous extrahepatic collateral routes, including periportal collateral vessels that arise from the gastroduodenal artery or pancreaticoduodenal arcade, right and left inferior phrenic arteries, right and left gastric arteries, pancreaticoduodenal arcade (which supplies the gastroduodenal and proper hepatic arteries), right and left internal mammary arteries and superior epigastric artery, intercostal artery, lumbar artery, adrenal arteries, capsular branches of the right renal artery, branches of the middle or right colic artery, and omental branches. The anastomosis between the right and left gastric arteries can serve as a collateral pathway to the liver after occlusion of the hepatic artery.[99] In anatomic variants in which the replaced LHA or lateral segmental artery arises from the LGA, when the LGA is occluded and HCC is supplied by these arteries, the route created by the

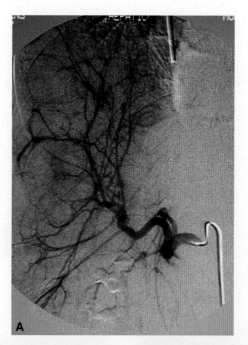

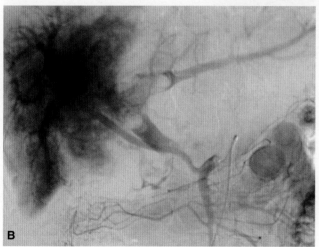

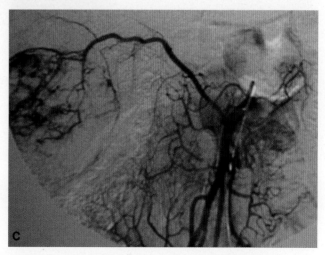

FIGURE 3.1 A. Digital subtraction angiographic image of a proper hepatic artery arising directly off the aorta. **B.** Digital subtraction angiographic image of an accessory right hepatic artery arising off the superior mesenteric artery, feeding a hypervascular tumor (hepatocellular carcinoma). **C.** Digital subtraction angiographic image of a replaced right hepatic artery arising off the superior mesenteric artery. Also shown in this angiogram are the arterioportal shunt (early depiction of the portal venous system) and thrombus in the main portal and splenic veins.

right and left gastric arteries can serve as an important pathway for intra-arterial therapies.

Stenosis or occlusion of the celiac axis is commonly associated with enlargement of the arteries of the pancreaticoduodenal arcade, which supply the distribution of the celiac axis by means of retrograde flow from the SMA (FIGURE 3.2A, B). Stenosis or occlusion of the celiac axis is easily seen at superior mesenteric arteriography as unopacified flow from the celiac axis. In nearly all cases of celiac axis stenosis and in some cases of celiac axis occlusion, chemoembolization or chemoinfusion can be performed via the CHA; if this is not possible, these procedures can be performed via the hypertrophic pancreaticoduodenal arcade.

Tumor neovascularization in the liver is commonly associated with the presence of arteriovenous shunts to the lungs and arterioportal shunts (APS), either at the level of the tumor or in nontumorous hepatic parenchyma. Arteriovenous shunting to the lungs is associated with tumor vascularity, tumor type, and tumor size.[100] APS associated with HCC have been reported in about 28.8% to 63.2% of HCCs.[101–103] APS have also been reported to occur with other types of metastases.[104] Their presence is considered a poor prognostic outcome factor, primarily caused by the rise in portal venous pressure, which increases the possibility for life-threatening complications, such as esophageal varices, ascites, and hepatic encephalopathy.[101,103,105]

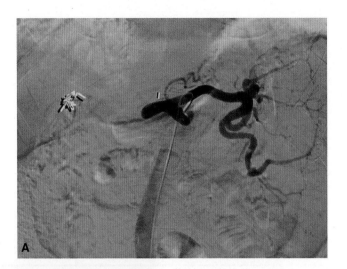

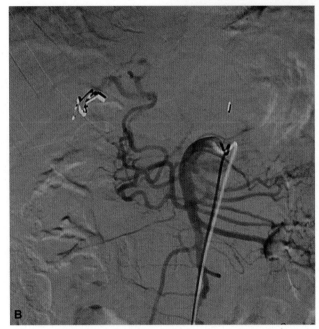

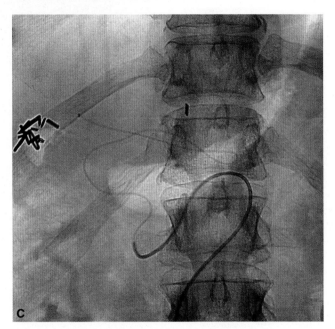

FIGURE 3.2 A. Digital subtraction angiographic image of the celiac axis showing miniscule flow to the common hepatic artery, which is highly stenotic, and enlargement of the arteries of the pancreaticoduodenal arcade. **B.** Digital subtraction angiographic image of the superior mesenteric artery with reconstitution of arterial flow to the tumor via a hypertrophied branch. **C.** Digital spot X-ray showing the course of the microcatheter inside the hypertrophied tumor-feeding artery that arises off the superior mesenteric artery.

Moreover, during TACE with ethiodized oil, the oily emulsion may bypass the intratumoral vasculature and be diverted into the portal vein branches and subsequently create an infarct to nontumorous hepatic tissue. At hepatic arteriography, a typical APS manifests as branching or dotlike vascular structures early in the arterial phase and, subsequently, as wedge-shaped focal parenchymal staining (FIGURE 3.3A–C). Its presence can be verified with selective injection of iodized oil and with follow-up imaging including iodized oil–enhanced computed tomography (CT). A grading of severity of arterioportal shunting has been proposed according to the extent of backflow to the portal vein into: shunt backflow to the segmental portal vein (grade 1), shunt backflow to the ipsilateral main portal vein of each lobe (grade 2), and shunt backflow to the contralateral lobe and/or the main portal vein (grade 3).[103] APS can be embolized before an intra-arterial therapy.[105–107] Gelatin sponge offers temporary occlusion with complete absorption of the embolized material and recanalization of the embolized vessels within a few weeks of the intervention.[107] PVA is not absorbable and it is more likely to produce a permanent occlusion.[108] Nontumorous APS may mimic hypervascular tumor at dynamic CT, magnetic resonance imaging (MRI), and hepatic angiography.[109] On CT or MR imaging, such an APS is typically wedge-shaped, enhanced on arterial-phase imaging, and becomes isoattenuating or isointense on portal-phase images.[109] Nontumorous APS can also be nodular rather than wedge-shaped on cross-sectional images.

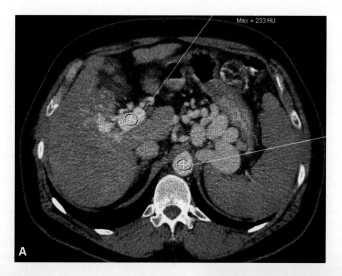

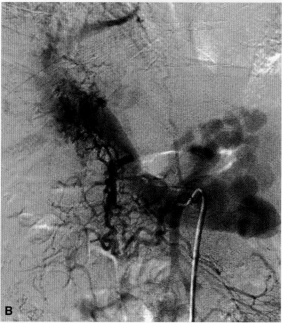

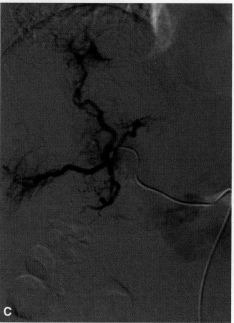

FIGURE 3.3 A. Axial contrast-enhanced CT image of the liver (arterial phase) showing early enhancement of the portal venous system caused by the presence of an arterioportal shunt. **B.** Digital subtraction angiographic image of the superior mesenteric artery showing the direct intratumoral communication of the arterial and portal venous systems (arterioportal shunting) with engorged gastric varices. The intratumoral arterioportal shunt was embolized with gelfoam pledgets. **C.** Digital subtraction angiographic image of the right hepatic artery demonstrating decreased shunting caused by prior embolization of the shunt with gelfoam. Additional gelfoam pledgets were injected to reduce shunting just prior to delivery of chemoembolization material.

Therefore, it is imperative to correlate these findings with hepatic arteriographic findings.

ASSESSMENT OF TUMOR RESPONSE TO INTRA-ARTERIAL THERAPY

The first criteria ever established for the recording and reporting of solid tumor response to therapy were the World Health Organization (WHO) criteria in 1979.[110] These criteria attempted to standardize the recording and reporting of response assessment for solid tumors so that response outcomes could be compared between research studies, clinical trials, and among institutions throughout the world. According to the WHO criteria, the response assessment is performed by measuring bidimensional tumor sizes. According to these criteria, complete response (CR) is defined as the disappearance of all signs of disease for at least 1 month and the lack of appearance of new lesions. Partial response (PR) is achieved with a 50% or more reduction in the sum of the tumor cross products. Stable disease (SD) indicates a decrease of less than 50% or an increase in tumor size of less than 25% over the original measurements. Progressive disease (PD) is considered a 25% or more increase in the sum of one or more of the tumor deposits or the appearance of new lesions.

In 1994, several organizations, including the European Organization for Research and Treatment of Cancer (EORTC), the National Cancer Institute of USA, and the National Cancer Institute of Canada, began to review the response assessment criteria with the intent of revising them. The revised system was called response evaluation criteria in solid tumors (RECIST) guidelines.[111] It used unidimensional measurements, which are less cumbersome to measure and calculate. In the initial RECIST guidelines, all measurable lesions up to a maximum of 5 lesions per organ and 10 lesions in total, representative of all involved organs, were identified and measured. A sum of the longest diameter for all target lesions was calculated and reported as the baseline sum longest diameter. To characterize the objective tumor response, the baseline sum longest diameter was used as the reference. CR is disappearance of all known lesion(s) confirmed at 4 weeks. PR is 30% or more decrease confirmed at 4 weeks. SD is when neither PR nor PD criteria are met. PD is 20% or more increase or new lesion(s). In the revised RECIST version 1.1 criteria of 2010, tumor size is measured as the sum of unidimensional diameters of up to two target lesions per organ.[112]

The relevance of the application of these WHO and RECIST criteria to intra-arterial therapies has been challenged because intra-arterial therapies lead to tumor ischemia and necrosis that may not always be paralleled by a reduction in size. In response to these concerns the EASL recommended measuring change in the area of tumor enhancement on contrast-enhanced imaging as the optimal method to assess treatment response. More recently the AASLD has proposed a formal amendment of the RECIST criteria to take into consideration changes in the degree of tumor arterial enhancement—the modified RECIST criteria (mRECIST).[113] According to the mRECIST, the following RECIST modifications have been proposed in the determination of tumor response for target lesions (Table 3.3). CR is considered the disappearance of any intratumoral arterial enhancement in all target lesions. PR is considered at least a 30% decrease in the sum of diameters of viable (contrast enhancement in the arterial phase) target lesions, taking as reference the baseline sum of the diameters of target lesions. PD is characterized as an increase of at least 20% in the sum of the diameters of viable (enhancing) target lesions, taking as reference the smallest sum of the diameters of viable (enhancing) target lesions recorded since the treatment started. SD includes any cases that do not qualify for either PR or PD.

Several investigators have raised the question whether it is "time" to move from anatomic unidimensional assessment of tumor burden to either volumetric anatomic assessment or to functional assessment (e.g., dynamic contrast-enhanced MRI or CT or [18] F-fluorodeoxyglucose positron emission tomographic [FDG-PET] techniques assessing tumor metabolism). The RECIST Working Group, however, believes that there is currently insufficient standardization and widespread availability to recommend adoption of these alternative assessment methods.[114] Moreover, the use of these promising newer approaches that could be employed either in addition or as substitutes for anatomic assessment requires appropriate and rigorous clinical validation studies.

FUTURE ROLE OF INTRA-ARTERIAL THERAPIES

Intra-arterial therapies have established their role primarily in the treatment of unresectable hepatic malignancies and continue to evolve. Because the ultimate goal of intra-arterial therapies is to offer a chance for liver cancer cure, it is highly likely that in the future current cytotoxic drugs will be routinely combined with molecular antiangiogenic or other novel drugs. Moreover, other novel drugs, acting on cancer metabolism, will be introduced into clinical practice. For instance, the novel agent 3-bromopyruvate, an alkylating agent and a potent inhibitor of glycolysis, is currently tested for intra-arterial delivery in

---

Table 3.3

Assessment of Tumor Response to Therapy: Comparison of the RECIST v.1.1 and mRECIST

RECIST	mRECIST for HCC
CR = Disappearance of all target lesions	CR = Disappearance of any intratumoral arterial enhancement in all target lesions
PR = At least a 30% decrease in the sum of diameters of target lesions, having as reference the baseline sum of the diameters of target lesions	PR = At least a 30% decrease in the sum of diameters of viable (enhancement in the arterial phase) target lesions, having as reference the baseline sum of the diameters of target lesions
SD = Any cases that do not qualify for either PR or PD	SD = Any cases that do not qualify for either PR or PD
PD = An increase of at least 20% in the sum of the diameters of target lesions, having as reference the smallest sum of the diameters of target lesions recorded since treatment started	PD = An increase of at least 20% in the sum of the diameters of viable (enhancing) target lesions, having as reference the smallest sum of the diameters of viable (enhancing) target lesions recorded since treatment started

mRECIST, modified Response Evaluation Criteria in Solid Tumors; CR, complete response; PR, partial response; SD, stable disease; PD, progressive disease.
Adapted from Lencioni R, Llovet JM. Modified RECIST (mRECIST) assessment for hepatocellular carcinoma. *Semin Liver Dis* 2010;30(1):52–60. Epub 2010/02/23.

a phase I study.[115] Because cancer cells depend on glycolysis for their energy requirements, 3-bromopyruvate seems a potent new antiglycolytic anticancer treatment option.[116] The primary mechanism of 3-bromopyruvate's action is thought to occur via preferential alkylation of glyceraldehyde-3-phosphate dehydrogenase (GAPDH), and 3-bromopyruvate mediated cancer cell death is linked to generation of free radicals, endoplasmic reticulum stress, and inhibition of global protein synthesis[117]; 3-bromopyruvate has been already successfully tested in many animal tumor models.[116]

It is also highly likely that imaging criteria used for characterization of tumor response to therapy will further adapt and better define tumor response on a molecular rather than morphologic level.

CONCLUSION

The described principles of intra-arterial therapies signify that these therapies have and combine medical and surgical aspects of clinical oncology, whereas a multidisciplinary approach is necessary for optimizing treatment strategies. With ongoing research, existing intra-arterial therapies will be further optimized. Combination of treatments, new technologies in imaging, and targeted drug delivery will ultimately improve the quality of life and survival of patients with unresectable hepatic malignancies.

REFERENCES

1. Forner A, Llovet JM, Bruix J. Hepatocellular carcinoma. *Lancet* 2012;379(9822):1245–1255. Epub 2012 Feb 23.
2. Liapi E, Geschwind JF. Transcatheter and ablative therapeutic approaches for solid malignancies. *J Clin Oncol* 2007;25(8):978–986. Epub 2007 Mar 14.
3. Liapi E, Kamel IR, Bluemke DA, et al. Assessment of response of uterine fibroids and myometrium to embolization using diffusion-weighted echoplanar MR imaging. *J Comput Assist Tomogr* 2005;29(1):83–86. Epub 2005 Jan 25.
4. Rohde S, Kovacs AF, Turowski B, et al. Intra-arterial high-dose chemotherapy with cisplatin as part of a palliative treatment concept in oral cancer. *AJNR Am J Neuroradiol* 2005;26(7):1804–1809. Epub 2005 Aug 11.
5. Liapi E, Geschwind JF. Chemoembolization for primary and metastatic liver cancer. *Cancer J* 2010;16(2):156–162. Epub 2010 Apr 21.
6. Vossen JA, Kamel IR, Buijs M, et al. Role of functional magnetic resonance imaging in assessing metastatic leiomyosarcoma response to chemoembolization. *J Comput Assist Tomogr* 2008;32(3):347–352. Epub 2008 Jun 4.
7. Liapi E, Geschwind JF, Vossen JA, et al. Functional MRI evaluation of tumor response in patients with neuroendocrine hepatic metastasis treated with transcatheter arterial chemoembolization. *AJR Am J Roentgenol* 2008;190(1):67–73. Epub 2007 Dec 21.
8. Cady B, Oberfield RA. Arterial infusion chemotherapy of hepatoma. *Surg Gynecol Obstet* 1974;138(3):381–384. Epub 1974 Mar 1.
9. Bern MM, McDermott W Jr, Cady B, et al. Intraarterial hepatic infusion and intravenous adriamycin for treatment of hepatocellular carcinoma: a clinical and pharmacology report. *Cancer* 1978;42(2):399–405. Epub 1978 Aug 1.
10. Clouse ME, Ahmed R, Ryan RB, et al. Complications of long term transbrachial hepatic arterial infusion chemotherapy. *AJR Am J Roentgenol* 1977;129(5):799–803. Epub 1977 Nov 1.
11. Stuart K. Chemoembolization in the management of liver tumors. *Oncologist* 2003;8(5):425–437. Epub 2003 Oct 8.
12. Lucas RJ, Tumacder O, Wilson GS. Hepatic artery occlusion following hepatic artery catheterization. *Ann Surg* 1971;173(2):238–243. Epub 1971 Feb 1.
13. Nakakuma K, Tashiro S, Hiraoka T, et al. Studies on anticancer treatment with an oily anticancer drug injected into the ligated feeding hepatic artery for liver cancer. *Cancer* 1983;52(12):2193–2200. Epub 1983 Dec 15.
14. Wheeler PG, Melia W, Dubbins P, et al. Non-operative arterial embolisation in primary liver tumours. *Br Med J* 1979;2(6184):242–244. Epub 1979 Jul 28.
15. Misra NC, Jaiswal MS, Singh RV, et al. Intrahepatic arterial infusion of combination of mitomycin-C and 5-fluorouracil in treatment of primary and metastatic liver carcinoma. *Cancer* 1977;39(4):1425–1429. Epub 1977 Apr 1.
16. Konno T, Tashiro S, Maeda H, et al. Intra-arterial injection of an oily antineoplastic agent in hepatic cancer [in Japanese]. *Gan To Kagaku Ryoho* 1983;10(2, pt 2):351–357. Epub 1983 Feb 1.
17. Yumoto Y, Jinno K, Tokuyama K, et al. Hepatocellular carcinoma detected by iodized oil. *Radiology* 1985;154(1):19–24. Epub 1985 Jan 1.
18. Llovet JM, Bruix J. Systematic review of randomized trials for unresectable hepatocellular carcinoma: chemoembolization improves survival. *Hepatology* 2003;37(2):429–442. Epub 2003 Jan 24.
19. Llovet JM, Real MI, Montana X, et al. Arterial embolisation or chemoembolisation versus symptomatic treatment in patients with unresectable hepatocellular carcinoma: a randomised controlled trial. *Lancet* 2002;359(9319):1734–1739. Epub 2002 Jun 7.
20. Lo CM, Ngan H, Tso WK, et al. Randomized controlled trial of transarterial lipiodol chemoembolization for unresectable hepatocellular carcinoma. *Hepatology* 2002;35(5):1164–1171. Epub 2002 May 1.
21. Fernandez M, Semela D, Bruix J, et al. Angiogenesis in liver disease. *J Hepatol* 2009;50(3):604–620. Epub 2009 Jan 23.
22. Thorgeirsson SS, Grisham JW. Molecular pathogenesis of human hepatocellular carcinoma. *Nat Genet* 2002;31(4):339–346. Epub 2002 Aug 1.
23. Folkman J. Tumor angiogenesis: therapeutic implications. *N Engl J Med* 1971;285(21):1182–1186. Epub 1971 Nov 18.
24. Breedis C, Young G. The blood supply of neoplasms in the liver. *Am J Pathol* 1954;30(5):969–977. Epub 1954 Sep 1.
25. Lien WM, Ackerman NB. The blood supply of experimental liver metastases: II, a microcirculatory study of the normal and tumor vessels of the liver with the use of perfused silicone rubber. *Surgery* 1970;68(2):334–340. Epub 1970 Aug 1.
26. Ackerman NB, Lien WM, Silverman NA. The blood supply of experimental liver metastases: 3, the effects of acute ligation of the hepatic artery or portal vein. *Surgery* 1972;71(4):636–641. Epub 1972 Apr 1.
27. Ridge JA, Bading JR, Gelbard AS, et al. Perfusion of colorectal hepatic metastases. Relative distribution of flow from the hepatic artery and portal vein. *Cancer* 1987;59(9):1547–1553. Epub 1987 May 1.
28. Sigurdson ER, Ridge JA, Kemeny N, et al. Tumor and liver drug uptake following hepatic artery and portal vein infusion. *J Clin Oncol* 1987;5(11):1836–1840. Epub 1987 Nov 1.
29. Frei E III, Canellos GP. Dose: a critical factor in cancer chemotherapy. *Am J Med* 1980;69(4):585–594. Epub 1980 Oct 1.
30. Brown DB, Nikolic B, Covey AM, et al. Quality improvement guidelines for transhepatic arterial chemoembolization, embolization, and chemotherapeutic infusion for hepatic malignancy. *J Vasc Interv Radiol* 2012;23(3):287–294. Epub 2012 Jan 31.
31. Covey AM, Maluccio MA, Schubert J, et al. Particle embolization of recurrent hepatocellular carcinoma after hepatectomy. *Cancer* 2006;106(10):2181–2189. Epub 2006 Apr 6.
32. Maluccio MA, Covey AM, Porat LB, et al. Transcatheter arterial embolization with only particles for the treatment of unresectable hepatocellular carcinoma. *J Vasc Interv Radiol* 2008;19(6):862–869. Epub 2008 May 28.
33. Laurent A, Beaujeux R, Wassef M, et al. Trisacryl gelatin microspheres for therapeutic embolization, I: development and in vitro evaluation. *AJNR Am J Neuroradiol* 1996;17(3):533–540.
34. Lewis AL, Adams C, Busby W, et al. Comparative in vitro evaluation of microspherical embolisation agents. *J Mater Sci Mater Med* 2006;17(12):1193–1204. Epub 2006 Dec 5.
35. Tadavarthy SM, Knight L, Ovitt TW, et al. Therapeutic transcatheter arterial embolization. *Radiology* 1974;112(1):13–16.
36. Link DP, Strandberg JD, Virmani R, et al. Histopathologic appearance of arterial occlusions with hydrogel and polyvinyl alcohol embolic material in domestic swine. *J Vasc Interv Radiol* 1996;7(6):897–905.
37. Laurent A, Wassef M, Chapot R, et al. Location of vessel occlusion of calibrated tris-acryl gelatin microspheres for tumor and arteriovenous malformation embolization. *J Vasc Interv Radiol* 2004;15(5):491–496.
38. Chuang VP, Wallace S. Hepatic artery embolization in the treatment of hepatic neoplasms. *Radiology* 1981;140(1):51–58. Epub 1981 Jul 1.
39. Jin B, Wang D, Lewandowski RJ, et al. Quantitative 4D transcatheter intraarterial perfusion MRI for standardizing angiographic chemoembolization endpoints. *AJR Am J Roentgenol* 2011;197(5):1237–1243. Epub 2011 Oct 25.
40. Geschwind J-FH, Ramsey DE, van der Wal BCH, et al. Transcatheter arterial chemoembolization of liver tumors: effects of embolization protocol on injectable volume of chemotherapy and subsequent arterial patency. *Cardiovasc Intervent Radiol* 2003;26(2):111.
41. Lewandowski RJ, Geschwind JF, Liapi E, et al. Transcatheter intraarterial therapies: rationale and overview. *Radiology* 2011;259(3):641–657. Epub 2011 May 24.

42. Marelli L, Stigliano R, Triantos C, et al. Transarterial therapy for hepato-cellular carcinoma: which technique is more effective? A systematic review of cohort and randomized studies. *Cardiovasc Intervent Radiol* 2007;30(1): 6–25. Epub 2006 Nov 15.

43. Schneider YJ, Baurain R, Zenebergh A, et al. DNA-binding parameters of daunorubicin and doxorubicin in the conditions used for studying the in-teraction of anthracycline-DNA complexes with cells in vitro. *Cancer Che-mother Pharmacol* 1979;2(1):7–10. Epub 1979 Jan 1.

44. Foglesong PD, Reckord C, Swink S. Doxorubicin inhibits human DNA topoisomerase I. *Cancer Chemother Pharmacol* 1992;30(2):123–125. Epub 1992 Jan 1.

45. Weiss RB. The anthracyclines: will we ever find a better doxorubicin? *Semin Oncol* 1992;19(6):670–686. Epub 1992 Dec 1.

46. Ballet F, Vrignaud P, Robert J, et al. Hepatic extraction, metabolism and biliary excretion of doxorubicin in the isolated perfused rat liver. *Cancer Chemother Pharmacol* 1987;19(3):240–245. Epub 1987 Jan 1.

47. Heibein AD, Guo B, Sprowl JA, et al. Role of aldo-keto reductases and other doxorubicin pharmacokinetic genes in doxorubicin resistance, DNA bind-ing, and subcellular localization. *BMC Cancer* 2012;12:381. Epub 2012 Sep 4.

48. Liapi E, Geschwind JF. Transcatheter arterial chemoembolization for liver cancer: is it time to distinguish conventional from drug-eluting chemoem-bolization? *Cardiovasc Intervent Radiol* 2011;34(1):37–49. Epub 2010 Nov 12.

49. Xiong YQ, Sun HC, Zhu XD, et al. Bevacizumab enhances chemosensi-tivity of hepatocellular carcinoma to adriamycin related to inhibition of survivin expression. *J Cancer Res Clin Oncol* 2011;137(3):505–512. Epub 2010 May 22.

50. Abou-Alfa GK, Johnson P, Knox JJ, et al. Doxorubicin plus sorafenib vs doxorubicin alone in patients with advanced hepatocellular carcinoma: a randomized trial. *JAMA* 2010;304(19):2154–2160. Epub 2010 Nov 18.

51. McCubrey JA, Steelman LS, Abrams SL, et al. Roles of the RAF/MEK/ERK and PI3K/PTEN/AKT pathways in malignant transformation and drug re-sistance. *Adv Enzyme Regul* 2006;46:249–279. Epub 2006 Jul 21.

52. Wakabayashi I, Groschner K. Vascular actions of anthracycline antibiotics. *Curr Med Chem* 2003;10(5):427–436. Epub 2003 Feb 7.

53. Robert J. Epirubicin. Clinical pharmacology and dose-effect relationship. *Drugs* 1993;45(suppl 2):20–30. Epub 1993 Jan 1.

54. Danesi R, Fogli S, Gennari A, et al. Pharmacokinetic-pharmacodynamic relationships of the anthracycline anticancer drugs. *Clin Pharmacokinet* 2002;41(6):431–444. Epub 2002 Jun 21.

55. Favelier S, Boulin M, Hamza S, et al. Lipiodol trans-arterial chemoembo-lization of hepatocellular carcinoma with idarubicin: first experience. *Car-diovasc Intervent Radiol* 2012. Epub 2012 Dec 12.

56. Boulin M, Guiu S, Chauffert B, et al. Screening of anticancer drugs for chemoembolization of hepatocellular carcinoma. *Anticancer Drugs* 2011;22(8):741–748. Epub 2011 Apr 14.

57. Go RS, Adjei AA. Review of the comparative pharmacology and clinical activity of cisplatin and carboplatin. *J Clin Oncol* 1999;17(1):409–422. Epub 1999 Aug 24.

58. Rosenberg B, Vancamp L, Krigas T. Inhibition of cell division in *Esch-erichia coli* by electrolysis products from a platinum electrode. *Nature* 1965;205:698–699. Epub 1965 Feb 13.

59. Ikeda M, Maeda S, Ashihara H, et al. Transcatheter arterial infusion chemo-therapy with cisplatin-lipiodol suspension in patients with hepatocellular carcinoma. *J Gastroenterol* 2010;45(1):60–67. Epub 2009 Aug 6.

60. Ono Y, Yoshimasu T, Ashikaga R, et al. Long-term results of lipiodol-transcatheter arterial embolization with cisplatin or doxorubicin for unresectable hepatocellular carcinoma. *Am J Clin Oncol* 2000;23(6): 564–568. Epub 2001 Feb 24.

61. Gaba RC. Chemoembolization practice patterns and technical methods among interventional radiologists: results of an online survey. *AJR Am J Roentgenol* 2012;198(3):692–699. Epub 2012 Feb 24.

62. Yukisawa S, Ishii H, Kasuga A, et al. A transcatheter arterial chemotherapy using a novel lipophilic platinum derivative (miriplatin) for patients with small and multiple hepatocellular carcinomas. *Eur J Gastroenterol Hepatol* 2012;24(5):583–588. Epub 2012 Feb 15.

63. Kaneko S, Furuse J, Kudo M, et al. Guideline on the use of new anticancer drugs for the treatment of Hepatocellular Carcinoma 2010 update. *Hepatol Res* 2012;42(6):523–542. Epub 2012 May 10.

64. Kimoto Y, Oota J, Nakano Y, et al. Intra-arterial infusion chemotherapy for metastatic hepatic tumor of colo-rectal cancer [in Japanese]. *Gan To Kagaku Ryoho* 1983;10(10):2205–2210. Epub 1983 Oct 1.

65. den Hartigh J, McVie JG, van Oort WJ, et al. Pharmacokinetics of mitomy-cin C in humans. *Cancer Res* 1983;43(10):5017–5021. Epub 1983 Oct 1.

66. Cerretani D, Roviello F, Pieraccini M, et al. Pharmacokinetics of intraarterial mitomycin C in hypoxic hepatic infusion with embolization in the treatment of liver metastases. *Vascul Pharmacol* 2002;39(1–2):1–6. Epub 2003 Mar 6.

67. Hoorn CM, Wagner JG, Petry TW, et al. Toxicity of mitomycin C to-ward cultured pulmonary artery endothelium. *Toxicol Appl Pharmacol* 1995;130(1):87–94. Epub 1995 Jan 1.

68. Gaba RC, Wang D, Lewandowski RJ, et al. Four-dimensional transcath-eter intraarterial perfusion MR imaging for monitoring chemoemboliza-tion of hepatocellular carcinoma: preliminary results. *J Vasc Interv Radiol* 2008;19(11):1589–1595. Epub 2008 Sep 27.

69. Liapi E, Lee KH, Georgiades CC, et al. Drug-eluting particles for interven-tional pharmacology. *Tech Vasc Interv Radiol* 2007;10(4):261–269. Epub 2008 Jun 24.

70. McNair AM. Using hydrogel polymers for drug delivery. *Med Device Tech-nol* 1996;7(10):16–22.

71. Peppas NA, Huang Y, Torres-Lugo M, et al. Physicochemical foundations and structural design of hydrogels in medicine and biology. *Annu Rev Biomed Eng* 2000;2:9–29.

72. Constantin M, Fundueanu G, Bortolotti F, et al. Preparation and charac-terisation of poly(vinyl alcohol)/cyclodextrin microspheres as matrix for inclusion and separation of drugs. *Int J Pharm* 2004;285(1–2):87–96.

73. Gish RG, Lencioni R, Di Bisceglie AM, et al. Role of the multidisciplinary team in the diagnosis and treatment of hepatocellular carcinoma. *Expert Rev Gastroenterol Hepatol* 2012;6(2):173–185. Epub 2012 Mar 2.

74. Georgiades CS, Hong K, Geschwind JF. Pre- and postoperative clinical care of patients undergoing interventional oncology procedures: a comprehen-sive approach to preventing and mitigating complications. *Tech Vasc Interv Radiol* 2006;9(3):113–124. Epub 2007 Jun 15.

75. Chung YE, Park MS, Park YN, et al. Hepatocellular carcinoma variants: radiologic-pathologic correlation. *AJR Am J Roentgenol* 2009;193(1): W7–W13. Epub 2009 Jun 23.

76. Mazzaferro V, Regalia E, Doci R, et al. Liver transplantation for the treatment of small hepatocellular carcinomas in patients with cirrhosis. *N Engl J Med* 1996;334(11):693–699. Epub 1996 Mar 14.

77. Thomas MB, Jaffe D, Choti MM, et al. Hepatocellular carcinoma: con-sensus recommendations of the National Cancer Institute Clinical Trials Planning Meeting. *J Clin Oncol* 2010;28(25):3994–4005. Epub 2010 Aug 4.

78. Investigators TCotLIPC. Prospective validation of the CLIP score: a new prognostic system for patients with cirrhosis and hepatocellular carcinoma. *Hepatology* 2000;31(4):840–845. Epub 2000 Mar 25.

79. American Joint Committee on Cancer. American Joint Committee on can-cer staging of hepatocellular carcinoma. In: Edge SB, Byrd DR, Compton CC, et al, eds. *American Joint Committee on Cancer Staging Manual*. 7th ed. New York, NY: Springer; 2010:175.

80. Llovet JM, Bru C, Bruix J. Prognosis of hepatocellular carcinoma: the BCLC staging classification. *Semin Liver Dis* 1999;19(3):329–338. Epub 1999 Oct 13.

81. Forner A, Reig ME, de Lope CR, et al. Current strategy for staging and treatment: the BCLC update and future prospects. *Semin Liver Dis* 2010;30(1):61–74. Epub 2010 Feb 23.

82. Okuda K, Ohtsuki T, Obata H, et al. Natural history of hepatocellular carci-noma and prognosis in relation to treatment. Study of 850 patients. *Cancer* 1985;56(4):918–928. Epub 1985 Aug 15.

83. Farinati F, Rinaldi M, Gianni S, et al. How should patients with hepatocel-lular carcinoma be staged? Validation of a new prognostic system. *Cancer* 2000;89(11):2266–2273. Epub 2001 Jan 9.

84. Huo TI, Huang YH, Lin HC, et al. Proposal of a modified Cancer of the Liver Italian Program staging system based on the model for end-stage liver disease for patients with hepatocellular carcinoma undergoing loco-regional therapy. *Am J Gastroenterol* 2006;101(5):975–982. Epub 2006 Apr 1.

85. Kaseb AO, Abbruzzese JL, Vauthey JN, et al. I-CLIP: improved stratifica-tion of advanced hepatocellular carcinoma patients by integrating plasma IGF-1 into CLIP score. *Oncology* 2011;80(5–6):373–381. Epub 2011 Aug 9.

86. Kaseb AO, Morris JS, Hassan MM, et al. Clinical and prognostic impli-cations of plasma insulin-like growth factor-1 and vascular endothelial growth factor in patients with hepatocellular carcinoma. *J Clin Oncol* 2011;29(29):3892–3899. Epub 2011 Sep 14.

87. Kudo M, Chung H, Haji S, et al. Validation of a new prognostic staging system for hepatocellular carcinoma: the JIS score compared with the CLIP score. *Hepatology* 2004;40(6):1396–1405. Epub 2004 Nov 27.

88. A comparison of lipiodol chemoembolization and conservative treat-ment for unresectable hepatocellular carcinoma. Groupe d'Etude et de Traitement du Carcinome Hepatocellulaire. *N Engl J Med* 1995;332(19): 1256–1261. Epub 1995 May 11.

89. Vauthey JN, Lauwers GY, Esnaola NF, et al. Simplified staging for hepatocellular carcinoma. *J Clin Oncol* 2002;20(6):1527–1536. Epub 2002 Mar 16.
90. Leung TW, Tang AM, Zee B, et al. Construction of the Chinese University Prognostic Index for hepatocellular carcinoma and comparison with the TNM staging system, the Okuda staging system, and the Cancer of the Liver Italian Program staging system: a study based on 926 patients. *Cancer* 2002;94(6):1760–1769. Epub 2002 Mar 29.
91. Vauthey JN, Dixon E, Abdalla EK, et al. Pretreatment assessment of hepatocellular carcinoma: expert consensus statement. *HPB (Oxford)* 2010;12(5):289–299. Epub 2010 Jul 2.
92. Pugh RN, Murray-Lyon IM, Dawson JL, et al. Transection of the oesophagus for bleeding oesophageal varices. *Br J Surg* 1973;60(8):646–649.
93. Khan KN, Nakata K, Kusumoto Y, et al. Evaluation of nontumorous tissue damage by transcatheter arterial embolization for hepatocellular carcinoma. *Cancer Res* 1991;51(20):5667–5671. Epub 1991 Oct 15.
94. Malinchoc M, Kamath PS, Gordon FD, et al. A model to predict poor survival in patients undergoing transjugular intrahepatic portosystemic shunts. *Hepatology* 2000;31(4):864–871.
95. Brown DB, Fundakowski CE, Lisker-Melman M, et al. Comparison of MELD and Child-Pugh scores to predict survival after chemoembolization for hepatocellular carcinoma. *J Vasc Interv Radiol* 2004;15(11):1209–1218.
96. Michels N. *Blood Supply and Anatomy of the Upper Abdominal Organs with a Descriptive Atlas.* Philadelphia, PA: Lippincott; 1955:64–69.
97. Lee KH, Sung KB, Lee DY, et al. Transcatheter arterial chemoembolization for hepatocellular carcinoma: anatomic and hemodynamic considerations in the hepatic artery and portal vein. *Radiographics* 2002;22(5):1077–1091. Epub 2002 Sep 18.
98. Hiatt JR, Gabbay J, Busuttil RW. Surgical anatomy of the hepatic arteries in 1000 cases. *Ann Surg* 1994;220(1):50–52. Epub 1994 Jul 1.
99. Chung JW, Kim HC, Yoon JH, et al. Transcatheter arterial chemoembolization of hepatocellular carcinoma: prevalence and causative factors of extrahepatic collateral arteries in 479 patients. *Korean J Radiol* 2006;7(4):257–266. Epub 2006 Dec 5.
100. Ho S, Lau WY, Leung WT, et al. Arteriovenous shunts in patients with hepatic tumors. *J Nucl Med* 1997;38(8):1201–1205. Epub 1997 Aug 1.
101. Ngan H, Peh WC. Arteriovenous shunting in hepatocellular carcinoma: its prevalence and clinical significance. *Clin Radiol* 1997;52(1):36–40. Epub 1997 Jan 1.
102. Okuda K, Musha H, Yamasaki T, et al. Angiographic demonstration of intrahepatic arterio-portal anastomoses in hepatocellular carcinoma. *Radiology* 1977;122(1):53–58. Epub 1977 Jan 1.
103. Kim YJ, Lee HG, Park JM, et al. Polyvinyl alcohol embolization adjuvant to oily chemoembolization in advanced hepatocellular carcinoma with arterioportal shunts. *Korean J Radiol* 2007;8(4):311–319. Epub 2007 Aug 4.
104. Heaston DK, Chuang VP, Wallace S, et al. Metastatic hepatic neoplasms: angiographic features of portal vein involvement. *AJR Am J Roentgenol* 1981;136(5):897–900. Epub 1981 May 1.
105. Huang MS, Lin Q, Jiang ZB, et al. Comparison of long-term effects between intra-arterially delivered ethanol and Gelfoam for the treatment of severe arterioportal shunt in patients with hepatocellular carcinoma. *World J Gastroenterol* 2004;10(6):825–829. Epub 2004 Mar 25.
106. Furuse J, Iwasaki M, Yoshino M, et al. Hepatocellular carcinoma with portal vein tumor thrombus: embolization of arterioportal shunts. *Radiology* 1997;204(3):787–790. Epub 1997 Sep 1.
107. Coldwell DM, Stokes KR, Yakes WF. Embolotherapy: agents, clinical applications, and techniques. *Radiographics* 1994;14(3):623–643; quiz 645–646. Epub 1994 May 1.
108. Doppman JL, Girton ME. Bile duct scarring following ethanol embolization of the hepatic artery: an experimental study in monkeys. *Radiology* 1984;152(3):621–626. Epub 1984 Sep 1.
109. Choi BI, Lee KH, Han JK, et al. Hepatic arterioportal shunts: dynamic CT and MR features. *Korean J Radiol* 2002;3(1):1–15. Epub 2002 Mar 29.
110. Miller AB, Hoogstraten B, Staquet M, et al. Reporting results of cancer treatment. *Cancer* 1981;47(1):207–214. Epub 1981 Jan 1.
111. Therasse P, Arbuck SG, Eisenhauer EA, et al. New guidelines to evaluate the response to treatment in solid tumors. European Organization for Research and Treatment of Cancer, National Cancer Institute of the United States, National Cancer Institute of Canada. *J Natl Cancer Inst* 2000;92(3):205–216. Epub 2000 Feb 3.
112. Eisenhauer EA, Therasse P, Bogaerts J, et al. New response evaluation criteria in solid tumours: revised RECIST guideline (version 1.1). *Eur J Cancer* 2009;45(2):228–247. Epub 2008 Dec 23.
113. Lencioni R, Llovet JM. Modified RECIST (mRECIST) assessment for hepatocellular carcinoma. *Semin Liver Dis* 2010;30(1):52–60. Epub 2010 Feb 23.
114. van Persijn van Meerten EL, Gelderblom H, Bloem JL. RECIST revised: implications for the radiologist. A review article on the modified RECIST guideline. *Eur Radiol* 2010;20(6):1456–1467. Epub 2009 Dec 25.
115. Ganapathy-Kanniappan S, Kunjithapatham R, Geschwind JF. Glyceraldehyde-3-phosphate dehydrogenase: a promising target for molecular therapy in hepatocellular carcinoma. *Oncotarget* 2012;3(9):940–953. Epub 2012 Sep 12.
116. Liapi E, Geschwind JF, Vali M, et al. Assessment of tumoricidal efficacy and response to treatment with 18F-FDG PET/CT after intraarterial infusion with the antiglycolytic agent 3-bromopyruvate in the VX2 model of liver tumor. *J Nucl Med* 2011;52(2):225–230.
117. Ganapathy-Kanniappan S, Kunjithapatham R, Torbenson MS, et al. Human hepatocellular carcinoma in a mouse model: assessment of tumor response to percutaneous ablation by using glyceraldehyde-3-phosphate dehydrogenase antagonists. *Radiology* 2012;262(3):834–845.

Principles of Locoregional Therapy: Thermoablative Techniques

MUNEEB AHMED and S. NAHUM GOLDBERG

INTRODUCTION

Image-guided tumor ablation is a minimally invasive strategy to treat focal tumors by inducing irreversible cellular injury through the application of thermal and, more recently, nonthermal energy or chemical injection. This approach has become a widely accepted technique and has been incorporated in the treatment of a range of clinical circumstances, including focal tumors in the liver, lung, kidney, bone, and adrenal glands.[1–6] Benefits of minimally invasive therapies compared to those of surgical resection include lesser mortality and morbidity, lower cost, and the ability to perform procedures on outpatients who are not good candidates for surgery.[7] Additional work is required, however, to improve outcomes and to overcome limitations in ablative efficacy, including the persistent growth of residual tumor at the ablation margin, the inability to effectively treat larger tumors, and the variability in complete treatment based on tumor location.[7]

Given the multiplicity of treatment types and potential complexity of paradigms in oncology and the wider application of thermal ablation techniques, a thorough understanding of the basic principles and recent advances in thermal ablation is a necessary prerequisite for its effective clinical use. These key concepts related to tumor ablation can be broadly divided into (1) those that relate to performing a clinical ablation, such as understanding the goals of therapy and mechanisms of tissue heating or tumor destruction, and (2) understanding the proper role of tumor ablation and the strategies that are being pursued to improve overall ablation outcome. These latter concepts include a systematic approach to technologic development, understanding and using the biophysiologic environment to maximize ablation outcome, combining tumor ablation with adjuvant therapies to synergistically increase tumor destruction, and improving tumor visualization and targeting through image navigation and fusion technology. Given that the greatest experimental and clinical experience exists for radiofrequency (RF)-based ablation, this is the representative model used to discuss many of these concepts. Many of these principles also apply when using alternative ablative modalities, as discussed in subsequent chapters.

GOALS OF MINIMALLY INVASIVE THERMAL TUMOR ABLATION

The overall goal of minimally invasive thermal tumor ablation for focal malignancies encompasses several specific objectives, regardless of the specific thermal ablative device used. The primary purpose of treatment is to completely eradicate all viable malignant cells within the target tumor. Based on tumor recurrence patterns in long-term studies in patients who have undergone surgical resection and, more recently, ablation, along with studies that have performed pathologic analysis of resection margins, there is often viable persistent microscopic tumor foci in a rim of apparently normal surrounding parenchymal tissue beyond the visible tumor margin. Therefore, tumor ablation therapies also attempt to include a 5- to 10-mm "ablative" margin of normal surrounding tissue in the target zone, although the required thickness of this margin is variable based on tumor and organ type.[8,9]

Given that appropriate and complete tumor destruction only occurs when the entire target tumor is exposed to favorable temperatures and, therefore, is determined by the pattern of tissue heating in the target tumor, for larger tumors (usually defined to be larger than 3 to 5 cm in diameter), a single ablation treatment may not be sufficient to entirely encompass the target volume.[3] Thus, an additional consideration is that multiple overlapping ablations or simultaneous use of multiple applicators may be required to successfully treat the entire tumor and achieve an ablative margin, although accurate targeting and probe placement can often be technically challenging (FIGURE 4.1).[10] Tumor biology can also affect ablation efficiency. Growth patterns of the tumor itself can influence overall treatment outcomes, with slow-growing tumors being more amenable to multiple treatment sessions over longer periods. These principles are applicable to a wide range of ablative technologies, including both thermal and nonthermal strategies.

Finally, although complete treatment of the target tumor is of primary importance, specificity and accuracy are also highly preferred with a secondary goal of incurring as little injury as possible to surrounding nontarget normal tissue. This ability to minimize damage to normal organ parenchyma is one of the significant advantages of minimally invasive percutaneous thermal ablation and can be critical in patients who have focal tumors in the setting of limited functional organ reserve. Examples of clinical situations where this is relevant include focal hepatic tumors in patients with underlying cirrhosis and limited hepatic reserve, patients with von Hippel-Lindau syndrome who have limited renal function and require treatment of multiple renal tumors, and patients with primary lung tumors with extensive underlying emphysema and limited lung function (FIGURE 4.2).[11–13] Many of these patients are not surgical candidates due to limited native organ functional reserve, placing them at a higher risk for postoperative complications or organ failure.

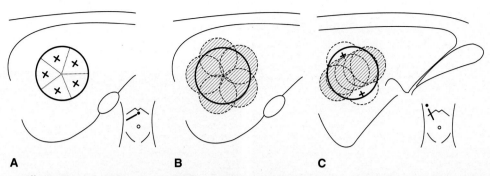

A   **B**   **C**

FIGURE 4.1 Illustration of performing multiple overlapping ablations to completely treat a large tumor, using a regular five-sided prism model. A. Maximum transverse view of the tumor: Five target sites are determined to guide electrode insertions. **B.** Same section as **A**: Five ablations are performed in the middle part of the tumor. **C.** The section perpendicular to **A**: Two additional ablations are performed at the two poles of the tumor. The tumor can be effectively ablated with seven ablation spheres × indicates the target site of the ablation—that is, the ablation sphere center.

Reprinted with permission from Chen M. *Radiology* 2004;232:260–271.

PRINCIPLES OF TISSUE HEATING IN THERMAL ABLATION

Ablative tissue heating occurs through two specific mechanisms. First, an applicator placed within the center of the target tumor delivers energy that interacts with tissue to generate focal heat immediately around it. This approach is similar for all thermal ablation strategies, regardless of the type of energy source used, although specific mechanisms of heat induction are energy specific.[14] For example, as RF current travels from the electrode applicator to the remote grounding pad, local tissue resistance to current flow results in frictional heat generation. In microwave-based systems, the needle antenna applies electromagnetic energy to the tissue, and as molecules with an intrinsic dipole moment (such as water) are forced to continuously align to the externally applied magnetic field, the kinetic energy that is generated results in local tissue heating, which extends deeper into tissues around the antennae (compared to, for example, RF energy). Laser ablation uses emission of laser energy from optic fibers to generate tissue heat immediately around the fiber tip. Ultrasound-based systems induce tissue heating by applying a focused beam of ultrasound energy with a high peak intensity, either directly around a percutaneously placed applicator (like for other ablative systems) or transcutaneously by directing several ultrasound beams of lower intensity from different directions so that they converge at the target tumor, where the ultrasound energy is absorbed by the tissue and converted to heat. The second mechanism of tissue heating in thermal ablation uses thermal tissue conduction.[15] Heat generated around the electrode diffuses through the tumor and results in additional high-temperature heating separate from the direct energy–tissue interactions that occur around the electrode. The contribution of thermal conduction to overall tissue ablation is determined by several factors. Tissue-heating patterns vary based on the specific energy source used—for example, microwave-based systems induce tissue heating at a much faster rate than RF-based systems and so thermal conduction contributes less to overall tissue heating.[15] Additionally, tumor and tissue characteristics also affect thermal conduction. As an example, primary hepatic

tumors (hepatocellular carcinoma) transmit heat better than the surrounding cirrhotic hepatic parenchyma.[3,16]

Regardless of the energy source used, the endpoint of thermal ablation is adequate tissue heating to induce coagulative necrosis throughout the defined target area. Relatively mild increases in tissue temperature above baseline (40° to 42°C) can be tolerated by normal cellular homeostatic mechanisms.[17] Low-temperature hyperthermia (42° to 45°C) results in reversible cellular injury, although this can increase cellular susceptibility to additional adjuvant therapies such as chemotherapy and radiation.[18,19] Irreversible cellular injury occurs when cells are heated to 46° to 48°C for 55 to 60 minutes and happens more rapidly as the temperature rises so that most cell types die in a few minutes when heated at 50°C (FIGURE 4.3).[20] Immediate cellular damage centers on protein coagulation of cytosolic and mitochondrial enzymes and nucleic acid-histone protein complexes, which triggers cellular death over the course of several days.[21] "Heat fixation" or "coagulation necrosis" is used to describe this thermal damage, even though ultimate manifestations of cell death may not fulfill strict histopathologic criteria of coagulative necrosis.[22] This has implications with regard to clinical practice because percutaneous biopsy and standard histopathologic interpretation may not be a reliable measure of adequate ablation.[22] Therefore, the optimal temperatures for ablation range likely exceed 50°C. On the other end of the temperature spectrum, tissue vaporization occurs at temperatures greater than 110°C, which, in turn, limits further current deposition in RF-based systems (as compared with, for example, microwave systems that do not have this limitation).

The exact temperature at which cell death occurs is multifactorial and tissue specific. Based on prior studies demonstrating that tissue coagulation can be induced by focal tissue heating to 50°C for 4 to 6 minutes,[23] this has become the standard surrogate endpoint for thermal ablation therapies in both experimental studies and in current clinical paradigms. Studies have shown, however, that depending on heating time, the rate of heat increase, and the tissue being heated, maximum temperatures at the edge of ablation are variable. For example, maximum temperatures at the edge of the ablation zone, known as the "critical temperature," have been shown to range from 30° to

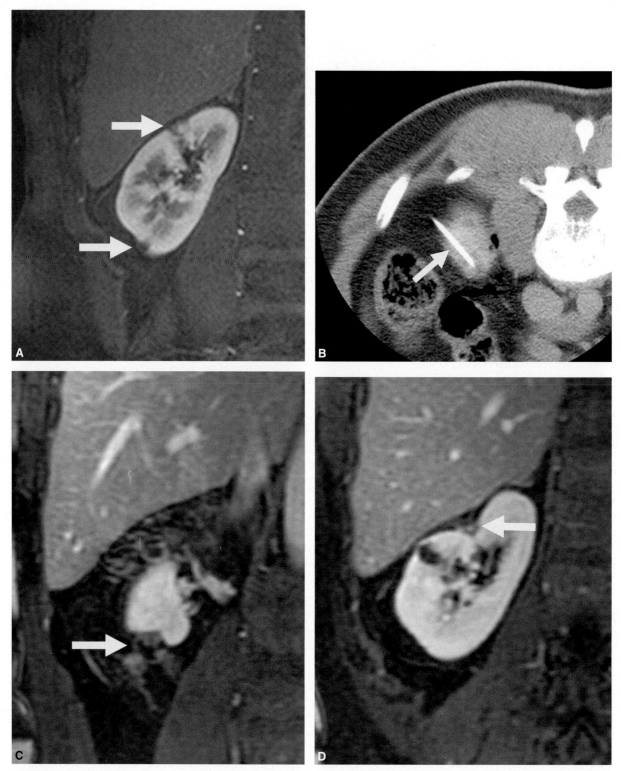

FIGURE 4.2 RF ablation as a nephron-sparing strategy in patients with multiple renal tumors. These are images from a 38-year-old male with von Hippel-Lindau disease, an autosomal dominant disease in which patients are at increased risk of developing multiple renal cell carcinomas (RCC). **A.** Two small RCC tumors (white arrows) are seen on this coronal contrast-enhanced T1-weighted MRI image. **B.** A CT fluoroscopic image demonstrates positioning of the RF electrode in one of the target tumors. **C, D.** Postablation contrast-enhanced coronal T1-weighted MRI images demonstrate successful ablation of two tumors in the right kidney.

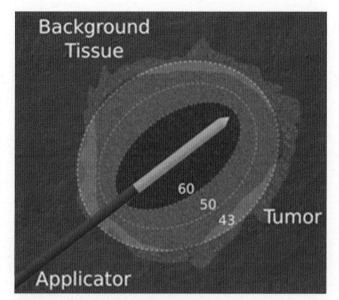

FIGURE 4.3 Schematic representation of focal thermal ablation therapy. Electrode applicators are positioned either with image-guidance or direct visualization within the target tumor, and thermal energy is applied via the electrode. This creates a central zone of high temperatures in the tissue immediately around the electrode (they can exceed 100°C) and surrounded by more peripheral zones of sublethal tissue heating (<50°C) and background liver parenchyma.

Reprinted with permission from Ahmed M. *Radiology* 2011;258:351–369.

77°C for normal tissues and from 41° to 64°C for tumor models (a 23°C difference).[24,25] Likewise, the total amount of heat administered for a given time, known as the thermal dose, varies significantly between different tissues.[24,25] Thus, the threshold target temperature of 50°C should be used only as a general guideline. This conceptual framework is also clearly applicable in determining optimal energy delivery paradigms for nonthermal energy sources as well.[26]

APPLYING THE PRINCIPLES OF THE BIOHEAT EQUATION TO ACHIEVE MEANINGFUL VOLUMES OF TUMOR ABLATION

Complete and adequate destruction by thermal ablation requires that the entire tumor (and usually an ablative margin) be subjected to cytotoxic temperatures. Success of thermal ablation is contingent on adequate heat delivery. The ability to heat large volumes of tissue in different environments depends on several factors encompassing both energy delivery and local physiologic tissue characteristics. The relationship between this set of parameters, as described by the Bioheat equation,[27] can be simplified to describe the basic relationship guiding thermal ablation induced coagulation necrosis as: "coagulation necrosis = (energy deposited × local tissue interactions) – heat loss."[28] Based on this relationship, a three-pronged approach to increase the ability to ablate larger tumors has been pursued. These encompass (1) technologic developments, including modification of energy input algorithms and electrode design to deposit more energy into the tissue; (2) improved understanding and

subsequent modification of the biophysiologic environment to increase tissue heating; and (3) incorporation of adjuvant therapies to increase uniformity of tumor cellular injury in the ablation zone, along with increasing cellular destruction in the nonlethal hyperthermic zone around the ablation. Although the RF ablation platform is the example used in the next section, this three-pronged approach serves as a successful model for the development of other ablation systems as well.

TECHNICAL DEVELOPMENTS TO IMPROVE ABLATIVE THERAPY

Most investigations to improve thermal ablation outcomes have focused on device development, much of which has been, as noted previously, for RF-based ablation systems. Technologic efforts to increase ablation size have focused on modifying energy deposition algorithms and electrode designs to increase both the amount of tissue exposed to the active electrode and the overall amount of energy that can be safely deposited into the target tissue.

Refinement of Energy Application Algorithms

The algorithm by which energy is applied during thermal ablation depends on the energy source, device, and type of electrode that is being used. Although initial power algorithms for RF-based systems were based on a continuous and constant high-energy input, tissue overheating and vaporization ultimately interfere with continued energy input caused by high impedance to current flow from gas formation. Therefore, several strategies to maximize energy deposition have been developed and, in some cases, incorporated into commercially available devices.

Applying high levels of energy in a pulsed manner, separated by periods of lower energy, is one such strategy that has been used with RF-based systems to increase the mean intensity of energy deposition (FIGURE 4.4).[29] If a proper balance between high- and low-energy deposition is achieved, preferential

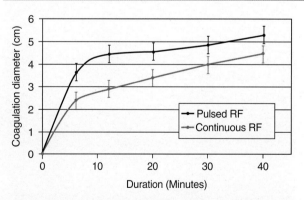

FIGURE 4.4 Increasing RF-induced tissue coagulation using a pulsing energy application compared to a continuous application. The diameter of coagulation necrosis obtained by applying continuous and pulsed RF to a 3-cm, internally cooled electrode for 6 to 40 minutes in ex vivo liver is presented. Continuous RF application was 750 mA, the maximum current applied with observing impedance rises. Pulsed RF technique followed a variable peak strategy. At all time points, greater coagulation is induced with pulsing technique.

Reprinted with permission from Goldberg SN. *JVIR* 1999;10:907–916.

tissue cooling occurs adjacent to the electrode during periods of minimal energy deposition without significantly decreasing heating deeper in the tissue. Thus, even greater energy can be applied during periods of high-energy deposition, thereby enabling deeper heat penetration and greater tissue coagulation.[30] Synergy between a combination of both internal cooling of the electrode and pulsing has resulted in even greater coagulation necrosis and tumor destruction than either method alone.[30] Pulsed-energy techniques have also been successfully used for microwave- and laser-based systems.

Another strategy is to slowly increase (or "ramp-up") the RF energy application in a continuous manner until the impedance to RF current flow increases prohibitively.[31,32] This approach is often paired with multitined expandable electrodes, which have a greater contact surface area with tissue, and in which the goal is to achieve smaller ablation zones around multiple small electrode tines. This algorithm is often combined with a staged expansion of the electrode system such that each small ablation occurs in a slightly different location within the tumor (with the overall goal being ablating the entire target region).

"Electrode switching" is an additional technique that is incorporated into pulsing algorithms to further increase RF tissue heating (FIGURE 4.5).[33] In this, multiple independently placed RF electrodes are connected to a single RF generator, and RF current is applied to a single electrode until an impedance spike is detected at which point current application is applied to the next electrode and so forth. Several studies have demonstrated significant increases in ablation zone size and a reduction in application time using this technique.[33,34] For example, Brace et al.[33] also show larger and more circular ablation zones with the switching application with more rapid heating being 74% faster than the sequential heating (12 vs. 46 minutes).

Finally, continued device development has also led to increases in the overall maximum amount of power that can be delivered.[35,36] For RF-based devices, the maximum amount of RF current that can be delivered depends on both the generator output and the electrode surface area because higher surface areas reduce the current density, and, therefore, adequate tissue heating around the electrode cannot be achieved. Whereas initial systems had maximum power outputs of less than 200 watts, subsequent investigation suggests that higher current output and larger ablation zones can be achieved if higher-powered generators are coupled with larger-surface area electrodes. For example, Solazzo et al.[36] used a 500-KHz (1,000-watt) high-powered generator in an in vivo porcine model and achieved larger coagulation zones with a 4-cm tip cluster electrode (5.2 ± 0.8 cm) compared with a 2.5-cm cluster electrode (3.9 ± 0.3 cm). Similar gains in ablation size have been seen in higher-powered versions of microwave-based systems.[37]

Electrode Modification

Development of ablation applicators (electrodes for RF, antennae for microwave, and diffuser tips for laser-based systems) has contributed significantly to the ability to achieve larger ablation zones reliably. Several strategies to increase the amount of energy deposition and the overall ablation size have been balanced with the need for smaller caliber electrodes to permit the continued use of these devices in a percutaneous and minimally invasive manner. These include the use of multiple electrodes simultaneously, either adjacent to each other or as part of an expandable device through a single introducer needle; the use of cooling systems to minimize tissue and electrode overheating; and the use of bipolar systems for RF ablation to increase tissue heating in the target zone.

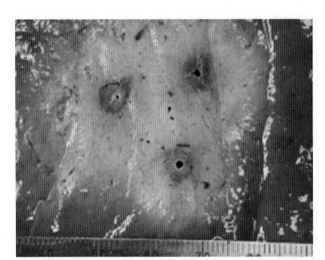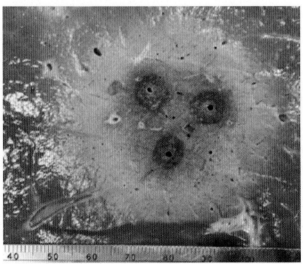

FIGURE 4.5 Example of using RF electrode "switching" to increase the size of the ablation zone. Representative ablations created in ex vivo bovine liver tissue by using sequential (left) and simultaneous (right) application of energy using three internally cooled (Cool-tip system, Covidien Inc., Boulder, CO) RF electrodes. Ablations created simultaneously were consistently larger and more circular in cross section, had better temperature profiles, and could be created much faster than those created sequentially. Scale is in millimeters.

Reprinted with permission from Brace CL. *JVIR* 2009;20:118–124.

Originally, simply lengthening the electrode tip increased coagulation in an asymmetric and preferentially longitudinal geometry. Use of a single electrode inserted multiple times to perform overlapping ablations requires significantly greater time and effort, making it impractical for routine use in a clinical setting. Therefore, the use of multiple electrodes simultaneously in a preset configuration represents a significant step forward in increasing overall ablation size. Initial work with multiple electrodes demonstrated that placement of several monopolar electrodes in a clustered arrangement (no more than 1.5 cm apart) with simultaneous RF application could increase coagulation volume by over 800% compared with a single electrode.[38] Subsequently, working to overcome the technical challenges of multiprobe application, multitined expandable RF electrodes have been developed.[39] These systems involve the deployment of a varying number of multiple thin, curved tines in the shape of an umbrella or more complex geometries from a central cannula.[40,41] This surmounts earlier difficulties by allowing easy placement of multiple probes to create large, reproducible volumes of necrosis. Leveen et al.,[42] using a 12-hook array, were able to produce lesions measuring up to 3.5 cm in diameter in in vivo porcine liver by administering increasing amounts of RF energy from a 50-watt RF generator for 10 minutes. More recently, Applebaum et al.,[43] using commercially available expandable electrodes with optimized stepped-extension and power input algorithms, were able to achieve greater than 5 cm of coagulation in in vivo porcine liver.

Although most conventional RF systems use monopolar electrodes (where the current runs to remotely placed grounding pads positioned on the patient's thighs to complete the circuit), several studies have reported results using bipolar arrays to increase the volume of coagulation created by RF application. In these systems, applied RF current runs from an active electrode to a second grounding electrode in place of a grounding pad. Heat is generated around both electrodes, creating elliptical lesions. McGahan et al.[44] used this method in ex vivo liver to induce necrosis of up to 4 cm in the long-axis diameter but could only achieve 1.4 cm of necrosis in the short diameter. Although this increases the overall size of coagulation volume, the shape of necrosis is unsuitable for actual tumors, making the gains in coagulation less clinically significant. Desinger et al.[45] have described another bipolar array that contains both the active and the return electrodes on the same 2-mm diameter probe. Lee et al.[46] used two multitined electrodes as active and return to increase coagulation during bipolar RF ablation. Finally, several studies have used a multipolar (more than two) array of electrodes (multitined and single internally cooled) during RF ablation to achieve even greater volumes of coagulation.[47,48]

One of the limitations for RF-based systems has been overheating surrounding the active electrode, leading to tissue charring, rising impedance, and RF circuit interruption, ultimately limiting overall RF energy deposition. One successful strategy to address this has been the use of internal electrode cooling, where electrodes contain two hollow lumens that permit continuous internal cooling of the tip with a chilled perfusate, and the removal of warmed effluent to a collection unit outside the body (FIGURE 4.6).[49] This reduces heating directly around the electrode, tissue charring, and rising impedance; allows greater RF energy deposition; and shifts the peak tissue temperature farther into the tumor, contributing to a broader depth of tissue heating from thermal conduction. In initial studies using cooling of 18-gauge single or clustered electrode needles using chilled saline perfusate, significant increases in RF energy deposition and ablation zone size were observed compared with conventional monopolar uncooled electrodes in ex vivo liver, with findings subsequently confirmed in in vivo large-animal models and clinical studies.[30,49] Similar results were observed when chilled saline was infused in combination with expandable electrode systems (referred to as an "internally cooled wet electrode"), although infusion of fluid around the electrode is more difficult to control and makes the reproducibility of results more variable.[50] Most recently, several investigators have used alternative cooling agents (e.g., argon or nitrogen gas) to achieve even greater cooling and, therefore, larger zones of ablation, around the RF

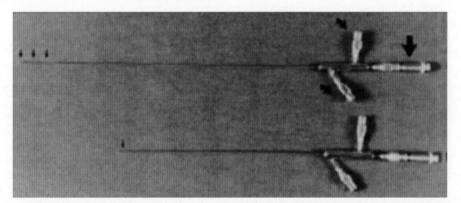

FIGURE 4.6 Example of an early perfused electrode. The shafts of these 18-gauge electrodes are electrically insulated, except for 1- to 3-cm exposed metallic tip (small arrows) from which RF waves emanate. There is a thin central RF electrode with a thermocouple embedded at the tip of the probe to allow for continuous temperature measurement (large arrow). Two central lumens extend to the electrode tip. One lumen is used to deliver 0°C saline to the tip of the probe, and the second returns the warmed saline effluent to a collection unit outside the body. In this closed system, no saline is deposited into the tissues.

Reprinted from Goldberg SN. *Acad Radiol* 1996;3:636–644.

electrode tip.[51] As for RF-based systems, cooling of the antennae shaft for microwave applicators has also been developed, reducing shaft heating (and associated complications such as skin burns) while allowing increased power deposition through smaller-caliber antennae.

Although many of these technologic advances have been developed independently of each other, they may often be used concurrently to achieve even larger ablation zones. Furthermore, although much of this work has been based on RF technology, specific techniques can be used for other thermal ablative therapies. For example, multiple electrodes and applicator cooling have been effectively applied in microwave-based systems as well.[52,53]

PRACTICAL APPLICATION OF TECHNOLOGIC DEVELOPMENTS: COMMERCIALLY AVAILABLE RF DEVICES

Several commercially available RF devices are commonly used and vary based on their energy application algorithms and electrode designs. This raises several issues to be addressed in turn.

Selecting an RF Ablation System—Is One System Better Than Another?

Three- to 5-cm zones of adequate thermal ablation can be achieved with most commercially available RF ablation devices when properly used, as described in the instructions for use. Although the specific size of the ablation zone and the time required to achieve adequate ablation will likely vary among different manufacturers and devices, a recent study by Lin et al. compared four separate and commonly used devices in over 100 patients with primary and secondary hepatic tumors and found little difference in ablation time and local tumor progression. [54]. Thus, it is important for operators to be completely familiar with their device of choice, including electrode shapes and deployment techniques, power-input algorithms, and common troubleshooting issues, to permit thorough treatment planning and maximize optimal clinical outcomes. In particular, familiarity with the anticipated ablation size and shape that can be achieved with the different devices when using their different electrode and parameter options is critical to planning a successful ablation and achieving an adequate ablative margin, especially for larger tumors. Yet, ultimately, good operator technique and careful patient selection contribute at least as much to treatment success as does the specific electrode choice.

Understanding the Principles/Algorithm of the Selected Device

The commonly used RF devices use different power application algorithms based on current flow, impedance, or time to deliver RF energy. Current electrode designs are paired to specific devices and companies, and RF power algorithms are also commonly tailored to specific electrode designs (such that operators cannot interchange many types of electrodes from one device to another, and the greatest efficiencies in use are likely found by following company-recommended application protocols). Several specific electrode designs are available, most commonly divided into those that are needlelike versus multitined

expandable. Specifically, practitioners should be familiar with the shape of the coagulation zone that each system generates. For example, some needlelike electrodes induce a more oval ablation zone parallel to the axis of the electrode, whereas some expandable electrodes generate ablation zones that are pancake-like and less oval-shaped perpendicular to the shaft of the electrode.

Examples of Commercially Available Systems

Several commercially available systems are described next. They represent examples of current clinically available systems (limited to the most commonly used devices that are approved by the Food and Drug Administration [FDA]) (FIGURE 4.7).

The Cool-tip RF ablation system (Covidien Inc., Boulder, CO) uses a pulsed application, which inputs high amounts of current alternating frequently with "off-periods" that are triggered by rises in impedance to reduce tissue overheating around the electrode, applied over a 12-minute time period. The Cool-tip RF system uses 17G needlelike electrodes as single, cluster, or multiple single electrodes that are internally cooled with ice water (to a temperature of less than 10°C). "Electrode switching" technology (described above) is currently only available with the Cool-tip RF system.

The Boston Scientific RF 300 ablation system (Boston Scientific, Natick, MA) employs two rounds of slowly increasing power to achieve tissue heating, which occurs until tissue impedance starts to rise, thereby limiting further current input to threshold levels, colloquially termed "roll-off"—the defined endpoint. The Boston Scientific RF system uses umbrella-shaped expandable electrodes with multiple (10 to 12) tines extending out from the needle shaft.

Finally, another commonly used device, the RITA system (Angiodynamics, Queensbury, NY), administers RF energy to set temperature endpoints (usually 105°C as measured by sensors within the electrode tips) combined with incremental extension of an expandable electrode system. The RITA system uses an expandable electrode system most often paired with slow saline drip infusion. It can create some of the largest zones of coagulation for a single RF electrode (5 to 7 cm), but this system tends to require relatively long periods of heating (30 to 45 minutes).[43]

MODIFICATION OF THE BIOPHYSIOLOGIC ENVIRONMENT

Although larger coagulation zones have been created by modifying electrode design in ablative procedures, there are limitations due to the tumor physiology itself. Recent investigations have centered on altering underlying tumor physiology as a means to improve thermal ablation. Current studies have focused on the effects of tissue characteristics in the setting of temperature-based therapies such as tissue perfusion, thermal conductivity, and system-specific characteristics such as electrical conductivity for RF-based ablation.

Tissue Perfusion

The leading factor constraining thermal ablation coagulation size in tumors continues to be tissue blood flow, which has two effects: a large vessel heat-sink effect and a microvascular perfusion mediated tissue cooling effect. First, larger-diameter blood

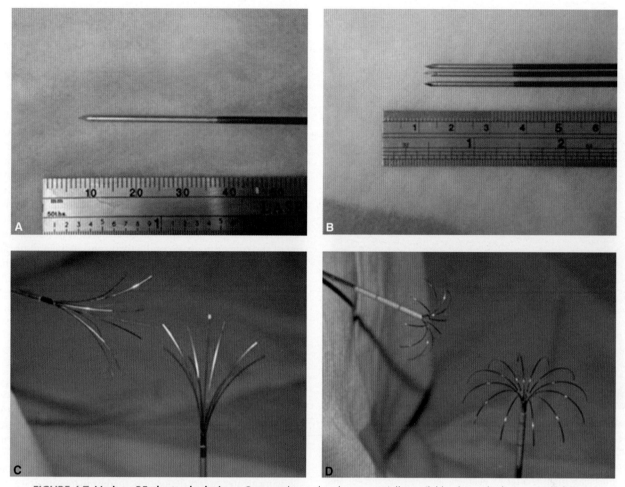

FIGURE 4.7 Various RF electrode designs. Commonly used and commercially available electrode designs, including **A.** a single internally cooled electrode with a 3-cm active tip (Cool-tip system, Valleylab, Boulder, CO), **B.** a cluster internally cooled electrode system with three 2.5-cm active tips (Cluster electrode system, Valleylab, Boulder, CO), and two variations of an expandable electrode system (**C.** Starburst [RITA Medical Systems, Mountain View, CA; **D.** LeVeen, Boston Scientific Corp, Natick, MA]).

Reprinted with permission from Ahmed M. *Radiology* 2011;258:351–369.

vessels with higher flow act as heat sinks, drawing away heat from the ablative area (FIGURE 4.8). Lu et al.[55] show this in an in vivo porcine model by examining the effect of hepatic vessel diameter on RF ablation outcome. Using computed tomography (CT) and histopathologic analysis, more complete thermal heating and a reduced heat-sink effect is seen when the heating zone was less than 3 mm in diameter. In contrast, vessels that are greater than 3 mm in diameter had higher patency rates, less endothelial injury, and greater viability of surrounding hepatocytes after RF ablation. Studies confirm the effect of hepatic blood flow on RF-induced coagulation in which increased coagulation volumes were obtained with decreased hepatic blood flow by embolotherapy, angiographic balloon occlusion, coil embolization, or the Pringle maneuver (total portal inflow occlusion).[56,57] The second effect of tissue vasculature is a result of perfusion-mediated tissue cooling (capillary vascular flow) that also functions as a heat sink. By drawing heat from the treatment zone, this effect reduces the volume of tissue that receives the required minimal thermal dose for coagulation. Targeted microvascular perfusion by using pharmacologic alteration of blood flow can also

improve overall RF ablation efficacy. Goldberg et al.[58] modulated hepatic blood flow using intra-arterial vasopressin and high-dose halothane in conjunction with RF ablation in in vivo porcine liver. Horkan et al.[59] has modulated the use of arsenic trioxide showing reduced blood flow and increased tumor destruction. More recently, another antiangiogenic drug, sorafenib, has been combined with RF ablation to increase overall tumor coagulation in small-animal models (FIGURE 4.9).[60] In this regard, newer nonthermal energy sources, such as irreversible electroporation (IRE), have been shown to be less affected by these effects and will likely provide an alternative in clinical situations where perfusion-mediated cooling impacts ablation outcome.[61]

Thermal Conductivity

Initial clinical studies using RF ablation for hepatocellular carcinoma in the setting of underlying cirrhosis noted an "oven" effect (i.e., increased heating efficacy for tumors surrounded by cirrhotic liver or fat, such as exophytic renal cell carcinomas), or altered thermal transmission at the junction of tumor tissue

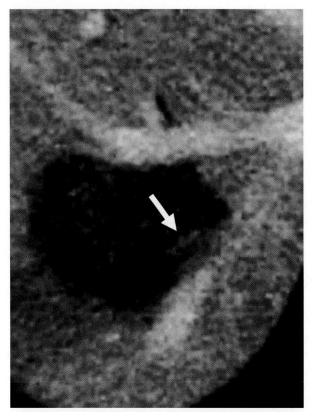

FIGURE 4.8 Example of local tumor progression at the edge of the RF ablation zone caused by the heat-sink effect. This is a clinical example in a patient who underwent focal RF tumor ablation of a single colorectal metastasis. Follow-up contrast-enhanced CT imaging 6 months after RF ablation demonstrates a focal area of local tumor progression (arrow) from incomplete treatment and persistently viable tumor cells caused by vessel-mediated cooling from the abutting adjacent right hepatic vein.

and surrounding tissue.[3] Subsequent experimental studies in ex vivo agar phantoms and bovine liver have confirmed the effects of varying tumor and surrounding tissue thermal conductivity on effective heat transmission during RF ablation and further demonstrated the role of "optimal" thermal conductivity characteristics on ablation outcome.[16,62] For example, very poor tumor thermal conductivity limits heat transmission centrifugally away from the electrode with marked heating in the central portion of the tumor and limited, potentially incomplete heating in peripheral portions of the tumor. In contrast, increased thermal conductivity (such as in cystic lesions) results in fast heat transmission (i.e., heat dissipation) with potentially incomplete and heterogeneous tumor heating. Furthermore, in agar phantom and computer modeling studies, Liu et al. demonstrated that differences in thermal conductivity between the tumor and surrounding background tissue (specifically, decreased thermal conductivity from increased fat content of surrounding tissue) result in increased temperatures at the tumor margin. However, heating was limited in the surrounding medium, making a 1-cm "ablative" margin more difficult to achieve.[62] An understanding of the role of thermal conductivity, and tissue and tumor-specific characteristics, on tissue heating may be useful when trying to predict ablation outcome in varying clinical settings (e.g., in exophytic renal cell carcinomas surrounded by perirenal fat, lung tumors surrounded by aerated normal parenchyma, or osseous metastases surrounded by cortical bone).[16]

Electrical Conductivity

The power deposition in RF-induced tissue heating strongly depends on the local electrical conductivity. The effect of local electrical conductivity can be divided into two main categories. First, altering the electrical activity environment immediately around the RF electrode with ionic agents can increase electrical conductivity prior to or during RF ablation. High local saline concentration increases the area of the active surface electrode, allowing greater energy deposition, thereby increasing the extent of coagulation necrosis.[63] Saline may be beneficial when ablating cavitary lesions, which might not have a sufficient current path. It should be noted, however, that saline infusion is not always a predictable process because fluid can migrate to unintended locations and cause complications if not used properly.[64] Second, different electrical conductivities between the tumor and surrounding background organ can affect tissue heating at the tumor margin. Several studies show increases in tissue heating at the tumor-organ interface when the surrounding medium is characterized by reduced lower electrical conductivity.[65] In

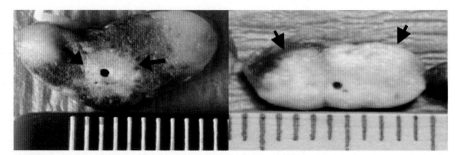

FIGURE 4.9 Reducing the negative effects of tumor microvascular perfusion on tissue heating by combining antiangiogenic therapy with RF ablation. RF ablation combined with antiangiogenic therapies, such as Sorafenib, a VEGF receptor inhibitor, results in significantly increased tumor coagulation (right image: 9 mm, black arrows) compared to RF ablation alone (4 mm, left image, black arrows) in this small-animal tumor model.

Reprinted with permission from Hakime et al. *Radiology* 2007;244:464–470.

certain clinical settings, such as treating focal tumors in either lung or bone, marked differences in electrical conductivity may result in variable heating at the tumor-organ interface and, indeed, limit heating in the surrounding organ, and may make obtaining a 1-cm ablative margin difficult. Lastly, electrical conductivity must be taken into account when using techniques such as hydrodissection to protect adjacent organs. Nonionic fluids can be used to protect tissues adjacent to the ablation zone (such as the diaphragm or bowel) from thermal injury. For this application, fluids with low ion content, such as 5% dextrose in water (D5W), should be used because they have been proven to electrically force RF current away from the protected organ, decrease the size and incidence of burns on the diaphragm and bowel, and reduce pain scores in patients treated with D5W when compared to ionic solutions, such as saline.[33,34] Ionic solutions like 0.9% saline should not be used for hydrodissection because, as noted above, they actually increase RF current flow.[66]

Tissue Fluid Content

Microwave-based systems use electromagnetic energy to forcibly align molecules with an intrinsic dipole moment (such as water) to the externally applied magnetic field, which generates kinetic energy and results in local tissue heating. Therefore, higher tissue water content influences the rates and maximum amounts of achievable tissue heating in these systems.[67] Incorporating tissue internal water content into computer modeling of tumor ablation to more accurately predict tissue heating has also been proposed.[68] In addition, Brace et al.[69] have demonstrated that greater dehydration (and resultant contraction of the ablation zone) occurs with microwave ablation compared with RF-based systems. Optimization of microwave heating by modulating the tissue fluid content is also being investigated.[70]

▍ COMBINING TUMOR ABLATION WITH ADJUVANT THERAPIES

Strategies to modify ablative systems and the biologic environment have been successful in improving the clinical utility of percutaneous ablation, but limitations in clinical efficacy persist. For example, with further long-term follow-up of patients undergoing ablation therapy, there has been an increased incidence of detection of persistent local tumor growth of ablated tumors, suggesting that there are residual foci of viable, untreated tumor tissue within and around the treatment zone.[3] As such, additional strategies are required to improve RF ablation efficacy by targeting these residual foci of viable malignant cells.

Currently, thermal ablation only takes advantage of temperatures that are sufficient by themselves to induce coagulation necrosis (greater than 50°C). Yet, based on the exponential decrease in RF tissue heating there is a steep thermal gradient in tissues surrounding an RF electrode. Hence, there is substantial flattening of the curve below 50°C with a much larger tissue volume encompassed by the 45°C isotherm. Modeling studies demonstrate that were the threshold for cell death to be decreased by as few as 5°C, tumor coagulation could be increased up to 1.5 cm (up to a 59% increase in spherical volume of the ablation zone).[65] Therefore, target tumors can be conceptually divided into three zones: (1) a central area, predominantly treated by thermal ablation, which undergoes heat-induced coagulation necrosis; (2) a peripheral rim, which undergoes reversible changes from sublethal hyperthermia; and (3) surrounding tumor or normal tissue that is unaffected by focal ablation although still exposed to adjuvant systemic therapies.

Several studies show that tumor destruction may be achieved by combining RF thermal ablation with adjuvant chemotherapy or radiation.[71-74] The goal of this combined approach is to increase tumor destruction that is occurring in the peripheral rim of sublethal temperatures (i.e., largely reversible cell damage induced by mildly elevating tissue temperatures to 41° to 45°C) surrounding the coagulation zone.[72] Heterogeneity of thermal diffusion with high-temperature heating (in the presence of vascularity) prevents adequate ablation. Because local control requires complete tumor destruction, ablation may be inadequate even if large zones of ablation that encompass the entire tumor are created. By killing tumor cells at lower temperatures, this combined paradigm will not only increase necrosis volume but may also create a more complete area of tumor destruction by filling in untreated gaps within the ablation zone. Combined treatment also has the potential to achieve equivalent tumor destruction with a concomitant reduction of the duration or course of therapy.

Combined Radiofrequency Ablation and Transarterial Chemoembolization

Although RF ablation and transarterial chemoembolization (TACE) are both independently and commonly used modalities for locoregional treatment of liver tumors such as hepatocellular carcinoma (HCC), several limitations to their optimal outcomes persist. For example, RF ablation is less effective in larger tumors and is difficult to use in specific locations or near larger blood vessels. In contrast, TACE can be used for larger tumors but rates of tumor necrosis are lower (30% to 90% compared with greater than 90% for RF ablation). There are several potential advantages with combining RF and TACE. This includes combined two-hit cytotoxic effects of exposure to nonlethal low-level hyperthermia in periablational tumor and adjuvant chemotherapy. Alterations in tumor perfusion can potentiate the effects of either RF ablation through preablation embolization of tumor vasculature or TACE with postablation peripheral hyperemia, increasing blood flow for TACE. Finally, performing TACE first can improve tumor visualization (through intratumoral iodized oil deposition) for RF ablation.[33]

RF ablation and TACE can be administered in varying paradigms, based on the sequence and time between therapies. Several studies have administered both therapies near concurrently. Mostafa et al.[57] demonstrated in VX2 tumors implanted in rabbit liver that the largest treatment volumes were obtained when TACE preceded RF ablation, compared with RF before TACE or either therapy alone. Ahrar et al.[75] investigated the effects of high-temperature heating on commonly used TACE agents (doxorubicin, mitomycin-C, and cisplatin) and found minimal change in the cytotoxic activity of the agents when exposed to clinically relevant durations of heating (greater than 100°C for less than 20 minutes). For HCC tumors invisible on ultrasound and unenhanced CT, Lee et al. reported that 71% of tumors could be adequately visualized for subsequent RF ablation [94]. Based on this, the optimal strategy for administration is likely performing TACE first, followed by RF ablation. This is confirmed in a recent randomized controlled study by Morimoto et al.,[76] comparing TACE-RF (on the same day) to RF alone for intermediate-sized HCC (3.1 to 5 cm in diameter), where TACE-RF resulted in lower rates of local tumor progression at 3 years.

Sequential or alternating administration represents another approach in combination therapy to primarily treat the target tumor with a single modality (either TACE or RF), followed by additional adjuvant treatments using either one or both modalities for residual disease. For example, RF ablation can be performed for an initial presentation of limited disease, followed by TACE performed at a later date for residual peripheral tumor, satellite nodules, or new foci. Likewise, TACE can be performed initially to control more extensive disease with subsequent RF directed at small foci of local recurrence or new small nodules (FIGURE 4.10).

Several studies using combination therapy have reported increases in ablation size and greater treatment efficacy with combination RF/TACE, particularly as the primary treatment of large (greater than 5 cm) unresectable tumors. For example, Yang et al.[77] treated 103 patients with recurrent unresectable HCC after hepatectomy and reported lower intrahepatic recurrence and longer 3-year survival compared with either therapy alone. The potential benefit of combining RF with TACE for small (less than 3 cm) tumors remains less clear because a recent meta-analysis of randomized-controlled studies reported no significant survival benefit for combination RF/TACE over RF alone.[78] Finally, tailoring treatment to each individual case remains important, because each modality can be adjuvantly used to "mop-up" residual disease after primary therapy.

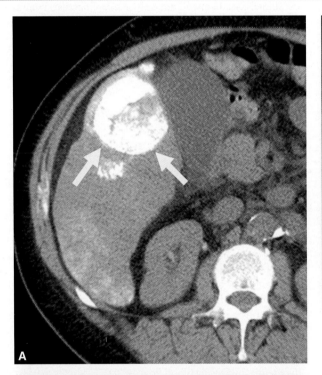

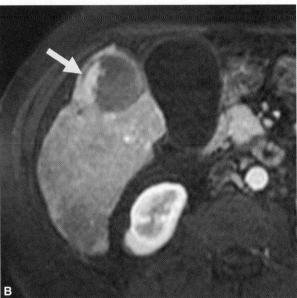

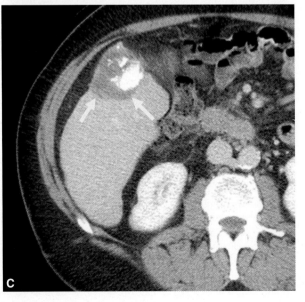

FIGURE 4.10 RF ablation of residual HCC after primary transarterial chemoembolization. Fifty-six-year-old man with a 4.8-cm vascular HCC, who underwent initial selective lipiodol-based TACE. **A.** Initial post-TACE, noncontrast CT demonstrates marked lipiodol uptake throughout the focal HCC. **B.** Axial contrast-enhanced subtracted T1-weighted MRI image during the arterial phase of contrast injection demonstrates a focal area of residual enhancing tumor along the lateral and inferior aspect of the tumor. **C.** Axial contrast-enhanced CT image immediately following RF ablation of the residual tumor demonstrates successful ablation without evidence of residual contrast enhancement.

Combined RF Ablation and Systemic Chemotherapies

Several studies have investigated the use of adjuvant chemotherapy (predominantly doxorubicin-based regimens) administered in close proximity of RF ablation. Combining ablative therapies with adjuvant direct intratumoral chemotherapy injection has not been particularly successful, given the many difficulties encountered in clinical practice, such as nonuniform drug diffusion and limited operator control on drug distribution. Although some benefit likely occurs with combining RF ablation with conventional intravenous systemic chemotherapy, there is limited published data quantifying this benefit to date. Rather, the focus of combination therapy has been on administered adjuvant liposomal or nanoparticle-based chemotherapies with RF ablation, which has demonstrated that combining RF ablation with chemotherapy encapsulated in nanoparticle delivery vehicles (such as liposomes) has several advantages. For example, liposome particles are completely biocompatible, cause very little toxic or antigenic reaction, and are biologically inert. Incorporation of polyethylene-glycol surface modifications minimizes plasma protein absorption on liposome surfaces and subsequent recognition and uptake of liposomes by the reticuloendothelial system, which further reduces systemic phagocytosis and results in prolonged circulation time, selective agent delivery through the leaky tumor endothelium (an enhanced permeability and retention effect), as well as reduced toxicity profiles.[79,80] In a pilot clinical study combining RF ablation (internally cooled electrode) with adjuvant liposomal doxorubicin, 10 patients with 18 intrahepatic tumors were randomized to receive either liposomal doxorubicin (20 mg Doxil) 24 hours prior to RF ablation or RF ablation alone (mean tumor size undergoing ablation was 4 ± 1.8 cm) (FIGURE 4.11).[74] Although no difference in the amount of tumor destruction was seen between groups immediately following RF, at 2 to 4 weeks, patients receiving liposomal doxorubicin had an increase in tumor destruction of 24% to 342% volumetric increase (median = 32%) compared to a decrease of 76% to 88% for patients who were treated with RF alone (a finding concordant with prior observations). Several additional and clinically beneficial findings were also observed only in the combination therapy group, including increased diameter of the treatment effect for multiple tumor types; improved completeness of tumor destruction, particularly adjacent to intratumoral vessels; and increased treatment effect, including the peritumoral liver parenchyma (suggesting a contribution to achieving an adequate ablative margin). Liposomal formulations containing other chemotherapy agents (such as cisplatin or paclitaxel) are also being developed, and some preliminary experimental studies have been performed combining these with RF ablation,[81,82] although determining which agents provide the greatest benefit remains to be seen and will likely vary in a tumor-specific manner. Finally, several "thermosensitive" liposomal formulations have also been developed that preferentially release their contents in hyperthermic conditions (42° to 45°C).[83] As a result, this doxorubicin-containing formulation is widely accepted for clinical practice. Several experimental studies combining RF ablation with adjuvant intravenous liposome-encapsulated chemotherapy (such as a commercially available doxorubicin-based agent, Doxil) increased tumor coagulation, intratumoral drug accumulation, and cellular cytotoxicity, and reduced tumor growth rates have all been reported.[72]

Combining Thermal Ablation with Adjuvant Radiation

Several studies have reported early investigation into combination RF ablation and radiation therapy with promising results.[71,73] The rationale for this combination of therapies include the known synergistic effects of combined external-beam radiation therapy and low-temperature hyperthermia.[84] Experimental animal studies have demonstrated increased tumor necrosis, reduced tumor growth, and improved animal survival with combined external beam radiation and RF ablation when compared to either therapy alone[71,85] Clinical studies in primary lung malignancies confirm the synergistic effects of these therapies.[73,86] For example, Grieco et al.[87] reported improved survival with combination therapy in 41 patients with inoperable stage I/II non–small-cell lung cancer treated with RF ablation and adjuvant radiation compared with either therapy alone. Potential causes for the synergy include the sensitization of the tumor to subsequent radiation due to the increased oxygenation resulting from hyperthermia-induced increased blood flow to the tumor.[88] Another possible mechanism, which has been seen in animal tumor models, is an inhibition of radiation-induced repair and recovery and increased free radical formation.[89] Future work is needed to identify the optimal temperature for ablation and optimal radiation dose, as well as the most effective method of administering radiation therapy (external-beam radiation therapy, brachytherapy, or yttrium microspheres), on an organ-by-organ basis.

Determining the Optimal Combination Therapy

Given the need to achieve complete eradication of all target tumor cells, including a 5- to 10-mm margin of seemingly normal surrounding tissue that may contain residual microscopic foci of disease, the argument for combining several modalities to achieve complete tumor cell death—similar to the multidisciplinary approach including surgery, radiation, and chemotherapy used for the treatment of most solid cancers—cannot be overstated. Approaching each case and individual tumor with the goal of using whatever options are available within the interventional armamentarium will likely provide the highest clinical yield. Several factors should be taken into consideration when planning combination therapy such that treatment is tailored to each case. First, tumor biology is a critical factor because certain tumors are more responsive to specific adjuvant therapies; for example, primary non–small-cell lung cancer is susceptible to external beam radiation compared with primary hepatocellular carcinoma. Marked tumor vascularity (such as is seen in HCC) limits RF tissue heating, and so optimal treatment likely includes performing adjuvant TACE first or administering adjuvant antiangiogenic therapy. Similarly, some vascular tumors (such as HCC or renal cell carcinoma) are more susceptible to antiangiogenic therapies and would likely benefit from combination therapy. Second, the overall disease burden (i.e., the size and number of tumors) is an important consideration when planning combination therapy. Smaller tumors (<3 cm) are often easily treated with a single modality (such as RF ablation), whereas larger tumors (>3.5 cm) require combination therapy. Similarly, multifocal tumors or the presence of satellite nodules around the primary tumor are also better suited to treatment

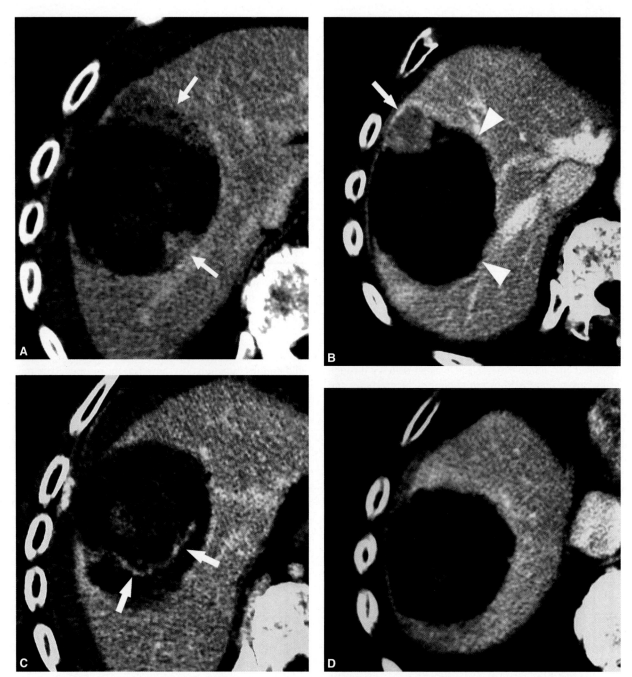

FIGURE 4.11 Increased tumor destruction with combined RF and liposomal doxorubicin. Eighty-two-year-old male with an 8.2-cm vascular hepatoma. **A.** CT image obtained immediately following RF ablation shows persistent regions of residual untreated tumor (white arrows) (black zone = ablated region). **B.** Two weeks following therapy, there is interval increase in coagulation as the 1.5-cm inferior region of residual tumor and the 1.2-cm anteromedial portion of the tumor no longer enhance (white arrowheads). A persistent nodule of viable tumor is identified (white arrow). This was successfully treated with a course of RF ablation. **C.** CT image obtained immediately following RF ablation demonstrates the persistence of a large vessel (white arrows) coursing through the nonenhancing ablated lesion. **D.** Two weeks post therapy, there is no enhancement throughout this region, and no vessel was seen on any of the three phases of contrast enhancement. No evidence of local tumor recurrence was identified at 48 months of follow-up.

Reprinted with permission from Goldberg SN, et al. *AJR* 2002;179:93–101.

with multiple modalities (e.g., RF ablation for the primary tumor and TACE for the residual peripheral satellite nodules). Finally, tumor accessibility and visibility (i.e., can it be easily seen and reached via a percutaneous approach) should also factor into any decision on combination therapy. For example, as was noted earlier in the chapter, tumors not visible on unenhanced CT or ultrasound for RF ablation can be treated with TACE first. Ultimately, as treatment options increase, many patients may receive multiple rounds of treatment in which various treatment options sequentially alternate based on the characteristics of residual tumor, as is commonly the case in patients with HCC who receive combinations of ablation, chemoembolization, and/or radioembolization.

IMPROVING IMAGE GUIDANCE AND TUMOR TARGETING

Thermal ablation is commonly performed with a percutaneous approach using imaging guidance with a single or combination of modalities (CT, ultrasound [US], or magnetic resonance imaging [MRI]). A successful ablation is contingent upon the operator's ability to visualize the tumor, position the electrode within the target, and accurately evaluate the treatment zone upon completion of the ablation. Several significant challenges to performing a successful ablation exist at each of these steps. For example, diagnostic imaging studies are often obtained with modalities that are separate from the modality being used for treatment (e.g., diagnostic MRI and ablation being performed with CT or US), positional variations between diagnostic and treatment imaging precludes an exact overlay of different imaging studies, and target tumors often have variable visibility with or without contrast on US, CT, and/or MRI. Electrode positioning often requires traversing a narrow course or window in a three-dimensional trajectory when only two-dimensional real-time imaging is available, often when the target is moving from respiratory motion. Finally, correlating the immediate postprocedure imaging to prior diagnostic imaging to determine adequacy of treatment, especially at the tumor margin, can often be difficult. All of these factors make treating some lesions extremely and technically challenging.[90]

Several technologies are being developed to address some of these difficulties.[90] Image-fusion software is now becoming commercially available to allow image overlay of two different imaging modalities for diagnostic interpretation. Multimodality image fusion for procedural guidance takes this further by pairing an existing data set from a prior diagnostic study to the "real-time" modality being used for the procedure. CT-US fusions systems often use a sensor in the US transducer and initial landmark localization to fuse a prior CT scan (which allows multiplanar reconstruction from the CT data set) with real-time US images. Finally, needle tracking systems are also been developed using either electromagnetic (EM) or optical (infrared-based) tracking technology.[91] In these systems, the needle tip is identified and localized in three-dimensional space and the needle trajectory overlays existing imaging. EM-based devices use a small field generator to create a rapidly changing magnetic field, in which a sensor coil in the needle tip creates an electrical current, allowing localization within three-dimensional space. Several of these devices have been tested for simple procedures, such as joint injection or biopsy, and can likely be applied to ablative procedures as well, especially when coupled with predictive modeling software[92,93]

CONCLUSION

Thermal ablation is being more widely accepted in clinical practices for the treatment of a range of tumors in various organ sites. A good conceptual framework that includes an understanding of the goals of tumor ablation and the mechanisms of tissue destruction that occur with ablation are a necessary prerequisite to its successful clinical application. The development of RF ablation serves as an excellent model for the evolution and development of additional ablation modalities (such as microwave, IRE, and cryotherapy-based systems). Several successful strategies have been used to improve thermal ablation efficacy including technologic advancements in ablation devices, such as electrode and navigation system developments, and modifications of tissue and tumor environment. Finally, thermal ablation has been successfully combined with adjuvant chemotherapy and radiation, and future investigation will explore tailoring specific adjuvant therapies based on a mechanistic rationale.

REFERENCES

1. Gervais DA, et al. Renal cell carcinoma: clinical experience and technical success with radio-frequency ablation of 42 tumors. *Radiology* 2003;226(2):417–424.
2. Kurup AN, Callstrom MR. Ablation of skeletal metastases: current status. *J Vasc Interv Radiol* 2010;21(suppl 8):S242–250.
3. Livraghi T, et al. Hepatocellular carcinoma: radiofrequency ablation of medium and large lesions. *Radiology* 2000;214:761–768.
4. Solbiati L, et al. Percutaneous radiofrequency ablation of hepatic metastases from colorectal cancer: long term results in 117 patients. *Radiology* 2001;221:159–166.
5. Venkatesan AM, et al. Percutaneous ablation of adrenal tumors. *Tech Vasc Interv Radiol* 2010;13(2):89–99.
6. Zemlyak A, Moore WH, Bilfinger TV. Comparison of survival after sublobar resections and ablative therapies for stage I non-small cell lung cancer. *J Am Coll Surg* 2010;211(1): 68–72.
7. Ahmed M, et al. Principles of and advances in percutaneous ablation. *Radiology* 2011;258(2):351–369.
8. Dodd GD 3rd, et al. Minimally invasive treatment of malignant hepatic tumors: at the threshold of a major breakthrough. *Radiographics* 2000;20(1):9–27.
9. Shimada K, et al. Role of the width of the surgical margin in a hepatectomy for small hepatocellular carcinomas eligible for percutaneous local ablative therapy. *Am J Surg* 2008;195(6):775–781.
10. Dodd GD 3rd, et al. Radiofrequency thermal ablation: computer analysis of the size of the thermal injury created by overlapping ablations. *AJR Am J Roentgenol* 2001;177(4):777–782.
11. Gervais DA, et al. Radiofrequency ablation of renal cell carcinoma: part 1, indications, results, and role in patient management over a 6-year period and ablation of 100 tumors. *AJR Am J Roentgenol* 2005;185(1):64–71.
12. Lencioni R, et al. Early-stage hepatocellular carcinoma in patients with cirrhosis: long-term results of percutaneous image-guided radiofrequency ablation. *Radiology* 2005 234(3):961–967.
13. Lencioni R, et al. Response to radiofrequency ablation of pulmonary tumours: a prospective, intention-to-treat, multicentre clinical trial (the RAPTURE study). *Lancet Oncol* 2008;9(7):621–628.
14. Goldberg SN, et al. Image-guided tumor ablation: standardization of terminology and reporting criteria. *J Vasc Interv Radiol* 2009;20(suppl 7):S377–390.
15. Schramm W, Yang D, Haemmerich D. Contribution of direct heating, thermal conduction and perfusion during radiofrequency and microwave ablation. *Conf Proc IEEE Eng Med Biol Soc* 2006;1:5013–5016.
16. Ahmed M, et al. Computer modeling of the combined effects of perfusion, electrical conductivity, and thermal conductivity on tissue heating patterns in radiofrequency tumor ablation. *Int J Hyperthermia* 2008;24(7):577–588.
17. Thrall DE, et al. A comparison of temperatures in canine solid tumours during local and whole-body hyperthermia administered alone and simultaneously. *Int J Hyperthermia* 1990;6(2):305–317.
18. Seegenschmiedt M, Brady L, Sauer R. Interstitial thermoradiotherapy: review on technical and clinical aspects. *Am J Clin Oncol* 1990;13:352–363.

19. Trembley B, Ryan T, Strohbehn J. Interstitial hyperthermia: physics, biology, and clinical aspects. In: *Hyperthermia and Oncology*, vol. 3. Utrecht, The Netherlands: VSP; 1992:11–98.

20. Larson T, Bostwick D, Corcia A. Temperature-correlated histopathologic changes following microwave thermoablation of obstructive tissues in patients with benign prostatic hyperplasia. *Urology* 1996;47:463–469.

21. Zevas N, Kuwayama A. Pathologic analysis of experimental thermal lesions: comparison of induction heating and radiofrequency electrocoagulation. *J Neurosurg* 1972;37:418–422.

22. Goldberg SN, et al. Treatment of intrahepatic malignancy with radiofrequency ablation: radiologic-pathologic correlation. *Cancer* 2000;88:2452–2463.

23. Goldberg SN, et al. Radiofrequency tissue ablation: importance of local temperature along the electrode tip exposure in determining lesion shape and size. *Acad Radiol* 1996;3:212–218.

24. Mertyna P, et al. Radiofrequency ablation: the effect of distance and baseline temperature on thermal dose required for coagulation. *Int J Hyperthermia* 2008;24(7):550–559.

25. Mertyna P, et al. Radiofrequency ablation: variability in heat sensitivity in tumors and tissues. *J Vasc Interv Radiol* 2007;18(5):647–654.

26. Daniels C, Rubinsky B. Electrical field and temperature model of nonthermal irreversible electroporation in heterogeneous tissues. *J Biomech Eng* 2009;131(7):071006.

27. Pennes H. Analysis of tissue and arterial blood temperatures in the resting human forearm. *J Applied Physiol* 1948;1:93–122.

28. Goldberg SN, Gazelle GS, Mueller PR. Thermal ablation therapy for focal malignancy: a unified approach to underlying principles, techniques, and diagnostic imaging guidance. *Am J Radiol* 2000;174:323–331.

29. Goldberg SN, et al. Percutaneous radiofrequency tissue ablation: optimization of pulsed-RF technique to increase coagulation necrosis. *JVIR* 1999;10:907–916.

30. Goldberg SN, et al. Large-volume tissue ablation with radiofrequency by using a clustered, internally-cooled electrode technique: laboratory and clinical experience in liver metastases. *Radiology* 1998;209:371–379.

31. Gulesserian T, et al. Comparison of expandable electrodes in percutaneous radiofrequency ablation of renal cell carcinoma. *Eur J Radiol* 2006;59(2):133–139.

32. McGahan JP, et al. Maximizing parameters for tissue ablation by using an internally cooled electrode. *Radiology* 2010;256(2):397–405.

33. Brace CL, et al. Radiofrequency ablation: simultaneous application of multiple electrodes via switching creates larger, more confluent ablations than sequential application in a large animal model. *J Vasc Interv Radiol* 2009;20(1):118–124.

34. Laeseke PF, et al. Multiple-electrode radiofrequency ablation creates confluent areas of necrosis: in vivo porcine liver results. *Radiology* 2006;241(1):116–124.

35. Brace CL, et al. Radiofrequency ablation with a high-power generator: device efficacy in an in vivo porcine liver model. *Int J Hyperthermia* 2007;23(4):387–394.

36. Solazzo SA, et al. High-power generator for radiofrequency ablation: larger electrodes and pulsing algorithms in bovine ex vivo and porcine in vivo settings. *Radiology* 2007;242(3):743–750.

37. Laeseke PF, et al. Microwave ablation versus radiofrequency ablation in the kidney: high-power triaxial antennas create larger ablation zones than similarly sized internally cooled electrodes. *J Vasc Interv Radiol* 2009;20(9):1224–1229.

38. Goldberg SN, et al. Radiofrequency tissue ablation using multiprobe arrays: greater tissue destruction than multiple probes operating alone. *Acad Radiol* 1995;2:670–674.

39. Bangard C, et al. Large-volume multi-tined expandable RF ablation in pig livers: comparison of 2D and volumetric measurements of the ablation zone. *Eur Radiol* 2010;20(5):1073–1078.

40. Rossi S, Buscarini E, Garbagnati F. Percutaneous treatment of small hepatic tumors by an expandable RF needle electrode. *AJR Am J Roentgenol* 1998;170:1015–1022.

41. Siperstein AE, et al. Laparoscopic thermal ablation of hepatic neuroendocrine tumor metastases. *Surgery* 1997;122:1147–1155.

42. Leveen RF. Laser hyperthermia and radiofrequency ablation of hepatic lesions. *Semin Interv Radiol* 1997;12:313–324.

43. Appelbaum L, et al. Algorithm optimization for multitined radiofrequency ablation: comparative study in ex vivo and in vivo bovine liver. *Radiology* 2010;254(2):430–440.

44. McGahan JP, et al. Hepatic ablation using bipolar radiofrequency electrocautery. *Acad Radiol* 1996;3(5):418–422.

45. Desinger K, et al. Interstitial bipolar RF-thermotherapy (REITT) therapy by planning by computer simulation and MRI-monitoring—a new concept for minimally invasive procedures. *Proc SPIE* 1999;3249:147–160.

46. Lee JM, et al. Bipolar radiofrequency ablation using wet-cooled electrodes: an in vitro experimental study in bovine liver. *AJR Am J Roentgenol* 2005;184(2):391–397.

47. Seror O, et al. Large (> or = 5.0-cm) HCCs: multipolar RF ablation with three internally cooled bipolar electrodes—initial experience in 26 patients. *Radiology* 2008;248(1):288–296.

48. Lee JM, et al. Multiple-electrode radiofrequency ablation of in vivo porcine liver: comparative studies of consecutive monopolar, switching monopolar versus multipolar modes. *Invest Radiol* 2007;42(10):676–683.

49. Goldberg SN, et al. Radiofrequency tissue ablation: increased lesion diameter with a perfusion electrode. *Acad Radiol* 1996;3:636–644.

50. Hsieh CL, et al. Effectiveness of ultrasound-guided aspiration and sclerotherapy with 95% ethanol for treatment of recurrent ovarian endometriomas. *Fertil Steril* 2009;91(6):2709–2713.

51. Hines-Peralta A, et al. Hybrid radiofrequency and cryoablation device: preliminary results in an animal model. *J Vasc Interv Radiol* 2004;15(10):1111–1120.

52. Tsai WL, et al. Review article: percutaneous acetic acid injection versus percutaneous ethanol injection for small hepatocellular carcinoma—a long-term follow-up study. *Aliment Pharmacol Ther* 2008.

53. He N, et al. Microwave ablation: an experimental comparative study on internally cooled antenna versus non-internally cooled antenna in liver models. *Acad Radiol* 2010;17(7):894–899.

54. Lin SM, Lin CC, Chen WT, Chen YC, Hsu CW. Radiofrequency ablation for hepatocellular carcinoma: a prospective comparison of four radiofrequency devices. *JVIR* 2007;18(9):1118–25. [PMID 17804774]

55. Lu DS, et al. Influence of large peritumoral vessels on outcome of radiofrequency ablation of liver tumors. *J Vasc Interv Radiol* 2003;14(10):1267–1274.

56. Patterson EJ, et al. Radiofrequency ablation of porcine liver in vivo: effects of blood flow and treatment time on lesion size. *Ann Surg* 1998;227(4):559–565.

57. Mostafa EM, et al. Optimal strategies for combining transcatheter arterial chemoembolization and radiofrequency ablation in rabbit VX2 hepatic tumors. *J Vasc Interv Radiol* 2008;19(12):1740–1748.

58. Goldberg SN, et al. Radio-frequency tissue ablation: effect of pharmacologic modulation of blood flow on coagulation diameter. *Radiology* 1998;209(3):761–767.

59. Horkan C, et al. Radiofrequency ablation: effect of pharmacologic modulation of hepatic and renal blood flow on coagulation diameter in a VX2 tumor model. *J Vasc Interv Radiol* 2004;15(3):269–274.

60. Hakime A, et al. Combination of radiofrequency ablation with antiangiogenic therapy for tumor ablation efficacy: study in mice. *Radiology* 2007;244(2):464–470.

61. Lee EW, et al. Advanced hepatic ablation technique for creating complete cell death: irreversible electroporation. *Radiology* 2010;255(2):426–433.

62. Liu YJ, et al. Thermal characteristics of microwave ablation in the vicinity of an arterial bifurcation. *Int J Hyperthermia* 2006;22(6):491–506.

63. Aube C, et al. Influence of NaCl concentrations on coagulation, temperature, and electrical conductivity using a perfusion radiofrequency ablation system: an ex vivo experimental study. *Cardiovasc Intervent Radiol* 2007;30(1):92–97.

64. Gillams AR, Lees WR. CT mapping of the distribution of saline during radiofrequency ablation with perfusion electrodes. *Cardiovasc Intervent Radiol* 2005;28(4):476–480.

65. Liu Z, et al. Radiofrequency tumor ablation: insight into improved efficacy using computer modeling. *AJR Am J Roentgenol* 2005;184(4):1347–1352.

66. Laeseke PF, et al. Use of dextrose 5% in water instead of saline to protect against inadvertent radiofrequency injuries. *AJR Am J Roentgenol* 2005;184(3):1026–1027.

67. Yang D, et al. Measurement and analysis of tissue temperature during microwave liver ablation. *IEEE Trans Biomed Eng* 2007;54(1):150–155.

68. Yang D, et al. Expanding the bioheat equation to include tissue internal water evaporation during heating. *IEEE Trans Biomed Eng* 2007;54(8):1382–1388.

69. Brace CL, et al. Tissue contraction caused by radiofrequency and microwave ablation: a laboratory study in liver and lung. *J Vasc Interv Radiol* 21(8):1280–1286.

70. Isfort P, et al. In vitro experiments on fluid-modulated microwave ablation. *Rofo* 2010;182(6):518–524.

71. Horkan C, et al. Reduced tumor growth with combined radiofrequency ablation and radiation therapy in a rat breast tumor model. *Radiology* 2005;235(1):81–88.

72. Ahmed M, Goldberg SN. Combination radiofrequency thermal ablation and adjuvant IV liposomal doxorubicin increases tissue coagulation and intratumoural drug accumulation. *Int J Hyperthermia* 2004;20(7):781–802.

73. Dupuy DE, et al. Radiofrequency ablation followed by conventional radiotherapy for medically inoperable stage I non-small cell lung cancer. *Chest* 2006;129(3):738–745.

74. Goldberg SN, et al. Radiofrequency ablation of hepatic tumors: increased tumor destruction with adjuvant liposomal doxorubicin therapy. *AJR Am J Roentgenol* 2002;179(1):93–101.

75. Ahrar K, et al. 2004 Dr. Gary J. Becker Young Investigator Award: relative thermosensitivity of cytotoxic drugs used in transcatheter arterial chemoembolization. *J Vasc Interv Radiol* 2004;15(9):901–905.

76. Morimoto M, et al. Midterm outcomes in patients with intermediate-sized hepatocellular carcinoma: a randomized controlled trial for determining the efficacy of radiofrequency ablation combined with transcatheter arterial chemoembolization. *Cancer* 2010;116(23):5452–5460.

77. Yang W, et al. Combination therapy of radiofrequency ablation and transarterial chemoembolization in recurrent hepatocellular carcinoma after hepatectomy compared with single treatment. *Hepatol Res* 2009;39(3):231–240.

78. Wang W, Shi J, Xie WF. Transarterial chemoembolization in combination with percutaneous ablation therapy in unresectable hepatocellular carcinoma: a meta-analysis. *Liver Int* 2010;30(5):741–749.

79. Vaage J, Barbara E. Tissue uptake and therapeutic effects of stealth doxorubicin. In: Lasic D, Martin F, eds. *Stealth Liposomes*. Boca Raton, FL: CRC Press; 1995.

80. Gabizon A, Shiota R, Papahadjopoulos D. Pharmacokinetics and tissue distribution of doxorubicin encapsulated in stable liposomes with long circulation times. *J Natl Cancer Inst* 1989;81:1484–1488.

81. Yang W, et al. Do liposomal apoptotic enhancers increase tumor coagulation and end-point survival in percutaneous radiofrequency ablation of tumors in a rat tumor model? *Radiology* 2010;257(3):685–696.

82. Ahmed M, et al. Combined radiofrequency ablation and adjuvant liposomal chemotherapy: effect of chemotherapeutic agent, nanoparticle size, and circulation time. *J Vasc Interv Radiol* 2005;16(10):1365–1371.

83. Negussie AH, et al. Formulation and characterisation of magnetic resonance imageable thermally sensitive liposomes for use with magnetic resonance-guided high intensity focused ultrasound. *Int J Hyperthermia* 2011;27(2):140–155.

84. Algan O, et al. External beam radiotherapy and hyperthermia in the treatment of patients with locally advanced prostate carcinoma. *Cancer* 2000;89(2):399–403.

85. Solazzo S, et al. RF ablation with adjuvant therapy: comparison of external beam radiation and liposomal doxorubicin on ablation efficacy in an animal tumor model. *Int J Hyperthermia* 2008;24(7):560–567.

86. Chan MD, et al. Combined radiofrequency ablation and high-dose rate brachytherapy for early-stage non-small-cell lung cancer. *Brachytherapy* 2011.

87. Grieco CA. et al. Percutaneous image-guided thermal ablation and radiation therapy: outcomes of combined treatment for 41 patients with inoperable stage I/II non-small-cell lung cancer. *J Vasc Interv Radiol* 2006;17(7):1117–1124.

88. Mayer R, et al. Hyperbaric oxygen and radiotherapy. *Strahlenther Onkol* 2005;181(2):113–123.

89. Solazzo S, et al. Liposomal doxorubicin increases radiofrequency ablation-induced tumor destruction by increasing cellular oxidative and nitrative stress and accelerating apoptotic pathways. *Radiology* 2010; 255(1): 62-74.

90. Wood BJ, et al. Navigation systems for ablation. *J Vasc Interv Radiol* 2010;21(suppl 8):S257–63.

91. Krucker J, et al. Electromagnetic tracking for thermal ablation and biopsy guidance: clinical evaluation of spatial accuracy. *J Vasc Interv Radiol* 2007;18(9):1141–1150.

92. Klauser AS, et al. Fusion of real-time US with CT images to guide sacroiliac joint injection in vitro and in vivo. *Radiology* 2010;256(2):547–553.

93. Khan MF, et al., Navigation-based needle puncture of a cadaver using a hybrid tracking navigational system. *Invest Radiol* 2006;41(10) 713–720.

94. Lee MW, Kim YJ, Park SW, Hwang JH, Jung SI, Jeon HJ, Kwon WK. Percutaneous radiofrequency ablation of small hepatocellular carcinoma invisible on both ultrasonography and unenhanced CT: a preliminary study of combined treatment with transarterial chemoembolization. *Br J Radiol* 2009;82(983): 908–15.

CHAPTER

5

Hepatocellular Carcinoma: Epidemiology, Staging, and Medical Management

ROBERT E. ROSES and JEAN-NICOLAS VAUTHEY

INTRODUCTION

Hepatocellular carcinoma (HCC) is the most common primary liver malignancy and the sixth most common cancer worldwide.[1] The majority of cases are diagnosed at an advanced stage and are fatal within months.[2] Eighty percent of new cases occur in developing countries, but the incidence is rising in economically developed regions, including Japan, Western Europe, and the United States.[3-6] Hepatic cirrhosis is the dominant risk factor.[7,8]

In the United States, where hepatitis C viral infection, alcohol use, and nonalcoholic fatty liver disease (NAFLD) are the most common causes of cirrhosis, the incidence of HCC doubled between 1975 and 1995 and continued to rise through 1998.[9,10] This trend will continue given the estimated four million hepatitis C seropositive individuals in the United States and the typical two- to three-decade period of latency between initial hepatitis C virus (HCV) infection and the development of HCC.[10] The incidence of NAFLD-associated cirrhosis is also increasing in the United States and will contribute further to this trend.[11,12]

Although the prognosis associated with HCC remains poor overall, progress has been made in the treatment of HCC. Surgical resection, transplantation, a variety of nonsurgical local-regional therapies, and systemic therapies have evolved considerably and increasing numbers of patients are candidates for treatment. The multidisciplinary nature of contemporary HCC therapy requires a thorough assessment of disease burden but also of the extent of chronic liver disease. Staging remains a challenge because no single staging system is applicable to all patients and a multitude of different staging systems serve complementary roles. It is, nonetheless, essential in selecting an appropriate treatment strategy. This chapter reviews the epidemiology and staging of HCC and touches on current medical therapies.

EPIDEMIOLOGY

HCC accounts for approximately 85% of all primary liver cancers and is the third leading cause of cancer-related death worldwide.[13,14] The distribution of HCC varies significantly by geography; it is endemic in parts of the world where hepatitis B (HBV) viral infection is also endemic. In Western countries,

HCV infection and alcoholic cirrhosis are the principal risk factors for HCC. The incidence of HCC is projected to increase fourfold by 2015, reflecting the rising incidence of HCV infection in American subpopulations.[10]

The incidence of HCC increases with age, although the age of peak incidence varies somewhat with geography. HCC is most commonly diagnosed between the fifth and sixth decades of life; however, HCC affects children and young adults in areas where HBV is endemic and perinatal infection is common. There is a strong male predominance in HCC incidence worldwide. In the United States, HCC affects males more than females with a male-to-female incidence ratio of 2.7 to 1; this difference is even greater in the low-risk populations of central and southern Europe.[15] HCC incidence rates are higher among African Americans than Caucasians (6.1 vs. 2.8 per 100,000 in men) and even higher in Hispanics, Asians, Pacific Islanders, and Native Americans.[4] Independent of HBV status, a family history of HCC in first-degree relatives is associated with a relative risk (RR) of 2.4 and overall risk (OR) of 2.9.[16]

RISK FACTORS

HCC usually develops in the setting of liver cell injury and resultant inflammation, hepatocyte regeneration, liver matrix remodeling, fibrosis, and cirrhosis. The major etiologies of liver cirrhosis include chronic HBV and HCV, alcohol consumption, hepatotoxic medications or other exposures, and genetic metabolic diseases. The mechanisms by which these varied etiologies lead to HCC are not fully understood.

Approximately four million Americans are infected with HCV.[17] Antibodies against HCV are detected in 90% of patients with HCC.[18] Risk factors for HCC in persons infected with HCV include: older age at the time of infection, male sex, coinfection with human immunodeficiency virus or HBV, diabetes, and obesity. Between 60% and 80% of anti-HCV-positive patients with HCC have cirrhosis.[19]

HCV exhibits significant genetic variability and has been classified into four major types based on nucleotide sequence homology. Types V and VI isolates have been reported provisionally based on partially sequenced genomes.[20,21] There is evidence that type II (genotype 1b), prevalent in Western countries and the Far

East, is more aggressive and is associated with progression to cirrhosis but also with HCC in the absence of cirrhosis.[22,23]

HBV accounts for approximately 50% of cases of HCC worldwide and nearly all cases in children. In endemic areas of Asia and Africa, where HBV is frequently transmitted from mother to newborn, the majority of infected individuals have a chronic course. As with HCV, most HCC develops in the setting of cirrhosis but can also arise independently. The risk of HCC in HBV-infected individuals is increased by male sex, older age, longer duration of infection, and alcohol use.

Heavy alcohol consumption is an important risk factor for HCC.[24] In the United States, alcoholic cirrhosis is associated with approximately 15% of HCC cases.[25,26] Alcohol use may further increase risk in patients with viral hepatitis because alcohol increases circulating HCV viral titers and HCC risk.[27] Other etiologies of cirrhosis and parenchymal liver diseases, including primary biliary cirrhosis, hemochromatosis, Wilson disease, alpha$_1$ antitrypsin deficiency, and glycogen storage disease, significantly increase HCC risk in alcohol drinkers.

Cigarette smoking is associated with HCC development, and synergistic relationships among tobacco use, alcohol consumption, and viral hepatitis may exist.[28–30] Oral contraceptive use has been linked to HCC in some studies although hormonal replacement was associated with protection against liver cancer in other studies.[31–33] Aflatoxins are secondary fungal metabolites (mycotoxins) often found in grains. Exposure to aflatoxins can result in liver necrosis and bile duct proliferation.[34] Aflatoxins can induce HCC in animals and exposure is associated with HBV carrier status. Relative risk of HCC is increased 3-fold after aflatoxin exposure, 9-fold in the setting of chronic HBV infection, and 59-fold with the combination of aflatoxin exposure and chronic HBV infection.

Obesity is associated with a spectrum of liver disease, including steatosis and cryptogenic cirrhosis. In the setting of steatosis, other genetic or environmental factors may lead to nonalcoholic steatohepatitis (NASH).[35,36] A direct relationship between obesity and primary liver tumors is suggested in the recent literature; however, obesity has not been definitively established as an independent risk factor for HCC.[37] There is more evidence implicating diabetes mellitus (DM) in the pathogenesis of HCC, independent of underlying chronic liver disease or cirrhosis. Moreover, the increased incidence of HCC corresponds to duration of DM, synergy between DM and other risk factors for HCC is apparent, and recurrence of HCC after resection or transplantation appears to be more common in patients with DM.[35,38–43] Hypothyroidism has a high prevalence in patients with NASH and has also been independently linked to HCC in a number of studies.[44–46]

Family aggregation of liver cancer has been reported but is difficult to verify given the coincident clustering of chronic HBV infection in families in most studies.[47,48] Despite this, a first-degree family history of HCC does appear to be a risk factor for HCC, independent of HBV and HCV infection, as demonstrated in America and European populations.[49] Hereditary hemochromatosis and alpha-1 antitrypsin deficiency lead to liver injury, often in concert with other factors such as HCV, and are associated with an increased risk of HCC.

PATHOLOGY

HCC can be classified into four types based on growth pattern: spreading, multifocal, encapsulated, and combined patterns.[50] The *spreading type* of HCC grows in nodular, pseudolobular,

or invasive patterns with poorly defined margins and develops in the setting of cirrhosis. It accounts for nearly 50% of cases in the United States. The *multifocal type* is characterized by the presence of multiple tumors of similar size. The hallmark of the *encapsulated type* is its tendency to compress rather than infiltrate surrounding liver tissue. It is the most common pattern in Asia and Africa but accounts for only 13% of cases in the United States. Combined patterns are seen in up to 25% of cases.

There are four histologic variants of HCC: cholangiocellular carcinoma (CCC), fibrolamellar hepatocellular carcinoma (FLHCC), clear cell HCC, and HCC with biliary differentiation. *CCC* shares features with cholangiocarcinoma and HCC. It occurs in the noncirrhotic liver and behaves more like a cholangiocarcinoma. It has a male predominance and is uniformly fatal. *FLHCC* is predominantly seen in the right hepatic lobe, accounts for 2% to 4% of HCCs, occurs equally in men and women, and typically occurs in adolescents and young adults without cirrhosis. It is characterized by the presence of fibrosis, arranged in a lamellar fashion, around HCC cells. FLHCC usually forms well-circumscribed large solitary lesions; alpha-fetoprotein (AFP) is frequently normal.[51] Imaging studies often reveal a heterogeneous mass with a central scar that may be confused with focal nodular hyperplasia (FNH). In comparison to classic HCC, FLHCC is more often resectable and is associated with a better survival. *Clear cell* HCC has a distinct histologic appearance and favorable prognosis. *HCC with biliary differentiation* has a rapid growth rate and decreased vascularity that renders it resistant to embolic therapy. The prognosis is poor.

IMAGING

Dual-phase (arterial and portal venous phases) or three-phase (arterial, portal venous, and delayed phases) imaging with dynamic intravenous contrast injection are invaluable for the detection and characterization of hepatocellular cancers. Moreover, arterial phase imaging allows delineation of vascular anatomy critical in patients who are candidates for transarterial chemoembolization (TACE), surgical resection, or liver transplantation. Computed tomography (CT) and magnetic resonance imaging (MRI) technologies are largely interchangeable in this regard although each has specific advantages. Advantages of CT include rapid image acquisition, wide availability, and high resolution.[52,53]

Recent advances in MRI technology and the development of newer contrast agents have enhanced the accuracy of liver MRI, which has now superseded CT as the most accurate noninvasive technique for HCC detection. Moreover, MRI does not involve exposure to ionizing radiation. MRI with extracellular or liver-specific contrast agents, such as superparamagnetic iron oxide (SPIO) particles or gadobenate dimeglumine, have been compared to CT imaging for HCC detection and are associated with similar or superior accuracy.[54–56] For example, Burrel and associates showed a per-lesion sensitivity of MRI of 76% versus 61% for CT. However, sensitivity of MRI for detection of small lesions is still low. In the same study, 100% of nodules greater than 2 cm were detected, compared to 84% for nodules between 1 and 2 cm, and 32% for nodules less than 1 cm.[55] The Food and Drug Administration (FDA) recently approved a liver-specific gadolinium contrast agent called gadolinium ethoxybenzyl diethylenetriamine penta-acetic acid (Gd-EOB-DTPA or gadoxetic acid disodium, Eovist [U.S.] or Primovist [Europe, Asia]) (Bayer

Healthcare) that is highly liver specific, with approximately 50% of the injected dose taken up by functioning hepatocytes and excreted in bile, compared with an uptake of 3% to 5% for gadobenate dimeglumine.[57–59] Results for detection of HCC using this agent are promising. Using both Gd-DTPA and SPIO, Bhartia and associates[60] demonstrated a sensitivity of 78%.

Additional information can be obtained using advanced MRI techniques including image subtraction, diffusion-weighted imaging (DWI), perfusion-weighted imaging (PWI), and magnetic resonance elastography (MRE). For example, DWI can detect tumor necrosis after TACE without the use of contrast media and DWI, PWI, and MRE can be used to identify background liver fibrosis and cirrhosis.[61–64]

▌ SEROLOGIC TESTS

Serum alpha-fetoprotein (AFP) is elevated in approximately 60% to 70% of cases of HCC in Caucasians and 80% to 90% of cases in Asians. AFP is normally produced by the fetal liver and yolk sac but falls to levels below 10 ng/mL in adult serum. A transient elevation of AFP level to 20 to 400 ng/mL may occur in the setting of hepatocyte regeneration, as in cirrhosis, active hepatitis, or partial hepatectomy. The positive predictive value of an AFP level of 400 ng/mL for HCC is over 95%, but normal AFP levels are not inconsistent with HCC if tumor burden is low. The lectin-reactive isoenzyme of AFP (AFP-L3) may be more sensitive than unfractionated AFP for the detection of HCC. Other markers such as gamma glutamyl transferase (GGT) isoenzymes, alkaline phosphatase, isoferritins, and monoclonal antibodies have not proven more useful than AFP.[65] Currently, the combination of serum AFP level and ultrasonography is the "gold standard" for HCC screening in high-risk populations.[66]

▌ STAGING

A variety of staging systems have been introduced in an effort to stratify patients based on prognosis and facilitate the selection of appropriate treatment strategies. At the time of a 2010 HCC consensus conference there were 18 internationally utilized staging systems.[67] None of the current systems is applicable to all patients and are all marked by geographic and disease stage performance variability. There are two general categories of staging systems: pathologic and clinical. Pathologic staging systems are directly applicable to patients undergoing transplantation or resection when pathologic assessment of the tumor is feasible. These include the Liver Cancer Study Group of Japan (LCSGJ) staging system, the Japanese Integrated Staging (JIS) score, the Chinese University Prognostic Index (CUPI), and the American Joint Committee on Cancer/International Union Against Cancer (AJCC/UICC) staging system. Clinical staging systems are useful for guiding the selection of therapies, particularly in patients with advanced disease, and include the Okuda staging system, the Cancer of the Liver Italian Program (CLIP) score, and the Barcelona Clinic Liver Cancer (BCLC) staging system.

Pathologic Staging Systems

The LCSGJ fourth edition was derived from analyses of 21,711 Japanese patients who underwent liver resection for HCC and follows the typical tumor-node-metastasis (TNM) schema common to most contemporary staging systems.[68] Tumor-specific factors considered include tumor number (solitary or multiple), size (<2 cm or >2 cm), and invasion of the portal vein, hepatic vein, or bile duct (present or not). Importantly, the presence of microvascular invasion, which has been demonstrated to have a prognostic power that outweighs that of lesion size, is not reflected in LCSGJ tumor score or overall stage.[51] The presence or absence of chronic liver disease is likewise not considered. Its applicability to the majority of patients with HCC who have cirrhosis is, therefore, limited.

The JIS score addresses this latter limitation by combining LCSGJ stage with Child-Pugh score.[69] Other limitations of the LCSGJ tumor scoring (most notably that microvascular invasion is not considered) remain. The first study of JIS score analyzed a cohort of 722 Japanese patients who underwent surgical or nonsurgical therapies for HCC; the findings were subsequently validated in a larger cohort of 4,525 patients.[69,70] This latter study has been criticized because no pathologic confirmation of HCC was performed in the majority of cases. It has, therefore, been suggested that many patients with dysplastic nodules rather than HCC were likely included in the group with small tumors and that the ability of JIS score to stratify patients has been exaggerated.

The CUPI was derived from data from 926 Chinese patients, a majority of whom received supportive care only.[71] It incorporated the fifth edition AJCC staging in combination with variables reflecting liver function (e.g., serum bilirubin and alkaline phosphatase level and the presence or absence of ascites). No advantage to the CUPI has been demonstrated in comparative studies of multiple staging systems.[72–74]

The AJCC/UICC staging system has recently been updated and is now in its seventh edition (Table 5.1). An advantage of AJCC/UICC is the use of central pathologic review. Tumor-related features considered include multifocality, size (in multifocal tumors only), and microscopic or major vascular invasion. Nodal and metastatic disease are characterized as present (N1, M1) or absent (N0, M0). Liver fibrosis and cirrhosis are graded and have prognostic significance within each T class. The staging system was based on outcomes from a cohort of patients in the East and West who underwent resection.[51,75] It has subsequently been validated in a cohort of Chinese patients, many of whom had HBV, and has likewise been shown to predict prognosis in patients undergoing liver transplantation.[76]

Clinical Staging Systems

The Okuda staging system was first introduced in 1985. Derived from data from 850 Japanese patients treated with surgical or nonsurgical therapies, the system stratifies patients based on four criteria: percent liver involvement by tumor (greater or less than 50% involved), ascites (present or absent), serum albumin (greater or less than 3 g/dL), and serum bilirubin (greater or less than 3 mg/dL).[77] The Okuda system is probably better for discriminating between patients with advanced disease than early disease. As is apparent from the criteria, patients with a range of tumors (i.e., all of those with tumors that involve less than 50% of the total liver volume) are grouped together, and, as a result, stratification of patients with lower tumor burden is suboptimal.

The CLIP score addresses some of the limitations of the Okuda system, adding additional tumor-related factors

Table 5.1

American Joint Committee on Cancer/International Union Against Cancer (AJCC/UICC) Staging System, Seventh Edition

	T classification		Stage
T1	Solitary with no vascular invasion	I	T1N0M0
T2	Solitary with vascular invasion or multifocal ≤5 cm	II	T2NoMo
T3a	Multiple tumors >5 cm	IIIA	T3aN0M0
T3b	Single tumor or multiple tumors of any size involving a major branch of the portal vein or hepatic vein	IIIB	T3bN0M0
T4	Invasion of adjacent organs (excluding the gallbladder) or perforation of visceral peritoneum	IIIC	T4N0M0
		IVA	Any T N1MN0
		IVB	Any T Any N M1

Data from Edge SB, Byrd DR, Compton CC, et al., eds. *AJCC Cancer Staging Manual.* 7th ed. New York, New York: Springer, 2010.

(e.g., solitary vs. multifocal and the presence or absence of portal vein thrombosis) as well as serum AFP level and stratifies patients into seven groups (Table 5.2).[78] The CLIP score has been validated in patients with a range of disease burden and outperformed Okuda in comparative studies.[78–80]

The BCLC staging system bears special emphasis because it has been validated as a prognostic tool in a variety of settings and is linked to a frequently referenced treatment algorithm widely utilized in clinical trial design.[81–83] The BCLC staging system incorporates liver function (Child-Pugh score), tumor characteristics (the number and size of nodules, the presence or absence of vascular invasion, and the presence or absence of extrahepatic spread), and, unlike any of the other clinical staging systems, performance status (Table 5.3).[84]

It is important to note that the BCLC treatment algorithm is based on a single institution experience. Moreover, it is fairly conservative with regard to the application of surgical therapy. Patients with larger singular tumors are not considered surgical candidates despite a growing experience with resection with acceptable outcomes in this group. Likewise, patient with multifocal disease that falls outside the Milan criteria and associated conditions who may benefit from resection or transplantation are excluded from these therapies.

Conspicuously absent from the BCLC staging system as well as all other current staging systems is the inclusion of molecular markers of disease biology. Work to establish such markers remains in a formative stage but some promising data have emerged. For example, Jonas and associates[85] reported that increased tumor DNA aneuploidy, expressed as an index, is a more powerful prognostic indicator than tumor size, Milan Criteria, or vascular invasion in cirrhotic patients with HCC following liver transplantation. Poon and associates[86] reported that pretreatment serum vascular endothelial growth factor (VEGF) levels independently predict overall and recurrence-free survival following radiofrequency ablation. Kaseb and associates[87] demonstrated a correlation between plasma IGF-1 levels and survival in patients with advanced HCC. Further advances in molecular approaches are expected to decrease the marked heterogeneity noted in current staging systems available. With these refinements, the more selective and scientific application of current therapies may be possible.

Table 5.2

Cancer of the Liver Italian Program (CLIP) Score

Variable	Point		
	0	1	2
Child-Pugh grade	A	B	C
Tumor morphology	Solitary and ≤50%	Multifocal and ≤50%	Massive or >50%
Serum ≤alpha-fetoprotein	<400 ng/mL	≥400 ng/dL	
Portal vein thrombosis	Absent	Present	

Data from A new prognostic system for hepatocellular carcinoma: a retrospective study of 435 patients: the Cancer of the Liver Italian Program (CLIP) investigators. *Hepatology.* 1998;28(3):751–755.

Table 5.3

Barcelona Clinic Liver Cancer (BCLC) Staging System

Stage	Performance status (PST)	Tumor extent	Liver disease	Therapy
A (early)	0	Solitary <5 cm		
A1			No portal hypertension	Resection
A2			Portal hypertension, normal bilirubin	
A3			Portal hypertension, abnormal bilirubin	Transplantation, radiofrequency ablation or ethanol injection
A4		Multifocal ≤3 and <3 cm	Child-Pugh A-B	
B (intermediate)		Multifocal >3 or ≥3 cm		Transarterial embolization
C (advanced)	1–2	Vascular invasion or extrahepatic spread		Investigational therapy
D (terminal)	3–4	Any	Child-Pugh C	Supportive care

Data from Llovet JM, Bru C, Bruix J. Prognosis of hepatocellular carcinoma: the BCLC staging classification. *Semin Liver Dis.* 1999;19:329–338.

MEDICAL THERAPY FOR HEPATOCELLULAR CARCINOMA

A discussion of the spectrum of local-regional therapies for HCC is beyond the scope of this chapter and these approaches are discussed in detail elsewhere in this volume. Unfortunately, a majority of patients with HCC present with advanced disease often coincident with advanced chronic liver disease. Few local-regional therapies are available to these patients. For this reason, increasing attention has been directed at the development of systemic therapies. In the past, the use of cytotoxic chemotherapy in HCC was associated with disappointing results. Progress in the elucidation of mechanisms of hepatocarcinogenesis and promising results with sorafenib have prompted interest in other targeted therapies and combination regimens.

Sorafenib is a polyvalent molecule that inhibits the serine-threonine kinase Raf-1 and tyrosine kinases including vascular endothelial growth factor receptor (VEGFR) 2, platelet-derived growth factor receptor (PDGFR), FLT3, Ret, and c-Kit. Two phase III studies, the SHARP trial and the Asia-Pacific trial, have compared sorafenib therapy with placebo in patients with advanced disease.[88,89] A modest survival advantage was demonstrated in both trials (median survival 10.7 months vs. 7.9 months in SHARP and 6.5 months vs. 4.2 months in Asia-Pacific). Building on this experience, a number of recent and ongoing trials are investigating combining multiple targeted agents or combinations of targeted and conventional cytotoxic therapeutics.[90,91]

REFERENCES

1. Parkin DM, Bray F, Ferlay J, et al. Estimating the world cancer burden: Globocan 2000. *Int J Cancer* 2001;94:153–156.
2. Thomas MB, Zhu AX. Hepatocellular carcinoma: the need for progress. *J Clin Oncol* 2005;23:2892–2899.
3. McGlynn KA, London WT. Epidemiology and natural history of hepatocellular carcinoma. *Best Pract Res Clin Gastroenterol* 2005;19:3–23.
4. Altekruse SF, McGlynn KA, Reichman ME. Hepatocellular carcinoma incidence, mortality, and survival trends in the United States from 1975 to 2005. *J Clin Oncol* 2009;27:1485–1491.
5. Taylor-Robinson SD, Foster GR, Arora S, et al. Increase in primary liver cancer in the UK, 1979–94. *Lancet* 1997;350:1142–1143.
6. Deuffic S, Poynard T, Buffat L, et al. Trends in primary liver cancer. *Lancet* 1998;351:214–215.
7. Smart RG, Mann RE, Suurvali H. Changes in liver cirrhosis death rates in different countries in relation to per capita alcohol consumption and Alcoholics Anonymous membership. *J Stud Alcohol* 1998;59:245–249.
8. Wong JB, McQuillan GM, McHutchison JG, et al. Estimating future hepatitis C morbidity, mortality, and costs in the United States. *Am J Public Health* 2000;90:1562–1569.
9. El-Serag HB, Davila JA, Petersen NJ, et al. The continuing increase in the incidence of hepatocellular carcinoma in the United States: an update. *Ann Intern Med* 2003;139:817–823.
10. El-Serag HB, Mason AC. Rising incidence of hepatocellular carcinoma in the United States. *N Engl J Med* 1999;340:745–750.
11. Ruhl CE, Everhart JE. Epidemiology of nonalcoholic fatty liver. *Clin Liver Dis* 2004;8:501–519, vii.
12. McCullough AJ. The clinical features, diagnosis and natural history of nonalcoholic fatty liver disease. *Clin Liver Dis* 2004;8:521–533, viii.
13. Parkin DM, Bray FI, Devesa SS. Cancer burden in the year 2000. The global picture. *Eur J Cancer* 2001;37(suppl 8):S4–66.
14. Parkin DM, Bray F, Ferlay J, et al. Global cancer statistics, 2002. *CA Cancer J Clin* 2005;55:74–108.
15. El-Serag HB, Rudolph KL. Hepatocellular carcinoma: epidemiology and molecular carcinogenesis. *Gastroenterology* 2007;132:2557–2576.
16. Shen FM, Lee MK, Gong HM, et al. Complex segregation analysis of primary hepatocellular carcinoma in Chinese families: interaction of inherited susceptibility and hepatitis B viral infection. *Am J Hum Genet* 1991;49:88–93.
17. Alter MJ, Kruszon-Moran D, Nainan OV, et al. The prevalence of hepatitis C virus infection in the United States, 1988 through 1994. *N Engl J Med* 1999;341:556–562.
18. Yoshizawa H. Hepatocellular carcinoma associated with hepatitis C virus infection in Japan: projection to other countries in the foreseeable future. *Oncology* 2002;62(suppl 1):8–17.
19. Freeman AJ, Dore GJ, Law MG, et al. Estimating progression to cirrhosis in chronic hepatitis C virus infection. *Hepatology* 2001;34:809–816.
20. Simmonds P. Variability of hepatitis C virus genome. *Curr Stud Hematol Blood Transfus* 1994;12–35.
21. Dusheiko G, Schmilovitz-Weiss H, Brown D, et al. Hepatitis C virus genotypes: an investigation of type-specific differences in geographic origin and disease. *Hepatology* 1994;19:13–18.

22. Nousbaum JB, Pol S, Nalpas B, et al. Hepatitis C virus type 1b (II) infection in France and Italy. Collaborative Study Group. *Ann Intern Med* 1995;122:161–168.

23. Silini E, Bono F, Cividini A, et al. Differential distribution of hepatitis C virus genotypes in patients with and without liver function abnormalities. *Hepatology* 1995;21:285–290.

24. Batey RG, Burns T, Benson RJ, et al. Alcohol consumption and the risk of cirrhosis. *Med J Aust* 1992;156:413–416.

25. Sorensen HT, Friis S, Olsen JH, et al. Risk of liver and other types of cancer in patients with cirrhosis: a nationwide cohort study in Denmark. *Hepatology* 1998;28:921–925.

26. Di Bisceglie AM, Rustgi VK, Hoofnagle JH, et al. NIH conference. Hepatocellular carcinoma. *Ann Intern Med* 1988;108:390–401.

27. Paronetto F. Immunologic reactions in alcoholic liver disease. *Semin Liver Dis* 1993;13:183–195.

28. Gandini S, Botteri E, Iodice S, et al. Tobacco smoking and cancer: a meta-analysis. *Int J Cancer* 2008;122:155–164.

29. Franceschi S, Montella M, Polesel J, et al. Hepatitis viruses, alcohol, and tobacco in the etiology of hepatocellular carcinoma in Italy. *Cancer Epidemiol Biomarkers Prev* 2006;15:683–689.

30. Mori M, Hara M, Wada I, et al. Prospective study of hepatitis B and C viral infections, cigarette smoking, alcohol consumption, and other factors associated with hepatocellular carcinoma risk in Japan. *Am J Epidemiol* 2000;151:131–139.

31. Maheshwari S, Sarraj A, Kramer J, et al. Oral contraception and the risk of hepatocellular carcinoma. *J Hepatol* 2007;47:506–513.

32. Persson I, Yuen J, Bergkvist L, et al. Cancer incidence and mortality in women receiving estrogen and estrogen-progestin replacement therapy—long-term follow-up of a Swedish cohort. *Int J Cancer* 1996;67:327–332.

33. Fernandez E, Gallus S, Bosetti C, et al. Hormone replacement therapy and cancer risk: a systematic analysis from a network of case-control studies. *Int J Cancer* 2003;105:408–412.

34. Ueno Y. The toxicology of mycotoxins. *Crit Rev Toxicol* 1985;14:99–132.

35. Tolman KG, Fonseca V, Tan MH, et al. Narrative review: hepatobiliary disease in type 2 diabetes mellitus. *Ann Intern Med* 2004;141:946–956.

36. Reddy JK, Rao MS. Lipid metabolism and liver inflammation. II. Fatty liver disease and fatty acid oxidation. *Am J Physiol Gastrointest Liver Physiol* 2006;290:G852–858.

37. Larsson SC, Wolk A. Overweight, obesity and risk of liver cancer: a meta-analysis of cohort studies. *Br J Cancer* 2007;97:1005–1008.

38. El-Serag HB, Hampel H, Javadi F. The association between diabetes and hepatocellular carcinoma: a systematic review of epidemiologic evidence. *Clin Gastroenterol Hepatol* 2006;4:369–380.

39. Bell DS, Allbright E. The multifaceted associations of hepatobiliary disease and diabetes. *Endocr Pract.* 2007;13:300–312.

40. Davila JA, Morgan RO, Shaib Y, et al. Diabetes increases the risk of hepatocellular carcinoma in the United States: a population based case control study. *Gut* 2005;54:533–539.

41. Veldt BJ, Chen W, Heathcote EJ, et al. Increased risk of hepatocellular carcinoma among patients with hepatitis C cirrhosis and diabetes mellitus. *Hepatology* 2008;47:1856–1862.

42. Yuan JM, Govindarajan S, Arakawa K, et al. Synergism of alcohol, diabetes, and viral hepatitis on the risk of hepatocellular carcinoma in blacks and whites in the U.S. *Cancer* 2004;101:1009–1017.

43. Komura T, Mizukoshi E, Kita Y, et al. Impact of diabetes on recurrence of hepatocellular carcinoma after surgical treatment in patients with viral hepatitis. *Am J Gastroenterol* 2007;102:1939–1946.

44. Liangpunsakul S, Chalasani N. Is hypothyroidism a risk factor for nonalcoholic steatohepatitis? *J Clin Gastroenterol* 2003;37:340–343.

45. Reddy A, Dash C, Leerapun A, et al. Hypothyroidism: a possible risk factor for liver cancer in patients with no known underlying cause of liver disease. *Clin Gastroenterol Hepatol* 2007;5:118–123.

46. Hassan MM, Kaseb A, Li D, et al. Association between hypothyroidism and hepatocellular carcinoma: a case-control study in the United States. *Hepatology* 2009;49:1563–1570.

47. Cai RL, Meng W, Lu HY, et al. Segregation analysis of hepatocellular carcinoma in a moderately high-incidence area of East China. *World J Gastroenterol* 2003;9:2428–2432.

48. Yu MW, Chang HC, Liaw YF, et al. Familial risk of hepatocellular carcinoma among chronic hepatitis B carriers and their relatives. *J Natl Cancer Inst* 2000;92:1159–1164.

49. Donato F, Gelatti U, Chiesa R, et al. A case-control study on family history of liver cancer as a risk factor for hepatocellular carcinoma in North Italy. Brescia HCC Study. *Cancer Causes Control* 1999;10:417–421.

50. Fong Y, Sun RL, Jarnagin W, et al. An analysis of 412 cases of hepatocellular carcinoma at a Western center. *Ann Surg* 1999;229:790–799; discussion 799–800.

51. Vauthey JN, Lauwers GY, Esnaola NF, et al. Simplified staging for hepatocellular carcinoma. *J Clin Oncol* 2002;20:1527–1536.

52. Iannaccone R, Laghi A, Catalano C, et al. Hepatocellular carcinoma: role of unenhanced and delayed phase multi-detector row helical CT in patients with cirrhosis. *Radiology* 2005;234:460–467.

53. Laghi A, Iannaccone R, Rossi P, et al. Hepatocellular carcinoma: detection with triple-phase multi-detector row helical CT in patients with chronic hepatitis. *Radiology* 2003;226:543–549.

54. Rode A, Bancel B, Douek P, et al. Small nodule detection in cirrhotic livers: evaluation with US, spiral CT, and MRI and correlation with pathologic examination of explanted liver. *J Comput Assist Tomogr* 2001;25:327–336.

55. Burrel M, Llovet JM, Ayuso C, et al. MRI angiography is superior to helical CT for detection of HCC prior to liver transplantation: an explant correlation. *Hepatology* 2003;38:1034–1042.

56. Kim HJ, Kim KW, Byun JH, et al. Comparison of mangafodipir trisodium- and ferucarbotran-enhanced MRI for detection and characterization of hepatic metastases in colorectal cancer patients. *AJR Am J Roentgenol* 2006;186:1059–1066.

57. Frericks BB, Loddenkemper C, Huppertz A, et al. Qualitative and quantitative evaluation of hepatocellular carcinoma and cirrhotic liver enhancement using Gd-EOB-DTPA. *AJR Am J Roentgenol* 2009;193:1053–1060.

58. Hammerstingl R, Huppertz A, Breuer J, et al. Diagnostic efficacy of gadoxetic acid (Primovist)-enhanced MRI and spiral CT for a therapeutic strategy: comparison with intraoperative and histopathologic findings in focal liver lesions. *Eur Radiol* 2008;18:457–467.

59. Jung G, Breuer J, Poll LW, et al. Imaging characteristics of hepatocellular carcinoma using the hepatobiliary contrast agent Gd-EOB-DTPA. *Acta Radiol* 2006;47:15–23.

60. Bhartia B, Ward J, Guthrie JA, et al. Hepatocellular carcinoma in cirrhotic livers: double-contrast thin-section MR imaging with pathologic correlation of explanted tissue. *AJR Am J Roentgenol* 2003;180:577–584.

61. Lee VS, Hecht EM, Taouli B, et al. Body and cardiovascular MR imaging at 3.0 T. *Radiology* 2007;244:692–705.

62. Mannelli L, Kim S, Hajdu CH, et al. Assessment of tumor necrosis of hepatocellular carcinoma after chemoembolization: diffusion-weighted and contrast-enhanced MRI with histopathologic correlation of the explanted liver. *AJR Am J Roentgenol* 2009;193:1044–1052.

63. Huwart L, Sempoux C, Vicaut E, et al. Magnetic resonance elastography for the noninvasive staging of liver fibrosis. *Gastroenterology* 2008;135:32–40.

64. Hagiwara M, Rusinek H, Lee VS, et al. Advanced liver fibrosis: diagnosis with 3D whole-liver perfusion MR imaging—initial experience. *Radiology* 2008;246:926–934.

65. Sutton FM, Russell NC, Guinee VF, et al. Factors affecting the prognosis of primary liver carcinoma. *J Clin Oncol* 1988;6:321–328.

66. Pateron D, Ganne N, Trinchet JC, et al. Prospective study of screening for hepatocellular carcinoma in Caucasian patients with cirrhosis. *J Hepatol* 1994;20:65–71.

67. Vauthey JN, Dixon E, Abdalla EK, et al. Pretreatment assessment of hepatocellular carcinoma: expert consensus statement. *HPB (Oxford)*; 2010;12:289–299.

68. Makuuchi M, Belghiti J, Belli G, et al. IHPBA concordant classification of primary liver cancer: working group report. *J Hepatobiliary Pancreat Surg* 2003;10:26–30.

69. Kudo M, Chung H, Osaki Y. Prognostic staging system for hepatocellular carcinoma (CLIP score): its value and limitations, and a proposal for a new staging system, the Japan Integrated Staging Score (JIS score). *J Gastroenterol* 2003;38:207–215.

70. Kudo M, Chung H, Haji S, et al. Validation of a new prognostic staging system for hepatocellular carcinoma: the JIS score compared with the CLIP score. *Hepatology* 2004;40:1396–1405.

71. Leung TW, Tang AM, Zee B, et al. Construction of the Chinese University Prognostic Index for hepatocellular carcinoma and comparison with the TNM staging system, the Okuda staging system, and the Cancer of the Liver Italian Program staging system: a study based on 926 patients. *Cancer* 2002;94:1760–1769.

72. Georgiades CS, Liapi E, Frangakis C, et al. Prognostic accuracy of 12 liver staging systems in patients with unresectable hepatocellular carcinoma treated with transarterial chemoembolization. *J Vasc Interv Radiol* 2006;17:1619–1624.

73. Chen TW, Chu CM, Yu JC, et al. Comparison of clinical staging systems in predicting survival of hepatocellular carcinoma patients receiving major or minor hepatectomy. *Eur J Surg Oncol* 2007;33:480–487.

74. Kondo K, Chijiiwa K, Nagano M, et al. Comparison of seven prognostic staging systems in patients who undergo hepatectomy for hepatocellular carcinoma. *Hepatogastroenterology* 2007;54:1534–1538.

75. Poon RT, Fan ST. Evaluation of the new AJCC/UICC staging system for hepatocellular carcinoma after hepatic resection in Chinese patients. *Surg Oncol Clin N Am* 2003;12:35–50, viii.

76. Vauthey JN, Ribero D, Abdalla EK, et al. Outcomes of liver transplantation in 490 patients with hepatocellular carcinoma: validation of a uniform staging after surgical treatment. *J Am Coll Surg* 2007;204:1016–1027; discussion 1027–1018.

77. Okuda K, Ohtsuki T, Obata H, et al. Natural history of hepatocellular carcinoma and prognosis in relation to treatment. Study of 850 patients. *Cancer* 1985;56:918–928.

78. A new prognostic system for hepatocellular carcinoma: a retrospective study of 435 patients: the Cancer of the Liver Italian Program (CLIP) investigators. *Hepatology* 1998;28:751–755.

79. Ueno S, Tanabe G, Sako K, et al. Discrimination value of the new western prognostic system (CLIP score) for hepatocellular carcinoma in 662 Japanese patients. Cancer of the Liver Italian Program. *Hepatology* 2001;34:529–534.

80. Levy I, Sherman M. Staging of hepatocellular carcinoma: assessment of the CLIP, Okuda, and Child-Pugh staging systems in a cohort of 257 patients in Toronto. *Gut* 2002;50:881–885.

81. Marrero JA, Fontana RJ, Barrat A, et al. Prognosis of hepatocellular carcinoma: comparison of 7 staging systems in an American cohort. *Hepatology* 2005;41:707–716.

82. Cillo U, Vitale A, Grigoletto F, et al. Prospective validation of the Barcelona Clinic Liver Cancer staging system. *J Hepatol* 2006;44:723–731.

83. Guglielmi A, Ruzzenente A, Pachera S, et al. Comparison of seven staging systems in cirrhotic patients with hepatocellular carcinoma in a cohort of patients who underwent radiofrequency ablation with complete response. *Am J Gastroenterol* 2008;103:597–604.

84. Llovet JM, Bru C, Bruix J. Prognosis of hepatocellular carcinoma: the BCLC staging classification. *Semin Liver Dis* 1999;19:329–338.

85. Jonas S, Al-Abadi H, Benckert C, et al. Prognostic significance of the DNA-index in liver transplantation for hepatocellular carcinoma in cirrhosis. *Ann Surg* 2009;250:1008–1013.

86. Poon RT, Lau C, Pang R, et al. High serum vascular endothelial growth factor levels predict poor prognosis after radiofrequency ablation of hepatocellular carcinoma: importance of tumor biomarker in ablative therapies. *Ann Surg Oncol* 2007;14:1835–1845.

87. Kaseb AO, Abbruzzese JL, Vauthey JN, et al. I-CLIP: Improved Stratification of Advanced Hepatocellular Carcinoma Patients by Integrating Plasma IGF-1 into CLIP Score. *Oncology* 2011;80:373–381.

88. Llovet JM, Ricci S, Mazzaferro V, et al. Sorafenib in advanced hepatocellular carcinoma. *N Engl J Med* 2008;359:378–390.

89. Cheng AL, Kang YK, Chen Z, et al. Efficacy and safety of sorafenib in patients in the Asia-Pacific region with advanced hepatocellular carcinoma: a phase III randomised, double-blind, placebo-controlled trial. *Lancet Oncol* 2009;10:25–34.

90. Thomas MB, Morris JS, Chadha R, et al. Phase II trial of the combination of bevacizumab and erlotinib in patients who have advanced hepatocellular carcinoma. *J Clin Oncol* 2009;27:843–850.

91. Zhu AX, Blaszkowsky LS, Ryan DP, et al. Phase II study of gemcitabine and oxaliplatin in combination with bevacizumab in patients with advanced hepatocellular carcinoma. *J Clin Oncol* 2006;24:1898–1903.

JANIVETTE ALSINA and TIMOTHY M. PAWLIK

CHAPTER 6

Surgical Management of Hepatocellular Carcinoma: Resection and Transplantation

INTRODUCTION

Hepatocellular carcinoma (HCC) is the third-leading cause of cancer-related deaths worldwide. The number of new cases has risen from 626,000 reported cases in 2002 to an estimated 748,000 new cases in 2008, making HCC the seventh most common cancer in the world. Overall 5-year survival for patients diagnosed with HCC can be as low as 5% depending on the stage of disease, prognostic factors, and whether the patient undergoes surgical treatment.[1,2] For patients who undergo potentially curative therapies including surgical resection, transplantation, and ablation, 5-year survival can range between 40% and 75%,[3] highlighting the need for accurate diagnosis and optimal treatment in this patient population.

The management approach to HCC is unique from other cancers in that both the tumor extent and the underlying hepatic reserve must be taken into consideration to select the best treatment strategy. This is because most patients with HCC present with end-stage liver disease.[4] Depending on a combination of factors that include tumor burden, baseline liver function, and the overall physiologic status of the patient, choices for complementary treatments include liver resection, liver transplantation, and the use of locoregional treatment options, such as radiofrequency ablation (RFA) and transcatheter arterial chemoembolization (TACE).

EPIDEMIOLOGY

A greater incidence in HCC has been noted in males and in patients from developing countries. The geographic variation is related in part to differences in the prevalence of risk factors for the development of HCC, namely hepatitis B and C infections, which are more common in Asia and in sub-Saharan Africa.[5,6] In fact, almost 80% of HCC cases in these regions are related to chronic hepatitis B virus (HBV) and hepatitis C virus (HCV) infections, which are more common than in the West.[7] These patients have a higher likelihood of developing HCC in the absence of cirrhosis[8] and are more likely to present at an earlier age probably because of the higher rates of HBV infection during childhood. For those patients with chronic hepatitis infection, the risk of developing HCC is 30 times higher among patients with chronic hepatitis B infection and 130 times higher for those coinfected with HBV and HCV.[9] Of note, among patients with chronic HBV, persistently high viral loads ($>1 \times 10^5$ copies/mL) are predictive of development of both cirrhosis, HCC, and of death from HCC.[10] In developed countries the most common risk factors for HCC are chronic hepatitis C infection, alcoholic liver disease, and nonalcoholic fatty liver disease (NAFLD). Of note, one in five patients diagnosed with HCC in the United States do not have an identifiable etiology.[6]

SURVEILLANCE

Regardless of the etiologic factors leading to the development of chronic liver disease, the most important risk factor associated with the development of HCC is the presence of cirrhosis. Once the diagnosis of cirrhosis is made the annual risk of developing HCC is approximately 1% to 8%.[11,12] Despite the use of surveillance strategies for high-risk groups, a significant number of patients with HCC present with advanced disease. Symptoms on presentation can include abdominal pain, weight loss, ascites, a palpable abdominal mass, and, sometimes, jaundice. Given the strong link between chronic HBV and HCV infection and the development of HCC, guidelines for surveillance have been proposed for patients considered to be at high risk (Table 6.1). Current recommendations include the use of liver ultrasound and alpha-fetoprotein (AFP) measurements every 6 months for hepatitis B carriers and for patients with known cirrhosis regardless of etiology.[13] Liver ultrasound has a reported 65% to 80% sensitivity and a 90% specificity for the detection of HCC lesions, whereas measurement of AFP levels is less sensitive (~60%) and less specific than ultrasound.[14] The finding of a liver mass in the context of cirrhosis should prompt evaluation of AFP levels, which are found to be elevated in 50% to 90% of HCC cases.[9]

Other testing, such as contrast-enhanced computed tomography (CT) or liver magnetic resonance imaging (MRI) is often used for surveillance as well as to obtain more detailed morphologic and anatomic information regarding lesions identified on ultrasonography. The size of the lesion is a useful parameter in deciding whether to pursue further diagnostic workup. Lesions smaller than 1 cm have a low likelihood of being HCC

Table 6.2
Child-Pugh Turcotte Classification System

Parameter	1 point	2 points	3 points
Albumin (g/dL)	>3.5	3.5–2.8	<2.8
Bilirubin (mg/dL)	<2.0	2.0–3.0	>3.0
INR	<1.7	1.7–2.3	>2.3
Ascites	Absent	Slight	Moderate
Hepatic encephalopathy	Absent	Mild (grade 1.0–2.0)	Chronic (grade 3–4)

Class A = 5–6 points, Class B = 7–9 points, Class C = 10–15 points.

and current recommendations are to offer surveillance every 3 months. This intensive surveillance should be continued for 18 to 24 months to rule out the possibility of a small, slow-growing HCC. Liver lesions greater than 1 cm with radiologic features characteristic of HCC (hypervascular on arterial phase with washout on venous delays) and AFP levels greater than 200 ng/mL do not require biopsy to confirm the diagnosis.[9] These patients should be referred for evaluation by a multidisciplinary team for potentially curative intervention.

In cases where the diagnosis is uncertain with inconclusive imaging, no underlying liver disease, and normal AFP levels, a percutaneous liver biopsy can be obtained to establish diagnosis.[6,15] It is important to point out that biopsy of small (<2 cm) lesions may be limited by both technical difficulties and the inability to discern between well-differentiated HCC and normal hepatocytes. There is no indication for a percutaneous biopsy in patients with lesions that have typical HCC characteristics on imaging (CT or MRI) and this practice should be discouraged because it can lead to complications, such as bleeding and, in rare cases, tumor seeding along the biopsy tract.[16]

FACTORS PREDICTIVE OF OUTCOME IN HEPATOCELLULAR CARCINOMA

Both intrinsic patient-related factors and tumor-related factors have an effect in the selection of management strategies and, ultimately, outcomes after treatment. Patient factors include any medical comorbidities that may preclude aggressive treatment given the high risk of complications. Additionally, the degree of baseline liver dysfunction determines the selection of management strategies. To better risk-stratify those patients at higher risk for liver dysfunction, multiple scoring systems have been developed. These include the Child-Pugh score, the Model for End-Stage Liver Disease (MELD) score, and the Ishak fibrosis score.

The Child-Pugh system (Table 6.2) provides an estimate of the liver's metabolic capacity by taking into account signs of liver failure (degree of ascites, presence of encephalopathy), levels of bilirubin, albumin, and the prothrombin time (or international normalized ratio [INR]) in patients with cirrhosis. The patients are risk-stratified into categories that range from compensated cirrhosis (class A) to decompensated cirrhosis (class B and C). The mortality caused by liver disease increases from 0% to 20% to 55% in patients with Child-Pugh class A, B, or C cirrhosis, respectively.[17] Resection, therefore, is most often reserved for only Child-Pugh class A patients. Given the increased risk in Child-Pugh B and C patients, most patients in these categories will not be candidates for resection but instead may be treated with nonresectional approaches including ablation and transplantation for patients who meet transplantation criteria (Table 6.3).

Another system for estimating the hepatic reserve is the MELD score, which uses three preoperative tests (INR, serum creatinine, and total serum bilirubin) to prognosticate outcomes in patients with cirrhosis. Although most often utilized to stratify the risk of death on the transplantation wait list, MELD can also be helpful to stratify risk of liver failure following hepatic resection. The use of MELD to quantitate perioperative risk of liver resection has been validated in liver resection studies and found to predict morbidity and mortality after HCC resection as well as long-term survival.[18,19] Specifically, for patients who undergo liver resection who have known cirrhosis and a MELD score greater than 9, the complication rate rises to 29% compared to 0% for patients with a MELD score that is less than 8.

Besides patient- and liver-related factors, tumor-related factors correlate with outcome following resection. Factors include overall tumor burden, tumor multifocality, and the presence of vascular invasion.[20,21] Some of these variables have been incorporated into various staging systems that aim to stratify patients into categories to both better predict prognosis and provide treatment guidelines.

Table 6.3
Milan Criteria for Liver Transplantation

Single lesion ≤5 cm, or

2–3 lesions none exceeding 3 cm, and

No vascular invasion and/or extrahepatic spread

Data from Mazzaferro V, Regalia E, Doci R, et al. Liver transplantation for the treatment of small hepatocellular carcinomas in patients with cirrhosis. *N Engl J Med* 1996;334:693–699.

STAGING

There are over 10 staging and scoring systems for HCC that have been developed and are in use worldwide. No single system accurately predicts the outcomes for all patients and this has prevented the acceptance and implementation of a universal staging system. Historically, staging approaches for HCC have included pathologic staging systems (AJCC, TNM/UICC), clinical systems (Okuda, CLIP), and transplant staging systems (University of California, San Francisco [UCSF] extended criteria, UNOS modified tumore-node-metastasis [TNM] staging system). The pathologic staging systems depend on removal of the primary tumor because these systems take into account the pathologic tumor characteristics. Many scoring systems take into account both pathologic data and clinical information in attempts to better risk-stratify patients.

Examples of pathologic systems include the Liver Cancer Study Group of Japan (LCSGJ), the Chinese University Prognostic Index (CUPI), and the American Joint Committee on Cancer/International Union Against Cancer (AJCC/UICC) system. The LCSGJ is a standard TNM system that aggregates vascular invasion, number of lesions, as well as size of the tumors in the T category.[22] This system does not take into account the underlying liver function and its accuracy has been questioned. The Japanese Integrated Staging Score (JIS) integrates the LCSGJ with the Child-Pugh system to address this deficiency. This system has been validated in Japan in terms of prognostic predictive power and stratification ability and has been proposed as a better prognostic model.[23]

First proposed in 1985, the Okuda staging system was the first system to include both tumor parameters and liver function parameters.[24] Scoring takes into account tumor burden greater than 50% of the liver, presence of ascites, hyperbilirubinemia (>3 mg/dL), and serum albumin levels (<3 g/dL). Given the number of tumor-related factors that are not taken into account in this system (vascular involvement, number of tumors, and total tumor volume) the Okuda system is outdated and more contemporary systems, such as the Cancer of the Liver Italian Program (CLIP) system, have replaced it.

The CLIP score was derived from a retrospective analysis and it incorporates tumor morphology, presence of portal vein thrombosis, levels of AFP, and Child-Pugh score.[25,26] The CLIP score has been reported to provide more accurate prognostic information than the Okuda system and better stratifies patients with advanced disease.[27] The ability of the CLIP system to risk-stratify patients with smaller tumors has, however, been questioned given its tumor burden cutoff of 50%.

Originally developed from a series of patients undergoing surgical resection of HCC, the Barcelona Clinic Liver Cancer (BCLC) system incorporates multiple patient and tumor parameters and two classification systems. The parameters include: performance status, uni- or multifocality of the tumor, the presence of vascular invasion, or portal hypertension. The staging systems incorporated are the Okuda stage and Child-Pugh classification.[28] The proponents of this staging system expanded it to include an algorithm for treatments based on each stage. This system has been validated with respect to its prognostic ability in multiple studies when compared to the Okuda system, CLIP, JIS, and the AJCC 6th edition,[29] but its recommendations for treatment options based on staging remain controversial.

The AJCC/UICC, 7th edition staging system was developed from a large patient cohort that underwent liver resection and is recommended as a better prognostic system, in particular for patients with early HCC and those with resected/transplanted disease (Table 6.4).[2,30] An expert consensus conference in 2003 suggested that no single system fulfilled all the requirements for accurately predicting outcomes in patients with HCC. The recommendation from this conference was that the CLIP staging system be used for prognosis and to guide treatment in patients with advanced HCC or liver disease.[31] This recommendation was recently updated[4] to include the use of the BCLC system as appropriate for the evaluation of medical patients with advanced liver disease who are not candidates for surgical intervention. For patients who qualify for surgical resection or transplantation, the AJCC/UICC system is favored.

Table 6.4

AJCC 7th Edition TNM Staging System for HCC

Primary tumor (T)

TX Primary tumor cannot be assessed

T0 No evidence of primary tumor

T1 Solitary tumor without vascular invasion

T2 Solitary tumor with vascular invasion or multiple tumors none more than 5 cm

T3a Multiple tumors more than 5 cm

T3b Single tumor or multiple tumors of any size involving a major branch of the portal vein or hepatic vein

T4 Tumor(s) with direct invasion of adjacent organs other than the gallbladder or with perforation of visceral peritoneum

Regional lymph nodes (N)

NX Regional lymph nodes cannot be assessed

N0 No regional lymph node metastasis

N1 Regional lymph node metastasis

Distant metastasis (M)

M0 No distant metastasis

M1 Distant metastasis

Fibrosis score (F)*

F0 Fibrosis score 0–4 (none to moderate fibrosis)

F1 Fibrosis score 5–6 (severe fibrosis or cirrhosis)

Anatomic stage/prognostic groups

Stage I T1 N0 M0

Stage II T2 N0 M0

Stage IIIA T3a N0 M0

Stage IIIB T3b N0 M0

Stage IIIC T4 N0 M0

Stage IVA Any T N1 M0

Stage IVB Any T Any N M1

*Fibrosis score.

Reprinted with permission from Edge SB, Byrd DR, Compton CC, et al, eds. *AJCC Cancer Staging Manual.* 7th ed. New York, NY: Springer; 2010.

PATIENT EVALUATION: PRETREATMENT IMAGING

Most HCCs develop in the setting of chronic liver disease with possible alterations in AFP levels and liver function tests, such as the total bilirubin. Some of these lesions are discovered during surveillance ultrasound in high-risk patients but most are detected during routine imaging. The use of multidetector row computer tomography (MDCT) and MRI are critical in characterizing extent of disease, which helps guide treatment decisions.

Detection of HCC using MDCT with contrast enhancement of both the arterial and portal venous phases has a sensitivity as high as 92.8%,[32] whereas studies using contrast-enhanced helical CT show a lower sensitivity in the range of 68%.[33] An advantage of using MDCT is the acquisition of the multiplanar reformations that aid in treatment planning by providing further information regarding the extent of disease, location relative to important vascular structures, and potential anatomic vascular variants that can affect treatment planning. The use of MDCT also allows for the assessment of any extrahepatic tumor extension.

In addition to CT, MRI of the liver with contrast helps in the detection of smaller HCC nodules (1 to 2 cm) that may be missed by CT[34] and aids in defining vessel patency and venous anatomy. The sensitivity of MRI is 89% with a specificity of 96% for lesions that demonstrate delayed hypodensity and a delayed outer rim in the portal venous phases.[35] Of note, both MDCT and MRI have limited sensitivity in the detection of nodules less than 1 cm given the inability to differentiate between cancerous lesions and nodules in a cirrhotic background.

PATIENT EVALUATION: SUITABILITY FOR RESECTION AND TRANSPLANTATION

The decision to treat HCC with operative modalities is based on the assessment of several factors: patient performance status, tumor extent, baseline functional liver reserve, and, for patients who are considered candidates for resection, the estimated functional liver remnant. For patients with HCC that is confined to the liver and amenable to surgical intervention the choice between offering liver resection or transplantation hinges on two main issues: the underlying hepatic functional reserve and whether the patient meets established transplantation criteria.

Determination of Hepatic Functional Reserve and Suitability for Resection

In the past, liver-directed treatments in patients with advanced liver disease were limited due to the high morbidity and mortality associated with the impaired function of the cirrhotic liver. The perioperative mortality rates after partial hepatectomy for HCC exceeded 10% in early series but new advances in surgical techniques, radiologic imaging, and anesthetic care have led to significant reductions in complications and deaths from liver resection down to less than 5% at high-volume hepatobiliary centers.[36,37]

Multiple studies have determined that the two most important issues to consider to minimize morbidity and mortality after liver resection is the patient's baseline liver function and predicted future liver remnant (FLR). The clinical assessment of liver function is commonly made by risk-stratifying patients using the Child-Pugh Turcotte classification system (Table 6.2) or the MELD score as discussed previously. Additional factors that can negatively affect outcomes after surgery include active hepatitis and the presence of portal hypertension. Those patients with underlying active hepatitis, as defined by elevated transaminases twice above the normal range, are poor surgical candidates due to a higher risk of postoperative liver failure, kidney failure, and an increased risk of intraoperative blood loss.[38] Portal hypertension caused by increased hepatic vascular resistance in cirrhosis is a known risk factor for liver decompensation after liver resection.[39] Methods to assess hepatic venous pressure preoperatively include invasive methods, such as hepatic venous pressure gradient (HVPG) measurements, and the use of indirect markers of portal hypertension, such as platelet number and clinical findings (varices, splenomegaly).[3]

HVPG measurements correlate with complications from portal hypertension including ascites, encephalopathy, and spontaneous bacterial peritonitis. Additionally, it predicts the development of HCC in patients with cirrhosis with an HVPG greater than 10 mm Hg being associated with a sixfold increase in the risk of developing HCC.[40] HPVG measurements are used by some centers to predict postoperative liver function and suitability of a patient for surgical resection[41] but this approach has not been widely adopted.

Evaluation of the Functional Liver Remnant Volume and Optimization Strategies

For those patients considered to be good candidates for resection, one of the main goals of preoperative planning is to minimize the risk of postoperative liver failure by leaving a sufficient volume of liver parenchyma after resection. One method used to estimate FLR volume uses volumetric imaging. The preoperative volumetric analysis can be performed using either three-dimensional CT or MRI (with the FLR volume standardized to the patient's total liver volume based on body surface area, which predicts its postoperative function).[42–44] For patients with chronic liver disease an estimated 40% FLR volume is a rough estimate of how much liver must be preserved to minimize the risk of postoperative liver failure but no absolute minimal FLR has been determined.[44]

For those patients who do not meet the criteria for an adequate FLR, portal vein embolization (PVE) may be used in an attempt to hypertrophy the future remnant. The basis of this approach, first described in 1986, is to induce atrophy of the embolized segments with a resulting compensatory hypertrophy of the FLR by redirecting the portal venous flow.[45] The use of PVE in patients with chronic liver disease leads to a significant decrease in the rate of postoperative complications including pulmonary complications, ascites, and liver failure. Patients who do not have hypertrophy of the FLR after PVE are generally not considered for major hepatic resections given the higher risk of postoperative liver dysfunction.[46]

Patient Evaluation: Transplantation Criteria

Early reports describing the use of transplantation strategies in the treatment of HCC were controversial given that the long-term results of this approach were not superior to surgical resection. Additionally, the increased cost, demands on a limited organ supply, and the need for lifetime immunosupression led many to believe that this approach was not justified. In 1996 a group from the University of Milan published their series on the use of liver transplantation for the treatment of HCC. An earlier study had suggested that patients with multinodular, large, diffuse, or unresectable tumors had worse outcomes.[47] Based on these results the Milan group examined their outcomes in patients with early disease. Their analysis suggested that transplantation should be reserved for those patients with either a single tumor less than 5 cm in diameter or no more than three tumor nodules, each smaller than 3 cm. Additional parameters included the absence of extrahepatic disease or vascular invasion.[48] Taken together these parameters came to be known as "The Milan Criteria" and became the standard for patient selection during the evaluation process for liver transplantation in HCC (Table 6.4).

Some groups have expanded these parameters to include larger tumors (UCSF criteria) with a maximum size of 6.5 cm for a single tumor or 4.5 cm for up to 3 nodules,[49] and increased number of tumors (Tokyo 5-5 criteria: 5 tumors up to 5 cm in diameter; Kyoto criteria: up to 10 nodules with a maximum size of 5 cm) but these systems have not been widely accepted. Using the Milan criteria to optimize patient selection 5-year survival has been reported as high as 83% at 4 years post-transplant.[48] This has led to the adaptation of the Milan criteria by the United Network for Organ Sharing (UNOS) as a condition for listing HCC patients in the transplant waiting list.

OUTCOMES OF LIVER RESECTION FOR HEPATOCELLULAR CARCINOMA

Improvements in perioperative care and careful patient selection using better imaging techniques and risk-stratification methods have led to a decrease in the complication rates after liver resection for patients with compensated cirrhosis (Childs A). For patients with disease limited to the liver and either no evidence of chronic liver disease or compensated cirrhosis, liver resection strategies offer a safe and effective alternative to liver transplantation. Arguments for the use of liver resection for the management of HCC as first-line therapy for HCC are based on its low morbidity and mortality, its reported 5-year survival of up to 75%,[50] and the limited supply of donor organs. Additionally, there are no tumor-related restrictions, such as tumor size or presence of vascular invasion, or a waiting period prior to intervention, making it more applicable than transplantation.

Outcomes for liver resection are best for patients with small, solitary tumors that are confined to the liver. Although an anatomic resection to remove the involved liver segment(s) was considered superior to nonanatomic resections in terms of disease-free survival and overall survival, multiple studies have shown that margin status is a better predictor of long-term outcomes than the extent of the hepatectomy. Resection with wide margins (1 to 2 cm) has been classically recommended based on data showing lower recurrence rates and improved overall survival for patients with small solitary tumors who underwent resection with a 2-cm margin (60% 5-year overall survival for 1-cm margin vs. 100% overall survival for 2-cm margins).[51] For patients with multifocal disease and limited liver reserve, the preservation of liver parenchyma takes precedence over wide resection margins.[52]

Another risk factor that negatively affects the overall survival in patients who undergo resection for HCC is the presence of major vascular invasion.[53] The 5-year overall survival and the median survival of patients with small tumors with and without vascular involvement have been reported to be 42% and 49 months versus 30% and 24 months, respectively.[21] Despite this some centers advocate resection even in the presence of major portal or hepatic vein invasion given the poor outcomes using nonsurgical approaches, either chemotherapy or RFA.[54] The long-term outcome following hepatic resection in the setting of major vascular invasion is very poor, however (FIGURE 6.1).

Other primary tumor characteristics including size and the number of lesions are strong prognostic factors for recurrence and overall survival but are not absolute contraindications to resection.[21] Patients with large (>5 cm) HCC who undergo resection have survival rates of 25% to 58% at 5 years,[20,54,55] and those with tumors larger than 10 cm have complication rates that are similar to reported rates in patients with smaller tumors[56] despite the technical challenges associated with the resection of large tumors (FIGURE 6.2). Based on these results and the lack of effective alternative strategies, some centers advocate the resection of large tumors to improve overall survival. Unfortunately, resection is rarely applicable to patients with large tumors because many of these patients present with concurrent advanced liver disease and therefore are not candidates for a major hepatic resection.

Worse overall survival and higher rates of recurrence are also associated with multinodular disease. Although patients with multinodular disease may theoretically be at an increased risk for postoperative liver failure due to the increased parenchymal volume that usually is resected to clear all lesions, a report from a multi-institutional study addressing the role of resection in multinodular disease found that these patients have complication rates similar to those with more limited disease. The overall survivals at 3 and 5 years were 50% and 39%, respectively, which are superior than alternative, nonsurgical therapies supports the role of surgical resection in patients with multinodular disease.[20] As such, surgical resection should be considered for patients with multinodular disease; however, most of these patients are probably better served with transplantation if they meet criteria.

Although vascular invasion, tumor size, and number of tumors are predictors of worse survival, none of these factors are absolute contraindications to liver resection for HCC. The only absolute contraindications for surgical resection of HCC include extrahepatic disease, decompensated cirrhosis, and an inadequate predicted FLR volume.

OUTCOMES OF LIVER TRANSPLANT FOR HEPATOCELLULAR CARCINOMA

The role of total hepatectomy and orthotopic liver transplantation (OLT) in the management of HCC has evolved from early attempts at transplanting those patients with advanced, unresectable disease to a more selective use of transplantation in patients with early disease. The use of transplant strategies offers the advantage of removing both the primary tumor and the cirrhotic liver that may predispose to future tumors. Outcomes from early studies at the University of Pittsburgh among patients with advanced HCC showed high rates of early recurrence with 13 of 23 patients recurring within 6 months after transplant and overall survival rates no better than the results obtained with liver resection.[57] In contrast, the landmark paper

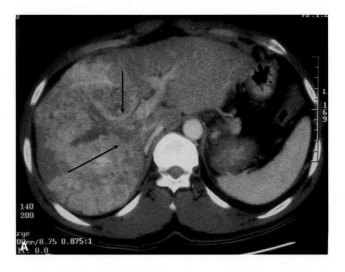

FIGURE 6.1 A. Computed tomography depicting a large HCC in the right liver associated with a hypervascular tumor thrombus extending into the main branch of the right portal vein (*arrows*). **B.** At a median follow-up of 93 months, the overall median survival for patients with HCC and major vascular invasion was 11 months. The 1-, 3-, and 5-year survival rates were 45%, 17%, and 10%, respectively.

Used with permission Pawlik TM, Poon RT, Abdalla EK, et al. Hepatectomy for hepatocellular carcinoma with major portal or hepatic vein invasion: results of a multicenter study. *Surgery* 2005;137(4):403–410.

by Mazzaferro and colleagues from the University of Milan reported a long-term survival that exceeded over 70% following OLT for early-stage HCC. Multiple subsequent studies comparing recurrence rates after OLT for HCC have shown lower recurrence rates after OLT (9% to 15%) than those after resection (37% to 59%).[53,58,59] Multiple centers have similarly reported 5-year survival in excess of 70% to 75% for patients undergoing transplantation for early-stage HCC and this has led to the acceptance of liver transplantation for HCC in cirrhotic patients (FIGURE 6.3).

The use of OLT as first-line treatment for early HCC, however, is not without some shortcomings. The incidence of disease progression while awaiting a graft is in the range of 10% to 23% and postoperative mortality rates after OLT are higher (9% to 22%) than those reported for liver resection (0% to 14%).[60,61] Additionally, issues with limited organ availability have led to dropout rates of up to 38% after 1 year on the transplant waiting list, leading some centers to report outcomes no better than resection when the dropouts are included in the analysis (54% at 2 years).[62] The median waiting time at one institution

was 7.7 months with a 21% dropout rate due to progression of disease (94%) or death (4%). Intention-to-treat analysis in this study showed no significant difference between patients who underwent resection and those treated with liver transplant (56% LR, 64% OLT).[53] In this study, the authors noted that the survival benefit of OLT over resection in the treatment of early HCC disappeared when the wait time was greater than 4 months.[53] Given the shortage of donor organs some centers have proposed live-donor liver transplantation strategies in an attempt to shorten the wait time and decrease the number of patients who progress on the wait list. This has led to shorter waiting times but analysis of the Adult-to-Adult Living Donor Liver Transplantation Cohort Study (A2ALL) showed higher rates of recurrences at 3 years when compared to deceased-donor transplantation (29% vs. 0%) with no difference in overall survival at 4 years.[63]

Another potential drawback of transplantation strategies includes the requirement for chronic immunosuppression, which places patients at higher risk for infections, potential nephrotoxicity, and HCC recurrence.[64]

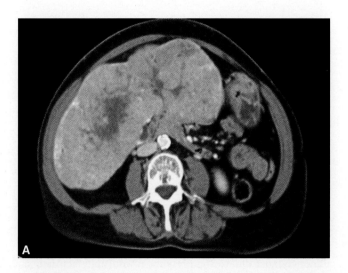

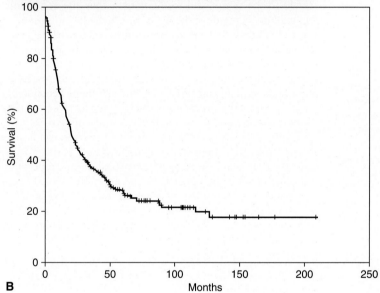

FIGURE 6.2 A. Computed tomography depicting a large HCC in the right inferior liver. **B.** At a median follow-up of 32 months (range, 0.2 to 208 months), the overall long-term median survival for patients with a hepatocellular carcinoma 10 cm in diameter or larger was 20.3 months.

Used with permission Pawlik TM, Poon RT, Abdalla EK, et al. Critical appraisal of the clinical and pathologic predictors of survival after resection of large hepatocellular carcinoma. *Arch Surg* (Chicago, IL: 1960) 2005;140:450–457; discussion 457–458.

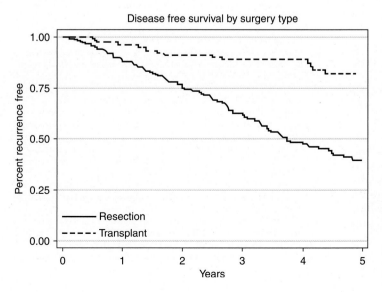

FIGURE 6.3 Disease-free survival was significantly better after liver transplantation (1, 3, and 5 years: 96%, 89%, and 82%, respectively) compared with liver resection (1, 3, 5 years: 88%, 62%, and 40%, respectively) (*p* < .001).

Used with permission Bellavance EC, Lumpkins KM, Mentha G, et al. Surgical management of early-stage hepatocellular carcinoma: resection or transplantation? *J Gastrointest Surg* 2008;12(10):1699–1708.

■ BRIDGES TO TRANSPLANTATION

The reported survival benefits for patients who undergo liver transplant have led to the use of liver-directed therapies to prevent disease progression while patients await transplantation. Strategies used as bridges to transplant include liver resection, intra-arterial approaches (transarterial embolization or transcatheter arterial chemoembolization, TAE/TACE), and ablative therapies (radiofrequency ablation or percutaneous ethanol injection, RFA/PEI).

Liver Resection

The use of liver resection prior to liver transplantation has been proposed as a treatment strategy while waiting for a suitable organ donor. Potential advantages of this approach over TACE and RFA include the availability of tissue for pathologic analysis and the potential superiority of resection over other systemic and liver-directed locoregional therapies. Although controversial due to the potential increased transplant operative risk after a partial hepatectomy, the goal of this approach is to transplant the patient prior to recurrence in the resected liver. Another problem with this approach in the United States includes the loss of HCC-related MELD score exception points for patients already listed on the transplant list.[8] A multi-institutional European study examined the outcomes of primary resection with secondary liver transplantation versus primary liver transplantation in the setting of cirrhosis. The results from this study showed higher rates of postoperative complications, intraoperative bleeding, and tumor recurrences when compared to patients who underwent liver transplantation as the first-line treatment.[65] Until further studies to determine which patients may benefit from using this strategy are completed, this approach remains controversial.

Nonoperative Therapies as Bridges to Transplantation: Radiofrequency Ablation and Transcatheter Arterial Chemoembolization

The use of TACE and RFA for treatment of HCC in the palliative setting has shown a survival advantage over no treatment. These findings have led to the use of these strategies to delay disease progression and in some cases attempt to downstage patients to qualify for transplantation. Advantages of TACE over RFA include the limitations of RFA for lesions larger than 3 cm and those near large vascular structures that lead to incomplete tumor necrosis after treatment.

The role of TACE in patients who subsequently undergo OLT has been examined in multiple studies. For patients who show disease progression after TACE the risk of disease recurrence is higher after OLT when compared with patients who do not progress. Among patients who did not progress following TACE several studies have reported a 5-year survival after transplantation of 80.9%[66,67] This patient population included patients with multinodular disease and angioinvasion; patients had undergone a median number of 5 TACE cycles with a median waiting time to OLT of 218 days. Outcomes from a different study showed that 23.7% of patients outside of the Milan criteria who were treated with TACE were downstaged to qualify for OLT and those who underwent transplant had

similar 2-year outcomes versus patients who initially met the Milan criteria.[68]

The use of RFA as a bridging therapy before liver transplantation has been investigated in small observational cohort studies. In one study, 54% of the tumors treated underwent complete necrosis after the first ablation, whereas the rest required repeated treatments while awaiting transplantation. In addition, 14% of those treated were noted to progress while waiting for an organ.[69] RFA treatment was found to decrease the wait list dropout rate when compared to no treatment for small HCC. Overall, there is limited evidence that it improves rates of recurrence after OLT or overall survival.

■ CONCLUSION

The management of HCC presents unique challenges to the oncologist due to the presence of multiple factors both related to the tumor and to the patient that affect decision making and outcomes. The decision of whether to pursue a surgical strategy first versus nonsurgical strategies depends on the patient's baseline physiologic status and the extent of the disease. In selecting patients for surgical resection versus transplantation, the current practice is to avoid liver resection in patients with advanced HCC in the setting of decompensated liver function and an insufficient hepatic reserve. For patients with disease limited to the liver and a noncirrhotic or Child-Pugh class A parenchymal disease, resection can be associated with good long-term outcomes. Those patients with early-stage HCC as defined by the Milan criteria and especially those with Child-Pugh B or C classes are better served with transplantation. The use of liver resection as a bridge to OLT remains controversial but the use of nonsurgical strategies, in particular, TACE, has shown to have improved outcomes and in selected cases can lead to downstaging that qualifies a patient for transplantation.

■ REFERENCES

1. Davila JA, Weston A, Smalley W, et al. Utilization of screening for hepatocellular carcinoma in the United States. *J Clin Gastroenterol* 2007;41(8):777–782.
2. Nathan H, Mentha G, Marques HP, et al. Comparative performances of staging systems for early hepatocellular carcinoma. *HPB (Oxford)* 2009;11:382–390.
3. Llovet JM, Schwartz M, Mazzaferro V. Resection and liver transplantation for hepatocellular carcinoma. *Semin Liver Dis* 2005;25(2):181–200.
4. Vauthey J-N, Dixon E, Abdalla EK, et al. Pretreatment assessment of hepatocellular carcinoma: expert consensus statement. *HPB (Oxford)* 2010;12:289–299.
5. Ferlay J, Shin HR, Bray F, et al. Estimates of worldwide burden of cancer in 2008: GLOBOCAN 2008. *Int J Cancer* 2010;127(12):2893–2917.
6. Yang JD, Harmsen WS, Slettedahl SW, et al. Factors that affect risk for hepatocellular carcinoma and effects of surveillance. *Clin Gastroenterol Hepatol* 2011;9(7):617–623.e1.
7. Perz JF, Armstrong GL, Farrington LA, et al. The contributions of hepatitis B virus and hepatitis C virus infections to cirrhosis and primary liver cancer worldwide. *J Hepatol* 2006;45(4):529–538.
8. Jarnagin W, Chapman WC, Curley S, et al. Surgical treatment of hepatocellular carcinoma: expert consensus statement. *HPB (Oxford)* 2010;12(5):302–310.
9. Sherman M. Hepatocellular carcinoma: epidemiology, surveillance, and diagnosis. *Semin Liver Dis* 2010;30(1):3–16.
10. Yeo W, Mo FK, Chan SL, et al. Hepatitis B viral load predicts survival of HCC patients undergoing systemic chemotherapy. *Hepatology* 2007;45(6):1382–1389.

11. Colombo M, de Franchis R, Del Ninno E, et al. Hepatocellular carcinoma in Italian patients with cirrhosis. *N Engl J Med* 1991;325(10):675–680.

12. Ganem D, Prince AM. Hepatitis B virus infection—natural history and clinical consequences. *N Engl J Med* 2004;350(11):1118–1129.

13. Bruix J, Sherman M. Management of hepatocellular carcinoma. *Hepatology* 2005;42(5):1208–1236.

14. Sherman M. Hepatocellular carcinoma: screening and staging. *Clin Liver Dis* 1011;15(2):323–334.

15. Bruix J, Sherman M. Diagnosis of small HCC. *Gastroenterology* 2005;129(4):1364.

16. Arii S, Sata M, Sakamoto M, et al. Management of hepatocellular carcinoma: Report of Consensus Meeting in the 45th Annual Meeting of the Japan Society of Hepatology (2009). *Hepatol Res* 2010;40:667–685.

17. Infante-Rivard C, Esnaola S, Villeneuve JP. Clinical and statistical validity of conventional prognostic factors in predicting short-term survival among cirrhotics. *Hepatology* 1987;7(4):660–664.

18. Teh SH, Christein J, Donohue J, et al. Hepatic resection of hepatocellular carcinoma in patients with cirrhosis: Model of End-Stage Liver Disease (MELD) score predicts perioperative mortality. *J Gastrointest Surg* 2005;9:1207–1215; discussion 1215.

19. Cucchetti A, Ercolani G, Vivarelli M, et al. Impact of model for end-stage liver disease (MELD) score on prognosis after hepatectomy for hepatocellular carcinoma on cirrhosis. *Liver Transpl* 2006;12(6):966–971.

20. Ng KK, Vauthey J-N, Pawlik TM, et al. Is hepatic resection for large or multinodular hepatocellular carcinoma justified? Results from a multi-institutional database. *Ann Surg Oncol* 2005;12:364–373.

21. Nathan H, Schulick RD, Choti MA, et al. Predictors of survival after resection of early hepatocellular carcinoma. *Ann Surg* 2009;249:799–805.

22. Makuuchi M, Belghiti J, Belli G, et al. IHPBA concordant classification of primary liver cancer: working group report. *J Hepatobiliary Pancreat Surg* 2003;10(1):26–30.

23. Kudo M, Chung H, Haji S, et al. Validation of a new prognostic staging system for hepatocellular carcinoma: the JIS score compared with the CLIP score. *Hepatology* 2004;40(6):1396–1405.

24. Okuda K, Ohtsuki T, Obata H, et al. Natural history of hepatocellular carcinoma and prognosis in relation to treatment. Study of 850 patients. *Cancer* 1985;56(4):918–928.

25. A new prognostic system for hepatocellular carcinoma: a retrospective study of 435 patients: the Cancer of the Liver Italian Program (CLIP) investigators. *Hepatology* 1998;28(3):751–755.

26. Llovet JM, Bruix J. Prospective validation of the Cancer of the Liver Italian Program (CLIP) score: a new prognostic system for patients with cirrhosis and hepatocellular carcinoma. *Hepatology* 2000;32(3):679–680.

27. Ueno S, Tanabe G, Sako K, et al. Discrimination value of the new western prognostic system (CLIP score) for hepatocellular carcinoma in 662 Japanese patients. Cancer of the Liver Italian Program. *Hepatology* 2001;34(3):529–534.

28. Llovet JM, Brú C, Bruix J. Prognosis of hepatocellular carcinoma: the BCLC staging classification. *Semin Liver Dis* 1999;19:329–338.

29. Cillo U, Vitale A, Grigoletto F, et al. Prospective validation of the Barcelona Clinic Liver Cancer staging system. *J Hepatol* 2006;44(4):723–731.

30. Kee K-M, Wang J-H, Lee C-M, et al. Validation of clinical AJCC/UICC TNM staging system for hepatocellular carcinoma: analysis of 5,613 cases from a medical center in southern Taiwan. *Int J Cancer* 2007;120:2650–2655.

31. Henderson JM, Sherman M, Tavill A, et al. AHPBA/AJCC consensus conference on staging of hepatocellular carcinoma: consensus statement. *HPB (Oxford)* 2003;5:243–250.

32. Iannaccone R, Laghi A, Catalano C, et al. Hepatocellular carcinoma: role of unenhanced and delayed phase multi-detector row helical CT in patients with cirrhosis. *Radiology* 2005;234(2):460–467.

33. Colli A, Fraquelli M, Casazza G, et al. Accuracy of ultrasonography, spiral CT, magnetic resonance, and alpha-fetoprotein in diagnosing hepatocellular carcinoma: a systematic review. *Am J Gastroenterol* 2006;101(3):513–523.

34. Burrel M, Llovet JM, Ayuso C, et al. MRI angiography is superior to helical CT for detection of HCC prior to liver transplantation: an explant correlation. *Hepatology* 2003;38(4):1034–1042.

35. Willatt JM, Hussain HK, Adusumilli S, et al. MR Imaging of hepatocellular carcinoma in the cirrhotic liver: challenges and controversies. *Radiology* 2008;247(2):311–330.

36. Bryant R, Laurent A, Tayar C, et al. Liver resection for hepatocellular carcinoma. *Surg Oncol Clin N Am* 2008;17(3):607–633, ix.

37. Wei AC, Tung-Ping Poon R, Fan ST, et al. Risk factors for perioperative morbidity and mortality after extended hepatectomy for hepatocellular carcinoma. *Br J Surg* 2003;90(1):33–41.

38. Farges O, Malassagne B, Flejou JF, et al. Risk of major liver resection in patients with underlying chronic liver disease: a reappraisal. *Ann Surg* 1999;229:210–215.

39. Bruix J, Castells A, Bosch J, et al. Surgical resection of hepatocellular carcinoma in cirrhotic patients: prognostic value of preoperative portal pressure. *Gastroenterology* 1996;111:1018–1022.

40. Ripoll C, Groszmann RJ, Garcia-Tsao G, et al. Hepatic venous pressure gradient predicts development of hepatocellular carcinoma independently of severity of cirrhosis. *J Hepatol* 2009;50(5):923–928.

41. Kanematsu T, Furui J, Yanaga K, et al. Measurement of portal venous pressure is useful for selecting the optimal type of resection in cirrhotic patients with hepatocellular carcinoma. *Hepatogastroenterology* 2005;52(66):1828–1831.

42. Ribero D, Abdalla EK, Madoff DC, et al. Portal vein embolization before major hepatectomy and its effects on regeneration, resectability and outcome. *Br J Surg* 2007;94(11):1386–1394.

43. Shoup M, Gonen M, D'Angelica M, et al. Volumetric analysis predicts hepatic dysfunction in patients undergoing major liver resection. *J Gastrointest Surg* 2003;7:325–330.

44. Vauthey J, Chaoui A, Do K, et al. Standardized measurement of the future liver remnant prior to extended liver resection: methodology and clinical associations. *Surgery* 2000;127:512–519.

45. Abdalla EK, Hicks ME, Vauthey JN. Portal vein embolization: rationale, technique and future prospects. *Br J Surg* 2001;88:165–175.

46. Farges O, Belghiti J, Kianmanesh R, et al. Portal vein embolization before right hepatectomy: prospective clinical trial. *Ann Surg* 2003;237:208–217.

47. Bismuth H, Chiche L, Adam R, et al. Liver resection versus transplantation for hepatocellular carcinoma in cirrhotic patients. *Ann Surg* 1993;218:145–151.

48. Mazzaferro V, Regalia E, Doci R, et al. Liver transplantation for the treatment of small hepatocellular carcinomas in patients with cirrhosis. *N Engl J Med* 1996;334:693–699.

49. Yao FY, Ferrell L, Bass NM, et al. Liver transplantation for hepatocellular carcinoma: expansion of the tumor size limits does not adversely impact survival. *Hepatology* 2001;33:1394–1403.

50. Izumi R, Shimizu K, Ii T, et al. Prognostic factors of hepatocellular carcinoma in patients undergoing hepatic resection. *Gastroenterology* 1994;106(3):720–727.

51. Shi M, Guo RP, Lin XJ, et al. Partial hepatectomy with wide versus narrow resection margin for solitary hepatocellular carcinoma: a prospective randomized trial. *Ann Surg* 2007;245(1):36–43.

52. Poon RT, Fan ST, Ng IO, et al. Significance of resection margin in hepatectomy for hepatocellular carcinoma: a critical reappraisal. *Ann Surg* 2000;231:544–551.

53. Shah SA, Cleary SP, Tan JCC, et al. An analysis of resection vs transplantation for early hepatocellular carcinoma: defining the optimal therapy at a single institution. *Ann Surg Oncol* 2007;14:2608–2614.

54. Pawlik TM, Poon RT, Abdalla EK, et al. Critical appraisal of the clinical and pathologic predictors of survival after resection of large hepatocellular carcinoma. *Arch Surg* (Chicago, IL: 1960) 2005;140:450–457; discussion 457–458.

55. Yang LY, Fang F, Ou DP, et al. Solitary large hepatocellular carcinoma: a specific subtype of hepatocellular carcinoma with good outcome after hepatic resection. *Ann Surg* 2009;249(1):118–123.

56. Liau KH, Ruo L, Shia J, et al. Outcome of partial hepatectomy for large (>10 cm) hepatocellular carcinoma. *Cancer* 2005;104(9):1948–1955.

57. Yokoyama I, Todo S, Iwatsuki S, et al. Liver transplantation in the treatment of primary liver cancer. *Hepatogastroenterology* 1990;37:188–193.

58. Margarit C, Escartín A, Castells L, et al. Resection for hepatocellular carcinoma is a good option in Child-Turcotte-Pugh class A patients with cirrhosis who are eligible for liver transplantation. *Liver Transpl* 2005;11:1242–1251.

59. Pierie JP, Muzikansky A, Tanabe KK, et al. The outcome of surgical resection versus assignment to the liver transplant waiting list for hepatocellular carcinoma. *Ann Surg Oncol* 2005;12:552–560.

60. Michel J, Suc B, Montpeyroux F, et al. Liver resection or transplantation for hepatocellular carcinoma? Retrospective analysis of 215 patients with cirrhosis. *J Hepatol* 1997;26:1274–1280.

61. Philosophe B, Greig PD, Hemming AW, et al. Surgical management of hepatocellular carcinoma: resection or transplantation? *J Gastrointest Surg* 1998;2:21–27.

62. Llovet JM, Fuster J, Bruix J. Intention-to-treat analysis of surgical treatment for early hepatocellular carcinoma: resection versus transplantation. *Hepatology* 1999;30:1434–1440.

63. Fisher RA, Kulik LM, Freise CE, et al. Hepatocellular carcinoma recurrence and death following living and deceased donor liver transplantation. *Am J Transplant* 2007;7:1601–1608.

64. Vivarelli M, Cucchetti A, La Barba G, et al. Liver transplantation for hepatocellular carcinoma under calcineurin inhibitors: reassessment of risk factors for tumor recurrence. *Ann Surg* 2008;248: 857–862.

65. Adam R, Azoulay D, Castaing D, et al. Liver resection as a bridge to transplantation for hepatocellular carcinoma on cirrhosis: a reasonable strategy? *Ann Surg* 2003;238:508–518; discussion 518–519.

66. Otto G, Heise M, Moench C, et al. Transarterial chemoembolization before liver transplantation in 60 patients with hepatocellular carcinoma. *Transplant Proc* 2007;39(2):537–539.

67. Otto G, Herber S, Heise M, et al. Response to transarterial chemoembolization as a biological selection criterion for liver transplantation in hepatocellular carcinoma. *Liver Transpl* 2006;12(8):1260–1267.

68. Chapman WC, Majella Doyle MB, Stuart JE, et al. Outcomes of neoadjuvant transarterial chemoembolization to downstage hepatocellular carcinoma before liver transplantation. *Ann Surg* 2008;248(4):617–625.

69. Brillet PY, Paradis V, Brancatelli G, et al. Percutaneous radiofrequency ablation for hepatocellular carcinoma before liver transplantation: a prospective study with histopathologic comparison. *AJR Am J Roentgenol* 2006;186(suppl 5):S296–305.

CHAPTER

7

Hepatocellular Carcinoma: Ablative Therapies, Intra-Arterial Therapies

RICCARDO LENCIONI, ELENI LIAPI, and JEAN-FRANÇOIS H. GESCHWIND

Ablative Therapies

INTRODUCTION

A careful multidisciplinary assessment of tumor characteristics, liver function, and physical status is required for proper therapeutic management of patients with hepatocellular carcinoma (HCC).[1,2] Candidates for resection must be carefully selected to minimize the risk of postoperative liver failure and improve long-term results. Access to liver transplantation has to be balanced between precise estimation of survival contouring individual tumor characteristics and organ availability. When surgical options are precluded, interventional locoregional therapies are recommended as the most appropriate therapeutic choice when the disease is isolated to the liver. Image-guided tumor ablation is recommended as the most appropriate therapeutic choice for nonsurgical patients with early-stage HCC and is considered a potentially radical treatment in properly selected candidates.[3] For patients presenting with more advanced or multinodular HCC and relatively preserved liver function, transcatheter arterial chemoembolization (TACE) is the current standard of care.[4]

ABLATIVE THERAPIES

Image-guided ablation is recommended for patients with early-stage HCC when surgical options are precluded.[1,2] Although tumor ablation procedures can be performed at laparoscopy or surgery, most procedures aimed at treating HCC are performed with a percutaneous approach. Hence, several authors refer to these procedures as percutaneous therapies. The concept of image guidance is stressed in the title to highlight that image guidance is critical to the success of these therapies.[5] Over the past 25 years, several methods for chemical or thermal tumor destruction have been developed and clinically tested.[6] More recently, a novel nonchemical, nonthermal ablation technique, irreversible electroporation (IRE), has been developed and is currently undergoing clinical investigation (Table 7.1).

Chemical Ablation

The seminal technique used for local ablation of HCC has been percutaneous ethanol injection (PEI). PEI is a well-established technique for the treatment of small, nodular-type HCC.[7] Its major limitation is the high local recurrence rate that may reach 33% in lesions smaller than 3 cm and 43% in lesions exceeding

Table 7.1
Percutaneous Methods for Image-Guided Ablation of Hepatocellular Carcinoma
Chemical ablation
Ethanol injection
Thermal ablation
Radiofrequency ablation
Microwave ablation
Laser ablation
Cryoablation
Irreversible electroporation

3 cm.[8,9] The injected ethanol does not always accomplish complete tumor ablation because of its inhomogeneous distribution within the lesion—especially in the presence of intratumoral septa—and the limited effect on extracapsular cancerous spread. The recent introduction of a specific device for single-session PEI, a multipronged needle with three retractable prongs, each with four terminal side holes (QuadraFuse; Rex Medical, Conshohocken, PA), has been shown to overcome some of these limitations by ensuring a more homogeneous ethanol perfusion throughout the whole tumor mass. In two recent studies, PEI performed with multipronged needles resulted in rates of sustained complete response ranging 80% to 90% in tumors smaller than 3 to 4 cm in diameter.[10,11] Hence, the technique seems still to be able to offer a valuable alternative to radiofrequency ablation (RFA), particularly for small lesions in an unfavorable location for thermal ablation.

Thermal Ablation

The thermal ablative therapies involved in clinical practice can be classified as either hyperthermic treatments—including RFA, microwave ablation (MWA), and laser ablation—or cryoablation. For adequate destruction of tumor tissue, the entire target volume and possibly an adequate tumor-free margin must be subjected to cytotoxic temperatures. Ideally, a 360°, 0.5- to 1-cm-thick ablative margin should be produced around the

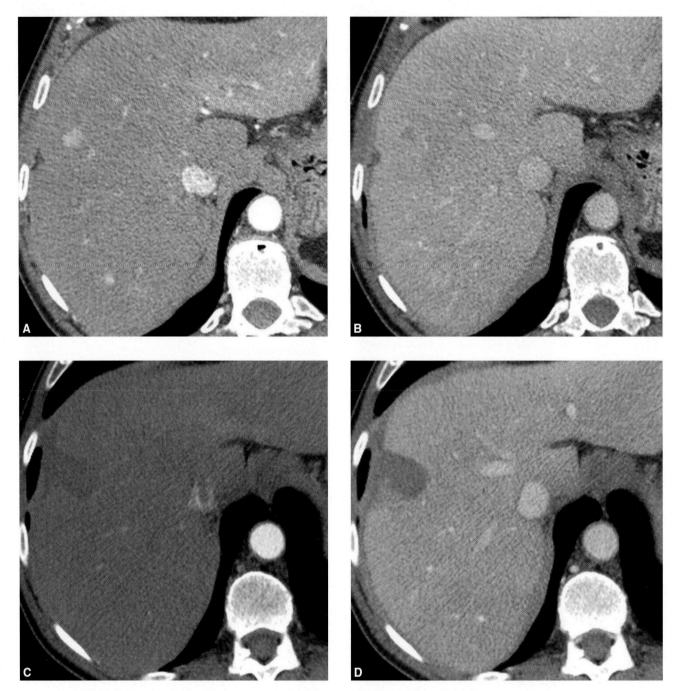

FIGURE 7.1 Complete response of small HCC after RFA. Pretreatment CT shows small hypervascular HCC with typical arterial phase enhancement (**A**) and portal venous phase washout (**B**). CT obtained 1 month after treatment shows larger unenhancing area in both the arterial (**C**) and the portal venous phase (**D**) replacing the tumor and consistent with complete ablation.

tumor. This cuff would ensure that the peripheral portion of the tumor as well as any microscopic invasions located in its close proximity have been eradicated (FIGURE 7.1).[12]

Radiofrequency Ablation

RFA has been the most widely assessed alternative to PEI for local ablation of HCC and is currently considered as the standard technique for local ablation of HCC.[3] Five randomized controlled trials (RCTs) have compared RFA versus PEI for the

treatment of early-stage HCC. These investigations consistently showed that RFA has a higher anticancer effect than PEI, leading to a better local control of the disease (Table 7.2).[13–17] The assessment of the impact of RFA on survival has been more controversial. Although a survival benefit was identified in the three RCTs performed in Asia, the two European RCTs failed to show statistically significant differences in overall survival (OS) between patients who received RFA and those treated with PEI, despite the trend favoring RFA (Table 7.2). In patients with early-stage

Table 7.2

Randomized Controlled Trials Comparing Radiofrequency Ablation Versus Ethanol Injection for the Treatment of Early-Stage Hepatocellular Carcinoma

Author and year	Initial CR	Treatment failure[a]	Overall survival (%)		
			1-year	3-years	P
Lencioni et al., 2003					
RFA (n = 52)	91%	8%	88	81	NS
PEI (n = 50)	82%	34%	96	73	
Lin et al., 2004					
RFA (n = 52)	96%	17%	82	74	0.014
PEI (n = 52)	88%	45%	61	50	
Shiina et al., 2005					
RFA (n = 118)	100%	2%	90	80	0.02
PEI (n = 114)	100%	11%	82	63	
Lin et al., 2005					
RFA (n = 62)	97%	16%	88	74	0.031
PEI (n = 62)	89%	42%	96	51	
Brunello et al., 2008					
RFA (n = 70)	96%	34%	88	59	NS
PEI (n = 69)	66%	64%	96	57	

CR, complete response; NS, not significant.

[a]Includes initial treatment failure (incomplete response) and late treatment failure (local recurrence).

HCC treated with percutaneous ablation, long-term survival is influenced by multiple different interventions, given that about 80% of the patients will develop recurrent intrahepatic HCC nodules within 5 years of the initial treatment and will receive additional therapies.[18] Nevertheless, three independent meta-analyses, including all RCTs, have confirmed that treatment with RFA offers a survival benefit as compared with PEI, particularly for tumors larger than 2 cm, thus establishing RFA as the standard percutaneous technique.[19–21] For studies that reported major complications, however, the incidence in RFA-treated patients was 4.1% (95% CI, 1.8% to 6.4%), compared to 2.7% (95% CI, 0.4% to 5.1%) observed in PEI-treated patients.[22] This difference was not statistically significant: nevertheless this safety profile should be taken into consideration as part of the overall risk/benefit profile in each individual case.

Recent reports on long-term outcomes of RFA-treated patients have shown that in patients with Child-Pugh class A and early-stage HCC, 5-year survival rates are as high as 51% to 64% and may reach 76% in patients who meet the Barcelona Clinic for Liver Cancer (BCLC) criteria for surgical resection (Table 7.3).[18,23–25] Therefore, an open question is whether RFA can compete with surgical resection as first-line treatment. Two RCTs have been reported with opposite results. Although the first one did not identify outcome differences, the second trial suggested a survival advantage for surgical resection.[26,27] Uncontrolled investigations have also reported similar results for

resection and RFA in very early stage tumors—that is, single HCC smaller than or equal to 2 cm in diameter.[28] Thus, at this point there are no unequivocal data to back up RFA as a replacement of resection as first-line treatment for patients with early-stage HCC.

The ability of RFA to achieve complete tumor eradication appears to depend on tumor size and location. In particular, histologic studies performed in liver specimens of patients who underwent RFA as bridge treatment to transplantation showed that the presence of large (3 mm or more) abutting vessels result in a drop of the rate of complete tumor necrosis to less than 50% because of the heat loss due to perfusion-mediated tissue cooling within the area to be ablated.[29] Other clinical experiences have suggested that treatment of HCC tumors in subcapsular location or adjacent to the gallbladder is associated with an increased risk of incomplete ablation and local tumor progression.[30,31] Treatment of tumors in such unfavourable locations has also been shown to result in a significant increase of major complications.[32,33]

To increase the efficacy of RFA, especially in tumors of intermediate size (3 to 7 cm), several authors have suggested the combined use of TACE and RFA. A combination including TACE followed by RFA has been used to minimize heat loss caused by perfusion-mediated tissue cooling and to increase the local therapeutic effect of RFA.[34–37] On the other hand, TACE with drug-eluting beads has been performed after an RFA procedure to increase tumor necrosis by exposing to high drug concentration the peripheral part of the tumor, where only

Table 7.3
Studies Reporting 5-Year Survival of Patients with Early-Stage Hepatocellular Carcinoma Who Received Radiofrequency Ablation as First-Line Nonsurgical Treatment

Author and year	Patients	Overall survival (%)		
		1-year	3-years	5-years
Lencioni et al., 2005				
Child-Pugh A	144	100	76	51
Child-Pugh B	43	89	46	31
Tateishi et al., 2005				
Child-Pugh A	221	96	83	63
Child-Pugh B-C*	98	90	65	31
Choi et al., 2007				
Child-Pugh A	359	NA	78	64
Child-Pugh B	160	NA	49	38
N'Kontchou et al., 2009				
BCLC resectable**	67	NA	82	76
BCLC unresectable	168	NA	49	27

NA, not available; BCLC, Barcelona Clinic for Liver Cancer.

*Only 4 of 98 patients had Child-Pugh C cirrhosis.

**BCLC criteria for resection include single tumor, normal bilirubin level (<1.5 mg/dL), and absence of significant portal hypertension.

sublethal temperatures may be achieved in a standard RFA treatment.[38] Other investigators have suggested the combined use of percutaneous approaches, such as ethanol injection and RFA.[39] Unfortunately, despite several investigations reporting promising results, no definitive proof of clinical efficacy was reached because no robust RCT comparing the survival outcomes achieved with such combinations of interventional techniques over those obtained with either therapy alone has been completed so far.

Microwave Ablation

MWA is emerging as a valuable alternative to RFA for thermal ablation of HCC. However, only one RCT has compared the effectiveness of MWA with that of RFA so far.[40] Although no statistically significant differences were observed with respect to the efficacy of the two procedures, a tendency favoring RFA was recognized in that study with respect to local recurrences and complications rates. It has to be pointed out, however, that MWA technology has evolved significantly since the publication of this trial. Newer devices seem to overcome the limitation of the small volume of coagulation that was obtained with a single probe insertion in early experiences.[41] An important advantage of MWA over RFA is that treatment outcome is not affected by vessels located in the proximity of the tumor.

Laser Ablation

To date, few data are available concerning the clinical efficacy of laser ablation because the treatment has been adopted by few centers worldwide. In particular, no RCTs to compare laser

ablation with any other treatment have been published thus far. In a recent multicenter retrospective analysis including nonsurgical patients with early-stage HCC, 5-year OS was 34% (41% in Child-Pugh class A patients).[42]

Cryoablation

Cryoablation had limited application in HCC.[43,44] The complication rate is not negligible, particularly because of the risk for "cryoshock," a life-threatening condition resulting in multiorgan failure, severe coagulopathy, and disseminated intravascular coagulation following cryoablation. There are currently no RCTs that support the use of hepatic cryoablation for HCC treatment.

Irreversible Electroporation

Electroporation is a technique that increases cell membrane permeability by changing the transmembrane potential and subsequently disrupting the lipid bilayer integrity to allow transportation of molecules across the cell membrane via nano-size pores. This process—when used in a reversible fashion—has been used in research for drug or macromolecule delivery into cells. IRE is a method to induce irreversible disruption of cell membrane integrity resulting in cell death without the need for additional pharmacologic injury (Lencioni et al. 2009).[45] The IRE system (NanoKnife, AngioDynamics, Queensbury, NY) consists of two major components: a generator and needlelike electrical probes. The generator can deliver up to 3,000 V of energy in a maximum of 100 pulses, which have a maximum pulse length of 100 μsec. The electrode probe is 19 gauge in diameter and has an active tip that can be exposed up to 4 cm. Two or more monopolar probes or a single bipolar probe must be used at a time. The number of monopolar probes that are used during an IRE procedure depends on the size and shape of the desired zone of tissue ablation. The treatment parameter for voltage depends on the distance between probes within the targeted tissue. IRE is administered under general anesthesia with administration of atracurium, cis-atracurium, pancuronium, or an equivalent neuromuscular blocking agent to prevent undesirable muscle contraction (Lencioni et al. 2009).[45]

IRE creates a sharp boundary between the treated and untreated area in vivo. This would suggest that IRE has the ability to sharply delineate the treatment area from the nontreated. Additionally, IRE can effectively create tissue death in micro- to millisecond ranges of treatment time compared to thermal ablation techniques, which require at least 20 minutes to hours. Moreover, because IRE is a nonthermal technique, there appears to be complete ablation to the margin of blood vessels without compromising their functionality. Therefore, issues associated with perfusion-mediated tissue cooling or heating (a significant challenge with thermal methods) are not relevant.

Preclinical investigation focused on HCC has shown promising results. In a recent study, HCC tumors were grown in rats that were divided into treatment and control groups.[46] For the treatment group, IRE electrodes were inserted and eight 100-μsec, 2,500-V pulses were applied to ablate the targeted tumor tissues.

Pathology correlation studies documented progression from poorly differentiated viable HCC tissues before treatment to extensive tumor necrosis and full regression in the treated rats. These findings suggest that IRE can be an effective strategy for targeted ablation of HCC and have prompted its clinical evaluation (FIGURE 7.2).

Intra-Arterial Therapies

▌ INTRODUCTION

HCC accounts for 85% to 90% of all primary liver cancers with high incidence rates in Southeast Asia and sub-Saharan Africa.[47] In the United States, HCC is currently the fastest growing cause of cancer-related death.[47] The incidence rates for HCC have tripled in the past two decades with the distribution shifting toward white younger individuals (45 to 60 years) and this increase is partially attributable to the rise in hepatitis C virus (HCV)-related HCC.[47]

Hepatocarcinogenesis is a complex multistep process in which many signaling cascades are involved and altered.[48] The most common mutations include the tumor suppressor gene TP53 (present in about 25% to 40% of HCC only, depending on tumor stage) and the gene for β catenin, CTNNB1 (present in about 25% only, primarily in HCV-related HCC). Several signaling cascades related to cell survival and proliferation are activated and have been investigated as therapeutic targets in preclinical and early clinical studies. Epithelial growth factor receptor (EGFR) and Ras signaling are activated in more than 50% of HCC tumors, whereas the mTOR (mammalian target of

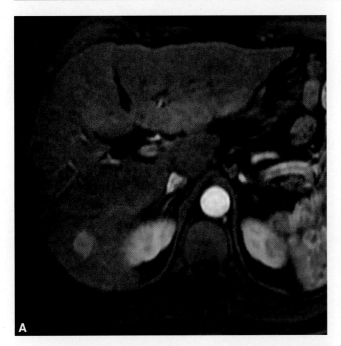
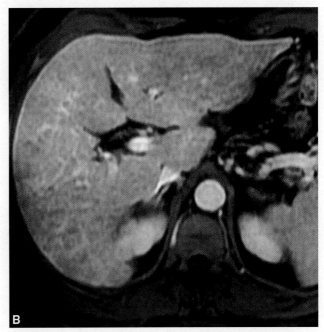

FIGURE 7.2 IRE of small HCC. Pretreatment dynamic MRI shows hypervascular tumor with arterial phase enhancement (**A**) and portal venous phase washout (**B**). The tumor is isointense on T2-weighted imaging (**C**) and slightly hyperintense on diffusion-weighted (DW) imaging obtained with b values of 500 (**D**). Its apparent diffusion coefficient (ADC) is 1.3 × 10^{-3} mm^2/second (**E**). On dynamic MRI performed 24 hours after IRE, a central hypodense area surrounded by an enhancing rim is depicted in the site of the tumor in both the arterial (**F**) and the portal venous phase (**G**). Note that the peripheral enhancing rim shows no washout. The rim is hyperintense on T2-weighted imaging (**H**), and DW imaging obtained with b values of 500 (**I**). The post-treatment ADC of the lesion is increased to 1.8 × 10^{-3} mm^2/second (**J**). *(continued)*

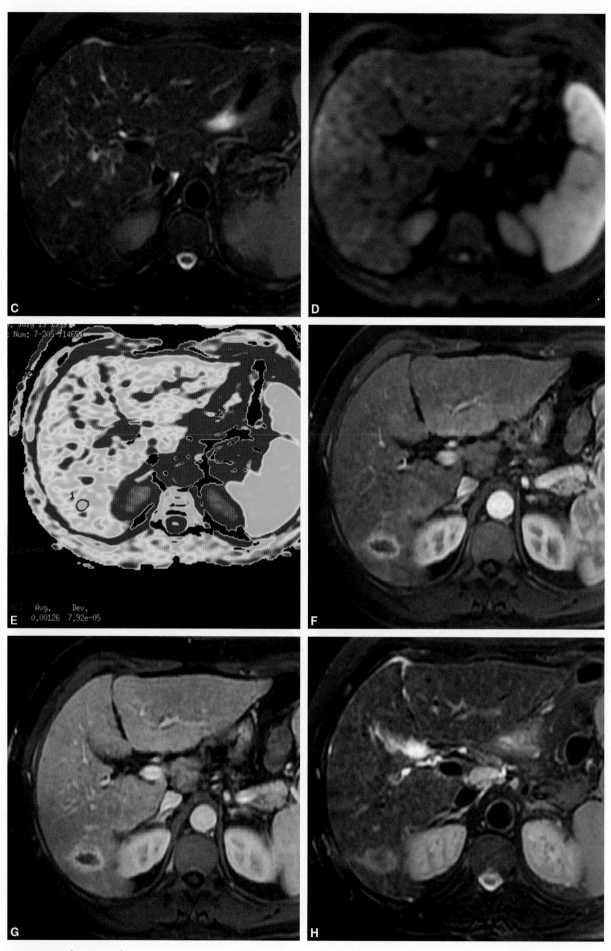

FIGURE 7.2 *(Continued)*

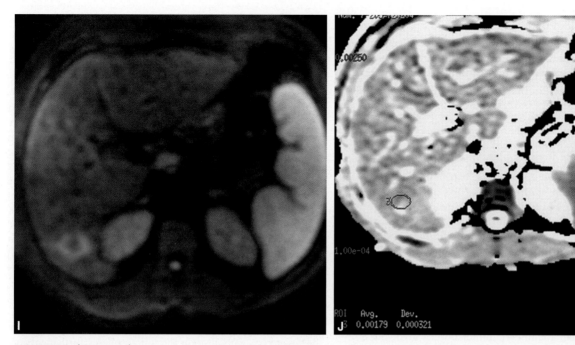

FIGURE 7.2 *(Continued)*

rapamycin) pathway is disrupted in 40% to 50% of liver cancers. Similarly, insulin-like growth factor receptor 1 (IGF1R) signaling is active in 20% of early HCCs, and deregulation of the hepatocyte growth factor (HGF) and c-MET pathway are commonly seen. Wingless (Wnt) signaling is activated in 30% of HCCs. HCC is considered a highly vascularized cancer and angiogenic activity through signaling of VEGFA, ANGPT2, and fibroblast growth factor (FGF) is a key event.[48]

Despite the diagnostic advances and surveillance modifications for early detection of HCC, most patients present with unresectable disease at the clinical visit. Up to 25% of patients have no symptoms at presentation and may be diagnosed by the presence of elevated liver function tests, elevated alpha-fetoprotein (AFP), or incidentally.[49] Assessment of prognosis is a crucial step in the management of patients with HCC. Contrary to other malignancies, long-term survival in these patients depends on the pathologic stage of the disease, the severity of underlying liver dysfunction, as well as the patient performance status. Any attempt to assess prognosis should account for tumor stage, degree of liver function, and clinical performance status. The BCLC staging system stratifies patients according to the outcome and simultaneously links outcome with recommended treatment.[50] The BCLC classification has been externally validated and establishes treatment recommendations for all stages of HCC.

Intra-arterial therapies for HCC are primarily intended for patients with unresectable liver cancer and preserved liver function.[51] Intra-arterial therapies for HCC have also been employed for down-staging prior to orthotopic liver transplantation (OLT) and prior to resection.[52] Very commonly, however, the therapeutic algorithm for management of patients with HCC is not straightforward and a multidisciplinary approach offers appropriate guidance from different experts in the field. Gastroenterologists, hepatologists, surgical oncologists, transplant surgeons, interventional and diagnostic radiologists, medical oncologists, radiation oncologists, and nuclear medicine physicians can all contribute to an integrative approach of this complex cancer.[53]

Most commonly performed intra-arterial therapies for HCC include transcatheter arterial chemoembolization with ethiodized oil (TACE), chemoembolization with drug-eluting beads (DEB-TACE), intra-arterial embolization (transarterial embolization [TAE]), and radioembolization with yttrium-90 microspheres. This chapter focuses on the use of these arterial directed therapies for HCC, including patient selection, techniques, and follow-up and clinical outcomes.

TRANSCATHETER ARTERIAL CHEMOEMBOLIZATION

Background

TACE with ethiodized oil (Lipiodol, Ultrafluide, Guerbet) for treatment of unresectable HCC was originally introduced in the 1980s.[54,55] TACE emerged as standard of care for unresectable HCC almost a decade ago, when two RCTs and a meta-analysis demonstrated a significant survival benefit in patients undergoing this procedure versus best supportive care.[56–58] Although years ago there were major discrepancies and heterogeneity in patients' selection and therapeutic algorithm, the current patient selection criteria, the indications for TACE, and the treatment protocols are better defined. The optimal population for TACE has been identified as BCLC B patients, and the technique has been improved.[59] Several areas of uncertainty exist as to which is the best embolic and/or chemotherapeutic agent, or what is the best follow-up and re-treatment strategy and to which extent TACE can be combined with other therapies. Many current clinical trials will most likely generate answers to these questions and further improve HCC patient outcomes.

Patient Selection

TACE with ethiodized oil, often referred to as oily chemoembolization, can be employed either for palliation of unresectable HCC or as an adjunctive therapy to liver resection or as a bridge to liver transplantation.[52,60,61] An important aspect in the selection of patients is the presence of adequate liver function. In patients with advanced liver disease (Child-Pugh C cirrhosis), treatment-induced liver failure may offset any potential benefit of the intervention. Predictors of outcome are related to tumor burden (tumor size, vascular invasion, and AFP levels), liver functional impairment (Child-Pugh, bilirubin, ascites), performance status (Karnofsky index, Eastern Cooperative Oncology Group [ECOG]), and response to treatment. The best candidates are asymptomatic patients with preserved liver function (Child-Pugh A or B cirrhosis) and with tumors that have not invaded the portal vein or metastasized beyond the liver.

Current absolute contraindications for TACE now include intractable systemic infection and extensive hepatic disease (Child-Pugh C). Relative contraindications include tumor resectability, serum bilirubin greater than 2 mg/dL, lactate dehydrogenase greater than 425 units/L, aspartate aminotransferase greater than 100 units/L, tumor burden involving more than 50% of the liver, presence of extrahepatic metastases, poor performance status, cardiac or renal insufficiency, ascites, encephalopathy, recent variceal bleeding, or significant thrombocytopenia, intractable arteriovenous fistula, surgical portocaval anastomosis, absence of hepatopedal blood flow and severe portal vein thrombosis (PVT), and tumor invasion to the inferior vena cava (IVC) and right atrium. PVT should not be considered a contraindication to TACE. In patients with PVT, the most important prognostic factor associated with improved survival is the Child-Pugh numerical score.[62] In cases of portal vein tumoral thrombosis, supraselective TACE can be performed if hepatopedal collateral flow is present.[51]

Transcatheter Arterial Chemoembolization Regimen

TACE involves the intra-arterial injection of a mixture of chemotherapeutic agent(s) with ethiodized oil, followed by arterial embolization of the tumor feeding vessel(s). The arterial embolization at the end of the procedure has two aims: (a) to induce tumor ischemia and subsequent tumor necrosis by reducing blood flow to the targeted tumor, and (b) to increase dwell time of injected cytotoxic agents in the tumor vicinity. Although complete arterial stasis is a valid endpoint for any embolization procedure, some residual antegrade flow, indicating patency of the tumor-feeding artery, at the end of TACE is desired and has been associated with improved survival benefit in patients with unresectable HCC.[4,63] Next we describe an overview of the most commonly administered components of TACE.

▌ ETHIODIZED OIL

Ethiodized or iodized oil (Lipiodol, Guerbet) is an iodinated ester derived from poppy seed oil that can be selectively taken up and retained by primary HCC and hepatic metastases. Ethiodized oil may carry both hydrophobic and hydrophilic chemotherapeutic agents and distally embolize small vessels. In contrast to its selective accumulation inside a tumor, when injected into the hepatic artery of nontumorous hepatic parenchyma, ethiodized oil is gradually cleared to the systemic circulation via the hepatic sinusoids or via phagocytosis by Kupffer cells. A single or multiple chemotherapeutic agents can be mixed with ethiodized oil through the use of a pumping method to prepare an emulsion. The stability, pharmacokinetics, and physical properties of ethiodized oil-chemotherapy mixture depend largely on the method of emulsion before injection. The stability of the emulsion can be influenced by the volume ratio between ethiodized oil and the contrast medium used to dissolve the chemotherapy, leading to higher stability for ethiodized oil and contrast medium when mixed at a ratio of 2 to 4:1.[54] When the volume of injected ethiodized oil is larger than the volume of contrast medium, the final end product is a water-in-oil emulsion with increased tumor uptake and less uptake by the lungs, compared to an oil-in-water-type emulsion. It is assumed that improved pharmacokinetic outcomes of TACE can be obtained by adjusting the mixing volume of ethiodized oil and doxorubicin to a 2 to 3:1 ratio (lipiodol/doxorubicin solution). Moreover, additional embolization with gelfoam has been shown to lead to minimal systemic drug toxicity.[64] Additionally, lipiodol microdroplets may reach the peritumoral portal veins, which cannot be targeted via embolization with microspheres, further enhancing the tumoricidal effect of the accompanying chemotherapy. Even though the use of lipiodol in TACE has been challenged over the past 5 years, there is substantial evidence confirming its efficacy.[65] Lipiodol is still widely adopted in TACE protocols.

▌ CHEMOTHERAPEUTIC AGENTS

Despite a long track of clinical research, the types and dosages of chemotherapeutic agents delivered during TACE have not been standardized.[65] To date, the most commonly used single chemotherapeutic drug worldwide is doxorubicin (36%), followed by cisplatin (31%) and epirubicin/doxorubicin (12%).[65] In the United States, the combination of 50 mg doxorubicin, 100 mg cisplatin, and 10 mg mitomycin C is the commonest drug combination administered during TACE.[66] This combination was first successfully tested in the 1990s in a phase I/II study of 51 patients with unresectable HCC.[67] In Japan, epirubicin (74%) is the most commonly used drug, followed by doxorubicin (9%), mitomycin C (9%), cisplatin (4%), and zinostatin stimalamer (SMANCS, 4%), primarily because the National Insurance System does not cover doxorubicin. Recently, another novel lipophilic cisplatin derivative has been commercially available in Japan, miriplatin, which mixes well with lipiodol and is released gradually to tumor cells.[68,69] All of these drugs exhibit preferential extraction when delivered intrahepatically, and they can achieve favorable tumor drug concentration with concurrent low systematic drug load. There is currently no clear evidence of advantageous properties of one agent over another and it is highly unlikely that, in the future, such evidence will be generated from RCTs.

▌ EMBOLIC MATERIALS

The intended purpose of intra-arterial embolization following the intra-arterial injection of chemotherapy is twofold: to prevent washout of the drug at the site of the tumor and to induce ischemic necrosis. This is achieved by injecting embolic materials into the targeted tumor feeding vessel(s) following the intra-arterial injection of lipiodol and chemotherapy. Several types of embolic agents have been utilized in conjunction with lipiodol for chemoembolization, including gelfoam powder and pledgets, polyvinyl alcohol (PVA), and starch microspheres or embospheres.

Gelatin bioabsorbable embolic agents, in the form of gelfoam sponge, pledgets, cubes, or powder, have been extensively used as an embolic agent for TACE. Gelatin sponge leads to transient blood vessel obstruction and is absorbed within 48 to 72 hours. Subsequent vascular recanalization occurs within 2 weeks.[70] It is one of the most commonly and currently employed material worldwide, especially in Japan.[70] Gelatin sponge causes a temporary vascular occlusion with recanalization occurring in approximately 2 weeks. When compared to powder, gelfoam sponge leads to more proximal arterial occlusion. Proximal occlusion may enhance the development of revascularization of treated lesions through recruited arterial collaterals, however, making it more difficult to re-treat patients if it becomes necessary. On the other hand, gelfoam powder can induce ischemic bile ducts necrosis. The use of gelatin sponge allows chemoembolization procedures to be repeated because it does not occlude the artery permanently, which is generally desirable.

PVA particles have been used extensively as an intravascular embolic agent for TACE.[71] PVA is a permanent, nonbiodegradable embolic agent, causing a variety of histologic responses to ischemia, from inflammatory and foreign body reactions to focal angionecrosis of the vessel wall.[72] The duration of the vascular occlusion induced by PVA is variable. Occlusions may last for several months as a result of organization of the thrombus with recanalization attributed to thrombus resorption and angioneogenesis.[72] In a study testing the effects of various embolization protocols on the injectable volume of chemotherapy and subsequent arterial patency, the type of chemoembolization protocol rather than the type of embolic material had a significant impact on the rate of arterial recanalization or arterial patency.[68]

PVA microspheres (Contour SE Microspheres, Boston Scientific, Natick, MA) and PVA hydrogel microspheres (Bead Block, Biocompatibles, Surrey, UK) are available for transcatheter use. Interestingly, compared to PVA particles, PVA microspheres have been found to cause a milder inflammatory response. Tris-acryl gel microspheres are made of synthetic, hydrophilic, and nonresorbable material. These were the first commercially available microspheres.[73] Colored and noncolored tris-acryl gelatin microspheres (Embogold and Embosphere Microspheres, Biosphere Medical, Rockland, MA) are commercially available. These microspheres are precisely calibrated, spherical, hydrophilic, microporous beads made of tris-acryl copolymer coated with gelatin. They come in a variety of sizes, ranging from 40 to 1,200 μm in diameter. Because of their smooth hydrophilic deformable surface, they tend to minimally aggregate, resulting in a lower rate of catheter occlusion and more distal penetration. When compared to PVA particles, they achieve a more distal penetration and embolization.[73] In a study comparing PVA particles and tris-acryl microspheres of similar size, the level of vascular occlusion with calibrated tris-acryl microspheres precisely correlated with particle size, where as the level of vascular occlusion with PVA particles did not.[73] Another study demonstrated that a greater number of embolized vessels were seen within the tumor tissue, compared to vessels located outside the tumor.[74] Tris-acryl gelatin microspheres have been mixed with carboplatin, mitomycin C, 5-fluorouracil, or pirarubicin for TACE, without altering their morphology and chemical properties.[75]

Technique

Next we describe the Johns Hopkins Hospital protocol, which consists of selective or supraselective TACE with the use of 50 mg doxorubicin, 100 mg cisplatin, and 10 mg of mitomycin C mixed with ethiodized oil, followed by the injection of embolic microspheres.

Following informed consent, the patient is brought to the interventional radiology suite, placed on the fluoroscopy table supine, and both groins are prepared in a sterile fashion. After peripheral venous access is obtained, hydration with 150 to 300 mL/hour of normal saline and administration of conscious sedation are initiated. Other premedications may include antiemetics, steroids, and/or antibiotic coverage for gram-negative enteric organisms. Antibiotic coverage is not universally endorsed; however, the risk of postembolization infection seems to be reduced by prolonged pre- and posttreatment antibiotic therapy. Also, pretreatment bowel preparation is not widely adopted. The procedural steps can be summarized as follows:

1. The single-wall Seldinger technique with an 18-gauge needle is used to access the right common femoral artery. A 5 French vascular sheath is then placed into the artery over a 0.035 glide wire. Under fluoroscopic guidance, a 5 French catheter (Simmons-1 or Cobra) is then used to select the superior mesenteric artery (SMA) and the celiac axis.

2. Selective SMA angiography: SMA angiography is essential to identify variant and hepatic accessory arteries (accessory or replaced hepatic artery), retrograde flow through the gastroduodenal artery (GDA), and visualize portal vein patency (FIGURES 7.3 and 7.4). Usually 30 mL of contrast agent is

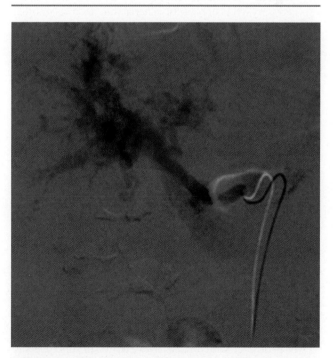

FIGURE 7.3 Digital subtraction angiographic image of a selective catheterization of the right hepatic artery with intratumoral arterioportal shunting and visualization of the portal vein during the arterial phase of intra-arterial injection of contrast medium.

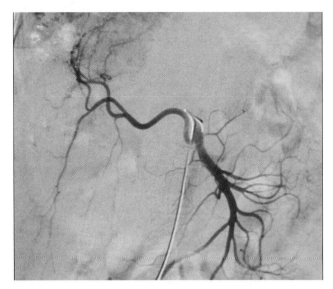

FIGURE 7.4 Digital subtraction angiographic image of a replaced right hepatic artery arising from the superior mesenteric artery.

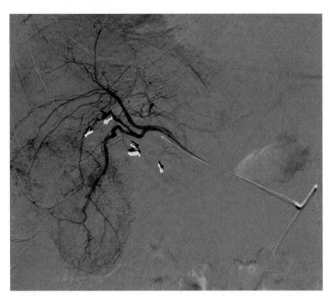

FIGURE 7.5 Digital subtraction angiographic image of a selectively catheterized right hepatic artery that feeds a hypervascular HCC tumor. Note the tumor hypervascularity, often called "tumor blush."

injected at a rate of 4 to 5 mL/second for visualization and identification of the portal vein.

3. Selective celiac angiography: This step adequately demonstrates hepatic branch anatomy, possible presence of replaced left hepatic artery, or other variant arteries. If possible, the right inferior phrenic artery should be interrogated to exclude extrahepatic collateral flow to the tumor. It is necessary that the injection rates used should balance adequate opacification of the targeted vessels without unnecessary reflux of contrast material into the aorta or other vessels proximal to the injection site. Usually, 8 to 12 mL of contrast agent is injected at a rate of 4 mL/second.

4. Selective hepatic artery angiography: Over the guide wire, the 5 French catheter is next advanced into the desired hepatic artery branch. Depending on tumor location, a selective hepatic arteriogram demonstrates the tumor "blush" (FIGURE 7.5). For evaluation of the left hepatic artery and arterial supply to hepatic segments II, III, IVA, and IVB, 4 to 8 mL of contrast agent is injected at a rate of 2 to 3 mL/second. For evaluation of the right hepatic artery and arterial supply to segments V, VI, VII, VIII, and I usually 8 to 10 mL of contrast medium is injected at a rate of 3 to 4 mL/second. The catheter should be advanced beyond the GDA (FIGURE 7.3). Special attention should be paid to identify the falciform (arising either from the middle or the left hepatic artery), phrenic, right, or accessory gastric arteries, and the supraduodenal, retroduodenal, retroportal, and cystic arteries to avoid nontarget embolization. Nontarget organ complications should be taken seriously and may include ischemic cholecystitis, splenic infarction, gastrointestinal mucosal lesions, pulmonary embolism and infarction, spinal cord injury, and ischemic skin lesions.[76–80] TACE can be performed with nonselective, selective, or supraselective catheterization of the hepatic arteries that feed a tumor. The use of microcatheters reduces vessel spasm and aids in negotiating highly tortuous vessels. In difficult cases with complex vascular anatomy, the utilization of cone beam CT

may help in minimizing procedure risks or complications and lead to a more effective tumor targeting[81] (FIGURE 7.4).

5. After the vessel of interest has been selected, a solution containing cisplatin 100 mg, doxorubicin 50 mg, and mitomycin C 10 mg in a 1:1 to 2:1 mixture with ethiodol is subsequently injected until stasis is achieved. Then, 15 to 20 mL of intra-arterial lidocaine is injected for immediate analgesia and to diminish postprocedural symptoms. This is followed by injection of 3 to 6 mL of a mixture containing tris-acryl gelatin microspheres (100 to 300 μm in size) suspended in a 1:1 ratio of contrast medium.

6. The technical endpoint of TACE is successful delivery of chemotherapy with targeted lipiodol deposition, reduction of arterial inflow to the tumor, and tumor devascularization (FIGURE 7.5). The threshold for technical success of chemoembolization is 98%.[61] Nonocclusive arterial embolization allows multiple subsequent sessions of TACE via the same hepatic arterial route and has been associated with improved OS.[4,63]

Complications

Major complications may occur in up to 10% of procedures with a 30-day mortality of approximately 1%.[61] A transient increase of liver enzymes for up to a month following the procedure is expected and has been well documented. Postembolization syndrome (PES), characterized by nausea, vomiting, abdominal pain, and fever, occurs in up to 90% of patients after the procedure and may last up to 3 days.[82] PES is thought to occur as a combination of tissue ischemia and an inflammatory response to chemoembolization or embolization.

The most common serious adverse events of TACE are liver abscess or liver infarction and cholecystitis, which occur in approximately 2% of the patients, despite antibiotic prophylaxis treatment and the absence of risk factors for abscess formation.

An intrahepatic abscess is likely to occur (30% to 80%) in patients with previous history of sphincter of Oddi dysfunction, sphincterectomy, or any type of biliary-enteric reconstructive surgery. Such patients have their biliary tree colonized by bacteria traveling freely from the gut. Because the hepatic artery also supplies the biliary plexus, the ischemic effects of TACE exacerbate the situation, trapping the bacteria within the biliary tree and causing abscess formation. Nontarget embolization (gastroduodenal, left or right gastric arteries, or other arteries) is a rare but serious complication. Variant vascular anatomy increases the risk of nontarget embolization, which may manifest as transient abdominal pain, ulcer, gastrointestinal bleeding, or ischemic mucosal necrosis.

Other possible complications include hepatic failure, main bile duct strictures, cerebral or pulmonary lipiodol embolism, or even death (1%). Hepatic failure after TACE is related to TACE-induced ischemic damage to the nontumorous liver tissue, and several risk factors have been identified including portal vein obstruction, the use of a high dose of anticancer drugs and lipiodol, a high basal level of bilirubin, a prolonged prothrombin time, and advanced Child-Pugh class. Because the definitions of TACE-induced hepatic failure vary across studies, the reported incidence of hepatic failure has varied widely from 0% to 49% with a median incidence of 8% (4). Irreversible hepatic damage has been described to occur in about 3% of patients.

Postoperative Care and Follow-Up Evaluation

After proper hemostasis is achieved, the patient is placed on patient-controlled analgesia (PCA) pump and intravenous (IV) hydration and sent to the recovery area. Frequent vital signs monitoring is only required for the first 4-hour postprocedure period, after which routine nursing checks are adequate. PRN medication should include (in addition to the morphine or fentanyl PCA) antinausea and additional pain medication for breakthrough pain. After the initial observation period, the patient is encouraged to ambulate under supervision. The use of a closure device can reduce the observation period to 2 hours.

When the patient is ambulatory, a noncontrast-enhanced CT scan of the liver is obtained to document the distribution of lipiodol in the liver and the degree of lipiodol uptake by the tumor.

Patients are advised to return for a follow-up clinical visit 4 to 6 weeks after treatment. During this visit, evaluation of liver function as well as a perfusion-diffusion magnetic resonance imaging (MRI) scan of the liver is performed. Decision to retreat is based on the combination of imaging and laboratory findings as well as the patient's performance status.

According to the World Health Organization (WHO) and the Response Evaluation Criteria in Solid Tumors (RECIST, version 1.1), reduction in tumor size is the optimal outcome of every chemoembolization. Because TACE and all other intra-arterial therapies produce tumor necrosis rather than change in tumor size within the first few months after treatment, the RECIST and WHO criteria may be inadequate or misleading in evaluating tumor response to therapy. In 2000, the European Association of the Study of the Liver (EASL) published guidelines that recommended taking into account tumor enhancement in determining tumor response to treatment. More recently, a group of experts from the American Association for the Study of Liver

Disease (AASLD) and the *Journal of the National Cancer Institute* convened to publish guidelines and formally modified the assessment of response based on the RECIST criteria according to tumor enhancement.[83] Computed tomography (CT) or MRI may adequately delineate such tumor enhancement and define tumor viability. The presence of lipiodol on CT scans after TACE may obscure tumor enhancement, however, and make image interpretation more difficult. The combination of perfusion and diffusion (diffusion-weighted imaging [DWI]) MRI can successfully overcome this limitation because lipiodol does not obscure gadolinium enhancement, and measurement of increased free water content within the tumor translates into cancerous cell death. Furthermore, diffusion MRI may prove useful in the immediate post-treatment period after TACE, when tumors are not expected to change in size despite the presence of necrosis[84] (FIGURE 7.5).

Lack of satisfactory response after the first session of TACE does not predict subsequent tumor response and repeated treatments targeting the same tumor(s) should be performed.[85] The emergence of any contraindications to TACE between consecutive procedures precludes re-treatment, thus prior to each procedure the relevant laboratory values should be obtained and the patient reevaluated.[84]

Clinical Outcomes

In 2002, two prospective randomized clinical trials showed a statistically significant survival advantage with the use of TACE versus best supportive care in selected patients with well-preserved liver functions.[56,57] Llovet et al.[56] prospectively studied the survival outcomes in patients treated with fixed interval (intention to treat) chemoembolization, embolization, and conservative measures. TACE was performed with doxorubicin (50 to 75 mg/m^2) and gelfoam in this study. The trial stopped when a statistically significant difference in OS was observed in the chemoembolization group. In a second RCT, Lo et al.[57] reported on 80 patients with unresectable HCC treated with TACE with cisplatin and gelatin sponge or supportive care and demonstrated that TACE significantly improves survival in select patients with unresectable HCC.

Since 2002, several series have been reported, confirming the efficacy of TACE.[69–72] The largest case-series (8,510 patients) of patients treated with TACE comes from Japan.[86] In this study, TACE was performed using an emulsion of lipiodol and a variety of anticancer agents (mostly epirubicin) followed by gelatin sponge particles. Median survival in this series was 34 months. Both the degree of liver damage and the tumor-node-metastasis (TNM) system proposed by the Liver Cancer Study Group of Japan demonstrated good stratification of survivals ($p = .0001$). In another recent large clinical study from Japan, 4,966 patients with HCC were treated with TACE and OS was evaluated based on tumor number, size, and liver function. Moreover, an algorithm for TACE based on liver damage, number of tumors, and tumor diameter was proposed and validated.[68] The overall median and 5-year survivals were 3.3 years and 34%, respectively. Multivariate analysis revealed that Child-Pugh class, tumor number, size, AFP, and des-gamma carboxy-prothrombin were independent predictors.

Initial meta-analyses demonstrated a survival benefit for patients treated with TACE over best supportive care.[58] One recent meta-analysis, however, stirred a lot of attention and criticism because it could not identify evidence to show that either TACE or TAE has a beneficial effect on survival in patients with unresectable HCC.[59,87] In this meta-analysis, the authors showed that additional patients might be needed to reach firm evidence to accept or refute the superiority of TAE/TACE over best supportive care. This Cochrane analysis had several controversial features, however.[59,88] It included a RCT undertaken in patients with early HCC in whom TAE (not TACE) was assessed in combination with standard treatment for those patients (ethanol or RFA). It also included a trial using absorbable gelatin powder with short follow-up. Furthermore, it excluded two trials that found improved survival because of risk of bias (according to Cochrane criteria). Finally, the Cochrane analysis had very stringent expectations for survival improvement (10%).

TACE has also been investigated as a tool for down-staging for OLT.[89–91] Overall, recent studies have described excellent post-transplantation outcomes in intermediate-advanced HCC patients after down-staging with 4-year cumulative survival rate up to 92% after down-staging. Interestingly, one study proposed that response to TACE might serve as a "biologic selection criterion" for OLT, irrespective of tumor size and number.[91] In this study, 50 patients exceeding the Milan criteria received OLT based on the criterion of objective response or minimal progression according to RECIST. Patients with objective response had a recurrence-free probability of 94.5%, which was significantly better than the 35.4% recurrence-free probability for the other patients with minimal tumor progression before OLT. The recurrence-free survival at 5 years was not significantly different between patients with tumor stage initially meeting Milan criteria and those exceeding these criteria (93.8% vs. 74.5%, respectively). In univariate and multivariate analysis, freedom from recurrence was strongly associated with response to TACE but was not influenced by the Milan criteria.

DRUG-ELUTING BEADS CHEMOEMBOLIZATION

Background

Chemoembolization with drug-eluting beads (DEB-TACE) was introduced to most interventional radiologists less than a decade ago. DEB-TACE offers simultaneous delivery of chemotherapy and embolization with sustained and controlled drug release over time.

Currently, there are two types of microspheres available for drug loading: LC Bead (DC Bead in Europe, Biocompatibles Ltd, UK) and superabsorbent polymer (SAP) QuadraSphere Microspheres (HepaSphere for Europe, Merit Medical Systems Inc, South Jordan, UT). LC Bead microspheres are nonbiodegradable microspheres comprising a PVA polymer hydrogel that has been modified by the addition of a sulfonic acid-containing component. LC Bead microspheres can be polymerized to formulate different-sized spheres, ranging in maximal diameter from 70 to 900 μm. They have received CE mark approval for the treatment of malignant hypervascular tumors and loading with doxorubicin. For DEB-TACE, the dose of doxorubicin is calculated based on either body surface (75 mg/m^2) or at a fixed dose of 150 mg per session. Precision Bead (Biocompatibles Ltd, UK) microspheres are the first factory-preloaded with doxorubicin (37.5 mg/vial) microspheres.

SAP QuadraSphere Microspheres (HepaSphere for Europe) are biocompatible, hydrophilic, absorbent, nonresorbable, acrylic copolymer microspheres, designed for hepatic arterial embolization. They can absorb fluids up to 64 times their dry state volume and subsequently expand with a rate that depends on the ionic concentration of their surrounding media. The size of dry particles ranges between 50 and 200 μm, corresponding to an expanded size range of 200 and 800 μm. The SAP microspheres can be loaded with doxorubicin, epirubicin, or cisplatin for drug delivery during DEB-TACE.[92] Initial in vitro and in vivo studies showed encouraging results, and these microspheres now have CE mark approval for TACE of HCC in combination with doxorubicin. Merit Medical has recently received 510(k) clearance for QuadraSphere Microspheres for use with doxorubicin for the treatment of primary liver cancer, and a multicenter RCT comparing DEB-TACE with SAP microspheres versus TACE is currently recruiting patients (ClinicalTrial.gov identifier: NCT01387932).

Patient Selection

DEB-TACE can be employed as a palliative option for unresectable HCC or as an adjunctive therapy to liver resection or as a bridge to liver transplantation as well as prior to or after RFA.[93–97] Drug-eluting beads in the United States may be used in trials approved by the Institutional Review Board (IRB) and Food and Drug Administration (FDA) Investigational Device Exemption (IDE).

Technique

Following, we describe the Johns Hopkins Hospital technique for DEB-TACE, which involves the injection of LC Bead microspheres (4 mL) in 1:1 ratio with contrast medium for a maximum doxorubicin dose of 150 mg:

1. Following the initial diagnostic angiographic steps of TACE for hepatic arterial characterization of the vascular anatomy and tumor vascularity, the DEBs (LC Bead, Biocompatibles Inc., Surrey, UK) that had been preloaded with 100 mg of doxorubicin in the central oncology pharmacy are suspended in equal volume of nonionic contrast medium (1:1) using a three-way stopcock and left for a few minutes to become homogeneously distributed within the syringe. This dilution is essential to avoid microsphere clustering and incontrollable tumor targeting.

2. A 2 French microcatheter is used for lobar or segmental/subsegmental positioning and DEB injection. Once the microcatheter is in place within the tumor-feeding artery, the DEBs are injected into the artery. For the segmental/subsegmental approach, the microcatheter is placed distally into the tumor-feeding vessel, ensuring sufficient forward flow. Catheter wedging should be avoided to prevent DEBs reflux. For the lobar approach, the catheter should be placed as selectively as possible in the right or left hepatic artery. Caution should be exercised in identifying the origin of the cystic artery as well as other arteries supplying flow to extrahepatic organs. If such collateral vessels are identified, they must be either embolized with coils or avoided by placing the catheter tip well beyond the origin of these vessels. Again, forward flow into the desired vessel must be maintained.[98]

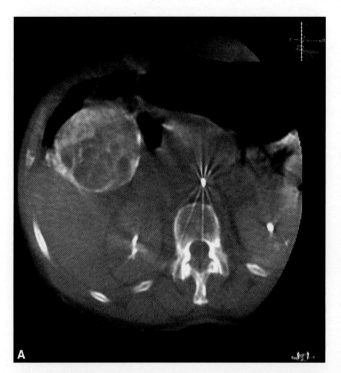 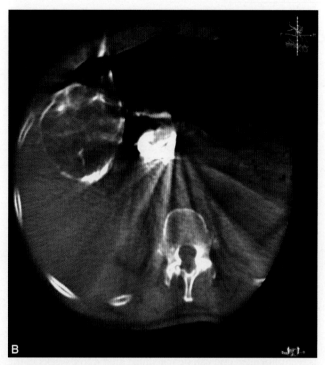

FIGURE 7.6 Cone beam CT axial images before (**A**) and after (**B**) selective chemoembolization with doxorubicin-eluting beads of a hypervascular HCC tumor with intra-arterial injection of contrast medium directly from the tumor-feeding artery (early arterial phase). Note the immediate devascularization, especially in the center of the tumor. Cone beam CT was performed using the Allura Xper FD20 angiographic system (Philips Healthcare, Best, The Netherlands), which is equipped with the XperCT option, enabling cone beam CT acquisition and volumetric image reconstruction. For each scan, the area of interest is positioned in the system isocenter, and over approximately 10 seconds, 312 projection images (30 frames per second) are acquired with the motorized C-arm covering a 200-degree clockwise arc at 20 degrees per second rotation speed.

3. The small size range of beads (100 to 300 μm) is currently preferred. The smaller size beads are thought to lead to more distal lodging, allowing, theoretically, greater delivery of drug to the tumor bed (FIGURE 7.6). DEBs (up to 4 mL) are administered by alternating injections of aliquots of the beads and contrast until complete delivery or when the blood flow of the feeding artery has slowed down substantially.

4. The injection of DEBs should be very slow. Alternating volumes of 1 mL of contrast medium to 1 mL of DEBs suspension per minute is recommended. Slow rotation of the syringe to avoid DEBs sedimentation is also recommended.

5. DEB-TACE does not involve the injection of lipiodol and does not require intra-arterial injection of lidocaine because the pain typically associated with the slow transit of the lipiodol-chemotherapy mixture through the arterial bed is not present when injecting the DEBs.

6. In our institution, substantial arterial flow reduction to the tumor is the technical endpoint, whereas complete occlusion is avoided to maintain the arterial tumor pathway for re-treatment. It is essential that forward flow exists at all times, as mentioned previously. If arterial stasis is seen before all DEBs are delivered, the injection must be stopped to avoid reflux of embolic material.

7. Intraprocedural C-arm dual-phase cone beam CT can be used immediately after DEB-TACE to verify successful tumor targeting. It has been recently demonstrated that intraprocedural C-arm dual-phase cone beam CT can predict tumor response obtained with MRI 1 month after DEB-TACE in patients with unresectable HCC.[99]

8. Repeated DEB-TACE sessions are recommended. In our institution, an average of two treatments (range: 1 to 3) per targeted tumor(s) is usually necessary to complete a DEB-TACE cycle. Regardless of the DEB-TACE protocol, it is important to ensure that the intended amount of drug be delivered to the tumor.

Complications

PES following DEB-TACE is not as intense as PES after TACE. A transient increase in liver function enzymes is commonly seen. Postprocedural increases in the liver enzymes aspartate aminotransferase (AST) and alanine aminotransferase (ALT) are less frequent in DEB-TACE compared to TACE, however. Interestingly, a recent randomized controlled study reported a 50% less increase in ALT after DEB-TACE compared to TACE and a 41% less increase in AST, similarly.[100] Cholecystitis and liver abscess may occur less frequently (2%). Periprocedural mortality is seen in less than 1% of cases with causes of mortality including myocardial infarction, progressive liver disease and failure, pulmonary embolism, and postoperative sepsis. Additional complications include mild asthenia, alopecia, hepatic infarction, pulmonary effusion, interstitial pneumonitis, gastric ulcer hemorrhage, variceal bleeding, spontaneous bacterial peritonitis, rash, and pancreatitis.[101,102]

Postoperative Care and Follow-Up Evaluation

Tumors targeted with DEB-TACE do not demonstrate lasting hyperdense changes that can obscure tumor enhancement, as seen with lipiodol. Therefore, a multiphase CT alone may adequately detect enhancement after DEB-TACE. It is important to remember that contrast medium can be retained in the tumor up to several days after bland TAE or DEB-TACE. Follow-up imaging with either CT or MR can be obtained 2 to 4 weeks after treatment to assess tumor response and to further tailor therapy. The use of the modified Response Evaluation Criteria in Solid Tumors (mRECIST) for HCC guideline for response classification can be employed for assessment of tumor response to therapy.[83] In patients with residual viable tumor, re-treatment is recommended and can be scheduled after 4 to 8 weeks in the absence of contraindications. Clinical and laboratory (including liver function tests) patient evaluation is essential before repeating treatment. In patients with complete response according to mRECIST, imaging follow-up can be scheduled every 2 to 3 months.[98]

Clinical Outcomes

DEB-TACE with doxorubicin-eluting beads (DC Beads, Biocompatibles, UK) was initially tested in a phase I/II study from China, where selected patients with unresectable HCC and Child-Pugh class A cirrhosis were treated with two sessions of DEB-TACE within 2 months interval. The phase I trial was a dose-escalating study starting from 25 to 150 mg doxorubicin in cohorts of 3 patients (total of 15 patients). No dose-limiting toxicity was observed for up to 150 mg doxorubicin, and this dose was used for 20 patients in the phase II study. The pharmacokinetic study showed a low peak plasma doxorubicin concentration (49.4 ± 23.7 ng/mL) without any evidence of systemic toxicity. Treatment-related complications were reported in 11.4% of cases with no treatment-related deaths. Among the 30 patients who completed two sessions of DEB-TACE, the partial and complete response rates were 50% and 0%, respectively, according to RECIST at 1 month after the second TACE. By mRECIST, taking into account the extent of tumor necrosis, 19 (63.3%) patients had a partial response and 2 (6.7%) had a complete response.

Following the phase I/II study from China, the BCLC reported on the efficacy of DEB-TACE in 27 Child-Pugh A patients (76% male, 59% HCV) with large/multifocal HCC. Doxorubicin dose was adjusted for bilirubin and body surface (range: 47 to 150 mg). Response rate, assessed by CT at 6 months, was 75% (66.6% on intention-to-treat). After a median follow-up of 27.6 months, 1- and 2-year survival was 92.5% and 88.9%, respectively. In a subsequent European study of 62 cirrhotic patients with single unresectable HCC,

DEB-TACE was repeated (maximum dose: 150 mg per session, 100 to 300 or 300 to 500 μm) every 3 months, for up to a total of three sessions. Overall objective response according to the EASL criteria was observed in 59.6%, 81.8%, and 70.8% across three treatments. At 9 months, an objective response was observed in 80.7%, progressive disease in 6.8%, and 12.2% showed stable disease. Severe procedure-related complications included cholecystitis and liver abscess and were seen in 3.2% of patients. The first U.S. prospective phase II study designed to evaluate safety and efficacy of DEB-TACE for unresectable HCC involved the treatment of 20 patients with preserved liver function (75% Child-Pugh A), good performance status, and rather large tumors (mean tumor size: 6.9 cm).[103] At 6-month follow-up, the disease control rate was 95% using RECIST. OS rates at 1 and 2 years were 65% and 55%, respectively; median OS was 26 months.

Complications of chemoembolization performed with DC Bead loaded with doxorubicin of diameters 100 to 300 μm and 300 to 500 μm were illustrated in a study of 237 patients.[104] Thirty-day mortality was 1.26% (3/237). Overall, grade 4 complications included irreversible liver failure and cholecystitis (5.48% of patients). Grade 2 liver function decline developed in 4.2% of patients. PES grade 1 or 2 was observed in up to 86.5%. Pleural effusion was seen in 8 patients (overall 3.37%; grade 1 in 1.8% to 3.7% across treatments; grade 3 in 0.42%). Grade 1 procedure-related laboratory pancreatitis was seen in 0.45%, and grade 2 gastrointestinal bleeding was seen in 0.84%. Procedure-associated skin erythema/grade 1 was seen in 0.84%. There was no correlation of liver failure or transient liver function deterioration with the diameter of the beads ($p = .25$ to $.37$ and $p = .14$ to $.89$, respectively). Stratifying with the diameter of the beads correlation values included: for cholecystitis ($p = .11$ to $.96$ across treatments), PES ($p = .35$ to $.83$), temporary/grade 1 elevation of liver enzymes ($p = .002$ to $.0001$), and bilirubin ($p = .04$ to $.99$).

The results from the PRECISION V trial, a prospective RCT comparing the efficacy of DEB-TACE versus TACE, were recently published.[100] A total of 212 patients were enrolled and received either TACE or DEB-TACE. DEB-TACE with doxorubicin showed a higher rate of complete response, objective response, and disease control compared with conventional TACE. Patients with Child-Pugh B, good performance status, bilobar disease, and recurrence following curative treatment benefited more significantly from the DEB-TACE procedure than they did from TACE as demonstrated by a significant increase in objective response ($p = .038$). There was a marked reduction in serious liver toxicities in patients treated with DEB-TACE.[103] Incidence rates for treatment-related complications were similar for both groups. Results about the survival benefits of each therapy were not reported in this study.

Results of a multicenter registry in Italy, using HepaSphere loaded with either doxorubicin or epirubicin for DEB-TACE in 50 patients with unresectable HCC, showed initial encouraging results.[105] No major complications occurred, except for a mild pancreatitis. PES was seen in 18% of patients. Thirty-day mortality was 0% and technical success rate was 100% with complete devascularization of the lesions at the end of all procedures. Six-month follow-up CT scans showed complete necrosis in 51.6% of patients, partial necrosis in 25.8%, and progressive disease in 22.6%.

TRANSCATHETER ARTERIAL EMBOLIZATION

Background

The anticancer effect of TAE relies on terminal arterial blockade and subsequent tumor ischemia, which, in turn, causes tumor necrosis. TAE was first described in the 1970s.[71] Several embolic agents have been used over the past four decades, such as gelatin sponge, acrylic copolymer gelatin, PVA, microspheres, or combinations of these.[106,107] Of note, TAE using microspheres is very different than TAE using absorbable gelatin sponge, large PVA, or other particles. When larger particles are used, proximal vessel blockade may induce transient ischemia and inadequate hypoxia, promoting cell survival through the expression of hypoxia-inducible factor 1. In case of severe hypoxia or anoxia, cell death can occur via a hypoxia-inducible factor 1–independent pathway.[108]

Patient Selection

In general, patients referred for TAE meet the following clinical criteria: bilirubin less than 2 mg/dL, tumor volume less than 50% of the liver volume, and the presence of a patent portal venous system.

Technique

Next we briefly describe the technique used at the Memorial Sloan-Kettering Cancer Center.[109] This technique is based on the notion that the primary effect of TACE is a result of terminal vessel ischemia rather than chemotherapy-induced cytotoxicity.[106]

Hepatic angiography is performed using a 4 or 5 French angiographic catheter to determine hepatic arterial anatomy. All vessels supplying the tumor are then catheterized as selectively as possible and embolized to stasis with PVA particles (size range: 50 to 100 μm; Cook, Bloomington, IN) and/or tris-acryl microspheres (size range: 40–120 to 100–300 μm; Embosphere, Biosphere Medical, Rockland, MA). Embolization is performed most often with the use of a microcatheter and until there is complete stasis in each vessel. Collateral vessels, such as the right phrenic artery, are also embolized. Staged procedures are performed in patients with bilobar disease or large (>10 cm) tumors.

Complications

PES consisting of pain, nausea, vomiting, and fever has been reported in up to 80% of patients, but most commonly PES does not require an extended hospital stay.[106] Splenic infarct (in combination with severely stenotic celiac axis) and transient hepatic failure have also been reported as rare complications of TAE.[106]

Postopertive Care and Follow-Up Evaluation

Postembolization tumor contrast agent retention has been shown to be a significant prognostic factor of tumor response to therapy. A postembolization noncontrast-enhanced CT scan can successfully demonstrate such retention. Like with other intra-arterial therapies, follow-up imaging with either CT or MR can be obtained 2 to 4 weeks after treatment. The use of mRECIST for HCC guideline for response classification can be employed to assess tumor response to therapy.[83]

Clinical Outcomes

Early studies on TAE reported the use of metallic coils, gelfoam (particles or powder), PVA, starch microspheres, or even autologous blood clots.[107,110–112] Metallic coils and autologous blood clots are now rarely used. Because of the unclear initial definition of TAE, many TAE studies in the 1990s and up to the beginning of 2000 included patients treated with TACE or TAE with lipiodol.[57,113–115] In studies that included a direct comparison of TAE and TACE, both procedures were shown to induce extensive tumor necrosis in more than 50% of the patients and with objective responses ranging between 16% and 60%.[57,58,107] However, an RCT that was published in 1998, comparing TAE to symptomatic treatment, reported a great antitumoral effect without difference in survival outcomes.[111]

Current data on clinical outcomes with the use of a standardized technique and contemporary embolic agents are limited for HCC. One retrospective analysis of 322 patients with HCC who underwent TAE between 1997 and 2004 was recently published.[109] Selective embolization of vessels feeding individual tumors was performed with small (in the range of 50 μm) PVA or spherical embolic particles (40 to 120 μm) intended to cause terminal vessel blockade. Repeat embolization was performed in cases of evidence of persistent viable tumor or development of new lesions. The median survival time was 21 months with 1-, 2-, and 3-year OS rates of 66%, 46%, and 33%, respectively. In patients without extrahepatic disease or portal vein involvement by tumor, the overall 1-, 2-, and 3-year survival rates increased to 84%, 66%, and 51%, respectively. Okuda stage, extrahepatic disease, diffuse disease ($\geq$5 tumors), and tumor size were independent predictors of survival on multivariate analysis. There were 90 complications (11.9%) in 75 patients, including eight deaths (2.5%), within 30 days of embolization. Interestingly, another retrospective study from this group of investigators reported that repeated TAE procedures in patients with unresectable HCC preserved patency of the hepatic arterial vasculature, despite the fact that embolization was carried out to complete stasis.[116] A recently published prospective, single center, RCT comparing DEB-TACE to TAE for unresectable HCC showed a longer time to progression (TTP) for the DEB-TACE group (p = .008); however, OS rates were not reported in this study.[117]

Bland arterial embolization has been shown to be an effective method of salvage therapy for patients with good liver function with recurrent HCC.[118] In a series of 45 patients with recurrent HCC, the median survival after TAE was 46 months with a median follow-up of 31 months. Patients who developed disease recurrence with a solitary lesion had a significantly improved survival (p = .03).

YTTRIUM-90 RADIOEMBOLIZATION FOR HEPATOCELLULAR CARCINOMA

Conventional external radiotherapy has been limited and unsatisfactory for HCC, primarily because the liver has a low irradiation tolerance.[119] The technique of radioembolization may overcome this limitation by delivering a high dose of radiation to the tumor while limiting the dose to nontumorous areas of the liver. Radioembolization combines delivery of internal radiation to the tumor with concomitant microembolization of its feeding artery. Most commonly used radioembolization materials are yttrium-90 (^{90}Y) radioactive glass or resin microspheres.

Background

^{90}Y is a pure β emitter (937 KeV), produced by bombardment of stable ^{89}Y with neutrons, that decays to stable ^{90}Zr with a half-life of 64.2 hours. The emitted electrons have an average tissue penetration of 2.5 mm (effective max 10 mm). One gigabecquerel (27 mCi) ^{90}Y/kg of tissue provides a dose of 50 Gy. The treatment of unresectable HCC with intra-arterial injection of ^{90}Y microspheres was initially approved in Canada in 1991.[120–122] Since the Humanitarian Device Exemption (HDE) was granted in 1999, the clinical application of ^{90}Y microspheres gradually expanded in the United States. Currently, there are two types of commercially available radioactive microspheres:

- ^{90}Y glass microspheres (TheraSphere, Nordion, Ottawa, Ontario, Canada)
- ^{90}Y glass resin-based microspheres (SIR-Spheres, Sirtex Medical Inc., Lake Forest, IL)

They both contain ^{90}Y as the active particle but differ in the type of carrier. ^{90}Y glass microspheres (TheraSphere) are non-biodegradable insoluble microspheres that contain ^{90}Y in an unbreakable glass matrix. TheraSphere microspheres have a mean diameter of 25 ± 10 μm and 1 mg contains between 22,000 and 73,000 microspheres. TheraSphere is supplied in 0.6 mL of sterile, pyrogen-free water contained in a 1-mL vee-bottom vial secured within a clear acrylic vial shield. TheraSphere is available in six dose sizes: 3 GBq (81 mCi), 5 GBq (135 mCi), 7 GBq (189 mCi), 10 GBq (270 mCi), 15 GBq (405 mCi), and 20 GBq (540 mCi). Each dose of ^{90}Y microspheres is supplied with an administration set that facilitates infusion of the microspheres from the dose vial (see later). The intended dose of radiation to the targeted area ranges between 125 and 150 Gy (12,500 and 15,000 rads). SIR-Spheres are biocompatible, nondegradable, resin-based ^{90}Y microspheres with a diameter of 29 to 35 μm and an average activity of 40 Bq per sphere. When compared to TheraSphere microspheres (specific activity of 2,467 Bq per glass microsphere), SIR-Spheres produce lower specific activity per sphere. SIR-Spheres were granted premarket approval by the FDA in 2002 for treating unresectable metastatic liver tumors from primary colorectal cancer with adjuvant floxuridine-based chemotherapy administered via the hepatic artery. SIR-Spheres have been evaluated for the treatment of unresectable HCC primarily in Australia, Hong Kong, and Europe.[123–125] The tissue penetration and decay characteristics of both microspheres are identical. The radioactivity of ^{90}Y delivered depends on the volume of the liver and is adjusted for shunting to the gastrointestinal tract and lungs based on estimates of flow from a ^{99}Tc-macroaggregated albumin scan. Following intra-arterial injection, TheraSphere microspheres embolize at distal the arteriolar level with increased and preferential accumulation along the vascular perimeter of a hepatic tumor.[126] Following intra-arterial hepatic injection, TheraSphere microspheres emit beta radiation that penetrates tissue a maximum effective 10 mm, thereby sparing the normal liver parenchyma beyond this limit. Radiation emission essentially ceases 10 days after the procedure, but even before that, this poses no threat to others.

Patient Selection

Patient eligibility can be determined in a multidisciplinary tumor board, consisting of interventional radiologists, medical and surgical oncologists, radiation oncologists, hepatologists, pathologists, and transplant surgeons. Pretreatment evaluation includes a routine clinical history, physical examination, complete blood count, blood biochemical analysis (including liver and renal function), and an AFP assay. Selection criteria are similar to those for TACE or DEB-TACE. Baseline clinical staging may be performed with the use of BCLC or Okuda staging system and Child-Pugh score. Functional status can be assessed by the ECOG or Karnofsky index performance status. Pretreatment imaging may include a triple-phase contrast-enhanced spiral CT scan of the abdomen, chest, and pelvis and/or contrast-enhanced MR scan of the abdomen and pelvis for identification of extrahepatic disease and calculation of tumor and liver volumes. At our institution, the standard imaging workup includes a baseline gadolinium-enhanced MRI scan of the liver and abdomen with diffusion/perfusion sequences for thoroughly assessing baseline tumor imaging characteristics and tumor staging.

Pretreatment Evaluation and Radiation Dosimetry

Unlike TACE or DEB-TACE, a pretreatment celiac and hepatic angiography is necessary for radioembolization. The purpose of this baseline angiography is to define the vascular anatomy, plan a tailored treatment, and detect possible extrahepatic shunting. Prophylactic coil embolization of the GDA and/or any other collateral vessel or gastric variant (such as the right gastric artery and its pancreaticoduodenal branches) that may result in microspheres being lodged into the gastrointestinal area is of no clinical consequence and highly recommended. Nontargeted delivery of ^{90}Y microspheres to the gastrointestinal tract may cause substantial morbidity. Exception to the recommendation for GDA embolization is the injection of radioactive microspheres either at the right or the left hepatic artery (lobar treatments) with the tip of the catheter placed very distally from the origin of the GDA.

Collateral or accessory tumor supply should also be readily identified because multiple injections may be necessary and the amount of radioactivity contributed by the injection from each vessel must be calculated respectively. For instance, a patient with an accessory right hepatic artery may receive three treatments (left hepatic [segments II to IV], right hepatic [segments V/VIII], and accessory right hepatic [segments VI/VII]). Direct arteriovenous intratumoral shunting is common in HCC, and ^{90}Y microspheres may shunt to the lungs, resulting in radiation-induced pneumonitis with significant morbidity and possible mortality when the total lung dose approaches 30 to 50 Gy. Therefore, baseline assessment of the degree of shunting to the lungs is essential. A ^{99m}Tc-macroaggregated albumin (^{99m}Tc-MAA) scan is performed after injecting ^{99m}Tc-MAA through the relevant hepatic artery (where treatment will be targeted) during the pretreatment angiography to calculate the percentage of radiation that might escape to the lungs. The size of these albumin microspheres is 30 to 50 μm, which closely resembles the size of ^{90}Y microspheres, and, therefore, their injection may be similar to the distribution of ^{90}Y microspheres. If activity is noted in the lungs, a shunt fraction is calculated as the ratio of the lung counts to the total counts. ^{99m}Tc-MAA scans cannot effectively demonstrate flow to the gastrointestinal tract and this drawback has been attributed to the much lower density of the MAA particles (approximately 1.3 g/cm^{-3}) than that of the glass microspheres (3.7 g/cm^{-3}). Overall, ^{99m}Tc-MAA provides a better simulation for the resin type of microspheres (density 1.6 g/cm^{-3}) rather than the glass type.

The radiation dose to the lungs can be estimated by assuming a uniform microsphere distribution according the following formula:

$$\text{Radiation dose (Gy)} = \frac{\text{Activity (GBq)} \times \text{Lung shunt fraction} \times 50}{\text{Mass of lungs (kg)}}$$

Total lung mass, including blood, is assumed to be 1 kg. The lung shunt fraction (LSF) is based on the ^{99m}Tc-MAA images and is calculated as:

$$\text{LSF} = \frac{\text{Number of counts in the lungs}}{\text{Number of counts in the lungs + the number of counts in the liver}}$$

Patients in whom the hepatopulmonary shunt fraction is greater than 10% of the injected dose with glass microspheres and greater than 20% with resin-based microspheres or in whom the shunt fraction indicates potential exposure of the lung to an absorbed radiation dose of more than 30 Gy should not be considered for treatment with ^{90}Y microspheres.

The final amount of radioactivity to be delivered to the tumor site is calculated by measuring the liver volume on cross-sectional imaging (CT and/or MRI). For maximal effect on the tumors, a dose of 100 to 150 Gy should be delivered to either lobe. Therefore, calculations of dose are based on the assumptions of a nominal target dose of 150 Gy/kg and a uniform distribution of microspheres throughout the liver volume. It is important to keep in mind that the dose is based on liver volume rather than tumor volume. The amount of radioactivity required to deliver the desired dose to the liver is calculated by using the following formula:

$$\text{Treatment activity required (GBq)} = \frac{\text{Desired dose (Gy)} \times \text{liver mass (kg)}}{50}$$

The liver mass is determined by measuring liver volume (mL) and using a conversion factor of 1.03 g/mL.

Calculation of the liver dose (Gy) delivered after injection is provided by the following formula:

$$\text{Injected dose (Gy)} = \frac{50 \times \text{Injected activity (GBq)} \times [1\text{-F*}]}{\text{Liver mass (kg)}}$$

*F is the fraction of injected activity localizing in the lungs, as measured by ^{99m}Tc-MAA SPECT. The upper limit of injected activity shunted to the lungs is F × A = 0.61 GBq.

Percentage of dose delivered to the patient can be calculated based on ion-chamber radiation detector measurements of the dose prior to administration, compared to measurements of the waste after administration. Before administration the acrylic shield containing the dose is measured at a distance of 30 cm from the detector. After administration the waste container inside the beta shield is measured at a distance of 30 cm from the detector at four rotational positions and these four measurements are averaged. The percentage of dose delivered to the patient can be calculated using the following equation:

$$\text{Percentage of dose delivered (\%)} = \frac{1 - \text{Waste measurement after administration}}{\text{Vial measurement befor administration}} \times 100 \text{ dose}$$

Note that the calculation of the dose to be delivered with the ^{90}Y resin microspheres is based on the extent of tumor involvement in the liver volume rather than on the assumption of a uniform distribution of radioactivity within the treated area. Two methods are currently used to calculate the actual dose with resin microspheres: the body surface area (BSA) method and an empirical one. The empirical method utilizes the percentage of liver tumor involvement to calculate the recommended dose and this dose can further be decreased, depending on the degree of arterioportal shunting on the ^{99m}Tc-MAA scan. According to the BSA method, the dose may be based on the BSA and the percentage of tumor involvement of the liver. The BSA is calculated in square meters as: $\text{BSA} = 0.20247 \times h^{0.725} \times w^{0.425}$, where h is height in meters and w is weight in kilograms. The percentage of tumor involvement of the liver (TI) is calculated as $\text{TI} = (\text{TV} \times 100)/(\text{TV} + \text{LV})$, where TV is the volume of the tumor and LV is the volume of the liver. The dose, then, may be calculated by using the following equation:

$$A_{\text{resin}} = (\text{BSA} - 0.2) + \left(\frac{\text{TI}}{100}\right)$$

where A_{resin} is the activity of the ^{90}Y content of the resin microspheres (in gigabecquerels).

Contraindications

^{90}Y microsphere radioembolization is contraindicated in patients with:

- Other concurrent malignancy
- Contraindications for arterial catheterization (vascular and bleeding abnormalities)
- Severe liver dysfunction (Child-Pugh C cirrhosis)
- Pulmonary insufficiency
- History of prior external beam radiation
- Evidence of any uncorrectable flow to the gastrointestinal tract
- Predicted risk of greater than 30 Gy (0.61 GBq; 16.5 mCi) from a single treatment or an accumulated dose of 50 Gy to be delivered to the lungs
- ECOG status greater than 2, or Karnofsky index performance status less than 60%

Pretreatment high risk factors include:

- Infiltrative type of tumor
- Tumor volume replacing at least 50% of hepatic parenchyma
- Serum albumin level less than 3 g/dL
- AST or ALT greater than 5 times the upper normal limit (UNL)
- Bilirubin greater than 2 mg/dL

Radioembolization with ^{90}Y microspheres can be used safely in patients with portal thrombosis of the first-order portal branches.[127] Prior intra-arterial therapy or systemic chemotherapy is not considered a contraindication to radioembolization. Radioembolization with ⁹⁰Y microspheres is currently tested either alone or in combination with sorafenib.

Technique

The catheterization set and delivery kit used for radioembolization should be carefully assembled because any error during the setup may lead to misadministration. It is very important to ensure that the connections to the saline bag, syringe, and inlet and outlet lines are tight so that the system is sealed and can maintain a constant pressure.

⁹⁰Y microspheres can be delivered through the hepatic artery of a segment or a lobe, depending on the distribution of HCC, making this approach suitable for focal and diffuse HCC as well as for patients with prior hepatectomy. Next we describe the radioembolization protocol with TheraSphere used at Johns Hopkins Hospital:

1. Following informed consent, access is achieved into the right (or left) common femoral artery, and an aortogram and celiac and superior mesenteric arteriograms are performed to delineate the vascular supply to the tumor and select the relevant feeding artery.

2. Like with TACE and DEB-TACE, the superior mesenteric arteriogram is carried well into the venous phase to check for patency of the portal vein. Anatomic variants, such as an accessory and/or replaced hepatic artery or a common origin of the left hepatic and left gastric artery, are commonly seen (up to 20% to 30%) and may become complicating factors because they increase the risk of nontarget embolization (FIGURE 7.7). Prophylactic coil embolization of these vessels should be considered if ⁹⁰Y microsphere treatment cannot be given safely.

3. After the catheter is positioned within the hepatic artery corresponding to the desired treatment target area, the ⁹⁰Y microspheres can be safely delivered. The use of a microcatheter is not encouraged because it may lead to excessive outflow resistance during injection, preventing adequate flow rates and particle suspension. Excessive resistance to flow in the administration system due to a smaller catheter diameter may additionally cause microspheres to be retained in the blue stopcock of the administration set and in the catheter.

4. The catheter should not occlude the vessel in which it is placed. Given the small volume of microspheres contained in a given dose of TheraSphere, the volume of saline solution required to infuse a vial of TheraSphere is around 20 mL and most of the microspheres have been infused after the first 20 mL of saline solution.[128] Radiation monitoring of the TheraSphere administration set and catheter must be used to verify when optimal delivery has been achieved. Radiation safety is always of utmost importance. Areas of increased vulnerability are the eyes, skin, and hands. Beta radiation from ⁹⁰Y can typically travel more than a meter in air but is substantially reduced by less than a centimeter of acrylic. Throughout the administration procedure, the ⁹⁰Y glass microspheres dose vial remains sealed within the clear acrylic vial shield in which it is supplied. Although the dose vial is shielded in acrylic, the outlet line and catheter are not. Typical surface radiation dose rates measured from patients are 4 to 12 mrem/hour. These dose ranges are well within the accepted radiation levels for outpatient radiation treatments, and no special precaution is necessary for either inpatients or outpatients.

Complications and Adverse Effects

The postradioembolization syndrome consists of fatigue, nausea, vomiting, anorexia, fever, abdominal discomfort, and cachexia. The most common adverse effects associated with

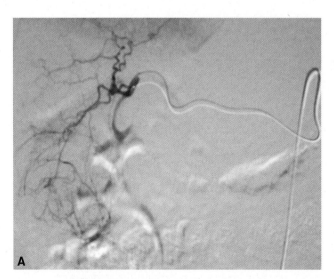 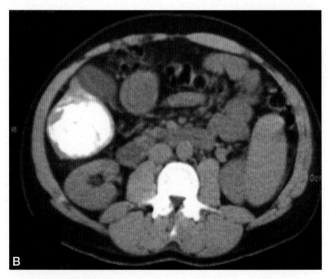

FIGURE 7.7 Digital subtraction angiographic image of a superselectively catheterized (with use of a microcatheter) tumor-feeding artery, supplying a hypervascular HCC tumor (**A**). Transcatheter chemoembolization (TACE) was subsequently performed with the use of doxorubicin, cisplatin, mitomycin C, mixed with lipiodol, followed by nonocclusive embolization with 100 to 300 μm sized microspheres. A noncontrast-enhanced CT scan of the liver was performed 24 hours following TACE, showing successful tumor targeting with homogenous intratumoral lipiodol deposition (**B**).

[90]Y microsphere treatment are elevation of bilirubin (34.7%), pain (17.4%), ascites (16.5%), hyperglycemia (16.5%), and transient elevations in liver enzyme levels (16.5%) as a result of tumor lysis with return to baseline within 2 to 3 weeks after treatment. Other adverse effects include hepatic decompensation and edema, decrease in platelet counts, gastrointestinal symptoms—including gastritis—and, occasionally, gastric and duodenal ulcerations (3.8% to 13%).[129] Most of the more serious adverse effects occur after whole-liver administration of ^{90}Y microspheres. Note that prophylactic therapy with gastric acid inhibitors on the day of treatment is highly recommended because it has resulted in a substantial reduction of associated gastrointestinal symptoms.

Postoperative Care and Follow-Up Evaluation

Following ^{90}Y microspheres embolization, patients are transferred to the recovery area for a 4- to 6-hour postangiogram observation and then to the floor for overnight admission. Mild pain and nausea may be controlled with medications and should not prevent the patients' discharge. Upon their discharge, patients are instructed on follow-up appointments, prescriptions, emergency and scheduling contact numbers, as well as radiation safety precautions. Prescripted medications include ciprofloxacin 500 mg bid × 7 days, compazine 5 to 10 mg every 8 hours as needed for nausea and vomiting, oxycodone 20 mg tablets one tablet po bid for pain, gastric acid inhibitors, and stool softeners. Mild and self-limiting liver enzyme elevation may be noted but usually is of no clinical significance. A physician assistant or research coordinator typically contacts the patients initially by phone 2 weeks after treatment. At approximately 4 to 6 weeks, the patient is asked to obtain a follow-up imaging study as well as laboratory and tumor marker tests. A brief clinical encounter is then scheduled to evaluate tumor response to treatment and assess the patient's liver function and performance status. The combination of tumor response, patient performance status, and liver function are the main factors dictating whether further treatment is necessary. Like with TACE and DEB-TACE, tumor response to treatment and tumor progression can be assessed by applying the WHO tumor response criteria,[130] the RECIST,[131] the EASL criteria,[132] and National Cancer Institute (NCI) amendments that define how to take tumor necrosis into consideration of response.[133]

Radiation-induced liver disease (RILD) usually occurs between 4 and 8 weeks after radioembolization with an incidence of up to 4%. Classic and nonclassic RILD may be seen after radioembolization. It has been shown that a single liver radiation dose of 150 Gy is associated with an increased risk of liver toxicities. The biochemical toxicity rates after radioembolization have ranged between 15% and 20%.[134]

A long-term complication of radioembolization is liver fibrosis, resulting in the contraction of the hepatic parenchyma and portal hypertension.[135] Liver fibrosis with concurrent portal hypertension is more evident radiologically rather than clinically because the clinical signs of portal hypertension, such as reduced platelet counts (<100,000/dL) or variceal bleeding, are rarely seen. This finding is more commonly seen with bilobar treatment, or in patients who had been previously treated with chemotherapy and have developed chemotherapy-associated steatohepatitis. The presence of preexisting cirrhosis leading to portal hypertension in most HCC patients makes them more susceptible to the aggravation of this complication. A long-term follow-up is therefore recommended for signs of evidence of portal hypertension.

Clinical Outcomes

In an initial U.S. multi-institutional, single arm, open-label study, patients classified as Okuda stage I and II had median OS of 628 and 384 days, respectively ($p = .02$).[136] An improved median survival was reported for a low mortality risk group of patients, compared to the high mortality risk group (hazard ratio, 6.0; 95% CI, 3.6 to 10.1; $p < .0001$).[137] Data from a European center on patients with unresectable HCC treated with ^{90}Y glass microsphere radioembolization demonstrated that the mean TTP was 10 months, whereas the median OS was 16.4 months.[138] A recent study reported similar median survival rates for radioembolization versus chemoembolization for HCC (20.5 vs. 17.4 months, respectively, $p = .232$) but with radioembolization resulting in longer TTP (13.3 months for radioembolization vs. 8.4 months for chemoembolization, $p = .046$) and less toxicity than chemoembolization.[139]

Factors predicting survival are baseline age, sex, ECOG performance status, presence of portal hypertension (but not PVT), tumor distribution, levels of bilirubin, albumin, AFP, and WHO/EASL response rate.[130] In this study, patients with thrombosis of the portal vein(s) and related segmental branches survived a median 216 days (95% CI, 126 to 423 days). Calculated from date of diagnosis, the median survival in this sample was 496 days (95% CI, 383 to 853 days).

In a retrospective study of patients exceeding the Milan criteria and treated with chemoembolization or radioembolization, radioembolization was shown to be more effective than chemoembolization for down-staging the disease to within transplant criteria.[140]

A retrospective comparison of radioembolization with chemoembolization showed that radioembolization and chemoembolization have similar effectiveness and safety profiles.[141] Similarly, another retrospective study of North American patients who had unresectable HCC concluded that both techniques are equivalent locoregional therapies for patients with unresectable HCC.[142] Another recent study comparing radioembolization to chemoembolization showed that radioembolization leads to longer TTP and less toxicity than chemoembolization with similar survival times.[139]

Radioembolization has been shown as a potential therapy bridging selected candidates to transplantation.[143] In a recent study, partial response, stable disease, and progressive disease rate in a group of 62 patients with HCC treated with ^{90}Y glass microsphere radioembolization using the conventional RECIST criteria after 3 months was 16%, 74%, and 10%, respectively.[138]

COMBINATION OF INTRA-ARTERIAL THERAPIES WITH ANTIANGIOGENIC THERAPIES

The introduction of antiangiogenic therapies, such as the multikinase inhibitor sorafenib, has recently changed the clinical management algorithm of patients with advanced HCC.[144]

Sorafenib (Nexavar, Bayer HealthCare Pharmaceuticals, Inc., Wayne, NJ) is a multikinase inhibitor that acts on vascular endothelial growth factor receptors (VEGFR-2 and VEGFR-3), platelet-derived growth factor receptor (PDGFR), c-kit, and RAF signaling, thus directly inhibiting cancer cell growth and angiogenesis. Two recent phase III trials (SHARP and Asia-Pacific Study) showed that sorafenib prolonged the survival of patients with advanced HCC.[144,145] In the SHARP trial, selected advanced HCC patients survived a median of 10.7 months.[144] These promising results boosted interest in evaluating sorafenib alone or in combination with other established treatments for HCC, such as TACE, DEB-TACE or radioembolization, and during the earlier stages of the disease. Several studies have now been published on the safety and efficacy of this combination and, not surprisingly, it seems that the schedule of sorafenib administration plays a key role in patient outcomes.

The first published, open-label phase I study of 14 patients who were treated with an uninterrupted continuous schedule of sorafenib (dose escalation from 200 to 400 mg bid) starting 7 days prior to TACE with doxorubicin (50 mg) showed that the continuous combination treatment regimen was tolerable and with an adverse event profile similar to that of sorafenib mono-therapy.[146] Another phase I study from Europe including 15 patients with primarily Child-Pugh A cirrhosis and HCC tumors of intermediate stage reported quite negative results, however, and stopped prematurely due to safety concerns, which included four TACE-related deaths.[147]

A double-blind placebo-controlled, phase III trial, conducted in Japan and South Korea, included 458 patients with unresectable HCC, Child-Pugh class A cirrhosis, and with equal or more than 25% tumor necrosis or shrinkage 1 to 3 months after one or two TACE sessions. Almost half of the patients received TACE with gelatin foam, lipiodol, and epirubicin. Patients were randomized 1:1 to sorafenib 400 mg bid or placebo and treated until progression/recurrence or unacceptable toxicity. Primary endpoint was time to radiologic progression (TTRP) and secondary endpoint was OS. The study failed to show an advantage of sorafenib over placebo with a median TTRP in the sorafenib and placebo groups of 5.4 and 3.7 months, respectively ($p = .252$). These results were attributed to the fact that 73% of patients had dose reductions and 91% had dose inter-ruptions, leading to a much lower than planned median daily dose of sorafenib (386 mg). This study was also criticized of the long delay in starting sorafenib after TACE with a median lag of 9.3 weeks between TACE and start of sorafenib therapy.[148]

In a single center randomized study that was conducted between 2007 and 2011, 62 HCV-positive patients with BCLC stage B HCC received either sorafenib (400 mg bid) or placebo 30 days after TACE.[149] TACE was performed with doxorubicin (30 mg), mitomycin C (10 mg), and 10 mL of lipiodol, followed by embolization with gelatin sponge pledgets. The median TTP was 9.2 months in the sorafenib group and 4.9 months in the placebo group (HR = 2.5; 95% CI, 1.66–7.56; $p < .001$).

The results from the first U.S. single center, single arm, prospective, phase II study on the continuous scheme of sorafenib administration combined with TACE were recently published.[150] In this study, 35 patients with unresectable HCC (mostly BCLC-stage C, Child Pugh score A) received TACE with doxorubicin-eluting beads (DEB-TACE) and sorafenib (400 mg bid). Although toxicities decreased during the second cycle, most patients experienced at least one grade 3 to 4 toxicity. Toxicities most commonly seen during the first cycle were fatigue (94%), anorexia (67%), increase in liver enzymes (64%), and dermato-logic adverse effects (48%). The combination of sorafenib and DEB-TACE was associated with a disease control rate of 95% according to RECIST and 100% according to the EASL criteria (FIGURES 7.8 to 7.11).

The results from the SPACE study (sorafenib or placebo in combination with TACE with doxorubicin-eluting beads [DEB-TACE] study), which is a global phase II randomized, double-blind, placebo-controlled study, were recently published. In this study, 307 patients with unresectable intermediate-stage HCC and Child-Pugh A cirrhosis were randomized to receive sorafenib (400 mg bid) or placebo in a continuous scheme, followed by DEB-TACE sessions.[151] All patients received DEB-TACE with 150 mg doxorubicin 3 to 7 days after the first dose of study drug and then on day 1 (±4 days) of cycles 3, 7, and 13, and every 6 cycles thereafter. Patients allowed optional DEB-TACE sessions between cycles 7 and 13 and cycles 13 and 19. There was a statistically significant advantage of sorafenib over placebo in TTP (median TTP: 169 days, HR: 0.797 [95% CI, 0.588, 1.080; $p = .072$]). There were no unexpected safety find-ings. Median treatment duration in the sorafenib and placebo groups was 4.8 and 6.3 months, respectively, and median daily dose of study drug was 566 and 791 mg, respectively.

The results from the START (Study in Asia of the Com-bination of TACE with Sorafenib in Patients with HCC) trial were recently reported.[152] In this phase II, single arm study, 166 patients (mostly hepatitis B positive) received TACE with doxorubicin (30 to 60 mg) with lipiodol and absorbable par-ticles. Sorafenib (400 mg bid) was stopped 3 days before and after TACE. TACE was performed on demand every 6 to 8 weeks and patients who were not candidates to receive further TACE continued on sorafenib monotherapy until disease progression or unacceptable toxicity occurred. The mean dose of sorafenib was 743.5 mg. The median TTP was 9 months and the median OS had not been reached at the time of the study results pre-sentation. The objective response rate was 53.8%, and 23.9% of patients experienced grade 3 adverse effects, most commonly hand-foot skin reaction (6.8%), neutropenia (6.1%), thrombo-cytopenia (3.4%), and ALT elevation (2%).

There are currently several clinical trials assessing molecular-targeting agents for intermediate and advanced HCC in com-bination with intra-arterial therapies: radioembolization and sorafenib or a combination of TACE with other agents, such as TSU-68 in phase II, or brivanib in a randomized, double-blind, multicenter phase III (BRISK TA) study.[153] Everolimus is also being tested in a phase II randomized, double-blind, multi-center Asian study with or without TACE in localized unresect-able HCC (The TRACER Study). All these global randomized control trials testing novel molecular agents with intra-arterial therapies show the drastic paradigm shift of treatment in HCC that is expected to occur within the next decade.

▌ CONCLUSION

Intra-arterial therapies for HCC have significantly evolved since their conception. Despite the technical and technologic peri-procedural advancements, their clinical success relies primarily on the appropriate patient selection. Patients most suitable for intra-arterial therapies are those with preserved liver function, limited tumor burden, and good clinical performance status.

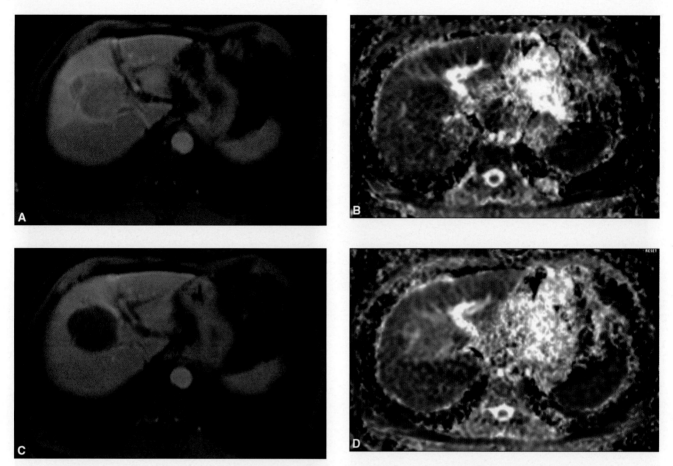

FIGURE 7.8 A. Axial T1-weighted gadolinium-enhanced MR image of the liver showing a highly vascular tumor before treatment with doxorubicin-eluting microspheres. **B.** Corresponding axial image of the apparent diffusion coefficient (ADC) map of this tumor (before treatment). **C.** Follow-up (2 months after DEB-TACE) axial T1-weighted gadolinium-enhanced MR image of the liver showing successful tumor targeting with significantly decreased enhancement after treatment with doxorubicin-eluting microspheres. **D.** Corresponding axial image of the ADC map of the treated tumor. Note the higher signal intensity of the tumor compared to **B**, signifying increased water mobility across cell membranes, which are now damaged by the cytotoxic therapy. Diffusion-weighted imaging was obtained with single-shot SE echo-planar diffusion sequences ($b = 0$ and 750 sec/mm^2).

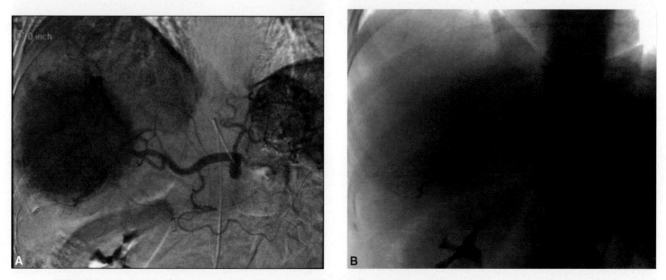

FIGURE 7.9 A. Digital subtraction angiographic image of the right hepatic artery feeding a hypervascular HCC tumor. Note the pretty significant "tumor blush." **B.** Digital subtraction angiographic image of the right hepatic artery showing minimal antegrade flow to the tumor, with almost complete devascularization of the tumor, after successful tumor targeting with doxorubicin-eluting beads (100 to 300 μm). **C.** Axial T1-weighted gadolinium-enhanced MR image of the liver showing a highly vascular tumor before treatment with doxorubicin-eluting microspheres. **D.** Follow-up (2 months after DEB-TACE) axial T1-weighted gadolinium-enhanced MR image of the liver showing successful tumor targeting with significantly decreased enhancement after treatment with doxorubicin-eluting microspheres. *(continued)*

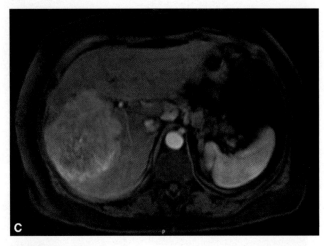

FIGURE 7.9 *(Continued)*

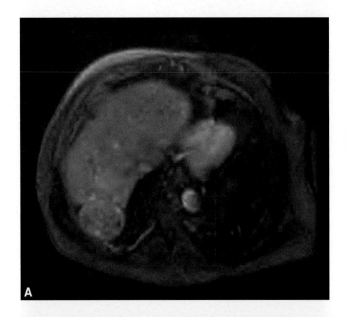

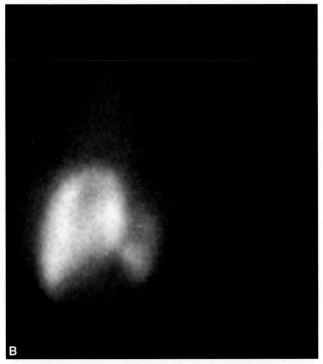

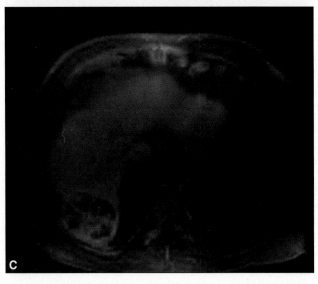

FIGURE 7.10 **A.** Axial T1-weighted gadolinium-enhanced MR image of the liver showing a highly vascular HCC tumor before treatment with yttrium-90 (^{90}Y) glass microspheres. **B.** ^{99m}Tc-macroaggregated albumin (^{99m}Tc-MAA) scan image shows minimal shunting to the lungs. This scan was performed after injecting ^{99m}Tc-MAA through the right hepatic artery during the baseline angiography to calculate the percentage of radiation that might escape to the lungs. **C.** Follow-up (2 months after treatment) axial T1-weighted gadolinium-enhanced MR image of the liver showing successful tumor targeting with decreased tumor enhancement after treatment with ^{90}Y glass microspheres.

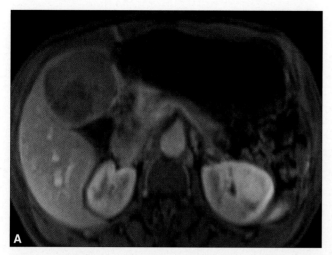 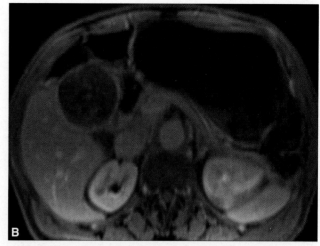

FIGURE 7.11 A. Axial T1-weighted gadolinium-enhanced MR image of the liver showing a highly vascular tumor before treatment with doxorubicin-eluting microspheres combined with sorafenib. **B.** Follow-up (2 months after DEB-TACE) axial T1-weighted gadolinium-enhanced MR image of the liver showing successful tumor targeting with decreased enhancement after treatment with doxorubicin-eluting microspheres and sorafenib. According to the RECIST criteria, there is little change in tumor size, corresponding to stable disease, whereas there is complete response according to mRECIST.

The efficacy and safety of all intra-arterial locoregional therapies for HCC additionally depend on multidisciplinary collaboration, technical expertise, and appropriate clinical follow-up and management. Current data suggest that intra-arterial therapies show clinical benefit in carefully selected patients with unresectable HCC. As new molecular targeted therapies enter the clinical arena, it is highly likely that combinations of intra-arterial and molecular therapies will be better defined and established in patients with unresectable HCC.

REFERENCES

1. Llovet JM, Di Bisceglie AM, Bruix J, et al; Panel of Experts in HCC-Design Clinical Trials. Design and endpoints of clinical trials in hepatocellular carcinoma. *J Natl Cancer Inst* 2008;100:698–711.
2. Bruix J, Sherman M; American Association for the Study of Liver Diseases. Management of hepatocellular carcinoma: an update. *Hepatology* 2011;53:1020–1022.
3. Lencioni R. Loco-regional treatment of hepatocellular carcinoma. *Hepatology* 2010;52:762–773.
4. Geschwind JF, et al. Transcatheter arterial chemoembolization of liver tumors: effects of embolization protocol on injectable volume of chemotherapy and subsequent arterial patency. *Cardiovasc Intervent Radiol* 2003;26(2):111–117.
5. Brown DB, Gould JE, Gervais DA, et al; Society of Interventional Radiology Technology Assessment Committee and the International Working Group on Image-Guided Tumor Ablation. Image-guided tumor ablation: standardization of terminology and reporting criteria. *J Vasc Interv Radiol* 2009;20(7 suppl):S377–S390.
6. Lencioni R, Crocetti L. Loco-regional treatment of hepatocellular carcinoma. *Radiology* 2012 Jan;262(1):43–58.
7. Lencioni R, Bartolozzi C, Caramella D, et al. Treatment of small hepatocellular carcinoma with percutaneous ethanol injection. Analysis of prognostic factors in 105 Western patients. *Cancer* 1995;76:1737–1746.
8. Khan KN, Yatsuhashi H, Yamasaki K, et al. Prospective analysis of risk factors for early intrahepatic recurrence of hepatocellular carcinoma following ethanol injection. *J Hepatol* 2000;32:269–278.
9. Koda M, Murawaki Y, Mitsuda A, et al. Predictive factors for intrahepatic recurrence after percutaneous ethanol injection therapy for small hepatocellular carcinoma. *Cancer* 2000;88:529–537.
10. Kuang M, Lu MD, Xie XY, et al. Percutaneous ethanol ablation of early-stage hepatocellular carcinoma by using a multi-pronged needle with single treatment session and high-dose ethanol injection. *Radiology* 2009;253:552–561.
11. Lencioni R, Crocetti L, Cioni D, et al. Single-session percutaneous ethanol ablation of early-stage hepatocellular carcinoma with a multipronged injection needle: results of a pilot clinical study. *J Vasc Interv Radiol* 2010;21:1533–1538.
12. Crocetti L, De Baere T, Lencioni R. Quality improvement guidelines for radiofrequency ablation of liver tumours. *Cardiovasc Intervent Radiol* 2010;33:11–17.
13. Lencioni R, Allgaier HP, Cioni D, et al. Small hepatocellular carcinoma in cirrhosis: randomized comparison of radiofrequency thermal ablation versus percutaneous ethanol injection. *Radiology* 2003;228:235–240.
14. Lin SM, Lin CJ, Lin CC, et al. Radiofrequency ablation improves prognosis compared with ethanol injection for hepatocellular carcinoma ≤ 4 cm. *Gastroenterology* 2004;127:1714–1723.
15. Shiina S, Teratani T, Obi S, et al. A randomized controlled trial of radiofrequency ablation versus ethanol injection for small hepatocellular carcinoma. *Gastroenterology* 2005;129:122–130.
16. Lin SM, Lin CJ, Lin CC, et al. Randomised controlled trial comparing percutaneous radiofrequency thermal ablation, percutaneous ethanol injection, and percutaneous acetic acid injection to treat hepatocellular carcinoma of 3 cm or less. *Gut* 2005;54:1151–1156.
17. Brunello F, Veltri A, Carucci P, et al. Radiofrequency ablation versus ethanol injection for early hepatocellular carcinoma: a randomized controlled trial. *Scand J Gastroenterol* 2008;43:727–735.
18. Lencioni R, Cioni D, Crocetti L, et al. Early-stage hepatocellular carcinoma in cirrhosis: long-term results of percutaneous image-guided radiofrequency ablation. *Radiology* 2005;234:961–967.
19. Orlando A, Leandro G, Olivo M, et al. Radiofrequency thermal ablation vs. percutaneous ethanol injection for small hepatocellular carcinoma in cirrhosis: meta-analysis of randomized controlled trials. *Am J Gastroenterol* 2009;104:514–524.
20. Cho YK, Kim JK, Kim MY, et al. Systematic review of randomized trials for hepatocellular carcinoma treated with percutaneous ablation therapies. *Hepatology* 2009;49:453–459.
21. Germani G, Pleguezuelo M, Gurusamy K, et al. Clinical outcomes of radiofrequency ablation, percutaneous alcohol and acetic acid injection for hepatocellular carcinoma: a meta-analysis. *J Hepatol* 2010;52:380–388.
22. Bouza C, López-Cuadrado T, Alcázar R, et al. Meta-analysis of percutaneous radiofrequency ablation versus ethanol injection in hepatocellular carcinoma. *BMC Gastroenterol* 2009;9:31.

23. Tateishi R, Shiina S, Teratani T, et al. Percutaneous radiofrequency ablation for hepatocellular carcinoma. *Cancer* 2005;103:1201–1209.

24. Choi D, Lim HK, Rhim H, et al. Percutaneous radiofrequency ablation for early-stage hepatocellular carcinoma as a first-line treatment: long-term results and prognostic factors in a large single-institution series. *Eur Radiol* 2007;17:684–692.

25. N'Kontchou G, Mahamoudi A, Aout M, et al. Radiofrequency ablation of hepatocellular carcinoma: long-term results and prognostic factors in 235 Western patients with cirrhosis. *Hepatology* 2009;50:1475–1483.

26. Chen MS, Li JQ, Zheng Y, et al. A prospective randomized trial comparing percutaneous local ablative therapy and partial hepatectomy for small hepatocellular carcinoma. *Ann Surg* 2006;243:321–328.

27. Huang J, Yan L, Cheng Z, et al. A randomized trial comparing radiofrequency ablation and surgical resection for HCC conforming to the Milan criteria. *Ann Surg* 2010;252:903–912.

28. Livraghi T, Meloni F, Di Stasi M, et al. Sustained complete response and complications rates after radiofrequency ablation of very early hepatocellular carcinoma in cirrhosis: is resection still the treatment of choice? *Hepatology* 2008;47:82–89.

29. Lu DS, Yu NC, Raman SS, et al. Radiofrequency ablation of hepatocellular carcinoma: treatment success as defined by histologic examination of the explanted liver. *Radiology* 2005;234:954–960.

30. Komorizono Y, Oketani M, Sako K, et al. Risk factors for local recurrence of small hepatocellular carcinoma tumors after a single session, single application of percutaneous radiofrequency ablation. *Cancer* 2003;97:1253–1262.

31. Kim SW, Rhim H, Park M, et al. Percutaneous radiofrequency ablation of hepatocellular carcinomas adjacent to the gallbladder with internally cooled electrodes: assessment of safety and therapeutic efficacy. *Korean J Radiol* 2009;10:366–376.

32. Llovet JM, Vilana R, Brú C, et al. Increased risk of tumor seeding after percutaneous radiofrequency ablation for single hepatocellular carcinoma. *Hepatology* 2001;33:1124–1129.

33. Teratani T, Yoshida H, Shiina S, et al. Radiofrequency ablation for hepatocellular carcinoma in so-called high-risk locations. *Hepatology* 2006;43:1101–1108.

34. Rossi S, Garbagnati F, Lencioni R, et al. Percutaneous radio-frequency thermal ablation of nonresectable hepatocellular carcinoma after occlusion of tumor blood supply. *Radiology* 2000;217:119–126.

35. Yamasaki T, Kurokawa F, Shirahashi H, et al. Percutaneous radiofrequency ablation therapy for patients with hepatocellular carcinoma during occlusion of hepatic blood flow. Comparison with standard percutaneous radiofrequency ablation therapy. *Cancer* 2002;95:2353–2360.

36. Veltri A, Moretto P, Doriguzzi A, et al. Radiofrequency thermal ablation (RFA) after transarterial chemoembolization (TACE) as a combined therapy for unresectable non-early hepatocellular carcinoma (HCC). *Eur Radiol* 2006;16:661–669.

37. Helmberger T, Dogan S, Straub G, et al. Liver resection or combined chemoembolization and radiofrequency ablation improve survival in patients with hepatocellular carcinoma. *Digestion* 2007;75:104–111.

38. Lencioni R, Crocetti L, Petruzzi P, et al. Doxorubicin-eluting bead-enhanced radiofrequency ablation of hepatocellular carcinoma: a pilot clinical study. *J Hepatol* 2008;49:217–222.

39. Zhang YJ, Liang HH, Chen MS, et al. Hepatocellular carcinoma treated with radiofrequency ablation with or without ethanol injection: a prospective randomized trial. *Radiology* 2007;244:599–607.

40. Shibata T, Iimuro Y, Yamamoto Y, et al. Small hepatocellular carcinoma: comparison of radio-frequency ablation and percutaneous microwave coagulation therapy. *Radiology* 2002;223:331–337.

41. Yu NC, Lu DS, Raman SS, et al. Hepatocellular carcinoma: microwave ablation with multiple straight and loop antenna clusters—pilot comparison with pathologic findings. *Radiology* 2006;239:269–275.

42. Pacella CM, Francica G, Di Lascio FM, et al. Long-term outcome of cirrhotic patients with early hepatocellular carcinoma treated with ultrasound-guided percutaneous laser ablation: a retrospective analysis. *J Clin Oncol* 2009;27:2615–2621.

43. Orlacchio A, Bazzocchi G, Pastorelli D, et al. Percutaneous cryoablation of small hepatocellular carcinoma with US guidance and CT monitoring: initial experience. *Cardiovasc Intervent Radiol* 2008;31:587–594.

44. Shimizu T, Sakuhara Y, Abo D, et al. Outcome of MR-guided percutaneous cryoablation for hepatocellular carcinoma. *J Hepatobiliary Pancreat Sci* 2009;16:816–823.

45. Lencioni R, Cioni D, Della Pina C, Crocetti L. Hepatocellular carcinoma: new options for image-guided ablation. *J Hepatobiliary Pancreat Sci* 2010;17:399–403.

46. Guo Y, Zhang Y, Klein R, et al. Irreversible electroporation therapy in the liver: longitudinal efficacy studies in a rat model of hepatocellular carcinoma. *Cancer Res* 2010;70:1555–1563.

47. El-Serag HB, Davila JA. Surveillance for hepatocellular carcinoma: in whom and how? *Therap Adv Gastroenterol* 2011;4(1):5–10.

48. Farazi PA, DePinho RA. Hepatocellular carcinoma pathogenesis: from genes to environment. *Nat Rev Cancer* 2006;6(9):674–687.

49. Taura N, et al. Relationship of alpha-fetoprotein levels and development of hepatocellular carcinoma in hepatitis C patients with liver cirrhosis. *Exp Ther Med* 2012;4(6):972–976.

50. Llovet JM, Bru C, Bruix J. Prognosis of hepatocellular carcinoma: the BCLC staging classification. *Semin Liver Dis* 1999;19(3):329–338.

51. Liapi E, et al. Transcatheter arterial chemoembolization: current technique and future promise. *Tech Vasc Interv Radiol* 2007;10(1):2–11.

52. Liapi E, Geschwind JF. Transcatheter and ablative therapeutic approaches for solid malignancies. *J Clin Oncol* 2007;25(8):978–986.

53. Gish RG, et al. Role of the multidisciplinary team in the diagnosis and treatment of hepatocellular carcinoma. *Expert Rev Gastroenterol Hepatol* 2012;6(2):173–185.

54. Nakamura H, et al. Transcatheter oily chemoembolization of hepatocellular carcinoma. *Radiology* 1989;170(3, pt 1):783–786.

55. Nakakuma K, et al. Studies on anticancer treatment with an oily anticancer drug injected into the ligated feeding hepatic artery for liver cancer. *Cancer* 1983;52(12):2193–2200.

56. Llovet JM, et al. Arterial embolisation or chemoembolisation versus symptomatic treatment in patients with unresectable hepatocellular carcinoma: a randomised controlled trial. *Lancet* 2002;359(9319):1734–1739.

57. Lo CM, et al. Randomized controlled trial of transarterial lipiodol chemoembolization for unresectable hepatocellular carcinoma. *Hepatology* 2002;35(5):1164–1171.

58. Llovet JM, Bruix J. Systematic review of randomized trials for unresectable hepatocellular carcinoma: chemoembolization improves survival. *Hepatology* 2003;37(2):429–442.

59. Forner A, Llovet JM, Bruix J. Hepatocellular carcinoma. *Lancet* 2012;379(9822):1245–1255.

60. Liapi E, Geschwind JF. Chemoembolization for primary and metastatic liver cancer. *Cancer J* 2010;16(2):156–162.

61. Brown DB, et al. Quality improvement guidelines for transhepatic arterial chemoembolization, embolization, and chemotherapeutic infusion for hepatic malignancy. *J Vasc Interv Radiol* 2012;23(3):287–294.

62. Georgiades CS, et al. Safety and efficacy of transarterial chemoembolization in patients with unresectable hepatocellular carcinoma and portal vein thrombosis. *J Vasc Interv Radiol* 2005;16(12):1653–1659.

63. Jin B, et al. Chemoembolization endpoints: effect on survival among patients with hepatocellular carcinoma. *AJR Am J Roentgenol* 2011;196(4):919–928.

64. Raoul JL, et al. Chemoembolization of hepatocellular carcinomas. A study of the biodistribution and pharmacokinetics of doxorubicin. *Cancer* 1992;70(3):585–590.

65. Marelli L, et al. Transarterial therapy for hepatocellular carcinoma: which technique is more effective? A systematic review of cohort and randomized studies. *Cardiovasc Intervent Radiol* 2007;30(1):6–25.

66. Gaba RC. Chemoembolization practice patterns and technical methods among interventional radiologists: results of an online survey. *AJR Am J Roentgenol* 2012;198(3):692–699.

67. Venook AP, et al. Chemoembolization for hepatocellular carcinoma. *J Clin Oncol* 1990;8(6):1108–1114.

68. Takayasu K, et al. Superselective transarterial chemoembolization for hepatocellular carcinoma. Validation of treatment algorithm proposed by Japanese guidelines. *J Hepatol* 2012;56(4):886–892.

69. Okusaka T, et al. Phase II trial of intra-arterial chemotherapy using a novel lipophilic platinum derivative (SM-11355) in patients with hepatocellular carcinoma. *Invest New Drugs* 2004;22(2):169–176.

70. Geschwind J-FH, et al. Transcatheter arterial chemoembolization of liver tumors: effects of embolization protocol on injectable volume of chemotherapy and subsequent arterial patency. *Cardiovasc Intervent Radiol* 2003;26(2):111.

71. Tadavarthy SM, et al. Therapeutic transcatheter arterial embolization. *Radiology* 1974;112(1):13–16.

72. Link DP, et al. Histopathologic appearance of arterial occlusions with hydrogel and polyvinyl alcohol embolic material in domestic swine. *J Vasc Interv Radiol* 1996;7(6):897–905.

73. Laurent A, et al. Trisacryl gelatin microspheres for therapeutic embolization, I: development and in vitro evaluation. *AJNR Am J Neuroradiol* 1996;17(3):533–540.

74. Laurent A, et al. Location of vessel occlusion of calibrated tris-acryl gelatin microspheres for tumor and arteriovenous malformation embolization. *J Vasc Interv Radiol* 2004;15(5):491–496.

75. Vallee J-N, et al. In vitro study of the compatibility of tris-acryl gelatin microspheres with various chemotherapeutic agents. *J Vasc Interv Radiol* 2003;14(5):621–628.

76. Inaba Y, et al. Right gastric artery embolization to prevent acute gastric mucosal lesions in patients undergoing repeat hepatic arterial infusion chemotherapy. *J Vasc Interv Radiol* 2001;12(8):957–963.

77. Hirakawa M, et al. Gastroduodenal lesions after transcatheter arterial chemo-embolization in patients with hepatocellular carcinoma. *Am J Gastroenterol* 1988;83(8):837–840.

78. Baysal T, et al. Supraumbilical dermal sclerosis and fat necrosis from chemoembolization of hepatocellular carcinoma. *J Vasc Interv Radiol* 1998;9(4):645–647.

79. Williams DM, et al. Hepatic falciform artery: anatomy, angiographic appearance, and clinical significance. *Radiology* 1985;156(2):339–340.

80. Lee KH, et al. Transcatheter arterial chemoembolization for hepatocellular carcinoma: anatomic and hemodynamic considerations in the hepatic artery and portal vein. *Radiographics* 2002;22(5):1077–1091.

81. Deschamps F, et al. Computed analysis of three-dimensional cone-beam computed tomography angiography for determination of tumor-feeding vessels during chemoembolization of liver tumor: a pilot study. *Cardiovasc Intervent Radiol* (2010) 33:1235–1242.

82. Leung DA, et al. Determinants of postembolization syndrome after hepatic chemoembolization. *J Vasc Interv Radiol* 2001;12(3):321–326.

83. Lencioni R, Llovet JM. Modified RECIST (mRECIST) assessment for hepatocellular carcinoma. *Semin Liver Dis* 2010;30(1):52–60.

84. Kamel IR, et al. Unresectable hepatocellular carcinoma: serial early vascular and cellular changes after transarterial chemoembolization as detected with MR imaging. *Radiology* 2009;250(2):466–473.

85. Georgiades C, et al. Lack of response after initial chemoembolization for hepatocellular carcinoma: does it predict failure of subsequent treatment? *Radiology* 2012;265(1):115–123.

86. Takayasu K, et al. Prospective cohort study of transarterial chemoembolization for unresectable hepatocellular carcinoma in 8510 patients. *Gastroenterology* 2006;131(2):461–469.

87. Oliveri RS, Wetterslev J, Gluud C. Transarterial (chemo)embolisation for unresectable hepatocellular carcinoma. *Cochrane Database Syst Rev* 2011(3):CD004787.

88. Ray CE, Jr., et al. The use of transarterial chemoembolization in the treatment of unresectable hepatocellular carcinoma: a response to the Cochrane Collaboration review of 2011. *J Vasc Interv Radiol* 2011;22(12):1693–1696.

89. Graziadei IW, et al. Chemoembolization followed by liver transplantation for hepatocellular carcinoma impedes tumor progression while on the waiting list and leads to excellent outcome. *Liver Transpl* 2003;9(6):557–563.

90. Bouchard-Fortier A, et al. Transcatheter arterial chemoembolization of hepatocellular carcinoma as a bridge to liver transplantation: a retrospective study. *Int J Hepatol* 2011;2011:974514.

91. Otto G, et al. Response to transarterial chemoembolization as a biological selection criterion for liver transplantation in hepatocellular carcinoma. *Liver Transpl* 2006;12(8):1260–1267.

92. de Luis E, et al. In vivo evaluation of a new embolic spherical particle (hepasphere) in a kidney animal model. *Cardiovasc Intervent Radiol* 2008; 31(2):367–376.

93. Aoki T, et al. Sequential preoperative arterial and portal venous embolizations in patients with hepatocellular carcinoma. *Arch Surg* 2004;139(7):766–774.

94. Llovet JM, Burroughs A, Bruix J. Hepatocellular carcinoma. *Lancet* 2003;362(9399):1907–1917.

95. Llovet JM. Treatment of hepatocellular carcinoma. *Curr Treat Options Gastroenterol* 2004;7(6):431–441.

96. Arii S, et al. Results of surgical and nonsurgical treatment for small-sized hepatocellular carcinomas: a retrospective and nationwide survey in Japan. The Liver Cancer Study Group of Japan. *Hepatology* 2000;32(6):1224–1229.

97. Livraghi T, et al. Multimodal image-guided tailored therapy of early and intermediate hepatocellular carcinoma: long-term survival in the experience of a single radiologic referral center. *Liver Transpl* 2004;10(2 suppl 1):S98–S106.

98. Lencioni R, et al. Transcatheter treatment of hepatocellular carcinoma with doxorubicin-loaded DC bead (DEBDOX): technical recommendations. *Cardiovasc Intervent Radiol* 2012;35(5):980–985.

99. Loffroy R, et al. Intraprocedural C-arm dual-phase cone-beam CT: can it be used to predict short-term response to TACE with drug-eluting beads in patients with hepatocellular carcinoma? *Radiology* 2013;266(2):636–648.

100. Lammer J, et al. Prospective randomized study of doxorubicin-eluting-bead embolization in the treatment of hepatocellular carcinoma: results of the PRECISION V study. *Cardiovasc Intervent Radiol* 2010;33(1):41–52.

101. Aladdin M, Ilyas M. Chemoembolization of hepatocellular carcinoma with drug-eluting beads complicated by interstitial pneumonitis. *Semin Intervent Radiol* 2011;28(2):218–221.

102. Liapi E, Geschwind JF. Transcatheter arterial chemoembolization for liver cancer: is it time to distinguish conventional from drug-eluting chemoembolization? *Cardiovasc Intervent Radiol* 2011;34(1):37–49.

103. Vogl TJ, et al. Liver, gastrointestinal, and cardiac toxicity in intermediate hepatocellular carcinoma treated with PRECISION TACE with drug-eluting beads: results from the PRECISION V randomized trial. *AJR Am J Roentgenol* 2011;197(4):W562–W570.

104. Malagari K, et al. Safety profile of sequential transcatheter chemoembolization with DC bead: results of 237 hepatocellular carcinoma (HCC) patients. *Cardiovasc Intervent Radiol* 2011;34(4):774–785.

105. Grosso M, et al. Transarterial chemoembolization for hepatocellular carcinoma with drug-eluting microspheres: preliminary results from an Italian multicentre study. *Cardiovasc Intervent Radiol* 2008;31(6):1141–1149.

106. Brown KT, et al. Particle embolization for hepatocellular carcinoma. *J Vasc Interv Radiol* 1998;9(5):822–828.

107. Bruix J, Sala M, Llovet JM. Chemoembolization for hepatocellular carcinoma. *Gastroenterology* 2004;127(5 suppl 1):S179–S188.

108. Papandreou I, et al. Anoxia is necessary for tumor cell toxicity caused by a low-oxygen environment. *Cancer Res* 2005;65(8):3171–3178.

109. Maluccio MA, et al. Transcatheter arterial embolization with only particles for the treatment of unresectable hepatocellular carcinoma. *J Vasc Interv Radiol* 2008;19(6):862–869.

110. Lin DY, et al. Hepatic arterial embolization in patients with unresectable hepatocellular carcinoma—a randomized controlled trial. *Gastroenterology* 1988;94(2):453–456.

111. Bruix J, et al. Transarterial embolization versus symptomatic treatment in patients with advanced hepatocellular carcinoma: results of a randomized, controlled trial in a single institution. *Hepatology* 1998;27(6):1578–1583.

112. Kwok PC, et al. A randomized clinical trial comparing autologous blood clot and gelfoam in transarterial chemoembolization for inoperable hepatocellular carcinoma. *J Hepatol* 2000;32(6):955–964.

113. Chang JM, et al. Transcatheter arterial embolization with or without cisplatin treatment of hepatocellular carcinoma. A randomized controlled study. *Cancer* 1994;74(9):2449–2453.

114. Kawai S, et al. Prospective and randomized trial of lipiodol-transcatheter arterial chemoembolization for treatment of hepatocellular carcinoma: a comparison of epirubicin and doxorubicin (second cooperative study). The Cooperative Study Group for Liver Cancer Treatment of Japan. *Semin Oncol* 1997;24(2 suppl 6):S6-38–S6-45.

115. Hatanaka Y, et al. Unresectable hepatocellular carcinoma: analysis of prognostic factors in transcatheter management. *Radiology* 1995;195(3):747–752.

116. Erinjeri JP, et al. Arterial patency after repeated hepatic artery bland particle embolization. *J Vasc Interv Radiol* 2010;21(4):522–526.

117. Malagari K, et al. Prospective randomized comparison of chemoembolization with doxorubicin-eluting beads and bland embolization with BeadBlock for hepatocellular carcinoma. *Cardiovasc Intervent Radiol* 2010;33(3):541–551.

118. Covey AM, et al. Particle embolization of recurrent hepatocellular carcinoma after hepatectomy. *Cancer* 2006;106(10):2181–2189.

119. Stillwagon GB, et al. 194 hepatocellular cancers treated by radiation and chemotherapy combinations: toxicity and response: a Radiation Therapy Oncology Group Study. *Int J Radiat Oncol Biol Phys* 1989;17(6):1223–1229.

120. Dancey JE, et al. Treatment of nonresectable hepatocellular carcinoma with intrahepatic 90Y-microspheres. *J Nucl Med* 2000;41(10):1673–1681.

121. Shepherd FA, et al. A phase I dose escalation trial of yttrium-90 microspheres in the treatment of primary hepatocellular carcinoma. *Cancer* 1992;70(9):2250–2254.

122. Lau WY, et al. Selective internal radiation therapy for nonresectable hepatocellular carcinoma with intraarterial infusion of [90]Yttrium microspheres. *Int J Radiat Oncol Biol Phys* 1998;40(3):583–592.

123. Lau WY, et al. Treatment of inoperable hepatocellular carcinoma with intrahepatic arterial yttrium-90 microspheres: a phase I and II study. *Br J Cancer* 1994;70(5):994–999.

124. Lim L, et al. Prospective study of treatment with selective internal radiation therapy spheres in patients with unresectable primary or secondary hepatic malignancies. *Intern Med J* 2005;35(4):222–227.

125. Popperl G, et al. Selective internal radiation therapy with SIR-Spheres in patients with nonresectable liver tumors. *Cancer Biother Radiopharm* 2005; 20(2):200–208.

126. Campbell AM, Bailey IH, Burton MA. Analysis of the distribution of intra-arterial microspheres in human liver following hepatic yttrium-90 microsphere therapy. *Phys Med Biol* 2000;45(4):1023–1033.

127. Salem R, et al. Use of yttrium-90 glass microspheres (TheraSphere) for the treatment of unresectable hepatocellular carcinoma in patients with portal vein thrombosis. *J Vasc Interv Radiol* 2004;15(4):335–345.

128. Salem R, Thurston KG. Radioembolization with ^{90}Yttrium microspheres: a state-of-the-art brachytherapy treatment for primary and secondary liver malignancies, part 1, technical and methodologic considerations. *J Vasc Interv Radiol* 2006;17(8):1251–1278.

129. Carretero C, et al. Gastroduodenal injury after radioembolization of hepatic tumors. *Am J Gastroenterol* 2007;102(6):1216–1220.

130. Salem R, et al. Radioembolization for hepatocellular carcinoma using yttrium-90 microspheres: a comprehensive report of long-term outcomes. *Gastroenterology* 2009;138(1):52–64.

131. Eisenhauer EA, et al. New response evaluation criteria in solid tumours: revised RECIST guideline (version 1.1). *Eur J Cancer* 2009;45(2):228–247.

132. Bruix J, et al. Clinical management of hepatocellular carcinoma. Conclusions of the Barcelona-2000 EASL conference. European Association for the Study of the Liver. *J Hepatol* 2001;35(3):421–430.

133. Llovet JM, et al. Design and endpoints of clinical trials in hepatocellular carcinoma. *J Natl Cancer Inst* 2008;100(10):698–711.

134. Sangro B, et al. Liver disease induced by radioembolization of liver tumors: description and possible risk factors. *Cancer* 2008;112(7):1538–1546.

135. Gaba RC, et al. Radiation lobectomy: preliminary findings of hepatic volumetric response to lobar yttrium-90 radioembolization. *Ann Surg Oncol* 2009;16(6):1587–1596.

136. Geschwind JF, et al. Yttrium-90 microspheres for the treatment of hepatocellular carcinoma. *Gastroenterology* 2004;127(5 suppl 1):S194–S205.

137. Goin JE, et al. Treatment of unresectable hepatocellular carcinoma with intrahepatic yttrium-90 microspheres: factors associated with liver toxicities. *J Vasc Interv Radiol* 2005;16(2):205–213.

138. Hilgard P, et al. Radioembolization with yttrium-90 glass microspheres in hepatocellular carcinoma: European experience on safety and long-term survival. *Hepatology* 2010;52(5):1741–1749.

139. Salem R, et al. Radioembolization results in longer time-to-progression and reduced toxicity compared with chemoembolization in patients with hepatocellular carcinoma. *Gastroenterology* 2011;140(2):497–507. e2.

140. Lewandowski RJ, et al. A comparative analysis of transarterial downstaging for hepatocellular carcinoma: chemoembolization versus radioembolization. *Am J Transplant* 2009;9(8):1920–1928.

141. Kooby DA, et al. Comparison of yttrium-90 radioembolization and transcatheter arterial chemoembolization for the treatment of unresectable hepatocellular carcinoma. *J Vasc Interv Radiol* 2010;21(2):224–230.

142. Carr BI, et al. Therapeutic equivalence in survival for hepatic arterial chemoembolization and yttrium 90 microsphere treatments in unresectable hepatocellular carcinoma: a two-cohort study. *Cancer* 2010;116(5): 1305–1314.

143. Kulik LM, et al. Yttrium-90 microspheres (TheraSphere) treatment of unresectable hepatocellular carcinoma: downstaging to resection, RFA and bridge to transplantation. *J Surg Oncol* 2006;94(7):572–586.

144. Llovet JM, et al. Sorafenib in advanced hepatocellular carcinoma. *N Engl J Med* 2008;359(4):378–390.

145. Cheng AL, et al. Efficacy and safety of sorafenib in patients in the Asia-Pacific region with advanced hepatocellular carcinoma: a phase III randomised, double-blind, placebo-controlled trial. *Lancet Oncol* 2009;10(1): 25–34.

146. Dufour JF, et al. Continuous administration of sorafenib in combination with transarterial chemoembolization in patients with hepatocellular carcinoma: results of a phase I study. *Oncologist* 2010;15(11): 1198–1204.

147. Sieghart W, et al. Conventional transarterial chemoembolisation in combination with sorafenib for patients with hepatocellular carcinoma: a pilot study. *Eur Radiol* 2012;22(6):1214–1223.

148. Kudo M, et al. Phase III study of sorafenib after transarterial chemoembolisation in Japanese and Korean patients with unresectable hepatocellular carcinoma. *Eur J Cancer* 2011;47(14):2117–2127.

149. Sansonno D, et al. Transarterial chemoembolization plus sorafenib: a sequential therapeutic scheme for HCV-related intermediate-stage hepatocellular carcinoma: a randomized clinical trial. *Oncologist* 2012;17(3): 359–366.

150. Pawlik TM, et al. Phase II trial of sorafenib combined with concurrent transarterial chemoembolization with drug-eluting beads for hepatocellular carcinoma. *J Clin Oncol* 2011;29(30):3960–3967.

151. Lencioni RL, et al. Sorafenib or placebo in combination with transarterial chemoembolization (TACE) with doxorubicin-eluting beads (DEBDOX) for intermediate-stage hepatocellular carcinoma (HCC): phase II, randomised, double-blind SPACE trial. In ASCO Gastrointestinal Cancers Symposium; 2012. *J Clin Oncol* 2012 *30 (Suppl. 04) LBA154*.

152. Chao YL, et al. START (Study in Asia of the combination of TACE (transcatheter arterial chemoembolization) with sorafenib in patients with hepatocellular carcinoma) Trial. Oral presentation presented at: ILCA Annual Conference; 2011.

153. Kudo M. Future treatment option for hepatocellular carcinoma: a focus on brivanib. *Dig Dis* 2011;29(3):316–320.

Colorectal Metastases: Medical Management

MARY F. MULCAHY

▍ INTRODUCTION

Colorectal cancer is the third most common cancer diagnosis in men and in woman and the third most common cause of cancer-related deaths overall in the United States. In 2013, there are expected to be 142,820 new cases of colorectal cancer diagnosed, which result in about 50,830 deaths.[1] When found at an early stage, cancer of the colon or rectum is highly curable with surgical resection and adjuvant therapy. Disease localized to the bowel is identifed in 39% of cases with a 5-year survival of 90%. Disease that has spread to regional lymph nodes is identifed in 37% of cases and demonstrates a 5-year survival of 70%. Colorectal cancer that has spread to distant sites is found 19% of the time at diagnosis with current 5-year survival of 12%. The most common site of metastases is the liver. Approximately 20% of patients diagnosed with liver-only coloreal metasteses are able to undergo surgical resection with 20% to 40% of these maintaining a long-term survival. Most patients with distant disease rely on systemic therapy to maintain control of the disease and improve survival and quality of life (QoL). The medical management of colorectal cancer metasteses has improved over the past decade with the development of multiple chemotherapy agents and active monoclonal antibodies.

▍ CLASSIFICATION OF THERAPY

Management of colorectal metastases has relied on systemic drug therapy. Agents used in the treatment of colorectal cancer fall into two categories: classic chemotherapy and tyrosine kinase inhibitors. The classic chemotherapy agents act by interfering with normal cellular functions, such as metabolism and cell division. The classic chemotherapy drugs used in the treatment of colorectal cancer include 5-fluorouracil (5-FU), irinotecan, and oxaliplatin. The tyrosine kinase inhibitors target abnormal cellular processes occurring within cancer cells. Tyrosine kinase inhibitors that have demonstrated efficacy are the vascular endothelial growth factor (VEGF) inhibitor bevacizumab, and the epidermal growth factor receptor (EGFR) inhibitors cetuximab and panitumumab. Most cases are managed by using these agents in combinations or sequentially. The regimen used will depend on physiologic considerations, toxicity considerations, and molecular characteristics of the tumor. Tumors may demonstrate de novo resistance to some of these agents and invariably develop resistance to each of them.

The activity of protein tyrosine kinases is tightly regulated because they function as mediators of cell growth, differentiation, and death. Numerous protein kinase genes have been identified as oncogenes associated with transforming retroviruses or human tumors. Protein tyrosine kinases are grouped based on structural similarities and cellular function as receptor tyrosine kinases and nonreceptor tyrosine kinases. Receptor tyrosine kinases have an extracellular and a cytoplasmic portion. The receptor tyrosine kinases include the receptors for epidermal growth factor (EGF), fibroblast growth factor (FGF), platelet-derived growth factor (PDGF), stem-cell factor (SCF), VEGF, and nerve growth factor (NGF). Nonreceptor tyrosine kinases lack receptor-like features but mediate critical cell signals of many cell surface receptors (e.g., growth factor receptor kinases, G-protein coupled receptors, B-cell receptor, T-cell receptor, and interferon gamma receptor). Protein tyrosine kinases catalyze the transfer of phosphate from adenosine triphosphate (ATP) to the hydroxyl group of a tyrosine residue in the protein substrate.

Fluoropyrimidine and Leucovorin

5-FU is a fluorinated pyrimidine and acts as an antimetabolite antineoplastic agent. It differs from the naturally occurring product, uracil, by the addition of a fluoride at position 5. 5-FU is converted to fluorinated uracil triphosphate (FUTP) through a series of normal kinase and phosphorylase enzymatic reactions. The FUTP is then incorporated into RNA and inhibits RNA activity and synthesis. 5-FU can also be converted to fluorodeoxyuridine monophosphate (FdUMP) through a different series of kinase and phosphorylase enzymatic reactions. FdUMP forms a tight, but reversible, covalent bond with thymidylate synthase (TS) in the presence of methylenetetrahydrofolate (CH_2-THF), a natural reduced folate. Binding of FdUMP to TS inhibits the formation of thymidylate from uracil. Thymidylate is the necessary precursor of thymidine triphosphate (dTTP), one of four deoxyribonucleotides required for synthesis of DNA. Thus, a deficiency of thymidylate leads to depletion of dTTP. FdUMP may be converted to fluorodeoxyuridine (FdUTP), which can be incorporated into DNA by DNA polymerase in place of dTTP. The selectivity of 5-FU for rapidly dividing cells is caused by the higher concentrations of TS in dividing cells, up to 20-fold, versus nonproliferating cells.

Leucovorin is a racemic mixture of the diastereoisomers of the 5-formyl derivative of tetrahydrofolic acid ((d,l)-5-formyltetrahydrofolate), a reduced form of folic acid. The isomers have different pharmacokinetics and activity. The biologically active component is the l-isomer and is also known as folinic acid. Folinic acid is the natural product, which on a molar basis is about twice as active as synthetic leucovorin. When given in combination with leucovorin, the DNA effects of 5-FU are enhanced through stabilization of the ternary complex of TS, FdUMP, and CH_2-THF.

5-FU may be delivered as an intravenous (IV) bolus injection, protracted infusion, oral prodrug, or hepatic artery infusion. The drug distributes widely throughout the body tissues and crosses the blood–brain barrier to a significant degree. Cerebral spinal fluid concentrations can be sustained for several hours. Fluorouracil also distributes well into ascites and pleural effusions; delayed elimination from these fluid reservoirs can prolong toxicity. A small portion of fluorouracil is converted to active metabolites (FdUMP, FUTP) in the tissues; the rest (85%) is catabolized via dihydropyrimidine dehydrogenase (DPD), the initial rate-limiting step, and other enzymes to the dihydropyrimidine form. DPD is widely distributed throughout the body including the liver, gastrointestinal (GI) mucosa, and peripheral white blood cells. The liver is the major site of 5-FU catabolism. During continuous infusion of 5-FU, however, the clearance of 5-FU exceeds liver blood flow, indicating significant extrahepatic metabolism. DPD plays a critical role in determining the amount of 5-FU available for anabolism and, therefore, may in part determine the efficacy and/or toxicity of 5-FU therapy. DPD exhibits significant interpatient variability in terms of activity. Individuals with low or nonexistent DPD activity experience severe toxicity when treated with conventional doses of 5-FU. It also appears this interpatient variability in DPD activity is responsible for the variable bioavailability following oral administration of 5-FU. Following IV administration of fluorouracil, the mean elimination half-life from plasma is 16 minutes (range: 8 to 20 minutes) and is dose dependent. In contrast to the parent compound, the intracellular nucleotides FdUMP and FUTP have prolonged half-lives. A small amount of unchanged 5-FU and primarily its metabolites are eliminated via the biliary and renal systems.

Resistance to 5-FU therapy may be caused by a variety of mechanisms due to the complex effects of 5-FU. Deletion or decreased activity of various activating enzymes, decreased availability of cofactors, competition with natural substrates (i.e., uracil triphosphate and dTTP), and increased activity of enzymes associated with the catabolism of 5-FU to inactive compounds (i.e., DPD) may all play a role in the development of chemotherapy resistance.

Adverse GI effects are common during systemic 5-FU therapy and include nausea/vomiting, diarrhea, and anorexia. Mild to moderate nausea and vomiting may be seen in up to 30% of patients, and these symptoms generally subside 2 or 3 days after cessation of therapy. Diarrhea and stomatitis are more common with constant infusions than with bolus therapy; however, both may be dose limiting regardless of administration. Life-threatening and sometimes fatal enterocolitis, dehydration, and diarrhea have occurred when high-dose 5-FU is given in combination with leucovorin, especially in elderly patients. Neutropenia, leukopenia, thrombocytopenia, and anemia can occur during systemic 5-FU therapy; however, the effects are usually reversible.

Bone marrow suppression is common with bolus 5-FU therapy and relatively uncommon with continuous infusions. Platelet and granulocyte nadirs usually occur 9 to 14 days after treatment; recovery is usually seen by day 30. Palmar-plantar erythrodysesthesia (hand and foot syndrome) occurs in roughly 24% to 40% of patients who receive an extended continuous IV infusion of 5-FU. Prolonged 5-FU infusions are more commonly associated with this syndrome than bolus injections. Hand and foot syndrome is characterized by a tingling sensation of the hands and feet when holding objects or walking, which may progress over several days. The palms and soles become symmetrically swollen with erythema and tenderness of the ends of the fingers and toes, possibly accompanied by desquamation. The syndrome will resolve over 5 to 7 days following cessation of 5-FU therapy.

Cardiotoxicity caused by systemic 5-FU therapy has been reported. Reported toxicities include angina, arrhythmias including ventricular tachycardia, cardiogenic shock, chest pain (unspecified), coronary vasospasm, electrocardiographic changes, myocardial infarction, palpitations, and sudden death. In general patients who have developed chest pain following 5-FU did so within several hours of receiving the third or fourth dose of drug. It is believed that fluorouracil causes vasospastic angina. Asymptomatic ST-T wave changes have been seen in up to 65% of monitored patients, which suggests cardiac ischemia. Continuous infusions of 5-FU, especially high doses, have been associated with an increased incidence of cardiac effects; although cardiotoxicity may occur after bolus injections as well. The chest pain responds to nitrates, calcium channel blockers, or beta blockers similar to other forms of angina. Thromboembolism, including pulmonary embolism, has also been reported with 5-FU therapy. Photosensitivity may develop following systemic or topical administration of fluorouracil, 5-FU. Skin rash (unspecified), maculopapular rash, and pruritus can develop even without sun exposure following systemic or topical 5-FU therapy.

Capecitabine is an orally administered prodrug of 5'-deoxy-5-fluorouridine (5'-DFUR), which generates 5-FU selectively in tumor cells. Diarrhea is a dose-limiting toxicity of capecitabine and occurs in roughly 50% to 57% of patients. The median time to first occurrence of grade 2 to 4 diarrhea is about 31 days (range: 1 to 322 days). Other GI side effects of capecitabine include nausea (44% to 53%), vomiting (26% to 37%), stomatitis (23% to 24%), abdominal pain (17% to 20%), constipation (9% to 15%), and dyspepsia (6% to 8%). In less than 5% of patients the following GI adverse reactions have been reported: GI obstruction, rectal bleeding, GI bleeding, esophagitis, gastritis, colitis, duodenitis, hematemesis, and necrotizing enterocolitis (typhlitis). Palmar-plantar erythrodysesthesia (hand and foot syndrome) has been reported in roughly 45% to 57% of patients receiving capecitabine therapy. In patients with either metastatic colon cancer or breast cancer receiving capecitabine 1,250 mg/m^2 PO twice daily as monotherapy, the incidence of grade 3/4 neutropenia, thrombocytopenia, and anemia was 3.2%, 1.7%, and 2.4%, respectively. Overall, the incidence of hyperbilirubinemia was 48% in colorectal cancer patients treated with capecitabine alone. Grade 3 or 4 hyperbilirubinemia (jaundice) has been reported in about 15.2% and 3.9%, respectively, of patients treated with capecitabine monotherapy in the overall clinical trial safety database. Grade 3 hyperbilirubinemia is defined as 1.5 to 3 times normal and grade 4 as greater than 3 times normal. Of 556 patients who had hepatic metastases at baseline and 309 patients without hepatic metastases at baseline, grade 3 or 4 hyperbilirubinemia occurred in 22.8% and 12.3%, respectively. Hepatic fibrosis, cholestatic hepatitis (cholestasis), and hepatitis have been reported in less than 5% of patients receiving capecitabine.

Irinotecan

Irinotecan (CPT-11) is one of many water-soluble derivatives of camptothecin (CPT), a cytotoxic plant alkaloid isolated from the Chinese tree *Camptotheca acuminata*. The activity of irinotecan is caused by the parent compound and the active metabolite 7-ethyl-10-hydroxycamptothecin (SN-38), which is about 1,000 times as potent as irinotecan. Irinotecan has activity in colorectal cancer similar to 5-FU and appears to be partially noncross resistant. All CPT analogs, including irinotecan and its metabolite SN-38, work by inhibiting topoisomerase I, a cellular enzyme involved in maintaining the topographic structure of DNA during translation, transcription, and mitosis.

Mechanisms of resistance to irinotecan include decreased conversion of irinotecan to SN-38, point mutations of topoisomerase I, reduced topoisomerase I activity, and decreased sensitivity of topoisomerase to topoisomerase inhibitors.

Irinotecan has anticholinesterase activity. Cholinergic effects including acute diarrhea appear to be caused by the parent compound alone. SN-38 does not have anticholinesterase activity at physiologic concentrations. Irinotecan is administered by IV infusion; although an oral formulation is under investigation. In plasma, both irinotecan and its active metabolite, SN-38, exist in an active lactone form and an inactive hydroxy acid anion form. The equilibrium between the two forms is pH dependent. An acid pH promotes the formation of the lactone form and a basic pH favors the hydroxy acid anion form. Plasma protein binding is roughly 30% to 68% for irinotecan, whereas SN-38 is approximately 95% bound. Both compounds are primarily bound to albumin.

Irinotecan is metabolized by carboxylesterase to SN-38 and via hepatic cytochrome P450 (CYP) 3A4 to aminopentane carboxylic acid (APC). SN-38 is further conjugated to form a glucuronide metabolite (SN-38G) by the enzyme UDP-glucuronosyl transferase 1A1 (UGT1A1). Both SN-38G and APC are 50 to 200 times less active than SN-38 in vitro and do not appear to contribute to the cytotoxic activity of irinotecan. Agents that induce CYP3A4 may increase metabolism of irinotecan to APC, however, decreasing the formation of the active metabolites. Individuals with a homozygous UGT1A1*28 allele (approximately 10% of the North American population) have a decreased ability to form the SN-38G metabolite and are, therefore, at increased risk for neutropenia.[2] Although no recommendations are available regarding testing for the UGT1A1*28 allele, laboratory tests are available. Correlation between irinotecan or SN-38 AUC (area under the concentration curve) and development of diarrhea is unclear due to conflicting study results. Excretion of irinotecan and its metabolites occurs primarily in the bile and feces and, to a lesser degree, through the kidneys. Urinary excretion of irinotecan accounts for 11% to 20% of the dose; SN-38, less than 1%; and SN-38G, 3%. It appears that SN-38 undergoes enterohepatic recirculation. The mean terminal elimination half-life is about 6 to 12 hours and 10 to 20 hours for irinotecan and SN-38, respectively.

Irinotecan and SN-38 AUC levels are higher in patients with liver metastasis and hepatic dysfunction compared to individuals with no liver metastasis or dysfunction. The effects secondary to the level increase is proportional to the degree of liver impairment, as measured by elevations in total bilirubin and transaminase concentrations. Specifically, increased neutropenia has been noted in patients with bilirubin levels greater than 1 to 2 mg/dL or elevated transaminase levels.

Hematologic adverse reactions associated with single-agent irinotecan therapy include anemia (60% to 97%), leukopenia (63% to 81%) (including lymphopenia), neutropenia (54% to 83%), and thrombocytopenia (32%); however, serious thrombocytopenia is uncommon. These adverse effects are dose limiting, dose related, and reversible.

Irinotecan therapy (single-agent or combination therapy) is associated with dose-limiting diarrhea, which occurs either early (during or within 24 hours of irinotecan administration) or late (more than 24 hours after administration). When given as a single agent, irinotecan-induced early diarrhea occurs in 43% of patients and late diarrhea occurs in 83% to 88% of patients; severe diarrhea occurred in 6% of patients with early-stage diarrhea and in 31% of patients with late-stage diarrhea. When given in combination with 5-FU and leucovorin, the incidence of early and late irinotecan-induced diarrhea is 43% and 72% to 85%, respectively. Elderly patients experienced a higher incidence of severe diarrhea than patients less than 65 years. Early diarrhea may be preceded by complaints of diaphoresis (16%) and abdominal pain/cramping (57%); however, the course is usually transient. Late diarrhea can be prolonged and life threatening and may lead to dehydration, electrolyte imbalance, or sepsis. The median time to onset of late diarrhea is 11 days following weekly administration and 5 days following 3-week regimens of irinotecan with a median duration of 3 to 7 days. It is proposed that the irinotecan metabolite, SN-38, is responsible for the late diarrhea because of biliary elimination of SN-38 and the GI metabolism of irinotecan by carboxylesterase. Irinotecan-induced nausea and vomiting usually occur during or shortly after its infusion. When given as a single agent, nausea and vomiting occur in 83% to 86% and 63% to 67% of patients, respectively. When combined with 5-FU and leucovorin, the incidence of nausea and vomiting is 67% to 80% and 45% to 60%, respectively. Regardless if irinotecan is given alone or in combination 5-FU/leucovorin, other GI adverse reactions occurring in 20% to 60% of patients include abdominal pain, anorexia, constipation, and stomatitis/mucositis.

Cholinergic symptoms including rhinitis, hypersalivation, sinus bradycardia, miosis, lacrimation, diaphoresis, flushing, and intestinal hyperstasis leading to abdominal cramping and early diarrhea may occur in some patients. If these symptoms occur, they manifest during or shortly after irinotecan infusion. These effects are thought to be related to the anticholinesterase activity of the parent compound and are expected to occur more frequently in patients receiving higher irinotecan doses. Prophylactic or therapeutic doses of atropine 0.25 to 1 mg IV or subcutaneously should be considered (unless clinically contraindicated) in patients experiencing cholinergic symptoms.

Oxaliplatin

Oxaliplatin (L-OHP) is a third-generation platinum analog. Oxaliplatin is a non–cell cycle specific, alkylating antineoplastic agent that inhibits DNA synthesis. Oxaliplatin contains a bulky carrier ligand, 1,2-diaminocyclohexane (DACH), not present in either cisplatin or carboplatin. It is the carrier ligand that determines the chemical reactivity and cytotoxicity of the platinum compound and influences the tissue distribution of the molecule. Oxaliplatin undergoes nonenzymatic conversion in blood and plasma to active derivatives via displacement of the labile oxalate ligand. Several transient reactive species are formed, including monoaquo-, monochloro-, dichloro-, and diaquo-DACH platinum, which covalently bind with various blood components or intracellular macromolecules. Potentially lethal bifunctional DNA-protein-Platinum (Pt) cross-links and inter- and intrastrand Pt-DNA cross-links are formed. Cross-links are formed between the N7 positions of two adjacent guanines (GG), adjacent adenine-guanines (AG), and guanines separated by an intervening nucleotide (GNG). These cross-links inhibit DNA replication and transcription. Cytotoxicity is cell cycle nonspecific. As compared to cisplatin, oxaliplatin produces fewer DNA cross-links and is less able to form these cross-links. Oxaliplatin is more efficient (potent) than cisplatin, however, and thus requires fewer DNA adducts to inhibit DNA chain elongation and produce cytotoxicity. Despite lower DNA reactivity than cisplatin, oxaliplatin exhibits similar or greater cytotoxicity in several human tumor cell lines. The DACH carrier ligand is thought to contribute to the enhanced cytotoxicity and lack of cross-resistance between oxaliplatin and cisplatin. The DACH ligand may also inhibit DNA repair by preventing or reducing the binding of repair proteins (e.g., the mismatch repair enzyme complex). Additionally, oxaliplatin has been shown to affect DNA integrity and induce apoptosis (programmed cell death), which may also contribute to the cytotoxicity of the drug.

Tumor cell resistance mechanisms to platinum compounds include reduced accumulation in cells, increased DNA repair mechanisms (e.g., changes in mismatch repair and enhanced replicative bypass), inactivation by conjugation with glutathione or sequestration involving metallothionine, and enhanced tolerance to platinum-DNA adducts. Changes in mismatch repair and enhanced replicative bypass do not appear to contribute to oxaliplatin resistance as compared to cisplatin or carboplatin.

Oxaliplatin is administered intravenously. Oxaliplatin undergoes rapid and extensive biotransformation in the blood, which makes pharmacokinetic monitoring of the parent or metabolite compound not feasible. Therefore, platinum pharmacokinetics rather than those of the parent compound or metabolite are discussed. In addition, the antitumor and toxic effects of oxaliplatin are caused by the platinum species present in the ultrafiltrable plasma fraction (non–protein-bound drug and biotransformation species); platinum bound to plasma proteins or erythrocytes is considered inactive. The decline of ultrafiltrable platinum levels following oxaliplatin administration is triphasic, characterized by two relatively short distribution phases (α-half-life 0.43 hour, β-half-life 16.8 hours) and a long terminal elimination phase (half-life 391 hours). As compared to cisplatin or carboplatin, oxaliplatin has a very large volume of distribution (582 L vs. 19.2 L and 17 L for cisplatin and carboplatin, respectively). This could be caused by the DACH moiety associated with oxaliplatin, which may confer some advantages in terms of enhanced tissue penetration due to altered cell membrane permeability. At the end of a 2-hour oxaliplatin infusion, roughly 15% of the administered platinum is present in the systemic circulation. The remaining 85% is rapidly distributed into tissues or is eliminated in the urine. Plasma protein binding of

platinum is irreversible and greater than 90%. The main binding proteins are albumin and gamma globulins. Platinum also binds irreversibly and accumulates (approximately twofold) in erythrocytes, where it appears to have no relevant activity. Intra-erythrocyte platinum does not act as a drug reservoir. Oxaliplatin does not undergo hepatic cytochrome P450 mediated metabolism. No hepatic enzyme-based or protein-binding–based drug interactions are predicted. Oxaliplatin appears to be cleared equally by tissue distribution and renal elimination. Renal clearance for oxaliplatin accounts for a little over half the total plasma clearance (54%); however, because tissue distribution is also important for oxaliplatin clearance, renal clearance alone is not a useful predictor of platinum exposure and toxicity after oxaliplatin administration.

The renal clearance of the ultrafiltrable platinum is significantly correlated with glomerular filtration rate (GFR). The AUC of platinum in the plasma ultrafiltrate increases as renal function decreases. The AUC (0 to 48 hours) of platinum in patients with mild (CrCl 50 to 80 mL/min), moderate (CrCl 30 to <50 mL/min), and severe (CrCl <30 mL/min) renal impairment is increased by about 60%, 140%, and 190%, respectively, compared to patients with normal renal function. In patients with renal impairment, further deterioration of renal function or increased toxicity was not reported with oxaliplatin administration.

Its activity and toxicity profiles differ from both cisplatin and carboplatin, and, thus, it lacks cross-resistance with these compounds. Oxaliplatin contains a bulky carrier ligand, DACH, not present in either cisplatin or carboplatin. Unlike cisplatin or carboplatin, it is not associated with significant renal or auditory toxicity, and hematologic toxicity is usually mild.

One type of neuropathy is an acute, reversible, primarily peripheral sensory neuropathy that occurs within hours to 1 to 2 days of dosing, resolves within 14 days, and frequently recurs with further dosing. These symptoms usually present as transient paresthesias, dysesthesia, and hypoesthesia in the hands, feet, perioral area, or throat. Jaw spasm, abnormal tongue sensation, dysarthria, ocular pain, and a feeling of chest pressure have also been observed. Acute neurosensory toxicity may be precipitated or exacerbated by exposure to cold temperatures or objects; ice should be avoided during the infusion. Also, instruct patients to avoid cold drinks and the use of ice and to cover exposed skin before exposure to cold temperature or cold objects. Prolongation of the oxaliplatin infusion time from 2 to 6 hours may mitigate acute toxicities. The second type of neuropathy is a persistent (>14 days), primarily peripheral neuropathy that is also characterized by paresthesias, dysesthesias, and hypoesthesias but may include deficits in proprioception that can interfere with daily activities (e.g., difficulty with fine motor skills, such as writing, buttoning, swallowing, and difficulty walking). Persistent neuropathy can occur without any prior acute neuropathy event. Most (80%) patients who developed grade 3 persistent neuropathy progressed from grade 1 or 2 events. The risk of developing function impairment was estimated to occur in 10% of patients receiving a cumulative oxaliplatin dose of 780 mg/m^2 and 50% at a cumulative dose of 1,170 mg/m^2.

Prevention or treatment of the neuropathies has been studied. Administering 1 g each of calcium gluconate and magnesium sulfate as a 30-minute infusion pre- and post-oxaliplatin may prevent or reduce neurotoxicity.[3] The Concept trial, a placebo-controlled study designed to assess the efficacy of calcium and magnesium in reducing oxaliplatin-induced neurotoxicity in colon cancer patients, was terminated early after an independent data monitoring committee determined that patients receiving calcium and magnesium had a significantly reduced response to chemotherapy. A subsequent central radiology review contradicted these findings, however, observing no difference in response to chemotherapy in patients receiving calcium and magnesium.[4] Gabapentin has been studied in the treatment of oxaliplatin-induced neurotoxicity. In a randomized trial, glutathione ($1,500$ mg/m^2 IV prior to oxaliplatin) demonstrated a protective effect against neuropathy without adversely affecting the efficacy of oxaliplatin. After 8 cycles, 9 of 21 patients treated with glutathione and 15 of 19 placebo patients developed neurotoxicity; grade 2 to 4 neurotoxicity was seen in 2 glutathione and 11 placebo patients.[5]

Hematologic adverse reactions were common during clinical trials of oxaliplatin plus 5-FU and leucovorin (LV). Thrombocytopenia (64% to 77%) occurred frequently. The incidence of grade 3/4 thrombocytopenia was 2% to 5% in patients with advanced colorectal cancer and about 2% in adjuvant therapy of colorectal cancer. Grade 3/4 hemorrhagic events (e.g., GI bleeding, hematuria, and epistaxis) were higher in those patients receiving oxaliplatin combination therapy as compared to 5-FU/LV in clinical trials. In the adjuvant trial, two patients died due to intracranial bleeding. Grade 3/4 GI bleeding was reported in 0.2% of adjuvant patients receiving oxaliplatin combination therapy. In previously untreated patients, the incidence of epistaxis was 10% in patients receiving oxaliplatin/5-FU/LV (range: 9% to 16% in all trials). Neutropenia occurred in 73% to 81% of patients with advanced colorectal cancer treated with oxaliplatin and infusional 5-FU/LV. Grade 3 and 4 neutropenia was reported in 35% and 18%, respectively, of previously untreated patients, and in 27% and 17%, respectively, of previously untreated patients. Neutropenia was commonly reported in patients receiving oxaliplatin/5-FU/LV as colorectal cancer adjuvant therapy with Grade 3 and 4 events reported in 29% and 12% of patients, respectively. The incidence of febrile neutropenia was 1% in previously treated patients receiving infusional 5-FU/LV arm compared to 6% in previously treated patients receiving oxaliplatin/5-FU/LV. In previously untreated patients, the incidence of febrile neutropenia was 4% in those receiving oxaliplatin/5-FU/LV as compared to 15% in patients receiving irinotecan/5-FU/LV. In the adjuvant trial, the incidence of febrile neutropenia was 0.7%. A higher incidence of anemia was reported in previously treated patients (81%, grade 3/4 2%) versus previously untreated patients (27%, grade 3/4 3%) receiving oxaliplatin/5-FU/LV. During the adjuvant therapy of colorectal cancer trial, anemia was reported in 76% (grade 3/4 1%) of patients treated with oxaliplatin/5-FU/LV. Leukopenia (76% to 85%, grade 3/4 19% to 20%) was reported in patients receiving oxaliplatin/5-FU/LV but was reported as greater than or equal to 2% to less than 5% in the adjuvant trial. The incidence of thromboembolism was 6% and 9% of patients previously untreated for advanced colorectal cancer and previously treated, respectively, receiving oxaliplatin/5-FU/LV. In patients receiving adjuvant therapy for colon cancer, the incidence of thromboembolism was 6% (1.8% grade 3/4) in the infusional 5-FU/LV arm and 6% (1.2% grade 3/4) in the oxaliplatin/5-FU/LV arm. Other hematologic adverse events reported include lymphopenia (6%), altered prothrombin time ($\geq$2% to <5%), rectal or vaginal hemorrhage ($\geq$2% to <5%), hemoptysis ($\geq$2% to <5%),

and melena ($\geq$2% to <5%). There have been reports both in clinical trials and from postmarketing reports of prolonged prothrombin time and international normalized ratio (INR) occasionally associated with hemorrhage in patients who received oxaliplatin/5-FU/LV while receiving anticoagulants. Hemolytic-uremic syndrome was also noted in the postmarketing report.

Grade 1 to 2 allergic or hypersensitivity reactions were noted in 7% to 10%, and grade 3 to 4 hypersensitivity reactions (2% to 3%) of colorectal patients in clinical trials; anaphylactoid reactions and anaphylactic shock to oxaliplatin were noted in 2% to 3% of patients. Postmarketing, immunoallergic hemolytic anemia, immunoallergic thrombocytopenia, anaphylactic shock, and angioedema have been reported. Allergic reactions, which can be fatal, can occur within minutes of oxaliplatin administration and during any cycle. The reactions were similar in nature and severity to those reported with other platinum-containing compounds (e.g., rash, urticaria, erythema, pruritus, and, rarely, bronchospasm, and low blood pressure). In previously untreated advanced colorectal patients, hypersensitivity symptoms included urticaria, pruritus, facial flushing, diarrhea associated with oxaliplatin infusion, shortness of breath, bronchospasm, diaphoresis, chest pain (unspecified), low blood pressure, disorientation, and syncope. These reactions were usually managed with standard epinephrine, corticosteroids, and antihistamines and require oxaliplatin discontinuation. Rechallenge is contraindicated; oxaliplatin is contraindicated for use in patients with known allergy to the drug or to other platinum compounds. Drug-related deaths associated with platinum compounds from anaphylaxis have been reported.[6]

Hepatotoxicity has been noted in patients receiving oxaliplatin plus 5-FU and LV. Elevated hepatic enzymes were reported in patients treated with oxaliplatin with or without 5-FU/LV. Overall increased transaminases were reported in 57% of patients with elevations noted in alkaline phosphatase (16% to 42%), alanine aminotransferase (ALT) (6% to 36%), and aspartate aminotransferase (AST) (17% to 54%). Hyperbilirubinemia was reported in 6% to 20% of patients. The incidence of elevated hepatic enzymes and hyperbilirubinemia was lower in previously untreated advanced colorectal patients receiving oxaliplatin/5-FU/LV as compared to previously treated patients. About 5% to 10% of patients in all treatment groups had some degree of elevation of serum creatinine. The incidence of grade 3/4 elevations in serum creatinine in the oxaliplatin/5-FU/LV arm was 1% in previously treated advanced colorectal patients. Changes noted on liver biopsies include peliosis hepatis, nodular regenerative hyperplasia or sinusoidal alterations, perisinusoidal fibrosis, and veno-occlusive disease (VOD).

Bevacizumab

Bevacizumab (rhuMAb-VEGF) is a humanized monoclonal antibody against VEGF, also known as vascular permeability factor (VPF or VEGF-A). It contains human framework regions and the complementarity-determining regions of the murine antibody, A4.6.1, against human (but not murine) VEGF (VEGF-A). Bevacizumab is produced in a Chinese hamster ovary cell system and has the same high-affinity and biologic properties as A4.6.1. Vascular targeting therapies are aimed at inhibiting tumor neovascularization and are not directly cytotoxic. Therefore, vascular targeting therapies used in cancer therapy usually need to be given in combination with traditional cytotoxic treatment modalities (e.g., chemotherapy, radiation therapy, or hormonal therapy). Bevacizumab binds to VEGF and prevents the binding of VEGF with its receptors, VEGFR-1 (Flt-1) and VEGFR-2 (Flk-1/KDR), found on the surface of endothelial cells. The role of VEGF is critical in angiogenesis, the formation of new blood vessels. In human cancers, the increased expression of VEGF is associated with increased microvascular density, tumor growth, metastasis, and a poor prognosis. Administration of bevacizumab to xenotransplant models of colon cancer in nude mice caused reduction of microvascular growth and inhibition of metastatic disease progression.

In the body, VEGF functions in angiogenesis by regulating both vascular proliferation and permeability. VEGF is unique due to its specificity and potency for vascular endothelium. Additionally, VEGF has antiapoptotic effects on cells in newly formed vessels by inducing bcl-2 and A1, antiapoptotic proteins. Other members of the VEGF gene family have been identified; however, their function has not been fully characterized. VEGF is expressed in tumor cells, macrophages, T-cells, smooth muscle cells, kidney cells, mesangial cells, keratinocytes, astrocytes, and osteoblasts. Expression of VEGF is regulated by differentiation, transformation, cytokines, hormones, and growth factors (e.g., EGF, transforming growth factor-β, keratinocyte growth factor, interleukin-1β, prostaglandin E$_2$, and insulin-like growth factor-1), and oxygen deprivation. Under hypoxic conditions, hypoxia-inducible factor-I activates transcription of the VEGF-A gene. VEGF-A promotes the proliferation of endothelial cells and chemotaxis of endothelial cells and monocytes. VEGF-A also can cause differentiation of monocytes into endothelial-like cells and inhibit the maturation of dendritic cells. These effects can deplete host immune cells and could lead to immunosuppression. VEGF-A also increases vascular permeability, leading to a leakage of plasma proteins that results in the formation of an extravascular fibrin gel. The increased vascular permeability results in increased intratumoral interstitial fluid pressure, which reduces the delivery of antineoplastic therapies. During fetal development and the early postnatal period, VEGF-A is critical for normal maturation; however, its function evolves with age. In mice, at about 4 weeks, vascularization becomes VEGF independent. In adult animals, VEGF-A inactivation has little effect on the vasculature although it is required during the development of the corpus luteum and for wound healing. Reduced levels of VEGF may cause neurodegeneration by impairing neural tissue perfusion.

Bevacizumab is administered as an IV infusion. The pharmacokinetic profile of bevacizumab was assessed using an assay that measured total bevacizumab levels (i.e., the assay did not differentiate between free bevacizumab and bound bevacizumab). Based on population pharmacokinetic analysis of 491 patients who received 1 to 20 mg/kg of bevacizumab weekly, every 2 weeks, or every 3 weeks, the estimated half-life of bevacizumab is about 20 days (range: 11 to 50 days). The predicted time to reach steady-state levels is 100 days.

The clearance of bevacizumab varies by body weight, gender, and by tumor burden. Patients with higher tumor burden (at or above median value of tumor surface area) had a higher bevacizumab clearance (0.249 vs. 0.199 L/day). In clinical trials, there has been no evidence of lesser efficacy in patients with higher tumor burden treated with bevacizumab as compared to patients with low tumor burden. The relationship between bevacizumab exposure and clinical outcomes has not been explored.

The incidence of hypertension and severe hypertension was increased in patients receiving chemotherapy plus bevacizumab as compared to those receiving chemotherapy alone. During clinical trials, 5% to 34% of bevacizumab recipients experienced hypertension (NCI CTC grades 1 to 5). The incidence of severe hypertension (NCI CTC grades 3 to 5) across all bevacizumab clinical trials ranged from 5% to 18%. In a study involving patients with metastatic colorectal cancer (mCRC), hypertension (grades 1 to 4) was reported in 23% of patients in the bolus-IFL (5-FU, leucovorin, and irinotecan) plus bevacizumab arm, 34% of patients in the 5-FU/LV plus bevacizumab arm, and 14% of patients receiving IFL alone.[7] Severe hypertension (grades 3 to 4) was reported in 12% of patients in the bolus-IFL plus bevacizumab arm and 2% of patients in the IFL alone arm of the trial. Among patients with severe hypertension in the bevacizumab arms, 51% had a diastolic reading greater than 110 mm Hg associated with a systolic reading less than 200 mm Hg. In another study involving patients with mCRC, grades 3 to 5 hypertension was reported in 9% of patients receiving treatment with bevacizumab plus FOLFOX4 and 2% of patients receiving FOLFOX4 alone.

Medication used for the management of grade 3 hypertension in patients receiving bevacizumab included angiotensin-converting enzyme inhibitors, beta blockers, diuretics, and calcium channel blockers. Development or worsening of hypertension can require hospitalization or require discontinuation of bevacizumab in 1.7% of patients. Hypertension can persist after discontinuation of bevacizumab therapy. Severe hypertension complicated by subarachnoid hemorrhage or hypertensive encephalopathy has been reported and, in some cases, has been fatal. In postmarket reports, acute increases in blood pressure have been associated with initial or subsequent infusions of bevacizumab; some cases were serious and were associated with clinical sequelae. Blood pressure monitoring every 2 to 3 weeks with medical treatment of hypertension is recommended during bevacizumab therapy. Temporary suspension of bevacizumab is recommended in patients with severe hypertension that is not controlled with medical management. Permanently discontinue bevacizumab in patients who develop hypertensive crisis or hypertensive encephalopathy.[8]

In clinical trials, proteinuria (defined as urine dipstick reading ≥1+) occurred more frequently and was more severe in patients receiving bevacizumab as compared to those receiving chemotherapy alone. The overall incidence of bevacizumab-associated proteinuria (all grades) during clinical studies was 20% with the incidence of severe proteinuria (grades 3 to 4) in bevacizumab-treated patients ranging from 0.7% to 7.4%. The median time to onset was 5.6 months and the median time to resolution was 6.1 months; 30% of patients experiencing bevacizumab-induced proteinuria required permanent drug discontinuation. In a study involving mCRC patients, proteinuria occurred in 24% of patients receiving bolus-IFL plus placebo, 36% receiving bolus-IFL plus bevacizumab, and in 36% of patients receiving 5-FU/LV plus bevacizumab. Grade 3 proteinuria (>3.5 g protein/24 hours) was reported in 2% (23 of 158) of patients receiving bolus-IFL plus bevacizumab and in 4% (2 of 50) of patients receiving 5-FU/LV plus bevacizumab. In a case series, kidney biopsy of six patients with proteinuria showed findings consistent with thrombotic microangiopathy. Monitor the development or worsening of proteinuria by serial dipstick urinalysis in patients receiving bevacizumab. Patients with a 2+ or greater urine dipstick reading should undergo further analysis with a 24-hour urine collection. Hold bevacizumab in patients with greater than or equal to 2 g of proteinuria per 24 hours and resume when less than 2 g of proteinuria per 24 hours. Postmarketing studies have shown poor correlation between urine protein/urine creatinine ratio and 24-hour urine protein. The safety of continued bevacizumab therapy or temporary suspension of the drug in patients with moderate to severe proteinuria has not been evaluated.

Nephrotic syndrome has been reported in less than 1% of patients receiving bevacizumab in any clinical trial. One patient died and one required dialysis. In three patients, proteinuria decreased in severity several months after discontinuation of bevacizumab; no patient had normalization of protein levels following discontinuation of bevacizumab. Bevacizumab should be permanently discontinued in patients with nephrotic syndrome.

Congestive heart failure (CHF) and left ventricular dysfunction (or left ventricular ejection fraction [LVEF] decline) has been reported with bevacizumab use in clinical trials. In a pooled analysis of all trials, NCI-CTC grade greater than or equal to 3 left ventricular dysfunction occurred in 1% of patients treated with bevacizumab compared with 0.6% of control patients.

Bleeding associated with the use of bevacizumab can be categorized based on the severity of the hemorrhagic event. Minor or moderate bleeding occurs more frequently in patients treated with bevacizumab versus those treated with chemotherapy alone. These events were generally mild and resolved without medical intervention and include epistaxis (16% to 35% vs. 10%), GI bleeding (24% vs. 6%), minor gum bleeding (2% vs. 0%), and vaginal bleeding (4% vs. 2%). Severe or fatal bleeding events, including hemoptysis, GI bleeding, hematemesis, central nervous system (CNS) bleeding, epistaxis, and vaginal bleeding, occurs up to five times more frequently in bevacizumab-treated patients versus patients treated with chemotherapy alone. Across all indications, severe (NCI-CTC grade ≥3) hemorrhagic events occurred in 1.2% to 4.6% of bevacizumab recipients.

Compared with chemotherapy alone, treatment with bevacizumab is associated with an increased risk of arterial and venous thromboembolism (VTE). The incidence of severe (grades 3 to 4) venous thrombotic events (i.e., deep venous thrombosis or intra-abdominal thrombosis) among 402 patients with metastatic colon cancer who received bevacizumab and chemotherapy was 15.1%, whereas 13.6% of 411 patients who received chemotherapy alone had the outcome. Additionally, in metastatic colon cancer patients, there is an increased risk of developing a second subsequent thromboembolic event with bevacizumab plus chemotherapy versus chemotherapy alone. Among mCRC patients who received warfarin for a venous thromboembolic event, 11 of 53 who had bevacizumab and chemotherapy had an additional thromboembolic event compared to 1 of 30 who had chemotherapy alone. In a second 4-arm study ($n = 1,401$) of mCRC patients, the overall first incidence of VTE was higher in the bevacizumab containing arms (13.5%) as compared to the chemotherapy-alone arms (9.6%). Among the 116 patients treated with anticoagulants after the initial VTE, the overall incidence of subsequent VTEs was higher in the bevacizumab arms ($n = 73$, 31.5%) as compared to the chemotherapy-alone arms ($n = 43$, 25.6%).

GI perforation complicated by intra-abdominal abscesses or fistula formation occurred more frequently in patients receiving bevacizumab as compared to controls during clinical trials

(range: 0.3% to 2.4%). Of the reported events, 30% were fatal. In colorectal clinical trials, including bevacizumab single-agent and combination chemotherapy, GI perforation, fistula formation, and/or intra-abdominal abscess incidence was 2.4. GI perforation, fistula (GI, enterocutaneous, esophageal, duodenal, rectal), and/or intra-abdominal abscess have also been reported during postmarket reports and trials for colorectal cancer and other types of cancer. Regardless of underlying cancer, patients with GI perforation typically presented with abdominal pain, nausea, vomiting, constipation, and fever. GI perforation occurred at various time points during treatment, ranging from 1 week to greater than 1 year from therapy initiation; most events occur within the first 50 days. The incidence of GI perforation with bolus-IFL (irinotecan, fluorouracil, leucovorin) and bevacizumab was 2% (6 of 392 patients) and with 5-fluorouracil/leucovorin (5-FU/LV) the incidence was 4% (4 of 109 patients).

Bevacizumab therapy should be permanently discontinued in patients with GI perforation, fistula formation in the GI tract, intra-abdominal abscess, or fistula formation involving an internal organ. Other serious GI adverse reactions reported in at least one patient during postmarketing surveillance include intestinal necrosis, mesenteric venous occlusion, and anastomotic ulceration. A meta-analysis of 12,294 patients in 17 randomized trials was conducted to determine the risk of GI perforation with bevacizumab treatment. Among 6,490 patients receiving bevacizumab, the incidence of GI perforation was 0.9%. The incidence of grade 5 (fatal) GI perforation was 0.3% with a mortality rate of 21.7% in patients receiving bevacizumab who developed a GI perforation. The relative risk of developing a GI perforation with bevacizumab compared to controls was 2.14 ($p = .011$). Patients with colorectal cancer and patients who received a dose equivalent to 5 mg/kg/week had a significantly increased risk of developing GI perforation. Consider the patient's history of ulcers or diverticulitis, radiation exposure, recent sigmoidoscopy or colonoscopy, resection of the primary tumor, GI obstruction, and current tumor presentation and placement. In the meta-analysis, most GI perforations occurred within the first 6 months of treatment.[9]

Bevacizumab therapy has been associated with impaired wound healing, wound bleeding, and wound dehiscence. In patients receiving either bolus-IFL or 5-FU/LV with bevacizumab, 1% developed wound dehiscence during the study period. Among patients requiring surgery on or within 60 days of treatment with bevacizumab, wound healing and/or bleeding complications occurred in 15% (6/39) of patients receiving bolus-ILF plus bevacizumab as compared to 4% of patients who received bolus-ILF alone. The appropriate interval between surgery and subsequent initiation of bevacizumab to avoid risks of impaired wound healing has not been determined; however, the manufacturer recommends holding bevacizumab therapy for at least 28 days and until the surgical incision has fully healed. There was one patient in whom anastomotic dehiscence occurred when bevacizumab therapy was started more than 2 months after surgery. The appropriate interval between termination of bevacizumab therapy and subsequent elective surgery also has not been determined. Bevacizumab has a half-life of approximately 20 days; therefore, it should be suspended at least 28 days prior to elective surgery. Permanently discontinue bevacizumab in patients with wound dehiscence requiring medical intervention.

Bevacizumab has been associated with the development of reversible posterior leukoencephalopathy syndrome (RPLS) (<0.1%) during clinical trials and postmarketing surveillance. RPLS is a disorder that can present with headache, seizures, lethargy, confusion, blindness, and other neurologic and visual disturbances. Mild to moderate hypertension may be present but is not necessary for the diagnosis. Diagnosis should be confirmed by magnetic resonance imaging (MRI). The onset of symptoms has been reported to occur from 16 hours to 1 year after initiation of bevacizumab treatment. Bevacizumab therapy should be discontinued in patients who develop RPLS, and hypertensive therapy initiated, if present. Symptoms usually resolve or improve within days, although neurologic sequelae have been noted in some patients. The safety of reinitiating bevacizumab in patients who experience RPLS is unknown.

Cetuximab

Cetuximab (IMC-C225) is a recombinant, human/mouse chimeric monoclonal antibody that binds specifically to the extracellular domain of the human EGFR. The EGFR is a transmembrane glycoprotein that is a member of a subfamily of type I receptor tyrosine kinases including EGFR (HER1), HER2, HER3, and HER4. EGFR is constitutively expressed in many normal epithelial tissues, including the skin and hair follicle. Overexpression of EGFR has been associated with poor prognosis, decreased overall survival (OS), and/or increased risk of metastasis.

Cetuximab is composed of the Fv regions of a murine anti-EGFR antibody with human IgG1 heavy and kappa light chain constant regions and has an approximate molecular weight of 152 kDa. Cetuximab is produced in a mammalian cell culture (i.e., murine myeloma). In June 2008, the results of two phase III trials in mCRC patients confirmed this association. In mCRC patients receiving cetuximab in combination with chemotherapy, no benefit was observed over chemotherapy alone in patients whose tumors expressed mutant K-RAS. In contrast, patients whose tumors expressed wild-type K-RAS showed significant improvement in efficacy endpoints over chemotherapy alone. K-RAS mutation status should be established prior to initiating therapy with cetuximab. Only patients with wild-type KRAS should be offered therapy with anti-EGFR agents. The Food and Drug Administration (FDA) approved cetuximab with irinotecan for EGRF-expressing mCRC refractory to irinotecan-based chemotherapy and as a single agent for EGRF-expressing mCRC in patients who are intolerant of irinotecan-based chemotherapy in February 2004; it was approved as monotherapy in October 2007 for EGRF-expressing mCRC after failure of both irinotecan- and oxaliplatin-based regimens.

Cetuximab is a monoclonal antibody that binds to and blocks the binding of ligands (e.g., EGF and tissue growth factor-α) to the EGFR (EGFR, HER1, c-ErbB-1) on the surface of normal and tumor cells. The binding of cetuximab to EGFR leads to internalization of the receptor, preventing further activation and blocks phosphorylation and activation of receptor-associated kinases, resulting in inhibition of cell growth, induction of apoptosis, and decreased matrix metalloproteinase and VEGF production. In vitro assays and in vivo animal studies have shown that cetuximab inhibits the growth and survival of cancer cells that overexpress EGFR. No antitumor effects of cetuximab were noted in human tumor xenographs lacking EGFR expression.

Additionally, signal transduction through the EGFR results in activation of wild-type K-RAS protein. In cells with activating K-RAS somatic mutations, the mutant K-RAS protein is continually active and appears independent of EGFR regulation.

Cetuximab may make cancer cells more vulnerable to other cancer chemotherapy agents and radiation therapy. Preclinical trials have suggested synergy between cetuximab and irinotecan, gemcitabine, and doxorubicin. The addition of cetuximab to irinotecan or irinotecan/5-FU chemotherapy in animal studies increased antitumor effects compared to chemotherapy alone. The mechanism of this synergy has not been established. It is thought that the blockage of EGFR signaling, which alone may be cytotoxic in some cell lines, may increase the vulnerability of cells to the cytotoxic effects of chemotherapy that may have only have been slightly effective without EGFR blockade. Although considered a cytostatic agent, cetuximab can cause tumor regression when given as a single agent. In some cancers, such as colorectal cancer, cells can activate the EGFR receptor through autocrine or paracrine mechanisms. These autocrine and paracrine mechanisms are necessary for cells to survive in a less than hospitable microenvironment around the tumor with low pH and pO_2 tension. These tumor cells may experience apoptosis when the autocrine and paracrine EGFR-activation is inhibited.

Cetuximab is administered as an IV infusion and exhibits nonlinear pharmacokinetics. Following a single 2-hour infusion of 400 mg/m², the mean elimination half-life was 97 hours (range: 41 to 213 hours). The mean steady-state half-life is 114 hours (range: 75 to 188 hours). The clearance of cetuximab decreases from 0.08 to 0.02 L/hour/m² as the dose is increased from 20 to 200 mg/m²; at doses of greater than 200 mg/m², cetuximab clearance appears to plateau. The volume of distribution seems to be independent of dose and approximates the vascular space of 2 to 3 L/m². Following a single 2-hour infusion of 400 mg/m² of cetuximab, the maximum mean serum concentration (C_{max}) of cetuximab was 184 mcg/mL (range: 92 to 327 mcg/mL). A 1-hour infusion of 250 mg/m² produced a C_{max} of 140 mcg/mL (range: 120 to 170 mcg/mL). Following the recommended dosing regimen in clinical trials, cetuximab concentrations reach steady-state levels by the third weekly infusion with mean peak and trough concentrations ranging from 168 to 235 mcg/mL and 41 to 85 mcg/mL, respectively. The area under the concentration time curve (AUC) increases in a greater than dose proportional manner as the dose is increased from 20 to 400 mg/m².

Cetuximab may cause serious infusion-related reactions that require medical intervention and immediate, permanent cetuximab discontinuation. Serious infusion reactions include rapid onset of airway obstruction, such as bronchospasm, stridor, hoarseness; hypotension; shock; loss of consciousness; myocardial infarction; and/or cardiac arrest. Approximately 90% of severe infusion reactions occurred with the first infusion despite premedication with antihistamines. Monitor patients for 1 hour after cetuximab infusions in a setting with resuscitation equipment and other agents necessary to treat anaphylaxis, such as epinephrine, corticosteroids, IV antihistamines, bronchodilators, and oxygen. For patients requiring treatment for infusion reactions, monitor them longer to confirm resolution of the event. For NCI CTC grade 1 or 2 and nonserious NCI CTC grades 3 to 4 infusion reactions, reduce the infusion rate by 50%. In clinical trials, serious infusion reactions (NCI CTC grades 3 and 4) occurred with cetuximab administration in 2% to 5% of 1,373 patients with fatal outcome reported in less than

1 in 1,000. In patients with colorectal cancer, infusion reactions occurred in 15% of patients treated with cetuximab alone. Infusion reaction was defined as any event infusion related, such as chills, rigors, dyspnea, sinus tachycardia, bronchospasm, chest tightness, swelling, urticaria, hypotension, flushing, rash, hypertension, nausea, angioedema, pain, pruritus, diaphoresis, tremor, shaking, cough, or visual disturbances. Fever of grades 1 to 2 severity occurred in 29% and of grades 3 to 4 severity in 1% of patients. Rigors or chills of grades 1 to 2 severity occurred in 13% and of grades 3 to 4 severity in less than 1% of patients.[10] Among 25 patients who had received cetuximab in the past and who had a hypersensitivity reaction after cetuximab receipt, 17 had immunoglobulin E (IgE) antibodies against the drug before treatment, whereas only 1 of 51 patients without a hypersensitivity reaction had IgE present. The IgE antibodies were specific for an oligosaccharide, galactose—1,3-galactose, which is present on the Fab portion of the cetuximab heavy chain. IgE antibodies against cetuximab were detected in several patients who never received cetuximab: 15 of 72 samples from control subjects in Tennessee, 3 of 49 samples from northern California, and 2 of 341 samples from Boston. Of the 8 patients who had received cetuximab in the past and had a hypersensitivity reaction but had negative results on the IgE assay, 7 had grade 1 or 2 reactions, and 1 had a grade 3 reaction. Five of the 8 patients were rechallenged; 1 had a second hypersensitivity reaction, and 4 completed treatment without further reactions.[11]

In clinical studies of cetuximab, acneiform rash was reported 76% to 88% of 1,373 patients and was severe in 1% to 17% of patients. Acneiform rash was defined as any event described as acne, rash (unspecified), maculopapular rash, pustular rash (vesicular rash), dry skin (xerosis), or exfoliative dermatitis. Acneiform rash usually developed within the first 2 weeks of therapy and resolved in most of the patients after treatment cessation, although in nearly half, the event continued beyond 28 days. Interruption of cetuximab receipt is needed if a grade 3 or 4 acneiform rash occurs; cetuximab dose modification is needed if the rash occurs a second or third time and improves with drug interruption, and cetuximab discontinuation is needed if the rash does not improve or if it occurs a fourth time. Instruct patients to limit sun exposure during cetuximab therapy. Paronychial inflammation, skin fissures, hypertrichosis, and inflammatory and infectious sequelae (e.g., blepharitis, cheilitis, cellulitis, conjunctivitis, keratitis, *Staphylococcus aureus* sepsis, and abscess formation) were also reported. Other dermatologic reactions seen in colorectal patients receiving cetuximab monotherapy included skin disorder (unspecified) (27%), pruritus (38%), rash (unspecified)/desquamation (77%), xerosis (49%), and nail changes (21%). Pruritus was of grades 3 to 4 severity in 2%, and rash/desquamation was of grades 3 to 4 severity in 12%. In head and neck cancer patients treated with cetuximab plus radiation, other dermatologic reactions reported included radiation dermatitis (grades 1 to 2 in 36%; grades 3 and 4 in 23%), radiation site reaction (18%), and pruritus (16%). In one clinical trial (*n* = 57 patients with mCRC), patients with a skin rash of any grade had a superior survival compared to patients with no skin rash. There was a trend toward improved survival with increasing grade of rash with patients with grade 3 rash appearing to have a longer survival as compared to patients with less severe skin rash.[12]

Cetuximab may cause several GI adverse events. Grades 1 to 2 diarrhea occurred in 37% of patients during colorectal cancer clinical trials; the incidence was 72% when cetuximab was used in combination with irinotecan. Grades 3 to 4 diarrhea occurred in 2% of patients receiving cetuximab and in 22% of patients receiving combination therapy.

Hypomagnesemia and accompanying electrolyte abnormalities have been reported to develop within days to months after the initiation of cetuximab. Periodically monitor patients for hypomagnesemia, hypocalcemia, and hypokalemia during and for at least 8 weeks after the completion of cetuximab. Replete electrolytes as necessary. In clinical trials, hypomagnesemia occurred in 55% of 365 patients; hypomagnesemia was severe (NCI-CTC grade 3 and 4) in 6% to 17% of patients. Cetuximab may impair magnesium reabsorption by blocking the EGFR, which is abundantly expressed in the kidney. A significant amount of filtered magnesium is reabsorbed at the ascending limb of the loop of Henle.[13]

Panitumumab

Panitumumab (ABX-EGF) is a fully human immunoglobulin (Ig) G2 antibody that binds with high affinity to the extracellular domain of the human EGFR.[14] Panitumumab is the first fully human monoclonal antibody directed against EGFR. The manufacturing process for panitumumab utilizes a genetically engineered XenoMouse system where the Ig genes of the mouse have been inactivated and functionally replaced by their human counterparts. XenoMouse system is purported to result in a rapid generation and production of a unique and reliable source of high-affinity fully human therapeutic monoclonal antibodies.[15] Panitumumab differs from cetuximab (Erbitux) in that it has a higher affinity for the receptor and it produces less hypersensitivity reactions.[16] Panitumumab has a similar mechanism of action to cetuximab, a monoclonal antibody that targets the ligand-binding domain of EGFR. Panitumumab is a fully human monoclonal antibody that binds specifically with high affinity to the EGFR, HER1, c-ErbB-1 on both normal and tumor cells.[17]

Panitumumab is administered as an IV infusion. Panitumumab clearance decreased from 30.6 to 4.6 mL/kg/day as the dose increased from 0.75 to 9 mg/kg. The mean clearance is 3.5 to 5.3 mL/kg/day, and elimination half-life is approximately 7.5 days (range: 3.6 to 10.9 days). When administered as a single agent, it exhibits nonlinear pharmacokinetics. Following a single-dose administration of panitumumab as a 1-hour infusion, the AUC increased in a greater than dose-proportional manner; however, at doses above 2 mg/kg, the AUC begins to increase in an approximately dose-proportional manner. Following the recommended dose regimen (6 mg/kg as a 1-hour infusion, administered once every 2 weeks), panitumumab concentrations reach steady-state levels by the third infusion with mean peak and trough concentrations of 154 to 272 mcg/mL and 25 to 53 mcg/mL, respectively.

▌ TREATMENT PLANNING

Treatment planning for the medical management of colorectal cancer metastases needs to take into consideration performance status (PS), organ physiology, and goals of therapy. Patients with a good PS will generally tolerate the side effects of combination chemotherapy so that they may achieve benefit. Patients with a marginal PS may be better served by a single-agent approach to chemotherapy. The benefits gained from chemotherapy may include a prolongation of survival, a delay in tumor progression, or the alleviation of cancer-related symptoms. These benefits have been measured and reported in cancer therapy clinical trials as median OS, progression-free survival (PFS), time to tumor progression (TTP), time to treatment failure (TTF), response rate (RR), and QoL. Measurements in tumor response and progression rely on radiographic imaging as defined using the Response Evaluation Criteria in Solid Tumor (RECIST). In addition, the side effect profile of particular regimens may be an important determinate in a patient's ability to tolerate and gain benefit from a chemotherapy regimen. The side effects of therapy regimens are reported using the standardized classification of the National Cancer Institute Common Terminology Criteria for Adverse Events (CTCAE). In the CTCAE, toxicities are evaluated by organ system and graded on a scale of 0 to 5 with 0 being no toxicity and 5 representing death related to the toxicity.

Colorectal cancer metastases will invariably develop a resistance pathway to therapy. Resistance may be determined by clinical signs and symptoms of progression of disease while on or shortly after therapy, or radiographic evidence of tumor growth or new tumor lesions. At the time that resistance is determined, patients may be considered for subsequent therapy using agents with a different cytotoxic or cytostatic mechanism. Each therapy regimen is generally referred to as a "line of therapy," but these lines are often blurred as patients' therapy is changed due to reasons other than resistance. Therapy may be changed or stopped as a result of progression of disease, cumulative side effects of therapy, or changes in the goals of care. Alternatively, patients with isolated colorectal metastases may demonstrate a response to therapy that allows them to proceed to the surgical resection or ablation of all disease. The multidisciplinary approach to colorectal metastases has led to a continuum of care.

First-Line Therapy

For a patient with a good PS and preserved organ function, the first line of therapy is often a combination of classic chemotherapy agents with a biologic agent. The standard therapy for colorectal metastases had long been 5-FU as a bolus injection potentiated by leucovorin administered for 5 days of a 28-day cycle or weekly for 6 weeks of an 8-week cycle.[18] A phase III clinical trial compared this standard regimen to the combination of 5-FU, leucovorin, and irinotecan (IFL) given on a weekly bolus schedule.[19] The combination therapy demonstrated an improved PFS (median, 7.0 vs. 4.3 months; $p = .004$), a higher rate of confirmed response (39% vs. 21%; $p < .001$), and longer OS (median, 14.8 vs. 12.6 months; $p = .04$). Grade 3 (severe) diarrhea was more common during treatment with IFL than during treatment with fluorouracil and leucovorin, but the incidence of grade 4 (life-threatening) diarrhea was similar in the two groups (<8%). Grade 3 or 4 mucositis, grade 4 neutropenia, and neutropenic fever were less frequent during treatment with IFL. Adding irinotecan to the regimen of fluorouracil and leucovorin did not compromise the QoL. Subsequent evaluation of studies using the IFL schedule found a greater toxicity risk, including mortality, than previously reported and this schedule soon fell out of favor.[20]

An alternate schedule of 5-FU and leucovorin had been studied with 5-FU delivered as both a bolus injection and a protracted infusion (LV5FU2) administered bimonthly.[21] When compared to the regimen of bolus 5-FU and leucovorin in the 5-day schedule, the LV5FU2 proved superior in terms of RR (32.6% vs. 14.5%), PFS (27.6 vs. 22.0 weeks), and toxicity (grade 3 or 4 in 11.1% vs. 22.9% patients), but not OS. The more favorable toxicity profile demonstrated on this schedule was felt to provide a safer and more effective backbone with which to build. The addition of oxaliplatin to the LV5FU2 regimen had significantly longer PFS (median, 9.0 vs. 6.2 months; $p = .0003$) and better RR (50.7% vs. 22.3%; $p = .0001$) when compared with the control arm.[22] The improvement in OS did not reach significance (median, 16.2 vs. 14.7 months; $p = .12$). LV5FU2 plus oxaliplatin gave higher frequencies of CTCAE grade 3/4 neutropenia (41.7% vs. 5.3% of patients), grade 3/4 diarrhea (11.9% vs. 5.3%), and grade 3 neurosensory toxicity (18.2% vs. 0%), but this did not result in impairment of QoL. Survival without disease progression or deterioration in global health status was longer in patients allocated to oxaliplatin treatment ($p = .004$).

Irinotecan with the LV5FU2 schedule had been evaluated in patients who had previously progressed on a 5-FU regimen demonstrating an improvement in PFS with a tolerable toxicity profile.[23] The combination of irinotecan and oxaliplatin (IrOx) was compared to irinotecan alone for patients who had previously progressed on a 5-FU containing regimen demonstrating a benefit in median TTP and improvement in tumor-related symptoms (TRS) for the combination therapy with a comparable toxicity profile.[24]

Attempts to determine the best first-line combination regimen for patients with colorectal metastases and good PS were undertaken. The standard of care at the time of the study enrollment was the IFL regimen and this was compared to a LV5FU2-oxaliplatin regimen (FOLFOX) and the IrOx regimen.[25] A median TTP of 8.7 months, RR of 45%, and median survival time of 19.5 months were observed for FOLFOX. These results were significantly superior to those observed for IFL (6.9 months, 31%, and 15.0 months, respectively) or for IrOx (6.5 months, 35%, and 17.4 months, respectively) for all endpoints for TTP, response, and survival. The FOLFOX regimen had significantly lower rates of severe nausea, vomiting, diarrhea, febrile neutropenia, and dehydration. Sensory neuropathy and neutropenia were more common with the regimens containing oxaliplatin. At the time that this study was conducted, oxaliplatin was not an available agent in the United States for patients to receive after progression on a non-oxaliplatin containing regimen. This was felt to be a confounding factor in the determination of OS in which some patients may have had all three agents available to them, whereas others only had 5-FU and irinotecan.

A study comparing the two drug regimens of 5-FU and oxaliplatin (FOLFOX) with 5-FU and irinotecan (FOLFIRI), and allowing for crossover so that all patients had access to all three proven active drugs, demonstrated median OS of 21.5 months in 109 patients allocated to FOLFIRI then FOLFOX versus 20.6 months in 111 patients allocated to FOLFOX then FOLFIRI ($p = .99$).[26] When taken together, these studies demonstrate equivalent OS for patients with a good PS, treated with a two-drug regimen on a bolus and infusion 5-FU schedule, with the choice of second agent used depending on the toxicity profile expected to be best tolerated for the particular patient.

In an attempt to minimize the cumulative oxaliplatin associated neurotoxicity without compromising efficacy, a number of studies have evaluated intermittent oxaliplatin administration.

In the OPTIMOX-1 study, previously untreated patients were randomly assigned to either FOLFOX administered every 2 weeks until progression (arm A) or FOLFOX for 6 cycles, maintenance without oxaliplatin for 12 cycles, and reintroduction of FOLFOX (arm B).[27] There were 620 patients enrolled, including an exploratory cohort of 95 elderly or poor prognosis patients. Median PFS and survival times were 9.0 and 19.3 months, respectively, in patients allocated to the continuous FOLFOX strategy (arm A) compared with 8.7 and 21.2 months, respectively, in patients allocated to the intermittent oxaliplatin strategy (arm B) (p = not significant). RRs were 58.5% with arm A and 59.2% with arm B. NCI CTCAE grade 3 or 4 toxicity was observed in 54.4% of the patients in arm A compared to 48.7% of patients in arm B. As expected, from cycle 7, fewer patients experienced grade 3 or 4 toxicity in arm B. Grade 3 sensory neuropathy was observed in 17.9% of the patients in arm A compared to 13.3% of patients in arm B (p = .12). In arm B, oxaliplatin was reintroduced in only 40.1% of the patients but achieved responses or stabilizations in 69.4% of these patients. The authors conclude that oxaliplatin can be safely stopped after 6 cycles in a FOLFOX regimen without a significant compromise of efficacy.

Given these results, a subsequent study to evaluate a complete break from therapy was pursued. The OPTIMOX-2 study was hampered by a change in the standard of care, forcing premature closure of the study and redesign of the endpoints.[28] This study compared chemotherapy discontinuation with maintenance therapy with leucovorin and fluorouracil after six cycles of FOLFOX chemotherapy in the first-line treatment of mCRC. In the study, 202 patients with untreated mCRC were randomly assigned to receive six cycles of FOLFOX followed by simplified leucovorin plus bolus and infusional fluorouracil until progression (arm 1 or maintenance arm, n = 98) or six cycles of FOLFOX before a complete stop of chemotherapy (arm 2 or chemotherapy-free interval [CFI] arm, n = 104). Reintroduction of FOLFOX was scheduled after tumor progression in both arms. The primary study endpoint was duration of disease control (DDC). The median DDC was 13.1 months in patients assigned to the maintenance arm and 9.2 months in patients assigned to the CFI arm (p = .046). Median PFS and OS were 8.6 and 23.8 months, respectively, in the maintenance arm and 6.6 and 19.5 months, respectively, in the CFI arm. Median duration of maintenance therapy (arm 1) and CFIs (arm 2) were 4.8 and 3.9 months, respectively. Overall RRs were 59.2% and 59.6% for the initial FOLFOX chemotherapy and 20.4% and 30.3% for FOLFOX reintroduction in arms 1 and 2, respectively. These results demonstrate a negative impact on DDC and PFS for a planned complete discontinuation of chemotherapy compared with the maintenance therapy strategy. Due to the premature closure of the study, it is underpowered to determine a statistically significant difference in OS; however, a trend to improved OS with continued maintenance therapy is identified.

Second-Line Therapy

At the time of progression of colorectal metastases on chemotherapy, patients maintaining a good PS may be considered for a second line of therapy. Second-line therapy was first explored with irinotecan after progression on a bolus schedule of 5-FU. There were 189 patients with proven mCRC, which had

progressed within 6 months of treatment with 5-FU, who were randomly assigned to either 300 to 350 mg/m^2 irinotecan every 3 weeks with supportive care or supportive care alone, in a 2:1 ratio.[29] Tumor-related symptoms were present in 134 (71%) patients and weight loss of more than 5% was seen in 15 (8%) patients. With a median follow-up of 13 months, the OS was significantly better in the irinotecan group (p = .0001), with 36.2% 1-year survival, versus 13.8% in the supportive care group. The survival benefit, adjusted for prognostic factors in a multivariate analysis, remained significant (p = .001). Survival without PS deterioration (p = .0001), without weight loss of more than 5% (p = .018), and pain-free survival (p = .003) were significantly better in the patients given irinotecan. In a QoL analysis, all significant differences, except for diarrhea score, were in favor of the irinotecan group.

A second study comparing irinotecan to an alternate form of 5-FU, with a presumed different mechanism, demonstrated a similar benefit.[30] In this study, 267 patients who had failed to respond to first-line bolus 5-FU or whose disease had progressed after treatment with first-line 5-FU were randomly assigned to irinotecan 300 to 350 mg/m^2 infused once every 3 weeks or 5-FU by continuous infusion. Treatment was given until disease progression, unacceptable toxic effects, or patient refusal to continue treatment. The primary endpoint was survival, whereas PFS, RR, symptom-free survival, adverse events, and QoL were secondary endpoints. Patients treated with irinotecan lived significantly longer than those on fluorouracil (p = .035). Survival at 1 year was increased from 32% in the 5-FU group to 45% in the irinotecan group. Median survival was 10.8 months in the irinotecan group and 8.5 months in the 5-FU group. Median PFS was longer with irinotecan (4.2 vs. 2.9 months for irinotecan and 5-FU, respectively; p = .030). The median pain-free survival was 10.3 and 8.5 months (p = .06) for irinotecan and 5-FU, respectively. Both treatments were equally well tolerated. QoL was similar in both groups. These studies taken together endorsed a role for second-line therapy for colorectal metastatic disease.

With the acceptance of irinotecan in combination with 5-FU as a first-line regimen, there was a need for further second-line therapies. In one study, 463 patients with mCRC who progressed after IFL therapy were randomly assigned to bolus and infusional 5-FU and leucovorin (LV5FU2), single-agent oxaliplatin, or the combination (FOLFOX).[31] A planned interim analysis evaluated objective RR, TTP, and alleviation of TRS in an initial cohort of patients. FOLFOX proved superior to LV5FU2 in all measures of clinical efficacy. Objective RRs were 9.9% for FOLFOX versus 0% for LV5FU2 (Fisher's exact test, p < .0001). Median TTP was 4.6 months for FOLFOX versus 2.7 months for LV5FU2 (two-sided, stratified log-rank test, p < .0001). Relief of TRS occurred in 33% of patients treated with FOLFOX versus 12% of patients treated with LVFU2 (chi-squared test, p < .001). Single-agent oxaliplatin was not superior to LV5FU2 in any measure of efficacy. Patients treated with FOLFOX experienced a higher incidence of clinically significant toxicities than patients treated with LV5FU2, but these toxicities were predictable and did not result in a higher rate of treatment discontinuation or 60-day mortality rate.

A subsequent study evaluated capecitabine plus oxaliplatin (XELOX) to FOLFOX as second-line therapy in mCRC in a randomized phase III noninferiority study after progression on an irinotecan-containing regimen.[32] A total of 627 patients were randomly assigned to receive XELOX or FOLFOX following disease progression/recurrence or intolerance to irinotecan-based chemotherapy. The primary endpoint was PFS. PFS for XELOX was noninferior to FOLFOX (hazard ratio [HR] = 0.97; 95% confidence interval [CI], 0.83 to 1.14). Median PFS was 4.7 months with XELOX versus 4.8 months with FOLFOX. The robustness of the primary analysis was supported by multivariate and subgroup analyses. Median OS was 11.9 months with XELOX versus 12.5 months with FOLFOX (HR = 1.02; 95% CI, 0.86 to 1.21). Treatment-related grade 3/4 adverse events occurred in 50% of XELOX- and 65% of FOLFOX-treated patients. Whereas grade 3/4 neutropenia (35% vs. 5% with XELOX) and febrile neutropenia (4% vs. <1%) were more common with FOLFOX, grade 3/4 diarrhea (19% vs. 5% with FOLFOX-4) and grade 3 hand-foot syndrome (4% vs. <1%) were more common with XELOX. XELOX is noninferior to FOLFOX-4 when administered as second-line treatment in patients with mCRC.

Sequential Single-Agent Compared to Combination Therapy

Given the added side effects experienced with combination therapy, patients with a suboptimal PS may not benefit from combination therapy. Studies evaluating combination therapy compared to sequential use of single-agent chemotherapy were undertaken to address this scenario. Through random assignment, 820 patients with advanced colorectal cancer received either first-line treatment with capecitabine, second-line irinotecan, and third-line capecitabine plus oxaliplatin (sequential treatment; $n = 410$) or first-line treatment with capecitabine plus irinotecan and second-line capecitabine plus oxaliplatin (combination treatment; $n = 410$).[33] The primary endpoint was OS. The median OS was 16.3 (95% CI, 14.3 to 18.1) months for sequential treatment and 17.4 (15.2 to 19.2) months for combination treatment ($p = .3281$). The HR for combination versus sequential treatment was 0.92 (95% CI, 0.79 to 1.08; $p = .3281$). The frequency of grades 3 to 4 toxicity over all lines of treatment did not differ significantly between the two groups, except for grade 3 hand-foot syndrome, which occurred more often with sequential treatment than with combination treatment (13% vs. 7%; $p = .004$). Interpretation combination treatment does not significantly improve OS compared with the sequential use of cytotoxic drugs in advanced colorectal cancer. Thus sequential treatment remains a valid option for patients with advanced colorectal cancer.

A second study enrolled 2,135 patients randomly assigned to three treatment strategies.[34] Strategy A (control group) was single-agent 5-FU (given with levofolinate over 48 hours every 2 weeks) until failure, then single-agent irinotecan. Strategy B was 5-FU until failure, then combination chemotherapy with either 5-FU and irinotecan (B-ir) or 5-FU and oxaliplatin (B-ox). Strategy C was combination chemotherapy from the outset with 5-FU and either irinotecan (C-ir) or oxaliplatin (C-ox). The primary endpoint was OS, analyzed by intention to treat. The median survival of patients allocated to control strategy A was 13.9 months, B-ir 15.0 months, B-ox 15.2 months, C-ir 16.7 months, and C-ox 15.4 months. Log-rank comparison of each group against control showed that only C-ir—the first-line combination strategy including irinotecan—satisfied the

statistical test for superiority ($p = .01$). Overall comparison of strategy B with strategy C was within the predetermined noninferiority boundary of HR equals 1.18 or less (HR = 1.06, 90% CI, 0.97 to 1.17). Taken together, these data challenge the assumption that, in this noncurative setting, maximum tolerable treatment must necessarily be used first line. The staged approach of initial single-agent treatment upgraded to combination when required is not worse than first-line combination and is an alternative option for discussion with patients.

The Continuum of Care

The study comparing FOLFOX to FOLFIRI and allowing for crossover[27] and the studies evaluating sequential therapy[33,34] provide further evidence of the benefits of multiple lines of therapy. Taken together, these results endorse a strategy of a continuum of care, in which the use of chemotherapy is tailored to the clinical setting and includes switching chemotherapy prior to disease progression, maintenance therapy, drug "holidays," and surgical resection of metastases in selected patients.[35] The continuum of care approach includes individualized planning, in which patients are given the opportunity to benefit from exposure to all active agents and modalities while minimizing unnecessary treatment and toxicity with the ultimate goal of improving survival as well as QoL. In this approach, the distinction between lines of therapy is no longer absolute using multiple lines of therapy for the benefit of patients with mCRC.

▌ TARGETED AGENTS

Bevacizumab

Bevacizumab, the monoclonal antibody against VEGF, had shown promising preclinical and clinical activity against mCRC, particularly in combination with chemotherapy. A phase III randomized study enrolling 813 patients compared the addition of bevacizumab to the combination chemotherapy regimen IFL, which was the standard of care at the time for mCRC.[7] The addition of bevacizumab to IFL demonstrated a median duration of survival of 20.3 months in the group given IFL plus bevacizumab, as compared with 15.6 months in the group given IFL plus placebo, corresponding to a HR for death of 0.66 ($p < .001$). The median duration of PFS was 10.6 months in the group given IFL plus bevacizumab, as compared with 6.2 months in the group given IFL plus placebo (HR for disease progression, 0.54; $p < .001$); the corresponding rates of response were 44.8% and 34.8% ($p = .004$). The median duration of the response was 10.4 months in the group given IFL plus bevacizumab, as compared with 7.1 months in the group given IFL plus placebo (HR for progression, 0.62; $p = .001$). Grade 3 hypertension was more common during treatment with IFL plus bevacizumab than with IFL plus placebo (11.0% vs. 2.3%) but was easily managed. This study established bevacizumab in the first line of therapy for mCRC, providing a statistically significant and clinically meaningful improvement in survival.

A subsequent study administered bevacizumab in combination with FOLFOX for previously treated mCRC.[36] In this study, 829 mCRC patients previously treated with 5-FU and irinotecan were randomly assigned to one of three treatment groups: FOLFOX with bevacizumab; FOLFOX without bevacizumab; or bevacizumab alone. The primary endpoint was OS with additional determinations of PFS, response, and toxicity. The median duration of survival for the group treated with FOLFOX and bevacizumab was 12.9 months compared with 10.8 months for the group treated with FOLFOX alone (corresponding HR for death = 0.75; p = .0011), and 10.2 months for those treated with bevacizumab alone. The median PFS for the group treated with FOLFOX in combination with bevacizumab was 7.3 months, compared with 4.7 months for the group treated with FOLFOX alone (corresponding HR for progression = 0.61; p < .0001), and 2.7 months for those treated with bevacizumab alone. The corresponding overall RR was 22.7%, 8.6%, and 3.3%, respectively (p < .0001 for FOLFOX with bevacizumab versus FOLFOX comparison). Bevacizumab was associated with an increase in hypertension, bleeding, and vomiting. The addition of bevacizumab to FOLFOX improves survival duration for patients with previously treated metastatic colorectal.

Bevacizumab was studied with oxaliplatin-based chemotherapy given with either infusion 5-FU (FOLFOX) or capecitabine (XELOX).[37] The original design of the study was to compare FOLFOX to XELOX in the first line of therapy for mCRC. When the results of the bevacizumab studies became available, a second randomization was undertaken to add bevacizumab or placebo and evaluate a primary endpoint of PFS. A total of 1,401 patients were randomly assigned in 2 × 2 factorial design, to XELOX versus FOLFOX, and then to bevacizumab versus placebo. Median PFS was 9.4 months in the bevacizumab group and 8.0 months in the placebo group (HR = 0.83; 97.5% CI, 0.72 to 0.95; p = .0023). Median OS was 21.3 months in the bevacizumab group and 19.9 months in the placebo group (HR = 0.89; 97.5% CI, 0.76 to 1.03; p = .077). RR, as assessed by investigators, was similar in the bevacizumab plus chemotherapy versus placebo plus chemotherapy groups (47% vs. 49%; odds ratio [OR], 0.90; 97.5% CI, 0.71 to 1.14; p = .31). Analysis of treatment withdrawals showed that, despite protocol allowance of treatment continuation until disease progression, only 29% and 47% of bevacizumab and placebo recipients, respectively, were treated until progression. The toxicity profile of bevacizumab was consistent with that documented in previous trials. The addition of bevacizumab to oxaliplatin-based chemotherapy significantly improved PFS in this first-line trial in patients with mCRC. OS differences did not reach statistical significance, and RR was not improved by the addition of bevacizumab. Treatment continuation until disease progression may be necessary to optimize the contribution of bevacizumab to therapy.

Cetuximab

The EGFR, which participates in signaling pathways that are deregulated in cancer cells, commonly appears on colorectal cancer cells. Cetuximab is a monoclonal antibody that specifically blocks the EGFR. Although most of the preclinical data with cetuximab alone has demonstrated primarily cytostatic activity, data combining cetuximab with marginally effective or ineffective cytotoxic chemotherapy have demonstrated marked synergy with dramatic improvement in antitumor activity for the combination.[38–41]

The efficacy of cetuximab in combination with irinotecan was compared with that of cetuximab alone in mCRC that was refractory to treatment with irinotecan.[42] Of those patients whose disease had progressed during or within 3 months after treatment with an irinotecan-based regimen, 329 were randomized to receive either cetuximab and irinotecan (at the same dose and schedule as in a prestudy regimen [218 patients]) or cetuximab monotherapy (111 patients). In cases of disease progression, the addition of irinotecan to cetuximab monotherapy was permitted. Immunohistochemical evidence of EGFR expression, either in the primary tumor or in at least one metastatic lesion, was required. The patients were evaluated radiologically for tumor response and were also evaluated for the TTP, survival, and side effects of treatment. The rate of response in the combination therapy group was significantly higher than that in the monotherapy group (22.9% [95% CI, 17.5 to 29.1] vs. 10.8% [95% CI, 5.7 to 18.1], p = .007). The median time to progression was significantly greater in the combination therapy group (4.1 vs. 1.5 months, p < .001 by the log-rank test). The median survival time was 8.6 months in the combination therapy group and 6.9 months in the monotherapy group (p = .48). Toxic effects were more frequent in the combination therapy group, but their severity and incidence were similar to those that would be expected with irinotecan alone. Cetuximab has clinically significant activity when given alone or in combination with irinotecan in patients with irinotecan-refractory colorectal cancer.

A phase III trial of cetuximab plus irinotecan as second-line therapy after fluoropyrimidine and oxaliplatin failure in patients with mCRC was conducted with a primary endpoint of survival.[43] This study randomly assigned 1,298 patients with EGFR-expressing mCRC who had experienced first-line fluoropyrimidine and oxaliplatin treatment failure to cetuximab plus irinotecan or irinotecan alone. Median OS was comparable between treatments: 10.7 months (95% CI, 9.6 to 11.3) with cetuximab/irinotecan and 10.0 months (95% CI, 9.1 to 11.3) with irinotecan alone (HR = 0.975; 95% CI, 0.854 to 1.114; p = .71). This lack of difference may have been caused by post-trial therapy: 46.9% of patients assigned to irinotecan eventually received cetuximab (87.2% of those who did received it with irinotecan). Cetuximab added to irinotecan significantly improved PFS (median, 4.0 vs. 2.6 months; HR = 0.692; 95% CI, 0.617 to 0.776; p ≤ .0001) and RR (16.4% vs. 4.2%; p < .0001), and resulted in significantly better scores in the QoL analysis of global health status (p = .047). Cetuximab did not exacerbate toxicity, except for acneiform rash, diarrhea, hypomagnesemia, and associated electrolyte imbalances. Neutropenia was the most common severe toxicity across treatment arms. Cetuximab and irinotecan improved PFS and RR and resulted in better QoL versus irinotecan alone. OS was similar between study groups, possibly influenced by the large number of patients in the irinotecan arm who received cetuximab and irinotecan poststudy.

Cetuximab was further evaluated as a component of first-line therapy for mCRC.[44] A total of 599 patients with EGFR expression by immunohistochemistry received cetuximab plus FOLFIRI, and 599 received FOLFIRI alone. The primary endpoint was PFS. The HR for PFS in the cetuximab-FOLFIRI group as compared with the FOLFIRI group was 0.85 (95% CI, 0.72 to 0.99; p = .048). There was no significant difference in OS between the two treatment groups (HR = 0.93; 95% CI, 0.81 to 1.07; p = .31). The following grade 3 or 4 adverse events were more frequent with cetuximab plus FOLFIRI than with FOLFIRI alone: skin reactions (which were grade 3 only) (in 19.7% vs.

0.2% of patients, $p < .001$), infusion-related reactions (in 2.5% vs. 0%, $p < .001$), and diarrhea (in 15.7% vs. 10.5%, $p = .008$).

Multiple reports had identified activity of cetuximab in tumors that did not express the EGFR by immunohistochemistry. Furthermore, mutation at key sites within the KRAS gene, which codes for the small G protein that links ligand-dependent receptor activation to intracellular pathways of the EGFR signaling cascade, causes constitutive activation of KRAS-associated signaling. Accumulation of evidence indicates that tumor KRAS mutation, commonly at codons 12 and 13, is associated with the inefficacy of cetuximab.[45–49] Further evaluation from the first-line study indicated a significant interaction between treatment group and KRAS mutation status for tumor response ($p = .03$) but not for PFS ($p = .07$) or OS ($p = .44$). The HR for PFS among patients with wild-type-KRAS tumors was 0.68 (95% CI, 0.50 to 0.94) in favor of the cetuximab-FOLFIRI group. The authors conclude that the first-line treatment with cetuximab plus FOLFIRI, as compared with FOLFIRI alone, reduced the risk of progression of mCRC. The benefit of cetuximab was limited to patients with KRAS wild-type tumors.

The role of cetuximab in combination with first-line therapy with FOLFOX for mCRC was evaluated in a randomized study with a primary endpoint of RR, and the results assessed by KRAS mutation status.[50] A total of 344 patients received FOLFOX with or without cetuximab. KRAS mutation status was assessed in the subset of 233 patients with assessable tumor samples. The confirmed RR for cetuximab plus FOLFOX was higher than with FOLFOX alone (46% vs. 36%). A statistically significant increase in the odds for a response with the addition of cetuximab to FOLFOX could not be established (OR = 1.52; $p = .064$). In patients with KRAS wild-type tumors, the addition of cetuximab to FOLFOX was associated with a clinically significant increased chance of response (RR = 61% vs. 37%; OR = 2.54; $p = .011$) and a lower risk of disease progression (HR = 0.57; $p = .0163$) compared with FOLFOX alone. Cetuximab plus FOLFOX was generally well tolerated. KRAS mutational status was shown to be a highly predictive selection criterion in relation to the treatment decision regarding the addition of cetuximab to FOLFOX for previously untreated patients with mCRC.

Cetuximab plus capecitabine and irinotecan (CAPIRI) compared with cetuximab plus capecitabine and oxaliplatin (CAPOX) as first-line treatment for patients with mCRC was evaluated with a primary endpoint of RR.[51] A total of 185 patients with mCRC were randomly assigned to cetuximab plus CAPIRI or CAPOX. In the intention-to-treat patient population ($n = 177$), RR was 46% (95% CI, 35 to 57) for CAPIRI plus cetuximab versus 48% (95% CI, 37 to 59) for CAPOX plus cetuximab. Analysis of the KRAS gene mutation status was performed in 81.4% of the intention-to-treat population. Patients with KRAS wild-type in the CAPIRI plus cetuximab arm showed an RR of 50.0%, a PFS of 6.2 months, and an OS of 21.1 months. In the CAPOX plus cetuximab arm, an ORR of 44.9%, a PFS of 7.1 months, and an OS of 23.5 months were observed. Although RR and PFS were comparable in KRAS wild-type and mutant subgroups, a trend toward longer survival was associated with KRAS wild-type. Both regimens had manageable toxicity profiles and were safe. This randomized trial demonstrates that the addition of cetuximab to CAPIRI or CAPOX is effective and safe in first-line treatment of mCRC. In the analyzed regimens, ORR and PFS did not differ according to KRAS gene mutation status.

The addition of cetuximab to oxaliplatin-based first-line combination chemotherapy for treatment of advanced colorectal cancer was further evaluated in a randomized phase III study with a primary endpoint of OS in patients with KRAS wild-type tumors.[52] A total of 729 patients with KRAS wild-type tumors received a fluoropyrimidine (capecitabine in 472 and infused fluorouracil plus leucovorin in 243) with oxaliplatin and were randomized to receive cetuximab or not. OS did not differ between treatment groups (median survival 17.9 months in the control group vs. 17.0 months in the cetuximab group; HR = 1.04; 95% CI, 0.87 to 1.23; $p = .67$). Similarly, there was no effect on PFS (8.6 months in the control group vs. 8.6 months in the cetuximab group; HR = 0.96; 0.82 to 1.12; $p = .60$). Overall RR increased from 57% ($n = 209$) with chemotherapy alone to 64% ($n = 232$) with addition of cetuximab ($p = .049$). Grade 3 and higher skin and GI toxic effects were increased with cetuximab (14 vs. 114 and 67 vs. 97 patients in the control group vs. the cetuximab group, respectively). This trial has not confirmed a benefit of addition of cetuximab to oxaliplatin-based chemotherapy in first-line treatment of patients with advanced colorectal cancer. Cetuximab increases RR, with no evidence of benefit in PFS or OS in KRAS wild type. The use of cetuximab in combination with oxaliplatin and capecitabine in first-line chemotherapy in patients with widespread metastases cannot be recommended.

Panitumumab

Panitumumab is a fully human monoclonal antibody directed against the EGFR. The activity of panitumumab plus best supportive care (BSC) was compared to that of BSC alone in patients with mCRC who had progressed after standard chemotherapy.[53] A total of 463 patients with 1% or more EGFR tumor cell membrane staining, measurable disease, and radiologic documentation of disease progression during or within 6 months of most recent chemotherapy were randomly assigned to panitumumab plus BSC ($n = 231$) or BSC alone ($n = 232$). Tumor assessments by blinded central review were scheduled from week 8 until disease progression. The primary endpoint was PFS. Secondary endpoints included objective response, OS, and safety. BSC patients who progressed could receive panitumumab in a cross-over study. Panitumumab significantly prolonged PFS (HR = 0.54; 95% CI, 0.44 to 0.66; $p < .0001$). Median PFS time was 8 weeks (95% CI, 7.9 to 8.4) for panitumumab and 7.3 weeks (95% CI, 7.1 to 7.7) for BSC. Mean (standard error) PFS time was 13.8 (0.8) weeks for panitumumab and 8.5 (0.5) weeks for BSC. Objective RRs also favored panitumumab over BSC; after a 12-month minimum follow-up, RRs were 10% for panitumumab and 0% for BSC ($p < .0001$). No difference was observed in OS (HR = 1.00; 95% CI, 0.82 to 1.22), which was confounded by similar activity of panitumumab after 76% of BSC patients entered the cross-over study. Panitumumab was well tolerated. Skin toxicities, hypomagnesemia, and diarrhea were the most common toxicities observed. No patients had grade 3/4 infusion reactions. Panitumumab significantly improved PFS with manageable toxicity in patients with chemorefractory colorectal cancer.

Panitumumab was evaluated with FOLFIRI combination chemotherapy as second-line therapy for mCRC in a randomized phase III study and prospectively analyzed by KRAS status.[54] A total of 1,186 patients with mCRC who had progressed on one chemotherapy regimen and had tumor specimen available for KRAS testing were randomized to receive FOLFIRI alone or FOLFIRI with panitumumab with a primary endpoint of PFS. KRAS status was available for 91% of patients: 597 (55%) with wild-type KRAS tumors and 486 (45%) with mutant KRAS tumors. In the wild-type KRAS subpopulation, when panitumumab was added to chemotherapy, a significant improvement in PFS was observed (HR = 0.73; 95% CI, 0.59 to 0.90; $p = .004$); median PFS was 5.9 months for panitumumab-FOLFIRI versus 3.9 months for FOLFIRI. A nonsignificant trend toward increased OS was observed; median OS was 14.5 months versus 12.5 months, respectively (HR = 0.85; 95% CI, 0.70 to 1.04; $p = .12$); RR was improved to 35% versus 10% with the addition of panitumumab. In patients with mutant KRAS, there was no difference in efficacy. Adverse event rates were generally comparable across arms with the exception of known toxicities associated with anti-EGFR therapy. Panitumumab plus FOLFIRI significantly improved PFS and is well tolerated as second-line treatment in patients with wild-type KRAS mCRC.

The efficacy and safety of panitumumab with FOLFOX as first-line therapy for mCRC was evaluated in a randomized phase III study with the primary endpoint of PFS and the results prospectively analyzed by KRAS status.[55] KRAS results were available for 93% of the 1,183 patients randomly assigned. In the wild-type KRAS stratum, panitumumab-FOLFOX significantly improved PFS compared with FOLFOX (median PFS, 9.6 vs. 8.0 months, respectively; HR = 0.80; 95% CI, 0.66 to 0.97; $p = .02$). A nonsignificant increase in OS was also observed for panitumumab-FOLFOX versus FOLFOX (median OS, 23.9 vs. 19.7 months, respectively; HR = 0.83; 95% CI, 0.67 to 1.02; $p = .072$). In the mutant KRAS stratum, PFS was significantly reduced in the panitumumab-FOLFOX4 arm versus the FOLFOX4 arm (HR = 1.29; 95% CI, 1.04 to 1.62; $p = .02$), and median OS was 15.5 months versus 19.3 months, respectively (HR = 1.24; 95% CI, 0.98 to 1.57; $p = .068$). Adverse event rates were generally comparable across arms with the exception of toxicities known to be associated with anti-EGFR therapy. Unlike the first-line study of cetuximab with fluoropyrimidine and oxaliplatin,[52] this study demonstrated that panitumumab-FOLFOX was well tolerated and significantly improved PFS in patients with wild-type KRAS tumors.

Combination Vascular Endothelial Growth Factor and Epidermal Growth Factor Receptor Inhibitor

Dual inhibition of VEGF and EGFR was evaluated in a randomized phase IIIB trial of chemotherapy (FOLFOX or FOLFIRI), bevacizumab, and panitumumab compared with chemotherapy and bevacizumab alone for the first-line treatment of mCRC.[56] Patients unselected by KRAS status were randomly assigned within each chemotherapy cohort to bevacizumab and chemotherapy with or without panitumumab. The primary endpoint was PFS within the oxaliplatin cohort. A total of 823 and 230 patients were randomly assigned to the oxaliplatin and irinotecan cohorts, respectively. Panitumumab was discontinued after a planned interim analysis of 812 oxaliplatin patients showed worse efficacy in the panitumumab arm. In the final analysis, median PFS was 10.0 and 11.4 months for the panitumumab and control arms, respectively (HR = 1.27; 95% CI, 1.06 to 1.52); median survival was 19.4 and 24.5 months for the

panitumumab and control arms, respectively. Grade 3/4 adverse events in the oxaliplatin cohort (panitumumab vs. control) included skin toxicity (36% vs. 1%), diarrhea (24% vs. 13%), infections (19% vs. 10%), and pulmonary embolism (6% vs. 4%). Increased toxicity without evidence of improved efficacy was observed in the panitumumab arm of the irinotecan cohort. KRAS analyses showed adverse outcomes for the panitumumab arm in both wild-type and mutant groups. The addition of panitumumab to bevacizumab and oxaliplatin- or irinotecan-based chemotherapy results in increased toxicity and decreased PFS. These combinations are not recommended for the treatment of mCRC in clinical practice.

A similar finding was identified with the dual inhibition of VEGF and EGFR using cetuximab and a capecitabine, oxaliplatin, and bevacizumab combination in the first line of therapy for mCRC.[57] A total of 755 patients were randomly assigned to determine a primary endpoint of PFS. The mutation status of the KRAS gene was evaluated as a predictor of outcome. The median PFS was 10.7 months in the chemotherapy and bevacizumab group and 9.4 in the chemotherapy, bevacizumab, and cetuximab group ($p = .01$). QoL scores were lower in the cetuximab group. OS and RR did not differ significantly in the two groups. Treated patients in the cetuximab group had more grade 3 or 4 adverse events, which were attributed to cetuximab-related adverse cutaneous effects. Patients treated with cetuximab who had tumors bearing a mutated KRAS gene had significantly decreased PFS as compared with cetuximab-treated patients with wild-type-KRAS tumors or patients with mutated KRAS tumors in the no cetuximab group. The addition of cetuximab to capecitabine, oxaliplatin, and bevacizumab resulted in significantly shorter PFS and inferior QoL. Mutation status of the KRAS gene was a predictor of poor outcome in the cetuximab group.

Conversion

A phase II trial of cetuximab in combination with FOLFOX in the first-line treatment of mCRC was undertaken in an unselected population to investigate the efficacy and safety of the combination.[58] In the clinical study, 43 patients were included. Confirmed RR was 72% with 95% disease control. Median PFS and median duration of response were 12.3 and 10.8 months, respectively. Ten patients (23%) underwent resection with curative intent of previously unresectable metastases. After a median follow-up of 30.5 months, median OS was 30.0 months. Cetuximab did not increase the characteristic toxicity of FOLFOX and was generally well tolerated. Cetuximab in combination with FOLFOX-4 is a highly active first-line treatment for mCRC, showing encouraging RR, median PFS, and median OS values. The treatment resulted in a high resectability rate, which could potentially result in an improved cure rate. This combination is under phase III development.

❚ CONCLUSION

The medical management of mCRC has improved the QoL and duration of life for a significant number of patients. At this time, with current therapy, the cure rate remains low. By incorporating the advances in medical management with surgical and interventional procedures, it is expected that more patients will enjoy a better survival.

REFERENCES

1. Siegel R, Naishadham D, Jemal A. Cancer statistics, 2013. *CA Cancer J Clin* 2013;63:11–30.
2. Innocenti F, Undevia SD, Iyer L, et al. Genetic variants in the UDP-glucuronosyltransferase 1A1 gene predict the risk of severe neutropenia of irinotecan. *J Clin Oncol* 2004;22:1382–1388.
3. Grothey A, Nikcevich DA, Sloan JA, et al. Intravenous calcium and magnesium for oxaliplatin-induced sensory neurotoxicity in adjuvant colon cancer: NCCTG N04C7. *J Clin Oncol* 2011;29:421–427.
4. Grothey A, Hochster H, Shpilsky A, et al. Effect of intravenous (IV) calcium and magnesium (Ca/Mg) versus placebo on response to FOLFOX+bevacizumab (BEV) in the CONcePT trial [abstract 208]. American Society of Clinical Oncology; 2008 Gastrointestinal Cancers Symposium.
5. Cascinu S, Catalano V, Cordella L, et al. Neuroprotective effect of reduced glutathione on oxaliplatin-based chemotherapy in advanced colorectal cancer: a randomized, double-blind, placebo-controlled trial. *J Clin Oncol* 2002;20:3478–3483.
6. Eloxatin (oxaliplatin) [package insert]. Bridgewater, NJ: Sanofi-Aventis U.S. LLC; 2009.
7. Hurwitz H, Fehrenbacher L, Novotny W, et al. Bevacizumab plus irinotecan, fluorouracil, and leucovorin for metastatic colorectal cancer. *N Engl J Med* 2004;350:2335–2342.
8. Avastin (bevacizumab) [package insert]. South San Francisco, CA: Genentech, Inc; 2011.
9. Hapani S, Chu D, Wu S. Risk of gastrointestinal perforation in patients with cancer treated with bevacizumab: a meta-analysis. *Lancet Oncol* 2009;10:559–568.
10. Erbitux (cetuximab) [package insert]. Branchburg, NJ: ImClone LLC; 2011.
11. Chung CH, Mirakhur B, Chan E, et al. Cetuximab-induced anaphylaxis and IgE specific for galactose-alpha-1,3-galactose. *N Engl J Med* 2008;358:1109–1117.
12. Saltz LB, Meropol NJ, Loehrer PJSr, et al. Phase II trial of cetuximab in patients with refractory colorectal cancer that expresses the epidermal growth factor receptor. *J Clin Oncol* 2004;22:1201–1208.
13. Schrag D, Chung KY, Flombaum C, et al. Cetuximab therapy and symptomatic hypomagnesemia. *J Natl Cancer Inst* 2005;97:1221–1224.
14. Crawford J, Sandler AB, Hammond LA, et al. ABX-EGF in combination with paclitaxel and carboplatin for advanced non-small cell lung cancer (NSCLC) [abstract 7083]. *Proc Am Soc Clin Oncol* 2004;23.
15. Yang XD, Jia XC, Corvalan JR, et al. Development of ABX-EGF, a fully human anti-EGF receptor monoclonal antibody, for cancer therapy. *Crit Rev Oncol Hematol* 2001;38:17–23.
16. Alekshun T, Garrett C. Targeted therapies in the treatment of colorectal cancers. *Cancer Control* 2005;12:105–110.
17. Cohen SJ, Cohen RB, Meropol NJ. Targeting signal transduction pathways in colorectal cancer—more than skin deep. *J Clin Oncol* 2005;23:5374–5385.
18. Buroker TR, O'Connell MJ, Wieand HS, et al. Randomized comparison of two schedules of fluorouracil and leucovorin in the treatment of advanced colorectal cancer. *J Clin Oncol* 1994;12:14–20.
19. Saltz LB, Cox JV, Blanke C, et al. Irinotecan plus fluorouracil and leucovorin for metastatic colorectal cancer. Irinotecan Study Group. *N Engl J Med* 2000;343:905–914.
20. Rothenberg ML, Meropol NJ, Poplin EA, et al. Mortality associated with irinotecan plus bolus fluorouracil/leucovorin: summary findings of an independent panel. *J Clin Oncol* 2001;19:3801–3807.
21. de Gramont A, Bosset JF, Milan C, et al. Randomized trial comparing monthly low-dose leucovorin and fluorouracil bolus with bimonthly high-dose leucovorin and fluorouracil bolus plus continuous infusion for advanced colorectal cancer: a French intergroup study. *J Clin Oncol* 1997;15:808–815.
22. de Gramont A, Figer A, Seymour M, et al. Leucovorin and fluorouracil with or without oxaliplatin as first-line treatment in advanced colorectal cancer. *J Clin Oncol* 2000;18:2938–2947.
23. Andre T, Louvet C, Maindrault-Goebel F, et al. CPT-11 (irinotecan) addition to bimonthly, high-dose leucovorin and bolus and continuous-infusion 5-fluorouracil (FOLFIRI) for pretreated metastatic colorectal cancer. GERCOR. *Eur J Cancer* 1999;35:1343–1347.
24. Haller DG, Rothenberg ML, Wong AO, et al. Oxaliplatin plus irinotecan compared with irinotecan alone as second-line treatment after single-agent fluoropyrimidine therapy for metastatic colorectal carcinoma. *J Clin Oncol* 2008;26:4544–4550.
25. Goldberg RM, Sargent DJ, Morton RF, et al. A randomized controlled trial of fluorouracil plus leucovorin, irinotecan, and oxaliplatin combinations in patients with previously untreated metastatic colorectal cancer. *J Clin Oncol* 2004;22:23–30.
26. Tournigand C, Andre T, Achille E, et al. FOLFIRI followed by FOLFOX6 or the reverse sequence in advanced colorectal cancer: a randomized GERCOR study. *J Clin Oncol* 2004;22:229–237.
27. Tournigand C, Cervantes A, Figer A, et al. OPTIMOX1: a randomized study of FOLFOX4 or FOLFOX7 with oxaliplatin in a stop-and-go fashion in advanced colorectal cancer—a GERCOR study. *J Clin Oncol* 2006;24:394–400.
28. Chibaudel B, Maindrault-Goebel F, Lledo G, et al. Can chemotherapy be discontinued in unresectable metastatic colorectal cancer? The GERCOR OPTIMOX2 Study. *J Clin Oncol* 2009;27:5727–5733.
29. Cunningham D, Pyrhonen S, James RD, et al. Randomised trial of irinotecan plus supportive care versus supportive care alone after fluorouracil failure for patients with metastatic colorectal cancer. *Lancet* 1998;352:1413–1418.
30. Rougier P, Van Cutsem E, Bajetta E, et al. Randomised trial of irinotecan versus fluorouracil by continuous infusion after fluorouracil failure in patients with metastatic colorectal cancer. *Lancet* 1998;352:1407–1412.
31. Rothenberg ML, Oza AM, Bigelow RH, et al. Superiority of oxaliplatin and fluorouracil-leucovorin compared with either therapy alone in patients with progressive colorectal cancer after irinotecan and fluorouracil-leucovorin: interim results of a phase III trial. *J Clin Oncol* 2003;21:2059–2069.
32. Rothenberg ML, Cox JV, Butts C, et al. Capecitabine plus oxaliplatin (XELOX) versus 5-fluorouracil/folinic acid plus oxaliplatin (FOLFOX-4) as second-line therapy in metastatic colorectal cancer: a randomized phase III noninferiority study. *Ann Oncol* 2008;19:1720–1726.
33. Koopman M, Antonini NF, Douma J, et al. Sequential versus combination chemotherapy with capecitabine, irinotecan, and oxaliplatin in advanced colorectal cancer (CAIRO): a phase III randomised controlled trial. *Lancet* 2007;370:135–142.
34. Seymour MT, Maughan TS, Ledermann JA, et al. Different strategies of sequential and combination chemotherapy for patients with poor prognosis advanced colorectal cancer (MRC FOCUS): a randomised controlled trial. *Lancet* 2007;370:143–152.
35. Goldberg RM, Rothenberg ML, Van Cutsem E, et al. The continuum of care: a paradigm for the management of metastatic colorectal cancer. *Oncologist* 2007;12:38–50.
36. Giantonio BJ, Catalano PJ, Meropol NJ, et al. Bevacizumab in combination with oxaliplatin, fluorouracil, and leucovorin (FOLFOX4) for previously treated metastatic colorectal cancer: results from the Eastern Cooperative Oncology Group Study E3200. *J Clin Oncol* 2007;25:1539–1544.
37. Saltz LB, Clarke S, Diaz-Rubio E, et al. Bevacizumab in combination with oxaliplatin-based chemotherapy as first-line therapy in metastatic colorectal cancer: a randomized phase III study. *J Clin Oncol* 2008;26:2013–2019.
38. Fan Z, Baselga J, Masui H, et al. Antitumor effect of anti-epidermal growth factor receptor monoclonal antibodies plus cis-diamminedichloroplatinum on well established A431 cell xenografts. *Cancer Res* 1993;53:4637–4642.
39. Baselga J, Pfister D, Cooper MR, et al. Phase I studies of anti-epidermal growth factor receptor chimeric antibody C225 alone and in combination with cisplatin. *J Clin Oncol* 2000;18:904–914.
40. Ciardiello F, Bianco R, Damiano V, et al. Antitumor activity of sequential treatment with topotecan and anti-epidermal growth factor receptor monoclonal antibody C225. *Clin Cancer Res* 1999;5:909–916.
41. Prewett MC, Hooper AT, Bassi R, et al. Enhanced antitumor activity of anti-epidermal growth factor receptor monoclonal antibody IMC-C225 in combination with irinotecan (CPT-11) against human colorectal tumor xenografts. *Clin Cancer Res* 2002;8:994–1003.
42. Cunningham D, Humblet Y, Siena S, et al. Cetuximab monotherapy and cetuximab plus irinotecan in irinotecan-refractory metastatic colorectal cancer. *N Engl J Med* 2004;351:337–345.
43. Sobrero AF, Maurel J, Fehrenbacher L, et al. EPIC: phase III trial of cetuximab plus irinotecan after fluoropyrimidine and oxaliplatin failure in patients with metastatic colorectal cancer. *J Clin Oncol* 2008;26:2311–2319.
44. Van Cutsem E, Kohne CH, Hitre E, et al. Cetuximab and chemotherapy as initial treatment for metastatic colorectal cancer. *N Engl J Med* 2009;360:1408–1417.
45. De Roock W, Piessevaux H, De Schutter J, et al. KRAS wild-type state predicts survival and is associated to early radiological response in metastatic colorectal cancer treated with cetuximab. *Ann Oncol* 2008;19:508–515.
46. Di Fiore F, Blanchard F, Charbonnier F, et al. Clinical relevance of KRAS mutation detection in metastatic colorectal cancer treated by cetuximab plus chemotherapy. *Br J Cancer* 2007;96:1166–1169.

47. Lievre A, Bachet JB, Boige V, et al. KRAS mutations as an independent prognostic factor in patients with advanced colorectal cancer treated with cetuximab. *J Clin Oncol* 2008;26:374–379.

48. Lievre A, Bachet JB, Le Corre D, et al. KRAS mutation status is predictive of response to cetuximab therapy in colorectal cancer. *Cancer Res* 2006;66:3992–3995.

49. Cervantes A, Macarulla T, Martinelli E, et al. Correlation of KRAS status (wild type [wt] vs. mutant [mt]) with efficacy to first-line cetuximab in a study of cetuximab single agent followed by cetuximab + FOLFIRI in patients (pts) with metastatic colorectal cancer (mCRC). *J Clin Oncol* 2008;26(suppl):2105.

50. Bokemeyer C, Bondarenko I, Makhson A, et al. Fluorouracil, leucovorin, and oxaliplatin with and without cetuximab in the first-line treatment of metastatic colorectal cancer. *J Clin Oncol* 2009;27:663–671.

51. Moosmann N, von Weikersthal LF, Vehling-Kaiser U, et al. Cetuximab plus capecitabine and irinotecan compared with cetuximab plus capecitabine and oxaliplatin as first-line treatment for patients with metastatic colorectal cancer: AIO KRK-0104—a randomized trial of the German AIO CRC study group. *J Clin Oncol* 2011;29:1050–1058.

52. Maughan TS, Adams RA, Smith CG, et al. Addition of cetuximab to oxaliplatin-based first-line combination chemotherapy for treatment of advanced colorectal cancer: results of the randomised phase 3 MRC COIN trial. *Lancet* 2011;377:2103–2114.

53. Van Cutsem E, Peeters M, Siena S, et al. Open-label phase III trial of panitumumab plus best supportive care compared with best supportive care alone in patients with chemotherapy-refractory metastatic colorectal cancer. *J Clin Oncol* 2007;25:1658–1664.

54. Peeters M, Price TJ, Cervantes A, et al. Randomized phase III study of panitumumab with fluorouracil, leucovorin, and irinotecan (FOLFIRI) compared with FOLFIRI alone as second-line treatment in patients with metastatic colorectal cancer. *J Clin Oncol* 2010;28:4706–4713.

55. Douillard JY, Siena S, Cassidy J, et al. Randomized, phase III trial of panitumumab with infusional fluorouracil, leucovorin, and oxaliplatin (FOLFOX4) versus FOLFOX4 alone as first-line treatment in patients with previously untreated metastatic colorectal cancer: the PRIME study. *J Clin Oncol* 2010;28:4697–4705.

56. Hecht JR, Mitchell E, Chidiac T, et al. A randomized phase IIIB trial of chemotherapy, bevacizumab, and panitumumab compared with chemotherapy and bevacizumab alone for metastatic colorectal cancer. *J Clin Oncol* 2009;27:672–680.

57. Tol J, Koopman M, Cats A, et al. Chemotherapy, bevacizumab, and cetuximab in metastatic colorectal cancer. *N Engl J Med* 2009;360:563–572.

58. Tabernero J, Van Cutsem E, Diaz-Rubio E, et al. Phase II trial of cetuximab in combination with fluorouracil, leucovorin, and oxaliplatin in the first-line treatment of metastatic colorectal cancer. *J Clin Oncol* 2007;25:5225–5232.

MARK G. VAN VLEDDER and MICHAEL A. CHOTI

CHAPTER

9

Colorectal Metastases: Surgical Management

▌ INTRODUCTION

Colorectal cancer is the third most common form of cancer in the United States with an estimated incidence of over 140,000 new cases each year and 50,000 deaths annually.[1] Approximately 50% of patients will have liver metastases at the time of presentation or will develop liver metastases during the course of their disease. Complete surgical resection of all metastatic deposits offers the only potential for definitive cure with reported 5-year survival rates exceeding 50% compared to a generally poor prognosis for those patients who are not surgical candidates.[2,3] Whereas in earlier years only patients with very limited (solitary or unilobar) liver metastases were considered for surgical therapy, the number of patients thought to be eligible for surgical therapy has increased based on encouraging results in those with more extensive disease. Yet, currently, only 20% to 30% of patients with liver-only metastases can be considered surgical candidates.[4–6] Improved systemic fluoropyrimidine-based chemotherapeutic regimens including oxaliplatin and irinotecan have improved survival and response rates. The addition of biologic therapies, such as bevacizumab, cetuximab, and panitumumab, have further improved the efficacy of combined-modality therapies for advanced colorectal cancer.[7] Also, strategies including preoperative hepatic preconditioning (e.g., partial portal vein embolization), staged liver resections, and resection combined with local tumor ablation have facilitated the treatment of patients with more extensive disease.[8,9] Chapter 9 reviews these advances in the surgical treatment of colorectal liver metastases (CRLM) and provides an overview of the developments and current outcomes of the surgical management of colorectal liver metastases.

▌ TECHNIQUES AND OUTCOME

Surgical Technique of Liver Resection

Improved surgical techniques as well as advances in pre- and postoperative care have allowed liver resection to be performed with relative safety and low morbidity. The main objective of every oncologic liver resection is to resect portions of the involved liver with adequate margins while preserving a sufficient amount of uninvolved parenchyma. Using resection planes as dictated by the surgical anatomy of the liver as described by Couinaud (FIGURE 9.1),[3,10] partial hepatectomy can be performed without affecting the function of the remaining liver or compromising large vascular structures.[11]

Liver resections can be classified as a major liver resection (greater than 3 contiguous segments) or as a minor resection (<3 segments). Major liver resections can be further classified as either left or right hepatectomy (hemihepatectomy) or extended hepatectomy with or without inclusion of the caudate lobe (segment 1). Minor resections can be divided into anatomic (segmental) or nonanatomic liver resections. Examples of anatomic resections include left lateral bisegmentectomy (segments 2/3), right posterior bisegmentectomy (sectorectomy or sectionectomy), or isolated segmental resection. Nonanatomic or subsegmental resections (wedge resection) can be especially helpful in the treatment of small superficial metastases to preserve hepatic parenchyma. The choice of resection depends on the size and number or tumor(s) identified and their position relative to the pedicles within the liver, provided complete margin negative removal is achieved.[12]

When performing a major hepatic resection, vascular structures supplying the region to be resected are typically isolated and secured extrahepatically prior to parenchymal dissection. Temporary clamping of the entire hepatic inflow (Pringle maneuver) can be used in some cases to reduce blood loss. Transection of the liver parenchyma is then conducted. Traditionally, the parenchyma is dissected using a blunt crushing technique (crush-clamp or finger-fracture technique), controlling intrahepatic vascular structures with clips or ties. More recently, a variety of newer devices and techniques have been developed to transect liver tissue, including the cavitron ultrasound aspirator (CUSA), saline-enhanced dissectors, bipolar energy sealing systems, ultrasonic coagulation, and thermal precoagulation techniques. Although some studies suggest that technical challenges and blood loss can be reduced with some of these devices, little data demonstrate superiority of any one technique over another. Therefore, the particular method of parenchymal dissection is largely left to the surgeon's experience and preference.

Typically, surgical access to the liver is obtained via open laparotomy. This approach allows for full mobilization, inspection, and palpation of the liver and ensures adequate exposure of all relevant anatomic structures. More recently, improved devices and techniques have allowed the expanded use of more minimally invasive surgical approaches. Specifically, laparoscopic approaches have been shown to be associated with

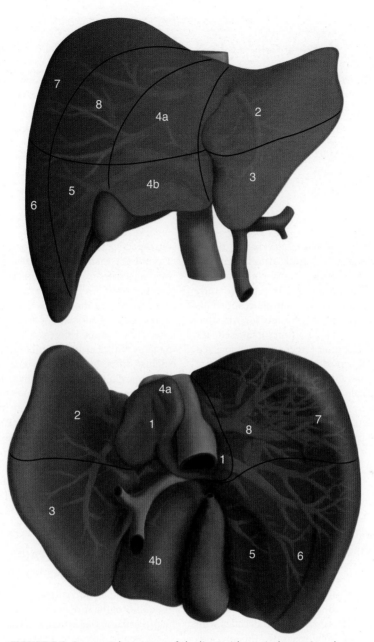

FIGURE 9.1 Segmental anatomy of the liver with surgical resection planes

less pain and more rapid recovery without compromise to oncologic success.[13] These advantages should be considered, however, in the light of a steep learning curve and a potentially increased risk of intraoperative complications caused by reduced vision. Moreover, intraoperative assessment of the liver might be challenged by difficulties in laparoscopic ultrasound and the inability to fully inspect and palpate the entire surface of the liver. Laparoscopic ultrasound probes can be difficult to use because of their limited degrees of freedom in movement. While open intraoperative ultrasound enables the detection of additional metastases in about 10-15% of patients, this might not be true for laparoscopic ultrasound.[14,15] Therefore, laparoscopic surgery for colorectal liver metastases should be reserved

for selected cases and performed by surgeons with experience in this technique.

Liver Resection: Morbidity and Mortality

Overall, the perioperative mortality of liver resection for colorectal metastases is less than 3% in most reported series. In high-volume centers, even major hepatic resections result in perioperative mortality of 1% or less (Table 9.1).[16] Complication rates similarly remain low, even following major resections. In a randomized controlled trial comparing outcomes following preoperative chemotherapy, overall mortality and morbidity were 1% and 20%, respectively.[17] While the amount of parenchyma

Table 9.1					
Studies Investigating Long-Term and Short-Term Outcomes After Curative-Intent Liver Resection for Colorectal Liver Metastases					
Author and year of publication	Number of patients included	Mortality	Morbidity	5-year disease-free survival	5-year overall survival
Nordlinger (1996)	1,568	2%	23%	15%	28%
Fong (1999)	1,001	3%	31%	Not reported	37%
Malik (2007)	700	3%	29.5%	31%	45%
de Jong (2009)	1,669	Not reported	Not reported	30%	47%

resected predominantly dictates the risk of developing major complications such as liver failure and death, Another important factor impacting the risk of postoperative complications and death is the presence of comorbidities. In a recent study by Breitenstein et al.,[18] the presence of multiple comorbidities (expressed as an increased American Society for Anesthesiologists score) was associated with a 1.5 times increased risk of major postoperative complications. Other factors associated with the development of major postoperative morbidity were the extent of liver resection and the preoperative transaminase level.[18] Selecting the appropriate patient for surgical therapy is important to reduce perioperative risk. Also, the potential for adverse outcome and the complexity of these operations justifies the recommendation that major liver resection be performed at high volume centers only.[19]

Liver Resection: Long-Term Outcomes and Predictors of Success

With increasing safety, improved imaging, and high efficacy of chemotherapeutic regimens, the prognosis of patients with liver metastases who are eligible for resection has markedly improved over the years with a median survival of up to 46 months and corresponding 5-year survival rates exceeding 50% (see Table 9.1). A study performed at Johns Hopkins found a clear trend toward improving survival over the recent decades with a 27% increase in 5-year survival in between two time periods (31% from 1984 to 1992 vs. 58% from 1993 to 1999). A systematic review by Simmonds et al.[20] including 30 studies showed slightly less optimistic but still encouraging results with an overall 5-year survival rate of approximately 30%.

Yet, still approximately two-thirds of patients will develop recurrent disease after liver resection, and, therefore, the percentage of patients who are actually cured is low.[21] In an attempt to identify those patients at the highest risk for recurrent disease and disease-associated death after curative-intent surgery, analyses have been performed to determine the prognostic indicators that could identify those patients who might benefit most from liver resection. Because more traditional scoring systems, such as the TNM and Dukes classification, have little or no prognostic value for patients with colorectal liver metastases, several clinical risk scores were introduced over the years in an attempt to stratify patients by their risk of recurrence and death prior to surgical intervention. In 1999, the Memorial Sloan Kettering Cancer Center group published its clinical risk score based on a retrospective review of 1,001 patients.[22] This risk score assigned 1 point for each of the following characteristics: disease-free interval less than 1 year, positive nodal status of primary tumor, preoperative CEA greater than 200 ng/mL, largest tumor greater than 5 cm, and more than five liver metastases. Stratifying by this score, patients with a score of 0 had a 60% chance to be alive after 5 years, whereas 5-year survival was not observed in patients with 5 points. Similarly, Nordlinger et al.[23] proposed a slightly different scoring system, which also incorporated surgical margin status and primary tumor stage. Although these risk scores offer some guidance to the clinician toward which patients might benefit most from liver resection, patients should not be excluded from resection based solely on these criteria because long-term survival can be derived even with poor prognostic indicators. These risk scores do not incorporate more direct measures of tumor biology, such as the responsiveness to preoperative chemotherapy, or of the mutational status of the primary tumor, such as Ki-67 or K-ras mutations, which might be more powerful predictors of recurrence and survival.[24–26]

DEFINING RESECTABILITY OF COLORECTAL METASTASES

The decision toward surgical resection should be made based on the ability of the surgeon to locally resect or ablate all disease with negative pathologic surgical margins as well as the absence of any extrahepatic disease that precludes curative treatment. Historically, only patients with very limited disease were considered to be candidates for liver resection, often excluding patients with more than three or bilateral metastases.[4] More recent studies have shown that high survival rates can be achieved even in patients with more extensive disease, and a high tumor number or the proximity of major vessels are no longer contraindications for surgical resection as long as negative pathologic margins can be obtained and enough functional liver parenchyma is left in situ.[6]

The paradigm toward complete resection of all disease has also shifted to the management of patients with liver metastases and concomitant extrahepatic metastases. Recent studies show that long-term survival can be obtained in patients with concomitant isolated lung metastases or even periportal lymph node metastases, although prognosis is generally less favorable when compared to patients without extrahepatic disease. In contrast, the presence of aortocaval lymph node metastases or multiple extrahepatic metastatic sites portends a poor prognosis and surgical resection should generally not be performed in these patients.[27,28]

PREOPERATIVE STAGING OF PATIENTS WITH COLORECTAL LIVER METASTASES

To assess the extent of intrahepatic tumor burden and the presence of extrahepatic disease, every patient who presents with potentially resectable CRLM should be subject to thorough preoperative evaluation. To save patients from futile laparotomy, accurate information should be obtained regarding the size, location, and number of all intrahepatic metastatic sites as well as their relation to surrounding vascular structures by contrast-enhanced, high-quality cross-sectional imaging. Although, as a standard, computed tomography (CT) is used more, and is adequate in most cases, emerging data suggest that magnetic resonance imaging (MRI) may have improved sensitivity compared to CT.[29,30] Enhanced MR imaging has been reported to be superior to CT, particularly for smaller lesions or following response to preoperative chemotherapy.[31] The actual impact of MR imaging over conventional multidetector computed tomography (MDCT) imaging in the management of patients is still controversial, however, and most centers will use MRI scans selectively in the evaluation of patients with CRLM.

Recently, 18-fluorodeoxyglucose positron emission tomography (18-FDG PET) was introduced in the preoperative evaluation of patients with CRLM. Whereas MR imaging, as well as CT imaging, relies on anatomic and vascular changes in the liver parenchyma as a result of tumor growth, FDG PET imaging visualizes the increased uptake of glucose in tumor cells and is, thus, a form of functional imaging. When combined with MDCT imaging, PET imaging can provide an even more accurate depiction of disease spread.[32] Although the exact role of PET imaging in the assessment of intrahepatic disease remains controversial, several studies have shown that PET imaging detects occult sites of extrahepatic disease in up to 27% of patients, significantly altering clinical management in the majority of cases.[33,34] Another study showed that the addition of PET to the preoperative workup significantly reduced the number of nontherapeutic laparotomies as a result of unsuspected intraoperative findings.[35] PET images should preferably be obtained prior to any preoperative chemotherapy because this alters the metabolic activity of tumor cells and thus decreases the sensitivity of PET scanning.

SURGICAL ASSESSMENT AND INTRAOPERATIVE ULTRASOUND

Before liver resection is initiated, a careful intraoperative assessment of the liver and abdominal cavity should be performed to evaluate the extent of intrahepatic disease and potential presence of unexpected extrahepatic disease, using visual inspection, manual palpation, and intraoperative ultrasound. To avoid patients from undergoing a nontherapeutic laparotomy, some

surgeons have advocated a diagnostic laparoscopy including intraoperative ultrasound in patients scheduled for liver resection to evaluate the extent of intra-abdominal disease.[36] With increasing accuracy of intraoperative staging modalities, the rate of nontherapeutic laparotomies has dramatically decreased over recent years and is currently as low as 4.7%. Therefore, the yield of routine diagnostic laparoscopy is considered to be low.[35]

Intraoperative ultrasound (IOUS) can be a major adjunct in the operative evaluation of patients undergoing planned liver resection. Not only does it provide valuable information with regard to the hepatic anatomy and aids the surgeon in the planning and executing the liver resection, IOUS can also detect additional intrahepatic metastases as small as 3 to 4 mm in size. A study from Johns Hopkins Hospital found that IOUS alone detects additional metastases in 10% of patients. In particular, the sensitivity of IOUS at detecting additional lesions was strongly impacted by the echogenicity of the known metastases, which can vary considerably (FIGURE 9.2). In fact, approximately 40% of patients will have hypoechoic tumors and another 20% will present with hyperechoic tumors, with an associated chance of finding additional metastases that is about three times higher when compared to patients with less conspicuous isoechoic tumors (40% of patients) (FIGURE 9.3).[14,37,38] Moreover, the echogenicity of liver metastases has been shown to be an independent predictor of overall survival, with patients with hyperechoic metastases having a significantly better prognosis when compared to patients with hypoechoic tumors.[39,40] IOUS should always be performed in a systematic way using a dedicated intraoperative probe and an experienced operator.

PERIOPERATIVE CHEMOTHERAPY

Converting Unresectable Disease to Resectable Disease

Currently, first-line chemotherapeutic regimens for metastatic colorectal cancer usually include 5-fluorouracil and leukovorin or capecitabine in combination with either irinotecan (FOLFIRI or XELIRI) or oxaliplatin (FOLFOX or XELOX) with response rates ranging up to 40% and a reported median survival ranging well over 20 months for patients with unresectable disease. The addition of biologic agents, such as monoclonal antibodies to vascular endothelial growth factor (bevacizumab) or epidermal growth factor receptor (cetuximab or panitumumab), has further increased response rates and overall survival even in patients with disease refractory to conventional first-line chemotherapy. Recently, Folprecht et al. reported that up to 30% of patients with initially unresectable disease and a nonmutated K-RAS oncogene became surgical candidates after first-line cetuximab combined with either FOLFOX or FOLFIRI.[41,42]

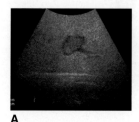

A

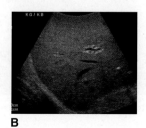

B

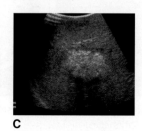

C

FIGURE 9.2 Ultrasound images of CRLM. **A.** Hypoechoic, **B.** Isoechoic, **C.** Hyperechoic

From van Vledder et al. *Ann Surg Oncol* 2010;17(10):2756–2763.

FIGURE 9.3 Bar graph demonstrating the correlation between the echogenicity of CRLM and the probability of finding additional metastases

From van Vledder et al. *Ann Surg Oncol* 2010;17(10):2756–2763.

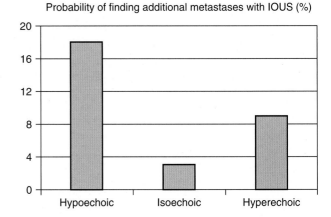

Probability of finding additional metastases with IOUS (%)

The goal of tumor downsizing with a chemotherapeutic response is to be able to remove the gross residual disease of all original sites of disease. Liver metastases located near major vascular pedicles that need to be salvaged are ideal candidates (FIGURE 9.4). Currently, it is estimated that approximately one-fourth of patients with liver-only metastases are initially resectable, and conversion from unresectable disease to resectable disease through tumor downsizing can be achieved in approximately 20% of those with initially considered unresectable disease.

Importantly, although patients with unresectable liver metastases would have a poor prognosis without surgery, salvage resection of initially unresectable disease can result in long-term survival or even cure. In a study by Adam et al.[43] investigating the fate of 154 patients who underwent liver resection of initially unresectable disease, the overall 5-year survival was 33%, which compared favorably to those who were initially resectable. Therefore, the conversion of unresectable disease to resectable disease is currently the main outcome variable in many trials investigating the efficacy of novel chemotherapeutic regimens for metastatic colon cancer initially not amenable for surgery.

Neoadjuvant and Adjuvant Chemotherapy in Initially Resectable Patients

Whereas the benefit of preoperative chemotherapy in patients with initially unresectable metastatic colon cancer is evident, the role and optimal sequencing of chemotherapy in patients with resectable disease is less clear. Chemotherapy can be administered

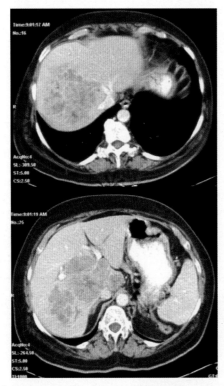
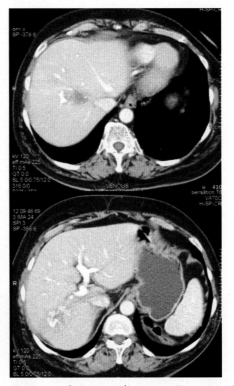

FIGURE 9.4 CT images of a patient with initially unresectable disease (left images) converted to resectable disease following preoperative chemotherapy (right images)

preoperatively as a neoadjuvant regimen, postoperatively as an adjuvant treatment, or pre- and postoperatively as a sandwich regimen. The main imperative for the administration of perioperative chemotherapy is to clear potential micrometastatic disease, prevent early recurrence, and thus prolong survival. Level 1 evidence to support this strategy is not abundant, however, and no data are available to compare the efficacy of preoperative chemotherapy with postoperative chemotherapy. A randomized controlled trial from France (EORTC 40983) investigating the impact of perioperative FOLFOX on long-term outcome in patients with resectable liver metastases showed an improved 3-year recurrence-free survival in the surgery-plus chemotherapy group (42% vs. 33%) when compared to the surgery-only group, although no benefit in overall survival was shown in this trial.[17] Another trial investigating the added value of adjuvant 5-fluorouracil and folinic acid showed an increase in 5-year disease-free survival in the chemotherapy group (33.5% vs. 26.7%), although no significant difference in overall survival was detected and the trial was much criticized for using a relatively inferior chemotherapeutic regimen.[44] Also, no level 1 evidence from phase III randomized controlled trials (RCTs) is available to show a beneficial effect of preoperative chemotherapy only. Although the exact value of neoadjuvant chemotherapy with regard to overall survival might not be clear, the application of preoperative chemotherapy may be associated with other benefits in terms of increased resection rates and improved preoperative patient selection. First, occult lesions might become apparent while on chemotherapy, thus allowing for timely alteration of patient management and preventing futile surgical intervention. Also, progression of tumor growth while on chemotherapy is a powerful predictor of dismal prognosis, and some have suggested that this might be a relative contraindication to surgical therapy. A French study showed that radiologic tumor progression while on chemotherapy was associated with poor postoperative outcome with a corresponding 5-year survival of only 8%,[45] although long-term survival is possible in nonresponders as long as an R0 resection can be performed.[46] Conversely, a major or even complete pathologic response to preoperative chemotherapy seems to be an extremely powerful predictor of good survival: Tanaka et al. showed that the presence of a complete pathologic response in one or more CRLM was associated

with a 70% chance to be alive 5 years after surgery, whereas only 8% of patients without such a response were alive after 5 years, and other studies have confirmed these results.[25,43,47] Unfortunately, predicting the pathologic response based on postchemotherapy imaging has proven to be challenging, and many studies have shown vast discrepancies between the observed radiologic response and the actual pathologic response.

Despite these potential advantages of preoperative chemotherapy, several less desirable effects have been reported as well. Apart from the "usual" systemic side effects associated with chemotherapy such as mucositis, neutropenia and neurologic toxicity, patients are exposed to a theoretical risk of disease progression to a point that their disease becomes unresectable although an R0 resection would have been possible if initiated at the time of diagnosis. Moreover, Perioperative chemotherapy has been associated with increased complication rates. In the EORTC 40983 trial, surgical morbidity increased from 16% to 25% when preoperative chemotherapy was administered compared to surgery alone. Other studies also described an association between preoperative chemotherapy and postoperative morbidity, most likely mediated by chemotherapy-associated liver injury (CALI), further defined as chemotherapy-associated steatosis or steatohepatitis and the sinusoidal obstructive syndrome.[48–50] For these reasons, it is generally recommended that no more than six cycles of preoperative chemotherapy should be administered in patients with resectable disease because little oncologic benefit is to be expected when chemotherapy is continued beyond this point, but the risk of liver injury and associated morbidity will continue to increase.[51] Advantages and disadvantages of preoperative chemotherapy are summarized in (Table 9.2).

Disappearing Metastases Following Chemotherapy

Another potential disadvantage of preoperative chemotherapy is related to the impact of chemotherapy on the accuracy of preoperative imaging. For instance, the presence of chemotherapy-associated steatosis can significantly affect the sensitivity of preoperative CT scanning in the detection of CRLM. In one study by Angelviel et al.,[52] discrepancies between preoperative CT images and histopathologic examination were observed in half of all patients treated

Table 9.2

Impact of Neoadjuvant Chemotherapy in Patients with Resectable Hepatic Colorectal Metastases

Potential advantages	Potential disadvantages
1. Allows time for additional and otherwise occult metastatic sites to appear	1. Tumors may progress to unresectable status
2. Allows for earlier therapy of occult micrometastatic disease	2. Discouraged compliance for subsequent therapy in case of chemotherapy associated morbidity
3. Allows for in vivo gauge of chemoresponsiveness, facilitating postoperative chemotherapy planning	3. Chemotherapy-associated hepatotoxicity
4. Response may allow for smaller resection	4. Potential for increased postoperative complications
5. Response is a prognostic factor	5. Response may hinder finding all sites of metastatic disease

with chemotherapy, whereas this was the case in less than one-third of the surgery-only patients. Moreover, small liver metastases can shrink and disappear while on chemotherapy, further complicating the management of these patients. Benoist et al.[53] found that although these lesions might become completely invisible on postchemotherapy CT scans, viable tumor cells are present in over 80% of these disappearing metastases. Other studies confirmed this discrepancy. A more recent study showed that viable tumor cells were present in approximately half of all disappearing lesions. In this study, disappearing metastases were common in patients undergoing preoperative chemotherapy with approximately one-fourth of patients having at least one lesion disappear. When carefully assessed intraoperatively, approximately 50% of these lesions were detected with IOUS. Moreover, overall survival was not significantly affected if some of these disappearing liver metastases were left surgically untreated possibly due to the opportunity of these patients to undergo repeat surgical intervention when a recurrence in these untreated lesions was observed during follow-up.[54] Regardless, It is generally recommended to completely resect or ablate all disease sites as known prior to chemotherapy to prevent early recurrence and the need for reoperation.

EXPANDING THE ROLE OF SURGICAL THERAPY FOR COLORECTAL LIVER METASTASES

Preoperative Liver Preconditioning to Achieve Remnant Liver Hypertrophy

Because of the remarkable regenerative capacities of the liver, up to 80% of the hepatic parenchyma can be resected in patients without underlying liver disease. In cases where the remnant volume is in question, it is important to measure the anticipated remnant liver volume using segmentation software and volumetric analysis. In cases in which the future liver remnant is too small to allow for safe resection, several strategies are available to completely clear the liver from all metastatic sites and preserve a sufficient amount of functional hepatic reserve. First, the volume of the remaining liver lobe can be increased by selective embolization or ligation of the portal vein branches of the involved hemiliver, eliciting compensatory hypertrophy of the contralateral liver.[55] After ligation or embolization, the increase in volume of the future liver remnant can be determined using repeat volumetric analysis.[56,57]

Two-Stage Hepatectomy

Another approach used in patients with bilateral metastases consists of two stages: a partial resection is performed in the first stage, followed by a second resection after hypertrophy to complete the metastectomy (FIGURE 9.5). Using this technique, one hemiliver is cleared of all macroscopic disease during a first operation by either resection or ablation. Most commonly, the smaller (sublobar) resection is performed first followed by the major resection to avoid gross disease in the hypertrophying liver. In some cases, the first operation can be combined with portal vein ligation (or postoperative embolization) of the contralateral liver lobe that will be resected later.[58] Several studies have yet shown that approximately two-thirds of patients will be able to complete both stages of the resection without disease progression and that prognosis of those patients who undergo complete eradication with a two-stage approach is comparable to that of a single-stage resection.[59]

Resection Combined with Ablation

In some situations, surgical resection can be combined with local ablative therapies to achieve complete local therapy of liver metastases. A wide variety of ablative methods are available, including cryoablation, microwave ablation, and radiofrequency ablation (RFA). RFA, the most commonly used ablation method, is

FIGURE 9.5 CT scan images of a patient who underwent a two-stage hepatectomy (FLR; Future Liver Remnant)

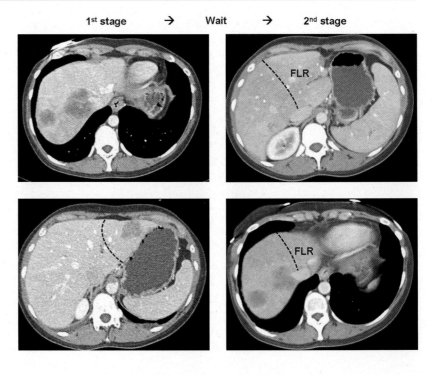

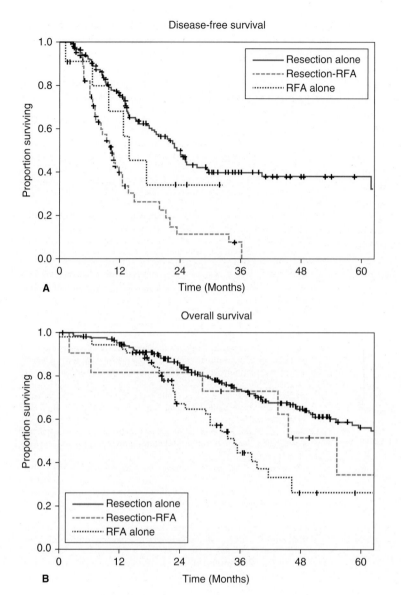

FIGURE 9.6 Kaplan Meyer curve showing overall survival in patients undergoing resection only, resection combined with ablation, or ablation only

From Gleisner et al. *Arch Surg* 2008 Dec;143(12):1204–1212.

a probe-based intratumoral therapy that relies on conductive heat generated by ionic agitation from alternating current. Most commonly, a monopolar system is employed with an active electrode and grounding pads. Direct local tissue heating results in tissue denaturation and cell death. As with resection alone, a curative-intent strategy that utilizes RFA requires the goal of complete "margin negative" ablation to achieve durable local control at the site. A preponderance of evidence is emerging that RFA is most successful in small tumors (less than 3 cm) and those away from major vascular structures.[60] Yet, it is often in such situations that the disease is unresectable. Local recurrence rates after ablation vary significantly in reported series, ranging from 4% to 40%. A systematic review and meta-analysis investigating factors associated with local recurrence after RFA found an overall local recurrence rate of 14.7% for CRLM treated with RFA.[61]

Outcomes regarding overall and disease-free survival following ablation, with or without resection, are difficult to compare to resection alone given the significant differences in patient selection and other biases. Indeed, Gleisner et al. reported that, although long-term survival was less favorable in patients undergoing surgical therapy including ablation of one or more metastases when compared to patients undergoing resection only (FIGURE 9.6), oncologic characteristics are significantly different, clearly impacting the ability to compare groups in any cohort study.[8,62]

▌ ADDITIONAL CONSIDERATIONS

Management of Synchronous Liver Metastases and Primary Tumor

Special consideration should be given to the patient with synchronous resectable liver metastases and a primary tumor that is still in situ. As with metachronous disease, adequate staging is critical to identify those patients who can be managed with curative intent and those who are initially resectable or may require a preoperative conversion strategy. The management goals remain the same—complete resection of all macroscopic metastatic disease, resection of the primary tumor, and integration of systemic or regional therapy. Traditionally, patients with synchronous metastases would undergo a resection of their primary tumor first, followed by a period to recuperate and potentially undergo systemic chemotherapy, and then followed by a subsequent staging and liver resection to address their metastases. More recently, initial systemic chemotherapy is often considered, particularly in the asymptomatic patient, to define tumor biology and chemotherapy responsiveness before embarking on surgical therapy. Combined liver and bowel resection has been shown to be safe in selected cases (particularly with less complicated hepatectomy and or colectomy).[63–67] Finally, a liver first-stage approach can be done.[68] Such a strategy can be advantageous in patients with resectable liver metastases and an asymptomatic primary rectal tumor, particularly when chemoradiation therapy is being considered prior to the proctectomy. Although no rigorous guidelines are advocated regarding the optimal management of patients with synchronous disease, any of these strategies can be considered and should be individuated based on multidisciplinary evaluation.

Repeat Liver Resection

Among the two-thirds of patients who will develop recurrence following apparently complete resection of CRLM, approximately 50% will recur again within the liver.[69] For these patients, repeat resection can be considered if again amenable to surgical therapy. As with the evaluation for initial resection, defining resectability should be based on the ability to achieve complete removal of macroscopic disease with preservation of sufficient functional liver parenchyma. If these criteria are followed, repeat hepatectomy is associated with an operative morbidity and mortality rate equal to those after primary liver surgery.[70] Importantly, several studies have shown that long-term outcome of repeat resection is comparable to initial resection, even with a third or even fourth liver resection.[21] Clearly, patients offered repeat resection are typically those with favorable biology and few comorbid conditions. In such cases, major resection is performed less commonly given the history of previous surgery, and tumor ablation is performed more frequently. The promising outcomes following repeat surgical therapy reinforce the need to consider an aggressive strategy in patients with recurrent CRLM.

■ CONCLUSION

Surgical therapy for hepatic colorectal metastases has been shown to be increasingly safe and effective therapy, resulting in more frequent and aggressive application of local therapies with curative intent. Preoperative and intraoperative assessment and planning are important to achieve safe and complete resection of all evident disease. Current methods for increasing the ability to offer liver resection include preoperative chemotherapy, preoperative portal vein embolization, staged resection, and ablative strategies. One can anticipate on the horizon an expanding use of local therapies of hepatic metastases, particularly as systemic chemotherapy improves. Minimally invasive approaches for resection, including laparoscopic and robotic resection, will likely be increasingly utilized as well as other nonresectional techniques. However, until the role of cytoreduction or incomplete local therapies is defined, complete, curative-intent therapy must be advocated.

■ REFERENCES

1. Jemal A, Siegel R, et al. Cancer statistics, 2010. *CA Cancer J Clin* 2010;60(5):277–300.
2. Rougier P, Milan C, et al. Prospective study of prognostic factors in patients with unresected hepatic metastases from colorectal cancer. Fondation Francaise de Cancerologie Digestive. *Br J Surg* 1995;82(10):1397–1400.
3. Choti MA, Sitzmann JV, et al. Trends in long-term survival following liver resection for hepatic colorectal metastases. *Ann Surg* 2002;235(6): 759–766.
4. Wilson SM, Adson MA. Surgical treatment of hepatic metastases from colorectal cancers. *Arch Surg* 1976;111(4):330–334.
5. Nordlinger B, Quilichini MA, et al. Hepatic resection for colorectal liver metastases. Influence on survival of preoperative factors and surgery for recurrences in 80 patients. *Ann Surg* 1987;205(3):256–263.
6. Pawlik TM, Abdalla EK, et al. Debunking dogma: surgery for four or more colorectal liver metastases is justified. *J Gastrointest Surg* 2006;10(2):240–248.
7. Adam R, Wicherts DA, et al. Patients with initially unresectable colorectal liver metastases: is there a possibility of cure? *J Clin Oncol* 2009;27(11):1829–1835.
8. de Jong MC, van Vledder MG, et al. Therapeutic efficacy of combined intraoperative ablation and resection for colorectal liver metastases: an international, multi-institutional analysis. *J Gastrointest Surg* 2011;15(2):336–344.
9. Wicherts DA, Miller R, et al. Long-term results of two-stage hepatectomy for irresectable colorectal cancer liver metastases. *Ann Surg* 2008;248(6):994–1005.
10. Malik HZ, Prasad KR, et al. Preoperative prognostic score for predicting survival after hepatic resection for colorectal liver metastases. *Ann Surg* 2007;246(5):806–814.
11. Couinaud. *Le Foie: Etudes anatomiques et chirugicales.* Paris, France: Masson; 1957.
12. Lalmahomed ZS, Ayez N, et al. Anatomical versus nonanatomical resection of colorectal liver metastases: is there a difference in surgical and oncological outcome? *World J Surg* 2010.
13. Kazaryan AM, Marangos IP, et al. Laparoscopic resection of colorectal liver metastases: surgical and long-term oncologic outcome. *Ann Surg* 2010;252(6):1005–1012.
14. van Vledder MG, Pawlik TM, et al. Factors determining the sensitivity of intraoperative ultrasonography in detecting colorectal liver metastases in the modern era. *Ann Surg Oncol* 2010;17(10):2756–2763.
15. Elias D, Sideris L, et al. Incidence of unsuspected and treatable metastatic disease associated with operable colorectal liver metastases discovered only at laparotomy (and not treated when performing percutaneous radiofrequency ablation). *Ann Surg Oncol* 2005;12(4):298–302.
16. Karoui M, Penna C, et al. Influence of preoperative chemotherapy on the risk of major hepatectomy for colorectal liver metastases. *Ann Surg* 2006;243(1):1–7.
17. Nordlinger B, Sorbye H, et al. Perioperative chemotherapy with FOLFOX4 and surgery versus surgery alone for resectable liver metastases from colorectal cancer (EORTC Intergroup trial 40983): a randomised controlled trial. *Lancet* 2008;371(9617):1007–1016.
18. Breitenstein S, DeOliveira ML, et al. Novel and simple preoperative score predicting complications after liver resection in noncirrhotic patients. *Ann Surg* 2010;252(5):726–734.
19. Choti MA, Bowman HM, et al. Should hepatic resections be performed at high-volume referral centers? *J Gastrointest Surg* 1998;2(1):11–20.
20. Simmonds PC, Primrose JN, et al. Surgical resection of hepatic metastases from colorectal cancer: a systematic review of published studies. *Br J Cancer* 2006;94(7):982–999.
21. de Jong MC, Mayo SC, et al. Repeat curative intent liver surgery is safe and effective for recurrent colorectal liver metastasis: results from an international multi-institutional analysis. *J Gastrointest Surg* 2009;13(12):2141–2151.
22. Fong Y, Fortner J, et al. Clinical score for predicting recurrence after hepatic resection for metastatic colorectal cancer: analysis of 1001 consecutive cases. *Ann Surg* 1999;230(3):309–318; discussion 318–321.

23. Nordlinger B, Guiguet M, et al. Surgical resection of colorectal carcinoma metastases to the liver. A prognostic scoring system to improve case selection, based on 1568 patients. Association Francaise de Chirurgie. *Cancer* 1996;77(7):1254–1262.

24. Allen PJ, Kemeny N, et al. Importance of response to neoadjuvant chemotherapy in patients undergoing resection of synchronous colorectal liver metastases. *J Gastrointest Surg* 2003;7(1):109–115; discussion 116–117.

25. Rubbia-Brandt L, Giostra E, et al. Importance of histological tumor response assessment in predicting the outcome in patients with colorectal liver metastases treated with neo-adjuvant chemotherapy followed by liver surgery. *Ann Oncol* 2007;18(2):299–304.

26. Nash GM, Gimbel M, et al. KRAS mutation correlates with accelerated metastatic progression in patients with colorectal liver metastases. *Ann Surg Oncol* 2010;17(2):572–578.

27. Adam R, de Haas RJ, et al. Concomitant extrahepatic disease in patients with colorectal liver metastases: when is there a place for surgery? *Ann Surg* 2011;253(2):349–359.

28. Pulitano C, Bodingbauer M, et al. Liver resection for colorectal metastases in presence of extrahepatic disease: results from an international multi-institutional analysis. *Ann Surg Oncol* 2010.

29. Nomura K, Kadoya M, et al. Detection of hepatic metastases from colorectal carcinoma: comparison of histopathologic features of anatomically resected liver with results of preoperative imaging. *J Clin Gastroenterol* 2007;41(8):789–795.

30. Blyth S, Blakeborough A, et al. Sensitivity of magnetic resonance imaging in the detection of colorectal liver metastases. *Ann R Coll Surg Engl* 2008;90(1):25–28.

31. Hekimoglu K, Ustundag Y, et al. Small colorectal liver metastases: detection with SPIO-enhanced MRI in comparison with gadobenate dimeglumine-enhanced MRI and CT imaging. *Eur J Radiol* 2009.

32. Kamel IR, Cohade C, et al. Incremental value of CT in PET/CT of patients with colorectal carcinoma. *Abdom Imaging* 2004;29(6):663–668.

33. Wiering B, Adang EM, et al. Added value of positron emission tomography imaging in the surgical treatment of colorectal liver metastases. *Nucl Med Commun* 2010;31(11):938–944.

34. Joyce DL, Wahl RL, et al. Preoperative positron emission tomography to evaluate potentially resectable hepatic colorectal metastases. *Arch Surg* 2006;141(12):1220–1226; discussion 1227.

35. Pawlik TM, Assumpcao L, et al. Trends in nontherapeutic laparotomy rates in patients undergoing surgical therapy for hepatic colorectal metastases. *Ann Surg Oncol* 2009;16(2):371–378.

36. Gholghesaei M, van Muiswinkel JM, et al. Value of laparoscopy and laparoscopic ultrasonography in determining resectability of colorectal hepatic metastases. *HPB* (Oxford) 2003;5(2):100–104.

37. Choti MA, Kaloma F, et al. Patient variability in intraoperative ultrasonographic characteristics of colorectal liver metastases. *Arch Surg* 2008;143(1):29–34; discussion 35.

38. van Vledder MG, Torbenson MS, et al. The effect of steatosis on echogenicity of colorectal liver metastases on intraoperative ultrasonography. *Arch Surg* 2010;145(7):661–667.

39. Gruenberger T, Jourdan JL, et al. Echogenicity of liver metastases is an independent prognostic factor after potentially curative treatment. *Arch Surg* 2000;135(11):1285–1290.

40. DeOliveira ML, Pawlik TM, et al. Echogenic appearance of colorectal liver metastases on intraoperative ultrasonography is associated with survival after hepatic resection. *J Gastrointest Surg* 2007;11(8):970–976; discussion 976.

41. Folprecht G, Gruenberger T, et al. Tumour response and secondary resectability of colorectal liver metastases following neoadjuvant chemotherapy with cetuximab: the CELIM randomised phase 2 trial. *Lancet Oncol* 2010;11(1):38–47.

42. Garufi C, Torsello A, et al. Cetuximab plus chronomodulated irinotecan, 5-fluorouracil, leucovorin and oxaliplatin as neoadjuvant chemotherapy in colorectal liver metastases: POCHER trial. *Br J Cancer* 2010;103(10):1542–1547.

43. Adam R, Wicherts DA, et al. Complete pathologic response after preoperative chemotherapy for colorectal liver metastases: myth or reality? *J Clin Oncol* 2008;26(10):1635–1641.

44. Portier G, Elias D, et al. Multicenter randomized trial of adjuvant fluorouracil and folinic acid compared with surgery alone after resection of colorectal liver metastases: FFCD ACHBTH AURC 9002 trial. *J Clin Oncol* 2006;24(31):4976–4982.

45. Adam R, Pascal G, et al. Tumor progression while on chemotherapy: a contraindication to liver resection for multiple colorectal metastases? *Ann Surg* 2004; 240(6):1052–1061; discussion 1061–1064.

46. Neumann UP, Thelen A, et al. Nonresponse to preoperative chemotherapy does not preclude long-term survival after liver resection in patients with colorectal liver metastases. *Surgery* 2009;146(1):52–59.

47. Tanaka K, Takakura H, et al. Importance of complete pathologic response to prehepatectomy chemotherapy in treating colorectal cancer metastases. *Ann Surg* 2009;250(6):935–942.

48. Pawlik TM, Olino K, et al. Preoperative chemotherapy for colorectal liver metastases: impact on hepatic histology and postoperative outcome. *J Gastrointest Surg* 2007;11(7):860–868.

49. Peppercorn PD, Reznek RH, et al. Demonstration of hepatic steatosis by computerized tomography in patients receiving 5-fluorouracil-based therapy for advanced colorectal cancer. *Br J Cancer* 1998;77(11):2008–2011.

50. Vauthey JN, Pawlik TM, et al. Chemotherapy regimen predicts steatohepatitis and an increase in 90-day mortality after surgery for hepatic colorectal metastases. *J Clin Oncol* 2006;24(13):2065–2072.

51. Kishi Y, Zorzi D, et al. Extended preoperative chemotherapy does not improve pathologic response and increases postoperative liver insufficiency after hepatic resection for colorectal liver metastases. *Ann Surg Oncol* 2010;17(11):2870–2876.

52. Angliviel B, Benoist S, et al. Impact of chemotherapy on the accuracy of computed tomography scan for the evaluation of colorectal liver metastases. *Ann Surg Oncol* 2009; 16(5):1247–1253.

53. Benoist S, Brouquet A, et al. Complete response of colorectal liver metastases after chemotherapy: does it mean cure? *J Clin Oncol* 2006;24(24):3939–3945.

54. van Vledder MG, de Jong MC, et al. Disappearing colorectal liver metastases after chemotherapy: should we be concerned? *J Gastrointest Surg* 2010;14(11):1691–1700.

55. Pamecha V, Glantzounis G, et al. Long-term survival and disease recurrence following portal vein embolisation prior to major hepatectomy for colorectal metastases. *Ann Surg Oncol* 2009;16(5):1202–1207.

56. Dello SA, Stoot JH, et al. Prospective volumetric assessment of the liver on a personal computer by nonradiologists prior to partial hepatectomy. *World J Surg* 2011;35(2):386–392.

57. Pamecha V, Levene A, et al. Effect of portal vein embolisation on the growth rate of colorectal liver metastases. *Br J Cancer* 2009;100(4):617–622.

58. Jaeck D, Oussoultzoglou E, et al. A two-stage hepatectomy procedure combined with portal vein embolization to achieve curative resection for initially unresectable multiple and bilobar colorectal liver metastases. *Ann Surg* 2004;240(6):1037–1049; discussion 1049–1051.

59. Tsai S, Marques HP, et al. Two-stage strategy for patients with extensive bilateral colorectal liver metastases. *HPB* (Oxford) 2010;12(4):262–269.

60. Mulier S, Ni Y, et al. Local recurrence after hepatic radiofrequency coagulation: multivariate meta-analysis and review of contributing factors. *Ann Surg* 2005;242(2):158–171.

61. Wong SL, Mangu PB, et al. American Society of Clinical Oncology 2009 clinical evidence review on radiofrequency ablation of hepatic metastases from colorectal cancer. *J Clin Oncol* 2010;28(3):493–508.

62. Gleisner AL, Choti MA, et al. Colorectal liver metastases: recurrence and survival following hepatic resection, radiofrequency ablation, and combined resection-radiofrequency ablation. *Arch Surg* 2008;143(12):1204–1212.

63. Tanaka K, Shimada H, et al. Outcome after simultaneous colorectal and hepatic resection for colorectal cancer with synchronous metastases. *Surgery* 2004;136(3):650–659.

64. van der Pool AE, de Wilt JH, et al. Optimizing the outcome of surgery in patients with rectal cancer and synchronous liver metastases. *Br J Surg* 2010;97(3):383–390.

65. Chen J, Li Q, et al. Simultaneous vs. staged resection for synchronous colorectal liver metastases: a metaanalysis. *Int J Colorectal Dis* 2011;26(2):191–199.

66. de Haas RJ, Adam R, et al. Comparison of simultaneous or delayed liver surgery for limited synchronous colorectal metastases. *Br J Surg* 2010;97(8):1279–1289.

67. Reddy SK, Pawlik TM, et al. Simultaneous resections of colorectal cancer and synchronous liver metastases: a multi-institutional analysis. *Ann Surg Oncol* 2007;14(12):3481–3491.

68. Mentha G, Roth AD, et al. 'Liver first' approach in the treatment of colorectal cancer with synchronous liver metastases. *Dig Surg* 2008;25(6):430–435.

69. de Jong MC, Pulitano C, et al. Rates and patterns of recurrence following curative intent surgery for colorectal liver metastasis: an international multi-institutional analysis of 1669 patients. *Ann Surg* 2009;250(3):440–448.

70. Shaw IM, Rees M, et al. Repeat hepatic resection for recurrent colorectal liver metastases is associated with favourable long-term survival. *Br J Surg* 2006;93(4):457–464.

CHAPTER

10

Colorectal Metastases: Ablative Techniques

LUIGI A. SOLBIATI

INTRODUCTION

Liver metastatic disease occurs in up to 50% of patients with colorectal cancer at some point during the course of their disease and is the most frequent cause of death of these patients. In the last 10 to 15 years, there have been significant advances in the treatment of liver metastatic colorectal cancer. More effective systemic or intra-arterial combination chemotherapy, with or without biologic therapy; more aggressive hepatic resection (even though still feasible in a minority of cases); chemoembolization; locally applied thermal ablation; and combined (systemic + local) treatments are continuously improving the outcome of patients.[1,2] Modern diagnostic imaging modalities, such as contrast-enhanced ultrasound, multidetector computed tomography (CT), magnetic resonance imaging (MRI), contrast-enhanced ultrasonography (CEUS), and positron emission tomography-computed tomography (PET-CT), allow to achieve early detection and accurate quantification of liver metastatic involvement and, consequently, to tailor therapy for each single patient.[3–7]

Hepatic resection remains the most effective treatment option, but patients who are eligible for resection are only a minority (20% to 35%).[1,8,9] Technically difficult and/or risky anatomic locations, new metastases or local postsurgical recurrences, multiple bilobar metastases, and comorbidities that increase anesthesiologic risk are still, at present, contraindications to resection and may on the contrary be the rationale for local thermal ablation. Actually, thermal ablation is (a) feasible in previously resected patients and nonsurgical candidates (due to the number and/or intrahepatic location of metastatic deposits, age, and comorbidity); (b) repeatable when incomplete and when local recurrence or development of new metachronous lesions occur; (c) applicable in combination with systemic or regional chemotherapy; (d) minimally invasive with limited complications rate and preservation of liver function; and (e) low cost.

Ablations can be performed by a percutaneous, a laparoscopic, or an open surgical approach. The technical aspects and results of mostly percutaneously performed ablations are discussed in this chapter.

TECHNICAL NOTES

Thermal ablations of liver metastases can be performed with radiofrequency (the most widely diffused modality), cryotherapy, and microwaves.[1,10] Few reports on the use of laser have been published.[11] Many aspects that are related to the interaction between the energy supplied and the histology of hepatic colorectal metastases are common among all the energy sources. Local ablation of liver metastases is generally more complex than that of hepatocellular carcinoma because of several reasons: Metastases do not have peripheral capsule, generally develop in noncirrhotic (i.e., regularly vascularized) liver parenchyma, have infiltrative growth, and develop peripheral satellite micronodules in the range of 5 to 10 mm from the margins in a large percentage of cases even when their size is less than 3 cm. Because of all these features, it is mandatory for ablation to achieve a 0.8- to 1-cm "safety halo" of necrosis of normal liver tissue at the periphery of the treated metastasis to decrease the risk of posttreatment local tumor progression (FIGURE 10.1). The "heat sink effect" caused by the presence of large venous vessels adjacent to metastatic tissue may also limit the diffusion of heating to the peripheral part of the metastases adjacent to the vascular structures. Considering all these problems, it is generally accepted that ablation of hepatic colorectal metastases is applicable to patients with no more than five to six metachronous liver metastases, each not exceeding 3.5 to 4 cm in its largest diameter.[12,13]

Temporary occlusion of the portal vein, intratumoral injection of saline solution during radiofrequency energy deposition, and pretreatment liposomal chemotherapy administration have been reportedly used to increase the volume of necrosis achieved by thermal energy.[14–16] More recently, stereotactic radiofrequency ablation with multiple probes inserted and regularly spaced around the periphery of the tumoral mass has been proposed as a successful modality of treatment of large metastatic lesions.[17]

Patient enrollment in the treatment process requires evaluation by an anesthesiologist. Laboratory tests include full blood count, coagulation screen, liver function test, and tumor markers.

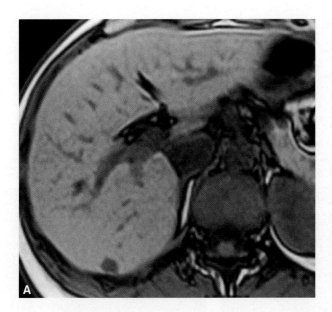 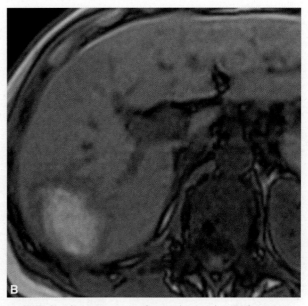

FIGURE 10.1 Small, subcapsular metastasis in segment VI **A.** ablated with microwaves. The resulting volume of coagulative necrosis is much larger than the lesion size. The thickness of the peripheral safety halo largely exceeds 10 mm **B.**

Percutaneous ablation of colorectal metastases is mostly performed under conscious sedation. General anaesthesia using endotracheal intubation and mechanical ventilation are used for treatments of lesions adjacent to the Glisson capsule (usually painful) or to risky anatomic structures and of large or multiple lesions that require many insertions of the energy device and a long period of treatment. As a result, international guidelines recommend that percutaneous ablations be performed in a dedicated operating room, where general anesthesia, endotracheal intubation, and mechanical ventilation can be optimally used if needed. Standard surgical asepsis rules must be strictly observed by the operating team. It is generally recommended to administer single-dose antibiotic prophylaxis prior to the treatment, whereas antihemetic and analgesic drugs may be needed postoperatively.

Percutaneous ablation is a minimally invasive procedure; thus there are few absolute contraindications to its use. Exclusion criteria include the presence of severe coagulopathy, liver failure, portal vein neoplastic thrombosis, and obstructive jaundice. Active extrahepatic disease is a contraindication to ablation, with the exception of coexisting small lung metastases, which generally have very slow growth (compared to the fast development of hepatic metastases) and do not interfere with the oncologic goal of ablation of liver lesions.

Caution has to be taken not to damage adjacent structures. Liver lesions adjacent to the hepatic hilum, gallbladder, stomach, and colon are potential candidates for ablation procedure yet require precise and careful planning. Adjacent vascular structures do not represent an obstacle alone. High blood flow in major hepatic vessels allow prompt dissipation of the warming effect secondary to the source of energy employed while the biliary system is vulnerable, especially if harboring bacteria. Gastric wall or bowel loop proximity to the area of treatment, considering the safety margin, may be a critical issue for treatment indications while selecting candidates. Perforations of

bowel loops by heating may occur many hours after ablation and may be clinically misleading, being usually less painful than perforations caused by inflammatory diseases. Relatively simple practical measures, such as positioning of the patient, selection of safe path to the target, and/or intraperitoneal injection of 500 mL of dextrose (if radiofrequency is employed) or saline solution (if microwaves are used) to create "artificial ascites," can provide adequate distance to avoid injury of critical structures.

Percutaneous ablations can be guided by sonography, CT, MRI, or PET-CT. Sonography is employed in most centers due to some favorable aspects including real-time control, low cost, and no use of ionizing radiations.[18] Sonography cannot assess the size of induced coagulation necrosis at the end of the planned energy deposition, however, and repositioning of the ablative device is made difficult by the hyperechogenic "cloud" of gas produced by heating. Accordingly, when sonography is utilized as a modality of guidance, the routine use of CEUS is nowadays considered fundamental for pretreatment planning, targeting of lesions undetectable in basal studies, and immediate control of early results of treatment because it enables rapid and precise assessment of the volume of necrosis achieved and detection of possibly remaining viable tumor that requires immediate additional treatment if performed a few minutes after withdrawal of the ablative device,[19-21] (FIGURE 10.2).

CT or MRI guidance is mandatory when sonographic targeting is not possible with significantly increased procedure time and greater complexity of the whole procedure. In general, all contrast-enhanced imaging modalities (CT, MRI, and CEUS) allow to detect the following:

- Actual number and size of the lesions to be treated, including the perilesional hypervascular halo with wash-out, which represents the most actively growing part of hepatic metastases
- Degree of enhancement and presence of areas of necrosis to facilitate the comparison of pre- and posttherapy patterns at the end of treatment

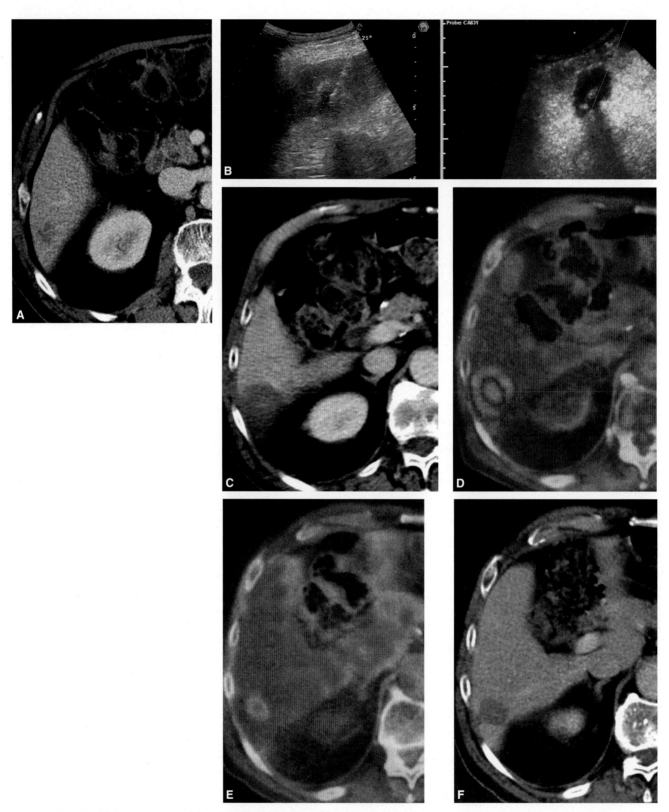

FIGURE 10.2 In a 64-year old patient with history of colon carcinoma single, 1.7 cm hepatic metastasis is detected in segment VI **A.** Ablation is performed with 6-minute insertion of 14G microwave antenna **B.** left. Few minutes after withdrawal of the device, CEUS is performed and large, oval, avascular volume of coagulative necrosis which indicates complete ablation is clearly visible. The 24-hour post-ablation CT study confirms the achievement of a volume of necrosis larger than the original metastasis **C.** while FDG-PET, performed 7 days after ablation shows the typical peripheral, ring-like uptake due to perilesional inflammatory reaction **D.** that completely disappears 3 months later **E.** Three years after ablation, the volume of necrosis is slightly smaller and no local tumor progression is detected **F.**

- Tumor margins, mostly for subcapsular and exophytic tumors, to thoroughly assess the relationships of tumors with surrounding structures and to adopt appropriate treatment strategies, reducing the risk of complications
- Zones of local tumor progression or residual tumors following previous locoregional or surgical treatments

Additionally, MRI can provide real-time assessment of the volume of necrosis during energy deposition due to the possibility to visualize the heating diffusion through thermal maps simultaneously with tissue necrotic changes.[22]

When sonography is the imaging modality used to guide ablation of colorectal metastases, its performances can be, at present, significantly improved employing real-time US-CT/MRI fusion imaging, the so-called virtual navigation systems, which combine real-time US with previously acquired contrast-enhanced CT or MRI volumetric scans multiplanarly reconstructed, transferred to the US machine, and coregistered through an electromagnetic tracking system.[23] Prior to performing the interventional procedure, the anticipated path of the interventional device and a virtual treatment volume based on the different dimensions and shape of the anticipated zone of ablation produced by the various ablation applicators can be drawn and overlapped on the real-time CT/MRI scans, simulating the needle placement and the ablation volume that is potentially achievable. This is of particular importance when multiple overlapped treatment volumes produced by a single applicator or the placement of multiple simultaneous applicators are needed to treat the entire tumor.

Real-time fusion imaging allows (a) to detect, in preprocedure planning, target lesions not visualized by B-mode US because of their small size or difficult anatomic location (FIGURE 10.3); (b) to target challenging lesions due to the visualization of the "virtual" ablative device (electrode, antenna, or cryoprobe) on the coregistered CT/MRI images; (c) to perform an adequate "control" of the treatment, repositioning the applicator immediately or modifying its effects (if needed) without having to wait for the reabsorption of gas bubbles before reinserting the applicator; (d) to precisely compare the volume of necrosis achieved with the pretreatment volume of the same lesion on contrast-enhanced CT or MRI.[24–27]

Ablation is considered successful when complete coagulative necrosis of the lesion and safety margin are obtained (Fig. 1,2). Posttreatment (at 24 hours or 1 month) contrast-enhanced cross-sectional imaging (CT or MRI) is crucial to assess completeness of treatment, exclude complications, and provide a baseline imaging for follow-up purposes. Contrast-enhanced

CT or MRI is performed on a routine basis in the long-term follow-up (Fig. 2F) in association with liver function tests and serum CEA levels to assess therapeutic response and to detect possible local tumor progression or new lesions promptly. Currently, contrast-enhanced and diffusion-weighted MRI is more accurate than contrast-enhanced CT for the detection of viable tumoral areas and local recurrences of colorectal metastases after ablation (FIGURE 10.4).[28–30]

The role of FDG PET-CT in the postablation workup has not been completely defined (Figs. 2D and 2E). In some reports it has shown sensitivity equivalent to that of MRI in the detection of areas of local tumor progression, characterized by abnormal FDG uptake.[31] Accordingly, PET-CT is being proposed as a complementary imaging modality in case of uncertain treatment response both in short-term (at 24 hours) and long-term follow-up.

RESULTS

Since the very first studies on local results[32] and long-term follow-up[33] after US-guided radiofrequency ablation of hepatic colorectal metastases published by our group, respectively, in 1997 and 2001, a large number of papers have been published on local control rate, complications, long-term follow-up, and survival following thermal ablation of hepatic colorectal metastases. Most studies deal with radiofrequency, cryotherapy, and microwave ablation, whereas very few have been performed with laser. In one of them,[11] local recurrence rates in 603 patients ranged from 1.9% for mets up to 2 cm in diameter to 4.4% for mets larger than 4 cm, and 3- and 5-year survival rates were 56% and 37%, respectively, with a median survival of 3.5 years. No major complications were reported. In a more recent paper,[34] the effectiveness rate in 87 patients was 85.6% and the local progression rate at 6 months was 10%. Median survival time was 54 months and survival rates were 72.4% at 3 years and 33.4% at 5 years.

As far as radiofrequency, cryotherapy, and microwave ablation are concerned, a systematic review of the papers published between January 1994 and January 2010 has recently been published.[10] In all, 226 potentially relevant studies were found, of which 75 met the inclusion criteria (minimum 1 year follow-up and more than 10 patients treated). Cryotherapy (26 studies) had a local tumor progression rate of 12% to 39%, with mean 1-, 3, and 5-year survival rates of 84%, 37%, and 17%, respectively, and a major complication rate ranging from 7% to 66%. Microwave ablation (13 studies) had a local tumor progression rate of 5% to 13%, with mean 1-, 3-, and 5-year survival rates of

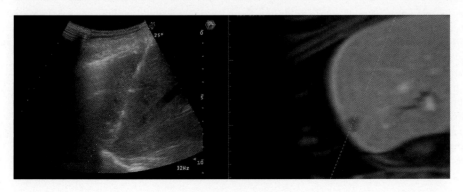

FIGURE 10.3 1.5 cm subdiaphragmatic metastasis from colon cancer almost undetectable with B-mode US, precisely targeted and ablated using real-time US / CT fusion imaging.

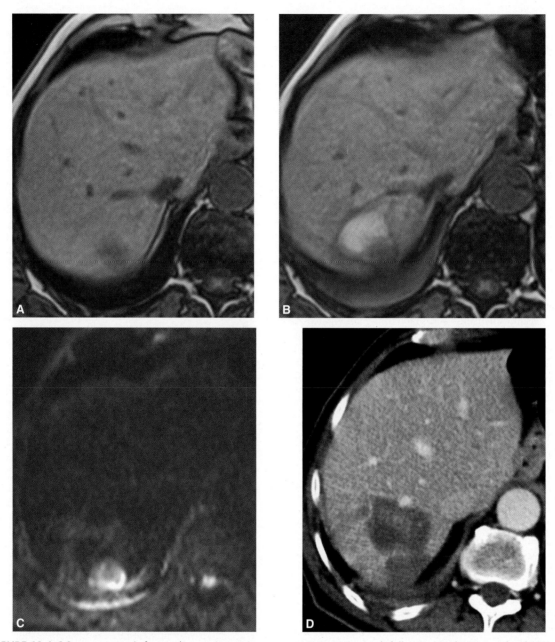

FIGURE 10.4 2.3 cm metastasis from colon carcinoma in segment VII **A.** At 4-month follow-up study, T1-weighted MRI **B.** and particularly diffusion-weighted MRI **C.** show an unablated area growing in the posterior portion of the metastasis. Re-treatment with microwaves is immediately performed and 24-hour post-ablation CT shows large, complete ablation **D.**

73%, 30%, and 16%, respectively, and a major complication rate ranging from 3% to 16%. Radiofrequency ablation (RFA) (36 studies) had a local tumor progression rate of 10% to 31%, with mean 1-, 3-, and 5-year survival rates of 85%, 36%, and 24%, respectively, and a major complication rate ranging from 0% to 33%. These data show that survival rates are similar between the ablative techniques although with wide variations between studies. Major complication rate is higher with cryotherapy, whereas the local tumor progression rate is lower after microwave ablation. Microwave ablation, although relatively new compared to RFA and cryotherapy, seems to be able to overcome two of the major limitations of RFA, that is, the size of the necrosis volume achievable and the significant decrease of the heat sink effect. Particularly, if the most updated high-power microwave generators are employed, microwaves allow to achieve larger volumes of necrosis in a markedly shorter time compared to RFA and to also treat adequately portions of tumors adjacent to large blood vessels without significant risks of thrombosis caused by heating (FIGURE 10.5). The majority of the studies available in the literature and included in the review[10] are single-arm, single-center retrospective and prospective studies, with wide variability in patient groups, adjuvant treatments, and management approach.

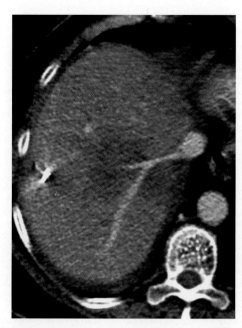

FIGURE 10.5 Large volume of coagulative necrosis, centrally located in the right hepatic lobe, achieved by microwaves, for single metastasis from colon carcinoma. The extent of coagulative necrosis also beyond the right hepatic vein demonstrates the lack of heat sink effect without thrombosis of the venous lumen.

Also in the recent review of the American Society of Clinical Oncology,[2] based exclusively on studies performed with RFA, a wide variability in the 5-year survival rate (14%–55%) and local tumor progression rate (3.6%–60%) is reported. In accordance with Mulier et al.,[35] in this review it is argued that time has come for randomized clinical trials in which thermal ablation is used as an alternative to resection in patients with colorectal hepatic metastases, but such trials are not currently being carried on. Several, single-center studies comparing the results of RFA and resection in two distinct populations of patients are available in the literature, but none of them can be accepted without criticism. As an example, in a series[36] of 348 patients treated with intention to cure, 190 had resection only, 101 had RFA and resection, and 57 had RFA alone. Recurrences were lowest with resection (52%), 64% for RFA and resection, and 84% for RFA alone. Liver-only recurrence after RFA was 44%. The 4-year survival rate was 65% for resection, 36% for resection and RFA, and 22% for RFA alone. Of course, RFA was usually a component of therapy when resection was not possible. Therefore, this is not a true comparison of RFA versus resection.

Taking into account the most recent and relevant single-center clinical studies,[37–43] mostly based on RFA, the following topics must be highlighted: relations between tumor size and local control rate, continuously improving outcome of patients, low complication rates, and use of thermal ablation during the "test of time."

Local control rates after RFA of colorectal hepatic metastases are strictly related to the size of the tumor. For tumors smaller than 2.5 cm, local control rates exceed 90% nowadays, in tumors between 2.5 and 3.5 cm they are in the 70% to 90% range, whereas for lesions between 3.5 and 5 cm the range is

between 50% and 70%.[39] It has been recently reported, however, that if stereotactic RFA is employed with multiple simultaneous electrodes placed under the guidance of optical stereotactical navigation system, local control rates for colorectal hepatic metastases can increase up to 88.9% for 3- to 5-cm lesions and to 82.6% for lesions larger than 5 cm.[17]

According to the latest literature reports, the outcome of patients undergoing thermal ablation of colorectal metastases is significantly improving with 5-year survival rates up to 48% at 5 years.[43] This may be caused by several factors: Modern imaging can detect and guide the targeting of very small lesions; larger volumes of necrosis are achievable, decreasing the risk of local progression; associated chemotherapy regimens are definitely more efficient than in past years; and initial local tumor progression can be precisely retargeted and treated. All these reasons can also explain the dramatic improvement in patient outcome achieved at our institution from the initial report[33] (14% survival rate at 5 years) to the most recent study.[44] In 99 patients with 202 metastases who have undergone RFA in combination with systemic chemotherapy and followed for up to 10 years, local tumor progression occurred in 11.9% of metastases and 54.2% of these were re-treated. Re-treatment increased survival over no re-treatment. Disease-free survival (including successful re-treatment) was 54.0%, 31.6%, 25.6%, 21.6%, and 15.8% (median: 13.1 months), and overall survival was 98%, 69.3%, 47.8%, 25%, and 18% (median: 53.2 months) at 1, 3, 5, 7, and 10 years, respectively. These survival rates are substantially equivalent to those of most surgical series reported in the literature.

Recently, additional indications to the use of thermal ablation for colorectal metastases that have been proposed are during the "test of time" before resection and when metastases develop after hepatectomy.

Not so long ago the "test of time" approach was proposed by surgeons to delay the resection of liver metastases to allow additional, still undetected lesions to develop and become identifiable, thus limiting the number of resections carried out in patients who may ultimately develop more metastases. On the one hand, RFA applied in this setting can significantly decrease the number of potential resections, hence resulting in complete tumor control in some of these patients, avoiding major surgery. Furthermore, offering a treatment option such as RFA to cancer patients rather than a "wait and see" behavior is favorable for these patients. In a recent study, using RFA as a "test of time" before resection in a group of 88 potentially operable patients with 134 metastases from colorectal carcinoma followed for a period of 18 to 75 months, RFA was successful in 60.2% of the patients, and 43.4% of these were disease-free at the period of the study. The remaining patients (56.6%) developed new untreatable intra- or extrahepatic metastases. RFA was unsuccessful in 39.8% of patients: 57.1% underwent resection, and the remaining 42.9% developed new untreatable metastases. No patients became untreatable because of the growth of incompletely ablated lesions. In summary, 50% of patients were spared surgery that would have been noncurative, whereas 26.1% additional patients avoided resection because of the curative result of RFA.[45]

In patients who have undergone hepatectomy, when new metastases develop, thermal ablation is preferred to repeat surgery because it is less invasive and can achieve complete ablation in over 90% of cases with very low complication rates and a 3-year overall survival rate of 41%.[46]

Literature reports have also demonstrated that RFA is a safe procedure with low rates of complications and mortality. Major complications such as hemorrhage, cholecystitis, or gastric or bowel wall involvement have been reported in a small percentage of cases ranging from 0.7% to 5.7%. Mortality rates reported ranged from 0.5% to 1.4%.[47,48]

CONCLUSION

Percutaneous ablation is an established therapeutic option for liver colorectal metastases, which may obviate the need for a major surgery and result in prolonged survival and chance for cure.

Accurate selection of patients and lesions to be treated and the use of state-of-the-art technology for guiding and performing ablations are of crucial importance for achieving good results.

Extensive operators' experience and technical advances provide larger coagulation volumes and, therefore, allow safe and effective treatment of medium- and, occasionally, even large-size metastases. In experienced hands, thermal ablation can achieve local control in up to 85% to 90% of treated lesions. Repeated thermal ablations for either local recurrences or new metastases are technically feasible and very often performed.

Results of RF ablation in terms of global and disease-free survival currently approach those reported for surgical metastasectomy. Adverse effect rates, costs, and hospitalization of thermal ablation are usually lower than those of surgical resection.

Recently increased awareness among referring oncologists, satisfactory results in long-term survival reported in scientific literature, and minimal invasiveness of RFA versus surgery contributed to the widely accepted status of valid therapeutic option for local treatment of patients with limited metastatic liver disease. In the future, the overlapping long-term outcome of both surgical resection and RFA will allow randomized studies comparing RFA versus resection for resectable metastatic liver tumors, which will enable a proper evaluation of the impact of RFA. RFA should not replace hepatic resection, whenever applicable, especially for large metastases because of the higher risk of local recurrence caused by residual viable tumor tissue within the necrotic area.

REFERENCES

1. Fahy BN, Jarnagin WR. Evolving techniques in the treatment of liver colorectal metastases: role of laparoscopy, radiofrequency ablation, microwave coagulation, hepatic arterial chemotherapy, indications and contraindications for resection, role of transplantation, and timing of chemotherapy. *Surg Clin North Am* 2006;86:1005–1022.
2. Wong SL, Mangu PB, Choti MA, et al. American Society of Clinical Oncology 2009 clinical evidence review on radiofrequency ablation of hepatic metastases from colorectal cancer. *J Clin Oncol* 2010;28:493–508.
3. Floriani I, Torri V, Rulli E, et al. Performance of imaging modalities in diagnosis of liver metastases from colorectal cancer: a systematic review and meta-analysis. *J Magn Reson Imaging* 2010;31:19–31.
4. Larsen LP, Rosenkilde M, Christensen H, et al. Can contrast-enhanced ultrasonography replace multidetector-computed tomography in the detection of liver metastases from colorectal cancer? *Eur J Radiol* 2009;69:308–313.
5. Maas M, Rutten IJ, Nelemans PJ, et al. What is the most accurate whole-body imaging modality for assessment of local and distant recurrent disease in colorectal cancer? A meta-analysis: imaging for recurrent colorectal cancer. *Eur J Nucl Med Mol Imaging* 2011;38:1560–1571.
6. Rappeport ED, Loft A, Berthelsen AK, et al. Contrast-enhanced FDG-PET/CT vs. SPIO-enhanced MRI vs. FDG-PET vs. CT in patients with liver metastases from colorectal cancer: a prospective study with intraoperative confirmation. *Acta Radiol* 2007;48:369–378.
7. Vriens D, de Geus-Oei LF, van der Graaf WT, et al. Tailoring therapy in colorectal cancer by PET-CT. *Q J Nucl Med Mol Imaging* 2009;53:224–244.
8. Adam R, Vinet E. Regional treatment of metastasis: surgery of colorectal liver metastases. *Ann Oncol* 2004;15(suppl 4):iv, 103–106.
9. Liu LX, Zhang WH, Jiang HC. Current treatment for liver metastases from colorectal cancer. *World J Gastroenterol* 2003;9:193–200.
10. Pathak S, Jones R, Tang JMF, et al. Ablative therapies for colorectal liver metastases: a systematic review. *Colorectal Disease* 2011;13:e252–e265.
11. Vogl TJ, Straub R, Eichler K, et al. Colorectal carcinoma metastases in liver: laser-induced interstitial thermotherapy—local tumor control rate and survival data. *Radiology* 2004;230:450–458.
12. Goldberg SN, Gazelle GS, Mueller PR. Thermal ablation therapy for focal malignancy. A unified approach to underlying principles, techniques, and diagnostic imaging guidance. *AJR Am J Roentgenol* 2000;174:323–331.
13. Goldberg SN, Solbiati L, Hahn PF, et al. Large-volume tissue ablation with radiofrequency by using a clustered, internally cooled electrode technique: laboratory and clinical experience in liver metastases. *Radiology* 1998;209:371–379.
14. DeBaere T, Bessoud B, Dromain C, et al. Percutaneous radiofrequency ablation of hepatic tumors during temporary venous occlusion. AJR 2002; 178: 53-59.
15. Goldberg SN, Kamel IR, Kruskal JB et al. Radiofrequency ablation of hepatic tumors: increased tumor destruction with adjuvant liposomal doxorubicin therapy. *AJR Am J Roentgenol* 2002;179:93–101.
16. Rhim H, Goldberg SN, Dodd GD 3rd, et al. Essential techniques for successful radio-frequency thermal ablation of malignant hepatic tumors. *Radiographics* 2001;21:S17–35.
17. Bale R, Widmann G, Schullian P, et al. Percutaneous stereotactic radiofrequency ablation of colorectal liver metastases. *Eur Radiol* 2012;22:930–937.
18. Tonolini M, Solbiati L. Ultrasound imaging in tumor ablation. In: vanSonnenberg E, McMullen W, Solbiati L, eds. *Tumor Ablation. Principles and Practice.* New York, NY: Springer; 2005:135–147.
19. Chen MH, Yang W, Yan K, et al. The role of contrast-enhanced ultrasound in planning treatment protocols for hepatocellular carcinoma before radiofrequency ablation. *Clin Radiol* 2007;62:752–760.
20. Andreana L, Kudo M, Hanataka K, et al. Contrast-enhanced ultrasound techniques for guiding and assessing response to locoregional treatments for hepatocellular carcinoma. *Oncology* 2010;78(suppl 1):68–77.
21. Miyamoto N, Hiramatsu K, Tsuchiya K, et al. Contrast-enhanced sonography-guided radiofrequency ablation for the local recurrence of previously treated hepatocellular carcinoma undetected by B-mode sonography. *J Clin Ultrasound* 2010;38:339–345.
22. Solomon SB, Silverman SG. Imaging in interventional oncology. *Radiology* 2010;257:624–640.
23. Wood BJ, Kruecker J, Abi-Jaoudeh N, et al. Navigation systems for ablation. *J Vasc Interv Radiol* 2010;21(8 suppl):S257–S263.
24. Hakime A, Deschamps F, De Carvalho EG, et al. Clinical evaluation of spatial accuracy of a fusion imaging technique combining previously acquired computed tomography and real-time ultrasound for imaging of liver metastases. *Cardiovasc Intervent Radiol* 2011;34(2):338–344.
25. Kisaka Y, Hirooka M, Koizumi Y, et al. Contrast-enhanced sonography with abdominal virtual sonography in monitoring radiofrequency ablation of hepatocellular carcinoma. *J Clin Ultrasound* 2010;38:138–144.
26. Liu FY, Yu XL, Liang P, et al. Microwave ablation assisted by a real-time virtual navigation system for hepatocellular carcinoma undetectable by conventional ultrasonography. *Eur J Radiol* 2012;81:1455–1459.
27. Solbiati L, Cova L, Ierace T. US-CT fusion for performing radiofrequency ablation of small or poorly visualized liver tumors. *Eur Radiol* 2005;15(suppl 3):C45.
28. Koh DM, Scurr E, Collins DJ, et al. Colorectal hepatic metastases: quantitative measurements using single-shot echo-planar diffusion-weighted MR imaging. *Eur Radiol* 2006;16:1898–1905.
29. Rempp H, Waibel L, Hoffmann R, et al. MR-guided radiofrequency ablation using a wide-bore 1.5-T MR system: clinical results of 213 treated liver lesions. *Eur Radiol* 2012, in press.
30. Vossen JA, Buijs M, Kamel IR. Assessment of tumor response on MR imaging after locoregional therapy. *Tech Vasc Interv Radiol* 2006;9:125–132.
31. Kuehl H, Antoch G, Stergar H, et al. Comparison of FDG-PET, PET/CT and MRI for follow-up of colorectal liver metastases treated with radiofrequency ablation: initial results. *Eur J Radiol* 2008;67:362–371.
32. Solbiati L, Goldberg SN, Ierace T, et al. Hepatic metastases: percutaneous radio-frequency ablation with cooled-tip electrodes. *Radiology* 1997;205:367–373.

33. Solbiati L, Livraghi T, Goldberg SN, et al. Percutaneous radiofrequency ablation of hepatic metastases from colorectal cancer: long-term results in 117 patients. *Radiology* 2001;221:159–166.

34. Puls R, Langner S, Rosenberg C, et al. Laser ablation of liver metastases from colorectal cancer with MR thermometry: 5-year survival. *J Vasc Interv Radiol* 2009;20:225–234.

35. Mulier S, Ni Y, Jamart J, et al. Radiofrequency ablation versus resection for resectable colorectal liver metastases: time for a randomized trial? *Ann Surg Oncol* 2008;15:144–157.

36. Abdalla EK, Vauthey JN, Ellis LM, et al. Recurrence and outcomes following hepatic resection, radiofrequency ablation and combined resection/ablation for colorectal liver metastases. *Ann Surg* 2004;239:818–827.

37. Abitabile P, Hartl U, Lange J, et al. Radiofrequency ablation permits an effective treatment for colorectal liver metastasis. *Eur J Surg Oncol* 2007;33:67–71.

38. Leen E, Horgan PG. Radiofrequency ablation of colorectal liver metastases. *Surg Oncol* 2007;16:47–51.

39. Pereira PL. Actual role of radiofrequency ablation of liver metastases. *Eur Radiol* 2007;17:2062–2070.

40. Gillams AR, Lees WR. Radio-frequency ablation of colorectal liver metastases in 167 patients. *Eur Radiol* 2004;14:2261–2267.

41. Jakobs TF, Hoffmann RT, Trumm C, et al. Radiofrequency ablation of colorectal liver metastases: mid-term results in 68 patients. *Anticancer Res* 2006;26:671–680.

42. Pereira PL. Actual role of radiofrequency ablation of liver metastases. *Eur Radiol* 2007;17:2062–2070.

43. Sorensen SM, Mortensen FV, Nielsen DT. Radiofrequency ablation of colorectal liver metastases: long-term survival. *Acta Radiol* 2007;48:253–258.

44. Solbiati L, Ahmed M, Cova L, et al. Small liver colorectal metastases treated with percutaneous radiofrequency ablation: local response rate and long-term survival with 10-year follow-up. *Radiology*, 2012;265:958–968.

45. Livraghi T, Solbiati L, Meloni F, et al. Percutaneous radiofrequency ablation of liver metastases in potential candidates for resection: the «test of time» approach. *Cancer* 2003;97:3027–3035.

46. Sofocleous CT, Petre EN, Gonen M, et al. CT-guided radiofrequency ablation as a salvage treatment of colorectal cancer hepatic metastases developing after hepatectomy. *J Vasc Interv Radiol* 2011;22:755–761.

47. DeBaere T, Risse O, Kuoch V, et al. Adverse events during radiofrequency treatment of 582 hepatic tumors. *AJR Am J Roentgenol* 2003;181:695–700.

48. Livraghi T, Solbiati L, Meloni MF, et al. Treatment of focal liver tumors with percutaneous radiofrequency ablation: complications encountered in a multicenter study. *Radiology* 2003;226:441–451.

CHAPTER

11

Colorectal Metastases: Intra-Arterial Therapies (Chemoembolization/ Radioembolization) and Portal Vein Embolization

KHAIRUDDIN MEMON, AHSUN RIAZ, DAVID C. MADOFF, ROBERT J. LEWANDOWSKI, and RIAD SALEM

INTRODUCTION

Colorectal cancer (CRC) is the fourth most common cancer diagnosed in men and the third most common in women; the highest incidence rates are seen in North America, Australia/New Zealand, Western Europe, and Japan.[1] Up to 1.23 million cases of CRC are diagnosed globally each year.[2] The liver is the most common site for colorectal metastases and it is estimated that 60% of patients diagnosed with CRC will experience hepatic metastases.[3] Surgical resection of liver-confined disease for patients with no evidence of disseminated disease, a resection strategy encompassing all liver disease with adequate remnant liver for recovery and medical fitness for laparotomy, is associated with a median overall survival of 44 months and a 5-year survival rate of 35%.[4] Unfortunately, bilateral tumor location, number and location of lesions, and inadequate hepatic reserve or comorbid conditions tend to limit an aggressive surgical approach in approximately 10% of patients presenting with liver metastases.[5] Thus, unresectable liver metastases continue to account for much of the morbidity and mortality in patients with CRC.[6,7]

For the majority of patients without resectable disease, the median overall survival is 22 months and rarely is associated with survival beyond 5 years.[8] Targeted nonsurgical approaches for liver-confined CRC metastases may offer survival advantages beyond that of systemic therapy alone. Numerous liver-directed therapies are available for treating unresectable liver metastases, including conformal radiation, radioembolization with yttrium-90 microspheres (^{90}Y), hepatic arterial infusion chemotherapy (HAC) with floxuridine (FUDR), transarterial chemoembolization, or radiofrequency ablation (RFA). These treatments are being studied with and without standard therapies, including fluoropyrimidines, irinotecan, oxaliplatin, tyrosine kinase inhibitors, and vascular endothelial growth factor- and epidermal growth factor-targeting agents.

Chemoembolization and radioembolization are novel intra-arterial therapies gaining widespread acceptance for the treatment of primary and secondary liver cancer.[9] These therapies enable the targeting of tumors directly without interfering with the normal hepatic parenchyma. These have displayed encouraging response rates, survival outcomes, and safe toxicity profile. On the other hand, portal vein embolization (PVE) is performed before surgery to minimize the risk of extensive resection in patients with small anticipated remnant livers.[10–13] PVE redirects portal blood flow to the future liver remnant (FLR) to hypertrophy the nonembolized segments and has been shown to improve the functional reserve of the FLR preoperatively. In appropriately selected patients, PVE has also been shown to reduce morbidity in the perioperative period and allow for safe, potentially curative hepatectomy for patients previously considered ineligible for resection based on anticipated small remnant livers.[14,15] For this reason, PVE is now performed routinely at many comprehensive hepatobiliary centers worldwide prior to major hepatectomy.

This chapter deals with intra-arterial therapies and PVE in two sections. The first section describes in detail the common clinical issues associated with intra-arterial therapies including patient selection, pretreatment evaluation, available devices, dose calculation, technical aspects of procedure, response assessment, and possible complications and their remedies. The second reviews the indications, techniques, and results of PVE and the potential complications that can occur from this procedure.

Section I: Intra-Arterial Therapies
GENERAL CONCEPTS

Both chemoembolization and radioembolization are based on the same general technique; that is, infusion of cytotoxic agent into the hepatic artery or its branches with the intent to targeting the tumor directly without involving surrounding hepatic parenchyma and the rest of the body. There are distinct differences, however, which are explored later. Both therapies require meticulous understanding of the vascular anatomy of the liver, diagnosing and staging of the tumor, and response evaluation.

HEPATIC VASCULAR ANATOMY

Hepatic malignancies have been the predominant target of interventional oncologists partly due to the favorable anatomy of the liver making image-guided approaches to tumors possible. The vascular supply of the tumors is predominantly by the hepatic artery. The normal parenchyma is supplied in contrast by the portal vein. This unique blood supply to the liver allows the hepatocytes to carry out their metabolic functions on the substrates absorbed from the gastrointestinal tract. It also predisposes the liver as a predominant site for metastases.[16–18]

An overview of the arterial supply of the liver is important to understand the use of transcatheter therapies for the treatment of liver malignancies. The celiac trunk is the first anterior branch of the abdominal aorta. It gives off the common hepatic artery, which becomes the proper hepatic artery that subsequently branches into the right and left hepatic arteries. These supply the corresponding lobes of the liver by giving off segmental branches. The cystic artery supplying the gallbladder usually arises from the right hepatic artery. Hepatic tumors are hypervascular structures predominantly supplied by parasitizing arterial flow from the surrounding tissue.

DIAGNOSIS OF HEPATIC METASTASES OF COLORECTAL CANCER

Unlike hepatocellular carcinoma (HCC), where a diagnosis can be made based on imaging criteria, no such criteria exist for colorectal metastases. Whenever a hepatic mass is identified in patients with primary CRC, pathologic evaluation is warranted.[19] Positron emission tomography (PET) scan plays an important role in diagnosing and staging of disease; however, it is more important is posttreatment follow-up.[19] Baseline 18[F] fluorodeoxyglucose-positron emission tomography (FDG-PET) imaging is encouraged but not considered necessary.[20] The presence of carcinoembryonic antigen (CEA) can substantiate the diagnosis; however, it is neither very sensitive nor specific.

PRETREATMENT EVALUATION

This includes a detailed patient history, physical examination, and laboratory evaluation. Any previous or concomitant chemotherapy is reviewed. Pretreatment angiography is performed for reviewing the vascular anatomy for the delivery of agent and to prevent its inadvertent spread to other tissues. Pretreatment angiography and technetium-99m labeled macroaggregated albumin (^{99m}Tc-MAA) scan are performed more meticulously for radioembolization and are covered in the relevant section of the chapter.

POSTTREATMENT RESPONSE ASSESSMENT

Tumor markers such as CEA may be used to compare posttreatment levels with pretreatment levels and this may be a way to assess response to therapy; however, radiologic monitoring remains the cornerstone of posttreatment response assessment.

Radiologic studies are performed 1 month posttreatment and then every 3 months to assess response to therapy, emergence of new lesions, or progression in treated lesions. Size criteria (WHO and RECIST guidelines) and necrosis criteria (EASL guidelines—usually for HCC) are used to assess response to therapy.[21–23] A 3-month follow-up 18 FDG-PET image may be obtained in patients who had a baseline FDG-PET study.

CHEMOEMBOLIZATION FOR HEPATIC COLORECTAL METASTASES

Conventional Transarterial Chemoembolization (TACE)

Introduction

TACE allows the delivery of a high dose of chemotherapeutic agents to the tumor with minimal systemic bioavailability. It has been used since the 1980s.[24,25] This is an inpatient procedure.

Patient Selection

Inclusion Criteria

TACE is best suited for patients with unresectable colorectal metastases to a liver with good performing status, preserved liver function, and no evidence of vascular invasion and extrahepatic metastasis.

Exclusion Criteria

In general, absolute contraindications to TACE include the absence of hepatopedal flow or compensatory collaterals, encephalopathy, and biliary obstruction. The relative contraindications include serum bilirubin (>2 mg/dL), lactate dehydrogenase (>425 U/L), aspartate aminotransferase (>100 U/L), tumor burden exceeding more than 50% of the liver, ascites, bleeding varices, thrombocytopenia, or cardiac or renal insufficiency.[26]

Procedure

After meticulous evaluation of the baseline characteristics and stage of the malignancy using clinical and radiologic data, angiography is performed to study the vascular anatomy of the region and the tumor. Doxorubicin alone as the chemotherapeutic is commonly used worldwide, whereas the combination of mitomycin C, doxorubicin, and cisplatin is preferred in the United States.[27] The chemotherapeutic drug is mixed with lipiodol and injected into the tumor feeding vessel during angiography. Lipiodol is a poppy seed oil containing 38% iodine by weight. It is a radio opaque substance and is visualized on posttreatment computed tomography (CT) scans in the target lesion. This is followed by the injection of bland embolic particles to prevent washout of the drug and to induce ischemic necrosis.[28]

Recent Studies on Chemoembolization for Colorectal Metastases

There are limited data on patients treated with chemoembolization for metastatic disease. Geschwind et al. demonstrated that chemoembolization can prolong survival of patients with colorectal metastases even in those who had not responded to systemic chemotherapy.[29] In a recent study, Albert et al. evaluated response and survival in 121 patients of unresectable hepatic colorectal metastases treated with chemoembolization with cisplatin, mitomycin C, ethiodized oil, and polyvinyl alcohol.

They observed partial response in 2%, stable disease in 41%, and progression in 57%. Median time to disease progression was 5 months. Median survival was 33 months from diagnosis of the primary colon cancer, 27 months from development of liver metastases, and 9 months from chemoembolization. They concluded that chemoembolization provides local disease control of hepatic metastases after 43% of treatment cycles.[30]

In a recent prospective study, Vogl et al. investigated repeated TACE with different drug combinations in the treatment of 463 patients with unresectable liver metastases of CRC. The local chemotherapy protocol consisted of mitomycin C alone (n = 243), mitomycin C with gemcitabine (n = 153), or mitomycin C with irinotecan (n = 67). According to RECIST guidelines, partial response, stable and progressive disease was demonstrated in 14.7%, 48.2%, and 37.1% of patients, respectively. After chemoembolization, the 1- and 2-year survival rates were 62% and 28%, respectively. There was no statistically significant difference between the three treatment protocols.[31]

Complications

Postembolization syndrome is seen after chemoembolization. It is usually not severe enough to require prolonged hospitalization.

Hepatobiliary Complications

Hepatic failure is a potential complication following chemoembolization, and proper patient selection (preserved liver function) is important for this procedure. Bilomas may form after chemoembolization. Bile duct injury may occur following this treatment and may lead to severe complications.[32] Up to 5.3% of patients may develop biliary complications following chemoembolization.[33] The occurrence of liver abscesses is rare but is possible after chemoembolization, especially in patients who have undergone biliary interventions.[32] They can be prophylactically managed with antibiotics and may require drainage if they occur.

Gastrointestinal Complications

There is the risk of inadvertent spread of the chemotherapeutic drug and the bland embolic material to the gastrointestinal tract. This may cause duodenal or gastric ulcers and may even lead to perforation in severe cases.[32]

Vascular Injury

Chemoembolization may lead to injury to the hepatic vasculature, leading to spasm. The intra-arterial approach increases the risk of vascular injury in all transcatheter techniques.[32] Chemotherapeutic agents may also have a role in causing this complication.[34]

Other Complications

There have been occurrences of tumor rupture (0.15%) following chemoembolization.[32] The time period between treatment and rupture was variable (0–45 days). Pulmonary artery embolism may occur and the patient may present with cough and dyspnea.[32]

TACE with Drug-Eluting Beads (DEB-TACE)

Introduction

The concept of DEBs is to load microspheres with chemotherapeutic agents and deliver them intra-arterially in a controlled manner. The unique properties of beads allow for fixed dosing and release of the drug in a sustained manner; this leads to a significant reduction in peak plasma concentration when compared with conventional TACE.[27]

Patient Selection and Procedure

Both inclusion and exclusion criteria for DEB-TACE are similar to conventional TACE. Procedural aspects are similar to conventional TACE; the microspheres are delivered to the tumor after angiographic evaluation of the vascular anatomy. The microspheres are composed of polyvinyl alcohol (PVA) polymers modified with sulfonate groups. By an ion exchange process, the sulfonate groups actively sequester doxorubicin from solution.[35]

Recent Studies

DEBs have been investigated for colorectal metastases to the liver. In a recent multicenter series of 55 patients with liver metastases of CRC with prior chemotherapy, Martin et al. investigated 99 treatment sessions with DEBIRI (drug-eluting bead, irinotecan). Adverse events occurred in 28%; response rates were 66% and 75% at 6 and 12 months, respectively; overall and progression-free survival was 19 and 11 months, respectively. The authors concluded that DEBIRI was safe/effective in metastatic colorectal cancer (MCC) refractory to multiple lines of systemic chemotherapy.[36] In another report, authors compared survival of patients treated with DEBIRI versus DEBs loaded with FOLFIRI in a 76-patient randomized phase III clinical trial. With a median follow-up of 24 months, they found a median survival and response rate of 48% and 70%, respectively, for DEBIRI versus 28% and 20%, respectively, for FOLFIRI. Cost per patient was 4,500 euros for DEBIRI and 10,250 euros for FOLFIRI.[37]

Bower et al. investigated the use of DEBIRI as a downstaging and neoadjuvant therapy in 55 patients with MCC in a single-arm multicenter study. They observed that 11 (20%) patients had significant response and downstaging of their disease or stable disease without extrahepatic disease progression, allowing resection, ablation, or resection and ablation. There were no postoperative deaths. Postoperative complications morbidity occurred in 18% of patients, with none of them hepatic related. They concluded that it is a safe and effective therapy in presurgical downstaging.[38]

Complications

The toxicity profile is similar to that seen after TACE, and preliminary data according to the PRECISION V trial may indicate that this is a safer therapy when compared to conventional TACE.

▮ RADIOEMBOLIZATION

Introduction

Radioembolization is the injection of micron-sized radioactive particles directly into the tumor via the arterial route, thus exposing the tumor to highly concentrated radiation and simultaneously sparing normal hepatic parenchyma. Flow dynamics and tumor hypervascularity allow the microspheres to preferentially travel to distal arterioles within the tumors, where beta emission from the isotope irradiates the tumor. External radiation has played an inconsequential role in liver malignancies due to the radiosensitivity demonstrated by hepatic tissue and consequent development of radiation-induced liver disease (RILD), a clinical syndrome of ascites, anicteric hepatomegaly, and elevation of liver enzymes upon exposure to doses greater than 35 Gray (Gy).[39,40] Besides, the dose given via external radiation is not sufficient to kill cancer cells. Radioembolization helps overcome both of these issues to a great extent. Many radioactive devices have been studied for radioembolization for HCC including iodine-131 labeled iodized oil (I-131 lipiodol), rhenium-188 HDD labeled iodized oil, phosphorus-32 glass microspheres, Milican/Holmium-166 microspheres (HoMS), and others, but the most commonly studied and used devices are yttrium-90 (^{90}Y) microspheres. There are two devices available for ^{90}Y infusion, TheraSphere (Nordion, Ottawa, Canada) and SIR-Spheres (Sirtex, Lane Cove, Australia). Of these, SIR-Spheres (resin microspheres) was granted premarket approval by the Food and Drug Administration (FDA) in 2002, defined as safe and effective for the approved indication. The indication is for the treatment of MCC to the liver with concomitant use of FUDR.

Technical Considerations before Yttrium-90 Radioembolization

Pretreatment Angiography

Given the propensity for arterial variants and hepatic tumors to exhibit arteriovenous shunting, all patients being evaluated for ^{90}Y must undergo pretreatment mesenteric angiography.[18,41] This, on one hand, allows for tailoring the treatment plan according to each patient's individual anatomy and, on the other, helps us assess any inadvertent spread of the microspheres to nontarget organs,[42] which can be controlled by prophylactic embolization.

The aortogram is performed to assess the tortuosity and the presence of atherosclerosis in the aorta. The superior mesenteric and celiac trunk angiograms allow interventional radiologists an opportunity to study the vascular anatomy of the liver. The patency of the portal vein and the presence of arterioportal shunting are also assessed. Prophylactic embolization of the gastroduodenal artery and right gastric artery is recommended as a safe and efficacious mode of minimizing the risks of hepatoenteric flow, particularly if using resin microspheres.[18,43,44] Other vessels that may need to be embolized are the falciform, inferior esophageal, left inferior phrenic, accessory left gastric, supraduodenal, and retroduodenal arteries.

Diagnostic angiography is essential to ensure that the blood supply to the tumor(s) has been adequately identified because incomplete identification of the blood supply to the tumor may lead to incomplete targeting and treatment. It also allows for accurate calculations of target volumes.[19]

Pulmonary Shunting and Technetium-99m Labeled Macroaggregated Albumin (^{99m}Tc-MAA) Scans

One of the angiographic features of liver tumors is direct arteriovenous shunting bypassing the capillary bed in contrast to metastatic tumors to the liver[45]; therefore, shunting of ^{90}Y microspheres to the lungs becomes a concern possibly resulting in radiation pneumonitis.[46] Because the size of a ^{99m}Tc-MAA particle closely mimics ^{90}Y, it is assumed that distribution of the two will be identical as well and this concept is utilized in assessing splanchnic and pulmonary shunting. It is important to correlate the findings of angiography to the findings of the ^{99m}Tc-MAA scan because the proximity of some portions of the gastrointestinal tract to the liver may confuse the findings of these nuclear medicine scans. Lung shunt fraction (LSF) is used to calculate the dose delivered to the lungs; appropriate adjustment for this parameter minimizes the risk of radiation pneumonitis.

Dosimetry

The technical considerations of dosimetry are beyond the scope of this chapter and are described in detail for both Sir-Spheres and TheraSphere.[19]

Patient Selection

Inclusion Criteria

(a) Unresectable colorectal metastases within the liver determined by the multidisciplinary team, (b) age greater than 18 years, (c) Eastern Cooperative Oncology Group (ECOG) performance status less than or equal to 2, (d) adequate pulmonary function test findings, (e) adequate hematologic parameters (granulocyte count $>1.5 \times 10^9$/L, platelet count $>50 \times 10^9$/L), renal function (serum creatinine level <2 mg/dL) and liver function (serum bilirubin level <1.5 mg/dL), (f) ability to undergo angiography and selective visceral catheterization, and (g) potentially resectable/transplantable by imaging.[20,47,48]

Exclusion Criteria

(a) Concurrent chemotherapy or radiotherapy, (b) evidence of uncorrectable flow to the gastrointestinal tract, (c) estimated radiation doses to the lungs greater than 30 Gy in a single administration or 50 Gy in multiple administrations, and (d) significant extrahepatic disease (life expectancy <3 months).

Yttrium-90 Radioembolization Procedure

The procedure for administering ^{90}Y should be followed with care and caution. The apparatus for the administration of ^{90}Y is designed to minimize radiation exposure to persons involved in the procedure. The tumor is approached under fluoroscopic guidance and the vial is injected into the vessel feeding the tumor. Tumor distribution guides for the selectivity of the treatment, that is, to one or more lobes/segments as required. A physicist should be present throughout the case to ensure that proper protocols are followed to minimize accidental radiation exposure. The details of the procedure and differences between the administration of Sir-Spheres and TheraSphere have been previously published.[19]

Recent Studies

Patients who have unresectable disease and are on systemic chemotherapy or have failed to respond to first- or second-line chemotherapeutic agents are considered as candidates for radioembolization. The combination of radioembolization with systemic chemotherapy has been shown to have a significantly better tumor response, a longer time to progression, survival benefit, and an acceptable safety profile.[49] The use of radioembolization alone has also been published in many series and has shown promising results.[50] Dose escalation studies have shown a better response with increasing doses.[51]

Cosimelli et al. investigated the use of ^{90}Y resin microspheres in a multicenter phase II trial in 50 patients with unresectable, chemotherapy refractory colorectal metastases in the liver. They observed early and intermediate (>48 hours) WHO G1-2 adverse events (mostly fever and pain) in 16% and 22% of patients, respectively, whereas two patients died due to renal failure at 40 days or liver failure at 60 days, respectively. Using RECIST criteria, 1 patient (2%) had a complete response, 11 (22%) partial response, 12 (24%) stable disease, and 22 (44%) progressive disease; 4 (8%) were nonevaluable. Median overall survival was 12.6 months (95% CI, 7.0–18.3); 2-year survival was 19.6%. They concluded that radioembolization produced meaningful response and disease stabilization.[52]

Sharma et al. performed a phase I study analyzing the combination of radioembolization with modified FOLFOX4 systemic chemotherapy in patients with unresectable CRC metastases in the liver in a series of 20 patients with the primary endpoint of toxicity.[53] Of these patients, 5 experienced National Cancer Institute (NCI; Bethesda, MD) grade 3 abdominal pain, 2 of whom had microsphere-induced gastric ulcers; grade 3 or 4 neutropenia was recorded in 12 patients; one episode of transient grade 3 hepatotoxicity was recorded. Partial responses were demonstrated in 18 patients and stable disease in 2 patients. Median progression-free survival was 9.3 months and median time to progression in the liver was 12.3 months. They concluded that this chemoradiation regime merits phase II–III trials.

In a recent multicenter phase III randomized trial comprising 46 patients with unresectable liver-limited MCC, Hendlisz et al. compared intravenous fluorouracil alone with a combination of radioembolization and intravenous fluorouracil. They concluded that combination therapy is well tolerated and significantly improves time-to-progression compared with fluorouracil alone and that this procedure was a valid therapeutic option for chemotherapy-refractory liver metastases of CRC.[54]

Complications

The postradioembolization syndrome (PRS) consists of the following clinical symptoms: fatigue, nausea, vomiting, anorexia, fever, abdominal discomfort, and cachexia. However, it occurs less commonly after radioembolization due to the small size of the particles and these seldom require hospitalization.[55–57] Complications have been described in detail by Riaz et al.[58]

Practical Advantages/Limitations of Intra-Arterial Therapies for Colorectal Metastases

Intra-arterial therapies have several advantages: (1) delivery of relatively high doses of toxic agent to small hepatic volume, (2) direct targeting of tumor tissue, (3) sparing the healthy hepatic tissue and the rest of the body from side effects and complications, (4) relatively low toxicity profile, (5) decision making not affected by lesional characteristics, (6) a sound therapeutic option for otherwise unresectable disease, (7) less hospital stay and faster recovery. There are, however, limitations: (1) the procedures do not target the entire disease simultaneously; therefore, repeat treatments are required: (2) absence of well-defined guidelines for response assessment following intra-arterial therapies; (3) lack of randomized trials comparing different intra-arterial therapies.

Section II: Portal Vein Embolization
▌ INDICATIONS AND CONTRAINDICATIONS

Several factors must be considered to determine if a particular patient will benefit from PVE. First, assessment for the presence of underlying hepatic disease is necessary to help determine if the FLR volume will be adequate for hepatic function after major hepatic resection. It is well known that a normal liver has a greater regenerative capacity, functions more efficiently, and tolerates injury better than a cirrhotic liver. Therefore, complications of a poorly functioning liver remnant are more common in cirrhotic patients compared with patients who have healthy livers and include ascites, fluid retention, and wound breakdown from poor protein synthesis. Patients with cirrhosis who have marginal liver remnants are also at increased risk for death from liver failure.[59] Consequently, most surgeons only consider patients with Child-Pugh Class A cirrhosis and normal liver function based on indocyanine green dye retention testing (<10%) as candidates for major hepatectomy.[60]

Other factors that must be considered prior to major hepatic resection include the following: (a) the extent and complexity of the planned resection and the likelihood that an associated extrahepatic surgery will be needed[61]; (b) the size of the patient because larger patients require larger FLRs than smaller patients[62]; (c) the presence of extrahepatic disease; and (d) whether or not the patient has had previous chemotherapy, which could cause hepatic injury.[63,64] These factors are considered in the setting of the patient's age and comorbidities (e.g., diabetes), which may affect hypertrophy.

The need for PVE is decided once the procedure type and extent of resection necessary to treat the patient have been determined. Liver volumetry using CT is used to aid in this decision. Guidelines for the minimal size of the FLR required prior to major hepatic resection have been established based on the presence or absence of underlying hepatic disease and patient size. Patients without underlying hepatic disease should undergo PVE only when the FLR is less than 20%.[65–67] PVE may also be indicated for patients with FLR less than 30% if they have received preoperative chemotherapy or if they have hepatic fibrosis or a severe hepatic injury.[64,68] It is typically recommended that patients with cirrhosis and FLR less than 40% should undergo PVE prior to major hepatectomy.[60] Failure to adhere to these well-established guidelines often result in excess use of PVE.[69]

With regard to complications, the only absolute contraindication to PVE is overt clinical portal hypertension such that the patient is not a surgical candidate.[13] All other contraindications are relative and include: (a) tumor invasion into the portal vein and/or FLR, (b) extrahepatic metastases including periportal adenopathy, (c) uncorrectable coagulopathy, (d) tumor precluding safe transhepatic access, (e) biliary dilation in the FLR that necessitates pre-PVE drainage, (f) mild portal hypertension that does not preclude resection, and (g) renal failure. In the presence of extensive portal vein invasion, PVE is contraindicated because portal flow is already redistributed. Tumor thrombus in small segmental portal branches, however, will not redistribute a considerable amount of flow. In this case, PVE may still be advised.

▌ TECHNICAL ASPECTS OF PORTAL VEIN EMBOLIZATION

To divert portal blood flow to the FLR, various embolic agents and three standard technical approaches have been described.[12,13] The goal is to achieve as complete embolization of the portal branches as possible to ensure sufficient hypertrophy of the FLR and avoid recanalization of the occluded veins. Embolization of all the portal branches supplying the area to be resected must be achieved to prevent formation of intrahepatic portoportal collateral vessels.[70]

A number of embolic agents have been used for PVE, including fibrin glue, gelatin sponge and thrombin, coils, n-butyl cyanoacrylate and ethiodized oil, microparticles, and absolute alcohol. No significant difference in degrees or rates of hypertrophy has been seen among these materials[71]; thus far, the major differences among agents are limited to their side-effect profiles.[72] Development of new agents to achieve more complete and permanent occlusions is ongoing in an effort to eliminate recanalization and thereby yield earlier and better hypertrophy.

The approach chosen is generally based on operator preference, the type of resection planned, and the embolic agent to be used. Access to the portal system may be achieved by the transhepatic contralateral, transhepatic ipsilateral, or transileocolic venous approach. The transhepatic contralateral technique involves percutaneously accessing the portal system through the FLR.[11,73,74] This method is the most widely used because it is considered by many to be technically easier; cannulation of the right portal venous branches is more direct from the left portal system. However, the contralateral technique carries with it the risk of injury to the FLR or to the left portal vein.[75] If this occurs, it can potentially make a patient previously considered resectable unresectable. Further, catheterization of segment 4 for embolization, if needed, may be difficult from the contralateral approach. An advantage of the transhepatic ipsilateral approach (i.e., through the liver to be resected) is that the FLR is not instrumented and therefore is not subjected to the same risks seen with the contralateral approach.[14,76,77] Catheterization of the right portal vein branches may be more difficult, however, due to the acute angulations between right portal branches, and the technique typically necessitates the use of reverse-curve catheters. In cases where right PVE is extended to segment 4 (i.e., if an extended right hepatectomy is planned), there is a small added risk of dislodging embolic material from the right lobe branches during embolization of segment 4 from catheter manipulation.[14,78] Therefore, in these cases, segment 4 should be embolized first. Another potential disadvantage is that embolic material may be displaced upon catheter removal, leading to nontarget embolization; however, this is exceedingly rare. Lastly, the ipsilateral access may be challenging in patients with large right hepatic tumors. In these circumstances, the contralateral approach can be used.

The transileocolic approach involves direct cannulation of the ileocolic vein during laparotomy with passage of a catheter into the portal system.[10] This approach was the original method for performing PVE and is still used by many surgeons in Asia. It is favored in centers without a dedicated interventional radiology suite, when percutaneous access is not considered possible, or when additional treatment is planned during the same surgery. This technique has the disadvantage of requiring general anesthesia and laparotomy, with their inherent risks, and the superior imaging equipment generally found in interventional radiology suites is frequently not available in operating suites.

As with any other procedure, technical complications of PVE have been reported. These include thrombosis of an unintended branch of the portal vein, migration of emboli into branches of the portal vein supplying the FLR, subcapsular hematoma, rupture of metastases, hemoperitoneum, transient hemobilia, transient liver failure, pneumothorax, and sepsis.[79,80] Vascular complications consist of pseudoaneurysm formation, arteriovenous fistula formation, and development of arterioportal shunts. Most complications occur in the punctured lobe, prompting

recommendations from Kodama et al. that the transhepatic ipsilateral approach be attempted first.[80]

■ RESULTS

Outcomes after PVE and hepatectomy vary depending on whether a patient has underlying liver disease or a healthy liver. In patients with chronic liver disease (i.e., chronic hepatitis, fibrosis, or cirrhosis), the increase in the FLR volumes after PVE varies (range, 28%–46%), and hypertrophy after PVE may not be complete until after 4 weeks because of slower regeneration rates.[81,82] In a 2005 study that included 40 patients with HCC in the setting of advanced liver fibrosis or cirrhosis, Denys and colleagues[83] found that only two factors significantly affected hypertrophy: mild degree of fibrosis (as indicated by Knodell histologic score[84] of less than F4), and a pre-PVE lower functional liver ratio as defined by the ratio between the left lobe (i.e., FLR) and the total liver volume minus tumor volume. Factors that did not correlate with improved hypertrophy included age, gender, history of diabetes, and prior TACE.

The important role of PVE in preparation of hepatectomy and of RPVE extended to segment 4 in preparation for extended hepatectomy in patients with normal underlying liver (e.g., colorectal hepatic metastases) and inadequate FLR volumes has also been well documented.[67,85–87] Ribero et al.[85] showed that in 85 patients without cirrhosis who underwent RPVE+4, the absolute FLR volume increased from an average of 16.6% before PVE to 25.8% after PVE, and the mean degree of hypertrophy (DH), defined as the difference between the sFLR before and after PVE, was 8.8%. Of the 21 patients without cirrhosis who underwent PVE without extension to segment 4, the sFLR increased from 28.1% to 43.7% with a median DH of 10.9%. The higher DH in patients who underwent RPVE compared to RPVE+4 was caused by substantial growth of segment 4. These results emphasize the importance of FLR size because both sFLR after PVE (≤20%) and DH (≤5%) are correlated with postoperative hepatic dysfunction. Combining the sFLR and DH values predicted hepatic dysfunction with high sensitivity and was associated with clinical outcomes. The importance of PVE in patients with sFLR less than or equal to 20% has subsequently been confirmed by the largest PVE outcomes study to date, which was conducted at M.D. Anderson Cancer Center.[67] These researchers analyzed 301 consecutive patients after extended right hepatectomy and found that rates of postoperative liver insufficiency and death from liver failure were comparable between patients with sFLR 20.1% to 30% and sFLR greater than or equal to 30% but higher in patients with sFLR less than or equal to 20% ($P < 0.05$).

No prospective randomized clinical trials to date have studied the efficacy of PVE and such trials are unlikely in the future because it would be considered by many unethical to deny preoperative PVE to patients with inadequate FLR size or function causing them to not qualify as surgical candidates.[71] A 2008 meta-analysis by Abulkhir et al.[15] concluded that PVE is safe and effective to induce hypertrophy of the remnant liver and decrease postoperative liver failure rates. Their study analyzed 37 publications on PVE using both percutaneous and transileocolic approaches that comprised 1,088 patients and found that major complications occurred in only 2.2% of patients. They also noted that the increase in the FLR volume was significantly greater in patients who underwent percutaneous PVE (11.9%) compared to those who underwent transileocolic PVE (9.7%).

The effects of neoadjuvant chemotherapy on liver regeneration after PVE have been investigated by different authors. Zorzi et al. retrospectively reviewed 65 patients treated with or without preoperative chemotherapy after PVE in preparation for hepatic resection of colorectal metastasis.[88] PVE was performed in 43 patients after chemotherapy, including 26 receiving concurrent bevacizumab, and in 22 without preprocedural chemotherapy. After 4 weeks, no statistically significant difference was observed in the volume of FLR and DH between the two groups. Another retrospective study compared 43 patients who were embolized during neoadjuvant chemotherapy to a second group of 57 patients who did not receive chemotherapy.[89] The two groups were also compared to 100 consecutive patients subjected to extended hepatectomies without preoperative PVE. There was no difference in liver growth between the two PVE groups. The PVE patients showed improved recovery after resection. Similar results were observed in a study by Goere et al. comparing live hypertrophy after PVE in two groups of 10 patients with colorectal carcinoma with and without neoadjuvant chemotherapy.[90] A separate small study compared liver volumes after PVE in 10 patients with colorectal carcinoma postchemotherapy and 5 patients without neoadjuvant chemotherapy. The patients exposed to prior chemotherapy exhibited significantly decreased liver hypertrophy. Despite the small sample size, the authors concluded that chemotherapy may reduce liver regeneration after PVE.[91]

Lastly, some studies have suggested accelerated tumor growth caused by increased cell replication following PVE.[92] Potential mechanisms include changes in cytokines or growth factors, alteration in hepatic blood supply, and an enhanced cellular host response.[93] Several small studies have shown increased growth of colorectal liver metastases following PVE, both in the embolized[94,95] and nonembolized liver, but comparison data of tumor growth prior to and following embolization are lacking. In addition, objective data have demonstrated no direct correlation between changes in tumor size and PVE.[93] Thus, although the benefits of PVE are clear, no true risk of clinically significant PVE-induced tumor growth has been established.

▌ CONCLUSION

Intra-arterial therapies can provide an innovative and minimally invasive alternate to a large group of patients of unresectable and/or chemorefractory hepatic colorectal metastases who are otherwise not a subject to curative therapies due to a number of reasons. These therapies have provided encouraging response rates and long-term outcomes including overall and progression-free survival. PVE is now advocated for those who have potentially resectable disease with marginal anticipated FLR volumes. It is hoped that further research and cooperation on international level will lead to enhancements in treatment modalities and consequently better patient outcomes.

▌ REFERENCES

1. Parkin DM BF, Ferlay J, Pisani P. Global cancer statistics, 2002. *CA Cancer J Clin* 2005;55:74–108.
2. Ferlay J, Shin HR, Bray F, et al. Estimates of worldwide burden of cancer in 2008: GLOBOCAN 2008. *Int J Cancer* 2010.
3. Sasson AR, Sigurdson ER. Surgical treatment of liver metastases. *Semin Oncol* 2002;29(2):107–118.
4. Tomlinson JS, Jarnagin WR, DeMatteo RP, et al. Actual 10-year survival after resection of colorectal liver metastases defines cure. *J Clin Oncol* 2007;25(29):4575–4580.
5. Kuebler JP. Radioembolization of liver metastases in patients with colorectal cancer: a nonsurgical treatment with combined modality potential. *J Clin Oncol* 2009;27(25):4041–4042.
6. Bengtsson G, Carlsson G, Hafstrom L, et al. Natural history of patients with untreated liver metastases from colorectal cancer. *Am J Surg* 1981;141(5):586–589.
7. Wagner JS, Adson MA, Van Heerden JA, et al. The natural history of hepatic metastases from colorectal cancer. A comparison with resective treatment. *Ann Surg* 1984;199(5):502–508.
8. Goldberg RM, Rothenberg ML, Van Cutsem E, et al. The continuum of care: a paradigm for the management of metastatic colorectal cancer. *Oncologist* 2007;12(1):38–50.
9. Riaz A, Salem R. Yttrium-90 radioembolization in the management of liver tumors: expanding the global experience. *Eur J Nucl Med Mol Imaging* 2010;37(3):451–452.
10. Makuuchi M, Thai BL, Takayasu K, et al. Preoperative portal embolization to increase safety of major hepatectomy for hilar bile duct carcinoma: a preliminary report. *Surgery* 1990;107(5):521–527.
11. de Baere T, Roche A, Vavasseur D, et al. Portal vein embolization: utility for inducing left hepatic lobe hypertrophy before surgery. *Radiology* 1993;188(1):73–77.
12. Madoff DC, Abdalla EK, Vauthey JN. Portal vein embolization in preparation for major hepatic resection: evolution of a new standard of care. *J Vasc Interv Radiol* 2005;16(6):779–790.
13. Avritscher R, Duke E, Madoff DC. Portal vein embolization: rationale, outcomes, controversies and future directions. *Expert Rev Gastroenterol Hepatol* 2010;4(4):489–501.
14. Madoff DC, Abdalla EK, Gupta S, et al. Transhepatic ipsilateral right portal vein embolization extended to segment IV: improving hypertrophy and resection outcomes with spherical particles and coils. *J Vasc Interv Radiol* 2005;16(2 pt 1):215–225.
15. Abulkhir A, Limongelli P, Healey AJ, et al. Preoperative portal vein embolization for major liver resection: a meta-analysis. *Ann Surg* 2008;247(1):49–57.
16. Salem R, Lewandowski RJ, Sato KT, et al. Technical aspects of radioembolization with 90Y microspheres. *Tech Vasc Interv Radiol* 2007;10(1):12–29.
17. Lewandowski RJ, Sato KT, Atassi B, et al. Radioembolization with (90)y microspheres: angiographic and technical considerations. *Cardiovasc Intervent Radiol* 2007;30(4):571–592.
18. Liu DM, Salem R, Bui JT, et al. Angiographic considerations in patients undergoing liver-directed therapy. *J Vasc Interv Radiol* 2005;16(7):911–935.
19. Salem R, Thurston KG. Radioembolization with 90 yttrium microspheres: a state-of-the-art brachytherapy treatment for primary and secondary liver malignancies: part 1: technical and methodologic considerations. *J Vasc Interv Radiol* 2006;17(8):1251–1278.
20. Mulcahy MF, Lewandowski RJ, Ibrahim SM, et al. Radioembolization of colorectal hepatic metastases using yttrium-90 microspheres. *Cancer* 2009;115(9):1849–1858.
21. World Health Organization. *WHO Handbook for Reporting Results of Cancer Treatment.* WHO Offset Publication. Geneva, Switzerland: World Health Organization; 1979:no.48.
22. Bruix J, Sherman M, Llovet JM, et al. Clinical management of hepatocellular carcinoma. Conclusions of the Barcelona-2000 EASL conference. European Association for the Study of the Liver. *J Hepatol* 2001;35(3):421–430.
23. Therasse P, Arbuck SG, Eisenhauer EA, et al. New guidelines to evaluate the response to treatment in solid tumors. European Organization for Research and Treatment of Cancer, National Cancer Institute of the United States, National Cancer Institute of Canada. *J Natl Cancer Inst* 2000;92(3):205–216.
24. Eksborg S, Cedermark BJ, Strandler HS. Intrahepatic and intravenous administration of adriamycin—a comparative pharmacokinetic study in patients with malignant liver tumours. *Med Oncol Tumor Pharmacother* 1985;2(1):47–54.
25. Ensminger W. Hepatic arterial chemotherapy for primary and metastatic liver cancers. *Cancer Chemother Pharmacol* 1989;23(suppl):S68–73.
26. Soulen MC. Chemoembolization of hepatic malignancies. *Oncology (Williston Park)* 1994;8(4):77–84; discussion 84, 89–90 passim.
27. Solomon B, Soulen MC, Baum RA, et al. Chemoembolization of hepatocellular carcinoma with cisplatin, doxorubicin, mitomycin-C, ethiodol, and polyvinyl alcohol: prospective evaluation of response and survival in a U.S. population. *J Vasc Interv Radiol* 1999;10(6):793–798.
28. Coldwell DM, Stokes KR, Yakes WF. Embolotherapy: agents, clinical applications, and techniques. *Radiographics* 1994;14(3):623–643; quiz 645–626.
29. Geschwind J, Hong K, Georgiades C. *Utility of Transcatheter Arterial Chemoembolization for Liver Dominant Colorectal Metastatic Adenocarcinoma in*

the Salvage Setting. American Society of Clinical Oncology Gastrointestinal Cancers Symposium. San Francisco, CA; January 26–28, 2006.

30. Albert M, Kiefer MV, Sun W, et al. Chemoembolization of colorectal liver metastases with cisplatin, doxorubicin, mitomycin C, ethiodol, and polyvinyl alcohol. *Cancer* 2011;117(2):343–352.

31. Vogl TJ, Gruber T, Balzer JO, et al. Repeated transarterial chemoembolization in the treatment of liver metastases of colorectal cancer: prospective study. *Radiology* 2009;250(1):281–289.

32. Xia J, Ren Z, Ye S, et al. Study of severe and rare complications of transarterial chemoembolization (TACE) for liver cancer. *Eur J Radiol* 2006.

33. Kim HK, Chung YH, Song BC, et al. Ischemic bile duct injury as a serious complication after transarterial chemoembolization in patients with hepatocellular carcinoma. *J Clin Gastroenterol* 2001;32(5):423–427.

34. Belli L, Magistretti G, Puricelli GP, et al. Arteritis following intra-arterial chemotherapy for liver tumors. *Eur Radiol* 1997;7(3):323–326.

35. Lencioni R, Crocetti L, Petruzzi P, et al. Doxorubicin-eluting bead-enhanced radiofrequency ablation of hepatocellular carcinoma: a pilot clinical study. *J Hepatol* 2008;49(2):217–222.

36. Martin RC, Joshi J, Robbins K, et al. Hepatic intra-arterial injection of drug-eluting bead, irinotecan (DEBIRI) in unresectable colorectal liver metastases refractory to systemic chemotherapy: results of multi-institutional study. *Ann Surg Oncol* 2010.

37. Fiorentini G. Trans-arterial Chemoembolization of Liver Metastases from Colorectal Carcinoma Adopting Drug Eluting-Beads Loaded with Irinotecan Compared to FOLFIRI: Results at Two Years of A Phase III Clinical Trial. Paper presented at: WCIO2011; New York, NY.

38. Bower M, Metzger T, Robbins K, et al. Surgical downstaging and neoadjuvant therapy in metastatic colorectal carcinoma with irinotecan drug-eluting beads: a multi-institutional study. *HPB (Oxford)* 2010;12(1):31–36.

39. Ingold JA, Reed GB, Kaplan HS, et al. Radiation hepatitis. *AJR J Roentgenol Radium Ther Nucl Med* 1965;93:200–208.

40. Geschwind JF, Salem R, Carr BI, et al. Yttrium-90 microspheres for the treatment of hepatocellular carcinoma. *Gastroenterology* 2004;127 (5 suppl 1):S194–205.

41. Salem R, Thurston KG, Carr BI, et al. Yttrium-90 microspheres: radiation therapy for unresectable liver cancer. *J Vasc Interv Radiol* 2002;13(9 pt 2):S223–229.

42. Covey AM, Brody LA, Maluccio MA, et al. Variant hepatic arterial anatomy revisited: digital subtraction angiography performed in 600 patients. *Radiology* 2002;224(2):542–547.

43. Murthy R, Nunez R, Szklaruk J, et al. Yttrium-90 microsphere therapy for hepatic malignancy: devices, indications, technical considerations, and potential complications. *Radiographics* 2005;25(suppl 1):S41–55.

44. Cosin O, Bilbao JI, Alvarez S, et al. Right gastric artery embolization prior to treatment with yttrium-90 microspheres. *Cardiovasc Intervent Radiol* 2007;30(1):98–103.

45. Chen JH, Chai JW, Huang CL, et al. Proximal arterioportal shunting associated with hepatocellular carcinoma: features revealed by dynamic helical CT. *AJR Am J Roentgenol* 1999;172(2):403–407.

46. Ho S, Lau WY, Leung TW, et al. Partition model for estimating radiation doses from yttrium-90 microspheres in treating hepatic tumours. *Eur J Nucl Med* 1996;23(8):947–952.

47. Wong CY, Salem R, Raman S, et al. Evaluating 90Y-glass microsphere treatment response of unresectable colorectal liver metastases by [18F] FDG PET: a comparison with CT or MRI. *Eur J Nucl Med Mol Imaging* 2002;29(6):815–820.

48. Wong CY, Salem R, Qing F, et al. Metabolic response after intraarterial 90Y-glass microsphere treatment for colorectal liver metastases: comparison of quantitative and visual analyses by 18F-FDG PET. *J Nucl Med* 2004;45(11):1892–1897.

49. Gray B, Van Hazel G, Hope M, et al. Randomised trial of SIR-Spheres plus chemotherapy vs. chemotherapy alone for treating patients with liver metastases from primary large bowel cancer. *Ann Oncol* 2001;12(12):1711–1720.

50. Kennedy A, Coldwell D, Nutting C, et al. Liver Brachytherapy for Unresectable Colorectal Metastases: US Results 2000–2004. Paper presented at: ASCO GI Symposium; January 27–29, 2005; Miami, Florida.

51. Goin JE, Dancey JE, Hermann GA, et al. Treatment of unresectable metastatic colorectal carcinoma to the liver with intrahepatic Y-90 microspheres: a dose-ranging study. *World J of Nuc Med* 2003;2:216–225.

52. Cosimelli M, Golfieri R, Cagol PP, et al. Multi-centre phase II clinical trial of yttrium-90 resin microspheres alone in unresectable, chemotherapy refractory colorectal liver metastases. *Br J Cancer* 2010;103(3):324–331.

53. Sharma RA, Van Hazel GA, Morgan B, et al. Radioembolization of liver metastases from colorectal cancer using yttrium-90 microspheres with concomitant systemic oxaliplatin, fluorouracil, and leucovorin chemotherapy. *J Clin Oncol* 2007;25(9):1099–1106.

54. Hendlisz A, Van den Eynde M, Peeters M, et al. Phase III trial comparing protracted intravenous fluorouracil infusion alone or with yttrium-90 resin microspheres radioembolization for liver-limited metastatic colorectal cancer refractory to standard chemotherapy. *J Clin Oncol* 2010;28(23):3687–3694.

55. Salem R, Lewandowski RJ, Atassi B, et al. Treatment of unresectable hepatocellular carcinoma with use of 90Y microspheres (TheraSphere): safety, tumor response, and survival. *J Vasc Interv Radiol* 2005;16(12):1627–1639.

56. Kennedy AS, Coldwell D, Nutting C, et al. Resin 90Y-microsphere brachytherapy for unresectable colorectal liver metastases: modern USA experience. *Int J Radiat Oncol Biol Phys* 2006;65(2):412–425.

57. Murthy R, Xiong H, Nunez R, et al. Yttrium 90 resin microspheres for the treatment of unresectable colorectal hepatic metastases after failure of multiple chemotherapy regimens: preliminary results. *J Vasc Interv Radiol* 2005;16(7):937–945.

58. Riaz A, Lewandowski RJ, Kulik LM, et al. Complications following radioembolization with yttrium-90 microspheres: a comprehensive literature review. *J Vasc Interv Radiol* 2009;20(9):1121–1130; quiz 1131.

59. Shirabe K, Shimada M, Gion T, et al. Postoperative liver failure after major hepatic resection for hepatocellular carcinoma in the modern era with special reference to remnant liver volume. *J Am Coll Surg* 1999;188(3):304–309.

60. Kubota K, Makuuchi M, Kusaka K, et al. Measurement of liver volume and hepatic functional reserve as a guide to decision-making in resectional surgery for hepatic tumors. *Hepatology* 1997;26(5):1176–1181.

61. Kawarada Y, Sanda M, Kawamura K, et al. Simultaneous extensive resection of the liver and the pancreas in dogs. *Gastroenterol Jpn* 1991;26(6):747–756.

62. Vauthey JN, Chaoui A, Do KA, et al. Standardized measurement of the future liver remnant prior to extended liver resection: methodology and clinical associations. *Surgery* 2000;127(5):512–519.

63. Elias D, Lasser P, Spielmann M, et al. Surgical and chemotherapeutic treatment of hepatic metastases from carcinoma of the breast. *Surg Gynecol Obstet* 1991;172(6):461–464.

64. Azoulay D, Castaing D, Krissat J, et al. Percutaneous portal vein embolization increases the feasibility and safety of major liver resection for hepatocellular carcinoma in injured liver. *Ann Surg* 2000;232(5):665–672.

65. Shoup M, Gonen M, D'Angelica M, et al. Volumetric analysis predicts hepatic dysfunction in patients undergoing major liver resection. *J Gastrointest Surg* 2003;7(3):325–330.

66. Abdalla EK, Barnett CC, Doherty D, et al. Extended hepatectomy in patients with hepatobiliary malignancies with and without preoperative portal vein embolization. *Arch Surg* 2002;137(6):675–680; discussion 680–671.

67. Kishi Y, Abdalla EK, Chun YS, et al. Three hundred and one consecutive extended right hepatectomies: evaluation of outcome based on systematic liver volumetry. *Ann Surg* 2009.

68. Adam R, Delvart V, Pascal G, et al. Rescue surgery for unresectable colorectal liver metastases downstaged by chemotherapy: a model to predict long-term survival. *Ann Surg* 2004;240(4):644–657; discussion 657–648.

69. Denys AL, De Baere T, Doenz F. Portal vein embolization: a plea for strict patient selection. *AJR Am J Roentgenol* 2006;187(1):W125; author reply 126.

70. Denys AL, Abehsera M, Sauvanet A, et al. Failure of right portal vein ligation to induce left lobe hypertrophy due to intrahepatic portoportal collaterals: successful treatment with portal vein embolization. *AJR Am J Roentgenol* 1999;173(3):633–635.

71. Abdalla EK, Hicks ME, Vauthey JN. Portal vein embolization: rationale, technique and future prospects. *Br J Surg* 2001;88(2):165–175.

72. Imamura H, Shimada R, Kubota M, et al. Preoperative portal vein embolization: an audit of 84 patients. *Hepatology* 1999;29(4):1099–1105.

73. Kinoshita H, Sakai K, Hirohashi K, et al. Preoperative portal vein embolization for hepatocellular carcinoma. *World J Surg* 1986;10(5):803–808.

74. de Baere T, Roche A, Elias D, et al. Preoperative portal vein embolization for extension of hepatectomy indications. *Hepatology* 1996;24(6):1386–1391.

75. Denys A, Madoff DC, Doenz F, et al. Indications for and limitations of portal vein embolization before major hepatic resection for hepatobiliary malignancy. *Surg Oncol Clin N Am* 2002;11(4):955–968.

76. Nagino M, Nimura Y, Kamiya J, et al. Selective percutaneous transhepatic embolization of the portal vein in preparation for extensive liver resection: the ipsilateral approach. *Radiology* 1996;200(2):559–563.

77. Madoff DC, Hicks ME, Abdalla EK, et al. Portal vein embolization with polyvinyl alcohol particles and coils in preparation for major liver resection for hepatobiliary malignancy: safety and effectiveness—study in 26 patients. *Radiology* 2003;227(1):251–260.

78. Kishi Y, Madoff DC, Abdalla EK, et al. Is embolization of segment 4 portal veins before extended right hepatectomy justified? *Surgery* 2008;144(5):744–751.

79. Di Stefano DR, de Baere T, Denys A, et al. Preoperative percutaneous portal vein embolization: evaluation of adverse events in 188 patients. *Radiology* 2005;234(2):625–630.

80. Kodama Y, Shimizu T, Endo H, et al. Complications of percutaneous transhepatic portal vein embolization. *J Vasc Interv Radiol.* 2002;13(12):1233–1237.

81. Shimamura T, Nakajima Y, Une Y, et al. Efficacy and safety of preoperative percutaneous transhepatic portal embolization with absolute ethanol: a clinical study. *Surgery* 1997;121(2):135–141.

82. Nagino M, Nimura Y, Kamiya J, et al. Changes in hepatic lobe volume in biliary tract cancer patients after right portal vein embolization. *Hepatology* 1995;21(2):434–439.

83. Denys A, Lacombe C, Schneider F, et al. Portal vein embolization with N-butyl cyanoacrylate before partial hepatectomy in patients with hepatocellular carcinoma and underlying cirrhosis or advanced fibrosis. *J Vasc Interv Radiol* 2005;16(12):1667–1674.

84. Knodell RG, Ishak KG, Black WC, et al. Formulation and application of a numerical scoring system for assessing histological activity in asymptomatic chronic active hepatitis. *Hepatology* 1981;1(5):431–435.

85. Ribero D, Abdalla EK, Madoff DC, et al. Portal vein embolization before major hepatectomy and its effects on regeneration, resectability and outcome. *Br J Surg* 2007;94(11):1386–1394.

86. Abdalla EK, Denys A, Chevalier P, et al. Total and segmental liver volume variations: implications for liver surgery. *Surgery* 2004;135(4):404–410.

87. Elias D, Cavalcanti A, de Baere T, et al. Long-term oncological results of hepatectomy performed after selective portal embolization [in French]. *Ann Chir* 1999;53(7):559–564.

88. Zorzi D, Chun YS, Madoff DC, et al. Chemotherapy with bevacizumab does not affect liver regeneration after portal vein embolization in the treatment of colorectal liver metastases. *Ann Surg Oncol* 2008;15(10):2765–2772.

89. Covey AM, Brown KT, Jarnagin WR, et al. Combined portal vein embolization and neoadjuvant chemotherapy as a treatment strategy for resectable hepatic colorectal metastases. *Ann Surg* 2008;247(3):451–455.

90. Goéré D, Farges O, Leporrier J, et al. Chemotherapy does not impair hypertrophy of the left liver after right portal vein obstruction. *J Gastrointest Surg* 2006;10(3):365–370.

91. Beal IK, Anthony S, Papadopoulou A, et al. Portal vein embolisation prior to hepatic resection for colorectal liver metastases and the effects of periprocedure chemotherapy. *Br J Radiol* 2006;79(942):473–478.

92. Pamecha V, Levene A, Grillo F, et al. Effect of portal vein embolisation on the growth rate of colorectal liver metastases. *Br J Cancer* 2009;100(4):617–622.

93. de Graaf W, van den Esschert JW, van Lienden KP, et al. Induction of tumor growth after preoperative portal vein embolization: is it a real problem? *Ann Surg Oncol* 2009;16(2):423–430.

94. Barbaro B, Di Stasi C, Nuzzo G, et al. Preoperative right portal vein embolization in patients with metastatic liver disease. Metastatic liver volumes after RPVE. *Acta Radiol* 2003;44(1):98–102.

95. Kokudo N, Tada K, Seki M, et al. Proliferative activity of intrahepatic colorectal metastases after preoperative hemihepatic portal vein embolization. *Hepatology* 2001;34(2):267–272.

Neuroendocrine Tumors: Medical and Surgical Management

PETER D. PENG, DAVID COSGROVE, and TIMOTHY M. PAWLIK

INTRODUCTION

Gastrointestinal neuroendocrine tumors are rare neoplasms that can be broadly subdivided into carcinoid and pancreatic islet cell tumors. Carcinoid tumors have an estimated population incidence of approximately 5 in 100,000,[1] whereas autopsy data put the incidence as high as 1.2% of the general populous in certain series.[2] Carcinoids are distributed throughout the gastrointestinal tract; they are most often found in the small bowel (42%), rectum (27%), and stomach (9%).[3] Pancreatic islet cell tumors have an estimated incidence of less than 1 in 100,000 but over 300 in 100,000 at autopsy.[4] Pancreatic neuroendocrine tumors arise from the pancreas and sometimes also involve the duodenum. Although usually indolent, neuroendocrine tumors have a well-documented metastatic potential, which depends on both primary location and hormonal secretion subtype. In one autopsy series, carcinoid metastases were identified in 29.4% of patients, the majority (61%) of whom had a small-bowel neuroendocrine primary tumor.[5] The most frequent site of metastatic disease was the liver (44%). Among patients with pancreatic islet cell tumors, hepatic metastasis is associated with histologic subtype. Among patients with insulinomas, hepatic metastasis occurs in about 10% of patients compared with about 40% to 95% of patients with glucagonomas or gastrinomas.

Even in the setting of metastatic disease to the liver, the natural history of neuroendocrine tumors is generally indolent as compared with metastatic adenocarcinoma. Patients with untreated metastatic disease can have 5-year survival ranging from 13% to 54%.[6,7] Patients with a significant liver tumor burden, however, are at risk of liver-related symptoms, liver failure, and potentially severe effects of hormonal oversecretion. Liver-directed therapy, such as resection, ablation, and chemoembolization, can improve both survival and control symptoms related to the metastatic disease. In fact, surgical resection of neuroendocrine liver metastasis remains the only potentially curative option for neuroendocrine liver metastases and has been associated with a 5-year survival ranging between 60% and 80%.[8–11] Other surgical options such as open radiofrequency ablation can sometimes be combined with resection to treat the entire intrahepatic tumor burden. Although still an investigational approach, liver transplantation for neuroendocrine liver metastasis has also been reported from several centers for patients with unresectable bilobar or miliary liver-only disease.

DIAGNOSIS/PREOPERATIVE CONSIDERATIONS

Neuroendocrine tumors are slow-growing neoplasms that can either present with subtle symptoms among patients with localized disease or more pronounced hormonal symptoms in the setting of metastatic disease. For carcinoid tumors, the traditional biochemical diagnosis is based on the measurement of serotonin metabolites in a 24-hour urine collection. Elevation of 5-hydroxyindoleacetic acid (HIAA) has high specificity (100%) and sensitivity (73%) in the diagnosis of carcinoid tumors.[12] Elevation of plasma chromogranin A levels has also been shown to have a high specificity (84% to 95%) and sensitivity (75% to 85%) in diagnosing carcinoid disease.[13] Pancreatic neuroendocrine tumors often are nonfunctioning, but a subset can produce hormones including insulin, glucagon, gastrin, and Vasoactive intestinal polypeptide (VIP), among others. In addition to biochemical tests, imaging studies should be obtained and these are outlined in Table 12.1. Computed tomography (CT) and magnetic resonance imaging (MRI) are the most common cross-sectional imaging studies utilized and can allow for the evaluation of extent of disease (local, liver metastasis, etc). CT and MRI have initially been reported to have only a sensitivity of 44% to 55% in the localization of carcinoid tumors; however, the advent of multidetector CT scanners now approximates 64% to 82% sensitivity.[14] Somatostatin receptor scintigraphy (Octreoscan) utilizes ^{111}In-labeled octreotide for scintigraphic localization of carcinoid tumors and has a sensitivity as high as 50% to 75% for carcinoid tumor localization.[15] Although metaiodobenzylguanidine (MIBG) scintigraphy has a low sensitivity (9% to 50%) and is not frequently utilized, it can be a useful complementary test if the octreotide scan is negative because it can identify about 10% of octreotide negative lesions.[16] Endoscopic ultrasound (EUS) may also be helpful in identifying and localizing pancreatic neuroendocrine tumors.

Table 12.1
Neuroendocrine Tumor Localization Studies

Study	Sensitivity	Notes
CT	64–82%	Improved with multidetector arterial phase imaging[14]
MRI	74–100%	T2-weighted images[14]
Octreoscan	61–96%	Lower for insulinomas[15]
MIBG	9–50%	Better for paragangliomas[16]

Neuroendocrine tumors can produce related hormones that can lead to an array of characteristic symptoms. Primary gastrointestinal carcinoid tumors release serotonin into the portal circulation that is inactivated by the liver into 5-HIAA. Hormonal production by hepatic metastasis accesses the systemic circulation directly via the hepatic veins, thereby allowing vasoactive mediators to bypass the liver degradation function. As such, patients with metastatic carcinoid to the liver can present with carcinoid syndrome, which can include cutaneous flushing, bronchoconstriction, diarrhea, and right-sided cardiac valvular disease. Patients with carcinoid syndrome should be treated preoperatively with somatostatin to decrease the risk of "carcinoid crisis" and subsequent intraoperative hemodynamic instability at the time of surgery due to tumor manipulation.[17] Pharmacologic syndromic control should not only be achieved preoperatively, but octreotide should also be available at the time of surgery for possible treatment of intraoperative symptoms attributable to carcinoid crisis such as hypotension or bronchospasm.

As noted, right-sided valvular disease is a well-reported phenomenon in patients with carcinoid syndrome. Although the mechanism is not fully understood, it is believed that serotonin initiates a fibrotic process in the heart leading most commonly to tricuspid regurgitation and pulmonary stenosis in up to 40% of patients with carcinoid syndrome.[18,19] As such, a high index of suspicion of cardiac/valvular involvement should be maintained among patients with metastatic carcinoid. A preoperative transthoracic echocardiography should be obtained to evaluate

the heart. Patients at risk for developing carcinoid heart disease should have an annual echocardiogram and evaluation by a cardiologist. Although patients with elevated 5-HIAA levels may benefit from octreotide therapy, carcinoid heart disease may progress even if 5-HIAA levels are carefully controlled.[20] Advanced valvular changes portend a poor prognosis and are the cause of death, rather than tumor progression, in up to one-third of patients.[21,22]

▌ SURGICAL CONSIDERATIONS

The goals of surgical resection for neuroendocrine tumors can either be curative or palliative, or a combination of both. In the setting of metastatic disease, patients with limited disease may benefit from complete extirpation of their disease to improve overall survival. For patients with advanced disease, most also benefit from tumor resection or debulking for symptom control and potential survival prolongation. For locoregional or limited metastatic disease, resection has been associated with improved long-term survival as outlined in Table 12.2.

One study from the Mayo Clinic retrospectively reviewed 74 patients who underwent resection of hepatic metastases from neuroendocrine tumors. Surgery involved hemi-hepatectomy (n = 36) or nonanatomic resections (n = 38) with an associated morbidity and mortality of 24% and 2.7%, respectively.[23] The 4-year survival was 73%, which was better than the 30% 5-year survival reported among patients who did not undergo resection.[6] An updated series from the same institution published in 2003 reported on 170 patients undergoing liver resection for neuroendocrine metastases, 120 of whom had carcinoid tumors.[10] In this series, 54% of patients underwent a major hepatectomy; the authors reported overall symptom control of 96% following surgery. The 5-year recurrence-free survival was 69%, whereas overall 5- and 10-year survival was 61% and 35%, respectively. The authors concluded that hepatic resection was associated with increased survival and improved quality of life when compared with untreated historic controls.

In a separate study from The University of Texas M.D. Anderson Cancer Center, patients (n = 177) undergoing hepatic resection for neuroendocrine liver metastases had a 5- and 10-year survival of 77% and 50%, respectively.[24] In a study from Australia, 74 patients underwent resection for hepatic metastasis

Table 12.2
Contemporary Series of Surgery for Neuroendocrine Liver Metastases

Study	Patient number	Curative intent (%)	Modality	Operative mortality (%)	Symptom control (%)	5-year survival (%)
Chamberlain et al. (2000)[9]	34	33	Resection	6	90	76
Sarmiento et al. (2003)[10]	170	44	Resection	1.2	96	61
Norton et al. (2003)[32]	16	100	Resection/Ablation	0	100	82
Mazzaglia et al. (2007)[29]	63		Ablation	0	92	48
Glazer et al. (2010)[24]	140		Resection/Ablation	0		77
Mayo et al. (2010)[8]	339	77	Resection/Ablation	1.5		74
Saxena et al. (2011)[25]	74	65	Resection	1		63

of neuroendocrine tumors with 38 patients undergoing synchronous cryablation.[25] Overall 5- and 10-year survival was 63% and 40%, respectively; the authors noted that histologic grade and extrahepatic disease were associated with overall survival. In the largest series reported to date, Mayo et al.[8] reported on an international, multi-institutional study of surgical management for hepatic neuroendocrine tumor metastasis, most of which were carcinoid in nature (53%). In this study, 339 patients underwent resection alone (78%), resection and ablation (19%), or ablation alone (3%).[8] Median survival was 125 months with overall 5- and 10-year survival being 74% and 51%, respectively. Although long-term survival was excellent, disease *recurrence* was almost universal (94%) at 5 years. Patients with hormonally functional neuroendocrine tumor (NET) who had an R0/R1 resection benefited the most from surgery (FIGURE 12.1). On multivariate analyses, synchronous disease, nonfunctional NET hormonal status, and extrahepatic disease remained predictive of worse survival. Of note, however, was the finding that there was no difference in the incidence of disease recurrence when comparing patients resected with negative versus positive surgical margins.

In addition to surgical resection, ablation may be utilized as a modality to treat oligo-metastatic disease in the liver either alone or in combination with hepatectomy. Ablation is generally most effective in treating smaller (<3 cm) lesions although larger lesions can be treated.[26] Laparoscopic and percutaneous approaches can allow for less invasive options, although open ablation can be combined with resection for more extensive disease. Ablation has been shown to be associated with improved survival and symptom control in several small series.[26,27] Siperstein and colleagues reported a 10-year experience with laparoscopic radiofrequency ablation (RFA) for neuroendocrine liver metastasis.[28–30] Perioperative morbidity was 5% and there were no perioperative deaths. Symptom relief was reported by 92% of patients and lasted a mean of 11 months. The authors reported a 5-year survival of 48% following initial RFA treatment. On multivariate analysis, liver tumor size was

associated with outcome because tumors greater than 3 cm were associated with a 3.3 times greater of worse long-term survival. As such, RFA may be appropriate when treating small, oligo-metastatic hepatic lesions. In another study that examined the role of ablation combined with resection, the authors noted that the use of ablation combined with resection was able to expand the number of patients eligible for complete surgical extirpation of all liver disease.[8] When complete surgical extirpation cannot be achieved, aggressive surgical debulking should generally only be undertaken when greater than 80% to 90% of the tumor can be resected or ablated because retrospective studies suggest improved symptom palliation and possible survival.[31,32]

Some centers have suggested that intra-arterial therapy (IAT) (including transarterial chemoembolization, bland transarterial embolization [TAE], drug-eluting beads, or yttrium-90) may be a better option as a primary therapy for neuroendocrine liver metastasis (NELM) compared with hepatic resection. The appeal of IAT is based on the fact that the blood supply for NELM is derived from the hepatic arteries. In a study from Memorial Sloan Kettering Cancer Center, 85 patients with neuroendocrine liver metastasis undergoing treatment with medical therapy (n = 18), hepatic artery embolization (n = 33), or hepatic resection (n = 34) were compared. The authors reported that hepatic resection was the only significant factor associated with prolonged survival on multivariate analysis.[9] Whereas 5-year survival following embolization was 50%, it was 76% among patients treated with surgical resection. Of the resected patients, however, 66% experienced disease recurrence. In a separate study by Mayo et al. that specifically investigated the role of surgical resection relative to IAT, 700 patients with NELM were examined (surgery, n = 339 vs. IAT, n = 414). The median and 5-year survival of patients treated with surgery was 123 months and 74% versus 34 months and 30% for IAT; however, the baseline clinicopathologic characteristics of the patients were vastly different. To account for these differences a propensity adjusted analysis

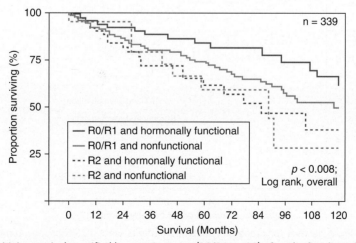

FIGURE 12.1 Kaplan–Meier survival stratified by margin status (R0/R1 vs. R2) after the first liver-directed operation and the hormonal function of the NET. Patients with hormonally functioning tumors who had R0/R1 resection had greater survival than other groups (*p* = 0.008).

Used with permission from Mayo SC, de Jong MC, Pulitano C, et al. Surgical management of hepatic neuroendocrine tumor metastasis: results from an international multi-institutional analysis. *Ann Surg Oncol* 2010;17(12):3129–3136.

model was utilized.[33] In the propensity-adjusted multivariate Cox model, asymptomatic disease was strongly associated with worse outcome. Although surgical management provided a survival benefit over IAT among symptomatic patients with greater than 25% hepatic tumor involvement, there was no difference in long-term outcome after surgery versus IAT among asymptomatic patients (FIGURE 12.2). Therefore, the authors concluded that asymptomatic patients with a large (>25%) burden of liver disease benefited least from surgical management and IAT may be a more appropriate treatment strategy. In general, surgical management of NELM should be reserved for patients with low-volume disease or for those patients with symptomatic high-volume disease.

Treatment of hepatic metastasis in the setting of a pancreaticoduodenectomy can represent a particular therapeutic challenge. Simultaneous presentation of hepatic metastasis and a pancreatic primary tumor has been reported to occur between 16% and 51% of the time.[8,34] Although resection or IAT may be warranted in this subset of patients, pancreaticoduodenectomy can complicate their treatment. Liver-directed therapy—resection, ablation, or IAT—can be associated with a higher incidence of liver-related complications such as hepatic abscess. The risk of abscess following liver-directed therapy in the setting of a pancreaticoduodenectomy is presumably caused by the biliary colonization after hepaticojejunostomy reconstruction.[35] In a dual center study of patients undergoing staged or simultaneous pancreaticoduodenectomy in association with liver-directed therapy, De Jong and colleagues[35] reported a significantly higher rate of hepatic abscess formation for staged procedures (pancreatectomy, then liver) when compared to simultaneous procedures. Therefore, the authors recommended that, in general, patients presenting with synchronous neuroendocrine disease in the pancreatic head and liver should be addressed either with a simultaneous resection or staged operation, with the liver operation preceding the pancreaticoduodenectomy. For patients with a previous pancreaticoduodenectomy who present with metachronous disease, ablation or IAT should generally be avoided because of the risk of abscess or it should be undertaken with caution.

Because the number of eligible patients for complete or greater than 80% to 90% debulking is low,[36,37] some investigators have suggested orthotopic liver transplantation as a potentially curative approach to bilateral unresectable liver metastasis. Although early single center reports suggested that patients receiving liver allografts for neuroendocrine liver metastasis had better outcomes when compared to other primary and secondary hepatic malignancies, allograft scarcity, impact of immunosuppression, and risk of recurrence have tempered enthusiasm for this therapeutic approach.[38–41] A retrospective multicenter French review of 31 cases of liver transplantation for neuroendocrine liver metastasis noted a 3- and 5-year overall survival to be 47% and 36%, respectively.[42] Carcinoid histology seemed to portend a better prognosis with a 5-year survival of 69%. In a separate study, Lehnert et al.[43] performed a systematic review of the published literature on liver transplantation for metastatic neuroendocrine carcinoma in 1998. Lehnert et al. identified 103 patients and noted a 2- and 5-year overall survival of 60% and 47%, respectively. Of note, however, was that 5-year disease-free was only 24%. In addition, extended operations, where transplantation was coupled with upper abdominal exenteration or pancreaticoduodenectomy, were associated with particularly poor outcomes. Taken together, neuroendocrine metastasis remains a limited indication for transplantation and is only performed at a limited number of centers.

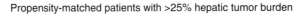
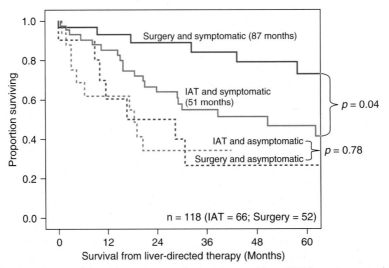

FIGURE 12.2 Kaplan-Meier survival for propensity matched patients with >25% hepatic tumor burden undergoing either intra-arterial therapy (IAT) or hepatic resection of neuroendocrine liver metastasis (NELM). Patients with high-volume symptomatic disease benefited the most from surgical management (median survival: surgery, 87 months vs. IAT, 51 months; $p = 0.04$).

Used with permission Mayo SC, de Jong MC, Bloomston M, et al. Surgery versus intra-arterial therapy for neuroendocrine liver metastasis: a multicenter international analysis. *Ann Surg Oncol* 2011.

MEDICAL MANAGEMENT

The mainstay of therapy for neuroendocrine tumors remains surgical resection and debulking in applicable cases. As noted, this has been augmented in recent years by other locoregional therapy options, including RFA, transarterial chemoembolization and radioembolization. To date, there is no evidence for additional benefit from systemic chemotherapy in the adjuvant setting, outside of select tumor types.[44]

Neuroendocrine tumors have traditionally exhibited very poor responses to conventional chemotherapy. One caveat to this mantra involves those tumors within the neuroendocrine spectrum that have a high proliferative index (Ki67 >20%) reflecting an aggressive tumor biology akin to that seen with small-cell cancers[45]; in such cases, cytotoxic chemotherapy is indicated as the primary mode of treatment because widespread metastases are common and local therapies typically do not impact the course of disease. Cisplatin-based doublet chemotherapy provides the best response rates, although the prognosis is typically grave. In general, carcinoid tumors appear to be particularly resistant to cytotoxic agents, with pancreatic NET occasionally evidencing encouraging results in early phase studies. Agents with some activity include streptozocin, doxorubicin, 5-fluorouracil, cisplatin, dacarbazine, and temozolomide.[46] Streptozocin, sanctioned for use in patients with advanced neuroendocrine tumors by the Food and Drug Administration (FDA) in 1982, is currently the only approved cytotoxic drug for the treatment of these neoplasms. It is an alkylating agent and has proven efficacy as a single agent or in combinations with 5-fluorouracil or doxorubicin or cisplatin.[47] The radiographic response rates in these studies are typically low, however (<20%), and the toxicity profile of this drug, or these combinations, is significant. More modern series have sought to further define the appropriate cytotoxic choice in advanced carcinoid tumors; in the largest such study, 249 patients were randomized to receive doxorubicin/5-fluorouracil, streptozocin/5-fluorouracil or streptozocin/dacarbazine.[48] Response rates were similar across treatment arms, about 15%, although overall survival appeared to favor the streptozocin/5-fluorouracil combination at 24.3 months. There was, however, significant renal toxicity noted in those patients receiving streptozocin. Although somewhat better response rates have been documented in small series of pancreatic NET,[49] this toxicity has certainly limited its

use in recent years, especially with the advent of newer cytotoxic agents.

Temozolomide is an orally bioavailable, alkylating agent, that shares an active metabolite with dacarbazine. Early, single-agent studies in patients with NET revealed response rates between 10% and 20%[50] with this agent and a considerably less toxic side effect profile. Recent studies have investigated combination therapy with other cytotoxic drugs and newer targeted agents. Some encouraging response rates and survival data have been generated by various combinations including temozolomide and bevacizumab, temozolomide and capecitabine, and temozolomide and thalidomide[51] as outlined in Table 12.3. Many practitioners would now consider this drug as the backbone of systemic chemotherapy options for advanced cases of neuroendocrine tumors. As outlined in most professional guidelines,[52] however, cytotoxic therapy should only be contemplated in these cases after other therapeutic avenues have been exhausted, especially with the advent of the targeted therapies.

Somatostatin analogs are widely used to control symptoms in patients with low-to-intermediate-grade NET, including carcinoid tumors. These agents act by binding to one of five somatostatin receptors, which tend to be overexpressed in most gastroenteropancreatic NET, and minimize hormone release. Numerous early phase studies of these agents have demonstrated some disease stabilization in patients with NET[53] with proposed mechanisms consisting of direct inhibition of proliferative pathways, including the MAP-kinase pathway, and indirect antitumor actions via inhibition of release of growth factors and hormones known to promote tumor growth, such as insulin-like growth factor 1 (IGF-1). These preclinical and early phase trial data prompted the development of a phase III study in Germany, known as the PROMID study (Placebo-controlled Prospective Randomized Study on the Antiproliferative Efficacy of Octreotide LAR in Patients with Metastatic Neuroendocrine Midgut Tumors).[54] In this trial 85 treatment-naïve patients with well-differentiated (Ki67 <2%) metastatic midgut NET and good performance status (KPS >60) were randomly assigned to either placebo or octreotide LAR (a depot form of this somatostatin analog) 30 mg intramuscular injection every month until tumor progression. Primary endpoint was time to progression (TTP), and secondary endpoints included survival time and tumor response; both functional and nonfunctional tumors were included. At the planned interim analysis,

Table 12.3

Phase II and III Trials of Cytotoxic Chemotherapy in Neuroendocrine Tumors

Regimen	Tumor type	Patients number	Response rate (%)	Median PFS	Median OS	Reference	Prospective
Streptozocin + 5-Fluorouracil	PNET	33	45	14 mo	16.8 mo	49	Y
Streptozocin + Doxorubicin	PNET	36	69	18 mo	26.4 mo	49	Y
Temozolomide + Capecitabine	PNET	30	70	18 mo	NA	64	N
Temozolomide + other agents	PNET	53	34	13.6 mo	35.3 mo	65	N
Streptozocin + 5-Fluorouracil	Carcinoid	249	16	NR	24.3 mo	48	Y
Doxorubicin + 5-Fluorouracil	Carcinoid	249	15.9	NR	15.7 mo	48	Y

PNET, pancreatic neuroendocrine tumor.

TTP in the octreotide LAR group was 14.3 months compared with 6 months in the placebo group (HR 0.34 (0.20–0.59); *p* = 0.000072), and the stable disease rate was 66.7% in the octreotide LAR group versus 37.2% in the placebo group after 6 months of treatment. Results were similar in patients with functional and nonfunctional tumors, and enrollment was stopped at this time. Because crossover to octreotide LAR was allowed at progression and the overall number of deaths was very low at the time of the interim analysis, survival data could not be assessed. The study did conclude, however, that octreotide LAR significantly lengthened median TTP compared with placebo in patients with well-differentiated metastatic midgut NET. Overall, treatment with octreotide LAR has proven successful in the control of symptoms of hormonal excess in functional NET, including carcinoid, and appears beneficial in inhibiting the proliferation of these tumors, whether functional or not. Novel somatostatin analogs have been developed and have exhibited at least comparable efficacy to octreotide in controlling symptoms of hormone excess. Lanreotide can be administered subcutaneously in the depot form[55] as opposed to the IM injection required for octreotide, whereas pasireotide has a markedly greater binding affinity to three of the five somatostatin receptors,[56] and early data suggest that it can achieve symptom control even in patients with inadequate control on octreotide LAR. It remains to be seen whether these encouraging data regarding symptom management will translate into disease control in future studies.

Interferon alpha can augment the efficacy of somatostatin analogs in controlling carcinoid syndrome symptoms, and a small number of trials documented biochemical and occasional radiographic responses in metastatic NET with this drug as a single agent.[57] Its unfavorable side effect profile has prevented the widespread adoption of interferon alpha in this patient population, and its future is likely limited, given the current focus on targeted therapy.

As noted above, the elucidation of various molecular pathways important to the proliferation of neuroendocrine tumors led to the investigation of targeted agents in this disease. Activation of the mammalian target of rapamycin (mTOR) signaling pathway, thought to be mediated through IGF-1, was proposed as one such pathway, and preclinical data suggested that inhibition of mTOR has a significant antiproliferative effect in pancreatic neuroendocrine cell lines.[58] Early phase clinical trials confirmed this hypothesis, and a prospective, randomized, placebo-controlled phase III trial was undertaken: the RAD001 in Advanced Neuroendocrine Tumors, third trial (RADIANT-3).[59] This study enrolled 410 patients with advanced, low-to-intermediate-grade pancreatic neuroendocrine tumors, who had evidence of radiographic progression within the previous 12 months. Patients were randomly assigned to everolimus (RAD001) 10 mg daily or placebo, and the primary endpoint was progression-free survival (PFS). Similar to PROMID, there was crossover allowed from the placebo group in the event of radiographic progression on study. Median PFS was 11 months in the everolimus group and 4.6 months in the placebo group (HR 0.35 (0.27–0.45); *p* < 0.001). These results led to the approval of everolimus for the first-line treatment of progressive pancreatic NET.

An important driver of angiogenesis in pancreatic neuroendocrine tumors is vascular endothelial growth factor (VEGF), acting through various cell surface receptors, many of which are expressed in these malignant cells. Sunitinib is a small molecule inhibitor of a number of these receptors, including VEGFR-2, VEGFR-3, and PDGFR-alpha and -beta. Early phase trials once again showed evidence of antitumor activity with sunitinib, leading to a randomized, double-blind, placebo-controlled phase III trial[60] in a similar patient population to that described above—advanced, well-differentiated pancreatic neuroendocrine tumors with evidence of disease progression within the previous 12 months. These 154 patients received either sunitinib 37.5 mg daily or placebo, and the primary endpoint was PFS. Secondary endpoints included overall survival, objective response rate, time to tumor response, and safety. Due to a higher number of deaths and serious adverse events in the placebo group, and a PFS difference favoring sunitinib, the trial was closed before planned enrollment was complete. Median PFS was 11.4 months in the sunitinib group, compared with 5.5 months in the placebo group (HR 0.42 (0.26–0.66); *p* < 0.001). The probability of PFS at 6 months in the sunitinib group was 71.3% versus 43.2% in the placebo arm. Sunitinib has also been approved for the treatment of progressive pancreatic NET and is typically used in sequence with everolimus. Numerous other agents targeting the VEGF pathway have undergone early phase trials in patients with NET, including bevacizumab,[61] sorafenib,[62] and pazopanib,[63] although response rates have been low in these small series and more work is clearly needed to identify the appropriate treatment population for these therapies.

Neither of the targeted therapy phase III trials noted above included patients with carcinoid tumors because, once again, carcinoid tumors had exhibited lower response rates in the early phase studies (Table 12.4). Those studies did document some activity in such tumors, however, and further elucidation of the relevant pathways will likely define the role of targeted therapy in this disease. As of now, most professional guidelines do not advocate for the use of these targeted therapies in patients with advanced carcinoid tumors but would still consider cytotoxic chemotherapy in suitable patients if no other local or regional approaches are available despite the low likelihood of radiographic or biochemical response.[52]

CONCLUSION

Gastrointestinal neuroendocrine tumors are rare neoplasms that can be broadly subdivided into carcinoid and pancreatic islet cell tumors. Even in the setting of metastatic disease to the liver, the natural history of neuroendocrine tumors is generally indolent as compared with metastatic adenocarcinoma. Preoperative workup should include relevant laboratory exams, cross-sectional imaging, as well as possible octreotide scan and/or EUS. In the setting of metastatic disease, some patients with limited disease may benefit from surgery to completely extirpate/debulk their disease. Surgery is associated with a long-term survival, but recurrence is near universal. IAT is another reasonable option for patients with extensive metastatic neuroendocrine disease to the liver. Data suggest that asymptomatic patients with a large (<25%) burden of liver disease benefited least from surgical management and IAT may be a more appropriate treatment strategy. In general, surgical management of NELM should be reserved for patients with low-volume disease or for those patients with symptomatic high-volume disease. New emerging targeted therapy for advanced neuroendocrine tumors includes octreotide analogs for carcinoid tumors and

Table 12.4

Selected Data Showing Response Rates and Median Time-to-Progression/Progression-Free Survival of Various Systemic Agents

Agent	Target/phase	Patients number	Tumor type	Response rate (%)	Median TTP/PFS	Reference
Everolimus + Octreotide LAR	mTOR, Ph II	30	Carcinoid	17	63 wk	66
		30	PNET	27	50 wk	
Everolimus (post chemotherapy)	mTOR, Ph II	115	PNET	9	9.7 mo	67
Temsirolimus	mTOR, Ph II	21	Carcinoid	5	6 mo	68
		15	PNET	7	10.6 mo	
Everolimus	mTOR, Ph III	410	PNET	NA	11 mo	59
Sunitinib	VEGFR-1, -2, -3; PDGFR-α, -β; KIT; RET, Ph II	41	Carcinoid	2	10.2 mo	69
		61	PNET	13	7.7 mo	
Sunitinib	VEGFR-1, -2, -3; PDGFR-α, -β; KIT; RET, Ph III	171	PNET	9.3%	11.4 mo	60
Sorafenib	VEGFR, PDGFR, BRAF, Ph II	50	Carcinoid	7	7.8 mo	62
		43	PNET	11	11.9 mo	
Pazopanib	VEGFR-1,-2,-3; PDGFR-α, -β; KIT, Ph II	22	Carcinoid	0	12.7 mo	63
		29	PNET	17	11.7 mo	

VEGFR, vascular endothelial growth factor receptor; PDGFR, platelet-derived growth factor receptor; KIT, kinase receptor; RET; BRAF.

everolimus as well as sunitinib for pancreatic neuroendocrine tumors. Patients with metastatic neuroendocrine tumors, therefore, benefit from a multidisciplinary approach that involves surgeons, interventional radiologists, medical oncologist, as well as endocrinologists.

REFERENCES

1. Lawrence B, Gustafsson BI, Chan A, et al. The epidemiology of gastroenteropancreatic neuroendocrine tumors. *Endocrinol Metab Clin North Am* 2011;40(1):1–18, vii.
2. Vosburgh E. Tumors of the diffuse neuroendocrine and gastroenteropancreatic endocrine system. *Cancer Medicine*. Beijing, P.R. China: People's Medical Publishing House - USA; 2010:940–958.
3. Modlin IM, Lye KD, Kidd M. A 5-decade analysis of 13,715 carcinoid tumors. *Cancer* 2003;97(4):934–959.
4. Kimura W, Kuroda A, Morioka Y. Clinical pathology of endocrine tumors of the pancreas. Analysis of autopsy cases. *Dig Dis Sci* 1991;36(7): 933–942.
5. Berge T, Linell F. Carcinoid tumours. Frequency in a defined population during a 12-year period. *Acta Pathol Microbiol Scand [A]* 1976;84(4):322–330.
6. Moertel CG. Karnofsky memorial lecture. An odyssey in the land of small tumors. *J Clin Oncol* 1987;5(10):1502–1522.
7. Thompson GB, van Heerden JA, Grant CS, et al. Islet cell carcinomas of the pancreas: a twenty-year experience. *Surgery* 1988;104(6):1011–1017.
8. Mayo SC, de Jong MC, Pulitano C, et al. Surgical management of hepatic neuroendocrine tumor metastasis: results from an international multi-institutional analysis. *Ann Surg Oncol* 2010;17(12):3129–3136.
9. Chamberlain RS, Canes D, Brown KT, et al. Hepatic neuroendocrine metastases: does intervention alter outcomes? *J Am Coll Surg* 2000;190(4):432–445.
10. Sarmiento JM, Heywood G, Rubin J, et al. Surgical treatment of neuroendocrine metastases to the liver: a plea for resection to increase survival. *J Am Coll Surg* 2003;197(1):29–37.
11. Touzios JG, Kiely JM, Pitt SC, et al. Neuroendocrine hepatic metastases: does aggressive management improve survival? *Ann Surg* 2005;241(5): 776–783; discussion 783–785.
12. Feldman JM, O'Dorisio TM. Role of neuropeptides and serotonin in the diagnosis of carcinoid tumors. *Am J Med* 22 1986;81(6B):41–48.
13. Campana D, Nori F, Piscitelli L, et al. Chromogranin A: is it a useful marker of neuroendocrine tumors? *J Clin Oncol* 2007;25(15):1967–1973.
14. Tamm EP, Kim EE, Ng CS. Imaging of neuroendocrine tumors. *Hematol Oncol Clin North Am* 2007;21(3):409–432; vii.
15. Ramage JK, Davies AH, Ardill J, et al. Guidelines for the management of gastroenteropancreatic neuroendocrine (including carcinoid) tumours. *Gut* 2005;54(suppl 4):iv, 1–16.

16. Kaltsas G, Korbonits M, Heintz E, et al. Comparison of somatostatin analog and meta-iodobenzylguanidine radionuclides in the diagnosis and localization of advanced neuroendocrine tumors. *J Clin Endocrinol Metab* 2001;86(2):895–902.

17. Kinney MA, Warner ME, Nagorney DM, et al. Perianaesthetic risks and outcomes of abdominal surgery for metastatic carcinoid tumours. *Br J Anaesth* 2001;87(3):447–452.

18. Gustafsson BI, Hauso O, Drozdov I, et al. Carcinoid heart disease. *Int J Cardiol* 2008;129(3):318–324.

19. Dero I, De Pauw M, Borbath I, et al. Carcinoid heart disease—a hidden complication of neuroendocrine tumours. *Acta Gastroenterol Belg* 2009;72(1):34–38.

20. Moller JE, Connolly HM, Rubin J, et al. Factors associated with progression of carcinoid heart disease. *N Engl J Med* 2003;348(11):1005–1015.

21. Westberg G, Wangberg B, Ahlman H, et al. Prediction of prognosis by echocardiography in patients with midgut carcinoid syndrome. *Br J Surg* 2001;88(6):865–872.

22. Oberg K. Neuroendocrine gastrointestinal tumors—a condensed overview of diagnosis and treatment. *Ann Oncol* 1999;10(suppl 2):S3–8.

23. Que FG, Nagorney DM, Batts KP, et al. Hepatic resection for metastatic neuroendocrine carcinomas. *Am J Surg* 1995;169(1):36–42; discussion 42–43.

24. Glazer ES, Tseng JF, Al-Refaie W, et al. Long-term survival after surgical management of neuroendocrine hepatic metastases. *HPB* 2010;12(6):427–433.

25. Saxena A, Chua TC, Sarkar A, et al. Progression and survival results after radical hepatic metastasectomy of indolent advanced neuroendocrine neoplasms (NENs) supports an aggressive surgical approach. *Surgery* 2011;149(2):209–220.

26. Berber E, Siperstein A. Local recurrence after laparoscopic radiofrequency ablation of liver tumors: an analysis of 1032 tumors. *Ann Surg Oncol* 2008;15(10):2757–2764.

27. Eriksson J, Stalberg P, Nilsson A, et al. Surgery and radiofrequency ablation for treatment of liver metastases from midgut and foregut carcinoids and endocrine pancreatic tumors. *World J Surg* 2008;32(5):930–938.

28. Akyildiz HY, Mitchell J, Milas M, et al. Laparoscopic radiofrequency thermal ablation of neuroendocrine hepatic metastases: long-term follow-up. *Surgery* 2010;148(6):1288–1293; discussion 1293.

29. Mazzaglia PJ, Berber E, Milas M, et al. Laparoscopic radiofrequency ablation of neuroendocrine liver metastases: a 10-year experience evaluating predictors of survival. *Surgery* 2007;142(1):10–19.

30. Mazzaglia PJ, Berber E, Siperstein AE. Radiofrequency thermal ablation of metastatic neuroendocrine tumors in the liver. *Curr Treat Options Oncol* 2007;8(4):322–330.

31. McEntee GP, Nagorney DM, Kvols LK, et al. Cytoreductive hepatic surgery for neuroendocrine tumors. *Surgery* 1990;108(6):1091–1096.

32. Norton JA, Warren RS, Kelly MG, et al. Aggressive surgery for metastatic liver neuroendocrine tumors. *Surgery* 2003;134(6):1057–1063; discussion 1063–1065.

33. Mayo SC, de Jong MC, Bloomston M, et al. Surgery versus intra-arterial therapy for neuroendocrine liver metastasis: a multicenter international analysis. *Ann Surg Oncol* 2011.

34. Elias D, Lasser P, Ducreux M, et al. Liver resection (and associated extrahepatic resections) for metastatic well-differentiated endocrine tumors: a 15-year single center prospective study. *Surgery* 2003;133(4):375–382.

35. De Jong MC, Farnell MB, Sclabas G, et al. Liver-directed therapy for hepatic metastases in patients undergoing pancreaticoduodenectomy: a dual-center analysis. *Ann Surg* 2010;252(1):142–148.

36. Carty SE, Jensen RT, Norton JA. Prospective study of aggressive resection of metastatic pancreatic endocrine tumors. *Surgery* 1992;112(6):1024–1031; discussion 1031–1032.

37. Ihse I, Persson B, Tibblin S. Neuroendocrine metastases of the liver. *World J Surg* 1995;19(1):76–82.

38. Arnold JC, O'Grady JG, Bird GL, et al. Liver transplantation for primary and secondary hepatic apudomas. *Br J Surg* 1989;76(3):248–249.

39. Dousset B, Saint-Marc O, Pitre J, et al. Metastatic endocrine tumors: medical treatment, surgical resection, or liver transplantation. *World J Surg* 1996;20(7):908–914; discussion 914–915.

40. Lang H, Oldhafer KJ, Weimann A, et al. Liver transplantation for metastatic neuroendocrine tumors. *Ann Surg* 1997;225(4):347–354.

41. Makowka L, Tzakis AG, Mazzaferro V, et al. Transplantation of the liver for metastatic endocrine tumors of the intestine and pancreas. *Surg Gynecol Obstet* 1989;168(2):107–111.

42. Le Treut YP, Delpero JR, Dousset B, et al. Results of liver transplantation in the treatment of metastatic neuroendocrine tumors. A 31-case French multicentric report. *Ann Surg* 1997;225(4):355–364.

43. Lehnert T. Liver transplantation for metastatic neuroendocrine carcinoma: an analysis of 103 patients. *Transplantation* 1998;66(10):1307–1312.

44. Iyoda A, Hiroshima K, Moriya Y, et al. Prospective study of adjuvant chemotherapy for pulmonary large cell neuroendocrine carcinoma. *Ann Thorac Surg* 2006;82(5):1802–1807.

45. Strosberg JR, Coppola D, Klimstra DS, et al. The NANETS consensus guidelines for the diagnosis and management of poorly differentiated (high-grade) extrapulmonary neuroendocrine carcinomas. *Pancreas* 2010;39(6):799–800.

46. Chan JA, Kulke MH. New treatment options for patients with advanced neuroendocrine tumors. *Curr Treat Options Oncol* 2011;12(2):136–148.

47. Moertel CG, Hanley JA. Combination chemotherapy trials in metastatic carcinoid tumor and the malignant carcinoid syndrome. *Cancer Clin Trials* 1979;2(4):327–334.

48. Sun W, Lipsitz S, Catalano P, et al. Phase II/III study of doxorubicin with fluorouracil compared with streptozocin with fluorouracil or dacarbazine in the treatment of advanced carcinoid tumors: Eastern Cooperative Oncology Group Study E1281. *J Clin Oncol* 2005;23(22):4897–4904.

49. Moertel CG, Lefkopoulo M, Lipsitz S, et al. Streptozocin-doxorubicin, streptozocin-fluorouracil or chlorozotocin in the treatment of advanced islet-cell carcinoma. *N Engl J Med* 1992;326(8):519–523.

50. Ekeblad S, Sundin A, Janson ET, et al. Temozolomide as monotherapy is effective in treatment of advanced malignant neuroendocrine tumors. *Clin Cancer Res* 2007;13(10):2986–2991.

51. Kulke MH, Stuart K, Enzinger PC, et al. Phase II study of temozolomide and thalidomide in patients with metastatic neuroendocrine tumors. *J Clin Oncol* 2006;24(3):401–406.

52. Clark OH, Benson AB, 3rd, Berlin JD, et al. NCCN clinical practice guidelines in oncology: neuroendocrine tumors. *J Natl Compr Canc Netw* 2009;7(7):712–747.

53. Arnold R, Trautmann ME, Creutzfeldt W, et al. Somatostatin analogue octreotide and inhibition of tumour growth in metastatic endocrine gastroenteropancreatic tumours. *Gut* 1996;38(3):430–438.

54. Rinke A, Muller HH, Schade-Brittinger C, et al. Placebo-controlled, double-blind, prospective, randomized study on the effect of octreotide LAR in the control of tumor growth in patients with metastatic neuroendocrine midgut tumors: a report from the PROMID Study Group. *J Clin Oncol* 2009;27(28):4656–4663.

55. O'Toole D, Ducreux M, Bommelaer G, et al. Treatment of carcinoid syndrome: a prospective crossover evaluation of lanreotide versus octreotide in terms of efficacy, patient acceptability, and tolerance. *Cancer* 2000;88(4):770–776.

56. Poll F, Lehmann D, Illing S, et al. Pasireotide and octreotide stimulate distinct patterns of sst2A somatostatin receptor phosphorylation. *Mol Endocrinol* 2010;24(2):436–446.

57. Oberg K, Eriksson B. The role of interferons in the management of carcinoid tumors. *Acta Oncol* 1991;30(4):519–522.

58. Couderc C, Poncet G, Villaume K, et al. Targeting the PI3K/mTOR pathway in murine endocrine cell lines: in vitro and in vivo effects on tumor cell growth. *Am J Pathol* 2011;178(1):336–344.

59. Yao JC, Shah MH, Ito T, et al. Everolimus for advanced pancreatic neuroendocrine tumors. *N Engl J Med* 2011;364(6):514–523.

60. Raymond E, Dahan L, Raoul JL, et al. Sunitinib malate for the treatment of pancreatic neuroendocrine tumors. *N Engl J Med* 2011;364(6):501–513.

61. Yao JC, Phan A, Hoff PM, et al. Targeting vascular endothelial growth factor in advanced carcinoid tumor: a random assignment phase II study of depot octreotide with bevacizumab and pegylated interferon alpha-2b. *J Clin Oncol* 2008;26(8):1316–1323.

62. Hobday TJ. MC044h, a phase II trial of sorafenib in patients with metastatic neuroendocrine tumors (NET): a phase II consortium (P2C) study. *J Clin Oncol* 2007;25(18S).

63. Phan A. A prospective, multi-institutional phase II study of GW786034 (pazopanib) and depot octreotide (sandostatin LAR) in advanced low grade neuroendocrine carcinoma (LGNEC). *J Clin Oncol* 2010;28(15S).

64. Strosberg JR, Fine RL, Choi J, et al. First-line chemotherapy with capecitabine and temozolomide in patients with metastatic pancreatic endocrine carcinomas. *Cancer* 2011;117(2):268–275.

65. Kulke MH, Hornick JL, Frauenhoffer C, et al. O6-methylguanine DNA methyltransferase deficiency and response to temozolomide-based therapy in patients with neuroendocrine tumors. *Clin Cancer Res* 2009;15(1):338–345.

66. Yao JC, Phan AT, Chang DZ, et al. Efficacy of RAD001 (everolimus) and octreotide LAR in advanced low- to intermediate-grade neuroendocrine tumors: results of a phase II study. *J Clin Oncol* 2008;26(26):4311–4318.

67. Yao JC, Lombard-Bohas C, Baudin E, et al. Daily oral everolimus activity in patients with metastatic pancreatic neuroendocrine tumors after failure of cytotoxic chemotherapy: a phase II trial. *J Clin Oncol* 2010;28(1):69–76.

68. Duran I, Kortmansky J, Singh D, et al. A phase II clinical and pharmacodynamic study of temsirolimus in advanced neuroendocrine carcinomas. *Br J Cancer* 2006;95(9):1148–1154.

69. Kulke MH, Lenz HJ, Meropol NJ, et al. Activity of sunitinib in patients with advanced neuroendocrine tumors. *J Clin Oncol* 2008;26(20):3403–3410.

Interventional Oncology in the Management of Neuroendocrine Tumor Metastases

TERENCE P. GADE and MICHAEL C. SOULEN

▌ INTRODUCTION

Once considered an exceedingly rare malignancy, the incidence and prevalence of neuroendocrine tumors (NETs) have increased rapidly, with a more than fivefold increase in incidence in the United States from 1973 to 2004 and a prevalence that is two to five times that of esophageal cancer, gastric cancer, pancreatic cancer, and hepatobiliary cancer (FIGURE 13.1).[1] This increasing prevalence has revealed the heterogeneity and complexities of neuroendocrine disease, spurred the development of new diagnostic tools (somatostatin receptor scintigraphy), and therapeutic options (somatostatin analogs, radioactive labeled octreotide, transarterial therapy, thermal ablation, and oral antiproliferative agents). A multidisciplinary approach involving oncology, gastroenterology, endocrinology, and surgery has resulted in improved outcomes.[2]

The typically long delay in diagnosis of NETs and their propensity for hepatic metastases create an important role for liver-directed therapies. Challenged by the shortage of physicians experienced in the diagnosis and management of this disease, these long-lived patients often access strong advocacy groups and web-based support sites that direct them to centers of excellence with physicians who offer a complete understanding of the spectrum of their disease. It is essential that interventional oncologists develop an intimate knowledge of the characteristics and management of NETs to know how and when best to apply the armamentarium of image-guided locoregional therapies and guide patients in integrating these with surgical, systemic, and supportive therapies.

▌ DEFINING NEUROENDOCRINE DISEASE

Terminology

Comprising a spectrum of epithelial neoplasms that originate from cells that synthesize peptide hormones released in response to a neuronal stimulus, neuroendocrine neoplasms may develop sporadically or as part of familial syndromes including multiple endocrine neoplasia, von Hippel-Lindau syndrome, and neurofibromatosis.[3] Neuroendocrine neoplasms were first reported by the German pathologist Siegfried Orbendorfer who described an unusual tumor growing within the small intestines that demonstrated benign growth characteristics. Given this benign behavior, Orbendorfer dubbed these tumors carcinoid or "carcinoma-like." The subsequent 100 years of experience with NETs have demonstrated that these neoplasms most often originate from the foregut gastroenteric, pancreatic, and pulmonary tissues but may arise from any organ given the widespread distribution of neuroendocrine cells within the body. They are not always benign with the potential to develop an invasive phenotype and metastasize.

The heterogeneity in origin and potential for malignancy of NETs has led to a heterogeneous nomenclature that can often be misleading because the applied terminology may imply prognosis and affect treatment decisions. Although several groups have examined the issue of classification of neuroendocrine neoplasms, none of these described systems has gained universal acceptance. The recently published World Health Organization (WHO) Classification of Tumors of the Digestive System of 2010 has addressed this issue with respect to the gastroenteropancreatic NETs (FIGURE 13.2).[4,5] This classification focuses on the major criteria determining malignant potential, including tumor histopathology or differentiation, grade, site, size, and stage, with the premise that all neuroendocrine neoplasms have malignant potential. Tumor differentiation describes the extent to which the neoplasm resembles its nonneoplastic counterpart. Tumor grade is based on proliferative activity, as determined by the number of mitoses per unit area of tumor (mitoses per 10 high-power microscopic fields or per 2 mm^2) or by the proliferative index (the percentage of cells immunolabeling for Ki-67). Grade 1 and grade 2 imply well-differentiated histopathology based on the proliferative index, with the term *carcinoma* restricted to NEC (neuroendocrine carcinoma) grade 3, which includes high-grade, poorly differentiated large-cell or small-cell neuroendocrine carcinomas.[4] The WHO classification system replaces previous terminology,

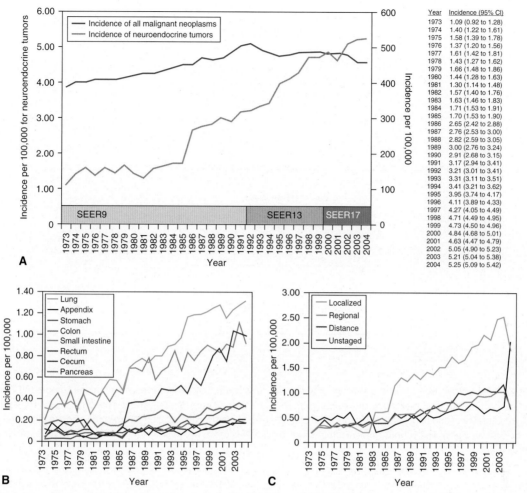

FIGURE 13.1 These graphs show the incidence of neuroendocrine tumors (NETs) over time by site and by disease stage. **A.** Annual age-adjusted incidence of NETs by year (1973 to 2004). The incidence is presented as the number of tumors per 100,000 (with 95% CIs) age adjusted for the 2000 U.S. standard population. Cases were selected from the Surveillance, Epidemiology, and End Results database (1973 to 2004) using International Classification of Diseases for Oncology histology codes 8150 to 8157, 8240 to 8246, and 8249. **B.** Time-trend analyses of the incidence of NETs by primary tumor site (1973 to 2004). Statistically significant increases in incidence at all sites are shown (P < .001). **C.** The incidence of NETs by disease stage at diagnosis. Statistically significant increases in incidence at all stages are shown (P < .001).

Yao et al. *J Clin Oncol* 2008;26:3063–3072.

including carcinoid and apudoma, as well as descriptions of embryonic origin.[6]

Demographics and Epidemiology

Analyses of NETs in the United States over the past 40 years within the Surveillance, Epidemiology and End Results (SEER) database of the National Cancer Institute provide a more complete index of the associated epidemiology.[1,7] These data reveal a significant increase in the age-adjusted incidence of NETs in the United States from 1.09 per 100,000 in 1973 to 5.25 per 100,000 in 2004.[1] Despite the relatively low incidence of NETs, they have a relatively high 29-year limited-duration prevalence estimated to be 103,312 cases or 35 per 100,000 as of January 1, 2004,[1] surpassing esophageal (28,644), gastric (65,836), pancreatic (32,353), and hepatobiliary cancer (21,427), underscoring the

indolent course of neuroendocrine neoplasms relative to other epithelial malignancies.[8]

The demographic distribution of neuroendocrine neoplasms demonstrates a slight female predominance, 52% to 55%, including neoplasms of gastric, colonic, appendiceal, bronchopulmonary, and gallbladder origin.[1,7] The population adjusted incidence reveals an overrepresentation of rectal and duodenal neuroendocrine neoplasms among African American patients.[7] The median and mean age at diagnosis have remained stable over the past 30 years at 63 and 62 years, respectively, with appendiceal and rectal neuroendocrine neoplasms having the youngest ages at diagnosis.[1] In their analysis of the most recent SEER registry encompassing data from 2000 to 2004, Yao et al. report that the gastrointestinal tract remains the primary site of origin of NETs, comprising 50.6% of all NETs with the jejunum/ileum (13.4%) and colon (17.2%) representing the

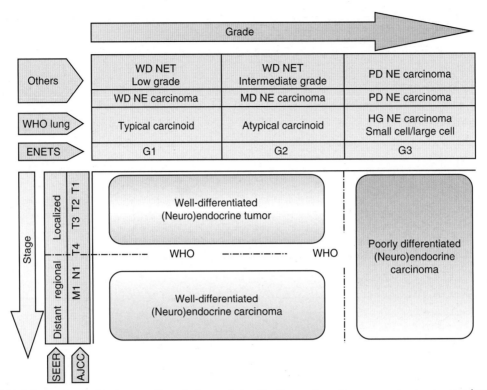

FIGURE 13.2 Comparison of various grading, staging, and classification systems for neuroendocrine tumors (NETs). The grading systems are displayed along the x-axis (top) and the staging systems along the y-axis (left). The WHO systems for gastrointestinal and pancreatic NETs include a combination of grading and staging information and are displayed with the box (lower right). The various nomenclature of each system is used. The overlaps between the different systems are approximate.

AJCC, American Joint Committee on Cancer; ENETS, European Neuroendocrine Tumors Society; HG, high grade; MD, moderately differentiated; NE, neuroendocrine; NET, neuroendocrine tumor; PD, poorly differentiated; SEER, Surveillance, Epidemiology, and End Results Program of the National Cancer Institute; WD, well differentiated; WHO, World Health Organization.

Klimstra et al. *Am J Surg Path* 2010;34:300–313.

most common sites of small- and large-bowel disease, respectively. Tracheobronchopulmonary neuroendocrine neoplasms represent the majority of extragastrointestinal disease, comprising 27% of all neuroendocrine neoplasms.

Diagnosis

Most neuroendocrine neoplasms are asymptomatic at their early stages and are discovered incidentally on imaging or surgery performed for unrelated disorders, leading to delayed diagnosis, which rarely occurs prior to metastasis.[9] The propensity for advanced disease at the time of diagnosis is underscored by the etiology of the presenting symptoms including local tumor mass effect, tumor-induced fibrosis, and tumor-secreted bioactive amines leading to emesis/abdominal pain, symptoms of mechanical bowel obstruction, weight loss/abdominal pain, and rectal bleeding/weight loss/abdominal pain, which are the most common symptoms of gastric, small-bowel, colon, and rectal neuroendocrine neoplasms, respectively.[10] The majority of patients with tracheobronchopulmonary neuroendocrine neoplasms are asymptomatic at presentation. The classical triad of cough, hemoptysis, and pneumonia are rarely seen. Although symptoms may vary based on the tumor cell of origin

and specific secreted hormone (serotonin, catecholamine, dopamine, histamine, gastrin, glucagon, prostaglandins) classical carcinoid syndrome resulting in cutaneous flushing (most common), diarrhea, bronchoconstriction, and right-sided heart failure is relatively uncommon. It has been reported with approximately 20% of small-bowel neuroendocrine neoplasms and less than 5% of extraenteric disease.[9] Symptoms relating to the secretion of bioactive amines generally coincide with the development of liver metastases because the liver normally metabolizes hormones secreted by gastropancreatic and midgut NETs. In the presence of hepatic metastases the frequency of carcinoid syndrome increases to 60%.[11] Carcinoid syndrome in the absence of liver metastases suggests a thoracic or ovarian origin, where the venous drainage is not filtered by the liver. The measurement of the serotonin breakdown product 5-hydroxyindole-3-acetic acid within urine has a specificity of 88% for serotonin-producing neuroendocrine neoplasms, which encompasses disease within the small intestine.

Confirmation of the diagnosis of a neuroendocrine neoplasm may be achieved using serum and urine biochemical studies. Measurements of relevant peptides and amines, which may include serotonin, substance P, chromogrannin A, histamine, gastrin, vasoactive intestinal peptide, glucagon, bradykinin, neurotensin, human chorionic gonadotrophin, neuropeptide K, neuropeptide L, and pancreatic polypeptide, can be guided by the patient's symptom complex. Among these, chromogrannin A is the most sensitive serum marker of neuroendocrine neoplasm with a sensitivity of 99% and a significant correlation of serum levels to tumor volume and burden; however, this glycoprotein is nonspecific and may be seen with small-cell lung and prostate cancer. False-positive elevations may occur in the setting of an atrophic gastritis and renal insufficiency.[9]

In addition to biochemical assays, diagnostic imaging plays an essential role in the management of patients with neuroendocrine neoplasms. A multimodality approach provides optimal evaluation of primary and metastatic disease including computed tomography (CT), magnetic resonance imaging (MRI), and scintigraphic imaging. Although a recent study suggests that MRI is more effective than CT in the detection of liver metastases, both triphasic contrast-enhanced CT and contrast-enhanced MR are recommended for initial evaluation and may provide complementary information regarding disease extent and vascular anatomy and facilitate posttreatment comparisons.[12] Nuclear medicine imaging approaches using tumor-specific radiolabeled receptor analogs or amine precursors provide an important adjunct to cross-sectional imaging and offer greater sensitivity and specificity. The most widely used single photon approach takes advantage of the fact that 70% to 90% of neuroendocrine neoplasms express multiple subtypes of somatostatin receptors to enable imaging with radioloabeled somatostatin analogs including ^{111}In-octreotide and ^{111}In-lantreotide with 93% and 87% sensitivity, respectively.[13] ^{111}In-octreotide demonstrates significantly higher sensitivity than other single photon somatostatin analogs including ^{123}I-metaiodobenzyl guanidine and has become the standard method of imaging NETs. This approach also provides predictive information regarding susceptibility to therapy with somatostain analogs.[14] Recently, promising positron emission tomography (PET) approaches have been demonstrated. The development of the universal chelator 1,4,7,10-tetra-azacyclodecane-1,4,7,10-tetra-acetic acid (DOTA) has facilitated the development of ^{68}Ga-DOTA-Tyr3 octreotide (DOTATOC) PET imaging for NETs. First described by Hoffman et al., ^{68}Ga-DOTATOC PET imaging NETs has demonstrated superior sensitivity and contrast as compared to ^{111}In-octreotide scintigraphy.[15,16] In addition, ^{11}C-5-hydroxytryptophan identified 98% of neoplasms and demonstrated greater sensitivity than scintigraphy and CT in a study of 42 patients with neuroendocrine neoplasms.[17,18] Finally, although highly differentiated tumors do not demonstrate increased uptake of [18]Fluoro-deoxyglucose (FDG), a recent study suggests that FDG-PET may be as or more sensitive than scintigraphy for imaging the subset of well-differentiated neuroendocrine neoplasms that are characterized by an aggressive phenotype with a high Ki-67 proliferative index.[19]

Prognosis

NETs generally evolve with a progressive and indolent growth. Patients typically develop symptoms with late-stage disease and frequently present with metastases involving the lymph nodes, bone, and/or liver. The staging of neuroendocrine neoplasms is based on the tumor-node-metastasis (TNM) notation recommended by the North American and the European Neuroendocrine Tumor Societies and the American Joint Committee on

Cancer. Although these staging systems are similar for intestinal tumors, they differ for early stage tumors arising in the pancreas or appendix.

There is a strong correlation between primary tumor site and stage of disease. The prevalence of distant metastases at diagnosis ranges from 5% for rectal neuroendocrine neoplasms to 39% for small-bowel disease and 64% for patients with pancreatic neuroendocrine neoplasms.[1] Histologic grade also correlates with the stage of disease with 21%, 30%, and 50% of patients with well-differentiated (G1), moderately differentiated (G2), and poorly differentiated (G3) tumors presenting with distant metastases, respectively. Hepatic metastases develop in an estimated 46% to 93% of patients with NETs.[11,20–22]

The median overall survival for patients with neuroendocrine neoplasms in the SEER registry from 1973 to 2004 was 75 months. The median survival was 124 and 64 months for patients with G1 and G2 disease, respectively, versus 10 months for patients with G3 and G4 disease.[1] Disease stage was an important predictor of survival with patients with G1 or G2 NETs with localized, regional, or distant metastatic disease demonstrating median survivals of 223, 111, and 33 months, respectively. In addition, the site of the primary tumor was a powerful predictor of survival. Interestingly, an examination of patient survival from 1973 to 2004 demonstrated no change for patients with localized or regional disease; however, a significant improvement in median survival was appreciated for patients with distant metastases beginning around 1988 corresponding with the introduction of the somatostatin analog octreotide.

THERAPEUTIC APPROACHES TO NEUROENDOCRINE NEOPLASMS

Surgery remains the only potentially curative therapy for patients with neuroendocrine neoplasms; however, curative resection of metastatic neuroendocrine neoplasms is possible in fewer than 10% of patients.[23] There is no consensus on the optimal management of metastatic disease for which a variety of approaches across several disciplines are applied including medical therapy with chemotherapeutics, surgical resection/cytoreduction, and minimally invasive locoregional therapies. These approaches, in combination with the indolent nature of NET progression allowing the application of multiple treatment strategies, underscore the importance of a multidisciplinary approach to the management of metastatic neuroendocrine neoplasms as well as the need for randomized controlled trials to compare the strategies.

Medical Management

The role of systemic therapy in the management of metastatic neuroendocrine neoplasms has undergone a dramatic evolution over the past 30 years, with the demonstration of the antiproliferative effects of somatostatin analogs representing the most important advance.[24] Somatostatin analogs were initially developed for the management of hormonal syndromes associated with neuroendocrine neoplasms.[25] The antiproliferative effects of octreotide were established in the landmark placebo-controlled, double-blind, prospective, randomized study on the effect of octreotide LAR in the control of tumor growth in patients with metastatic neuroendocrine midgut tumors, or PROMID study.[26] The PROMID study demonstrated a statistically significant prolongation in median time to progression in patients with metastatic midgut NETs from 6 months in the placebo arm to 14.3 months in the octreotide LAR arm (FIGURE 13.3). The benefit was independent of the presence of a carcinoid syndrome and of chromogrannin A levels. This response, in combination with the low toxicity, clearly establishes the role of somatostatin analog therapy in all patients with metastatic midgut NETs.

Interferon-alpha therapy was applied prior to the introduction of somatostatin analogs and demonstrated improvement in hormonal symptoms due to the upregulation of somatostatin receptors. Studies investigating combination therapy involving interferon-alpha and somatostatin analogs have reported symptomatic improvement with an increased duration of disease stability; however, the data assessing a potential survival benefit remain inconclusive.[27]

Two new agents were approved in 2011 by the Food and Drug Administration for treatment of metastatic pancreatic NETs. Everolimus (Affinitor), is an inhibitor of the serine/threonine kinase mammalian target of rapamycin (mTOR). The RADIANT-2 phase III trial of everolimus in patients with well or moderately differentiated metastatic NET with carcinoid symptoms demonstrated an improvement in progression-free survival of 5 months and a statistically significant 40% reduction in risk of progression for patients receiving everolimus plus octreotide LAR as compared to patients receiving placebo plus octreotide.[28] The RADIANT-3 study of everolimus in patients with metastatic pancreatic NETs demonstrated an improvement in progression-free survival of 7 months with an associated 65% reduction in risk of progression for patients receiving everolimus as compared to placebo (FIGURE 13.4).[29]

Sunitinib (Sutent), is a multityrosine kinase receptor inhibitor of vascular endothelial growth factor (VEGF) receptors 1, 2, and 3, and platelet-derived growth factor (PDGF). A double-blind, placebo-controlled phase III clinical trial of sunitinib demonstrated a 7-month improvement in progression-free survival for patients with metastatic, well-differentiated pancreatic NETs.[30]

Early results of a phase II clinical trial investigating combination therapy for metastatic NETs of the gut using the multikinase inhibitor sorafenib, which blocks VEGF and PDGF, with

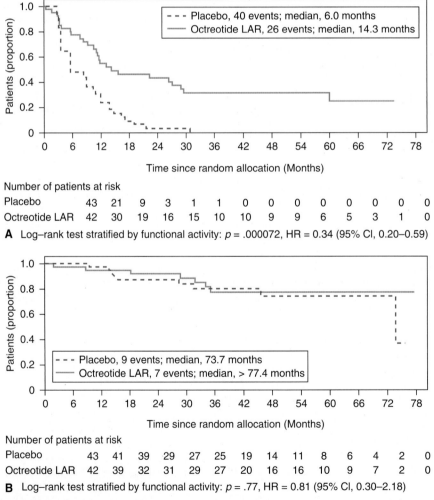

FIGURE 13.3 A. Conservative intent-to-treat analysis of time to progression or tumor-related death. **B.** Intent-to-treat analysis of overall survival.

HR, hazard ratio.

Rinke et al. *J Clin Oncol* 2009;27:4656–4663.

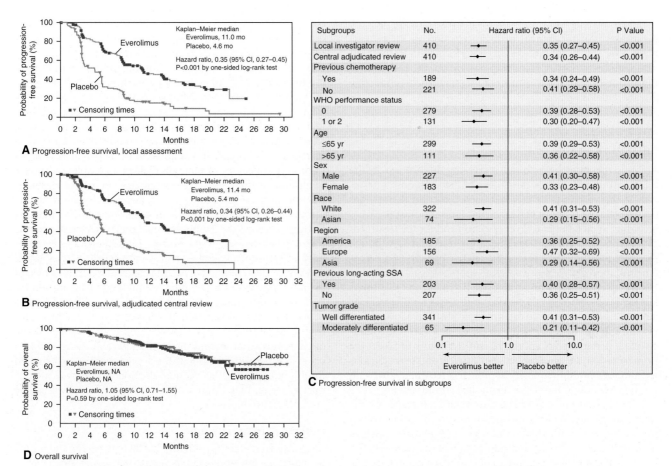

FIGURE 13.4 Progression-free and Overall Survival. Kaplan–Meier curves are shown for progression-free survival as assessed by local investigators (Panel A) and by adjudicated central review (Panel B). A forest plot (Panel C) shows the effect of study treatment on progression-free survival in patient subgroups. Kaplan–Meier curves are also shown for overall survival (Panel D).

NA, not available; SSA, somatostatin analog.

Yao et al. *N Engl J Med* 2011;364:514–523.

bevacizumab, a monoclonal against VEGF, showed a median progression-free survival of 12.4 months with moderate side effects including hand-foot syndrome.[31] Phase II clinical trials of combination therapy with temozolomide and the antivascular agent thalidomide or the antimetabolite capecitabine have demonstrated response rates of 45% as compared to 7% in metastatic midgut neuroendocrine neoplasm and 70% response rate with an 18-month progression-free survival in metastatic pancreatic neuroendocrine neoplasms, respectively.[32,33] The oral regimen of temozolomide and capecitabine has achieved this remarkable objective response rates with minimal toxicity.

Surgical Management

Surgical resection remains the only potentially curative therapy for neuroendocrine neoplasms and should be considered for all affected patients despite the absence of randomized-controlled studies comparing surgery to other interventions.[34] Resection of the primary tumor and local lymph nodes is the treatment of choice for patients with grade 1-2 neuroendocrine neoplasms without distant metastases or extensive local invasion.[35,36]

Surgery also remains an important consideration for potentially resectable advanced NETs, including hepatic metastases with 5-year survival rates of 50% to 85% and should be considered in all patients.[37–40]

Although surgery is the treatment of choice for resectable disease, resection of the primary tumor and subtotal resection (debulking) of liver metastases may have an important role in metastatic neuroendocrine disease. Retrospective data regarding resection of nonpancreatic primary tumors in patients with metastases suggest a survival benefit and underscore the need for randomized-controlled trials.[37,41] The role of resection of pancreatic primaries is less clear. Similarly, there are limited data for the role of cytoreduction in patients with unresectable metastases. Defined as resection of 90% of the tumor or metastasis, debulking has been advocated in the surgical literature based on retrospective case studies; however, the absence of randomized-controlled studies demonstrating improved response to chemotherapy following cytoreduction in combination with the efficacy of modern antisecretory medications in controlling symptoms have been cited as arguments against cytoreduction.[37,40–47]

Based on the slow growth of neuroendocrine hepatic metastases and the benefit of liver resection in their treatment, liver transplantation has been performed in select cases. Although the reported experience has grown, the role of liver transplantation for the treatment of metastatic neuroendocrine disease remains unclear.[48]

Locoregional Therapy

Ablative Therapy

Ablative therapies have found increasing application in the treatment of malignancy due to established response rates as well as the versatility of this approach. Ablation therapy has been developed for both percutaneous and surgical approaches including as an adjunct to liver resection and for the treatment of patients who are not candidates for resection.[49] Although there are no studies examining the relative benefits of a percutaneous approach versus a surgical approach, each technique has its advantages and disadvantages. Percutaneous ablation is less invasive, relatively inexpensive, and allows for direct image guidance, whereas open or laparoscopic ablation allows direct visualization of disease extent, access to locations not conducive to a percutaneous approach, and the ability to resect the primary lesion. In selecting between surgical and percutaneous techniques a multidisciplinary approach is recommended with careful attention to the above-mentioned considerations.

The application of percutaneous ablative therapy for the treatment of neuroendocrine metastases to the liver evolved from experience with ablation of other malignancies, such as hepatocellular carcinoma and colorectal metastases, which defined limitations based on tumor size and anatomic location. Percutaneous ablative therapies are therefore primarily utilized for palliation of carcinoid symptoms and management of recurrent disease following resection or prior ablation in patients with fewer than four to five metastatic lesions, each of which measures less than 3 cm in maximal diameter.[50] Radiofrequency (RF) ablation is the most frequent percutaneous ablative technology reported for the treatment of hepatic metastases of NETs and may be performed using MR, CT, or ultrasonography (US) guidance. This technique produces thermal injury by a high-frequency alternating current passed from an uninsulated electrode into surrounding tissues, resulting in frictional heating of tissue surrounding the electrodes leading to cellular injury. Given the demonstrated release of vasoactive hormones during ablation, patients should be premedicated with somatostatin analogs prior to ablation to avoid carcinoïd crisis.[51] Like with chemoembolization, bilioenteric anastomosis is a risk factor for the development of liver abscess following thermal ablation, and liver abscesses have been reported to occur despite prolonged antibiotherapy in four of nine patients with a bilioenteric anastomosis 13 to 62 days after RF ablation.[52] The results for RF ablation of neuroendocrine metastases to the liver have been encouraging. In the largest reported series of RF ablation for metastases of NETs, Berber et al.[53] reported a local efficacy of 97%, which is higher than that reported for other liver tumors. In this series, RF ablation was performed during laparoscopy in 34 patients bearing 234 metastases with a mean size of 2.3 cm. Symptom relief was complete in 63% and partial in 32%. The mean size of tumors that could not be ablated completely was 4.2 cm, confirming the limited efficacy of RF ablation in treating large tumors. Symptomatic response to RF ablation is well

established and has been effective for the control of symptoms in patients unresponsive to hepatic artery embolization.[54] More recently, Karabulut et al.[55] reported decreased morbidity for RF ablation in comparison to embolization and resection in their multimodality study of neuroendocrine liver metastases.

Additional ablative techniques have been applied for the treatment of neuroendocrine liver metastases on a more limited basis including ethanol injection and cryoablation. Rarely effective for treatment of metastases from other malignancies, Livraghi et al.[56] reported that ablation using percutaneous, intratumoral injection of ethanol affected a complete response in all four of the treated neuroendocrine hepatic metastases. Cryoablation applies freezing and thawing cycles following the intratumoral injection of liquid nitrogen or expansive argon gas through a cryoprobe. Tumor destruction is affected during the freezing and thawing cycles wherein intracellular and extracellular ice forms in a region known as the "iceball." Cryoablation therapy for the treatment of hepatic metastases is well-known in the intraoperative setting but has found limited application for percutaneous therapy. Although there are no published reports of percutaneous cryoablation of metastatic NETs, the recent introduction of smaller, argon-based cryoprobes enabling the use of conscious sedation and the ability to sculpt the iceball to a prescribed size should facilitate the development of cryoablation for this indication. Other thermal ablation technologies include microwave and laser application systems, all of which can be applied to NET metastases.

Hepatic Arterial Therapy

Intra-arterial therapy is primarily a palliative therapy and is used for patients with unresectable disease that is not amenable to resection or ablation. The two primary indications for intra-arterial therapy are palliation for hormone-related symptoms that are uncontrolled with somatostatin analogs and progression of unresectable hepatic metastases that threaten liver function. The most effective timing of the intervention with respect to disease burden has not been clearly defined and approaches differ considerably among centers. Liver metastases of NETs are sometimes very slow growing and can remain stable for several years. It is generally agreed that in the case where tumor burden of the liver is low (<25% of the liver volume), progression of the tumor must be documented on two subsequent imaging studies prior to starting intra-arterial therapy (or any other treatment). Even with documented progressive disease, some centers will not initiate liver-directed therapy in asymptomatic patients with normal liver function until the tumor burden reaches 25% to 50% of the liver volume. The rationale for this conservative approach is that even progressive disease may take years before it threatens liver function, and embolization therapies can only be applied a finite number of times in a patient's lifetime and hence should only be employed when there is a clinical indicator. Extensive tumor burden within the liver at the time of diagnosis is an indication for prompt and aggressive therapy because it is now established in several studies that extensive liver involvement limits the likelihood of success and increases the risk of complication of intra-arterial therapy.[57] Intra-arterial therapy is considered to be the first-line therapy for liver-dominant low-grade NETs.[58] Extrahepatic disease to the lungs, bones, or lymph nodes do not constitute a contraindication to intra-arterial therapy as long as the disease predominates within the liver and the prognosis is primarily dependent on the natural history of the hepatic metastases. Intra-arterial therapy may be combined with systemic chemotherapy in cases of distant metastases. Systemic chemotherapy is preferred in high-grade tumors. These high-grade tumors are usually fast growing, with a significant extra-hepatic tumor burden at diagnosis, and tend to respond less to embolization than low-grade carcinoid. This lower response rate might be caused by the lower arterialization in high-grade tumor compared to low-grade ones.

The rationale for intra-arterial therapy of hepatic metastases of neuroendocrine neoplasms is based on the vascular biology of metastatic disease to the liver, which derive 80% to 100% of their blood supply from the hepatic artery, as compared to the normal hepatic parenchyma, which receives two-thirds of its blood supply from the portal venous system.[59] The dependence of metastases on the arterial blood supply has been exploited with two primary forms of locoregional therapy including intra-arterial infusion of chemotherapeutics and embolic occlusion of the selected artery to induce ischemia. Approaches focusing on the intra-arterial infusion of chemotherapeutics alone or in combination with systemic chemotherapy have proven ineffectual in the treatment of neuroendocrine metastases to the liver with response rates of 21% and 22% to doxorubicin and streptozocin/5-fluorouracil, respectively.[60] Given its limited efficacy, the infusion-only approach has been supplanted by embolic approaches, which often include arterial infusion of a chemotherapeutic prior to embolization. Initially achieved through surgical ligation of arteries supplying the liver with response rates as high as 60% and durations of up to 12 months, catheter-based delivery of embolics with or without coincident administration of chemotherapeutics is now the standard of care for inducing ischemia in metastatic neuroendocrine neoplasms to the liver.[61,62]

Bland embolization was initially applied in the 1970s with a variety of embolics including gelfoam slurry with[63] and without lipiodol,[64] gelfoam powder,[64,65] polyvinyl alcohol (PVA) particles,[66] and tris-acryl particles. Chemoembolization combining intra-arterial chemotherapy with embolics developed in the 1980s. A variety of agents have been used for chemoembolization in aqueous or lipid-based formulations without a significant difference in response rates.[67] The two most commonly reported regimens include doxorubicin alone (50 mg/m²) or a combination of cisplatin (100 mg), adriamycin (50 mg), and mitomycin-C (10 mg). The use of streptozocin, known to have some efficacy against NETs after IV delivery, has not demonstrated superiority to other agents and is associated with a poor side effect profile including pain upon injection.[68] Chemoembolization classically involves injection of an emulsion of the selected agent with ethiodized oil (Lipiodol, Guerbet Group LLC, Bloomington, IN) followed by particle embolization until near-stasis is achieved. The selected chemotherapeutic is mixed with ethiodized oil to maximize delivery based on this agent's propensity to be selectively taken up and retained by the tumor feeding vessels.[69] Ethiodized oil increases dwell time of the chemotherapeutic within the tumor due to vascular slackening induced by the agent's viscosity and permeation of the abnormal tumor vasculature.[70,71]

More recently, a non–oil-based platform for drug delivery using drug-eluting embolic beads has been translated for clinical application in patients with metastatic gastrointestinal NETs, with early data demonstrating promising response rates.[72] Drug-eluting beads combine arterial embolization with

the sustained release of chemotherapy drugs into adjacent tissue.[73,74] The beads consist of microspheres that range from 100 to 900 µm in diameter and are composed of biocompatible polymers, such as PVA hydrogel, that have been sulphonated to enable the binding of chemotherapy and are loadable with up to 100 mg of chemotherapeutic. Once loaded with chemotherapeutic, the microspheres are mixed with iodinated contrast and injected intra-arterially to allow visualization of delivery under fluoroscopy. If stasis is not reached with administration of up to 4 g of microspheres then the treatment can be completed with bland microspheres. The microspheres release the drug over 14 days with a peak of intratumoral concentration at 3 days reaching levels that are 400 times higher than when the drug is injected intra-arterially without loading.[74] The systemic pharmacokinetic profile achieved with drug-eluting beads has been demonstrated to be more favorable than that seen with conventional chemoembolization with decreased serum levels of chemotherapeutic expected to decrease systemic side effects.[75] Two recent reports highlight an unexpectedly high rate of liver and biliary necrosis following drug-eluting bead embolization of neuroendocrine neoplasm metastases, however, with a relative risk ratio of 8:1 compared to oily chemoembolization, indicating the need for caution in applying this new technology in such patients.[76,77]

In evaluating patients with hepatic metastases from NETs for bland or chemoembolization, patient anatomy as well as the extent of disease must be assessed. With respect to patient anatomy, the patency of the portal vein is of paramount importance because hepatic artery occlusion in patients with portal vein thrombosis may lead to liver failure. Embolization may be performed in patients with portal vein thrombosis that involves two or fewer hepatic segments. Of note, intra-arterial infusion of a chemotherapeutic without subsequent embolization may offer a safe alternative in patients with portal vein thrombosis. To avoid injury to the gut or pancreas, it is important to carefully identify nontarget branches, such as the right gastric artery, that may arise from the hepatic artery proper or its left-sided branches, supraduodenal branches of the right hepatic artery, omental, and falciform arteries, which typically arises from the left hepatic artery. Catheterization should try to pass beyond the origin of the cystic artery to lower postembolization pain. Bile duct dilation is a relative contraindication due to the risk of biliary necrosis and biloma formation in these patients. Of greater concern are patients with a bilioenteric anastomosis, a finding that is not uncommon in patients with islet cell carcinoma, who are at high risk for severe infectious complications following hepatic artery embolization.[78] If hepatic artery embolization is performed in patients with a bilioenteric anastomosis, a tailored regimen of antibiotic prophylaxis should be administered. A recommended regimen includes 500 mg of oral levofloxacin daily and 500 mg of oral metronidazole twice daily initiated 48 hours before the procedure as well as 1 gram of oral neomycin (Teva) and 1 gram of oral erythromycin administered at 1 PM, 2 PM, and 11 PM on the day prior to the procedure. Intravenous levofloxacin and metronidazole should then be continued on the same schedule while the patient is in the hospital and should be resumed using preprocedure oral regimen for 2 weeks following discharge.[79] Although this regimen has been demonstrated to decrease the incidence of sepsis in patients with a history of bilioenteric anastomosis, postprocedural sepsis is still more frequent than in patients without bilioenteric anastomosis.[79]

The extent and number of hepatic metastases is an essential consideration in planning embolization. In the case where the patient's disease is located in a single hepatic lobe or where selective catheterization of individual tumors is possible, direct targeting each tumor is recommended. When there is a bilobar disease with multiple tumors, a two-stage approach is recommended wherein half of the liver is treated in each session with each session separated by 4 to 8 weeks' time. Whereas patients with preserved liver function are not at risk for posttreatment liver insufficiency, those with the constellation of more than 50% of liver involvement, lactate dehydrogenase (LDH) greater than 425 international units per liter, AST greater than 100 international units per liter, or bilirubin greater than 2 mg/dl are at risk for posttreatment liver failure. Segmental or lobar embolization should be repeated according to clinical and biologic tolerance until the entire tumor burden is treated.

Patients selected for intra-arterial therapy must be prepared for the procedure with somatostatin analog therapy (octreotide 500 mcg subcutaneously or intravenously) to reduce the risk of inducing carcinoid crisis. Patients should receive vigorous intravenous hydration (200 cc/hour) and receive corticoid and antiemetic therapy that will help mitigate postembolization syndrome. Follow-up imaging is performed 4 weeks following treatment. Although too early to evaluate treatment response, this scan is used to assess the completeness of the treatment and identify potential complications such as nontarget embolization, hepatic necrosis, or liver abscesses. CT is the most commonly used technique for follow-up imaging; however, there is growing interest in the use of MRI for follow-up imaging given its application of nonionizing radiation among a patient population that will receive many scans over their lifetime, as well as recent data suggesting MRI is the more sensitive for identifying hepatic metastases of NETs.[12] If lipiodol has been used, a high degree of lipiodol uptake by the tumors on CT is associated with improved efficacy. Although there are limited data on follow-up of patients following drug-eluting bead chemoembolization, a report of CT perfusion performed as early as 4 days after therapy demonstrated a significant prolongation of the median transit time (MTT) from 3.2sec before treatment to 5.7sec, and a decrease in mean blood flow from 476 mL/100 g/min before treatment to 285 mL/100 g/min after treatment, which was predictive of late tumor response in 8 of 10 responders.[80]

There are clear data that intra-arterial therapies provide a therapeutic benefit over systemic therapies. Touzios et al.[22] reported significantly better 5-year survival rates after chemoembolization (50%) than after medical therapies (25%) in patients with metastatic gastrointestinal NETs. Similarly, Chamberlain et al.[20] reported a 76% and 39% survival at 1 and 3 years, respectively, following medical therapy as compared to 94%, 83%, and 50% at 1, 3, and 5 years, respectively, after bland embolization. Roche et al.[81] reported complete symptom relief in 53 and partial relief in 25 of 64 patients with gastrointestinal NETs treated with chemoembolization. A decrease in tumor burden was achieved in 74% of patients, whereas disease remained stable in 15%. Several studies demonstrate superior response rates for extrapancreatic NETs as compared to pancreatic NETs of the gastrointestinal system, including Gupta et al., who reported significantly higher morphologic response rates and longer progression-free survival for extrapancreatic

neuroendocrine neoplasms (66.7% and 22.7 months, respectively) than for islet cell carcinoma (35.2% and 16.1 months, respectively).[57,82,83] Although a review of the literature demonstrates chemoembolization to be the preferred technique for intra-arterial therapy of neuroendocrine metastases to the liver, there are no definitive data demonstrating the relative superiority of chemoembolization over bland embolization or vice versa. Although Gupta et al. found no difference in the response rates for patients with hepatic metastases of extrapancreatic gastrointestinal NETs, the authors reported longer overall survival (31.5 months vs. 18.2 months) and improved response (50% vs. 25%) for patients with hepatic metastases of islet cell tumors treated with chemoembolization versus bland embolization, noting that these data did not reach statistical significance.[57] Ruutaianen et al.[84] reported a retrospective review of 67 patients with hepatic metastases of NETs who underwent 219 embolization procedures and concluded that chemoembolization demonstrated improvement in time to progression (TTP), symptom control, and overall survival. Except for TTP among patients with carcinoid tumors, statistical significance was not achieved for the other outcome measures due to the small cohort and crossover between treatment modalities, emphasizing the need for a multicenter prospective randomized trial. The limited clinical experience with drug-eluting bead chemoembolization is encouraging with Gaur et al.[72] reporting a median TTP of 419 days in patients with hepatic metastases of gastrointestinal NETs.

Selective Internal Radiation

There are two approaches for the selective delivery of internal radiation: (1) selective intra-arterial embolization of feeding hepatic arteries with microspheres loaded with radioactive yttrium-90 (^{90}Y) and (2) intravenous administration of a somatostatin analog labeled with a beta-emitting isotope. Initially applied for the treatment of hepatocellular cancers and hepatic metastases for colorectal cancer, the application of radioembolotherapy with ^{90}Y microspheres for treatment of hepatic metastases of NETs is growing. This approach involves the loading of nondegradable glass or resin microspheres with the pure β-emitter ^{90}Y, which has a half-life of 2.67 days, has an energy level of 0.94 MeV, and demonstrates a mean soft tissue penetration of 2.5 mm.[85] ^{90}Y loaded microspheres are commercially available in two formulations including TheraSpheres in which the isotope is embedded within glass spheres (TheraSphere; MDS Nordion, Inc., ON, Canada) or SIR-Spheres in which the isotope is bonded to the surface of the resin microsphere through sulfonyl group activation (SIR-Spheres; SIR-Tex Medical Limited, Sydney, Australia). Importantly, there is no clinically significant leaching of the ^{90}Y from either type of microsphere. A standard dose of approximately 4 million glass spheres has an activity of ranging from 3 to 10 GBq. A standard dose of approximately 50 million resin spheres constitutes an activity of 0.75 to 3.03 GBq. Although Rhee et al.[86] reported that a statistically significant greater median radiation dose was delivered to patients with hepatic metastases of NETs using glass microspheres, no difference in response was appreciated. Studies reporting the application of ^{90}Y radioembolotherapy for the treatment of hepatic metastases of NETs have increased over the past several years and suggest that this technique offers similar benefits to chemoembolization, with the largest series reported by Kennedy et al.[87] demonstrating stable disease in

22.7%, partial response in 60.5%, complete response in 2.7%, and progression of disease in 4.9% based on imaging criteria with a median survival of 70 months. Antitumoral effect is demonstrated by local tumor control, decreased tumor marker levels, and improved clinical symptoms.[88] A notable exception to these findings is a study by Whitney et al.,[89] who reported a significantly lower response rate after 12 months of follow-up in patients treated with ^{90}Y radioembolotherapy as compared with patients treated with drug-eluting beads. In contrast to the severe side effect profile typically associated with chemoembolization, ^{90}Y radioembolotherapy is an outpatient procedure and does not result in significant toxicities in liver synthetic parameters; however, ^{90}Y radioembolotherapy may be associated with a flare phenomenon that involves a spike in tumor markers immediately following treatment.[90] This finding may correspond with the timing of postprocedural abdominal pain with exacerbation of carcinoid and neuroendocrine symptoms. The comparable efficacy of ^{90}Y radioembolization in combination with the more benign toxicity profile compared to chemoembolization has led to studies examining the integration of this technique into the treatment paradigm for patients with metastatic NETs.[91] Randomized controlled studies are needed in order to elucidate the role of ^{90}Y radioembolization relative to chemoembolization including cost-benefit and quality of life analyses.[89]

Although a complete discussion of the intravenous injection of somatostatin analog-based intravenous radiotherapy is beyond the scope of this chapter, it is a therapy that provides disease control in the majority of patients with systemic metastases, and interventional oncologists participating in the care of NET patients should make themselves familiar with the relevant literature because this topic frequently is brought up by patients who are seeking information on all possible treatment options. It should be noted that this approach has been adapted for intra-arterial therapy. McStay et al.[92] reported that intra-arterial injection of yttrium-90-tetra-azacyclododecane tetra-acetic acid (DOTA) lantreotide provided a partial response in 16% of patients with stable disease reported for 63% of treated patients. Clinical improvement was reported by 61% of 23 patients treated. Similarly, intra-arterial delivery of ^{131}I-labeled methyliodobenzylguanidine (MIBG), an established nuclear medicine therapy for the treatment of NETs, has been reported, with Brogsitter et al.[93] reporting an up to fourfold increase tumor uptake compared to intravenous injection. Reports of the application of this approach for metastatic NETs is limited, but it is noteworthy that it has been utilized in patients who developed progressive disease following intra-arterial therapy with relief of patient symptoms in 80% of treated patients.[94]

CONCLUSION

Neuroendocrine tumors are a complex group of malignancies whose high prevalence is second only to colon cancer among patients with hepatic malignancies. Their indolent course leads to a variety of interventions over many years, such that this disease will grow to occupy a substantial portion of a liver oncology practice. Interventional oncologists should be familiar with all aspects of the care of these patients and assemble a team of specialists with similar expertise to provide optimal care to this often misunderstood population.

REFERENCES

1. Yao JC, Hassan M, Phan A, et al. One hundred years after "carcinoid": epidemiology of and prognostic factors for neuroendocrine tumors in 35,825 cases in the United States. *J Clin Oncol* 2008;26:3063–3072.
2. Singh S, Law C. Multidisciplinary reference centers: the care of neuroendocrine tumors. *J Oncol Pract* 2010;6:e11–16.
3. Zikusoka MN, Kidd M, Eick G, et al. The molecular genetics of gastroenteropancreatic neuroendocrine tumors. *Cancer* 2005;104:2292–2309.
4. Bosman FT, Carneiro F, Hruban RH, et al. *WHO Classification of Tumours of the Digestive System.* 4th ed. Lyon, France: IARC Press; 2010.
5. Klimstra DS, Modlin IR, Adsay NV, et al. Pathology reporting of neuroendocrine tumors: application of the Delphic consensus process to the development of a minimum pathology data set. *Am J Surg Pathol* 2010;34:300–313.
6. Volante M, Righi L, Berruti A, et al. The pathological diagnosis of neuroendocrine tumors: common questions and tentative answers. *Virchows Arch* 2011;458:393–402.
7. Modlin IM, Lye KD, Kidd M. A 5-decade analysis of 13,715 carcinoid tumors. *Cancer* 2003;97:934–959.
8. Surveillance, Epidemiology and End Results Program. *Cancer Statistics Review 1975–2004.* Bethesda, MD: National Cancer Institute; 2004.
9. Gustafsson BI, Kidd M, Modlin IM. Neuroendocrine tumors of the diffuse neuroendocrine system. *Curr Opin Oncol* 2008;20:1–12.
10. Modlin IM, Kidd M, Latich I, et al. Current status of gastrointestinal carcinoids. *Gastroenterology* 2005;128:1717–1751.
11. Blonski WC, Reddy KR, Shaked A, et al. Liver transplantation for metastatic neuroendocrine tumor: a case report and review of the literature. *World J Gastroenterol* 2005;11:7676–7683.
12. Dromain C, de Baere T, Lumbroso J, et al. Detection of liver metastases from endocrine tumors: a prospective comparison of somatostatin receptor scintigraphy, computed tomography, and magnetic resonance imaging. *J Clin Oncol* 2005;23:70–78.
13. Rodrigues M, Traub-Weidinger T, Li S, et al. Comparison of ^{111}In-DOTA-DPhe1-Tyr3-octreotide and 111In-DOTA-lanreotide scintigraphy and dosimetry in patients with neuroendocrine tumours. *Eur J Nucl Med Mol Imaging* 2006;33:532–540.
14. Janson ET. Treatment of neuroendocrine tumors with somatostatin analogs. *Pituitary* 2006;9:249–256.
15. Frilling A, Sotiropoulos GC, Radtke A, et al. The impact of ^{68}Ga-DOTATOC positron emission tomography/computed tomography on the multimodal management of patients with neuroendocrine tumors. *Ann Surg* 2010;252:850–856.
16. Hofmann M, Maecke H, Borner R, et al. Biokinetics and imaging with the somatostatin receptor PET radioligand (68)Ga-DOTATOC: preliminary data. *Eur J Nucl Med* 2001;28:1751–1757.
17. Carrasquillo JA, Chen CC. Molecular imaging of neuroendocrine tumors. *Semin Oncol* 2010;37:662–679.
18. Orlefors H, Sundin A, Garske U, et al. Whole-body (11)C-5-hydroxytryptophan positron emission tomography as a universal imaging technique for neuroendocrine tumors: comparison with somatostatin receptor scintigraphy and computed tomography. *J Clin Endocrinol Metab* 2005;90:3392–3400.
19. Abgral R, Leboulleux S, Deandreis D, et al. Performance of (18)fluorodeoxyglucose-positron emission tomography and somatostatin receptor scintigraphy for high Ki67 (>/=10%) well-differentiated endocrine carcinoma staging. *J Clin Endocrinol Metab* 2011;96:665–671.
20. Chamberlain RS, Canes D, Brown KT, et al. Hepatic neuroendocrine metastases: does intervention alter outcomes? *J Am Coll Surg* 2000;190:432–445.
21. Knox CD, Anderson CD, Lamps LW, et al. Long-term survival after resection for primary hepatic carcinoid tumor. *Ann Surg Oncol* 2003;10:1171–1175.
22. Touzios JG, Kiely JM, Pitt SC, et al. Neuroendocrine hepatic metastases: does aggressive management improve survival? *Ann Surg* 2005;241:776–783; discussion 83–85.
23. McEntee GP, Nagorney DM, Kvols LK, et al. Cytoreductive hepatic surgery for neuroendocrine tumors. *Surgery* 1990;108:1091–1096.
24. Sun W, Lipsitz S, Catalano P, et al. Phase II/III study of doxorubicin with fluorouracil compared with streptozocin with fluorouracil or dacarbazine in the treatment of advanced carcinoid tumors: Eastern Cooperative Oncology Group Study E1281. *J Clin Oncol* 2005;23:4897–4904.
25. Kvols LK, Moertel CG, O'Connell MJ, et al. Treatment of the malignant carcinoid syndrome. Evaluation of a long-acting somatostatin analogue. *N Engl J Med* 1986;315:663–666.

26. Rinke A, Muller HH, Schade-Brittinger C, et al. Placebo-controlled, double-blind, prospective, randomized study on the effect of octreotide LAR in the control of tumor growth in patients with metastatic neuroendocrine midgut tumors: a report from the PROMID Study Group. *J Clin Oncol* 2009;27:4656–4663.

27. Strosberg JR, Cheema A, Kvols LK. A review of systemic and liver-directed therapies for metastatic neuroendocrine tumors of the gastroenteropancreatic tract. *Cancer Control* 2011;18:127–137.

28. Yao JC, Hainsworth JD, Baudin E, et al. Everolimus plus octreotide LAR (E+O) versus placebo plus octreotide LAR (P+O) in patients with advanced neuroendocrine tumors (NET): Updated results of a randomized, double-blind, placebo-controlled, multicenter phase III trial (RADIANT-2). *J Clin Oncol* 2011;29.

29. Yao JC, Shah MH, Ito T, et al. Everolimus for advanced pancreatic neuroendocrine tumors. *N Engl J Med* 2011;364:514–523.

30. Raymond E, Dahan L, Raoul JL, et al. Sunitinib malate for the treatment of pancreatic neuroendocrine tumors. *N Engl J Med* 2011;364:501–513.

31. Castellano E, Capdevila J, Salazar R, et al. Sorafenib and bevacizumab combination targeted therapy in advanced neuroendocrine tumor: A phase II study of the Spanish Neuroendocrine Tumor Group (GETNE0801). *J Clin Oncol* 2011.

32. Kulke MH, Stuart K, Enzinger PC, et al. Phase II study of temozolomide and thalidomide in patients with metastatic neuroendocrine tumors. *J Clin Oncol* 2006;24:401–406.

33. Strosberg JR, Fine RL, Choi J, et al. First-line chemotherapy with capecitabine and temozolomide in patients with metastatic pancreatic endocrine carcinomas. *Cancer* 2011;117:268–275.

34. Gurusamy KS, Ramamoorthy R, Sharma D, et al. Liver resection versus other treatments for neuroendocrine tumours in patients with resectable liver metastases. *Cochrane Database Syst Rev* 2009:CD007060.

35. Rindi G, de Herder WW, O'Toole D, et al. Consensus guidelines for the management of patients with digestive neuroendocrine tumors: why such guidelines and how we went about it. *Neuroendocrinology* 2006;84: 155–157.

36. Rindi G, de Herder WW, O'Toole D, et al. Consensus guidelines for the management of patients with digestive neuroendocrine tumors: the second event and some final considerations. *Neuroendocrinology* 2008;87:5–7.

37. Capurso G, Bettini R, Rinzivillo M, et al. Role of resection of the primary pancreatic neuroendocrine tumour only in patients with unresectable metastatic liver disease: a systematic review. *Neuroendocrinology* 2011;93:223–229.

38. Chen H, Hardacre JM, Uzar A, et al. Isolated liver metastases from neuroendocrine tumors: does resection prolong survival? *J Am Coll Surg* 1998;187:88–92; discussion 92–93.

39. Coppa J, Pulvirenti A, Schiavo M, et al. Resection versus transplantation for liver metastases from neuroendocrine tumors. *Transplant Proc* 2001;33:1537–1539.

40. Yao KA, Talamonti MS, Nemcek A, et al. Indications and results of liver resection and hepatic chemoembolization for metastatic gastrointestinal neuroendocrine tumors. *Surgery* 2001;130:677–682; discussion 682–685.

41. Hellman P, Lundstrom T, Ohrvall U, et al. Effect of surgery on the outcome of midgut carcinoid disease with lymph node and liver metastases. *World J Surg* 2002;26:991–997.

42. Musunuru S, Chen H, Rajpal S, et al. Metastatic neuroendocrine hepatic tumors: resection improves survival. *Arch Surg* 2006;141:1000–1004; discussion 1005.

43. Norton JA, Kivlen M, Li M, et al. Morbidity and mortality of aggressive resection in patients with advanced neuroendocrine tumors. *Arch Surg* 2003;138:859–866.

44. Oberg KE, Reubi JC, Kwekkeboom DJ, et al. Role of somatostatins in gastroenteropancreatic neuroendocrine tumor development and therapy. *Gastroenterology* 2010;139:742–753, 753 e1.

45. Osborne DA, Zervos EE, Strosberg J, et al. Improved outcome with cytoreduction versus embolization for symptomatic hepatic metastases of carcinoid and neuroendocrine tumors. *Ann Surg Oncol* 2006;13: 572–581.

46. Rindi G, Wiedenmann B. Neuroendocrine neoplasms of the gut and pancreas: new insights. *Nat Rev Endocrinol* 2011.

47. Sarmiento JM, Que FG. Hepatic surgery for metastases from neuroendocrine tumors. *Surg Oncol Clin N Am* 2003;12:231–242.

48. Mathe Z, Tagkalos E, Paul A, et al. Liver transplantation for hepatic metastases of neuroendocrine pancreatic tumors: a survival-based analysis. *Transplantation* 2011;91:575–582.

49. Gamblin TC, Christians K, Pappas SG. Radiofrequency ablation of neuroendocrine hepatic metastasis. *Surg Oncol Clin N Am* 2011;20: 273–279, vii–viii.

50. Solbiati L, Ierace T, Tonolini M, et al. Radiofrequency thermal ablation of hepatic metastases. *Eur J Ultrasound* 2001;13:149–158.

51. Wettstein M, Vogt C, Cohnen M, et al. Serotonin release during percutaneous radiofrequency ablation in a patient with symptomatic liver metastasis of a neuroendocrine tumor. *Hepatogastroenterology* 2004;51:830–832.

52. Elias D, Di Pietroantonio D, Gachot B, et al. Liver abscess after radiofrequency ablation of tumors in patients with a biliary tract procedure. *Gastroenterol Clin Biol* 2006;30:823–827.

53. Berber E, Flesher N, Siperstein AE. Laparoscopic radiofrequency ablation of neuroendocrine liver metastases. *World J Surg* 2002;26:985–990.

54. Henn AR, Levine EA, McNulty W, et al. Percutaneous radiofrequency ablation of hepatic metastases for symptomatic relief of neuroendocrine syndromes. *AJR Am J Roentgenol* 2003;181:1005–1010.

55. Karabulut K, Akyildiz HY, Lance C, et al. Multimodality treatment of neuroendocrine liver metastases. *Surgery* 2011;150:316–325.

56. Livraghi T, Vettori C, Lazzaroni S. Liver metastases: results of percutaneous ethanol injection in 14 patients. *Radiology* 1991;179:709–712.

57. Gupta S, Johnson MM, Murthy R, et al. Hepatic arterial embolization and chemoembolization for the treatment of patients with metastatic neuroendocrine tumors: variables affecting response rates and survival. *Cancer* 2005;104:1590–1602.

58. Roche A, Girish BV, de Baere T, et al. Trans-catheter arterial chemoembolization as first-line treatment for hepatic metastases from endocrine tumors. *Eur Radiol* 2003;13:136–140.

59. Bierman HR, Byron RL, Jr., Kelley KH, et al. Studies on the blood supply of tumors in man. III. Vascular patterns of the liver by hepatic arteriography in vivo. *J Natl Cancer Inst* 1951;12:107–131.

60. Engstrom PF, Lavin PT, Moertel CG, et al. Streptozocin plus fluorouracil versus doxorubicin therapy for metastatic carcinoid tumor. *J Clin Oncol* 1984;2:1255–1259.

61. Moertel CG, Johnson CM, McKusick MA, et al. The management of patients with advanced carcinoid tumors and islet cell carcinomas. *Ann Intern Med* 1994;120:302–309.

62. Nobin A, Mansson B, Lunderquist A. Evaluation of temporary liver dearterialization and embolization in patients with metastatic carcinoid tumour. *Acta Oncol* 1989;28:419–424.

63. Schell SR, Camp ER, Caridi JG, et al. Hepatic artery embolization for control of symptoms, octreotide requirements, and tumor progression in metastatic carcinoid tumors. *J Gastrointest Surg* 2002;6:664–670.

64. Pueyo I, Jimenez JR, Hernandez J, et al. Carcinoid syndrome treated by hepatic embolization. *AJR Am J Roentgenol* 1978;131:511–513.

65. Lunderquist A, Ericsson M, Nobin A, et al. Gelfoam powder embolization of the hepatic artery in liver metastases of carcinoid tumors. *Radiologe* 1982;22:65–70.

66. Ajani JA, Carrasco CH, Charnsangavej C, et al. Islet cell tumors metastatic to the liver: effective palliation by sequential hepatic artery embolization. *Ann Intern Med* 1988;108:340–344.

67. Madoff DC, Gupta S, Ahrar K, et al. Update on the management of neuroendocrine hepatic metastases. *J Vasc Interv Radiol* 2006;17:1235–1249; quiz 1250.

68. Dominguez S, Denys A, Madeira I, et al. Hepatic arterial chemoembolization with streptozotocin in patients with metastatic digestive endocrine tumours. *Eur J Gastroenterol Hepatol* 2000;12:151–157.

69. de Baere T, Dufaux J, Roche A, et al. Circulatory alterations induced by intra-arterial injection of iodized oil and emulsions of iodized oil and doxorubicin: experimental study. *Radiology* 1995;194:165–170.

70. de Baere T, Denys A, Briquet R, et al. Modification of arterial and portal hemodynamics after injection of iodized oils and different emulsions of iodized oils in the hepatic artery: an experimental study. *J Vasc Interv Radiol* 1998;9:305–310.

71. Imaeda T, Yamawaki Y, Seki M, et al. Lipiodol retention and massive necrosis after lipiodol-chemoembolization of hepatocellular carcinoma: correlation between computed tomography and histopathology. *Cardiovasc Intervent Radiol* 1993;16:209–213.

72. Gaur SK, Friese JL, Sadow CA, et al. Hepatic arterial chemoembolization using drug-eluting beads in gastrointestinal neuroendocrine tumor metastatic to the liver. *Cardiovasc Intervent Radiol* 2011;34:566–572.

73. Carter S, Martin Ii RC. Drug-eluting bead therapy in primary and metastatic disease of the liver. *HPB* (Oxford) 2009;11:541–550.

74. Hong K, Khwaja A, Liapi E, et al. New intra-arterial drug delivery system for the treatment of liver cancer: preclinical assessment in a rabbit model of liver cancer. *Clin Cancer Res* 2006;12:2563–2567.

75. Varela M, Real MI, Burrel M, et al. Chemoembolization of hepatocellular carcinoma with drug eluting beads: efficacy and doxorubicin pharmacokinetics. *J Hepatol* 2007;46:474–481.

76. Reyes D, Kamel C, Georgiades C, et al. *Prospective, Phase II Study of Chemoembolization with Drug-eluting Beads for Hepatic Neuroendocrine Metastases: Interim Analysis.* Chicago, IL: Society for Interventional Radiology; 2011: S4–S5.

77. Guiu B, Deschamps F, Aho S, et al. Liver/biliary injuries following chemoembolisation of endocrine tumours and hepatocellular carcinoma: Lipiodol vs. drug-eluting beads. *J Hepatol* 2011.

78. de Baere T, Roche A, Amenabar JM, et al. Liver abscess formation after local treatment of liver tumors. *Hepatology* 1996;23:1436–1440.

79. Patel S, Tuite CM, Mondschein JI, et al. Effectiveness of an aggressive antibiotic regimen for chemoembolization in patients with previous biliary intervention. *J Vasc Interv Radiol* 2006;17:1931–1934.

80. Coenegrachts K, De Baere T, Abdel Rehim M, et al. *Transarterial Chemoembolization (TACE) of Neuroendocrine Hepatic Metastases Using Drug Eluting Beads.* Chicago, IL: Radiological Society of North America; 2005.

81. Roche A, Girish BV, de Baere T, et al. Prognostic factors for chemoembolization in liver metastasis from endocrine tumors. *Hepatogastroenterology* 2004;51:1751–6.

82. Eriksson BK, Larsson EG, Skogseid BM, et al. Liver embolizations of patients with malignant neuroendocrine gastrointestinal tumors. *Cancer* 1998;83:2293–2301.

83. Stokes KR, Stuart K, Clouse ME. Hepatic arterial chemoembolization for metastatic endocrine tumors. *J Vasc Interv Radiol* 1993;4:341–345.

84. Ruutiainen AT, Soulen MC, Tuite CM, et al. Chemoembolization and bland embolization of neuroendocrine tumor metastases to the liver. *J Vasc Interv Radiol* 2007;18:847–855.

85. Kennedy A, Nag S, Salem R, et al. Recommendations for radioembolization of hepatic malignancies using yttrium-90 microsphere brachytherapy: a consensus panel report from the radioembolization brachytherapy oncology consortium. *Int J Radiat Oncol Biol Phys* 2007;68:13–23.

86. Rhee TK, Lewandowski RJ, Liu DM, et al. 90Y radioembolization for metastatic neuroendocrine liver tumors: preliminary results from a multi-institutional experience. *Ann Surg* 2008;247:1029–1035.

87. Kennedy AS, Dezarn WA, McNeillie P, et al. Radioembolization for unresectable neuroendocrine hepatic metastases using resin 90Y-microspheres: early results in 148 patients. *Am J Clin Oncol* 2008;31:271–279.

88. Paprottka PM, Schmidt GP, Trumm CG, et al. Changes in normal liver and spleen volume after radioembolization with (90)y-resin microspheres in metastatic breast cancer patients: findings and clinical significance. *Cardiovasc Intervent Radiol* 2011;34:964–972.

89. Whitney R, Valek V, Fages JF, et al. Transarterial chemoembolization and selective internal radiation for the treatment of patients with metastatic neuroendocrine tumors: a comparison of efficacy and cost. *Oncologist* 2011;16:594–601.

90. Liu DM, Kennedy A, Turner D, et al. Minimally invasive techniques in management of hepatic neuroendocrine metastatic disease. *Am J Clin Oncol* 2009;32:200–215.

91. Kennedy A, Coldwell D, Sangro B, et al. Integrating radioembolization into the treatment paradigm for metastatic neuroendocrine tumors in the liver. *Am J Clin Oncol* 2011.

92. McStay MK, Maudgil D, Williams M, et al. Large-volume liver metastases from neuroendocrine tumors: hepatic intraarterial 90Y-DOTA-lanreotide as effective palliative therapy. *Radiology* 2005;237:718–726.

93. Brogsitter C, Pinkert J, Bredow J, et al. Enhanced tumor uptake in neuroendocrine tumors after intraarterial application of 131I-MIBG. *J Nucl Med* 2005;46:2112–2116.

94. Gupta S, Krishnamurthy S, Broemeling LD, et al. Small (</=2-cm) subpleural pulmonary lesions: short- versus long-needle-path CT-guided biopsy—comparison of diagnostic yields and complications. *Radiology* 2005;234:631–637.

Biliary Tract Cancers: Intrahepatic Cholangiocarcinoma

KELVIN HONG

INTRODUCTION

Cholangiocarcinoma is a rare primary liver malignancy with an incidence of 1 to 2 per 100,000 in the United States, but rates are higher in Japan and Southeast Asia.[1] Although the perception is that cholangiocarcinomas are rare, cancer statistics suggest that they are becoming more common and more lethal, very concerning combined with poor prognosis (FIGURE 14.1).[2] From 1975 to 2000, the age-adjusted incidence of intrahepatic cholangiocarcinoma (ICC) in the United States has increased from 0.32 to 0.85 per 100,000 and an accelerating increase in age-adjusted incidence (165%) and overall annual incidence increase (9.11%).[2] Prognosis is almost universally poor, with no improvement in survival over the last 25 years despite new drugs and surgical and nonsurgical treatments. The 1- and 5-year survival rates in 1975 were 15.8% and 2.6%, respectively. In 2000 the 1-, 2- and 5-year survival have essentially remained unchanged at 25%, 13%, and 3.5%, respectively.[1,2] Annual mortality from ICCs has increased slightly faster than the incidence (+9.4%). Although surgical resection offers the only chance for cure, only approximately 30% of patients with cholangiocarcinoma are eligible for resection because of the advanced nature of the disease at the time of diagnosis.[2] However, even for surgically resectable patients, survival prognosis is modest with postsurgical 1-, 3-, and 5-year survival at 58%, 33%, and 33%, respectively.[3,4] The prognosis for patients with unresectable disease (70%) is even more dismal (5- to 8-month survival), making up the bulk of patients presenting with this disease.[1–4] ICC generally presents in a more insidious advanced state than extrahepatic cholangiocarcinomas (ECCs), so prognosis is even worse comparatively. Systemic chemotherapy and radiation has been disappointing in regard to its efficacy with most regimens resulting in a median survival of 6 to 12 months.[5] No randomized studies have shown a significant improvement in overall survival compared to the best of supportive care.[6] Side effects are common and often limit patients' tolerance of the therapy and their quality of life. There has been growing interest in other modalities for treatment of cholangiocarcinoma because of these poor results with standard systemic therapy. The rarity of this disease, however, coupled with small patient populations typically studied (few case series greater than 100 patients), make it difficult to accrue robust data to support any particular new therapy.

CLASSIFICATION

Using the most basic definition, ICC refers to the 10% of bile duct cancers that arise from the epithelial cells of the intrahepatic bile ducts. The other 90% of cholangiocarcinomas arise from the epithelial cells of the extrahepatic bile ducts and are referred to as ECC with the majority located near the bifurcation of the common hepatic duct.[1] Although this definition appears straightforward, development of different definitions and systems of classification by various groups has led to confusion. In the literature, ICC also is referred to as "peripheral," based on its location in the liver, or "mass forming," based on its morphologic growth pattern. The delineation of ICC is a relatively recent phenomenon, with the earliest case reports and series in the 1970s and 1980s.[2,3] Because of these inconsistencies in definition and the relatively small numbers of cases reported by each group, there is currently no consensus on classification. ECC has been further subdivided into several categories including hilar, perihilar, distal, and diffuse.[4,5] Hilar cholangiocarcinoma, also called a Klatskin tumor, is used to describe tumors that involve the bifurcation of the common hepatic duct (FIGURE 14.2).[7]

ANATOMIC PATHOPHYSIOLOGY

Anatomically, a majority (approximately 70%) of cholangiocarcinomas occurs at or by the time of diagnosis, involves the biliary confluence, and is thus termed *Klatskin-type neoplasms*. Another 10% to 15% involve the common hepatic/bile duct (CH/BD) alone, whereas the remaining 15% to 20% are of the intrahepatic type (ICC). Cholangiocarcinomas, in general, represent only 10% to 15% of primary liver cancers with ICCs comprising only about 15% of those. ICCs are primary liver cancers with cholangiocytic molecular and histopathologic characteristics located peripheral to the biliary ductal confluence/hilum.[1,7,8] Advances in pathophysiology and morphology have been able

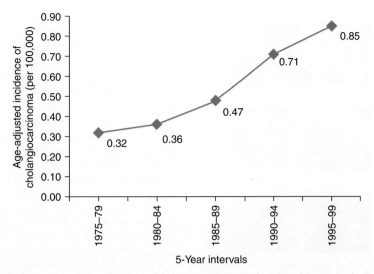

FIGURE 14.1 Graph depicting rising age-adjusted incidence rate of ICC in the United States in the last three decades.

Reprinted with permission from Shaib YH, Davila JA, McGlynn K, et al. Rising incidence of intrahepatic cholangiocarcinoma in the United States: a true increase? *J Hepatol* 2004 Mar; 40(3):472–477.

to identify different subtypes of ICC. This is important because ICC subtype and survival appear to correlate. To choose the most appropriate treatment modalities, it is important to understand the behavior of ICC and its subtype, location, physiologic, and imaging features in context within the patient's overall performance status. The main subtypes of ICC are (FIGURE 14.3) as follows:

1. Mass forming: homogeneous, low-attenuating masses with capsular retraction with peripheral irregularly enhancing rim post contrast (comprising 50%)
2. Periductal infiltrating: periductal enhancement or thickening and/or enhancement with irregularly dilated intrahepatic ducts (10%)
3. Intraductal: diffuse and marked ductasia, with or without a papillary mass, an intraductal cast-like lesion (10%)
4. Mixed: mass forming and periductal infiltrating (30%)

Morphologic mass-forming cancers therefore comprise the majority of ICCs (up to 70% to 80%). [1,7]

RISK FACTORS

Risk factors for cholangiocarcinoma are mainly conditions that result in chronic inflammation or chronic cholestasis.[1] The majority of patients, however, will have no identifiable risk factor (Table 14.1). Recent evidence suggests that the ICC type is potentially pathophysiologically and genotypically different from the rest of cholangiocarcinoma.[9] Phenotypically, primary nonstromal hepatic neoplasms can be hepatic, cholangitic, or the rare mixed hepatic-cholangitic type. Genotypic aberrations (such as the *p53* mutation) have been reported in patients with ICC-complicated cirrhosis, suggesting that ICC and HCC may arise from the same hepatic precursor cells.[10] Recent studies have suggested that ICCs are different from hepatocellular carcinomas (HCCs) in energy metabolism: HCCs appear to upregulate hexokinase II (HKII), whereas ICCs show no increase in HKII but generate energy via the pentose phosphate pathway.[9,10] Noninflammatory conditions, especially familial cholestatic diseases, have also been implicated in carcinogenesis.[1] The majority of patients, however,

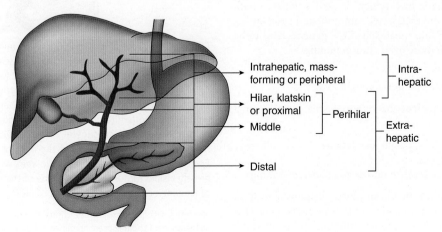

FIGURE 14.2 Classification of cholangiocarcinoma

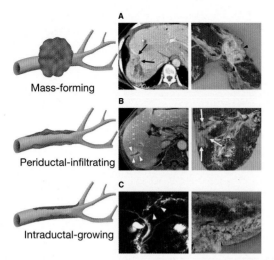

FIGURE 14.3 A. Mass-forming ICC: contrast-enhanced CT and photograph of the gross specimen showing a large, low-attenuated mass (arrows and arrowheads) with surrounding parenchymal atrophy, capsular retraction, and bile duct dilatation. **B.** Periductal-infiltrating ICC: T1-weighted MR image and photograph of the gross specimen showing periductal enhancement/tumor around the irregularly dilated intrahepatic duct (arrowheads and arrows). **C.** Intraductal-growth ICC: T2-weighted MRCP image showing the mildly dilated duct with irregularities that mimic impacted stones (arrowheads). Photograph of the gross specimen reveals a dilated bile duct with innumerable small polypoid lesions representing tubular carcinomas. Reprinted with permission from Chung YE, Kim MJ, Park YN, et al. Varying appearances of cholangiocarcinoma: radiologic-pathologic correlation. *Radiographics* 2009;29(3):683–700.

have no risk factors at presentation. Despite such recent advances in the genetics and energy metabolism pathways of ICCs, therapy options remain very limited: surgery offered for the few surgical candidates or for the remaining majority, palliation.

▌DIAGNOSIS

Cholangiocarcinoma is thought to present with jaundice, which is true of ECC. In contradistinction, the clinical presentation of patients with ICC can be insidious with advanced disease at presentation. Lymphatic involvement is early compared with HCC, with intrahepatic metastases common, and vascular invasion can be seen. Symptomatically, ECC patients tend to be identified earlier with more overt clinical findings[11]:

- Pruritus and jaundice
- With abdominal pain, anorexia, weight loss

In comparison, ICC patients have more vague constitutional symptoms and signs:

- Upper abdominal pain, weight loss, fatigue
- Frequently asymptomatic
- Their liver mass frequently found as an incidental finding

There is no blood test that is absolutely diagnostic of ICC, although liver function tests and serum tumor markers of cancer antigen 19-9 (CA 19-9), carcinoembryonic antigen (CEA), and α-fetoprotein typically are used. Elevated liver function

tests (LFTs) with alanine amino transferase (ALT) and aspartate aminotransferase (AST) are frequently abnormal at presentation. Hyperbilirubinemia is rarer because the peripheral nature of ICC causes only focal and minimal to no biliary ductal dilatation.[11,12] ICC is known to be the "intrahepatic tumor in the absence of jaundice."[12] Various types of imaging are used to diagnose cholangiocarcinoma including ultrasound, computed tomography (CT) scan, magnetic resonance imaging (MRI), MRI cholangiography, CT cholangiography, endoscopic retrograde cholangiopancreatography (ERCP), and endoscopic ultrasound. However, contrast-enhanced CT or MRI is required to determine resectability, treatment planning, and response to treatment (FIGURES 14.3, 14.4, 14.5). On gross pathology the tumor can appear dense, fibrous, and minimally necrotic; however, it tends to encircle vessels and other structures with minimal distortion (FIGURE 14.4A) and does not tend to cause portal vein thrombosis (in contradistinction to HCC).[7] On imaging, the peripheral, mass-forming lesion subtype (FIGURE 14.3A) usually presents earlier due to volume-related symptoms. The periductal infiltrating subtype (FIGURE 14.3B), which can spread along the Glisson sheath with a propensity to spread and metastasize earlier yet present symptomatically later.

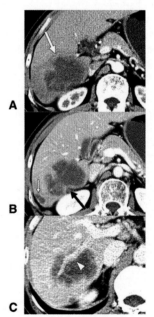

FIGURE 14.4 Typical features of mass-forming cholangiocarcinoma on contrast CT scan. (**A**) Arterial phase CT scan shows a tumor with ragged rim enhancement at the periphery (arrow). (**B**) Axial portal venous phase CT scan shows gradual centripetal enhancement of the tumor with capsular retraction (black arrow). A satellite nodule is also seen (white arrow). (**C**) Three-minute delayed phase CT scan shows gradual centripetal enhancement with tumor encasement of the posterior branch of the right portal vein (arrowhead). Encasement of a portal or hepatic vein without formation of a grossly visible tumor thrombus is one of the distinguishing features of cholangiocarcinoma as opposed to HCC.

Reprinted with permission from Chung YE, Kim MJ, Park YN, et al. Varying appearances of cholangiocarcinoma: radiologic-pathologic correlation. *Radiographics* 2009;29(3):683–700.

DIFFERENTIAL DIAGNOSIS

The differential diagnosis includes other primary liver cancers, such as HCC and ICC, and metastatic tumors, especially of colorectal origin. Once detected on imaging, the conclusive diagnosis of ICC may be elusive and ultimately be one of "diagnosis by exclusion." There are no reliable immunohistologic chemical stains that are diagnostic or specific for ICC. Percutaneous liver biopsy can be done for diagnostic sampling, although it may be pathologically nonspecific. It can be difficult to differentiate ICC from a metastatic adenocarcinoma, or an HCC with cholangiocellular features. Workup can include other studies, such as a mammogram, CT scan chest, upper and lower intestinal endoscopy, or positron emission tomography (PET) scan, to rule out an extrahepatic primary adenocarcinoma. There is controversy on the usefulness of cancer markers for the diagnosis of ICC. A third of patients will have a mildly elevated CEA at the time of presentation (19). Also, AFP may be elevated, especially in poorly differentiated cholangiocarcinomas, because both hepatocytes and cholangiocytes differentiate from the same progenitor cells. The incidence of elevated CEA and alpha fetoprotein (AFP) in patients with ICC is too low, however, to be of diagnostic significance or to be used for surveillance in a reliable manner.

STAGING

Several staging systems have been proposed to consider ICC as distinctly separate from HCC and ECC. Because of their inherent disease differences, cholangiocarcinoma is the only

Table 14.1
Risk Factors for Cholangiocarcinoma

Definitive Risk Factors:
- Sclerosing cholangiatis
- Biliary malformation (e.g., choledocal cysts)
- Thoratrast
- Liver fluke infection (*Opisthorchis viverrini*)
- Hepatolithiasis

Probable Risk Factors:
- Liver fluke infection (*Clonorchis sinensis*)
- Hepatitis C
- Cirrhosis
- Toxins (dioxin, polyvinyl chloride)

malignancy that has subtypes with completely different staging systems (ECC vs. ICC). Difficulty with utilizing earlier staging systems was caused by the inclusion of combined prognostic outcomes from other primary liver tumors, such as HCC, that have led to proposed changes to the staging system specific for ICC. Okabayashi et al.[13] proposed a specific ICC staging system that has been the basis for further refinement, leading to the most current proposed system (Table 14.2) based on the TMN tumor nomenclature, in the American Joint Committee on Cancer seventh edition staging for ICC.[14] The American Joint Committee on Cancer/International Union Against Cancer

Table 14.2	
American Joint Committee on Cancer Seventh Edition Staging for ICC (AJCC/UICC 2010)	
TMN classification	
T1	Solitary tumor without vascular invasion[a]
T2a	Solitary tumor with vascular invasion[b]
T2b	Multiple tumors, with or without vascular invasion[a]
T3	Tumor perforating the visceral peritoneum or involving local extrahepatic structures by direct invasion
T4	Tumor with periductal invasion[b]
N0	No regional lymph node metastasis
N1	Regional lymph node metastasis[c]
M0	No distant metastasis
M1	Distant metastasis
Stage	
Stage I	T1 N0 M0
Stage II	T2 N0 M0
Stage III	T3 N0 M0
Stage IVA	T4 N0 M0, Any T N1 M0
Stage IV B	Any T, Any N M1

[a] Includes major vascular (portal or hepatic vein) and microvascular invasion.
[b] Includes tumors with periductal-infiltrating or mixed mass-forming and periductal-infiltrating growth pattern.
[c] Nodal involvement of the celiac, periaortic, or caval lymph nodes is considered to be distant metastasis (M1).
AJCC/UICC, American Joint Committee on Cancer (AJCC), International Union Against Cancer (UICC).

(AJCC/UICC) system recognizes three distinct morphologic groups of ICC: mass forming, periductal infiltrating, and mixed mass forming and periductal infiltrating. The presence of any periductal-infiltrating component is used to define a T4 staging. ICC staging uses tumor number and the presence of vascular invasion, but not tumor size. Other important prognostic factors include lymph node metastasis and resection margin status. The National Cancer Institute, National Cancer Registrars Association, Commission on Cancer, and the AJCC all currently use the AJCC seventh edition staging system. Its purpose is predominantly prognostic, however, and it will require subsequent validation. A staging system providing treatment guidance has not been developed and is needed for guidance on therapy selection.

TREATMENT MODALITIES

Surgery

Although surgical resection offers the only chance for cure, only approximately 30% of patients with cholangiocarcinoma are eligible for resection because of the advanced nature of the disease at the time of diagnosis.[2] Even for surgically resectable patients, survival prognosis is modest, however, with postsurgical 1-, 3-, and 5-year survival at 58%, 33%, and 33%, respectively.[14-15] The range of 5-year survival rates after successful surgical resection are between 14% and 40%, with up to 50% recurring locally, with the most common site of recurrence after resection in the liver.[14] The prognosis for patients with unresectable disease (70%) is even more dismal (5- to 8-month survival), making up the bulk of patients presenting with this disease[1-4] ICC generally presents in a more insidious advanced state than ECC, so prognosis is even worse comparatively as ECC.

Nonsurgical Treatments

Patients with unresectable ICC have a median survival of between 5 and 8 months.[14] There is a need, therefore, for more effective palliative therapies to treat patients with inoperable disease. Results from traditional systemic chemotherapy and external beam radiation have been disappointing in the past. Interventional treatments that have been used successfully in other primary liver tumors, notably HCC, have gained traction in the treatment of unresectable ICC. Given the positive impact these therapies have made on HCC patient survival, there has been a growing interest in using them for ICC. Although cholangiocarcinoma is not necessarily considered to be as hypervascular as HCC, it still derives its blood supply directly from the hepatic artery, making intra-arterial therapy an attractive treatment modality (FIGURE 14.5). These therapies may be classified into chemotherapy- and radiotherapy-based treatments and percutaneous thermal ablation. Chemotherapy-based treatments include transarterial chemoembolization, transcatheter arterial chemoinfusion and drug-eluting beads chemoembolization. Radiotherapy-based treatments include radioembolization with yttrium-90. Interpreting the results of studies involving intra-arterial therapies for unresectable ICC is difficult to perform because of the lack of large series, the heterogeneity of the patient population and study criteria, as well as the lack of accepted primary and secondary end points when dealing with intra-arterial locoregional therapies. Thermal ablations application in ICC have been anecdotal and modest to date due to the relative large sizes of most ICC at presentation and the technical

size limitations in available thermal ablation devices. Overall, treatment algorithms for nonsurgical patients with ICC have not reached national nor international consensus, and treatment choices currently are generally local and regionally based.

Systemic Chemotherapy

There are no standardized recommendations for systemic chemotherapy in unresectable ICC. Due to the relative small number of patients and the heterogeneous patient population in biliary tract cancers, randomized phase III studies examining systemic chemotherapy have been lacking. Phase II results with 5-fluorouracil (5-FU) has approximately a 10% to 15% response rate when provided alone.[16] Combination chemotherapy with 5-FU showed response rates between 15% and 55% and a median survival rate of 6 to 12 months. Gemcitabine showed a 30% response rate when used as a single agent. Gemcitabine combined with a platinum compound yielded a 30% to 50% response rate and 10- to 15-month survival.[17,18] Systemic chemotherapy trials include advanced bile duct cancers (ECC, hilar, and ICC), and studies frequently do not stratify response rates and overall survival by location of the bile duct pathology. When stratified specifically for ICC, six studies show results that differentiated ICC from other biliary tract cancers (Table 14.3). These studies reported response rates of 5.9% to 30% and overall survival from 5 to 10.3 months (from date of diagnosis).[19-26]

Transcatheter Arterial Chemoembolization

The concept of locoregional delivery of chemotherapy via the artery directly to tumors is quite attractive and has been used in the management of patients with colorectal cancer metastatic to the liver as well as patients with HCC. The rationale for transcatheter arterial chemoembolization (TACE) relies on the fact that tumors draw most of their blood supply from the hepatic artery and therefore can be targeted more effectively by using an intra-arterial approach. In this way, high doses of chemotherapy can be delivered directly to the cancer cells without damaging surrounding healthy liver tissue (supplied mostly by the portal vein). First described by Yamada in 1980, TACE exploits this dual blood supply of the liver for the treatment of liver tumors.[26] Additionally, embolic agents are then injected to further decrease drug washout by reducing arterial inflow to increase bioavailability of the drugs. Lipiodol, when injected intra-arterially (emulsified with cytotoxic agents), remains for a longer period in the tumor than in normal liver tissue because of the absence of Kupffer cells within the tumor cells and simultaneously acts as an emulsion carrier for the cytotoxic agents, thereby prolonging contact time between the drugs and the tumor cells.[27] Worldwide, doxorubicin is the most widely used single chemotherapeutic agent with this technique, yet in the United States the combination of cisplatin, doxorubicin, and mitomycin is the preferred drug regimen.[27] Current evidence includes seven studies (Table 14.4) utilizing TACE for the treatment of unresectable ICC. Controversy persists regarding the ideal cytotoxic agent and embolic agent. Given these encouraging results in HCC, TACE became the logical treatment of other primary liver cancers, such as unresectable ICC, which led to the publication of early series by Tanaka et al. (chemoinfusion)[28] and Burger et al. (conventional TACE).[29] One of the earliest groups to adopt conventional TACE (doxorubicin, cisplatin, and mitomycin C, Embospheres) was Burger et al.,[30] who treated 17 jconsecutive

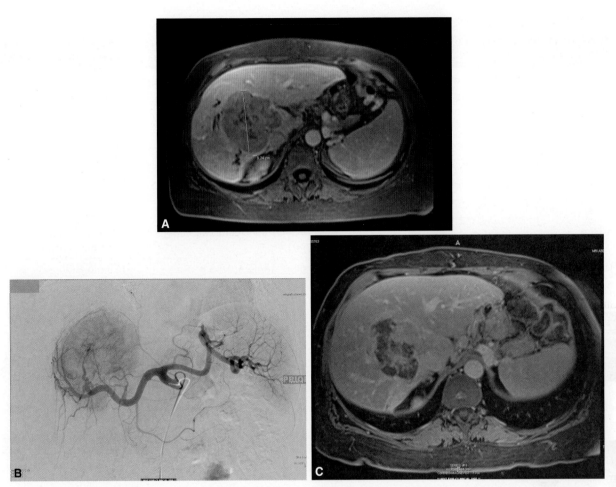

FIGURE 14.5 A. Gadolinium-enhanced postcontrast T1-weighted MRI through the liver showing a heterogenous mass in the right lobe of the liver with resultant left lobe atrophy and a mass distending the liver capsule. **B.** Intraprocedural chemoembolization angiographic image showing hepatic artery hypervascular tumor blush, consistent with a mass seen on MRI. **C.** Posttreatment early follow-up MRI after 4 weeks postchemoembolization showing a mass with loss of enhancement postgadolinium (EASL criteria >75%), comprising necrotic nonviable tissue, and reduction of size and mass effect.

Table 14.3				
Published Series for ICC Patients Treated with Systemic Chemotherapy				
Investigators	Number of patients	Regimen	Response rates (CR+PR)	Overall survival (OS)
Lee et al. (2004)	20	Epirubicin, cisplatin, ?5-FU	10	5
Feisthammel et al. (2007)	17	Irinotecan + 5-FU	5.9%	5.5
Kim et al. (2008)	38	Gemcitabine ± platinums	16.7	7.6
		vs		
	54	Fluoropyrimidines ± platinums	19.5	7.6
Takezako et al. (2008)	39	Cisplatin, epirubicin + 5-FU	10	9.1
Nehls et al. (2008)	18	Capecitabine + oxaliplatin	0	5.2
Sasaki et al. (2009)	14	Gemcitabine + S-1	28.6	10.3

S-1 is an oral fluoropyrimidine prodrug, which is widely used for various solid tumors. 5-FU, 5-fluorouracil.

	Number of		Patient factors: child-pugh	
Investigators	patients	Treatment	score/ECOG	Median survival
Burger et al. (2005)	17	Doxorubicin, cisplatin, mitomycin C	88% (15/17) A 12% (2/17) B	23 mo (from diagnosis)
Kirchoff et al. (2005)	8	Cisplatin, doxorubicin, starch microspheres + systemic chemotherapy (gemcitabine)		12 mo 7 mo TTP
Vogl et al. (2006)	8	IA chemotherapy (gemcitabine) and IA starch microspheres	17 ICC 7 pancreatic cancer	20.2 mo 6.8 mo TTP (No spheres = 13.5 mo , 4.2 mo)
Herber et al. (2007)	15	Lipiodol and mitomycin C – no embolic agents	14/15 A, 1/15 B	16.3 mo
Gusani et al. (2008)	42	Gemcitabine + cisplatin, oxaliplatin/combinations	42% extrahepatic disease	9.1 mo
Kim et al. (2008)	36[1]	Cisplatin and lipiodol	82% A 9% B	12 mo
Soulen et al. (2011)	62	Doxorubicin, cisplatin, mitomycin C	ECOG 0 = 89% ECOG 1 = 10% ECOG 2 = 1%	20 mo (from diagnosis) 15 mo (from TACE) Combined systemic chemotherapy vs. TACE alone = 28 mo vs. 16 mo

Table 14.4

Published Evidence from After Conventional Chemoembolization Treatment (TACE) for ICC

TTP, time to progression.

patients with unresectable ICC. The majority of the patients had preserved liver functions (15/17 Child A, 2/17 B) and performance status (14/17 ECOG 0-1). The median survival for 17 patients treated with TACE was 23 months and TACE was well-tolerated overall. Moreover, tumors were noted to be hypervascular (FIGURES 14.1 through 14.3), confirming ICC as a suitable target for intra-arterial therapies.

In one of the largest TACE studies to date, Soulen et al. utilized 3 conventional drug techniques on 62 consecutive ICC patients.[30] Overall they achieved median survival of 20 months (from date of diagnosis), with mean time to progression of 8 months and 28% free of progression at 12 months, and 1-, 2-, and 5-year survival of 75%, 39%, and 17%, respectively. Interestingly, the subgroup who received systemic chemotherapy had improved overall survival (median 28 months vs. 16 months) when compared to the TACE-alone group and suggesting potential synergy between TACE and systemic chemotherapy. Overall, evidence to date suggests that TACE confers survival benefits from 9 to 23 months.[30–35]

Chemoinfusion

Transcatheter arterial chemoinfusion (TACI) describes catheter-based intra-arterial therapy that delivers high concentrations of chemotherapeutic agents directly to liver tumor tissues followed by no embolization, which differentiates it from traditional TACE and systemic chemotherapy. TACI is analogous

to arterial port infusion therapy previously popularized for the treatment of hepatic arterial infusion (HAI) in liver colorectal metastases. Tanaka et al.[29] reported the first experience using intra-arterial approach to treating ICC in 2002. The results of this study provided credence for the concept of delivering chemotherapeutic drugs via the hepatic artery in ICC. An arterial chemotherapeutic infusion therapy was used via a percutaneous implanted port system (femoral or subclavian access) with the tip of the catheter embedded in the hepatic artery or gastroduodenal artery. Fixation of the catheter tip required complex coil or glue embolization to ensure safe fixation. In total, 11 patients with unresectable ICC were treated with a port infusion of fluorouracil-based regimen combined with a variety of other agents (doxorubicin, mitomycin C, cisplastin). Indeed, by achieving a mean survival of 26 months (cumulative 1-, 2-, and 3-year, 91%, 51%, and 20%, respectively). Because this study used mean survival rather than median survival, a direct comparison with other studies in the literature is difficult. Approximately three other chemoinfusion series have been published (Table 14.5), resulting in survival benefits ranging between 12 and 26 months.[37–39]

Chemoembolization with Drug-Eluting Beads

The emergence of new concepts in drug delivery has led to significant improvements in chemoembolotherapy. In 2005, a new type of drug-eluting microsphere allowing controlled

Table 14.5

Published Studies for Treatment of ICC with Arterial Chemoinfusion Therapy

Investigator	Number of patients	Treatment	Patient factors: child-pugh score/ ECOG	Radiologic response CR+PR	Median survival
Tanaka et al. (2002)	11	5-FU, with adriamycin, epirubicin, cisplatin	7/11 extrahepatic	64% WHO	26 mo (mean) 14.5 mo PFS
Vogl et al. (2006)	9	IA chemotherapy (gemcitabine) and IA starch microspheres	17 ICC 7 pancreatic cancer		20.2 mo 6.8 mo TTP (No spheres = 13.5 mo, 4.2 mo)
Kim et al. (2008)	36[1]	Cisplatin and lipiodol	82% A 9% B	10/42 (23%) RECIST 17/42 (40%) EASL	12 mo
Shitara et al. (2008)	20	Mitomycin C and starch microspheres ports	ECOG 0/1/2 3/12/5	50% RECIST	14.1 mo TTP = 8.3 mo

PFS, progression-free survival.

drug release was launched. The drug-eluting properties of these microspheres allow prolonged and controlled release of the chemotherapeutic agent into the tumor bed, thereby achieving greater drug concentration within the tumor and minimizing systemic toxicity.[39] The potential benefits of such spheres are great because a sustainable release of chemotherapy over time could have a greater effect on tumor kill. There are currently two main types of microspheres: DC Bead microspheres (Biocompatibles, UK) and Quadrasphere (Hepaspher for Europe) microspheres (Biosphere Medical, Inc). These microspheres are nonbiodegradable polyvinyl alcohol (PVA) microspheres that are CE mark approved for the treatment of malignant hypervascular tumors and loaded with doxorubicin. Since its introduction, TACE with drug-eluting beads has shown encouraging results in the treatment of unresectable HCC.

There have been three small studies to date using this improved concept of TACE with DEB in the treatment of ICC, loading different chemotherapy agents (doxorubicin, oxaliplatin, irinotecan) in the reported studies. Despite the small sample sizes, there were impressive response rates,

and overall outcomes ranged between 13 and 30 months.[40,41] The most recent series by Schiffman et al. (irinotecan loaded DEB-TACE)[42] treated 24 patients with bulky tumors (mean size 11.5 cm) who achieved median overall survival (OS) of 30 months. In this cohort, patients who had previously received systemic chemotherapy were compared with historical controls who were treated with chemotherapy alone. The favorable outcome for the combination DEB+ chemotherapy group (30 months vs. 12.7 months for chemotherapy alone) again suggests that there may be a potential synergistic action between intra-arterial therapies and systemic chemotherapy. It is becoming apparent that the drug-eluting technology could play an increasing role in the management of patients with ICC (Table 14.6).

Radioembolization with Ytrium-90 Microspheres

Traditionally, whole-liver external-beam radiation therapy hashad limited use in the treatment of primary liver cancers because the liver parenchyma is radiation sensitiveand is unable to tolerate the radiation dose required to achievetumoricidal effects. The concept of radioembolization forliver cancer

Table 14.6

Published Evidence from After Drug-Eluting Chemoembolization (DEB-TACE) For ICC

Investigator	Number of patients	Treatment	Patient factors: child-pugh score/ECOG	Median survival (OS)
Aliberti et al. (2008)	11	Doxorubicin-eluting beads		13 mo
Poggi et al. (2009)	9/11	Oxaliplatin-eluting beads + chemo vs chemo alone	A 77%, B 13% A 81%, B 9%, C 9%	30 mo (DEB + chemotherapy) 12.7 mo (chemotherapy alone)
Schiffmann et al. (2011)	24	Irinotecan-eluting beads	Median size = 11.5 cm	17.5 mo

Table 14.7

Published Evidence for Treatment of ICC with ^{90}Y Radioembolization

Investigator	Number of patients	Patient Factors: child-pugh score/ECOG	Radiologic response CR+PR	Median survival
Ibrahim et al. (2008)	24	ECOG 0%–42%, 1%–50%, 2%–8%	27% WHO 77% EASL	14.9 mo
Saxena et al. (2009)	25	ECOG 0%–60%, 1%–28%, 2%–12%	24% RECIST	9.3 mo

consists of delivering internal radiation selectively and deeply within the tumor bed to maximize the efficacy of the treatment and to avoid injuring the normal liver parenchyma. Radioembolization delivers small radioactive (yttrium-90) particles deeply within the tumor bed. There are two available types of radioactive microspheres: ^{90}Y-impregnated glass microspheres (Theraspheres, MDS Nordion, Ottawa, Ontario, Canada; diameter 25±10 mm) and resin-based microspheres (SIR-Spheres, SIRtex, New South Wales, Australia; diameter 29 to 35 mm). Based on promising results obtained in other types of liver cancer, radioembolization has also been used in a limited fashion to treat patients with ICC.[43,44] Two groups recently reported their respective experiences with ^{90}Y radioembolization in the treatment of ICC. Ibrahim et al. treated 24 patients with unresectable ICC with glass-based ^{90}Y microspheres (TheraSpheres) with a target dose of 120 Gray, using a bilobar approach with two separate treatments 1 to 2 months apart. The overall median survival was 14.9 months (from the time of the first procedure). Objective tumor response rates (WHO) were documented in 19 patients (86%). Using resin-based ^{90}Y microspheres (SIR-Spheres), Saxena et al. treated 25 patients with unresectable ICC. The overall median survival from the time of the first procedure was 9.3 months (20.4 months from diagnosis), and 1-, 2-, and 3-year survival of 40%, 27%, and 13%, respectively, was

reported. Factors associated with improved survival included good performance status and peripheral tumor type. A radiologic response (RECIST) was seen in 72% of the patients. The most common clinical toxicities were fatigue (64%) and self-limiting abdominal pain (40%) (Table 14.7).

Thermal Ablation

The use of percutaneous thermal ablation in ICC is limited. In patients who are not candidates for surgical resection due to poor liver function or prohibitive comorbidities, thermal ablation initially appears to be a good option. Ffor thermal ablation to be considered, however, the ICC lesion needs to be small (≤3–5 cm) and located away from major vascular or biliary structures. Most patients with ICC, however, will usually either be candidates for surgical resection or will present with large tumors. Three recently published thermal ablation studies in ICC patients (two with radiofrequency ablation [RFA], one with microwave) (Table 14.8),[46–48] albeit with small cohorts, show promising outcomes (10–38 months mean overall survival). These results represent a carefully selected group of ICC, however, with very small primary lesions (1.9–3.4 cm mean diameter). Typically, ICC patients present with much larger lesions and more advanced stages. The largest of the three series, Kim et al.[47] report their experience with treating 13 ICC patients

Table 14.8

Published Evidence from After Thermal Ablation for ICC

Investigator	Number of patients	Treatment	Patient factors: stage/tumor/ECOG	Median survival (OS)
Carrafiello et al. (2010)	6 17 tumors	RFA	Mean size = 3.4 cm	OS = 20 mo
Kim et al. (2011)	13 17 tumors	RFA	Mean size = 1.9 cm 88% < 5 cm; 59% < 3 cm Extrahepatic = 7% (1/13) Stage 1 (61%) Stage 2 (23%), 3 (7%), 4 (7%)	OS = 38.5 mo MTP = 32.2 mo 1, 3, 5 mo = 85%, 51%, 15%
Yu et al. (2011)	15 24 tumors	Microwave ablation	Mean size = 3.2 cm 40% extrahepatic disease	OS = 10 mo 6, 12, 24 mo = 78%, 60%, 60%

MTP,

(17 lesions), with mean size of 1.9 cm (59% less than 3 cm), and early disease presentation (84% stage 1 or 2), median overall survival (38.5 months), and 1-, 3-, and 5-year survival of 85%, 51%, and 51%, respectively. Ablations for ICC may play a future greater role in the treatment of ICC although widespread adoption is uncertain.

CONCLUSION/FUTURE

ICC remains a relatively poorly understood malignancy despite its recent increase in incidence and this increase is expected to continue. Some progress has been made in unlocking the differences of ICC as compared to hilar cholangiocarcinoma, ECC, and HCC. The greater understanding of the pathophysiology, its risk factors, genotypes, phenotypes, and recent formulation of its own staging system hopefully will allow clinicians greater tools to improve the outcomes of a dismal disease. Coupled with the advent of still-palliative but effective treatment methods, such as TACE, DEB-TACE, ^{90}Y, and ablation, has provided viable palliative treatment alternatives to patients who, thus far, if unresectable, were offered few options. ICC remains a complex disease that presents the clinician with a host of diagnostic and therapeutic challenges and is therefore best managed by a multidisciplinary team (oncology, gastrointestinal surgery, transplant surgery, diagnostic and interventional radiology). Combination therapies may provide some future strategies to further improve the outcomes of ICC patients.

REFERENCES

1. Shaib Y, El-Serag HB. The epidemiology of cholangiocarcinoma. *Semin Liver Dis* 2004;24(2):115–125.
2. Shaib YH, Davila JA, McGlynn K, et al. Rising incidence of intrahepatic cholangiocarcinoma in the United States: a true increase? *J Hepatol* 2004;40(3):472–477.
3. Patel T. Increasing incidence and mortality of primary intrahepatic cholangiocarcinoma in the United States. *Hepatology* 2001;33(6):1353–1357.
4. Uenishi T, Hirohashi K, Kubo S, et al. Clinicopathological factors predicting outcome after resection of massforming intrahepatic cholangiocarcinoma. *Br J Surg* 2001;88(7):969–974.
5. Thongprasert S. The role of chemotherapy in cholangiocarcinoma. *Ann Oncol* 2005;16(suppl 2):ii, 93–96.
6. Mazhar D, Stebbing J, Bower M. Chemotherapy for advanced cholangiocarcinoma: what is standard treatment? *Future Oncol* 2006;2(4): 509–514.
7. Chung YE, Kim MJ, Park YN, et al. Varying appearances of cholangiocarcinoma: radiologic-pathologic correlation. *Radiographics* 2009;29(3):683–700.
8. Parkin DM, Ohshima H, Srivatanakul P, et al. Cholangiocarcinoma: epidemiology, mechanisms of carcinogenesis and prevention. *Cancer Epidemiol Biomarkers Prev* 1993;2(6):537–544.
9. Nomoto K, Tsuneyama K, Cheng C, et al. Intrahepatic cholangiocarcinoma arising in cirrhotic liver frequently expressed p63-positive basal/stem-cell phenotype. *Pathol Res Pract* 2006;202(2):71–76.
10. Lee JD, Yang WI, Park YN, et al. Different glucose uptake and glycolytic mechanisms between hepatocellular carcinoma and intrahepatic mass-forming cholangiocarcinoma with increased (18)F-FDG uptake. *J Nucl Med* 2005;46(10):1753–1759.
11. Chen M-F. Peripheral cholangiocarcinoma (cholangiocellular carcinoma): clinical features, diagnosis and treatment. *J Gastroenterol Hepatol* 1999;14:1144–1148.
12. Poultsides GA, Zhu AX, Choti MA, et al. Intrahepatic cholangiocarcinoma. *Surg Clin North Am* 2010;90(4):817–837.
13. Okabayashi T, Yamamoto J, Kosuge T, et al. A new staging system for massforming intrahepatic cholangiocarcinoma: analysis of preoperative and postoperative variables. *Cancer* 2001;92(9):2374–2383.
14. Edge S, Byrd D, Compton C, et al. *AJCC Cancer Staging Manual.* 7th ed. New York, NY: Springer-Verlag; 2010.
15. Tamandl D, Herberger B, Gruenberger B, et al. Influence of hepatic resection margin on recurrence and survival in intrahepatic cholangiocarcinoma. *Ann Surg Oncol* 2008;15(10):2787–2794.
16. Nathan H, Aloia TA, Vauthey JN, et al. A proposed staging system for intrahepatic cholangiocarcinoma. *Ann Surg Oncol* 2009;16(1):14–22.
17. Eckel F, Schmid RM. Chemotherapy in advanced biliary tract carcinoma: a pooled analysis of clinical trials. *Br J Cancer* 2007;96(6):896–902.
18. Aljiffry M, Walsh MJ, Molinari M. Advances in diagnosis, treatment and palliation of cholangiocarcinoma: 1990–2009. *World J Gastroenterol* 2009;15:4240–4262.
19. Valle J, Wasan H, Palmer DH, et al. Cisplatin plus gemcitabine versus gemcitabine for biliary tract cancer. *N Engl J Med* 2010;362:1273–1281.
20. Rao S, Cunningham D, Hawkins RE, et al. Phase III study of 5FU, etoposide and leucovorin (FELV) compared to epirubicin, cisplatin and 5FU (ECF) in previously untreated patients with advanced biliary cancer. *Br J Cancer* 2005;92:1650–1654.
21. Feisthammel J, Schoppmeyer K, Mossner J, et al. Irinotecan with 5-FU/FA in advanced biliary tract adenocarcinomas: a multicenter phase II trial. *Am J Clin Oncol* 2007;30:319–324.
22. Lee MA, Woo IS, Kang JH, et al. Epirubicin, cisplatin, and protracted infusion of 5-FU (ECF) in advanced intrahepatic cholangiocarcinoma. *J Cancer Res Clin Oncol* 2004;130:346–350.
23. Nehls O, Oettle H, Hartmann JT, et al. Capecitabine plus oxaliplatin as first-line treatment in patients with advanced biliary system adenocarcinoma: a prospective multicentre phase II trial. *Br J Cancer* 2008;98:309–315.
24. Sasaki T, Isayama H, Nakai Y, et al. Multicenter, phase II study of gemcitabine and S-1 combination chemotherapy in patients with advanced biliary tract cancer. *Cancer Chemother Pharmacol* 2010;65(6):1101–1107.
25. Sasaki T, Isayama H, Nakai Y, et al. Multicenter, phase II study of gemcitabine and S-1 combination chemotherapy in patients with advanced biliary tract cancer. *Cancer Chemother Pharmacol* 2010;65(6):1101–1107.
26. Takezako Y, Okusaka T, Ueno H, et al. Phase II study of cisplatin, epirubicin and continuous infusion of 5-fluorouracil in patients with advanced intrahepatic cholangiocellular carcinoma (ICC). *Hepatogastroenterology* 2008;55:1380–1384.
27. Yamada R, Nakatsuka H, Nakamura K, et al. Hepatic artery embolization in 32 patients with unresectable hepatoma. *Osaka City Med J* 1980;26(2):81–96.
28. Geschwind JF. Chemoembolization for hepatocellular carcinoma: where does the truth lie? *J Vasc Interv Radiol* 2002;13:991–994.
29. Tanaka N, Yamakado K, Nakatsuka A, et al. Arterial chemoinfusion therapy through an implanted port system for patients with unresectable intrahepatic cholangiocarcinoma—initial experience. *Eur J Radiol* 2002;41:42–48.
30. Burger I, Hong K, Schulick R, et al. Transcatheter arterial chemoembolization (TACE) in unresectable cholangiocarcinoma—initial experience in a single institution. *J Vasc Interv Radiol* 2005;16(3):339–345.
31. Kiefer MV, Albert M, McNally M, et al. Chemoembolization of intrahepatic cholangiocarcinoma with cisplatinum, doxorubicin, mitomycin C, ethiodol, and polyvinyl alcohol: a 2-center study. *Cancer* 2011;117(7):1498–1505.
32. Kirchhoff T, Zender L, Merkesdal S, et al. Initial experience from a combination of systemic and regional chemotherapy in the treatment of patients with nonresectable cholangiocarcinoma in the liver. *World J Gastroenterol* 2005;11(8):1091–1095.
33. Vogl TJ, Schwarz W, Eichler K, et al. Hepatic intraarterial chemotherapy with gemcitabine in patients with unresectable cholangiocarcinomas and liver metastases of pancreatic cancer: a clinical study on maximum tolerable dose and treatment efficacy. *J Cancer Res Clin Oncol* 2006;132(11):745–755.
34. Herber S, Otto G, Schneider J, et al. Transarterial chemoembolization (TACE) for inoperable intrahepatic cholangiocarcinoma. *Cardiovasc Intervent Radiol* 2007;30(6):1156–1165.
35. Gusani NJ, Balaa FK, Steel JL, et al. Treatment of unresectable cholangiocarcinoma with gemcitabine-based transcatheter arterial chemoembolization (TACE): a single-institution experience. *J Gastrointest Surg* 2008;12(1):129–137.
36. Kim JH, Yoon HK, Sung KB, et al. Transcatheter arterial chemoembolization or chemoinfusion for unresectable intrahepatic cholangiocarcinoma: clinical efficacy and factors influencing outcomes. *Cancer* 2008;113(7):1614–1622.
37. Vogl TJ, Schwarz W, Eichler K, et al. Hepatic intraarterial chemotherapy with gemcitabine in patients with unresectable cholangiocarcinomas and liver metastases of pancreatic cancer: a clinical study on maximum tolerable dose and treatment efficacy. *J Cancer Res Clin Oncol* 2006;132(11):745–755.

38. Kim JH, Yoon HK, Sung KB, et al. Transcatheter arterial chemoembolization or chemoinfusion for unresectable intrahepatic cholangiocarcinoma: clinical efficacy and factors influencing outcomes. *Cancer* 2008;113(7):1614–1622.

39. Shitara K, Ikami I, Munakata M, et al. Hepatic arterial infusion of mitomycin C with degradable starch microspheres for unresectable intrahepatic cholangiocarcinoma. *Clin Oncol* 2008;20(3):241–246.

40. Hong K, Khwaja A, Liapi E, et al. New intra-arterial drug delivery system for the treatment of liver cancer: pre-clinical assessment in a rabbit model of liver cancer. *Clin Cancer Res* 2006;1298:2563–2567.

41. Aliberti C, Benea G, Tilli M, et al. Chemoembolization (TACE) of unresectable intrahepatic cholangiocarcinoma with slow-release doxorubicin-eluting beads: preliminary results. *Cardiovasc Intervent Radiol* 2008;31(5):883–888.

42. Poggi G, Amatu A, Montagna B, et al. OEM-TACE: a new therapeutic approach in unresectable intrahepatic cholangiocarcinoma. *Cardiovasc Intervent Radiol* 2009;32(6):1187–1192.

43. Schiffman SC, Metzger T, Dubel G,et al. Precision hepatic arterial irinotecan therapy in the treatment of unresectable intrahepatic cholangiocellular carcinoma: optimal tolerance and prolonged overall survival. *Ann Surg Oncol* 2011;18(2):431–438.

44. Ibrahim SM, Mulcahy MF, Lewandowski RJ, et al. Treatment of unresectable cholangiocarcinoma using yttrium-90 microspheres: results from a pilot study. *Cancer* 2008;113(8):2119–2128.

45. Saxena A, Bester L, Chua TC, et al. Yttrium-90 radiotherapy for unresectable intrahepatic cholangiocarcinoma: a preliminary assessment of this novel treatment option. *Ann Surg Oncol* 2009.

46. Carrafiello G, Laganà D, Cotta E, et al. Radiofrequency ablation of intrahepatic cholangiocarcinoma: preliminary experience. *Cardiovasc Intervent Radiol* 2010;33(4):835–839.

47. Carrafiello G, Laganà D, Cotta E, et al. Radiofrequency ablation of intrahepatic cholangiocarcinoma: preliminary experience. *Cardiovasc Intervent Radiol* 2010;33(4):835–839.

48. Yu MA, Liang P, Yu XL,et al. Sonography-guided percutaneous microwave ablation of intrahepatic primary cholangiocarcinoma. *Eur J Radiol* 2011;80(2):548–552.

CHAPTER 15

Biliary Tract Cancers: Extrahepatic Management

TARUN SABHARWAL and ANDREAS ADAM

INTRODUCTION

Interventional radiologists first became involved in the management of malignant obstruction of the biliary tree in the late 1960s, when Kaude et al.[1] introduced nonsurgical biliary drainage. Since then, improved diagnostic imaging techniques, significant developments in interventional radiology, and the results of clinical trials have revolutionized and clearly defined the role of percutaneous biliary interventions.

Percutaneous transhepatic cholangiography (PTC) is now rarely employed for purely diagnostic purposes and has been largely replaced by noninvasive imaging techniques, such as ultrasonography (US), computed tomography, magnetic resonance cholangiography (MRC), and endoscopic retrograde cholangiography (ERC). PTC is now reserved for problematic cases and as a prelude to percutaneous intervention.

BILIARY DRAINAGE FOR MALIGNANT STRICTURES

Biliary obstruction is potentially fatal because of the adverse pathologic effects including depressed immunity, impaired phagocytic activity, reduced Kupffer cell function, and paucity of bile salts reaching the gut, with consequent endotoxemia, septicemia, and renal failure. Most patients with malignant obstructive jaundice caused by carcinoma of the gallbladder, carcinoma of the pancreas, and cholangiocarcinoma present with advanced disease[2,3] and only 20% to 30% of such tumors are resectable at the time of diagnosis.[2,4] Palliation of the malignant obstruction relieves the patient of itching and jaundice, reduces the risk of infection and septicemia, and generally improves the quality of life. Surgical, endoscopic, and interventional radiologic (IR) percutaneous techniques are available for biliary drainage. Because of the lower morbidity and mortality associated with ERC and percutaneous transhepatic biliary drainage (PTBD) compared to surgical methods, surgery is now rarely employed for palliative purposes.

Because most patients undergo endoscopic retrograde cholangiopancreaticogram (ERCP) during the diagnostic workup for obstructive jaundice endoscopic insertion of biliary endoprostheses is performed more often than percutaneous drainage. If ERCP demonstrates a malignant stricture, an endoprosthesis can be inserted immediately after cholangiography. In patients with strictures below the hilum of the liver, endoscopic drainage

achieves a high rate of success, is associated with fewer complications than percutaneous intervention, and avoids the discomfort of a percutaneous biliary catheter.

The majority of strictures of the mid and lower common bile ducts, which are mainly caused by carcinoma of the head of the pancreas, can be drained effectively by the endoscopic approach.[5] Many hilar biliary strictures are difficult to treat endoscopically, however, and are best dealt with interventional radiologic techniques.[6] The indications for PTBD are summarized in Table 15.1.

Preoperative Percutaneous Transhepatic Biliary Drainage

The practice of PTBD prior to surgery is controversial. It has not been shown to decrease surgical morbidity or mortality. It is advocated by some surgeons in certain circumstances before curative resection, however, as a method of correcting metabolic derangements produced by biliary obstruction prior to surgery. Either internal/external biliary drainage catheters or more plastic stents are inserted 2 to 6 weeks prior to elective surgery. Some surgeons favor PTBD because the biliary catheters are easy to locate at surgery, particularly during difficult dissections of lesions at the hepatic hilum.[6]

ROLE OF IMAGING BEFORE PALLIATIVE BILIARY DRAINAGE

Because the method of management of malignant biliary obstruction depends on the resectability of the underlying tumor, patients should undergo accurate staging of the disease. One of the important goals of preoperative imaging is establishing whether there is vascular invasion by a tumor at the hepatic hilum. Previously, angiography was used to identify the vascular anatomy prior to surgery in carcinoma gallbladder[7] and hilar cholangiocarcinoma.[8–10] Recently, dual-phase helical computed tomography (CT) has been used to evaluate vascular invasion in hilar tumors[11,12] and may soon be able to provide all the information required to comprehensively evaluate each patient for resectability.[2]

High-quality three-dimensional (3D) reconstruction images made possible by helical CT are uniquely suitable for the depiction of the complex anatomy of the biliary tree.

Table 15.1
Indications for Percutaneous Transheptic Biliary Drainage
1. To manage infectious complications of biliary obstruction, such as cholangitis and sepsis
2. To relieve obstructive jaundice when an endoscopic retrograde approach fails or is not indicated
3. Preoperative decompression and stent placement to assist in surgical manipulation (controversial)
4. To gain access to the biliary system to perform other bile duct interventions, such as biopsy, stent placement, and transhepatic brachytherapy for cholangiocarcinoma

Three-dimensional reconstructions can be produced successfully by taking advantage of the negative contrast effect of low-attenuation bile in the dilated ducts relative to the adjacent enhanced liver[13] and can determine the level and cause of biliary obstruction.[14,15] CT is very helpful in the identification of variant ductal anatomy and in the selection of the most appropriate duct for drainage (FIGURE 15.1).

Magnetic resonance imaging (MRI) performs as well as CT in the demonstration of direct spread of the tumor to the liver and in the detection of hepatic metastases. Visualization of intrahepatic bile ducts on MRI depends on the size of the ducts, the concentration of bile, motion artifact, and periportal high signal. CT and US are more sensitive than MRI in detecting intrahepatic bile duct dilatation. Magnetic resonance cholangiopancreaticography (MRCP) has been a very useful development for imaging the biliary tree.[16–18] MRCP can accurately define the extent of ductal involvement in patients with malignant hilar and perihilar obstruction. Ductal dilatation, strictures, and anatomic variation are well depicted by this technique and this ability makes this modality well suited for planning the optimal therapeutic approach for patients with biliary obstruction.

In suspected malignant biliary obstruction, percutaneous fine-needle aspiration (FNA) or biopsy can used for cytologic or histologic confirmation of the presence of a malignant tumor. Cytologic study is positive in roughly 50% of the patients with cholangiocarcinoma, although the reported sensitivity varies widely.

If FNA fails, percutaneous biopsy can be done by cholangiographic or US guidance. Alternatively the cholangiographic tract could also be used to obtain brushings or a biopsy using forceps, or a cardiac bioptome (FIGURE 15.2).

Preparation for PTBD

Blood Tests

Coagulation profile: The International normalized ratio (INR) should be less than 1.5. Vitamin K, fresh frozen plasma, and platelets (as needed) should be administered to correct any coagulopathy.

Liver function tests: Serum bilirubin and alkaline phosphatase levels should be checked to obtain baseline values (an elevated alkaline phosphatase level, even in the setting of a near-normal bilirubin indicates a low-grade obstruction).

Baseline renal function: Blood urea and creatinine should be checked, especially before administering preprocedure nephrotoxic antibiotics. IV fluids should be administered during drainage as a prophylactic measure against hepatorenal failure.

Informed Consent

The procedure should be explained completely to the patient, outlining the risks with specific attention to sepsis and bleeding.

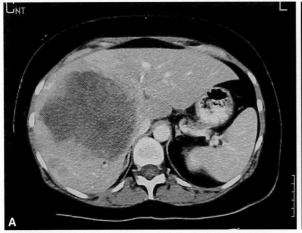 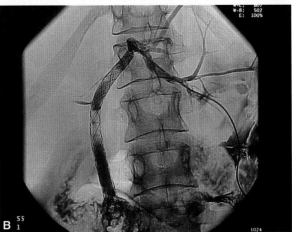

FIGURE 15.1 A. CT scan shows a large right-sided tumor and therefore the left lobe was chosen for PTC. **B.** Poststenting the left duct.

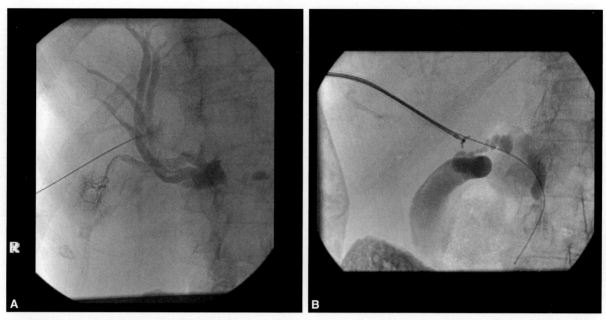

FIGURE 15.2 A. Percutaneous cholangiogram in a suspected cholangiocarcinoma patient. **B.** Myocardial biopsy needle used via PTC route and through 7 French sheath

Prophylactic Antibiotics

Appropriate antibiotics are administered to avoid biliary sepsis because of the high incidence of bacterial colonization of obstructed biliary systems. The spectrum of antibiotic coverage must include both gram-positive and gram-negative organisms. *Escherichia coli* is the most common organism involved; enterococci, klebsiella species, and *Streptococcus viridans* are other frequently observed organisms. The antibiotics should be continued for 24 to 72 hours following the procedure. Antibiotic therapy should be modified according to the results of positive bile or blood cultures.

Sedation/Analgesia

Biliary procedures are most often performed under conscious sedation (midazolam and fentanyl) with liberal infiltration of local anesthetic at the site and up to the capsule of the liver. Use of longer-acting local anesthetics may help to provide long postprocedure pain relief. Intercostal blocks have also been used and in some cases general anaesthetic is required.

Skin Preparation

It is best to prepare a wide area, which will permit access to the biliary system from the left and right sides, as needed.Contraindications for PTBD are summarized in Table 15.2.

Biliary Drainage Procedure

Technique

External Drainage

A percutaneous transhepatic cholangiogram (PTC) is performed prior to biliary drainage to define the biliary anatomy. A 22-gauge needle is inserted into the liver immediately anterior to the midaxillary line and advanced horizontally to the lateral

Table 15.2
Contraindications for Percutaneous Transheptic Biliary Drainage

- Uncorrectable bleeding diathesis.

- Large volume of ascites (relative; procedure may be difficult with potential for bile peritonitis. Consider a left-sided approach and/or insert an ascitic drain).

- Segmental isolated intrahepatic obstructions that do not cause significant symptoms should not be drained. Bacterial contamination usually occurs when an isolated ductal system is accessed. As a consequence of this contamination, it is often impossible to withdraw drainage even if the drainage is not required clinically. Thus a patient could be left with a permanent, unwanted, and potentially problematic drainage catheter.

- Patients with multiple obstructed and isolated biliary segments, often caused by numerous hepatic metastases. In these patients, drainage is often ineffective in relieving symptoms and can therefore be avoided.

- Unsafe access route because of either interposed bowel or lung.

border of the vertebral column (FIGURE 15.3). Dilated ducts are located by withdrawing the needle and injecting contrast medium or aspirating until bile is obtained. The aspiration method has the advantage of avoiding a large stain of parenchymal contrast if several passes are required. If the ducts are not dilated, the aspiration method is less effective and the injection method should be used. Some radiologists puncture the bile ducts using ultrasound guidance. Once a duct has been located, undiluted contrast medium is injected until the obstructed biliary system is outlined (FIGURE 15.4). A tilting table is helpful to convey contrast to the lower common bile duct (CBD). In many patients with obstruction of the CBD, flow of contrast medium may appear to stop immediately below the hilum, creating a false impression of hilar obstruction; tilting the fluoroscopy table is the best way of demonstrating the lower CBD in such cases.

Although it may be possible to use the duct catheterized by the PTC needle for drainage, the duct is usually at an angle to the needle track, which causes difficulty in cathetermanipulations, or is close to the liver hilum, which increases the risk of complications (vascular injury). In most cases it is best to perform a second, peripheral puncture of a suitable duct with a horizontal course (FIGURE 15.5). Lateral screening using a C-arm is very helpful, although not essential, for localization of the duct in the anterior-posterior plane.

Although bile duct catheterization can be achieved with standard 18-gauge needles and guidewires, most radiologists use one of several minimally invasive access sets, such as the Accustick set (Meditech, Boston Scientific Corp, MA) (FIGURE 15.6) or the Neff set (William Cook, Europe), for this purpose. These systems allow the radiologist to drain the biliary tree using an initial puncture with a 21- or 22-gauge needle followed by sequential changes of increasingly larger guidewires and catheters.[19] The use of suchsystems enables small ducts to beselected for drainage and probably reduces the risk of complications, such as hemobilia and bile leakage. The final result of either method is the

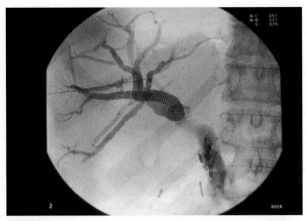

FIGURE 15.4 Undiluted contrast medium injected until the obstructed biliary system is outlined

placement of a catheter with several side holes deep in the biliary tree. At this stage the tip of the catheter lies above the obstructing lesion, which is referred to as external biliary drainage. The catheter is connected to a gravity drainage bag and the tube is secured to the skin to prevent inadvertent removal.

External-Internal Drainage

External-internal drainage refers to percutaneous catheter drainage of the bile ducts with the catheter passed through the stricture so that side holes are placed above and below the obstructing lesion. This offers increased stability compared with external drainage and also allows drainage of bile into the duodenum with the advantages of improved fluid and electrolyte balance. For these reasons, most radiologists aim for internal-external drainage if possible at the time of initial PBD. Most strictures can be catheterized with modern angled-tip catheters and hydrophilic guidewires. Occasionally, a stricture is so tight that it cannot be traversed. In this situation, an external catheter should be inserted. After a few days of external drainage, a channel through the stricture usually appears due to resolution of tissue edema, which can be negotiated by the radiologist at a second session.

Some patients are managed for long periods with internal-external catheters. This type of biliary drainage, however, is

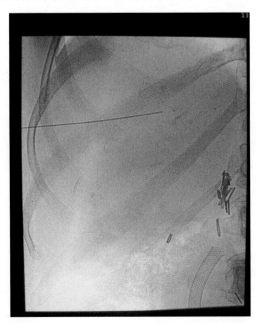

FIGURE 15.3 PTC with 22-gauge needle placed immediately anterior to the midaxillary line and advanced horizontally to the lateral border of the vertebral column

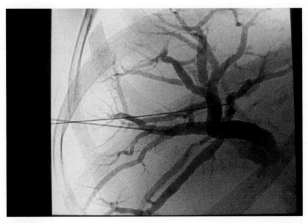

FIGURE 15.5 Second puncture of a more peripheral and better angled duct is chosen

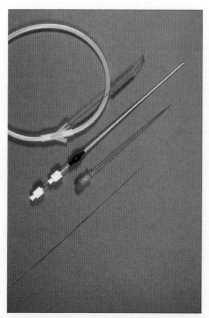

FIGURE 15.6 Minimally invasive access set (Accustick, Boston Scientific)

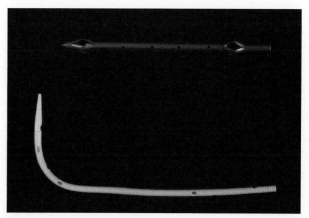

FIGURE 15.7 Plastic endoprostheses. (Top, Miller stent, COOK, with double mushroom either end; and bottom, the Carey-Coons stent, Boston Scientific)

associated with bile leaks, infection, patient discomfort, and psychological problems connected with catheters protruding through the skin. If possible, internal-external catheters should be exchanged for endoprostheses.

Internal Drainage

Endoprostheses. Endoprostheses enable internal drainage of bile across the obstructing lesion and avoid the need for external catheters. There are two types of endoprostheses available for use in the biliary tract, plastic and metallic. Both types may be inserted using either the percutaneous or endoscopic route. Metallic stents are not indicated for benign strictures. Therefore, if the diagnosis of malignancy is uncertain, the procedure should be delayed until histologic proof of disease is obtained.

Plastic endoprostheses consist of plastic or Teflon hollow tubes 8 to 14 cm long with end holes (e.g., Carey-Coons, Boston Scientific Corp., Galway, Ireland), and in some cases side holes (Cook prosthesis, W. Cook Europe) (FIGURE 15.7) to allow drainage of bile from above a stricture to the duodenum. As previously mentioned, plastic stents are more easily deployed by the endoscopists. The caliber of radiologic plastic stents varies from 8 to 12 French. Ideally the largest size should always be used to provide optimal biliary drainage and reduce problems of occlusion by bile encrustation. As a result, a relatively large transhepatic track is required for percutaneous insertion. Because of the increased risk of pain, bleeding and perihepatic bile leakage, which may be caused by the creation of a 12 French hole in the liver, insertion of plastic endoprostheses is generally carried out as a two-stage procedure. PBD isperformed and an 8F biliary drainage catheter is inserted. After a few days, the patient is brought back to the interventional radiology suite and the biliary catheter is removed over a guidewire. The transhepatic track is dilated from 8 French to 12 French followed by insertion of the plastic endoprosthesis across the stricture so that the upper

end is above the stricture and the lower end projects through the ampulla into the duodenum. It is usual to insert a temporary external biliary catheter, which is removed 24 hours later after check cholangiography (FIGURE 15.8).

Self-expanding metallic endoprostheses are metallic springs 6 to 10 cm long, which are introduced into the bile ducts in a compressed state and expand to a much larger diameter (8 to 12 mm) when the stents are released from their introducer (FIGURE 15.9). The main advantage of metallic stents is that they achieve a much larger diameter than plastic stents when deployed, which allows more efficient biliary drainage. Because they are inserted in a compressed state, the transhepatic track required for metallic stent insertion is generally smaller (5 to 7 French) than for plastic stents (10 to 12 French). This means that metallic stents can be inserted during the same procedure as PBD, which avoids the necessity for a period of external biliary drainage.

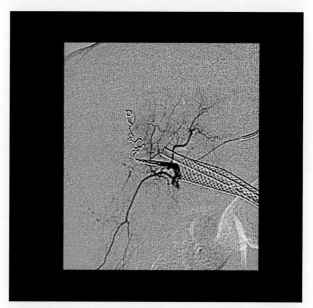

FIGURE 15.8 Check cholangiography shows satisfactory position of Carey-Coons stent with proximal end lying above the stricture and the distal end projects through the ampulla into the duodenum

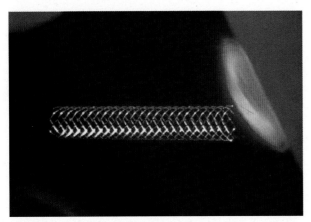

FIGURE 15.9 Self-expanding metallic endoprostheses in a deployed state (10 mm in diameter and 7 cm long)

Percutaneous biliary drainage is performed and a catheter is manipulated across the stricture. Instead of inserting a biliary drainage catheter, the stricture is predilated to 10 mm using a balloon catheter to facilitate rapid expansion of the metallic stent. After predilation, the stent on its introducer system is advanced across the lesion and is deployed so that the lower end projects through the ampulla and the upper end is well above the stricture. After stent deployment, a temporary small catheter is inserted foraccess in case of complications and is removed the next day after cholangiography. Postprocedure management instructions following biliary drainage are summarized in Table 15.3.

Technical Approach: Entry from Right or Left Side and Principles for Drainage

According to the Bismuth classification system,[20] a type 1 obstruction occurs distal to the confluence of the right and left hepatic ducts (primary confluence); type 2 involves the primary

Table 15.3
Postprocedure Management Instructions Following Biliary

- Patients should be hospitalized for at least 24 hours following biliary drainage and monitored for sepsis and vital signs.
- An appropriate antibiotic combination should be continued after drainage is established.
- The internal-external biliary drainage catheter should be used for external drainage for the first 12 to 24 hours. If the catheter permits drainage of bile into the bowel, then the drainage catheter can be capped to allow internal drainage. If the patient is able to tolerate internal drainage for 8 to 12 hours, then he/she can be discharged. If internal drainage is not possible, then external bag drainage must be maintained. Bile output can range from 400 to 800 mL/day. With external drainage, dehydration can occur, unless adequate steps are taken to replace the lost fluids.
- Biliary drainage catheters should be forward flushed with normal saline every 48 hours. This helps prevent debris from accumulating in the catheter and causing it to occlude.
- If patients are to be sent home on internal drainage, they should not be discharged until the ability to have their bile drained internally is demonstrated adequately without evidence of sepsis or pericatheter leakage.
- Complete instructions for tube care are given prior to discharge. Patients should be instructed to flush the tube gently with 10 cc of saline once or twice per day to keep it debris free. They should be instructed to call if they experience pain, chills, fever, or nausea or vomiting. Any malposition of the tube, bleeding within it, or leakage around the tube should also be taken seriously.
- The dressing around the drainage catheter should be changed at least every 48 hours and bathing avoided. Also, the biliary drainage catheters should be changed every 3 to 4 months.
- Pericatheter leakage is the result of catheter kinking, occlusion, or displacement. Fluoroscopic evaluation is essential for determining and correcting this problem depending on the causes as mentioned. Sometimes upsizing the catheter is the only solution.
- Serum bilirubin values may be followed as an indicator of adequate drainage. Depending on the size and type of drain, it takes, on an average, 10 to 15 days for the bilirubin levels to drop by 50%. If the bilirubin level starts rising, catheter occlusion should be suspected.
- After adequate drainage, biliary sepsis should be relieved. If sepsis remains a problem, then additional studies should be performed to determine the cause, which can be catheter occlusion or undrained biliary ducts. A thorough cholangiogram with special attention to the ductal anatomy can sometimes identify a missing ductal segment, indicating an isolated undrained system. Alternatively, an MRCP or a CT cholangiogram can be performed.
- Late sepsis, manifesting as fever several days or weeks after the patient has been adequately drained, is usually indicative of obstruction of the drainage catheter. If the patient has a capped biliary catheter, the tube should be uncapped to allow the bile to drain externally. If externalizing the drainage catheter resolves the infection, then fluoroscopic evaluation of the catheter can be performed electively. If fever persists after externalization, however, then an emergency catheter evaluation should be performed. If catheter obstruction is not the source of sepsis, then the patient should be evaluated for undrained ductal segments.

confluence but not the secondary confluence; type 3 involves the primary confluence and, additionally, either right (3a) or left (3b) secondary confluence; and type 4 involves the secondary confluence of both the right and left hepatic ducts.

Strictures in the common hepatic duct or the CBD can be treated with a single stent. In the case of a type 1 lesion, there are two advantages in approaching from the right side: the angle of approach to the point of obstruction is 90° or greater, making for easy catheter insertion; and the radiologist's hands are well away from the x-ray beam. Care should be taken to avoid the pleural reflection so as not to breach the pleural space.

The advantage of using the left-sided approach is that US can be utilized for the initial puncture and avoids the accidental breach of pleural space. With left-sided drains, patients have less catheter-related discomfort (the right intercostal approach being more painful) and they can more easily manage the catheter when it exits out from the midline, rather than the midaxillary line. The left-sided approach is also preferable when there is ascites because the risk of peritoneal leak is reduced. For left-sided approach, the operator needs to ensure that the catheter enters the medial, rather than the lateral, ducts. The lateral ducts are more posterior and, therefore, the catheter pathway will be directed posteriorly and then anteriorly, thus affecting the pushability, while negotiating the more distal obstruction.

Hilar strictures may be treated by a single stent or by bilateral stents, depending on the pattern of biliary obstruction. If there is free communication between the left and right systems, unilateral stenting is sufficient. If both the right and left ducts are obstructed, bilateral stents may be necessary (FIGURE 15.10).

Bilateral stenting is performed usually using a side-by-side or Y configuration. If only unilateral biliary drainage has been performed, but it is necessary to drain both lobes, bilateral drainage

can still be accomplished if metallic stents are used. A metallic stent is placed from one hepatic duct to the other across the hepatic duct confluence, followed by placement of a second long stent from the ipsilateral lobe to the duodenum (FIGURE 15.11). Although this T configuration achieves drainage of both liver lobes, the Y configuration is preferable because it allows easier intervention if the stents become occluded. Biliary side branches covered by the uncovered stents during placement are not associated with branch occlusion.

It is important to be aware of the anatomy of the right and left hepatic ducts. The right hepatic duct is short, unlike the left, which is 2 to 3 cm long, until its bifurcation into the segmental ducts. Thus a catheter placed in the right system initially drains a greater part of the liver because of the size difference between the lobes. Once the tumor grows, the situation reverses because the catheter placed in the right side now drains only one segment, whereas the left-sided catheter drains the entire left lobe. Thus, for type 2 lesions either the right anterior system or the left system is chosen (left is chosen if the left lobe of the liver is of good size). For type 3a lesions, if there is extensive involvement of the right secondary confluence, we do either a single left-sided drainage or ideally combine it with right anterior or posterior drainage (keeping in mind the cost of the procedure, life expectancy and the subjective assessment of the amount of liver to be drained as seen on CT). It has been shown that drainage of 25% of the liver volume using a single catheter/endoprosthesis may be sufficient.[21] An endoscopic study has shown that draining both lobes in patients with hilar lesions prolongs life expectancy.[22] For type 3b lesions the approach is similar. For type 4 lesions one should use at least two drains. Lobes and segments that are atrophic or have extensive tumor burden are not drained unless they are infected. Another approach in type 4

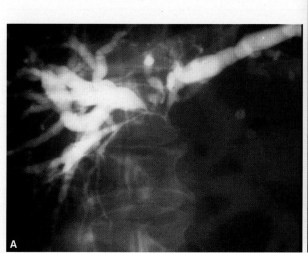
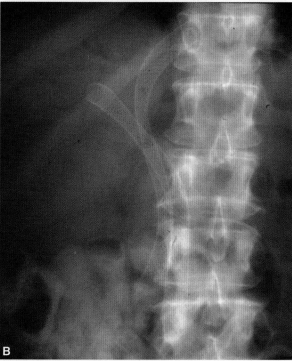

FIGURE 15.10 Right and left hepatic duct to CBD metallic stents (Y configuration)

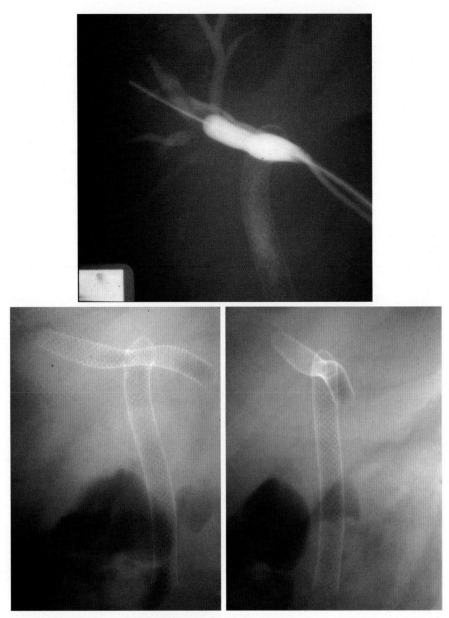

FIGURE 15.11 T-stent configuration

lesions is to perform T (chi configuration) stenting, which allows drainage of the entire major segmental ducts.[23] One stent extends from the left duct through the hilar stricture to the right anterior duct; the other stent is placed across the right posterior segmental duct through the hilar stricture into the CBD or through the papilla into the duodenum. Stent deployment should be performed simultaneously. Ultimately the two stents form a chi-shaped configuration.[23]

It is generally advisable to have the distal end of the stent project just through the ampulla into the duodenum.[6] This is because the rigid nature of the stent can sometimes cause kinking of the lower part of the CBD, which may cause obstruction (with the newer flexible nitinol stents, this may probably be unnecessary). Additionally, it is easier to cannulate them endoscopically for clearance or for additional endoprosthesis insertion. If the

stent projects too far into the duodenum, it can cause erosion of the opposite wall.[24]

Metallic or plastic stents?   Both types of stents provide good palliation of malignant obstructive jaundice. Plastic stents are placed by many endoscopists because of their acceptable patency rates, retrievability, low cost, and the ability of the endoscopist to insert plastic stents in a single-stage procedure.

Metallic stents are more expensive than plastic endoprostheses and there has been considerable debate since metallic stents were introduced as to whether the results of metallic stents compared with plastic devices justify their additional costs.[24] Although most retrospective studies suggest that both types of stents produce acceptable palliation,[25] the results of randomized trials indicate that metallic stents have significantly longer patency rates than plastic stents.[26–28] These trials reported that metallic stents are, in fact, more cost effective than plastic devices because of the reduced number of reinterventions required for the patients with metallic stents compared with plastic stents and the shorter stay in hospital.[26–28] As a result of these data and the smaller introducer systems of metallic stents, most interventional radiologists choose metallic endoprosteses for internal biliary drainage.[29]

Percutaneous management of the occluded stent. Plastic stents are prone to occlusion by bile encrustation. The main cause of occlusion of metallic stents is tumor ingrowth or overgrowth; bile encrustation seldom occurs. The best method of treatment of blocked biliary stents is endoscopic replacement, in the case of plastic endoprostheses, or endoscopic insertion of a plastic stent inside a metallic endoprosthesis. Percutaneous evaluation and therapy of occluded stents is usually reserved for patients in whom endoscopy has been unsuccessful or is not possible. The percutaneous method involves an initial PTC to confirm stent occlusion and to define the biliary anatomy, followed by catheterization of a suitable duct. If the occluded stent is plastic, the stent must be removed before a new endoprosthesis is inserted. Plastic stents can be removed either by withdrawing them through the transhepatic track by grasping them with a wire loop snare or balloon catheter, or by pushing them into the duodenum and allowing them to pass through the digestive tract.

Most metallic stents cannot be removed (there are a new generation of retrievable metallic stents now available). Occlusion of metallic stents is managed percutaneously by inserting a new metallic endoprosthesis coaxially within the first stent. If the cause of occlusion is overgrowth of tumor, the new device must extend beyond the upper limit of the tumor.

Access loops. Surgeons often affix the afferent loop of jejunum to the parietal peritoneum at the time of the creation of the bilioenteric anastomosis to allow easy percutaneous access to the biliary tree if a stricture occurs at a later date. The apex of the loop is marked by a circle of metallic clips, enabling the entry site of the loop to be visualized on fluoroscopy. If an access loop is present, it can be punctured with a fine needle under fluoroscopic guidance. Contrast medium is injected to opacify the loop and identify the route to the bilioenteric anastomosis. A minimally invasive access set (e.g., Accustick) is used to dilate the percutaneous track and to pass a catheter and guidewire to the site of the anastomosis. The catheter is advanced across the stricture into the biliary tree and a stiff guidewire is inserted into the intrahepatic ducts. This method of access allows repeated percutaneous dilatation of the stricture without the discomfort of the transhepatic route.

Covered biliary stents. Covered stents represent an evolution of bare stents and are aimed mainly to prevent obstruction caused by tumor ingrowth within the stent lumen.[30] The first clinical studies of polyurethane-covered Wallstents showed that these stents can be safely implanted.[30,31] The 6-month patency rate was found to be inferior to that of noncovered Wallstents (46.8% vs. 67%), however, partly because of a breach in the covering membrane that allowed tumor

ingrowth.[31] It was concluded that such a type of covered stent had no significant advantages versus bare stents.[31,32] Now polytetrafluoroethylene and fluorinated ethylene propylene (ePTFE/FEP)–covered metallic stents have been introduced. The stent consists of an inner ePTFE/FEP lining and an outer supporting structure of nitinol wire. Multiple wire sections elevated from the external surface provide anchoring. Stents are available in two versions, with or without holes in the proximal stent lining. Holes should provide drainage of the cystic duct or biliary side branches when covered by the proximal stent end. They are more effective than polyurethane-covered Wallstents.[33,34] In 10% of cases, however, one can still get branch duct obstruction.[34,35] These early studies are promising; however, significant improvements in patency would be still desirable.

COMBINED BILIARY AND DUODENAL OBSTRUCTION

In some advanced cases of pancreatic cancer, metastasis or malignant lymphadenopathy patients can present with both biliary and duodenal obstruction. As a palliative procedure the combined stenting of both the biliary stricture and duodenal stricture can be performed in one sitting by the radiologist. The biliary stent is placed from the percutaneous route as described previously, whereas the duodenal stent can be placed via the transoral route. There are essentially two ways for these placement, that is, placing the duodenal stent first and then the biliary stent just through the mesh of the duodenal stent (FIGURE 15.12) or placing both stents side to side within the duodenal lumen.

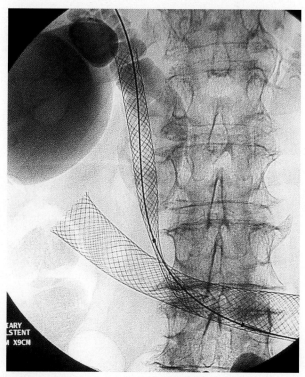

FIGURE 15.12 Transoral duodenal and percutaneous biliary stent placements in a patient with pancreatic carcinoma

Combined Transhepatic Endoscopic Approach (Rendezvous Procedure)

Transhepatic placement of a catheter of small diameter across the obstructed duct and into the duodenum offers a second chance for the endoscopist. This arrangement is very useful when the endoscopist has initially failed to negotiate the obstruction at an earlier attempt,[36] and it is not advisable to create a large transhepatic track because of the risk of bile leakage into the peritoneum, or in patients with coagulopathy. With a transhepatically inserted 4 or 5 French catheter negotiated across the obstruction into the duodenum, a 450-cm exchange guidewire, such as Zebra (Microvasive), is inserted into the catheter. The patient is placed in the prone oblique position for the insertion of the endoscope. The endoscopist grasps the lower end of the guidewire with a snare or biopsy forceps and brings it out of the proximal end of the endoscope biopsy channel while the radiologist keeps feeding the wire at the skin entry site. The transhepatic catheter is now withdrawn so that its tip lies in the intrahepatic portion of the biliary tree above the malignant stricture. The endoscopist now proceeds with the placement of a large-bore biliary endoprosthesis in the standard fashion while the guidewire is held taut between the endoscopic and percutaneous ends. When the endoprosthesis is in position and free egress of bile is documented, the transhepatic catheter can be removed. If adequacy of decompression is questionable, the transhepatic catheter may be retained for observation and reintervention, if required.

▌ COMPLICATIONS

Complications of percutaneous biliary interventions can be divided into early, that is, procedural complications and late complications.[6] Most procedural complications are related to the initial biliary drainage with mortality ranging from 0% to 2.8%[37,38] and major complications occurring in 3.5% to 9.5%.[39,40] Also, higher procedure-related deaths have been reported for malignant diseases (3%) compared to benign diseases (0%).[41,42] This is also true of procedure-related complications (7% vs. 2%). Minor complications, such as mild self-limiting hemobilia, fever, and transient bacteremia, occur in up to 66% of patients.[43]

Immediate Complications

These may be the following:

1. Sedation: Problems may occur if care is not taken to constantly monitor patients during and after the procedure for complications of cardiorespiratory depression. Pulse oximetry should be used for monitoring all patients undergoing procedures involving conscious sedation.
2. Hemorrhage: Mild hemobilia is common, occurring in up to 16% of cases.[38] More severe bleeding requiring transfusion occurs in approximately 3% of patients.[44] Hemorrhage is minimized by the correction of coagulation defects and avoidance of percutaneous intervention in patients with severe incorrectable coagulopathies. It is usually self-limited and seldom requires treatment. If bleeding is mild and venous in origin, repositioning the catheter so that the trailing side holes are located within the biliary tree and not within the hepatic parenchyma, and, if required, upsizing the catheter to tamponade the bleeding point usually suffices. The catheter should be regularly irrigated with saline

to maintain its patency and to clear any thrombus from the bile ducts (FIGURE 15.13). If hemobilia does not resolve with these measures or is severe, vascular embolization should be performed through the transhepatic track or by hepatic arteriography (FIGURE 15.14).
3. Sepsis: Manipulation of catheters and guidewires within an infected biliary tract can produce rapid bacteremia, which may progress to septicemic shock if antibiotic coverage is not administered prior to the procedure. Intravenous antibiotics should be continued following biliary drainage until the catheter is removed.
4. Pericatheter leak in approximately 15% of the patients.[45]
5. Pancreatitis (0%–4%).[45]
6. Pneumothorax, hemothorax, bilothorax (<1%).[46,47]
7. Contrast reaction (<2%).[45]

Delayed Complications

These include the following:

1. Cholangitis: Approximately 50% of bile cultures will be positive when obtained at initial puncture.[41] When an internal-external drainage is performed with an 8F catheter, recurrent cholangitis secondary to inadequate drainage is possible. The rate of sepsis will decrease if this is replaced by a 10 to 12 French drain.[44]
2. Catheter dislodgment (approximately 15%–20%).[38,48]
3. Peritonitis (1%–3%).[45]
4. Hypersecretion of bile (0%–5%)[42]: This can cause significant fluid and electrolyte imbalance and is usually seen within several days of drainage.
5. Cholecystitis caused by blockage of the cystic duct by covered stents. To address this complication, holes in the proximal stent lining are made, which should hypothetically allow for drainage of cystic or branch biliary ducts when their orifice is covered by the stent.[39,40] But still, this complication may be seen, for which percutaneous cystic duct stent placement,[49] percutaneous cholecystostomy, or cholecystectomy may be required.
6. Biliopleural fistula.[46]
7. Skin infection, irritation.
8. Intrahepatic/perihepatic abscess.
9. Metastatic seeding of the serosa or tract with cholangiocarcinoma[42] and pancreatic carcinoma[38,50] has been reported.

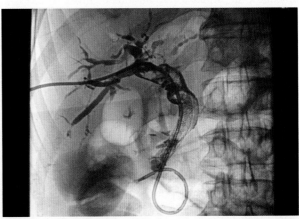

FIGURE 15.13 Cholangiogram demonstrating significant filling defects consistent with hemobilia

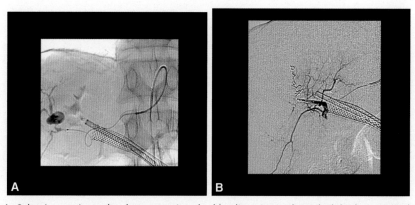

FIGURE 15.14 A. Selective angiography demonstrating the bleeding site in the right lobe liver. **B.** Coils placed through a microcatheter. Note that coiling is performed beyond and proximal to pseudoaneurysm/hemorrhage site to close the front and back doors.

Some routine precautions that help in significantly reducing the incidence of complications are provided in Table 15.4.

CLINICAL RESULTS AND PATIENT SURVIVAL

In general, the technical success rate has varied from 86% to 100% with successful drainage rates of 81% to 96%. The 30-day mortality rate has been 1% to 49% and complication rate of 6% to 58%.[48,51–57] This marked variation in results is probably caused by differences in the criteria for patient selection, the experience and expertise of different operators, and the criteria used to define success and complications.

Patient survival after metallic stent placement is difficult to estimate and compare among various reports and this would be attributable to variations in population, additional treatment, patient selection, and the stage of the tumor. In the literature, patients receiving this treatment have been reported to live 93 to 420 days longer.[58,59] In patients with hilar obstruction, longer survival rates have been observed after both lobes have been drained as compared to those who had one lobe drained.[59,60,61] This may be attributable to the higher septic complications that may occur in patients with unilateral drainage. The drawbacks for multisegment drainage, however, are increased cost, longer procedure time, and greater technical difficulty.

Table 15.4	
Methods of Reducing Frequency of Common Complications	
Sepsis	Antibiotic prophylaxis
Hemorrhage	Minimal manipulation
Bile leak	Restrict volume of contrast injected and aspirate bile prior to contrast injection
Cholangitis	Normalize coagulation factors
Catheter dislodgment	Fine-needle coaxial technique
	Peripheral duct puncture
	Careful positioning of side holes to avoid communication with an intrahepatic vessel
	Avoid puncture of extrahepatic ducts
	Single puncture site in liver capsule
	Careful positioning of side holes
	Ensure adequate drainage by careful positioning of side holes
	Irrigation of catheter with sterile saline
	Large-diameter catheters (12 French) for long drainage
	Routine tube exchange every 2 to 3 months
	Safety stitch method
	Self-retaining (pigtail) catheter

■ REFERENCES

1. Kaude JV, Weidenmier CH, Agee OF. Decompression of the bile ducts with the percutaneous technique. *Radiology* 1969;93:69–71.
2. Kumaran V, Gulati MS, Paul SB, et al. The role of dual phase helical CT in assessing resectability of carcinoma of the gallbladder. *Eur Radiol* 2002;12:1993–1999.
3. Blumgart LH. Cholangiocarcinoma. In: Blumgart LH (ed.). *Surgery of the Liver and Biliary Tract.* Edinburgh, UK: Churchill Livingstone; 1998;1:721–753.
4. Pillai VAK, Shreekumar KP, Prabhu NK, et al. Utility of MR cholangiography in planning transhepatic biliary interventions in malignant hilar obstructions. *Indian J Radiol Imaging* 2002;12:37–42.
5. Speer AG, Russel CG, Hatfield ARW. Randomised trial of endoscopic versus percutaneous stent insertion in malignant obstructive jaundice. *Lancet* 1987;11:57–62.
6. Morgan RA, Adam A. Percutaneous management of biliary obstruction. In: Gazelle GS, Saini S, Mueller PR (eds.). *Hepatobiliary and Pancreatic Radiology Imaging and Intervention.* New York, NY: Thieme;1998:677–709.
7. Kersjes W, Koster O, Heuer M, et al. A comparison of imaging procedures in the diagnosis of gallbladder and bile duct carcinomas. *Rofo Fortschr Geb Rontgenstr Neuen Bildgeb Verfahr* 1990;153:174–180.
8. Gulliver DJ, Baker ME, Cheng CA, et al. Malignant biliary obstruction: efficacy of thin section dynamic CT in determining resectability. *AJR Am J Roentgenol* 1992;159:503–507.
9. Choi BI, Lee JH, Han MC, et al. Hilar cholangiocarcinoma: comparative study with sonography and CT. *Radiology* 1989;172:689–692.
10. de Aretxabala X, Roa I, Burgos L, et al. Gallbladder cancer in Chile. A report on 54 potentially resectable tumours. *Cancer* 1992;69:60–65.
11. Cha JH, Han JK, Kim TK, et al. Preoperative evaluation of Klatskin tumour: accuracy of spiral CT in determining vascular invasion as a sign of unresectability. *Abdom Imaging* 2000;25:500–507.
12. Feydy A, Vilgrain V, Denys A, et al. Helical CT assessment in hilar cholangiocarcinoma: correlation with surgical and pathologic findings. *AJR Am J Roentgenol* 1999;172:73–77.
13. Van Beers BE, Lacrosse M, Trigaux JP, et al. Non invasive imaging of the biliary tree before or after laparoscopic cholecystectomy: use of three dimensional spiral CT cholangiography. *AJR Am J Roentgenol* 1994;162:1331–1335.
14. Kwon AH, Uetsuji S, Yamada O, et al. Three dimensional reconstruction of the biliary tract using spiral computed tomography. *Br J Surg* 1995;82:260–263.
15. Zeman RK, Berman PM, Silverman PM, et al. Biliary tract: three dimensional helical CT without cholangiographic contrast material. *Radiology* 1995;196:865–867.
16. Rao NDLV, Gulati MS, Paul SB, et al. Three-dimensional helical CT cholangiography with minimum intensity projection in gallbladder carcinoma patients with obstructive jaundice: comparison with magnetic resonance cholangiography and percutaneous transhepatic cholangiography. *J Gastroenterol Hepatol* 2005;20:304–308.
17. Park SJ, Han JK, Kim TK, et al. Three-dimensional spiral CT cholangiography with minimum intensity projection in patients with suspected obstructive biliary disease: comparison with percutaneous transhepatic cholangiography. *Abdom Imaging* 2001;26(3):281–286.
18. Adamck HE, Albert J, Lietz M, et al. A prospective evaluation of magnetic resonance cholangiography in patients with suspected bile duct obstruction. *Gut* 1998;43:680–683.
19. Cope C. Conversion from small (0.018 inch) to large (0.038 inch) guide wires in percutaneous drainage procedures. *AJR Am J Roentgenol* 1982;138:170–171.
20. Bismuth H, Corlette MB. Intrahepatic cholangioenteric anastomosis in carcinoma of the hilus of the liver. *Surg Gynecol Obstet* 1975;140:170–178.
21. Polydorou AA, Chisholm EM, Romanos AA, et al. A comparison of right versus left hepatic duct endoprosthesis insertion in malignant hilar biliary obstruction. *Endoscopy* 1989;21:266–271.
22. Chang WH, Kortan P, Haber GB. Outcome in patients with bifurcation tumors who undergo unilateral versus bilateral hepatic duct drainage. *Gastrointest Endosc* 1998;47:354–362.
23. Lee KH, Lee DY, Kim KW. Biliary intervention for cholangiocarcinoma. *Abdom Imaging* 2004;29:581–589.
24. Morgan RA, Adam A. Metallic stents in the treatment of patients with malignant biliary obstruction. *Semin Intervent Radiol* 1996;13:229–240.
25. Rossi P, Bezzi M, Rossi M, et al. Metallic stents in malignant biliary obstruction: results of a multicenter European study of 240 patients. *J Vasc Interv Radiol* 1994;5:279–285.
26. Davids PHP, Groen AK, Rauws EAJ, et al. Randomised trial of self-expanding metal stents versus polyethylene stents for distal malignant biliary obstruction. *Lancet* 1992;340:1488–1492.
27. Knyrim K, Wagner H-J, Pausch J, et al. A prospective, randomised controlled trial of metal stents for malignant obstruction of the common bile duct. *Endoscopy* 1993;25:207–212.
28. Lammer J, Hausegger KA, Fluckiger F, et al. Common bile duct obstruction due to malignancy: treatment with plastic versus metal stents. *Radiology* 1996;201:167–172.
29. Adam A, Roddie ME, Jackson JE, et al. Wallstent endoprostheses for biliary malignancy: what is the verdict after 7 years use? *Radiology* 1994; 193(P):327.
30. Shim CS, Lee JH, Cho JD, et al. Preliminary results of a new covered biliary metal stent for malignant biliary obstruction. *Endoscopy* 1998;30: 345–350.
31. Rossi P, Bezzi M, Salvatori FM, et al. Clinical experience with covered Wallstents for biliary malignancies: 23-month follow-up. *Cardiovasc Intervent Radiol* 1997;20:441–447.
32. Hausegger KA, Thurnher S, Bodendorfer G, et al. Treatment of malignant biliary obstruction with polyurethane-covered Wallstents. *AJR Am J Roentgenol* 1998;170:403–408.
33. Bezzi M, Zolovkins A, Cantisani V, et al. New ePTFE/FEP–covered stent in the palliative treatment of malignant biliary obstruction. *J Vasc Interv Radiol* 2002;13:581–589.
34. Schoder M, Rossi P, Uflacker R, et al. Malignant biliary obstruction: treatment with ePTFE-FEP–covered endoprostheses—initial technical and clinical experiences in a multicenter trial. *Radiology* 2002;225:35–42.
35. Nicholson DA, Cheety N, Jackson J. Patency of side branches after peripheral placement of metallic biliary endoprosthesis. *J Vasc Interv Radiol* 1992;3:127–130.
36. Wayman J, Mansfield JC, Mathewson K, et al. Combined percutaneous and endoscopic procedures for bile duct obstruction: simultaneous and delayed techniques compared. *Hepatogastroenterol* 2003;50:915–918.
37. Ferrucci JT, Jr, Mueller PR, Harbim WP. Percutaneous transhepatic biliary drainage: technique, results and applications. *Radiology* 1980;135:1–13.
38. Hamlin JA, Friedman M, Stein MG, et al. Percutaneous biliary drainage: complications of 118 consecutive catheterizations. *Radiology* 1986;158:199–202.
39. Lamaris JS, Stoker J, Dees J, et al. Nonsurgical palliative treatment of patients with malignant biliary obstruction—the place of endoscopic and percutaneous drainage. *Clin Radiol* 1987;38:603–608.
40. Clark RA, Mitchell SE, Colley DP, et al. Percutaneous catheter biliary decompression. *AJR Am J Roentgenol* 1981;137:503–509.
41. Yee AC, Ho CS. Complications of transhepatic biliary drainage: benign vs malignant diseases. *AJR Am J Roentgenol* 1987;148:1207–1209.
42. Carrasco CH, Zornoza J, Bechtel WJ. Malignant biliary obstruction: complications of percutaneous biliary drainage. *Radiology* 1984;152: 343–346.
43. Berquist TH, May GR, Johnson CM, et al. Percutaneous biliary decompression: internal and external drainage in 50 patients. *AJR Am J Roentgenol* 1981;136:901–906.
44. Mueller PR, vanSonnenberg E, Ferrucci JT, Jr. Percutaneous biliary drainage: technical and catheter related problems in 200 procedures. *AJR Am J Roentgenol* 1982;138:17–23.
45. Rosenblatt M, Aruny JE, Kandarpa K. Transhepatic cholangiography, biliary decompression, endobiliary stenting, and cholecystostomy. In: Kandarpa K, Aruny JE (eds.). *Handbook of Interventional Radiology Procedures.* Philadelphia, PA: Lippincott Williams & Wilkins;2002:302–331.
46. Strange C, Allen ML, Freedland PN, et al. Biliopleural fistula as a complication of percutaneous biliary drainage: experimental evidence for pleural inflammation. *Am Rev Respir Dis* 1988;137:959–961.
47. Dawson SL, Neff CC, Mueller PR, et al. Fatal hemothorax after inadvertent transpleural biliary drainage. *AJR Am J Roentgenol* 1983;141:33–34.
48. Gazzaniga GM, Faggioni A, Bondanza G, et al. Percutaneous transhepatic biliary drainage—twelve years experience. *Hepatogastroenterology* 1991;38:154–159.
49. Sheiman RG, Stuart K. Percutaneous cystic duct stent placement for the treatment of acute cholecystitis resulting from common bile duct stent placement for malignant obstruction. *J Vasc Interv Radiol* 2004;15:999–1001.

50. Cutherell L, Wanebo HJ, Tegtmeyer CJ. Catheter tract seeding after percutaneous biliary drainage for pancreatic cancer. *Cancer* 1986;57:2057–2060.

51. Wittich GR, VanSonnertberg E, Simeone JF. Results and complications of percutaneous drainage. *Semin Interv Radiol* 1985;2:39–49.

52. Pereiras RV, Jr, Rheingold OJ, Huston D, et al. Relief of malignant obstructive jaundice by percutaneous insertion of a permanent prosthesis. *Ann Intern Med* 1978;89:589–593.

53. Vorgeli DR, Gummy AB, Weese JL. Percutaneous transhepatic cholangiography, drainage and biopsy in patients with malignant biliary obstruction. An alternate to surgery. *Am J Surg* 1985;150:243–247.

54. Joseph PK, Bizer LS, Sprayregan SS, et al. Percutaneous transhepatic biliary drainage. Results and complications in 81 patients. *JAMA* 1986;255:2763–2767.

55. Lammer J, Neurager K. Biliary drainage endoprosthesis: experience with 201 patients. *Radiology* 1986;159:625–629.

56. Schild H, Klose KJ, Staritz M, et al. The results and complications of 616 percutaneous transhepatic biliary drainages. *Rofo Fortschr Geb Rontgenstr Neuen Bildgeb Verfahr* 1989;151(3):289–293.

57. Murai R, Hashiguchi F, Kusuyama A, et al. Percutaneous stenting for malignant biliary stenosis. *Surg Endosc* 1991;5:140–142.

58. Rieber A, Brambs HJ. Metallic stents in malignant biliary obstruction. *Cardiovasc Intervent Radiol* 1997;20:43–49.

59. Cowling MG, Adam AN. Internal stenting in malignant biliary obstruction. *World J Surg* 2001;25:355–361.

60. Deviere J, Baize M, de Toeuf J, et al. Long-term follow-up of patients with hilar malignant stricture treated by endoscopic internal biliary drainage. *Gastrointest Endosc* 1988;34:95–101.

61. Motte S, Deviere J, Dumonceau JM, et al. Risk factors for septicemia following endoscopic biliary stent. *Gastroenterology* 1991;101:1374–1381.

CHAPTER
16

Renal Cell Carcinoma: Medical, Surgical, and Image-Guided Therapies

RONALD RODRIGUEZ and CHRISTOS GEORGIADES

■ INTRODUCTION

Epidemiology

Renal cell carcinoma (RCC) (also known as hypernephroma or renal adenocarcinoma) is primary cancer of the kidney arising from the renal tubular epithelium. It has unique clinicopathologic characteristics that present both opportunities and challenges. For example, low-grade cancers have a low metastatic potential and slow growth rate, making RCC a curable disease for many, if not most, patients. On the other hand, renal function preservation is very important because RCC patients are at an increased risk for metachronous lesions and some present with already diminished renal function. Treatment planning, taking these factors into account, must aim at cure while preserving as much renal parenchyma as possible. The World Health Organization (WHO) has divided RCC into distinct histopathologic subgroups (Table 16.1). Each subgroup demonstrates distinct histology, molecular biology, and prognosis.[1,2] RCC is the 10th most common cancer worldwide, accounting for about 2% to 3% of all cancers, and the 5th most common solid, nonskin cancer. Its incidence is highest in the Western world. Specifically, the incidence of RCC in the United States is approximately 59,000 (2009), up sharply from 32,000 in 2003 (FIGURE 16.1), whereas the age-adjusted incidence and mortality currently stand at 13.5 and 4.1 per 100,000, respectively, with a lifetime risk of 1.43%.[3–7] The current annual mortality rate of RCC in the United States is approximately 12,000 with a 5-year all-cause survival of 50%.[4,5] The recent sharp increase in the incidence of RCC is to a small extent attributable to an increase in its main recognized risk factors, that is, cigarette smoking and obesity. Most of the increase in incidence of RCC is a result of the incidental detection of renal masses secondary to the increased utilization of computed tomography (CT), magnetic resonance imaging (MRI), and ultrasonography (US).[4,5]

Staging

The current tumor-node-metastasis (TNM) staging of RCC is shown in Table 16.2. The recognition of the varied histologic types and the unpredictable behavior even within the

Table 16.1

Histologic Subtypes of Renal Cell Carcinoma According to the World Health Organization

Disease behavior and patient prognosis depends to a certain extent on the histologic subtype of RCC. For example, a chromophobe subtype portends a better prognosis, and treatment should be tailored accordingly. Follow-up may indeed be the best option for an elderly patient with a 1-cm chromophobe RCC and severe cardiac disease.

	Histologic subtype of renal cell carcinoma	Prevalence
1	Clear cell	70%
2	Papillary	10–15%
3	Chromophobe	5–9%
4	Multilocular cystic	1%
5	Collecting duct	1%
6	Medullary	1%
7	Mucinous tubular	1%
8	Spindle	1%
9	Neuroblastoma associated	1%
10	Xp11.2 translocation-TFE3	1%
11	Unclassified	4–7%

same subtype is compelling researchers to expand staging to include histology, nuclear grading, and other nonmorphologic tumor characteristics.[8] This new TNM staging system was introduced to highlight the correlation between 10-year cause-specific survival and tumor size for patients undergoing radical nephrectomy (<4 cm, >4 to ≤7 cm, and >7 cm, 90%, 71%, and

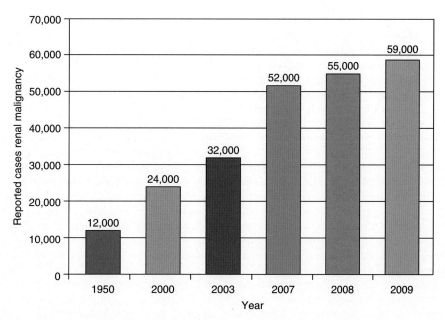

FIGURE 16.1 The incidence of renal cell carcinoma in the United States. Many factors, including the increase in associated risk factors (obesity and smoking) as well as the increased utilization of cross-sectional imaging, have resulted in a significant increase in the incidence of RCC. A positive outcome is that most RCC are localized and relatively small in size at the time of diagnosis and therefore potentially curable.

62%, respectively).[8] Although repeat surgery for residual disease and metastasectomy have been shown to improve survival, cure is unlikely in patients with metastases.

Background

Nephron sparing surgery (NSS) has been shown to have the same local tumor recurrence rate and provide the patient with the same life expectancy as radical nephrectomy for disease confined to the kidney.[4] Since its introduction in 1990, laparoscopic partial nephrectomy has become an increasingly popular NSS choice for organ-confined disease with more and more urologists offering this option. The utilization of laparoscopy (either transperitoneal or retroperitoneal) for radical or partial nephrectomy has more than doubled in the last decade and, more recently, trained surgeons are more likely to offer this procedure compared to older ones.[9] Outcome studies have shown that for T1 to T3a disease (i.e., disease confined within Gerota's fascia) laparoscopic partial nephrectomy has a disease-free survival similar

Table 16.2

TNM Staging of Renal Cell Carcinoma

In the Western world, more than 75% of RCC are detected at stage 1A or 1B. This enables the physician to discuss a number of treatment options ranging from radical nephrectomy to percutaneous ablation. Although ablation has been used to treat stage 1B RCC (4 to 7 cm or even larger), such lesions are best suited for surgery unless there is a contraindication.

T		N		M	
1a	≤4 cm, limited to kidney	X	Cannot be assessed	X	Cannot be assessed
1b	>4 to ≤7 cm, limited to kidney	0	No lymph nodes	0	No distant metastases
2	>7 cm, limited to kidney	1	1 node	1	Distant metastases
3a	Perinephric or adrenal extension, but within Gerota's	2	>1 node		
3b	Renal vein or IVC, rest within Gerota's				
3c	Vena cava above diaphragm				
4	Outside Gerota's				

to that of radical nephrectomy.[4] The next evolutionary step in NSS was laparoscopic ablation. Early results after cryoablation are quite encouraging and for selected patients it appears to offer benefits similar to those of surgical resection. For tumors up to 4 cm in diameter laparoscopic cryoablation has been shown to have a nearly 100% cancer-specific-free 3-year survival.[10,11] A literature analysis grouping all published series at the time on laparoscopic cryoablation[5] showed a 97% to 100% cancer-specific 5-year survival for lesions smaller than 3 cm.

Image-guided, percutaneous cryoablation offers the latest in minimally invasive nephron sparing surgery (MINSS). This has been made possible by the introduction of thinner cryoprobes and advances in imaging guidance, specifically CT, MRI, and US. Early results show a primary efficacy of 80% to 100% and a secondary efficacy of near 100%.[5,12–14] The main limitations of the percutaneous approach include technical difficulties with central/anterior lesions and risk of collateral injury to adjacent organs and limitations due to lesion size. On the other hand, there are significant advantages to the percutaneous approach, such as being the least invasive procedure, having the quickest recovery, and offering visualization of the whole "ice-ball" in real time (CT and MRI).

The use of traditional systemic chemotherapies has long been proven ineffective and abandoned. However, during the last decade a number of targeted agents have been shown to improve survival in the setting of metastatic disease. Because of the high cure rates of surgical treatments and the low metastatic potential, systemic chemotherapy is currently not indicated in early stage disease.

■ SURGICAL THERAPIES

The range of options for localized renal masses includes observation, radical nephrectomy, nephron sparing resection, or ablation. Of these, the surgical options of radical and NSS depend in large part on the characteristics of the mass, the general health of the patient, the surgeon's preference (primarily a function of experience), and the patient's preference when the options are clearly laid out. Never have there been so many different options available, and making a final decision is now more involved than ever before. We present, however, our own preferences for assisting with this decision making.

Radical Nephrectomy

For lesions that appear to be locally extensive with potential involvement of neighboring organs, open surgery is still preferred. This is particularly true if a colectomy, splenectomy, or distal pancreatectomy is anticipated. In addition, local adenopathy or tumor thrombus invading into the renal vein and vena cava may also be a relative indication for consideration of open surgery as opposed to laparoscopy. We have on occasions been able to accomplish a laparoscopic resection, however, even with tumor thrombus extending into the vena cava, provided that the thrombus just enters the cava and can be manipulated back into the renal vein with certain maneuvers. Large tumors are also often best approached in open fashion. On some occasions even tumors as large as 20 cm can be approached laparoscopically, given the right local anatomy. Specifically, if the colon can be seen in its entirety from a medial camera

placement and there is enough space anteriorly to maneuver and reflect the colon and its attachments medially, then we are usually able to resect the kidney laparoscopically, even with large renal masses, provided no other structures are involved. When open surgery is required, the choice of surgical approach is also dictated by the surgeon's training and experience and the location and extent of disease. Tumors with thrombus extending into the inferior vena cava (IVC) above the level of the hepatic veins are usually performed with a midline incision to allow extension to a sternotomy, if required. On some occasions, however, when patients are particularly obese an anterior midline approach is suboptimal and we have been able to perform a veno-venous bypass (with thrombus extending to the atria) from an eighth interspace thoracoabdominal incision with super obese patients. Tumors with thrombus extending into the IVC but below the hepatic veins are most easily approached by a thoracoabdominal approach although many prefer chevron for such situations. We find the thoracoabdominal approach obviates the need for mobilization of the liver on the right side, and it has become our approach of choice for most cases with tumor thrombus. For other less extensive tumors, laparoscopy is the preferred approach when nephrectomy is deemed necessary. Laparoscopy has gained widespread popularity because it is less morbid than open surgery and results in a faster convalescence. Recently, there have been several developments in laparoscopic surgery that have become popularized. Notably, there has been a tendency toward minimizing port size and location. Most surgeons have moved away from the "hand" assisted method of laparoscopy to favor pure laparoscopic ports. Single port surgery has gained popularity in major laparoscopic centers as a means of improving the cosmetic impact of surgery. Such single port approaches require specialized equipment (which can bend around corners), however, and markedly complicate an already complex operation, such that the increase in risk often seems at odds with the perceived benefits. Nonetheless, single port surgery (LESS, for laparoendoscopic single site surgery) has become a viable option for patients with favorable body habitus and a relatively straightforward renal mass. The most extreme form of this trend is the so-called NOTES approach (for natural orifice transluminal endoscopic surgery). This approach uses a natural orifice instead of a transabdominal port. It has been accomplished primarily in animals as a proof of principle, and transvaginal nephrectomy with a single transabdominal port has been accomplished at several institutions, including our own. The true utility of such strategies, however, has yet to be determined. The vast majority of patients for whom such complicated strategies could be employed are also in fact eligible for NSS, and, increasingly, this is the strategy employed by most physicians charged with treating RCC.

Cytoreductive Nephrectomy

About one-third of patients diagnosed with RCC present with metastatic disease and around 50% of patients will develop metastasis after initial diagnosis. Cytoreductive surgery with systemic therapy has been shown to decrease the sequelae of metastatic disease (paraneoplastic syndrome) and also increase survival. In March 2004, the South West Oncology Group (SWOG) published the results of their randomized trial of cytoreductive nephrectomy + adjuvant immunotherapy versus immunotherapy alone for metastatic RCC. The results of that trial confirmed earlier, but less rigorously performed studies, that there was a survival benefit to cytoreductive nephrectomy—especially in the appropriately selected patient. The patients benefiting the most from this approach are those with metastases limited to the lungs and an excellent performance status. In such patients, survival is improved by 13.6 months. Risk and benefits need to be weighed in the decision, however, to perform a cytoreductive surgery. Patients with poor performance status and with a large metastatic disease burden are less likely to derive much benefit from surgery. Frequently, we find that patients with metastatic disease can undergo resection laparoscopically and this is always preferred when technically feasible because it allows a shorter recovery interval until starting systemic therapy.

Although the SWOG was able to demonstrate a survival benefit when combining cytoreductive surgery with immunotherapy, these strategies predated the current era of targeted chemotherapy for RCC. Since 2007, at least five new drugs have been approved by the Food and Drug Administration (FDA) for the treatment of RCC: sunitinib, sorafenib, everolimus, temsirolimus, and pazopanib. These drugs primarily target tyrosine kinase and protein kinase pathways as well as mTOR pathways and are targeted specifically to disrupt vascular endothelial growth factor/hypoxia-inducible factor (VEGF/HIF) pathway signaling, which is known to be particularly active in RCC. In this new era of targeted chemotherapy, it is unknown whether or not the same degree of survival benefit occurs when cytoreductive nephrectomy is performed in combination with these new agents as an adjuvant. Our own personal anecdotal experience has been that the combination of cytoreduction with these new agents can often result in markedly improved disease control, frequently to the point of NED (no evidence of disease) on subsequent imaging, even when preoperative imaging suggested widespread metastatic disease. Hence, we continue to believe that there is a significant role for cytoreductive nephrectomy and minimizing disease burden prior to initiating adjuvant chemotherapy. An interesting corollary to this strategy is the ability sometimes to accomplish cytoreduction with interventional approaches, such as percutaneous cryoablation. We have, in fact, performed this approach on multiple occasions with reasonable results and believe that a larger multicenter trial may be necessary to answer the question as to whether or not cytoreductive cryoablation with adjuvant chemotherapy improves clinical outcomes in patients with advanced disease.

Nephron Sparing Surgery

Indications for NSS for the treatment of RCC have included conditions, such as unilateral renal agenesis, horseshoe kidney, or bilateral RCC, in which radical nephrectomy would leave the patient anephric, resulting in the need for immediate dialysis. Additional relative indications include unilateral RCC with a diseased contralateral kidney, placing the patient at risk for significantly diminished renal function. Examples of these conditions include diabetes, hypertensive nephrosclerosis, renal artery stenosis, renal calculi, and chronic pyelonephritis. Tumors less than 4 cm in size have also been considered good candidates for NSS provided that the renal artery or vein did not appear to be involved. More recently, there has been a

tendency to extend the indication to include tumors of larger size but typically only in cases where there is an expectation that the function of the contralateral kidney may not be optimal. The treatment options for NSS have increased significantly in recent years. Namely, although open partial nephrectomy remains the gold standard by which surgical outcomes should be measured, minimally invasive methods are gaining widespread popularity. Laparoscopic partial nephrectomy techniques have evolved to the point that most centers are able to offer this approach for many patients. Even more recently, there has been a very strong movement toward the use of the DaVinci robot for partial nephrectomies to allow minimally invasive treatment of tumors that otherwise would normally be treated with open techniques. The strength of the DaVinci robot is that it markedly facilitates the ability to rapidly and accurately perform intracorporeal suturing while the renal vessels are clamped. Ischemia under such conditions is purely warm ischemia, however, as opposed to open surgery where cold ischemia is employed. In those conditions, speed is of the essence because any ischemia beyond 20 to 30 minutes will result in irreversible injury to the kidney. Open partial nephrectomy in our own center is preferred when more than one mass requires resection, when the mass is complex with the need for collecting system repair, and when the resection is deep, central, and possibly involves the renal vessels. In some cases, we will also prefer an open approach when there is a unilateral kidney because cold ischemia can be employed, minimizing the potential loss of renal function. Tumors that are more exophytic, lateral, or smaller are ideal for laparoscopic partial nephrectomy and the use of the DaVinci has allowed larger or deeper tumors to be approached, when open surgery might otherwise be more commonly used. Long-term outcomes from partial nephrectomy done with robotic techniques are not yet available and will take many years to mature, although there is no reason a priori to believe that they will be fundamentally different than other series. Although it is clear that open partial nephrectomy will always remain the gold standard for nephron sparing management of renal masses, increasingly alternative methods are being utilized because the open approach is considered morbid with an extended recovery time.

▌ IMAGE-GUIDED THERAPIES

Cryoablation and Radiofrequency Ablation

Image-guided, percutaneous radiofrequency ablation (RFA) and cryoablation are becoming increasingly popular treatment options, especially for patients who are not surgical candidates. RFA (FIGURE 16.2) for RCC was introduced in 1997 and has since proven to be an effective means of local tumor treatment, albeit long-term follow-up is lacking still. Short-term local tumor control rates are in the range of 90% to 95%[15–19] although for smaller tumors only. Published results have shown that RFA is particularly effective in treating renal tumors smaller than 3 cm. Gervais et al.[16] found RFA to be 100% and 81% effective in the treatment of renal tumors less than or equal to 3 cm and greater than 3 cm, respectively. Varkarakis et al.[20] showed 100% success in treating tumors smaller than 3 cm and 78% success in those tumors 3 cm or larger. Zagoria et al.[18] were also 100% successful in treating smaller tumors, but success dropped to 60% in the treatment of tumors over 3 cm in size. In a study

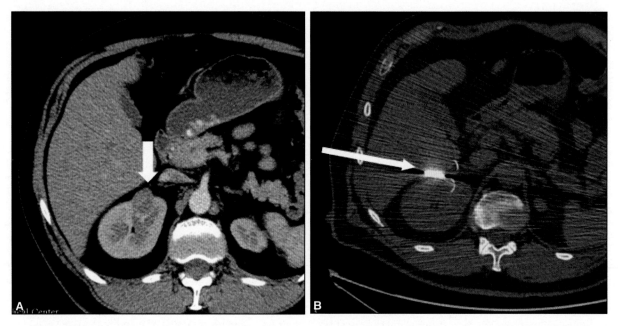

FIGURE 16.2 Radiofrequency ablation (RFA) of an anterior right renal tumor (*short white arrow*). There is no demonstrated difference in the efficacy between cryoablation and RFA for RCC. Certain differences, however, do exist. Cryoablation is much less painful and it provides real-time feedback because the ice-ball is visible. On the other hand, RFA has a slightly lower risk of hemorrhage because it coagulates damaged blood vessels. **A.** Right medial solid renal mass, with liver obstructing access. **B.** A transhepatic approach (*thin white arrow*) as shown above is thus theoretically safer with RFA.

Courtesy of Dr. Paul Harrod-Kim.

encompassing the work of two centers, Gupta et al. reported data on 163 tumors in 151 treated patients. At mean follow-up of 1.5 years, 153 of the 163 (94%) tumors showed no evidence of recurrence. Long-term outcomes following RFA were recently published by Levinson et al.[21] Looking at a consecutive cohort of patients with 5.1 years of follow-up, 27 of 31 tumors (87%) showed no evidence of recurrence/residual tumor. Of the four treatment failures, three were successfully re-treated with ablation and one was surgically resected, yielding a disease-specific survival of 100% at a mean follow-up of 57 months. Major complications following RFA are rare (3% to 8%) and primarily include bleeding and urothelial injury.[16,18]

With the introduction of argon-based cryoablation equipment and smaller diameter cryoprobes, percutaneous cryoablation became practicable (FIGURES 16.3 and 16.4). The published intraoperative experience has demonstrated the durability of this cold-based mechanism of tissue destruction with 3-year follow-up data showing 96% local control.[22] Additional reports of surgical cryoablation outcomes show 5-year local control rates as high as 94%.[23] Two large percutaneous cryoablation studies have demonstrated excellent short-term local control rates. Littrup et al.[24] treated 49 tumors in 48 patients. At a mean follow-up of 1.6 years, local control was achieved in 45 of 49 (92%) tumors. Atwell et al.[25] published their results in the treatment of 115 tumors in 110 patients. At a mean follow-up of 1.1 years, three patients were known to have local treatment failure (97% local control). Complications associated with cryoablation appear to be similar to RFA, occurring in up to 6% of patients.[24,25] In conclusion, the rate of significant complications of percutaneous ablation is about 6% and the efficacy about 90% to 95%

for both RFA and cryoablation. Despite the excellent short-term outcomes, however, both modalities suffer from lack of long-term results.

Although there is lack of prospective, randomized studies comparing ablative modalities with the reference standard of NSS, multiple single arm studies have demonstrated high efficacy and an acceptable safety profile for both RFA and cryoablation. Reported efficacy is around 95% to 98% for stage IA and lower for stage IB disease. The risk of significant complications is around 4% to 6% for both modalities.[16,18,25,26] Studies demonstrating these high-efficacy rates for both modalities are prone to the same criticism, that is, lack of long-term follow-up.

Microwave ablation has been reported to have certain theoretical advantages compared to other ablative modalities for treating cystic tumors or tumors adjacent to heat sinks. There is even less published data on its efficacy and safety regarding treatment of RCC.[27] In summary, there is no demonstrated difference in safety or efficacy between the ablative modalities or ablation systems available. Subsequently, the selection of the ablative modality or ablation system depends mostly on the operator's experience, which is the variable most strongly associated with good outcomes.

Complications of Percutaneous Ablation

When ablation is chosen, there are some precautions we have found useful, which are not necessarily well documented in the literature. Namely, percutaneous ablation can result in nerve injury and neuralgia—primarily involving the intercostal nerves but also the gentifemoral and lateral femoral cutaneous nerves

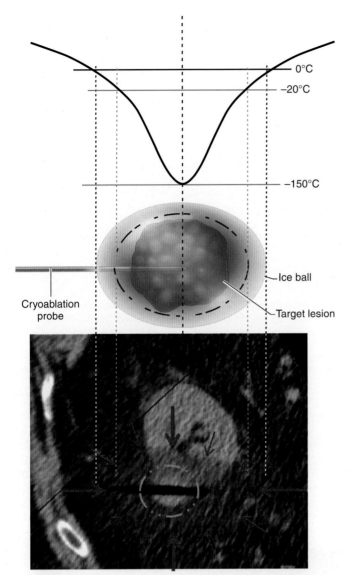

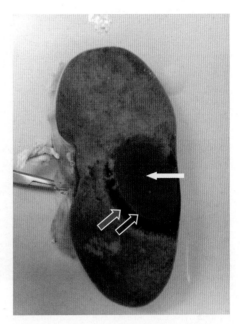

FIGURE 16.4 In vitro appearance of a swine kidney after percutaneous cryoablation. At the end of the freezing cycle the renal artery was injected with methylene blue, staining the perfused portion (non-ice-ball) of the kidney. The hypervascular ring (*blue arrow*) around the ice-ball is stained by methylene blue significantly more than the surrounding renal parenchyma. The nonperfused (and thus not stained) ice-ball demonstrates a red hue (*red arrow*). The cryoprobe defect is seen in the center of the defect (*white arrow*).

FIGURE 16.3 Principles of cryoablation. The visible ice-ball demarcates the 0°C isotherm (*red arrows*). This temperature is not lethal and, therefore, the ice-ball should cover the target lesion (*blue circle*) plus a safety margin beyond it. Lethal temperature for mammalian tissue is −20°C and is found approximately 5 mm inside the visible ice-ball. The black line represents the void left after removal of the cryoprobe because the tissues are still frozen.

(FIGURE 16.5). When performing these procedures, care should be taken to minimize the risk of injury to these structures. Hydro- or air-dissection via a spinal needle may protect the nerve, or any nontarget structure for that matter, including the pancreas and colon (FIGURE 16.6). Occasionally, we have found that temporary use of pregabalin may help ameliorate these symptoms when opioids are inadequate, but in the vast majority of cases, the neuralgia is self-limited and resolves spontaneously without intervention. Patients with two or more risk factors for cardiac disease, or with known history of cardiac disease, are counseled to initiate periprocedural beta blockers, typically ceasing their use within a month after ablation. Patients with lesions near or involving the adrenal gland are counseled to take alpha- and beta-blocking agents to prevent a catecholamine surge during the ablation from precipitating a cardiac event. Finally, lesions that are in close proximity to the ureter (FIGURE 16.7) are best treated by placing a ureteral stent prior to ablation and leaving in situ for at least a month after the ablation to facilitate complete healing without stricture. Although no formal studies have been conducted to determine the precise utility of these maneuvers, we have found that our initial experience was overrepresented for cardiac arrhythmias and ureteral strictures until these steps were taken. Now such complications are exceedingly rare.

The imaging appearance of RCC on follow-up imaging after ablation varies but in general it shows as a devascularized mass on short-term follow-up that gradually shrinks long term (FIGURE 16.8). A hypervascular and sometimes permanent ring may appear representing fibrosis and should not be confused with residual tumor.

▌ MEDICAL THERAPIES

Because most RCC are detected at an early stage (70% to 80%), the primary treatment objective is cure. This can be achieved in most cases with nephrectomy, NSS, or MINSS. Systemic chemotherapy (or radiation for that matter) offers no additional benefit in patients without established metastatic disease. On the other hand, approximately 20% to 30% of patients with RCC have advanced disease at presentation. Some of those with localized

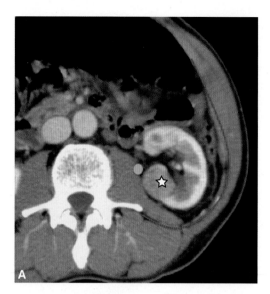
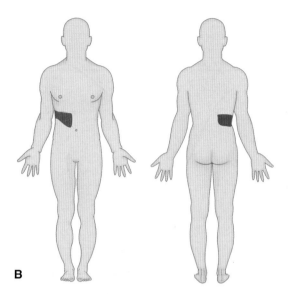

FIGURE 16.5 The intercostal (*red*) and genitofemoral (*yellow*) nerves subpart **A** are frequently at risk during renal ablation. If injured, symptoms involve the dermatomes depicted in subpart **B** and may take weeks to months to resolve. Hydro- or air-dissection with a spinal needle can help minimize the risk of nerve injury. Potential nerve injury should not be a contraindication to treatment.

disease will develop metastases at some point, raising the lifetime risk of metastatic RCC (mRCC) to 40% to 50%. The 5-year survival of patients with mRCC is reported to be 0% to 18%. Approximately 92% of patients with mRCC present with only one or two metastases of which 45% to 64% are pulmonary metastases with the rest involving lymph nodes, bone, nephrectomy site, liver, adrenal, pancreas, brain, thyroid, and subcutaneous tissues.[28] The fact that the majority of patients present with oligometastatic

disease presents an opportunity to improve life expectancy. The surgical literature suggests that metastasectomy improves the 5-year survival to approximately 40% to 50%[29] from the 0% to 18% without treatment. Cytoreductive nephrectomy appears to impart an independent survival benefit[30] for patients with mRCC.

In addition to the survival benefit imparted by surgical cytoreduction, a number of targeted chemotherapeutic agents have shown promise in further improving life expectancy. The

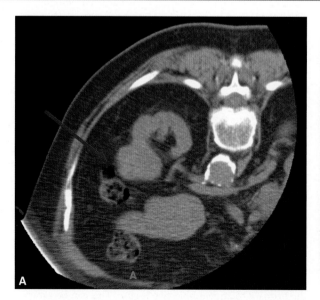
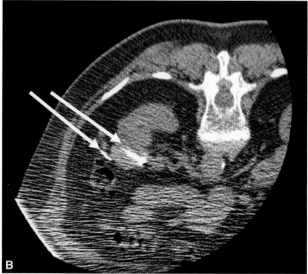

FIGURE 16.6 **A.** Occasionally, a nontarget organ may be in close proximity to the tumor (*red arrow, colon*). It is always worth attempting ablation because by placing the patient prone, the anatomy may change and allow for safe treatment. Air- or hydro-dissection are almost always effective in separating the nontarget organ (colon above) from the lesion. **B.** A spinal needle is usually placed between the two (*lower white arrow*); air or water are infused and the ablation probe (*upper white arrow*) can then be safely placed for treatment.

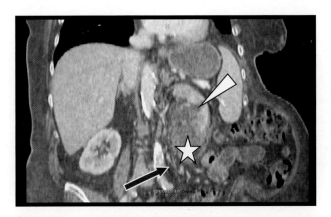

FIGURE 16.7 During ablation of an anterior, inferior RCC (*star*) the ureter (*red arrow*) was inadvertently injured. This was manifested as hydronephrosis (*white arrowhead*) that required prolonged drainage via percutaneous nephrostomy tube. Placement of a double-J ureteral stent prior to ablating RCC near the ureter mitigates this risk.

advent of these targeted agents has indeed changed the treatment paradigm for mRCC. The tyrosine kinase inhibitors (TKI) sunitinib and pazopanib, as well as the anti-VEGF antibody bevacizumab in combination with interferon alpha (INF-a), are now approved for first-line use in patients with mRCC. Sunitinib has been shown to prolong progression-free-survival from 5 to 11 months compared to standard INF-a. In addition, sunitinib results in a better objective response (31% versus 6%, $p < .001$).[31] The mTOR inhibitor temsirolimus has also been approved as a first-line treatment in high-risk patients. It has been shown to improve the 3-month survival of patients with mRCC. Everolimus is FDA approved as a second-line therapy after progression on prior TKI therapy and has shown efficacy across risk groups. In summary, in the majority of patients, systemic chemotherapies are indicated only for advanced disease. The first of these agents was approved in 2007, and hence the long-term experience with these new drugs is unknown. Anecdotally, many patients have responded far more favorably to these new agents than was originally predicted by the registrations of clinical trials, which led to their approval. Long-term outcomes, however, are still pending analysis.

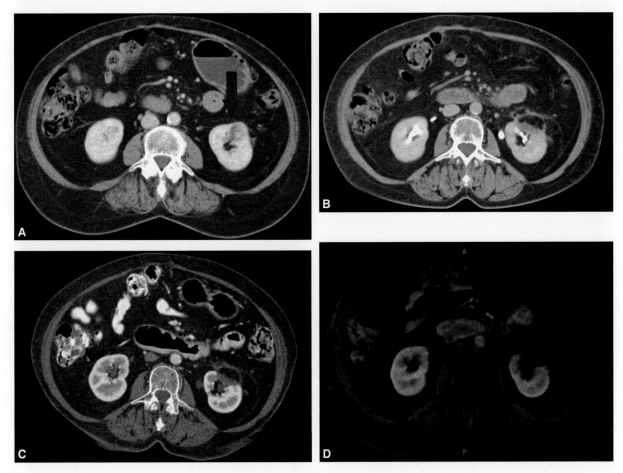

FIGURE 16.8 Appearance of an RCC at yearly intervals after ablation. Baseline (*red arrow*) shows a solid, 2.5-cm mass. Follow-up shows a shrinking, nonenhancing scar and a persistent thin hypervascular ring at the margin of the cryoablation ice-ball, representing fibrosis. This should not be confused with residual tumor. Pre-ablation **A**, 12-month post-ablation **B**, 24-month post-ablation **C** and 36-month post-ablation **D**.

DISCUSSION

Decision Making in Approaching a Renal Mass

With the rapid proliferation of techniques for treating renal masses, decision making regarding treatment has become more complex. There is no universally accepted algorithm for approaching a renal mass. Instead, we generally offer the patient counseling and tailor treatment according to their individual needs. Patients who are elderly with significant comorbid conditions and for whom life expectancy is not expected to exceed 3 years are usually counseled to consider observation and expectant management. In those cases, we generally counsel that intervention should only be undertaken if the cancer appears to be aggressive and the risk of inaction would likely result in a terminal condition. Such a decision is usually best made by initial frequent monitoring with imaging every 3 months for up to 1 year. Once relative stability is established, monitoring frequency can be decreased to every 4- to 6-month intervals. If during such monitoring the tumor is growing significantly (>1 cm between each set of imaging) then intervention may be more compelling. For patients in whom intervention is deemed desirable and/or necessary but whose underlying health is still significantly compromised, ablation is our preferred approach. Not all lesions can be approached by ablation. Cystic lesions are usually better suited to observation or surgical resection and we only rarely recommend ablation for such lesions. Lesions larger than 4 cm have a much higher failure rate with ablation and, therefore, are typically avoided. However, in many instances in which surgery is just not feasible, we have successfully ablated very large lesions by performing "staged" ablations with several treatment sessions, typically spaced apart by 1 month intervals to allow recovery and to assess the residual disease to be ablated. In most cases, we can complete treatment in two sessions, and even with very large lesions, we can usually achieve a complete treatment within three sessions. Local regional anatomy, however, plays a significant role in planning such "staged" procedures because adjacent organs can often limit our ability to fully ablate a lesion without collateral injury.

Lesions that are smaller (4 cm) and amenable to surgical intervention in an otherwise healthy individual are usually counseled that partial nephrectomy is the gold standard, although ablation may still be reasonable. In such cases, we always emphasize the need for continued long-term follow-up because the 5- and 10-year outcomes of ablation are not yet clearly established. When partial nephrectomy is chosen, the modality of partial nephrectomy (open, laparoscopic, or robotic) depends primarily on the size, location, and choice of the treating surgeon. Large lesions in patients with otherwise good kidney function are typically recommended for radical nephrectomy. Most radical nephrectomies can be performed laparoscopically, provided no other structures are involved and the size of the lesion is not prohibitive. FIGURE 16.9 shows the current types and relative rates of treatment currently in the United States. When other structures are involved (e.g., tumor thrombus, or involvement of the colon, pancreas, or spleen), then an open approach is preferred.

Immunologic Implications of Cryosurgery

There are multiple theories to the mechanism of action of cryoablative surgery. The most accepted is a combination of two synergistic mechanisms of action: one being direct cellular injury leading to coagulative necrosis, and the second indirect injury

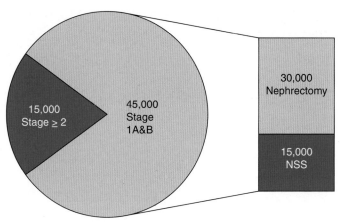

RCC incidence in USA = 60,000

FIGURE 16.9 Of the nearly 60,000 Americans who are diagnosed every year (as of 2010) with RCC, approximately 75% (45,000) have stage 1A or 1B, which is considered curable disease. Despite the excellent long-term outcomes of partial nephrectomy, the majority of these patients are treated with nephrectomy. Eventually, only 1:3 of patients with stage 1A or 1B disease is treated with nephron sparing surgery (NSS). This is likely caused by lack of necessary expertise outside larger medical centers.

by vascular thrombosis leading to apoptosis along the edge of the ablation zone. Once cells and tissue have been destroyed, the immune system is activated to assist in the healing process. Interleukin 6 levels are known to rise substantially after cryoablation (personal observation by our own measurements). The innate immune system is stimulated to help clear out the local debris and form a mature scar. The mature scar often takes as long as a year to form, and if there is intralesional hemorrhage, dense calcification may also form along the ablation zone (typically near the center of the ablation). Historically, many groups have reported anecdotal evidence of enhanced survival in patients with metastatic disease treated by cryoablation.[32] No clear evidence exists, however, to substantiate that cryoablation alone can result in a significant anti-tumor immunity in the absence of any other stimulus. In contrast, at least two different groups have found that additional adjuvant treatments, either with toll-like receptor agonists or with T-reg down-regulators, are able to result in the generation of systemic antitumor immunity[33] and our own.[34] As a result of such preclinical studies, several groups (including our own) are actively involved in clinical trials combining immune stimulation with cryoablation for patients with advanced disease. In the future, such strategies may have profound implications for the treatment of kidney cancer, even with localized disease. For instance, if local treatments are combined with an adjuvant, it may be possible to prevent subsequent recurrences in the future, or enhance the efficacy of local treatment in those patients who might otherwise have recurred at a later date.

CONCLUSION

Treatment of the patient with RCC is optimized with a multidisciplinary team effort. Because of RCC's unique clinic-pathologic characteristics and behavior the patient's own life expectancy, comorbid conditions, and personal preferences play a major

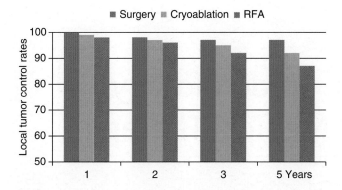

FIGURE 16.10 Local tumor control rates (Y-axis) after surgery, cryoablation and RFA for stage 1A RCC. Surgery (and especially partial nephrectomy) remains the gold standard despite the very similar outcomes. The reason is that surgery still has the longest and most robust follow-up data. The choice of treatment, however, depends on many factors, including comorbid conditions, tumor morphology, and patient preference.

role is choosing the specific treatment. Patients with comorbid conditions, single kidneys, compromised renal function, or syndromes that predispose them to multiple RCC should be considered for ablation. For the majority of patients, however, and until long-term data are forthcoming for local treatments, partial nephrectomy remains the best treatment option (FIGURE 16.10). Finally, some patients will require combination treatments and concerted efforts by both urology and interventional radiology to ensure the best chance for cure and renal function preservation.

▌ REFERENCES

1. Prasad SR, Humphrey PA, Catena JR, et al. Common and uncommon histologic subtypes of renal cell carcinoma: imaging spectrum with pathologic correlation. *Radiographics* 2006;26:1795–1806.
2. Reuter VE. The pathology of renal epithelial neoplasms. *Semin Oncol* 2006;33:534–543.
3. McLaughlin JK, Lipworth L, Tarone RE. Epidemiologic aspects of renal cell carcinoma. *Semin Oncol* 2006;33:527–533.
4. Kuczyk MA, Anastasiadis AG, Zimmermann R, et al. Current aspects of the surgical management of organ-confined, metastatic and recurrent renal cell cancer. *BJU Int* 2005;96:721–727.
5. Hafron J, Kaouk JH. Cryosurgical ablation of renal cell carcinoma. *Cancer Control* 2007;14:211–217.
6. Lipworth L, Tarone RE, McLaughlin JK. The epidemiology of renal cell carcinoma. *J Urol* 2006;176:2353–2358.
7. Horner MJ, Ries LAG, Krapcho M, et al. *SEER Cancer Statistics Review, 1975–2006*. Bethesda, MD: National Cancer Institute.
8. Ficarra V, Galfano A, Mancini M, et al. TNM staging systems for renal cell carcinoma: current status and future perspectives. *Lancet Oncol* 2007;8:554–558.
9. Best S, Ercole B, Lee C, et al. Minimally invasive therapy for renal cell carcinoma: is there a new community standard? *Urology* 2004;64:22–25.
10. Weld KJ, Figenshau RS, Venkatesh R, et al. Laparoscopic cryoablation for small renal masses: three-year follow-up. *Urology* 2007;69:448–451.
11. Wyler SF, Sulser T, Ruszat R, et al. Intermediate-term results of retroperitoneoscopy-assisted cryotherapy for small renal tumors using multiple ultrathin cryoprobes. *Eur Urol* 2007;51:971–979.
12. Aron M, Gill IS. Minimally invasive nephron-sparing surgery (MINSS) for renal tumors: part II, probe ablative therapy. *Eur Urol* 2007;51:348–357.
13. Shingleton WB, Sewell PE, Jr. Cryoablation of renal tumours in patients with solitary kidneys. *BJU Int* 2003;92:237–239.
14. Georgiades CS, Hong K, Marx J, et al. Percutaneous cryoablation for renal tumors: safety and short term follow up. Presented at: CIRSE Annual Meeting; September 2007; Athens, Greece. Available at: http://www.cirse.org/files/File/cirse2007_final_web72_reduzierte%20groesse(2).pdf. Accessed Sept 2007.
15. Farrell MA, Charboneau WJ, DiMarco DS, et al. Image-guided radiofrequency ablation of solid renal tumors. *Am J Roentgenol* 2003;180(6):1509–1513.
16. Gervais DA, McGovern FJ, Arellano RS, et al. Radiofrequency ablation of renal cell carcinoma: part 1, indications, results, and role in patient management over a 6-year period and ablation of 100 tumors. *AJR Am J Roentgenol* 2005;185(1):64–71.
17. Hegarty NJ, Gill IS, Desai MM, et al. Probe-ablative nephron-sparing surgery: cryoablation versus radiofrequency ablation. *Urology* 2006;68(suppl 1):7–13.
18. Zagoria RJ, Traver MA, Werle DM, et al. Oncologic efficacy of CT-guided percutaneous radiofrequency ablation of renal cell carcinomas. *AJR Am J Roentgenol* 2007;189(2):429–436.
19. Gupta A, Raman JD, Leveillee RJ, et al. General anesthesia and contrast enhanced computed tomography to optimize renal percutaneous radiofrequency ablation: multi-institutional intermediate-term results. *J Endourol* 2009;23(7):1099–1105.
20. Varkarakis IM, Allaf ME, Inagaki T, et al. Percutaneous radio frequency ablation of renal masses: results at a 2-year mean followup. *J Urol* 2005;174(2):456–460; discussion 460.
21. Levinson AW, Su LM, Agarwal D, et al. Long-term oncological and overall outcomes of percutaneous radio frequency ablation in high risk surgical patients with a solitary small renal mass. *J Urol* 2008;180(2):499–504; discussion 504.
22. Gill IS, Remer EM, Hasan WA, et al. Renal cryoablation: outcome at 3 years. *J Urol* 2005;173(6):1903–1907.
23. Stein RJ, Kaouk JH. Renal cryotherapy: a detailed review including a 5-year follow-up. *BJU Int* 2007;99(5 pt B):1265–1270.
24. Littrup PJ, Ahmed A, Aoun HD, et al. CT-guided percutaneous cryotherapy of renal masses. *J Vasc Interv Radiol* 2007;18(3):383–392.
25. Atwell TD, Farrell MA, Leibovich BC, et al. Percutaneous renal cryoablation: experience treating 115 tumors. *J Urol* 2008;179(6):2136–2140; discussion 2140–2141.
26. Breen DJ, Rutherford EE, Stedman B, et al. Management of renal tumors by image-guided radiofrequency ablation: experience in 105 tumors. *Cardiovasc Intervent Radiol* 2007;30(5):936–942.
27. Lark PE, Woodruff RD, Zagoria RJ, et al. Microwave ablation of renal parenchymal tumors before nephrectomy: phase I study. *AJR Am J Roentgenol* 2007;188(5):1212–1214.
28. Naito S, Yamamoto N, Takayama T, et al. Prognosis of Japanese metastatic renal cell carcinoma patients in the cytokine era: a cooperative group report of 1463 patients. *Eur Urol* 2010;57:317–325.
29. Hofmann HS, Neef H, Krohe K, et al. Prognostic factors and survival after pulmonary resection of metastatic renal cell carcinoma. *Eur Urol* 2005;48:77–81.
30. Russo P, O'Brien MF. Surgical intervention in patients with metastatic renal cancer: metastasectomy and cytoreductive nephrectomy. *Urol Clin North Am* 2008;35:679–686.
31. Motzer RJ, Hutson TE, Tomczak P. Sunitinib versus interferon alfa in metastatic renal-cell carcinoma. *N Engl J Med* 2007;356:115–124.
32. Sidana A, Chowdhury WH, Fuchs EJ, et al. Cryoimmunotherapy in urologic oncology. *Urology* 2010;75(5):1009–1014.
33. den Brok MH, Sutmuller RP, Nierkens S, et al. Synergy between in situ cryoablation and TLR9 stimulation results in a highly effective in vivo dendritic cell vaccine. *Cancer Res* 2006;66(14):7285–7292.
34. Levy MY, Sidana A, Chowdhury WH, et al. Cyclophosphamide unmasks an antimetastatic effect of local tumor cryoablation. *J Pharmacol Exp Ther* 2009;330(2):596–601.

CHAPTER
17
Lung Cancer: Epidemiology, Staging and Medical Therapy

MARJORIE G. ZAUDERER, ALEXANDER D. DRILON, and LEE M. KRUG

INTRODUCTION

Lung cancer is a lethal disease. Despite recent insights into its biology and an expansion of therapeutic options, approximately 160,000 people continue to die from lung carcinoma each year in the United States. Worldwide, it is the leading cause of death from cancer, accounting for more mortality than breast, prostate, and colorectal cancer combined.[1]

EPIDEMIOLOGY

Lung cancer is undoubtedly one of the most preventable malignancies affecting modern society. Prior to the increased prevalence of smoking in the early 1900s, lung cancer was a rare malignancy. With the advent of widespread manufacturing of cigarettes in 1910, the number of deaths from lung cancer rose dramatically. This was first noted in men in the 1930s, and later in women in the 1960s, with a 20-year lag-time observed between the rise in smoking rates and the increase in mortality (FIGURE 17.1).[2] It was only in the late 1950s, however, that a causal relationship between the two was established, largely through the efforts of epidemiologists such as Doll and Hill and their work on the British Doctors Study. Despite this, it took several more years until the United States Surgeon General's Warning was released in 1964. Fortunately, the mortality from lung cancer in men has decreased since the early 1990s, likely reflecting a reduction in tobacco usage. Mortality in women has begun to plateau and will hopefully decrease in the years to come.[1]

Today, about 220,000 individuals in the United States are diagnosed with lung cancer each year.[1,3] The incidence peaks between the ages of 65 and 85 and varies by ethnic and racial groups, with the highest age-adjusted rates in the United States among African American men. Incidence among Asian, Hispanic, and Native Americans is approximately 40% to 50% of those of Caucasians.[3]

ETIOLOGIES

Approximately 85% of lung cancer cases are attributable to smoking. The risk is closely associated with the number of pack-years smoked and the age at which smoking is initiated. Compared with never-smokers, the relative risk of developing the malignancy is between 10- and 20-fold higher for active smokers and up to 2-fold higher for people exposed to passive smoke.

The risk decreases by roughly 75% after 10 to 15 years of abstinence, but never approaches zero, with about half of all lung cancers in the US occurring in former smokers.[4]

About 55 carcinogens and approximately 4,000 other compounds are present in the particulate phase of cigarette smoke.[5] The two predominant classes of nicotine-related carcinogens are the N-nitrosamines and the polycyclic aromatic hydrocarbons. Both groups of compounds are metabolized by the p450 enzyme system and result in the development of DNA adducts. These by-products have been postulated to lead to the development of lung tumors in several animal models.

Lung cancer has also been associated, albeit to a lesser degree, with other exposures such as asbestos and radon. *Asbestos* is a term for a group of naturally occurring fibers composed of silicates that are commonly used for construction and insulation due to their physical properties. Exposure to the fibers has been associated with the development of pulmonary asbestosis, mesothelioma, and lung cancer. The risk for the latter is dramatically increased by a concomitant history of smoking.[6]

Cumulative exposure to radon, a radioactive, odorless gas that occurs naturally as a product of uranium decay, has been associated with the development of lung cancer. Although most of the models of exposure have been based on uranium miner studies, residential exposure secondary to accumulation in insufficiently ventilated buildings has been proposed.[7] Other risk factors for lung cancer include exposure to radiation, nickel, chromium, beryllium, and air pollution.

SCREENING

The grim prognosis associated with lung cancer is, in part, related to the fact that most patients present with advanced disease. Attempts to detect the disease at an earlier and potentially more curable stage, therefore, seem intuitive. The major interventions that have been examined in this respect include chest radiography, sputum cytology, and low-dose helical computed tomography (CT) scans.

In the 1980s, Johns Hopkins, Memorial Sloan-Kettering, and Mayo Clinic conducted studies, each involving about 10,000 participants, who were randomized to screening with chest x-rays and/or sputum cytology. Although these studies found an increase in earlier-stage disease and an improvement in overall survival, no differences were noted in lung cancer specific mortality.[8–11] This led to a long-standing recommendation against using these

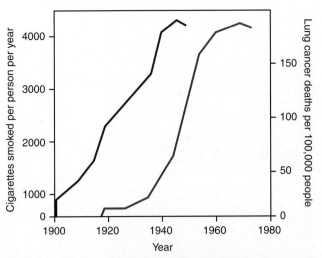

FIGURE 17.1 Lung cancer and smoking association. Twenty-year time lag between smoking and lung cancer. The incidence of lung cancer in men rose in 1910. It was only in 1930 that the mortality from lung cancer began to rise in a fashion virtually parallel to the increase in cigarettes smoked per person per year.

Adapted from the NIH.gov website

modalities as routine screening tools. Of note, these studies were conducted in an era where squamous cell carcinoma represented the most common non–small-cell lung cancer histology.

More recently, several series have examined the role of low-dose helical CT as a screening tool for lung cancer given its higher sensitivity for detecting smaller tumors that would be at an earlier stage compared to chest radiography. The International Early Lung Cancer Project (I-ELCAP) undertook an observational study screening 31,567 high-risk individuals with annual low-dose helical CT scans. Of the 484 patients who were diagnosed with lung cancer, 85% had clinical stage I disease. The estimated 10-year survival in this group was 88% overall and 92% in those who were able to undergo resection within a month. Although these numbers were higher in comparison to a reported 8-year survival rate of 75% by the National Cancer Institute Surveillance, Epidemiology, and End Results (SEER) database, the major criticism of this study was the lack of a control group, subjecting the results to length-time, lead-time, and overdiagnosis bias. [12]

To address this, the National Lung Screening Trial was initiated where 53,454 heavy or former smokers (defined as 30 pack-years) between the ages of 55 and 74 were randomized to either chest radiography or low-dose helical CT annually for a total of 3 screens. There were 247 deaths from lung cancer per 100,000 person-years in the low-dose CT group and 309 deaths per 100,000 person-years in the radiography group, representing a relative reduction in mortality from lung cancer with low-dose CT screening of 20%. All-cause mortality was reduced as well by 6.7% when the two groups were compared. [13]

These findings strongly support the role of CT screening in the early detection of lung cancer in patients with a heavy smoking history. As with any screening modality, the socioeconomic implications of this move demand close scrutiny. These concerns need to be weighed, however, against the fact that the 20% reduction in lung cancer mortality is comparable to a 21% reduction in breast

cancer mortality achieved by annual mammography [14] —a practice that has achieved widespread use. Of course, smoking cessation and prevention remain the optimal ways to prevent lung cancer.

PATHOLOGY

Lung carcinomas are broadly divided into two categories: non–small-cell lung cancer (NSCLC) and small-cell lung cancer (SCLC). The former accounts for 87% of cases, whereas the latter accounts for 13%. [15] NSCLC is further subdivided into squamous cell carcinoma, adenocarcinoma, and large-cell carcinoma. Pathologic classification is based on the latest World Health Organization (WHO) classification of lung tumors from 2004.

Non–Small-Cell Lung Cancer

Adenocarcinoma. Adenocarcinoma (AC) (FIGURE 17.2A) has emerged as the most common histologic subtype of NSCLC over the last 20 years, accounting for 40% to 50% of cases of NSCLC. The exact etiology of this shift is unclear but may be related to changes in smoking patterns and the use of filtered or low-tar cigarettes. Histologically, the tumor can be characterized by the presence of acini or glands, papillary or micropapillary structures, mucin formation, and solid areas. A large proportion of adenocarcinomas show a mixture of these patterns. [16] Adenocarcinomas tend to arise from the periphery of the lung and in scar tissue and have a propensity to present with metastatic disease. Nonsmokers are more likely to develop adenocarcinoma, although the majority of patients with the disease are smokers.

Bronchioloalveolar carcinoma (BAC) is separated out as a subset of pulmonary adenocarcinomas in the 2004 WHO classification. Pure *bronchioloalveolar carcinoma* is defined as a noninvasive neoplasm with a characteristic lepidic growth pattern. This distinction was made based on earlier studies that demonstrated a favorable prognosis for this subgroup. More commonly, however, BAC is found admixed with areas of invasive disease of varying proportions. Recently, there has been a move to replace the terms *BAC* and *mixed subtype adenocarcinoma* with terms such as *adenocarcinoma in situ* and *minimally invasive adenocarcinoma*. [17]

Squamous cell carcinoma. Squamous cell carcinoma (SCC) (FIGURE 17.2B) accounts for approximately 30% to 35% of NSCLC. It is thought to arise from a sequence of changes in normal bronchial epithelium, resulting in the development of metaplasia, dysplasia, carcinoma in situ, and, finally, invasive carcinoma. [18] Of the non–small-cell histologies, squamous cell carcinoma is the most highly associated with smoking. Well-differentiated tumor cells form keratin and intracellular bridges with infiltrating nests of cells and central necrosis that often results in cavitary disease. The tumors have a predilection for the central airways, causing obstruction of the bronchi and its attendant consequences, pneumonia and atelectasis. SCC is associated with a paraneoplastic syndrome of PTHrP secretion that results in hypercalcemia. Prior to the late 1980s, it represented the most prevalent subtype of NSCLC.

Large-cell carcinoma. Large-cell carcinoma (FIGURE 17.2C) accounts for approximately 10% of cases of NSCLC. Histologically, the tumor is characterized by large sheets of poorly differentiated

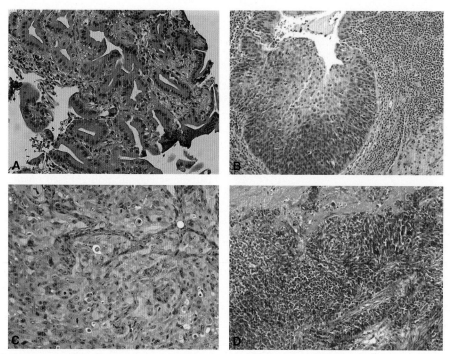

FIGURE 17.2 Lung cancer histology. A. Adenocarcinoma with notable acinar differentiation. **B.** Squamous cell carcinoma showing keratinization. Intercellular bridges are noted at higher magnification. **C.** Large-cell carcinoma with large, undifferentiated cells and no noticeable squamous or adenocarcinoma differentiation. **D.** Small-cell carcinoma with oval- and spindle-shaped cells, scant cytoplasm, and finely granular chromatin.

Courtesy of Dr. Andre Moreira, Memorial Sloan-Kettering Pathology Department

malignant cells with glandular, papillary, squamous, or small-cell features, often with areas of necrosis.[16] With improvements in histologic technique, cases of large-cell carcinoma have been reclassified as poorly differentiated adenocarcinoma or squamous cell carcinoma. Large-cell neuroendocrine carcinoma (LCNEC) is an aggressive malignancy occurring mainly in smokers characterized by neuroendocrine features both histologically and by immunohistochemistry. LCNEC has a prognosis intermediate between well-differentiated NSCLC and SCLC.

Small-Cell Lung Cancer

Small-cell carcinomas of the lung (FIGURE 17.2D) are histologically and biologically distinct neoplasms. In comparison to NSCLC, these tumors have a different natural history and prognosis. Biologically, SCLCs are characterized by a high-growth fraction, rapid doubling time, the early development of metastasis, and a propensity for recurrence after initial therapy.

Histologically, the malignancy is characterized by small round or oval cells with scant cytoplasm, nuclear molding, finely granular chromatin, and inconspicuous nucleoli. Tumor cells are often arranged in patterns forming trabeculae, rosettes, or peripheral palisading characteristic of neuroendocrine malignancies. Immunohistochemical stains are usually positive for CD56, synaptophysin, and chromogranin.[16] SCLC can be found mixed with large cells or with other NSCLC histologies. Differential diagnoses include poorly differentiated NSCLC, typical and atypical carcinoid, Merkel cell carcinoma, sarcoma with small-cell features such as synovial sarcoma, and lymphoma.

MOLECULAR BIOLOGY

The molecular landscape of lung cancer has shifted dramatically in the last decade. Specifically, we have come to understand the role of key mutations in the pathogenesis of disease and in the development of resistance to therapy. These alterations evolve in the presence of multiple other abnormalities, both genetic and epigenetic, that characterize the malignant phenotype.

Oncogenes

Alterations in epidermal growth factor receptor (EGFR) signaling have played a major role in redefining lung cancer therapeutics over the last few years. The receptor is a cell surface protein that binds extracellular ligands important for cell growth. This in turn results in receptor dimerization, intracellular kinase phosphorylation, and a cascade of downstream signaling involved in cell cycling, proliferation, and survival (FIGURE 17.3). Overexpression of EGFR secondary to an increase in gene copy number has been described in up to 50% of NSCLC and is thought to be a negative prognostic factor.[19]

Activating mutations of the tyrosine kinase domain of *EGFR* are present in approximately 10% to 15% of adenocarcinomas. The incidence of these alterations is enriched in a selected cohort of individuals, notably never-smokers, and particularly those from East Asia.[20] The most common molecular changes involve deletions in exon 19 and the L858R mutation in exon 21, both of which confer sensitivity to tyrosine kinase

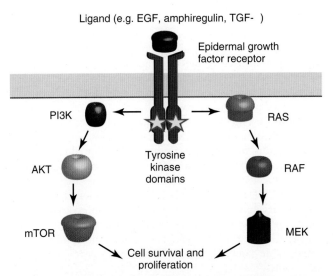

FIGURE 17.3 Epidermal growth factor receptor (EGFR) pathway. Activation mutations of the tyrosine kinase domain lead to increased ligand-independent downstream signaling in tumor cells. This results in the activation and maintenance of prosurvival pathways.

inhibition. The T790M mutation, on the other hand, confers resistance to tyrosine kinase inhibitors and is often developed in refractory disease after an initial response to therapy.[21] Amplification of the *MET* oncogene has been described as a separate major mechanism of acquired resistance to EGFR tyrosine kinase inhibition.[22]

RAS proteins are downstream components of growth factor receptor pathways such as EGFR. *KRAS* mutations are the most common oncogenic driver mutations in NSCLC. These alterations are found in 20% to 30% of adenocarcinomas and take the form of missense mutations that introduce an amino acid substitution at positions 12, 13, or 61.[23] *KRAS* mutations have been associated with tobacco-related carcinogens and confer resistance to EGFR tyrosine kinase inhibitors.

Recent work has uncovered the presence of the *EML4-ALK* fusion gene in approximately 3% to 7% of adenocarcinomas, and this, too, occurs primarily in patients without a history of smoking. The translocation results in the formation of a constitutively active tyrosine kinase with downstream effects on cell proliferation and survival. In a manner similar to EGFR mutations, tumor cells become highly reliant or "oncogene addicted" to increased ALK signaling, making them sensitive to tyrosine kinase inhibition.[24]

Gene amplification and gene product overexpression of *Myc* lead to increased oncogenesis via dysregulation of apoptosis, proliferation, and differentiation. *Myc* amplification is noted in 10% of NSCLCs and 20% of SCLCs and is more common in cell lines from previously treated patients.[25]

Tumor Suppressor Genes

Mutation of *p53* is the most common genetic alteration in NSCLCs. It occurs in up to 70% of adenocarcinomas and squamous cell carcinomas. The *p53* gene has been described as the "guardian of the genome." Mutations have been shown to interfere with the regulation of cell division, growth regulation, DNA repair, and apoptosis. In SCLC, mutated *p53* is more prevalent, occurring in up to 90% of cases.[26]

Alterations in the retinoblastoma gene, or *Rb,* are also common in lung cancer, with mutations occurring in up to 10% of NSCLC and 90% of SCLC. The gene encodes a protein product that is important for the regulation of cell cycling. *CDKN2A* or *p16* inactivation is present in 60% of NSCLC and in less than 5% of SCLC.[27]

Angiogenesis

Vascular endothelial growth factor (VEGF) is a key regulator involved in the migration and proliferation of endothelial cells responsible for tumor blood vessel formation. High expression of VEGF has been associated with increased microvessel density and poor prognosis in NSCLC. An increase in VEGF expression has been reported in approximately 60% of early stage NSCLC and serves as a biologic rationale for monoclonal antibody inhibition of the ligand.[28]

▌ CLINICAL PRESENTATION

The presenting symptoms of lung cancer vary according to the primary tumor's anatomic location and degree of spread. For patients with central lesions, common symptoms include cough, increased sputum production, hemoptysis, wheezing, shortness of breath, and obstructive pneumonia. Patients with peripheral lesions may present with pleuritic chest pain. Weight loss, anorexia, fatigue, and low-grade fever are common symptoms regardless of location.

A tumor in the pulmonary apex, also known as a Pancoast tumor, often leads to a variety of clinical manifestations. Invasion of the brachial plexus can result in significant shoulder and arm pain in an ulnar distribution that is referred to as the Pancoast syndrome. Compression of sympathetic ganglia or nerves often leads to Horner's syndrome, characterized by unilateral ptosis, miosis, anhidrosis, and enophthalmos. Involvement of the recurrent laryngeal nerve can cause hoarseness secondary to unilateral vocal cord paralysis.

Superior vena cava syndrome occurs secondary to a large tumor obstructing the superior vena cava. Symptoms include shortness of breath, facial edema, venous distention in the chest and neck, and upper extremity swelling.

The majority of patients who are diagnosed with lung cancer present with advanced disease. More than half of patients with NSCLC are diagnosed with stage III or IV disease, and up to half of adenocarcinomas can present with metastatic disease. In SCLC, 60% to 70% of patients present with extensive stage disease.

Metastatic disease has a propensity for involvement of a number of organs, notably the adrenals, liver, bones, and brain. Symptoms depend on the organ of involvement, such as pain caused by bony metastases or seizures caused by brain metastases. Pleural effusions can cause progressive shortness of breath and may require drainage by a thoracentesis, talc pleurodesis, or placement of a pleural catheter. Patients with pericardial effusions can present with symptoms of tamponade requiring a pericardial drainage or window procedure.

A small subset of patients present with paraneoplastic manifestations. These symptoms are usually secondary to ectopic hormone production.[29] Hypercalcemia of malignancy is often associated with squamous etiology and occurs due to the production of PTH-related protein. Hypertrophic pulmonary osteoarthropathy is associated with adenocarcinomas and results in pain in the upper and lower extremities secondary to long-bone periostitis.

Small-cell lung carcinoma, in particular, has been linked to a variety of paraneoplastic syndromes. The Syndrome of Inappropriate Diuretic Hormone secretion, or SIADH, is a classic association and is characterized by hyponatremia, hyposmolarity, and, if very severe, mental status changes. Cushing syndrome develops secondary to ectopic ACTH secretion and results in hypertension, hypokalemia, metabolic alkalosis, and hyperglycemia. The Lambert-Eaton syndrome is diagnosed clinically in the setting of proximal weakness that improves with repeated activity. These neurologic symptoms are produced by antibodies to voltage-gated calcium channels on presynaptic neurons. Although much more rare, paraneoplastic abnormalities such as cerebellar degeneration, limbic encephalopathy, optic neuritis, and dementia have been associated with both SCLC and NSCLC. Anti-Hu antibodies, in particular, can be found in SCLC and result in encephalomyelitis involving the cerebellum, cortex, limbic system, and brainstem.

▌WORKUP AND STAGING

Staging is a critical component of lung cancer management. Accurate staging serves to guide therapy decisions and determine prognosis.

The initial evaluation of a patient involves a thorough history and exam. This includes an assessment of performance status and weight loss. In terms of diagnostic tests, a CT of the chest and upper abdomen with visualization of the adrenals and blood work including a complete blood count and serum chemistries are often ordered. Magnetic resonance imaging (MRI) of the brain is recommended in patients with small-cell histology, or with non–small-cell histology and disease that is at least stage II or more advanced.[30] Positron emission tomography (PET) scanning is utilized to detect tumor physiology. As a single modality, it has been found to be more sensitive than computed tomography in detecting mediastinal nodal disease. Sensitivity is increased further when combined with CT scanning. Patients who undergo a PET scan do not require a bone scan due to adequate evaluation of bony disease in the former.

Evaluation of the mediastinum is an essential component of staging. This is particularly important in NSCLC where surgery plays a pivotal role. Patients with nodes that are larger than 1 cm on a CT scan require pathologic evaluation regardless of fluorodeoxyglucose uptake on PET. Mediastinoscopy was classically thought of as the gold standard in this respect. However, transbronchial, transthoracic, and endoscopic approaches to lymph node sampling have been shown to have comparable sensitivities.[31]

The TNM staging system has recently been revised by the International Association for the Study of Lung Cancer and adopted by the International Union Against Cancer and the American Joint Committee on Cancer (Tables 17.1 and 17.2). Major revisions include the subdivision of T1 and T2 based on size and reclassification of tumors larger than 7 cm as T3. Satellite nodules in the same lobe were downgraded from T4 to T3, as were satellite nodules in a different ipsilateral lobe from M1 to T4. M staging was redefined as well, with satellite nodules in the opposite lung and pleural and pericardial effusions reclassified as M1a disease and distant metastases classified as M1b disease.[32]

Another revision has been the application of the TNM system to small-cell carcinoma of the lung.[33] Traditional staging has followed the two-stage Veterans' Affairs Lung Study Group schema that separates SCLC into limited- or extensive-stage disease. Limited-stage disease is determined by whether or not the disease can be encompassed in one radiation port.[34]

Table 17.1

International System for Staging Lung Cancer Stage TNM Descriptors

Primary Tumor (T)	
	T0 No primary tumor

	T1 Tumor ≤3 cm, surrounded by lung or visceral pleura, not more proximal than lobar bronchus
	  T1a tumor ≤2 cm
	  T1b tumor >2 cm but ≤3 cm

	T2 Tumor >3 cm but ≤7 cm or with any of the following: invades visceral pleura, involves main bronchus ≥2 cm distal to the carina, atelectasis or obstructive pneumonia extending to hilum but not involving entire lung
	  T2a tumor >3 but ≤5 cm
	  T2b tumor >5 but ≤7 cm

	T3 Tumor >7 cm; directly invading chest wall, diaphragm, phrenic nerve, mediastinal pleura, or parietal pericardium; tumor in the main bronchus or <2 cm distal to the carina, or atelectasis/obstructive pneumonitis of entire lung; separate tumor nodules in same lobe
	T4 Tumor of any size with invasion of heart, great vessels, trachea, recurrent laryngeal nerve, esophagus, vertebral body, or carina; separate tumor nodules in different ipsilateral lobe

Table 17.1

International System for Staging Lung Cancer Stage TNM Descriptors (*Continued*)

Regional Lymph Nodes (N)	N0 No regional lymph node metastasis
	N1 Metastasis in ipsilateral peribronchial and/or perihilar lymph nodes and intrapulmonary nodes, including involvement by direct extension
	N2 Metastasis in ipsilateral mediastinal and/or subcarinal lymph nodes
	N3 Metastasis in contralateral hilar, ipsilateral or contralateral scalene, or supraclavicular lymph nodes
Distant Metastasis (M)	M0 No distant metastasis
	M1a Separate tumor nodules in a contralateral lobe or tumor with pleural nodules or malignant pleural dissemination
	M1b Distant metastasis

Table 17.2

International System for Staging Lung Cancer Stage Groups According to TNM Descriptor and Subgroups

Lung Cancer Stage Groups

T/M	Subgroup	N0	N1	N2	N3
T1	T1a	Ia	IIa	IIIa	IIIb
	T1b	Ia	IIa	IIIa	IIIb
T2	T2a	Ib	IIa	IIIa	IIIb
	T2b	IIa	IIb	IIIa	IIIb
T3	T3$_{>7}$	IIb	IIIa	IIIa	IIIb
	T3$_{inv}$	IIb	IIIa	IIIa	IIIb
	T3$_{satell}$	IIb	IIIa	IIIa	IIIb
T4	T4$_{inv}$	IIIa	IIIa	IIIb	IIIb
	T4$_{ipsi nod}$	IIIa	IIIa	IIIb	IIIb
M1	M1a$_{contr nod}$	IV	IV	IV	IV
	M1a$_{pl dissem}$	IV	IV	IV	IV
	M1b	IV	IV	IV	IV

NSCLC Therapies

A simplified paradigm for the management of NSCLC based on stage is displayed in FIGURE 17.4. Whenever possible, surgical resection is performed because it offers the best chance for long-term cure. With early stage NSCLC (stages I and II), complete resection is usually feasible. Postoperative chemotherapy is recommended for patients with stage II disease. Patients with N2 lymph node involvement (stage IIIA) have even greater risk of relapse, and additional therapies such as neoadjuvant or adjuvant chemotherapy and/or postoperative radiation therapy are needed in addition to surgery.

If surgery is not possible, either because of the extent of disease with N3 lymph nodes and/or T4 tumors (stage IIIB) or the patient does not have adequate cardiopulmonary reserve to tolerate resection, concurrent chemotherapy and radiation therapy is utilized. In advanced (stage IV) disease when cure is not possible, chemotherapy alone is the mainstay of therapy.

Surgery

Surgical resection is the primary treatment for early stage disease. Careful preoperative assessment is required not only to accurately stage the disease but also to assess medical operability. Lobectomy, the removal of a single lobe of the lung, is the standard of care. In a trial conducted by the Lung Cancer Study Group, limited pulmonary resection compared to lobectomy has a 30% increase in the death rate ($p = 0.08$), a 75% increase in recurrence rates ($p = 0.02$), and a tripled local recurrence rate ($pv = 0.008$).[35] However, this study was conducted 20 years ago, and, with the change in histology and staging techniques since then, the use of wedge resections or segmentectomies is being reconsidered for very small tumors. Wedge resections may be required in select situations—for example, to preserve lung function in patients with limited cardiopulmonary reserve, or in cases with multiple pulmonary nodules. To reduce surgical morbidity, closed surgical procedures, such as video-assisted thoracoscopic surgery (VATS), are used but up to 25% of cases require conversion to an open procedure, usually for difficulty in dissecting lymph nodes from the vascular structures.[36]

For proximal tumors not amenable to lobectomy, a pneumonectomy may be performed, but this carries a greater risk of complications and mortality, particularly with right-sided pneumonectomies and after induction therapy.[37] Sleeve resections, in which a lobe may be spared by reconstructing the bronchus or trachea, are preferred over pneumonectomies if feasible because they are associated with equivalent survival outcomes but fewer complications.[38] In more advanced disease, when tumors invade adjacent structures such as the chest wall, diaphragm, or mediastinum, *en bloc* resection with the involved structures is performed. Outcomes are variable and depend on the completeness of resection, extent of invasion, and lymph node status.[39,40]

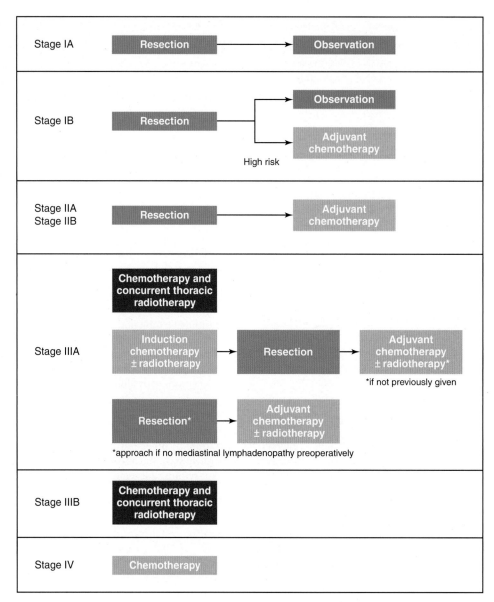

FIGURE 17.4 Treatment schema for NSCLC

Mediastinal lymph node resection is performed at the time of surgery. Based on a randomized trial of 532 stage IA to III patients, which showed a statistically significant improvement in median overall survival to 59 months with systematic lymph node dissection (SND) versus 34 months with mediastinal lymph node sampling (MLS), SND is preferred.[41] This approach improves the accuracy of clinical staging and helps reduce unnecessary surgical resections in patients with more advanced disease.

Radiation Therapy

Definitive Radiation

Among patients who are unable or unwilling to undergo resection, conventional fractionated radiation to a dose of at least 54 Gy may be used as a definitive treatment modality.[42] Various approaches have been studied to improve the efficacy of standard radiation. For example, the hyperfractionation of radiation into multiple daily doses demonstrated an approximate increase in survival of 9 months among patients with early stage disease in one trial,[43] but this approach suffers from logistical inconveniences as well as lack of additional confirmatory studies. On the other hand, stereotactic body radiation therapy (SBRT), which delivers a single or very limited number of high-dose fractions of radiation (FIGURE 17.5), is more in vogue because the sophisticated treatment plans enable higher doses to be administered with tighter margins.

Concurrent Chemoradiotherapy

Although radiation is effective in treating a primary tumor, patients with NSCLC are at high risk for developing metastatic disease, and, thus, systemic treatment with chemotherapy is an essential component, particularly for patients with locally advanced disease. Several trials have established

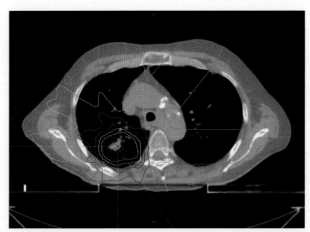

FIGURE 17.5 SBRT treatment plan. This is a prototypical treatment plan for early stage NSCLC using SBRT with 3 fractions of 1800 cGy.

Courtesy of Andreas Rimner, Memorial Sloan-Kettering Cancer Center

chemoradiotherapy as a standard definitive therapy option for patients with stage III disease.[44–46] Dillman's phase III trial established that the addition of chemotherapy improved survival over treatment with radiation alone.[47] That study administered chemotherapy first followed by radiation in a sequential fashion, but subsequent studies demonstrated that concurrent treatment is actually more effective.[48–51] For patients with stage IIIA disease treated with definitive chemoradiation, the addition of surgery has unclear benefits. Chemotherapy along with 45 Gy of radiation followed by resection was compared to chemotherapy with 61 Gy of radiation in 429 stage IIIA patients. Median survival based on intent to treat was 23.6 and 22.2 months, respectively (no statistically significant difference).[44] Surgical mortality was exceptionally high for patients who underwent pneumonectomy after induction therapy. When those patients were excluded in a subgroup analysis, a small survival benefit was seen if only a lobectomy was performed.

Postoperative Radiation Therapy

Although postoperative radiation therapy (PORT) decreases local tumor recurrence after surgical resection,[52,53] overall survival is not improved. In fact, a meta-analysis demonstrated an association between PORT and shorter survival (hazard ratio (HR) 1.18) and this negative effect was most dramatic among those with stage I and II disease.[52] However, a SEER database analysis demonstrated an association between PORT and improved survival in stage III patients (HR 0.855).[54] PORT is recommended in patients at high risk of local recurrence, such as those with mediastinal lymph node involvement or positive resection margins.

Chemotherapy

Adjuvant Chemotherapy

Multiple randomized trials have established that the administration of cisplatin-based chemotherapy after surgical resection of stage II to IIIA disease improves survival.[55–57] This was initially demonstrated in the International Adjuvant Lung Cancer trial in which treatment with etoposide or a Vinca alkaloid plus cisplatin improved the 5-year survival from 40% to 45% (HR 0.86, $p < 0.03$).[55] A study conducted by the National Cancer Institute

of Canada confirmed an even greater benefit using adjuvant vinorelbine and cisplatin, with the 5-year survival improving from 54% to 69%.[57] The variation in the magnitude of benefit is likely due to the heterogeneity of study designs, such as differences in the stages of disease included in the various trials. The "LACE" meta-analysis summarized the results of multiple such studies and showed a 5-year absolute benefit in risk of death of 5.4% (HR 0.89; 95% CI, 0.82–0.96; $p = 0.005$).[58] The benefit was greatest for stage II and III disease (HR 0.83; 95% CI, 0.73–0.95; and HR 0.83; 95% CI, 0.72–0.94, respectively) compared to stage IA and IB (HR 1.40; 95% CI, 0.95–2.06; and HR 0.93; 95% CI, 0.78–1.10, respectively). One study did suggest a benefit for patients with stage IB disease if the tumor size was greater than 4 cm.[59]

Neoadjuvant Chemotherapy

There are several theoretical advantages to administering chemotherapy prior to surgical resection: treatment of microscopic metastatic disease; improved tolerance of therapy prior to surgery; and reduction of tumor volume prior to surgery. Most importantly, neoadjuvant chemotherapy improves survival for patients with stage IIIA NSCLC, as evidenced by two classic randomized studies reported in 1994.[60,61] Neoadjuvant chemotherapy may also be considered for patients with stage II disease, or even stage I disease with large tumors. The Southwest Oncology Group led an Intergroup trial that attempted to study this.[62] Patients with stage IB to IIIA disease were randomized to neoadjuvant chemotherapy with three cycles of paclitaxel/carboplatin, or surgery alone. The median survival was 41 months in the surgery-only arm and 62 months in the preoperative chemotherapy arm. Despite this large numerical difference, the results did not reach statistical significance; this is likely because the trial was forced to close early as the data regarding the benefit of adjuvant chemotherapy emerged.

Neoadjuvant Chemoradiotherapy

Three small randomized phase III trials comparing induction chemotherapy to induction chemoradiotherapy have been reported. In one of these trials, 96 patients with IIIA or IIIB disease were randomized to chemoradiotherapy followed by surgery versus chemotherapy followed by surgery. Five-year survival was 31% in the group that received chemoradiotherapy and only 15% in the chemotherapy group. Combining chemoradiation prior to surgery, however, may result in the administration of suboptimal doses of chemotherapy and, as discussed above, may increase surgical risk, particularly if a pneumonectomy is required. As such, utilization of induction chemoradiotherapy varies by institution. For Pancoast tumors, which arise in the apex of the lung invading the first rib and brachial plexus and have a lower risk of distant metastatic spread, neoadjuvant chemoradiotherapy is the standard approach because it offers improved survival compared to induction radiation alone.[63] Among 110 patients with T3-4, N0-1 disease, 5-year survival was encouraging relative to historical controls at 44% for all patients and 54% for those who had complete resection.[63]

First-line Therapy for Metastatic Disease

Several trials and meta-analyses have demonstrated that doublet platinum-based chemotherapy improves survival and quality of life, and it is therefore the standard of care for good performance status patients.[64] Multiple platinum-based regimens have shown similar efficacy (Table 17.3). An Eastern Cooperative Oncology Group (ECOG) trial compared four regimens (carboplatin and

Table 17.3

Phase III Trials Comparing Platinum-Based Chemotherapy Regimens

Agents	N	Response Rate	Median Overall Survival	1-year survival	Reference
Gemcitabine-Cisplatin	135	40.6%	8.7 months	32%	Cardenal[100]
versus		$p = 0.02$	$p = 0.18$		
Etoposide-Cisplatin		21.9%	7.2 months	26%	
Docetaxel-Cisplatin	1218	31.6%	11.3 months	46%	Fossella[70]
versus		$p = 0.03$	$p = 0.04$		
Docetaxel-Carboplatin		24.5%	10.1 months	41%	
Vinorelbine-Cisplatin	444	28%	8.1 months	36%	Kelly[101]
versus		NS	$p = 0.87$		
Paclitaxel-Carboplatin		25%	8.6 months	38%	
Paclitaxel-Cisplatin	1207	21%	7.8 months	31%	Schiller[65]
versus		NS	NS		
Gemcitabine-Cisplatin		22%	8.1 months	36%	
versus		NS	NS		
Docetaxel-Cisplatin		17%	7.4 months	31%	
versus		NS	NS		
Paclitaxel-Carboplatin		17%	8.1 months	34%	
Paclitaxel-Carboplatin	618	25%	8.5 months	33%	Rosell[102]
versus		$p = 0.45$	$p = 0.02$		
Paclitaxel-Cisplatin		28%	9.8 months	38%	
Gemcitabine-Cisplatin	612	30%	9.8 months	37%	Scagliotti[66]
versus		NS	NS		
Vinorelbine-Cisplatin		30%	9.5 months	37%	
versus		NS	NS		
Paclitaxel-Carboplatin		32%	9.9 months	43%	
Paclitaxel-Cisplatin	480	31.8%	8.1 months	35.9%	Smit[103]
versus		$p = 0.36$	$p = 0.67$		
Gemcitabine-Cisplatin		36.8%	8.9 months	33.1%	
Etoposide-Cisplatin	369	15%	274 days	37%	Belani[104]
versus		$p = 0.06$	$p = 0.09$		
Paclitaxel-Carboplatin		23%	233 days	32%	
Pemetrexed-Cisplatin	1725	30.6%	10.3 months	43.5%	Scagliotti[68]
versus		NI	NI		
Gemcitabine-Cisplatin		28.2%	10.3 months	41.9%	

NS, nonsignificant; NI, noninferior.

paclitaxel, cisplatin and docetaxel, cisplatin and gemcitabine, and cisplatin and paclitaxel) and found no significant differences in response rate (17%–22%, overall 19%) and median overall survival (7.4–8.1 months, overall 7.9 months; 95% CI, 7.3–8.5).[65] Another trial comparing cisplatin and gemcitabine, carboplatin and paclitaxel, and cisplatin and vinorelbine did not demonstrate any significant differences in overall response rates (30%–32%) or median overall survival (9.5–9.9 months).[66] A meta-analysis of eight randomized trials comparing cisplatin and carboplatin regimens demonstrated a higher response rate associated with cisplatin regimens but no statistically significant survival advantage.[67] Therefore, the selection of particular agents should be based on the side effect profile that will be most tolerable in a particular patient.

Only recently has histology been shown to impact the outcomes with specific chemotherapy regimens. In a phase III trial comparing pemetrexed/cisplatin to gemcitabine/cisplatin,[68] a subset analysis of patients with adenocarcinoma and large-cell carcinoma histology showed that overall survival was statistically superior with cisplatin/pemetrexed compared to cisplatin/gemcitabine (12.6 vs. 10.9 months). Among those with squamous histology, survival was improved with cisplatin/gemcitabine compared to cisplatin/pemetrexed (10.8 vs. 9.4 months).

Second-line Therapy

All patients with advanced NSCLC who are treated with a first-line chemotherapy regimen will ultimately develop progression of disease. At that point, switching to a second-line therapy may be considered and has been demonstrated to improve survival in randomized trials. Docetaxel was compared to best-supportive care in patients with progression of disease after at least one platinum-based chemotherapy regimen. There were statistically significant improvements in time to progression (10.6 vs. 6.7 weeks) and median overall survival (7.0 vs. 4.6 months) with docetaxel.[69] Another trial comparing docetaxel to vinorelbine or ifosfamide confirmed the benefits of second-line docetaxel.[70] The role of pemetrexed was established in a study comparing second-line pemetrexed to second-line docetaxel.[71] No statistically significant differences were detected in response rate (9.1% pemetrexed vs. 8.8% docetaxel), median progression-free survival (2.9 months for both), or median overall survival (8.3 months for pemetrexed and 7.9 months for docetaxel). However, several toxicities including grade 3 or 4 neutropenia, febrile neutropenia, neutropenia with infections, and hospitalizations for neutropenic fevers were less frequent with pemetrexed, thereby establishing it as an equally efficacious but less toxic second-line therapy.

Maintenance Therapy

Maintenance therapy with pemetrexed may be considered for patients who have stable disease or response to their initial four cycles of platinum-based chemotherapy. In a randomized trial, maintenance pemetrexed improved progression-free and overall survival compared to best supportive care (4.3 vs. 2.6 months and 13.4 vs. 10.6 months).[72]

Novel Agents

Epidermal Growth Factor Receptor

The discovery of EGFR and its importance in lung cancer spawned the development and study of two small molecular tyrosine kinase inhibitors of EGFR, gefitinib and erlotinib. Interest in this class of drugs escalated as phase I and II trials in patients

with NSCLC showed that these agents could induce tumor shrinkage[73–75] and this was particularly dramatic in a small subset of patients. Eventually, a phase III trial was conducted comparing erlotinib to placebo in patients with previously treated NSCLC who showed improved progression-free survival and overall survival compared to placebo (progression-free survival 2.2 vs. 1.8 months; overall survival 6.7 vs. 4.7 months).[76] The response rate for erlotinib in this unselected group of patients was 9%. Further analysis of patients who responded well to erlotinib across various studies revealed certain clinical characteristics, namely, adenocarcinoma histology, Asian descent, and a history of never smoking. Ultimately, tumor samples from patients with robust responses were found to harbor mutations in the EGFR gene.[77–79] In single-arm studies enrolling patients preselected to have NSCLC with an EGFR mutation, 65% to 80% of patients respond to EGFR tyrosine kinase inhibitors.[80–82] The importance of this finding was further highlighted by the phase III "IPASS" trial, which compared gefitinib to standard chemotherapy (carboplatin and paclitaxel) in the first-line setting for East Asian nonsmoking or former light-smoking patients with advanced lung adenocarcinoma.[83] Gefitinib was superior with respect to progression-free survival (HR 0.74; 95% CI, 0.65–0.85). Among the subgroup of patients whose tumors had mutations in EGFR, the progression-free survival benefit was significantly longer with gefitinib (HR 0.48; 95% CI, 0.36–0.64). Additionally, among those without the mutation, progression-free survival was worse with gefitinib (HR 2.85; 95% CI, 2.05–3.98). Thus, for patients whose tumor has an EGFR mutation, treatment with an EGFR tyrosine kinase inhibitor is preferred as first-line therapy, whereas chemotherapy is preferred in the absence of a mutation.

Unfortunately, all patients who initially respond to EGFR tyrosine kinase inhibition eventually develop disease progression. The causes of acquired resistance are under active investigation, and two mechanisms have so far been identified: secondary EGFR mutations (T790M) and MET oncogene amplification. Strategies and drugs to overcome this resistance are an active area of current investigation.

Angiogenesis

Bevacizumab is a monoclonal antibody that binds to VEGF. In a phase III trial, patients with metastatic NSCLC received first-line treatment with paclitaxel/carboplatin plus bevacizumab or placebo. The addition of bevacizumab improved the response rate from 15% to 35%, time to progression from 4.5 to 6.2 months, and median overall survival from 10 to 12 months.[84] Notably, squamous histology, clinically significant hemoptysis, and untreated brain metastases are contraindications to bevacizumab because of an increased risk of bleeding.

SCLC Therapies

As with NSCLC, the treatment of SCLC depends on the stage of disease at the time of diagnosis (FIGURE 17.6). The use of surgery in the treatment of SCLC is quite rare and restricted to patients with very limited disease and no lymph node involvement. For all other patients with limited-stage SCLC (disease confined to the chest within one radiation therapy field), concurrent chemoradiotherapy is the standard of care. For extensive-stage disease (disease beyond the chest), chemotherapy alone is the primary treatment.

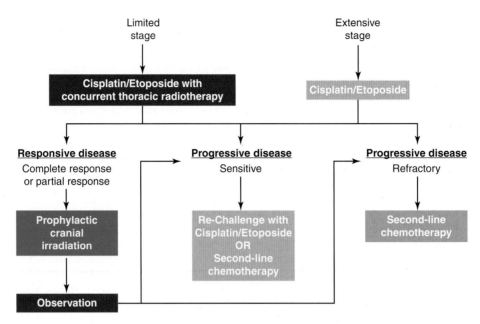

FIGURE 17.6 Treatment schema for small-cell lung carcinoma

Cisplatin and etoposide was established as the standard of care through three randomized trials comparing this regimen to cyclophosphamide, an anthracycline, and vincristine.[85–87] The largest trial randomized 436 patients to cisplatin and etoposide (EP) or cyclophosphamide, epirubicin, and vincristine (CEV). Two- and 5-year survival was improved with EP compared to CEV (14% and 5% vs. 6% and 2%). Median overall survival was also improved with EP in the limited-stage patients (14.5 vs. 9.7 months). No statistically significant survival difference between the treatment regimens was noted in the extensive-stage patients. Because of similar efficacy and less toxicity, carboplatin can be used in those who are unable to tolerate cisplatin.

For limited-stage disease, concurrent radiation therapy is begun with the first or second cycle of chemotherapy. A meta-analysis of 2,100 patients with limited-stage SCLC who were randomized to receive either chemotherapy alone or in combination with radiation therapy demonstrated a 14% reduction in death rate with the combination of chemotherapy and radiation.[88] This survival benefit was confirmed in a second meta-analysis.[89] Additional meta-analyses demonstrated the benefit of beginning radiation therapy prior to the third cycle of chemotherapy. Among 1,524 patients, there was a small but statistically significant improvement in 2-year survival for patients who began radiation therapy within 9 weeks of starting chemotherapy.[90] Different fractionations of thoracic radiation have also been studied. A randomized trial of 417 patients compared twice-daily radiotherapy to once-daily radiotherapy.[91] Five-year survival was improved with twice-daily fractionation (26% vs. 16%, $p = 0.04$). However, the interpretation of these results is challenging because both arms in this study received 45Gy of radiation, even though the bioequivalent doses are not the same. Given patient preference and logistical constraints, many patients continue to receive once-daily fractionated radiation to a dose of at least 60Gy.

Brain metastases occur in up to 25% of patients and are as common as 50% to 80% in patients who survive 2 years.[92] Because the brain lesions are sometimes the sole site of relapse and are often disabling, prophylactic cranial irradiation (PCI) has been recommended in those who are initially free of central nervous system involvement. In a meta-analysis that included 7 trials and 987 patients mainly with limited-stage SCLC who were randomized to receive PCI or not after achieving a complete response, PCI decreased the risk of brain metastases by more than 50% and also improved 3-year survival from 15% to 21%.[93] A European Organisation for Research and Treatment of Cancer (EORTC) randomized trial with 286 patients demonstrated a survival advantage with PCI even for patients with extensive-stage SCLC who responded to chemotherapy.[94] PCI decreased the incidence of symptomatic brain metastases at 1 year from 40% to 15% and improved 1-year survival from 13% to 27%.

If recurrence occurs more than 3 months after completing initial therapy, patients are considered to have "sensitive" relapse and can be rechallenged with a platinum-based regimen or receive second-line therapy. However, if recurrence occurs within 3 months or there was no response to initial therapy, patients are considered to have "refractory" disease and should receive different agents from their initial therapy. Few large trials have been conducted in the relapsed setting. A phase II trial with topotecan in 101 relapsed patients showed a response rate of 38% in sensitive patients and 6% in refractory patients, and median survival was 6.9 and 4.7 months, respectively.[95] Another trial randomized 211 relapsed patients to topotecan versus CAV (cyclophosphamide, doxorubicin, and vincristine). There was no statistically significant difference in response rate (24% and 18%, respectively, for topotecan and CAV) or median overall survival (25 and 24.7 weeks, respectively, for topotecan and CAV). Based on the decrease in symptom burden documented in this trial, topotecan was approved as second-line therapy for SCLC. Oral topotecan use has also been examined in the relapsed setting. A trial with 141 patients with relapsed SCLC not considered candidates for standard intravenous therapy were randomized to topotecan with best supportive care or to best supportive care alone.[96] Median overall survival was improved from 13.9 weeks to 25.9 weeks with oral topotecan. Additionally, patients receiving oral topotecan had greater symptom control and a slower deterioration in quality of life. The response rate was low with no complete responses, 7% partial responses, and 44% stable disease.

Disease Surveillance and Monitoring

For NSCLC there are no randomized trials to guide disease surveillance and monitoring in patients with early stage or locally advanced disease who have completed their planned therapies. Two retrospective reviews suggest that there is no survival benefit associated with the detection of asymptomatic recurrence.[97,98] However, a prospective study of 192 patients demonstrated longer median survival after the diagnosis of recurrence in asymptomatic compared to symptomatic patients.[99] Because this finding is likely confounded by lead-time bias, no clear benefit for intensive screening has been established. Currently, the National Comprehensive Cancer Network (NCCN) recommends a history, physical examination, and chest CT every 4 to 6 months for the first 2 years and then annually. Of course, if new or worrisome symptoms arise, evaluation should proceed as medically indicated.

For SCLC, after recovery from therapy, the NCCN guidelines recommend a history, physical, chest imaging, and blood work as clinically indicated at each visit every 3 to 4 months during the first 2 years and then every 6 months for the next 3 years. After 5 years, follow-up can occur annually.

▌ REFERENCES

1. Jemal A, Bray F, Center MM, et al. Global cancer statistics. *CA Cancer J Clin* 2011;61:69–90.
2. Peace LR. A time correlation between cigarette smoking and lung cancer. *J R Statist Soc D (The Statistician)* 1985;34:371–381.
3. *SEER Stat Fact Sheets: Lung and Bronchus.* 2010. Available at: http://seer .cancer.gov/statfacts/html/lungb.html. Accessed 2010.
4. Garfinkel L SE. Lung cancer and smoking trends in the United States over the past 25 years. *CA Cancer J Clin* 1991;41:137–145.
5. Smith C, Perfetti TA, Garg R, et al. IARC carcinogens reported in cigarette mainstream smoke and their calculated log P values. *Food Chem Toxicol* 2003;41:807.
6. Mossman BT, Lippmann M, Hesterberg TW, et al. Pulmonary endpoints (lung carcinomas and asbestosis) following inhalation exposure to asbestos. *J Toxicol Environ Health B Crit Rev* 2011;14:76–121.
7. Osann KE. Epidemiology of lung cancer. *Curr Opin Pulm Med* 1998;4:198–204.
8. Frost JK, Ball WC, Jr., Levin ML, et al. Early lung cancer detection: results of the initial (prevalence) radiologic and cytologic screening in the Johns Hopkins study. *Am Rev Respir Dis* 1984;130:549–554.
9. Marcus PM, Bergstralh EJ, Fagerstrom RM, et al. Lung cancer mortality in the Mayo Lung Project: impact of extended follow-up. *J Natl Cancer Inst* 2000;92:1308–1316.
10. Melamed MR, Flehinger BJ, Zaman MB, et al. Screening for early lung cancer. Results of the Memorial Sloan-Kettering study in New York. *Chest* 1984;86:44–53.
11. Patz EF, Jr., Goodman PC, Bepler G. Screening for lung cancer. *N Engl J Med* 2000;343:1627–1633.
12. Henschke CI, Yankelevitz DF, Libby DM, et al. Survival of patients with stage I lung cancer detected on CT screening. *N Engl J Med* 2006;355: 1763–1771.
13. National Lung Screening Trial Research Team. Reduced lung-cancer mortality with low-dose computed tomographic screening. N Engl J Med 2011;365(5):395–409.
14. Nystrom L, Andersson I, Bjurstam N, et al. Long-term effects of mammography screening: updated overview of the Swedish randomised trials. *Lancet* 2002;359:909–919.
15. Govindan R, Page N, Morgensztern D, et al. Changing epidemiology of small-cell lung cancer in the United States over the last 30 years: analysis of the surveillance, epidemiologic, and end results database. *J Clin Oncol* 2006;24:4539–4544.
16. World Health Organization. Pathology and genetics of tumors of the lung, pleura, thymus and heart. In: Travis WD, Brambilla E, Muller-Hermelink H, et al., eds. World Health Organization Classification of Tumors. Lyon: IARC Press; 2004:38.
17. Travis WD, Brambilla E, Noguchi M, et al. International Association for the Study of Lung Cancer, American Thoracic Society, European Respiratory Society International Multidisciplinary Classification of Lung Adenocarcinoma. *J Thorac Oncol* 2011;6:244–285.
18. Ishizumi T, McWilliams A, MacAulay C, et al. Natural history of bronchial preinvasive lesions. *Cancer Metastasis Rev* 2010;29:5–14.
19. Hirsch FR, Varella-Garcia M, Bunn PA, Jr., et al. Epidermal growth factor receptor in non-small-cell lung carcinomas: correlation between gene copy number and protein expression and impact on prognosis. *J Clin Oncol* 2003;21:3798–3807.
20. Cataldo VD, Gibbons DL, Perez-Soler R, et al. Treatment of non-small-cell lung cancer with erlotinib or gefitinib. *N Engl J Med* 2011;364:947–955.
21. Balak MN, Gong Y, Riely GJ, et al. Novel D761Y and common secondary T790M mutations in epidermal growth factor receptor-mutant lung adenocarcinomas with acquired resistance to kinase inhibitors. *Clin Cancer Res* 2006;12:6494–6501.
22. Bean J, Brennan C, Shih JH, et al. MET amplification occurs with or without T790M mutations in EGFR mutant lung tumors with acquired resistance to gefitinib or erlotinib. Proc Natl Acad Sci U S A 2007;104(52):20932–7.
23. Riely GJ, Marks J, Pao W. KRAS mutations in non-small cell lung cancer. *Proc Am Thorac Soc* 2009;6:201–205.
24. Shaw AT, Yeap BY, Mino-Kenudson M, et al. Clinical features and outcome of patients with non-small-cell lung cancer who harbor EML4-ALK. *J Clin Oncol* 2009;27:4247–4253.
25. Ozkara HA, Ozkara S, Topcu S, et al. Amplification of the c-myc oncogene in non-small cell lung cancer. *Tumori* 1999;85:508–511.
26. Sun Y. p53 and its downstream proteins as molecular targets of cancer. *Mol Carcinog* 2006;45:409–415.
27. Choong NW, Salgia R, Vokes EE. Key signaling pathways and targets in lung cancer therapy. *Clin Lung Cancer* 2007;8 Suppl 2:S52–60.
28. Yano T, Tanikawa S, Fujie T, et al. Vascular endothelial growth factor expression and neovascularisation in non-small cell lung cancer. *Eur J Cancer* 2000;36:601–609.
29. Campanella N, Moraca A, Pergolini M, et al. Paraneoplastic syndromes in 68 cases of resectable non-small cell lung carcinoma: can they help in early detection? *Med Oncol* 1999;16:129–133.
30. NCCN. Clinical Practice Guidelines in Oncology: Non-Small Cell Lung Cancer Version 1.2013.
31. Deslauriers J, Gregoire J. Clinical and surgical staging of non-small cell lung cancer. *Chest* 2000;117:96S–103S.
32. Detterbeck FC, Boffa DJ, Tanoue LT. The new lung cancer staging system. *Chest* 2009;136:260–271.
33. Vallieres E, Shepherd FA, Crowley J, et al. The IASLC Lung Cancer Staging Project: proposals regarding the relevance of TNM in the pathologic staging of small cell lung cancer in the forthcoming (seventh) edition of the TNM classification for lung cancer. *J Thorac Oncol* 2009;4: 1049–1059.
34. Zelen M. Keynote address on biostatistics and data retrieval. *Cancer Chemother Rep 3* 1973;4:31–42.
35. Ginsberg RJ, Rubinstein LV. Randomized trial of lobectomy versus limited resection for T1 N0 non-small cell lung cancer. Lung Cancer Study Group. *Ann Thorac Surg* 1995;60:615–622; discussion 22–23.
36. Sagawa M, Sato M, Sakurada A, et al. A prospective trial of systematic nodal dissection for lung cancer by video-assisted thoracic surgery: can it be perfect? *Ann Thorac Surg* 2002;73:900–904.
37. Kappers I, van Sandick JW, Burgers SA, et al. Surgery after induction chemotherapy in stage IIIA-N2 non-small cell lung cancer: why pneumonectomy should be avoided. *Lung Cancer* 2010;68:222–227.
38. Ferguson MK, Lehman AG. Sleeve lobectomy or pneumonectomy: optimal management strategy using decision analysis techniques. *Ann Thorac Surg* 2003;76:1782–1788.
39. Downey RJ, Martini N, Rusch VW, et al. Extent of chest wall invasion and survival in patients with lung cancer. *Ann Thorac Surg* 1999;68:188–193.

19

42

79

40. Voltolini L, Rapicetta C, Luzzi L, et al. Lung cancer with chest wall involvement: predictive factors of long-term survival after surgical resection. *Lung Cancer* 2006;52:359–364.

41. Wu Y, Huang ZF, Wang SY, et al. A randomized trial of systematic nodal dissection in resectable non-small cell lung cancer. *Lung Cancer* 2002;36:1–6.

42. Rowell NP, Williams CJ. Radical radiotherapy for stage I/II non-small cell lung cancer in patients not sufficiently fit for or declining surgery (medically inoperable). *Cochrane Database Syst Rev* 2001:CD002935.

43. Jeremic B, Milicic B. From conventionally fractionated radiation therapy to hyperfractionated radiation therapy alone and with concurrent chemotherapy in patients with early-stage nonsmall cell lung cancer. *Cancer* 2008;112:876–884.

44. Albain KS, Swann RS, Rusch VW, et al. Radiotherapy plus chemotherapy with or without surgical resection for stage III non-small-cell lung cancer: a phase III randomised controlled trial. *Lancet* 2009;374:379–386.

45. Johnstone DW, Byhardt RW, Ettinger D, et al. Phase III study comparing chemotherapy and radiotherapy with preoperative chemotherapy and surgical resection in patients with non-small-cell lung cancer with spread to mediastinal lymph nodes (N2); final report of RTOG 89-01. Radiation Therapy Oncology Group. *Int J Radiat Oncol Biol Phys* 2002;54:365–369.

46. van Meerbeeck JP, Kramer GW, Van Schil PE, et al. Randomized controlled trial of resection versus radiotherapy after induction chemotherapy in stage IIIA-N2 non-small-cell lung cancer. *J Natl Cancer Inst* 2007;99:442–450.

47. Dillman RO, Seagren SL, Propert KJ, et al. A randomized trial of induction chemotherapy plus high-dose radiation versus radiation alone in stage III non-small-cell lung cancer. *N Engl J Med* 1990;323:940–945.

48. Auperin A, Le Pechoux C, Rolland E, et al. Meta-analysis of concomitant versus sequential radiochemotherapy in locally advanced non-small-cell lung cancer. *J Clin Oncol* 2010;28:2181–2190.

49. Fournel P, Robinet G, Thomas P, et al. Randomized phase III trial of sequential chemoradiotherapy compared with concurrent chemoradiotherapy in locally advanced non-small-cell lung cancer: Groupe Lyon-Saint-Etienne d'Oncologie Thoracique-Groupe Francais de Pneumo-Cancerologie NPC 95-01 Study. *J Clin Oncol* 2005;23:5910–5917.

50. Furuse K, Fukuoka M, Kawahara M, et al. Phase III study of concurrent versus sequential thoracic radiotherapy in combination with mitomycin, vindesine, and cisplatin in unresectable stage III non-small-cell lung cancer. *J Clin Oncol* 1999;17:2692–2699.

51. Zatloukal P, Petruzelka L, Zemanova M, et al. Concurrent versus sequential chemoradiotherapy with cisplatin and vinorelbine in locally advanced non-small cell lung cancer: a randomized study. *Lung Cancer* 2004;46:87–98.

52. Effects of postoperative mediastinal radiation on completely resected stage II and stage III epidermoid cancer of the lung. The Lung Cancer Study Group. *N Engl J Med* 1986;315:1377–1381.

53. Feng QF, Wang M, Wang LJ, et al. A study of postoperative radiotherapy in patients with non-small-cell lung cancer: a randomized trial. *Int J Radiat Oncol Biol Phys* 2000;47:925–929.

54. Lally BE, Zelterman D, Colasanto JM, et al. Postoperative radiotherapy for stage II or III non-small-cell lung cancer using the surveillance, epidemiology, and end results database. *J Clin Oncol* 2006;24:2998–3006.

55. Arriagada R, Bergman B, Dunant A, et al. Cisplatin-based adjuvant chemotherapy in patients with completely resected non-small-cell lung cancer. *N Engl J Med* 2004;350:351–360.

56. Douillard JY, Rosell R, De Lena M, et al. Adjuvant vinorelbine plus cisplatin versus observation in patients with completely resected stage IB-IIIA non-small-cell lung cancer (Adjuvant Navelbine International Trialist Association [ANITA]): a randomised controlled trial. *Lancet Oncol* 2006;7:719–727.

57. Winton T, Livingston R, Johnson D, et al. Vinorelbine plus cisplatin vs. observation in resected non-small-cell lung cancer. *N Engl J Med* 2005;352:2589–2597.

58. Pignon JP, Tribodet H, Scagliotti GV, et al. Lung adjuvant cisplatin evaluation: a pooled analysis by the LACE Collaborative Group. *J Clin Oncol* 2008;26:3552–3559.

59. Strauss GM, Herndon JE, 2nd, Maddaus MA, et al. Adjuvant paclitaxel plus carboplatin compared with observation in stage IB non-small-cell lung cancer: CALGB 9633 with the Cancer and Leukemia Group B, Radiation Therapy Oncology Group, and North Central Cancer Treatment Group Study Groups. *J Clin Oncol* 2008;26:5043–5051.

60. Rosell R, Gomez-Codina J, Camps C, et al. A randomized trial comparing preoperative chemotherapy plus surgery with surgery alone in patients with non-small-cell lung cancer. *N Engl J Med* 1994;330:153–158.

61. Roth JA, Fossella F, Komaki R, et al. A randomized trial comparing perioperative chemotherapy and surgery with surgery alone in resectable stage IIIA non-small-cell lung cancer. *J Natl Cancer Inst* 1994;86:673–680.

62. Pisters KM, Vallieres E, Crowley JJ, et al. Surgery with or without preoperative paclitaxel and carboplatin in early-stage non-small-cell lung cancer: Southwest Oncology Group Trial S9900, an intergroup, randomized, phase III trial. *J Clin Oncol* 2010;28:1843–1849.

63. Rusch VW, Giroux DJ, Kraut MJ, et al. Induction chemoradiation and surgical resection for superior sulcus non-small-cell lung carcinomas: long-term results of Southwest Oncology Group Trial 9416 (Intergroup Trial 0160). *J Clin Oncol* 2007;25:313–318.

64. Azzoli CG, Baker S, Jr., Temin S, et al. American Society of Clinical Oncology Clinical Practice Guideline update on chemotherapy for stage IV non-small-cell lung cancer. *J Clin Oncol* 2009;27:6251–6266.

65. Schiller JH, Harrington D, Belani CP, et al. Comparison of four chemotherapy regimens for advanced non-small-cell lung cancer. *N Engl J Med* 2002;346:92–98.

66. Scagliotti GV, De Marinis F, Rinaldi M, et al. Phase III randomized trial comparing three platinum-based doublets in advanced non-small-cell lung cancer. *J Clin Oncol* 2002;20:4285–4291.

67. Hotta K, Matsuo K, Ueoka H, et al. Meta-analysis of randomized clinical trials comparing cisplatin to carboplatin in patients with advanced non small-cell lung cancer. *J Clin Oncol* 2004;22:3852–3859.

68. Scagliotti GV, Parikh P, von Pawel J, et al. Phase III study comparing cisplatin plus gemcitabine with cisplatin plus pemetrexed in chemotherapy-naive patients with advanced-stage non-small-cell lung cancer. *J Clin Oncol* 2008;26:3543–3551.

69. Shepherd FA, Dancey J, Ramlau R, et al. Prospective randomized trial of docetaxel versus best supportive care in patients with non-small-cell lung cancer previously treated with platinum-based chemotherapy. *J Clin Oncol* 2000;18:2095–2103.

70. Fossella FV, DeVore R, Kerr RN, et al. Randomized phase III trial of docetaxel versus vinorelbine or ifosfamide in patients with advanced non-small-cell lung cancer previously treated with platinum-containing chemotherapy regimens. The TAX 320 Non-Small Cell Lung Cancer Study Group. *J Clin Oncol* 2000;18:2354–2362.

71. Hanna N, Shepherd FA, Fossella FV, et al. Randomized phase III trial of pemetrexed versus docetaxel in patients with non-small-cell lung cancer previously treated with chemotherapy. *J Clin Oncol* 2004;22:1589–1597.

72. Ciuleanu T, Brodowicz T, Zielinski C, et al. Maintenance pemetrexed plus best supportive care versus placebo plus best supportive care for non-small-cell lung cancer: a randomised, double-blind, phase 3 study. *Lancet* 2009;374:1432–1440.

73. Fukuoka M, Yano S, Giaccone G, et al. Multi-institutional randomized phase II trial of gefitinib for previously treated patients with advanced non-small-cell lung cancer (The IDEAL 1 Trial) [corrected]. *J Clin Oncol* 2003;21:2237–2246.

74. Kris MG, Natale RB, Herbst RS, et al. Efficacy of gefitinib, an inhibitor of the epidermal growth factor receptor tyrosine kinase, in symptomatic patients with non-small cell lung cancer: a randomized trial. *JAMA* 2003;290:2149–2158.

75. Perez-Soler R, Chachoua A, Hammond LA, et al. Determinants of tumor response and survival with erlotinib in patients with non–small-cell lung cancer. *J Clin Oncol* 2004;22:3238–3247.

76. Shepherd FA, Rodrigues Pereira J, Ciuleanu T, et al. Erlotinib in previously treated non-small-cell lung cancer. *N Engl J Med* 2005;353:123–132.

77. Lynch TJ, Bell DW, Sordella R, et al. Activating mutations in the epidermal growth factor receptor underlying responsiveness of non-small-cell lung cancer to gefitinib. *N Engl J Med* 2004;350:2129–2139.

78. Paez JG, Janne PA, Lee JC, et al. EGFR mutations in lung cancer: correlation with clinical response to gefitinib therapy. *Science* 2004;304:1497–1500.

79. Pao W, Miller V, Zakowski M, et al. EGF receptor gene mutations are common in lung cancers from "never smokers" and are associated with sensitivity of tumors to gefitinib and erlotinib. *Proc Natl Acad Sci U S A* 2004;101:13306–13311.

80. Sequist LV, Martins RG, Spigel D, et al. First-line gefitinib in patients with advanced non-small-cell lung cancer harboring somatic EGFR mutations. *J Clin Oncol* 2008;26:2442–2449.

81. Inoue A, Suzuki T, Fukuhara T, et al. Prospective phase II study of gefitinib for chemotherapy-naive patients with advanced non-small-cell lung cancer with epidermal growth factor receptor gene mutations. *J Clin Oncol* 2006;24:3340–3346.

82. Sunaga N, Tomizawa Y, Yanagitani N, et al. Phase II prospective study of the efficacy of gefitinib for the treatment of stage III/IV non-small cell lung cancer with EGFR mutations, irrespective of previous chemotherapy. *Lung Cancer* 2007;56:383–389.

83. Mok TS, Wu YL, Thongprasert S, et al. Gefitinib or carboplatin-paclitaxel in pulmonary adenocarcinoma. *N Engl J Med* 2009;361:947–957.

84. Sandler A, Gray R, Perry MC, et al. Paclitaxel-carboplatin alone or with bevacizumab for non-small-cell lung cancer. *N Engl J Med* 2006;355:2542–2550.

85. Fukuoka M, Furuse K, Saijo N, et al. Randomized trial of cyclophosphamide, doxorubicin, and vincristine versus cisplatin and etoposide versus alternation of these regimens in small-cell lung cancer. *J Natl Cancer Inst* 1991;83:855–861.

86. Roth BJ, Johnson DH, Einhorn LH, et al. Randomized study of cyclophosphamide, doxorubicin, and vincristine versus etoposide and cisplatin versus alternation of these two regimens in extensive small-cell lung cancer: a phase III trial of the Southeastern Cancer Study Group. *J Clin Oncol* 1992;10:282–291.

87. Sundstrom S, Bremnes RM, Kaasa S, et al. Cisplatin and etoposide regimen is superior to cyclophosphamide, epirubicin, and vincristine regimen in small-cell lung cancer: results from a randomized phase III trial with 5 years' follow-up. *J Clin Oncol* 2002;20:4665–4672.

88. Pignon JP, Arriagada R, Ihde DC, et al. A meta-analysis of thoracic radiotherapy for small-cell lung cancer. *N Engl J Med* 1992;327:1618–1624.

89. Warde P, Payne D. Does thoracic irradiation improve survival and local control in limited-stage small-cell carcinoma of the lung? A meta-analysis. *J Clin Oncol* 1992;10:890–895.

90. Fried DB, Morris DE, Poole C, et al. Systematic review evaluating the timing of thoracic radiation therapy in combined modality therapy for limited-stage small-cell lung cancer. *J Clin Oncol* 2004;22:4837–4845.

91. Turrisi AT, 3rd, Kim K, Blum R, et al. Twice-daily compared with once-daily thoracic radiotherapy in limited small-cell lung cancer treated concurrently with cisplatin and etoposide. *N Engl J Med* 1999;340:265–271.

92. Komaki R, Cox JD, Whitson W. Risk of brain metastasis from small cell carcinoma of the lung related to length of survival and prophylactic irradiation. *Cancer Treat Rep* 1981;65:811–814.

93. Auperin A, Arriagada R, Pignon JP, et al. Prophylactic cranial irradiation for patients with small-cell lung cancer in complete remission. Prophylactic Cranial Irradiation Overview Collaborative Group. *N Engl J Med* 1999;341:476–484.

94. Slotman B, Faivre-Finn C, Kramer G, et al. Prophylactic cranial irradiation in extensive small-cell lung cancer. *N Engl J Med* 2007;357:664–672.

95. Ardizzoni A, Hansen H, Dombernowsky P, et al. Topotecan, a new active drug in the second-line treatment of small-cell lung cancer: a phase II study in patients with refractory and sensitive disease. The European Organization for Research and Treatment of Cancer Early Clinical Studies Group and New Drug Development Office, and the Lung Cancer Cooperative Group. *J Clin Oncol* 1997;15:2090–2096.

96. O'Brien ME, Ciuleanu TE, Tsekov H, et al. Phase III trial comparing supportive care alone with supportive care with oral topotecan in patients with relapsed small-cell lung cancer. *J Clin Oncol* 2006;24:5441–5447.

97. Walsh GL, O'Connor M, Willis KM, et al. Is follow-up of lung cancer patients after resection medically indicated and cost-effective? *Ann Thorac Surg* 1995;60:1563–1570; discussion 70–72.

98. Younes RN, Gross JL, Deheinzelin D. Follow-up in lung cancer: how often and for what purpose? *Chest* 1999;115:1494–1499.

99. Westeel V, Choma D, Clement F, et al. Relevance of an intensive postoperative follow-up after surgery for non-small cell lung cancer. *Ann Thorac Surg* 2000;70:1185–1190.

100. Cardenal F, Lopez-Cabrerizo MP, Anton A, et al. Randomized phase III study of gemcitabine-cisplatin versus etoposide-cisplatin in the treatment of locally advanced or metastatic non-small-cell lung cancer. *J Clin Oncol* 1999;17:12–18.

101. Kelly K, Crowley J, Bunn PA, Jr., et al. Randomized phase III trial of paclitaxel plus carboplatin versus vinorelbine plus cisplatin in the treatment of patients with advanced non-small-cell lung cancer: a Southwest Oncology Group trial. *J Clin Oncol* 2001;19:3210–3218.

102. Rosell R, Gatzemeier U, Betticher DC, et al. Phase III randomised trial comparing paclitaxel/carboplatin with paclitaxel/cisplatin in patients with advanced non-small-cell lung cancer: a cooperative multinational trial. *Ann Oncol* 2002;13:1539–1549.

103. Smit EF, van Meerbeeck JP, Lianes P, et al. Three-arm randomized study of two cisplatin-based regimens and paclitaxel plus gemcitabine in advanced non-small-cell lung cancer: a phase III trial of the European Organization for Research and Treatment of Cancer Lung Cancer Group—EORTC 08975. *J Clin Oncol* 2003;21:3909–3917.

104. Belani CP, Lee JS, Socinski MA, et al. Randomized phase III trial comparing cisplatin-etoposide to carboplatin-paclitaxel in advanced or metastatic non-small cell lung cancer. *Ann Oncol* 2005;16:1069–1075.

CHAPTER 18

Ablation of Primary and Secondary Lung Cancers

BRADLEY B. PUA and STEPHEN B. SOLOMON

In 2010, the American Cancer Society estimated that of newly diagnosed cancers, lung cancer remained the leading cause of death in both men and women, accounting for 28% of all cancers deaths.[1] Primary lung cancers are broadly divided into two main histologic subtypes: non–small-cell lung cancer (NSCLC) and small-cell lung cancer (SCLC) accounting for 85% to 90% and 10% to 15% of diagnoses, respectively. SCLC is diagnosed at advanced stages and as such is often associated with lower survival rates compared to NSCLC. Systemic therapies remain the mainstay for patients with SCLC with only a small subset qualifying for local salvage therapies. Comparatively, NSCLC is more often diagnosed at early stages, allowing therapy with curative intent.

Surgical resection remains the standard of therapy for patients with early stage primary lung cancer. Controversy exists over whether these patients should undergo lobectomy or sublobar resection, prompting multiple investigations and a study sponsored by the National Cancer Institute.[2,3] Primary strategies for treatment of patients with early stage lung cancer who are not surgical candidates include ablative therapies, external beam radiation, and systemic chemotherapy.

Metastatic disease to the lungs is common, owing to the lung's filtration ability. Autopsies demonstrate that up to 50% of cancer patients have lung metastasis. It has been demonstrated that in the United States, pulmonary metastasis can be found in up to 30% of patients with colorectal cancer.[4] Surgical resection for pulmonary metastasis (pulmonary metastatectomy) is a debated topic secondary to lack of randomized, controlled clinical trials.[5] Nevertheless, surgical metastatectomy is an accepted and widespread treatment for these patients with survival rates of 36% at 5 years and 26% at 10 years after complete metastatectomy.[6] Information gathered from multiple retrospective trials indicate that the patients who experience the most benefit from pulmonary metastatectomy are those with a long disease-free interval from initial resection of the primary tumor, patients without extrathoracic metastasis, and those for whom an R0 (complete microscopic resection) resection can be achieved.[7] Recent literature suggests that with concurrent adjuvant therapy, patients with metastatic renal cell cancer is conferred a survival benefit even with incomplete resection.[8] Similar to treatment of primary lung cancers, ablative therapies in metastatic disease is currently reserved for patients who are not ideal surgical candidates.

▌ ABLATION

Image-guided ablation in the pulmonary system currently refers to destruction of cells, typically targeted tumor cells, utilizing thermal energy (heating or cooling). The most common techniques of thermal ablation are radiofrequency ablation (RF ablation), microwave ablation, and cryoablation, for which RF ablation is the most studied and serves as a benchmark for the performance of microwave and cryoablation.

Radiofrequency Ablation

Radiofrequency ablation is a minimally invasive technology that has proven useful in patients with unresectable liver cancer.[9] In 2000, Dupuy et al.[10] first reported use of percutaneous RF ablation of small lung malignancies, spurring a large number of investigations as to its utility in primary lung cancer as well as in treatment of metastatic lung lesions. A prospective, intention to treat, multicenter clinical trial, the Radiofrequency Ablation of Pulmonary Tumors Response Evaluation (RAPTURE) trial, showed that in 106 patients with 183 primary or secondary lung tumors (<3.5 cm), treated with RF ablation, cancer-specific survival for patients with NSCLC was 92% at 1 year and 73% at 2 years. Patients with colorectal metastasis had a cancer-specific survival of 93% at 1 year and 67% at 2 years.[11] Another study with longer follow-up reports a 27%, 5-year overall survival rate after RF ablation of stage I NSCLC.[12] It should be noted that the aforementioned study was an early retrospective study and, therefore, survival analysis was not disease specific. Additionally, a proportion of their patients were being treated concomitantly with systemic chemotherapy and/ or radiation and patients treated with RF ablation may be negatively affected by lead-time bias (some patients followed up to 1 year before RF ablation), which could potentially underestimate actual survival. Results from an open-labeled prospective trial of RF ablation for treatment of lung metastasis in nonsurgical candidates demonstrated 3- and 5-year survivals of 60% and 45%, respectively.[13] Although these figures are promising, they remain inferior to optimal surgical resection when it comes to early primary disease and further randomized studies need to be performed to evaluate efficacy in treatment of metastasis[14-16] (Table 18.1).

Table 18.1	
Treatment Specific Lung Cancer Survival	
Treatment	NSCLC–5-year survival
Surgical[14,15]	Stage IA (lobectomy)–up to 80% survival
	Stage I (VATS)–63.6% survival
Radiofrequency ablation[12]	Stage I–27%
No treatment[16]	All stages–14%

RF ablation is a technique that utilizes frictional energy created by oscillating tissue ions from an alternating current, thereby supplying destructive heat to the target tissue. This current is generated by a voltage gradient created between an electrode placed within the target lesion and dispersive electrodes placed on the patient's skin (monopolar system). Depending on the protocol used, the applied power ranges from 10 to 200 W with the frequency of the alternating current being in the region of radio waves (400 kHz). The strength of the electric field and the resultant area of tissue heating is predicted with the bioheat transfer equation.[17]

Therapeutic RF ablation strives to heat tissues in the range of 60° to 100°C, where protein denaturation and enzymatic deactivation occurs, leading to near instantaneous cell death.[18] It has been found that as tissues are heated, cells undergo coagulation necrosis with temperatures greater than 50°C for at least 5 minutes.[19]

Common to most ablative technologies is its decreased effectiveness when in close proximity to large vessels. This is often termed *the heat sink effect*, referring to removal of heat energy from the target tissues by flowing blood. Investigators have demonstrated that proximity of the target tumor to vessels larger than 3 mm can result in incomplete treatment if a revision of ablation algorithm/strategy is not made[20] (FIGURE 18.1).

Percutaneous RF ablation in the lung is generally performed with computed tomography (CT) guidance.

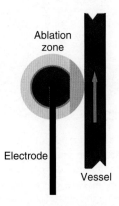

FIGURE 18.1 The temperature of blood, approximately 37°C, flowing close to the ablation zone, will decrease the temperature in the immediate surrounding region, which may affect ablation efficacy. It is important to be aware of this phenomenon, especially with vessels greater than 3 mm in size.

The three main systems currently being used in the United States for RF ablation are the LeVeen system (Boston Scientific, Watertown, MA), the StarBurst System (Angiodynamics, Queensbury, NY), and the Cooltip Electrode (Covidien, Boulder, CO). All these systems are monopolar and vary with the way energy is delivered, their electrode properties and shapes, as well as their mechanisms to ensure adequate tumor ablation. Although studies have been performed comparing these systems, results remain disparate. Some studies demonstrate no difference in terms of regions of necrosis and local tumor progressions, whereas others demonstrate system specific advantages.[21,22] Until more definitive studies can be performed, the system of choice is often based on operator comfort.

Briefly, the LeVeen system detects circuit impedance and follows a protocol that increases the power incrementally until a dramatic rise in the impedance (roll off) occurs. The StarBurst system is a temperature-based system capable of monitoring surrounding tissue temperature until a target temperature is reached. A type of StarBurst electrode also allows perfusion of a small amount of saline into the surrounding tissue, thought to provide tine cooling and allow for more effective heating of the target area. The Cool-tip system is another impedance-based system with an additional thermocouple at the tip that measures local temperature to ensure adequate ablation. The delivered power of the system is incrementally increased until there is a detected impedance increase of 20 ohms, prompting the system to decrease power delivery and continue ablation for a set period. At the completion of ablation, a target temperature of greater than 60°C is required.

Microwave Ablation

Like RF ablation, microwave ablation has been explored in the treatment of hepatic malignancies.[23] Although clinical experience with microwave ablation in the lung is small, some theoretical advantages exist, which include: higher intratumoral temperatures, larger ablation volumes, and reduced treatment times.[24] An animal study suggests improved performance of microwave versus RF ablation in regions abutting blood vessels up to 2 mm.[25] Preliminary survival data in treatment of both primary and metastatic lung cancers has yielded actuarial survival at 1, 2, and 3 years to be 65%, 55%, and 45%, respectively.[26]

Microwave ablation is a fairly new technology and will require additional investigation as to its clinical effectiveness and safety. Although similar to RF ablation with respect to utilization of heat energy, investigators have already found many differences in the way this energy is dispersed, which may alter techniques that have been modeled after RF ablation. RF ablation relies on thermal conductivity and, therefore, air-filled alveolar spaces of the lungs can limit the size of effective ablation, termed the *oven effect* by Liu et al.[27] Although microwave technology is still in its infancy, it is thought that it may not be similarly hindered.[28]

Cryoablation

Cryoablation depends on a rapid freeze-thaw cycle that causes cell membrane rupture and subsequent cell death. Cryoablation probes (cryoprobes) are based on propelling inert gas (argon) through a small area (probe) and releasing it into a larger area; this change from a small (high-pressure area) to a large (low-pressure area) causes gaseous expansion, resulting in a decrease in surrounding tissue temperatures. The use of cold rather than heat may confer some advantages. Cryoablation has been shown to be associated with a low procedural morbidity when used near mediastinal structures.[29] In fact, very early studies demonstrated that the collagen architecture of central bronchi is preserved after cryoablation.[30]

Few reported studies exist with long-term follow-up of patients after cryoablation. A small study with mean follow-up time of 21 months reported a 1-year survival of 89.4% and a 20% local progression rate. Advantages of cryoablation over RF ablation include the ability to monitor ice ball formation on imaging, potentially larger ablation volumes, and less procedural pain.[31] Although the ice ball is easily visualized as a 40 to 60 HU decrease from preablation attenuation, we caution that the ice ball does not necessarily correlate with the actual region of coagulative necrosis.[32] As with microwave ablation, additional studies need to be performed to evaluate this technique.

▌ SELECTION

RF ablation, and by extension other ablative techniques, is useful in patients who are not ideal surgical candidates or for use as adjunctive salvage therapy (Table 18.2). Nonsurgical candidates include patients who are too high risk for surgery based on pulmonary functional reserve or with other medical comorbidities. Goals of ablation include potential cure, increased length of survival, or symptomatic palliation.

In treatment of **early stage primary lung cancer,** the pretreatment size of the lesion has significant impact of risk of local tumor recurrence and survival. Early investigators have determined that in RF ablation of lesions less than 3 cm in size, complete tumor necrosis can be achieved in 69% of the lesions, whereas complete tumor necrosis could only be achieved in 39% of ablated lesions larger than 3 cm.[33] Median time to progression for tumors less than or equal to 3 cm has been determined to be 45 months, whereas for tumors greater than 3 cm, 12 months.[12] In 2009, the American Joint Committee on Cancer suggested multiple changes to staging of lung cancers.[34] One of these changes included separation of stage Ia lesions to T1a and T1b, based on lesion size greater than or less than 2 cm. These

changes are likely reflective of recent surgical literature suggesting that tumor size less than 2 cm independently confers a survival advantage regardless of surgical and/or adjuvant treatment strategy (lobectomy, segmentectomy, or wedge resection; open or video assisted).[35–37] Although it remains to be seen whether this new size criteria advantage will translate to ablated lesions, recent data have suggested that ablation of a lesion smaller than 2 cm is associated with lower risk of tumor progression.[38]

Local tumor progression after surgical resection with adjuvant brachytherapy can be as high as 6%.[39] These therapies often alter remaining lung parenchyma and pleura, rendering repeat resection difficult, leading to increased surgical morbidity and secondary recurrence rates.[40] It is in this subset where image-guided ablation may be utilized for **salvage therapy** (FIGURE 18.2). Ablation can also be utilized for salvage after radiation, chemotherapy, and for treatment of a chemotherapeutic resistant clone.

In applying ablation to treatment of **metastasis**, a "test of time" paradigm has been suggested.[41] In theory, with a "test of time," a subset of patients with oligometastasis (localized metastasis) will go on to develop new extensive metastatic lesions. If these patients were to be initially treated with ablation, those with successful ablations will be spared surgery and those who subsequently develop new metastatic disease would have been spared noncurative surgery. This paradigm was first suggested in treatment of colorectal metastasis to the liver where patients were treated with RF ablation, in which 98% of patients were spared surgical resection; 44% of those because they remained free of disease, and 56% secondary to development of disease progression.

Table 18.2
Current Indications for Ablation
Early stage cancer
1. Nonsurgical candidates (medically inoperable or refusing surgery)
2. Local tumor progression with prior surgery or radiation precluding repeat surgery
Metastatic disease
1. Test of time
2. Nonsurgical candidates
3. Single enlarging focus in the setting of well-controlled widespread disease
Salvage
1. Prior surgery and/or radiation
2. Palliation: Pain

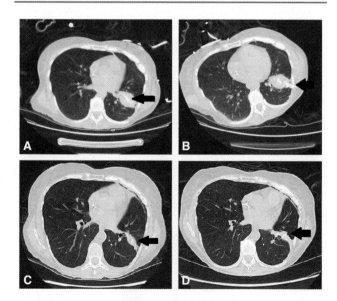

FIGURE 18.2 **A.** CT scan of a patient with metastatic disease and local tumor recurrence in an area of prior resection (*solid arrow*). Although the size of the lesion dramatically decreases the chance of a complete ablation (A0 ablation), ablation can be performed for cytoreduction—to diminish bulk tumor burden. **B.** Two RF electrodes were used to increase the ablation zone (*solid arrow*). **C.** 2 years after ablation, with concurrent adjuvant chemotherapy, the treated region (*solid arrow*) demonstrated a significant reduction in size. **D.** 3 years after ablation, the treated area (*solid arrow*) continued to display no size increase.

For widespread pulmonary metastasis, no data currently exist in regard to the number of metastasis to treat. It may be reasonable to limit treatment to patients with fewer than four metastatic lesions, similar to the limitations placed on surgical metastatectomy, as suggested in traditional surgical literature.[6] Currently, sequential surgical metastatectomy has been suggested and may be another arena where ablation can be utilized.[42,43]

Patients with metastatic disease of lung primary are often treated with systemic targeted chemotherapy and followed with repeated imaging studies. Should these tumors progress, a different chemotherapeutic regimen is often warranted. A subset of these patients will present with stable or decreasing metastatic burden, secondary to response to their chemotherapeutic regimen, however, with a single enlarging focus. An important example of this phenomenon is in treatment of certain metastatic NSCLCs. Certain NSCLCs are known to overexpress receptors, such as epidermal growth factor receptor (EGFR).[44] EGFR tyrosine kinase inhibitors, such as gefitinib, have been used with much success in this group of patients.[45] Unfortunately, some of these tumors develop a second mutation rendering it resistant to this drug, as evidenced by a single enlarging tumor despite improvement of other metastasis.[46] Rather than change the chemotherapeutic treatment, which appears effective against the bulk of the disease, this single enlarging lesion could be targeted by ablative therapy, which is indiscriminate of tumor genetics[47] (FIGURE 18.3).

Although a diminished pulmonary function may limit surgical resection, it has been determined that these restrictions may not be applied to ablation. It has been demonstrated that forced vital capacity (FVC) and forced expiratory volume in 1 second (FEV1) are not significantly diminished when measured at 3 months after RF ablation.[48] Although RF ablation has been successfully performed in post pneumonectomy patients, caution is always advised.[49]

With rapid improvements in ablative technologies, surgical techniques, and chemotherapeutic and radiation treatments, it will be imperative to discuss oncologic patients in a multidisciplinary setting, such as a tumor board. Each representative from their respective disciplines will be able to share and discuss the most up-to-date treatment strategies in their fields, rendering optimal patient care.

PREPROCEDURAL EXAMINATION

Even after discussion in a multidisciplinary setting, it is imperative that the physician performing the ablation do a thorough history and physical examination, preferably in a clinic setting well in advance of the procedure. Details such as a history of bleeding diathesis, potential concurrent cardiopulmonary compromise (which may affect choice of sedation), concurrent infections, as well as medications, such as anticoagulants and bronchodilators, should be sought.

Histologic sampling via image-guided biopsy is preferred prior to the date of the procedure. Although some practitioners have performed the biopsy on the same date, interval preprocedural biopsy confers several advantages. Often, after percutaneous biopsy, a small amount of hemorrhage may be created, which can hinder proper placement of the ablation electrode and may lead to inadequate ablation. Additionally, unexpected histologic diagnoses such as infection will change the course of therapy.

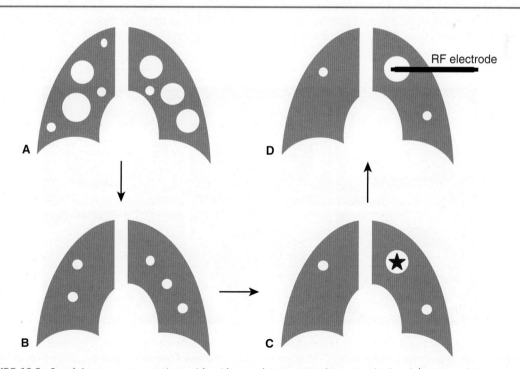

FIGURE 18.3 Panel **A** represents a patient with widespread metastatic disease in the lungs (tumors–white circular lesions). These patients are generally managed with chemotherapy and/or radiation therapy. Panel **B** demonstrates interval response at midcycle of the chemotherapy. Upon further follow-up, Panel **C** demonstrates that in a small percentage of these patients, the bulk of the disease will continue to respond; however, it may have one single enlarging focus of disease (*starred*), presumably secondary to an additional mutation, rendering this focus resistant to systemic chemotherapy. This single enlarging focus can be the target of ablation because ablation is indiscriminant of tumor genetics (Panel **D**).

Caution should be taken with any conductive metallic objects in close proximity to the electrode array. A device manufacturer warns that localized burns may be induced with electrical current being carried through these objects.[50] Although patients with implantable cardioverters-defibrillators (ICD) have had RF ablation performed without incident, it is recommended that in patients who are pacemaker dependent, a cardiology consultation be obtained and these devices be deactivated.[51]

A recent staging imaging study, such as CT or positron emission tomography/computed tomography (PET/CT), is important in assessing tumor characteristics, such as target tumor size, concurrent nodal involvement, and proximity to neighboring vital structures. Preprocedural imaging also plays a role in planning access trajectory, applicator (electrodes, antennas, or cryoprobes) choice, and the use of adjunctive imaging modalities, such as CT fluoroscopy or ultrasound.

An intimate knowledge of the ablation shape and diameter of each type of ablation applicator is extremely important to ensure adequate ablation. Some RF electrodes that consist of a single insulated needle with a noninsulated tip will create a more oblong ablation zone versus a multitined electrode, which may create a more spherical shape. Additionally, tumors that are irregular in shape or are larger than the known effective ablation zone may require multiple ablations to cover the area. This problem is usually solved by either ablating with one applicator in multiple positions or utilizing multiple applicators.

▍ TECHNIQUE

It is our practice to administer antibiotics 1 hour prior to the procedure directed toward skin flora. Although prophylactic antibiotics have not been proven to be of benefit, it is theorized that the ablated devitalized tissue can serve as a nidus for potential infection.

Once consent is obtained, the patient is positioned on the CT. Patient positioning is of utmost importance because inadequate patient padding may lead to nerve injury secondary to pressure, such as has been reported with brachial plexus injuries.[52] If possible, patient arms should be kept at their sides.

Ablation may be performed under general anesthesia or conscious sedation. Performing these procedures under general anesthesia may confer certain advantages, such as the ability to control the airway, ventilation rate, and tidal volume, all of which can aid in lesion targeting in an otherwise anatomically difficult region. For example, a modest change in patient tidal volume may allow increased separation between a peripherally based lesion and the chest wall, lowering the risk to chest wall structures.

Correct placement of dispersive grounding pads, equidistant from the target, will diminish the risk of skin damage. Patient temperature should be monitored throughout the procedure because energy may be transferred through the grounding circuit. It is recommended that the positioning of the groundings pads be checked routinely after manipulating the patient, prior to and during the ablation.

Needle/applicator positioning, access trajectory, and access sites are determined based on considerations similar to those made for lung biopsies: limiting the number of fissures traversed and choice of trajectory to limit the risk of injury to adjacent organs. Routine use of 3D reconstructions as well as reformations in the coronal and sagittal planes in addition to the standard axial imaging can be helpful to optimize electrode placement.

Adjunctive techniques have been reported that may be of utility during ablation. Advanced separation techniques, such as creating an artificial pneumothorax, has been used in treating lesions abutting the chest wall or mediastinum[53] (FIGURE 18.4). Single lung ventilation with selective bronchial occlusion has

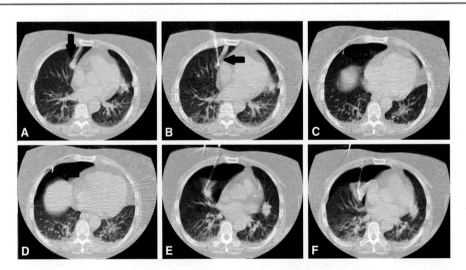

FIGURE 18.4 A. Target tumor is the pulmonary nodule within the right middle lobe (*solid arrow*), adjacent to the pericardium. **B.** A cryoablation probe is advanced into the target tumor (*solid arrow*). The proximity to the pericardium precludes safe and effi cacious ablation in this position. **C.** A small 21G needle (*hollow arrow*) is advanced lower in the thorax and a pneumothorax is created. **D.** The tip of the 21G needle (*hollow arrow*) is noted in the lower thorax and more air is injected into the right hemithorax, expanding the pneumothorax. **E.** The air separation helps to collapse the lung away from the pericardium. Additionally, lateral torque can be applied to the ablation probe by carefully pulling the probe medially to help pull the lung away from the pericardium. **F.** Ablation can commence safely with minimal risk to the pericardium and adjacent structures, such as the phrenic nerve.

also shown some benefit. In an animal model, Oshima et al.[54] reports that RF ablation of a lesion in a collapsed lung (bronchus has been occluded) can yield a greater thermal volume and higher mean temperatures. These findings were corroborated in another animal model utilizing microwave energy.[55]

Currently, there is no accepted standard or ablation protocol. Some authors utilize the electrode manufacturer's ablation settings, whereas others have modified these settings according to experience. Overall, the objective of the modifications is to balance ablation size and efficacy while diminishing the insulator effects of the surrounding charred tissue. In general, lung protocols begin at lower power settings and are performed over longer periods as compared to liver protocols. In our practice, we generally start at a lower power (20 to 30 W) when treating lesions within lung tissue versus treating lesions in solid organs. Additional thermocouples could also be used and directed at the periphery of the ablation zone to monitor for proper temperatures. These devices may also be placed near critical structures abutting the ablation zone to ensure that these structures are not damaged by the ablative energy (FIGURE 18.5).

POSTPROCEDURE

An immediate postprocedure CT is useful to evaluate the ablation zone for complications, such as hemorrhage, pneumothorax, and collateral damage to adjacent structures. Data from CT-guided lung biopsies have demonstrated that manual aspiration after lung biopsy may have potential to prevent worsening pneumothoraces and diminish the need for chest tube placement. The same group reports that the rate of chest tube placement was statistically higher in patients with more than 543 mL of air aspirated.[56]

Although ablation procedures may be performed on an ambulatory, same-day basis, a subset of patients may be admitted for overnight observation. This is heavily dependent on associated medical comorbidities, postprocedure requirements (pain control, oxygenation), or any complications. The most common complaint in the postprocedure setting is pleuritic pain, which is generally well controlled with over-the-counter analgesics. We routinely counsel patients that they may have transient minimal hemoptysis after the procedure.

Postprocedure chest radiographs are performed immediately after the procedure and at 2 hours postprocedure.[57] Acute symptoms should prompt an earlier radiograph. For patients remaining overnight for reasons other than pneumothorax, a repeat chest radiograph is obtained prior to discharge.

COMPLICATIONS

Complications after RF ablation in the thorax are well established.[58] The most common include pneumothorax, hemoptysis, pleural effusions, and pain. A lesser known potential complication is nerve injury. A more comprehensive list of potential side effects and complications is listed in Table 18.3.

The most common complication of RF ablation is development of a pneumothorax with reports ranging from 83% in earlier studies to as low as 9%.[59,60] More recent retrospective and prospective reviews place the rate closer to 16.5% to 32% with only a minority requiring thoracostomy tube treatment.[58,61] Risk factors associated with development of a pneumothorax include treatment of central tumors, treatment of patients without prior lung surgery (scar being presumably protective), and patients with prior radiation therapy. Degree of emphysema, treatment of large tumors, number of electrode passes, and electrode/trocar size have not been associated with risk.[61,62] Delayed or recurrent pneumothorax, although rare, has also been reported to occur. It is suggested that up to 40.2% of pneumothoraces can be delayed or recurrent with the mean duration to confirmation being 24 ± 66.4 hours. Fortunately, this group found that only 12% of the patients with delayed or recurrent pneumothorax required treatment.[63] There is very little known about this entity and how this may affect current postprocedural follow-up. Presumably, necrotic tissue at the lung periphery, along the electrode tract, may give way to delayed pneumothoraces.

Occasionally, the question of the time interval to safely resume air travel is raised, more specifically, if the changes in

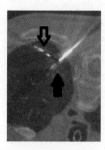

FIGURE 18.5 CT scan during ablation demonstrating an ablation applicator with surrounding ablation ground glass opacity (*solid arrow*). A thermocouple is situated with its tip at the periphery of the lesion to monitor for adequate temperature at the ablation margins (*hollow arrow*).

Table 18.3	
Complications of Ablation	
Side effects/complications	Rate[a]
Pneumothorax	16.5–32%
Pneumothorax requiring chest tube	3.5%
Hemoptysis/death from massive hemorrhage	3–16.1%/0.4%
Hemoptysis (cryoablation)	36–62%
Subcutaneous emphysema	16%
Abscess	5%
Pain	46%
Pleural effusions	13%
Air embolism	Rare
Nerve Injury	Rare

[a]Rates refer to risk after RF ablation unless otherwise specified. [58, 59, 61, 65, 66, 68]

barometric pressure could otherwise cause sealed air leaks to reopen or small pneumothoraces to enlarge and become symptomatic. Although local standards apply, the Air Transport Medicine Committee of the Aerospace Medical Association asserts that a pneumothorax should be considered a contraindication for flight and that air travel should wait for 2 to 3 weeks after radiographic resolution of the pneumothorax.[64]

The incidence of hemoptysis ranges from 3% to 16.1%.[59,65] Death from massive hemoptysis is exceedingly rare. It should be stressed that this entity is usually self-limiting, requiring no further intervention. The incidence of hemoptysis after cryoablation appears to be slightly higher, 36% to 62%.[66,67] It is uncertain whether or not this is secondary to hemostatic/coagulative effects of heat energy or the relative infancy of the procedure.

Underscoring the importance of a clear knowledge of anatomy, thermal injury to the intercostals and phrenic nerves as well the brachial plexus have been reported in treatment of tumors in an apical or paramediastinal location.[68,69] Ablation close to the chest wall without using separation techniques may lead to intercostals nerve injury, resulting in neuropathy and paresthesias or pleuritic pain. The course of such an injury is variable with symptomatic improvement over time. We have found use of antiseizure medications such as pregabalin (Lyrica) or gabapentin (Neurontin) helpful.

Interestingly, microbubble formation after RF ablation, as detected by carotid ultrasound, has been reported.[70] Fortunately, the investigators were unable to find any clinical sequelae or changes on head CT. These findings were further confirmed by another group utilizing magnetic resonance imaging (MRI) with diffusion weighted imaging and they also failed to detect changes related to cerebral infarction or neurologic deficit.[71]

▌ IMAGING FOLLOW-UP

Owing to the variability of the natural course of primary lung cancers and metastasis, local practices for imaging follow-up may vary. It may be reasonable to perform the first follow-up imaging (not inclusive of the immediate postprocedure CT) within a 3-month period. In 2009, the Technology Assessment Committee of the Society of Interventional Radiology, in its guidelines for reporting standards for thermal ablation of lung cancers, suggested that a CT follow-up should be performed every 3 months after an early scan (1 to 3 months) documents absence of viable tumor, which sets a baseline for follow-up imaging comparison.[72]

Computed Tomography

The expected appearance of the immediate postablation CT image is that of ground glass opacity surrounding the ablated tumor. It is believed that the area of surrounding ground glass opacity may be predictive of efficacy of therapy.[73,74] Some believe that a postablation area four times larger than the initial tumor size is predictive of complete treatment, whereas others suggest that a minimum of a 5-mm margin of ground glass opacity surrounding the tumor is required.[75,76] Most importantly, the region lacking of ground glass opacity correlated with the site of future progression. This region of surrounding ground glass usually resolves in 1 month. Associated pleural effusions, pleural

thickening, and, occasionally, cavitation, may also be seen, which is expected to resolve as well.[77]

Contrast-enhanced CT studies can be helpful in determining the extent of tumor necrosis. Early animal studies have determined that a 10 HU increase between the pre- and postcontrast images suggest a region of viable tumor.[72] Surrounding inflammation can often enhance; therefore, utilizing the enhancement pattern rather than a threshold value may be of more utility.[78]

Because postablation inflammation and hemorrhage usually resolve with postablation size returning to preablation size at 3 months, it may be reasonable to obtain the follow-up CT at this interval to assess for growth that would be highly suspicious for local tumor progression or recurrence.[79] An earlier baseline is often obtained from which follow-up imaging is compared.

Positron Emission Tomography/Computed Tomography

PET/CT is rapidly becoming a popular method for staging and has growing utility in determining adequacy of ablation and monitoring local tumor progression. There is currently no consensus regarding optimal time for PET/CT follow-up or a recommendation on a maximum standardized uptake value (SUVmax), which would suggest recurrence. Higaki et al.,[80] in evaluating the optimum time point for postprocedural PET/CT, determined that at 3 to 9 months after RF ablation, lesions with SUVmax of at least 1.5 were suspicious for locoregional recurrence with 77.8% sensitivity and 85.7% to 90.5% specificity (an abnormal contrast-enhanced CT was used to determine locoregional recurrence). Although we consider any nodular area with SUVmax of greater than 3.0 suspicious for recurrence, the characteristics of the radiotracer uptake is more important.

Six distinctive patterns of fludeoxyglucose (FDG) uptake have been evaluated: diffuse, focal, heterogeneous, rim, and rim plus focal uptake, with focal uptake either at the site of the original tumor or at a different site. It is known that rim uptake is favorable and likely corresponds to surrounding inflammation, which can persist for months.[81] Other patterns that were favorable included diffuse, heterogeneous, and rim with focal uptake if that focal uptake did not correspond to the initial site of the tumor. If rim with focal uptake is identified with the area of focal uptake corresponding to the original tumor site, this correlated with local recurrence.[82] Of course, any areas demonstrating new or increasing regions of FDG uptake should be considered suspicious and prompt consideration for percutaneous biopsy. The optimum timepoint to obtain a PET/CT is 3 months after the ablation. This timepoint diminishes the false positive rate associated with inflammation.[83]

Interestingly, a group has observed that FDG uptake may be seen in mediastinal lymph nodes or at the needle path even at 3 months; all these regions normalized on further follow-up, suggesting areas of inflammation.[83] This could potentially complicate identification of disease progression to nodal stations.

Magnetic Resonance Imaging

Traditionally, MRI is not utilized for lung imaging secondary to long acquisition times. This renders it susceptible to motion artifacts caused by cardiac pulsation and numerous air-tissue interfaces. Newer sequences with shorter acquisition times are being investigated to determine its utility in both diagnosis of lung neoplasm and staging.[84,85] A pilot study utilizing apparent diffusion coefficient (ADC) demonstrated that there was a significant difference in the ADC of postablation patients who eventually developed local tumor progression, as determined by a mean 6-month CT follow-up.[86] As sequences become more refined, there is a potential for MRI to play a larger role in pre treatment and post treatment planning as well as to guide the intervention.

❚ REFERENCES

1. American Cancer Society. *Cancer Facts and Figures 2010*. Atlanta, GA: American Cancer Society; 2010.
2. Ginsberg RJ, Rubinstein LV. Randomized trial of lobectomy versus limited resection for T1 N0 nonsmall cell lung cancer. Lung Cancer Study Group. *Ann Thorac Surg* 1995;60:615–622.
3. Altorki N. *A Randomized Phase III Trial of Lobectomy Versus Sublobar Resection for Small (<2 Cm) Peripheral Non-small Cell Lung Cancer*. CALGB (Cancer and Leukemia Group B) study #140503.
4. McCormack PM. Ginsberg RJ. Current management of colorectal metastases to lung. *Chest Surg Clin N Am* 1998;8:119–126.
5. Treasure T. Pulmonary metastasectomy: a common practice based on weak evidence. *Ann R Coll Surg Engl* 2007;89:744–748.
6. Long-term results of lung metastasectomy: prognostic analyses based on 5206 cases. The International Registry of Lung Metastases. *J Thorac Cardiovasc Surg* 1997;113:37–49.
7. Pastorino U, Buyse M, Friedel G, et al. Long-term results of lung metastasectomy: prognostic analyses based on 5206 cases. *J Thorac Cardiovasc Surg* 1997;113:37–49.
8. Vogl UM, Zehetgruber H, Dominkus M, et al. Prognostic factors in metastatic renal cell carcinoma: metastasectomy as independent prognostic variable. *Br J Cancer* 2006;95:691–698.
9. Curley SA, Izzo F, Delrio P, et al. Radiofrequency ablation of unresectable primary and metastatic hepatic malignancies: results in 123 patients. *Ann Surg* 1999;230:1–8.
10. Dupuy DE, Zagoria RJ, Akerley W, et al. Percutaneous radiofrequency ablation of malignancies in the lung. *Am J Roentgenol* 2000;174:57–59.
11. Lencioni R, Crocetti L, Cioni R, et al. Response to radiofrequency ablation of pulmonary tumours: a prospective, intention-to-treat, multicentre clinical trial (the RAPTURE study). *Lancet* 2008;9:621–628.
12. Simon CJ, Dupuy DE, DiPetrillo TA, et al. Pulmonary radiofrequency ablation: long term safety and efficacy in 153 patients. *Radiology* 2007;243:268–275.
13. Chua TC, Sarkar A, Saxena A, et al. Long-term outcome of image-guided percutaneous radiofrequency ablation of lung metastases: an open-labeled prospective trial of 148 patients. *Annals Oncol* 2010;21:2017–2011.
14. Thomas P, Rubinstein L; and the Lung Cancer Study Group. Cancer recurrence after resection: t1 n0 non-small cell lung cancer. *Ann Thorac Surg* 2009;49:242–247.
15. Roviaro G, Varoli F, Vergani C, et al. Long-term survival after videothoracoscopic lobectomy for stage I lung cancer. *Chest* 2004;126:725–732.
16. Munden RF, Swisher SS, Stevens CW, et al. Imaging of the patient with non-small cell lung cancer. *Radiology* 2005;237:803–818.
17. Goldberg SN, Gazelle GS, Mueller PR. Thermal ablation therapy for focal malignancy: a unified approach to underlying principles, techniques, and diagnostic imaging guidance. *Am J Roentgenol* 2000;174:323–331.
18. Goldberg SN, Dupuy DE. Image-guided radiofrequency tumor ablation: challenges and opportunities—part I. *J Vasc Interv Radiol* 2001;12:1021–1032.
19. Goldberg SN, Ahmed M, Gazelle GS, et al. Radio-frequency thermal ablation with NaCl solution injection: effect of electrical conductivity on tissue heating and coagulation-phantom and porcine liver study. *Radiology* 2001;219:157–165.
20. Lu DS, Raman SS, Limanond P, et al. Influence of large peritumoral vessels on outcome of radiofrequency ablation of liver tumors. *J Vasc Interv Radiol* 2003;14:1267–1274.
21. Hiraki T, Sakurai J, Tsuda T, et al. Risk factors for local progression after percutaneous radiofrequency ablation of lung tumors: evaluation based on a preliminary review of 342 tumors. *Cancer* 2006;107:2873–2880.

22. Lin SM, Lin CC, Chen WT, et al. Radiofrequency ablation for hepatocellular carcinoma: a prospective comparison of four radiofrequency devices. *J Vasc Interv Radiol* 2007;18:1118–1125.
23. Le MD, Chen JW, Xie XY, et al. Hepatocellular carcinoma: US-guided percutaneous microwave coagulation therapy. *Radiology* 2001;221:167–172.
24. Brace CL, Hinshaw JL, Laeseke PF, et al. Pulmonary thermal ablation: comparison of radiofrequency and microwave devices by using gross pathologic and CT findings in a swine model. *Radiology* 2009;251:705–711.
25. Crocette L, Bozzi E, Favina P, et al. Thermal ablation of lung tissue: in vivo experimental comparison of microwave and radiofrequency ablation. *Cardiovasc Interv Radiol* 2010;33:818–827.
26. Wolf FJ, Grand DJ, Machan JT, et al. Microwave ablation of lung malignancies: effectiveness, CT findings, and safety in 50 patients. *Radiology* 2008;247:871–879.
27. Liu Z, Ahmed M, Weinstein Y, et al. Characterization of the RF ablation-induced "oven effect": the importance of background tissue thermal conductivity on tissue heating. *Int J Hyperthermia* 2006;22:327–342.
28. Brace CL. Radiofrequency and microwave ablation of the liver, lung, kidney and bone: what are the differences? *Curr Prob Diagn Radiol* 2009;38:135–143.
29. Wang H, Littrup PJ, Duan Y, et al. Thoracic masses treated with percutaneous cryotherapy: initial experience with more than 200 procedures. *Radiology* 2005;235:289–298.
30. Carpenter RJ, Neel HB, Sanderson DR. Cryosurgery of bronchopulmonary structures. An approach to lesions inaccessible to the rigid bronchoscope. *Chest* 1977;72:279–284.
31. Dupuy DE, Shulman M. Current status of thermal ablation treatments for lung malignancies. *Semin Interv Radiol* 2010;27:268–275.
32. Permpongkosol S, Nicol TL, Link RE, et al. Differences in ablation size in porcine liver and lung after cryoablation using the same ablation protocol. *Am J Roentgenol* 2007;188:1028–1032.
33. Akeboshi M, Yamakado K, Nakatsuka A, et al. Percutaneous radiofrequency ablation of lung neoplasms: initial therapeutic response. *J Vasc Interv Radiol* 2004;15:463–470.
34. American Joint Committee on Cancer (AJCC). *Cancer Staging Manual*. 7th ed. Edge SB, Byrd DR, Carducci MA, et al., eds. New York, NY: Springer; 2009.
35. Fernando HC, Santos RS, Benfield JR, et al. Lobar and sublobar resection with and without brachytherapy for small stage IA non-small cell lung cancer. *J Thorac Cardiovasc Surg* 2005;129:261–267.
36. Okada M, Nishio W, Sakamoto T, et al. Effect of tumor size on prognosis in patients with non-small cell lung cancer: the role of segmentectomy as a type of lesser resection. *J Thorac Cardiovasc Surg* 2005;129:87–93.
37. Shigemura N, Akashi A, Funaki S, et al. Long term outcomes after a variety of video-assisted thoracoscopic lobectomy approaches for clinical stage IA lung cancer: a multi-institutional study. *J Thorac Cardiovasc Surg* 2006;132:507–512.
38. Okuma T, Matsuoka T, Yamamoto A, et al. Determinants of local progression after computed tomography-guided percutaneous radiofrequency ablation for unresectable lung tumors: 9-year experience in a single institution. *Cardiovasc Interv Radiol* 2009;33:787–793.
39. Lee W, Daly BD, DiPetrillo TA, et al. Limited resection for non-small cell lung cancer: observed local control with implantation of I-125 brachytherapy seeds. *Ann Thorac Surg* 2003;75:237–242.
40. Fernando HC. Radiofrequency ablation to treat non-small cell lung cancer and pulmonary metastases. *Ann Thorac Surg* 2008;85:S780–S784.
41. Livraghi T, Solbiati L, Meloni F, et al. Percutaneous radiofrequency ablation of liver metastases in potential candidates for resection: the "test-of-time approach". *Cancer* 2003;97:3027–3035.
42. Bath OF, Kaklamanos IG, Moffat FL, et al. Metastasectomy as a cytoreductive treatment of isolated pulmonary and hepatic metastases from breast cancer. *Surg Oncol* 1999;8:35–42.
43. Russo P, O'Brien MF. Surgical intervention in patients with metastatic renal cancer: metastasectomy and cytoreductive nephrectomy. *Urol Clin North Am* 2008;35:679–686.
44. Bunn PA Jr, Franklin W. Epidermal growth factor receptor expression, signal pathway, and inhibitors in non-small cell lung cancer. *Semin Oncol* 2002;29:38–44.
45. Mitsudomi T, Kosaka T, Endoh H, et al. Mutations of the epidermal growth factor receptor gene predict prolonged survival after gefitinib treatment in patients with non–small-cell lung cancer with postoperative recurrence. *J Clin Oncol* 2005;23:2513–2520.
46. Guix M, Faber AC, Wang SE, et al. Acquired resistance to EGFR tyrosine kinase inhibitors in cancer cells is mediated by loss of IGF-binding proteins. *J Clin Invest* 2008;118:2609–2619.

47. Hiraki T, Gobata H, Mimura H, et al. Does tumor type affect local control by radiofrequency ablation in the lungs? *Eur J Radiol* 2010;74:136–141.

48. Ambrogi MC, Lucchi M, Dini P, et al. Percutaneous radiofrequency ablation of lung tumours: results in the mid-term. *Eur J Cardiothorac Surg* 2006;30:177–183.

49. Ambrogi MC, Fanucchi O, Lencioni R, et al. Pulmonary radiofrequency ablation in a single lung patient. *Thorax* 2006;61:828–829.

50. LeVeen Needle Electrode [prescriptive information]. Malborough, MA: Boston Scientific; 2011.

51. Hayes DL, Charboneau JW, Lewis BD, et al. Radiofrequency treatment of hepatic neoplasms in patients with permanent pacemakers. *Mayo Clin Proc* 2001;76:950–952.

52. Shankar S, Vansonnenberg E, Silverman SG, et al. Brachial plexus injury from CT-guided RF ablation under general anesthesia. *Cardiovasc Interv Radiol* 2005;28:646–648.

53. Solomon SB, Thornton RH, Dupuy DE, et al. Protection of the mediastinum and chest wall with an artificial pneumothorax during lung ablations. *J Vasc Interv Radiol* 2008;19:610–615.

54. Oshima F, Yamakado K, Akeboshi M, et al. Lung radiofrequency ablation with and without bronchial occlusion: experimental study in porcine lungs. *J Vasc Interv Radiol* 2004;15:1451–1456.

55. Santos RS, Gan J, Ohara CJ, et al. Microwave ablation of lung tissue: impact of single-lung ventilation on ablation size. *Ann Thorac Surg* 2010;90:1116–1119.

56. Yamagami T, Terayama K, Yoshimatsu R, et al. Role of manual aspiration in treating pneumothorax after computed tomography-guided lung biopsy. *Acta Radiol* 2009;50:1126–1133.

57. Pua BB, Solomon SB. Radiofrequency ablation of pulmonary tumors. In: Kandarpa K, Machan L, eds. *Handbook of Vascular & Interventional Radiologic Procedures.* 4th ed. Philadelphia, PA: Lippincott Williams & Wilkins; 2010.

58. Zhu JC, Yan TD, Glenn D, et al. Radiofrequency ablation of lung tumors: feasibility and safety. *Ann Thorac Surg* 2009;87:1023–1028.

59. Suh RD, Walace AB, Sheehan RE, et al. Unresectable pulmonary malignancies: CT-guided percutaneous radiofrequency ablation–preliminary results. *Radiology* 2003;229:821–829.

60. Belfiore G, Moggio G, Tedeschi E, et al. CT-guided radiofrequency ablation: a potential complementary therapy for patients with unresectable primary lung cancer—a preliminary report of 33 patients. *Am J Roentgen* 2004;183:1003–1011.

61. Okuma T, Matsuoka T, Yamamoto A, et al. Frequency and risk factors of various complications after computed tomography-guided radiofrequency ablation of lung tumors. *Cardiovasc Interv Radiol* 2008;31:122–130.

62. Hiraki T, Tajiri N, Mimua H, et al. Pneumothorax, pleural effusion, and chest tube placement after radiofrequency ablation of lung tumors: incidence and risk factors. *Radiology* 2006;241:275–283.

63. Yoshimatsu R, Yamagami T, Terayama K, et al. Delayed and recurrent pneumothorax after radiofrequency ablation of lung tumors. *Chest* 2009;135:1002–1009.

64. Air Transport Medicine Committee, Aerospace Medical Association. Medical guidelines for air travel. *Aviat Space Environ Med* 1996;67(suppl):Bl–B8.

65. Nour-Eldin NE, Naguib NN, Mack M, et al. Pulmonary hemorrhage complicating radiofrequency ablation, from mild hemoptysis to life-threatening pattern. *Eur Radiol* 2011;21:197–204. doi: 10.1007/s00330-010-1889-1891.

66. Wang H, Littrup PJ, Duan Y, et al. Thoracic masses treated with percutaneous cryotherapy: initial experience with more than 200 procedures. *Radiology* 2005;235:289–298.

67. Kawamura M, Izumi Y, Tsukada N, et al. Percutaneous cryoablation of small pulmonary malignant tumors under computed tomographic guidance with local anesthesia for nonsurgical candidates. *J Thorac Cardiovasc Surg* 2007;131:1007–1013.

68. Hiraki T, Gobara H, Mimura H, et al. Brachial nerve injury caused by percutaneous radiofrequency ablation of apical lung cancers: a report of four cases. *J Vasc Interv Radiol* 2010;21:1129–1133.

69. Thornton RH, Solomon SB, Dupuy DE, et al. Phrenic nerve injury resulting from percutaneous ablation of lung malignancy. *Am J Roentgenol* 2008;191:565–568.

70. Rose SC, Fotoohi M, Levin DL, et al. Cerebral microembolization during radiofrequency ablation of lung malignancies. *J Vasc Interv Radiol* 2002;13:1051–1054.

71. Yamamoto A, Matsuoka T, Toyoshima M, et al. Assessment of cerebral microembolism during percutaneous radiofrequency ablation of lung tumors using diffusion-weighted imaging. *Am J Roentgenol* 2004;183:1785–1789.

72. Rose SC, Dupuy DE, Gervais DA, et al. Research reporting standards for percutaneous thermal ablation of lung neoplasms. *J Vasc Radiol* 2009;20:S474–S485.

73. Lee JM, Jin GY, Goldberg SN, et al. Percutaneous radiofrequency ablation for inoperable non-small cell lung cancer and metastases: preliminary report. *Radiology* 2004;230:125–134.

74. Goldberg SN, Gazclle GS, Compton CC, et al. Radio-frequency tissue ablation of VX2 tumor nodules in the rabbit lung. *Acad Radiol* 1996;3:929–935.

75. Anderson EM, Lees WR, Gillams AR. Early indicators of treatment success after percutaneous radiofrequency of pulmonary tumors. *Cardiovasc Interv Radiol* 2009;32:478–483.

76. de Baere T, Palussiere J, Auperin A, et al. Midterm local efficacy and survival after radiofrequency ablation of lung tumors with minimum follow-up of 1 year: prospective evaluation. *Radiology* 2006;240:587–596.

77. Bojarski JD, Dupuy DE, Mayo-Smith WW. CT imaging findings of pulmonary neoplasms after treatment with radiofrequency ablation: results in 32 tumors. *Am J Roentgenol* 2005;185:466–471.

78. Jin GY, Lee JM, Lee YC, et al. Primary and secondary lung malignancies treated with percutaneous radiofrequency ablation: evaluation with follow-up helical CT. *AJR Am J Roentgenol* 2004;183:1013–1020.

79. Nguyen C, Scott WJ, Goldberg M. Radiofrequency ablation of lung malignancies. *Ann Thorac Surg* 2006;82:365–371.

80. Higaki F, Okumura Y, Sato S, et al. Preliminary retrospective investigation of FDG-PET/CT timing in follow-up of ablated lung tumor. *Ann Nucl Med* 2008;22:157–163.

81. Kang S, Luo R, Liao W, et al. Single group study to evaluate the feasibility and complications of radiofrequency ablation and usefulness of post treatment positron emission tomography in lung tumours. *World J Surg Oncol* 2004;2:30–35.

82. Singnurkar A, Solomon SB, Gönen M, et al. 18F-FDG PET/CT for the prediction and detection of local recurrence after radiofrequency ablation of malignant lung lesions. *J Nucl Med* 2010;51:1833–1840.

83. Deandreis D, Leboulleux S, Dromain C, et al. Role of FDG PET/CT and chest CT in the follow-up of lung lesions treated with radiofrequency ablation. *Radiology* 2011;258:270–276.

84. Zhang TT, Li ZY, Wu JL. Status and progress on therapeutic evaluation of targeted therapy, radiotherapy and chemotherapy in lung carcinoma using new MRI techniques. *Int J Med Radiol* (Chinese) 2009;32:453–456.

85. Li Z, Zhang T, Xu B, et al. Usefulness of DWI in the evaluation of pulmonary isolated lesion. *Chinese German J Clin Oncol* 2010;9:P388–P390.

86. Okuma T, Matsuoka T, Yamamoto A, et al. Assessment of early treatment response after CT-guided radiofrequency ablation of unresectable lung tumours by diffusion-weighted MRI: a pilot study. *Br J Radiol* 2009;82:989–994.

Bone/Musculoskeletal Tumors: Painful Metastases

A. NICHOLAS KURUP and MATTHEW R. CALLSTROM

BACKGROUND

Over the past two decades, image-guided percutaneous ablation methods have been applied to metastatic disease beyond the liver and lung. Specifically, percutaneous ablation techniques have proven effective for palliation of painful metastases to bone and soft tissue. Tumor ablation in bone was initially described in the treatment of benign osteoid osteomas.[1] The success of that treatment, which has now become standard of care for osteoid osteomas,[2] led to the application of ablative technology in the treatment of limited metastatic disease to bone and soft tissue. Various ablative technologies, including radiofrequency ablation (RFA), cryoablation, microwave ablation, laser ablation, focused ultrasound (FUS), and ethanol, have been applied in the treatment of bone and soft-tissue metastases. These ablations have been augmented with cement instillation in bone (cementoplasty) in many reported cases.

The application of ablative methods to bone and soft-tissue metastases has been driven by the significant need for focal therapy applied to cancer-related bone pain. Up to 85% of patients with the three most common types of cancer—lung, breast, and prostate—develop metastases to bone.[3] Bone metastases may lead to significant morbidity from pain, pathologic fracture, or compression of adjacent neural structures. Painful skeletal metastases are frequently undertreated with up to 79% of patients experiencing severe pain before effective palliative therapy is pursued.[4] Patients with metastases to bone have a poor prognosis overall with a median survival of 3 years or less, although 5-year survival may range from 5% to 40%, depending on tumor histology and extent.[5,6] Multidisciplinary teams treating these patients have a number of therapeutic options to treat the pain from skeletal metastases.

Patients with widespread metastatic disease are typically treated systemically. Opioids offer pain relief albeit with side effects, including sedation, nausea, and constipation.[7] Bisphosphonate medications are an important class of antiosteoclastic agents, which are evolving into standard of care for painful widespread metastases.[8–11] Targeted pharmacologic agents, including chemotherapeutics, hormonal modulators, and radiopharmaceuticals, have limited application for most painful skeletal metastases.

Patients with limited but painful metastatic disease to bone are treated with external beam radiation therapy as standard of care. Radiation therapy achieves pain reduction in most patients.[12] This pain relief may take weeks to occur and is transient more than half the time. Moreover, 20% to 30% of patients show no

pain relief, and of those who do respond, almost half have recurrent pain at a median of 16 weeks following treatment.[13–17] Unfortunately, repeat radiation therapy of a previously irradiated painful metastasis to bone or soft tissue is frequently not possible due to limitations in normal tissue tolerance.

Surgery for bone metastases is usually reserved for those lesions at significant risk of impending pathologic fracture and less commonly to achieve local control in patients with oligometastatic disease. The expected poor natural history of bone or nonvisceral soft-tissue metastases as well as comorbidities and postoperative length of recovery limit the application of surgery in these patients.

INDICATIONS AND CONTRAINDICATIONS

Image-guided percutaneous ablation of painful metastases to bone and soft tissue is performed in three main patient populations. The first group of patients has limited metastatic disease with pain refractory to conventional therapies. Alternatively, patients who refuse conventional therapy for painful metastases may be appropriate for ablation. The second group is patients with limited metastatic disease, which, based on tumor location or extent, places them at risk for further morbidity without local treatment. Lesions in these patients may be at risk of pathologic fracture or compromise of an adjacent critical structure, most often neural tissues. These tumors are most commonly in the axial skeleton, often in the vertebrae or periacetabular regions. Finally, patients with limited metastatic disease who are poor surgical candidates may benefit from ablation. These patients with oligometastatic disease may benefit from percutaneous ablation to achieve local control or disease remission regardless of whether their metastases are symptomatic. Similarly, localized therapy with percutaneous ablation may be appropriate in patients with relatively stable metastatic disease but with a limited number of progressing skeletal or soft-tissue metastases.

Absolute contraindications to percutaneous ablation of painful metastases are limited. These include uncorrectable bleeding diathesis, inability to tolerate the level of anesthesia required for the procedure, and absence of safe percutaneous access to the painful lesion(s). Relative contraindications are more common. Most importantly, patients with widespread painful metastases are unlikely to benefit meaningfully from local therapy, including percutaneous ablation. Likewise, tumor ablation is less effective in improving upon mild pain. Additionally, effective treatment of painful metastases that are in close proximity to critical structures may be difficult or impossible. Various maneuvers to displace vital structures from target lesions or techniques to monitor function of adjacent nerves may assist in overcoming some of these challenges, but some tumors cannot be safely treated with percutaneous ablation in spite of these methods.

■ PATIENT SELECTION

Proper patient selection is crucial to the successful treatment of painful metastases with percutaneous ablation (FIGURE 19.1). Appropriate patients have moderate to severe pain, typically considered to be patients who self-report worst pain in a 24-hour

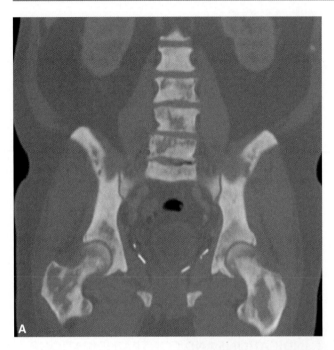
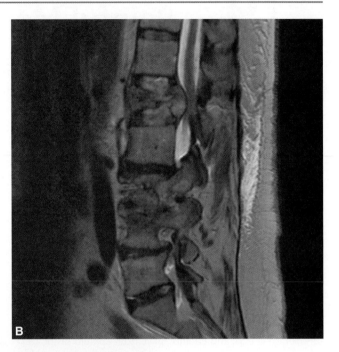
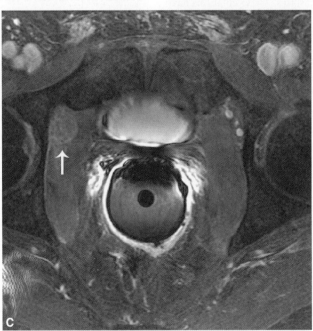

FIGURE 19.1 Poor candidates for percutaneous ablation of musculoskeletal metastases. **A.** Diffuse osteoblastic metastases from prostate carcinoma in this 68-year-old man would be better served with systemic therapy. Pain is typically difficult to localize to one or a few metastases to target for local therapy in these patients. **B.** A large L1 vertebral body metastasis from breast carcinoma with pathologic compression in a 49-year-old woman has a significant epidural component compressing the spinal cord. This lesion is not amenable to percutaneous ablation due to risk of dural and spinal cord injury, and surgical decompression and stabilization are indicated. **C.** A small soft-tissue prostate carcinoma metastasis (*arrow*) at the right obturator foramen in a 50-year-old man would require sacrifice of the obturator nerve for adequate treatment. This patient was treated with hormonal deprivation with good response.

period as 4 or greater on a 10-point pain scale. Percutaneous ablation to palliate pain in patients with mild pain levels, scored as less than 4/10, is not as effective. In these cases, it is difficult to improve upon mild pain, and this level of pain can usually be managed effectively with oral analgesics. Moreover, the number of painful metastases targeted should be limited, usually between one and three lesions. The location of a patient's pain should correlate with a focal abnormality on cross-sectional imaging. Patients with more numerous metastases are better served with a systemic, rather than a focal, approach, because localization for directed therapy is difficult in these patients. Although all types of skeletal metastases may be amenable to ablative therapy, osteolytic lesions, mixed osteolytic/osteoblastic lesions, or predominantly soft-tissue lesions are often best suited to percutaneous ablation. Osteoblastic metastases are frequently diffuse within the skeletal system and may be challenging during placement of the ablative device due to access through intact bone. Finally, the target lesion or lesions should be separated or possibly displaced from critical structures. Ideally, a 1-cm margin between the target lesion and a critical structure allows for safe treatment. If such separation is not possible, accurate monitoring of the ablation zone and sufficient operator experience becomes even more crucial.

▌ TECHNIQUE

General

Anesthesia

Percutaneous tumor ablation may be performed under general anesthesia or with conscious sedation, and choice of anesthesia level may depend on local preference and ablative system employed. General anesthesia allows for maximal control of a patient's hemodynamics, airway, respiration, and positioning. Conscious sedation allows for shorter procedure time and less expense. Lower levels of sedation may also permit functional monitoring of neural structures near the targeted lesion. Complexity of the particular case, which incorporates lesion size, accessibility, and nearness to vulnerable critical structures, often dictates the level of anesthesia required. Because ice formation is relatively painless, lower levels of anesthesia may be possible with cryoablation.

Image Guidance

Safe and effective percutaneous ablation of painful metastases to bone and soft tissue requires appropriate image guidance. The imaging modality used depends on its ability to visualize the targeted lesion for device placement and ablation monitoring. Fluoroscopic guidance affords high spatial and temporal resolution. It is most commonly used for needle placement in vertebroplasty performed in pathologically fractured vertebral bodies, but it is inadequate for tumor ablation itself because it cannot target small tumors and provides no information for monitoring the ablation zone. Ultrasound guidance offers good spatial and excellent temporal resolution for placement of applicators. It is most useful in superficial soft-tissue tumors or markedly osteolytic skeletal metastases. However, it has limited value in targeting deep lesions or those with intact cortical bone. Moreover, ultrasound cannot be used to monitor ablation zones during treatment because of limited visualization through the gas produced from heat-based techniques and the ice produced in cryoablation. Computed tomography (CT) is

the most commonly used imaging modality to guide musculoskeletal tumor ablation procedures. It provides good resolution of most bone and soft-tissue tumors, affords the best global imaging of the lesion relative to its local environment, is widely available, and allows relatively quick placement of applicators under CT fluoroscopy. Moreover, serial intraprocedural unenhanced CT imaging allows excellent visualization of the growing ice ball during cryoablation. Data acquired with multidetector CT scanners may be rapidly reconstructed to provide multiplanar evaluation of device placement and ablation zone coverage. Radiation dose to patients with metastatic disease is of limited clinical concern. Finally, magnetic resonance imaging (MRI) has superior bone and soft-tissue contrast resolution. Real-time imaging and temperature monitoring sequences are now available for application during MRI-guided ablations, allowing intraprocedural monitoring of both heat- and cold-based thermal ablative techniques. These procedures can be time-consuming, MRI-compatible ablation devices remain limited, and access to MRI scanners for intervention is restricted or not practical in most clinical practice settings.

Anatomic Considerations

Safe percutaneous ablation of bone and soft-tissue metastases requires complete understanding of the anatomy surrounding any targeted lesion (FIGURE 19.2). Critical normal structures in proximity to metastases may include the central nervous system, major peripheral nerves, artery of Adamkiewicz, bowel, bladder, or skin. The spinal cord, nerve roots, and major motor nerves are the most crucial structures to consider, given the frequency of metastases arising in the axial skeleton. These structures may need to be visibly or physiologically monitored, thermally insulated from the ablation energy, and/or displaced from the metastasis. Intact cortical bone provides some protection against thermal damage to adjacent soft tissue with heat-based systems.[18] Moreover, nearby major vessels should be noted because they may serve as a source of perfusion-mediated tissue cooling or heating during thermal ablation procedures, thereby preserving adjacent tumor.[19,20] Although a 1-cm margin between vital structure and targeted metastasis is generally considered necessary to allow for safe ablation, the allowable distance in practice depends on the visibility of the tumor, normal structure, and ablation zone; the predictability of the ablation zone; temperature monitoring usage; and experience of the interventional radiologist.

Additionally, the tumor's internal or local anatomy should be considered. For palliation of pain, the bone/tumor interface should be targeted as the source of pain rather than the central portion of the tumor.[21] Complete coverage of the tumor with a sufficient margin of treated normal tissue is required to achieve local control of a tumor. The internal structure of tumors may affect device placement; specifically, deliberate spacing of applicators within tumors with substantial central necrosis can be difficult and may require additional applicators to be placed for adequate tumor coverage.

Finally, access to sclerotic lesions or those deep to thick, intact cortical bone may require additional bone access devices. Ablation applicators may be placed directly into metastases that are completely or predominantly soft tissue, lytic metastases with only a thin rim of remaining bone, or metastases in very osteopenic patients with little difficulty. A sterile bone drill with Steinmann pins or a bone biopsy needle (often 11 or 13 gauge) may be needed to penetrate superficial bone and create a course through which thermal ablation applicators may be placed.

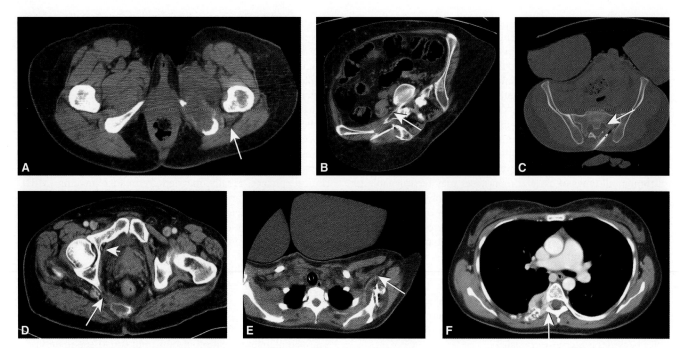

FIGURE 19.2 Common areas of concern for ablation of bone and soft-tissue metastases. **A.** A metastasis in the left inferior pubic ramus is in close proximity to the sciatic nerve (*arrow*). **B.** A cryoprobe is partially visualized in a metastasis in the right iliac bone with the lumbar plexus (*arrow*) along the anterior aspect of the sacrum. **C.** A cryoprobe is in place in the posterior left sacrum. The S1 nerve root (*arrow*) is in close proximity. **D.** An osteolytic metastasis is present in the inferior sacrum. The pudendal nerve (*long arrow*) is in close proximity. The obturator nerve (*short arrow*) is well separated from the tumor. **E.** Two cryoprobes are partially imaged in a tumor involving the scapula with a surrounding ice ball approaching the brachial plexus (*arrow*). **F.** Ablation of a paravertebral tumor (*arrow*) that extends to the edge of the vertebral body and foramen should consider the potential adjacency of the artery of Adamkiewicz. This blood vessel, which provides blood supply to the ventral cord, originates from a segmental artery arising from the abdominal aorta.

Reproduced with permission from Kurup AN, Callstrom MR. Ablation of skeletal metastases: current status. *J Vasc Interv Radiol* 2010;21(suppl 8):S242–S250.

Adjunctive Procedures

Several techniques have been developed to monitor tumor ablation intraprocedurally and to protect at-risk adjacent structures (FIGURE 19.3). Thermocouples may be placed along critical structures to ensure that damaging temperatures are not reached. Electrophysiologic monitoring with motor-evoked potentials can provide timely feedback on the functional status of adjacent nerves during ablation. Limited physical examination can similarly provide information regarding intact nerve function. Displacement of vital structures with fluid ("hydrodisplacement"), angiography balloons, or gas (typically CO_2) is commonly performed to prevent collateral damage. Sterile 5% dextrose in water is usually used instead of saline for hydrodisplacement when performing RFA to prevent the theoretical extension of thermal injury through ion-containing fluid.[22] Placement of tepid water in a sterile glove at the skin surface may minimize the risk of dermal injury with cryoablation of a superficial lesion.

Radiofrequency Ablation

RFA is the most widely accepted and studied method of percutaneous tumor ablation (FIGURE 19.4). Originally applied to the treatment of benign osteoid osteomas in bone, RFA is now routinely used to treat bone and soft-tissue metastases. High-frequency (RF, 450 to 600 kHz) alternating current produces ionic agitation within the tumor cells and intracellular space, leading to lethal temperatures, typically greater than 60°C. Grounding pads are placed on the patient's skin, typically along the upper thighs, to complete the electrical circuit and dissipate the energy applied.

Multiple manufacturers produce RF generators and applicators, called electrodes. RFA electrodes are generally 17 gauge in caliber and manufactured in different shapes, including single linear electrodes, cluster electrodes, and expandable or deployable umbrella-shaped electrodes. The uninsulated tip of an electrode is placed within the tumor. For deployable devices, expandable tines are advanced to the margins of the soft-tissue portion of the tumor. The exposed length of the tines controls the size of the resulting ablation zone. With these devices, once the target temperature up to 100°C (or impedance limit for impedance-controlled systems) is reached, the ablation is treated for 5 to 15 minutes. A single ablation may be sufficient for a lesion less than or equal to 3 cm, but larger lesions require treatment using multiple deployments. Single or cluster electrodes internally cooled with chilled water may be placed in the soft-tissue portion of the tumor with tips usually near the bone/tumor interface. RF energy is applied at maximum current with these internally cooled systems.[23] Up to three probes may be used simultaneously with switching generator technology.[24]

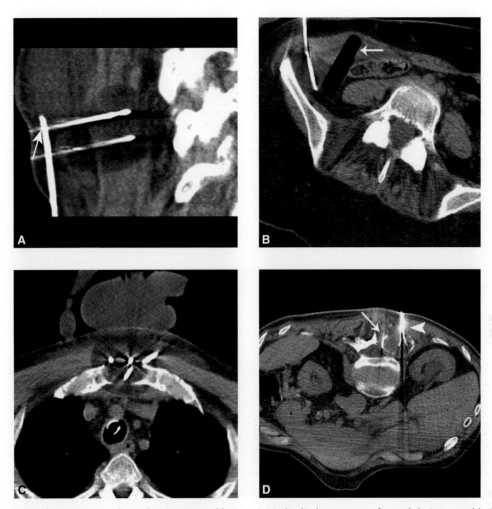

FIGURE 19.3 Adjunctive procedures during tumor ablation. **A**. Hydrodisplacement performed during cryoablation of a paraspinal esophageal carcinoma metastasis. Sagittal reformatted image shows 5% dextrose in water instilled through a 5 French Yueh catheter (*arrow*). **B**. Esophageal dilatation balloon (*arrow*) inflated to displace adjacent colon during cryoablation of a parailiac ovarian carcinoma metastasis. **C**. Sterile glove containing tepid water placed for skin protection during cryoablation of a sternal metastasis from lung carcinoma. **D**. Thermocouple used to monitor temperature adjacent to the spinal canal during radiofrequency ablation of a rectal carcinoma metastasis in an L1 transverse process. The thermocouple (*arrow*) was placed medially compared to the multitined RFA electrode (*arrowhead*) placed centrally within the tumor.

Other Heat-Based Percutaneous Therapies

Microwave ablation devices may have a role in treating larger lesions. In fact, given the low electrical and thermal conductivity of bone, microwave energy may be better suited to treat bone tumors.[25] However, no systematic description of this application currently exists in the literature with only small series described.[26,27] Similarly, laser ablation has been described in the treatment of osteosarcoma and soft-tissue sarcoma with no large series of treatment of bone and soft-tissue metastases.[28]

Cryoablation

Tissue freezing has a long history of use in the treatment of tumors, but historically it has been limited to intraoperative use either with direct application of liquid nitrogen to the surgical field or insertion of large caliber, uninsulated cryoablation probes. Modern percutaneous cryoablation devices employ room temperature, pressurized argon and helium gases for tissue cooling and heating, respectively. Expansion of argon gas as it passes from a smaller, inner cannula into a larger, outer cannula within a cryoprobe results in rapid cooling, reaching −100°C within a few seconds. A visible ice ball is produced along the uninsulated distal shaft of the probe, appearing low in attenuation on CT and as a signal void on MRI. The outer ice ball margin marks the 0°C isotherm with irreversible tissue destruction occurring at −20°C to −40°C, typically 3 to 5 mm deep to the margin.[29,30]

Two cryoablation systems are currently available, one produced by Endocare, Inc. (division of HealthTronics, Austin, TX) allowing up to 8 cryoprobes to operate independently, and one manufactured by Galil Medical (Arden Hills, MN) with a maximum of 25 cryoprobes distributed across five independently operating channels. Cryoprobes measure 1.5 to 2.4 mm in diameter (about 11- to 15-gauge calibers) with the larger probes generating ice balls of about 3.5 cm in maximal diameter and 5.5 cm

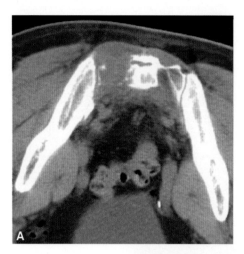
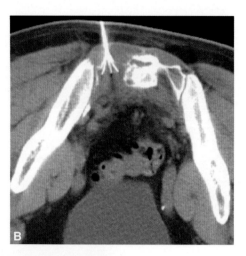
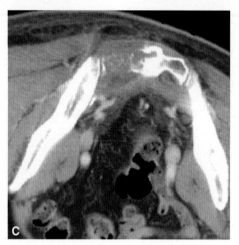

FIGURE 19.4 Radiofrequency ablation (RFA) of a painful sacral metastasis. **A**. Large destructive metastasis in the upper sacrum. **B**. Multitined RFA electrode in the metastasis. Treatment required multiple overlapping ablations. **C**. Postcontrast CT shows a nonenhancing ablation zone encompassing the tumor.

in length. With multiple cryoprobes synchronously activated, large tumors may be treated with ice balls measuring over 8 cm in diameter (FIGURE 19.5). Cryoprobes are generally placed in parallel arrangement within the tumor, but alternate configurations may be used to contour the ice to cover irregularly shaped tumors and avoid vulnerable structures. To eliminate nonlethal temperatures in regions of overlap or at the tumor margin, cryoprobes should be within about 2 cm of each other and 1 cm of the margin. Treatment is usually performed with two 10-minute freezes separated by a 5-minute passive thaw, although freeze cycle length may be increased or decreased depending on the adequacy of tumor coverage and proximity of adjacent critical structures. Using unenhanced CT imaging with body window and level settings (W400, L40), the ice ball may be monitored as frequently as every 2 minutes during each freeze.[31,32] Active thaw with helium for several minutes is necessary to allow removal of cryoprobes once treatment is completed.

Focused Ultrasound

FUS, also called high-intensity focused ultrasound (HIFU), is a completely noninvasive thermal ablation method. It uses FUS energy to heat and destroy internal tissue without placement of percutaneous applicators. Bone is an appropriate target for this therapy given its high acoustic absorption. Heating at the skeletal surface likely results in palliation of pain due to destruction of periosteal innervation.[33,34] MRI, including MR thermometry sequences, is used for tumor targeting and monitoring energy deposition. FUS has been used to treat benign and malignant tumors located in the uterus, breast, liver, prostate, and brain.[35,36] Tissues reach ablative temperatures of greater than 65°C. This technology is limited to treatment of lesions with an acoustic window, and interposed bowel or nerves can be injured if contained within the path of the transducer to the target lesion.

Ethanol Ablation

Simple and inexpensive, ethanol instillation leads to cellular dehydration, vascular thrombosis, tissue ischemia, and necrosis. Ninety-five percent ethanol mixed with dilute contrast material is directly injected into the tumor through a fine needle (20 to 25 gauge). Lidocaine may be added to the mixture for local anesthesia. Unpredictable diffusion of the ethanol within and around the tumor limits this technique's effectiveness and, potentially, its safety.[37]

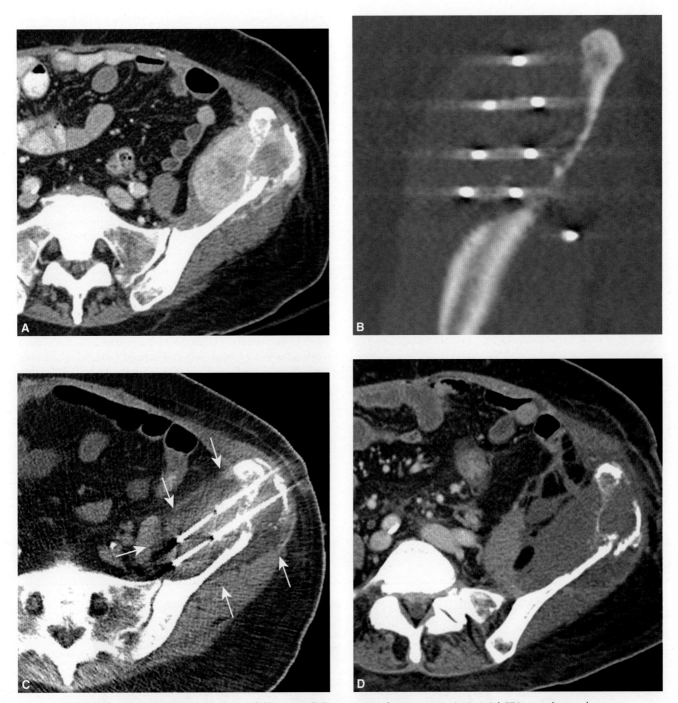

FIGURE 19.5 Cryoablation of a large painful hepatocellular carcinoma bone metastasis. **A.** Axial CT image shows a heterogeneously enhancing 5 × 8 × 6 cm metastasis in the left iliac wing of a 66-year-old woman. **B.** Oblique sagittal reformatted CT image shows 8 Perc-24 cryoprobes systematically placed within the mass. **C.** Axial CT image shows the ice ball (*arrows*) encompassing the metastasis. **D.** Axial contrast-enhanced CT image 3 months after cryoablation shows complete absence of enhancement consistent with tumor necrosis.

Reproduced with permission from Kurup AN, Callstrom MR. Ablation of skeletal metastases: current status. *J Vasc Interv Radiol* 2010;21(suppl 8):S242–S250.

Cementoplasty

Cement instillation into axially loaded bone at risk for fracture is called cementoplasty, osteoplasty, or vertebroplasty when applied in the spine. The cement likely has a direct effect on

nociceptors as well as stabilizes painful microfractures within metastases.[38] Painful metastases subject to axial loading, including those in the vertebral bodies, periacetabular regions, and proximal femurs, are candidates for cementoplasty. When performed in combination with percutaneous ablation of a painful metastasis, cementoplasty is usually performed the following day (FIGURE 19.6). This allows for more complete thawing of the tumor after cryoablation. Cementoplasty also may be performed with conscious sedation. Bone biopsy needles, 11 to 13 gauge in caliber, may be placed into the metastasis, usually through the same access site created during the ablation procedure. When two are used, polymethylmethacralate (PMMA) cement is slowly injected into one needle under fluoroscopy or CT fluoroscopy, and the second needle may serve initially as a vent. Frequent imaging is necessary to ensure proper filling of the tumor cavity and minimize the risk of cement intravasation or extension outside of bone, particularly in periarticular or perineural locations. The bone access needles should be removed with care to avoid leakage of cement along the access tracts. Patients may be assessed for weight-bearing after 1 hour under direct supervision, and limits to ambulation may be determined by patient pain and degree of underlying bone destruction.

▌OUTCOMES/RESULTS

Radiofrequency Ablation

Two major trials have shown excellent results in palliating of painful skeletal metastases. The first single-arm, prospective, multicenter trial, included 62 patients treated with the multitined RITA device (AngioDynamics, Lathum, NY).[21,39] This trial showed a clinically significant decrease (≥2 points on an 11-point scale) in worst pain in a 24-hour period in 59 of 62 patients (95%). Serious adverse events occurred in four patients (6.5%), including increase in tumor-cutaneous fistulae in three patients, likely caused by increased pressure from necrotic tissue in the ablation cavity, as well as a pathologic fracture of a large treated acetabular metastasis in one patient. A second American College of Radiology Imaging Network (ACRIN) supported, single-arm, prospective, multicenter trial included 55 patients treated with the Radionics Cool-tip electrode system

(Covidien, Boulder, CO).[23] Using a 100-point pain scale, this trial showed decreased pain at 1 month (16.9 point drop, 14.0 odds ratio) and at 3 months (14.2 point drop, 8.0 odds ratio). Serious toxicities occurred in three patients (5%), including solitary cases of local pain, neuropathic pain, and foot drop. Several smaller, single-center studies also confirm the efficacy of RFA of painful metastases with acceptably low complication rates.

Despite these results, RFA has some limitations. Intraprocedural monitoring remains challenging because the ablation zone cannot be visualized with CT or ultrasound, although it can be estimated with MR thermometry. In addition, although three RFA electrodes may be used simultaneously, overlapping ablations are needed to treat large lesions. Finally, significantly increased pain and narcotic requirements in the immediate postablation period are common following RFA compared to cryoablation.[40]

Cryoablation

A single-arm, single-institution, prospective trial of cryoablation in 14 patients with painful skeletal metastatic disease showed encouraging results.[41] Using an 11-point scale, mean score for worst pain in a 24-hour period decreased from 6.7 to 3.8 over 4 weeks. Pain relief was durable through the 24-week follow-up period in 80% of the patients who reported excellent pain relief at the immediate postablation time point. Furthermore, eight of eight patients who were prescribed opioid analgesics prior to the procedure reduced their doses following cryoablation. No serious complication was seen.

Focused Ultrasound

Recent studies have shown effective pain palliation for skeletal metastases treated with FUS. A prospective, multicenter trial of 36 FUS treatments of 32 bone metastases in 31 patients showed significant reduction in pain (≥2 points on the Visual Analog Scale)

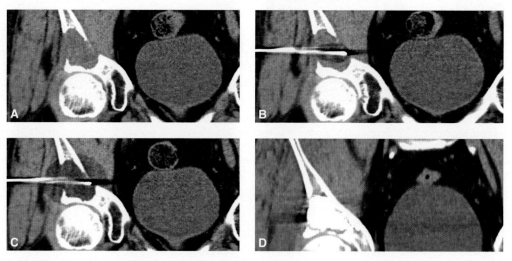

FIGURE 19.6 Combination cryoablation and cementoplasty. **A.** Coronal reformatted CT image shows a 4-cm right periacetabular renal cell carcinoma metastasis in a 71-year-old man. A low attenuation ice ball surrounds the tip of one of two cryoprobes early (**B**) and late (**C**) during treatment of the tumor. **D.** Cementoplasty was performed to add structural support to this important weight-bearing region.

in 18 (72%) of 25 patients with follow-up of at least 3 months.[42,43] Nine patients reported complete elimination of pain, six had no response, and one had increased pain. Mean visual analog scores (VAS) decreased from 5.9 to 1.8. No significant complication occurred, although two patients terminated treatment prematurely due to sonication-related pain. A separate single-center trial of 12 skeletal metastases treated in 11 patients showed decreased VAS pain scores from mean of 6.0 to 0.5 at 3 months.[44] All patients decreased analgesia use, including seven patients who ceased using analgesics altogether. No adverse events occurred.

Ethanol Ablation

In a series of 27 painful bone metastases treated in 25 patients with one to three doses of 3 to 25 mL of 95% ethanol, Gangi and colleagues[45] reported complete pain relief in 3 patients, 75% reduction in analgesics in 10 patients, 25% to 50% reduction in 5 patients, and minimal or no relief in 7 patients as measured 24 to 48 hours following the procedure. Pain relief was rapid and lasted 10 to 27 weeks in this series. One serious complication occurred, specifically weakness after treatment of a vertebral metastasis extending into the brachial plexus.

Cementoplasty

Cementoplasty may be performed as solitary treatment or in combination with ablative therapy in the treatment of painful metastatic disease involving bone.[46–54] Anselmetti and colleagues[46] treated 50 patients with painful extraspinal osteolytic metastases with cementoplasty, including 7 patients treated in combination with RFA for tumors greater than 7 cm.[46] Mean VAS for pain decreased from 9.1/10 to 2.1/10 within 3 months and remained

reduced during the 2-year follow-up period. Allowing for the small sample size, no significant difference in pain relief was identified between those treated with RFA and cementoplasty compared with cementoplasty alone. Munk and colleagues[51] treated 25 previously irradiated, painful metastatic lesions in 19 patients with combined RFA and cementoplasty. Mean pain scores decreased from 7.9/10 to 3.8/10 in 6 weeks with 18 patients reporting increased mobility. A small study of five patients by Hierholzer and colleagues[54] found cementoplasty alone to significantly reduce pain from skeletal metastases, including three patients with tumors in nonaxial skeletal locations.

▌ COMPLICATIONS AND MANAGEMENT

The complications of thermal ablation include injury to normal structures during needle device placement, thermal damage to adjacent structures, and insufficiency/instability with pathologic fracture of the treated bone (FIGURE 19.7). The risks during device placement are similar to other percutaneous needle insertion procedures, allowing for the relatively large caliber of bone access needles or drills. Thermal damage to the normal structures described previously may result in nerve dysfunction, bowel or bladder perforation, infection, skin burns, or tumor/fistula formation. These complications are minimized through measures to displace or insulate critical structures as well as intraprocedural monitoring with imaging and thermocouples.

▌ SUMMARY

Patients with painful metastases to bone and soft tissue have an unmet need for localized therapy when conventional therapies, including radiation therapy or surgery, fail or are clinically

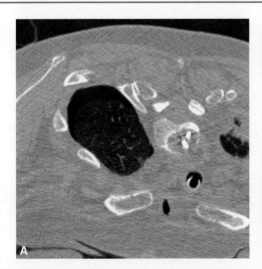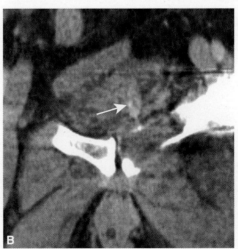

FIGURE 19.7 Complications following ablation and/or cementoplasty of musculoskeletal metastases. **A**. Small pneumothorax during cryoablation of T2 vertebral body metastasis from renal cell carcinoma in a 51-year-old man required small-caliber chest tube drainage overnight. **B**. Active contrast extravasation (*arrow*) into a moderate-sized prevesical hematoma immediately following cryoablation of a pubic body metastasis from papillary thyroid carcinoma in a 59-year-old man. The bleeding stopped, and the patient remained stable with no intervention. **C**. Femoral neuropathy in a 58-year-old woman resulted from cryoablation of a psoas muscle metastasis from melanoma during which the ice ball encompassed the femoral nerve (*arrow*). The patient recovered over a few months. **D**. Cement extravasation following combined ablation and cementoplasty of a painful periacetabular metastasis from renal cell carcinoma in a 71-year-old man. Fortunately, the cement remained asymptomatic within the gluteal musculature. *(continued)*

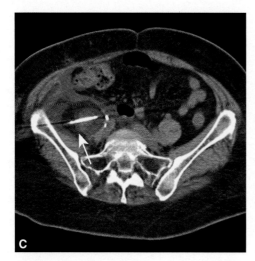 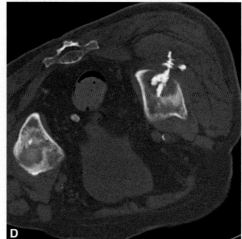

FIGURE 19.7 *(Continued)*

unsuitable. Percutaneous thermal and chemical ablative therapies can effectively treat these metastases in carefully selected patients. Choice of ablative technology depends on lesion size, visibility, and location. Cementoplasty is a useful adjunct in treating lesions at risk for pathologic fracture caused by axial loading and may even have direct analgesic effects when used alone. Several adjunctive techniques allow safe treatment of metastases even in relative proximity to normal critical structures.

REFERENCES

1. Rosenthal DI, Alexander A, Rosenberg AE, et al. Ablation of osteoid osteomas with a percutaneously placed electrode: a new procedure. *Radiology* 1992;183:29–33.
2. Rosenthal DI, Hornicek FJ, Wolfe MW, et al. Percutaneous radiofrequency coagulation of osteoid osteoma compared with operative treatment. *J Bone Joint Surg Am* 1998;80(6):815–821.
3. Nielsen OS, Munro AJ, Tannock IF. Bone metastases: pathophysiology and management policy. *J Clin Oncol* 1991;9:509–524.
4. Janjan N. Bone metastases: approaches to management. *Semin Oncol* 2001; 28(4 suppl 11):28–34.
5. Coleman RE. Skeletal complications of malignancy. *Cancer* 1997;80(suppl 8): 1588–1594.
6. Tubiana-Hulin M. Incidence, prevalence and distribution of bone metastases. *Bone* 1991;12(suppl 1):S9–S10.
7. Hara S. Opioids for metastatic bone pain. *Oncology* 2008;74(suppl 1):52–54.
8. Conte PF, Latreille J, Mauriac L, et al. Delay in progression of bone metastases in breast cancer patients treated with intravenous pamidronate: results from a multinational randomized controlled trial. The Aredia Multinational Cooperative Group. *J Clin Oncol* 1996;14(9):2552–2559.
9. Ernst DS, Brasher P, Hagen N, et al. A randomized, controlled trial of intravenous clodronate in patients with metastatic bone disease and pain. *J Pain Symptom Manage* 1997;13(6):319–326.
10. Robertson AG, Reed NS, Ralston SH. Effect of oral clodronate on metastatic bone pain: a double-blind, placebo-controlled study. *J Clin Oncol* 1995;13(9):2427–2430.
11. Wong R, Wiffen PJ. Bisphosphonates for the relief of pain secondary to bone metastases. *Cochrane Database Syst Rev* 2002;(2):CD002068.
12. Tong D, Gillick L, Hendrickson FR. The palliation of symptomatic osseous metastases: final results of the Study by the Radiation Therapy Oncology Group. *Cancer* 1982;50(5):893–899.
13. Cole DJ. A randomized trial of a single treatment versus conventional fractionation in the palliative radiotherapy of painful bone metastases. *Clin Oncol (R Coll Radiol)* 1989;1:59–62.
14. Gaze MN, Kelly CG, Kerr GR, et al. Pain relief and quality of life following radiotherapy for bone metastases: a randomised trial of two fractionation schedules. *Radiother Oncol* 1997;45(2):109–116.
15. Jeremic B, Shibamoto Y, Acimovic L, et al. A randomized trial of three single-dose radiation therapy regimens in the treatment of metastatic bone pain. *Int J Radiat Oncol Biol Phys* 1998;42(1):161–167.
16. Price P, Hoskin PJ, Easton D, et al. Prospective randomised trial of single and multifraction radiotherapy schedules in the treatment of painful bony metastases. *Radiother Oncol* 1986;6(4):247–255.
17. Spiegel D, Sands S, Koopman C. Pain and depression in patients with cancer. *Cancer* 1994;74:2570–2578.
18. Dupuy DE, Hong R, Oliver B, et al. Radiofrequency ablation of spinal tumors: temperature distribution in the spinal canal. *AJR Am J Roentgenol* 2000;175:1263–1266.
19. Bitsch RG, Rupp R, Bernd L, et al. Osteoid osteoma in an ex vivo animal model: temperature changes in surrounding soft tissue during CT-guided radiofrequency ablation. *Radiology* 2006;238(1):107–112.
20. Chang I, Mikityansky I, Wray-Cahen D, et al. Effects of perfusion on radiofrequency ablation in swine kidneys. *Radiology* 2004;231(2): 500–505.
21. Callstrom MR, Charboneau JW, Goetz MP, et al. Image-guided ablation of painful metastatic bone tumors: a new and effective approach to a difficult problem. *Skeletal Radiol* 2006;35(1):1–15.
22. Laeseke PF, Sampson LA, Winter TC III, et al. Use of dextrose 5% in water instead of saline to protect against inadvertent radiofrequency injuries. *AJR Am J Roentgenol* 2005;184(3):1026–1027.
23. Dupuy DE, Liu D, Hartfeil D, et al. Percutaneous radiofrequency ablation of painful osseous metastases: a multicenter American College of Radiology Imaging Network trial. *Cancer* 2010;116(4):989–997.
24. Weisbrod AJ, Atwell TD, Callstrom MR, et al. Percutaneous radiofrequency ablation with a multiple-electrode switching-generator system. *J Vasc Interv Radiol* 2007;18(12):1528–1532.
25. Brace CL. Radiofrequency and microwave ablation of the liver, lung, kidney, and bone: what are the differences? *Curr Probl Diagn Radiol* 2009;38(3):135–143.
26. Simon CJ, Dupuy DE, Mayo-Smith WW. Microwave ablation: principles and applications. *Radiographics* 2005;25:S69–S84.
27. Grieco CA, Simon CJ, Mayo-Smith WW, et al. Image-guided percutaneous thermal ablation for the palliative treatment of chest wall masses. *Am J Clin Oncol* 2007;30(4):361–367.
28. Gebauer B, Tunn PU. Thermal ablation in bone tumors. *Recent Results Cancer Res.* 2006;167:135–146.
29. Chosy SG, Nakada SY, Lee FT Jr, et al. Monitoring renal cryosurgery: predictors of tissue necrosis in swine. *J Urol* 1998;159(4):1370–1374.
30. Littrup PJ, Jallad B, Vorugu V, et al. Lethal isotherms of cryoablation in a phantom study: effects of heat load, probe size, and number. *J Vasc Interv Radiol* 2009;20(10):1343–1351.
31. Lee FT Jr, Chosy SG, Littrup PJ, et al. CT-monitored percutaneous cryoablation in a pig liver model: pilot study. *Radiology* 1999;211(3):687–692.

32. Sandison GA, Loye MP, Rewcastle JC, et al. X-ray CT monitoring of iceball growth and thermal distribution during cryosurgery. *Phys Med Biol* 1998;43(11):3309–3324.

33. Mercadante S, Fulfaro F. Management of painful bone metastases. *Curr Opin Oncol* 2007;19(4):308–314.

34. Ripamonti C, Fulfaro F. Malignant bone pain: pathophysiology and treatments. *Curr Rev Pain* 2000;4(3):187–196.

35. Stewart EA, Gostout B, Rabinovici J, et al. Sustained relief of leiomyoma symptoms by using focused ultrasound surgery. *Obstet Gynecol* 2007;110 (2, pt 1):279–287.

36. Jolesz FA. MRI-guided focused ultrasound surgery. *Annu Rev Med* 2009; 60:417–430.

37. Gangi A, Dietemann JL, Schultz A, et al. Interventional radiologic procedures with CT guidance in cancer pain management. *Radiographics* 1996;16(6): 1289–1304; discussion 1304–1306.

38. Sabharwal T, Katsanos K, Buy X, et al. Image-guided ablation therapy of bone tumors. *Semin Ultrasound CT MR* 2009;30(2):78–90.

39. Goetz MP, Callstrom MR, Charboneau JW, et al. Percutaneous image-guided radiofrequency ablation of painful metastases involving bone: a multicenter study. *J Clin Oncol* 2004;22(2):300–306.

40. Thacker PG, Callstrom MR, Curry TB, et al. Palliation of painful metastatic disease involving bone with imaging-guided treatment: comparison of patients' immediate response to radiofrequency ablation and cryoablation. *AJR Am J Roentgenol* 2011;197(2):510–515.

41. Callstrom MR, Atwell TD, Charboneau JW, et al. Painful metastases involving bone: percutaneous image-guided cryoablation—prospective trial interim analysis. *Radiology* 2006;241(2):572–580.

42. Catane R, Beck A, Inbar Y, et al. MR-guided focused ultrasound surgery (MRgFUS) for the palliation of pain in patients with bone metastases—preliminary clinical experience. *Ann Oncol* 2007;18(1):163–167.

43. Liberman B, Gianfelice D, Inbar Y, et al. Pain palliation in patients with bone metastases using MR-guided focused ultrasound surgery: a multicenter study. *Ann Surg Oncol* 2009;16(1):140–146.

44. Gianfelice D, Gupta C, Kucharczyk W, et al. Palliative treatment of painful bone metastases with MR imaging—guided focused ultrasound. *Radiology* 2008;249(1):355–363.

45. Gangi A, Kastler B, Klinkert A, et al. Injection of alcohol into bone metastases under CT guidance. *J Comput Assist Tomogr* 1994;18:932–935.

46. Anselmetti GC, Manca A, Ortega C, et al. Treatment of extraspinal painful bone metastases with percutaneous cementoplasty: a prospective study of 50 patients. *Cardiovasc Intervent Radiol* 2008;31(6):1165–1173.

47. Basile A, Giuliano G, Scuderi V, et al. Cementoplasty in the management of painful extraspinal bone metastases: our experience. *Radiol Med (Torino)* 2008;113(7):1018–1028.

48. Belfiore G, Tedeschi E, Ronza FM, et al. Radiofrequency ablation of bone metastases induces long-lasting palliation in patients with untreatable cancer. *Singapore Med J* 2008;49(7):565–570.

49. Hoffmann RT, Jakobs TF, Trumm C, et al. Radiofrequency ablation in combination with osteoplasty in the treatment of painful metastatic bone disease. *J Vasc Interv Radiol* 2008;19(3):419–425.

50. Masala S, Manenti G, Roselli M, et al. Percutaneous combined therapy for painful sternal metastases: a radiofrequency thermal ablation (RFTA) and cementoplasty protocol. *Anticancer Res* 2007;27(6C): 4259–4262.

51. Munk PL, Rashid F, Heran MK, et al. Combined cementoplasty and radiofrequency ablation in the treatment of painful neoplastic lesions of bone. *J Vasc Interv Radiol* 2009;20(7):903–911.

52. Schaefer O, Lohrmann C, Herling M, et al. Combined radiofrequency thermal ablation and percutaneous cementoplasty treatment of a pathologic fracture. *J Vasc Interv Radiol* 2002;13(10):1047–1050.

53. Toyota N, Naito A, Kakizawa H, et al. Radiofrequency ablation therapy combined with cementoplasty for painful bone metastases: initial experience. *Cardiovasc Intervent Radiol* 2005;28(5):578–583.

54. Hierholzer J, Anselmetti G, Fuchs H, et al. Percutaneous osteoplasty as a treatment for painful malignant bone lesions of the pelvis and femur. *J Vasc Interv Radiol* 2003;14(6):773–777.

CHAPTER
20

Vascular Access: Venous and Arterial Ports

THIERRY DE BAÈRE and ERIC DESRUENNES

▌ HEPATIC INTRA-ARTERIAL PORT

Indications

Because Hepatic Arterial Infusion Chemotherapy (HAIC) is a locoregional treatment, it is most often used in cases of liver cancer without extrahepatic disease, or in patients with predominant hepatic disease. Such treatment has been used mostly as salvage therapy after failure of standard of care systemic therapies. Additionally, this treatment is also being considered because response rates remain largely positive even in situations when the same drug that was used systemically and failed to elicit any kind of response is used intra-arterially. Due to the high response rate of (HAIC), recent reports and ongoing studies using it as first-line therapy exist. The goal of such therapies in first line, typically referred to as induction therapy, is to obtain the highest response as early as possible in the disease to downstage a nonsurgical candidate to a surgical candidate. Indeed, it has been demonstrated that the increase in response rate of colorectal liver metastases (CRLM) to treatment is correlated linearly with an increase in resection rate and, consequently, with an increase chance of cure.[1] Such induction chemotherapy targeting the liver specifically is obviously even more interesting in patients with liver-limited disease that demonstrated a steeper slope of the linear correlation between response and downstaging from nonoperable to surgical candidates. HAIC used in an adjuvant setting after liver resection has been demonstrated to increase survival.[2]

For primary tumors, namely, hepatocellular carcinoma (HCC), (HAIC) is less commonly used due to the high efficacy of transarterial chemoembolization (TACE). Indications may include patients who have not responded to TACE or patients considered noncandidates for TACE due to portal vein thrombosis or advanced liver insufficiency.[3,4]

Rationale

Colorectal cancer is the most common type of cancer in the Western world. The most common cause of death from this cancer is hepatic metastases. CRLM will occur in 50% to 75% of patients during the course of the disease. At the time of diagnosis 20% are present and 30% to 50% will appear later in the course of the disease. Even if surgery is the best treatment option for liver metastases, it will be possible in only 20% of patients. Furthermore, 70% of patients who underwent surgery will develop new CRLM. Consequently, it is not surprising that systemic chemotherapy is the dominant form of therapy for

patients with liver metastases. Despite a real improvement in the response rate of systemic chemotherapy from 10% to 20% with 5-fluorouracil (5-FU) alone to 16% to 40% with a combination of 5-FU and folinic acid, and even better results with the latter regimen including 5-FU-oxaliplatin and 5-FU-irinotecan, there are still patients who do not respond who could benefit from HAIC, especially because HAIC has been shown to provide excellent responses in patients who previously did not respond to systemic chemotherapy. The main advantage of HAIC is to deliver markedly higher drug concentrations in tumors, thus resulting in a significant increase in response rates because these tumors typically display a steep dose-response curve. The advantage of such an intra-arterial approach is directly related to the first-pass extraction of the drug by the liver and inversely proportional to the body clearance of the drug. Consequently, the choice of the drug is of utmost importance. Floxuridine (FUDR) has been extensively used for HAIC because it is extracted by the liver at more than 95% during the first pass with an increase of exposure of the liver 100 to 300 times higher than with a systemic perfusion. When compared to systemic administration, the estimated increase in liver exposure by HAIC is approximately 20-fold for THP adriamycin, 5- to 10-fold for 5-FU, 4- to 7-fold for cisplatin, 6- to 8-fold for mitomycin, 4-fold for oxaliplatinum, and only 2-fold for doxorubicin. All clinical trials using 5-FU or FUDR have demonstrated a better response rate with HAIC than with a systemic approach. Yet, despite such data, few trials have demonstrated a survival benefit.[5,6] Intra-arterial chemotherapy was more or less abandoned at the time systemic irinotecan and oxaliplatinum proved to give equivalent response rate to intra-arterial 5-FU. A recent French multicenter trial, which used these new drugs intra-arterially (HAIC)—100 mg/m^2 oxaliplatinum repeated every second week—reported an overall response rate of 64% (95% CI: 44% to 81%) in patients who had been heavily pretreated.[7] Additionally, new drug combinations including HAIC plus systemic oxaliplatinum and irinotecan allowed as high as 88% tumor response.[8]

Given the fact that such treatment required an injection every second week, it was clearly not convenient to have to repeat peripheral arterial access and hepatic artery catheterization for each subsequent course of HAIC. As a result, a permanent and easy access route had to be obtained using a port linked to an intra-arterial catheter. In the past, implantation of ports for HAIC required a laparotomy. Recently, a laparoscopic approach has been reported in a small series.[9] In the past, a percutaneous approach was needed to place a catheter in the hepatic artery for infusional chemotherapy with the need for repeated peripheral arterial access and hepatic artery catheterization for each subsequent planned course of HAIC.[10] Today, a minimally invasive technique using image guidance allows easy placement of catheter/port systems for HAIC without the need for open surgery or repeated catheterization.

Technique

Access Route

The catheter is usually introduced through the axillary or femoral artery.[11–13] The intercostal artery route was reported in only one series.[14] Since the first report by Arai et al.[15] in 1982, the axillary route has been much more described than the femoral route. It was preferred because it allowed easier insertion of the catheter in the hepatic artery due to the naturally descending orientation of the initial part of the celiac trunk, thus avoiding the sharp angulation encountered when using the femoral access. Disadvantages of the axillary route include a higher rate of overall complications, some severe, such as 3% of aneurysm formation requiring arterial stenting, axillary artery thrombosis,[13] and 0.5% to 1% of stroke.[10,12] Aneurysms are generally the result of the difficult access into and manual compression of the axillary artery itself. These issues have led some to access the axillary artery through a surgical cut-down of a small branch, typically the thoracic-acromial artery.[12] Strokes are caused by the formation of emboli as a result of the body of the catheter, which rests across the takeoff of the left vertebral artery. The retrieval or exchange of such catheters is risky enough that it is recommended that such a maneuver be performed through a femoral access.[12] Using the femoral artery for catheter port insertion is technically more challenging but can be achieved in most

patients due to improvement in endovascular material design. Furthermore, a femoral access will most often be needed for endovascular flow remodeling, even if the indwelling catheter is inserted through the axillary arterial route.

Arterial Flow Remodeling

Flow remodeling is nearly always needed before indwelling catheter insertion because HAIC requires whole liver perfusion with chemotherapy through a single artery (FIGURE 20.1). First, anatomically replaced hepatic arteries should be occluded proximally with stainless steel coils, a form of endovascular "surgical ligation," to allow perfusion of the whole liver through a single artery and a single catheter (FIGURE 20.2). Second, those arteries not providing flow to the liver (such as those feeding the stomach, duodenum, or pancreas) that arise between the perfusion hole in the catheter and the liver must be permanently occluded to avoid toxicity resulting from extrahepatic drug perfusion. In clinical practice, the gastroduodenal artery and the right gastric artery are the more frequent arteries requiring endovascular occlusion because it is rarely possible to place the perfusion hole of the catheter downstream of these two arteries. Occlusion of the right gastric artery is considered to be critically important to minimize toxicity from the infused drug to the liver as discussed in the results section. Such a procedure is also one of the most technically challenging aspects of any HAIC catheter insertion procedure. First, it is sometimes difficult to visualize the right gastric artery on hepatic artery angiography; second, it can arise from several places between the common hepatic artery and the distal part of the left branch of the hepatic artery. When its origin cannot be seen on the hepatic artery angiogram, it is often useful to perform selective angiography of the left gastric artery. In most instances, contrast will reflux into the right gastric artery, which

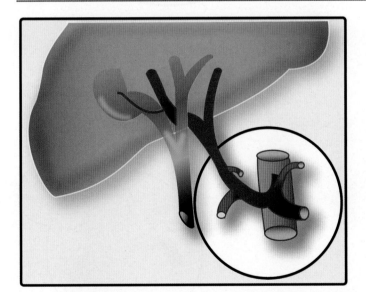 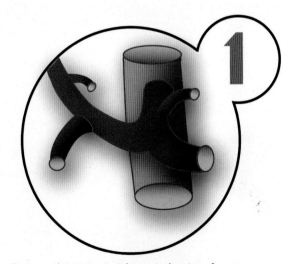

FIGURE 20.1 Schematic drawing of the three different techniques of catheter implantation. **A.** Schematic drawing of steps needed for implantation of an intra-arterial catheter with distal tip in the gastroduodenal artery. Normal anatomy (*1*), coil inserted in the right gastric artery (*2*), indwelling catheter in place with side hole in the distal part of the common hepatic artery (*3*), coils in the gastroduodenal artery around the catheter (*4*), flow of chemotherapy through the implanted catheter (*5*). **B.** Schematic drawing of a free-floating catheter implanted in the hepatic artery proper after coil occlusion of the gastroduodenal and right gastric arteries. **C.** Schematic drawing of a catheter implanted distally in a peripheral branch of the hepatic artery after coil occlusion of the gastroduodenal and right gastric arteries. *(continued)*

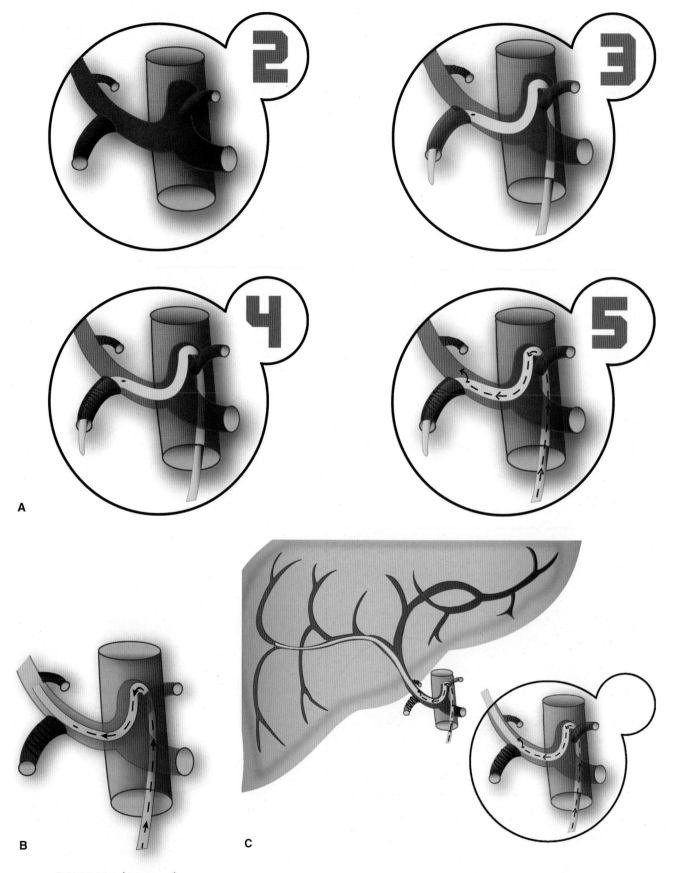

FIGURE 20.1 (Continued)

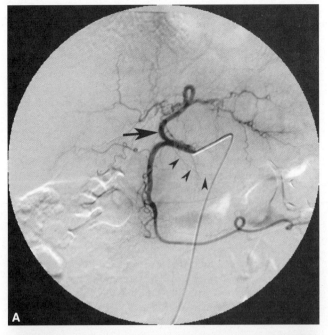

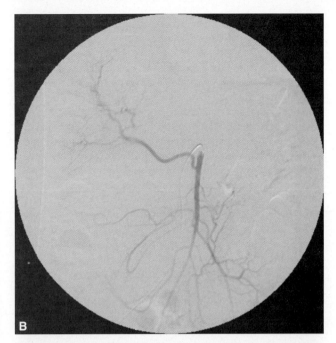

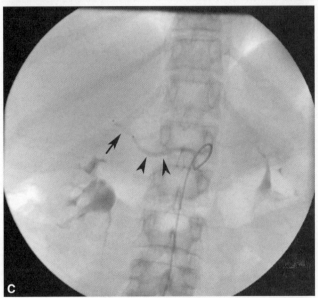

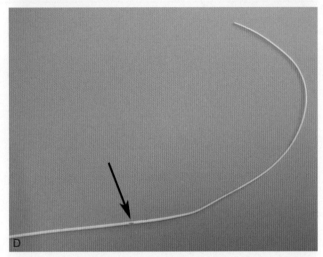

Study Date: 25/09/2003
Study Time: 00:00:00
MRN: 200308272EM

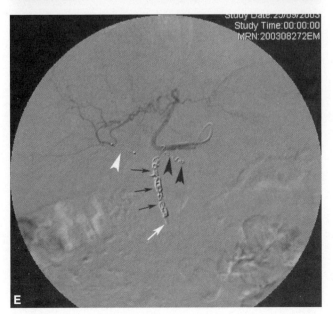

FIGURE 20.2 Angiograms during implantation of an intra-arterial hepatic catheter with distal tip in the gastroduodenal artery. **A.** Angiogram obtained after injection in the middle hepatic artery shows a branch for the left liver (*arrow*) and the gastroduodenal artery. The right gastric artery can be faintly seen (*arrowheads*). **B.** Angiogram obtained after injection in the superior mesenteric artery shows a replaced right hepatic artery. **C.** After occlusion of the replaced right hepatic artery with an endovascular occluding device (*arrow*) the contrast medium is seen in the proximal part of the replaced right hepatic artery (*arrowheads*). **D.** Distal part of the 5 French indwelling catheter demonstrating a side hole (*arrow*). By shortening the catheter, distance from the side hole to the tip will be customized for each patient according to the anatomy. Usually the side hole is between 7 and 10 cm from the tip. **E.** The right gastric artery has been occluded with coils (*black arrowheads*) and the tip of the indwelling catheter (*white arrow*) has been placed in the gastroduodenal artery, which has also been occluded with coils (*arrows*). Injection of contrast medium in the femoral-implanted port opacifies the complete hepatic vascularization and only hepatic arteries through side hole of the catheter. Note the collateral arterial pathways through the liver hilum that vascularized the right hepatic artery distal to the occluding device (*white arrowhead*).

223

will help determine the exact location of its origin (FIGURE 20.3). Sometimes, it may be possible to perform superselective catheterization of the left gastric followed by retrograde catheterization of the right gastric to embolize it with coils (FIGURE 20.3). The absence of reported toxicities affecting the gallbladder makes it unnecessary to systematically embolize the cystic artery or other vessels providing flow to the gallbladder. If a very large cystic artery exists, however, it probably should be embolized.

Catheter Positioning

The HAIC catheter can be left floating in the hepatic artery lumen but with significant risks of migration and thus is not favored. The catheter tip can be stabilized by inserting the catheter deeply into the gastroduodenal artery (or when impossible in a distal branch of the hepatic artery). A side hole can then be created in the indwelling catheter within the hepatic artery upstream of its first bifurcation. After the catheter tip is placed within the gastroduodenal artery, coils or/and cyanoacrylate glue are carefully delivered around it to both affix the catheter and occlude the gastroduodenal artery. In this manner, the distal portion of the catheter, between the side hole, which will be used for the delivery of the chemotherapy, and the end hole, will spontaneously occlude within a few minutes to a few hours after the procedure (clotting). Practically, after initial angiography and embolization of the replaced hepatic and right gastric arteries, the gastroduodenal artery is catheterized as distally as possible down to the distal right epiploic artery. Then, a stiff 0.018 guide wire is advanced, allowing over-the-wire insertion of the indwelling catheter. The most commonly used indwelling catheter is tapered from 5 French to 2.7 French (ST-305C, B. Braun Medical, Center Valley, PA). Then, occlusion of the gastroduodenal artery around the indwelling catheter can be obtained with a second catheter introduced through a contralateral femoral puncture. A different method consists of inserting another microcatheter through the indwelling catheter and its side hole before being advanced to the gastroduodenal artery,

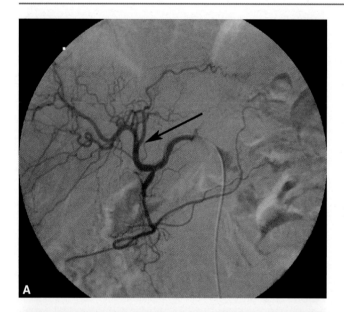

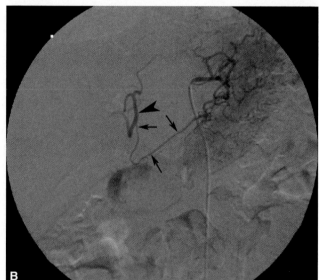

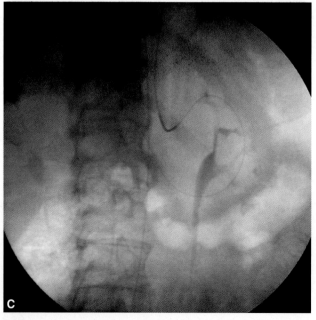

FIGURE 20.3 The reverse technique for occlusion of the right gastric artery. **A.** Angiogram obtained after injection in the middle hepatic artery shows a usual anatomy with right, left branches to the liver and gastroduodenal artery. The right gastric artery (*arrow*) can be faintly seen arising from the left branch of the hepatic artery. This branch could not be catheterized through the left hepatic artery. **B.** Injection in the left gastric artery demonstrates the entire artery from the small curvature of the stomach (*arrows*) and reverse opacification of the right gastric to the left branch of the hepatic artery (*arrowhead*). **C.** A 0.018 guide wire has been inserted from the celiac trunk through the left gastric then the right gastric to reach the left branch of the hepatic artery and will allow coiling of the origin of the right gastric.

where it can be embolized using 0.018 coils. Once secured and in place, the infusion catheter is tunneled and attached to a port placed either in the chest or pelvic wall depending on the access route (axillary or femoral). Catheter maintenance consists of flushing with heparin solution (500 international units/10 mL) after the completion of each chemotherapy course. Catheter positioning should be checked routinely angiographically or via injection of radionuclide (Tc-MAA) every two courses to ensure patency and adequate perfusion of the liver.

Contraindications

It is obvious that the hepatic artery must be patent to allow for HAIC. Therefore, occlusion or severe stenosis of the hepatic artery constitutes absolute contraindications. In the same manner retrograde flow caused by severe stenosis of the celiac trunk does not allow for port-catheter placement. The artery chosen for access (femoral or axillary) must be patent and free of any stenosis or severe atherosclerotic disease to avoid thrombosis after insertion of the indwelling catheter. Because a port will be implanted, to avoid local sepsis, the patient must not have signs of local or general infection before catheter placement. Patency of the portal system is not mandatory. One should be aware, however, that in cases where the portal vein patency is compromised, hepatic necrosis could occur if the indwelling catheter also induces hepatic artery thrombosis.

Results

Port/Catheter Placement

Technical success of catheter insertion is very high and close to 100% in most series.[12] In our experience, the initial success rate of the femoral approach at a first attempt was 92% (48/52), and the overall success of catheter implantation was 98% (51/52), including three patients with a second attempt, two through the femoral artery and one through the subclavian artery.[16] Catheter infusion hole migration is significantly higher for a free-floating catheter (50%) as compared to when the catheter tip is placed and secured within the gastroduodenal artery (14%, $p = .032$) or in a distal hepatic artery branch (0%, $p = .024$) without any significant difference between the latter two options.[16]

A large series of percutaneously implanted ports revealed patency rates of 91%, 81%, and 58% at 6 months, 1 year, and 2 years, respectively, allowing 3 to 102 courses of chemotherapy (mean = 35).[12] A study comparing percutaneously to surgically placed catheter/ports reported an overall incidence of device-related complication causing temporary or definitive suppression of HAIC in 42.7% of percutaneous placement and 7.1% of surgical ones.[17] But the rate of complication was the same provided that the 35.7% rate of tip migration in the percutaneous group was not taken into account. Indeed, such migration would have not occurred had the catheter tip been secured within the gastroduodenal artery instead of being left free floating within the hepatic artery. Hospital stay and analgesic requirement were both significantly lower in the percutaneous group (1.8 ± 0.7 days and 2 ± 0.9 doses, respectively) than in the surgical group (8.2 ± 22 days and 9.7 ± 3.2 doses, respectively). Interestingly gastroduodenal complications related to chemotherapy toxicity in the case of extrahepatic perfusion were lower in the percutaneous (7.1%) than in the surgical group (17.8%).[17] In a comparative study, the success rates of implantation were 97% (65/67) for percutaneous placement and 98% (58/59) for surgical implantation.[18] Among 107 patients, there was no significant

difference in the primary functionality of the catheter between percutaneous placement ($n = 4.80$ courses) and surgical implantation ($n = 4.82$ courses), but functionality after revision was significantly higher for percutaneous than for surgical placement (9.18 vs. 5.95 courses, $p = .004$). This increase in secondary functionality is due to the fact that revision of a percutaneously placed port is much easier than that of a surgically placed port. The rates of discontinuation of HAIC related to complications of the port-catheters were 21% for percutaneous and 34% for surgical implantation.[18]

The most serious (and feared) complication of HAIC is gastroduodenal ulceration caused by the delivery of chemotherapy to an extrahepatic feeder that remains patent beyond the location of the catheter tip. The main artery responsible for such complication is the right gastric artery. This is why it should be embolized if at all possible. Indeed, the rate of gastroduodenal ulcerations is significantly lower ($p = .019$) when the right gastric artery is embolized than when it is not, 5%.[16] The success rate of right gastric artery embolization significantly improved due to the learning curve of the interventional radiologists as it went from 17% for the first 23 patients to 66% ($n = 16$) for the latter 24 ($p = .0006$).[16] As mentioned earlier, embolization of the cystic artery is not mandatory because the reported incidence of cholecystitis is extremely low. In three series including a total of 153 patients who had percutaneously implanted catheter/ports, only 8 patients required a cholecystectomy.[11,13,17] Thrombosis of the hepatic artery is rare and seems to be related to the size of the indwelling catheter, specifically when a catheter larger than 5 French is placed in the hepatic artery. Infection of the actual port and femoral artery thrombosis are reported to be less than 2%.

Chemotherapy

In the past when the combination of 5-FU and folinic acid was the standard regimen for systemic chemotherapy in CRLM, clinical trials demonstrated a better response rate with HAIC than with systemic therapy using 5-FU or FUDR. Only a few trials managed to show a survival benefit with HAIC, however.[5,6] More recently, HAIC using oxaliplatin combined with systemic 5-FU demonstrated an overall response rate of 62% among the 39 assessable patients including 17, 12, and 12 patients who had failed to respond to prior systemic chemotherapy with FOLFIRI or FOLFOX, or both, respectively.[19] In that study, further R0 surgical resection and radiofrequency ablation were performed in 18 and 2% of initially unresectable CRLM, respectively. A triple combination consisting of HAIC with FUDR and systemic oxaliplatin and irinotecan yielded a 90% tumor response.[8] More recently, 49 patients with unresectable CRLM (53% previously treated with chemotherapy) were enrolled in a phase I protocol with HAIC consisting of 5-FU and dexamethasone plus systemic chemotherapy with oxaliplatin and irinotecan.[20] In that study, 73% of patients had more than five liver tumors, 98% had bilobar disease, and 86% had six segments or more involved. Ninety-two percent of the 49 patients had complete (8%) or partial (84%) response, and 47% (23/49) were able to undergo resection despite the fact that this group of patients had extensive disease. For chemotherapy naïve and previously treated patients, the median survival from the start of HAIC therapy was 50.8 and 35 months, respectively. In our center, 36 patients who presented with extensive unresectable CRLM (≥4 liver tumors in 86%; bilobar disease in 91%) were treated using HAIC with oxaliplatin (100 mg/m² in 2 hours) plus systemic

5-FU-leucovorin (LV, 400 mg/m^2 in 2 hours; FU, 400 mg/m^2 bolus then 2,400 mg/m^2 in 46 hours) and cetuximab (400 mg/m^2 then 250 mg/m^2/week, or 500 mg/m^2 every 2 weeks) as first-line treatment.[21] The overall response rate was 90% (95% CI, 70 to 99) and the disease control rate was 100% (95% CI, 84 to 100). Forty-eight percent of patients were downstaged to undergo R0 resection and/or radiofrequency ablation. After a median follow-up of 11 months, median progression-free survival (PFS) was 20 months (median overall survival [OS], not reached; 12- and 18-month OS, 100%).

It is clear from all the available data that HAIC is an effective therapy when used judiciously. With better drugs, it could be even more impactful and potentially lead to significant improvement in survival.

VENOUS CATHETER AND PORTS

Externalized central venous catheters and implantable central venous access ports system are widely used to improve venous access reliability in patients receiving prolonged courses of cytotoxic therapy, anti-infectious therapy, or long-term parenteral nutrition. Totally implantable venous access port systems have several advantages over externalized catheters, including reliable venous access, low incidence of infection, absence of maintenance, and fewer restrictions on activities, such as bathing and sports. Ports are usually inserted by surgeons, anesthesiologists, or radiologists.

Description

These devices consist of a port made of titanium or plastic with a self-sealing septum, accessible by percutaneous needle puncture, and a radiopaque catheter usually made in a well-tolerated long-term material, typically silicone or polyurethane. Most of the ports are single lumen, but there are others with dual lumen for separate administration of incompatible drugs. The connection between the catheter and the port can either be sealed during manufacturing or made at the time of placement. Most of the ports are now validated for high-pressure injection of contrast media with a maximum pressure of 300 psi, which correspond to flow rates of up to 5 mL/second.[22]

Indications

The main indications for port insertion are cytotoxic chemotherapy for solid tumors and long-term antibiotic therapy (e.g., cystic fibrosis), whereas externalized catheters are more generally used in hematologic diseases and for long-term parenteral nutrition. Blood sampling is possible with ports provided that large flushing is performed after the blood draw.

Preoperative Assessment

Platelet count should be more than 50,000/mm^3, white cells more than 1,000, and international normalized ratio (INR) less than 1.5. A preoperative chest radiograph is not mandatory but useful in case of pulmonary disease, lymphoma, and ear-nose-throat (ENT) tumors. In such cases and when a mediastinal invasion, compression, or thrombosis is suspected, a chest computed tomography (CT) scan is necessary to verify the absence of superior vena cava occlusion or partial thrombosis.

Vitamin K antagonists should be replaced by low molecular weight heparin (LMWH). A reduced dose of LMWH should be administered the day before implantation and none the morning of the implantation. When possible, antiplatelet therapy should be discontinued 5 days before implantation except in patients who had recent coronary or arterial stenting. There is no need to stop low-dose aspirin as well as nonsteroid anti-inflammatory drugs.

Access Route

Ultrasound imaging and guidance are part of the standard technique for central venous access in our institution (2,000 indwelling catheters implanted each year). The internal jugular vein accounts for 50% of the central venous access, the brachio-cephalic vein via a supraclavicular approach for 35%, the axillary or subclavian vein via an infraclavicular approach for 10%, and the femoral vein for 5%.

The percutaneous subclavian access was the first method described. Access to the subclavian vein is usually easy and rapid because of reliable anatomic landmarks, especially bony landmarks. It can be approached by an infra- or supraclavicular route. When anatomic landmarks are used, there is a low incidence of pneumothorax (1% to 5%) and a risk of compression between the clavicle and first rib (pinch-off syndrome) concerning long-term catheters inserted via the infraclavicular route. Pinch-off syndrome occurs in 1% of cases and may lead to the fracture of the catheter (FIGURE 20.4) and the embolization of a fragment into the cardiac chambers or the pulmonary

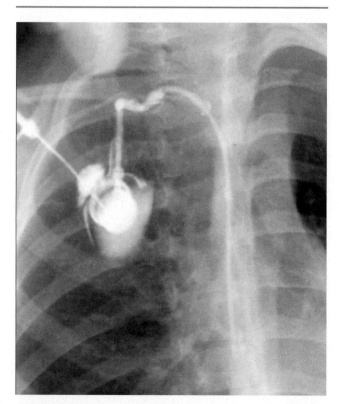

FIGURE 20.4 Fracture of catheter and extravasation of contrast in the costoclavicular space of an 18-month-old infant (pinch-off syndrome).

arteries.[23,24] For these reasons subclavian infraclavicular access using an anatomic landmark is not the best access for long-term central venous catheters and should be replaced by ultrasound-guided infraclavicular access of the axillary/subclavian vein (FIGURE 20.5) or by ultrasound-guided supraclavicular access of the brachiocephalic vein (FIGURE 20.6).

Percutanous access of the internal jugular vein has recently gained popularity because of the absence of pneumothorax and pinch-off syndrome. The relatively high rate of inadvertent carotid puncture becomes nearly irrelevant (incidence close to zero) when ultrasound guidance is used.[25,26] The right internal jugular vein is in direct line with the superior vena cava and the right atrium and is therefore ideally suited for long-term access. On the other hand, the cosmetic aspect is not always perfect because the catheter is sometimes clearly visible around the neck area. For cosmetic reasons, the best approach for jugular vein catheterization is probably a low and posterior approach behind the clavicular head of the sternocleidomastoid muscle (FIGURE 20.7).

The external jugular vein is not used very often because its junction with the brachiocephalic trunk is sometimes acute and will not always allow the passage of the catheter.

The cut-down approach of the cephalic vein is often used by surgeons. Here, a cosmetic advantage is evident, particularly in women, but it also has some disadvantages, such as 5% to 10% failures because the vein is either too small or tortuous to be successfully catheterized,[27] thereby causing more venous thromboses than when the other methods are used.

The brachial and forearm veins may also be used for central venous access, either via a cut-down or through a percutaneous vein puncture guided by venography or ultrasound.[28]

Percutaneous access of the femoral vein is specifically indicated when the following conditions are present: mediastinal compression or invasion of the superior vena cava in lung cancer or lymphoma, superior vena cava thrombosis, impossibility to puncture neck or chest veins due to local tumor invasion, infection, and postradiation therapy stenosis. Provided that

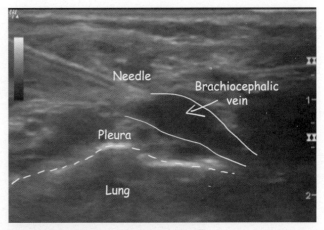

FIGURE 20.6 Ultrasound-guided supraclavicular access of the brachiocephalic vein in a 3-year-old infant.

the technique is well applied and the tip is close to the right atrium, infectious and thrombotic complications are comparable to those seen after subclavian or jugular access.[29,30] Because of the frequency of lung cancer and the mediastinal location of lymphoma, femoral access should represent around 5% of all implanted ports (FIGURE 20.8).

Catheter Tip Location

All recent studies have shown that the position of the tip of central venous devices is a significant factor for predicting catheter dysfunction and catheter-related venous thrombosis. When the tip is located in the last third of the superior vena cava or the right atrium, the rate of venous thrombosis is between 3% and 5%, compared with 42% and 46% when the tip lies in the proximal third of the vena cava or in the brachiocephalic vein.[31,32] Recommendations from a French multidisciplinary working group in 2008 are that the optimal tip position for central venous catheters and ports is the distal third of the superior vena cava or the proximal right atrium.[33] This last position does not conform to manufacturers and Food and Drug Administration guidelines, although no complications have been observed with long-term Silastic central venous lines where the tip rests in the right atrium.

Update on Vein Thrombosis Prophylaxis and Treatment

Symptomatic deep venous thrombosis of the upper limbs develops in 2.4% of patients when ultrasound guidance is used for central venous access.[34] The presence of mediastinal lymph nodes has been shown to be a risk factor for catheter-related venous thrombosis,[35] and one should carefully examine the chest CT scan before implanting a central venous device in patients suffering from lung cancer, lymphoma, and other diseases, such as advanced ENT or thyroid cancer. Patients with catheters that are too short and who suffer from gastrointestinal cancers or extended metastatic diseases have a higher incidence and risk of deep venous thrombosis as well.

For patients with catheter-related deep venous thrombosis and cancer, treatment with LMWH for at least 3 to 6 months

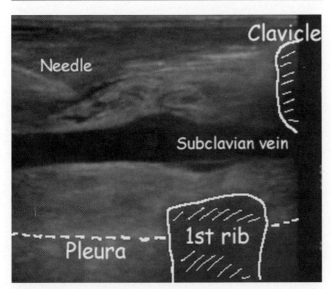

FIGURE 20.5 Ultrasound-guided infraclavicular access of the subclavian vein with the needle "in plane."

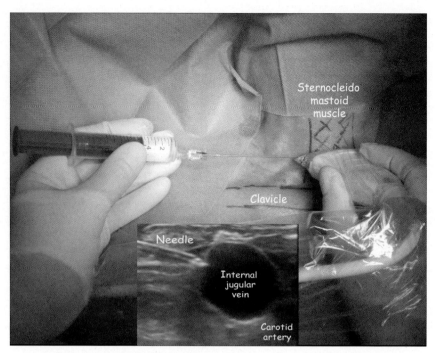

FIGURE 20.7 Ultrasound-guided posterior access of the internal jugular vein.

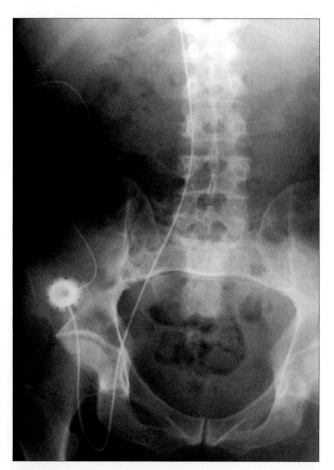

FIGURE 20.8 Femoral long-term access; the port is implanted on the abdominal wall in front of the iliac bone.

is recommended.[33,36] If the tip of the catheter is in the correct location and the port is functioning well, it is possible to keep it in place and to avoid retrieving it.

Recent studies failed to show any benefit from prophylaxis with warfarin or LMWH compared to placebo for the prevention of catheter-related thrombosis.[37,38] Based on these findings the American College of Chest Physicians Conference on Antithrombotic and Thrombolytic Therapy and the French working group both suggested that the risk of clinically important catheter-related venous thrombosis may be too low to warrant routine prophylaxis and have recommended that clinicians do not routinely use prophylaxis in cancer patients.[33,39]

Catheter-Related Infection

Minor temporary local infection should be treated with local antiseptics and possibly oral antibiotics. Nevertheless, the port should be explanted in case of local swelling or purulent drainage.

Systemic infection is defined as fever, chills, and a positive blood culture. Methods of diagnosing catheter-related infection without removing the catheter consist of comparison of paired blood cultures drawn simultaneously via the port and from a peripheral venous site. Quantitative blood cultures or measurement of differential time to germ growth are used for this purpose.[40] After a port infection has been proved, the port should be removed in the presence of severe neutropenia or septic shock, or *Staphylococcus aureus, Pseudomonas* and *Stenotrophomonas,* and *Candida* species are isolated from blood culture. Parenteral then oral antibiotic therapy should be prescribed for at least 10 days in case of bacteremia. Antibiotic-lock technique without removing the port is a possible alternative when *Staphylococcus epidermidis, Escherichia coli,* or other digestive microorganisms are isolated.[41] Local antibiotic locks consist of 2 mL of highly concentrated amikacin or vancomycin (15 mg/mL) that are changed every day for at least 10 days, after which blood cultures should be performed a few days after the end of the treatment to confirm the success or the failure of this treatment.

▌REFERENCES

1. Folprecht G, Grothey A, Alberts S, et al. Neoadjuvant treatment of unresectable colorectal liver metastases: correlation between tumour response and resection rates. *Ann Oncol* 2005;16:1311–1319.
2. Kemeny N, Huang Y, Cohen A, et al. Hepatic arterial infusion of chemotherapy after resection of hepatic metastases from colorectal cancer. *N Engl J Med* 1999;341:2039–2048.
3. Seki H, Kimura M, Yoshimura N, et al. Hepatic arterial infusion chemotherapy using percutaneous catheter placement with an implantable port: assessment of factors affecting patency of the hepatic artery. *Clin Radiol* 1999;54:221–227.
4. Hwang JY, Jang BK, Kwon KM, et al. Efficacy of hepatic arterial infusion therapy for advanced hepatocellular carcinoma using 5-fluorouracil, epirubicin and mitomycin-C [in Korean]. *Korean J Gastroenterol* 2005;45:118–124.
5. Meta-Analysis Group in Cancer. Reappraisal of hepatic arterial infusion in the treatment of nonresectable liver metastases from colorectal cancer. *J Natl Cancer Inst* 1996:252–258.
6. Kemeny NE, Niedzwiecki D, Hollis DR, et al. Hepatic arterial infusion versus systemic therapy for hepatic metastases from colorectal cancer: a randomized trial of efficacy, quality of life, and molecular markers (CALGB 9481). *J Clin Oncol* 2006;24:1395–1403.
7. Boige V, Lacombe S, de Baere T. Hepatic arterial infusion of oxaliplatin combined with 5FU and folinic acid in non resectable liver metastasis of colorectal cancer: a promising option for failures to systemic chemotherapy. *J Clin Oncol* 2003;22:291.
8. Kemeny N, Jarnagin W, Paty P, et al. Phase I trial of systemic oxaliplatin combination chemotherapy with hepatic arterial infusion in patients with unresectable liver metastases from colorectal cancer. *J Clin Oncol* 2005;23:4888–4896.
9. Franklin ME Jr, Gonzalez JJ Jr. Laparoscopic placement of hepatic artery catheter for regional chemotherapy infusion: technique, benefits, and complications. *Surg Laparosc Endosc Percutan Tech.* 2002 Dec;12(6):398–407.
10. Habbe TG, McCowan TC, Goertzen TC, et al. Complications and technical limitations of hepatic arterial infusion catheter placement for chemotherapy. *J Vasc Interv Radiol* 1998;9:233–239.
11. Herrmann KA, Waggershauser T, Sittek H, et al. Liver intraarterial chemotherapy: use of the femoral artery for percutaneous implantation of catheter-port systems. *Radiology* 2000;215:294–299.
12. Tanaka T, Arai Y, Inaba Y, et al. Radiologic placement of side-hole catheter with tip fixation for hepatic arterial infusion chemotherapy. *J Vasc Interv Radiol* 2003;14:63–68.
13. Zanon C, Grosso M, Clara R, et al. Combined regional and systemic chemotherapy by a mini-invasive approach for the treatment of colorectal liver metastases. *Am J Clin Oncol* 2001;24:354–359.
14. Castaing D, Azoulay D, Fecteau A, et al. Implantable hepatic arterial infusion device: placement without laparotomy, via an intercostal artery. *J Am Coll Surg* 1998;187:565–568.
15. Arai Y, Kamimura N, Suyama K. A method to retain subcutaneously the catheter end connected to a new silicone reservoir in intraarterial infusion chemotherapy. *Gan To Kagaku Ryoho* 1982; 9:1838–43.
16. Deschamps F, Rao P, Teriitehau C, et al. Percutaneous femoral implantation of an arterial port catheter for intraarterial chemotherapy: feasibility and predictive factors of long-term functionality. *J Vasc Interv Radiol* 2010;21:1681–1688.
17. Aldrighetti L, Arru M, Angeli E, et al. Percutaneous vs. surgical placement of hepatic artery indwelling catheters for regional chemotherapy. *Hepatogastroenterology* 2002;49:513–517.
18. Deschamps F, Elias D, Goere D, et al. Intra-arterial hepatic chemotherapy: a comparison of percutaneous versus surgical implantation of port-catheters. *Cardiovasc Intervent Radiol* 2010;9:9.
19. Boige V, Malka D, Elias D, et al. Hepatic arterial infusion of oxaliplatin and intravenous LV5FU2 in unresectable liver metastases from colorectal cancer after systemic chemotherapy failure. *Ann Surg Oncol* 2008;15:219–226.
20. Kemeny NE, Melendez FD, Capanu M, et al. Conversion to resectability using hepatic artery infusion plus systemic chemotherapy for the treatment of unresectable liver metastases from colorectal carcinoma. *J Clin Oncol* 2009;27:3465–3471.
21. Malka D, Paris E, Caramella C, et al. Combined hepatic oxaliplatin, intravenous LV5FU2 and erbitux [abstract]. *Pro Am Soc Clin Oncol* 2010:abstract 3558.
22. Wieners G, Redlich U, Dudeck O, et al. First experiences with intravenous port systems authorized for high pressure injection of contrast agent in multiphasic computed tomography [in German]. *Rofo* 2009;181:664–668.
23. Aitken DR, Minton JP. The "pinch-off sign": a warning of impending problems with permanent subclavian catheters. *Am J Surg* 1984;148:633–636.
24. Ouaknine-Orlando B, Desruennes E, Cosset MF, et al. The pinch-off syndrome: main cause of catheter embolism [in French]. *Ann Fr Anesth Reanim* 1999;18:949–955.
25. Leonard KR, Hinders MK. Guided wave helical ultrasonic tomography of pipes. *J Acoust Soc Am* 2003;114:767–774.
26. Karakitsos D, Labropoulos N, De Groot E, et al. Real-time ultrasound-guided catheterisation of the internal jugular vein: a prospective comparison with the landmark technique in critical care patients. *Crit Care* 2006;10:R162.
27. Biffi R, Orsi F, Pozzi S, et al. Best choice of central venous insertion site for the prevention of catheter-related complications in adult patients who need cancer therapy: a randomized trial. *Ann Oncol* 2009;20:935–940.
28. Marcy PY, Magne N, Castadot P, et al. Radiological and surgical placement of port devices: a 4-year institutional analysis of procedure performance, quality of life and cost in breast cancer patients. *Breast Cancer Res Treat* 2005;92:61–67.
29. Bertoglio S, Disomma C, Meszaros P, et al. Long-term femoral vein central venous access in cancer patients. *Eur J Surg Oncol* 1996;22:162–165.
30. Wolosker N, Yazbek G, Munia MA, et al. Totally implantable femoral vein catheters in cancer patients. *Eur J Surg Oncol* 2004;30:771–775.
31. Luciani A, Clement O, Halimi P, et al. Catheter-related upper extremity deep venous thrombosis in cancer patients: a prospective study based on Doppler US. *Radiology* 2001;220:655–660.
32. Cadman A, Lawrance JA, Fitzsimmons L, et al. To clot or not to clot? That is the question in central venous catheters. *Clin Radiol* 2004;59:349–355.
33. Debourdeau P, Kassab Chahmi D, Le Gal G, et al. 2008 SOR guidelines for the prevention and treatment of thrombosis associated with central venous catheters in patients with cancer: report from the working group. *Ann Oncol* 2009;20:1459–1471.
34. Cavanna L, Civardi G, Vallisa D, et al. Ultrasound-guided central venous catheterization in cancer patients improves the success rate of cannulation and reduces mechanical complications: a prospective observational study of 1,978 consecutive catheterizations. *World J Surg Oncol* 2010;8:91.
35. Labourey JL, Lacroix P, Genet D, et al. Thrombotic complications of implanted central venous access devices: prospective evaluation. *Bull Cancer* 2004;91:431–436.
36. Buller HR, Agnelli G, Hull RD, et al. Antithrombotic therapy for venous thromboembolic disease: the Seventh ACCP Conference on Antithrombotic and Thrombolytic Therapy. *Chest* 2004;126:401S–428S.
37. Couban S, Goodyear M, Burnell M, et al. Randomized placebo-controlled study of low-dose warfarin for the prevention of central venous catheter-associated thrombosis in patients with cancer. *J Clin Oncol* 2005;23(18):4063–4069.
38. Karthaus M, Kretzschmar A, Kroning H, et al. Dalteparin for prevention of catheter-related complications in cancer patients with central venous catheters: final results of a double-blind, placebo-controlled phase III trial. *Ann Oncol* 2006;17:289–296.
39. Geerts WH, Bergqvist D, Pineo GF, et al. Prevention of venous thromboembolism: American College of Chest Physicians Evidence-Based Clinical Practice Guidelines (8th Edition). *Chest* 2008;133:381S–453S.
40. Blot F, Nitenberg G, Chachaty E, et al. Diagnosis of catheter-related bacteraemia: a prospective comparison of the time to positivity of hub-blood versus peripheral-blood cultures. *Lancet* 1999;354:1071–1077.
41. Messing B, Peitra-Cohen S, Debure A, et al. Antibiotic-lock technique: a new approach to optimal therapy for catheter-related sepsis in home-parenteral nutrition patients. *JPEN J Parenter Enteral Nutr* 1988;12:185–189.

Palliative Care and Symptom Management

SEAN M. MARKS, DREW A. ROSIELLE, and WILLIAM S. RILLING

INTRODUCTION

Advanced cancers are devastating and debilitating diseases that lead to worsening symptom burden as the cancer progresses. Through the natural course of illness, patients experience functional impairments that damage their independence and lead to significant emotional and psychological distress.[1] As cancer progresses,[2] disease-modifying or even life-prolonging interventions become less available. Instead, the scope of the medical care becomes increasingly focused on symptom relief, psychosocial and family support, and aligning patients' treatments with realistic care goals rooted in an understanding of their expected course.

Palliative care describes any form of medical care or treatment that concentrates on reducing the severity of disease symptoms, rather than striving to halt, delay, or reverse progression of the disease itself or provide a cure. Optimally, palliative care utilizes an interdisciplinary team of physicians, nurses, chaplains, psychologists, social workers, and speech, physical, and occupational therapists to provide symptom relief and maximize quality of life. It has been defined by the World Health Organization as care *[T]hat improves the quality of life of patients and their families facing the problems associated with life-threatening illness, through the prevention and relief of suffering by means of early identification and impeccable assessment and treatment of pain and other problems, physical, psychosocial and spiritual.*[3]

Palliative care should be provided to patients and their families throughout the course of any advanced illness, even while patients are receiving disease-modifying treatments. Much of the care patients with cancer receive can be described as palliative, and many patients do not receive specialist palliative care services, either because specialist palliative care services are unavailable or patients' palliative care needs are straight-forward. Instead, patients often receive palliative care from their cancer providers or primary care physicians. Therefore, it is imperative that nonspecialist clinicians are competent in managing common cancer-related symptoms.

SYMPTOM PREVALENCE IN PATIENTS WITH ADVANCED CANCER

Acknowledging a full spectrum of individual variability,[3] investigators from the National Hospice Study (NHS) described a pathway of symptom progression that occurs for most patients with advanced cancer at the end stage of disease.[4] Termed the *terminal cancer syndrome*, this constellation of signs and symptoms was found in patients independent of age, sex, histologic type, and metastatic pattern of disease and is identified by a moribund functional status, organ failure, cachexia, leading to death.[4] Even with advancements in cancer therapeutics, most advanced cancer patients experience an inevitable and steep decline in function in the last 3 months of life in which they can become progressively disabled and dependent on others and have escalating and distressing symptoms. It is imperative that cancer providers recognize these signs and symptoms of a short prognosis and factor in the patient's prognosis in their medical care plan. Evidence suggests that cancer patients' desire for prognostic information approaches nearly 100% as prognosis decreases.[5] Not receiving a prognosis is a common reason families say they are dissatisfied with end-of-life care because prognostic information can allow patients and families to set goals, priorities, and realistic expectations for care. Advanced cancer patients who had early discussions about end-of-life care with their physicians were more likely to receive less ineffectual care at the end of life, had longer lengths of stay in hospice, had better quality of life, and were no more depressed or anxious than patients who did not have such discussions.[6]

Unfortunately, despite relatively well-established prognostic guidelines for cancer patients, physicians are generally poor prognosticators. Most studies have shown that physicians often overestimate the prognosis of terminally ill cancer patients by a factor of three to five.[7,8] Many reasons have been put forward as to why physicians overestimate prognosis, but perhaps the most important factor is acknowledging this practice pattern. Experts recommend that clinicians ask him or herself *"Would I be surprised if the patient died within a year?"* Answering no should compel clinicians to consider the patient's immediate and long-term future and care plan. It also advised that clinicians offer the chance to share this prognostic information with patients and their families.

SYMPTOM PREVALENCE IN ADVANCED CANCER AT EARLIER STAGES OF ILLNESS

Although patients with cancer at the very end of life may have a more uniform constellation of symptoms, evidence suggests that at earlier stages of the disease a patient's symptom profile can be more varied. Table 21.1[10,11] lists the prevalence of common symptoms among patients with advanced cancer.

Although much of the clinical practice of symptom management for cancer patients is based more on clinical experience than on well-controlled clinical trials, experience has shown that most cancer-related symptoms can be effectively treated such that patients dying from cancer can maintain an acceptable quality of life.

When managing a patient's symptom, it is best to consider a wide differential diagnosis and pursue a problem-focused

Table 21.1	
Prevalence of Common Symptoms among Patients with Advanced Cancer[9,10]	
Fatigue	51–100%
Psychological distress	50%
Pain	33–57%
Anorexia	36–70%
Weakness	51%
Nausea	21–45%
Dyspnea	31–39%
Constipation	23–90%
Insomnia	9%
Weight loss	39%
Xerostomia	42%
Cough	37%
Taste alterations	37%

evaluation. New or progressive symptoms in the advanced cancer patient most often occur as a result of the cancer. Therefore, when assessing a cancer-related symptom many palliative care experts suggest beginning with the medical evaluation of the cancer.

The following sections discuss the most common and distressing symptoms cancer patients face and describe general management principles.

▌ PAIN

Pain is a complex neurocognitive experience that occurs within the context of a patient's life.[12] Pain can be influenced by the meaning of the pain to the patient, its duration, its impact on a patient's vocational, familial, and social life,[13] as well as a patient's attitudes, expectations, and beliefs.[14] Because the intensity of a patient's pain is subjective, current guidelines state that pain must be assessed and documented regularly through standardized pain assessment tools. Several pain rating scales have been validated in cancer-related pain including the visual analogue scale,[15] the numerical rating scale,[16] and the verbal rating scale.[17] It is recommended that clinicians document a patient's self-report of pain using one of these validated scales consistently to guide their management decisions (FIGURE 21.1).

Although at least three quarters of end-stage cancer patients will experience significant pain,[18] the vast majority of patients' pain can be effectively treated with appropriate management.[19] Among the most frequently cited reason for poorly controlled pain is knowledge deficits among health care providers.[20] Common knowledge deficits surrounding opioids include risk of addiction, routes of administration, calculation of equianalgesic doses, titration of doses, and management of side effects.[21] It is also essential for clinicians to understand when to initiate opioids for cancer-related pain.

For the initial management of mild to moderate cancer-related pain, providers should provide prompt oral administration of nonopioid pain relievers such as nonsteroidal anti-inflammatory drugs (NSAIDs), acetaminophen, and weak-opioids such as tramadol.[22] For moderate to severe cancer-related pain, however, all nonopioid medications have dose-limiting side effects and ceiling effects. Because opioids do not have ceiling effects and are proven to be safe in cancer-related pain, they are the drugs of choice for moderate to severe pain. If safe, nonopioids, such

---

Visual analogue scale

No pain _____ Worst imaginable pain

Numerical rating scale

No pain   Worst imaginable pain

0   1   2   3   4   5   6   7   8   9   10

Verbal rating scale

  0   No pain

  1   Mild pain

  2   Moderate pain

  3   Severe pain

FIGURE 21.1 Pain scales.

Table 21.2

Opioid Equianalgesic Table

Drug	Parenteral	PO	Parenteral: PO ratio	Duration of action (hr)
Morphine IR	10	30	1:3	3–4
Hydromorphone (Dilaudid)	1.5	7.5	1:5	3–4
Oxycodone IR	N/A in U.S.	20–30	—	3–4
Codeine	130	200	1:1.5	3–4
Hydrocodone	—	30	—	3–4
Fentanyl	0.1	—	—	1–3

Data from Cherny NI. Opioid analgesics: comparative features and prescribing guidelines. Drugs 1996; 51(5): 713–737; McCaffery, M., & Pasero, C. Pain: Clinical Manual, 2nd ed. St. Louis: Mosby. 1999.

as NSAIDs, should be used in conjunction with opioids even in patients with moderate to severe pain.

Two of the key concepts in opioid pharmacology for clinicians to understand are potency and equianalegesia. Potency refers to the intensity of analgesic effect for a given dose and is determined by opioid binding affinity to opioid receptors in the brain and spinal cord. Although different opioids may have different potencies, potency is not the same as the efficacy of the drug. Because pure opioid agonist medications have the same mechanism of action and do not have a ceiling effect, they can be dosed to be equally efficacious in treating moderate to severe pain.[23] This concept of equal effectiveness is called equianalgesia. Evidence supports this pharmacodynamic concept because no opioid is proven to more effective than another. Furthermore, the general side effect profile among pure opioid agonists is also quite similar with the exception of meperidine, codeine, and propoxyphene, which are known to be associated with more neuroexcitatory side effects and delirium, especially in patients with renal insufficiency.[24]

Therefore, in determining which opioid to initiate pain management, it is important to consider cost of medication, available routes, familiarity, and formulation. Opioids are formulated into two different classes—short acting and long acting. In general, short-acting formulations are used for "breakthrough" or as-needed pain flares. Typically, short-acting oral opioids have an onset of analgesia in 30 minutes, with peak effect at 60 to 90 minutes, and provide 3 to 4 hours of analgesia. Therefore, they

are often used in initiation of therapy in opioid naïve patients, because their short half life may make them less risky if the patient has a dose-limiting side effect such as somnolence. Long-acting formulations of opioids are typically manufactured to provide a steady level of pain relief for 8 to 72 hours. It is recommended that patients with continuous moderate to severe pain be managed with a combination of long-acting and short-acting opioids. Tables 21.2 and 21.3 list commonly available short- and long-acting opioids along with their equianalgesic dose. Pain experts have expressed concern regarding the accuracy and consistency of published opioid dose conversion tables[24a] and their effect on patient safety[24b] considering the considerable intra-individual variability in opioid pharmacoly. Therefore, equianalgesic tables provided in tables 21.2 and 21.3 should only serve as a general guideline for clinicians and should not be used as a substitute for clinical judgment in the application to any individual patient situation. For most patients, morphine is considered the first opioid of choice because of its low cost and familiarity of use. It should be used cautiously, however, in patients with renal failure.

Another key component to cancer pain management is frequent reassessment of pain after dose initiation or dose changes. When titrating opioids, it is best to increase doses by percentages and not by dose values. Experts recommend that opioids be increased 25% to 50% for ongoing mild to moderate pain and 50% to 100% for moderate to severe pain.

"Adjuvants" are a heterogeneous group of additional medications that can be added to a patient's pain management regimen

Table 21.3

Commonly Available Long-Acting Opioids

Long-acting opioid	Strengths available	Duration (hr)
Morphine ER aka MS Contin[a]	15, 30, 60, 100, 200 mg	8–12
Oxycodone ER aka Oxycontin[a]	10, 20, 40, 80 mg	8–12
Fentanyl patch	12, 25, 50, 75, 100 mcg/hr	48–72
Kadian (morphine)[b]	10, 20, 30, 50, 60, 80, 100, 200 mg	12–24

[a]Must be given as intact pills, cannot be crushed or used in G or J tubes.
[b]Capsule can be opened and sprinkled in food (oral or G-tubes).

along with the principal opioid or nonopioid analgesics. The most commonly used and best studied class of adjuvant medications is anticonvulsant therapy, such as gabapentin or pregabalin, or an antidepressant medication, such as amitriptyline, nortriptyline, or duloxetine.

Besides drug therapy, all patients with cancer-related pain should be evaluated for the potential use of nondrug therapies. These include education, counseling, physical modalities, and physical/occupational therapy. Patient education in itself can be a powerful analgesic intervention because it can give patients a greater sense of control and empowerment by understanding their treatment options. Simple counseling techniques can include normalization of symptoms and relaxation techniques. Physical modalities can include application of heat, cold, and massage.

Prompt referral to specialist providers is recommended when routine treatments fail to adequately manage a patient's pain. Palliative care and pain management teams are available at many institutions. Interventional pain management specialists may be needed to assess for interventions such as nerve blocks or steroid injections that can improve pain control. Analgesic interventional radiology procedures are an important and emerging modality for cancer-related pain and are discussed elsewhere in this text.

NAUSEA AND VOMITING

Nearly 60% of advanced cancer patients experience nausea.[25] Nausea remains one of the primary detriments to quality of life for patients undergoing cancer therapy,[26] and it also aggravates weight loss and lead to electrolyte disturbances and aspiration pneumonia.

The pathophysiology of nausea and vomiting is complex and is coordinated in the brainstem vomiting center (VC). The VC receives sensory input primarily from the chemoreceptor trigger zone (CTZ) located in the base of the fourth ventricle. The CTZ acts as a sampling port for emetogenic toxins in the blood and cerebrospinal fluid. Chemotherapy, opioids, uremic toxins from renal failure, and metabolic disturbances can all trigger the VC via this mechanism. Because the mechanisms of nausea can be so varied, it is important to consider a wide differential diagnosis and pursue a diagnostic workup that is focused to the most likely cause.

Two of the most common etiologies for nausea in cancer patients are chemotherapy and opioid induced. For chemotherapy-induced nausea, there are well-established prophylactic drug regimens. Most regimens use a combination of dexamethasone and an antagonist of the serotonin receptor subtype-3 (5HT3), such as ondansetron or granisetron.[27] Chemotherapy-induced nausea can also be delayed or persist for several days to a few weeks after chemotherapy, especially with certain regimens that are known to be highly emetogenic. For the treatment of delayed chemotherapy-induced nausea, dopamine blockers, glucocorticoids, and aprepitant, a neurokinin-1 inhibitor, all have demonstrated efficacy.[28,29]

Nausea is an expected side effect of opioids and is not an allergic reaction.[30] It usually occurs at the initiation of opioid therapy or following a dose increase. It is exacerbated by constipation; therefore, evaluation and appropriate management of constipation is advised. For most patients, nausea is self-limiting within a few days and does not require a dose adjustment. Some patients idiosyncratically have more nausea with some opioids over others. Therefore, if nausea persists or is particularly severe, a trial of an alternative opioid may be reasonable. Pharmacologic treatment of opioid-induced nausea is empiric with antidopaminergic antiemetics (e.g., prochlorperazine) being most commonly used as a first-line agent.

Dopamine antagonists are a good first choice for the symptomatic treatment of nonspecific nausea in advanced cancer patients due to low cost, availability, and favorable side effect profile. Metoclopramide, in particular, is well studied in advanced cancer.[31] Other agents in this class include prochlorperazine, haloperidol, droperidol, and chlorpromazine. Table 21.4 lists some other common etiologies of nausea and common therapies.

CONSTIPATION

Constipation is a distressing symptom that is estimated to occur in 40% to 90% of cancer patients.[32] As a subjective complaint it can describe inadequate passage of stool, increased hardness of stool, decreased frequency of stool, or decreased size of stool. It can impact a patient's health by contributing to discomfort, anorexia, weight loss, obstipation, bowel obstruction, and delirium in the medically frail.[33] Etiologies of constipation in the cancer patient include metabolic causes, such as hypercalcemia and uremia; mechanical causes, such as bowel obstruction and fecal impaction; oncologic causes, such as spinal cord compression and cauda equina syndrome; and drug-induced from medications including opioids, serotonin antagonists, anticholinergic agents, iron, and certain chemotherapeutic agents, such as the vinca alkaloids.

Of particular concern is opioid-induced constipation. Over half of all patients treated with opioids experience constipation,[34] and it does not attenuate with duration of therapy. Opioids lead to constipation by inhibiting peristalsis, decreasing gastrointestinal secretions, and increasing sphincter tone.

The best treatment for opioid-induced constipation is prophylaxis. Rarely, decreasing the opioid dose is necessary if pain is well controlled and constipation is severe. Rotation to a different

Table 21.4	
Common Etiologies of Nausea and Vomiting in Cancer and Their Potential Therapies	
Etiology of nausea	**Proposed therapy**
Vestibular disturbance	Antihistamines or promethazine
Bowel obstruction	Octreotide; anticholinergics, such as scopolamine or glycopyrrolate
Cerebral edema	Corticosteroids, such as dexamethasone
Anticipatory nausea or anxiety	Benzodiazepines
Chemotherapy/serum toxins	D2 blockers, 5HT3 blockers

opioid is unlikely to be of much benefit insofar as all opioids are constipating and patients typically do not develop tolerance to this side effect. There is some evidence that transdermal fentanyl is less constipating than oral opioids.[35]

Pharmacologic strategies for managing and preventing constipation are largely empiric. There are four general categories of pharmacologic treatments: stimulants, bulk-forming agents, osmotic, and surfactant laxatives. Stimulants, such as senna or bisacodyl, are often used in the prevention and treatment of opioid-induced constipation. They appear to work by stimulating the myenteric plexus to increase peristalsis. Many experts recommend scheduling these medications whenever a patient is placed on a long-acting opioid to prevent constipation from becoming severe.

Bulk-forming agents, such as fiber and psyllium, have a limited role in opioid-induced constipation. Although they increase stool mass and water content, they do not promote motility so are not effective as monotherapy. There is no defined role for oral surfactant agents, such as docusate, in patients with advanced illness.[36]

Osmotic laxatives contain poorly absorbable salts or carbohydrates, which osmotically retain fluid in the intestinal lumen, leading to laxation. Saline-based laxatives usually contain magnesium salts and can be used safely long term in lower doses. They are often used as an added agent to a stimulant laxative in opioid-induced constipation. They should be used cautiously in patients with renal failure due to concern for hypermagnesemia. Common carbohydrate-based osmotic laxatives are lactulose and sorbitol. They can be poorly tolerated because of their sweet taste but are generally felt to be effective as an as-needed agent. Polyethylene glycol 3350 is a nonabsorbable polymer that comes as a powder patients dissolve in liquid. Most patients with serious medical illnesses require higher doses than the approved 17 g daily; PEG 3350 causes catharsis at doses of several hundred grams a day. All laxatives can cause cramping, bloating, flatulence, nausea, and electrolyte disturbances.

Rectal therapies, such as enemas and suppositories, are most often reserved for refractory constipation. Enemas cause colonic distention, which stimulates rectal contraction and fecal evacuation. Suppositories can have either a stimulant effect (e.g., bisacodyl) or a surfactant effect (e.g., glycerin). In patients with fecal impaction, manual disimpaction along with large-volume enemas may be necessary.

Methylnaltrexone is a newer agent that has been approved by the Food and Drug Administration (FDA) for opioid-induced constipation in patients with advanced illness who have not responded to traditional laxatives. It is a subcutaneously injectable quaternary derivative of naltrexone with restricted ability to cross the blood–brain barrier.[37] Therefore, it acts as peripheral opioid antagonist and does not cause withdrawal or reverse analgesia. Multiple studies have demonstrated its efficacy in treating opioid-induced constipation.[38,39] It is contraindicated in patients with bowel obstructions, which should be ruled out with a careful history and physical examination and, if needed, plain-film radiography prior to administering methylnaltrexone.

■ CONSTITUTIONAL SYMPTOMS

Fatigue, anorexia, and weight loss are disturbing manifestations of cancer for the patient and family that often progress in intensity as the underlying cancer progresses. Anorexia occurs in up to 70% of cancer patients and more than half of cancer patients experience unintended weight loss throughout the course of their illness.[40] Anorexia and weight loss can be particularly distressing to patients and families because they can be a source of social isolation and conflict between family members or the health team regarding issues of nutrition and oral intake. Education and emotional support are the best first step in alleviating fears of starvation. When appropriate, health professionals can assist patients and families by shifting the focus on anorexia away from the patient and back on the cancer. Nutritional counseling is a commonly used intervention; however, research has not shown any significant long-term benefit.[41]

There are several orexigenic drugs that have been shown to increase appetite, caloric intake, and weight. Unfortunately, there are limited data to suggest that they can improve patients' quality of life, energy level, muscle mass, or survival. Furthermore, the increase in weight is likely due to an increase in fat mass and many of these agents are associated with limiting side effects. Therefore, they are best used to alleviate persistent *distress* related to low appetite, but not with the expectation they will be disease-modifying in any way. Table 21.5 lists commonly available orexigenic therapies, common dosing, and potential side effects.

Fatigue is the most frequently cited symptom from cancer and its treatments, occurring in nearly 100% of patients with

Table 21.5

Common Pharmacotherapies for Anorexia and Cachexia

Class	Drug	Dose	Potential risks
Progesterone	Megestrol	Start at 80–160 mg PO qday and titrate up to 800 mg/day	Peripheral edema, increased risk of thromboembolic events
	Medroxyprogesterone acetate	400 mg PO qday and titrate to 400 mg PO bid	
Glucocorticoid	Dexamethasone	2–4 mg oral once to twice a day	Myopathy, thrush, peripheral edema, hyperglycemia, Cushingnoid syndrome
	Prednisone	20–40 mg PO daily	
Cannabinoids	Dronabinol	2.5 mg orally after meals	Psychotomimetic side effects

advanced cancer.[42] Cancer-related fatigue is distinct from exercise-induced fatigue, in that the symptoms are disproportionate to activity and are not ameliorated by rest.[43] The pathophysiology of cancer-related fatigue is likely similar to cancer-related anorexia and weight loss in that research suggests it is related to inflammatory cytokines and neurohormonal disruption that accompanies the cancer.[44]

The first step in the treatment of cancer-related fatigue is to address any underlying causes that may be amenable to intervention, such as anemia or depression. Moderate aerobic exercise is recommended because research suggests it can improve the severity of the symptoms.[45] Psychostimulants, such as methylphenidate or modafinil, have also been used for the treatment of cancer-related fatigue, although their effectiveness in controlled studies has been mixed.[46–48] Psychostimulants are also useful in the management of depression, especially when the prominent symptom is psychomotor retardation.[49] They usually begin their effectiveness within 2 days and are often dosed twice daily.

Education and support should be offered to all patients complaining of cancer-related fatigue. If a patient's function is affected, helping him or her establish realistic expectations and goals can be necessary if the fatigue cannot be ameliorated.

PSYCHIATRIC SYMPTOMS

Psychiatric symptoms, such as depression and anxiety, are underdiagnosed and yet often treatable in cancer patients. Although only a minority of cancer patients develop depression, it is much more common in cancer patients than in the general population and its prevalence increases as the burden of illness worsens.[50] Diagnosis of depression can be challenging and complicated in cancer due to an overlap of the somatic symptoms of depression with the common symptoms of cancer (e.g., fatigue, anorexia, weight loss, sleep disturbance). Furthermore, clinicians often erroneously accept depression as being a normal part of having cancer because feelings of grief, sadness, and loss are common in cancer patients and not usually pathologic.

Pervasive and persistent feelings of guilt, shame, anhedonia, worthlessness, hopelessness, helplessness, and suicidality are not characteristic of the normal emotional adjustments to a life-threatening diagnosis, however, and instead are strongly suggestive of major depression.[51] A simple bedside intervention of asking "Are you feeling down, depressed, or hopeless most of the time over the last 2 weeks?" has shown excellent reliability and validity in screening cancer patients for depression.[52]

Pharmacologic and nonpharmacologic therapies are recommended in the treatment of depression because together these therapies have been shown to be more efficacious than either alone.[53,54] Referral to a psychologist, clinical social worker, primary care physician, palliative care physician, and/or psychiatrist when appropriate is advised.

Three main classes of pharmacologic agents are available: (1) tricyclic (and related) antidepressants, (2) selective serotonin reuptake inhibitors (SSRIs) and serotonin and noradrenaline reuptake inhibitors (SNRIs), and (3) psychostimulants. No class of antidepressants has superior efficacy over any other.[54]

Anxiety occurs commonly in cancer patients with prevalence between 30% and 50%.[55] Temporary anxiousness surrounding specific medical events, such as a test result or a procedure, is common and not pathologic. If a patient's anxiety is pervasive and interrupts his or her ability to participate in necessary medical care or activities of daily living, it should be assessed and treated.

Anxiety responds to nonpharmacologic therapies including cognitive and psychotherapeutic interventions, such as relaxation techniques. Pharmacologic treatment can be useful for both incidental and pervasive anxiety. For incidental symptoms (e.g., before a procedure) cognitive interventions and/or pretreatment with a short-acting benzodiazepine are the mainstay of care. For longer-term treatment of anxiety, referral to the patient's primary care provider, a palliative medicine team, or a mental health professional may be necessary. Scheduled, low-dose long-acting benzodiazepines, such as clonazepam, are effective but are associated with the risk of sedation, abuse, and delirium. SSRIs and SNRIs are effective for generalized anxiety disorder. Buspirone is a nonbenzodiazepine anxiolytic that functions as a partial serotonin receptor agonist. It has minimal abuse potential and proven efficacy; however, like SSRIs, it can take several weeks to be effective.[56]

PALLIATIVE MEDICINE AND HOSPICE CARE

Although patient preferences for medical care at the end of life can be varied, evidence suggests that as patients near the end of their life, symptom management and honest disclosure of medical information and options are important themes in the concept of a "good death."[57] Because the symptoms of cancer often progress as the patient's underlying cancer progresses, palliative care, or care that manages the symptoms and side effects of cancer and its treatment, may become more of the focus of the patient's medical treatment plan (FIGURE 21.2).

Whereas palliative care refers to management of symptoms related to an underlying illness, palliative medicine refers to a newly recognized medical subspecialty. Besides expert symptom assessment and treatment, palliative medicine physicians and palliative care interdisciplinary teams can offer assistance in determining prognosis, breaking bad news to patients and families, establishing goals of medical care, and planning for the future in the face of a life-threatening illness. Many major medical institutions now have palliative medicine physicians and palliative care teams. The scope of practice may vary from institutions but commonly include: (1) inpatient consultative palliative care services, (2) outpatient palliative care clinics, (3) acute inpatient palliative care wards, (4) nursing home palliative care services, and (5) home palliative care services including home hospice.

Hospice care has the same philosophy and multidisciplinary approach as palliative care but has some distinct features. Hospice can be thought of as a specific set of palliative care services for a specific patient population with short prognoses. Hospice care is largely defined by the Medicare Hospice Benefit (MHB) in the United States. State government insurers, such as Medicaid and private insurers, generally cover hospice services commensurate with the MHB. The MHB requires physician certification that a patient has an expected prognosis of 6 months or less if the disease runs its expected course. Medically eligible patients can elect to enroll into the hospice benefit if their goals of care are for comfort.

The vast majority of hospice care is provided in patients' homes. The MHB provides payment and access to skilled home health aides, nursing support, volunteer visits, durable medical equipment, pharmacologic therapies related to the terminal diagnosis, respite care, physical and occupational therapy, social work, chaplaincy services, and bereavement follow-up.[58] Additionally, Medicare-certified hospice agencies must be able to provide acute, inpatient level care for severe symptom control or

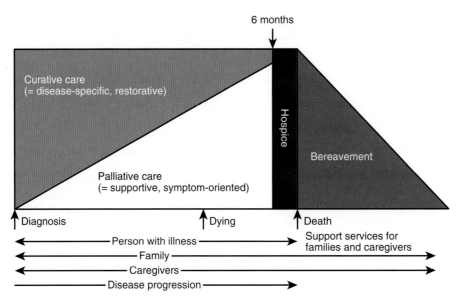

FIGURE 21.2 Schematic showing the integration of palliative care and hospice as a serious, non-curable illness progresses.

imminent death, although the MHB does not cover room and board fees for long-term facilities, such as a residential hospice.[59]

Open and honest discussions with patients and their families that accurately acknowledge the patients' prognosis and future burden of illness are necessary to appropriately determine their goals of care and preferences for treatment at the end of life. Once goals of care have been established, referral to a hospice agency may be helpful in managing the physical and psychological symptoms that an advanced cancer patient will face at the end of life.

COORDINATING CARE IN PATIENTS WITH ADVANCED CANCER

Patients with advanced cancer and multiple cancer-related symptoms require coordinated multidisciplinary management to optimize care. As one of the many specialists who will be involved in the care of these patients, interventional oncologists have an opportunity and responsibility to help coordinate care. Many different practice models exist and the responsibilities of the interventional oncologist physician will vary from patient to patient and will depend on individual expertise and clinical resources available. In some patients, the interventional oncologist may be the patient's primary physician coordinating care and symptom management. In others, the palliative care physician, medical oncologist, surgical oncologist, or hepatologist may be coordinating care with the interventional oncologist in a consultant role. These roles often vary as the patient progresses through multimodality therapeutic regimens. Whatever the role assumed in a particular patient, communication among the managing physicians is critical and the patient needs to know who to contact when problems and questions arise.

CONCLUSION

Palliative care is focused on symptom relief and maximizing patient function without necessarily impacting the natural history of the underlying disease. As the field of interventional oncology matures, interventional oncology physicians caring for patients with advanced cancer will need to be comfortable with the management of common cancer-related symptoms. Interventional radiologists (IRs) will need to feel comfortable with communicating prognosis and other critical information to patients and their families. Working in concert with colleagues in other clinical cancer specialties, interventional oncologists will be able to offer therapeutic options that will maximize quantity and quality of life and help to optimally manage the many common symptoms in this challenging and rewarding patient population.

REFERENCES

1. Lunney JR, Lynn J, Foley DJ, et al. Patterns of functional decline at the end of life. *JAMA* 2003;289(18):2387–2392.
2. Teno JM, Weitzen S, Fennel ML, et al. Dying trajectory in the last year of life: does cancer trajectory fit other diseases? *J Palliat Med* 2001;4:457–464.
3. World Health Organization. WHO definition of palliative care. Available at: http://www.who.int/cancer/palliative/definition/en. Accessed March 11, 2011.
4. Busch H. The complexity of the cancer problem. *Fed Proc* 1979;38:94–96.
5. Wachtel T, Allen-Masterson S, Reuben D, et al. The end stage cancer patient: terminal common pathway. *Hospice J* 1988;4:43–80.
6. Wright AA, Zhang B, Ray A, et al. Associations between end-of-life discussions, patient mental health, medical care near death, and caregiver bereavement adjustment. *JAMA* 2008;300(14):1665–1673.
7. Glare P, Virik K, Jones M, et al. A systematic review of physicians' survival predictions in terminally ill cancer patients. *Br Med J* 2003;327:195–201.
8. Christakis NA, Lamont EB. Extent and determinants of error in doctors' prognoses in terminally ill patients: prospective cohort study. *Br Med J* 2000;320:469–473.
9. Mitchell AJ. Reluctance to disclose difficult diagnoses: a narrative review comparing communication by psychiatrists and oncologists. *Support Care Cancer* 2007;15:819–828.
10. Vainio A, Auvinen A; with members of Symptom Prevalence Group. Prevalence of symptoms among patients with advanced cancer: an international collaborative study. *J Pain Symptom Manage* 1996;12(1):3–10.
11. Yalçin B, Büyükçelik A, Şenler FC, et al. Frequency of symptoms in patients with advanced cancer. *Turk J Cancer* 2005;35(4):177–180.
12. Serlin RC, Mendoza TR, Nakamura Y, et al. When is cancer pain mild, moderate or severe? Grading pain severity by its interference with function. *Pain* 1995;61:277–284.

13. Turk DC, Melzack R. The measurement and assessment of people in pain. In: Turk DC, Melzack R, eds. *Handbook of Pain Assessment*. New York, NY: The Guildford Press; 1992:3–12.

14. Williamson A, Hoggart B. Pain: a review of the three commonly used pain rating scales. *J Clin Nurs* 2005;14:798–804.

15. Ahles TA, Ruckdeschel JC, Blancard EB. Cancer related pain: II, assessment with the visual analogue scale. *J Psychosom Res* 1984;28(2):121–124.

16. Paice JA, Cohen FL. Validity of a verbally administered numeric rating scale to measure cancer pain intensity. *Cancer Nurs* 1997;20(2):88–93.

17. Lara-Munoz C, De Leon SP, Feinstein AR, et al. Comparison of three rating scales for measuring subjective phenomena in clinical research: I, use of experimentally controlled auditory stimuli. *Arch Med Res* 2004;35:43–48.

18. Lussier D, Huskey AF, Portenoy RK. Adjuvant analgesics in cancer pain management. *Oncologist* 2004;9:571–591.

19. Mercadante S, Portenoy RK. Opioid poorly-responsive cancer pain: part 1, clinical considerations. *J Pain Symptom Manage* 2001;21:144–150.

20. VanRoenn JH, Cleeland CS, Gonin R, et al. Physician attitudes and practice in cancer pain management. *Ann Intern Med* 1993;119:121–126.

21. Gordon DB, Stevenson KK, Griffie J, et al. Opioid equianalgesic calculations. *J Palliat Med* 1999;2(2):209–218.

22. World Health Organization. WHO's pain ladder. Available at: http://www.who.int/cancer/palliative/painladder/en/. Accessed February 23, 2011.

23. Inturrisi CE, Hanks F. Opioid analgesic therapy. In: Doyle D, Hanks GWC, MacDonald N, eds. *Oxford Textbook of Palliative Medicine*. Oxford, New York, Toronto: Oxford University Press; 1993:166–182.

24. Weissman DE. Fast facts and concepts #71: meperidine for pain: what's all the fuss? June 2002. End-of-Life Physician Education Resource Center. Available at: http://www.eperc.mcw.edu. Accessed March 11, 2011.

24a. Shaheen PE, Walsh D, Lasheen W, Davis MP, Lagman RL. Opioid equianalgesic tables: are they all equally dangerous? *J Pain Symptom Management* 2009;38(3):409–17.

24b. Webster LR, Fine PG. Overdose deaths demand new paradigm for opioid rotation. Pain Med 2012; 13(4): 571–574.

25. Davis MP, Walsh D. Treatment of nausea and vomiting in advanced cancer. *Support Care Cancer* 2000;8:444–452.

26. de Boer-Dennert M, de Wit R, Schmitz PI, et al. Patient perceptions of the side-effects of chemotherapy: the influence of 5HT3 antagonists. *Br J Cancer* 1997;76:1055–1061.

27. Aapro M. 5-HT3-receptor antagonists in the management of nausea and vomiting in cancer and cancer treatment. *Oncology* 2005;69:97–109.

28. Hesketh PJ, Grunberg SM, Gralla RJ, et al. The oral neurokinin-1 antagonist aprepitant for the prevention of chemotherapy-induced nausea and vomiting: a multinational, randomized, double-blind, placebo-controlled trial in patients receiving high-dose cisplatin—the Aprepitant Protocol 052 Study Group. *J Clin Oncol* 2003;21:4077–4080.

29. Herrstedt J, Muss HB, Warr DG, et al. Efficacy and tolerability of aprepitant for the prevention of chemotherapy-induced nausea and emesis over multiple cycles of moderately emetogenic chemotherapy. *Cancer* 2005;104:1548–1555.

30. Campora E, Merlini L, Bruzzone M, et al. The incidence of narcotic-induced emesis. *J Pain Symptom Manage* 1991;6:428–430.

31. Glare P, Pereira G, Kristjanson LJ, et al. Systematic review of the efficacy of antiemetics in the treatment of nausea in patients with far-advanced cancer. *Support Care Cancer* 2004;12:432–440.

32. Mancini I, Bruera E. Constipation in advanced cancer patients. *Support Care Cancer* 1998;6:356–364.

33. Fallon M, O'Neill B. ABC of palliative care: constipation and diarrhoea. *Br Med J* 1997;315:1293–1296.

34. Tamayo AC, Diaz-Zuluaga PA. Management of opioid-induced bowel dysfunction in cancer patients. *Support Care Cancer* 2004;12:613–618.

35. Allan L, Richarz U, Simpson K, et al. Transderman fentanyl versus sustained release oral morphine in strong-opioid naïve patients with chronic low back pain. *Spine* 2005;30:2484–2490.

36. Librach SL, Bouvette M, De Angelis C, et al. Consensus recommendations for the management of constipation in patients with advanced, progressive illness. *J Pain Symptom Manage* 2010;40(5):761–773.

37. Yuan CS. Methylnaltrexone mechanisms of action and effects on opioid bowel dysfunction and other opioid adverse effects. *Ann Pharmacother* 2007;41(6):984–993.

38. Thomas J, Karver S, Cooney GA, et al. Methylnaltrexone for opioid-induced constipation in advanced illness. *N Engl J Med* 2008;358(22):2332–2343.

39. Portenoy RK, Thomas J, Moehl Boatwright ML, et al. Subcutaneous methylnaltrexone for the treatment of opioid-induced constipation in patients with advanced illness: a double-blind randomized, parallel group, dose-ranging study. *J Pain Symptom Manage* 2008;35(5):458–468.

40. Yavuzsen T, Davis MP, Walsh D, et al. Systematic review of the treatment of cancer-associated anorexia and weight loss. *J Clin Oncol* 2005;23:8500–8511.

41. MacDonald N. Is there evidence for earlier intervention in cancer-associated weight loss? *J Support Oncol* 2003;1:279–286.

42. Ahlberg K, Ekman T, Gaston-Johansson F, et al. Assessment and management of cancer-related fatigue in adults. *Lancet* 2003;362:640–650.

43. Adamsen L, Midtgaard J, Andersen C, et al. Transforming the nature of fatigue through exercise: qualitative findings from a multidimensional exercise programme in cancer patients undergoing chemotherapy. *Eur J Cancer Care* 2004;13:362–370.

44. Sood A, Moynihan TJ. Cancer related fatigue: an update. *Curr Oncol Rep* 2005;7:277–282.

45. Dimeo FC, Stieglitz RD, Novelli-Fischer U, et al. Effects of physicial activity on the fatigue and psychologic status of cancer patients during chemotherapy. *Cancer* 1999;85:2273–2277.

46. Bruera E, Driver L, Barnes EA. Patient-controlled methylphenidate for the management of fatigue in patients with advanced cancer: a preliminary report. *J Clin Oncol* 2003;21:4439–4443.

47. Carroll JK, Kohli S, Mustian KN, et al. Pharmacologic treatment of cancer related fatigue. *Oncologist* 2007;12(suppl):43–51.

48. Morrow GR, Jean-Pierre P, Roscoe JA, et al. A phase III randomized, placebo-controlled, double-blind trial of a eugeroic agent in 642 cancer patients reporting fatigue during chemotherapy: a URCC CCOP Study [abstract]. *J Clin Oncol* 2008;26(suppl): 9512.

49. Pereira J, Bruera E. Depression with psychomotor retardation: diagnostic challenges and the use of psychostimulants. *J Palliat Med* 2001;4: 15–21.

50. Pirl WF. Evidence report on the occurrence, assessment, and treatment of depression in cancer patients. *J Natl Cancer Inst Monogr* 2004;32:32–39.

51. Periyakoil VJ. *Fast Facts and Concepts #43: Is It Grief or Depression?* 2nd ed. End-of-Life Physician Education Resource Center; 2005. Available at: http://www.eperc.mcw.edu. Accessed March 11, 2011.

52. Chochinov HM, Wilson KG, Enns M, et al. "Are you depressed?" Screening for depression in the terminally ill. *Am J Psychiatry* 1997;154:674–676.

53. Sheard T, Maguire P. The effect of psychological interventions on anxiety and depression in cancer patients: results of two meta-analyses. *Br J Cancer* 1999;80:1770–1780.

54. Thase ME, Greenhouse JB, Frank E, et al. Treatment of major depression with psychotherapy or psychotherapy-pharmacotherapy combinations. *Arch Gen Psychiatry* 1997;54:1009–1015.

55. Chochinov HM. Depression in cancer patients. *Lancet Oncol* 2001;2:499–505.

56. Burgess C, Cornelius V, Love S, et al. Depression and anxiety in women with early breast cancer: five year observational cohort study. *Br Med J* 2005;330:702.

57. Bottomley A. Anxiety and the adult cancer patient. *Eur J Cancer Care* 1998;7:217–224.

58. Steinhauser KE, Clipp EC, McNeilly M, et al. In search of a good death: observations of patients, families, and providers. *Ann Intern Med* 2000;132(10):825–832.

59. Morrison RS, Meier D. Palliative care. *N Engl J Med* 2004;350:2582–2590.

SECTION II

Gynecology and Male Fertility

Management Options for Uterine Fibroids

JUSTIN S. LEE and JAMES B. SPIES

INTRODUCTION

Uterine myomas (otherwise known as fibroids) are the most common benign tumors of the female genitourinary tract. The incidence is estimated to be between 5.4% and 77% in reproductive age women.[1,2] The exact etiology for the formation of fibroids is unknown; however, their growth is known to be hormonally influenced.[3] Fibroids may present as a solitary mass but more commonly present as multiple growths within the uterus. The most common symptom is menorrhagia. Fibroids can be responsible for dysmenorrhea, chronic pelvic pain, urinary tract symptoms, constipation, and infertility.

Fibroid location is directly linked to symptomatology. Myomas are classified by their location relative to the endometrial cavity. Submucosal fibroids lie just beneath the endometrium and distort the endometrial cavity. Intramural fibroids are within the muscular myometrium and enlarge the uterus. Subserosal fibroids are covered by the uterine serosa and grow exophytically from the myometrium. Transmural fibroids are a subtype of intramural fibroids in that they span the myometrium with a deeper submucosal portion and a superficial subserosal component. Pedunculated fibroids are attached to the myometrium by a thin stalk of smooth muscle and can be subclassified as intracavitary, if they are in the endometrial cavity, or exophytic, if they are protruding off the uterus. In general, fibroids that exert mass effect on the endometrial cavity, such as submucosal or pedunculated intracavitary fibroids, tend to produce abnormal bleeding symptoms. Fibroids that enlarge the uterus and push on adjacent structures produce bulk symptoms.

The decision whether to treat fibroids is clinically based on the patient's symptoms and their impact on quality of life. Fibroid related symptoms have been shown to negatively impact the quality of life of reproductive age women.[4] It is unusual, however, for fibroids to cause any life-threatening sequela. Patients with menorrhagia may develop symptomatic anemia, and large fibroids may produce hydronephrosis of one or both kidneys. Left untreated, symptomatic fibroids are unlikely to disappear. Studies in which patients with symptomatic fibroids were part of an observational placebo group generally found no changes in symptoms over time.[5,6]

Depending on the age of a patient and the severity of her symptoms, observation alone may be an option. Women approaching menopause who have declining estrogen levels and cessation of their menstrual cycles may achieve improvement in their symptoms without intervention. Despite the lack of new fibroid growth after menopause, large fibroids can take time to shrink, causing persistent bulk symptoms. For these patients, intervention must have the goal of reducing fibroid volume or removing them altogether.

MEDICAL MANAGEMENT

Estrogen and Progesterone

Fibroid growth is mainly influenced by estrogen and progesterone, which explains why symptoms are most pronounced in women of reproductive age and tend to regress after menopause. In vitro studies suggest that estrogen and progestin stimulate myoma cell growth.[7] Supportive evidence is that fibroids have been observed to enlarge during high hormonal states, such as pregnancy.[8] Despite these findings, oral contraceptive pills (OCPs) containing varying levels of estrogen and progestin are a common first-line treatment to control menorrhagia and dysmenorrhea.[9] Surprisingly, this use of low-dose hormones does not result in fibroid growth.[10,11]

In a prospective study of 87 women with fibroids, 55 who were given low-dose monophasic OCPs were compared with 32 controls.[12] In the OCP group, there was a statistically significant decrease in menstrual duration from 5.8 to 4.4 days and an increase in mean hematocrit level from 35.8% to 37.8%. There was no difference in mean uterine size between the groups.

A levonorgestrel-releasing intrauterine contraceptive device (LR-IUD) (MIrena, Bayer Healthcare Pharmaceuticals, Pittsburgh, PA) also has been used to treat menorrhagia associated with fibroids with similar results.[13] Levonorgestrel is a progesterone analog, which when combined with an IUD releases low levels of the hormone locally. A systematic review of the literature, reveals 11 prospective, noncomparative studies evaluating the use of LR-IUDs for fibroid-related menorrhagia. All 11 studies found a decrease in bleeding; however, expulsion of IUDs tended to be higher in patients with fibroids, although the difference was not statistically significant.[14]

Progestin-only treatments have been used to diminish the size of fibroids. Medroxyprogesterone (Depo-Provera, Pfizer, New York, NY) administered to 20 premenopausal women with fibroids produced amenorrhea in 30%, improvement in bleeding symptoms in 70%, and a 48% reduction in mean uterine size and 33% reduction in fibroid volumes.[15] Unfortunately, similar studies demonstrated the opposite effect, with increased growth of fibroids in response to progesterone.[16] In vitro data also have shown an increase in mitotic activity with progestin-only therapy, whereas with combination estrogen-progestin therapy there was no increase in cell activity compared with controls.[17]

Overall, estrogen-progesterone therapy may help control menorrhagia in patients with fibroids. However, these medical therapies do not address the underlying fibroids themselves. A strategy of watchful waiting plus OCPs may be suitable for patients approaching menopause depending on symptom severity. Common side effects of hormone therapy are weight gain, nausea, variations in menstrual flow, breast tenderness, discomfort or swelling, depression or mood disturbances, decreased sexual desire or response, and acne. Rare serious side effects include deep vein thrombosis, liver adenomas, and gallstones. Older women, particularly those with hypertension, and smokers have a 20% to 40% increased risk of stroke, and use of the pill is contraindicated in these patients.[18]

Gonadotropin-Releasing Hormone Agonists

Gonadotropin-releasing hormone agonists (GNRH agonists) are the most established medical therapy for the treatment of fibroid symptoms. The mechanism of action involves manipulation of the hypothalamic-pituitary axis, leading to decreased circulating levels of estrogen and progesterone. GNRH is secreted from the hypothalamus and acts on receptors in the anterior pituitary to stimulate the release of the gonadotropins leutinizing hormone (LH) and follicle-stimulating hormone (FSH). GNRH agonists diminish the number of available receptors on the anterior pituitary, leading to decreased LH and FSH levels, thereby inducing a hypoestrogenic state. Patients thus experience a menopause-like state with amenorrhea and decrease in fibroid size. GNRH agonists also cause a local decrease in the fibroids' estrogen levels by suppressing aromatase P450, and thus promoting degeneration, decrease in cell size and cell number, and, most importantly, decrease in uterine blood flow.[19,20]

Early studies, such as the multicentered Leuprolide study, a double-blind randomized controlled trial, found that patients treated with leuprolide (a GNRH agonist) had reductions of uterine volume of 36% at 12 weeks and 45% at 24 weeks. Placebo patients had no significant reduction in uterine volume.[6] Similar studies were repeated using various strategies for administering GNRH agonists, such as daily subcutaneous injections and monthly injections. A 30% reduction in fibroid size and overall uterine size reduction of 35% can be achieved in as little as 8 weeks.[21–23] Menorrhagia symptoms also respond, resulting in significant elevation of hematocrit levels.[23] Unfortunately, after discontinuation of treatment, the effects of GNRH agonists reverse to pretreatment levels. In the Leuprolide study, each patient in the treatment group had a return to pretreatment uterine size by 24 weeks. Patients generally return to menses in 4 to 8 weeks. Despite a rapid return to size, however, patients may remain asymptomatic for up to a year after cessation of GNRH agonist treatment.[24]

Long-term GNRH agonist use is limited by its side effect profile, which is usually poorly tolerated. As many as 95% of patients treated with GNRH agonists should be expected to experience side effects related to the hypoestrogenic state.[6] The most common side effect is vasomotor flushing or "hot flashes" similar to those associated with menopause. Other less common side effects are arthralgias, insomnia, emotional lability, decreased libido, and vaginal dryness.[25] In the Leuprolide study, these symptoms led 8% of patients to stop GNRH agonist therapy.

Long-term GNRH agonists also are associated with a loss of bone density.[26] In otherwise healthy young women who can expect a natural loss of bone density after menopause, premature

loss with long-term use is particularly problematic. The hypoestrogenic state causes an increase in bone resorption versus formation. Several strategies have been proposed using combination therapies, in which GNRH agonists are used in conjunction with low-dose estrogens and progesterone in a so-called add-back protocol. In a prospective, randomized, double-blind, placebo-control trial specifically evaluating calcium metabolism in patients treated with GNRH agonists, all patients showed increased bone turnover.[26] When adding medroxyprogesterone, however, the rate of bone turnover slowed. Recent long-term studies using GNRH agonists and a similar add-back protocol for the treatment of endometriosis has yielded mixed results.[27]

Another add-back strategy using tibolone, a synthetic estrogen alternative, reduced the side effects of GNRH agonists and showed no difference in bone density between patients treated versus controls.[28] Tibolone is not available in the United States. Lastly, women treated with GNRH agonists and raloxifene, a selective estrogen modulator, had similar reduction in uterine and fibroid volumes without changes in bone density.[29] Patients did experience the usual menopausal side effects.

In summary, GNRH agonists are a potent medical therapy for patients with fibroids that will decrease fibroid size, uterine volume, and uterine blood flow. Unfortunately, long-term use is limited by a high side effect profile. Add-back strategies utilizing low-dose hormones to diminish these unwanted side effects as well as limit the loss of bone density have been employed with mixed results. Therefore, GNRH agonists cannot be considered as a long-term fibroid therapy.

▌ SURGICAL OPTIONS

Hysterectomy

Surgical excision of fibroids has been the cornerstone for definitive treatment of patients with symptomatic fibroids. Hysterectomy has long stood as the gold standard for the treatment of heavy menstrual bleeding, especially for women finished having children or beyond their reproductive years.[30] Fibroids were responsible for roughly one-third of the 598,000 hysterectomies performed in the United States in 1999.[31]

Hysterectomy is the only fibroid treatment that has close to 100% efficacy for the treatment of fibroid-related menorrhagia and bulk symptoms. The Maine Women's Health Study demonstrated that 72% of women experienced improvement of their symptoms after hysterectomy, whereas only 3% reported a psychological impact from the removal of their uterus.[32] In a multicentered, randomized trial comparing hysterectomy to medical therapy for abnormal uterine bleeding from 1997 to 2000, patients in the hysterectomy group reported greater improvement in symptoms and health-related quality of life as scored in the 36-item Short Form Health Survey (SF-36).[33] At the end of the study, 53% of women in the medical treatment group requested hysterectomy.

Hysterectomy for fibroids is most often performed through an abdominal incision. However, other minimally invasive approaches, such as laparoscopic and vaginal hysterectomy, exist. The advantages of these less-invasive approaches are a decreased hospital stay and quicker recovery. The eVALuate study—a parallel, multicenter, randomized control trial—compared 937 women undergoing a hysterectomy for benign conditions. Patients were randomized to groups comparing a laparoscopic approach with open hysterectomy and a laparoscopic approach to vaginal hysterectomy. The primary endpoints of the study were major complications, such as blood loss requiring transfusion and hematoma requiring reintervention. Secondary endpoints were pain as measured on a visual analog score, analgesic requirement, assessment of sexual activity, body image, and quality of life. Overall, the study demonstrated the advantages of laparoscopic and vaginal approaches over open hysterectomy with decreased pain, short hospital stay, and improved quality of life at 6 weeks.[34] The study did show that laparoscopic hysterectomy had a higher complication rate compared to the open approach. The rate of severe hemorrhage was 4.6% in the laparoscopic group and 2.4% in the open group. Ureteral injury only occurred in the laparoscopic group. Uplanned conversion to an open procedure was the second most common complication.

Despite studies showing clear advantages in the less invasive methods for hysterectomy, these options still represent a small percentage of hysterectomies performed. In a 2003 study that examined hysterectomy technique, of the 538,722 hysterectomies performed, 66.1% were performed open, 21.8% were transvaginal, and only 11.8% were performed laparoscopically.[35] The explanation for this finding is multifactorial. For one, patients with large uteri have been shown to have an increased risk of bleeding complications with increasing uterine size.[36] Laparoscopic techniques also have been shown to increase operative time. In addition, laparoscopic skills vary amongst gynecologists and their comfort with laparoscopy.[37] Despite these factors, due to the growing patient preference for minimally invasive techniques, it is likely that the proportion of hysterectomies performed using minimally invasive techniques will increase in the future.

Interestingly, there are other factors, including age, race, geographic, socioeconomic, and health care provider bias, that influence a varying rate of hysterectomy in the United States.[38] Epidemiologic studies have shown that the rate of hysterectomy is higher in the southeastern parts of the country, and that hysterectomy rates are higher in patients with lower education level.[35,39] Nevertheless, as more minimally invasive treatments become widely available, additional studies will show a decrease in these trends.

Myomectomy

Myomectomy is the uterine-sparing surgical option for fibroid treatment. The goal of a myomectomy is to remove some or all of the fibroids from the uterus. Despite the preservation of the uterus, studies have not shown a significant decrease in the perioperative morbidity between myomectomy and hysterectomy.[40] Traditional open myomectomy remains the most common approach. Laparoscopic and hysteroscopic myomectomy are increasingly available with experienced laparoscopic gynecologists and fibroids that are appropriately accessible through minimally invasive techniques.

The advantages of myomectomy are the preservation of the uterus as well as the ability to totally remove the symptomatic fibroids. The disadvantages are surgical recovery time, blood loss at the time of surgery, postoperative distortion of the uterus, postoperative adhesions, and the potential risk of unplanned hysterectomy while performing the myomectomy. Although there is no strict definition of which patient is most appropriate for myomectomy, a patient with multiple small intramural fibroids scattered throughout the uterus is not the best candidate. On the other hand, a patient with individual fibroids that, are felt to contribute specifically to the patient's symptoms, may be more appropriate for myomectomy. These would include fibroids that are distorting the endometrial cavity, which has been presumed to contribute to infertility. Location has not been shown to contribute specifically to fertility, however, and a debate about fibroid location and its impact continues.[41]

Myomectomy does represent a less invasive surgical option for treatment. A retrospective study comparing myomectomy to hysterectomy found that operative times were longer in the myomectomy group but that estimated blood loss was greater in the hysterectomy group. There was no difference in perioperative morbidity between the groups.[40]

In a study of perioperative morbidity in patients undergoing multiple versus single myomectomy, estimated blood loss was significantly higher for patients with multiple fibroids excised compared to those who had a single fibroid removed. Despite this, the length of hospital stay of about 5 days was not significantly different between the two groups.[42]

Perioperative hemorrhage is the most common complication associated with myomectomy. Several preoperative strategies exist that attempt to limit intraoperative blood loss. One approach is the use of recombinant erythropoietin to increase preoperative hemoglobin prior to surgery. In a prospective, randomized trial, the use of preoperative erythropoietin 3 weeks prior to surgery was associated with a significant reduction in transfusion rates compared to controls.[43] GNRH agonists have also been used to treat menorrhagia and decrease fibroid and uterine size prior to myomectomy and hysterectomy. Several studies have been published describing this strategy with improved hemoglobin concentrations and decreased blood loss.[44,45]

Adhesion formation after myomectomy is another significant postoperative complication that is difficult to predict and prevent. In a small study of 26 patients who underwent laparoscopy 6 weeks after myomectomy, as many as 93% of patients had formed adnexal adhesions.[46] The rate of adhesion formation was greater for fibroids removed from the posterior aspect of the uterus versus the anterior surface. The impact of adhesion formation is unknown, but adhesions are associated with small-bowel obstruction, increase the difficulty of future abdominal surgery, and may have an impact on fertility.[47]

Laparoscopic myomectomy was introduced to reduce the postoperative recovery associated with open myomectomy. A meta-analysis comparing laparoscopic to open myomectomy suggests that a laparoscopic approach is associated with decreased transfusion requirement, decreased postoperative pain, decreased hospital stay, and shorter recovery times.[48] The widespread application of a laparoscopic approach for myomectomy is limited, however, by surgical experience, uterine size, and fibroid location. In general, anterior fundal fibroids are easier to remove compared with posterior fibroids, which may be low in the cul-de-sac and in close proximity to the rectum.[49] Some published criteria for the upper limits of laparoscopy are a single fibroid less than 15 cm or no more than three fibroids with a size of 5 cm.[50] These size limits depend on the individual laparoscopist's skill.

Robot-assisted laparoscopic surgical devices have recently been approved for use in the United States for gynecologic surgery. widespread application is limited, however, by the large capital cost and annual maintenance costs of the robotic devices.[51] Additionally, the introduction of robot-assisted laparoscopic surgery in postgraduate training is highly variable. A meta-analysis of the safety and effectiveness of robotic-assisted laparoscopic surgery that included 22 studies concluded that the available nonrandomized data show limited evidence that robot-assisted surgery conferred any benefit compared to conventional laparoscopy in myomectomy patients.[52]

Hysteroscopic Myomectomy

Submucosal fibroids distorting the endometrial cavity are postulated to cause problems with fertility and contribute to menorrhagia. A meta-analysis of women with submucosal fibroids found a significantly lower rate of pregnancy and higher rate of miscarriage.[53] Patients who had submucosal fibroids removed had a significant increase in pregnancy rates.[54] There is a similar response in menorrhagia after submucosal resection.[55] The need for future reintervention was found to be high in long-term follow-up studies, however.

Hysteroscopic myomectomy is reserved for the resection of submucosal fibroids. Successful resection depends on the percentage of the fibroid that is submucosal and its size. A system has been created to classify the resectability of submucosal fibroids based on the extent of the fibroid within the endometrial cavity.[56] There are three types of fibroids according to the classification scheme. A type 0 fibroid is entirely within the endometrial cavity off a stalk. A type I fibroid has greater than 50% of the fibroid within the endometrial cavity, and a type II has less than 50% of the fibroid within the endometrial cavity.

Recurrence After Myomectomy

An issue related to any uterine-preserving intervention is fibroid recurrence. Recurrence leads to additional procedures and, often, hysterectomy. Understanding and quantifying a rate of fibroid recurrence is difficult due to the many variables associated with the development and detection of new fibroids. Additionally, it is sometimes impossible to ascertain if the new symptoms are a result of fibroids that were not removed during the initial myomectomy or if they are newly formed. Factors, such as age and hormonal status, certainly contribute. Fauconnier et al.[57] published a literature review of fibroid recurrence from 1966 to 1999. Although the authors admit that there some limitations based on the variability in calculating recurrence between the studies, they found that the cumulative risk of recurrence for myomectomy was approximately 10% over 5 years. Specifically, the risk of recurrence was significantly higher for patients who underwent laparoscopic myomectomy, those with multiple fibroids removed at the time of myomectomy, and those who had previously been treated with GNRH agonists.

In a more recent population-based study of women enrolled in a Washington State health maintenance organization (HMO) who underwent myomectomy and were followed for 11 years, that 21.8% underwent a second surgery[58] and almost 75% of these surgeries were hysterectomies. The cumulative incidence of a second surgery was 23.5% at 5 years with an annual incidence of surgery of 4.6%. As expected, women over the age of 50 had a 50% decreased risk for subsequent surgery.

Uterine Artery Occlusion or Ligation

Uterine artery occlusion is another less well-studied uterine sparing option for the treatment of symptomatic fibroids. The procedure involves ligation of the uterine arteries with bipolar coagulation or a surgically placed clamp. The procedure is performed either laparoscopically or transvaginally with Doppler ultrasound guidance. The ligation or occlusion of the artery is usually permanent, but pilot studies have been performed to evaluate the use of a temporary transvaginal device.[59]

There are few randomized studies evaluating uterine artery occlusion, but studies showing short-term symptom relief have been published. A single-arm prospective study showed symptom improvement in 89% of patients with an average reduction in fibroid volume assessed by ultrasound of 76% at 10 months.[60] Results of other studies have not been as dramatic, however.

A randomized comparative trial of uterine artery embolization (UAE) versus laparoscopic uterine artery occlusion in 66 women over 48 months found a 48% rate of symptom recurrence in the uterine artery occlusion patients versus 17% in the UAE group.[61] A 33% reduction in fibroid volume was seen in the uterine artery occlusion group. Complete fibroid infarction as assessed by contrast-enhanced magnetic resonance imaging (MRI) was only seen in 23% of the patients treated with uterine artery occlusion versus 100% of the UAE patients. Greater reduction of fibroid volume with complete devascularization occurred in the UAE group.

Endometrial Ablation

Endometrial ablation is a treatment for menorrhagia reserved for women who have plans for future pregnancy. Ablation is performed using many different modalities including microwave energy, cryotherapy, electrocautery, and thermal balloons. Endometrial ablation can be performed in conjunction with hysteroscopic myomectomy; however, nonhysteroscopic techniques also are widely available. Endometrial ablation is an attractive option for the treatment of menorrhagia because it is less invasive than traditional surgeries. Endometrial ablation is effective at controlling bleeding but may be less effective in patients with submucosal fibroids. In a retrospective review of 246 patients treated with an office-based ablation technique, 53.4% reported postprocedure amenorrhea, 26.8% reported light periods or spotting, 9.1% had normal menses, 6.5% reported menorrhagia, and 5.2% of the patients went on to hysterectomy for further bleeding.[62] Patients who had submucosal fibroids had lower rates of amenorrhea compared with those who had normal endometrial cavities. Patients with fibroids also were more likely to go on to hysterectomy.

A meta-analysis of endometrial ablation versus hysterectomy found better control of heavy menstrual bleeding in the hysterectomy patients with improved long-term satisfaction rates.[63] Length of procedure, duration of hospital stay, and recovery time were all increased for hysterectomy patients. Hysterectomy was a more durable procedure, however. Patients in the ablation group were more likely to require either repeat ablation or hysterectomy after the initial procedure compared to hysterectomy.

❚ NONSURGICAL OPTIONS

Uterine Artery Embolization

UAE, which is discussed at length in subsequent chapters, has been shown to be a durable, minimally invasive procedure that can provide significant symptom reduction and improved quality of life.[64] There have been three prominent prospective randomized trials comparing UAE to hysterectomy and/or myomectomy, which have all shown faster recovery times and shorter hospital stays with UAE.[65–67] Complication rates are low with both procedures. The most common complications in UAE are postembolization pain and fever, groin hematoma, and vaginal discharge, whereas common complications for hysterectomy are blood transfusion, wound infections, and injury to adjacent pelvic structures.[68]

Currently, there are several controversies surrounding UAE. The most debated is the impact of embolization on future fertility. A meta-analysis of the literature found that the miscarriage rate was higher in UAE, but that other problems, such as intrauterine growth retardation, preterm delivery, and malpresentation, were not increased in UAE compared to other fibroid therapies.[69]

A second concern is the impact of UAE on ovarian function. There have been concerns that an unknown amount of nontarget embolization occurs, resulting in some degree of ovarian ischemia. A 60-month prospective cohort study of ovarian function in which 36 women ages 26 to 39 undergoing UAE were compared to 36 controls found no difference in ovarian reserve as measured by serum hormonal levels between the two groups.[70]

Finally, uterine size and fibroid size have been a concern for critics of UAE due to incomplete embolization of larger fibroids. In a recently published retrospective study of 431 UAE patients, 71 were identified as having a large fibroid burden, defined as either a dominant fibroid greater than 10 cm in diameter or a uterine volume of greater than 700 cm^3.[71] During a 48-month follow-up period there was a 14% rate of hysterectomy and a mean volume reduction rate of 44%. The authors concluded that a large fibroid volume does not change the efficacy of UAE or increase the rate of adverse events.

A multicenter, retrospective cohort study comparing the safety and cost-effectiveness of hysterectomy and UAE (the HOPEFUL study) evaluated 972 patients who underwent UAE and found that 18% of UAE-treated patients went on to have additional treatments for their fibroid symptoms, including hysterectomy.[72] As with all uterine sparing procedures, similar rates of recurrence after UAE have been demonstrated in randomized control trials.[66] Nevertheless, economic analysis found that UAE was less expensive than hysterectomy even after the need for additional procedures was factored into the analysis. The authors correctly acknowledge that younger women have a greater risk of developing recurrent fibroids, indicating that UAE may not be cost-effective in younger patient populations.

UAE is a safe and effective uterine-sparing option for patients with symptomatic fibroids. A successful bilateral UAE should effectively treat all fibroids with one procedure. As with all treatments, it requires a thorough patient evaluation and appropriate patient selection to obtain maximal favorable outcomes. UAE is also cost-effective when compared to traditional surgical options.

Magnetic Resonance Imaging–Guided Focused Ultrasound

MRI-guided focused ultrasound (MRgFU) is an ablative technique that uses focused ultrasound energy to produce heat, causing cell death. Real-time MRI is employed to guide the treatment in three-dimensions, allowing for precise targeting of tissues and monitoring of tissue temperature during treatment.[73]

The ultrasound system is composed of multiple elements operating at frequencies in the range of 1.0 to 1.35 MHz. The convergence of multiple ultrasound beams on a single focused point causes heat, leading to protein denaturation and, ultimately, cell death. The advantage of MRgFU is that it is completely noninvasive. There are no skin incisions, allowing patients to have a rapid recovery with very little postprocedure morbidity. The procedure is currently not recommended for patients who desire future fertility and also is limited in its widespread availability due to the high cost of MRI and limited reimbursement. Clinical trials approved by the Food and Drug Administration (FDA) are ongoing.

A prospective study of 91 women with 141 fibroids treated with MRgFU followed over 24 months with the primary endpoint of fibroid volume change and severe symptom scores found that a reduction of about 40% was achievable with improvement in the symptom severity score.[74] The average procedure time was 2 hours, 50 minutes ± 1 hour, 36 minutes, and 82 patients required reintervention of some form over the 24-month follow-up period. A limitation of MRgFU is the variable response seen in fibroids with differing imaging characteristics. Funaki et al. make a distinction in fibroid type based on the pretreatment signal characteristics on MRI. Type 1 fibroids demonstrate T2 signal lower than skeletal muscle. Type 2 fibroids have T2 signal greater than skeletal muscle but signal lower than myometrium, and type 3 have signal greater than the surrounding myometrium. Overall, type 3 fibroids do not respond as well as type 1 or 2 with higher rates of reintervention. The reintervention rate for type 1 or 2 fibroids over 24 months was 14%, whereas the rate was 21.6% for patients with type 3 fibroids.[74] Similar prospective studies have shown high rates of reintervention of around 19% within 6 months of MRgFU treatment.[75]

In summary, MRgFU is a novel noninvasive approach to treat symptomatic fibroids. Its main advantage is an almost nonexistent recovery and minimally invasive approach. Unfortunately, its widespread application is hampered by the limitations of the technique. It is best suited for patients with a single dominant fibroid. The size of the fibroid impacts the length and, subsequently, the cost of the procedure. Certain fibroids show unfavorable response to the treatment and thus a thorough evaluation with a preprocedural MRI is necessary. There are also other limitations. MRgFU cannot be done through abdominal scars due to the deposition of heat in the scar and overlying skin. The technology is currently limited to 15 cm of depth, which may prevent treatment in some morbidly obese patients. Finally, because of the length of time needed to treat a fibroid, patients with large and multiple fibroids are less than ideal candidates.

▌CONCLUSION

There are many treatment options available for patients who suffer from symptomatic uterine fibroids. Choosing the most appropriate treatment plan is based on the individual patient symptoms, her preferences for therapy, and the extent of the fibroids. Patient age, fertility status, fibroid burden, fibroid type and location, imaging characteristics, and desire for uterine preservation must all be taken into consideration.

Asymptomatic patients can safely be followed with periodic assessment of their symptoms. Symptomatic patients should be evaluated for the extent of symptoms and their impact on quality of life. Imaging, such as MRI, should evaluate the location and mass effect of fibroids on the endometrial cavity. In some women, medical therapy may be a good option. Patients with dominant submucosal or pedunculated submuscosal fibroids should be considered for hysteroscopic myomectomy. Patients with multiple fibroids, anemia, and no plans for future fertility are ideal candidates for UAE or hysterectomy.

Patients with fewer fibroids, who seek a uterine sparing procedure, should be considered for myomectomy, particularly those with infertility thought to be related to fibroids. Patients with bulk-related symptoms can be treated with UAE, myomectomy, or hysterectomy depending on realistic goals for intervention. Currently, MRgFU is limited in its availability and may be recommended for patients with no future fertility plans with a few fibroids that meet imaging criteria.

The choices of therapy have dramatically expanded over the past decade and patients can now be active participants in treatment selection. Uterine fibroids can be treated in most cases through minimally invasive means, and a great advance in the care of this common condition.

▌ REFERENCES

1. Wallach EE, Vlahos NF. Uterine myomas: an overview of development, clinical features, and management. *Obstet Gynecol* 2004;104:393–406.
2. Lethaby A, Vollenhoven B. Fibroids (uterine myomatosis, leiomyomas). *Am Fam Physician* 2005;71:1753–1756.
3. Marsh EE, Bulun SE. Steroid hormones and leiomyomas. *Obstet Gynecol Clin North Am* 2006;33:59–67.
4. Stewart EA. Uterine fibroids. *Lancet* 2001;357:293–298.
5. Carlson KJ, Miller BA, Fowler FJ. The Maine Women's Health Study: II, outcomes of nonsurgical management of leiomyomas, abnormal bleeding, and chronic pelvic pain. *Obstet Gynecol* 1994;83:566–572.
6. Friedman AJ, Hoffman DI, Comite F, et al. Treatment of leiomyomata uteri with leuprolide acetate depot: a double-blind, placebo-controlled, multicenter study. The Leuprolide Study Group. *Obstet Gynecol* 1991;77:720–725.
7. Walker CL. Role of hormonal and reproductive factors in the etiology and treatment of uterine leiomyoma. *Recent Prog Horm Res* 2002;57:277–294.
8. Chavez NF, Stewart EA. Medical treatment of uterine fibroids. *Clin Obstet Gynecol* 2001;44:372–384.
9. ACOG Committee on Practice Bulletins-Gynecology. ACOG Practice Bulletin. The use of hormonal contraception in women with coexisting medical conditions. Number 18, July 2000. *Int J Gynaecol Obstet* 2001;75:93–106.
10. Chiaffarino F, Parazzini F, La Vecchia C, et al. Use of oral contraceptives and uterine fibroids: results from a case-control study. *Br J Obstet Gynaecol* 1999;106:857–860.
11. Parazzini F, Negri E, La Vecchia C, et al. Oral contraceptive use and risk of uterine fibroids. *Obstet Gynecol* 1992;79:430–433.
12. Friedman AJ, Thomas PP. Does low-dose combination oral contraceptive use affect uterine size or menstrual flow in premenopausal women with leiomyomas? *Obstet Gynecol* 1995;85:631–635.
13. Grigorieva V, Chen-Mok M, Tarasova M, et al. Use of a levonorgestrel-releasing intrauterine system to treat bleeding related to uterine leiomyomas. *Fertil Steril* 2003;79:1194–1198.
14. Zapata LB, Whiteman MK, Tepper NK, et al. Intrauterine device use among women with uterine fibroids: a systematic review. *Contraception* 2010;82:41–55.
15. Venkatachalam S, Bagratee JS, Moodley J. Medical management of uterine fibroids with medroxyprogesterone acetate (Depo Provera): a pilot study. *J Obstet Gynaecol* 2004;24:798–800.
16. Ishikawa H, Ishi K, Serna VA, et al. Progesterone is essential for maintenance and growth of uterine leiomyoma. *Endocrinology* 2010;151:2433–2442.
17. Cramer SF, Robertson AL, Ziats NP, et al. Growth potential of human uterine leiomyomas: some in vitro observations and their implications. *Obstet Gynecol* 1985;66:36–41.
18. Lobo RA. The risk of stroke in postmenopausal women receiving hormonal therapy. *Climacteric* 2009;12(suppl 1):81–85.
19. Kang JL, Wang DY, Wang XX, et al. Up-regulation of apoptosis by gonadotropin-releasing hormone agonist in cultures of endometrial cells from women with symptomatic myomas. *Hum Reprod* 2010;25:2270–2275.
20. Rutgers JL, Spong CY, Sinow R, et al. Leuprolide acetate treatment and myoma arterial size. *Obstet Gynecol* 1995;86:386–388.
21. Carr BR, Marshburn PB, Weatherall PT, et al. An evaluation of the effect of gonadotropin-releasing hormone analogs and medroxyprogesterone acetate on uterine leiomyomata volume by magnetic resonance imaging: a prospective, randomized, double blind, placebo-controlled, crossover trial. *J Clin Endocrinol Metab* 1993;76:1217–1223.
22. Van Leusden HA. Impact of different GnRH analogs in benign gynecological disorders related to their chemical structure, delivery systems and dose. *Gynecol Endocrinol* 1994;8:215–222.
23. Lethaby A, Vollenhoven B, Sowter M. Pre-operative GnRH analogue therapy before hysterectomy or myomectomy for uterine fibroids. *Cochrane Database Syst Rev* 2000:CD000547.
24. Healy DL, Vollenhoven BJ. The role of GnRH agonists in the treatment of uterine fibroids. *Br J Obstet Gynaecol* 1992;99(suppl 7):23–26.
25. Rackow BW, Arici A. Options for medical treatment of myomas. *Obstet Gynecol Clin North Am* 2006;33:97–113.
26. Carr BR, Breslau NA, Peng N, et al. Effect of gonadotropin-releasing hormone agonist and medroxyprogesterone acetate on calcium metabolism: a prospective, randomized, double-blind, placebo-controlled, crossover trial. *Fertil Steril* 2003;80:1216–1223.
27. Takeuchi H, Kobori H, Kikuchi I, et al. A prospective randomized study comparing endocrinological and clinical effects of two types of GnRH agonists in cases of uterine leiomyomas or endometriosis. *J Obstet Gynaecol Res* 2000;26:325–331.
28. Palomba S, Morelli M, Di Carlo C, et al. Bone metabolism in postmenopausal women who were treated with a gonadotropin-releasing hormone agonist and tibolone. *Fertil Steril* 2002;78:63–68.
29. Palomba S, Orio F, Russo T, et al. Long-term effectiveness and safety of GnRH agonist plus raloxifene administration in women with uterine leiomyomas. *Hum Reprod* 2004;19:1308–1314.
30. Munro MG. Management of heavy menstrual bleeding: is hysterectomy the radical mastectomy of gynecology? *Clin Obstet Gynecol* 2007;50:324–353.
31. Farquhar CM, Steiner CA. Hysterectomy rates in the United States 1990–1997. *Obstet Gynecol* 2002;99:229–234.
32. Carlson KJ, Miller BA, Fowler FJ. The Maine Women's Health Study: I, outcomes of hysterectomy. *Obstet Gynecol* 1994;83:556–565.
33. Kuppermann M, Varner RE, Summitt RL, et al. Effect of hysterectomy vs medical treatment on health-related quality of life and sexual functioning: the medicine or surgery (Ms) randomized trial. *JAMA* 2004;291:1447–1455.
34. Garry R, Fountain J, Mason S, et al. The eVALuate study: two parallel randomised trials, one comparing laparoscopic with abdominal hysterectomy, the other comparing laparoscopic with vaginal hysterectomy. *Br Med J* 2004;328:129.
35. Wu JM, Wechter ME, Geller EJ, et al. Hysterectomy rates in the United States, 2003. *Obstet Gynecol* 2007;110:1091–1095.
36. Unger JB, Paul R, Caldito G. Hysterectomy for the massive leiomyomatous uterus. *Obstet Gynecol* 2002;100:1271–1275.
37. Wattiez A, Cohen SB, Selvaggi L. Laparoscopic hysterectomy. *Curr Opin Obstet Gynecol* 2002;14:417–422.
38. Kramer MG, Reiter RC. Hysterectomy: indications, alternatives and predictors. *Am Fam Physician* 1997;55:827–834.
39. Palmer JR, Rao RS, Adams-Campbell LL, et al. Correlates of hysterectomy among African-American women. *Am J Epidemiol* 1999;150:1309–1315.
40. Sawin SW, Pilevsky ND, Berlin JA, et al. Comparability of perioperative morbidity between abdominal myomectomy and hysterectomy for women with uterine leiomyomas. *Am J Obstet Gynecol* 2000;183:1448–1455.
41. Donnez J, Jadoul P. What are the implications of myomas on fertility? A need for a debate? *Hum Reprod* 2002;17:1424–1430.
42. Kunde K, Cortes E, Seed P, et al. Evaluation of perioperative morbidity associated with single and multiple myomectomy. *J Obstet Gynaecol* 2009;29:737–741.
43. Sesti F, Ticconi C, Bonifacio S, et al. Preoperative administration of recombinant human erythropoietin in patients undergoing gynecologic surgery. *Gynecol Obstet Invest* 2002;54:1–5.
44. Lethaby A, Vollenhoven B, Sowter M. Efficacy of pre-operative gonadotrophin hormone releasing analogues for women with uterine fibroids undergoing hysterectomy or myomectomy: a systematic review. *Br J Obstet Gynaecol* 2002;109:1097–1108.

45. Palomba S, Morelli M, Noia R, et al. Short-term administration of tibolone plus GnRH analog before laparoscopic myomectomy. *J Am Assoc Gynecol Laparosc* 2002;9:170–174.

46. Tulandi T, Murray C, Guralnick M. Adhesion formation and reproductive outcome after myomectomy and second-look laparoscopy. *Obstet Gynecol* 1993;82:213–215.

47. Nezhat C. The "cons" of laparoscopic myomectomy in women who may reproduce in the future. *Int J Fertil Menopausal Stud* 1996;41:280–283.

48. Jin C, Hu Y, Chen XC, et al. Laparoscopic versus open myomectomy—a meta-analysis of randomized controlled trials. *Eur J Obstet Gynecol Reprod Biol* 2009;145:14–21.

49. Luciano AA. Myomectomy. *Clin Obstet Gynecol* 2009;52:362–371.

50. Agdi M, Tulandi T. Endoscopic management of uterine fibroids. *Best Pract Res Clin Obstet Gynaecol* 2008;22:707–716.

51. Amodeo A, Linares Quevedo A, Joseph JV, et al. Robotic laparoscopic surgery: cost and training. *Minerva Urol Nefrol* 2009;61:121–128.

52. Reza M, Maeso S, Blasco JA, et al. Meta-analysis of observational studies on the safety and effectiveness of robotic gynaecological surgery. *Br J Surg* 2010;97:1772–1783.

53. Pritts EA, Parker WH, Olive DL. Fibroids and infertility: an updated systematic review of the evidence. *Fertil Steril* 2009;91:1215–1223.

54. Shokeir T, El-Shafei M, Yousef H, et al. Submucous myomas and their implications in the pregnancy rates of patients with otherwise unexplained primary infertility undergoing hysteroscopic myomectomy: a randomized matched control study. *Fertil Steril* 2010;94:724–729.

55. Polena V, Mergui JL, Perrot N, et al. Long-term results of hysteroscopic myomectomy in 235 patients. *Eur J Obstet Gynecol Reprod Biol* 2007;130:232–237.

56. Cohen LS, Valle RF. Role of vaginal sonography and hysterosonography in the endoscopic treatment of uterine myomas. *Fertil Steril* 2000;73:197–204.

57. Fauconnier A, Chapron C, Babaki-Fard K, et al. Recurrence of leiomyomata after myomectomy. *Hum Reprod Update* 2000;6:595–602.

58. Reed SD, Newton KM, Thompson LB, et al. The incidence of repeat uterine surgery following myomectomy. *J Womens Health* (Larchmt) 2006;15:1046–1052.

59. Hald K, Kløw NE, Qvigstad E, et al. Treatment of uterine myomas with transvaginal uterine artery occlusion: possibilities and limitations. *J Minim Invasive Gynecol* 2008;15:631–635.

60. Liu WM, Ng HT, Wu YC, et al. Laparoscopic bipolar coagulation of uterine vessels: a new method for treating symptomatic fibroids. *Fertil Steril* 2001;75:417–422.

61. Hald K, Noreng HJ, Istre O, et al. Uterine artery embolization versus laparoscopic occlusion of uterine arteries for leiomyomas: long-term results of a randomized comparative trial. *J Vasc Interv Radiol* 2009;20:1303–1310; quiz 1311.

62. Glasser MH, Heinlein PK, Hung YY. Office endometrial ablation with local anesthesia using the HydroThermAblator system: comparison of outcomes in patients with submucous myomas with those with normal cavities in 246 cases performed over 5(1/2) years. *J Minim Invasive Gynecol* 2009;16:700–707.

63. Lethaby A, Shepperd S, Cooke I, et al. Endometrial resection and ablation versus hysterectomy for heavy menstrual bleeding. *Cochrane Database Syst Rev* 2000:CD000329.

64. Goodwin SC, Spies JB, Worthington-Kirsch R, et al. Uterine artery embolization for treatment of leiomyomata: long-term outcomes from the FIBROID Registry. *Obstet Gynecol* 2008;111:22–33.

65. Pinto I, Chimeno P, Romo A, et al. Uterine fibroids: uterine artery embolization versus abdominal hysterectomy for treatment—a prospective, randomized, and controlled clinical trial. *Radiology* 2003;226:425–431.

66. Edwards RD, Moss JG, Lumsden MA, et al. Uterine-artery embolization versus surgery for symptomatic uterine fibroids. *N Engl J Med* 2007;356:360–370.

67. Hehenkamp WJ, Volkers NA, Birnie E, et al. Symptomatic uterine fibroids: treatment with uterine artery embolization or hysterectomy—results from the randomized clinical Embolisation versus Hysterectomy (EMMY) Trial. *Radiology* 2008;246:823–832.

68. Van Voorhis B. A 41-year-old woman with menorrhagia, anemia, and fibroids: review of treatment of uterine fibroids. *JAMA* 2009;301:82–93.

69. Homer H, Saridogan E. Uterine artery embolization for fibroids is associated with an increased risk of miscarriage. *Fertil Steril* 2010;94:324–330.

70. Tropeano G, Di Stasi C, Amoroso S, et al. Long-term effects of uterine fibroid embolization on ovarian reserve: a prospective cohort study. *Fertil Steril* 2010;94:2296–2300.

71. Smeets AJ, Nijenhuis RJ, van Rooij WJ, et al. Uterine artery embolization in patients with a large fibroid burden: long-term clinical and MR follow-up. *Cardiovasc Intervent Radiol* 2010;33:943–948.

72. Hirst A, Dutton S, Wu O, et al. A multi-centre retrospective cohort study comparing the efficacy, safety and cost-effectiveness of hysterectomy and uterine artery embolisation for the treatment of symptomatic uterine fibroids. The HOPEFUL study. *Health Technol Assess* 2008;12:1–248, iii.

73. Hesley GK, Felmlee JP, Gebhart JB, et al. Noninvasive treatment of uterine fibroids: early Mayo Clinic experience with magnetic resonance imaging-guided focused ultrasound. *Mayo Clin Proc* 2006;81:936–942.

74. Funaki K, Fukunishi H, Sawada K. Clinical outcomes of magnetic resonance-guided focused ultrasound surgery for uterine myomas: 24-month follow-up. *Ultrasound Obstet Gynecol* 2009;34:584–589.

75. Marret H, Bleuzen A, Guérin A, et al. French first results using magnetic resonance-guided focused ultrasound for myoma treatment [in French]. *Gynecol Obstet Fertil* 2011;39:12–20.

CHAPTER 23

Uterine Artery Embolization: Indications and Imaging

HOWARD B. CHRISMAN, SABEEN DHAND, and ROBERT L. VOGELZANG

INTRODUCTION

First being reported by Ravina et al.[1] in 1995, uterine artery embolization (UAE) has been a very popular nonsurgical alternative to uterine hysterectomy or myomectomy for symptomatic uterine leiomyomata. Multiple large studies have demonstrated the efficacy in reducing or eliminating major symptoms with success rates approaching up to 90%.[2–11] Given the emphasis on rigorous patient workup and management, UAE takes advantage of the progressive trend of the active clinical role of a radiologist. This chapter focuses on the clinical indications and imaging requirements for patients undergoing UAE.

INDICATIONS

Patient Selection

The primary criteria for patient selection are symptomatic leiomyomata, also referred to as fibroids. Clinical signs and symptoms depend on the size, location, and number of fibroids with the most common clinical presentation being abnormal vaginal bleeding and pelvic pain. Other common bulk symptoms include pelvic pressure, bloating, back pain, and urinary frequency/urgency.[12,13]

Patients often present with a combination of both abnormal bleeding and bulk symptoms. Because many of these symptoms are overall nonspecific and can be caused by a multitude of diseases, proper clinical workup is necessary to confirm a causal relationship of the presenting symptoms to the fibroids alone. Therefore, a thorough medical and physical evaluation is necessary to appropriately select patients for a successful embolization. This includes a detailed general medical history with emphasis on gynecologic details, including pregnancy, pelvic infection, results of Papanicolaou testing, medications, and other coexistent medical conditions. Basic laboratory values, such as a complete blood count, prothrombin times with international normalized ratio, and blood urea nitrogen and/or serum creatinine levels, are recommended, and additional labs should be obtained based on the individual's history.[12]

After a thorough evaluation, imaging is always required to confirm the presence of fibroids, demonstrate viability by enhancement, and exclude other pathology.[12,13] In fact, Omary et al.[14] showed that magnetic resonance imaging (MRI) actually changed the initial diagnoses of interventional radiologists in one in every five patients suspected of having fibroids based on history and physical exam alone while increasing the mean diagnostic confidence of a diagnosis of symptomatic fibroids for the remaining patients by 22%.

After the patient's symptoms can be attributed to leiomyomata, the patient should be informed of all treatment options, ranging from medical therapy, UAE, myomectomy, and hysterectomy,

among others. Finally, before the final scheduling of the UAE, consultation with the treating gynecologist should be performed.

Important Considerations in Patient Selection

Although not the focus of this chapter, adenomyosis is a well-known condition defined as ectopic endometrial glands and stroma within the myometrium with smooth muscle hyperplasia, resulting in enlargement of the uterus (FIGURE 23.1). It is a common condition discovered in the population seeking UAE because the presenting symptoms can mimic that of fibroids. Adenomyosis can be both of the focal or diffuse form. Previously considered a cause of failure, recent literature suggests that UAE may also be an effective treatment with improvement of symptoms in up for 70% of patients with adenomyosis. Even though this success rate is less than the 90% reported at the beginning of this chapter, UAE still offers an attractive alternative to surgery to more than half of the patients with coexistent adenomyosis.[15,16] Therefore, during the patient selection process, it is also important to identify this disease process so that the patient may be well informed of accurate treatment outcomes.

A desire to maintain fertility is a common clinical concern for younger patients. Therefore, an understanding of this patient population is important before offering UAE as an option. The patient whose primary concern is fertility should be directed to a

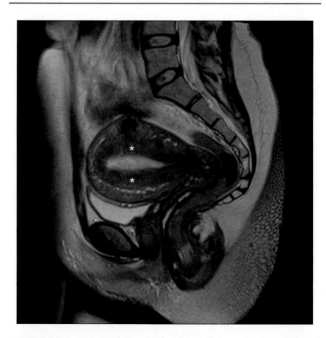

FIGURE 23.1 A sagittal T2-weighted MRI demonstrates a widened junctional zone (*) typical of adenomyosis.

246

fertility specialist. For the young patient whose main concern is symptoms but still wants to maintain possibility of future fertility, embolization should be discussed. In general, most studies and reports have demonstrated uncomplicated deliveries after the procedure.[17–19] In fact, the multicenter ONTARIO trial in 2005 suggested equal outcomes for UAE when compared to alternatives with respect to full-term deliveries but suggested a possible trend to abnormal placentation in those who were treated with embolization.[19] More recently, however, a few studies comparing UAE and myomectomy found superior reproductive outcomes after myomectomy in early follow-up.[20,21] Therefore, at the time of this publication, myomectomy is still considered by some as the standard of care for preserving fertility in the setting of fibroids.[13] Regardless, UAE should still be considered in young patients of reproductive age, especially those who are not good surgical candidates due to other medical problems.

Another commonly encountered patient is one with dominant fibroid disease resulting in uterine size greater than 24 weeks' gestation (FIGURE 23.2). Although this patient population clearly responds to UAE, with uterine volume reductions ranging from 20% to 45%, the baseline size of the uterus does limit outcomes of the procedure because endpoint volumes of large fibroids/uteri are still, in fact, large. This concept can be best described by understanding spherical (or near spherical) volume measurements, calculated by $4/3\pi r^3$. Imagine, for example, a patient with an 18-cm spherical uterus, where the volume is approximately 3,050 cm^3 but a 16-cm sphere has 30% less volume at approximately 2,140 cm^3. Therefore, a patient with abdominal fullness who is undergoing UAE with the expectation of a flat abdomen may well be disappointed if such a large uterus remains. Thus, for an individual patient, decreasing the bulk of a large uterus to a noticeable dimension may be difficult. The limitations of size reduction for this population should be clearly discussed with the patient prior to performing UAE.

Absolute contraindications to UAE include pregnancy and active, untreated infection of the pelvic viscera. Additionally, if leiomyosarcoma or other pelvic malignancy is suspected (FIGURE 23.3), UAE is generally avoided unless the procedure is being performed for palliation or as an adjunct to surgery. As with any other angiographic procedure, relative contraindications include coagulopathy, severe contrast allergy, and renal impairment. Other relative contraindications include immunocompromise, prior pelvic radiation/surgery, or chronic

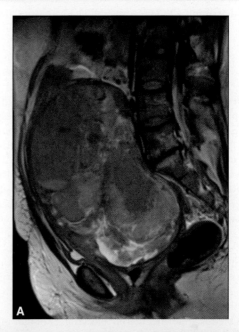
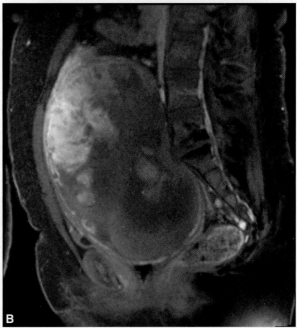

FIGURE 23.3 **A.** A sagittal T2-weighted image demonstrates a markedly enlarged uterus with heterogenous signal, (**B**) with an enhancement pattern not typical of fibroids. The patient had metastatic disease in the chest at the time of this scan, and biopsy confirmed the diagnosis of leiomyosarcoma.

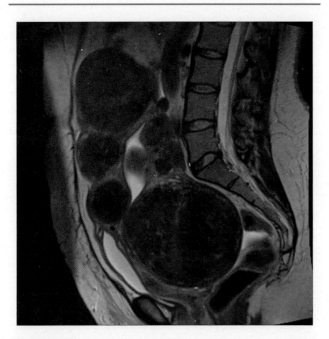

FIGURE 23.2 A sagittal T2-weighted image demonstrates multiple large fibroids, resulting in a massively enlarged uterus at approximately 25 weeks' gestation.

endometritis because these processes can interfere with the postprocedural healing process. Finally, attention to the use of gonadotropin-releasing agonists, such as leuprolide, is important because these agents may cause diffuse vasospasm, limiting the technical success of the embolization.[12,13]

■ IMAGING: BEFORE THE PROCEDURE

As mentioned previously, all patients who are being considered for UAE must undergo confirmatory imaging prior to therapy. In current practice, ultrasound and MRI are widely accepted modalities for determining the presence and characteristics of uterine fibroids.[12,13] Given its extensive availability, ultrasound is a well-accepted, first-line method for many patients.[22–24] In fact, most current gynecologists and other referring physicians use ultrasound as the initial diagnostic test when fibroids are suspected. However, the superior level of soft tissue characterization and less operator-dependency make MRI a much more powerful tool in the pre procedural assessment of uterine leiomyomata, especially for those patients considering embolization. Although some studies find that transvaginal ultrasonography (US) is as effective as MRI in the detection of fibroids,[25] MRI outperforms ultrasound in the evaluation of the location, number, and size of leiomyomas. MRI allows the accurate evaluation of the entire female pelvis for other causes of pain or contraindications to the procedure, increasing a practitioner's diagnostic confidence of treatment success for symptomatic fibroids. Therefore, MRI is now considered the gold standard for preprocedural evaluation for UAE.[14,23,26]

Furthermore, imaging greatly facilitates the practitioner's ability to establish a causal relationship between fibroids and the patient's symptoms. For example, given the relative location to the endometrial cavity, submucosal fibroids are usually responsible for abnormal uterine bleeding, although intramural fibroids can still encroach on the cavity and produce similar symptoms. In contrast, large intramural or subserosal leiomyomas usually result in mass effect upon adjacent organs and nerve plexi, resulting in symptoms of pain, urinary frequency, urgency, or constipation.[23,27]

The fibroid location type also plays a significant role in patient selection. It has been suggested that owing to preferential vascular flow to the inner aspects of the uterus, submucosal fibroids respond to embolization of the uterine vasculature better than intramural or subserosal fibroids.[28,29,36] Careful consideration has to be given to large submucosal fibroids, however, because treatment of these types of fibroids with UAE may result in increased sloughing, prolonged discharge, and infection.[30] Another example includes pedunculated fibroids with an attachment point measuring less than half the diameter of the fibroid itself, which after embolization can undergo stalk infarction with risk of detachment of the fibroid mass into the peritoneum (FIGURE 23.4).[31] Other limited data also suggest a higher incidence of collateral supply from neighboring structures, such as the ovaries, to pedunculated fibroids, also limiting the success of the procedure.[32]

Ultrasound

On ultrasound, fibroids appear as well-defined, hypoechoic masses in the uterus with relatively poor through acoustic transmission (FIGURE 23.5). Focal or generalized uterine enlargement, a lobulated uterine wall contour, and disruption of the endometrial lining are common additional findings but vary with the location the fibroids. Calcification frequently develops within

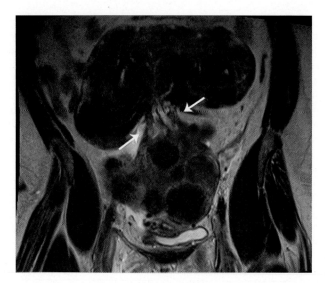

FIGURE 23.4 A T2-weighted coronal image of the uterus demonstrates a large pedunculated fibroid arising from the superior aspect of a fibroid uterus from a discrete stalk measuring approximately 4 cm (*arrows*).

a fibroid as a result of degeneration, necrosis, or hemorrhage (FIGURE 23.6). To better evaluate the extent of disease, additional techniques can also be used, including pelvic ultrasound, with its higher detail to delineate the location of the fibroids, and sonohysterography, which aids in differentiating submucosal fibroids from endometrial polyps.[23] Other, less widely used techniques are Doppler flow, as McLucas et al.[33] have shown, that a high peak systolic velocity of the uterine artery (>64 cm per second) prior to embolization to be a significant predictor of UAE failure.

Ultrasound may also be helpful in identifying other pelvic pathology. Careful attention to the above-mentioned contraindications, such as adnexal masses, malignancy, or pregnancy, is inherently dependent on the technical skills of the sonographer. One should always keep in mind the possibility of coexistent adenomyosis, which may appear as overall decreased or heterogeneous echogenicity of the uterus caused by the tiny irregular cystic spaces in the myometrium, ill-defined or heterogeneous echotexture of the myometrium, and a lobular or asymmetrically

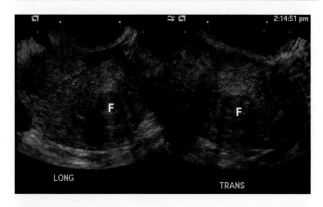

FIGURE 23.5 Sagittal (or longitudinal) and transverse endovaginal ultrasound demonstrate a hypoechoic mass within the uterus with poor acoustic transmission typical of a fibroid (*F*).

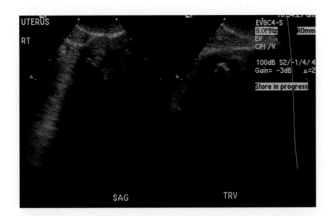

FIGURE 23.6 Sagittal and transverse endovaginal ultrasound demonstrating a heavily calcified fibroid.

enlarged uterus. At the author's institution, however, we generally find ultrasound to be of little or no value in prospectively identifying adenomyosis; over the past 15 years, we have evaluated well over 5,000 patients for UAE and cannot recall any in whom ultrasound made the initial diagnosis of adenomyosis. Other findings include apparent widening of the endometrium or poor definition of the endomyometrial junction, which are more clearly defined on transvaginal sonography (FIGURE 23.7).[23,34,35]

Preprocedural: Magnetic Resonance Imaging

Nondegenerated uterine leiomyomas are usually well-circumscribed and have a homogeneously decreased signal intensity on T2-weighted images compared with the outer myometrium and are isointense on T1-weighted images relative to the myometrium (FIGURES 23.8A and B). The tumors typically demonstrate significant contrast enhancement compared with normal myometrium, related to their high vascularity, making embolization such an effective treatment (FIGURE 23.8C).[36]

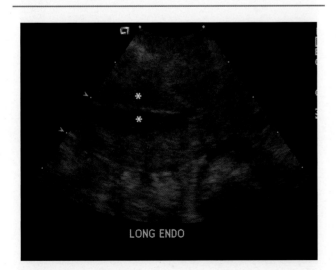

FIGURE 23.7 A longitudinal view of the uterus with endovaginal ultrasound demonstrating an apparent widening of the endometrium or poor definition of the endomyometrial junction (*), compatible with adenomyosis.

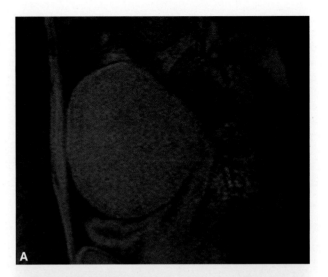

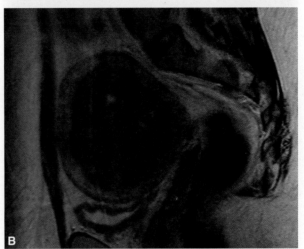

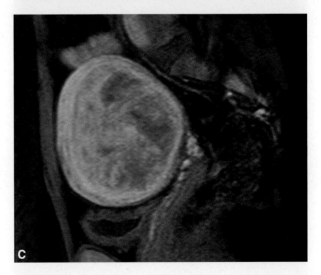

FIGURE 23.8 A. A sagittal T1-weighted image demonstrates an enlarged, lobulated uterine fundus secondary to an isointense mass that is difficult to distinguish from normal myometrium. **B.** A sagittal T2-weighted image at the same position demonstrates this mass to have decreased T2 signal typical of a fibroid. **C.** Contrast-enhanced MRI at the same position confirms that this fibroid enhances heterogenously.

It is important to keep in mind that leiomyomas can also have a variable appearance depending on the presence of a cellular-type leiomyoma and degeneration. Cellular-type leiomyomas demonstrate higher T2 signal intensity as a result of more compact smooth muscle cells with little to no collagen (FIGURE 23.9). Leiomyomas with hyaline and calcified degeneration demonstrate similar low T2 signal as nondegenerated fibroids, but those with cystic and myxoid degeneration will demonstrate high T2 signal intensity with little or no

enhancement in the degenerated regions (FIGURES 23.10 and 23.11). Fibroids with hemorrhage are the most variable, often with diffuse or peripheral high signal on T1-weighted images, and variable signal intensity with or without a low-signal intensity rim on T2-weighted images (FIGURES 23.12A and B). [24,36–38,48] Hemorrhagic fibroids typically do not demonstrate enhancement secondary to the loss of blood supply, subsequently resulting in a poor response to UAE (FIGURE 23.12C). [37–39] The opposite is true for a fibroid with high intrinsic T2 signal because the increased cellularity and vascularity within these fibroids characteristically respond well to embolization. [37–39]

Again not the focus of this chapter, but important to keep in mind when reviewing imaging for fibroids, is adenomyosis

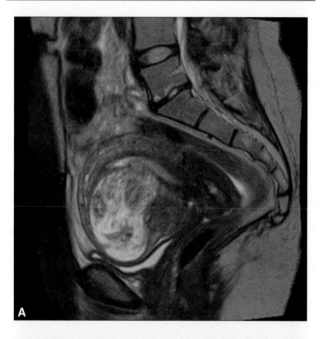

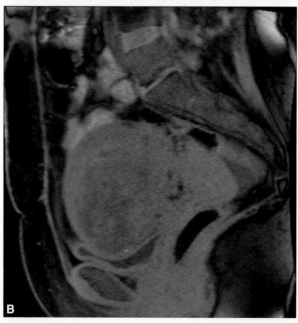

FIGURE 23.9 A. A sagittal T2-weighted image of the uterus demonstrates higher intrinsic T2 signal typical of a cellular fibroid. B. T1-weighted MRI at the same position show expected low signal in the regions of T2 hyperintensity.

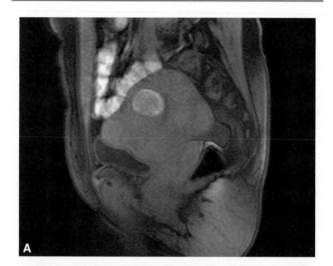

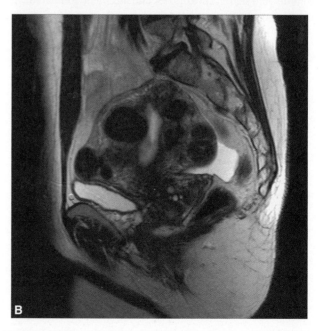

FIGURE 23.10 A. Sagittal T1-weighted images through the uterus demonstrate high signal characteristic of calcification. B. The high signal corresponds to a diffusely low T2 signal on the T2-weighted sequence, confirming a calcified fibroid.

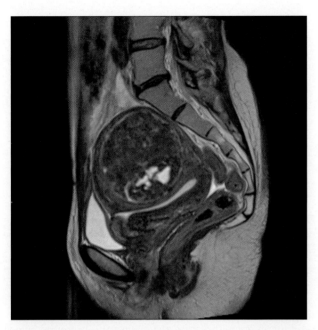

FIGURE 23.11 A sagittal T2-weighted image of the uterus demonstrates several areas of high T2 signal intensity within the postero-inferior aspect of a round T2 hypointense mass, compatible with a cystic fibroid.

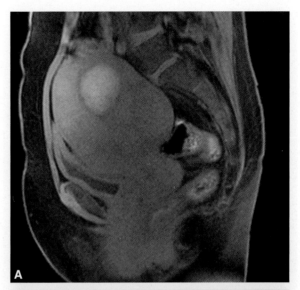

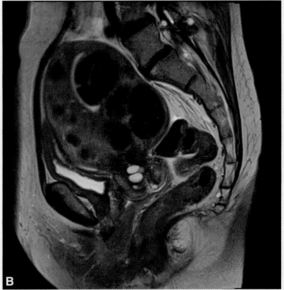

(FIGURE 23.13). Adenomyosis is diagnosed on MR by the presence of low signal on T2-weighted imaging, producing a focal or diffuse widening of the junctional zone with a thickness greater than 12 mm, increasing the accuracy of diagnosis. Several T2 bright foci in the myometrium can be seen and correspond to heterotropic endometrial tissue, cystic dilatation of glands, or hemorrhagic foci. Linear striations of hyperintensity on T2-weighted images represent invasion of the endometrium into the myometrium and can sometimes result in a pseudowidening of the endometrium.[34]

▍IMAGING: AFTER THE PROCEDURE

According to the most recent care guidelines by the Task Force on UAE and the Standards Division of the Society of Interventional Radiology, follow-up imaging is indicated 3 to 6 months after the procedure to quantify fibroid infarction by volume reduction of both the uterus and treated fibroids (commonly calculated by the ellipse formula: length × width × depth × 0.5233).[12] Short- and long-term complications of the procedure have been well described, and imaging provides a method for the early detection and assessment of these unforeseen circumstances. Additionally, sequential follow-up postprocedural imaging allows the ability to determine increase in baseline leiomyoma volume, which can indicate leiomyosarcoma.[12]

Expected reductions in volume are approximately 40% for uterine volume and up to 70% for dominant fibroids. The majority of volume reduction occurs within a 6-month period following embolization with even further reduction occurring 6 to 12 months.[1,6,19,40–44] Therefore, at most institutions, routine follow-up imaging is performed at 3 and 6 months for an accurate gauge of response to therapy.

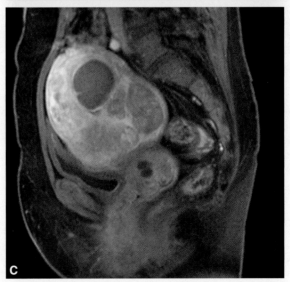

FIGURE 23.12 A–C. Sagittal T1-, T2-, and contrast-enhanced images of the uterus demonstrates a hemorrhagic fibroid that does not enhance.

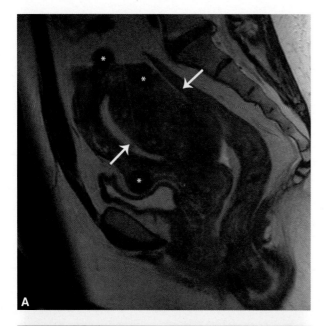

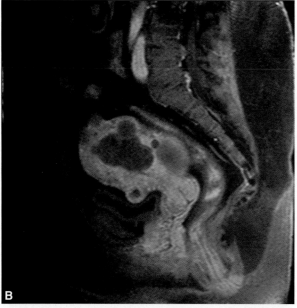

FIGURE 23.13 A. A sagittal T2-weighted image of the uterus demonstrates a focal region of junction zonal widening with foci of T2 hyperintensity typical of focal adenomyosis (*arrows*). The T2 hypointense masses are fibroids that are present concurrently with focal adenomyosis (*denote a few of the several fibroids present on the selected image). **B.** Postembolization, contrast-enhanced T1-weighted sequence demonstrates successful treatment of the fibroids and the region of tissue previously affected by focal adenomyosis.

Postprocedural Ultrasound

Embolic agents may be seen within the uterine arteries immediately following embolization, usually as echogenic areas within a clot in the embolized arteries. In contrast, fibroids have a varied and complex sonographic appearance after embolization. The majority of fibroids show a heterogeneous increase in echogenicity, although for some, there may be a decrease in

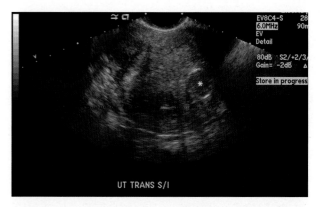

FIGURE 23.14 Postembolization sonography of the uterus demonstrates a peripherally calcified, degenerated fibroid known as the "fetal head sign."

echogenicity.[23,45] As early as 1 month following embolization, air may fill potential spaces left by tissue infarction and desiccation, resulting in gas with "dirty" shadowing on ultrasound, which can be confused with infection in the absence of any history.[23]

At 6 months to 1 year following embolization, a hyperechoic rim around an increasingly hypoechoic fibroid is frequently referred to as the "fetal head sign" and represents peripheral calcification (FIGURE 23.14). This peripheral location of calcification differs from that of the dystrophic calcification that may be seen centrally with natural degeneration of fibroids described earlier.[23,46] On color Doppler flow, there is an expected decrease in the blood flow to fibroids after embolization, but the perifibroid vascularity usually remains patient after embolization.[47]

Postprocedural Magnetic Resonance Imaging

Fortunately, fibroids have a much more common imaging pattern on postembolization MRI follow-up. Just hours after the procedure, fibroids demonstrated increased T2-weighted signal and decreased delineation between the tumor and myometrium secondary to edema. Contrast-enhanced images will show an immediate reduction of blood flow to both the treated fibroid and adjacent myometrium.[48,49] Just after 3 days, however, there is reperfusion to the myometrium and progressive increase of signal intensity on T1-weighted MR images and decrease of signal intensity on T2-weighted images after embolization. This combination of T1 hyperintensity and T2 hypointensity are typical of blood products from expected hemorrhagic infarction and often referred to as a "bag of blood products" by some diagnosticians (FIGURE 23.15).[24,37,38,48]

The initial volume reduction that occurs after embolization may mask residual viable tissue that may still grow, and additional collateral arterial supply or arterial spasm resulting in inadequate embolization may result in areas of residual perfusion to the tumor.[50] Therefore, volume measurements alone are not adequate to assess long-term outcome of the procedure, and administration of contrast provides additional information to quantify the amount of residual perfusion. Residual perfusion can be calculated by taking the volume of enhancing tissue relative to the total volume of the fibroid. Pelage et al.[50] showed that 60% of patients with fibroids demonstrating more than 10% of residual perfusion on follow-up imaging had continued growth

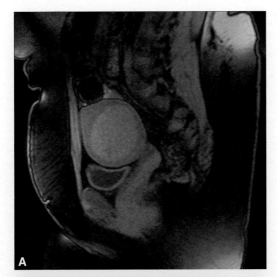

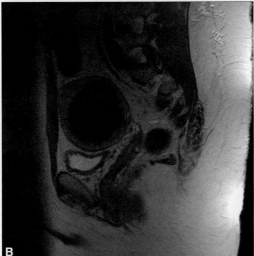

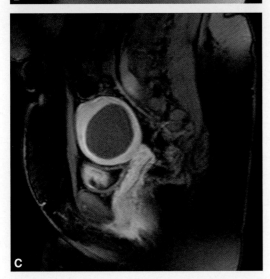

FIGURE 23.15 Approximately 3 months after embolization of the patient shown in FIGURE 23.8 demonstrates (**A**) increased T1 signal; (**B**) decreased T2 signal; and (**C**) no residual perfusion on the contrast-enhanced images typical of a "bag of blood products" seen in a technically successful embolization. The overall volume of the degenerating fibroid has also decreased in size.

of leiomyomas and were symptomatic 3 years after the procedure. The study also revealed that all patients whose fibroids had less than 10% residual perfusion (referred to as complete infarction) were found to have persistent minimal to no perfusion after the 3-year study period. Therefore, determining residual perfusion on follow-up imaging is currently the best prognostic factor in determining successful long-term embolization outcome.

IMAGING OF COMPLICATIONS

Although rare, there are a number of known complications associated with UAE. They include nonspecific periprocedural conditions, such as hematoma, pseudoaneurysm, arteriovenous fistula, as well as other major, specific complications including ovarian dysfunction, passage of fibroids, infection of necrotic fibroids and/or the uterus, uterine ischemia, and even death.[51] Fortunately, imaging aids in the early diagnosis of many of these conditions and the imaging appearance of a selected few are discussed in this section.

Because there is no specific arterial supply to a fibroid, it is expected that a small degree of uterine ischemia occurs in all UAEs, although the ischemia is usually neither severe nor long lasting.[52] There have been a few reports of diffuse uterine necrosis following embolization.[53–55] In a pathologically proven report of uterine necrosis following UAE, an MRI performed less than 24 hours after the procedure revealed a homogeneously dark uterus on T1-weighted images and diffuse nonenhancement of the uterus after contrast enhancement. This was related to global hypoperfusion, which was greater than expected for an uncomplicated embolization.[53]

There has been a reported rate of up to 3% for transcervical expulsion of fibroids.[56–58] There is a greater risk of fibroid passage for fibroids that are in contact with the endometrial surface.[51] In patients who present with persistent uterine contractions, pain, or heavy vaginal bleeding following embolization, ultrasound is a helpful, quick, and low-cost method to examine the pelvis, although in clinical practice we find that MR reveals far more information than ultrasound. Depending on the time course of the expulsion, sonography can demonstrate a heterogeneous to hypoechoic mass within the endometrial canal.[23] On MRI, a T1 hyperintense, T2 hypointense fibroid can be identified distending the endometrium canal and often dilating the cervix (FIGURE 23.16). Cervical extension of fibroid fragments should be particularly noted because this finding is often associated with endometritis and may require careful clinical observation and initiation of antibiotics. Contrast-enhanced MRI is especially useful to demonstrate any viable attachment to the uterine wall.[51] Occasionally, resection under hysteroscopy or dilatation and curettage is required for those that remain partially attached to the wall.

Finally, another uncommon complication of embolization includes infection, such as endometritis, with prevalence of up to 2% to 3%.[27,44,56,59] The sonographic appearance of endometritis may be normal, but findings may also include an enlarged uterus with thickened, heterogenous endometrium, which may even have fluid within the endometrial canal or gas within the myometrium. On MRI, the uterus will be enlarged and demonstrate high T1 signal fluid representing intracavitary hematoma. Foci of T1- and T2 signal voids are compatible with gas secondary to gas-forming organisms (FIGURE 23.17).[51] In contrast to diffuse uterine infection, a rare postembolization complication includes a necrotic, infected fibroid, known as a pyomyoma.[44]

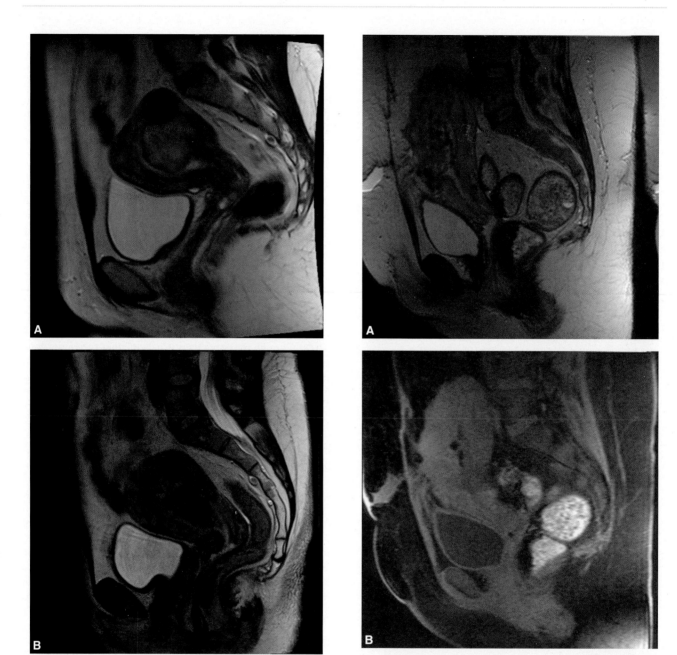

FIGURE 23.16 A. A sagittal T2-weighted image demonstrates an intrinsically high T2 intense fibroid before embolization. **B.** A few months after embolization, the fibroid is noted within the endometrial canal approximating the proximal cervical canal.

FIGURE 23.17 A and **B.** Sagittal T2- and T1-weighted images demonstrate signal voids compatible with air, and the T2-weighted sequence shows high signal within the canal consistent with fluid in expected endometritis.

The sonographic appearance of pyomyomas includes nonspecific findings, such as internal echoes and reverberation artifact from foci of air.[51] In a recent report of a large pyomyoma, MR findings included a multiseptated cystic mass with some solid enhancing components as well as normal uterine morphology, simulating a mucinous cystadenocarcinoma.[60] In that case, the authors used F18-2-deoxyglucose (FDG) positron emission tomography (PET) to exclude malignancy based on the tumors' only mild metabolic activity. Given the rare occurrence of such large pyomyomas, there is limited evidence available currently on the diagnostic value of molecular imaging in these specific cases.

▌ REFERENCES

1. Ravina JH, Herbreteau D, Ciraru-Vigneron N, et al. Arterial embolisation to treat uterine myomata. *Lancet* 1995;346:671–672.
2. Goodwin SC, Spies JB, Worthington-Kirsch R, et al. Uterine artery embolization for treatment of leiomyomata: long-term outcomes from the FIBROID registry. *Obstet Gynecol* 2008;111:22–33.
3. Bradley E, Reidy J, Forman R, et al. Transcatheter uterine artery embolisation to treat large uterine fibroids. *Br J Obstet Gynaecol* 1998;105:235–240.
4. Worthington-Kirsch RL, Popky GL, Hutchins FL. Uterine arterial embolization for the management of leiomyomas: quality-of-life assessment and clinical response. *Radiology* 1998;208:625–629.
5. Goodwin SG, McLucas B, Lee M, et al. Uterine artery embolization for the treatment of uterine leiomyomata: midterm results. *J Vasc Interv Radiol* 1999;10:1159–1165.

6. Spies JB, Scialli AR, Jha RC, et al. Initial results from uterine fibroid embolization for symptomatic leiomyomata. *J Vasc Interv Radiol* 1999;10:1149–1157.

7. Hutchins FL Jr, Worthington-Kirsch RL, Berkowitz RP. Selective uterine artery embolization as primary treatment for symptomatic leiomyomata uteri. *J Am Assoc Gynecol Laparosc* 1999;6:279–284.

8. Walker WJ, Green A, Sutton C. Bilateral uterine artery embolisation for myomata—results, complications and failures. *Min Invas Ther Allied Technol* 1999;8:449–454.

9. Pelage JP, Le Dref O, Soyer P, et al. Fibroid-related menorrhagia: treatment with superselective embolization of the uterine arteries and mid-term follow-up. *Radiology* 2000;215:428–431.

10. Brunereau L, Herbreteau D, Gallas S, et al. Uterine artery embolization in the primary treatment of leiomyomas. *AJR Am J Roentgenol* 2000;175:1267–1272.

11. Andersen PE, Lund N, Justesen P, et al. Uterine artery embolization of symptomatic uterine fibroids. *Acta Radiol* 2001;42:234–238.

12. Andrews RT, Spies JB, Sacks D, et al. Patient care and uterine artery embolization for leiomyomata. *J Vasc Interv Radiol* 2009;20:S307–S311.

13. Stokes LS, Michael JW, Godwin RB. Quality improvement guidelines for uterine artery embolization for symptomatic leiomyomas. *J Vasc Interv Radiol* 2010;21:1153–1163.

14. Omary RA, Vasireddy S, Chrisman HB, et al. The effect of pelvic MR imaging on the diagnosis and treatment of women with presumed symptomatic uterine fibroids. *J Vasc Interv Radiol* 2002;13:1149–1153.

15. Lohle PNM, De Vries J, Klazen CAH, et al. Uterine artery embolization for symptomatic adenomyosis with or without uterine leiomyomas with the use of calibrated trisacryl gelatin microspheres: midterm clinical and MR imaging follow-up. *J Vasc Interv Radiol* 2007;18:835–841.

16. Goldberg J. Uterine artery embolization for adenomyosis: looking at the glass half full [letter]. *Radiology* 2005;236:1111–1112.

17. Holub Z, Mara M, Kuzel D, et al. Pregnancy outcomes after uterine artery occlusion: prospective multicentric study. *Fertil Steril* 2008;90:1886–1891.

18. Walker WJ, McDowell SJ. Pregnancy after uterine embolization for leiomyomata: a series of 56 completed pregnancies. *Am J Obstet Gynecol* 2006;195:1266–1271.

19. Pron G, Mocarski E, Bennett J, et al. Pregnancy after uterine artery embolization for leiomyomata: the Ontario multicenter trial. *Obstet Gynecol* 2005;105(1):67–76.

20. Usadi R, Marshburn PB. The impact of uterine artery embolization on fertility and pregnancy outcome. *Curr Opin Obstet Gynecol* 2007;19:279–283.

21. Goldberg J, Pereira L. Pregnancy outcomes following treatment for fibroids: uterine fibroid embolization versus laparoscopic myomectomy. *Curr Opin Obstet Gynecol* 2006;18:402–406.

22. Tranquart F, Brunereau L, Cottier JP, et al. Prospective sonographic assessment of uterine artery embolization for the treatment of fibroids. *Ultrasound Obstet Gynecol* 2002;19:81–87.

23. Ghai S, Dheeraj RK, Benjmain MS, et al. Uterine artery embolization for leiomyomas: pre- and postprocedural evaluation with US. *Radiographics* 2005;25:1159–1176.

24. Vedantham S, Sterling KM, Goodwin DC, et al. Uterine fibroid embolization: preprocedural assessment. *Tech Vasc Interv Radiol* 2002;5(1):2–16.

25. Dueholm M, Lundorf E, Hansen ES, et al. Accuracy of magnetic resonance imaging and transvaginal ultrasonography in the diagnosis, mapping, and measurement of uterine myomas. *Am J Obstet Gynecol* 2002;186:409–415.

26. Ascher SM, Arnold LL, Patt RH, et al. Adenomyosis: prospective comparison of MR imaging and transvaginal sonography. *Radiology* 1994;190:803–806.

27. Hovsepian DM, Siskin GP, Bonn J, et al. Quality improvement guidelines for uterine artery embolization for symptomatic leiomyomata. *J Vasc Interv Radiol* 2009;20:S193–S199.

28. Aziz A, Petrucco OSM, Makinoda S, et al. Transarterial embolization of the uterine arteries: patient reactions and effects on uterine vasculature. *Acta Obstet Gynecol Scand* 1998;77:334–340.

29. Sampson J. The blood supply of uterine myomata. *Surg Gynecol Obstet* 1912;14:215.

30. Verma SK, Bergin D, Gonsalves CF, et al. Submucosal fibroids becoming endocavitary following uterine artery embolization: risk assessment by MRI. *AJR Am J Roentgenol* 2008;190:1220–1226.

31. Goodwin SC, Wong GC. Uterine artery embolization for uterine fibroids: a radiologist's perspective. *Clin Obstet Gynecol* 2001;44:412–424.

32. Nikolic B, Spies JB, Abbara S, et al. Ovarian artery supply of uterine fibroids as a cause of treatment failure after uterine artery embolization: a case report. *J Vasc Interv Radiol* 1999;10:1167–1170.

33. McLucas B, Perrella R, Goodwin S, et al. Role of uterine artery Doppler flow in fibroid embolization. *J Ultrasound Med* 2002;21:113–120.

34. Reinhold C, Tafazoli F, Mehio A, et al. Uterine adenomyosis: endovaginal US and MR imaging features with histopathologic correlation. *Radiographics* 1999;19(spec no):S147–S160.

35. Atri M, Reinhold C, Mehio AR, et al. Adenomyosis: US features with histologic correlation in an in vitro study. *Radiology* 2000;215:783–790.

36. Murase E, Siegelman ES, Outwater EK, et al. Uterine leiomyomas: histopathologic features, MR imaging findings, differential diagnosis, and treatment. *Radiographics* 1999;19:1179–1197.

37. Jha RC, Ascher SM, Imaoka I, et al. Symptomatic fibroleiomyomata: MR imaging of the uterus before and after uterine arterial embolization. *Radiology* 2000;217:228–235.

38. Burn PR, McCall JM, Chinn RJ, et al. Uterine fibroleiomyoma: MR imaging appearances before and after embolization of uterine arteries. *Radiology* 2000;214:729–734.

39. Yamashita Y, Torashima M, Takahashi M, et al. Hyperintense uterine leiomyoma at T2-weighted MR imaging: differentiation with dynamic enhanced MR imaging and clinical implications. *Radiology* 1993;189:721–725.

40. Goodwin SC, Vedantham S, McLucas B, et al. Preliminary experience with uterine artery embolization for uterine fibroids. *J Vasc Interv Radiol* 1997;8:517–526.

41. Bradley EA, Reidy JF, Forman RG, et al. Transcatheter uterine artery embolisation to treat large uterine fibroids. *Br J Obstet Gynaecol* 1998;105:231–234.

42. Worthington-Kirsch RL, Hutchins FL,

43. Popky GL. Uterine artery embolization for the management of symptomatic fibroids: current experience with 125 patients with follow-up of up to one year [abstract]. *Radiology* 1998;206:575.

44. Walker WJ, Pelage JP. Uterine artery embolisation for symptomatic fibroids: clinical results in 400 women with imaging follow up. *Br J Obstet Gynaecol* 2002;109:1262–1272.

45. Weintraub JL, Romano WJ, Krisch MJ, et al. Uterine artery embolization: sonographic imaging findings. *J Ultrasound Med* 2002;21:633–637.

46. Nicholson TA, Pelage JP, Ettles DF. Fibroid calcification after uterine artery embolization: ultrasonographic appearance and pathology. *J Vasc Interv Radiol* 2001;12:443–446.

47. Tranquart F, Brunerear L, Cottier JP, et al. Prospective sonographic assessment of uterine artery embolization for the treatment of fibroids. *Ultrasound Obstet Gynecol* 2002;19:81–87.

48. Kroncke TJ. Imaging before and after uterine artery embolization [in German]. *Radiologe* 2008;48(7):639–648.

49. deSouza NM, Williams AD. Uterine arterial embolization for leiomyomas: perfusion and volume changes at MR imaging and relation to clinical outcome. *Radiology* 2002;222:367–374.

50. Pelage JP, Guaou Guaou N, Jha RC, et al. Uterine fibroid tumors: long-term MR imaging outcome after embolization. *Radiology* 2004;230:803–809.

51. Kitamura Y, Ascher S, Cooper C, et al. Imaging manifestations of complications associated with uterine artery embolization. *Radiographics* 2005;25:S119–S132.

52. Sterling KM, Volgelzang RL, Chrisman HB, et al. V. Uterine fibroid embolization: management of complications. *Tech Vasc Interv Radiol* 2002;5:56–66.

53. Gabriel H, Pinto CM, Kumar M, et al. MRI detection of uterine necrosis after uterine artery embolization for fibroids. *AJR Am J Roentgenol* 2004;183:733–736.

54. Godfrey CD, Zbella EA. Uterine necrosis after uterine artery embolization for leiomyoma. *Obstet Gynecol* 2001;98:950–952.

55. Cottier JP, Fignon A, Tranquart F, et al. Uterine necrosis after arterial embolization for postpartum hemorrhage. *Obstet Gynecol* 2002;100:1074–1077.

56. Spies JB, Spector A, Roth AR, et al. Complications after uterine artery embolization for leiomyomas. *Obstet Gynecol* 2002;100:873–880.

57. Laverge F, D'Angelo A, Davies NJ, et al. Spontaneous expulsion of three large fibroids after uterine artery embolization. *Fertil Steril* 2003;80:450–452.

58. Abbara S, Spies JB, Scialli AR, et al. Transcervical expulsion of a fibroid as a result of uterine artery embolization for leiomyomata. *J Vasc Interv Radiol* 1999;10:409–411.

59. Fedele L, Bianchi S, Dorta M, et al. Transvaginal ultrasonography versus hysteroscopy in the diagnosis of uterine submucous myomas. *Obstet Gynecol* 1991;77:745–748.

60. Lee SR, Kim BS, Moon HS. Magnetic resonance imaging and positron emission tomography of a giant multiseptated pyomyoma simulating an ovarian cancer. *Fertil Steril* 2010;94:1900–1902.

Uterine Artery Embolization for Symptomatic Fibroids: Clinical Presentation, Techniques, and Management

DOUGLAS B. YIM, DARREN D. KIES, and HYUN S. KIM

INTRODUCTION

Uterine fibroids (leiomyomas) are common benign tumors present in women typically of childbearing age. One study has shown age-related prevalence of uterine fibroids to be 4% in women 20 to 30 years of age, 11% to 18% in women 30 to 40 years of age, and 33% in women 40 to 60 years of age based on ultrasound detection.[1] In general, as women grow older, many will develop uterine fibroids. Depending on the population studied or the diagnostic method used, as many as 77% of women are diagnosed with uterine leiomyomas.[1,2] Fortunately, most of these women are asymptomatic and no treatment is needed. Up to 30% can present with significant morbidity, however, such that they will go on to have a hysterectomy by age 60 at an annual cost to the U.S. health care system of $1.2 billion.[3,4]

In 1995, a novel application of a minimally invasive technique called uterine fibroid embolization (UFE) was first described in France as a primary treatment for managing the symptoms associated with uterine fibroids.[5] Awareness of this initial European experience made its way to the United States, and U.S. investigators published their results in 1997.[6] Eventually, considerable interest by interventional radiologists and then gynecologists gained momentum, such that now UFE is a well-accepted, safe alternative to surgery for the treatment of symptomatic uterine fibroids, endorsed by both the Society of Interventional Radiology (SIR) and the American College of Obstetrics and Gynecology (ACOG).[7]

Although the equipment and techniques used for UFE are very familiar to most interventional radiologists, the preprocedural workup may be less familiar. Despite the high prevalence of uterine fibroids among women, most are asymptomatic and their fibroids are only found incidentally on a routine gynecologic exam and ultrasound. These patients may present to the practitioner's office looking for treatment options despite their lack of symptoms just because they were told they had fibroids. Therefore, appropriate patient selection becomes important to achieve the desired outcomes. Because many options, both surgical and nonsurgical, are available, a clear idea of the indications for offering UFE will allow the interventionalist to help guide the patient to achieve her desired goal. This is particularly important becasue there are no well-established guidelines for patient selection due to the lack of long-term comparative outcomes for the various therapies.[8]

The symptoms related to uterine fibroids can be categorized into either those related to menstrual irregularities or to bulk symptoms. Severe menorrhagia is the most common symptom that brings a patient into the practitioner's office for consultation. The patient may also suffer from menometrorrhagia, metrorrhagia, and dymenorrhea. She may complain of fatigue secondary to the resultant iron deficiency anemia. While obtaining a detailed menstrual history, it becomes apparent the tremendous lifestyle challenges patients experience with heavy menstrual bleeding, requiring frequent changing of pads and tampons, as often as every 2 hours, for several days during their cycle. This becomes very problematic for women in the modern workplace. So the negative impact on lifestyle alone should be enough to undertake UFE, especially because this procedure is well suited for treating menorrhagia. The lack of iron deficiency anemia should not be an exclusion criterion for treatment because many women treat this effectively with iron supplementation.

The second most common set of complaints are those related to bulk symptoms from large fibroids (FIGURE 24.1). From sheer uterine mass effect, the patient may experience pelvic pressure, bloating, heaviness, and dull ache made worse with exercise, bending over, or sexual intercourse. Large fibroids may also cause rectal pressure and pain with associated feelings of urgency to have a bowel movement (FIGURE 24.2). The patient may complain of urinary frequency, urgency, nocturia, and occasional incontinence. Sometimes the enlarged uterus may exert mass effect on the ureters, causing asymptomatic hydronephrosis.

Apart from clinical symptoms, the size, location, and vascularity of the fibroids characterized on magnetic resonance imaging (MRI) play an important role in proper patient selection. Typically, well-vascularized fibroids and those with a uterus less than 20 weeks' size have the greatest degree of fibroid shrinkage (FIGURES 24.3A and B). Some advocate not treating patients with a uterus greater than 24 weeks' size because, at best, embolization achieves 40% to 70% volume loss and this may not be enough to reduce the bulk symptoms in this subset of patients.[9–11] Furthermore, the location of the fibroids is a consideration in properly selecting patients for UFE, because there is evidence in the literature suggesting that the location of fibroids may impact successful treatment outcome.[12]

Having a clear idea of the indications also means having a clear idea of the contraindications to UFE such that poor

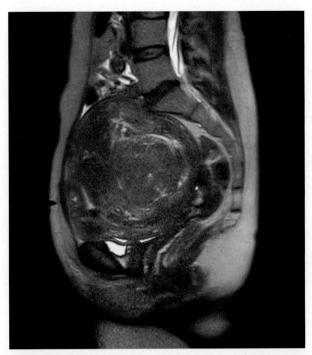

FIGURE 24.1 T2 Sag MRI shows a very large intramural fibroid occupying most of the pelvis.

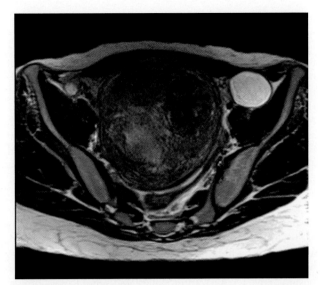

FIGURE 24.2 T2 Axial image shows the same fibroid with significant mass effect upon the rectum.

outcomes and poor patient satisfaction are minimized. UFE is contraindicated for patients who are pregnant or have suspected pregnancy. Until further data are accumulated, the desire for future fertility is also a contraindication. Any suspicion for malignancy as a cause of the patients' symptoms, such as endometrial cancer, is a contraindication to embolization. This would require further investigation, preferably by a gynecologist, with an endometrial biopsy and/or a hysteroscopy.

Adenomyosis can mimic the symptoms of fibroids exactly and may even present itself on examination as a uterine mass caused by a palpable adenomyoma.[13] Few reports have described short-term efficacy with uterine artery embolization in treating adenomyosis; however, no long-term data exist and currently embolization is not indicated in treating the symptoms caused by adenomyosis.[14] An abnormal adnexal mass on physical exam or imaging obviously requires further investigation to rule out malignancy before embarking on UFE. Sometimes, the question of malignancy is not clear by imaging with either ultrasound or MRI. Changes within a leiomyoma caused by benign hyaline or hemorrhagic degeneration may show suspicious signal characteristics on MRI indistinguishable from malignant

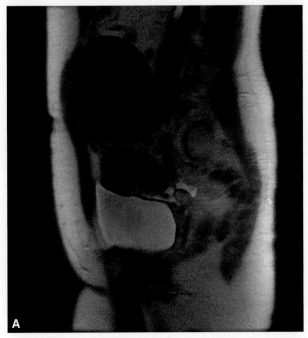

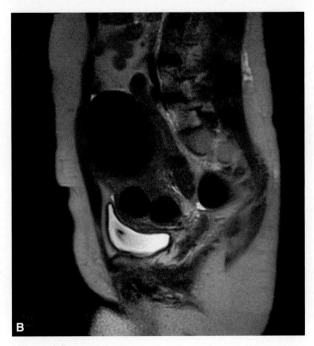

FIGURE 24.3 T2 Sag MRI of a fibroid uterus before (**A**) and 3 months after (**B**) embolization.

degeneration.[15] Luckily, sarcomatous transformation of a leiomyoma is extremely rare, that being 0.1% to 0.8%.[16] Nonetheless, if an MRI does show a large necrotic mass arising from the uterus and there is clinical suspicion of rapid growth, one must be suspicious of a malignant process. Postmenopausal bleeding is unlikely due to fibroids, and these patients require further workup with an endometrial biopsy and/or a hysteroscopy to rule out endometrial cancer. Premenopausal women with significant persistent metrorrhagia, irregular intermenstrual bleeding, or prolonged bleeding greater than 10 days should also be considered for endometrial biopsy because this pattern of bleeding may be caused by endometrial hyperplasia, polyps, and endometrial cancer.[17]

Even when significant contraindications to uterine embolization are not present, some anatomic subtypes of fibroids may easily lend themselves to surgical treatment. Serosal, subserosal, and intramural fibroids are easily treated with myomectomy, both open and laparoscopic, the latter even associated with less postoperative recovery. Intracavitary and submucosal fibroids, especially when they are small (less than 3 cm) can be easily removed hysteroscopically. Controversy still lingers around the safety of embolizing pedunculated fibroids. There are reports showing efficacy and safety in treating pedunculated fibroids with embolization if the stalk diameter is equal to or greater than 2 cm.[18–20] Ultimately, the decision rests with the patient because both surgical and nonsurgical treatments are available, safe, and effective.

The principles of particle embolization for uterine fibroids have essentially remained the same since the mid-1990s. The particle material has evolved over time, however, and several studies have tried to determine the best embolic agents to achieve complete and durable infarction of uterine fibroids. Still, no large, double-blinded, prospective, randomized controlled studies exist to definitively answer which embolic agents achieve the best results in treating uterine fibroids. If used properly, most available embolic agents are similarly effective.[21,22] Those agents include gelfoam, poly vinyl alcohol (PVA) particles, spherical polyvinyl alcohol particles (sPVA), and tris-acryl gelatin microspheres (TAGM) (FIGURE 24.4). Shortly after the introduction of sPVA, a randomized comparison of sPVA and TAGM was undertaken and prematurely ended due to poor fibroid infarction rates from sPVA when compared to TAGM.[23] Others have found similar less than desirable infarction rates with sPVA.[24]

So the typical recommendation for TAGM is to start with 500 to 700 micron-size particles. If stasis has not been achieved following injection of two vials of 500 to 700 micron particles, increase to 700 to 900 micron particles for the remainder of the embolization in the same uterine artery. Once stasis is achieved, this procedure is repeated on the contralateral side, again starting with 500 to 700 micron particles. For PVA, use 355 to 500 micron-size particles. The newer sPVA is recommended at 700 to 900 micron-size particles.[25,26] During arterial embolization experiments with sheep uteri using PVA and TAGM, French investigators found that larger particles greater than 500 micron size were associated with significantly less uterine necrosis.[27]

Once arterial access is obtained, most commonly at the right common femoral artery for a single access approach or at both groins for a bilateral approach, an initial pelvic arteriogram is performed with the pigtail catheter at or just below the level of the renal arteries. This is done to map the pelvis, determine the size of the uterine arteries, assess the vascularity of the fibroid(s), and detect any variant anatomy. Additionally, the initial angiogram is useful to look for ovarian arterial supply to the fibroid(s) (FIGURE 24.5).

The internal iliac artery bifurcates to an anterior and posterior division with the uterine artery usually the first branch off the anterior division (FIGURE 24.6). The uterine artery may come off as part of a true trifurcation in 40% of the population (FIGURE 24.7). The uterine artery may be found arising directly from the hypogastric artery 5% of the time (FIGURE 24.8). Additionally, the uterine artery may be the second or third branch arising from the anterior division (FIGURE 24.9). The cervicovaginal artery will branch from the second and third portions of the uterine artery approximately 53% of the time, whereas the rest of time it branches directly off the internal pudendal artery.[28]

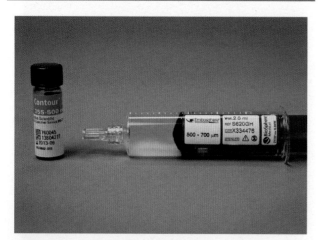

FIGURE 24.4 Contour PVA Particles 355–500 μm (Boston Scientific) and Embosphere TAGM particles 500–700 μm (Biosphere medical).

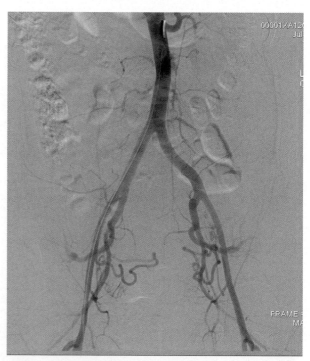

FIGURE 24.5 Initial pelvic angiogram displays typical arterial anatomy with normally tortuous uterine arteries.

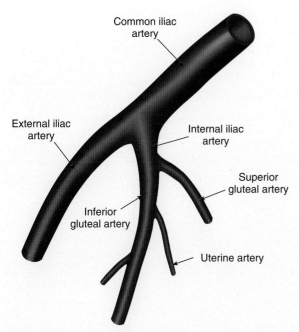

FIGURE 24.6 Illustration depicts typical first takeoff branching pattern of the uterine artery from the anterior division of the internal iliac artery.

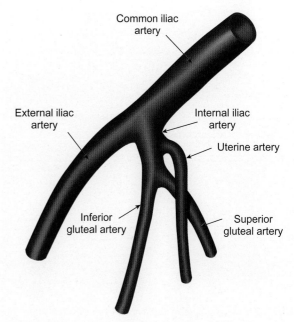

FIGURE 24.8 Illustration depicts the uterine artery arising directly off the internal iliac artery in 5% of the population.

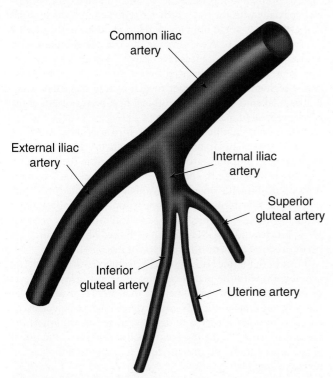

FIGURE 24.7 Illustration depicts true trifurcation of the internal iliac artery in 40% of population.

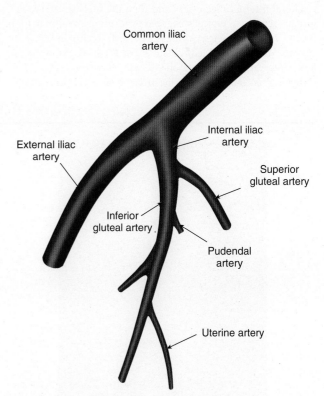

FIGURE 24.9 Illustration depicts the uterine artery as the third branch off the anterior division.

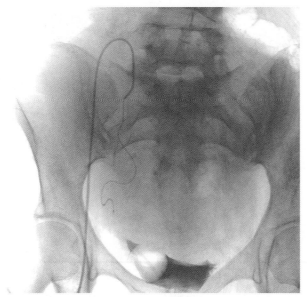

FIGURE 24.10 Angiogram displays the typical "Waltman loop" configuration to select out the ipsilateral uterine artery.

A 4 French or 5 French angled angiographic catheter and wire is used to select the uterine artery. Over the wire, the angled catheter is advanced over the aortic bifurcation to select the contralateral internal iliac artery and then the uterine artery. The ipsilateral artery is typically engaged by forming a Waltman loop (FIGURE 24.10). Catheters with a preformed "Waltman loop" are available from Cook Medical and Merit Medical (FIGURE 24.11). Some interventionalists embolize directly through the 4- or 5-Fr catheter, especially if the uterine artery is large and the catheter

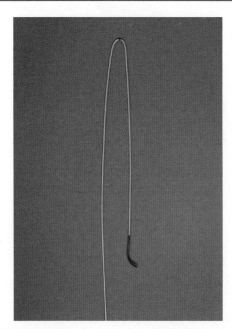

FIGURE 24.11 Image of a manufactured "Waltman loop" into a catheter (Cook Medical).

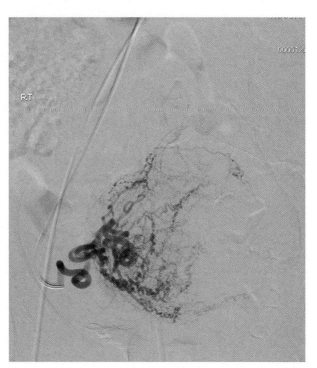

FIGURE 24.12 Direct cannulation without the use of a microcatheter.

does not restrict forward blood flow (FIGURE 24.12). But this is the exception, and most use a large inner diameter microcatheter coaxially with the outer catheter retracted into the internal iliac artery so as not to limit forward blood flow into the uterine artery (FIGURE 24.13). We always use this coaxial technique with a microcatheter because it is less likely to induce vessel spasm. The microcatheter is advanced over a microwire to the horizontal segment, past the major medial turn of the artery. Care is always taken to advance the catheter beyond the origin of the cervicovaginal branch (FIGURE 24.14).

Whichever embolic agent is chosen to use, there are typically two approaches to how much embolic to administer. Two angiographic endpoints are typically described in the literature. One might embolize to complete occlusion and stasis or subtotal occlusion with sluggish flow, giving a "pruned tree" appearance to the uterus.[29] Most comparison studies indicate that neither of these endpoints show statistical differences between PVA particles and TAGM in regard to desired fibroid infarction, periprocedural pain, or other aspects of recovery.[22]

Once both uterine arteries have been embolized, a final pelvic arteriogram with the pigtail catheter at or just below the level of the renal arteries can be helpful to assess for ovarian arterial contributions to the fibroids or other unanticipated vascular contributions as well as to detect early recanalization of the uterine arteries.[30] Some interventionalists will forgo the initial pelvic arteriogram and only perform a final postembolization pelvic angiogram.

Durable symptomatic relief after UFE will be achieved for most of the patients, but 10% to 15% of them will not improve due to several reasons. In young women less than 40 years of age, repeat embolization can be needed in as high as 25% of patients.[31] The most common cause is technical failure to catheterize the uterine artery. This sometimes happens in one or

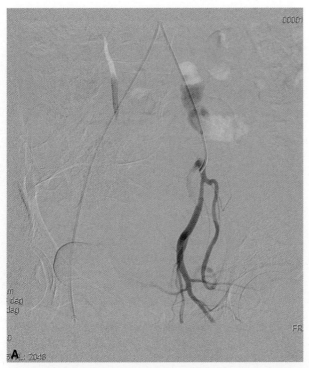
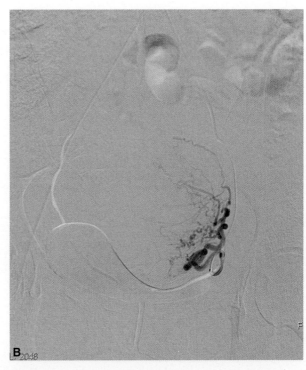

FIGURE 24.13 **A.** The 5F RUC catheter is positioned near the origin of the uterine artery. **B.** With the microcatheter engaged in the uterine artery, the 5F catheter is repositioned proximal to the origin of uterine artery not to restrict forward blood flow.

both arteries either due to vasospasm or challenging anatomy. Sometimes, the origin of one or both uterine arteries may be at an acute angle, thus making cannulation with a typical angled catheter very difficult (FIGURE 24.15). One trick is to use a 4 French or 5 French TC catheter (Cook Medical), which has a tight radius 180-degree curve (FIGURE 24.16). Over a wire, advance the tip beyond the origin of the difficult uterine artery. Then after removing the guide wire, gently inject contrast while retracting the catheter until the reverse facing tip engages the

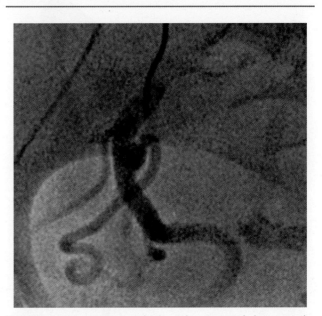

FIGURE 24.14 Magnified image of a microcatheter engaged well beyond the horizontal portion of the uterine artery.

FIGURE 24.15 Angiogram displays the mismatch between the direction of the catheter tip and the acute angle of the origin of the uterine artery.

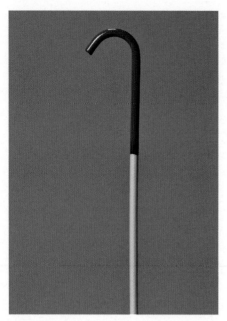

FIGURE 24.16 Image of a TC Slip Cath (Cook Medical), 180-degree tight radius.

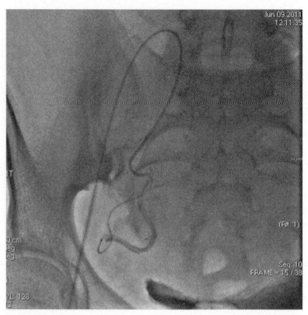

FIGURE 24.18 TC Slip Cath with coaxial microcatheter in the uterine artery.

origin of the uterine artery (FIGURES 24.17A and B). The continuous injection of contrast not only opacifies the origin of the uterine artery but also serves to prevent the catheter tip from dissecting the vessel. Once the catheter tip engages the origin, a microcatheter and microwire can be coaxially advanced into the uterine artery (FIGURE 24.18).

Another useful technique to consider is to wait a few minutes after embolization and then check blood flow with contrast injection to ensure that there has not been early recanalization of the artery, which could lead to inadequate fibroid infarction. By doing this shortly after embolization, time is saved because additional embolization can be easily performed to

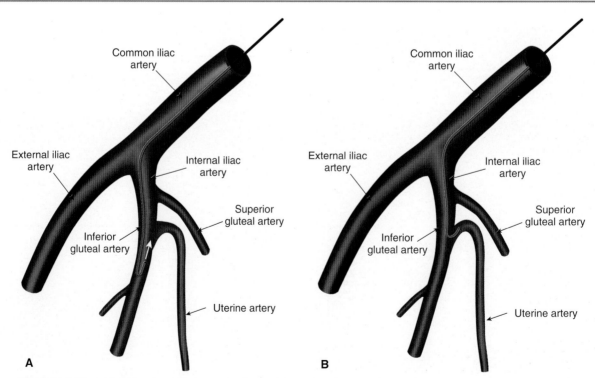

FIGURE 24.17 A. The TC catheter tip is position beyond the origin of an acutely branching uterine artery. **B.** The TC catheter tip has been pulled back to engage the acutely branching uterine artery.

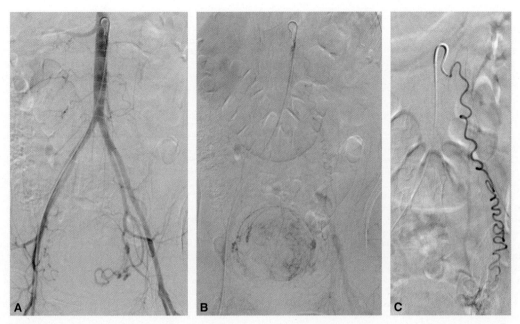

FIGURE 24.19 A, B. Serial images from a postembolization angiogram show faint appearance of the left uterine artery. **C.** Once cannulated the enlarged left ovarian artery and its collateral supply to the uterus are demonstrated.

achieve fibroid infarction before moving on to the opposite uterine artery.

Finally, the ovarian artery may provide partial blood supply to fibroids. In 5% to 10% of cases, the ovarian artery can contribute to fibroid perfusion (FIGURES 24.19A–C) and this may lead to incomplete infarction from uterine artery embolization alone.[32] The evidence in the medical literature, although limited, suggests that embolizing the contributing ovarian artery is effective in completing the infarction of fibroids.[33] Nonetheless, there is still debate over the most effective method of ovarian artery embolization.

Now after the procedure, a thoughtful care plan should be initiated to deal with the symptoms of postembolization syndrome that all patients will experience to varying degrees and to monitor for possible complications of the procedure.[34] Typically, patients are admitted overnight and discharged the next morning. There are some practitioners who perform UFE as a "same-day" procedure in an outpatient setting.[35] But for most who are admitted overnight, they are placed on a patient-controlled analgesia (PCA) pump—morphine sulfate or Dilaudid typically. Additionally, Toradol 30 mg IV is administered every 6 hours to provide nonsteroidal anti-inflammatory pain control.

For nausea, various medications are available for use. We use Zofran 4 to 8 mg intravenously as needed every 6 hours. Other typical medications include Reglan 5 to 10 mg intravenously every 4 to 6 hours or suppositories like Tigan 200 mg per rectum every 6 to 8 hours. Phenergan 25 mg can be taken orally every 4 to 6 hours. These antiemetics can be taken prophylactically or as needed. Some have used scopolamine patches preprocedure as a way to control the onset of nausea with good success.

In the morning of discharge, the PCA pump and all intravenous medications are discontinued and switched to oral equivalents. If the patient had a Foley catheter placed prior to the procedure, it is discontinued in the morning. The patient should be tolerating POs, voiding on her own, and in reasonable pain control on oral medication. The discharge medications include narcotics, nonsteroidal anti-inflammatory drugs (NSAIDs), and antiemetics. Some practitioners prescribe a short course of antibiotics. The patient is instructed to follow up in 4 to 6 weeks and plan on obtaining a postembolization MRI in 3 to 6 months to assess fibroid devascularization.

❚ REFERENCES

1. Lurie S, et al. Age-related prevalence of sonographicaly confirmed uterine myomas. *J Obstet Gynaecol* 2005;25(1):42–44.
2. Myers ER, et al. Management of uterine leiomyomata: what do we really know? *Obstet Gynecol* 2002;100(1):8–17.
3. Whiteman MK, et al. Inpatient hysterectomy surveillance in the United States, 2000–2004. *Am J Obstet Gynecol* 2008;198(1):34.e1–34.e7.
4. Lepine LA, et al. Hysterectomy surveillance—United States, 1980–1993. *MMWR CDC Surveill Summ* 1997;46(4):1–15.
5. Ravina JH, et al. Arterial embolisation to treat uterine myomata. *Lancet* 1995;346(8976):671–672.
6. Goodwin SC, et al. Preliminary experience with uterine artery embolization for uterine fibroids. *J Vasc Interv Radiol* 1997;8(4):517–526.
7. ACOG Committee Opinion. Uterine artery embolization. *Obstet Gynecol* 2004;103(2):403–404.
8. Viswanathan M, et al. Management of uterine fibroids: an update of the evidence. *Evid Rep Technol Assess* (Full Rep) 2007;(154):1–122.
9. Jha RC, et al. Symptomatic fibroleiomyomata: MR imaging of the uterus before and after uterine arterial embolization. *Radiology* 2000;217(1):228–235.
10. Pelage JP, et al. Uterine fibroid tumors: long-term MR imaging outcome after embolization. *Radiology* 2004;230(3):803–809.
11. Burn PR, et al. Uterine fibroleiomyoma: MR imaging appearances before and after embolization of uterine arteries. *Radiology* 2000;214(3):729–734.
12. Spies JB, et al. Leiomyomata treated with uterine artery embolization: factors associated with successful symptom and imaging outcome. *Radiology* 2002;222(1):45–52.
13. Tahlan A, Nanda A, Mohan H. Uterine adenomyoma: a clinicopathologic review of 26 cases and a review of the literature. *Int J Gynecol Pathol* 2006;25(4):361–365.

14. Bratby MJ, Walker WJ. Uterine artery embolisation for symptomatic adenomyosis—mid-term results. *Eur J Radiol* 2009;70(1):128–132.

15. Cornfeld D, et al. MRI appearance of mesenchymal tumors of the uterus. *Eur J Radiol* 2010;74(1):241–249.

16. Amant F, et al. Clinical management of uterine sarcomas. *Lancet Oncol* 2009;10(12):1188–1198.

17. Casablanca Y. Management of dysfunctional uterine bleeding. *Obstet Gynecol Clin North Am* 2008;35(2):219–234, viii.

18. Katsumori T, Akazawa K, Mihara T. Uterine artery embolization for pedunculated subserosal fibroids. *AJR Am J Roentgenol* 2005;184(2):399–402.

19. Margau R, et al. Outcomes after uterine artery embolization for pedunculated subserosal leiomyomas. *J Vasc Interv Radiol* 2008;19(5):657–661.

20. Smeets AJ, et al. Safety and effectiveness of uterine artery embolization in patients with pedunculated fibroids. *J Vasc Interv Radiol* 2009;20(9):1172–1175.

21. Katsumori T, et al. Uterine artery embolization using gelatin sponge particles alone for symptomatic uterine fibroids: midterm results. *AJR Am J Roentgenol* 2002;178(1):135–139.

22. Spies JB, et al. Polyvinyl alcohol particles and tris-acryl gelatin microspheres for uterine artery embolization for leiomyomas: results of a randomized comparative study. *J Vasc Interv Radiol* 2004;15(8):793–800.

23. Spies JB, et al. Spherical polyvinyl alcohol versus tris-acryl gelatin microspheres for uterine artery embolization for leiomyomas: results of a limited randomized comparative study. *J Vasc Interv Radiol* 2005;16(11):1431–1437.

24. Golzarian J, et al. Higher rate of partial devascularization and clinical failure after uterine artery embolization for fibroids with spherical polyvinyl alcohol. *Cardiovasc Intervent Radiol* 2006;29(1):1–3.

25. Kroencke TJ, et al. Acrylamido polyvinyl alcohol microspheres for uterine artery embolization: 12-month clinical and MR imaging results. *J Vasc Interv Radiol* 2008;19(1):47–57.

26. Worthington-Kirsch RL, et al. Comparison of the efficacy of the embolic agents acrylamido polyvinyl alcohol microspheres and tris-acryl gelatin microspheres for uterine artery embolization for leiomyomas: a prospective randomized controlled trial. *Cardiovasc Intervent Radiol* 2011;34(3):493–501.

27. Pelage JP, et al. Uterine artery embolization in sheep: comparison of acute effects with polyvinyl alcohol particles and calibrated microspheres. *Radiology* 2002;224(2):436–445.

28. Hughes LA, Worthington-Kirsch RL. Uterine artery embolization—vascular anatomic considerations and procedure techniques. In: Tulandi T, ed. *Uterine Fibroids.* Cambridge, UK: Cambridge University Press; 2003:83–90.

29. Spies JB, et al. Initial experience with use of tris-acryl gelatin microspheres for uterine artery embolization for leiomyomata. *J Vasc Interv Radiol* 2001;12(9):1059–1063.

30. White AM, et al. Uterine fibroid embolization: the utility of aortography in detecting ovarian artery collateral supply. *Radiology* 2007;244(1):291–298.

31. Kim HS, Paxton BE, Lee JM. Long-term efficacy and safety of uterine artery embolization in young patients with and without uteroovarian anastomoses. *J Vasc Interv Radiol* 2008;19(2, pt 1):195–200.

32. Matson M, Nicholson A, Belli AM. Anastomoses of the ovarian and uterine arteries: a potential pitfall and cause of failure of uterine embolization. *Cardiovasc Intervent Radiol* 2000;23(5):393–396.

33. Scheurig-Muenkler C, et al. Ovarian artery embolization in patients with collateral supply to symptomatic uterine leiomyomata. *Cardiovasc Intervent Radiol* 2011;34(6):1199–1207.

34. Ganguli S, et al. Postembolization syndrome: changes in white blood cell counts immediately after uterine artery embolization. *J Vasc Interv Radiol* 2008;19(3):443–445.

35. Siskin GP, et al. Outpatient uterine artery embolization for symptomatic uterine fibroids: experience in 49 patients. *J Vasc Interv Radiol* 2000;11(3):305–311.

Uterine Artery Embolization: Outcome from Therapy

JAMES B. SPIES

INTRODUCTION

For generations, the mainstay of therapy for uterine fibroids has been hysterectomy. In the early 1990s, interest grew among patients for alternatives that would be effective for symptom control but that would spare the uterus. Myomectomy had long been the primary uterine-sparing therapy for fibroids, but it remained a major operative procedure with significant bleeding risk.[1] The desire for less-invasive therapies began to grow.

Also beginning in the early 1990s, Drs. Jacques Ravina and Jean Jacques Merland of the Hospital Lariboissiere in Paris, France, were evaluating the use of preoperative embolization of the uterus to reduce blood loss during myomectomy. They were surprised when some patients had their symptoms resolved while awaiting surgery. They followed the progress of 16 such patients and reported this experience in 1995.[2] This was the first report in the English language medical literature of uterine artery embolization (UAE) as a sole therapy for managing symptoms from uterine fibroids.

That report of uterine embolization led Drs. Goodwin and McLucas[3] at UCLA to evaluate this treatment. They published their initial results in 1997, which created considerable interest among the lay press and other investigators in the United States. These early reports led to subsequent investigations by others, resulting in the ultimate acceptance of UAE by the American College of Obstetricians and Gynecologists as a "safe and effective alternative to hysterectomy."[4]

Uterine embolization is now offered in hundreds of hospitals across the world and there is growing interest in this treatment by both interventionalists and gynecologists. With such widespread interest, there is a need for a review of the outcomes from UAE for practicing physicians. This chapter is intended to serve that purpose, summarizing the outcome from therapy, including changes in symptoms, imaging, and quality of life, as well as reproductive outcomes and complications. Before discussing UAE outcomes, however, some background on fibroids will be helpful to place this therapy in context.

UTERINE FIBROIDS

Uterine fibroids, also called myomas or leiomyomas, are benign muscular tumors and are the most common tumors of the female reproductive tract.[5] Forty percent of women still menstruating beyond the age of 50 years have fibroids.[6] In the United States, 30% of women will have had a hysterectomy by age 60 and 60% of these will be for fibroids.[5] The cost to the health care system is enormous with annual expenditures for hysterectomy for fibroids alone at $2 billion.[7] There are several factors that predispose to the development of fibroids, including African American ethnicity, early menarche, and high body mass index.[8]

Fibroids are named according to their position in the uterus, as shown in FIGURE 25.1. The three primary types are submucosal, intramural, and serosal, with the position of the center of the fibroid dictating the name. Both submucosal and serosal fibroids may be pedunculated and the degree to which they are attached to the body of the uterus is often considered in determining whether UAE is the best therapeutic choice. Fibroids may be transmural, extending from the serosal surface of the uterus to the endometrial surface. Rarely, they may also arise in the broad ligament and the role of embolization in this rare subset of fibroids is unknown.

Symptoms associated with fibroids generally relate to their position in the uterus with heavy menstrual bleeding occurring most commonly in uteri where fibroids distort the endometrial surface (submucosal and intramural). Bulk symptoms, such as pressure, heaviness, pain, or urinary symptoms, relate more to the overall size of the uterus. Uterine enlargement is most commonly caused by intramural and serosal fibroids and depends on their size and number. Pedunculated serosal fibroids also are likely to cause pressure symptoms by compressing adjacent organs, such as the rectum, or extend into the flank, where they may cause localized symptoms related to their size and position.

OUTCOME FROM UTERINE EMBOLIZATION

Early Case Series

Between 1998 and 2003, six case series of 100 patients or larger were published[9–14] and provided the basis of our early understanding of UAE. Those results are summarized in Table 25.1.

This experience demonstrated that symptoms improved in most of the patients. Between 81% and 94% of patients showed improvement in their menorrhagia with most experiencing significant improvement. For the bulk-related symptoms caused by fibroids, which include pelvic pain, pressure and bloating, and urinary frequency, 64% to 96% of patients improved. The variability in outcome relates in part to the means of assessment of outcome. In most of these series, the symptom follow-up was obtained via questionnaire with patients initially rating their symptom change 3 to 6 months after treatment. Although many of these studies were limited to a single follow-up, the duration of follow-ups varied from 6 to 29 months. One limitation of the early era of UAE is that there were no long-term studies on a large cohort of patients published and this slowed the acceptance of UAE by referring physicians.

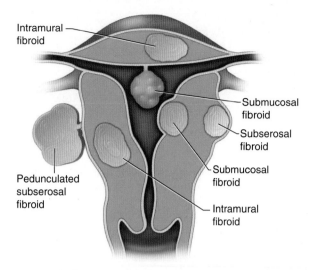

Intramural fibroid

Submucosal fibroid

Subserosal fibroid

Submucosal fibroid

Pedunculated subserosal fibroid

Intramural fibroid

FIGURE 25.1 Illustration of different anatomic locations of fibroids.

Health-Related Quality of Life Outcomes

A broader assessment of health status and outcome from therapy is possible using a quality of life questionnaire. This type of questionnaire assesses overall health status, including broad categories, such as general health perception, mental status, bodily pain, vitality, emotional status, self-image, and sexual functioning. An early pilot study using a proprietary fibroid-specific quality of life questionnaire to assess outcome from fibroid embolization has been published,[15] and it demonstrated statistically significant improvement in all the general health scales at both month 3 and month 6 with marked improvement in general health perception, comparative health perception, physical functioning, energy, mental health, sexual functioning, and self-image. There were corresponding decreases in the three measures of restricted activity, difficulty with activity, pain, and health distress. All the symptom-specific measures significantly improved by month 3 and all but one (backaches) improved by month 6. These findings suggested that health-related quality of life (HRQL) is substantially improved by UAE.

However, the questionnaire used in that study was proprietary with limited validation. It became clear that better tools were needed to evaluate UAE outcomes and those of other fibroid therapies. The Society of Interventional Radiology (SIR) Foundation sponsored the creation of the UFS-QOL, a fibroid-specific symptom and quality of life questionnaire.[16] The goal was to create a questionnaire that could be used to assess patient status before and after fibroid treatment and, therefore, estimate improvement. The symptom score from that questionnaire is the primary outcome measure with scores ranging from 0

Table 25.1

Early Case Series of the Outcome from Uterine Artery Embolization for Fibroids (Inclusion Criteria: Series Including a Minimum of 100 Patients)

Reference number	Number of patients	Mean follow-up	Menorrhagia % improved	Pressure/pain % improved	Mean fibroid volume reduction	Reported complications (number)
10	305	12 mo	86% at 3 mo	64% at 3 mo	—	Puncture site hematoma, 4
			85% at 6 mo	77% at 6 mo		Hysterectomy, 1
			92% at 12 mo	92% at 12 mo		Readmission for pain, 2
9	188	29 mo	90%	—	50–100% in 87% of patients at 6 mo	Fibroid expulsion, 6
						Hysterectomy for uterine necrosis and bowel obstruction, 1
14	167	6 mo	82% at 6 mo	—	49% at 6 mo	Fibroid passage, 5%
					52% at 12 mo	Hysterectomy for infection, 1
12	200	21 mo	86% at 3 mo	93% at 3 mo	42% at 3 mo	Hysterectomies, 0
			88% at 6 mo	93% at 6 mo	60% at 1 y	Endometrial infection, 2
			90% at 1 y	91% at 1 y		Fibroid expulsion, 1
						Pulmonary embolus, 1
						DVT, 1
13	400	16.7 mo	84%	79%	73% at mean of 9.7 mo	Hysterectomies, 3 (3 for infection), Amenorrhea, 7%
						Fibroid expulsion/ hysteroscopy, 3.5%
11	550	8.9 mo (median)	83%	77%	42% at 3 mo	—

(no symptoms) to 100 (very severe symptoms). The questionnaire also yields a HRQL score with the score inversed (100, perfect quality of life; 0, extremely poor quality of life). The UFS-QOL was first used in the FIBROID Registry and has become a tool commonly used for assessing comparative outcomes of fibroid treatments. Those initial results are presented in the next section.

The FIBROID Registry

In 1999, the SIR Foundation (at that time known as the Cardiovascular and Interventional Radiology Research and Education Foundation or CIRREF) organized a cooperative effort of SIR members, industry sponsors, and the Food and Drug Administration (FDA). The intent was to enroll a cohort of patients treated with UAE and to determine short- and long-term outcomes. The first patient was enrolled in December 2000 and the registry was closed at the end of 2002. With 72 contributing sites, a total of 3,160 patients were enrolled.[17] This is the largest single study of UAE outcomes. The initial report was the short-term outcomes,[18] which focused primarily on the safety of the procedure. The major in-hospital complication rate was 0.66% and major adverse events within the first 30 days postdischarge occurred in 4.8% of patients. The most common of these complications was pain, requiring either prolongation of hospital stay or readmission for management. Additional surgical intervention was required in 1% of patients with three patients (0.1%) requiring a hysterectomy. The adverse events of the registry are summarized later in this chapter and in Table 25.2.

The 1-year outcomes from the registry were published in 2005.[19] At 6 months after therapy, the mean symptom score had diminished from 58.6 to 19.9 and was maintained at 12 months (mean 19.2). The HRQL score had a similar magnitude of improvement with mean scores improving from 46.9 to 85 at 6 months and 86.7 at 12 months. By way of comparison, normal women have a mean symptom score of 15.3 and a mean quality of life score of 92.8.[20] Patient satisfaction among registry patients was high with 82% of patients agreeing that they would recommend the procedure to a friend. The study identified several factors associated with a greater improvement in symptoms. These included a primary symptom of heavy menstrual bleeding, multiple fibroids (versus single), smaller fibroids, and submucosal dominant fibroids. Increasing age was associated with poorer improvement in symptom score. The only technical factor that was associated with failure was unilateral embolization, which usually indicated that the procedure could not be completed on one-half of the uterus—a partial technical failure.

The 3-year results were also published[21] and confirmed the durability of UAE as a fibroid treatment. Mean symptom score at 24 months after therapy was 18.2 and at 3 years it was 16.5, indicating continued symptom control for most of the patients. The cumulative rate of subsequent surgical interventions was reported and included myomectomy in 2.8%, hysterectomy in 9.8%, and repeat UAE in 1.8%. Subsequent hospitalizations were recorded in intervals: 2.9% from 0 to 6 months, 2.2% from 6 to 12 months, 3.8% from 12 to 24 months, and 4.2% from 24 to 36 months after treatment. Patient satisfaction remained high with 85.7% of women agreeing that they would recommend the

Table 25.2

Summary of Complications from the FIBROID Registry

In-hospital adverse events n = 3,041			Post-hospital discharge adverse events n = 2,729		
Complication	*Number*	*%*	*Complication*	*Number*	*%*
None	**2,952**	**97**	**None**	**2,019**	**74**
Major events	**20**	**0.6**	**Major events**	**135**	**4.1**
Prolonged pain	6	0.2	Recurrent pain	65	2.4
Nausea	4	0.2	Fibroid expulsion	19	0.7
Vessel injury	3	0.1	Infection	17	0.6
Other	7	0.2	Persistent bleeding	7	0.2
			Thromboembolism	4	0.15
			Other	23	0.8
Minor events	**74**	**2.3**	**Minor events**	**848**	**22**
Groin hematoma	22	0.7	Pain	264	9.8
Vessel injury	13	0.4	New hot flashes	156	5.7
Urinary retention	11	0.4	Fibroid passage	123	4.5
Drug reaction	5	0.2	Infection	82	3.0
Contrast reaction	3	0.1	Bleeding	55	1.8
Nontarget embolization	1	0.03	Headache	18	0.6
Device-related	1	0.03	Other	150	5.4
Other	18	0.6			

Adapted from the FIBROID Registry Short Term outcomes, with major events defined as SIR Class C–F, minor events SIR class A and B.

procedure to a friend. This final report from the registry also presented the results of multivariable analyses. Clinical factors associated with improved symptom and quality of life outcomes were use of prior medication (for control of menstrual bleeding), heavy bleeding as a presenting symptom, and submucosal fibroid location. Other factors associated with better 3-year outcomes included older age, lower body mass index, and lower initial symptom scores. Lower uterine segment or cervical position of the dominant fibroid was associated with a worse quality of life score at 3 years compared to others.

Long-Term Outcome of UAE

Several investigators completed long-term follow-up studies, and the major series with 5-year data are included in Table 25.3.[22–26] These studies demonstrate a substantial degree of uniformity in symptom control with an average of about 80% of women maintaining symptom control. Still, subsequent hysterectomy rates were variable, ranging from 5% to 28%. Subsequent interventions were also variable. A study of repeat uterine embolization is of interest in that it sheds light on the causes of reintervention.[27] In that small series, the reinterventions were most likely caused by a combination of initially incompletely treated fibroids and new fibroids. Patients with a longer interval between initial and subsequent treatment tended to have a greater proportion of new fibroids.

Quantitative Assessment of Menstrual Bleeding Improvement

There also have been studies that focus on other outcomes, primarily menstrual bleeding, in an attempt to semiquantitatively estimate the impact of UAE on menstrual blood loss. One approach is a menorrhagia questionnaire, which is a series of questions that can be scored to estimate menstrual bleeding severity,[28] and pictorial blood loss assessment charts, in which the woman marks a pictogram of menstrual pads and tampons with varying degrees of saturation.[29] There has been at least one study that used both these methods to assess outcome.[30] The menorrhagia questionnaire estimated that menstrual blood loss was diminished from baseline by 46.8% at 3 months, 56.6% by 6 months, and 61.3% at 12 months. The pictorial blood loss

assessment chart noted a similar magnitude change of 55% by 3 months and 58.1% by 6 months.

The "gold standard" for measuring menstrual blood loss is the actual elution of menstrual blood from soiled menstrual pads and tampons with analysis using the alkaline haematin method.[31] The definition of menorrhagia is blood loss of 80 mL or greater during a menstrual cycle. One study assessed menstrual blood loss before and after UAE using the alkaline haematin method.[32] At baseline, median menstrual blood loss was 162 mL and it diminished to 60 mL at 3 months, 70 mL at 6 to 9 months, 37 mL at 12 to 24 months, 18 mL at 24 to 36 months, and 41 mL at 36 to 48 months, demonstrating durable control of menstrual bleeding.

Taken together, these data confirm the effectiveness of UAE in reducing menstrual bleeding and providing durable relief of menorrhagia.

Imaging Outcome

One follow-up examination by magnetic resonance imaging (MRI) or ultrasound has been routinely done at 3 to 6 months after embolization in most of the reported case series. This has been the basis of most of the reports of uterine and fibroid volume decrease after embolization. These findings are summarized in Table 25.1 with volume reductions ranging from 20% to 73% depending on the interval of imaging after embolization. This has been one measure of outcome success with the implication that greater shrinkage likely indicates a more successful outcome.

Having said that, the degree to which the fibroid shrinks does not appear to correlate well with outcome. In an analysis of the impact of baseline and short-term imaging outcome, there was no clear association of symptom improvement and the degree of shrinkage.[33] The study did indicate that larger dominant leiomyoma volume was associated with smaller percent reduction in volume at 3 months ($p = .03$). Submucosal leiomyoma location was associated with a greater volume reduction at 3 months than other locations ($p = .02$), but that difference did not persist at 12 months ($p = .09$). After adjusting for other variables, the odds of improved bleeding and bulk-related symptoms were not higher for greater fibroid volume reduction or fibroid location.

Not only does the degree of shrinkage not predict symptom improvement in the short run, it is unlikely to predict the

Table 25.3					
Long-Term Follow-Up after Uterine Artery Embolization for Fibroids					
Study	N	Duration of follow-up	% with symptom control	Hysterectomy rate	Recurrence rate*
Five-year follow-up					
Lohle et al.[23]	100	54 mo (median)	90%	11%	23%
Spies et al.[24]	200	60 mo (minimum)	73%	13.7%	20%
Walker and Barton-Smith[26]	172	60–72 mo	>80%	5%	16%
Gabriel-Cox et al.[22]	562	58 mo	80%	19.7%	Not reported
Van der Kooij et al.[25]	88	60 mo	75.9%	28.4%	31%

*Recurrence defined as subsequent need for hysterectomy, myomectomy, or repeat uterine embolization.

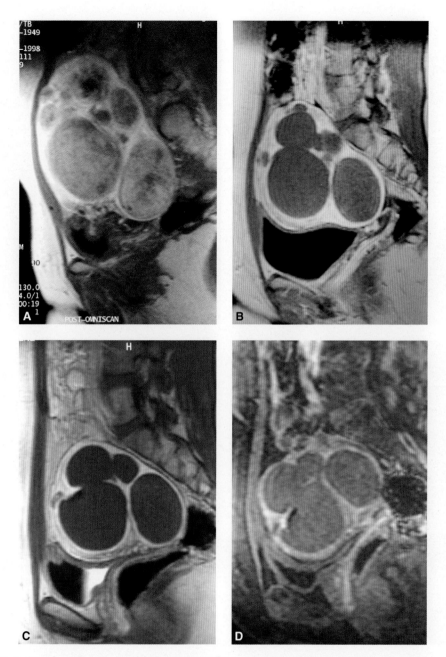

FIGURE 25.2 Series of sagittal T1-weighted contrast-enhanced images of the pelvis before and after embolization. **A.** Pre-embolization image showing enhancing fibroids. **B.** Image 3 months after embolization, revealing no enhancement of the fibroids. **C and D.** Images at 1 and 3 years, respectively, after treatment, demonstrating continued decrease in the fibroid volume.

long-term outcome. Complete infarction of all the fibroids, in general, results in excellent long-term outcomes with no recurrence of fibroids at 3 years in most cases (FIGURE 25.2).[34] The question of the frequency of recurrence of fibroids (either fibroids not completely treated or new fibroids) is not yet clear, but there is evidence that incomplete fibroid infarction does result in regrowth over time with recurrence of symptoms (FIGURE 25.3). This can be predicted by using MRI with contrast enhancement. Even with short-term symptomatic improvement, the presence of persisting viable fibroid tissue on MRI is likely to lead to early recurrence. Based on the limited data

available[27] repeat embolization appears to be effective in treating the fibroids and relieving symptoms.

Comparing Therapies for Fibroids

Among the first studies to compare outcomes of UAE with those of other therapies was a comparative retrospective review by Broder et al.[35] Fifty-nine patients underwent embolization and 30 patients had abdominal myomectomy. The patient groups were identified retrospectively with a minimum of 3 years since therapy and, as a result, the groups were not comparable at

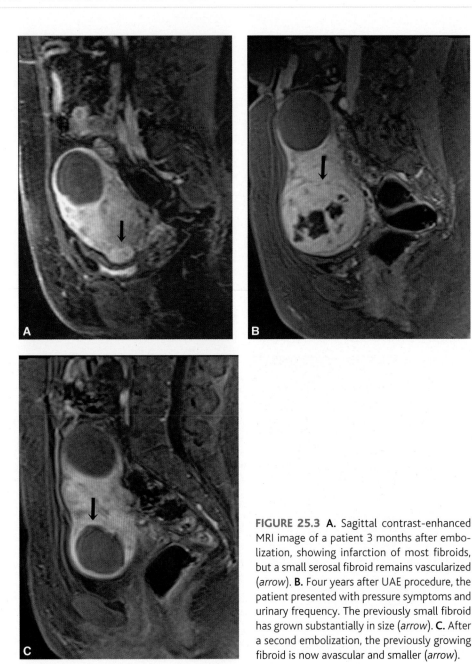

FIGURE 25.3 A. Sagittal contrast-enhanced MRI image of a patient 3 months after embolization, showing infarction of most fibroids, but a small serosal fibroid remains vascularized (*arrow*). **B.** Four years after UAE procedure, the patient presented with pressure symptoms and urinary frequency. The previously small fibroid has grown substantially in size (*arrow*). **C.** After a second embolization, the previously growing fibroid is now avascular and smaller (*arrow*).

baseline with the embolization patients being, on average, older and having greater severity of fibroid disease. The key finding of that study was that this group of myomectomy patients was significantly less likely to have subsequent fibroid interventions (3% versus 29%, $p = .004$), suggesting that myomectomy was more durable. In another small study of similar retrospective design, Razavi and coworkers found nearly opposite outcomes with embolization patients much more likely to be improved in terms of menorrhagia (92% versus 64%, $p < .05$) and pelvic mass effect (91% versus 76%, $p < .05$).[36] These authors also found that in myomectomy patients, there were higher complication rates, longer use of postoperative narcotics, and longer hospitalization and recovery times.

Both of these studies share similar limitations. Both identified the cohorts months or years after therapy. Baseline variables were not controlled and even the indications for therapy may have been different. For these reasons, conclusions favoring one or the other of the therapies cannot be considered definitive based on these retrospective reviews.

A much larger retrospective cohort study was the HOPE-FUL study, a multicenter comparison of hysterectomy and UAE completed in the United Kingdom under the auspices of the National Health Service.[37] Among patients treated at 18 centers, 649 UAE patients and 459 hysterectomy patients were identified as having completed treatment by 2002 and having data available. Minimum follow-up was 8.6 years for hysterectomy and 4.6 years for UAE. They found lower complication rates for UAE (UAE 17.6% versus 26.1% hysterectomy, OR 0.48) with an even lower odds ratio (OR) of 0.25 for UAE when considering major or severe complications. There was a higher rate of fibroid symptom relief with hysterectomy (89% for hysterectomy versus 80% for UAE, $p < .0001$) but a greater percentage of UAE patients would recommend the procedure to a friend compared to hysterectomy patients (86% UAE versus 70% hysterectomy, $p = .007$). The subsequent hysterectomy rate for UAE patients was 11.2% and, overall, 18.3% of UAE patients needed one or more additional fibroid treatment with a cumulative rate of reintervention adjusted for differential follow-up of 23%.

Subsequently, two prospective comparative studies were completed, although neither was a randomized design. The first was a prospective nonrandomized study comparing uterine embolization to hysterectomy.[30] The study reported on 102 embolization patients and 50 hysterectomy patients. Both groups had similar short-term outcomes on nonbleeding symptoms, although hysterectomy had an advantage for controlling pelvic pain 12 months after therapy ($p = .021$). UAE also was effective in improving menstrual bleeding. Most complications were minor, but the frequency of complications after embolization was half that of hysterectomy (27.5% versus 50%, $p = .01$). A second prospective nonrandomized study compared the outcome from myomectomy and embolization[38] comparing 149 UAE patients and 60 myomectomy patients. In this study, the UAE patients had a shorter hospital stay, shorter recovery, and lower rate of complications (22.1% UAE versus 40.1% myomectomy). Both treatment groups had similar levels of symptom control and improvement in quality of life. The menorrhagia questionnaire used in the study showed a 49.2% decrease in bleeding score at 3 months and 55.2% at 6 months. The myomectomy group had a 43% decrease in bleeding score at 3 months and 46.1% at 6 months. There was no statistically significant difference in the bleeding scores between the two groups.

A recent larger prospective cohort study compared the outcomes of UAE, hysterectomy, and myomectomy to normal controls.[20] A total of 375 patients participated: 101 normal subjects, 107 UAE patients, 61 myomectomy patients, and 106 hysterectomy patients. The primary outcome measure was the symptom score of the UFS-QOL and secondary measures were the quality of life score of the UFS-QOL and the SF-36, a well-established general HRQL questionnaire. The study's importance was the comparison of outcomes with normal subjects without uterine fibroids. Although the mean symptom scores of the three fibroid therapy groups indicated substantial symptoms prior to treatment, there was marked improvement of all three with symptoms reduced into the range of normal. The change with therapy for myomectomy and UAE were the same for both procedures, although hysterectomy patients had fewer symptoms than the normal subjects—primarily because they no longer had menstrual bleeding. There was no difference in rates of complications among the groups.

Randomized Trials

In the past several years, a number of randomized trials comparing UAE to other therapies have been completed. There have been three trials comparing UAE to conventional surgery (hysterectomy or myomectomy) for symptom control and two comparing it to minimally invasive therapies. An additional randomized comparison of UAE versus myomectomy is reviewed in the following section on reproductive outcomes.

The first randomized comparison published[39] was a small study (40 UAE patients, 20 hysterectomy) and found the length of stay was shorter for UAE. Six months after therapy, 31 of 36 embolization patients had improved bleeding, with 3 failures undergoing hysterectomy. The study was too small to provide definitive assessment of relative outcomes.

The EMMY trial was a multicenter randomized trial in the Netherlands comparing uterine embolization and hysterectomy.[40,41] Patient satisfaction and improvements in quality of life were similar for both groups. Both groups had similar rates of at least moderate satisfaction (UAE 92%, versus hysterectomy 90%), although hysterectomy patients had a greater degree of satisfaction with outcome ($p = .02$). At 2 years, 24% of the embolization patients had recurrence of symptoms that led to hysterectomy. The 5-year follow-up from this study has recently been published and confirmed the effectiveness of UAE with a 5-year hysterectomy rate among the UAE patients of 28%.[25] The hysterectomy group required additional intervention in 8% of patients.

The REST trial was a multicenter study from the United Kingdom that randomized patients in a 2:1 ratio, 106 UAE patients and 51 surgical patients.[42] The key finding was that surgery and embolization are similarly effective in improving symptoms and HRQL. Having said that, with a median follow-up of 32 months, the likelihood of reintervention was much higher in UAE patients (21 for UAE versus 1 for surgery, $p < .001$). Ten of these interventions occurred in the first year, primarily due to failure of symptom control, and 11 occurred during subsequent follow-up. Recently, the results of this trial at 5 years were presented and will soon be published.

UAE has also sparked interest among gynecologists for a "surgical UAE" procedure, leading to the development of laparoscopic ligation or occlusion of the uterine arteries, with the claim that this provides comparable outcomes to uterine embolization. To date, there have been two randomized comparisons of the two procedures. One was a study of 20 patients randomly assigned to either UAE or laparoscopic occlusion of the uterine arteries.[43] There was less pain in recovery for the laparoscopic group and the initial results suggested comparable clinical outcomes. However, contrast-enhanced MRI follow-up was not used in this study and thus the conclusions that can be reached regarding fibroid infarction rates are limited. The second study published is larger (58 patients), had longer follow-up (median 48 months), and included follow-up with contrast-enhanced MRI.[44] This study demonstrated a clear advantage for UAE over laparoscopic occlusion. Clinical failure and symptom recurrence was significantly greater with laparoscopic occlusion than with UAE (laparoscopic occlusion 48% versus UAE 17%, $p = .02$). Complete fibroid infarction was found on MRI in all 26 of the UAE patients but in only 5 of the 22 laparoscopic occlusion patients who had imaging follow-up. These findings strongly suggest that laparoscopic uterine artery occlusion is less effective in the long term than UAE.

Reproductive Outcomes

The sole randomized study that has addressed the question of fertility was a study from Prague by Mara et al.,[45] comparing myomectomy and UAE in women seeking to become pregnant. In the study, 121 patients were randomly assigned to either UAE ($n = 58$) or myomectomy ($n = 63$). Although early symptomatic improvement was similar in both groups, there were substantially more reinterventions in the UAE group. This was in part due to the study design, which called for any UAE patients left with fibroids larger than 5 cm 6 months or later after embolization to undergo a myomectomy This increased the number of reinterventions, 33% in the UAE group, but also confounded the results to some degree because this subgroup underwent both UAE and myomectomy, limiting the interpretability of the reproductive outcomes.

The initial report from this trial indicated similar levels of symptom control for both. There was no difference in the impact of the two procedures on serum follicle-stimulating hormone (FSH) levels. A second report from the study presented the initial reproductive results (RR) 2 years after treatment.[46] These favor myomectomy. UAE patients had a greater likelihood of not getting pregnant (RR 2.22), of not delivering (RR 1.54), and of aborting spontaneously (RR 2.79). Having said that, in the first 2 years, this study did show that 50% of the UAE patients who attempted to become pregnant did so, despite the fact that 15 of the UAE patients had to undergo secondary myomectomy for a large residual fibroid. The average interval for the repeat surgery was just over 12 months and this paper presents 2-year outcomes. Those who had both a UAE and a myomectomy were asked not to attempt pregnancy for 12 of the 24 months of follow-up. Longer-term reproductive outcomes from this study will be perhaps a better indicator of UAE reproductive outcomes.

Whereas the Prague trial focused on pregnancy rates and delivery rates, Homer and Saridogan[47] recently published a systematic review of pregnancy risks after UAE to determine whether UAE increases the likelihood of pregnancy complications. This review summarized all the reported UAE patients in the literature at the time ($n = 227$) and compared them to controls culled from a variety of studies with the number of controls ranging from 961 to 4,322 subjects. The results are summarized in Table 25.4. The review found, among UAE patients, increased odds of miscarriage (OR 2.8, $p < .0001$), cesarean section (OR 2.1, $p < .0001$), and postpartum hemorrhage (OR 6.4, $p < .0001$) with no increased odds of preterm delivery, malpresentation, or intrauterine growth retardation. Although it is quite likely that these increased odds reflect real increases in risk, this study has limitations. First, the controls were asymptomatic infertile women. Because of their lack of symptoms, they likely had on average smaller and fewer fibroids than the UAE group. There is also a greater likelihood of prior fibroid surgeries in the UAE group and the reported UAE

patients were among the first ever treated with the procedure. The authors also recognize that the increased rate of postpartum hemorrhage may be caused by the higher cesarean section rates rather than the UAE procedure. Most of the cesarean sections were reported to have been elective rather than after a trial of labor. Although the potential for confounding is significant in this type of case control design, this is the best evidence currently available and patients who become pregnant after UAE should be monitored for these potential complications.

Although the Prague trial provides some initial data on likelihood of pregnancy, our understanding of the frequency of pregnancy and its complications is still very limited. In the absence of more definitive data, myomectomy may be preferred for those who have a high priority for future pregnancy. Having said that, it is clear that women can become pregnant and safely deliver after UAE and the extent of fibroid disease, prior surgical history, comorbidities, and patient preference all have to be considered when recommending therapy in this group of patients. Thus, UAE may be recommended in those patients in whom other, more established therapies have failed, are likely to reduce fertility further, or which are at increased risk of adverse event. In any case, the uncertainty regarding future fertility after any fibroid therapy should be discussed with each patient.

Potential Impact of UAE on the Reproductive Tract

In the absence of definitive data on pregnancy rates and outcomes, one may consider the impact of UAE on the reproductive system as a surrogate for reproductive outcomes. In other words, does UAE harm the ovaries, the endometrium, and uterine function? Although a clear answer to the question is not yet available, there are data to begin to answer it.

There are several ways that reproductive structure may be affected by UAE. During the procedure, some of the flow in the uterine arteries is decreased at least temporarily. It is uncertain what effect this will have on the uterine function. It appears that in most patients, the arteries reopen to the normal portions of the uterus after UAE and it is rare for there to be a permanent ischemic injury to the uterus. Uterine wall defects have been described,[48] however, and this may weaken the wall and potentially interfere with implantation of a fetus. This would appear to be most likely with large fibroids that span the entire wall of the uterus. Fibroids

Table 25.4

Comparative Reproductive Outcomes: UFE Versus Fibroid Controls

Complication	UFE (%)	Controls (%)	Odds ratio	95% CI	p value
Miscarriage	35.2	16.5	2.8	2.0–3.8	<.0001
Preterm delivery	14	16	0.9	0.5–1.5	.69
Malpresentation	10.4	13	0.8	0.4–1.5	.56
IUGR	7.3	11.7	0.6	0.3–1.3	.24
Cesarean section	66%	48.5	2.1	1.4–2.9	<.0001
PP hemorrhage	13.9	2.5	6.4	3.5–11.7	<.0001

UFE, uterine fibroid embolization; CI, confidence interval; PP, post-partum; IUGR, intra-uterine growth retardation.
Reprinted with permission from Homer H, Saridogan E. Uterine artery embolization for fibroids is associated with an increased risk of miscarriage. *Fertil Steril* 2010;94:324–330.

compress the normal uterine tissue adjacent to them and as they shrink, normal tissue usually is restored to a more normal configuration. For any individual, it is difficult to predict whether the uterus will be weakened sufficiently to cause a problem during labor. At the time pregnancy is confirmed, a sonogram should be performed to assess the site of implantation relative to the residual fibroid tissue and the overall integrity of the uterine wall.

Maintaining the integrity of the uterus is also essential for future childbearing. There is relatively little known about the impact of UAE on the endometrium. There are reports of endometrial atrophy after UAE,[49] although the true incidence is unknown. One interesting study of hysteroscopy in a group of UAE patients showed a relatively high incidence of abnormalities with only 37% having completely normal hysteroscopic findings.[50] The study noted intracavitary protrusion of fibroids in 37%, yellowish coloration of the endometrium in 28%, intrauterine or cervical adhesions in 4%, and communication between the myoma and the uterine cavity in five cases (10%). A normal, functional endometrium was histologically verified in 44 women of 49 (90%) who could be evaluated. Therefore, although focal abnormalities were found in many patients, the significance of these findings was not clear and most women had normal endometrial biopsies.

There have been several studies published evaluating the potential impact of UAE on ovarian function. In an early study, basal (third day of menstrual cycle) serum FSH was measured in a group of women before and after embolization.[51] FSH levels are an indirect measure of ovarian reserve and commonly used in infertility practice as a predictor of successful in vitro fertilization. Among the 35 women in the study under the age of 45, there was no permanent change in FSH. None of the women in that study had cessation of menstrual periods. A second study by Ahmad and coworkers[52] found similar results. Tulandi et al.[53] did see a trend toward an increase in FSH levels and suggested that there may be a subclinical effect on ovarian function. All of these studies were completed early in the experience of UAE. A more recent assessment by the EMMY investigators using serum antimullerian hormone demonstrated a similar magnitude decrease in levels compatible with diminished ovarian reserve for both uterine embolization and hysterectomy.[54] The opposite was found by the REST investigators in a very recent assessment with no difference detected in changes in serum FSH between UAE and surgery or in the frequency of the onset of amenorrhea.[55]

■ COMPLICATIONS

To date, UAE has been remarkably safe with few serious complications. As experience with the procedure has grown, however, a variety of complications have been identified and some can be quite serious. There have been several deaths reported as a result of UAE. These include two deaths caused by sepsis,[56,57] two from pulmonary embolus,[58,59] and one from apparent misembolization to the left side of the heart via uterine atrioventricular (AV) shunting and a patent foramen ovale.[60] The potential for such tragic outcomes underscores the need for recognition and prompt management of complications.

For convenience, the complications from UAE may be divided into several categories, which include arteriographic complications, allergic and other adverse drug reactions, misembolization, fibroid expulsion (with or without associated endometritis), uterine infection or injury, and thromboembolic

complications. With the publication of the FIBROID Registry, we have a clearer picture of the frequency than we have had in the past and those results are presented in Table 25.2. There have also been additional large case series from which the relative frequency of complications have been presented and these confirm the relative safety of UAE.[13,37,61,62]

Arteriographic Complications

Perhaps because UAE is usually performed on women in their 30s and 40s, arteriographic complications are very unusual and usually are directly related to the puncture site. Hematoma is the most common complication in this group, occurring in 0.7% of registry patients. However, it is rare that a patient might require prolonged hospitalization or operative intervention for hematoma.

More serious puncture site complications occur even more rarely. There have been reports of arterial dissection or perforation during embolization[62] and arterial thrombosis.[61] It appears that this type of injury occurs in well less than 1% of patients.

Allergic and Drug Reactions

Although difficult to anticipate and avoid, allergic reactions to medications or other drug intolerances and reactions are relatively common in this patient population. Of the minor complications requiring some therapy, this class is among the more common, as noted in the Ontario trial.[62] The most common manifestation is periprocedural urticaria. Other drug reactions are not unique to uterine embolization. Nausea and epigastric pain secondary to gastritis related to the use of nonsteroidal anti-inflammatories do occasionally occur. The routine use of prophylactic antibiotics is common but has the potential to cause complications. There have been with two confirmed cases of C. difficile infections reported after just one preprocedure dose of antibiotics,[61] raising a question about the benign nature of antibiotic prophylaxis. These are the only reports to date.

Misembolization

Although this complication is always feared with any embolization procedure, it has rarely occurred after UAE (except to the ovary). For a misembolization to occur to another part of the pelvis, particles would have to reflux into another branch, be directly embolized into a nonuterine vessel, or pass through communicating vessels to an artery supplying a different structure. There has been a report of transient labial ischemic ulcer after UAE, which resolved in several days with conservative management.[63] There was a more clinically severe misembolization resulting in a large buttock ulcer requiring surgical management[64] and there are a few anecdotes of sciatic nerve injury and at least one case of distal ureteral stricture as a result of UAE. As noted earlier, there has been one death caused by misembolization through shunts to the heart.

Amenorrhea

Although technically misembolization of the ovaries, ovarian dysfunction is not the result of injection of embolic into the wrong vessel and it may be unavoidable in most cases. It is caused by passage of embolic material into ovarian vessels via communicating tubal arteries.

Amenorrhea may be the result and its incidence ranges from 2% to 15% of cases.[3,12,13,65] In the registry, the incidence was 7%. Most cases of amenorrhea have occurred in women over the age of 45. In only one series has the incidence been reported higher than 7%.[65] The authors of that report investigated the potential cause and demonstrated that ovarian vessels do become occluded after embolization in the majority of cases, at least when using polyvinyl alcohol (PVA) particles to complete stasis.[66] These imaging findings have been confirmed in at least one case, in which embolic material was discovered in ovarian vessels.[67] The potential effect on ovarian function is discussed earlier in the section on potential impact on reproductive function.

As a final note, not all cases of amenorrhea are caused by ovarian injury; there are reports of amenorrhea resulting from endometrial atrophy, which is believed to be caused by excessive myometrial ischemia.[68] In one of the cases, small-size PVA particles (150 to 250 micron) were used and may have caused excessive deep myometrial injury.

Fibroid Expulsion

Perhaps the most common complication requiring additional gynecologic intervention is fibroid expulsion, often associated with either bleeding or infection.[13,61,69–71] When a fibroid is completely expelled after embolization, it has been viewed by some as a desirable event and not a complication. In our experience, if a fibroid is passing, there usually is significant cramping pain and an infection or unusual bleeding can occur. Because this is an uncontrolled event with an unpredictable outcome, it has to be considered an adverse event. In approximately 3% of patients, a dilatation and curettage (D & C), hysteroscopic resection, or short hospitalization has been necessary for fibroid expulsion[61] and it may necessitate hysterectomy. In our experience, hysterectomy is necessary in approximately 1 in 200 cases with half of these caused by fibroid expulsion.

Given the potential severity of the secondary complications of fibroid passage, we monitor these patients closely. They should have a pelvic examination initially to determine whether the cervix is open or to see if there is extruding tissue (FIGURE 25.4). Both of these findings suggest that an infection is likely to develop unless the fibroid is removed. The pelvic examination also will allow the physician to determine if there is uterine tenderness or pain with cervical motion, which would indicate more generalized infection of the uterus. We obtain a complete blood count, urinalysis, urine culture, and cervical cultures if a discharge is present. If the patient is toxic, blood cultures are also obtained. Although low-grade fever is common in the first few days after UAE, fever arising more than a week after treatment is usually associated with infection.

Patients who appear toxic should be admitted and treated with intravenous antibiotics. Empiric therapy for both gram-negative organisms and anaerobes is suggested. Inpatient management is also indicated for those with heavy bleeding and severe pain. In these patients, an MRI of the pelvis to assess the status of the uterine cavity and the fibroids is very helpful. Often the migration of the fibroid into the uterine cavity and toward the lower uterine segment is evident, confirming the diagnosis (FIGURE 25.5). After initiation of antibiotics, we usually observe the patient for a brief time (up to 48 hours). If the fibroid does not spontaneously pass within 48 hours of onset of symptoms, we favor early intervention by a gynecologist with D & C, hysteroscopic resection, or manual extraction of the expelling fibroids.

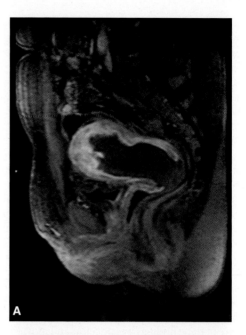

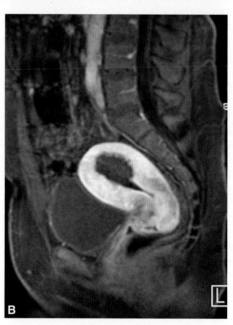

FIGURE 25.4 A. Sagittal contrast-enhanced MRI image of the patient 4 months after embolization with fibroid expulsion and a widely dilated cervix. **B.** After extraction, there is a near-normal uterus with a minimal residual fibroid.

Complications Leading to Hysterectomy after Embolization

Whereas a minor endometrial infection may be controlled with oral or intravenous antibiotics, left unchecked it might progress to pyometritis, uterine rupture, or sepsis.[3,13,56,57] Hysterectomy may be the inevitable consequence of uncontrolled infection and thus early intervention is important. Similarly, off-cycle and severe bleeding may occur during fibroid passage. Although

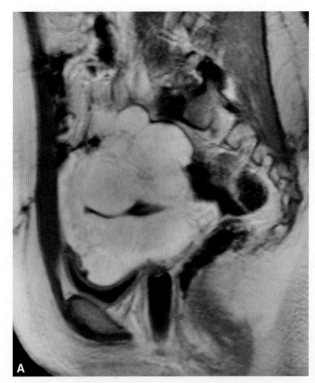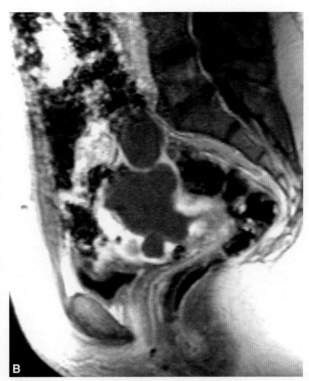

FIGURE 25.5 A. Sagittal contrast-enhanced MRI image revealing several enhancing fibroids. **B.** Two months after embolization, the patient developed 3 days of cramping pain with follow-up MRI revealing all the fibroids devascularized but with migration into the lower uterine segment compatible with impending fibroid passage.

reembolization may be possible, its efficacy in this circumstance is not known. If bleeding is not controlled, hysterectomy may be needed.

Although rare, there have been cases of severe ischemic uterine injury without generalized uterine infection.[72,73] Although the published literature is sparse on uterine injuries after UAE, there have been a few patients who have required hysterectomy for persisting severe pain after uterine embolization.[74] The etiology of the pain is not clear but appears to be persisting ischemia of the normal myometrium and this has been confirmed on pathologic examination.

In all cases where there is concern of myometrial injury or pyometrium, MRI may clarify the diagnosis. If the MRI were to show evidence of diffuse uterine abnormality, suggesting infection and the patient septic and not responding to initial resuscitation, then emergency hysterectomy is indicated.

There have been rare late complications that have led to hysterectomy as well. These include ischemic uterine rupture 3 months after embolization,[75] uterine necrosis requiring hysterectomy 2 months after embolization,[76] vesicouterine fistula developing after embolization,[77] and adhesion formation leading to bowel obstruction.[78] Although rare, these cases highlight the need to consider a uterine injury when atypical symptoms present weeks or months after embolization.

Thromboembolic Complications

Deep venous thrombosis (DVT), pulmonary embolus, and thrombosis of the arterial puncture site have all been reported as complications of UAE, including the two deaths mentioned

earlier in the chapter. In a review of thromboembolic complications after UAE, an incidence of pulmonary embolus of 1 in 400 was noted with occasional isolated DVT as well.[79]

Like many operative interventions, UAE results in tissue injury and this can activate the clotting cascade. In a study that measured several prothrombotic factors before and after embolization,[80] there was clearly an increase that suggested moderate transient hypercoagulability. Although the factors increased, it was to a lesser extent than seen in many surgical procedures and the extent of the clinical risk relative to surgery appears low.

There are other known predisposing factors to thromboembolic disease. In the population undergoing UAE, the use of birth control pills and other exogenous hormones is a known risk factor for the development of venous thrombus, but the benefit of stopping hormones to reduce perioperative risk is unclear.[81] Any attempt to routinely discontinue oral contraceptives prior to embolization will need to be begun 4 to 6 weeks before the procedure to ensure normalization of clotting factors and must be weighed against the risk of an unwanted pregnancy in the interim.

Regardless of predisposing factors, there are some measures that may reduce the risk of thrombosis. Early ambulation after UAE may decrease the chance of DVT. We use automated venous compression devices after UAE in all our patients. For those at increased risk, including those with a personal or family history of venous thrombosis or hypercoagulability, we will use prophylactic low-molecular-weight heparin in the postprocedure period.

The key to detecting venous thromboembolic disease is vigilance. Symptoms suggesting either arterial or venous thrombus need immediate evaluation and appropriate management.

FUTURE DIRECTIONS

Although there has been a remarkable growth in our knowledge of UAE since its introduction in the mid-1990s, there remain some unanswered questions. One of the key issues that remains unresolved is a full understanding of the potential impact of UAE on the reproductive system and just as importantly the impact of other uterine sparing therapies for fibroids. The choice of therapies for women seeking future pregnancy is not clear and may vary considerably depending on the extent of the fibroids, prior therapies, and age.

Beyond that a better understanding and refinement of uterine embolization technique is needed. This includes refinement of endpoint, development of more advanced embolics, including temporary agents, and improved periprocedural care. Finally, greater refinement of patient selection criteria would be helpful, particularly predicting who is likely to have poor symptomatic improvement or who might be at greater risk of complications.

CONCLUSION

Uterine embolization for fibroids is effective, both in terms of symptom control and also in improving HRQL. Complications are infrequent and usually minor and serious complications are rare. There are now considerable data of outcomes compared with more conventional fibroid therapies and also of the long-term outcomes of UAE. Clearly, the safety and effectiveness of UAE is now well established and the procedure can take its place among standard therapies for fibroids.

REFERENCES

1. Parker WH. Uterine myomas: management. *Fertil Steril* 2007;88:255–271.
2. Ravina J, Herbreteau D, Ciraru-Vigneron N, et al. Arterial embolisation to treat uterine myomata. *Lancet* 1995;346:671–672.
3. Goodwin S, Vedantham S, McLucas B, et al. Preliminary experience with uterine artery embolization for uterine fibroids. *J Vasc Interv Radiol* 1997;8:517–526.
4. ACOG practice bulletin. Alternatives to hysterectomy in the management of leiomyomas. *Obstet Gynecol* 2008;112:387–400.
5. Agency for Healthcare Research and Quality. Management of uterine fibroids. Evidence report. Technology assessment: number 34. Agency for Healthcare Research and Quality. 2000. http://www.ahrq.gov. Accessed December 15, 2011.
6. Zhao S, Wong J, Arguelles L. Hospitalization costs associated with leiomyomas. *Clin Ther* 1999;21:563–575.
7. Flynn M, Jamison M, Datta S, et al. Health care resource use for uterine fibroid tumors in the United States. *Am J Obstet Gynecol* 2006;195:955–964.
8. Faerstein E, Szklo M, Rosenshein N. Risk factors for uterine leiomyoma: a practice-based case-control study: I, African-American heritage, reproductive history, body size, and smoking. *Am J Epidemiol* 2001;153:1–10.
9. Ravina J, Ciraru-Vigneron N, Aymard A, et al. Uterine artery embolisation for fibroid disease: results of a 6 year study. *Min Invas Ther Allied Technol* 1999;8:441–447.
10. Hutchins FL Jr, Worthington-Kirsch R, Berkowitz RP. Selective uterine artery embolization as primary treatment for symptomatic leiomyomata uteri. *J Am Assoc Gynecol Laparosc* 1999;6:279–284.
11. Pron G, Bennett J, Common A, et al. The Ontario uterine fibroid embolization trial: part 2, uterine fibroid reduction and symptom relief after uterine artery embolization for fibroids. *Fertil Steril* 2003;79:120–127.
12. Spies J, Ascher S, Roth AR, et al. Uterine artery embolization for leiomyomata. *Obstet Gynecol* 2001;98:29–34.
13. Walker WJ, Pelage J. Uterine artery embolisation for symptomatic fibroids: clinical results in 400 women with imaging follow up. *Br J Obstet Gynaecol* 2002;109:1262–1272.
14. McLucas B, Adler L, Perella R. Uterine fibroid embolization: nonsurgical treatment for symptomatic fibroids. *J Am Coll Surg* 2001;192:95–105.
15. Spies J, Warren E, Mathias S, et al. Uterine fibroid embolization: measurement of health-related quality of life before and after therapy. *J Vasc Interv Radiol* 1999;10:1293–1303.
16. Spies J, Coyne K, Guaou Guaou N, et al. The UFS-QOL, a new disease-specific symptom and health-related quality of life questionnaire for leiomyomata. *Obstet Gynecol* 2002;99:290–300.
17. Myers E, Goodwin S, Landow W, et al. Prospective data collection of a new procedure by a specialty society: The FIBROID Registry. *Obstet Gynecol* 2005;106:44–51.
18. Worthington-Kirsch R, Spies J, Myers E, et al. The Fibroid Registry for outcomes data (FIBROID) for uterine artery embolization: short term outcomes. *Obstet Gynecol* 2005;106:52–59.
19. Spies J, Myers ER, Worthington-Kirsch R, et al. The FIBROID Registry: symptom and quality-of-life status 1 year after therapy. *Obstet Gynecol* 2005;106:1309–1318.
20. Spies J, Bradley L, Guido R, et al. Outcomes for leiomyoma therapies: comparison with normal controls. *Obstet Gynecol* 2010;116:641–652.
21. Goodwin SC, Spies JB, Worthington-Kirsch R, et al. Uterine artery embolization for treatment of leiomyomata: long-term outcomes from the FIBROID Registry. *Obstet Gynecol* 2008;111:22–33.
22. Gabriel-Cox K, Jacobson GF, Armstrong MA, et al. Predictors of hysterectomy after uterine artery embolization for leiomyoma. *Am J Obstet Gynecol* 2007;196:588.e1–588.e6.
23. Lohle PN, Voogt MJ, De Vries J, et al. Long-term outcome of uterine artery embolization for symptomatic uterine leiomyomas. *J Vasc Interv Radiol* 2008;19:319–326.
24. Spies J, Bruno J, Czeyda-Pommersheim F, et al. Long-term outcome of uterine artery embolization of leiomyomas. *Obstet Gynecol* 2005;106:933–939.
25. van der Kooij S, Hehenkamp WJ, Volkers NA, et al. Uterine artery embolization vs hysterectomy in the treatment of symptomatic uterine fibroids: 5-year outcome from the randomized EMMY trial. *Am J Obstet Gynecol* 2010;203:e1–e13.
26. Walker WJ, Barton-Smith P. Long-term follow up of uterine artery embolisation—an effective alternative in the treatment of fibroids. *Br J Obstet Gynaecol* 2006;113:464–468.
27. Yousefi S, Czeyda-Pommersheim F, White AM, et al. Repeat uterine artery embolization: indications and technical findings. *J Vasc Interv Radiol* 2006;17:1923–1929.
28. Ruta DA, Garratt AM, Chadha YC, et al. Assessment of patients with menorrhagia: how valid is a structured clinical history as a measure of health status? *Qual Life Res* 1995;4:33–40.
29. Higham JM, O'Brien PM, Shaw RW. Assessment of menstrual blood loss using a pictorial chart. *Br J Obstet Gynaecol* 1990;97:734–739.
30. Spies J, Cooper J, Worthington-Kirsch R, et al. Outcome from uterine embolization and hysterectomy for leiomyomas: results of a multi-center study. *Am J Obstet Gynecol* 2004;191:22–31.
31. Fraser IS, Warner P, Marantos PA. Estimating menstrual blood loss in women with normal and excessive menstrual fluid volume. *Obstet Gynecol* 2001;98:806–814.
32. Khaund A, Moss JG, McMillan N, et al. Evaluation of the effect of uterine artery embolisation on menstrual blood loss and uterine volume. *Br J Obstet Gynaecol* 2004;111:700–705.
33. Spies J, Roth A, Jha R, et al. Uterine artery embolization for leiomyomata: factors associated with successful symptomatic and imaging outcome. *Radiology* 2002;222:45–52.
34. Pelage J, Guaou Guaou N, Jha R, et al. Long-term imaging outcome after embolization for uterine fibroid tumors. *Radiology* 2004;230:803–809.
35. Broder M, Goodwin S, Chen G, et al. Comparison of long-term outcomes of myomectomy and uterine artery embolization. *Obstet Gynecol* 2002;100:864–868.
36. Razavi MK, Hwang G, Jahed A, et al. Abdominal myomectomy versus uterine fibroid embolization in the treatment of symptomatic uterine leiomyomas. *AJR Am J Roentgenol* 2003;180:1571–1575.
37. Hirst A, Dutton S, Wu O, et al. A multi-centre retrospective cohort study comparing the efficacy, safety and cost-effectiveness of hysterectomy and uterine artery embolisation for the treatment of symptomatic uterine fibroids. The HOPEFUL study. *Health Technol Assess* (Winchester, England) 2008;12:1–248, iii.
38. Goodwin SC, Bradley LD, Lipman JC, et al. Uterine artery embolization versus myomectomy: a multicenter comparative study. *Fertil Steril* 2006;85:14–21.
39. Pinto I, Chimeno P, Romo A, et al. Uterine fibroids: uterine artery embolization versus abdominal hysterectomy for treatment—a prospective randomized and controlled clinical trial. *Radiology* 2003;226:425–431.
40. Hehenkamp WJ, Volkers N, Donderwinkel P, et al. Uterine artery embolization versus hysterectomy in the treatment of symptomatic uterine fibroids (EMMY trial): peri- and postprocedural results from a randomized controlled trial. *Am J Obstet Gynecol* 2005;193:1618–1629.

41. Hehenkamp WJ, Volkers NA, Birnie E, et al. Symptomatic uterine fibroids: treatment with uterine artery embolization or hysterectomy—results from the randomized clinical Embolisation versus Hysterectomy (EMMY) trial. *Radiology* 2008;246:823–832.

42. Edwards RD, Moss JG, Lumsden MA, et al. Uterine-artery embolization versus surgery for symptomatic uterine fibroids. *N Engl J Med* 2007;356:360–370.

43. Ambat S, Mittal S, Srivastava DN, et al. Uterine artery embolization versus laparoscopic occlusion of uterine vessels for management of symptomatic uterine fibroids. *Int J Obstet Gynecol* 2009;105:162–165.

44. Hald K, Noreng HJ, Istre O, et al. Uterine artery embolization versus laparoscopic occlusion of uterine arteries for leiomyomas: long-term results of a randomized comparative trial. *J Vasc Interv Radiol* 2009;20:1303–1310.

45. Mara M, Fucikova Z, Maskova J, et al. Uterine fibroid embolization versus myomectomy in women wishing to preserve fertility: preliminary results of a randomized controlled trial. *Eur J Obstet Gynecol Reprod Biol* 2006;126:226–233.

46. Mara M, Maskova J, Fucikova Z, et al. Midterm clinical and first reproductive results of a randomized controlled trial comparing uterine fibroid embolization and myomectomy. *Cardiovasc Intervent Radiol* 2008;31:73–85.

47. Homer H, Saridogan E. Uterine artery embolization for fibroids is associated with an increased risk of miscarriage. *Fertil Steril* 2010;94:324–330.

48. De Iaco P, Golfieri R, Ghi T, et al. Uterine fistula induced by hysteroscopic resection of an embolized migrated fibroid: a rare complication after embolization of uterine fibroids. *Fertil Steril* 2001;75:818–820.

49. Walker WJ, Carpenter TT, Kent AS. Persistent vaginal discharge after uterine artery embolization for fibroid tumors: cause of the condition, magnetic resonance imaging appearance, and surgical treatment. *Am J Obstet Gynecol* 2004;190:1230–1233.

50. Mara M, Fucikova Z, Kuzel D, et al. Hysteroscopy after uterine fibroid embolization in women of fertile age. *J Obstet Gynaecol Res* 2007;33:316–324.

51. Spies JB, Roth AR, Gonsalves SM, et al. Ovarian function after uterine artery embolization for leiomyomata: assessment with use of serum follicle stimulating hormone assay. *J Vasc Interv Radiol* 2001;12:437–442.

52. Ahmad A, Qadan L, Hassan N, et al. Uterine artery embolization treatment of uterine fibroids: effect on ovarian function in younger women. *J Vasc Interv Radiol* 2002;13:1017–1020.

53. Tulandi T, Sammour A, Valenti D, et al. Ovarian reserve after uterine artery embolization for leiomyomata. *Fertil Steril* 2002;78:197–198.

54. Hehenkamp WJ, Volkers NA, Broekmans FJ, et al. Loss of ovarian reserve after uterine artery embolization: a randomized comparison with hysterectomy. *Hum Reprod* 2007;22:1996–2005.

55. Rashid S, Khaund A, Murray L, et al. The effects of uterine artery embolisation and surgical treatment on ovarian function in women with uterine fibroids. *Br J Obstet Gynaecol* 2010;17:985–989.

56. de Blok S, de Vries C, Prinssen HM, et al. Fatal sepsis after uterine artery embolization with microspheres. *J Vasc Interv Radiol* 2003;14:779–783.

57. Vashisht A, Studd J, Carey A, et al. Fatal septicaemia after fibroid embolisation. *Lancet* 1999;354:307–308.

58. Hamoda H, Tait P, Edmonds D. Fatal pulmonary embolus after uterine artery fibroid embolisation. *Cardiovasc Intervent Radiol* 2009;32:1080–1082.

59. Lanocita R, Frigerio L, Patelli G, et al., eds. A fatal complication of percutaneous transcatheter embolization for treatment of uterine fibroids [abstract]. SMIT/CIMIT 11th Annual Scientific Meeting; 1999; Boston, Massachusetts.

60. Anonymous. Fatal nontarget embolization via an intrafibroid arterial venous fistula during uterine fibroid embolization. *J Vasc Interv Radiol* 2009;20:419–420.

61. Spies J, Spector A, Roth A, et al. Complications after uterine artery embolization for leiomyomata. *Obstet Gynecol* 2002;100:873–880.

62. Pron G, Bennett J, Common A, et al. Technical results and effects of operator experience on uterine artery embolization for fibroids: the Ontario uterine fibroid embolization trial. *J Vasc Interv Radiol* 2003;14:545–554.

63. Yeagley TJ, Goldberg J, Klein TA, et al. Labial necrosis after uterine artery embolization for leiomyomata. *Obstet Gynecol* 2002;100:881–882.

64. Dietz DM, Stahlfeld KR, Bansal SK, et al. Buttock necrosis after uterine artery embolization. *Obstet Gynecol* 2004;104:1159–1161.

65. Chrisman HB, Saker MB, Ryu RK, et al. The impact of uterine fibroid embolization on resumption of menses and ovarian function. *J Vasc Interv Radiol* 2000;11:699–703.

66. Ryu R, Chrisman H, Omary RA, et al. The vascular impact of uterine artery embolization: prospective sonographic assessment of ovarian arterial circulation. *J Vasc Interv Radiol* 2001;12:1071–1074.

67. Payne JF, Robboy SJ, Haney AF. Embolic microspheres within ovarian arterial vasculature after uterine artery embolization. *Obstet Gynecol* 2002;100:883–886.

68. Tropeano G, Litwicka K, SiStasi C, et al. Permanent amenorrhea associated with endometrial atrophy after uterine artery embolization for symptomatic uterine fibroids. *Fertil Steril* 2003;79:132–135.

69. Berkowitz R, Hutchins F, Worthington-Kirsch R. Vaginal expulsion of submucosal fibroids after uterine artery embolization: a report of three cases. *J Reprod Med* 1999;44:373–376.

70. Abbara S, Spies J, Scialli A, et al. Transcervical expulsion of a fibroid as a result of uterine artery embolization for leiomyomata. *J Vasc Interv Radiol* 1999;10:409–411.

71. Pelage J, LeDref O, Soyer P, et al. Fibroid-related menorrhagia: treatment with superselective embolization of the uterine arteries and midterm follow-up. *Radiology* 2000;215:428–431.

72. Siskin G, Stainken B, Dowling K, et al. Outpatient uterine artery embolization for symptomatic uterine fibroids: experience in 49 patients. *J Vasc Intervent Radiol* 2000;11:305–311.

73. Torigian D, Siegelman E, Terhune K, et al. MRI of uterine necrosis after uterine artery embolization for treatment of uterine leiomyomata. *AJR Am J Roentgenol* 2005;184:555–559.

74. Pron G, Mocarski E, Cohen M, et al. Hysterectomy for complications after uterine artery embolization for leiomyoma: results of a Canadian multicenter clinical trial. *J Am Assoc Gynecol Laparosc* 2003;10:99–106.

75. Shashoua AR, Stringer NH, Pearlman JB, et al. Ischemic uterine rupture and hysterectomy 3 months after uterine artery embolization. *J Am Assoc Gynecol Laparosc* 2002;9:217–220.

76. Godfrey CD, Zbella EA. Uterine necrosis after uterine artery embolization for leiomyoma. *Obstet Gynecol* 2001;98:950–952.

77. Sultana CJ, Goldberg J, Aizenman L, et al. Vesicouterine fistula after uterine artery embolization: a case report. *Am J Obstet Gynecol* 2002;187:1726–1727.

78. Payne JF, Haney AF. Serious complications of uterine artery embolization for conservative treatment of fibroids. *Fertil Steril* 2003;79:128–131.

79. Czeyda-Pommersheim F, Magee ST, Cooper C, et al. Venous thromboembolism after uterine fibroid embolization. *Cardiovasc Intervent Radiol* 2006;29:1136–1140.

80. Nikolic B, Kessler CM, Jacobs HM, et al. Changes in blood coagulation markers associated with uterine artery embolization for leiomyomata. *J Vasc Interv Radiol* 2003;14:1147–1153.

81. Oakes J, Hahn P, Lillicrap D, et al. A survey of recommendations by gynecologists in Canada regarding oral contraceptive use in the perioperative period. *Am J Obstet Gynecol* 2002;187:1539–1543.

Pelvic Congestion Syndrome

R. TORRANCE ANDREWS

▌INTRODUCTION

Varices of the ovary and broad ligament are the female equivalent of their better-known male counterpart, the scrotal varicocele. Both conditions are caused by valvular incompetence and/or reflux in the gonadal veins, which are in turn secondary to the unusual anatomy of the gonadal venous pathway (as discussed later). When associated with postural pelvic pain and other symptoms, female pelvic varices are the *sine qua non* of a sometimes disabling condition called pelvic congestion syndrome (PCS, also known as pelvic venous incompetence or PVI). Although female pelvic varices and the scrotal varicocele share a common etiology and list of treatment options, their presentation, diagnosis, and even acknowledgment by the medical community are quite different.

The condition known today as PCS appears to have had its initial description in 1829. While writing about pelvic pain, which he ascribed to the "irritable uterus," Robert Gooch gave the account of a patient whose pain was "so much increased by sitting up and walking about as to compel her to confine herself entirely to the recumbent posture."[1] He noted that the condition of irritable uterus might "be subdivided into several classes, in one of which congestion is an essential part."[2] In 1888, Dudley described a nearly identical pattern of symptoms caused by "varicocele of the broad ligament," a condition that he attributed to, among other things, "an absence of valves in the veins, allowing of blood-pressure from gravity."[3] Having thus proposed an association between venous pathology and pelvic pain, Dudley went on to describe the successful treatment of congestive pelvic pain by salpingectomy and resection of pelvic varices in four cases. In one of these, pathologic evaluation of the resected tissue showed "chronic congestion of the veins."

Despite this promising start, the topic of pelvic venous congestion essentially disappeared from the literature for the next several decades. In 1921, Emge lamented that "no other subject in the large field of gynecology has been treated so negligently as the one on varicose veins of the female pelvis."[4] Similarly concerned, Fothergill reminded his students in the same year that "congestion and oedema of the ovaries are constantly observed" in patients with varices of the broad ligament.[5] Both authors described in detail the positional nature of pelvic pain associated with such varices. Nonetheless, it was not until 1949 that Taylor—the author most closely associated with PCS (and by whose name many subsequent authors have referred to the condition)—for the first time specifically attributed pelvic congestion to "a disorder of the pelvic circulation" and suggested that the resulting symptoms constituted a unique syndrome.[6-9] In a series of papers written that year, Taylor indicated the role of reflux-induced vascular dilatation and stasis in the syndrome and attributed these conditions, in part, to anatomic defects and gravity.

Not all practitioners are convinced of the legitimacy of Taylor's proposed syndrome. Chronic pelvic pain was (and still is) felt by many to have a significant psychological/psychosomatic overlay and little validity,[10-14] and Taylor's attempt to authenticate one aspect of the condition was viewed by some with scorn: Atlee,[12] in 1966, referred to the concept of PCS as "diagnostic garbage" and accused those who make the diagnosis of being ignorant barbers in serious need of self-examination. Less antagonistic but no less dubious, Fry et al.[13] offered the alternate explanation that "a disturbance in the father-daughter dyad . . . may predispose to the later development of personality traits and patterns of social interactions that contribute to the development of pelvic venous congestion." Also highly doubtful, Levitan et al.[14] proposed that all women with chronic pelvic pain and a normal pelvic examination undergo psychological assessment and treatment before being offered laparoscopy or other invasive testing.

In defense of those who doubt the existence of PCS, it should be noted that that pain in the lower abdomen and pelvis is a common manifestation of many organic conditions. For example, Howard[15] listed 70 possible etiologies for pelvic pain, including genitourinary, gastroenteric, musculoskeletal, neurological, psychiatric, and hematologic processes. Furthermore, dilated ovarian veins and pelvic varices are frequently seen in asymptomatic women, especially those who are multiparous.[16-20] Thus, their presence alone cannot be viewed as pathognomonic for PCS. Additionally, it should be recalled that bimanual pelvic examination and diagnostic studies like computed tomography (CT), magnetic resonance imaging (MRI), and ultrasound are performed with the patient recumbent—a position in which the pelvic veins are decompressed. Laparoscopy, considered by most gynecologists to be the definitive test for pelvic pathology, is done with the patient recumbent or in Trendelenburg position, and with the abdomen distended by pressurized gas. In such a configuration, venous structures in the pelvis are both passively and actively compressed and might not be recognized as abnormal. Given the manifold etiologies for pelvic pain and the overlap between asymptomatic patients with dilated pelvic veins and symptomatic patients whose dilated veins are not easily recognized, one must acknowledge the grounds for skepticism.

Perhaps the best evidence that can be offered in support of the PCS concept is its male counterpart. Scrotal varicocele is a universally accepted medical condition, the presentation, natural history, and treatment options of which are well known. So, too, are the embryology and vascular supply of the testicle, which are essentially identical to those of the ovary. Yet although varicoceles are quite common, affecting up to 15% of the male population,[21] only 2% to 10% of men with varicocele experience pain.[22] Most men who seek treatment for varicocele suffer instead from decreased fertility or testicular atrophy. Nonetheless, men treated for pain by ligation or embolization of the refluxing gonadal vein experience symptomatic improvement in over 80% of cases.[22-25] One can readily extrapolate from this experience that a subset of women with both pelvic pain and adnexal varices will experience relief with treatment of their venous pathology.

In 1985 and 1990, respectively, Lechter and Alvarez[26] and Hobbs[27] confirmed this supposition, each reporting technical and clinical success in treating PCS by eliminating reflux with surgical ligation of the ovarian vein using techniques previously applied to the testicular vein for the treatment of varicocele. Citing their work, and building upon the existing experience with transcatheter occlusion of the testicular vein, Edwards et al.[28] performed the first ovarian vein embolization for PCS in 1993. His patient had presented with typical symptoms and laparoscopic findings of a prominent vein in the broad ligament. After bilateral coil embolization of her ovarian veins, she experienced resolution of pain, and this was sustained over the recorded 6-month follow-up interval. More than a dozen authors have subsequently validated Edward's results (Table 26.1).

ANATOMY

Ovarian venous drainage begins in the pampiniform plexus of the broad ligament, which in turn communicates with both the uterine plexus and the ovarian veins. The former empties through the internal iliac system, whereas the latter travel cephalad from the pelvis. Inferiorly, the ovarian vein frequently exists as a complex of intertwined channels, which merge as they rise from the pelvis into a single discrete vessel. Classically, the left ovarian vein empties into the left renal vein lateral to the aorta, whereas the right empties into the anterolateral aspect of the inferior vena cava approximately 3 cm caudal to the right renal vein (FIGURE 26.1). However, numerous variations to these patterns, including duplication of the veins and anomalous insertions, have been described (Table 26.2).[29]

The ovarian veins usually contain valves in their cranial segments, which serve to direct venous flow against gravity and also interrupt the otherwise continuous column of blood bearing down on the adnexae. Surprisingly, however, valves are absent in up to 6% of the right, and 15% of the left, ovarian veins, and when present are incompetent in 35% to 41% of cases.[30]

The normal ovarian vein has a diameter of less than 4 mm, trending larger with increasing parity.[30,31] On the other hand, there is no universal agreement regarding a diameter beyond which pathology can be said to exist. Various authors have used diameters of as little as 5 mm[32] and as great as 10 mm[33] as an indicator of disease. Nonetheless, as already discussed, the isolated anatomic finding of dilated veins (however they are defined) is meaningless in the absence of the constellation of symptoms that constitute the pelvic congestion syndrome.

PHYSIOLOGY

The symptoms of PCS are attributed to increased venous pressure in the ovary and adnexa, which causes dilatation of the venules, decreased clearance of blood, local hypoxia and acidemia, and compromise of microcirculatory function.[34] It is postulated that the most common cause of this cascade of events is the absence or incompetence of valves in the ovarian veins. With such a defect, ovarian venous outflow is compromised and renal or caval blood can flow retrograde through the ovarian veins to pool in the adnexae. Because the valves cannot be replaced or

repaired, the only mechanical option for treatment is to interrupt this reflux pathway.

Another cause of elevated pressure that is unique to the *left* ovarian vein is dysfunction of the left renal vein into which it flows. When the left renal vein is excessively compressed between the aorta and the superior mesenteric artery or follows an anomalous path between the aorta and the spine, its outflow can be severely compromised. In this condition, which is known as "Nutcracker syndrome," the left ovarian vein may even be recruited to serve as a collateral drainage pathway, carrying renal blood retrograde through the pampiniform plexus and the uterine plexus to the internal iliac vein. A similar "overflow" situation can develop in cases of portal hypertension: with portal outflow compromised, splenorenal shunts can develop with a resulting increase in left renal vein flow. Again, the left ovarian vein is overpressurized and can begin flowing retrograde, serving as a collateral drainage pathway (FIGURE 26.2). The treatment for these two conditions is to address the renal venous stenosis or the portal hypertension, respectively, as discussed elsewhere in this text; embolization of the ovarian vein, as discussed in this chapter, would be appropriate only if the patient continues to experience PCS symptoms thereafter.

PATIENT SELECTION FOR EMBOLOTHERAPY

As has already been discussed, the presence of dilated ovarian and/or adnexal veins is not uncommon, especially among multiparous women, and often occurs without symptoms. Therefore, the anatomic finding of varices is not by itself indicative of PCS. Rather, it is the combination of these varices with a specific set of symptoms that constitutes the syndrome. Even then, PCS is a diagnosis of exclusion, meaning that other potential causes of pain should be excluded before one settles on the diagnosis of PCS.

PCS is suggested by a history of deep, aching pelvic pain and tenderness that is exacerbated by upright posture and relieved by recumbency. Many women feel the pain more significantly on one side than the other, whereas others report that the location of pain is shifting. Other commonly reported symptoms include abnormal menstrual bleeding, abnormal vaginal leukorrhea, dysmenorrhea, and dyspareunia, especially with deep penetration and intercourse occurring after periods of being upright. Although there is no definite relationship between symptoms and the phase of the menstrual cycle, some women do report an increase just before their menses.

Physical examination may reveal varices on the labia, the perineum, or the thighs, especially after the patient has been standing (although absence of these findings does not contradict the diagnosis). Abdominal palpation may elicit marked tenderness over the ovarian point. In fact, Beard et al.[35] reported that the combination of ovarian tenderness to palpation and a history of postcoital ache had a sensitivity and specificity of 94% and 77%, respectively, for PCS.

Noninvasive imaging findings in PCS include dilated ovarian veins, varices in the adnexa, and dilated arcuate veins across the myometrium.[36] These anatomic abnormalities are readily identified by routine transvaginal ultrasound (TVUS), CT, or MRI (FIGURES 26.3 to 26.5). Physiologic pathology, in the form of ovarian vein reflux, can be documented by abdominal duplex ultrasound, multidetector CT, or time-resolved MRI.[19,37] Abdominal and transvaginal duplex imaging may furthermore demonstrate variable waveforms with Valsalva.[36]

Table 26.1

Peer-Reviewed Reports of Transcatheter Occlusion of the Ovarian and Iliac Veins for Pelvic Congestion

Year	Author	Patients	Technique and target	Follow-up	Results	Complications
1993	Edwards et al.[28]	1	Coils BO	Clinical; 6 months	Significant relief	None
1994	Sichlau et al.[33]	3	Coils BO 3 (100%)	Clinical; at least 14 months	100% with initial significant improvement; 1 with recurrent symptoms at 14 months	None
1997	Capasso et al.[48]	19	Glue, coils, or both LO 13 (68%); BO 6 (32%)	Clinical and U/S; mean 15.4 months (range 10–32)	Complete relief in 11 (57%), partial in 3 (16%), and no change in 5 (26%). 5 patients (26%) had recurrent symptoms and underwent repeat embolization	None
1997	Tarazov et al.[50]	6	Coils LO 5 (83%); BO 1 (17%)	Clinical; 12–48 months	Resolution of pelvic pain in all cases	None
1998	Cordts et al.[53]	9	Coils BO 4 (44%); LO 4 (44%); left obturator vein 1 (11%)	Clinical; mean 13.4 months	8/9 patients (88%) had >80% immediate relief. Overall and individual symptom relief varied from 40% to 100%. Two women had a mild to moderate return of the symptoms at 6 and 22 months	None
2000	Maleux et al.[52]	41	Glue (40); glue and coils (1) LO 32(78%); BO 9 (22%)	Clinical; mean 19.9 months (range 1–61)	Technical success 98%; partial relief of symptoms in 4 patients (9.7%) and total relief of symptoms in 24 (58.5%); of 9 patients (22%) treated for bilateral reflux, 5 (55%) had partial or complete relief	Minor glue embolism to pulmonary artery in 2 cases, both with transient pain and hemoptysis but otherwise asymptomatic
2002	Venbrux et al.[42]	56	Coils, gelfoam, and sclerosant BO 56 (100%); BI 43 (77%)	Clinical; mean 22.1 months (range 6–38)	Technical success 100%; improvement or elimination of symptoms in 54/56 (96%)	Pulmonary embolization of coils in 2 cases; both patients asymptomatic and coils successfully retrieved
2003	Pisco et al.[51]	5	Sclerosant LO 5	Clinical; 9–12 months	All patients with resolution of symptoms	None
2003	Bachar et al.[47]	6	Coils LO 3; BO 3	Clinical; 7.3 months	3 (50%) complete relief; 2 (33%) had partial or complete relief	None
2003	Pieri et al.[44]	33	Sclerosant LO 11 (33%); RO 1 (1%); BO 21 (64%)	Clinical at 1 and 12 months; TVUS at 6 and 12 months	Symptoms improved or resolved in 20 (61%), persistent in 13 (39%). Reduced size and extent of varices	None

Year	Study	N	Treatment	Follow-up	Results	Complications
2003	Chung and Huh[57]	52	Coils LO 43; RO 4; BO 5	Clinical mean 26.6 ± 5.2 months	Statistically significant reduction in pain score, which continued to improve over the follow-up period	Embolization of coils to the lung (1) and the left renal vein (1); both removed without incident
2006	Kwon et al.[54]	67	Coils LO 64; RO 1; BO 2	Clinical; mean 44.8 months (range 3–72)	55 (82%) had improvement or resolution of symptoms, 10 (15%) had no change, 2 (3%) progressed	Embolization of coils to the pulmonary artery (1) and left renal vein (1); both removed without incident
2006	Kim et al.[43]	127[a]	Coils, sclerosant, and gelfoam BO 106; LO 20; BI 108 (85%)	Clinical; mean 45 ± 18 months	Technical success 100%. 30 patients were not available for follow-up. 80 (83%) had significant improvement; 13 (13%) nsc, 4 (3%) were worse	Pulmonary embolization of coils in 2 cases; both patients were asymptomatic and coils were successfully retrieved[b]
2007	Creton et al.[55]	24	Coils LO 18; RO 0; LI 7; R I5; BI 1	36 months	23 (96%) had improvement or resolution of symptoms; 1 patient did not improve significantly	Embolization of a coil to the pulmonary artery; left in place without sequelae
2008	Ratnam et al.[39]	218	Coil embolization LO 170 (78%); RO 92 (42.2%); LI 123 (56.4%); RI 141 (64.7%)	TVUS at 6 wk	Of 193 patients available for study, mild reflux was still present in 16 (8.3%): 6 (2.8%) had marked persistent reflux, and 3 (1.4%) patients had new reflux. These 9 underwent repeat embolization with success	Pulmonary embolization of coils in 2 cases; 1 was asymptomatic and 1 was successfully retrieved. 1 misplaced coil protruding into the common femoral vein, not requiring treatment. 1 patient with perineal thrombophlebitis.
2008	Tropeano et al.[56]	20	Sclerosant LO 17; BO 3	Clinical; mean 15.1 months (range 12–18)	15 (88%) had marked to complete relief and 2 had mild to moderate relief; 3 patients with residual symptoms underwent repeat sclerotherapy at 3 months and became asymptomatic	None
2008	Gandini et al.[58]	38	Sclerosant LO 32 (84%); BO 6 (16%)	Clinical and TVUS at 1, 3, 6, and 12 months	Statistically significant clinical improvement in all measurements and reduced size and number of varices	None

[a]56 previously reported by Venbrux et al. (2002).

[b]Both previously reported by Venbrux et al. (2002).

LO, left ovarian vein; RO, right ovarian vein; BO, bilateral ovarian vein; LI, left internal iliac vein; RI, right internal iliac vein; BI, bilateral internal iliac vein; TVUS, transvaginal ultrasound; U/S, ultrasound; nsc, no significant change.

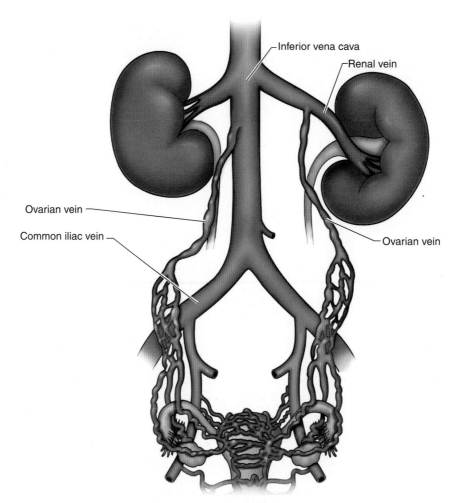

FIGURE 26.1 The anatomy of PCS: Classically, the left ovarian vein inserts upon the left renal vein and the right ovarian vein inserts upon the infrarenal vena cava. Failure of the valves in these vessels or increased pressure in the left renal vein allows blood to flow retrograde, causing the veins of the adnexae and myometrium to dilate and become overpressurized. Reflux can also occur through the internal iliac veins.

As has been mentioned, the sensitivity of CT and MRI studies in detecting the abnormalities of PCS may be somewhat compromised by the recumbent posture of patients being studied, in which position gravity-mediated venous pooling in the pelvis is minimized. Although TVUS is limited in its ability to visualize the full course of the ovarian vein, it has the advantage of being able to image the adnexa in patients both supine and upright, thus allowing the effect of gravity to be demonstrated.[38,39]

Although noninvasive techniques are continually improving, catheter venography has been the gold standard for evaluating ovarian vein function since its first description.[40] This is so because of the unparalleled information it provides regarding the anatomy of the ovarian vein and its collaterals and also because venography can unequivocally confirm reflux in real time. Furthermore, having demonstrated reflux, the operator can proceed immediately to treatment of that condition.

It can be argued that catheter venography, because of its invasiveness, should not be performed except as part of an embolization procedure. Thus, if a patient is to undergo diagnostic ovarian venography because noninvasive techniques have been unable to document reflux despite a highly suggestive clinical history, the patient should be consented for both diagnostic venography and embolization. Conversely, it can also be argued that a planned embolization procedure should be terminated if the operator is unable to document reflux by injecting contrast at the ostia of the ovarian veins prior to selectively catheterizing those vessels. Valsalva or tilting of the procedure into reverse Trendelenburg position may enhance the detection of this finding.

PLANNING THE PROCEDURE

Ovarian and iliac venography and embolization are low-risk procedures that require little in the way of preparation. Of course, one should observe the usual precautions for use of iodinated contrast, for bleeding risks, and for contrast and medication allergies, but there is no specific medical or preoperative therapy regimen that must be completed prior to intervention. Many patients ask whether the procedure should be timed to correlate with any particular point in their menstrual cycles, but there is no evidence to support the value of such efforts.

Medications

The procedure can be readily accomplished with local anesthetic and conscious sedation; general anesthesia is not indicated.

Table 26.2

Pattern of Gonadal Venous Drainage in 100 Adult Cadavers

Right gonadal venous anatomy			Left gonadal venous anatomy		
Number of gonadal veins identified	*Incidence*	*Insertion sites of 115 individual right gonadal veins*	*Number of gonadal veins identified*	*Incidence*	*Insertion site of 122 individual left gonadal veins*
1	85	IVC (84) Right renal vein (1)	1	82	
2	15	IVC (23) Angle of right renal vein/IVC (7)	2	15	Left renal vein (122)
3	0	NA	3	2	
4	0	NA	4	1	
Incidence of collateral flow to the bowel - 21%			Incidence of collateral flow to the bowel - 32%		

IVC, inferior vena cava; NA, not applicable.
Data from Favorito LA, Costa WS, Sampaio FJ. Applied anatomic study of testicular veins in adult cadavers and in human fetuses. *Int Braz J Urol* 2007; 33(2):176–180.

Infection is not reported, but some operators administer a single dose of antibiotic therapy at the outset of the procedure to cover skin flora (e.g., a first-generation cephalosporin). Although ovarian vein embolization can be performed on an outpatient basis, many operators routinely keep their patients overnight for postprocedure observation and pain management. Those who do so generally order in advance a patient-controlled analgesia (PCA) pump with morphine, dilaudid, fentanyl, or similar narcotic agent. Antiemetics may also be valuable, especially if a PCA is to be employed. Phenergan, ondansetron, and others are

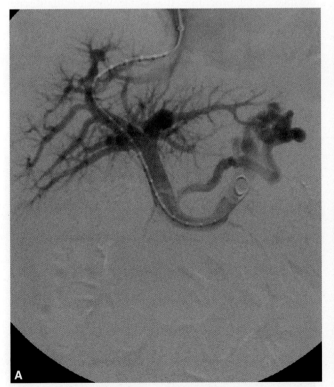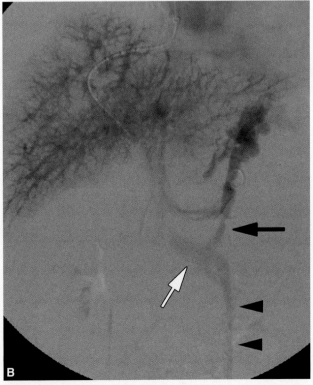

FIGURE 26.2 Ovarian reflux due to portal hypertension. Early (**A**) and late (**B**) images from a direct portogram performed during creation of a transjugular intrahepatic portsystemic shunt show a splenorenal shunt (*black arrow*) opacifying the left renal vein (*white arrow*) and causing retrograde flow through the left ovarian vein (*arrowheads*).

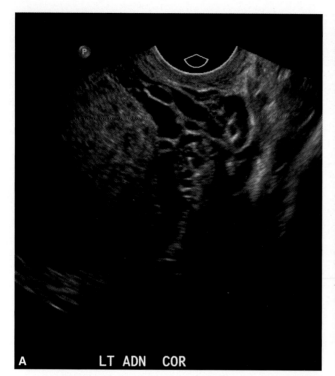
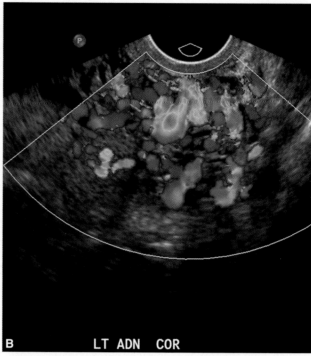

FIGURE 26.3 Endovaginal ultrasound in PCS. Gray-scale imaging (**A**) shows a cluster of anechoic tubular structures in the left adnexa that with color Doppler (**B**) demonstrate vigorous blood flow.

effective but require repeated doses. The author prefers to use a scopolamine transdermal patch, which is placed immediately before embolization and provides a stable delivery of antiemetic for 72 hours with that single application.

Imaging Equipment

Because the percutaneous treatment of PCS uses ionizing radiation to target the pelvis, there is a small but unavoidable risk of radiation-induced injury to the ovaries and other pelvic

contents. It is important that the imaging chain be of high quality and that it be adjusted to reduce the dose to the lowest level possible for the procedure. If available, low-dose fluoroscopy should be utilized and the pulse rate should be as low as possible without compromising the examination. The image intensifier should be kept close to the patient and the use of magnification and oblique views limited. Most importantly, the operator should refrain from acquiring extraneous images because the dose associated with each fixed image is roughly equivalent to that of 49 seconds of fluoroscopy.[41]

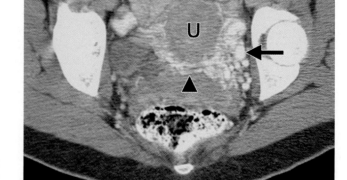

FIGURE 26.4 CT in PCS. High-density tubular structures in the left adnexa (*arrow*) and crossing midline (*arrowhead*) behind the fundus of the uterus (*U*) are typical of pelvic varices in contrast-enhanced CT.

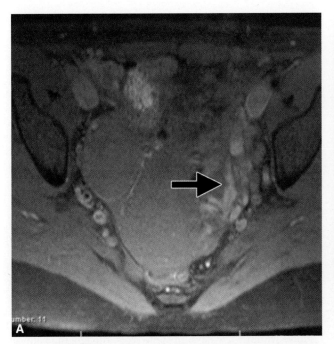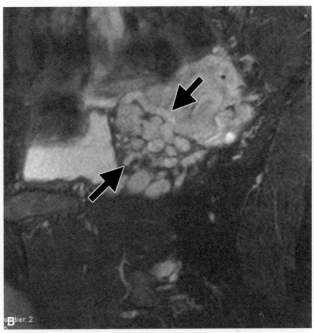

FIGURE 26.5 MRI in PCS. Axial (**A**) and oblique (**B**) sagittal views of the pelvis demonstrate high-signal tubular structures in the left adnexa.

It is helpful, although not mandatory, that the imaging table be capable of tilting. Placing the patient in reverse Trendelenburg position may enhance the visualization of reflux during venography and may also reduce the risk of complications during embolization (as discussed next). A power injector is useful, but hand injection of contrast is generally adequate for the procedure.

TECHNIQUE

The premise of treatment for PCS is that its symptoms can be alleviated by eliminating the reflux pathways that generate abnormal hydrostatic pressure on the ovary and adnexa. Thus, the goal of endovascular therapy is to occlude both the major channels of ovarian reflux and any branch vessels that might provide a mechanism for recurrence through collateral flow. Because such branches can be both numerous and difficult to visualize, the likelihood of recurrence is reduced by occluding the ovarian veins as close to the ovary as possible; simply embolizing the left and right ovarian veins at the level of their confluence with the left renal vein or the vena cava, respectively, is ill-advised. Deep catheterization and embolization of the ovarian veins and their branches may require coaxial microcatheter technique but is critical for long-term clinical success.

In addition to treating the ovarian vein, some authors also routinely seek out and, if found, embolize branches of the internal iliac veins that communicate with pelvic varices or with the ovarian veins.[39,42,43] Venbrux and Kim use balloon-occlusion venography to evaluate for such channels and to perform sclerotherapy of those that are identified. Their practice is to perform iliac embolization 3 to 6 weeks after ovarian embolization although they do not present a rationale for this delay. Ratnam bases the decision to embolize iliac branches on TVUS findings and uses coils to treat

internal iliac branches concurrent with ovarian vein embolization. A review of literature does identify any study comparing patients treated by ovarian vein embolization alone to those treated by combined ovarian and iliac vein embolization.

Ovarian Vein Embolization

The ovarian veins can be approached from femoral, jugular, or even upper extremity access sites.[44] Femoral access may be preferred if the operator plans to use reverse Trendelenburg positioning during venography or embolization, but the insertion angle of the ovarian veins on the left renal vein and the right side of the IVC is such that an approach from above the diaphragm may facilitate their stable catheterization.

Femoral Approach

The left renal vein can be readily catheterized from the groin with a cobra-shaped catheter, which can then be advanced without difficulty into the left ovarian vein. Once the ovarian vein has been catheterized, many operators place a long curved sheath into the vessel to provide stability for subsequent manipulation of an angiographic catheter caudally into the pelvis.

The right ovarian vein is best entered from the groin using a recurved catheter, such as a Simmons 2. A similarly shaped catheter with a smaller radius in its primary curve may not have adequate wall contact to engage the vein. From the groin approach, deep catheterization of the right ovarian vein generally requires a coaxial microcatheter.

Jugular Approach

Both the left renal vein and the right ovarian vein can be identified and catheterized from above the diaphragm with a simple angled-tip catheter. A multipurpose shape, with its elongated distal segment, enhances engagement of the venous ostia. After having engaged the right ovarian vein, the catheter can generally be advanced well into the pelvis without additional manipulation. On the left, however, one must first engage the renal vein and then rotate the catheter some 90 degrees to engage the ovarian ostium. Long sheaths or those with curved shapes are generally not required.

Embolic Delivery

Gonadal embolization has been performed with detachable balloons, coils, plugs, liquid sclerosants, glue, and various combinations of these agents with gelfoam and with each other. An advantage to the use of liquid or polymer agents like sclerosants or glue is their ability to treat branch vessels concurrently with the dominant channel even if these branches are not clearly seen or readily catheterized. If coils, plugs, or detachable balloons are used without such agents, it is important that collateral branches be identified and coiled individually. Failure to do so will increase the risk of reflux through collateral pathways. On the other hand, liquid agents have their own risks: carelessly handled, these agents may inadvertently flow through naturally occurring anastomoses to the mesentery, which are not uncommon (Table 26.2),[29] creating a risk for bowel injury. The specific technique employed will vary by operator experience.

A typical approach to embolization of the ovarian vein once it has been deeply catheterized is to first evaluate the capacitance of the adnexal varices by slowly injecting contrast and watching for it to spill back along the catheter. Having thereby determined how much fluid the varices will hold, one can safely instill this same volume of sclerosant. Alternatively, the sclerosant can be mixed with contrast, thus rendering it radiopaque, and simply injected under continuous fluoroscopy. The injection is halted when backflow along the catheter is seen. The author prefers the latter technique, using a contrast and gelfoam slurry to dilute 3% sodium tetradecyl sulfate to concentrations of approximately 1%. Having treated the most caudal area of reflux, the operator withdraws the catheter to approximately the level of the sacral promontory and performs coil embolization. This process is repeated, if necessary, in any large parallel ovarian venous channels that may exist in the pelvis. Once the pelvic vessels are occluded, the catheter is serially withdrawn by distances of approximately 5 cm with additional sclerosant and coils delivered at each level. Ultimately, one creates an alternating "sandwich" of sclerosant and coils that spans the full length of the ovarian vein. Care must of course be taken to ensure that neither the sclerosant nor the coils enter the left renal vein or the vena cava. Valsalva and reverse Trendelenburg positioning can decrease this risk.

Iliac Vein Embolization

As with the ovarian veins, the internal iliac veins can be catheterized from the femoral or jugular approach. Ratnam et al.[39] used jugular access for all cases, whereas Venbrux et al.[42] and Kim et al.[43] used femoral access. Catheter selection for these different access sites is similar to that described previously. The technique of Venbrux et al.[42] and Kim et al.[43] is to perform venography and, if necessary, embolization, through the endhole of an inflated balloon occlusion catheter, the positioning of which is facilitated by use of a long sheath. This may be difficult to accomplish in the ipsilateral internal iliac vein when using the femoral approach, a

problem that can be overcome by using bilateral femoral access and treating each internal iliac vein from the contralateral side.

Initial diagnostic injection is made into the internal iliac vein and pelvic varices or ovarian collaterals are identified. The catheter is then repositioned superselectively into the venous branches that supply these structures and embolization performed. As indicated, Venbrux and Kim use an occlusion balloon for venography and sclerotherapy. These authors use a slurry of gelfoam and liquid sclerosant, keeping the balloon inflated for 5 minutes after delivery of the agent to prevent its reflux into nontarget venous structures. Ratnam uses coils alone.

Postprocedure Care

The pelvic varices associated with PCS can be quite capacious. As a result, the amount of thrombus generated by embolization can be quite extensive. This, in turn, creates the potential for symptomatic aseptic pelvic thrombophlebitis. The likelihood of symptoms is increased by the use of sclerosing agents, which are designed to cause a direct injury to the endothelium. Patients will generally note an aching pain within a few hours of treatment. For most, the symptoms will be relatively mild and will resolve within a few days. In some cases, though, the pain can be quite debilitating. Venbrux et al.[42] and Kim et al.[43] routinely admit their patients for overnight observation and PCA.

Following discharge, patients are usually managed with nonsteroidal anti-inflammatory agents (NSAIDs) and, in some cases, oral narcotic agents. Antiemetics may be prescribed as well. As mentioned, the author prescribes a scopolamine transdermal patch, which provides for the constant delivery of antiemetic for 72 hours. Postprocedural antibiotics are not indicated.

Patients may continue to experience inflammatory pain for several weeks after ovarian and/or iliac vein embolization. In some cases, they may manifest the typical symptoms of postembolization syndrome.[45] NSAIDs are the mainstay of postprocedure care, but it may be useful to add a short steroid pulse—such as a medrol dosepack—in severe cases.

▎ COMPLICATIONS

In addition to the usual host of complications inherent to endovascular procedures (access site hematoma, contrast reaction, nephrotoxicity, vascular injury, etc.), embolotherapy for PCS carries the unique risk of treatment material migration. Twelve such events are reported among the cases listed in Table 26.1. Two of these involved glue embolizing to the pulmonary artery. Both patients experienced transient pain and hemoptysis but did not require treatment. Ten other cases involved coils with seven of those embolizing to the pulmonary artery. Five pulmonary coils and two coils in renal veins were retrieved using endovascular snares. Two pulmonary coils and one in the external iliac vein were asymptomatic and were left in place. Six of the 10 coil embolizations (60%) occurred during embolization of the internal iliac veins.

The risk of coils or other agents migrating during embolotherapy is always present and cannot be entirely eliminated. The key factors in reducing this risk are (1) matching the size of a coil to that of the target vessel or the polymerization rate of glue or similar agents to its flow rate, (2) appropriately positioning the delivery catheter, and (3) providing support adequate to prevent the catheter from being pushed out of position during delivery of the embolic material. As a result of their experiences with migration events, Venbrux discontinued the use of coils for iliac embolization and Ratnam no longer embolizes large trunk branches, instead placing coils only within refluxing tributary branches.

Because PCS often occurs in young women, its treatment by embolotherapy might raise concerns regarding fertility. Specifically, it can be postulated that manipulation of ovarian venous outflow might impact ovarian function. As already noted, however, the most common indication for gonadal vein embolization in male patients is diminished fertility, and rather than impairing testicular function, the treatment has been clearly shown to improve sperm quality among subfertile men.[46] Venbrux et al.[42] specifically addressed the issue of ovarian function after endovascular PCS treatment in 2002 and found no menstrual changes in any of his 56 patients. Kim et al.[43] identified no significant differences in follicle-stimulating hormone, luteinizing hormone, or estradiol when measured at day 3 of the menstrual cycle before embolotherapy, 6 months after embolotherapy, and then yearly. Two of his patients became pregnant during the follow-up interval. So, too, did a patient of Bachar et al.[47] and three of four patients treated by Capasso et al.[48] who were not using birth control.

Another concern regarding ovarian vein embolization is that it unavoidably exposes the ovaries to ionizing radiation, which might increase the risk of malignancy or lead to genetic anomalies in future pregnancies. Radiation risk has not been investigated with specific regard to ovarian vein embolization. Uterine artery embolization (UAE), a similar procedure that requires even more focused targeting of the pelvis than does ovarian vein embolization, has been the subject of several publications in this regard, however. It has been shown that, with careful technique, the radiation risk during UAE is minimal.[41]

❚ OUTCOMES

Published results for the treatment of PCS with embolotherapy are summarized in Table 26.1. Technical success—defined as occlusion of refluxing gonadal and/or internal iliac veins—is nearly 100%. Clinical success—defined as a durable subjective improvement in the presenting symptoms—is also quite high but is difficult to compare among manuscripts. In 2010, the Society of Interventional Radiology published reporting standards for the outcome of endovascular treatment for PCS,[49] but no such standardization existed prior to that document (a period that included all of the studies currently available for review). Thus, although these patients have clearly done well as a group, it is not always possible to determine the degree to which individual women experienced symptom relief. In fact, the large study published by Ratnam et al.[39] does not report clinical response at all.

Clinical Response

Edwards et al.,[28] Tarazov et al.,[50] and Pisco et al.[51] reported 100% resolution of symptoms in all of their cases, although with a combined total of just 12 patients. Capasso et al.,[48] Maleux et al.,[52] and Bachar et al.,[47] with a total of 76 patients, reported complete resolution of symptoms in 58%, 58%, and 50% of their subjects, respectively, with 16%, 10%, and 33%, respectively, experiencing partial relief (overall clinical response rates of 74%, 68%, and 83%). Sichlau et al.,[33] Cordts et al.,[53] Kwon et al.,[54] Kim et al.,[43] Creton et al.,[55] and Tropeano et al.[56] reported improvement *or* resolution of symptoms in 82% to 100% of their combined 250 patients but did not specifically

subdivide these responses. Only two authors described patients whose symptoms were worse after embolotherapy: Kim et al.[43] (n = 4, or 3% of his cohort) and Kwon et al.[54] (n = 2; 3%).

Chung and Huh[57] and Gandini et al.[58] did not discuss individual patient responses, but instead reported cumulative pain scores in a total of 90 patients. Using a visual analog scale, Chung's patients recorded a decrease in pain score from 7.8 ± 1.2 at baseline to 3.2 ± 0.9 one year after embolization (p < .05). Gandini's patients began at 7.8 ± 1.8 and dropped to 2.7 ± 2.8 over the same interval (p < .05). He also reported statistically significant improvement in dyspareunia, urinary urgency, and dysmenorrhea.

Time Course

Reported response times are widely varied with subjective improvement noted as early as 1 week after treatment in one study but requiring as many as 3 months in another.[42,47,48,54] These differences may very well represent variations in study design and, in particular, the follow-up intervals employed. Most authors have given no information at all regarding the timeline of response, and those who have done so have not correlated these data with patient variables (parity, patient age, number of veins treated, etc.). It is therefore difficult to determine a pattern. Kwon et al.[54] noted that patients who had not experienced any improvement by 3 months did not improve thereafter.

Recurrence of symptoms among patients who had initially experienced improvement was noted infrequently and by a minority of authors.[42,48,53,56] When this event occurred, it was most often seen after greater than 12 months and was generally responsive to repeat embolization of recanalized veins.

Prognostic Considerations

Dyspareunia

Capasso noted that all 5 of the patients in his study who failed to respond to embolotherapy had presented with dyspareunia, and that only 2 of 10 patients with dyspareunia achieved complete symptom relief. He concluded that this symptom might predict a poor outcome. No subsequent author has noted a similar correlation, however, and both Maleux et al.[52] and Creton et al.[55] reported that dyspareunia was entirely unrelated to outcome in their patient populations.

Parity and Anatomy

Several authors have reported nulliparous patients among their cohorts, contradicting a historic impression that PCS is a consequence of prior pregnancy. Although these patients were in the minority, Capasso et al.,[48] Maleux et al.,[52] Bachar et al.,[47] Kwon et al.,[54] and Kim et al.[43] each noted that the clinical response to therapy was independent of parity. Capasso et al.[48] and Maleux et al.[52] also noted that patients having bilateral reflux did not respond differently than did those with unilateral reflux if all refluxing veins were treated.

Prior Hysterectomy

The patient cohort described by Kim was unique in that it included 25 patients who had previously undergone hysterectomy for chronic pelvic pain. These 25 patients were analyzed as a subgroup and were found to have experienced a reduction in overall pain score from 7.9 ± 0.9 to 2.7 ± 2.7 (p < .001) and a trend toward decreased urinary frequency.

FAILURES

The persistence of symptoms after embolization therapy—allowing for recovery from the procedure itself and the resolution of any phlebitis—indicates either untreated reflux or a nonvascular etiology for those symptoms (that is, a diagnosis other than PCS), whereas recurrence after an initially positive clinical response is suggestive of recanalization. In either case, a repeat evaluation of the venous system is warranted. Noninvasive venous imaging may be appropriate if reflux had been clearly demonstrated by noninvasive means prior to the embolization procedure. Its absence thereafter would be a strong evidence of technical success. On the other hand, catheter venography remains the gold standard for demonstrating reflux and should be considered if noninvasive studies are equivocal or if there remains a high index of suspicion for reflux despite a normal noninvasive study.

Ongoing reflux may be caused by incomplete embolization of previously targeted veins. Alternatively, reflux may be occurring through channels not previously studied or at a rate that limits its detection. In the search for ongoing reflux, each previously embolized vein should be studied again. Reflux, if identified, should be re-treated. If a sclerosing agent or gelfoam was not used initially, the use of such additive agents should be strongly considered at the time of re-embolization. In addition, one should consider performing a vena cavagram to identify previously occult venous collaterals or duplications and using reverse Trendelenburg position and the Valsalva maneuver during both selective and nonselective injections to enhance the visualization of reflux (Pieri et al.[44] reported an increase of 22% in the diameter of ovarian veins with Valsalva). If the initial treatment did not include venography of the internal iliac system, such an evaluation should be pursued in the face of ongoing symptoms with embolization performed if reflux is demonstrated.

As already mentioned, reflux into the left ovarian vein can be exacerbated by left renal venous hypertension. The presence of a splenorenal shunt in a patient with portal hypertension or of extrinsic compression of the left renal vein by midline arterial structures may increase the likelihood of recanalization of the embolized left renal vein and should be addressed as described elsewhere in this text.

RELATIVE THERAPEUTIC EFFECTIVENESS COMPARED TO MEDICAL AND SURGICAL MANAGEMENT

Medical Management

As already noted, PCS is a diagnosis of exclusion, meaning that all other etiologies for its symptoms should be ruled out before it is diagnosed. For many patients, this equates to years of treatment for other conditions that are associated with pelvic pain, such as uterine fibroids, endometriosis, and irritable bowel syndrome. Because the medical treatment for those conditions frequently overlaps with that of PCS, most patients ultimately diagnosed with PCS will already have been exposed to and failed a wide range of medical management strategies.

Aside from analgesics and nonsteroidal anti-inflammatory agents, the medical therapies most commonly employed for PCS are based on hormonal suppression. Numerous agents have been used in this regard, including combined oral contraceptives, oral and subcutaneously implanted progestins, and gonadotropin-releasing hormone agonists.[59–61] There have been, to date, no published studies directly comparing any of these therapies to embolization of the ovarian vein, but their efficacy versus placebo or no therapy appears to be roughly similar to that of embolization. These are palliative therapies that require chronic use. Long-term compliance and cost can be problematic, and the agents are associated with significant side effects that include weight gain, acne, hot flashes, and vaginal dryness.

Another medical strategy uses a phlebotropic agent to enhance venous tone. Daflon, a micronized purified flavonoid fraction, has shown some value in the management of hemorrhoids and lower extremity venous insufficiency. Two randomized, blinded studies compared daflon to placebo in a total of 30 women with laparoscopically diagnosed PCS and found a statistically significant reduction in pain.[62,63] As with the hormonal agents discussed previously, however, long-term benefit requires chronic use. Neither daflon nor diosmin, its major ingredient, is approved by the United States Food and Drug Administration at the time of this writing.

Surgical Management

Whereas medical therapy is palliative for PCS, the goal of surgical therapy is to offer a definitive cure. Surgical therapies fall into two broad strategies: the interruption of reflux by ligation of the ovarian vein, and resection of the symptomatic ovary and fallopian tube, often in association with hysterectomy.

Ovarian Vein Ligation

Surgical ligation of the ovarian vein is similar in concept to ovarian embolization. Lechter and Alvarez[26] and Hobbs[27] demonstrated the efficacy of ovarian vein ligation in the treatment of PCS using open surgical techniques in 1985 and 1990, respectively. In 2003, Gargiulo described laparoscopic ligation of the ovarian veins in 23 women and reported complete resolution of pain in 18 (78%) with marked reduction of pain in the others. All patients demonstrated a positive clinical response at 6 months.[64] Among 17 patients who were available for follow-up at 12 months—all of whom had experienced completion remission of symptoms by 6 months—the results were durable.

Further evidence supporting the utility of surgical ligation of the ovarian vein is provided by Belenky, who described a group of 22 patients who were incidentally noted to have ovarian reflux during arteriography performed prior to renal donation. Among these women, 13 had reported symptoms of PCS. Of these 13 patients, 7 (54%) experienced complete relief and 3 (23%) experienced improvement of those symptoms after donation nephrectomy with concurrent ligation of the ovarian vein.[20]

Oophorectomy and Hysterectomy

There are many who view hysterectomy and/or oophorectomy as being the definitive treatment for PCS, including Taylor, the author most closely associated with the condition. In fact, this therapy is often used as the ultimate step when embolotherapy has failed. There is evidence, however, that the value of these techniques may be overstated.

In a randomized prospective study, Chung and Huh[57] compared embolization of the ovarian veins ($n = 52$) with hysterectomy and symptomatic ipsilateral ($n = 27$) or bilateral salpingo-oophorectomy ($n = 27$). At 3-, 6-, and 12-month follow-up, patients treated with embolization had a statistically significantly greater reduction in pain using a visual analog scale than did either of the other patient groups.

Interestingly, as already mentioned, the embolotherapy patient cohort described by Kim included 25 women who remained symptomatic after having undergone hysterectomy for pelvic pain. Following embolization, these patients experienced a statistically significant reduction in pain and a trend toward decreased urinary frequency. There has been no subsequent study confirming the value of embolotherapy as a rescue technique after failure of hysterectomy/oophorectomy to control pelvic pain, and the physiology of this response is not clear, but the experience of this patient group may call into question the role of surgical intervention as the definitive treatment option.

CONCLUSION

Pelvic congestion syndrome (PCS), a clinical entity viewed with skepticism by some, is a diagnosis of exclusion in the etiology of female pelvic pain. There is compelling and reproducible, if somewhat sparse, evidence that the elimination of reflux in ovarian and internal iliac veins can provide relief of PCS symptoms in most affected women, and that definitive control can be achieved with percutaneous embolotherapy. The rates of complication and of symptom recurrence after embolotherapy appear to be quite low, which suggests that an attempt at symptom control with such means should be strongly considered prior to more invasive surgical intervention.

REFERENCES

1. Gooch R. *An Account of Some of the Most Important Diseases Peculiar to Women.* London, England: John Murray; 1829:341.
2. Gooch R. *An Account of Some of the Most Important Diseases Peculiar to Women.* London, England: John Murray; 1829:343.
3. Dudley AP. Varicocele in the female: what is its influence on the ovary? *N Y Med J* 1888;48:147–149.
4. Emge LA. Varicose veins of the female pelvis. *Surg Gynecol Obstet* 1921;32(2):133–138.
5. Fothergill WE. A lecture on varicocele in the female; given to graduates at St. Mary's Hospital, Manchester, November, 1921. *Br Med J* 1921;2(3179):925–926.
6. Taylor HC. Vascular congestion and hyperemia; their effect on structure and function in the female reproductive system. *Am J Obstet Gynecol* 1949;57(2):211–230.
7. Taylor HC. Vascular congestion and hyperemia; their effect on function and structure in the female reproductive organs; the clinical aspects of the congestion-fibrosis syndrome. *Am J Obstet Gynecol* 1949;57(4):637–653.
8. Taylor HC. Vascular congestion and hyperemia; their effect on function and structure in the female reproductive organs; etiology and therapy. *Am J Obstet Gynecol* 1949;57(4):654–668.
9. Taylor HC. Life situations, emotions and gynecologic pain associated with congestion. *Res Publ Assoc Res Nerv Ment Dis* 1949;29:1051–1056.
10. Snaith L, Ridley B. Gynaecological psychiatry; a preliminary report on an experimental clinic. *Br Med J* 1948;2(4573):418–421.
11. Benson RC, Hanson KH, Matarazzo JD. Atypical pelvic pain in women: gynecologic-psychiatric considerations. *Am J Obstet Gynecol* 1959;77(4):806–825.
12. Atlee HB. *Acute and Chronic Iliac Pain in Women; A Problem in Diagnosis.* Springfield, IL: Thomas; 1966:135–137.
13. Fry RPW, Beard RW, Crisp AH, et al. Sociopsychological factors in women with chronic pelvic pain with and without pelvic venous congestion. *J Psychosom Res* 1997;42(1):71–85.
14. Levitan Z, Eibschitz I, De Vries K, et al. The value of laparoscopy in women with chronic pelvic pain and a "normal pelvis." *Int J Gynaecol Obstet* 1985;23:71–74.
15. Howard FM. Chronic pelvic pain. *Obstet Gynecol* 2003;101(3):594–611.
16. Rozenblit AM, Ricci ZJ, Tuvia J, et al. Incompetent and dilated ovarian veins: a common CT finding in asymptomatic parous women. *AJR Am J Roentgenol* 2001;176:119–122.
17. Nascimento AB, Mitchell DG, Holland G. Ovarian veins: magnetic resonance imaging findings in an asymptomatic population. *J Magn Reson Imaging* 2002;15(5):551–556.
18. Halligan S, Campbell D, Bartram CI, et al. Transvaginal ultrasound examination of women with and without pelvic venous congestion. *Clin Radiol* 2000;55(12):954–958.
19. Hiromura T, Nishioka T, Nishioka S, et al. Reflux in the left ovarian vein: analysis of MDCT findings in asymptomatic women. *AJR Am J Roentgenol* 2004;183(5):1411–1415.
20. Belenky A, Bartal G, Atar E, et al. Ovarian varices in healthy female kidney donors: incidence, morbidity, and clinical outcome. *AJR Am J Roentgenol* 2002;179:625–627.
21. Mohammed A, Chinegwundoh F. Testicular varicocele: an overview. *Urol Int* 2009;82:373–379.
22. Peterson AC, Lance RS, Ruiz HE. Outcomes of varicocele ligation done for pain. *J Urol* 1998;159:1565–1567.
23. Yaman Ö, Özdiler E, Anafarta K, et al. Effect of microsurgical subinguinal varicocele ligation to treat pain. *Urology* 2000;55:107–108.
24. Altunoluk B, Soylemez H, Efe E, et al. Duration of preoperative scrotal pain may predict the success of microsurgical varicocelectomy. *Int Braz J Urol* 2010;36:55–59.
25. Yeniyol CO, Tuna A, Yener H, et al. High ligation to treat pain in varicocele. *Int Urol Nephrol* 2003;35:65–68.
26. Lechter A, Alvarez A. Pelvic varices and gonadal veins. In: Negus D, Jantet G, eds. *Phlebology '85.* London, England: John Libbey;1986:225–228.
27. Hobbs JT. The pelvic congestion syndrome. *Br J Hosp Med* 1990;43:200–206.
28. Edwards RD, Robertson IR, MacLean AB, et al. Case report: pelvic pain syndrome—successful treatment of a case by ovarian vein embolization. *Clin Radiol* 1993;47(6):429–431.
29. Favorito LA, Costa WS, Sampaio FJ. Applied anatomic study of testicular veins in adult cadavers and in human fetuses. *Int Braz J Urol* 2007;33(2):176–180.
30. Ahlberg NE, Bartley O, Chidekel N. Right and left gonadal veins: an anatomic and statistical study. *Acta Radiol* 1966;4(6);593–601.
31. Pavkov ML, Koebke J, Notermans HP, et al. Quantitative evaluation of the utero-ovarian venous pattern in the adult human female cadaver with plastination. *World J Surg* 2004;28(2):201–205.
32. Beard RW, Highman JH, Pearce S, et al. Diagnosis of pelvic varicosities in women with chronic pelvic pain. *Lancet* 1984;10:946–949.
33. Sichlau MJ, Yao JS, Vogelzang RL. Transcatheter embolotherapy for the treatment of pelvic congestion syndrome. *Obstet Gynecol* 1994;83(5 pt 2):892–896.
34. Foong LC, Gamble J, Sutherland IA, et al. Microvascular changes in the peripheral microcirculation of women with chronic pelvic pain due to congestion. *BJOG* 2002;109:867–873.
35. Beard RW, Reginald PW, Wadsworth J. Clinical features of women with chronic lower abdominal pain and pelvic congestion. *Br J Obstet Gynaecol* 1988;95(2):153–161.
36. Park SJ, Lim JW, Ko YT. Diagnosis of pelvic congestion syndrome using transabdominal and transvaginal sonography. *AJR Am J Roentgenol* 2004;182:683–688.
37. Kim CY, Miller MJ Jr, Merkle EM. Time-resolved MR angiography as a useful sequence for assessment of ovarian vein reflux. *AJR Am J Roentgenol* 2009;193(5):W458–W463.
38. Giacchetto C, Cotroneo GB, Marincolo F, et al. Ovarian varicocele: ultrasonic and phlebographic evaluation. *J Clin Ultrasound* 1990;18(7):551–555.
39. Ratnam LA, Marsh P, Holdstock JM, et al. Pelvic vein embolisation in the management of varicose veins. *Cardiovasc Intervent Radiol* 2008;31(6):1159–1164. Epub 2008 Aug 28.
40. Ahlberg NE, Bartley O, Chidekel N, et al. Roentgenological diagnosis of pelvic varicosities in women. *Acta Obstet Gynecol Scand* 1965;43(suppl 7):120–121.
41. Andrews RT, Brown PH. Uterine arterial embolization: factors influencing patient radiation exposure. *Radiology* 2000;217(3):713–722.
42. Venbrux AC, Chang AH, Kim HS. Pelvic congestion syndrome (pelvic venous incompetence): impact of ovarian and internal iliac vein embolotherapy on menstrual cycle and chronic pelvic pain. *J Vasc Interv Radiol* 2002;13(2):171–178.
43. Kim HS, Malhotra AD, Rowe PC, et al. Embolotherapy for pelvic congestion syndrome: long-term results. *J Vasc Interv Radiol* 2006;17(2, pt 1):289–297.

44. Pieri S, Agresti P, Morucci M, et al. Percutaneous treatment of pelvic congestion syndrome. *Radiol Med* 2003;105(1-2):76–82.

45. Monedero JL, Ezpeleta SZ, Castro JC, et al. Embolization treatment of recurrent varices of pelvic origin. *Phlebology* 2006;21(1):3–11.

46. Nabi G, Asterlings S, Greene DR, et al. Percutaneous embolization of varicoceles: outcomes and correlation of semen improvement with pregnancy. *Urology* 2004;63(2):359–363.

47. Bachar GN, Belenky A, Greif F, et al. Initial experience with ovarian vein embolization for the treatment of chronic pelvic pain syndrome. *Isr Med Assoc J* 2003;5(12):843–846.

48. Capasso P, Simons C, Trotteur G, et al. Treatment of symptomatic pelvic varices by ovarian vein embolization. *Cardiovasc Intervent Radiol* 1997;20(2):107–111.

49. Black CM, Thorpe K, Venbrux AC, et al. Research reporting standards for endovascular treatment of pelvic venous insufficiency. *J Vasc Interv Radiol* 2010;21(6):796–803.

50. Tarazov PG, Prozorovskij KV, Ryzhkov VK. Pelvic pain syndrome caused by ovarian varices. Treatment by transcatheter embolization. *Acta Radiol* 1997;38(6):1023–1025.

51. Pisco JM, Alpendre J, Santos DD. Sclerotherapy of female varicocele. *Acta Med Port* 2003;16(1):9–12.

52. Maleux G, Stockx L, Wilms G, et al. Ovarian vein embolization for the treatment of pelvic congestion syndrome: long-term technical and clinical results. *J Vasc Interv Radiol* 2000;11(7):859–864.

53. Cordts PR, Eclavea A, Buckley PJ, et al. Pelvic congestion syndrome: early clinical results after transcatheter ovarian vein embolization. *J Vasc Surg* 1998;28(5):862–868.

54. Kwon SH, Oh JH, Ko KR, et al. Transcatheter ovarian vein embolization using coils for the treatment of pelvic congestion syndrome. *Cardiovasc Intervent Radiol* 2007;30(4):655–661.

55. Creton D, Hennequin L, Kohler F, et al. Embolisation of symptomatic pelvic veins in women presenting with non-saphenous varicose veins of pelvic origin—three-year follow-up. *Eur J Vasc Endovasc Surg* 2007;34(1):112–117.

56. Tropeano G, Di Stasi C, Amoroso S, et al. Ovarian vein incompetence: a potential cause of chronic pelvic pain in women. *Eur J Obstet Gynecol Reprod Biol* 2008;139(2):215–221.

57. Chung MH, Huh CY. Comparison of treatments for pelvic congestion syndrome. *Tohoku J Exp Med* 2003;201:131–138.

58. Gandini R, Chiocchi M, Konda D, et al. Transcatheter foam sclerotherapy of symptomatic female varicocele with sodium-tetradecyl-sulfate foam. *Cardiovasc Intervent Radiol* 2008;31(4):778–784.

59. Cheong Y, William Stones R. Chronic pelvic pain: aetiology and therapy. *Best Pract Res Clin Obstet Gynaecol* 2006;20:695–711.

60. Shokeir T, Amr M, Abdelshaheed M. The efficacy of Implanon for the treatment of chronic pelvic pain associated with pelvic congestion: 1-year randomized controlled pilot study. *Arch Gynecol Obstet* 2009;280:437–443.

61. Soysal ME, Soysal S, Vicdan K, et al. A randomized controlled trial of goserelin and medroxyprogesterone acetate in the treatment of pelvic congestion. *Hum Reprod* 2001;16:931–939.

62. Taskin O, Uryan I I, Buhur A, et al. The effects of Daflon on pelvic pain in women with Taylor syndrome. *J Am Assoc Gynecol Laparosc* 1996;3(4, suppl):S49.

63. Simsek M, Burak F, Taskin O. Effects of micronized purified flavonoid fraction (Daflon) on pelvic pain in women with laparoscopically diagnosed pelvic congestion syndrome: a randomized crossover trial. *Clin Exp Obstet Gynecol* 2007;34:96–98.

64. Gargiulo T, Mais V, Brokaj L, et al. Bilateral laparoscopic transperitoneal ligation of ovarian veins for treatment of pelvic congestion syndrome. *J Am Assoc Gynecol Laparosc* 2003;10(4):501–504.

Postpartum Pelvic Hemorrhage

KHASHAYAR FARSAD and JOHN A. KAUFMAN

Postpartum hemorrhage remains a major cause of significant maternal morbidity and mortality worldwide according to the World Health Organization, contributing to approximately one-quarter of cases of maternal mortality.[1] Postpartum hemorrhage may either occur acutely within 24 to 48 hours after delivery, or present in a delayed fashion from days to several weeks after delivery. The definition of postpartum hemorrhage can vary from 500 cc blood loss with a vaginal delivery, 1,000 cc blood loss with a cesarean section, greater than 10% drop in hematocrit after any delivery, or need for blood transfusion after any delivery.[2,3] No matter the standard by which postpartum hemorrhage is defined, however, most patients will be treated accordingly if there is any significant change in hemodynamic status during the immediate postpartum period.

ETIOLOGY OF POSTPARTUM HEMORRHAGE

The most common etiology of postpartum hemorrhage is uterine atony, affecting up to 1 in 20 deliveries, and representing over 50% of cases of postpartum hemorrhage.[2–4] Another source of postpartum hemorrhage is abnormality of placentation, including placenta previa, placenta accreta, and placenta percreta. Abnormal placentation significantly increases in frequency with subsequent cesarean deliveries.[5,6] Antenatal screening for abnormal placentation in certain countries has been implemented to prepare for potential hemorrhagic delivery complications. Iatrogenic causes also contribute to postpartum hemorrhage, including lacerations to the cervix and/or vagina.[7,8] Furthermore, cesarean section has been associated with vascular malformations and pseudoaneurysms.[9] Uterine rupture is a dramatic and fortunately rare cause of postpartum hemorrhage. Other etiologies of postpartum hemorrhage include retained placental tissue, congenital vascular anomalies, and coagulopathies.

TREATMENT OF POSTPARTUM HEMORRHAGE

Medical Management

Treatment for postpartum hemorrhage is very effective and can include medical management, surgical management, and endovascular management. Medical management typically involves a protocol of supportive measures with fluid resuscitation, blood volume resuscitation, uterotonic medication, visual inspection for perineal and cervical trauma, and uterine massage. Repair of recognized lacerations to the cervix and vagina are usually included in this scheme. This form of intervention works in most cases with reported failure rates of between 8% and 40%.[2,4,10] For cases that fail this initial management, escalation of care is required to either operative management or endovascular

treatment. Many centers have set protocols for massive transfusion adapted for obstetrics care, usually modified from trauma protocols. Some centers have devised a scoring system to predict who may ultimately require these advanced interventions based on known abnormalities of placental implantation, early signs of hemodynamic compromise, and evidence of coagulopathy.[4] These paradigms of treatment are becoming a recognized part of high-level obstetrics care in many centers.

Operative Management

Operative treatment of postpartum hemorrhage involves a variety of possible maneuvers.[8,10,11] Ligation of the internal iliac arteries and/or uterine arteries can be performed to decrease perfusion to the bleeding uterus, although this is known to carry a failure rate of approximately 50% due to collateral circulation.[2] A compression (B-Lynch) suture or intrauterine balloon may be employed to attempt to tamponade the bleeding using external or internal compression, respectively. Finally, intra-abdominal packing or hysterectomy may be ultimately required to stop a life-threatening hemorrhage. Despite these attempts, failure of all of these methods, including hysterectomy, has been reported.[2,4,12]

Endovascular Management

Endovascular treatment has recently become a major part of advanced intervention for the treatment of postpartum hemorrhage. The first described case involved persistent uncontrolled bleeding in a patient who had undergone both bilateral internal iliac artery ligation and hysterectomy in futile attempts to stop the bleeding.[13] At angiography, a bleeding collateral branch to the pelvis from the medial circumflex femoral artery was found and embolized, stabilizing the patient.[13] Since then, several reports have been published describing transcatheter embolization of the internal iliac arteries and uterine arteries and embolization of various collateral branches as means to adequately control postpartum hemorrhage.[2,3,14–21] Newer-generation materials and product designs, from catheters, guide wires, and embolic agents, have enabled highly selective treatment of a bleeding source while preserving potentially important collateral vessels.

ANATOMY AND ANGIOGRAPHY

The uterine arteries are most frequently paired branches of the anterior division of the internal iliac arteries, although variant anatomy is also seen, including a unilateral uterine artery and total uterine arterial supply from ovarian arteries. The uterine arteries comprise an initial descending segment coursing anterolaterally along the pelvic wall, a horizontal segment, and an ascending segment, which courses to the uterine fundus.[22,23] This ascending segment gives rise to arcuate branches, which penetrate the myometrium and anastomose with contralateral arcuate arteries. Cervicovaginal branches typically arise from the horizontal segment of the uterine artery.[23] Ovarian and tubal anastomoses are common and comprise the terminal branches of the uterine arteries as they pass into the broad ligament, connecting intramural segments with the ovarian arteries from the aorta.[22–24] The uterine arteries are typically 2 to 5 mm in diameter and become markedly hypertrophied during pregnancy with brisk flow (FIGURE 27.1).[23] As the uterus grows, the intramural segments of the uterine arteries will course high into the abdomen.

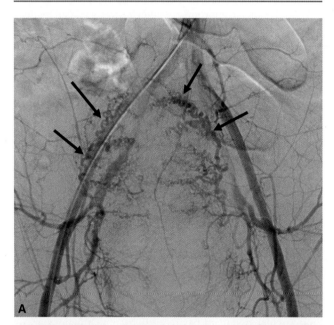

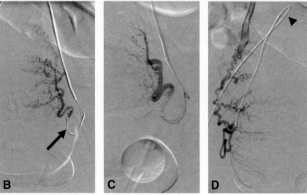

FIGURE 27.1 Postpartum hemorrhage with uterine atony. **A.** Pelvic angiogram demonstrates markedly hypertrophied uterine arteries with significant displacement caused by the gravid uterus (*arrows*). **B.** Selective catheterization of the anterior division of the left internal iliac artery with microcatheter subselection of the left uterine artery (*arrow*). **C.** After gelatin sponge embolization of the left uterine artery, the previously hypertrophied vessels are significantly pruned. **D.** Creation of a Waltman loop (*arrow head*) in the abdominal aorta with the base catheter allows for selection of the ipsilateral internal iliac and uterine arteries for embolization.

Collateral arterial supply to the uterus is abundant and is often the source of persistent bleeding after operative or endovascular intervention for postpartum hemorrhage.[25,26] As described previously, collaterals from the ovarian arteries can be a major source of persistent uterine hemorrhage after ligation or embolization of the uterine arterial supply from the internal iliac arteries and, thus, should actively be sought in this setting.[25] Additional sources of collaterals include other ipsilateral or contralateral anterior division branches of the internal iliac arteries, lumbar segmental arteries, the median sacral artery, the inferior epigastric artery, extremity branches from the medial and lateral circumflex femoral arteries, the inferior mesenteric artery, and the round ligament artery.[22,27] Systematic interrogation of all possible sources of collateral supply to the uterus may be required after a failed operation or embolization to prevent ongoing hemorrhage.

▌ TECHNIQUE

Endovascular treatment utilizes equipment that should be readily available in most interventional radiology (IR) suites equipped for standard arterial procedures. Access is typically via the common femoral artery, either unilaterally or bilaterally. Performing a pelvic angiogram is good practice to identify the predominant bleeding site, bleeding vessel, and possible associated collaterals. In particular, external iliac artery branches with collateral supply to the uterus may be identified early in this way. Abdominal aortography and selective ovarian arteriography may be necessary to identify significant collateral supply from ovarian artery branches.[25] Although this may be performed prior to the initial pelvic angiogram and embolization, some interventionalists may choose to perform this after embolization to identify recruited collateral supply. After the initial pelvic angiogram, the internal iliac arteries are selected for more detailed angiography and possible treatment. Typical equipment includes either a 4 French or a 5 French base catheter and a hydrophilic guide wire. With selection of the anterior division trunk of the internal iliac artery, more detailed angiography may be performed to identify the bleeding source. Depending on the nature of bleeding identified and the stability of the patient, a microcatheter system may be employed for selective embolization of the uterine arteries or for subselective embolization of a bleeding branch (FIGURE 27.1). In the absence of obvious arterial contrast extravasation, the microcatheter may be placed in the uterine artery for empiric embolization. Positioning the microcatheter in the horizontal segment of the uterine artery prior to embolization would spare the cervicovaginal branches.[23]

Catheterization of both internal iliac arteries may be performed from the same arterial access site by choosing a curved catheter to select the contralateral internal iliac artery and then employing a Waltman loop in the abdominal aorta to select the ipsilateral internal iliac artery (FIGURE 27.1).[28] Some interventionalists utilize a Roberts preshaped uterine catheter (Cook Medical) to select both the contralateral and ipsilateral common iliac arteries without the need to fashion a Waltman loop. With either of these approaches, a unilateral arteriotomy will suffice to access both internal iliac arteries in many situations. Bilateral common femoral artery access may also be utilized if selection of the ipsilateral internal iliac artery becomes challenging, if the patient is very unstable and requires simultaneous bilateral

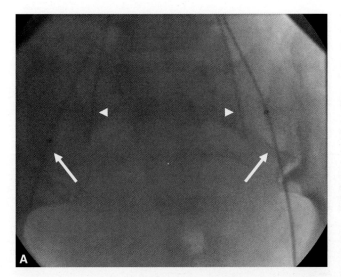
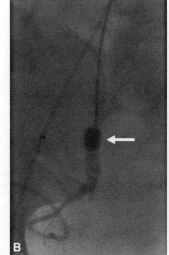
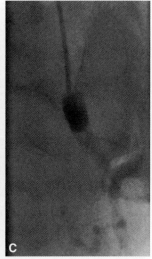

FIGURE 27.2 Preoperative bilateral internal iliac artery balloon occlusion catheter placement. **A.** Access to the common femoral arteries maintained via 6 French sheaths bilaterally (*arrows*), through which 5 French balloon occlusion catheters are placed in each of the contralateral internal iliac arteries (*arrowheads*). **B** and **C.** Inflation of balloons with contrast (B, *arrow*) determines the occlusive volume, and injection of the catheters with contrast confirms appropriate location.

treatment, or if the procedure is anticipated in advance and bilateral access is used for simultaneous embolization or balloon occlusion (FIGURE 27.2).

Embolic Agents

Embolization most commonly is performed using absorbable gelatin sponge (FIGURES 27.1 and 27.3). This is ideally performed from the uterine arteries but may also be performed more proximally either at the origin of the anterior division of the internal iliac artery or at the origin of the main internal iliac artery. The condition of the patient usually determines the degree of selectivity the interventionalist may afford without compromising further hemodynamic function. In most cases, empiric gelatin sponge embolization of the uterine arteries bilaterally is the most effective initial endovascular treatment of choice. The gelatin sponge is cut into 1- to 2-mm pieces and mixed with diluted contrast. The gelatin sponge and diluted contrast is then formed into a slurry by passing the mixture between two syringes through a three-way stopcock. Finer pieces of gelatin sponge or powdered gelatin can predispose to tissue infarction due to very distal embolization.

When a clearly injured artery is identified at angiography, coil embolization may be attempted if the patient's hemodynamic status can tolerate the additional time investment required for subselective embolization (FIGURE 27.4). Coil embolization of the internal iliac arteries is also a viable option to decrease arterial pressure and hemorrhage. Coiling may also be a solution to exclude a pseudoaneurysm from the native circulation.[22,29] Gelatin sponge may be added in combination with coiling to augment the thrombotic effect. Permanent particulate embolic agents may be used for recurrent or persistent bleeding or in the posthysterectomy setting.[22] Furthermore, liquid embolic agents may have a role in embolizing arteriovenous malformations or pseudoaneurysms.[22,29]

Preemptive Endovascular Approaches

In some cases, when a high risk of postpartum hemorrhage can be anticipated, particularly based on antenatal assessment of abnormal placentation, a preemptive endovascular approach may be undertaken. One method employs preoperative bilateral access to the internal iliac arteries or uterine arteries in anticipation of postpartum endovascular embolization.[30,31] The patient then undergoes cesarean delivery and hysterectomy, followed by immediate transfer to the IR suite for pelvic or uterine artery embolization. Another method involves preoperative placement of bilateral internal iliac artery balloon occlusion catheters for subsequent intraoperative inflation to control hemorrhage during cesarean delivery and hysterectomy.[32–34] In this procedure, the bilateral common femoral arteries are accessed in the IR suite or in the operating room (OR) with C-arm fluoroscopic guidance. At the authors' institution, 6 French sheaths are introduced, through which 5 French occlusion balloon catheters are placed in the bilateral internal iliac arteries (FIGURE 27.2). The volume of contrast solution required to fill the balloons to occlusion is recorded, and syringes with these preset volumes are drawn and connected to the balloon port. The catheters and sheaths are sutured in place, and a saline flush solution is connected to the sheaths and catheters to maintain patency. In most circumstances, the occlusion catheters are inflated with the prefilled syringes to their appropriate volume after cesarean delivery and cord clamping to help control subsequent intraoperative blood loss. It is important to note that balloon occlusion of the internal iliac arteries will not cease blood flow to the pelvis but rather will decrease the perfusion pressure to theoretically lessen blood loss during the anticipated procedure. Perfusion to the pelvis will persist via extensive collateral branches, such as from the external iliac arteries, the inferior mesenteric artery, segmental lumbar aortic branches, and the ovarian arteries. The balloons are deflated just prior to closure to ensure hemostasis, and the access sheaths may be left in place connected to flush solution in the

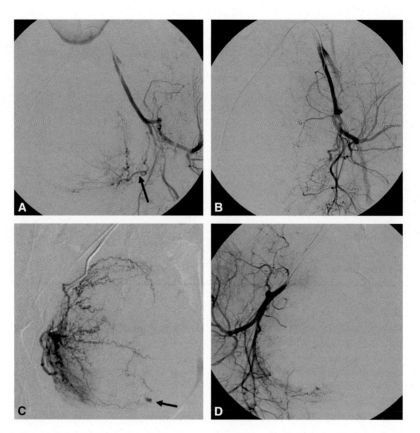

FIGURE 27.3 Delayed postpartum hemorrhage after cesarean delivery. **A.** Catheterization and angiography of the left internal iliac artery with a 5 French catheter from a right femoral approach demonstrates a hypertrophied left uterine artery (*arrow*). **B.** After gelatin sponge embolization, significant pruning of uterine artery branches is noted. **C.** Selection of the ipsilateral uterine artery in the same patient with a 3 French microcatheter again demonstrates marked vascularity of the uterus with a focus of focal contrast extravasation (*arrow*). **D.** After gelatin sponge embolization, vascularity has significantly decreased.

event subsequent emergent embolization is required.[32] Some authors have used an approach combining bilateral internal iliac artery occlusion catheter placement with gelatin sponge embolization to control intraoperative blood loss in the setting of abnormal placentation.[35]

OUTCOMES AFTER ENDOVASCULAR TREATMENT

Control of Hemorrhage

Success rates of endovascular treatment for postpartum hemorrhage have been reported at 78% to 100% with most published results reporting between 90% and 100% success at stopping the hemorrhage.[2,15,20] Most series report a reembolization rate for rebleeding of between 5% and 10%.[2,14,20,26] Most rebleeding episodes are adequately managed with repeat embolization, often addressing either a bleeding collateral not previously recognized or recanalization of an embolized vessel.[25,26] Abdominal aortography may be necessary at re-treatment for persistent postpartum bleeding to identify ovarian artery collaterals. Hysterectomy is occasionally required to stop persistent hemorrhage after endovascular therapy with a reported range between

4% and 25% of cases depending on the particular series.[2,12,26,36] Importantly, hysterectomy may not be the definitive procedure to stop bleeding as previously discussed.[2]

Abnormalities in placentation, particularly placenta percreta, may carry a higher risk of requiring ultimate hysterectomy compared with other causes of postpartum hemorrhage, such as uterine atony, according to some series.[9,10,12,36] This may be important for preprocedural counseling and planning, especially in making the decision for a preemptive internal iliac artery catheterization prior to delivery. The studies looking at the effectiveness of preemptive internal iliac artery catheterization for prophylactic pelvic artery embolization have primarily been based on case reports or small case control retrospective series.[19,30,31] A study by Diop et al.[31] compared 17 patients with placenta accreta, 6 of whom had preemptive bilateral common femoral artery sheaths placed for immediate transfer to the IR suite after cesarean section for pelvic artery embolization, and 11 patients who were taken to the IR suite for embolization after bleeding became a clinical problem. In the six patients with empiric embolization, the placenta was left in situ for spontaneous involution over time. The authors reported a significant decrease in time to treat and decrease in estimated blood loss in the preemptively treated group compared with the

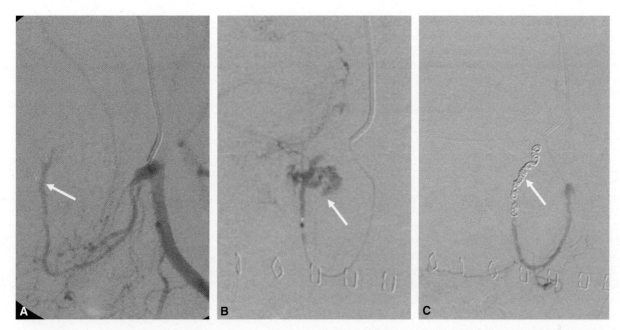

FIGURE 27.4 Postpartum hemorrhage after cesarean delivery. **A.** Angiogram with a 5 French catheter in the anterior division of the left internal iliac artery from a right femoral approach demonstrates amorphous contrast emanating from the distal aspect of a uterine artery branch (*arrow*). **B.** Microcatheter subselection and angiography demonstrates active extravasation of contrast from a lacerated vessel (*arrow*). **C.** Coil embolization through the microcatheter successfully stops the hemorrhage (*arrow*).

11 patients treated after postpartum hemorrhage became clinically manifest.[31] Some authors have advocated bilateral uterine artery embolization with either placement of sutures in the placental bed or compression of the placental bed as a successful management option avoiding hysterectomy in cases with known abnormal placentation.[37] As stated earlier, the abnormally implanted placenta may be left to involute in situ after uterine artery embolization.[38]

Data with respect to preemptive catheterization for intraoperative balloon occlusion are also primarily based on case reports or small retrospective series, and prospective data with an adequately powered number of patients are lacking. Although some reports suggest efficacy with this approach,[33,34] others have not demonstrated substantive differences in estimated blood loss or transfusion requirements compared to noncatheterized control subjects.[39–41] Thus, more definitive studies are needed if a preoperative endovascular approach is to become a universally accepted practice for patients with known abnormal placentation and a high suspected risk of intraoperative hemorrhage.

Fertility after Embolization

Whereas transient alteration in menses has been described after pelvic embolization for postpartum hemorrhage, early menopause has not been reported to be a significant sequela in the available studies.[42–46] This finding is further supported by the literature from uterine and ovarian artery embolization for symptomatic fibroids demonstrating resumption of normal menses in most cases.[47] The data on fertility outcomes after pelvic embolization for postpartum hemorrhage are difficult to assess because they are often either retrospective or based on

survey. Moreover, it is necessarily difficult to tease out the relationship of infertility with embolization rather than possible underlying obstetric issues leading to postpartum hemorrhage. Nevertheless, a retrospective study comparing 53 women with postpartum hemorrhage who were embolized with 106 women treated conservatively found no statistically significant difference in incidence of subsequent pregnancy after embolization.[46] A separate 10-year retrospective review evaluating the French and English literature reporting fertility follow-up on a total of 168 women undergoing embolization for postpartum hemorrhage found an embolization success rate of 92%, with need of subsequent hysterectomy in 7 patients (4%), and 4 deaths (2%).[48] Forty-five subsequent pregnancies were identified with a miscarriage rate of 18% and a cesarean section rate of 62%.[48] Six of the pregnancies that came to term (19%) were significant for recurrent postpartum hemorrhage, of which two underwent hysterectomy.[48] This and other reports suggest higher rates of pregnancy abnormalities after uterine artery embolization, including postpartum hemorrhage and need for cesarean delivery, although long-term data with enough statistical power are not available to fully identify all potential sequelae with respect to future pregnancy.[43,45]

Additional Complications

Additional complications from pelvic embolization for postpartum hemorrhage are relatively low. Access site complications, such as groin hematoma, arterial dissection, pseudoaneurysm, or arteriovenous fistula formation, are expected to be generally less than 5%. Postembolization uterine necrosis and abscess formation has been described in rare instances, as has adnexal and bladder necrosis.[49–51] Lower extremity ischemia as a result of nontarget embolism from the embolization procedure can occur.[52] Isolated reports describing extremity thromboembolism following balloon occlusion of the internal iliac arteries have also been described.[53,54] The risk of maternal and fetal radiation exposure poses an additional concern for an endovascular procedure; however, this can be minimized by use of pulsed fluoroscopy, use of low magnification, tightly coning the field of view, and limiting oblique imaging to decrease radiation doses.[55]

■ CONCLUSION

Endovascular treatment of postpartum hemorrhage is an effective, minimally invasive option to manage a potentially life-threatening situation while hopefully preserving normal uterine and ovarian function. Many centers have placed endovascular therapy as a first-line treatment in the algorithm of patients who fail initial conservative measures. Prophylactic embolization or balloon occlusion catheter placement, although still somewhat controversial, is an accepted practice in some centers in the setting of an anticipated postpartum hemorrhage, such as from abnormal placentation. Rebleeding can occur and is often the result of additional collateral vessels not appreciated at the time of the initial embolization. Although long-term follow-up with large numbers of patients is relatively lacking, outcomes with respect to resumption of menses and future fertility after endovascular treatment for postpartum hemorrhage have thus far been very encouraging.

■ REFERENCES

1. World Health Organization (WHO). *WHO Recommendations for the Prevention of Postpartum Haemorrhage.* Geneva, Switzerland: World Health Organization; 2007:116.
2. Vegas G, Illescas T, Munoz M, et al. Selective pelvic arterial embolization in the management of obstetric hemorrhage. *Eur J Obstet Gynecol Reprod Biol* 2006;127:68–72.
3. Gonsalves M, Belli A. The role of interventional radiology in obstetric hemorrhage. *Cardiovasc Intervent Radiol* 2010;33:887–895.
4. Gayat E, Resche-Rigon M, Morel O, et al. Predictive factors of advanced interventional procedures in a multicentre severe postpartum haemorrhage study. *Intensive Care Med* 2011;37:1816–1825.
5. Publications Committee, Society for Maternal-Fetal Medicine, Belfort MA. Placenta accreta. *Am J Obstet Gynecol* 2010;203:430–439.
6. Silver RM, Landon MB, Rouse DJ, et al. Maternal morbidity associated with multiple repeat cesarean deliveries. *Obstet Gynecol* 2006;107:1226–1232.
7. Yamashita Y, Takahashi M, Ito M, et al. Transcatheter arterial embolization in the management of postpartum hemorrhage due to genital tract injury. *Obstet Gynecol* 1991;77:160–163.
8. Ledee N, Ville Y, Musset D, et al. Management in intractable obstetric haemorrhage: an audit study on 61 cases. *Eur J Obstet Gynecol Reprod Biol* 2001;94:189–196.
9. Ganguli S, Stecker MS, Pyne D, et al. Uterine artery embolization in the treatment of postpartum uterine hemorrhage. *J Vasc Interv Radiol* 2011;22:169–176.
10. Zwart JJ, Dijk PD, van Roosmalen J. Peripartum hysterectomy and arterial embolization for major obstetric hemorrhage: a 2-year nationwide cohort study in the Netherlands. *Am J Obstet Gynecol* 2010;202:150.e1–150.e7.
11. Doumouchtsis SK, Papageorghiou AT, Arulkumaran S. Systematic review of conservative management of postpartum hemorrhage: what to do when medical treatment fails. *Obstet Gynecol Surv* 2007;62:540–547.
12. Sentilhes L, Gromez A, Clavier E, et al. Predictors of failed pelvic arterial embolization for severe postpartum hemorrhage. *Obstet Gynecol* 2009;113:992–999.
13. Brown BJ, Heaston DK, Poulson AM, et al. Uncontrollable postpartum bleeding: a new approach to hemostasis through angiographic arterial embolization. *Obstet Gynecol* 1979;54:361–365.
14. Deux JF, Bazot M, Le Blanche AF, et al. Is selective embolization of uterine arteries a safe alternative to hysterectomy in patients with postpartum hemorrhage? *AJR Am J Roentgenol* 2001;177:145–149.
15. Gilbert WM, Moore TR, Resnik R, et al. Angiographic embolization in the management of hemorrhagic complications of pregnancy. *Am J Obstet Gynecol* 1992;166:493–497.
16. Greenwood LH, Glickman MG, Schwartz PE, et al. Obstetric and nonmalignant gynecologic bleeding: treatment with angiographic embolization. *Radiology* 1987;164:155–159.
17. Hansch E, Chitkara U, McAlpine J, et al. Pelvic arterial embolization for control of obstetric hemorrhage: a five-year experience. *Am J Obstet Gynecol* 1999;180:1454–1460.
18. Merland JJ, Houdart E, Herbreteau D, et al. Place of emergency arterial embolisation in obstetric haemorrhage about 16 personal cases. *Eur J Obstet Gynecol Reprod Biol* 1996;65:141–143.
19. Mitty HA, Sterling KM, Alvarez M, et al. Obstetric hemorrhage: prophylactic and emergency arterial catheterization and embolotherapy. *Radiology* 1993;188:183–187.
20. Pelage JP, Le Dref O, Mateo J, et al. Life-threatening primary postpartum hemorrhage: treatment with emergency selective arterial embolization. *Radiology* 1998;208:359–362.
21. Yamashita Y, Harada M, Yamamoto H, et al. Transcatheter arterial embolization of obstetric and gynaecological bleeding: efficacy and clinical outcome. *Br J Radiol* 1994;67:530–534.
22. Salazar GM, Petrozza JC, Walker TG. Transcatheter endovascular techniques for management of obstetrical and gynecologic emergencies. *Tech Vasc Interv Radiol.* 2009;12:139–147.
23. Pelage JP, Le Dref O, Soyer P, et al. Arterial anatomy of the female genital tract: variations and relevance to transcatheter embolization of the uterus. *AJR Am J Roentgenol* 1999;172:989–994.
24. Razavi MK, Wolanske KA, Hwang GL, et al. Angiographic classification of ovarian artery-to-uterine artery anastomoses: initial observations in uterine fibroid embolization. *Radiology* 2002;224:707–712.
25. Wang MQ, Liu FY, Duan F, et al. Ovarian artery embolization supplementing hypogastric-uterine artery embolization for control of severe postpartum hemorrhage: report of eight cases. *J Vasc Interv Radiol* 2009;20:971–976.
26. Bros S, Chabrot P, Kastler A, et al. Recurrent bleeding within 24 hours after uterine artery embolization for severe postpartum hemorrhage: are there predictive factors? *Cardiovasc Intervent Radiol* 2012;35:508–514.
27. Saraiya PV, Chang TC, Pelage JP, et al. Uterine artery replacement by the round ligament artery: an anatomic variant discovered during uterine artery embolization for leiomyomata. *J Vasc Interv Radiol* 2002;13:939–941.
28. Pelage JP, Soyer P, Le Dref O, et al. Uterine arteries: bilateral catheterization with a single femoral approach and a single 5-F catheter—technical note. *Radiology* 1999;210:573–575.
29. Soyer P, Fargeaudou Y, Morel O, et al. Severe postpartum haemorrhage from ruptured pseudoaneurysm: successful treatment with transcatheter arterial embolization. *Eur Radiol* 2008;18:1181–1187.
30. Alvarez M, Lockwood CJ, Ghidini A, et al. Prophylactic and emergent arterial catheterization for selective embolization in obstetric hemorrhage. *Am J Perinatol* 1992;9:441–444.
31. Diop AN, Chabrot P, Bertrand A, et al. Placenta accreta: management with uterine artery embolization in 17 cases. *J Vasc Interv Radiol* 2010;21:644–648.
32. Tan CH, Tay KH, Sheah K, et al. Perioperative endovascular internal iliac artery occlusion balloon placement in management of placenta accreta. *AJR Am J Roentgenol* 2007;189:1158–1163.
33. Shih JC, Liu KL, Shyu MK. Temporary balloon occlusion of the common iliac artery: new approach to bleeding control during cesarean hysterectomy for placenta percreta. *Am J Obstet Gynecol* 2005;193:1756–1758.
34. Weeks SM, Stroud TH, Sandhu J, et al. Temporary balloon occlusion of the internal iliac arteries for control of hemorrhage during cesarean hysterectomy in a patient with placenta previa and placenta increta. *J Vasc Interv Radiol* 2000;11:622–624.
35. Dubois J, Garel L, Grignon A, et al. Placenta percreta: balloon occlusion and embolization of the internal iliac arteries to reduce intraoperative blood losses. *Am J Obstet Gynecol* 1997;176:723–726.
36. Soyer P, Morel O, Fargeaudou Y, et al. Value of pelvic embolization in the management of severe postpartum hemorrhage due to placenta accreta, increta or percreta. *Eur J Radiol* 2011;80:729–735.
37. Park JK, Shin TB, Baek JC, et al. Failure of uterine artery embolization for controlling postpartum hemorrhage. *J Obstet Gynaecol Res* 2011;37:971–978.

38. Timmermans S, van Hof AC, Duvekot JJ. Conservative management of abnormally invasive placentation. *Obstet Gynecol Surv* 2007;62:529–539.
39. Levine AB, Kuhlman K, Bonn J. Placenta accreta: comparison of cases managed with and without pelvic artery balloon catheters. *J Matern Fetal Med* 1999;8:173–176.
40. Bodner LJ, Nosher JL, Gribbin C, et al. Balloon-assisted occlusion of the internal iliac arteries in patients with placenta accreta/percreta. *Cardiovasc Intervent Radiol* 2006;29:354–361.
41. Shrivastava V, Nageotte M, Major C, et al. Case-control comparison of cesarean hysterectomy with and without prophylactic placement of intravascular balloon catheters for placenta accreta. *Am J Obstet Gynecol* 2007;197:402.e1–402.e5.
42. Salomon LJ, deTayrac R, Castaigne-Meary V, et al. Fertility and pregnancy outcome following pelvic arterial embolization for severe post-partum haemorrhage. A cohort study. *Hum Reprod* 2003;18:849–852.
43. Berkane N, Moutafoff-Borie C. Impact of previous uterine artery embolization on fertility. *Curr Opin Obstet Gynecol* 2010;22:242–247.
44. Delotte J, Novellas S, Koh C, et al. Obstetrical prognosis and pregnancy outcome following pelvic arterial embolisation for post-partum hemorrhage. *Eur J Obstet Gynecol Reprod Biol* 2009;145:129–132.
45. Goldberg J, Pereira L, Berghella V. Pregnancy after uterine artery embolization. *Obstet Gynecol* 2002;100:869–872.
46. Hardeman S, Decroisette E, Marin B, et al. Fertility after embolization of the uterine arteries to treat obstetrical hemorrhage: a review of 53 cases. *Fertil Steril* 2010;94:2574–2579.
47. Hu NN, Kaw D, McCullough MF, et al. Menopause and menopausal symptoms after ovarian artery embolization: a comparison with uterine artery embolization controls. *J Vasc Interv Radiol* 2011;22:710–715.e1.
48. Chauleur C, Fanget C, Tourne G, et al. Serious primary post-partum hemorrhage, arterial embolization and future fertility: a retrospective study of 46 cases. *Hum Reprod* 2008;23:1553–1559.
49. Coulange L, Butori N, Loffroy R, et al. Uterine necrosis following selective embolization for postpartum hemorrhage using absorbable material. *Acta Obstet Gynecol Scand* 2009;88:238–240.
50. Porcu G, Roger V, Jacquier A, et al. Uterus and bladder necrosis after uterine artery embolisation for postpartum haemorrhage. *Br J Obstet Gynaecol* 2005;112:122–123.
51. Chassang M, Novellas S, Baudin G, et al. Uterine necrosis complicating embolization with resorbable material for postpartum hemorrhage. *J Radiol* 2011;92:725–728.
52. Maassen MS, Lambers MD, Tutein Nolthenius RP, et al. Complications and failure of uterine artery embolisation for intractable postpartum haemorrhage. *Br J Obstet Gynaecol* 2009;116:55–61.
53. Chouliaras S, Hickling DJ, Tuck JS. Thromboembolism of the leg following prophylactic balloon occlusion of the uterine arteries. *Br J Obstet Gynaecol* 2009;116:1278–1279.
54. Bishop S, Butler K, Monaghan S, et al. Multiple complications following the use of prophylactic internal iliac artery balloon catheterisation in a patient with placenta percreta. *Int J Obstet Anesth* 2011;20:70–73.
55. Nikolic B, Spies JB, Campbell L, et al. Uterine artery embolization: reduced radiation with refined technique. *J Vasc Interv Radiol* 2001;12:39–44.

CHAPTER

28

Varicocele

ANDREW S. AKMAN, ALI ALBAYATI, and ANTHONY C. VENBRUX

HISTORY

In 1955 Tulloch reported improvement of semen parameters following varicocelectomy in an azospermic male that led to a successful pregnancy.[1] This report sparked interest in varicoceles as a potentially treatable cause of male infertility. As new treatment methods were devised, researchers sought to clarify the cause of varicoceles and their link to male infertility. The results to this point have been inconclusive and somewhat controversial, but treatment of varicoceles continues and varicocele embolization remains an important procedure within interventional radiology.

Testicular varicoceles are found in approximately 4% to 23% of the general population.[2–6] In the late 19th century, researchers began to link varicoceles with male infertility. In 1885, Barwell[7] published data on the treatment of dilated veins of 100 patients by ligating them with a wire loop. Four years later, Bennett[8] described improved semen quality following treatment in a patient with a bilateral varicocele. In 1965, 10 years after Tulloch's case report, MacLeod[9] published a study of 200 men with varicoceles and low sperm counts, demonstrating a large percentage experienced increasing counts and improved sperm motility following spermatic vein ligation.[9] He also noted that the number of cells demonstrating stress pathology or abnormal morphology significantly decreased following surgical ligation. As the link between the varicocele and infertility continued to solidify, new treatment methods were developed. The first endovascular techniques for spermatic vein ligation were reported in 1977 and 1978 and used sclerosing agents to occlude the spermatic vein.[10,11] In 1981, detachable balloons and coils were introduced as means of embolizing the internal spermatic vein (ISV).[12,13] Although further improvements in both surgical ligation and endovascular occlusion have led to increasing procedural success rates, research conclusively linking varicocele repair to improved fertility has not yet appeared.

PATHOPHYSIOLOGY

Varicoceles are characterized by abnormal distention of the pampiniform venous plexus.[14] In addition to the pampiniform plexus, the ISV can be dilated to the level of the renal vein on the left and the inferior vena cava (IVC) on the right. Most varicoceles are left-sided (90%) with isolated right-sided varicoceles being extremely rare (0.4% to 9%).[2,3,5,6,15]

Varicoceles can be classified as primary or secondary. Secondary varicoceles most frequently result from external venous compression secondary to an abdominal mass.[16–18] Right-sided varicoceles have also been described in patients with situs inversus.[19] An isolated right-sided varicocele is a rare finding with an incidence of 0.4% and should initiate a workup for an abdominal mass.[15]

Most varicoceles, including those found in patients with infertility, are primary in nature. There are three main anatomic explanations for the development of a varicocele: valvular incompetence, the angle of insertion of the left gonadal vein on the left renal vein, and chronic compression secondary to adjacent vascular structures.[20] Valvular incompetence has been theorized to lead to venous insufficiency; however, varicoceles do not form in all patients without valves. A study of 659 men with varicoceles demonstrated that 73% had an absence of valves.[21] Although there is clearly an association with valvular incompetence and varicocele, critics have suggested that valve dysfunction may occur secondary to venous dilation.[22]

The second theory of primary varicocele formation relates to the relationship of the left spermatic vein with the left renal vein. Buch and Cromie[23] postulated that the acute angle of entry that the left spermatic vein makes with the high-pressure left renal vein creates a hydrostatic column of pressure against which venous drainage from the testes must flow. Over time, the veins dilate and venous flow reverses.

Compression by adjacent vascular structures, described as a "nutcracker effect," has also been hypothesized as a contributing factor to varicocele formation. An increase in pressure of the left renal vein as it passes between the aorta and superior mesenteric artery creates the nutcracker effect and the resulting increased hydrostatic pressure in the left renal vein extends into the gonadal vein.[24]

Although the exact pathology of varicocele has not been completely explained, the end result is dilation of the pampiniform plexus and ISV eventually leading to reversal of flow. Data suggest that varicocele is a progressive condition because there is a direct relationship between varicocele prevalence and age.[25,26]

RELATIONSHIP TO INFERTILITY

Multiple theories have been proposed to explain the relationship of varicocele and infertility; however, research has yielded mixed results to this point. Current theories link increased temperature, decreased testosterone levels, elevated venous pressure, reactive oxygen species (ROS), and toxic substances with varicoceles and infertility.

It has been accepted that optimal temperature for sperm production is several degrees below body temperature. The pampiniform plexus is thought to act as a heat sink to decrease the temperature of arterial blood to the testes.[27] It is postulated that slow or stagnant blood flow within the pampiniform plexus in a patient with a varicocele does not provide adequate heat exchange, leading to increased testicular temperature and disruption of spermatogenesis.[20] Investigators have described elevated temperature of the testes in patients with varicocele and low sperm quality[28] and linked increased temperature to dysfunction of the seminiferous epithelium and decrease in spermatocytes and spermatids.[29] Increased temperature has also been linked to decreased DNA synthesis in germ cells and protein synthesis in Sertoli cells.[30,31] Despite these findings, the exact impact of testicular temperature on spermatogenesis has not been demonstrated.

Reflux of toxic metabolites from the left kidney and adrenal gland has also been postulated as contributing to infertility. Elevated levels of these metabolites are thought to cause arteriolar vasoconstriction, which leads to chronic hypoperfusion and epithelial dysfunction.[32] Cadmium in particular has been implicated, with studies showing a link between cadmium levels and disruption of spermatogenesis and sperm dysfunction.[33] Increased cadmium concentrations have been described in men with varicoceles.[33]

Another mechanism by which varicoceles are postulated to lead to infertility is by elevated venous pressures. It is suggested that elevated venous pressures cause chronic arterial vasoconstriction in an effort to limit blood flow to the testes. The chronic hypoperfusion then leads to impaired fertility. This model has not been conclusively proven because studies in animal models have demonstrated both increased and decreased blood flow in varicoceles.[4,34]

At normal levels, ROS are important for normal sperm function and attachment to the oocyte. At increased levels ROS have been shown to cause damage to the sperm membrane and DNA. Studies have demonstrated elevated levels of ROS in infertile men with varicoceles.[35,36] Investigators have since demonstrated improvement in DNA damage and ROS levels following varicocele repair.[37,38]

Several studies have noted decreased testosterone levels in infertile males with varicoceles, leading to speculation that varicoceles cause Leydig cell dysfunction. In a 1992 study conducted by the World Health Organization, investigators noted that males over 30 with varicoceles had lower testosterone levels than their counterparts who are less than 30 years of age. This was in contradistinction to patients without varicoceles who did not exhibit a difference in testosterone levels between the two age groups. This led to the conclusion that varicoceles lead to progressive Leydig cell dysfunction over time.[39]

▍ ANATOMY[40]

There are multiple pathways for venous drainage of the testes (FIGURE 28.1). The spermatic venous plexus or pampiniform plexus is formed by multiple tortuous venous sinuses with an approximate diameter of 5 mm. Approximately at the level of the femoral head, the sinuses join to form the ISV, functioning as the major route of drainage. Most commonly, the left ISV drains into the left renal vein and the right ISV drains directly into the infrarenal IVC (FIGURE 28.2). Additional routes of venous drainage from the left testes include the external pudendal, vasal, and cremasteric veins. The external pudendal vein (superficial external pudendal vein) originates from the plexus at the level of the inferior pubic ramus and travels superiolaterally to terminate in the great saphenous vein and, subsequently, the femoral vein. The vasal vein (ductus deferens vein) arises near the testis and passes upward where it empties into the internal iliac vein via the inferior or superior vesical

veins. The cremasteric vein (external spermatic vein) empties into the external iliac vein via the inferior epigastric vein. After embolization or ligation, the external pudendal vein most often provides the major drainage from the scrotum followed by the cremasteric vein.[40]

Several investigators have described the spermatic venous anatomy using postmortem specimens or venography; however, considerable differences exist in the description of venous collaterals, the existence of cross-scrotal collaterals, and venous valves. Lechter et al.[41] analyzed 200 spermatic veins from 100 cadavers and found that the classic pattern was present 78% of the time on the right and 79% of the time on the left (FIGURE 28.3). The spermatic vein may terminate in the right renal vein in 8% of the cases, and in 16% of the cases multiple right-sided terminations may be present. On the left, a double termination is present 19% of the time, a triple system 1% of the time, and, rarely, branches may terminate directly into the IVC (FIGURE 28.3).

The ISV usually demonstrates one to six trunks that coalesce as they ascend. In some cases, one trunk can split into additional trunks as it ascends (FIGURES 28.4 and 28.5).

Collateral vessels around the spermatic vein anastamose with the systemic circulation via the cremasteric, pudendal, vasal, retroperitoneal, ureteral, peritoneal, renal, right testicular, adrenal veins, and IVC. They also connect to the portal system through the splenic, superior mesenteric, and sigmoid colonic veins. Lechter et al.[41] found that 67% of the left-side veins and 49% of the right-side veins demonstrated collaterals with those in the upper third of the vein coming from Gerota's fascia and the lower third coming from the retroperitoneum. Examining autopsy specimens, Wishashi noted that the spermatic vein divided at L4 into medial and lateral divisions (FIGURE 28.6). The medial division was the largest, terminating in the renal vein on the left and the IVC on the right. After dividing, multiple small branches extend from the medial division to anastamose with the veins of the bladder, ureter, and renal pelvis. The lateral division terminates in the perinephric fat. Multiple small branches extend from the lateral division and join the renal capsular vessels and the colonic veins.[42] Wishashi[42] did find cadaver evidence of communication at the L3 level between the medial spermatic vein divisions in 55% of the cases. Others have demonstrated scrotal cross-collaterals.

Marsman[43] noted in 17% to 19% of cases the presence of collateral pathways that bypass the ISVs and form aberrantly fed varicoceles, making successful percutaneous embolization more difficult with a lower technical success rate. Typically, high parallel or renal collaterals cause recurrences for patients treated with embolization, and midvessels and low vessels cause recurrences for patients treated with surgical ligation.[40] Other causes of recurrence were because of transscrotal collaterals.[40]

▍ PATIENT SELECTION

Varicoceles are most commonly diagnosed by palpation on physical exam. The grading system designed by Dubin and Amelar in 1978 remains the most commonly used classification system. A grade 1 varicocele is palpable with a valsalva maneuver, a grade 2 varicocele is palpable without valsalva, and a grade 3 varicocele is visible without palpation. A grade 0 varicocele is not palpable and considered subclinical.[44] Evaluation of subclinical varicoceles is most commonly performed with duplex and color

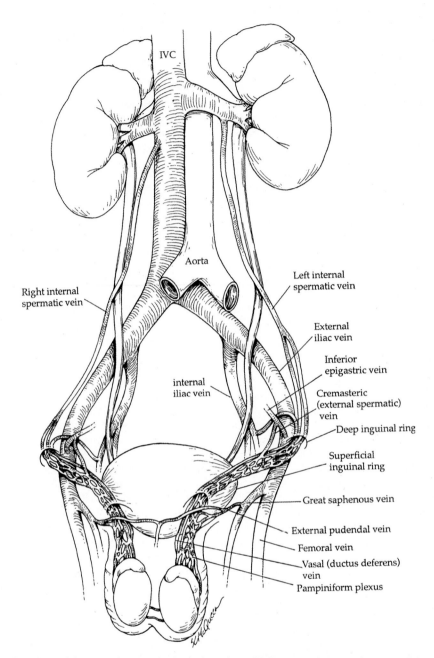

FIGURE 28.1 Classic gonadal venous drainage for both the right and left testes. The main drainage of the testes involves several veins that originate from the pampiniform plexus as the spermatic, cremasteric, pudendal, and vasal veins. The left gonadal vein enters the left renal vein, whereas the right renal vein enters the inferior vena cava below the right renal vein.

Doppler ultrasound, which shows dilation of the pampiniform plexus to greater than 2 mm.

Given that multiple studies have failed to link subclinical varicoceles to infertility, the American Urologic Association currently recommends using only the physical exam for detection of varicoceles in infertile men.[45] Ultrasound is suggested for use only if the physical exam is inconclusive.

Following detection of a varicocele, there are essentially three indications for treatment: infertility, testicular atrophy in adolescent or pediatric patients, and pain. In infertility associated patients several criteria must be met to recommend treatment. The varicocele must be palpable, the couple must have

documented infertility with the female having normal or correctable infertility, and the male must have abnormal semen parameters or sperm function.[45] Males with palpable varicoceles and abnormal semen parameters who desire to conceive in the future should also be offered treatment. Adolescent or pediatric patients with palpable varicoceles and testicular atrophy should also be treated because embolization or ligation has been shown to increase testicular volume.[46–48] In adolescent patients with normal testicular volume and a palpable varicocele, surveillance of testicular size and/or semen parameters should be performed. If either becomes abnormal, treatment should be offered. A small percentage (2% to 14%) of patients with varicocele present

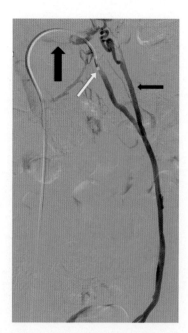

FIGURE 28.2 Catheterization of the left internal spermatic vein. A Hopkins Hook catheter is positioned with the tip (*white arrow*) at the origin of the left internal spermatic vein and the body of the hook in the left renal vein (*large black arrow*), which is minimally opacified. Note the presence of an accessory trunk (*small black arrow*), which drains into a branch of the left renal vein. This is an incompetent vein with flow primarily directed toward the testis.

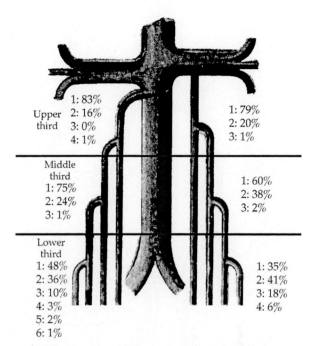

FIGURE 28.4 Number of venous trunks as they ascend from the pampiniform plexus with the percentage seen in 200 gonadal veins.

From Lechter A, Lopez G, Martinez C, et al. Anatomy of the gonadal veins: a reappraisal. *Surgery* 1991;109:735–739.

with pain most commonly described as a dull, aching pain that increases with exercise.[49]

TECHNIQUE

Patients are typically treated on an outpatient basis with IV conscious sedation. If there is concern for vagal reaction, atropine may be administered provided there is no history of heart

disease.[50] Radiation shielding is used over the gonadal and buttock areas.[50] Additional care is made to minimize radiation dose by opting for fluoroscopic image saves instead of digitial substraction angiography or single exposures when possible. Vascular access is typically obtained from the right common

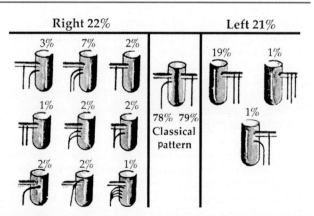

FIGURE 28.3 Anatomic variation in the termination of the right and left gonadal veins with the percentages of each variation as seen in 200 gonadal veins as determined by Lechter et al.

From Lechter A, Lopez G, Martinez C, et al. Anatomy of the gonadal veins: a reappraisal. *Surgery* 1991;109:735–739.

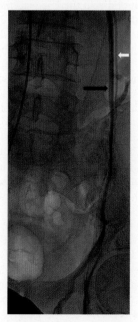

FIGURE 28.5 Left internal spermatic venogram. There is a large main trunk (*black arrow*) with a smaller accessory trunk (*white arrow*).

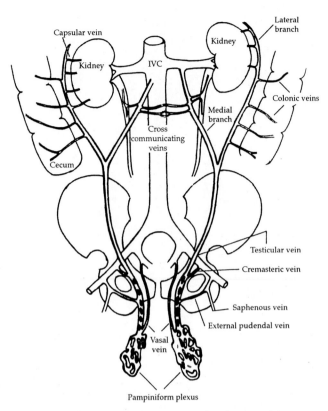

FIGURE 28.6 Anatomy of the left and right gonadal vein as described by Wishashi. There are medial and lateral divisions as well as collaterals to both the portal and systemic venous systems.

From Wishashi M. Detailed anatomy of the internal spermatic vein and ovarian vein. Human cadaver study and operative spermatic venography: clinical aspects. *J Urol* 1991;145:780–784.

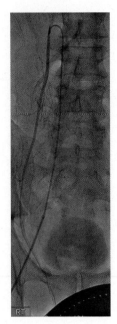

FIGURE 28.7 Right internal spermatic venogram in a patient with testicular atrophy and a varicocele. A Simmons 1 catheter has been used to select the right gonadal vein.

femoral vein or right internal jugular vein. After access of the right common femoral vein there is placement of a 7 French to 9 French vascular sheath. A 7 French or 8 French Hopkins curve catheter (modified Cobra catheter) is then used to selectively catheterize the left renal vein and then the orifice of the left ISV (FIGURE 28.2).[50] From the right jugular approach a 5 French sheath is placed and a 5 French angled tip catheter, such as a JB1 or H1H, is used to select the left renal vein and ISV.

For right-sided varicoceles treated from a femoral approach, a Simmons 1 catheter is used to select the origin of the right ISV, which is usually located on the right anterolateral surface of the cava just below the right renal vein (FIGURE 28.7).[50] Rarely, the origin of this vessel is found along the inferior surface of the right renal vein[50]. From the jugular approach the 5 French angled tip catheter used for the left side can also be used to select the right ISV.

With the ISV orifice engaged, an injection of approximately 10 to 20 cc of contrast is made while the patient performs a valsalva maneuver.[50] Images are then obtained, extending from the level of the orifice of the ISV to the pubic symphysis. The techniques described previously are used to minimize the testicular radiation dose. If reversal of flow is found to be present in the ISV, treatment may proceed.[50]

Both mechanical and pharmacologic methods have been used to occlude the ISV. Mechanical agents include embolization coils, microcoils, tissue adhesives, Ivalon plugs (Ivalon,

Inc., San Diego, CA), and woven nitinol wire plugs (Amplatzer vascular plug, St. Jude Medical, St. Paul, MN). Sclerosing agents include sodium tetradecyl sulfate 3% (sotradecol), sodium morrhuate (no longer available in the United States), absolute ethanol, and boiling contrast. Recent trials with Polytetrafluoroethylene(PTFE)-covered self-expanding nitinol occlusion devices (ArtVentive Medical Group, Carlsbad, CA) have also shown promising results, although these devices are not yet commercially available in the United States.

When using coils, a 5 French end-hole catheter is advanced through the guide catheter into the distal ISV just above the pubic symphysis.[50] Coil embolization then extends from this level to the ISV origin. The endpoint is occlusion of the ISV and its collaterals (FIGURE 28.8). When large collateral veins are present, selective catheterization and embolization is recommended (FIGURE 28.9).[50] Once the left ISV has been occluded, an attempt should be made to catheterize the right ISV. If there is reflux present, embolization should be performed even in the absence of a clinically apparent varicocele on this side.[50] If the 5 French catheter cannot be advanced into the right ISV, a microcatheter can be used coaxially. Coil embolization then proceeds in an identical manner to the left.

Collaterals may make embolization challenging.[50] Small collateral pathways may become more apparent following embolization of the main ISV and if accessible these should subsequently be catheterized and coil embolized (FIGURE 28.10).

Multiple techniques have been described with sclerosing agents. The main goal is to limit flow of the sclerosent into the scrotum to avoid pampiniform plexus phlebitis. One technique is occlusion of the distal vein with coils prior to infusion of the sclerosing agent. To further reduce the risk of reflux of sclerosant into the pampiniform plexus, during injection and for approximately 10 minutes after, manual compression of the inguinal canal with a leaded glove is performed.[50]

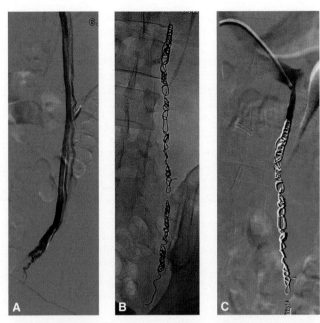

FIGURE 28.8 A. Left internal spermatic venogram shows a large primary vein with multiple smaller trunks. **B.** Coils are deployed throughout the course of the main spermatic vein across the origins of the additional trunks. **C.** Magnified postembolization venogram with injection at the origin of the left internal spermatic vein demonstrates cessation of flow through the primary vein without filling of smaller collaterals.

PROCEDURAL COMPLICATIONS

Complications associated with varicocele embolization are infrequent, occurring in up to 11% of patients.[51–53] The majority are mild and not specific to the procedure, but rather to any procedure involving percutaneous venous access. These include venous injury or severe spasm, allergic reaction to contrast media, and localized hematomas at the access site. There is the possibility of nontarget embolization or coil migration. Incorrectly sized coils can migrate centrally into the pulmonary arteries, possibly necessitating retrieval. If using sclerosing agents, pampiniform plexus thrombophlebitis has been reported to occur about 0.5% of the time.[54] It can be treated with anti-inflammatories and antibiotics. Equally rarely, scleroscent can leak into the renal vein, leading to renal vein thrombosis.

If care is taken to minimize radiation to the gonads with collimation and shielding, radiation exposure is minimal. In 2000, Chalmers et al. published a retrospective series of patients in whom radiation dose to the gonads was measured, and lifetime cancer risk was estimated to be 0.1%. In a small prospective series of patients, the authors found that they were able to lower the radiation dose by sevenfold with careful attention to exposure during the procedure.[55]

OUTCOMES

Endovascular varicocele repair has reported technical success rates, ranging from 90% to 97%.[44,56,57] Recurrence following embolization usually results from gradual enlargement of small

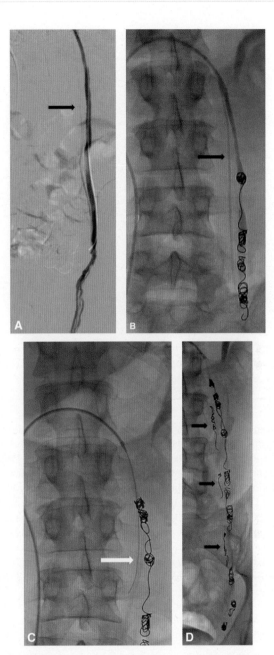

FIGURE 28.9 A. Left internal spermatic venogram with a faintly visible collateral (*black arrow*). **B.** Following coil embolization of the primary vein, the collateral vessel is more completely opacified (*black arrow*). **C.** A hydrophilic wire (*white arrow*) is advanced into the collateral vessel over which a 5 French catheter can be passed **D.** Coils (*black arrows*) have been deployed throughout the course of the collateral vessel.

collateral branches over time. The reported rate of recurrence ranges from 2% to 12%.[51,58,59]

When assessing successful treatment of infertility, results are more controversial secondary to the paucity of randomized controlled studies. The Cochrane Database published a report in 2009, which searched for randomized controlled trials that reported pregnancy rate as an outcome of varicocele repair, and found eight studies meeting this criterion. The combined odds ratio that was constructed found no significant change in pregnancy rate

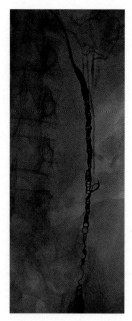

FIGURE 28.10 Left internal spermatic venogram following embolization of the main trunk depicts multiple collateral branches extending toward the renal capsule and branches of the renal vein.

between varicocele repair and expectant management.[60] One of the criticisms of this report, however, was that patients with subclinical varicoceles and normal semen parameters were included. Despite the conclusion of the Cochrane report, promising results from additional studies have been published. A recent study by Abdel-Meguid et al.[61] followed 145 subjects and showed a significant difference, 32.9% versus 13.9%, in the rate of spontaneous pregnancy between treated patients and untreated patients, respectively.

Treatment of adolescent patients with varicocele and testicular hypotrophy has shown promising results with "catch-up growth" of the affected testis in approximately 80% of patients.[64,65]

In patients with painful varicoceles, 83% to 93% experience partial resolution of symptoms with 70% to 88% reporting complete resolution of symptoms.[1,49,62,63]

CONCLUSION

Varicocele embolization remains an important procedure within interventional radiology. The prospect of short recovery time and minimal morbidity offers an appealing alternative to surgery for patients. Indications for treatment include infertility, pain, and testicular atrophy. Despite evidence that suggests a link between varicocele and infertility, the relationship remains controversial secondary to lack of randomized controlled trials.

KEY REFERENCES

American Urological Association; American Society for Reproductive Medicine. *Report on Varicocele and Infertility.* Linthicum, MD: American Urological Association; 2001.
Dubin L, Amelar R. Varicocele. *Urol Clin North Am* 1978;5(3):563–572.

Evers J, Collins J, Clarke J. Surgery or embolization for varicoceles in subfertile men. *Cochrane Database of Systematic Reviews* 2009;1–23.
Abdel-Meguid T, Al-Sayyad A, Tayib A, et al. Does varicocele repair improve male infertility? An evidence-based perspective from a randomized, controlled trial. *Eur Urol* 2011;59(3):455–461.

REFERENCES

1. Tulloch W. Varicocele in subfertility: results of treatment. *Br Med J* 1955;2:356.
2. Turner T. Varicocele: still an enigma. *J Urol* 1983;129:695–699.
3. Steeno O, Knops J, DeClerck L, et al. Prevention of fertility disorders by detection and treatment of varicocele at school and college. *Andrologia* 1976;8:47–53.
4. Saypol D. Varicocele. *J Androl* 1981;2:61–71.
5. Meacham R, Townsend R, Rademacher D, et al. The incidence of varicoceles in the general population when evaluated by physical examination, grayscale sonography, and color Doppler sonography. *J Urol* 1994;151:1535–1538.
6. Comhaire F. Varicocele infertility: an enigma. *Int J Androl* 1983;6:401–404.
7. Barwell R. One hundred cases of varicocele treated by subcutaneous wire loop. *Lancet* 1885;1:978.
8. Bennett W. Varicocele: particularly with reference to its radical cure. *Lancet* 1889;1:261–265.
9. MacLeod J. Seminal cytology in the presence of varicocele. *Fertil Steril* 1965;16:735–757.
10. Iaccarino V. Trattamento conservativo del varicocele: flebografia selettiva escleroterapia delle vene gonadiche. *Riv Radiol* 1977;17:107–117.
11. Lima S, Castro M, Costa O. A new method for the treatment of varicocele. *Andrologia* 1978;10:103–106.
12. White RJ, Kaufman S, Barth K, et al. Balloon occlusion of the internal spermatic vein for the treatment of varicoceles. *JAMA* 1981;246(15):1701–1702.
13. Weissbach L, Thelen M, Adolphs H. Treatment of idiopathic varicoceles by transfemoral testicular vein occlusion. *J Urol* 1981;126:354–356.
14. Bittles M, Hoffer E. Gonadal vein embolization: treatment of varicocele and pelvic congestion syndrome. *Semin Intervent Radiol* 2008;25(3):261–270.
15. Diamond D. Adolescent varicocele: emerging understanding. *BJU Int* 2003;92:48–51.
16. Roy CI, Wilson T, Raife M, et al. Varicocele as the presenting sign of an abdominal mass. *J Urol* 1989;141(3):597–599.
17. Shaji S, Steele C, Qasim A, et al. Right testicular varicocele: an unusual presentation of cecal adenocarcinoma. *Am J Gastroenterol* 2003;98:701–703.
18. Thomas AJ, Geisinger MA. Current management of varicoceles. *Urol Clin North Am* 1990;17(4):893–907.
19. Wilms G, Oyen R, Casselman J, et al. Solitary or predominantly right-sided varicocele: a possible sign of situs inversus. *Urol Radiol* 1988;9(1):243–264.
20. Eisenberg M, Lipshultz L. Varicocele-induced infertility: newer insights into its pathophysiology. *Indian J Urol* 2011;27(1):58–64.
21. Braedel H, Steffens J, Ziegler M, et al. A possible ontogenic etiology for idiopathic left varicocele. *J Urol* 1994;151(1):62–66.
22. Verstoppen G, Steeno O. Varicocele and the pathogenesis of the associated subfertility: a review of the various theories: II, results of surgery. *Andrologia* 1977;9(4):293–305.
23. Buch J, Cromie W. Evaluation and treatment of the preadolescent varicocele. *Urol Clin North Am* 1985;12(1):3–12.
24. Mali W, Oei H, Arndt J, et al. Hemodynamics of the varicocele: part II, correlation among the results of renocaval pressure measurements, varicocele scintigraphy and phlebography. *J Urol* 1986;135(3):489–493.
25. Canales B, Zapzalka D, Ercole C, et al. Prevalence and effect of varicoceles in an elderly population. *Urology* 2005;66(3):627–631.
26. Raman J, Walmsley K, Goldstein M. Inheritance of varicoceles. *Urology* 2005;65(6):1186–1189.
27. Dahl E, Herrick J. A vascular mechanism for maintaining testicular temperature by counter-current exchange. *Surg Gynecol Obstet* 1959;108:697–705.
28. Goldstein M, Eid J. Elevation of intratesticular and scrotal skin surface temperature in men with varicocele. *J Urol* 1989;142(3):743–745.
29. Mieusset R, Bujan L. Testicular heating and its possible contributions to male infertility: a review. *Int J Androl* 1995;18(4):169–184.
30. Steinberger A. Effect of temperature on the biochemistry of the testis. In: Zorgniotti A, ed. *Temperature and Environmental Effects on the Testis.* Vol 286. New York, NY: Plenum Press; 1991:33–37.

31. Fujisawa M, Yoshida S, Matsumoto O, et al. Deoxyribonucleic acid polymerase activity in the testes of infertile men with varicocele. *Fertil Steril* 1988;50(5):795–800.
32. Miyaoka R, Esteves S. A critical appraisal on the role of varicocele in male infertility. *Adv Urol* 2012;2012(Article ID 597495):1–9.
33. Chia S, Xu B, Ong C, et al. Effect of cadmium and cigarette smoking on human semen quality. *Int J Fertil Menopausal Stud* 1994;39(5):292–298.
34. Hsu H, Chang L, Chen M, et al. Decreased blood flow and defective energy metabolism in the varicocele-bearing testicles of rats. *Eur Urol* 1994;25(1):71–75.
35. Agarwal A, Prabakaran S, Allamaneni S. Relationship between oxidative stress, varicocele and infertility: a meta-analysis. *Reprod Biomed Online* 2006;12(5):630–633.
36. Blumer C, Restelli A, Giudice P, et al. Effect of varicocele on sperm function and semen oxidative stress. *BJU Int* 2012;109(2):259–265.
37. Smit M, Romijn J, Wildhagen M, et al. Decreased sperm DNA fragmentation after surgical varicocelectomy is associated with increased pregnancy rate. *J Urol* 2010;183(1):270–274.
38. Dada R, Shamsi M, Venkatesh S, et al. Attenuation of oxidative stress & DNA damage in varicocelectomy: implications in infertility management. *Indian J Med Res* 2010;132:728–730.
39. World Health Organization. The influence of varicocele on parameters of fertility in a large group of men presenting to infertility clinics. *Fertil Steril* 1992;57(6):1289–1293.
40. Shlansky-Goldberg R, Solomon JA. Perspectives on varicocele management. In: Baum S, Pentecost M, eds. *Abrams' Angiography Interventional Radiology*. Philadelphia, PA: Lippincott Williams & Wilkins; 2006:776–800.
41. Lechter A, Lopez G, Martinez C, et al. Anatomy of the gonadal veins: a reappraisal. *Surgery* 1991;109:735–739.
42. Wishashi M. Detailed anatomy of the internal spermatic vein and ovarian vein. Human cadaver study and operative spermatic venography: clinical aspects. *J Urol* 1991;145:780–784.
43. Marsman J. The aberrantly fed varicocele: frequency, venographic appearance, and results of transcatheter embolization. *AJR Am J Roentgenol* 1995;164:649–657.
44. Dubin L, Amelar R. Varicocele. *Urol Clin North Am* 1978;5(3):563–572.
45. American Urological Association; American Society for Reproductive Medicine. *Report on Varicocele and Infertility*. Linthicum, MD: American Urological Association; 2001.
46. Lund L, Tang Y, Roebuck D, et al. Testicular catch-up growth after varicocele correction in adolescents. *Pediatr Surg Int* 1999;15(3–4):234–237.
47. Laven J, Haans L, Mali W, et al. Effects of varicocele treatment in adolescents: a randomized study. *Fertil Steril* 1992;58(4):756–762.
48. Sayfan J, Siplovich L, Koltun L, et al. Varicocele treatment in pubertal boys prevents testicular growth arrest. *J Urol* 1997;157(4):1456–1457.
49. Kim S, Jung H, Park K. Outcomes of microsurgical subinguinal varicocelectomy for painful varicoceles. *J Androl* 2012;33(5):872–875.
50. Grieme B, Venbrux A. Management of male varicocele. In: Mauro M, Murphy K, Thomson K, et al., eds. *Image-Guided Intervention*. Philadelphia, PA: Elsevier; 2008:887–891.
51. Reyes B, Trerotola S, Venbrux A, et al. Percutaneous embolotherapy of adolescent varicocele: results and long-term follow-up. *J Vasc Interv Radiol* 1994;5(1):131–134.
52. Shlansky-Goldberg R, VanArsdalen K, Rutter C, et al. Percutaneous varicocele embolization versus surgical ligation for the treatment of infertility: changes in seminal parameters and pregnancy outcomes. *J Vasc Interv Radiol* 1997;8(5):759–767.
53. Nabi G, Asterlings S, Greene D, et al. Percutaneous embolization of varicoceles: outcomes and correlation of semen improvement with pregnancy. *Urology* 2004;63(2):359–363.
54. Wunsch R, Efinger K. The interventional therapy of varicoceles amongst children, adolescents, and young men. *Eur J Radiol* 2005;53:46–56.
55. Chalmers N, Hufton A, Jackson R, et al. Radiation risk estimation in varicocele embolization. *Br J Radiol* 2000;73(867):293–297.
56. Evers J, Collins J. Assessment of efficacy of varicocele repair for male subfertility: a systematic review. *Lancet* 2003;361(9371):1849–1852.
57. Alqahtani A, Yazbeck S, Dubois J, et al. Percutaneous embolization of varicocele in children: a Canadian experience. *J Pediatr Surg* 2002;37(5):783–785.
58. Pryor J, Howards S. Varicocele. *Urol Clin North Am* 1987;14(3):499–513.
59. Zuckerman A, Mitchell S, Venbrux A, et al. Percutaneous varicocele occlusion: long-term follow-up. *J Vasc Interv Radiol* 1994;5(2):315–319.
60. Evers J, Collins J, Clarke J. Surgery or embolization for varicoceles in subfertile men. *Cochrane Database of Systematic Reviews* 2009;1–23.
61. Abdel-Meguid T, Al-Sayyad A, Tayib A, et al. Does varicocele repair improve male infertility? An evidence-based perspective from a randomized, controlled trial. *Eur Urol* 2011;59(3):455–461.
62. Yaman O, Ozdiler E, Anafarta K, et al. Effect of microsurgical subinguinal varicocele ligation to treat pain. *Urology* 2000;55(1):107–108.
63. Karademir K, Senkul T, Baykal K, et al. Evaluation of the role of varicocelectomy including external spermatic vein ligation in patients with scrotal pain. *Int J Urol* 2005;12(5):484–488.
64. Kass EJ, Belman AB. Reversal of testicular growth failure by varicocele ligation. *J. Urol.* 1987;137(3):475–476.
65. Salzhauer EW, Sokol A, Glassberg KI. Paternity after adolescent varicocele repair. *Pediatrics.* 2004;114(6):1631–1633.

Vascular Anomalies: Hemangiomas and Vascular Malformations

Classification/Terminology

AYLIN TEKES and SALLY E. MITCHELL

INTRODUCTION

Vascular anomalies represent a wide spectrum of lesions that can present in any part of the body with the head and neck being the most common. Most vascular anomalies can be diagnosed and classified according to physical exam and history; however, radiologic evaluation is needed to (1) confirm the diagnosis, (2) prove the diagnosis in challenging cases where physical exam and history are not sufficient, (3) define the full anatomic detail of the vascular anomaly, (4) help target areas that need treatment, and (5) monitor treatment response. Accurate classification is crucial because morbidity and treatment differ significantly between different groups of vascular anomalies.

Longstanding confusion in classification of vascular anomalies stems from ignorance of their pathophysiology. Understanding the pathophysiology of these lesions has been revolutionized by the landmark article by Drs. Mulliken and Glowacki in 1982,[1] revealing the biologic behavior of vascular anomalies. In this first biologic classification, vascular anomalies were divided into two major groups: vascular tumors (with cellular proliferation and hyperplasia) and vascular malformations (focal defects of vascular morphogenesis). Vascular malformations were subdivided further into lesions consisting of capillary, venous, arterial, lymphatic, and fistulous networks.

Since 1982, classification of vascular anomalies has been an area of growing awareness. Burrows and colleagues[2] initially characterized the angiographic flow patterns in 1983. Building on this classification system, Jackson and colleagues[3] proposed a complimentary classification system in 1993 that considered flow rate as a variable determining diagnosis and treatment. In this flow rate–based classification, vascular anomalies were divided into hemangiomas, vascular malformations (low-flow venous malformations [VMs] and high-flow arteriovenous malformations [AVMs]), and lymphatic malformations (LMs). Meanwhile, Belov[4] introduced a classification system in 1990, focusing on the embryologic site of origin of the defect that led to the development of each particular malformation. In this classification system, each malformation was subdivided into two basic anatomopathologic forms: truncular and extratruncular. The truncular form was more severe and resulted from a relatively late embryologic defect or event arising within a differentiated vascular trunk. The extratruncular form was often less severe and resulted from a relatively early embryonal dysplasia within the primitive undifferentiated capillary network.

Each classification system has brought clarifications to our current understanding of vascular anomalies. The International Society of Study of Vascular Anomalies (ISSVA) was founded by Mulliken and Young in 1976, and the ongoing developments

in the classification systems were discussed biannually. A final classification of vascular anomalies based on cellular features, vascular flow characteristics, and clinical behavior was refined and updated during the 1992 meeting and adopted by ISSVA in 1996 (Table 29.1). This classification system defines the common language in the evaluation of vascular anomalies and should be used by all disciplines involved in the care of these lesions.

Historically, vascular anomalies were named and categorized after their gross appearance, location, fluid content, and an overlapping clinical course, resulting in redundant, ambiguous, and sometimes misleading terms. Nomenclature of vascular anomalies have evolved from "angiomas" to "vascular birthmarks" to the general name for the group "vascular anomalies" in the past few decades. The term *hemangioma* has incorrectly served as a generic word to describe most of these vascular anomalies. To avoid errors in diagnosis and management, as well as improve communication between multiple different clinical disciplines involved in the care of vascular anomalies, certain terms should be abandoned for more appropriate terms. The term *strawberry or capillary hemangioma* should be replaced by *infantile hemangioma*; *cavernous hemangioma* should be replaced by *venous malformation*; previously called *port-wine stains*

Table 29.1

Vascular Anomalies

Vascular tumors	Vascular malformations
Infantile hemangiomas	Slow-flow malformations -VM, -LM, -CM
Congenital hemangiomas -RICH, -NICH	High-flow vascular malformations -AVM, -AVF
Others: Kaposiform hemangioendothelioma Tufted angioma Pyogenic granuloma	Combined vascular malformations -CLV (Klippel-Trenaunay) -CV with AV shunting (Parkes-Weber)

VM, venous malformation; LM, lymphatic malformation; CM, capillary malformation; RICH, rapidly involuting congenital hemangioma; NICH, noninvoluting congenital hemangioma; AVM, arteriovenous malformation; AVF, arteriovenous fistula; CLV, capillary lymphatic venous malformation; CV with AV shunting, capillary venous with arteriovenous shunting.
Adapted and simplified from International Study of Society of Vascular Anomalies (ISSVA) 1996.

are known to represent "capillary malformations." The suffix "-oma" implies tumoral growth; therefore *lymphangioma* is a misnomer because LMs are not vascular tumors but vascular malformations. The terms *lymphangioma* and *cystic hygroma* should be replaced by the term *lymphatic malformation*.

DIAGNOSTIC EVALUATION STRATEGIES AND RECOMMENDATIONS

Multidisciplinary approach integrating the clinical presentation and imaging findings is mandatory in the diagnostic evaluation of vascular anomalies. Soft-tissue vascular anomalies are congenital and may present anywhere in the body from head to toe, most commonly in the head and neck region, followed by extremities,[5] presenting generally during infancy or childhood, although they may not be noticed until adulthood. Infantile hemangiomas (IHs) often involute during childhood, whereas vascular malformations persist through adulthood. Skin discoloration with or without a palpable mass, pain, bleeding, cosmetic concern, or malfunction are the leading presenting symptoms. The complex and variable nature of vascular anomalies requires diagnosis and care by a team involving but not limited to dermatologists, interventional radiologists, pediatric radiologists, musculoskeletal radiologists, plastic surgeons, and head and neck surgeons. Most vascular tumors and vascular malformations are recognized on clinical basis. Presenting age, softness of the palpable lesion, and extent and distribution in the involved body part provide critical clinical information. For example, a teenager presenting with a new, soft palpable mass in the neck most likely presents a vascular malformation. The chance of an infantile hemangioma is unlikely in this clinical setting because IHs present during infancy and commonly involute before the teenage years.

Various imaging modalities including gray scale ultrasonography (US), Doppler US, computed tomography (CT), magnetic resonance imaging (MRI), and conventional angiography have been used in the evaluation of vascular anomalies. MRI plays a major role given the multiplanar imaging capability and multiple different tissue contrasts.

What Imaging Modality First, When and How?

Each diagnostic imaging study should be tailored to provide an answer to the clinical question. Therefore, appropriate communication between the radiologist and ordering physician is very important. US with Doppler imaging is often the initial imaging modality sought for evaluation of vascular anomalies in pediatric patients because of its portability, accessibility, lack of ionizing radiation, and limited need/no need for sedation. Gray scale imaging defines the extent and compressibility of the lesion and determines whether a lesion is cystic or solid. Spectral and color Doppler are used to identify flow characteristics[6] and to differentiate arterial from venous flow. The interrogation of superficial and small vascular lesions, which may be inconspicuous on MRI, can be well performed with US with a high-frequency transducer. US is an operator-dependent modality; therefore, unless it is evaluated by a trained technologist and monitored by the radiologist, reliability of the US imaging findings may be questionable. Full anatomic extent of the vascular anomaly may be difficult in large lesions.

Use of CT is highly limited in the evaluation of vascular anomalies given the high radiation and relatively limited soft-tissue contrast compared to MRI. It is, however, useful in cases where assessment of osseous involvement is crucial, such as the sinuses, skull base, cranium, mandible.[7]

The radiologist is required to define the anatomic extent of the vascular anomaly in detail in regard to depth and size and its relationship/proximity to major arteries, veins, and nerves. Classification of the vascular anomaly based on ISSVA guidelines and evaluation of response to treatment can be most accurately and reliably assessed by MRI because of its superior soft-tissue resolution and multiplanar imaging capabilities. Contrast-enhanced MRI and magnetic resonance angiography (MRA) are suitable for the evaluation of most vascular anomalies. "As low as reasonably achievable" (ALARA) radiation protection paradigm and the image gentle campaign was introduced 10 years ago to limit radiation as much as possible to children. A radiation-free diagnostic evaluation is especially important in children, requiring repeated monitoring and treatment follow-up, as in the case of vascular anomalies, because digital subtraction angiography (DSA) or computed tomography angiography (CTA) may incur significant radiation exposure.

Utilization/combination of more than one imaging modality may be necessary to obtain all necessary information.

Magnetic Resonance Imaging Protocol in the Evaluation of Vascular Anomalies

Contrast-enhanced MRI of vascular anomalies must be combined with MRA, ideally a time-resolved 3D dynamic contrast-enhanced MRA (DCE-MRA). No vascular anomaly protocol with MRI is complete without a DCE-MRA. Structural information provided by the conventional T1-weighted (T1-W) and T2-weighted (T2-W) imaging is complemented with the dynamic enhancement information. The radiologist should check each case ideally immediately after the acquisition of the first set of T2-W image to determine whether or not the field of view is comprehensive enough to include the entire vascular anomaly, as well upon completion of the exam to check adherence to the protocol, and image quality.

MRI starts with fat-saturated or suppressed T2-W imaging performed in all three orthogonal planes. Fat suppression or saturation is crucial because almost all vascular anomalies present with increased T2 signal. Anatomic extent of the lesion can be best evaluated in this sequence. This is followed by an axial precontrast T1-W image. Upon administration of contrast, DCE-MRA is performed followed by postcontrast T1-W imaging with fat saturation in all three orthogonal planes. Depending on the vendor and the experience of the radiologist, T1-W imaging can be performed using a 2D or a 3D technique. Three-dimensional technique enables multiplanar reconstruction of the pre- and postcontrast imaging, thus it can reduce the scanning time.

DCE-MRA is a 3D gradient echo (GRE) time-resolved MRA technique used to dynamically assess the timing of contrast enhancement and define the arterial feeders and venous drainage of a vascular anomaly.[8,9] Most vascular anomalies show some degree of contrast enhancement, and it is impossible to determine the timing/phase (arterial, capillary, or venous) of enhancement in postcontrast T1-W images.

DCE-MRA is performed in a single orthogonal plane that depicts the vascular anomaly the best, and coronal plane is generally the default choice. DCE-MRA offers high temporal resolution in the order of seconds[10] and provides functional data about the dynamics of contrast enhancement, which is invaluable in the diagnosis of vascular anomalies. Multiphase studies, comprising arterial, capillary, venous, and delayed venous phases, can be optimized by selecting enhancement phases with optimal characteristics on the workstation. Rapid DCE-MRA data acquisition is based on a combination of parallel imaging and k-space undersampling.[11] View-sharing and keyhole techniques are used by fully sampling the central k-space during each acquisition, whereas only a small fraction of the k-space periphery is acquired at the same time. A full k-space periphery is generated for each image by adding information from previous and subsequent acquisition to obtain a sharp, high-resolution image with good image contrast. The high-resolution components encoded in the k-space periphery are relatively stable over time, whereas the low-frequency k-space center carries the significant contrast changes during bolus passage. Spatial resolution is relatively low compared to conventional 3D MRA techniques.

Image quality and spatial resolution of the data can be further enhanced with the use of blood-pool MR contrast agents, which reversibly binds to serum albumin with high affinity with a binding fraction of approximately 90%.[12] Therefore, it is strongly restricted to the blood pool in which it remains for a prolonged period, thus the limited/minimal enhancement of soft tissues surrounding the vascular anomaly. The albumin binding reduces the tumbling speed of the contrast agent molecules, thus leading to an up to sixfold increase in R1 relaxivity and signal compared to freely diffusible contrast agents, such as gadobenate dimeglumine.[13] Advantages over traditional contrast agents include higher intravascular concentration of contrast over a longer time period and increased relaxivity, giving better signal-to-noise (SNR) and contrast-to-noise ratios (CNR) for imaging.[11] Children have a much faster circulation time than adults and lower doses are used and injection times are longer, resulting in higher contrast dilution.[11] Blood-pool contrast agents can be administered at an approximately threefold lower dose than diffusible contrast agents while achieving an SNR gain, leading to a more compact bolus facilitating the separation of contrast enhancement phases. Both arterial and venous enhancement persists over a prolonged time, making contrast timing less critical: bolus tracking is not required. These are highly advantage points that make them preferable in the evaluation of vascular anomalies in children. Blood-pool contrast agents have slower excretion from the blood pool and thus may increase the risk for nephrogenic systemic fibrosis (NSF) in pediatric patients with immature kidney function.[11] Contrarily, lower concentrations in the interstitial space, lower dose, a biliary excretion of approximately 10%, and an ionic molecular structure may lower the risk.[11] NSF has not been found in patients younger than 6 years,[14] although high-contrast doses have been used in children with immature kidneys.[15]

Accurate diagnosis and classification can often be provided by contrast-enhanced MRI and DCE-MRA, progressively limiting the need for DSA in the initial diagnosis.

MRI diagnosis is made with the information combining the T1 and T2 signal characteristics and, most importantly, the dynamic enhancement pattern. Dynamic enhancement information provides major decision support in the appropriate classification of these lesions and is further discussed in each vascular anomaly separately.

▌ VASCULAR ANOMALIES

Vascular Tumors

Infantile Hemangiomas

IHs make up at least 90% of all vascular tumors. IHs are the most common vascular tumors of infancy, more common in white caucasian infants with the highest incidence in preterm infants weighing less than 1,000 g.[16] Low birth weight is the single most important predictor of IH with the risk of IH increasing by 40% for every 500 g decrease in birth weight.[17] IHs often are inapparent at birth and most appear in the first 6 weeks of life with a typical triphasic evolution: proliferation, plateau, and involution. Most hemangiomas double in size in the first 2 months of life, and approximately 80% reach their maximum size between 3 and 5 months of age.[18] IHs are positive for immunohistochemical markers, such as GLUT-1, that help differentiate congenital hemangiomas from vascular malformations. Morphologically, IHs can be divided into superficial, deep, and mixed types.[19] They can further be classified as focal, segmental, and indeterminate. Segmental and deep hemangiomas are known to have a longer proliferation phase. Segmental hemangiomas are important to recognize because they can be part of PHACE syndrome: posterior fossa malformation, hemangiomas, arterial anomalies, coarctation of the aorta, and eye abnormalities. Imaging is not required for the majority of IHs but may be required to confirm the suspected diagnosis in atypical lesions and to determine anatomic extent for deep lesions. Imaging might be required in excluding other atypical vascular tumors, or soft-tissue malignancies, and vascular malformations.[19] Surgical planning and response to treatment can be best evaluated by MRI.

The evolutionary phase of the hemangioma determines the imaging features. Regardless of the modality of choice, IH is visualized as a well-defined, focal, soft-tissue mass. Although infiltration of more than one tissue plane/adjacent organ may be observed, IHs generally present as a mass enlarging from a center in a single tissue plane.

US shows variable echogenicity within a solid mass with increased color flow within the mass and low resistance in spectral analysis. Either arterial feeder and venous drainage can be visualized with Doppler US.

MRI reveals a T2 bright, T1 isointense mass with homogenous avid contrast enhancement. Best diagnostic clue is a soft-tissue mass that shows avid, homogenous, "arterial" contrast enhancement noted in the DCE-MRA (FIGURE 29.1).

In T2-W spin echo (SE) imaging arterial feeder and venous drainage can be depicted as serpiginous flow voids, giving the clue that these are vessels, not phleboliths. Typically, no perilesional edema is observed. A common misnomer is that "phleboliths" are seen in hemangiomas. The term *phlebolith* refers to "calcification in a vein" and is commonly seen in venous malformations, not hemangiomas. Presence of calcification in a vascular soft-tissue mass should raise the possibility of congenital vascular hemangiomas, or hemangioendotheliomas, not an IH.

Unlike congenital forms, arteriovenous shunting is rare in IH; however, it is a possibility.[6] During regression, the number of vessels and size of the lesion decrease, but the high-frequency

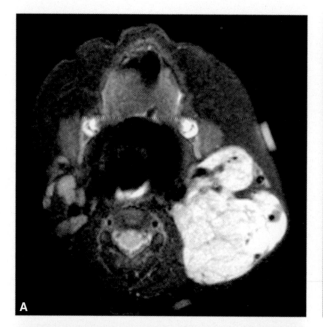

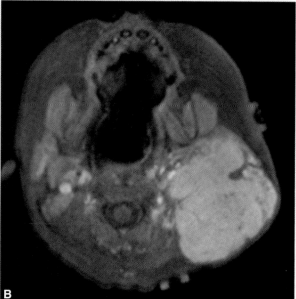

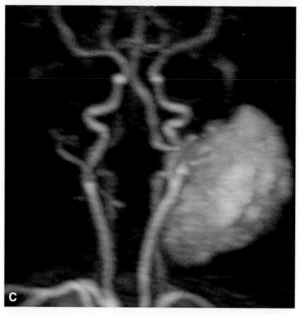

FIGURE 29.1 Six-month-old female with a palpable soft mass in the left lateral neck, an infantile hemangioma (IH). **A.** Axial T2-W image with fat saturation demonstrates a well-defined hyperintense soft-tissue mass in the left neck with few internal serpiginous flow voids. **B.** Postcontrast T1-weighted image with fat saturation demonstrates avid, homogenous internal contrast enhancement of the solid vascular mass. **C.** Time-resolved dynamic contrast-enhanced MRA (DCE-MRA) in the arterial phase demonstrates that the avid homogenous enhancement of the IH starts in the arterial phase (note that only the arteries are enhanced, no veins visualized) from a feeding artery taking off from the left external carotid artery. Serpiginous flow voids noted in A was demonstrated to represent the feeding arteries and draining veins of the IH. This is not to be confused with phleboliths seen in venous malformations. Phleboliths are round or oval shaped and do not elongate or appear as serpiginous.

Doppler shifts representing the vascular supply may remain stable.[20] During the involution phase, areas of fibro-fatty transformation can be recognized within the mass, which may reveal itself as areas of nonenhancing tissue. Approximately 40% of IHs in the head and neck region involute with fat replacement.

If the soft-tissue mass shows few arteries or veins, and spectral analysis reveals high resistance and an MRI depicts perilesional edema, other tumoral lesions, such as sarcoma, neuroblastoma, myofibromatosis, or hemangiopericytoma, should be considered.[21]

Congenital Hemangiomas

Congenital hemangiomas are divided into noninvoluting congenital hemangioma (NICH) and rapidly involuting congenital hemangioma (RICH).[22] Unlike IH, congenital hemangiomas

are fully formed at birth with clinically little or no growth after birth. There is no gender predilection and, clinically. it is difficult to differentiate NICH from RICH in the neonatal time period—retrospectively differentiation is made. RICH involutes by 12 months of age, whereas NICH involutes partially or none and may require surgical excision. Ultimate diagnosis and differentiation is made based on the natural history of the lesion. Imaging findings are similar to IH with some differences like possible vascular aneurysms, higher likelihood of arteriovenous shunting, and intravascular thrombus (never present in IH).

Kaposiform Hemangioendothelioma

These are rare vascular tumors that typically present in the first 2 to 3 years of life. Unlike IH, they are rare in the head and neck region and commonly present in the extremities. US reveals an ill-defined mass with variable echogenicity. Calcifications can be observed (never present in IH). MRI shows an ill-defined T2 hyperintense mass with heterogeneous enhancement. Unlike IH, they can be locally aggressive, crossing tissue planes. The most common, and potentially life-threatening complication, is Kassabach-Merritt phenomenon.

Vascular Malformations

Vascular malformations can be seen anywhere in the body from head to toe with variable size and depth. They are believed to represent developmental dysmorphogenesis in angiogenesis and vasculogenesis between the 4th and 10th weeks of intra-uterine life. Molecular discoveries indict genes expressed in endothelial cells and involved in receptor signaling.[23] They are present at birth, although they may not become visible until childhood and, rarely, until adulthood. Vascular malformations grow commensurately with the child, and exacerbations may follow after trauma, infection, or hormonal changes. Typically, they do not regress spontaneously, unlike IH. Isolated forms of vascular malformations are far more common than mixed types (involving more than one vessel type such as capillary-lympho-venous). Mixed-complex types of vascular malformations can be seen in some syndromes, such as Klippel-Trenaunay, Parkes-Weber, Blue Rubber Bleb Nevus, or Mafucci.

They are classified based on the involved vessel type and flow rate: Low-flow vascular malformations; such as (VM), LM, capillary malformations (CM), and high-flow vascular malformations; such as (AVM).

Low-Flow Vascular Malformations
Venous Malformation

VMs are the most common type of vascular malformation and present as soft, compressible lesions. VMs are commonly infiltrative in nature and violate multiple tissue planes, such as the subcutaneous fat and muscle. Focal, noninfiltrating presentations can be seen. The lesions vary in size from very small to extensive, involving multiple body parts. Generally even when large, VMs tend to be continuous in nature. Multifocality may suggest familial predisposition.[24] They tend to extend within the muscle groups of extremities, along the nerves and major arteries or veins.

US reveals a lesion with usually low echogenicity, with no detectable flow, or monophasic low-velocity flow. Most of the time Doppler flow is difficult to obtain because of below-threshold flow or thrombosis. Valsalva or manual compression might be helpful during US imaging because they may induce flow.[21] Also, manual compression can reveal the easily compressed venous spaces in a VM. Phleboliths can be seen as areas of calcification within the lesion.

MRI is the best modality to define the full anatomic extent of VMs. VMs are serpiginous T2 hyperintense lesions, which often show phleboliths. Hemorrhage, thrombosis, or phleboliths may reveal variable degrees of T1 hyperintensity. Some degree of fat tissue or muscle tissue may be observed interspersed between the venous channels.

Presence of phleboliths and internal enhancement in the venous phase of DCE-MRA are the best diagnostic clue

in diagnosis of VM. Phleboliths can be identified as well-demarcated, focal, round- or oval-shaped areas that reveal dark signal on T2-W imaging with surrounding high T2 signal (FIGURE 29.2). This surrounding rim of high T2 signal is thought to represent the venous blood between the phlebolith and vessel wall. Variable degrees of internal contrast enhancement can be seen, depending on the presence of internal thrombosis, phleboliths, and prior embolization (FIGURE 29.2). VMs do not have arterial feeders and may communicate with systemic veins, which is crucial to note before embolization. DCE-MRA

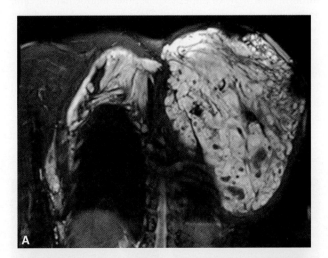

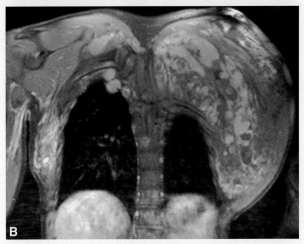

FIGURE 29.2 Seventeen-year-old male with a large venous malformation (VM) infiltrating the subcutaneous fat of the back and chest wall with multiple previous embolizations. **A.** Coronal T2-W fat-saturated image demonstrates a large, lobular T2 hyperintense VM infiltrating the bilateral chest wall on the left worse than the right. Multiple round/oval T2 dark foci are noted within the VM representing phleboliths. Note the T2 bright signal surrounding the phleboliths representing the venous blood. **B.** Coronal T1-weighted image with fat saturation: heterogenous contrast enhancement within the venous malformation is in part secondary to the presence of thrombus and phleboliths and in part secondary to delayed enhancement in this large VM.

demonstrates presence of flow within the lesion in the venous phase only with gradual increase.

Peripheral lesions can lead to bone thinning, demineralization with possible pathologic fracture, and limb underdevelopment. They may also lead to skeletal hypertrophy or remodeling and muscle contracture from infiltration of the malformation or secondary to sclerotherapy treatment.[25,26] They have been associated with muscle atrophy and subcutaneous fat prominence.[27]

Dysplastic/anomalous veins or persistent embryonic veins can be observed, especially in the setting of syndromes, such as Klippel-Trenaunay (FIGURE 29.3). It is critical that the venous anatomy be clearly delineated in Klippel-Trenaunay to determine if treatment of superficial venous malformations and anomalous veins is possible. If the deep venous system is absent or severely hypoplastic, then treatment to ablate superficial malformations may not be possible.

Lymphatic Malformations

LMs are present as a soft, nonpulsatile mass commonly located in the head and neck region and can also be seen in the trunk, extremities, axilla, mediastinum, or peritoneal cavity/mesentery.

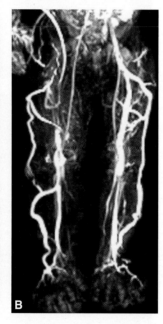

FIGURE 29.3 Three-year-old girl with enlargement of the right lower extremity: Klippel-Trenaunay syndrome. **A.** Coronal T2-W image with fat saturation shows asymmetric enlargement of the right lower extremity including the subcutaneous fat and muscle. Focal area of lobular increased T2 signal in the right vastous medialis muscle represents a venous malformation. Also note enlargement in the bilateral feet on the right worse than the left. **B.** Steady-state subtracted contrast-enhanced MRA coronal MIP of the bilateral lower extremities demonstrate presence of bilateral embryonic veins in the lateral calf, draining into the popliteal vein and anomalous deep femoral artery on the right, and draining into the left common femoral vein on the left. Note that overall the venous system is enlarged/patulous.

They are the second most common type of vascular malformations after VMs.[28] Sudden enlargement can be observed secondary to internal bleeding or infection. Morphologically, they can present as macrocystic, microcystic, or mixed. Variable size and trans-spatial infiltration can be observed.

US reveals a cystic mass with lobulations and septations. Although these are slow-flow lesions, Doppler US may reveal small arteries at the level of septations.

LMs are commonly T2 hyperintense and high T1 signal can be seen in the presence of internal hemorrhage/high protein content.

Fluid-fluid level can be seen in LM likely reflecting debris from inflammation or hemorrhage; however, it should be noted that fluid-fluid level is a sign of slow-flow malformation and can sometimes be seen in VMs as well. Therefore, it should not be taken as a sole diagnostic criterion in the diagnosis of LM.

The lymphatic cysts do not show internal enhancement after intravenous contrast administration, which is the most decisive finding on MR in the differentiation from other vascular anomalies (FIGURE 29.4). Septal or wall enhancement, however, is commonly observed. In patients with diffuse microcystic involvement, enhancing walls may challenge the interpretation because they may appear as areas of relatively solid enhancement.

Capillary Malformations

CMs are limited to superficial layers of the skin; however, over time they can become nodular and thicker. Previously called "port wine stains," CMs can be seen in Sturge-Weber syndrome, Klippel-Trenaunay, or Parkes-Weber syndrome. They are diagnosed on clinical basis. A high-frequency US transducer might be helpful in the delineation of these lesions. Given the superficial involvement MRI has limited value.

High-Flow Vascular Malformations
Arteriovenous Malformations

AVMs are high-flow lesions characterized by direct connections between arteries and veins without an intervening capillary bed. They are considered as the most aggressive type of vascular malformations. They are most common in the head and neck region, and nearly 70% involve the midface.

AVMs are made of multiple feeding arteries with increased diastolic flow and increased venous return with systolic/diastolic flow. They present with ill-defined borders with no soft-tissue mass. Most of the time, fat tissue can be seen around the AVM. Unlike hemangiomas, there is always arterialization of all the draining veins (i.e., pulsatile flow) in AVMs.

MRI examination allows evaluation of the extension into adjacent structures, especially bone involvement. Bone infiltration is most commonly seen in AVMs among all vascular malformations. MRI findings include dilated feeding arteries and draining veins with no surrounding tissue matrix.[29] Tangles of serpiginous signal voids are typically observed in AVMs on both T1- and T2-W SE sequences, whereas increased signal is observed on GRE and angiographic sequence, indicating a high-flow lesion.[30] DCE-MRA typically shows early venous filling in the arterial phase. Systemic arteries feeding the AVM and draining veins can also be assessed in DCE-MRA (FIGURE 29.5).[31]

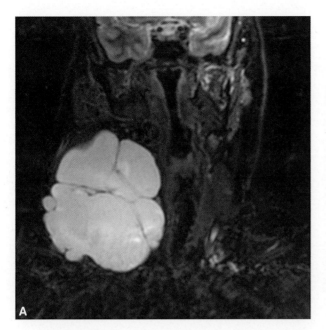
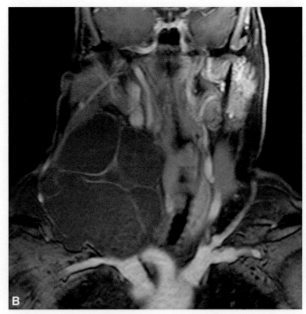

FIGURE 29.4 Sixty-six-year-old female with a soft palpable right neck mass: lymphatic malformation. Patient first presented at 46 years of age, delayed presentation of vascular malformation in adulthood is possible. **A.** Axial T2-W image with fat saturation demonstrates a large, lobular, multicystic/septated hyperintense mass in the right neck representing a macrocystic lymphatic malformation. **B.** Note that only peripheral cyst wall/septation enhancement is noted in this coronal T1-W image with fat saturation. Lymph fluid does not show enhancement after intravenous contrast administration. The airway is patent, although there is minimal leftward shift.

Syndromes with Slow-Flow and High-Flow Vascular Malformations

Syndromes with Slow-Flow Malformations

Sturge-Weber syndrome is a nonheritable disorder that typically presents with a capillary malformation in the V1 distribution of trigeminal. Typically an ipsilateral leptomeningeal malformation is seen in the parieto-occipital region that may eventually result in atrophy and calcifications in the subjacent cerebral cortex likely secondary to steal phenomenon. Patients may present with seizures and variable degree of mental retardation.[32]

Klippel-Trenaunay syndrome may present with mixed type slow-flow malformation, capillary venolymphatic malformation (CLVM) with limb overgrowth.[33,34] MRI demonstrates venous varicosities mainly in the superficial aspect of the subcutaneous fat, which are deformed, insufficient, or absent valves. The pathognomonic marginal vein of Servelle is often identified in the subcutaneous fat of the lateral calf and thigh and can communicate with the deep venous system at various levels. The lower limb is more frequently involved. DCE-MRA can be used to assess the route of drainage of the venous system and to determine the varicosities that may benefit from sclerotherapy or resection. It is critical to clearly define the deep venous system in this syndrome in which 50% may present with absent or hypoplastic or aneurysmal segments of deep veins.

Blue rubber bleb nevus syndrome is a sporadic disease characterized by multiple VMs of the skin with multiple gastrointestinal VMs.[35]

Proteus syndrome consists mainly of lymphatic venous malformations (LVM), hemihypertrophy, pigmented nevi, gigantism involving the extremities (hand, foot), intra-abdominal lipomatosis, and macrocephaly.[36]

Bannayan-Riley-Ruvalcaba syndrome is an autosomal-dominant condition associated with phosphatase and tensin homolog (PTEN) gene mutation on chromosome 10q. Clinical features include macrocephaly, pseudopapilloedema, pigmented maculas on the penis, gastrointestinal polyposis, visceral lipoma, thyroiditis, and capillary and combined malformations.

Glomovenous malformation is an autosomal-dominant condition, also known as glomangioma. It is characterized by multiple, often tender, blue nodular dermal lesions in the skin. US imaging features are similar to those of VM with the exception that the lesion cannot be completely emptied by compression. The lesions are considered to be VMs with the presence of glomus cells.

Syndromes with High-Flow Malformations

Parkes-Weber syndrome involves a combination of arteriovenous fistulas (AVFs), congenital varicose veins, and a cutaneous capillary malformation associated with limb hypertrophy.[37]

Osler-Weber-Rendu syndrome (hereditary hemorrhagic telangiectasia) manifests as diffuse mucosal telangiectasia involving the nasopharynx, gastrointestinal tract, and sometimes the urinary and genital mucosa. AVMs involving the pulmonary hepatic and cerebral arteries may be present.[38]

Capillary malformation–AVM syndrome is a hereditary disorder characterized by cutaneous capillary malformation associated with AVM or AVF.

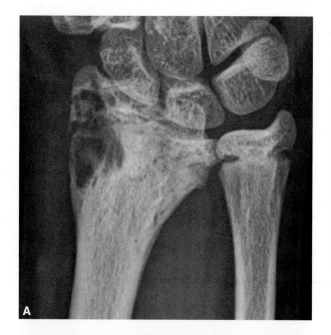

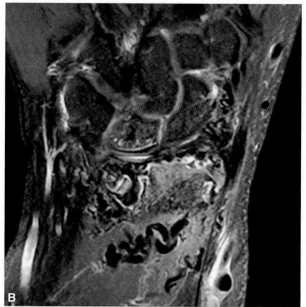

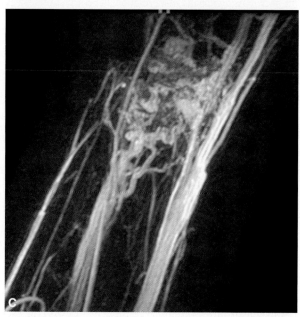

FIGURE 29.5 Thirteen-year-old male with swelling, erythema, and bruit over the volar aspect of the left wrist and an arteriovenous malformation (AVM). **A**. AP view of the left wrist demonstrates mild deformity and enlargement in the distal left radius and focal area of lucency on the medial aspect of the distal metaphysis and epiphysis. **B**. Coronal T1-weighted image demonstrates that deformity in the distal left radius is from a tangle of flow voids in the distal wrist without a soft-tissue component representing the AVM. Note the involvement in the lunate bone. **C**. Time-resolved DCE-MRA in the arterial phase demonstrates a tangle of vessels in the wrist joint with arterial filling from the interosseous and radial artery and early venous drainage to the median antecubital vein and radial veins, which are enlarged.

Cobb syndrome is a rare nonhereditary syndrome where a cutaneous capillary malformation is associated with AVM of the spinal cord.

CONCLUSION

A multidiciplinary team approach is necessary to provide accurate diagnosis and management of vascular anomalies. It is crucial that all specialists should communicate with a uniform standardized terminology as suggested by ISSVA classification. Vascular anomalies can present anywhere in the body, and rather than choosing a body part protocol, dedicated vascular anomaly protocols should be used, ideally optimized for that body part. Dynamic contrast-enhanced MRA is a crucial part of the protocol because enhancement pattern and timing is a key feature in the classification.

REFERENCES

1. Mulliken JB, Glowacki J. Hemangiomas and vascular malformations in infants and children: a classification based on endothelial characteristics. *Plast Reconstr Surg* 1982;69(3):412–422.
2. Burrows PE, Mulliken JB, Fellows KE, et al. Childhood hemangiomas and vascular malformations: angiographic differentiation. *AJR Am J Roentgenol* 1983;141(3):483–488.
3. Jackson IT, Carreno R, Potparic Z, et al. Hemangiomas, vascular malformations, and lymphovenous malformations: classification and methods of treatment. *Plast Reconstr Surg* 1993;91(7):1216–1230.
4. Belov S. Classification of congenital vascular defects. *Int Angiol* 1990;9(3):141–146.
5. Werner JA, Dunne AA, Folz BJ, et al. Current concepts in the classification, diagnosis and treatment of hemangiomas and vascular malformations of the head and neck. *Eur Arch Otorhinolaryngol* 2001;258(3):141–149.
6. Dubois J, Garel L. Imaging and therapeutic approach of hemangiomas and vascular malformations in the pediatric age group. *Pediatr Radiol* 1999;29(12):879–893.

7. Choi DJ, Alomari AI, Chaudry G, et al. Neurointerventional management of low-flow vascular malformations of the head and neck. *Neuroimaging Clin N Am* 2009;19(2):199–218.

8. Ohgiya Y, Hashimoto T, Gokan T, et al. Dynamic MRI for distinguishing high-flow from low-flow peripheral vascular malformations. *AJR Am J Roentgenol* 2005;185(5):1131–1137.

9. van Rijswijk CS, van der Linden E, van der Woude HJ, et al. Value of dynamic contrast-enhanced MR imaging in diagnosing and classifying peripheral vascular malformations. *AJR Am J Roentgenol* 2002;178(5):1181–1187.

10. Hadizadeh DR, Gieseke J, Beck G, et al. View-sharing in keyhole imaging: partially compressed central k-space acquisition in time-resolved MRA at 3.0T. *Eur J Radiol* 2011;80(2):400–406.

11. Prince MR, Pearson GD, Zhang HL, et al. Advantages of blood pooling in pediatric MR angiography. *JACC Cardiovasc Imaging* 2010;3(5):514–516.

12. Lauffer RB, Parmelee DJ, Dunham SU, et al. MS-325: albumin-targeted contrast agent for MR angiography. *Radiology* 1998;207(2):529–538.

13. Ersoy H, Jacobs P, Kent CK, et al. Blood pool MR angiography of aortic stent-graft endoleak. *AJR Am J Roentgenol* 2004;182(5):1181–1186.

14. Prince MR, Zhang HL, Roditi GH, et al. Risk factors for NSF: a literature review. *J Magn Reson Imaging* 2009;30(6):1298–1308.

15. Bahrami S, Raman SS, Sauk S, et al. Ten-year experience with nephrogenic systemic fibrosis: case-control analysis of risk factors. *J Comput Assist Tomogr* 2009;33(6):819–823.

16. Amir J, Metzker A, Krikler R, et al. Strawberry hemangioma in preterm infants. *Pediatr Dermatol* 1986;3(4):331–332.

17. Drolet BA, Swanson EA, Frieden IJ, et al. Infantile hemangiomas: an emerging health issue linked to an increased rate of low birth weight infants. *J Pediatr* 2008;153(5):712–715, 715.e1.

18. Chang LC, Haggstrom AN, Drolet BA, et al. Growth characteristics of infantile hemangiomas: implications for management. *Pediatrics* 2008;122(2):360–367.

19. Puttgen KB, Pearl M, Tekes A, et al. Update on pediatric extracranial vascular anomalies of the head and neck. *Childs Nerv Syst* 2010;26(10):1417–1433.

20. Dubois J, Garel L, Grignon A, et al. Imaging of hemangiomas and vascular malformations in children. *Acad Radiol* 1998;5(5):390–400.

21. Dubois J, Alison M. Vascular anomalies: what a radiologist needs to know. *Pediatr Radiol* 2010;40(6):895–905.

22. Enjolras O, Mulliken JB, Boon LM, et al. Noninvoluting congenital hemangioma: a rare cutaneous vascular anomaly. *Plast Reconstr Surg* 2001;107(7):1647–1654.

23. Vikkula M, Boon LM, Mulliken JB. Molecular genetics of vascular malformations. *Matrix Biol* 2001;20(5–6):327–335.

24. Boon LM, Mulliken JB, Vikkula M, et al. Assignment of a locus for dominantly inherited venous malformations to chromosome 9p. *Hum Mol Genet* 1994;3(9):1583–1587.

25. Upton J, Mulliken JB, Murray JE. Classification and rationale for management of vascular anomalies in the upper extremity. *J Hand Surg Am* 1985;10(6, pt 2):970–975.

26. Upton J, Coombs CJ, Mulliken JB, et al. Vascular malformations of the upper limb: a review of 270 patients. *J Hand Surg Am* 1999;24(5):1019–1035.

27. Rak KM, Yakes WF, Ray RL, et al. MR imaging of symptomatic peripheral vascular malformations. *AJR Am J Roentgenol* 1992;159(1):107–112.

28. Marler JJ, Mulliken JB. Current management of hemangiomas and vascular malformations. *Clin Plast Surg* 2005;32(1):99–116, ix.

29. Hovius SE, Borg DH, Paans PR, et al. The diagnostic value of magnetic resonance imaging in combination with angiography in patients with vascular malformations: a prospective study. *Ann Plast Surg* 1996;37(3):278–285.

30. Siegel MJ. Magnetic resonance imaging of musculoskeletal soft tissue masses. *Radiol Clin North Am* 2001;39(4):701–720.

31. Ziyeh S, Strecker R, Berlis A, et al. Dynamic 3D MR angiography of intra- and extracranial vascular malformations at 3T: a technical note. *AJNR Am J Neuroradiol* 2005;26(3):630–634.

32. Enjolras O, Riche MC, Merland JJ. Facial port-wine stains and Sturge-Weber syndrome. *Pediatrics* 1985;76(1):48–51.

33. Delis KT, Gloviczki P, Wennberg PW, et al. Hemodynamic impairment, venous segmental disease, and clinical severity scoring in limbs with Klippel-Trenaunay syndrome. *J Vasc Surg* 2007;45(3):561–567.

34. Jacob AG, Driscoll DJ, Shaughnessy WJ, et al. Klippel-Trenaunay syndrome: spectrum and management. *Mayo Clin Proc* 1998;73(1):28–36.

35. Moodley M, Ramdial P. Blue rubber bleb nevus syndrome: case report and review of the literature. *Pediatrics* 1993;92(1):160–162.

36. Samlaska CP, Levin SW, James WD, et al. Proteus syndrome. *Arch Dermatol* 1989;125(8):1109–1114.

37. Enjolras O. Classification and management of the various superficial vascular anomalies: hemangiomas and vascular malformations. *J Dermatol* 1997;24(11):701–710.

38. Guttmacher AE, Marchuk DA, White RI Jr. Hereditary hemorrhagic telangiectasia. *N Engl J Med* 1995;333(14):918–924.

Medical and Surgical Management

KATHERINE B. PUTTGEN, RICHARD J. REDETT, and SALLY E. MITCHELL

The great heterogeneity in vascular tumors and vascular malformations makes discussion of uniform management guidelines difficult. Patients are optimally managed with a multidisciplinary approach. Management strategy depends on age of the patient, location of the tumor or malformation, threat to function (e.g., threat to vision, airway, feeding, ambulation), presence of ulceration and pain associated with the vascular anomaly, and degree of disfigurement. This chapter addresses the current medical and surgical management of infantile hemangioma (IH), the most common vascular tumor of infancy,[1] and of capillary, venous, lymphatic, and arteriovenous malformations (AVMs). Treatment of IH is primarily medical during the proliferative phase, except in the most dramatic and life threatening of lesions. Management of vascular malformations typically involves a combination of medical, surgical, and, often, primarily interventional, techniques, which is addressed in Chapter 31, Interventional Techniques.

INFANTILE HEMANGIOMA

Most IHs present as innocuous lesions that require only education, reassurance, and expectant management. Most appear within the first month of life with many presenting with a nascent telangiectatic patch on the skin at birth. Most IHs, 60%, occur on the head and neck, followed by the trunk (25%) and extremities (15%).[2] In the first 2 months of life, most IHs double in size, and the majority reach 80% of their maximum size between 3 and 5 months of age.[3] The proliferative phase is generally complete and maximum size achieved by 9 months, although deep hemangiomas (those without any epidermal change and which appear as compressible bluish nodules beneath the skin surface), segmental IHs (those that occupy a developmental unit), and larger IHs tend to have a longer proliferative phase.[3,4] After a plateau, involution occurs over a period of years. An important principle useful in guiding management of IH is that complete involution of the IH does not equate with complete resolution because up to 50% of patients will have some degree of scarring comprising a fibrofatty residuum, residual telangiectasias, or atrophy of the overlying skin.[5] Any degree of ulceration will leave a scar.

IHs may be divided morphologically into those that are segmental (appearing to arise from a developmental unit and which tend to be larger in size), those that are localized (appearing to arise from a single point), or indeterminate (not clearly falling into either category). In a study of over 1,000 infants with IH, segmental IH was 11 times more likely to have a complication and 8 times more likely to require treatment than nonsegmental (i.e., localized) IH. In addition to segmental IH, large IHs and those located on the face more often experience complications and require treatment.[6] Periocular and airway IHs commonly require treatment because of associated visual compromise

(i.e., astigmatism or visual axis occlusion) or acute airway obstruction.[7] Nasal tip IH may affect nasal growth through destruction of nasal cartilage and also may require more urgent treatment.[8] The concept of segmental IH is most important because it pertains to PHACE syndrome, an acronym for *p*osterior fossa malformations, *h*emangiomas, *a*rterial anomalies, *c*oarctation of the aorta, and *e*ye abnormalities. Sternal cleft and supraumbilical raphe can also be seen, and the disorder is sometimes referred to PHACES. Formal diagnostic criteria have recently been described.[9] Neurologic sequelae of PHACE are the most common and ominous associated finding, which present as structural brain and cerebral vasculature anomalies or as progressive stenotic or occluded cerebral arteries. Both moya-moya like vasculopathy and arterial ischemic strokes have been reported.[10–12] The most common intracranial arterial anomalies in PHACE are dysgenesis, abnormal origin or course, stenosis, and absence of vessels. The internal cerebral artery (ICA) and the embryonic branches of the ICA are most commonly involved. Abnormal vessels are ipsilateral to the cutaneous IH in almost all cases.[12]

Ulceration is the most common complication of IH, seen in almost 16% of patients in a tertiary referral population. Treatment options include barrier creams and wound dressings, such as Duoderm (ConvaTec) or Aquacel Ag (ConvaTec), pulsed dye laser (PDL),[13] becaplermin gel,[14] topical timolol,[15,16] and the systemic treatments outlined next. When treatment is necessary, most IHs are treated medically during the proliferative phase and often into the plateau and early involutional phases.

The traditional first-line therapy for IH for several decades has been high-dose corticosteroids—generally 2 to 3 mg/kg/day, although some practitioners use up to 5 mg/kg/day. Response rates reported in the literature vary from 30%[17] to 100%.[18,19] Most publications are retrospective case reports or case series, making it difficult to draw clear conclusions. One study showed induction of regression in one-third of treated patients, stabilization in one-third, and no effect on growth in the remaining third.[17] A meta-analysis found that 84% of patients exhibited stabilization or shrinkage of treated IH and suggested that response is likely dose dependent.[20] Side effects of oral corticosteroids are well known and include growth retardation, hypertension, cardiomyopathy, immunosuppression, decreased bone density, aseptic hip necrosis, hypothalamic-pituitary-adrenal axis suppression, gastrointestinal irritation, glaucoma, cataracts, diabetes, irritability, disturbance of sleep, and behavioral change. Several studies suggest that the majority of side effects experienced during treatment for infants with IH are short lived and that even children who experience growth retardation return to pretreatment growth curves after treatment is complete.[21] Oral histamine receptor blockers should be used during corticosteroid therapy to prevent gastric upset. Children must also be monitored carefully for development of infections, particularly for *Pneumocystis carinii* pneumonia (PCP).[22,23] Although not accepted as standard practice, some physicians advocate for concomitant PCP prophylaxis in all infants taking corticosteroids for IH. Live virus vaccines should not be administered to patients treated with corticosteroids.

Intralesional corticosteroids have also been used, primarily in the treatment of localized IH. Multiple injections are typically necessary. The ability to spare patients from systemic side effects is often given as a justification for intralesional treatment. Infants can develop sustained adrenal suppression and growth retardation from intralesional injection of corticosteroid, however, just as can occur with oral corticosteroid.[24] Complications in periocular IH treated with intralesional steroids include skin necrosis and possible retinal artery occlusion and blindness because the pressure of injection typically exceeds systemic arterial pressure.[25–27] If performed, this treatment must be done by an experienced ophthalmologist. Because better alternative treatments exist, the authors do not recommend this therapy. Vincristine is a second-line therapy for severe function- or life-threatening IH. Administration requires an indwelling catheter, and onset of response is slower than that of alternative therapies. Neuropathy and immunosuppression are significant potential side effects. Reports are limited to small case reports and case series. One such case series reports a 90% response rate.[28] Because of potentially irreversible spastic diplegia in up to 20% of infants treated with interferon-α, this treatment has fallen out of favor. The risk of neurologic damage is higher in infants younger than 12 months of age, and it is this age group that most often requires therapy, making this agent less desirable.[29–31]

The most significant advance in the therapy of IH in the last three decades has been the discovery of propranolol, a nonselective beta blocker, as an effective and apparently safe therapeutic option for treatment of IH. Its use was initially reported by Léauté-Labrèze and colleagues[32] after the serendipitous discovery of response of a large facial segmental IH in a patient who required propranolol after development of hypertrophic cardiomyopathy from high-dose corticosteroid treatment. Multiple case reports and case series document successful treatment with propranolol.[33–47] It is important to note that at the time of writing, data from randomized controlled trials are currently lacking, although trials are currently underway. Reports of complications with propranolol therapy including hypoglycemia, hypoglycemic seizures, hyperkalemia,[48–51] lack of response to therapy,[52] and bronchospasm are evidence that this newer therapy must be given with supervision and respect for potential complications. A uniform protocol for drug initiation, monitoring, and taper does not exist. The authors initiate therapy for children under 8 weeks of age in an inpatient setting over 48 hours, starting at 1 mg/kg/day and increase to 2 mg/kg/day dosing, divided three times a day. Blood pressure and heart rate are monitored 1 hour after each dose. For infants treated as outpatients, dose escalation occurs more slowly, over approximately 2 weeks. Pretreatment electrocardiogram is only necessary in patients with a personal or family history of congenital heart disease or arrhythmia. In such cases, cardiology consultation should be obtained. Routine echocardiogram is not necessary. Therapy is necessary for approximately 6 months or until maximum clinical benefit is achieved and the proliferative phase has ended.

The use and optimal timing of PDL in IH is somewhat controversial. Because of its relatively superficial depth of penetration (maximum less than 2 mm),[53] it has no role, in the authors' opinion, in the treatment of proliferating IH, with the exception of those complicated by ulceration. In the case of ulceration, PDL can encourage ulcer healing through mechanisms that are not fully understood; PDL does, however, carry the possible risk of worsening ulceration. Once involuted, residual erythema and telangiectasias can be treated effectively with PDL.[54]

During the proliferative phase, treatments aside from medication include percutaneous or endolesional laser,[55,56] embolization, percutaneous injection of sclerosants, and surgery. These treatments are often utilized in an effort to debulk large lesions, treat lesions that interfere with function (especially around the eye or nasal tip) or those that are life threatening, and those not responding adequately to medical therapy. Surgery during the proliferative phase is much less common and generally not recommended except in cases of failure of medical therapy, severe ulceration requiring skin grafting, or presence of a lesion that will ultimately need excision and the anticipated scar would be similar if removed early or late.[57] Risk of increased blood loss and inferior cosmetic result is higher if surgery is performed earlier, and early surgical intervention may increase the need for multiple surgeries. Surgery is most often necessary to treat residual scarring and excess tissue left behind after regression or partial regression of IH.[58] The decision to intervene during early involution (ages 1 to 3) versus late involution (ages 3 to 10 or older) depends on the anticipated psychological morbidity associated with a visible disfiguring birthmark, which may benefit from treatment prior to the establishment of memory and development of self-image and the anticipated scar based on lesion size and location.[57] Surgical technique depends on location, size, and age of the patient. Caution should be used when resecting lesions close to the lower eyelid or corner of the mouth to prevent ectropion or commissure elevation, respectively. IH acts as a natural tissue expander, making primary closure possible in many cases. Purse string closure is a technique that allows for significant decrease in the size of the final scar achieved and is often preferable, especially on the face. It is designed to be a two-staged procedure in which the puckered purse string closure of the first stage is removed in a small lenticular reexcision in the second. Many families opt to forego the second stage, however, because of acceptable cosmetic results after the first.[59–61]

Treatment options for nasal tip hemangiomas in infants remain controversial.[62] Larger, more complex lesions can irreversibly distort or prevent normal development of the underlying lower lateral cartilages and septum and cause nasal airway obstruction, thereby prompting early intervention.[63] A multidisciplinary approach using early medical and surgical treatment offers the best chance of a satisfactory result. Propranolol or corticosteroids can be used to hasten the proliferative phase and potentially improve the aesthetic result from surgery.

The surgical approach to nasal tip hemangiomas depends on the location of the lesion (superficial or deep) and whether or not there is significant skin involvement or redundancy (FIGURES 30.1A, C, D). Deeper hemangiomas with little or no redundant skin can be excised using an external rhinoplasty approach through a transcolumellar incision. After resection of the subcutaneous hemangioma and fibrofatty tissue, the lower lateral cartilages can be approximated using a resorbable suture.

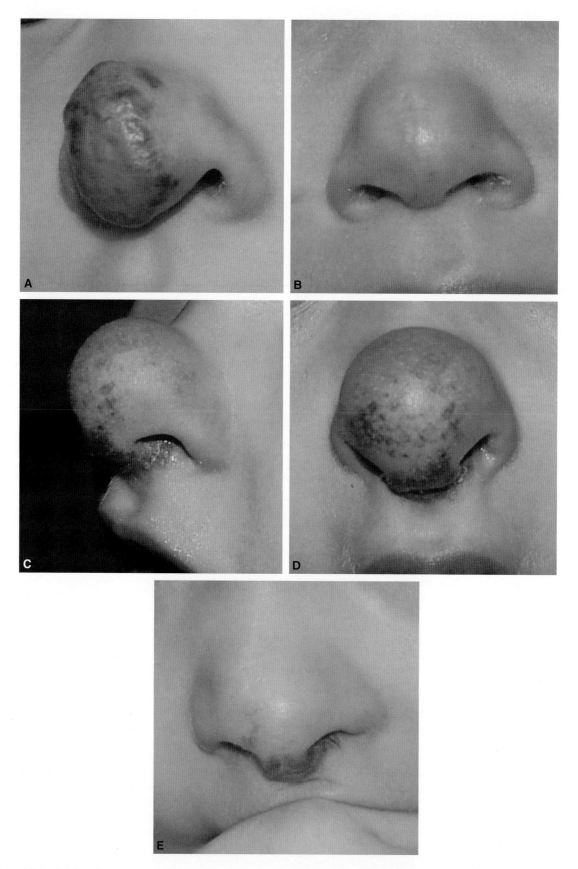

FIGURE 30.1 Panels **A**, **C**, and **D** show two preoperative nasal tip IHs. Panels **B** and **E** show the postoperative outcome following direct excision, which was necessary in both cases given the significant superficial IH present in these mixed (superficial and deep) IHs.

The external rhinoplasty approach provides excellent exposure to the surgical site and leaves a barely perceptible scar across the columella (FIGURE 30.1B and E). A direct excision on the dorsum of the nose is sometimes required for those hemangiomas with a significant superficial portion that involves the overlying nasal skin. It is important to remove as much of the overlying skin as possible while preserving all of the vestibular lining to prevent scar contracture and distortion of the nasal rim.[62]

Congenital hemangiomas are significantly less common than IHs and are divided into rapidly involuting (RICH) and noninvoluting (NICH) (Chapter 29). Both RICH and NICH lesions typically require surgical resection—the former because of significantly fibrofatty residuum and the latter because of a mass component and lack of involution (FIGURE 30.2).

CAPILLARY MALFORMATION

Capillary malformations (CMs) present at birth as flat pink to red patches on the skin and persist in this fashion throughout childhood. In adulthood, however, CMs often become darker purple, thicker, nodular, and disfiguring. CMs have traditionally been referred to as "port wine stains," but in keeping with the classification scheme of the International Society for the Study of Vascular Anomalies (ISSVA),[2] outlined in detail in Chapter 29, they are referred to herein as CM. CMs occur in 0.3% of newborns[1] and can be isolated or occur in conjunction with venous, lymphatic, or arteriovenous malformation or arteriovenous fistulae. Underlying malformations should be ruled out with physical exam and imaging if necessary. When CMs occur on the face in a V1, and to a lesser extent V2 or V3, distribution of the trigeminal nerve, Sturge-Weber syndrome (SWS), characterized by ipsilateral ocular and leptomeningeal anomalies, may be present and needs to be ruled out by ophthalmologic and neurologic examination and imaging. Up to 25% of infants with characteristic facial CM will have SWS.[64] Medical therapy of CM, exclusive of treatment of any underlying abnormalities, consists of treatment with PDL, either 585 or 595 nm, which is considered the gold standard therapy. Studies are conflicting as to whether the 585 or 595 nm is more effective in lightening CM.[65,66] Multiple treatments are necessary to obtain optimal results, often between 10 and 15 treatments. The ideal interval between laser sessions is unknown, but the majority of practitioners treat every 6 to 12 weeks. One study suggests that a 2-week interval may be more beneficial.[67] Many authors suggest that treatment early in life beginning in infancy is more effective than treatment in older children and adults, although the optimal age to begin therapy remains unknown.[68,69] The primary limitations of PDL are the inability to cause complete or acceptable lightening of CM for many patients. Other lasers suggested for treatment of resistant CM include the 755-nm long pulsed Alexandrite laser, 810-nm Diode laser, and the 1064-nm neodymium:yttrium-aluminum-garnet laser, and intense pulse light systems.[70,71] Recurrence of CM after acceptable lightening is another problem with therapy, and recurrence has been reported more than 10 years after successful treatment.[72,73] Adverse effects are minimal when appropriate patients are selected and appropriate settings are employed and include scabbing, blistering, hyper- and hypo-pigmentation, and scar.[74] Tissue expansion can be used to treat smaller CMs, especially those that are darker, nodular, and more disfiguring.

VENOUS MALFORMATIONS

The treatment of venous malformations (VMs), although once primarily surgical, has evolved such that sclerotherapy alone (Chapter 31) or sclerotherapy coupled with subsequent surgical excision is now the primary modality for management. Combined percutaneous sclerotherapy or glue embolization prior to

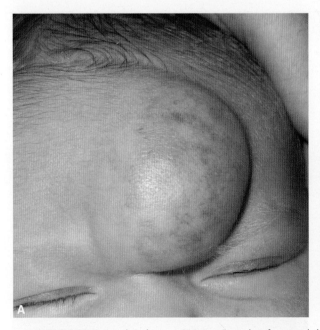
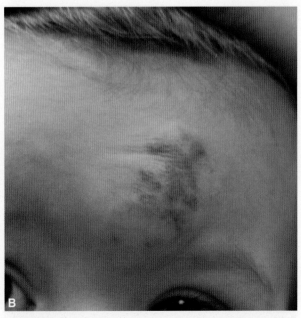

FIGURE 30.2 Panel **A** shows a RICH at 2 weeks of age and the significant, but far from total, involution by 11 months of age in panel **B**. Note the marked fibrofatty residuum, which will require surgical intervention.

surgery can help reduce the size of the eventual resection and better define the extent of the lesion. A combined approach can be particularly useful in the head and neck region where aesthetic and functional outcomes are so dependent on the size and location of the resection (FIGURE 30.3).

LYMPHATIC MALFORMATIONS

There is a limited role for medical management in most microcystic and macrocystic lymphatic malformations (LMs) aside from compression to the affected limb in those who are good candidates. Compression can help to minimize pain and swelling and can decrease risk of infection. Physical therapy and use of pneumatic compression therapy can be helpful for management of chronic lymphedema in diffuse LMs.[75] For microcystic LM, carbon dioxide laser can be used with temporary improvement in drainage from superficial lesions located both intraorally and on the skin surface, but recurrence of weeping and drainage is the rule.[76] Intraoral use of yttrium-aluminum-garnet and potassium-titanyl-phosphate lasers have also been reported, as has radiofrequency ablation.[77]

Sirolimus has been reported for treatment of complex vascular anomalies, including diffuse microcystic LMs and the vascular tumor, kaposiform hemangioendothelioma (KHE).[78,79] Clinical trials are currently underway and at this stage only case reports and small case series document experience. Hammill et al.[79] reported a series of six patients, five of whom had LM, in which all patients demonstrated marked improvement with sirolimus after failure of multiple standard therapies including sclerotherapy, surgical intervention, and medical management. Average time to response was 25 days (range, 8 to 65 days). Side effects included known side effects of mucositis, hypercholesterolemia, headache, transaminitis, and neutropenia. It should be noted that there are reports of lymphedema being induced in transplant patients on sirolimus therapy for immunosuppression.[80] This medication may represent a significant advance in the treatment options for patients with complicated LM and other VMs and tumors, but further study is necessary. Its use at this stage should only be considered after patients fail more standard therapies.

The surgical treatment of LMs is difficult because the lesions are often infiltrative and have a high risk of recurrence if incompletely excised (FIGURE 30.4). LMs of the head and neck are particularly difficult to excise because of their frequent proximity to cranial nerves. Permanent postoperative nerve damage can be as high as 33% after excision of head and neck LMs.[81] Surgery is probably best reserved for microcystic lesions or those lesions that do not respond to sclerotherapy.

ARTERIOVENOUS MALFORMATIONS

There is little role for medical management in the treatment of most AVMs (FIGURE 30.5). Many case series document improvement with embolization or embolization combined with surgical resection, but progression is the rule with this most aggressive vascular malformation. A recent retrospective review of 272 patients found that surgery, either alone or coupled with embolization, for AVMs that were more localized or of lower stage (Chapter 29) had better outcomes.[82] A smaller study by Jeong et al.[83] suggests similarly that surgery with sclerotherapy provides higher likelihood of resolution or long-term improvement, but that the risk of permanent surgical complications is greater than 15%. AVMs of the ear represent a special site and the literature suggests that once AVMs progress to stage III with destruction, pain, ulceration, and bleeding, embolization preoperatively followed by subtotal or total auricular amputation results in good outcomes for AVMs of the ear. In high stage AVMs, it is unlikely that embolization alone will be sufficient for optimal control.[84]

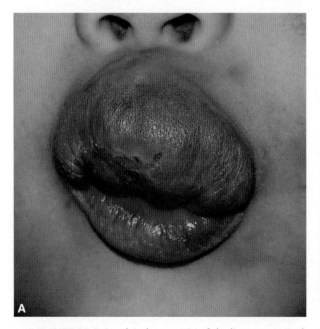
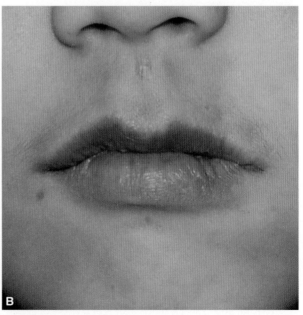

FIGURE 30.3 ■ Panel **A** shows a VM of the lip preoperatively, and panel **B** shows the postoperative result.

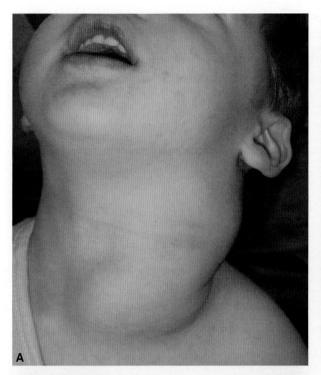

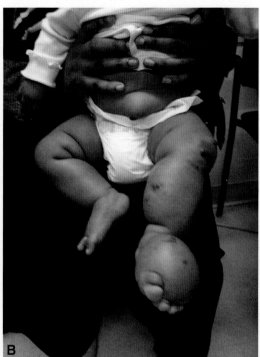

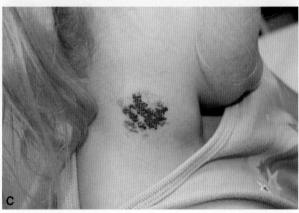

FIGURE 30.4 Panel **A** shows a macrocystic LM of the left lateral neck prior to sclerotherapy. Panel **B** shows a diffuse, infiltrative, microcystic LM of the left lower extremity prior to surgical debulking. Panel **C** shows a microcystic LM located in the skin and superficial subcutaneous tissue of the right neck.

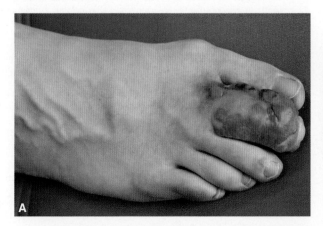

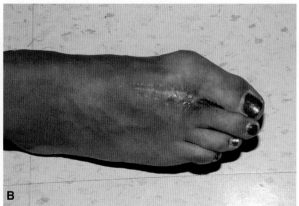

FIGURE 30.5 An AVM of the right second toe before **A** and after **B** surgical resection with ray amputation.

Panel **B**, courtesy of Anthony Tufaro, MD.

REFERENCES

1. Jacobs AH, Walton RG. The incidence of birthmarks in the neonate. *Pediatrics* 1976;58(2):218–222.
2. Finn MC, Glowacki J, Mulliken JB. Congenital vascular lesions: clinical application of a new classification. *J Pediatr Surg* 1983;18(6):894–900.
3. Chang LC, Haggstrom AN, Drolet BA, et al. Growth characteristics of infantile hemangiomas: implications for management. *Pediatrics* 2008;122(2):360–367.
4. Brandling-Bennett HA, Metry DW, Baselga E, et al. Infantile hemangiomas with unusually prolonged growth phase: a case series. *Arch Dermatol* 2008;144(12):1632–1637.
5. Mulliken JB, Fishman SJ, Burrows PE. Vascular anomalies. *Curr Probl Surg* 2000;37(8):517–584.
6. Haggstrom AN, Drolet BA, Baselga E, et al. Prospective study of infantile hemangiomas: clinical characteristics predicting complications and treatment. *Pediatrics* 2006;118(3):882–887.
7. O TM, Alexander RE, Lando T, et al. Segmental hemangiomas of the upper airway. *Laryngoscope* 2009;119(11):2242–2247.
8. Hamou C, Diner PA, Dalmonte P, et al. Nasal tip haemangiomas: guidelines for an early surgical approach. *J Plast Reconstr Aesthet Surg* 2010;63(6):934–939.
9. Metry D, Heyer G, Hess C, et al. Consensus statement on diagnostic criteria for PHACE syndrome. *Pediatrics* 2009;124(5):1447–1456.
10. Heyer GL, Millar WS, Ghatan S, et al. The neurologic aspects of PHACE: case report and review of the literature. *Pediatr Neurol* 2006;35(6):419–424.
11. Drolet BA, Dohil M, Golomb MR, et al. Early stroke and cerebral vasculopathy in children with facial hemangiomas and PHACE association. *Pediatrics* 2006;117(3):959–964.
12. Hess CP, Fullerton HJ, Metry DW, et al. Cervical and intracranial arterial anomalies in 70 patients with PHACE syndrome. *AJNR Am J Neuroradiol* 2010;31(10):1980–1986.
13. David LR, Malek MM, Argenta LC. Efficacy of pulse dye laser therapy for the treatment of ulcerated haemangiomas: a review of 78 patients. *Br J Plast Surg* 2003;56(4):317–327.
14. Metz BJ, Rubenstein MC, Levy ML, et al. Response of ulcerated perineal hemangiomas of infancy to becaplermin gel, a recombinant human platelet-derived growth factor. *Arch Dermatol* 2004;140(7):867–870.
15. Pope E, Chakkittakandiyil A. Topical timolol gel for infantile hemangiomas: a pilot study. *Arch Dermatol* 2010;146(5):564–565.
16. Guo S, Ni N. Topical treatment for capillary hemangioma of the eyelid using beta-blocker solution. *Arch Ophthalmol* 2010;128(2):255–256.
17. Enjolras O, Riche MC, Merland JJ, et al. Management of alarming hemangiomas in infancy: a review of 25 cases. *Pediatrics* 1990;85(4):491–498.
18. Zarem HA, Edgerton MT. Induced resolution of cavernous hemangiomas following prednisolone therapy. *Plast Reconstr Surg* 1967;39(1):76–83.
19. Brown SH, Neerhout RC, Fonkalsrud EW. Prednisone therapy in the management of large hemangiomas in infants and children. *Surgery* 1972;71(2):168–173.
20. Bennett ML, Fleischer AB, Chamlin SL, et al. Oral corticosteroid use is effective for cutaneous hemangiomas: an evidence-based evaluation. *Arch Dermatol* 2001;137(9):1208–1213.
21. Boon LM, MacDonald DM, Mulliken JB. Complications of systemic corticosteroid therapy for problematic hemangioma. *Plast Reconstr Surg* 1999;104(6):1616–1623.
22. Aviles R, Boyce TG, Thompson DM. *Pneumocystis carinii* pneumonia in a 3-month-old infant receiving high-dose corticosteroid therapy for airway hemangiomas. *Mayo Clin Proc* 2004;79(2):243–245.
23. Maronn ML, Corden T, Drolet BA. *Pneumocystis carinii* pneumonia in infant treated with oral steroids for hemangioma. *Arch Dermatol* 2007;143(9):1224–1225.
24. Weiss AH. Adrenal suppression after corticosteroid injection of periocular hemangiomas. *Am J Ophthalmol* 1989;107(5):518–522.
25. Egbert JE, Paul S, Engel WK, et al. High injection pressure during intralesional injection of corticosteroids into capillary hemangiomas. *Arch Ophthalmol* 2001;119(5):677–683.
26. Ruttum MS, Abrams GW, Harris GJ, et al. Bilateral retinal embolization associated with intralesional corticosteroid injection for capillary hemangioma of infancy. *J Pediatr Ophthalmol Strabismus* 1993;30(1):4–7.
27. Reyes BA, Vazquez-Botet M, Capo H. Intralesional steroids in cutaneous hemangioma. *J Dermatol Surg Oncol* 1989;15(8):828–832.
28. Enjolras O, Brevière GM, Roger G, et al. Vincristine treatment for function- and life-threatening infantile hemangioma [in French]. *Arch Pediatr* 2004;11(2):99–107.
29. Wörle H, Maass E, Köhler B, et al. Interferon alpha-2a therapy in haemangiomas of infancy: spastic diplegia as a severe complication. *Eur J Pediatr* 1999;158(4):344.
30. Deb G, Jenkner A, Donfrancesco A. Spastic diplegia and interferon. *J Pediatr* 1999;134(3):382.
31. Barlow CF, Priebe CJ, Mulliken JB, et al. Spastic diplegia as a complication of interferon alfa-2a treatment of hemangiomas of infancy. *J Pediatr* 1998;132(3, pt 1):527–530.
32. Léauté-Labrèze C, Dumas de la Roque E, Hubiche T, et al. Propranolol for severe hemangiomas of infancy. *N Engl J Med* 2008;358(24):2649–2651.
33. Sans V, de la Roque ED, Berge J, et al. Propranolol for severe infantile hemangiomas: follow-up report. *Pediatrics* 2009;124(3):e423–e431.
34. Jadhav VM, Tolat SN. Dramatic response of propranolol in hemangioma: report of two cases. *Indian J Dermatol Venereol Leprol* 2010;76(6):691–694.
35. Schiestl C, Neuhaus K, Zoller S, et al. Efficacy and safety of propranolol as first-line treatment for infantile hemangiomas. *Eur J Pediatr* 2010. Available at: http://www.ncbi.nlm.nih.gov/pubmed/20936416. Accessed December 21, 2010.
36. Mazereeuw-Hautier J, Hoeger PH, Benlahrech S, et al. Efficacy of propranolol in hepatic infantile hemangiomas with diffuse neonatal hemangiomatosis. *J Pediatr* 2010;157(2):340–342.
37. Muthamilselvan S, Vinoth PN, Vilvanathan V, et al. Hepatic haemangioma of infancy: role of propranolol. *Ann Trop Paediatr* 2010;30(4):335–338.
38. Maturo S, Hartnick C. Initial experience using propranolol as the sole treatment for infantile airway hemangiomas. *Int J Pediatr Otorhinolaryngol* 2010;74(3):323–325.
39. Theletsane T, Redfern A, Raynham O, et al. Life-threatening infantile haemangioma: a dramatic response to propranolol. *J Eur Acad Dermatol Venereol* 2009;23(12):1465–1466.
40. Arneja JS, Pappas PN, Shwayder TA, et al. Management of complicated facial hemangiomas with beta-blocker (propranolol) therapy. *Plast Reconstr Surg* 2010;126(3):889–895.
41. Blanchet C, Nicollas R, Bigorre M, et al. Management of infantile subglottic hemangioma: acebutolol or propranolol? *Int J Pediatr Otorhinolaryngol* 2010;74(8):959–961.
42. Holmes WJM, Mishra A, Gorst C, et al. Propranolol as first-line treatment for rapidly proliferating infantile haemangiomas. *J Plast Reconstr Aesthet Surg* 2010. Available at: http://www.ncbi.nlm.nih.gov/pubmed/20797926. Accessed December 21, 2010.
43. Buckmiller L, Dyamenahalli U, Richter GT. Propranolol for airway hemangiomas: case report of novel treatment. *Laryngoscope* 2009;119(10):2051–2054.
44. Buckmiller LM, Munson PD, Dyamenahalli U, et al. Propranolol for infantile hemangiomas: early experience at a tertiary vascular anomalies center. *Laryngoscope* 2010;120(4):676–681.
45. Fay A, Nguyen J, Jakobiec FA, et al. Propranolol for isolated orbital infantile hemangioma. *Arch Ophthalmol* 2010;128(2):256–258.
46. Taban M, Goldberg RA. Propranolol for orbital hemangioma. *Ophthalmology* 2010;117(1):195–195.e4.
47. Leboulanger N, Fayoux P, Teissier N, et al. Propranolol in the therapeutic strategy of infantile laryngotracheal hemangioma: a preliminary retrospective study of French experience. *Int J Pediatr Otorhinolaryngol* 2010;74(11):1254–1257.
48. Breur JMPJ, de Graaf M, Breugem CC, et al. Hypoglycemia as a result of propranolol during treatment of infantile hemangioma: a case report. *Pediatr Dermatol* 2010. Available at: http://www.ncbi.nlm.nih.gov/pubmed/20738795. Accessed December 21, 2010.
49. Holland KE, Frieden IJ, Frommelt PC, et al. Hypoglycemia in children taking propranolol for the treatment of infantile hemangioma. *Arch Dermatol* 2010;146(7):775–778.
50. Bonifazi E, Acquafredda A, Milano A, et al. Severe hypoglycemia during successful treatment of diffuse hemangiomatosis with propranolol. *Pediatr Dermatol* 2010;27(2):195–196.
51. Pavlakovic H, Kietz S, Lauerer P, et al. Hyperkalemia complicating propranolol treatment of an infantile hemangioma. *Pediatrics* 2010;126(6):e1589–e1593.
52. Canadas KT, Baum ED, Lee S, et al. Case report: treatment failure using propanolol for treatment of focal subglottic hemangioma. *Int J Pediatr Otorhinolaryngol* 2010;74(8):956–958.
53. Frieden IJ. Which hemangiomas to treat—and how? *Arch Dermatol* 1997;133(12):1593–1595.

54. Marler J, Mulliken J. Current management of hemangiomas and vascular malformations. *Clin Plast Surg* 2005;32(1):99–116.

55. Angiero F, Benedicenti S, Benedicenti A, et al. Head and neck hemangiomas in pediatric patients treated with endolesional 980-nm diode laser. *Photomed Laser Surg* 2009;27(4):553–559.

56. Angiero F, Benedicenti S, Romanos GE, et al. Treatment of hemangioma of the head and neck with diode laser and forced dehydration with induced photocoagulation. *Photomed Laser Surg* 2008;26(2):113–118.

57. Greene AK. Management of hemangiomas and other vascular tumors. *Clin Plast Surg* 2011;38(1):45–63.

58. Greene AK, Rogers GF, Mulliken JB. Management of parotid hemangioma in 100 children. *Plast Reconstr Surg* 2004;113(1):53–60.

59. Mulliken JB, Rogers GF, Marler JJ. Circular excision of hemangioma and purse-string closure: the smallest possible scar. *Plast Reconstr Surg* 2002;109(5):1544–1554; discussion 1555.

60. Vlahovic A, Simic R, Kravljanac D. Circular excision and purse-string suture technique in the management of facial hemangiomas. *Int J Pediatr Otorhinolaryngol* 2007;71(8):1311–1315.

61. Wu JK, Rohde CH. Purse-string closure of hemangiomas: early results of a follow-up study. *Ann Plast Surg* 2009;62(5):581–585.

62. Arneja JS, Chim H, Drolet BA, et al. The Cyrano nose: refinements in surgical technique and treatment approach to hemangiomas of the nasal tip. *Plast Reconstr Surg* 2010;126(4):1291–1299.

63. Pitanguy I, Machado BH, Radwanski HN, et al. Surgical treatment of hemangiomas of the nose. *Ann Plast Surg* 1996;36(6):586–592; discussion 592–593.

64. Ch'ng S, Tan ST. Facial port-wine stains—clinical stratification and risks of neuro-ocular involvement. *J Plast Reconstr Aesthet Surg* 2008;61(8):889–893.

65. Frohm Nilsson M, Passian S, Wiegleb Edstrom D. Comparison of two dye lasers in the treatment of port-wine stains. *Clin Exp Dermatol* 2010;35(2):126–130.

66. Greve B, Raulin C. Prospective study of port wine stain treatment with dye laser: comparison of two wavelengths (585 nm vs. 595 nm) and two pulse durations (0.5 milliseconds vs. 20 milliseconds). *Lasers Surg Med* 2004;34(2):168–173.

67. Tomson N, Lim SPR, Abdullah A, et al. The treatment of port-wine stains with the pulsed-dye laser at 2-week and 6-week intervals: a comparative study. *Br J Dermatol* 2006;154(4):676–679.

68. Chapas AM, Eickhorst K, Geronemus RG. Efficacy of early treatment of facial port wine stains in newborns: a review of 49 cases. *Lasers Surg Med* 2007;39(7):563–568.

69. Minkis K, Geronemus RG, Hale EK. Port wine stain progression: a potential consequence of delayed and inadequate treatment? *Lasers Surg Med* 2009;41(6):423–426.

70. Izikson L, Anderson RR. Treatment endpoints for resistant port wine stains with a 755 nm laser. *J Cosmet Laser Ther* 2009;11(1):52–55.

71. Jasim ZF, Handley JM. Treatment of pulsed dye laser-resistant port wine stain birthmarks. *J Am Acad Dermatol* 2007;57(4):677–682.

72. Nelson JS, Geronemus RG. Redarkening of port-wine stains 10 years after laser treatment. *N Engl J Med* 2007;356(26):2745–2746; author reply 2746.

73. Ozluer SM, Barlow RJ. Partial re-emergence of a port-wine stain following successful treatment with flashlamp-pumped dye laser. *Clin Exp Dermatol* 2001;26(1):37–39.

74. Wareham WJ, Cole RP, Royston SL, et al. Adverse effects reported in pulsed dye laser treatment for port wine stains. *Lasers Med Sci* 2009;24(2):241–246.

75. Gloviczki P, Driscoll DJ. Klippel-Trenaunay syndrome: current management. *Phlebology* 2007;22(6):291–298.

76. Glade RS, Buckmiller LM. CO_2 laser resurfacing of intraoral lymphatic malformations: a 10-year experience. *Int J Pediatr Otorhinolaryngol* 2009;73(10):1358–1361.

77. Edwards PD, Rahbar R, Ferraro NF, et al. Lymphatic malformation of the lingual base and oral floor. *Plast Reconstr Surg* 2005;115(7):1906–1915.

78. Blatt J, Stavas J, Moats-Staats B, et al. Treatment of childhood kaposiform hemangioendothelioma with sirolimus. *Pediatr Blood Cancer* 2010;55(7):1396–1398.

79. Hammill AM, Wentzel M, Gupta A, et al. Sirolimus for the treatment of complicated vascular anomalies in children. *Pediatr Blood Cancer* 2011;57(6):1018–1024.

80. Desai N, Heenan S, Mortimer PS. Sirolimus-associated lymphoedema: eight new cases and a proposed mechanism. *Br J Dermatol* 2009;160(6):1322–1326.

81. Emery PJ, Bailey CM, Evans JN. Cystic hygroma of the head and neck. A review of 37 cases. *J Laryngol Otol* 1984;98(6):613–619.

82. Liu AS, Mulliken JB, Zurakowski D, et al. Extracranial arteriovenous malformations: natural progression and recurrence after treatment. *Plast Reconstr Surg* 2010;125(4):1185–1194.

83. Jeong H-S, Baek C-H, Son Y-I, et al. Treatment for extracranial arteriovenous malformations of the head and neck. *Acta Otolaryngol* 2006;126(3):295–300.

84. Wu JK, Bisdorff A, Gelbert F, et al. Auricular arteriovenous malformation: evaluation, management, and outcome. *Plast Reconstr Surg* 2005;115(4):985–995.

Interventional Techniques

STEVEN L. HSU, CLIFFORD R. WEISS, and SALLY E. MITCHELL

INTRODUCTION

For a variety of reasons, clinicians have struggled with the diagnosis and classification of these vascular anomalies. Vascular anomalies can be associated with significant morbidity and mortality, thus knowledge of the proper categorization, diagnosis, and management of these entities is essential. A classification system of vascular anomalies proposed by Mulliken and Glowacki in 1982 has gained wide acceptance and facilitated an organized approach to understanding these lesions.[1] In their classification system, they divided all vascular anomalies into two primary groups: hemangiomas and vascular malformations. They further characterized the vascular malformations into low-flow and high-flow lesions. Both hemangiomas and vascular malformations are discussed further in the following sections.

HEMANGIOMAS

Hemangiomas are benign neoplasms of endothelial cells that ordinarily line the lumen of blood vessels. They are the most common benign tumor of infancy, occurring in approximately 12% of infants.[2] Hemangiomas occur more commonly in Caucasians, premature infants, and females with a female-to-male predominance of approximately 3:1 to 5:1.[2–6] Several descriptors have been applied to hemangiomas that add unnecessary complexity and confusion to their classification and understanding. Hemangiomas are typically absent at birth but appear within the first few months of life.[4,5] These hemangiomas have been referred to as infantile hemangiomas. On rare occasion, hemangiomas may be fully formed at birth and these are referred to as congenital hemangiomas.[6,7] Two types of congenital hemangiomas exist: rapidly involuting congenital hemangioma (RICH) and noninvoluting congenital hemangioma (NICH).[6,8]

Embolization of Hemangiomas

It is rare for embolization to be used in the management of hemangiomas. Embolization of hemangiomas can be directed at the proliferating hemangioma that is causing significant complications. Once embolotherapy has resolved the associated complication, the hemangioma may regress with no future interventions.[9,10] Embolotherapy can also promote definitive surgical resection by reducing tumor bulk and intraoperative blood loss, thus decreasing surgical morbidity.[10–13] When hemangiomas are embolized, they are mostly approached from the arterial side. The most prevalent example is arterial embolization of hepatic hemangiomas that are causing high-output cardiac failure.[9,14] A combined arterial and venous embolization of hepatic hemangiomas involving both arterial feeders and draining veins has been described with resolution of high-output cardiac failure and subsequent regression of the tumor without

the need for additional interventions.[10] Interventional radiologic interventions have also been performed in the case of hemangiomas, resulting in Kasabach-Merritt syndrome. Kasabach-Merritt syndrome is a complication of large hemangiomas or Kaposiform hemangioendotheliomas with development of thrombocytopenia and consumptive coagulopathy and is associated with a 14% mortality rate.[13] Hemangiomas complicated by Kasabach-Merritt syndrome can occur anywhere in the body, and transarterial embolization of these hemangiomas can improve pain and thrombocytopenia within hours of intervention.[10,13]

VASCULAR MALFORMATIONS

Vascular malformations are characterized by deformities of vascular channels resulting from abnormal development of vessel elements during the embryogenic or fetal stages of life.[1,2,4,6] Vascular malformations are not defined by cellular proliferation, as in the case of hemangiomas,[1–4,6] and unlike hemangiomas vascular malformations are present at birth and enlarge proportionally to the growth of the child.[1,2,4] There is an equal distribution of vascular malformations in both genders.[3] Although vascular malformations can be compartmentalized into histologic categories, a more useful classification is the classification of vascular malformations into low-flow or high-flow lesions.[2–4,6] Low-flow lesions include venous malformations (VMs), lymphatic malformations (LMs), and mixed lesions. High-flow vascular malformations include arteriovenous malformations (AVMs) and arteriovenous fistulas (AVFs). We begin with a discussion of low-flow vascular malformations.

VENOUS MALFORMATIONS

VMs are the most common type of vascular malformation and are composed of dysplastic venous vessels.[2,4,6,15,16] Histology reveals dilated vascular channels of variable size associated with an abnormal smooth muscle architecture, which is suspected to be the major contributing culprit in the gradual expansion of VMs over time.[4,6,15,17] The dilated venous channels can communicate with draining veins.[4] Like all vascular malformations, VMs are present at birth and grow proportionally with the growth of the individual; however, they may remain asymptomatic or may manifest clinically at any age, typically during late childhood or early adulthood.[1,2,4,17] When symptoms arise, patients typically complain of pain, often caused by phlebothrombosis or filling with blood and distension in a dependent position. VMs can also impair function and can cause significant cosmetic deformity.[6,17] VMs rarely regress.[4] As mentioned previously in the hemangioma section, deep hemangiomas have been labeled cavernous hemangiomas.[18] Unfortunately, the term *cavernous hemangioma* has also been used improperly to refer to VMs. Such confusing and overlapping labels of antiquity should be eradicated from clinical vernacular.[1,2,17]

Diagnosis

Similar to hemangiomas, most VMs can be diagnosed by clinical history and physical examination alone.[19] VMs can occur anywhere on the body, most commonly in the head and neck (47%), extremities (40%), and trunk (13%).[18,19] Approximately 90% of VMs are solitary, and the remainder are multiple.[6,17,19] When multiple VMs are encountered, inheritable conditions of VMs should be considered including glomuvenous malformation, cutaneomucosal VM, cerebral cavernous VM, and blue rubber bleb nevus syndrome.[17,19]

A family history of VMs should be investigated with each patient seen in the clinic. VMs can be localized to a particular anatomic area or extensive in distribution.[6,17] VMs occur in the skin and subcutaneous tissues; however, there is frequent involvement of the underlying musculature, joint structures, abdominal viscera, and central nervous system.[6,17] When superficial enough to be seen on physical examination, they typically appear bluish in coloration and are soft, compressible, and nonpulsatile to palpation, but the appearance can vary relative to the extensiveness of the VM.[3,6,17] When localized, VMs can appear as small varicosities, but when extensive they can appear as blue nodular masses (FIGURES 31.1 and 31.2).[6,17] VMs expand when the affected area is dependant or following the Valsalva maneuver when the lesions are in the head and neck or trunk.[3,6,17] As such, many patients will describe pain or discomfort at the end of the day, particularly after prolonged standing or physical exertion or upon awakening in the morning due to the effects of stasis and swelling within the VMs.[3,6,17] Although clinical history and physical examination can provide the diagnosis of a VM in greater than 90% cases, imaging is often used to determine the extent of the VMs and their underlying structural involvement.[19] Again, the two most useful modalities employed are ultrasonography and magnetic resonance imaging (MRI). Prior to imaging, it is helpful to keep in mind the varied imaging appearances of VMs as they relate to the types of VMs recently proposed by Puig and colleagues.[20,21] Typically, ultrasound examination is performed first given its rapid assessment of the VM, relative low cost, and noninvasive nature.[22,23] Ultrasound examination of VMs typically reveal hypoechoic collection of vessels with slow internal flow manifesting as mobile low-level echogenicities that can be associated with thickening of overlying subcutaneous tissues and phleboliths.[23,24] Ultrasonography can confirm the diagnosis of a VM; however, unless the VM is superficial, ultrasonography cannot assess the entire extent and involvement of deeper structures. Thus, MRI is the preferred imaging modality. MRI examination of VMs demonstrates T1 isointense or hypointense, T2 hyperintense space(s) of variable size often infiltrating into adjacent musculature, joints, nerves, and organs.[2,24] Phleboliths can manifest themselves as focal hypointensities on gradient-recalled echo images.[2,24] Delayed postcontrast MR imaging will show variable enhancement.[2,17,24] MR venography is a useful imaging tool to elucidate the presence of draining veins. Direct venography is unnecessary to diagnosing VMs; however, angiographic examination may demonstrate draining veins not visualized with other modalities and is essential prior to sclerotherapy (FIGURE 31.2).[2,19]

Clinical Management and Interventions

It is important to note that most VMs are asymptomatic.[25] VMs, however, can also produce significant pain and discomfort.[4] When VMs are extensive or involve critical structures, the resulting mass effect can lead to cosmetic or functional impairments.[6,17] Treatment is indicated for VMs that produce pain or cause functional or cosmetic impairments.[3,6,17] Prior to initiation of treatment, coagulation studies should be sought in all patients with VMs due to their association with localized intravascular coagulopathy (LIC).[25] The slow flow and stagnation of blood within VMs promote continuous coagulation activation, consumption of coagulation factors, and elevation of D-dimer levels.[6,17,25–27] LIC is characterized by this persistent elevation of D-dimer levels, and in the setting of VM there is an associated variable decrease in both fibrinogen and platelet levels.[6,17,25,26] LIC, however, should be entirely differentiated from Kasabach-Merritt syndrome, which is marked by profound thrombocytopenia.[6,17,25,26] The clinical significance of LIC is causation of pain secondary to local thrombotic events and potential conversion to disseminated intravascular coagulopathy (DIC) in the setting of surgical/nonsurgical interventions, or trauma. With DIC hemostatic ability is overwhelmed by consumption of coagulation factors.[25–27] Therefore, all patients with VMs need evaluation of hemoglobin, hematocrit, thrombin time, platelets, D-dimer, and fibrinogen. Patients with an elevated D-dimer and low fibrinogen are evaluated by hematology and receive low-molecular-weight heparin (LMWH) therapy for 10 days prior to and 10 days postsclerotherapy or surgery. This will correct the LIC consumption of fibrinogen, improving the patient's coagulation for the procedure.

Elastic Compression Garments

Elastic compression garments should be prescribed to patients with VMs, particularly if extensive, involving a limb.[3,4,6,17,19] Compression garments can minimize volume within the VM and decrease blood stagnation while the patient is in an upright position, thus decreasing associated pain.[6,19]

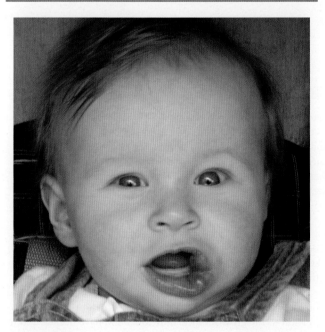

FIGURE 31.1 Child with venous malformation localized to the left corner of the mouth.

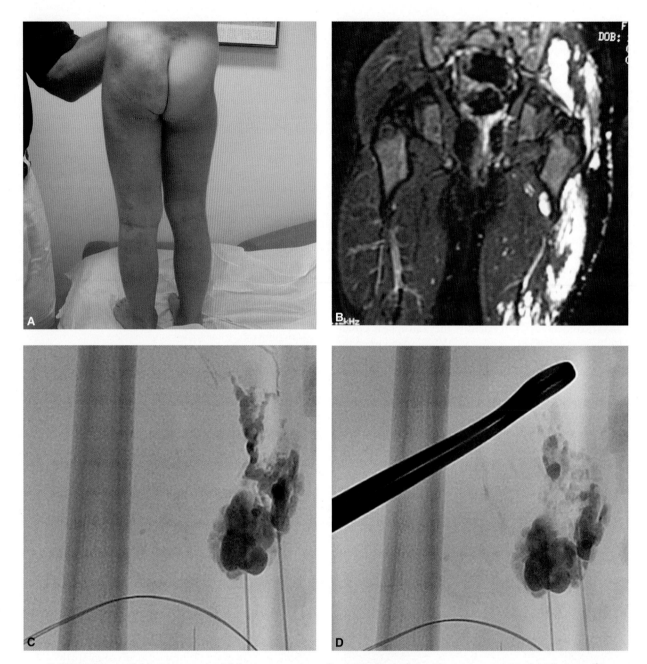

FIGURE 31.2 A. Child with extensive left lower extremity unilateral limb venous malformation. **B.** MRI of thigh shows T2 Fat Sat images demonstrating extensive venous malformation in the thigh musculature as well as the subcutaneous VM. **C.** Percutaneous venogram. Note needles used to access VM under ultrasound guidance. Contrast injection demonstrates the saccular stagnant VM and some normal draining veins connecting to the deep venous system. **D.** Clamp compression of draining veins connecting to deep venous system during ethanol infusion in order to isolate the venous malformation. Compression is held for approximately 2 to 5 minutes after injection as well.

Pharmacotherapy

In patients with recurrent pain related to phlebothrombosis, prophylactic aspirin may be administered on a daily basis to prevent local thrombosis.[6,19] When LIC is a complicating feature of VMs, LMWH has been employed to reduce painful recurrent thromboses and improve coagulation profile.[25–27] LMWH treatment has the potential of reducing D-dimer and normalizing fibrinogen levels.[25–27] In addition, LMWH has been recommended as a prophylactic treatment in patients with severe LIC at risk for developing DIC whether or not interventions are planned.[19,25–27]

One line of pharmacotherapy requiring further study is the use of oral contraceptives. Vascular malformations grow in proportion to the growth of the individual and have been found to enlarge most rapidly during the period of puberty. This suggests a role of sex hormones in the growth of these malformations.[19,28]

It has been demonstrated that high-dose estrogen administration results in rapid endometrial endothelial proliferation, whereas progesterone administration in combination with low-dose estrogen results in a relatively reduced rate of endometrial endothelial proliferation.[29] Hence, some have advocated the use of progesterone-only oral contraceptives in women with VMs. Further studies proving the definitive efficacy of progesterone on VMs and further studies delineating the types of VMs that can be treated in this manner are still needed.[19] For example, progesterone receptors, but not estrogen receptors, have been identified in head and neck VMs.[27] Additional research is necessary to investigate the presence of estrogen and progesterone receptors on VMs located in other sites. Without such research, the administration of progesterone-only contraceptives or various combinations of oral contraceptives may not only be inefficacious, but may also prove detrimental to the treatment of these lesions.

Sclerotherapy

Sclerotherapy is the first-line therapy for VMs.[6,17,19] Sclerosants are directly injected into the malformation, which results in inflammation, endothelial injury, and thrombosis.[3,19,30] Various sclerosants have been used for treatment of VMs including absolute ethanol, sodium tetradecyl sulfate (STS), sodium morrhuate, polidocanol, alcoholic solution of zein, bleomycin, and ethanolamine oleate.[3,19] Absolute ethanol is the most common sclerosing agent used for VMs, is considered to be the most effective, and is associated with the lowest recurrence rate.[6,30] When absolute ethanol is selected as the sclerosant, meticulous attention should be made to both the dose and the rate of administration. To avoid critical complications, such as cardiopulmonary collapse, arrhythmia, and hemolysis-related renal failure, the maximum dose of absolute alcohol should not exceed 1 mL/kg and should not be administered in aliquots exceeding 0.1 mL/kg given every 5 minutes with good hydration.[19]

Under ultrasound guidance, the VM is accessed with a 21- or 22-gauge needle. Following confirmation of venous return, a syringe/tubing combination is attached to the needle, and digital subtraction angiography (DSA) is performed to visualize the accessed portion of the VM, to estimate the capacity, and to assess the associated draining veins (FIGURE 31.2C).[3,19] If access is fully within the VM and DSA demonstrates extravasation of contrast, it is imperative to redirect the needle into the VM. If there is a large associated draining vein manual compression or a tourniquet can be applied prior to injection of sclerosant to prevent rapid transit into the systemic circulation (FIGURE 31.2D).[17,19] Also, coils and glue have been used for occlusion of connecting veins prior to sclerotherapy of the VM. Double needle technique may also be employed to minimize risk of systemic complications. With this technique two needles are placed into an isolated VM, allowing for simultaneous sclerotic administration through one needle and decompression/drainage through the other.[3,21,31] Following injection of the sclerosant, it is left to dwell in the VM for a specified period, typically 20 minutes. During this period of dwell, other portions of the VM may be targeted under ultrasound guidance with 21- or 22-gauge needles and the previous steps repeated. The amount of sclerosant in each portion of the VM should be carefully recorded by the interventional radiologist and confirmed by technologists and nursing staff. Following adequate dwell time, the syringe is disconnected from the needle at each injection site and careful observation of venous return is made. If venous return is noted, DSA should be performed again and another dose of

sclerosant should be administered under fluoroscopic guidance and allowed to dwell for another 10 to 20 minutes. Care should be taken to note new venous drainage that occurs because of ongoing thrombosis and altered flow in the malformation. The absence of venous return correlates with adequate volume of injected sclerosant and suggests successful endothelial damage/ongoing thrombosis of the VM. When there is no return, the needle is then removed and the overlying skin cleaned and bandaged.

The overall rate of complications from percutaneous sclerotherapy is approximately 12%.[32] It is helpful to classify complications into local and systemic. The most common complications are local and involve skin blistering and ulceration, particularly when the VM is located superficially in the dermis.[19,30] When skin pallor or color changes are observed following sclerosant injection, suggesting skin irritation or ischemia, cold sterile saline may be applied to reduce the risk of blistering and ulceration.[31] Postprocedural blistering and ulceration are managed with regular application of antibiotic ointment and sterile dressings.[30] For superficial VMs, the use of STS has been advocated, which is considered to be less toxic compared to absolute ethanol.[30] Serious local complications include larger and deeper ulcerations and transient or permanent nerve injury.[6,17,19,30] Often, the authors will arrange intraprocedural nerve monitoring when the VM is observed to be in proximity to large nerves.

Systemic complications, such as hemolysis, hemoglobinuria, renal injury, and cardiac arrest secondary to arrhythmias, have been reported with the use of the most common sclerosing agents, which are ethanol and STS.[6,17,19,30] These systemic complications are more common when extensive VMs are treated.[19] To prevent renal injury, good hydration during the procedure is recommended. Also, sodium bicarbonate can be administered in addition to twice the rate of maintenance fluid for the first several hours following sclerotherapy.[19] Systemic complications can be minimized by limiting total dose administered per treatment, by limiting the rate of administration during a treatment, and by partitioning treatments into multiple sessions.[30,31]

Most patients who receive sclerotherapy are admitted for overnight observation and pain control following the procedure. When the treated VM involves a limb, it is helpful to document the patency of the deep venous system via ultrasound examination postprocedurally, particularly when large draining veins are visualized prior to sclerosant injection.

Interval Follow-Up Plan/Strategies

Multiple sclerotherapy sessions are often necessary, particularly when managing extensive VMs. The endpoint of treatment is the cessation of pain, cosmetic and functional improvement, or when all available portions of the VM are obliterated. Patients can be advised that sclerotherapy often alleviates pain and/or decreases the size of VMs in approximately 75% to 90% of cases.[19,32] Following discharge from the hospital, the patients should return to clinic in 1 week and then at approximately 6 weeks for clinical and imaging (MRI) reassessment and to plan for reintervention. After the VM is under control, annual visits and MRI assessments are helpful for interval follow-ups.

Treatments on the Horizon

The future involves increased usage of magnetic resonance (MR)-guided percutaneous sclerotherapy of vascular malformations.[31,33] At present, certain academic medical centers, including the authors' own, are performing MR-guided percutaneous sclerotherapy. VMs are capable of causing significant patient pain and discomfort even when they are small. When small VMs are buried within subcutaneous fat, or when VMs are "hidden" by overlying anatomic structures or by scar from prior sessions, localization under ultrasound can be challenging. In these cases the lesions are amenable to MR visualization and MR-guided intervention. A great deal of startup effort is required to perform MR-guided interventions because both ancillary staff and interventional radiologists require familiarity and training in the usage of MR-compatible equipment. In addition, assistance from MR physicists is necessary to devise specific imaging sequences. These prerequisites are key to widespread usage of this immensely useful modality for therapy.

LYMPHATIC MALFORMATIONS

LMs are vascular malformations derived from abnormal development of lymphatic channels.[24] They consist of irregular spaces of varying size filled with chylous fluid.[4] LMs are classified as macrocystic, microcystic, or mixed.[2,6,17,24,34] In the past, macrocystic LMs have been referred to as cystic hygromas, and macro or microcystic LMs have been termed lymphangiomas.[6] Part of the challenge in understanding and managing vascular malformations is becoming familiar with and recognizing prior nomenclatures. As with other outdated labels previously mentioned, the terms *lymphangiomas* and *cystic hygromas* should be avoided and replaced completely with the term *lymphatic malformations*. Macrocystic LMs have cystic spaces measuring at least 2 cm³; microcystic LMs have cystic spaces measuring less than 2 cm³; and mixed LMs have cystic spaces that measure both greater than and less than 2 cm³.[34,35] Histology of these lesions demonstrates vessels of variable thicknesses comprising malformed smooth and skeletal muscle elements associated with collections of lymphocytes and germinal centers.[17]

LMs are present at birth but may not be noted until 2 years of age.[4,6,17] In fact, large LMs may be detected on prenatal ultrasound examination.[6,17] As with all vascular malformations, LMs grow proportionally to the growth of the child; however, LMs may also enlarge abruptly due to either intralesional hemorrhage or infection within the LM or elsewhere in the body.[6,17] Often LMs can distort a patient's appearance and impair normal function, particularly when they are located in the head and neck. LMs tend to occur in the head and neck in approximately 75% of cases and in the axilla/chest in 25% of cases.[4] Other locations where LMs can occur commonly are the mediastinum, retroperitoneum, buttock, and perineum.[2,6,17]

Diagnosis

The diagnosis of LM can be made on history and clinical examination alone.[34] Typically parents describe the presence of a mass discovered immediately at birth or noted before the age of 2 years, usually located in a characteristic region for LM, such as the head and neck or axillary/chest. They also describe rapid lesion expansion and often pain during periods of illness. On physical examination, LMs are nonpulsatile, soft, and rubbery to palpation.[2,35] The overlying skin is typically normal, although a bluish hue has been described, especially when intralesional hemorrhage has occurred.[6,17] With dermal involvement, small vesicles and skin puckering may be visible in addition to clear or sanguinous drainage from the vesicles.[6,17] When LMs occur

within the oral cavity, affecting the tongue, white vesicles can be seen on its mucosal surface.[35] When intralesional hemorrhage occurs within these mucosal or dermal LMs, the small vesicles will develop a dark red or maroon color (FIGURE 31.3).[6]

Although the clinical history and physical examination can provide the diagnosis of LM, imaging studies help delineate the extent of the LMs and their involvement of underlying structures. Ultrasound examination can help to classify LMs into the macrocystic, microcystic, or mixed categories.[2,24] Macrocystic LMs appear as a simple single cystic space or a multilocular cystic structure separated by intervening thin septations.[24] Ultrasound examination of microcystic LMs will demonstrate cystic spaces measuring less than 2 cm³, and mixed LMs will have cystic spaces that measure both greater than and less than 2 cm³. The septa separating the cystic spaces can demonstrate internal color flow. MRI is again the preferred imaging modality for visualizing LMs in their entirety, for determining the involvement of and proximity to critical structures, and for determining the LM type.[17] MRI examination of LMs demonstrates T1 hypointense, T2 hyperintense spaces that may be macrocystic, microcystic, or mixed in size.[24] If intralesional hemorrhage has occurred, characteristic T1 and T2 signals will vary depending on the age of the blood. Three salient features relevant to LMs are the presence of fluid-fluid levels, lack of respect for fascial planes, and enhancement of the LM septa.[2,4,17,24] Enhancement of the LM septa serves best to differentiate LMs from VMs. When the LMs are microcystic, the MR examination may fail to resolve the small cysts, thus reveal a T2 hyperintense solid mass.[4,24] Microcystic LMs can prove problematic because it is imperative that the clinician consider other solid masses in the diagnostic differential.[24] Ultrasound may be of utility in these cases given the improved spatial resolution to permit visualization of microcysts. Occasionally, a lymphangiogram may be useful, particularly in LMs associated with chylous leak.[17]

Clinical Management and Interventions

Treatment of LMs is directed toward managing the potential complications that may be caused by these lesions, which include hemorrhage, infection, compromise to anatomic or physiologic function, and distorted appearance.[6,36] Management can consist of observation/conservative management, surgery, intralesional sclerotherapy, or a combination of these therapies. When the LM is small and does not result in functional or aesthetic compromise, observation for possible involution may be warranted.[36] LMs can dramatically increase in size secondary to infection or intralesional hemorrhage. Infections anywhere in the body can result in enlargement of the LM. LM enlargement secondary to infections is thought to occur as a consequence to alterations in lymphatic flow or changes in the composition of leukocytes.[17] When LM enlargement is secondary to infection elsewhere in the body, the management can be conservative; however, when the infection involves the LM itself (lesional cellulitis), rapid administration of antibiotics should be initiated.[6,17] Cellulitis of LMs occurs commonly, particularly in LMs involving the cervicofacial region and perineum.[6,17,37] Intralesional hemorrhage resulting in LM enlargement can occur spontaneously or due to trauma and happens in approximately 8% to 12.6% of LMs.[37] Hemorrhage can be differentiated from infection by the development of a bluish or dark reddish hue to the LM and by the lack of localized erythema (suggesting lesional cellulitis) and by the

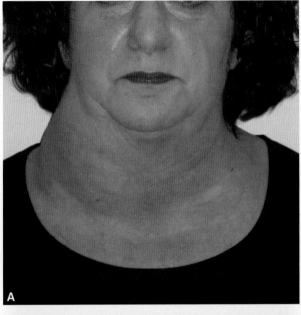

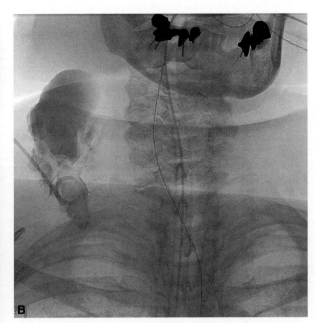

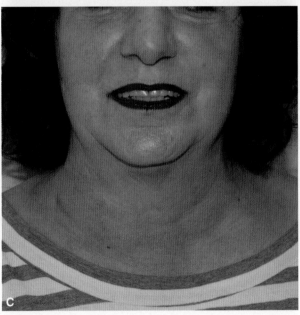

FIGURE 31.3 A. Lymphatic malformation pretreatment. (See MRI on the same patient, Chapter 32, FIGURES 32.4A and B). **B.** 6 French pigtail catheter placed in lymphatic malformation for doxycycline sclerotherapy. Contrast fills the LM sac. **C.** LM after doxycycline sclerotherapy at 6-week follow-up.

lack constitutional signs and symptoms of infection. Rest and pain control are all that is required; however, if the intralesional hemorrhage is large, prophylactic antibiotics are recommended to prevent infection.[6,17] Parents can be provided a prescription of antibiotics to be initiated at the first signs of infection.[6]

Sclerotherapy

As in the treatment of VMs, sclerosants are directly injected into cystic spaces of LMs to induce endothelial injury.[38] Typically, sclerotherapy is performed under general anesthesia, and depending on the location of treatment, some patients may require overnight hospital stay for pain control and observation. The technical aspects of the percutaneous sclerotherapy procedure are similar to VM. Under ultrasound guidance, the LM is accessed with a 21- or 22-gauge needle. Fluid returned or aspirated from the

needle must be closely examined to verify access into the LM and proper diagnosis. The fluid returned should be chylous in nature, that is, light in color and thin in viscosity; however, this may not be entirely reliable, particularly if intralesional hemorrhage has occurred.[36] To maximize sclerosant effectiveness, the LM should be entirely aspirated prior to delivery of the sclerosant to limit dilution of the administered sclerosant.[36] Various sclerosants have been used for treatment of LMs including absolute ethanol, picinabil (OK-432), STS, bleomycin, and doxycycline.[6,17,36] The particulars of each sclerosant are discussed separately.

Doxycycline

Doxycycline has been discovered as a useful sclerosant, following its use in pleurodesis and pericardiodesis.[39] Doxycycline is used at a concentration of 5 to 20 mg/mL with a maximum total of 200 mg doxycycline injected into each cyst.[39,40] There is no consensus on the sclerosant dwell time. When the estimated cyst diameter is less than 3 cm at the authors' institution, doxycycline is usually injected via the access needle and left to dwell for approximately 15 minutes. When the cyst diameter is greater than 3 cm, then a pediatric drainage catheter is placed and doxycycline is infused periodically over a period of days.[36] Some groups recommend a dwell time of 6 hours followed by drainage of the sclerosant through the drainage catheter daily for 3 days prior to removal of the catheter.[36] At the authors' institution, doxycycline is initially administered. If the overall dose limit is not reached, we typically administer 50% to 75% of the volume drained from the lesion. The doxycycline is typically permitted to dwell for approximately 6 hours, after which the lesion is allowed to drain for 4 to 8 hours. This volume is measured, and again doxycycline at 50% to 75% of the drained volume is administered. Typically we repeat this cycle twice a day for 3 to 7 days until the output volume decreases to minimal or no drainage, at which time the drain is pulled and infusions are stopped.

Picinabil (OK-432)

OK-432 is a product derived from group A *Streptococcus pyogenes,* which has been successfully used as a sclerosant in pleurodesis for malignant pleural effusions.[35,39] Similar to doxycycline, given the success of OK-432 for pleurodesis, it has been applied OK-432 to the treatment of LMs with favorable outcomes.[41,42] A later study performed by Ogita et al.[43] demonstrated complete resolution or marked reduction in the size of LMs in 67% of patients when OK-432 was used as the primary therapy versus less than 30% when OK-432 was administered as an adjunctive treatment following partial surgical resection or initial bleomycin administration. This has prompted the recommendation that OK-432 should be used as the primary therapy for LMs, particularly for macrocystic LMs.[35,43] Follow-up studies have continued to demonstrate the efficacy and safety of OK-432 in treatment of macrocystic LMs.[39,44] Technically, following access with a small-gauge needle(s), the needle is replaced with a small drainage catheter and the cyst is drained.[35] Contrast is again injected through the catheter to visualize lack of contrast extravasation and estimate cyst volume. Then 100% of the volume is injected into the cyst with OK-432 prepared with 0.1 mg of OK-432 dissolved in 10 mL of normal saline.[35,42] The dose should not exceed 0.2 mg of OK-432 per session, corresponding to 20 mL.[35,42] As with all sclerotherapy sessions, the sclerosant is subsequently drained after a defined dwell time. Serious adverse events that can arise secondary to OK-432 administration include airway obstruction specifically with regard to treatment of LMs involving the upper airway.[44] Airway obstruction and other adverse events often can be anticipated and planned for based on preprocedure imaging and assessment of the LM's proximity to critical structures (such as the airway) and the knowledge that OK-432 induces significant inflammation.[44] Otherwise, OK-432 is a safe sclerosant for LM treatment.[44] Given numerous reports of OK-432 efficacy and safety, research is currently underway in the United States to gain FDA approval for clinical use.

Bleomycin

Bleomycin is another sclerosant that can be used for the treatment of LMs. It is administered at a concentration of 1 mg/mL normal saline.[39] The dose limit is 0.3 to 0.6 mg/kg with approximately 1 to 5 mg of bleomycin injected into each cyst.[34,45]

Bleomycin sclerotherapy has high efficacy with complete or near-complete response rate of 40% and marked response to treatment of 30%.[39,45] The two most serious side effects of bleomycin treatment are pulmonary fibrosis and interstitial pneumonia.[34–36,39] There is an increase in these side effects with an increase in the dose.[34] Recently bleomycin foam therapy of LMs has been described. Foaming decreased the total volume of bleomycin used. Its advantages include less swelling postsclerotherapy, which is an advantage for lesions, especially in the orbit or in the tongue and airway.

ETOH/STS

In some groups, absolute ethanol is recommended for select LMs, specifically extratruncular LMs that have failed OK-432 treatment or extratruncular LMs that are located deeply, given the multitude of side effects as previously mentioned in the VM section.[6,17,19,30,36,46,47] Absolute ethanol is sometimes used in conjunction with STS.[36] Following endothelial injury with absolute ethanol and STS, promotion of LM collapse is facilitated by leaving intralesional drainage catheters in place for 3 days.[44] When absolute ethanol/STS combination was used for macrocystic LM, the efficacy rate was reported at 100% with complete ablation of the LM.[48,49]

Interval Follow-Up Plan/Strategies

Each clinic should adhere to a reasonable timetable for follow-up. At our institution patients are recommended to return to the clinic 1 week following discharge for assessment of postprocedural complications and then to return to the clinic in approximately 6 weeks after receiving an MRI of the involved region. LMs with minimal or partial response to a sclerosant may be treated a second time with the same sclerosant or with a different sclerosing agent. Microcystic LMs, which are less responsive to sclerotherapy, can be considered for surgical resection. At all stages of the process, a multidisciplinary approach should be instituted for collaborative effort and best treatment outcomes.

Treatments on the Horizon

The future of LM interventions involves use of sophisticated imaging modality for LM access, discovery of potentially more efficacious sclerosants, and the utilization of molecular modulators. MR-guided sclerotherapy may facilitate treatment of LMs that are located deeply or in difficult-to-access locations. Potentially more efficacious sclerosants with minimal adverse event profiles may emerge, which may be effective when used on both macrocystic and microcystic LMs. As investigators further our understanding of the molecular biology of LMs, various signal regulators may be discovered that may be useful to halt proliferation of LMs and induce their regression.

▌ ARTERIOVENOUS MALFORMATIONS

High-flow vascular malformations are rare and consist of AVMs and AVFs.[4,24] AVMs are composed of niduses/abnormal collections of vessels forming abnormal connections between arteries and veins, bypassing the normal intervening capillaries.[50,51] Like all vascular malformations, they are present at birth and may remain asymptomatic until they emerge clinically due to sequelae of arteriovenous shunting. These sequelae can include

Table 31.1	
Schobinger Staging of Arteriovenous Malformations	
Stage I (quiescence)	Pink-bluish stain, warmth, and arteriovenous shunting by way of Doppler examination
Stage II (expansion)	Same as stage I, plus enlargement, pulsations, thrill, bruit, and tense/tortuous veins
Stage III (destruction)	Same as stage II, plus dystrophic skin changes, ulceration, tissue necrosis, bleeding, or persistent pain
Stage IV (decompensation)	Same as stage III, plus cardiac failure

From Fishman SJ, et al. Gastrointestinal manifestations of vascular anomalies in childhood: varied etiologies require multiple therapeutic modalities. *J Pediatr Surg* 1998;33(7):1163–1167.

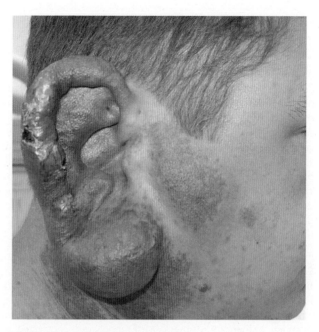

FIGURE 31.4 AVM involving the right ear.

pain, bleeding, ulcerations, and cardiac failure or the appearance of an enlarging mass with resultant cosmetic distortion or impairment of function.[4,6,17,51] AVMs grow proportionally to the growth of the individual; however, sex hormones likely play a role in their growth, given their rapid progression during puberty and pregnancy.[4,6,17,51] Trauma can also result in enlargement of AVMs likely secondary to production of local hypoxia and resultant stimulation of angiogenic factors.[6,17,24,51] AVMs can be clinically classified according to the Schobinger staging for AVMs (Table 31.1).[6,51] The Schobinger staging for AVMs categorizes AVMs based on their behavior and clinical effect, beginning with stage 1, quiescent stage, to stage 4, decompensation stage.[6,51] In order of decreasing frequency, AVMs tend to occur in the central nervous system, limbs, trunk, and viscera.[6,17]

Diagnosis

In 90% of the cases, the diagnosis of AVM can be made on history and clinical examination alone.[52] The mass of an AVM is typically present at birth and is often mistaken for a hemangioma.[6,17,52] On physical examination, AVMs can present as a warm palpable mass with overlying reddish hue and an associated palpable thrill and bruit (FIGURE 31.4).[6,17,50,52] Although the clinical history and physical examination can provide the diagnosis, imaging studies are used to confirm the diagnosis and again help delineate the extent of the AVMs.[6,17] Ultrasound examinations demonstrate hypoechoic tortuous feeding arteries without an associated soft tissue mass and increased (arterialized) diastolic flow, given unimpeded communication between arteries and veins through abnormal vascular channels.[24] The corresponding draining veins demonstrate arterialized high-velocity flow.[24] MRI is again the preferred imaging modality for visualizing AVMs in their entirety to determine full extent, anatomic involvement, and proximity to critical structures, and to assist in treatment planning.[6,17,52] MRI examination of AVMs demonstrates the presence of T1, T2, and GRE hypointense serpentine flow voids.[24,50,52] Although AVMs are not associated with

a soft tissue mass, the adjacent tissues, such as the muscle, may demonstrate T1 hypointensity and T2 hyperintensity compatible with edema with variable enhancement.[24,50] There may be an increase in adjacent subcutaneous fat and bony changes, such as sclerosis.[50] MRA and 3D reconstructed images can render an even fuller representation of the lesion.

Clinical Management and Intervention

Treatment options for AVMs include surgical resection or embolization procedures, or a combination of both.[6,17,52] Complete surgical resection is rarely achievable, given the extensive nature of AVMs.[51,52] Embolization requires therapy directed at the nidus, at the site of shunting from the artery to the vein. Given the difficulties of treating some AVMs, the goal of treatment should be directed toward managing the potential sequelae of AVMs and toward controlling symptoms that may arise.[3,52]

AVMs have been noted to enlarge during puberty and pregnancy, likely stimulated by the increased concentration of sex hormones in their chemical milieu. Preventive counsel can be made to women with AVMs who may consider pregnancy. Liu and colleagues[51] have reported that pregnant women with nonproblematic stage I AVMs did not have an increased risk of progression of their AVMs compared to nonpregnant patients. Pregnant women with stage II through IV AVMs were not studied; therefore, it is unclear whether these higher-stage AVMs will progress during pregnancy. Regardless, these patients should be informed of the potential risk of AVM progression with pregnancy.[51]

Treatment of stages I and II AVMs results in better long-term control than treated AVMs of higher stages.[51] Often stages III and IV AVMs need to be treated. Because of improved long-term control of treated AVMs of lower stages, some are advocating the treatment of lower-stage AVMs even when the lesions are located in nonaesthetically critical or functional locations to prevent their progression to higher-stage lesions.[51]

Surgical Excision and Related Issues

Surgical resection of AVMs offers improved long-term control of the AVMs or reduced recurrence rate if the AVM nidus can be removed completely, especially for AVMs localized in noncritical areas in which function and appearance are not affected. It is important for surgical excision to be complete and to avoid simply ligating feeding arteries because other arterial feeders will pick up perfusion of the AVM nidus immediately. Preoperative embolization 24 to 48 hours prior to surgical resection can aid in defining the contours of the AVM and reduce blood loss.[6,17,51,52] Even when the goal is directed toward complete surgical resection, most AVMs recur.[51,52]

Embolization

Because AVMs are often not resectable, embolization can improve the patient's symptomology by reducing the AVM size and shunt[52] and, sometimes, in very skilled hands, can result in complete obliteration of the AVM. Embolization is directed at the site of arteriovenous shunting within the AVM. It can be difficult with extensive AVMs to find the exact site of the original congenital shunt because of subsequent tortuosity of multiple feeding arteries that overlap the site of the shunt. It is critical, however, that the AVM be shut down at this site and not proximally to obtain the best long-term result. Also treating AVMs at the site of shunting only can help to avoid complications that are most often caused by nontarget nutrient vessel embolization. Technically, AVMs can be treated from the arterial side, from the venous side, or percutaneously directly into the shunt site. It is important to realize and to prepare the patient that multiple embolizations are usually required to obtain long-term success in embolization of AVMs.[53]

From the arterial side, the AVM main feeder is selected, usually with a 5 French catheter, through which a microcatheter is advanced to subselect the distal feeding branches. The goal is to direct the microcatheter beyond any normal vessels into a very distal feeder just proximal to the arteriovenous site of shunting. Ideally, the embolic agent is placed into the nidus to the point of the draining veins.[52] Treatment of AVMs is done with liquid embolic agents including n-butyl cyanoacrylate Onyx and absolute ethanol (FIGURE 31.5).[52,53] Absolute ethanol is considered by many to be the best agent for permanently closing down AVMs.[54] Ethanol must be used with caution to avoid infusing any nutrient into normal vessels and requires accessing very distally to the site of arteriovenous abnormal connection.

From the venous side, the AVM can be treated, especially if there is a single draining vein or a venous sac on the venous side of the arteriovenous shunting (FIGURE 31.6). (If there are multiple veins, this approach is unlikely to be successful.) For treatment from the venous side, a balloon occlusion catheter can be useful for occluding outflow and injecting liquid embolic into the AV shunt site. Ethanol can be injected into the venous side. Coils are often used to slow down the flow on the venous side or to occlude the venous sac in a more saccular AVM. Glue may be used alone or added to coils to help occlude the venous sac. It is critical to prevent coils or glue from traveling into the normal venous system from this approach. If the venous approach can be used, it is often a safer approach to AVM treatment due to the avoidance of nutrient

arterial embolization (to nerves, skin, normal structures) from the arterial approach. Often the venous approach results in a dramatic decrease in arterial feeders once the venous side of the AVM is occluded, thus a better chance at a "curative" embolization.[55]

At times, direct percutaneous access into the AVM can be performed if there is lack of sufficient arterial or venous access, often caused by a difficult intravascular route or occluded proximal arterial feeders.[6,17,52] Usually ethanol or glue is used in the percutaneous approach at the site of arteriovenous shunting, although coils can also be delivered through percutaneous needles if treating into a venous sac.

Embolization can be performed as primary treatment or as a preoperative measure for planned future resection.[3,6,17,51,52] Care must be taken to deploy embolic agents selectively and not within proximal arterial feeders because embolization of proximal arteries can eliminate access for future embolic therapy. Furthermore, the local ischemia induced by proximal embolization stimulates recruitment of collateral vessels and can worsen the AVM.[6,17,52] A common complication of embolic therapy is ulceration caused by distal migration of embolic material and resulting ischemia.[52] When ulceration has occurred, fastidious wound care must be applied and permit healing by secondary intention.[52]

Interval Follow-Up Plan/Strategies

It has been reported that approximately 57% of patients who undergo surgical resection and embolic therapy will have AVM recurrence within the first year following treatment.[51,52] Approximately 98% of AVMs will enlarge/recur within 5 years following treatment.[51,52] Therefore, the absence of reexpansion within 5 years indicates favorable long-term outcomes, and patients who have undergone surgical and/or embolic therapy should be followed for at least 5 years with an increased frequency of clinic visits if symptoms recur or if there is enlargement of AVMs.

Treatments on the Horizon

The future of AVM interventions is similar to that of LMs, requiring elucidation of the molecular biology of vascular malformations and the signal regulators that may induce regression or halt growth. In the more immediate future, development of newer embolic agents may result in more favorable long-term outcomes with reduction in 1- or 5-year recurrence rates.[52]

Special Consideration

Hereditary hemorrhagic telangiectasia (HHT) is otherwise referred to as Osler-Weber-Rendu disease. It is an autosomal dominant entity characterized by the presence of AVMs in multiple organ systems including the brain, lung, liver, and gastrointestinal tract.[17,56] Patients typically present with epistaxis by 12 years of age. Cerebral AVMs can be managed with transarterial embolization, stereotactic radiation, surgery, or a combination of these.[56] Transarterial embolization is the treatment of choice for pulmonary AVMs (PAVMs), and such intervention should be performed using retrievable permanent embolics at an HHT center of excellence.[56] PAVMs with feeding arteries measuring 2mm or more in diameter should be treated, although modern microcatheters and wire allow for treatment of even smaller lesions. Gastrointestinal AVMs are managed with endoscopic cauterization, iron

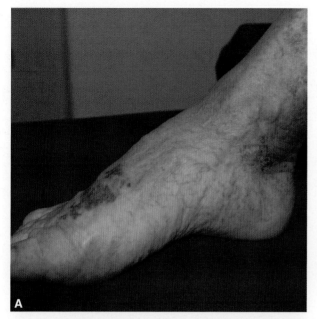

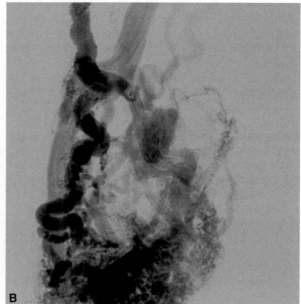

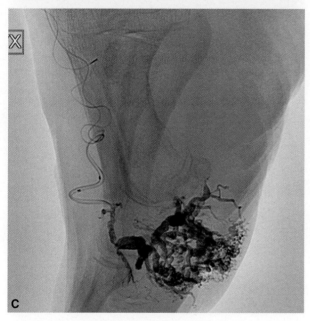

FIGURE 31.5 **A.** Patient with foot AVM and venous hypertension. **B.** Arteriogram of the foot AVM demonstrating a 5 French catheter in the enlarged dorsalis pedis artery, the nidus at the ball of the foot, and early draining veins. **C.** Microcatheters extending from the 5 French catheter into the main feeder of the AVM for onyx delivery. Although it was difficult to avoid onyx within the proximal AVM feeding vessel, onyx flowed into the nidus at the ball of the foot. Patient's venous hypertension greatly improved with good healing of venous ulcerations of the leg. More ideal embolization would have been to deliver embolic material only in the distal shunting regions of the AVM.

supplementation for anemia, and consideration for hormonal or antifibrinolytic therapy.[56]

ARTERIOVENOUS FISTULAS

An AVF is a direct communication of an artery and vein without the presence of a nidus or abnormal intervening vascular channels between arteries and veins.[3] AVFs can be congenital or acquired. When discussing AVFs as vascular malformations, only the congenital type of AVF is considered. Congenital AVFs can occur anywhere in the body.[50] The clinical sequelae of AVF include high-output heart failure, ischemia distal to the arteriovenous shunt, and development of increased local venous pressure. In the legs, distal to an AVF or AVM, a patient may develop claudication, rest pain, deep venous thromboses of the lower extremities, and varicose veins.[3]

Diagnosis

On physical examination, AVF may be pulsatile with palpation and a bruit may be auscultated. Ultrasound examination will demonstrate high velocity on the arterial side proximal to the location of the fistula with low-resistance waveforms. The draining vein will demonstrate arterialized flow. There can be an associated perivascular thrill. Magnetic resonance angiography (MRA) is more useful than conventional MR, given the ability to visualize early filling of a draining vein compatible with the presence of an AVF.

Clinical Management and Intervention

With regard to management of AVFs, most acquired AVFs spontaneously resolve within a few months; thus conservative management with interval imaging and clinical surveillance is

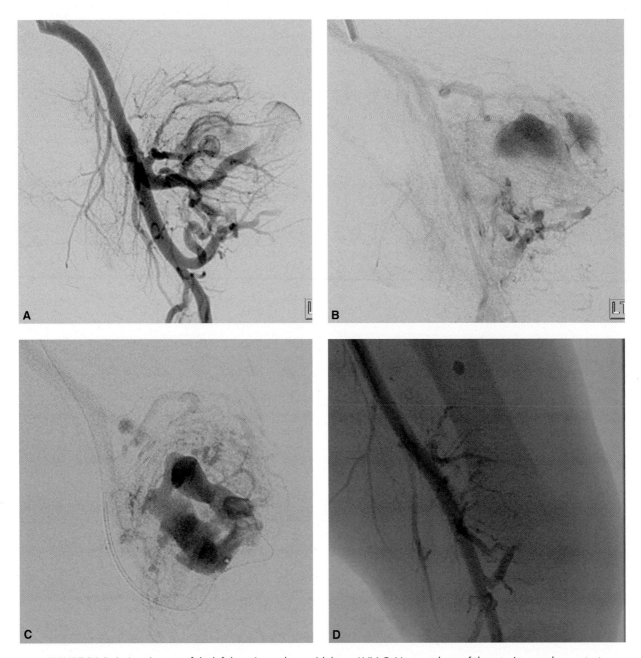

FIGURE 31.6 A. Arteriogram of the left knee in newborn with large AVM. **B.** Venous phase of the arteriogram demonstrating large venous sacs filling from arteriovenous shunts from branches of the superficial femoral artery. Note the draining veins of AVM into the deep venous system. **C.** Selective microcatheter from the artery through the arteriovenous fistula and into the venous sacs. Venous sacs embolized with ethanol and glue at two settings. **D.** Angiogram of the left knee 2 years later, showing no recurrence of AVM.

recommended. When the fistulous connection is large or there are other clinical sequelae, early treatment is the rule. Interventions include surgical or endovascular repair of the fistula.[3] With regard to endovascular repair, a covered stent can be deployed to cover the fistula and eliminate the arteriovenous shunt while preserving distal arterial flow. Alternatively when the fistula is of sufficient length between the artery and the vein, embolization, often with coils, may be performed to obliterate the fistula.[57]

OTHER SYNDROMES INVOLVING VASCULAR MALFORMATIONS

Klippel-Trénaunay Syndrome

Klippel-Trénaunay syndrome (KTS) is a combined vascular malformation involving lymphatic, venous, and capillary elements, otherwise referred to as a capillary lymphaticovenous malformation (CLVM). Typically, the vascular malformation

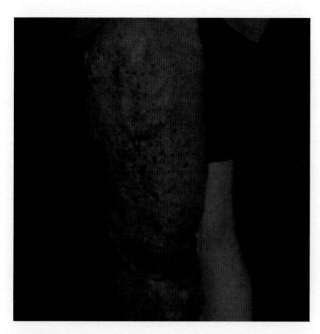

FIGURE 31.7 KTS involving the left lower extremity.

involves a limb, particularly the lower extremity, in 95% of the cases.[24] In most cases in which there is involvement of a limb, there is also associated limb overgrowth.[4,24,50] Patients with KTS may have enlarged superficial varices that are often valveless and result in swelling and pain (FIGURE 31.7). Although the deeper LMs and VMs may be treated with percutaneous sclerotherapy, the superficial varices often have patent connections into the deep system. At our institution, we use intravenous laser therapy for occluding these large superficial varices. Deep venous anomalies in KTS may include aplasia, hypoplasia, stenosis, and aneurysmal disease. Therefore, one must be sure that the patient with KTS has a patent deep venous system before occluding superficial varices to avoid a swollen, poorly draining limb.[58]

Parkes Weber Syndrome

Parkes Weber syndrome (PWS) no longer is considered part of KTS. PWS includes capillary malformation, hemihypertrophy, and diffuse skin level AVMs.[3,6,17] Similar to KTS, there is predominant involvement of the extremities with higher localization to the lower extremities than the upper extremities.[6,17]

■ CONCLUSION

Vascular anomalies include hemangiomas and vascular malformations. Hemangiomas are differentiated from vascular malformations by their endothelial proliferation and characteristic lifecycle. Vascular malformations can be fully understood by classifying them into low-flow and high-flow vascular malformations. Low-flow vascular malformations include VMs, LMs, and mixed malformations. High-flow malformations include AVMs and AVFs. Specific clinical considerations are applied to each entitiy with particular management goals and profiles.

■ REFERENCES

1. Mulliken JB, Glowacki J. Hemangiomas and vascular malformations in infants and children: a classification based on endothelial characteristics. *Plast Reconstr Surg* 1982;69(3):412–422.
2. Burrows PE, et al. Cerebral vasculopathy and neurologic sequelae in infants with cervicofacial hemangioma: report of eight patients. *Radiology* 1998;207(3):601–607.
3. Baum S, Pentecost MJ, eds. *Abrams' Angiography: Interventional Radiology.* 2nd ed. Philadelphia, PA: Lippincott Williams & Wilkins; 2006:1264.
4. Donnelly LF, Adams DM, Bisset GS 3rd. Vascular malformations and hemangiomas: a practical approach in a multidisciplinary clinic. *AJR Am J Roentgenol* 2000;174(3):597–608.
5. Fishman SJ, et al. Gastrointestinal manifestations of vascular anomalies in childhood: varied etiologies require multiple therapeutic modalities. *J Pediatr Surg* 1998;33(7):1163–1167.
6. Marler JJ, Mulliken JB. Current management of hemangiomas and vascular malformations. *Clin Plast Surg* 2005;32(1):99–116, ix.
7. Boon LM, Enjolras O, Mulliken JB. Congenital hemangioma: evidence of accelerated involution. *J Pediatr* 1996;128(3):329–335.
8. Greene AK. Management of hemangiomas and other vascular tumors. *Clin Plast Surg* 2011;38(1):45–63.
9. Enjolras O, Gelbert F. Superficial hemangiomas: associations and management. *Pediatr Dermatol* 1997;14(3):173–179.
10. Kretschmar O, Knirsch W, Bernet V. Interventional treatment of a symptomatic neonatal hepatic cavernous hemangioma using the Amplatzer vascular plug. *Cardiovasc Intervent Radiol* 2008;31(2):411–414.
11. Akamatsu N, et al. Giant liver hemangioma resected by trisectorectomy after efficient volume reduction by transcatheter arterial embolization: a case report. *J Med Case Reports* 2010;4:283.
12. Kato S, et al. Surgical management of aggressive vertebral hemangiomas causing spinal cord compression: long-term clinical follow-up of five cases. *J Orthop Sci* 2010;15(3):350–356.
13. Wolfe SQ, et al. Transarterial embolization of a scalp hemangioma presenting with Kasabach-Merritt syndrome. *J Neurosurg Pediatr* 2009;4(5):453–457.
14. Enjolras O, et al. Management of alarming hemangiomas in infancy: a review of 25 cases. *Pediatrics* 1990;85(4):491–498.
15. Fernandez-Pineda I. Vascular tumors and malformations of the colon. *World J Gastroenterol* 2009;15(41):5242–5243.
16. Flis CM, Connor SE. Imaging of head and neck venous malformations. *Eur Radiol* 2005;15(10):2185–2193.
17. Mulliken JB, Fishman SJ, Burrows PE. Vascular anomalies. *Curr Probl Surg* 2000;37(8):517–584.
18. Boon LM, et al. Glomuvenous malformation (glomangioma) and venous malformation: distinct clinicopathologic and genetic entities. *Arch Dermatol* 2004;140(8):971–976.
19. Greene AK, Alomari AI. Management of venous malformations. *Clin Plast Surg* 2011;38(1):83–93.
20. Puig S, et al. Classification of venous malformations in children and implications for sclerotherapy. *Pediatr Radiol* 2003;33(2):99–103.
21. Puig S, et al. Vascular low-flow malformations in children: current concepts for classification, diagnosis and therapy. *Eur J Radiol* 2005;53(1):35–45.
22. Dubois J, Alison M. Vascular anomalies: what a radiologist needs to know. *Pediatr Radiol* 2010;40(6):895–905.
23. Paltiel HJ, et al. Soft-tissue vascular anomalies: utility of US for diagnosis. *Radiology* 2000;214(3):747–754.
24. Arnold R, Chaudry G. Diagnostic imaging of vascular anomalies. *Clin Plast Surg* 2011;38(1):21–29.
25. Dompmartin A, et al. Association of localized intravascular coagulopathy with venous malformations. *Arch Dermatol* 2008;144(7):873–877.
26. Martin LK, Russell S, Wargon O. Chronic localized intravascular coagulation complicating multifocal venous malformations. *Australas J Dermatol* 2009;50(4):276–280.
27. Mazoyer E, et al. Coagulation disorders in patients with venous malformation of the limbs and trunk: a case series of 118 patients. *Arch Dermatol* 2008;144(7):861–867.
28. Duyka LJ, et al. Progesterone receptors identified in vascular malformations of the head and neck. *Otolaryngol Head Neck Surg* 2009;141(4):491–495.
29. Heryanto B, Rogers PA. Regulation of endometrial endothelial cell proliferation by oestrogen and progesterone in the ovariectomized mouse. *Reproduction* 2002;123(1):107–113.
30. Berenguer B, et al. Sclerotherapy of craniofacial venous malformations: complications and results. *Plast Reconstr Surg* 1999;104(1):1–11; discussion 12–15.
31. Choi DJ, et al. Neurointerventional management of low-flow vascular malformations of the head and neck. *Neuroimaging Clin N Am* 2009;19(2):199–218.

32. Burrows PE, Mason KP. Percutaneous treatment of low flow vascular malformations. *J Vasc Interv Radiol* 2004;15(5):431–445.

33. Nanz D, et al. Contrast material-enhanced visualization of the ablation medium for magnetic resonance-monitored ethanol injection therapy: imaging and safety aspects. *J Vasc Interv Radiol* 2006;17(1):95–102.

34. Sanlialp I, et al. Sclerotherapy for lymphangioma in children. *Int J Pediatr Otorhinolaryngol* 2003;67(7):795–800.

35. Giguere CM, Bauman NM, Smith RJ. New treatment options for lymphangioma in infants and children. *Ann Otol Rhinol Laryngol* 2002;111(12, pt 1):1066–1075.

36. Perkins JA, et al. Lymphatic malformations: review of current treatment. *Otolaryngol Head Neck Surg* 2010;142(6):795–803, 803.e1.

37. Tran Ngoc N, Tran Xuan N. Cystic hygroma in children: a report of 126 cases. *J Pediatr Surg* 1974;9(2):191–195.

38. Alomari AI, et al. Percutaneous sclerotherapy for lymphatic malformations: a retrospective analysis of patient-evaluated improvement. *J Vasc Interv Radiol* 2006;17(10):1639–1648.

39. Renton JP, Smith RJ. Current treatment paradigms in the management of lymphatic malformations. *Laryngoscope* 2011;121(1):56–59.

40. Nehra D, et al. Doxycycline sclerotherapy as primary treatment of head and neck lymphatic malformations in children. *J Pediatr Surg* 2008;43(3):451–460.

41. Ogita S, et al. OK-432 therapy for unresectable lymphangiomas in children. *J Pediatr Surg* 1991;26(3):263–268; discussion 268–270.

42. Ogita S, et al. Intracystic injection of OK-432: a new sclerosing therapy for cystic hygroma in children. *Br J Surg* 1987;74(8):690–691.

43. Ogita S, et al. OK-432 therapy in 64 patients with lymphangioma. *J Pediatr Surg* 1994;29(6):784–785.

44. Smith MC, et al. Efficacy and safety of OK-432 immunotherapy of lymphatic malformations. *Laryngoscope* 2009;119(1):107–115.

45. Sung MW, et al. Bleomycin sclerotherapy in patients with congenital lymphatic malformation in the head and neck. *Am J Otolaryngol* 1995;16(4):236–241.

46. Lee BB, et al. Current concepts in lymphatic malformation. *Vasc Endovascular Surg* 2005;39(1):67–81.

47. Narkio-Makela M, et al. Treatment of lymphatic malformations of head and neck with OK-432 sclerotherapy induce systemic inflammatory response. *Eur Arch Otorhinolaryngol* 2011;268(1):123–129.

48. Shiels WE 2nd, et al. Percutaneous treatment of lymphatic malformations. *Otolaryngol Head Neck Surg* 2009;141(2):219–224.

49. Shiels WE 2nd, et al. Definitive percutaneous treatment of lymphatic malformations of the trunk and extremities. *J Pediatr Surg* 2008;43(1):136–139; discussion 140.

50. Burrows PE, et al. Diagnostic imaging in the evaluation of vascular birthmarks. *Dermatol Clin* 1998;16(3):455–488.

51. Liu AS, et al. Extracranial arteriovenous malformations: natural progression and recurrence after treatment. *Plast Reconstr Surg* 2010;125(4):1185–1194.

52. Greene AK, Orbach DB. Management of arteriovenous malformations. *Clin Plast Surg* 2011;38(1):95–106.

53. Rockman CB, et al. Transcatheter embolization of extremity vascular malformations: the long-term success of multiple interventions. *Ann Vasc Surg* 2003;17(4):417–423.

54. Do YS, et al. Ethanol embolization of arteriovenous malformations: interim results. *Radiology* 2005;235(2):674–682.

55. Jackson JE, Mansfield AO, Allison DJ. Treatment of high-flow vascular malformations by venous embolization aided by flow occlusion techniques. *Cardiovasc Intervent Radiol* 1996;19(5):323–328.

56. Faughnan ME, et al. International guidelines for the diagnosis and management of hereditary haemorrhagic telangiectasia. *J Med Genet* 2011;48(2):73–87.

57. Waigand J, et al. Percutaneous treatment of pseudoaneurysms and arteriovenous fistulas after invasive vascular procedures. *Catheter Cardiovasc Interv* 1999;47(2):157–164.

58. Delis KT, et al. Hemodynamic impairment, venous segmental disease, and clinical severity scoring in limbs with Klippel-Trenaunay syndrome. *J Vasc Surg* 2007;45(3):561–567.

Transjugular Intrahepatic Portosystemic Shunts

ZIV J. HASKAL and BERTRAND JANNE D'OTHÉE

INTRODUCTION

As with many innovations, a groundbreaking concept long precedes the ability to realize it. Nearly 20 years elapsed between Drs. Rosch and Hanafee's first report of the creation of percutaneous portosystemic canine shunts in 1969[1] and the modern implementation. In 1982, Colapinto reported the first human application of the technique, using prolonged balloon inflation in an attempt to create a durable liver shunt tract.[2] The first human transjugular intrahepatic portosystemic shunt (TIPS) lined with a metal stent was described by Richter et al.[3] in 1988. Those procedures rapidly evolved from ones requiring mapping angiography, transhepatic targeting baskets, and other guiding methods into today's routine TIPS, which may require less than an hour to create.[3] Tens of thousands of TIPS have been created to help treat the many complications of portal hypertension and more than 2,000 relevant scientific papers have been published in the English language alone. The current literature of TIPS is a mature one; the number of prospective controlled trials involving TIPS exceeds those of many other endovascular interventions.

TIPS FORMATION

The stereotypic TIPS is created in several steps: (a) catheterizing and mapping a suitable hepatic vein, typically the largest caudally directed right hepatic vein; (b) passing a long curved needle from within the hepatic vein through the hepatic parenchyma to puncture a branch of the intrahepatic portal vein; (c) passing catheters across this parenchymal tract into the portal venous system, performing venograms and hemodynamic assessments; (d) dilating the hepatic parenchymal tract between the portal and hepatic veins; (e) lining the tract and outflow of the hepatic vein with a stent or stent-graft; (f) performing progressive dilatation of these devices until the desired degree of partial portal decompression has been achieved (FIGURE 32.1).

There are many variations in the instrument sets, stents, and techniques used to fashion a TIPS, although basic principles remain the same. Most variations aim to make the portal vein puncture easier or address anatomic abnormalities. Shunts can be created using fluoroscopic guidance alone, combined external ultrasound,[4] intravascular ultrasound guidance,[5,6] computed tomography (CT) guidance,[7,8] directly from the inferior vena cava (transcaval), retrograde transmesenteric surgical approaches,[9,10] and others. Most procedures are still performed using fluoroscopic guidance alone under conscious sedation and require only an overnight stay in the hospital.

PATIENT SELECTION

The *contraindications* to TIPS creation can be classified as anatomic or physiologic. Relative anatomic contraindications (i.e., ones that make TIPS formation more complex but do not preclude it) include portal venous system thromboses, hepatic malignancies, polycystic liver disease, and biliary obstruction. Physiologic contraindications include severely impaired hepatic function or encephalopathy such that diversion of portal flow would lead to unacceptably worsening liver function or failure; heart failure or pulmonary hypertension, or intracardiac shunts that limit the ability to tolerate the increased cardiac output and work as well as the increased and atrial pressures that follow any portosystemic shunt; uncorrectable coagulopathies; and perhaps sepsis.[11]

In elective TIPS patients with impaired hepatic synthetic function (e.g., total serum bilirubin >3 mg/dL), elevated Mayo End-Stage Liver Disease (MELD) scores, baseline encephalopathy, or cardiac impairment or pulmonary hypertension require careful consultations with referring hepatologists and cardiologists to both agree on the medical necessity of the procedure, the possibility of accelerated time to transplant, strategies to optimize TIPS outcome, and a more conservative approach or initially creating a smaller shunt to assess patient tolerance and symptomatic improvement (with the ability to further enlarge the shunt at a later date).

The potential technical *complications* of TIPS are numerous, although in experienced hands they should be very infrequent. Because some of the steps mimic those of a transhepatic liver biopsy (performed in a cephalocaudal direction), similar liver injury can occur, particularly with prolonged attempts at puncturing the portal vein. Indeed, it is arguable that, unless one maintains a regular competency in shunt formation, elective procedures should be referred to experienced centers to reduce risks of liver injury and the patient radiation dose that can accompany a lengthy procedure. The Society of Interventional Radiology TIPS Quality Improvement document described a list of the more common important complications, dividing them into minor and major severities, with the following incidences for each[12]:

- Minor complications (4%): encephalopathy controlled by medical therapy, 10% to 25%; transient contrast-induced renal failure, 2%; fever, 2%; entry site hematoma, 2%; transient pulmonary edema, 1%
- Major complications (3%): hemobilia, 2%; hepatic artery injury, 1%; gallbladder puncture, 1%; stent malposition, 1%; hemoperitoneum, 0.5%; hepatic infarction, 0.5%; renal failure requiring chronic dialysis, 0.25%; radiation skin burn, 0.1%

Mortality rates attributable to intraprocedural complications should not exceed 1%. The reported incidence of new or worsened encephalopathy ranges from 15% to 31% and largely depends on the severity of preexisting liver disease and encephalopathy.[13–15] Careful patient selection, improved measures for control of encephalopathy, and calibrated shunt diameters allow experienced operators to lessen the incidence. Patients treated for refractory ascites or hydrothoraces often have more baseline encephalopathy and worse liver function compared to patients with variceal hemorrhage, and thus may experience more worsened encephalopathy after TIPS. Naturally, controlled trials have shown higher encephalopathy rates in TIPS patients compared to those treated with large-volume paracentesis (LVP) or endoscopic sclerotherapy or band ligation. With proper patient selection, postprocedure lactulose or rifaximin therapy, and judicious initial creation of smaller shunts in higher-risk

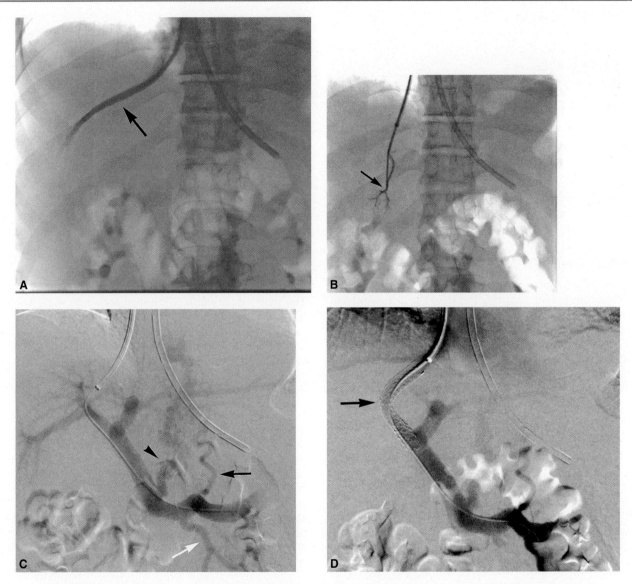

FIGURE 32.1 TIPS creation in a 42-year-old man with alcoholic cirrhosis and acute massive variceal hemorrhage. An uninflated balloon tamponade catheter is in place. **A.** A narrow right hepatic vein (*arrow*) is used for shunt construction. **B.** A small peripheral branch of the portal vein (*arrow*) was punctured using a Colapinto needle from with the Haskal TIPS set. A hydrophilic wire was manipulated through this branch into the splenic vein. **C.** Initial portal venography demonstrates hepatofugal flow in coronary (*arrow head*), short gastric (*black arrow*), and inferior mesenteric veins (*white arrow*). **D.** After shunt creation, the portosystemic gradient was reduced from 23 to 11 mm Hg. A Viatorr TIPS endograft (*arrow*) lines the shunt (WL Gore and Associates, Flagstaff, AZ). **E.** Residual variceal flow was embolized to stasis using a combination of platinum coils (*arrow*) and absolute alcohol. **F.** Five months later, his TIPS was intentionally narrowed due to continued grade 1 encephalopathy, despite lactulose and rifaximin therapy. A 10-mm diameter by 50-mm long polyethylene teraphthalate covered Wallgraft (Boston Scientific, Natick, MA), constrained in an hourglass shape (*arrow*) using a 6-0-ePTFE suture (WL Gore and Associates). The portosystemic gradient was increased from 12 to 18 mm Hg. His encephalopathy disappeared. *(continued)*

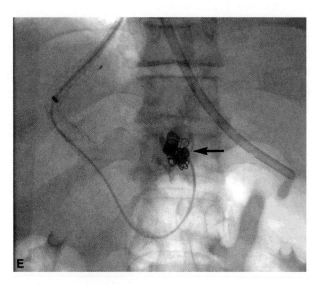
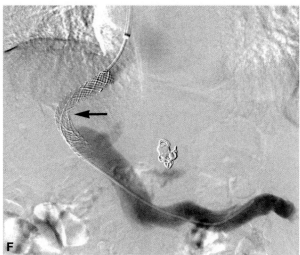

FIGURE 32.1 *(Continued)*

patients, shunt reduction or intentional occlusion is rarely needed.[16–21] Prudence is warranted when intentionally occluding a shunt because it has been reported to initiate hepatorenal syndrome (HRS) in a small number of patients.[22]

OUTCOMES BY INDICATION

The ability to reduce portal venous pressures in a completely percutaneous fashion has vastly increased the indications and numbers of patients treated as well as largely superseded open surgical portosystemic shunt formation. Among reported indications for TIPS are acute uncontrolled or recurrent esophageal, gastric or ectopic variceal bleeding, portal gastropathy, refractory ascites, hepatic hydrothorax, Budd-Chiari syndrome (BCS), and HRS.

Acute Esophageal Variceal Bleeding Refractory to Medical Treatment

Most patients with actively bleeding esophageal varices, that is, "acute bleeding," can be controlled with first-line pharmacologic and/or endoscopic means by using band ligation or injection sclerotherapy. Failure of these treatments is an indication for portal decompression (or potentially accelerated transplantation in appropriate candidates). Most reports of emergency surgical shunt creation in the acute setting describe mortalities of 30% to 77%.[23,24] One report of pooled data from 509 acutely bleeding patients treated with TIPS described excellent control of variceal bleeding in 93.6 ± 6.7% (mean ± SD) with an early rebleeding rate of 12.4 ± 6.1%. Despite this, 35.8 ± 16% of patients died in the hospital or within 6 weeks, reflecting the severe comorbidities (e.g., liver failure, adult respiratory distress syndrome, aspiration pneumonia, multiorgan failure) that plague these critically ill patients.[25] Prognostic factors predicting survival after TIPS have been extensively studied. Significant factors include MELD scores,[26–31] Child-Pugh class or score,[32] pre-TIPS APACHE II scores,[33–37] preprocedure total serum bilirubin (>3 mg/dL),[34] emergent indications for TIPS, and endotracheal

intubation.[38,39] In 2010, however, Garcia-Pagan et al. reported a controlled trial evaluating the early use of TIPS in patients with esophageal variceal hemorrhage, in which patients were assigned to TIPS or endoscopic therapy and vasoactive medications within 24 hours of admission. At 14 months follow-up, both the rates of rebleeding and transplant-free survival were significantly better in patients randomized to early TIPS ($p = .001$ and $p < .001$, respectively). Further, ICU days were higher in the non-TIPS group. This study, one in which ePTFE stent grafts were used, is one of the first to demonstrate a survival benefit for patients referred sooner for TIPS.[40] Thus, salvage therapy with TIPS is important in the acute setting but may not increase midterm survival in some of these severely ill patients.

Recurrent Esophageal Variceal Bleeding

Once an esophageal variceal hemorrhage has occurred, the risk of rebleeding is at least 50%. Portal decompression, be it surgically or interventionally achieved, lowers rebleeding risks far more than endoscopic treatments, although the incidence of subsequent hepatic encephalopathy is almost always higher. In one meta-analysis of 811 patients, rebleeding rates for endoscopic therapies was 47% versus 19% for TIPS, respectively.[41] More than 12 randomized trials have compared secondary prevention of variceal bleeding using TIPS versus endoscopic sclerotherapy or band ligation.[42–54] In nine trials, the median rebleeding rate for TIPS was 16% versus 44% for endoscopic therapy. Survival was rarely improved,[48] emphasizing the progressive nature of advanced liver disease and the need for transplant evaluation.

TIPS has been compared to medical therapy in a small number of patients. In one series of 91 patients the risk of rebleeding was 39% at 2 years for those treated with pharmacologic therapy versus 13% in those receiving a TIPS.[55] Encephalopathy developed in 14% of those receiving medical therapy and 38% of TIPS patients. Child-Pugh class improved in 72% of the drug group but in only 45% of the TIPS group. The 2-year survival rate was the same in both groups, 72%. The cost of therapy in the TIPS group was twice that of the medical group.[55] Of note, in some of the trials, the patients referred for TIPS were medical failures, whereas in others they had a single index bleed before randomization.

Finally, there is no evidence to support the use of TIPS for primary prophylaxis of variceal bleeding, that is, at initial diagnosis of varices but prior to any bleeding. Until controlled trials appear, primary prophylaxis is achieved with medical therapy and, occasionally, endoscopic means.

Gastric Varices

TIPS has proven efficacious for controlling gastric variceal bleeding in multiple nonrandomized trials.[56–60] It appears that TIPS is equally effective in controlling gastric and esophageal variceal bleeding. Further controlled trials are needed to compare endoscopic glue injections versus TIPS for acute or recurrent gastric variceal bleeding. In the authors' opinion, TIPS is extremely useful for control of gastric variceal bleeding, although procedural endpoints can be different than those for esophageal varices. Lower final portosystemic gradients may be needed, which are often combined with liquid transcatheter sclerosis of varices and embolization.

Another alternative to TIPS and embolization of gastric varices is balloon-occluded retrograde transvenous obliteration (BRTO).[61–79] This technique, pioneered in Japan, involves retrograde catheterization of the gastric variceal outflow into the left renal vein, isolation of collateral veins (e.g., phrenic and lumbar veins by embolization), and endovascular sclerotherapy of the gastric varices. It has proven reproducible and effective for obliteration of gastric varices and, in some cases, improving liver function and reducing hepatic encephalopathy. The procedure is increasingly offered in the Western Hemisphere because use of agents other than ethanolamine has proven fruitful. Of note is that BRTO is often performed in Japan in patients for primary prophylaxis, that is, prior to an index bleed. There may also be a role for controlled trials comparing TIPS versus BRTO in acute or recurrent gastric variceal bleeding. One 20-patient trial comparing endoscopic sclerotherapy to transvenous obliteration reported results mimicking endoscopic therapy but using less sclerosants. In another, 1-year follow-up endoscopies revealed variceal decrease or disappearance in 81% of patients. Some authors have suggested that portal perfusion and liver function can be improved by occlusion of competing splenorenal shunt in such patients.[80]

Ectopic Varices

Duodenal, intestinal, stomal, and anorectal varices are relatively uncommon but appear to respond well to TIPS and possible adjunctive embolization.[81–96] It is worth emphasizing the need for clinical suspicion of intestinal varices in patients with liver disease and occult lower gastrointestinal bleeding. Diagnostic visceral angiography (with careful attention to the venous phase) should be considered because CT or magnetic resonance imaging (MRI) can miss the varices. These varices often develop within adhesions related to prior abdominal surgery and they may decompress into more unusual venous channels, such as the gonadal or ovarian veins. Capsule endoscopy may also be useful in establishing the diagnosis. Finally, BRTO has also been used for the treatment of ectopic varices.[74,77,97,98]

Portal Hypertensive Gastropathy and Gastric Antral Vascular Ectasia

These two entities are distinct, yet can either coexist or be difficult to distinguish during endoscopy. The mucosa in portal hypertensive gastropathy (PHG) can show a mosaic-like pattern, usually within the fundus or body of the stomach. Gastric antral vascular ectasia (GAVE) is characterized by linear or diffuse red patches within the antrum. PHG is limited to patients with portal hypertension, whereas GAVE can be seen in a variety of conditions.[99] The effect of TIPS on PHG and GAVE has been examined in several series.[100–105] In one report 75% of 54 patients with severe PHG showed both endoscopic improvement and a decrease in the need for transfusions after TIPS creation.[105] In another, 9/10 patients showed endoscopic improvement in PHG following TIPS.[106] In the authors' experience, TIPS is very useful in controlling blood loss caused by portal gastropathy or its similar manifestations within the duodenum or small bowel. In contrast, bleeding from GAVE in patients with cirrhosis was unaffected by TIPS. GAVE is not an indication for TIPS. It is best treated with endoscopic ablation using argon plasma coagulation, lasers, or heater probes. For patients with severe recurrent bleeding or uncontrollable acute bleeding from GAVE, an antrectomy with Billroth I anastomosis may be needed.

Refractory Ascites

In the early 1990s the lead indication for TIPS was variceal bleeding. As experience has grown and, perhaps, endoscopic therapies evolved, refractory ascites has become the lead indication for TIPS at many transplant centers. Ascites is considered refractory to medical treatment when it is unresponsive to or intolerant of sodium restriction and high doses of diuretics (400 mg/day spironolactone and 160 mg/day furosemide).[107,108] Once refractory ascites develops (i.e., in 5% to 10% of cirrhotic patients with ascites), the patient has a poor prognosis with approximately 50% mortality at 12 months.[109,110] Although far fewer randomized trials comparing TIPS to paracentesis exist, compared to those for variceal bleeding, conclusions can still be drawn. TIPS can clearly reduce the incidence of cirrhotic ascites and reduce the need for diuretic use and LVP. Pooling the data from four controlled trials encompassing 264 patients, the mean incidence of improvement in ascites at 3 to 4 months was 57.8% for TIPS, compared with 19% for LVP.[111–114] The number of subsequent paracentesis was lower in the TIPS group. Improvements in creatinine clearance and reduced diuretic requirements were described in survivors. Encephalopathy was somewhat greater in the TIPS groups, at 34.0 ±19.8%, as compared to the LVP groups, 18.5 ± 12.0%. Somewhat surprisingly there was no difference in the quality of life between the two groups in one of the studies.[113] Cost-effectiveness was not examined in any of the studies. A transplant-free survival benefit for TIPS was seen in two trials[112,115] but not on others.[113–114] Overall survival was not improved in the NASTRA trial (North American Study for the Treatment of Refractory Ascites), although a 6-month mean survival difference was seen in the TIPS patients—arguably notable in a patient population in whom survival without transplant is typically limited. In 2007, Salerno et al.[116] performed a meta-analysis of individual patient data from these preceding randomized trials comparing TIPS with paracentesis. A total of 305 patients were analyzed, evenly split among the groups. The actuarial likelihood of transplant-free survival was significantly better within the TIPS group (p = .035). Hepatic encephalopathy episodes were significantly greater in the TIPS group (p = .006). Increasing age, serum total bilirubin, and serum sodium levels were also independently associated with survival.

One prospective study randomized patients with refractory ascites to TIPS or pleuroperitoneal (Denver) shunts.[117] Primary median shunt patencies were similar (TIPS 4.4 months, Denver 4.0 months), although assisted patencies were 31 months for TIPS compared with 13 months for the Denver shunts. Survival in the TIPS groups was also longer, 28.7 versus 16 months. These findings favor the use of TIPS in refractory ascites patients who can tolerate portal decompression.

The technical challenges of creating a TIPS in patients with refractory ascites are greater because the liver and donor hepatic veins are more shrunken than in typical variceal bleeding patients. Technical tricks in these settings include the use of carbon dioxide wedged portography to visualize the portal system (leading to reduced iodinated contrast volumes), exaggerated curves upon the portal access needles, vein exit sites that lie more dorsal and closer to the junction with the inferior vena cava, use of transmesenteric techniques, or intravascular ultrasound guidance for transcaval shunt construction.

Refractory Hepatic Hydrothorax

Hepatic hydrothorax can develop in patients with cirrhotic ascites when diaphragmatic pores allow fluid to pass between the peritoneal and pleural spaces. In most patients the defect is in the diaphragm that overlies the dome of the liver. Hepatic hydrothorax is estimated to occur in approximately 5% of cirrhotic patients with or without concomitant ascites. In a series of studies, the effect of TIPS has been relatively uniform; that is, resolution of the hepatic hydrothorax or a decrease in the need for thoracentesis.[118–125] Because alternatives are few for these patients (e.g., pleuro-peritoneal shunts), TIPS provides important first-line care when diuresis fails.

Hepatorenal Syndrome

HRS is a feared complication of liver disease whose development often brings a poor prognosis. It is characterized by activation of the renin-angiotensin and sympathetic systems, renal vasoconstriction, low systemic and splanchnic vascular resistance, and high cardiac output. HRS exists in two forms. Type 1 is a rapidly progressive form (2 weeks) of renal failure, whereas type 2 HRS 2 is characterized by a more insidious onset of renal failure. The prognosis for patients with type 1 HRS is significantly worse than for those with type 2 HRS.[126,127] The treatment of choice of HRS is liver transplantation, which addresses both the hepatic and renal diseases; while awaiting transplant, supportive management may include medical therapy, dialysis, and TIPS. TIPS has been used in a number of patients with HRS, yielding reports of improved glomerular filtration rates, renal plasma flow, and urine sodium handling, and reduction of serum creatinine and plasma aldosterone levels.[128–135] Although survival in type I HRS after TIPS appears improved compared with historical expectations, none of the trials were randomized and no comparative survival benefits have been shown. In one series, only 20% of the patients with type 1 HRS

were alive 1 year after TIPS insertion, whereas approximately 45% patients with type 2 HRS survived at 1 year.[128,135] In the four controlled trials in which TIPS was compared to LVP in the control of refractory cirrhotic ascites discussed previously, there was no consistent improvement in renal function with TIPS compared to LVP, although one did find a reduced incidence of HRS in those receiving a TIPS.[113] Pre-TIPS bilirubin levels were predictive of survival in these patients as well.[135] TIPS needs to be compared to other therapies, such as terlipressin, before its widespread role in the treatment of the HRS is determined.

Budd-Chiari Syndrome

Budd-Chiari syndrome (BCS) results from obstructed egress of the blood from the liver caused by either hepatic vein thrombosis or obstruction of the inferior vena cava.[136,137] Liver injury, fibrosis, and cirrhosis result from unremitting hepatic congestion, a condition unmitigated by anticoagulation. Surgical shunts have long proven useful in preventing or stabilizing liver disease in BCS patients, although their prothrombotic tendencies and caval compression have required more extensive surgeries, including mesoatrial shunts. Accordingly, it is logical that TIPS could afford the same benefits in properly selected BCS patients. Although numerous case series[138–156] have described the beneficial use of TIPS in acute and chronic BCS, no long-term or prospective controlled trials have compared TIPS to medical or surgical therapies. Liver transplant-free survival rates of 88% at 1 year and 78% at 5 years have been reported in a single arm cohort).[157] The reintervention rate has been reported to be higher in BCS patients undergoing TIPS,[150,158] which is likely related to underlying hypercoagulability or anatomic factors related to the TIPS. Indeed, it must be noted that TIPS construction in BCS patients can be significantly more demanding that in cirrhotic patients (FIGURES 32.2 and 32.3). In BCS patients, the liver is swollen in both posteroanterior and cephalocaudal dimensions (the opposite of often shrunken liver seen in ascites patients), the liver parenchyma may be "soft" (making it easier to disrupt with needle passes), and extensive hepatic vein collateral may provide near-continuous confusing return of blood into the puncture needle during its slow withdrawal, adding to the complexity of TIPS formation. The underlying prothrombotic tendencies may require heavy doses of anticoagulation to prevent acute thrombosis of bare stents. Finally, in the absence of hepatic vein remnants, shunt must be constructed from the vena cava, raising the risk of inadvertent right atrial or intraperitoneal puncture. In the authors' decades-long experience of treating acute and chronic BCS patients with TIPS, these technical challenges have proven significant and warrant adjustments in conventional techniques, including the use of adjunctive imaging, such as external ultrasound, routine use of coaxial fine-needle systems, percutaneous cholangiography-type injections of contrast (for portal localization), and antiplatelet agents. With these modifications, however, shunts can be constructed safely and expeditiously. Nevertheless, in the authors' experience, only one BCS patient in 10 years treated with TIPS has undergone liver transplantation—a patient with preexisting established Child C cirrhosis. Annual biopsies of these patients have shown regression of sinusoidal congestion after TIPS and absence of developing fibrosis.[137]

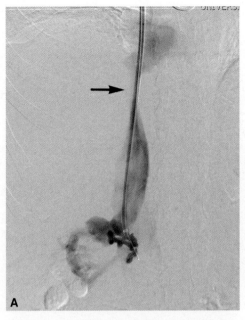

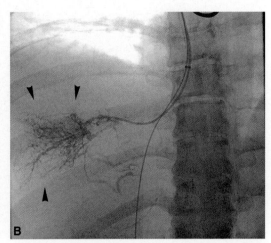

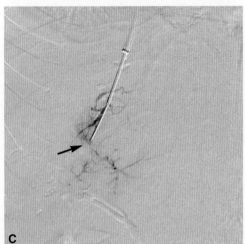

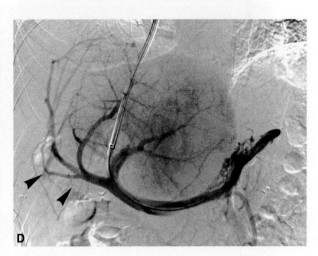

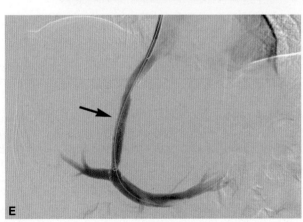

FIGURE 32.2 TIPS creation in a 43-year-old patient with chronic Budd Chiari syndrome. **A.** Initial cava gram demonstrates compression of the vena cava by the congested liver (*arrow*). **B.** The typical "spider web" pattern of hepatic vein collaterals is seen during wedged contrast injection (*arrowheads*). **C.** A coaxial fine-needle system is advanced through the vena cava (through the Colapinto needle) to puncture a tiny peripheral branch of the portal vein (*arrow*). This branch was catheterized using a 0.018-inch guide wire and manipulated into the main portal vein. **D.** Initial splenic venography demonstrated splaying of the portal vein (*arrow heads*) and enlargement of the caudate vessels (and preferential filling). The absolute portal pressure was 32 mm Hg. **E.** After creation of the transcaval shunt (*arrow*), the final portosystemic gradient was reduced from 27 to 13 mm Hg.

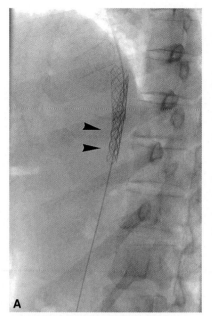

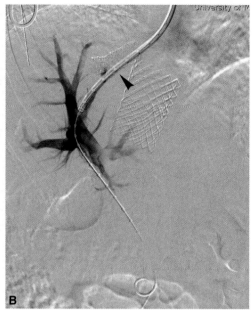

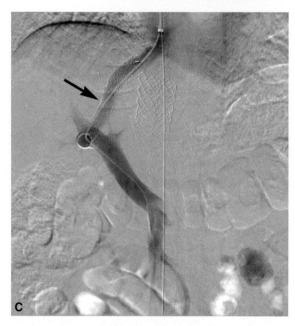

FIGURE 32.3 TIPS in a patient with Budd-Chiari syndrome. A 42-year-old man with longstanding Budd-Chiari syndrome and increasing ascites. Caval and hepatic vein stents had been placed at an outside hospital. **A.** The balloon expandable caval stent had become completely flattened by the continued compression from the congested, swollen liver (*arrow heads*). The right atrial pressure was 7 mm Hg; the free hepatic vein pressure was 18 mm Hg. **B.** The right portal vein was punctured through the mesh of the preexisting hepatic vein stent (*arrow head*). The initial portal vein pressure was 40 mm Hg (portosystemic gradient of 33 mm Hg). **C.** The TIPS was created using a Viatorr endograft (*arrow*). The portal pressure was reduced to 32 mm Hg and the atrium pressure increased to 16 mm Hg (final portosystemic gradient was 16 mm Hg). Five weeks later, he returned for scheduled shunt venography and transcaval liver biopsy. The intravascular pressures had dropped to 3 mm Hg in the right atrium, 10 mm Hg in the portal vein, and a portosystemic gradient of 7 mm Hg. His ascites had resolved.

SURVEILLANCE AND SHUNT PATENCY

Surveillance Modalities

As TIPS use spread in the early 1990s, it became clear that stenoses and occlusions developed frequently, placing patients at risk of potentially serious or life-threatening recurrent complications. Numerous studies described the phenomenon and rates of TIPS dysfunction, ranging from 18% to 78%.[42,45-47,49-51,159,160] Undoubtedly, these variations reflect differences in sampling intervals and relative accuracies of surveillance techniques. Most physicians have utilized Doppler sonography to assess shunt patency.[161-182] Indeed, many early reports described very high accuracies, although these retrospective case series suffered from inconsistent patency standards, lack of gold-standard comparisons with catheter venography, and, arguably, lack of clinically relevant definitions of patency. Further, some larger later studies were flawed because sonographic criteria of shunt dysfunction were used to trigger gold-standard venography; however, when sonography suggested no shunt dysfunction, patency was assumed without venographic proof.[175,183] Sonography is limited in its ability to characterize shunt patency because minimum lumen diameter and percent diameter stenosis do not directly correlate with clinically relevant measures. Maintenance of a low portosystemic pressure gradient is the goal—a measure that inconsistently follows percent diameter stenosis.[174]

One prospective study compared 151 Doppler sonograms with TIPS venograms and assessments of portal pressure. Using the definition of a portosytemic gradient of less than 15 mm HG for success and greater than or equal to 15 mm Hg for failure, sonography provided a sensitivity and specificity of only 86%

and 48%, respectively.[174] Thus, an abnormal Doppler ultrasound is predictive of occlusion or stenosis, whereas a normal ultrasound does not exclude TIPS dysfunction.[174,179,180,184-186] Logically, the best indicator of TIPS dysfunction is a recurrence of the condition for which the TIPS was originally inserted; for example, variceal bleeding, hepatic hydrothorax, or ascites. If recurrent varices are identified by upper endoscopy then the TIPS is most likely insufficient. Documentation of patency can only be achieved with certainty by recatheterization of the shunt, venography, and hemodynamic assessments. Interestingly, though, as device developments improve primary shunt patency and physician confidence increases, sonography may become increasingly useful because absolute accuracy will be less necessary.

Pathogenesis of Shunt Stenosis and Occlusion

The histopathology of TIPS thrombosis and stenosis has been characterized.[187-194] In 1991, LaBerge et al.[189] first described the histology of TIPS in seven patients who had undergone liver transplantation. At 4 days after TIPS, fresh clot adhered to the mesh of the wallstents lining the tracts. By 3 weeks, the shunt lumen was lined with a 400- to 600-μm-thick layer of pseudointimal tissue. At 3 months, the stents were enveloped within a layer of dense collagen. We have also performed analyses of the histopathologic response of humans and swine to TIPS creation. Human livers from necropsy and liver transplantation containing TIPS that had been in place 10 to 1,089 days were evaluated using a variety of histologic stains, including hematoxylin and eosin, trichrome, and immunohistochemical stains for smooth muscle cell actin, high-molecular-weight cytokeratins, and factor VIII. The parenchymal tracts of the shunts were lined with circumferential layers of myofibroblasts and collagen matrix. The cells appeared to originate from the liver surface (by proliferating nuclear cell antibody studies) and grew to entirely encapsulate the stents. The shunt lumina were lined with a single cell layer that stained positive for factor VIII, indicating that a neoendothelium had formed.

An experiment by Teng et al.[193] sheds light on the role of bile in acute shunt thrombosis. In culturing smooth muscle cells with bile, serum and bile, and serum alone, they found that bile was a powerful inhibitor of smooth muscle cell proliferation. These findings suggest that TIPS failure associated with bile leaks is probably caused by the thrombogenic effect of bile combined with its inhibitory effect on endothelialization and healing of the TIPS tract. Thus bile plays a prominent, partial role in the mechanism of TIPS stenosis. In cases of rapid and recurring stenosis, bile duct transection may be the prime mover, whereas in other cases the proliferative fibroblast layers may simply represent a healing response to the massive local liver injury that occurs with stretching and tearing of liver parenchyma during tract angioplasty and stent placement. Because fibroblasts are scattered throughout the liver, it is not surprising that they proliferate in response to shunt creation.

The outflow hepatic vein represents a separate site of shunt stenosis (FIGURE 32.4).[159,199] In one prospective study of TIPS, all hepatic veins shrank an average of 50% in diameter in response to TIPS, accounting for the flow-limiting lesions in most cases.[160] Typically this process begins within 3 to 6 months after the shunt creation. The proliferating smooth muscle cells that narrow the hepatic vein are identical and continuous with those that line the parenchymal tract.[187-198] This intimal hyperplasia mimics the standard biologic response seen at many surgical graft anastomoses, including dialysis access grafts, coronary bypasses, or lower extremity bypass grafts. Bile leaks have no apparent role in the remote hepatic vein stenosis in TIPS—the

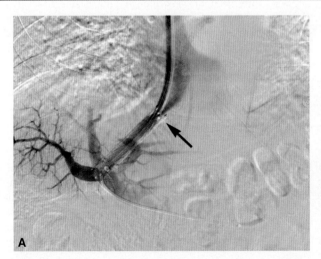
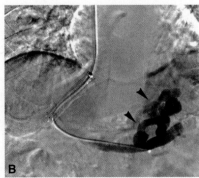

FIGURE 32.4 Balloon retrograde transvenous obliteration (BRTO) of varices for treatment of refractory encephalopathy. A 65-year-old man had previously undergone TIPS formation for treatment of esophageal varices. He was referred from an outside facility for evaluation of continued grade 2 encephalopathy and potential shunt reduction. Also notable was chronic anemia attributed to gastropathy and periodic melena. He required dual antiplatelet therapy because of implanted coronary stents. **A.** Initial TIPS venography demonstrated a shunt lined by a stent that was already flow limited due to hepatic vein stenosis (*arrow*). Despite this stenosis, the portosystemic gradient was 7 mm Hg. **B.** Splenic venography demonstrated the reason for the low portosystemic gradient, revealing a large spleno-gastro-renal shunt (*arrow heads*). The presence of this native shunt explained his continued gastrointestinal oozing, low gradient, and encephalopathy. *(continued)*

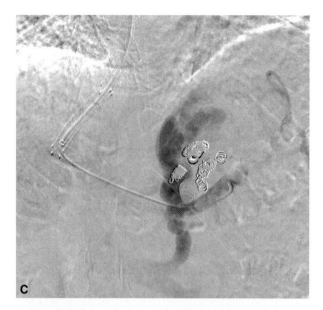

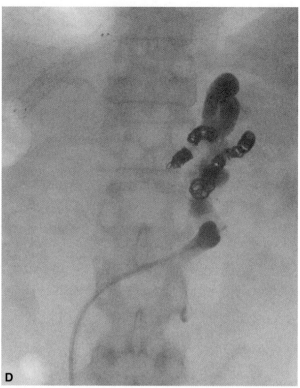

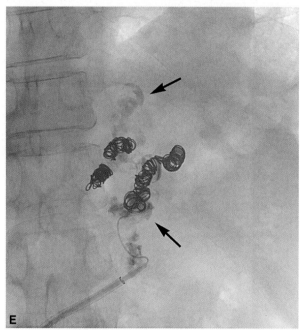

FIGURE 32.4 (*Continued*) **C.** As a provocative test, numerous embolization coils were placed into the varices, raising the gradient by 7 mm Hg. At 1-week follow-up, his encephalopathy had slightly, but noticeably, improved. He was admitted for BRTO. **D.** Using a retrograde, transfemoral approach, a balloon occlusion catheter was introduced into the left adrenal vein (the outflow of the gastrorenal shunt), inflated, and venography performed. The patent varix is shown. Sotradecol foam (3%) was injected into the static varix through a microcatheter advanced deeply into it (not shown). It was allowed to dwell for several hours. The balloon was deflated and variceal stasis was confirmed. **E.** Final venography demonstrated successful varix thrombosis (*arrows*). At 2-week follow-up, he was, for the first time since TIPS, completely free of hepatic encephalopathy and able to drive. Repeat endoscopy demonstrated no gastric varices. At 6 months, he had had no further requirement for blood transfusion.

latter is likely related to phenomena implicated in intimal hyperplasia elsewhere, including shear stress.

Anticoagulation might not be expected to affect secondary hepatic vein stenosis due to intimal hyperplasia, but it might reduce early shunt thrombosis related to bile or other unknown local or systemic factors. Sauer et al.[200] evaluated this question by randomizing 49 patients with variceal bleeding to prophylactic anticoagulation after TIPS. During the 3 months of post-TIPS anticoagulation, five shunt occlusions developed in the control group with none in the treatment group. During subsequent months of follow-up, there was no difference in the rate of shunt stenosis between the two groups. It is unknown whether any of the occlusions were related to bile leaks. Siegerstetter et al.[201] randomized 84 patients to receive standard heparin treatment or a combination of trapidil, a drug with anti-platelet-derived growth

factor (PDGF) activity, and ticlopidine, a platelet aggregation inhibitor. Their findings suggest that the incidence of hepatic vein stenosis could be reduced by combined inhibition of platelet aggregation and anti-PDGF activity. Certainly it is clear that TIPS failure occurs at multiple sites and for multiple reasons. Treatments intended to prolong shunt patency must address all causes.

Management of Shunt Failure: The Use of Stent Grafts

Research into improving TIPS patency moved in many directions, including brachytherapy (single doses with afterloaders and fractionated doses via radioactive stents), external-beam irradiation, oral medications (e.g., anticoagulants, antiplatelet agents), and local delivery of antiproliferative drugs into the

TIPS tract. Most investigations were directed toward combining porous stent skeletons with biocompatible graft materials. TIPS stent-grafts proved the next step in TIPS device evolution.

The porcine model is well suited to TIPS formation and device testing because shunt formation is achieved using the identical techniques and equipment used in humans, and the porcine pathologic response is similar to that seen in human TIPS, that is, fibroblast proliferation and extracellular matrix deposition within the parenchymal tract, followed by hepatic vein stenoses at a later stage.[202] Unlike humans, however, the model provides a very accelerated rate of shunt stenosis, typically occurring within 2 to 4 weeks of TIPS formation. Fortunately, porcine TIPS stenoses develop in the absence of portal hypertension—an advantage because inducing durable portal hypertension in pigs has proven extremely difficult.[203,204]

A variety of graft materials and coatings have been studied in both swine and human TIPS in an attempt to prolong TIPS patency, including silicone, polytetrafluoroethylene (PTFE), polyethylene terephthalate (PET), composite polyurethane-coated Dacron-covered stents, and polycarbonate urethane covered stents. Swine TIPS lined with expanded PTFE (ePTFE) have shown marked improvements in shunt patency when compared to bare stent controls. In 1995, Nishimine et al.[202] published the first animal investigation evaluating the efficacy of covered stents for TIPS. They compared the results of 13 swine TIPS lined with bare stents with 13 swine TIPS lined with handmade PTFE stent-grafts. At 4 weeks, one control TIPS was patent (8%), whereas 9/13 (69%) of the PTFE stent-grafts demonstrated a stenosis of less than 50%. By 3 months, 6 of the 13 stent-grafts remained patent (defined as <50% shunt stenosis). In five cases, hepatic vein stenoses contributed to loss of graft patency. In 1997, these results were expanded upon using an encapsulated ePTFE stent-graft designed specifically for TIPS.[205] Eight TIPS were created in eight pigs by using this stent-graft. All but one shunt were patent at 1, 3, 4, and 5-month explant and venography. In contrast, the wallstent control group developed occlusions or stenoses of 45% to 85% within 4 weeks. The observed histologic responses mimicked those of humans.

In humans, Saxon et al.[206] published the results of an important pilot study evaluating stent-grafts for revisions of TIPS stenoses and occlusions. Six patients with an initial mean primary TIPS patency duration of 50 days (range, 9 to 100 days) had their TIPS lined with a modified Z-stent endoskeleton supporting 4 mm Gore PTFE graft (W.L. Gore) that had been dilated to 14 mm in diameter. Once delivered, the PTFE was sandwiched against the shunt lumen with a standard wallstent. Three patients had initially demonstrable biliary fistulae. Of five surviving patients, three remained patent at a mean venographic follow up of 315 days. One shunt occluded and one became stenotic due to graft misplacement. The authors concluded that PTFE-covered stent-grafts were effective for revision of TIPS in patients with tract stenosis and occlusion. Subsequently, Ferral et al.[207] reported the use of a modified Cragg Endopro System I stent-graft (Mintec, Bahamas), a polyester fabric-coated nitinol stent, for creation of TIPS in 13 patients. Using unspecified sonographic criteria, one shunt was deemed stenotic at an unspecified follow-up interval, whereas two shunts were found occluded at 2- and 3-month follow-up. Although performance of shunt venography, the gold-standard exam for evaluating the degree of shunt stenosis, was described as having been performed, the results of these portograms were not;

this technical note focused largely on the acute and short-term results of the devices in a TIPS application. A small series later described repeated acute shunt thrombosis in TIPS patients lined with PET-covered wallstents, all of which were successfully salvaged using PTFE stent-grafts.[208] Why polyester stent-grafts incite thrombosis in de novo TIPS in contrast to their desirable properties in arterial applications is unclear. Whether they are equally thrombotic in revision TIPS applications is also unknown.

Expanding on the promising results with animal and pilot studies with PTFE, numerous case reports and series reporting patency improvements with homemade PTFE TIPS stent-grafts appeared.[5,208–213] In 2000, the Viatorr TIPS endoprosthesis (W.L. Gore and Associates) became available in Europe. Since then several thousand TIPS stent-grafts have been implanted for de novo or revision applications and reports of outcome are rapidly appearing in publication.[30,214–220] In one series typifying the results described in other retrospective Viatorr series, Hausegger et al.[218] reported primary patencies of 87% and 80% at 6 and 12 months, respectively, using sonographic or venographic criteria. Notably, the mean initial post-TIPS portosystemic gradient of 6 mm Hg was almost unchanged in those patients undergoing 6-month venography—arguably one of the most critical endpoints in shunt function. In a retrospective case-matched series of bare stent TIPS versus stent-grafts, Angermayr et al.[30] reported statistically significant survival improvements in patients receiving PTFE grafts.

In 1999, the multicenter U.S. pivotal randomized trial comparing de novo TIPS created with the wallstent and Viatorr was begun. This was completed in 2004, after enrolling 253 patients. At 6-month venography, percent diameter TIPS stenosis was significantly lower in the Viatorr group (16% versus 42%, $p < .001$). By Kaplan Meyer analysis, time to reinterventions was also significantly shorter in the wallstent group ($p = .007$). Expanded PTFE TIPS endografts marked a dramatic and inarguable improvement in primary TIPS patency and reduction in need for subsequent invasive interventions and vigilant patency surveillance. It is estimated that greater than 80% of TIPS created worldwide are lined with ePTFE endografts, and that this percentage continues to rise. Studies comparing TIPS and endoscopic therapies bear repetition, and controlled trials of smaller caliber might yet prove useful in selected populations by minimizing the negative effects of portal decompression upon liver perfusion.[40,215,217,221–231]

▌ CONCLUSION

TIPS has been extensively studied in both animal and clinical research since its introduction more than two decades ago. Major technical improvements, such as the introduction of covered stents, have translated into improved clinical outcomes and broader use. These advances have helped TIPS to become a crucial and routine therapy in the management of portal hypertension.

▌ REFERENCES

1. Rosch J, Hanafee WN, Snow H. Transjugular portal venography and radiologic portacaval shunt: an experimental study. *Radiology* 1969;92(5):1112–1114.
2. Colapinto RF, Blendis LM. Liver biopsy through the transjugular approach. Modification of instruments. *Radiology* 1983;148(1):306.

3. Richter GM, Palmaz JC, Noldge G, et al. The transjugular intrahepatic portosystemic stent-shunt. A new nonsurgical percutaneous method [in German]. *Radiologe* 1989;29(8):406–411.

4. Roeren T, Richter GM, Limberg B, et al. Ultrasound guided puncture of the portal vein in transjugular intrahepatic portasystemic stent shunt (TIPSS) [in German]. *Radiologe* 1996;36(9):677–682.

5. Petersen B, Uchida BT, Timmermans H, et al. Intravascular US-guided direct intrahepatic portacaval shunt with a PTFE-covered stent-graft: feasibility study in swine and initial clinical results. *J Vasc Interv Radiol* 2001;12(4):475–486.

6. Petersen B. Intravascular ultrasound-guided direct intrahepatic portacaval shunt: description of technique and technical refinements. *J Vasc Interv Radiol* 2003;14(1):21–32.

7. Bloch R, Fontaine A, Borsa J, et al. CT-guided transfemoral portocaval shunt creation. *Cardiovasc Intervent Radiol* 2001;24(2):106–110.

8. Quinn SF, Sheley RC, Semonsen KG. Creation of a portal vein to inferior vena cava shunt using CT guidance and a covered endovascular stent. *AJR Am J Roentgenol* 1997;169(4):1159–1160.

9. Rozenblit G, Del Guercio LR. Combined transmesenteric and transjugular approach for intrahepatic portosystemic shunt placement. *J Vasc Interv Radiol* 1993;4(5):661–666.

10. Rozenblit G, Del Guercio LR, Savino J, et al. Splenic venous hypertension presenting as variceal hemorrhage caused by portal hypertension. *J Am Coll Surg* 1996;182(1):63–68.

11. Azoulay D, Castaing D, Dennison A, et al. Transjugular intrahepatic portosystemic shunt worsens the hyperdynamic circulatory state of the cirrhotic patient: preliminary report of a prospective study. *Hepatology* 1994;19(1):129–132.

12. Haskal ZJ, Martin L, Cardella JF, et al. Quality improvement guidelines for transjugular intrahepatic portosystemic shunts. SCVIR Standards of Practice Committee. *J Vasc Interv Radiol* 2001;12(2):131–136.

13. Jalan R, Elton RA, Redhead DN, et al. Analysis of prognostic variables in the prediction of mortality, shunt failure, variceal rebleeding and encephalopathy following the transjugular intrahepatic portosystemic stent-shunt for variceal haemorrhage. *J Hepatol* 1995;23(2):123–128.

14. Sanyal AJ, Freedman AM, Shiffman ML, et al. Portosystemic encephalopathy after transjugular intrahepatic portosystemic shunt: results of a prospective controlled study. *Hepatology* 1994;20(1, pt 1):46–55.

15. Somberg KA, Riegler JL, LaBerge JM, et al. Hepatic encephalopathy after transjugular intrahepatic portosystemic shunts: incidence and risk factors. *Am J Gastroenterol* 1995;90(4):549–555.

16. Haskal ZJ, Middlebrook MR. Creation of a stenotic stent to reduce flow through a transjugular intrahepatic portosystemic shunt. *J Vasc Interv Radiol* 1994;5(6):827–829; discussion 9–30.

17. Brophy D, Haskal ZJ. Simpler ways to deliver the stenotic stent for reducing TIPS flow. *J Vasc Interv Radiol* 1998;9(6):1032–1033.

18. Hauenstein KH, Haag K, Ochs A, et al. The reducing stent: treatment for transjugular intrahepatic portosystemic shunt-induced refractory hepatic encephalopathy and liver failure. *Radiology* 1995;194(1):175–179.

19. Kerlan RK Jr, LaBerge JM, Baker EL, et al. Successful reversal of hepatic encephalopathy with intentional occlusion of transjugular intrahepatic portosystemic shunts. *J Vasc Interv Radiol* 1995;6(6):917–921.

20. Haskal ZJ, Cope C, Soulen MC, et al. Intentional reversible thrombosis of transjugular intrahepatic portosystemic shunts. *Radiology* 1995;195(2):485–488.

21. Forauer AR, McLean GK. Transjugular intrahepatic portosystemic shunt constraining stent for the treatment of refractory postprocedural encephalopathy: a simple design utilizing a Palmaz stent and Wallstent. *J Vasc Interv Radiol* 1998;9(3):443–446.

22. Paz-Fumagalli R, Crain MR, Mewissen MW, et al. Fatal hemodynamic consequences of therapeutic closure of a transjugular intrahepatic portosystemic shunt. *J Vasc Interv Radiol* 1994;5(6):831–834.

23. Sarfeh IJ, Rypins EB, Mason GR. A systematic appraisal of portacaval H-graft diameters. Clinical and hemodynamic perspectives. *Ann Surg* 1986;204(4):356–363.

24. Sarfeh IJ, Rypins EB. The emergency portacaval H graft in alcoholic cirrhotic patients: influence of shunt diameter on clinical outcome. *Am J Surg* 1986;152(3):290–293.

25. Vangeli M, Patch D, Burroughs AK. Salvage tips for uncontrolled variceal bleeding. *J Hepatol* 2002;37(5):703–704.

26. Schepke M, Roth F, Fimmers R, et al. Comparison of MELD, Child-Pugh, and Emory model for the prediction of survival in patients undergoing transjugular intrahepatic portosystemic shunting. *Am J Gastroenterol* 2003;98(5):1167–1174.

27. Salerno F, Merli M, Cazzaniga M, et al. MELD score is better than Child-Pugh score in predicting 3-month survival of patients undergoing transjugular intrahepatic portosystemic shunt. *J Hepatol* 2002;36(4):494–500.

28. Rosado B, Kamath PS. Transjugular intrahepatic portosystemic shunts: an update. *Liver Transpl* 2003;9(3):207–217.

29. Kamath PS, Wiesner RH, Malinchoc M, et al. A model to predict survival in patients with end-stage liver disease. *Hepatology* 2001;33(2):464–470.

30. Angermayr B, Cejna M, Karnel F, et al. Child-Pugh versus MELD score in predicting survival in patients undergoing transjugular intrahepatic portosystemic shunt. *Gut* 2003;52(6):879–885.

31. Alessandria C, Gaia S, Marzano A, et al. Application of the model for end-stage liver disease score for transjugular intrahepatic portosystemic shunt in cirrhotic patients with refractory ascites and renal impairment. *Eur J Gastroenterol Hepatol* 2004;16(6):607–612.

32. LaBerge JM, Somberg KA, Lake JR, et al. Two-year outcome following transjugular intrahepatic portosystemic shunt for variceal bleeding: results in 90 patients. *Gastroenterology* 1995;108(4):1143–1151.

33. Rubin RA, Haskal ZJ, O'Brien CB, et al. Transjugular intrahepatic portosystemic shunting: decreased survival for patients with high APACHE II scores. *Am J Gastroenterol* 1995;90(4):556–563.

34. Rajan DK, Haskal ZJ, Clark TW. Serum bilirubin and early mortality after transjugular intrahepatic portosystemic shunts: results of a multivariate analysis. *J Vasc Interv Radiol* 2002;13(2, pt 1):155–161.

35. Brensing KA, Horsch M, Textor J, et al. Hemodynamic effects of propranolol and nitrates in cirrhotics with transjugular intrahepatic portosystemic stent-shunt. *Scand J Gastroenterol* 2002;37(9):1070–1076.

36. Aggarwal A, Ong JP, Younossi ZM, et al. Predictors of mortality and resource utilization in cirrhotic patients admitted to the medical ICU. *Chest* 2001;119(5):1489–1497.

37. LaBerge JM, Ring EJ, Gordon RL, et al. Creation of transjugular intrahepatic portosystemic shunts with the wallstent endoprosthesis: results in 100 patients. *Radiology* 1993;187(2):413–420.

38. Chalasani N, Clark WS, Martin LG, et al. Determinants of mortality in patients with advanced cirrhosis after transjugular intrahepatic portosystemic shunting. *Gastroenterology* 2000;118(1):138–144.

39. Patch D, Nikolopoulou V, McCormick A, et al. Factors related to early mortality after transjugular intrahepatic portosystemic shunt for failed endoscopic therapy in acute variceal bleeding. *J Hepatol* 1998;28(3):454–460.

40. Garcia-Pagan JC, Caca K, Bureau C, et al. Early use of TIPS in patients with cirrhosis and variceal bleeding. *N Engl J Med* 2010;362(25):2370–2379.

41. Papatheodoridis GV, Goulis J, Leandro G, et al. Transjugular intrahepatic portosystemic shunt compared with endoscopic treatment for prevention of variceal rebleeding: a meta-analysis. *Hepatology* 1999;30(3):612–622.

42. Cabrera J, Maynar M, Granados R, et al. Transjugular intrahepatic portosystemic shunt versus sclerotherapy in the elective treatment of variceal hemorrhage. *Gastroenterology* 1996;110(3):832–839.

43. Sauer P, Theilmann L, Stremmel W, et al. Transjugular intrahepatic portosystemic stent shunt versus sclerotherapy plus propranolol for variceal rebleeding. *Gastroenterology* 1997;113(5):1623–1631.

44. Merli M, Salerno F, Riggio O, et al. Transjugular intrahepatic portosystemic shunt versus endoscopic sclerotherapy for the prevention of variceal bleeding in cirrhosis: a randomized multicenter trial. Gruppo Italiano Studio TIPS (G.I.S.T.). *Hepatology* 1998;27(1):48–53.

45. Cello JP, Ring EJ, Olcott EW, et al. Endoscopic sclerotherapy compared with percutaneous transjugular intrahepatic portosystemic shunt after initial sclerotherapy in patients with acute variceal hemorrhage. A randomized, controlled trial. *Ann Intern Med* 1997;126(11):858–865.

46. Sanyal AJ, Freedman AM, Luketic VA, et al. Transjugular intrahepatic portosystemic shunts compared with endoscopic sclerotherapy for the prevention of recurrent variceal hemorrhage. A randomized, controlled trial. *Ann Intern Med* 1997;126(11):849–857.

47. Garcia-Villarreal L, Martinez-Lagares F, Sierra A, et al. Transjugular intrahepatic portosystemic shunt versus endoscopic sclerotherapy for the prevention of variceal rebleeding after recent variceal hemorrhage. *Hepatology* 1999;29(1):27–32.

48. Pomier-Layrargues G, Villeneuve JP, Deschenes M, et al. Transjugular intrahepatic portosystemic shunt (TIPS) versus endoscopic variceal ligation in the prevention of variceal rebleeding in patients with cirrhosis: a randomised trial. *Gut* 2001;48(3):390–396.

49. Jalan R, Forrest EH, Stanley AJ, et al. A randomized trial comparing transjugular intrahepatic portosystemic stent-shunt with variceal band ligation in the prevention of rebleeding from esophageal varices. *Hepatology* 1997;26(5):1115–1122.

50. Rossle M, Deibert P, Haag K, et al. Randomised trial of transjugular-intrahepatic-portosystemic shunt versus endoscopy plus propranolol for prevention of variceal rebleeding. *Lancet* 1997;349(9058):1043–1049.

51. Sauer P, Hansmann J, Richter GM, et al. Endoscopic variceal ligation plus propranolol vs. transjugular intrahepatic portosystemic stent shunt: a long-term randomized trial. *Endoscopy* 2002;34(9):690–697.

52. Meddi P, Merli M, Lionetti R, et al. Cost analysis for the prevention of variceal rebleeding: a comparison between transjugular intrahepatic porto-systemic shunt and endoscopic sclerotherapy in a selected group of Italian cirrhotic patients. *Hepatology* 1999;29(4):1074–1077.

53. Rosemurgy AS, Serafini FM, Zweibel BR, et al. Transjugular intrahepatic portosystemic shunt vs. small-diameter prosthetic H-graft portacaval shunt: extended follow-up of an expanded randomized prospective trial. *J Gastrointest Surg* 2000;4(6):589–597.

54. Rosemurgy AS 2nd, Goode SE, Camps M. The effect of small-diameter H-graft portacaval shunts on portal blood flow. *Am J Surg* 1996;171(1):154–156; discussion 6–7.

55. Escorsell A, Banares R, Garcia-Pagan JC, et al. TIPS versus drug therapy in preventing variceal rebleeding in advanced cirrhosis: a randomized controlled trial. *Hepatology* 2002;35(2):385–392.

56. Chau TN, Patch D, Chan YW, et al. "Salvage" transjugular intrahepatic portosystemic shunts: gastric fundal compared with esophageal variceal bleeding. *Gastroenterology* 1998;114(5):981–987.

57. Barange K, Peron JM, Imani K, et al. Transjugular intrahepatic portosystemic shunt in the treatment of refractory bleeding from ruptured gastric varices. *Hepatology* 1999;30(5):1139–1143.

58. Rees CJ, Nylander DL, Thompson NP, et al. Do gastric and oesophageal varices bleed at different portal pressures and is TIPS an effective treatment? *Liver* 2000;20(3):253–256.

59. Tripathi D, Therapondos G, Jackson E, et al. The role of the transjugular intrahepatic portosystemic stent shunt (TIPSS) in the management of bleeding gastric varices: clinical and haemodynamic correlations. *Gut* 2002;51(2):270–274.

60. Chikamori F, Kuniyoshi N, Shibuya S, et al. Eight years of experience with transjugular retrograde obliteration for gastric varices with gastrorenal shunts. *Surgery* 2001;129(4):414–420.

61. Takaji R, Kiyosue H, Matsumoto S, et al. Partial thrombosis of gastric varices after balloon-occluded retrograde transvenous obliteration: CT findings and endoscopic correlation. *AJR Am J Roentgenol* 2011;196(3):686–691.

62. Kiyosue H, Tanoue S, Kondo Y, et al. Balloon-occluded retrograde transvenous obliteration of complex gastric varices assisted by temporary balloon occlusion of the splenic artery. *J Vasc Interv Radiol* 2011;22(7):1045–1048.

63. Kasuga A, Mizumoto H, Matsutani S, et al. Portal hemodynamics and clinical outcomes of patients with gastric varices after balloon-occluded retrograde transvenous obliteration. *J Hepatobiliary Pancreat Sci* 2010;17(6):898–903.

64. Kiyosue H, Matsumoto S, Onishi R, et al. Balloon-occluded retrograde transvenous obliteration (B-RTO) for gastric varices: therapeutic results and problems [in Japanese]. *Nippon Igaku Hoshasen Gakkai Zasshi* 1999;59(1):12–19.

65. Choi YH, Yoon CJ, Park JH, et al. Balloon-occluded retrograde transvenous obliteration for gastric variceal bleeding: its feasibility compared with transjugular intrahepatic portosystemic shunt. *Korean J Radiol* 2003;4(2):109–116.

66. Ibukuro K, Mori K, Tsukiyama T, et al. Balloon-occluded retrograde transvenous obliteration of gastric varix draining via the left inferior phrenic vein into the left hepatic vein. *Cardiovasc Intervent Radiol* 1999;22(5):415–417.

67. Kim ES, Park SY, Kwon KT, et al. The clinical usefulness of balloon occluded retrograde transvenous obliteration in gastric variceal bleeding [in Korean]. *Taehan Kan Hakhoe Chi* 2003;9(4):315–323.

68. Tanoue S, Kiyosue H, Matsumoto S, et al. Development of a new coaxial balloon catheter system for balloon-occluded retrograde transvenous obliteration (B-RTO). *Cardiovasc Intervent Radiol* 2006;29(6):991–996.

69. Ibukuro K, Sugihara T, Tanaka R, et al. Balloon-occluded retrograde transvenous obliteration (BRTO) for a direct shunt between the inferior mesenteric vein and the inferior vena cava in a patient with hepatic encephalopathy. *J Vasc Interv Radiol* 2007;18(1, pt 1):121–125.

70. Takao H, Ohtomo K. Balloon-occluded retrograde transvenous obliteration of gastric varices using three-dimensional rotational angiography. *Br J Radiol* 2009;82(975):e55–e57.

71. Tanaka R, Ibukuro K, Abe S, et al. Treatment of hepatic encephalopathy due to inferior mesenteric vein/inferior vena cava and gonadal vein shunt using dual balloon-occluded retrograde transvenous obliteration. *Cardiovasc Intervent Radiol* 2009;32(2):390–393.

72. Tanihata H, Minamiguchi H, Sato M, et al. Changes in portal systemic pressure gradient after balloon-occluded retrograde transvenous obliteration of gastric varices and aggravation of esophageal varices. *Cardiovasc Intervent Radiol* 2009;32(6):1209–1216.

73. Araki T, Hori M, Motosugi U, et al. Can balloon-occluded retrograde transvenous obliteration be performed for gastric varices without gastrorenal shunts? *J Vasc Interv Radiol* 2010;21(5):663–670.

74. Hashimoto N, Akahoshi T, Yoshida D, et al. The efficacy of balloon-occluded retrograde transvenous obliteration on small intestinal variceal bleeding. *Surgery* 2010;148(1):145–150.

75. Janne d'Othee B, Walker TG, Marota JJ, et al. Splenic venous congestion after balloon-occluded retrograde transvenous obliteration of gastric varices. *Cardiovasc Intervent Radiol* 2012;35(2):434-438.

76. Sabri SS, Swee W, Turba UC, et al. Bleeding gastric varices obliteration with balloon-occluded retrograde transvenous obliteration using sodium tetradecyl sulfate foam. *J Vasc Interv Radiol* 2011;22(3):309–316; quiz 16.

77. Teo TK, Sabri SS, Turba UC, et al. Obliteration of bleeding peristomal varices with balloon-occluded retrograde transvenous obliteration using sodium tetradecyl sulfate foam. *J Vasc Interv Radiol* 2011;22(7):1049–1051.

78. Yamagami T, Tanaka O, Yoshimatsu R, et al. Successful balloon-occluded retrograde transvenous obliteration for large gastric varices in combination with temporary occlusion of the splenic artery. *J Vasc Interv Radiol* 2011;22(9):1343–1345.

79. Uehara H, Akahoshi T, Tomikawa M, et al. Prediction of improved liver function after balloon-occluded retrograde transvenous obliteration: relation to hepatic vein pressure gradient. *J Gastroenterol Hepatol* 2012;27(1):137–141.

80. Baik GH, Kim DJ, Lee HG, et al. Therapeutic efficacy of balloon-occluded retrograde transvenous obliteration in the treatment of gastric varices in cirrhotic patients with gastrorenal shunt [in Korean]. *Korean J Gastroenterol* 2004;43(3):196–203.

81. Bernstein D, Yrizarry J, Reddy KR, et al. Transjugular intrahepatic portosystemic shunt in the treatment of intermittently bleeding stomal varices. *Am J Gastroenterol* 1996;91(10):2237–2238.

82. Johnson PA, Laurin J. Transjugular portosystemic shunt for treatment of bleeding stomal varices. *Dig Dis Sci* 1997;42(2):440–442.

83. Kishimoto K, Hara A, Arita T, et al. Stomal varices: treatment by percutaneous transhepatic coil embolization. *Cardiovasc Intervent Radiol* 1999;22(6):523–525.

84. Labori KJ, Carlsen E. Treatment of bleeding peristomal varices. *Eur J Surg* 2002;168(11):654–656.

85. Lashley DB, Saxon RR, Fuchs EF, et al. Bleeding ileal conduit stomal varices: diagnosis and management using transjugular transhepatic angiography and embolization. *Urology* 1997;50(4):612–614.

86. Lagier E, Rousseau H, Maquin P, et al. Treatment of bleeding stomal varices using transjugular intrahepatic portosystemic shunt. *J Pediatr Gastroenterol Nutr* 1994;18(4):501–503.

87. Shibata D, Brophy DP, Gordon FD, et al. Transjugular intrahepatic portosystemic shunt for treatment of bleeding ectopic varices with portal hypertension. *Dis Colon Rectum* 1999;42(12):1581–1585.

88. Toumeh KK, Girardot JD, Choo IW, et al. Percutaneous transhepatic embolization as treatment for bleeding ileostomy varices. *Cardiovasc Intervent Radiol* 1995;18(3):179–182.

89. Weinberg GD, Matalon TA, Brunner MC, et al. Bleeding stomal varices: treatment with a transjugular intrahepatic portosystemic shunt in two pediatric patients. *J Vasc Interv Radiol* 1995;6(2):233–236.

90. Wong RC, Berg CL. Portal hypertensive stomapathy: a newly described entity and its successful treatment by placement of a transjugular intrahepatic portosystemic shunt. *Am J Gastroenterol* 1997;92(6):1056–1057.

91. Haskal ZJ, Scott M, Rubin RA, et al. Intestinal varices: treatment with the transjugular intrahepatic portosystemic shunt. *Radiology* 1994;191(1):183–187.

92. Demirel H, Pieterman H, Lameris JS, et al. Transjugular embolization of the inferior mesenteric vein for bleeding anorectal varices after unsuccessful transjugular intrahepatic portosystemic shunt. *Am J Gastroenterol* 1997;92(7):1226–1227.

93. Fantin AC, Zala G, Risti B, et al. Bleeding anorectal varices: successful treatment with transjugular intrahepatic portosystemic shunting (TIPS). *Gut* 1996;38(6):932–935.

94. Godil A, McCracken JD. Rectal variceal bleeding treated by transjugular intrahepatic portosystemic shunt. Potentials and pitfalls. *J Clin Gastroenterol* 1997;25(2):460–462.

95. Katz JA, Rubin RA, Cope C, et al. Recurrent bleeding from anorectal varices: successful treatment with a transjugular intrahepatic portosystemic shunt. *Am J Gastroenterol* 1993;88(7):1104–1107.

96. Ory G, Spahr L, Megevand JM, et al. The long-term efficacy of the intrahepatic portosystemic shunt (TIPS) for the treatment of bleeding anorectal varices in cirrhosis. A case report and review of the literature. *Digestion* 2001;64(4):261–264.

97. Akasaka T, Shibata T, Isoda H, et al. Septic complication after balloon-occluded retrograde transvenous obliteration of duodenal variceal bleeding. *Cardiovasc Intervent Radiol* 2010;33(6):1257–1261.

98. Minami S, Okada K, Matsuo M, et al. Treatment of bleeding stomal varices by balloon-occluded retrograde transvenous obliteration. *J Gastroenterol* 2007;42(1):91–95.

99. Burak KW, Lee SS, Beck PL. Portal hypertensive gastropathy and gastric antral vascular ectasia (GAVE) syndrome. *Gut* 2001;49(6):866–872.

100. Dagher L, Burroughs A. Variceal bleeding and portal hypertensive gastropathy. *Eur J Gastroenterol Hepatol* 2001;13(1):81–88.

101. Garcia N, Sanyal AJ. Portal hypertensive gastropathy and gastric antral vascular ectasia. *Curr Treat Options Gastroenterol* 2001;4(2):163–171.

102. Mezawa S, Homma H, Ohta H, et al. Effect of transjugular intrahepatic portosystemic shunt formation on portal hypertensive gastropathy and gastric circulation. *Am J Gastroenterol* 2001;96(4):1155–1159.

103. Panes J, Pique JM. Therapeutic options for bleeding portal hypertensive gastropathy. *J Gastroenterol Hepatol* 1998;13(10):977–979.

104. Sarin SK, Agarwal SR. Gastric varices and portal hypertensive gastropathy. *Clin Liver Dis* 2001;5(3):727–767, x.

105. Kamath PS, Lacerda M, Ahlquist DA, et al. Gastric mucosal responses to intrahepatic portosystemic shunting in patients with cirrhosis. *Gastroenterology* 2000;118(5):905–911.

106. Urata J, Yamashita Y, Tsuchigame T, et al. The effects of transjugular intrahepatic portosystemic shunt on portal hypertensive gastropathy. *J Gastroenterol Hepatol* 1998;13(10):1061–1067.

107. Runyon BA, Committee APG. Management of adult patients with ascites due to cirrhosis: an update. *Hepatology* 2009;49(6):2087–2107.

108. Runyon BA; Practice Guidelines Committee AAftSoLD. Management of adult patients with ascites due to cirrhosis. *Hepatology* 2004;39(3):841–856.

109. Gines P, Cardenas A, Arroyo V, et al. Management of cirrhosis and ascites. *N Engl J Med* 2004;350(16):1646–1654.

110. Gines P, Guevara M, Perez-Villa F. Management of hepatorenal syndrome: another piece of the puzzle. *Hepatology* 2004;40(1):16–18.

111. Lebrec D, Giuily N, Hadengue A, et al. Transjugular intrahepatic portosystemic shunts: comparison with paracentesis in patients with cirrhosis and refractory ascites: a randomized trial. French Group of Clinicians and a Group of Biologists. *J Hepatol* 1996;25(2):135–144.

112. Rossle M, Ochs A, Gulberg V, et al. A comparison of paracentesis and transjugular intrahepatic portosystemic shunting in patients with ascites. *N Engl J Med* 2000;342(23):1701–1707.

113. Sanyal AJ, Genning C, Reddy KR, et al. The North American Study for the treatment of refractory ascites. *Gastroenterology* 2003;124(3):634–641.

114. Gines P, Uriz J, Calahorra B, et al. Transjugular intrahepatic portosystemic shunting versus paracentesis plus albumin for refractory ascites in cirrhosis. *Gastroenterology* 2002;123(6):1839–1847.

115. Salerno F, Merli M, Riggio O, et al. Randomized controlled study of TIPS versus paracentesis plus albumin in cirrhosis with severe ascites. *Hepatology* 2004;40(3):629–635.

116. Salerno F, Camma C, Enea M, et al. Transjugular intrahepatic portosystemic shunt for refractory ascites: a meta-analysis of individual patient data. *Gastroenterology* 2007;133(3):825–834.

117. Rosemurgy AS, Zervos EE, Clark WC, et al. TIPS versus peritoneovenous shunt in the treatment of medically intractable ascites: a prospective randomized trial. *Ann Surg* 2004;239(6):883–889; discussion 9–91.

118. Siegerstetter V, Deibert P, Ochs A, et al. Treatment of refractory hepatic hydrothorax with transjugular intrahepatic portosystemic shunt: long-term results in 40 patients. *Eur J Gastroenterol Hepatol* 2001;13(5):529–534.

119. Gordon FD, Anastopoulos HT, Crenshaw W, et al. The successful treatment of symptomatic, refractory hepatic hydrothorax with transjugular intrahepatic portosystemic shunt. *Hepatology* 1997;25(6):1366–1369.

120. Haskal ZJ, Zuckerman J. Resolution of hepatic hydrothorax after transjugular intrahepatic portosystemic shunt (TIPS) placement. *Chest* 1994;106(4):1293–1295.

121. Lazaridis KN, Frank JW, Krowka MJ, et al. Hepatic hydrothorax: pathogenesis, diagnosis, and management. *Am J Med* 1999;107(3):262–267.

122. Spencer EB, Cohen DT, Darcy MD. Safety and efficacy of transjugular intrahepatic portosystemic shunt creation for the treatment of hepatic hydrothorax. *J Vasc Interv Radiol* 2002;13(4):385–390.

123. Strauss RM, Boyer TD. Hepatic hydrothorax. *Semin Liver Dis* 1997;17(3):227–232.

124. Degawa M, Hamasaki K, Yano K, et al. Refractory hepatic hydrothorax treated with transjugular intrahepatic portosystemic shunt. *J Gastroenterol* 1999;34(1):128–131.

125. Cardenas A, Kelleher T, Chopra S. Review article: hepatic hydrothorax. *Aliment Pharmacol Ther* 2004;20(3):271–279.

126. Gines P, Guevara M, Arroyo V, et al. Hepatorenal syndrome. *Lancet* 2003;362(9398):1819–1827.

127. Runyon BA. Treatment of patients with cirrhosis and ascites. *Semin Liver Dis* 1997;17(3):249–260.

128. Brensing KA, Textor J, Strunk H, et al. Transjugular intrahepatic portosystemic stent-shunt for hepatorenal syndrome. *Lancet* 1997;349(9053):697–698.

129. Cardenas A, Arroyo V. Hepatorenal syndrome. *Ann Hepatol* 2003;2(1):23–29.

130. Guevara M, Gines P, Bandi JC, et al. Transjugular intrahepatic portosystemic shunt in hepatorenal syndrome: effects on renal function and vasoactive systems. *Hepatology* 1998;28(2):416–422.

131. Jalan R, Forrest EH, Redhead DN, et al. Reduction in renal blood flow following acute increase in the portal pressure: evidence for the existence of a hepatorenal reflex in man? *Gut* 1997;40(5):664–670.

132. Lerut J, Goffette P, Laterre PF, et al. Sequential treatment of hepatorenal syndrome and posthepatic cirrhosis by intrahepatic portosystemic shunt (TIPSS) and liver transplantation. *Hepatogastroenterology* 1995;42(6):985–987.

133. Sturgis TM. Hepatorenal syndrome: resolution after transjugular intrahepatic portosystemic shunt. *J Clin Gastroenterol* 1995;20(3):241–243.

134. Wong F, Pantea L, Sniderman K. Midodrine, octreotide, albumin, and TIPS in selected patients with cirrhosis and type 1 hepatorenal syndrome. *Hepatology* 2004;40(1):55–64.

135. Brensing KA, Textor J, Perz J, et al. Long term outcome after transjugular intrahepatic portosystemic stent-shunt in non-transplant cirrhotics with hepatorenal syndrome: a phase II study. *Gut* 2000;47(2):288–295.

136. Bilbao JI, Pueyo JC, Longo JM, et al. Interventional therapeutic techniques in Budd-Chiari syndrome. *Cardiovasc Intervent Radiol* 1997;20(2):112–119.

137. Cura M, Haskal Z, Lopera J. Diagnostic and interventional radiology for Budd-Chiari syndrome. *Radiographics* 2009;29(3):669–681.

138. Perello A, Garcia-Pagan JC, Gilabert R, et al. TIPS is a useful long-term derivative therapy for patients with Budd-Chiari syndrome uncontrolled by medical therapy. *Hepatology* 2002;35(1):132–139.

139. Mancuso A, Fung K, Mela M, et al. TIPS for acute and chronic Budd-Chiari syndrome: a single-centre experience. *J Hepatol* 2003;38(6):751–754.

140. Ochs A, Sellinger M, Haag K, et al. Transjugular intrahepatic portosystemic stent-shunt (TIPS) in the treatment of Budd-Chiari syndrome. *J Hepatol* 1993;18(2):217–225.

141. Peltzer MY, Ring EJ, LaBerge JM, et al. Treatment of Budd-Chiari syndrome with a transjugular intrahepatic portosystemic shunt. *J Vasc Interv Radiol* 1993;4(2):263–267.

142. Rogopoulos A, Gavelli A, Sakai H, et al. Transjugular intrahepatic portosystemic shunt for Budd-Chiari syndrome after failure of surgical shunting. *Arch Surg* 1995;130(2):227–228.

143. Richard HM 3rd, Cooper JM, Ahn J, et al. Transjugular intrahepatic portosystemic shunts in the management of Budd-Chiari syndrome in the liver transplant patient with intractable ascites: anatomic considerations. *J Vasc Interv Radiol* 1998;9(1, pt 1):137–140.

144. Strunk HM, Textor J, Brensing KA, et al. Acute Budd-Chiari syndrome: treatment with transjugular intrahepatic portosystemic shunt. *Cardiovasc Intervent Radiol* 1997;20(4):311–313.

145. Nicoll A, Fitt G, Angus P, et al. Budd-Chiari syndrome: intractable ascites managed by a trans-hepatic portacaval shunt. *Australas Radiol* 1997;41(2):169–172.

146. Kuo PC, Johnson LB, Hastings G, et al. Fulminant hepatic failure from the Budd-Chiari syndrome. A bridge to transplantation with transjugular intrahepatic portosystemic shunt. *Transplantation* 1996;62(2):294–296.

147. Hastings GS, O'Connor DK, Pais SO. Transjugular intrahepatic portosystemic shunt placement as a bridge to liver transplantation in fulminant Budd-Chiari syndrome. *J Vasc Interv Radiol* 1996;7(4):616.

148. Uhl MD, Roth DB, Riely CA. Transjugular intrahepatic portosystemic shunt (TIPS) for Budd-Chiari syndrome. *Dig Dis Sci* 1996;41(7):1494–1499.

149. Blum U, Rossle M, Haag K, et al. Budd-Chiari syndrome: technical, hemodynamic, and clinical results of treatment with transjugular intrahepatic portosystemic shunt. *Radiology* 1995;197(3):805–811.

150. Ryu RK, Durham JD, Krysl J, et al. Role of TIPS as a bridge to hepatic transplantation in Budd-Chiari syndrome. *J Vasc Interv Radiol* 1999;10(6):799–805.

151. Avenhaus W, Ullerich H, Menzel J, et al. Budd-Chiari syndrome in a patient with factor V Leiden—successful treatment by TIPSS placement followed by liver transplantation. *Z Gastroenterol* 1999;37(4):277–281.

152. Sanyal AJ. Budd-Chiari syndrome: is TIPS tops? *Am J Gastroenterol* 1999;94(3):559–561.

153. Brunerova L, Bartakova H, Jankovska M, et al. The Budd-Chiari syndrome in a patient with primary thrombocythemia treated with interferon alfa and transjugular portosystemic shunt [in Czech]. *Cas Lek Cesk* 2004; 143(3):198–201.

154. Rossle M, Olschewski M, Siegerstetter V, et al. The Budd-Chiari syndrome: outcome after treatment with the transjugular intrahepatic portosystemic shunt. *Surgery* 2004;135(4):394–403.

155. Das HS, Punamiya S, Kalokhe S, et al. Budd-Chiari syndrome treated with transjugular intrahepatic portosystemic shunt. *J Assoc Physicians India* 2003;51:309–310.

156. Blokzijl H, de Knegt RJ. Long-term effect of treatment of acute Budd-Chiari syndrome with a transjugular intrahepatic portosytemic shunt. *Hepatology* 2002;35(6):1551–1552.

157. Garcia-Pagan JC, Heydtmann M, Raffa S, et al. TIPS for Budd-Chiari syndrome: long-term results and prognostics factors in 124 patients. *Gastroenterology* 2008;135(3):808–815.

158. Cejna M, Peck-Radosavljevic M, Schoder M, et al. Repeat interventions for maintenance of transjugular intrahepatic portosystemic shunt function in patients with Budd-Chiari syndrome. *J Vasc Interv Radiol* 2002; 13(2, pt 1):193–199.

159. Saxon RS, Ross PL, Mendel-Hartvig J, et al. Transjugular intrahepatic portosystemic shunt patency and the importance of stenosis location in the development of recurrent symptoms. *Radiology* 1998;207(3):683–693.

160. Haskal ZJ, Pentecost MJ, Soulen MC, et al. Transjugular intrahepatic portosystemic shunt stenosis and revision: early and midterm results. *AJR Am J Roentgenol* 1994;163(2):439–444.

161. Bodner G, Peer S, Fries D, et al. Color and pulsed Doppler ultrasound findings in normally functioning transjugular intrahepatic portosystemic shunts. *Eur J Ultrasound* 2000;12(2):131–136.

162. Wachsberg RH. Doppler ultrasound evaluation of transjugular intrahepatic portosystemic shunt function: pitfalls and artifacts. *Ultrasound Q* 2003;19(3):139–148.

163. Ferguson JM, Jalan R, Redhead DN, et al. The role of duplex and colour Doppler ultrasound in the follow-up evaluation of transjugular intrahepatic portosystemic stent shunt (TIPSS). *Br J Radiol* 1995;68(810):587–589.

164. Longo JM, Bilbao JI, Rousseau HP, et al. Color Doppler-US guidance in transjugular placement of intrahepatic portosystemic shunts. *Radiology* 1992;184(1):281–284.

165. Chong WK, Malisch TA, Mazer MJ, et al. Transjugular intrahepatic portosystemic shunt: US assessment with maximum flow velocity. *Radiology* 1993;189(3):789–793.

166. Ferral H, Foshager MC, Bjarnason H, et al. Early sonographic evaluation of the transjugular intrahepatic portosystemic shunt (TIPS). *Cardiovasc Intervent Radiol* 1993;16(5):275–279.

167. Foshager MC, Ferral H, Finlay DE, et al. Color Doppler sonography of transjugular intrahepatic portosystemic shunts (TIPS). *AJR Am J Roentgenol* 1994;163(1):105–111.

168. Ralls PW, Egan RT, Katz MD, et al. Color Doppler sonography to evaluate transjugular intrahepatic portacaval stent shunt. *J Ultrasound Med* 1993;12(8):487–489.

169. Surratt RS, Middleton WD, Darcy MD, et al. Morphologic and hemodynamic findings at sonography before and after creation of a transjugular intrahepatic portosystemic shunt. *AJR Am J Roentgenol* 1993;160(3):627–630.

170. Talavera A, Artaza T, Gomez R, et al. Usefulness of Doppler sonography in monitoring transjugular intrahepatic portosystemic shunts. *J Clin Ultrasound* 1994;22(2):137–140.

171. Lind CD, Malisch TW, Chong WK, et al. Incidence of shunt occlusion or stenosis following transjugular intrahepatic portosystemic shunt placement. *Gastroenterology* 1994;106(5):1277–1283.

172. Foshager MC, Ferral H, Nazarian GK, et al. Duplex sonography after transjugular intrahepatic portosystemic shunts (TIPS): normal hemodynamic findings and efficacy in predicting shunt patency and stenosis. *AJR Am J Roentgenol* 1995;165(1):1–7.

173. Dodd GD 3rd, Zajko AB, Orons PD, et al. Detection of transjugular intrahepatic portosystemic shunt dysfunction: value of duplex Doppler sonography. *AJR Am J Roentgenol* 1995;164(5):1119–1124.

174. Haskal ZJ, Carroll JW, Jacobs JE, et al. Sonography of transjugular intrahepatic portosystemic shunts: detection of elevated portosystemic gradients and loss of shunt function. *J Vasc Interv Radiol* 1997;8(4):549–556.

175. Kanterman RY, Darcy MD, Middleton WD, et al. Doppler sonography findings associated with transjugular intrahepatic portosystemic shunt malfunction. *AJR Am J Roentgenol* 1997;168(2):467–472.

176. Kimura M, Sato M, Kawai N, et al. Efficacy of Doppler ultrasonography for assessment of transjugular intrahepatic portosystemic shunt patency. *Cardiovasc Intervent Radiol* 1996;19(6):397–400.

177. Feldstein VA, Patel MD. Doppler ultrasonography of transjugular intrahepatic portosystemic shunts. *West J Med* 1996;165(1–2):56–57.

178. Chong WK, Mazer MJ. Doppler velocity criteria for transjugular intrahepatic portosystemic shunt (TIPS) stenosis. *AJR Am J Roentgenol* 1996;166(1):215–216.

179. Murphy TP, Beecham RP, Kim HM, et al. Long-term follow-up after TIPS: use of Doppler velocity criteria for detecting elevation of the portosystemic gradient. *J Vasc Interv Radiol* 1998;9(2):275–281.

180. Menzel J. Duplex ultrasonography of TIPS: how useful is it? *Gastroenterology* 1999;116(5):1272–1273.

181. Zizka J, Elias P, Krajina A, et al. Value of Doppler sonography in revealing transjugular intrahepatic portosystemic shunt malfunction: a 5-year experience in 216 patients. *AJR Am J Roentgenol* 2000;175(1):141–148.

182. Benito A, Bilbao J, Hernandez T, et al. Doppler ultrasound for TIPS: does it work? *Abdom Imaging* 2004;29(1):45–52.

183. Feldstein VA, Patel MD, LaBerge JM. Transjugular intrahepatic portosystemic shunts: accuracy of Doppler US in determination of patency and detection of stenoses. *Radiology* 1996;201(1):141–147.

184. Eloubeidi M, Trotter JF, Rockey DC. Ultrasonography or venography for the diagnosis of TIPS malfunction? *Gastroenterology* 1998;115(6):1604; author reply 5–6.

185. LaBerge J, Feldstein VA. Ultrasound surveillance of tips—why bother? *Hepatology* 1998;28(5):1433–1434.

186. Owens CA, Bartolone C, Warner DL, et al. The inaccuracy of duplex ultrasonography in predicting patency of transjugular intrahepatic portosystemic shunts. *Gastroenterology* 1998;114(5):975–980.

187. Sanyal AJ, Contos MJ, Yager D, et al. Development of pseudointima and stenosis after transjugular intrahepatic portasystemic shunts: characterization of cell phenotype and function. *Hepatology* 1998;28(1):22–32.

188. LaBerge JM, Ferrell LD, Ring EJ, et al. Histopathologic study of stenotic and occluded transjugular intrahepatic portosystemic shunts. *J Vasc Interv Radiol* 1993;4(6):779–786.

189. LaBerge JM, Ferrell LD, Ring EJ, et al. Histopathologic study of transjugular intrahepatic portosystemic shunts. *J Vasc Interv Radiol* 1991;2(4):549–556.

190. Saxon RR, Mendel-Hartvig J, Corless CL, et al. Bile duct injury as a major cause of stenosis and occlusion in transjugular intrahepatic portosystemic shunts: comparative histopathologic analysis in humans and swine. *J Vasc Interv Radiol* 1996;7(4):487–497.

191. Terayama N, Matsui O, Kadoya M, et al. Transjugular intrahepatic portosystemic shunt: histologic and immunohistochemical study of autopsy cases. *Cardiovasc Intervent Radiol* 1997;20(6):457–461.

192. Ducoin H, El-Khoury J, Rousseau H, et al. Histopathologic analysis of transjugular intrahepatic portosystemic shunts. *Hepatology* 1997; 25(5):1064–1069.

193. Teng GJ, Bettmann MA, Hoopes PJ, et al. Transjugular intrahepatic portosystemic shunt in a porcine model: histologic characteristics at the early stage. *Acad Radiol* 1998;5(8):547–555.

194. Sanyal AJ, Mirshahi F. Endothelial cells lining transjugular intrahepatic portasystemic shunts originate in hepatic sinusoids: implications for pseudointimal hyperplasia. *Hepatology* 1999;29(3):710–718.

195. Cohen GS, Young HY, Ball DS. Stent-graft as treatment for TIPS-biliary fistula. *J Vasc Interv Radiol* 1996;7(5):665–668.

196. Stout LC, Lyon RE, Murray NG, et al. Pseudointimal biliary epithelial proliferation and Zahn's infarct associated with a 6 1/2-month-old transjugular intrahepatic portosystemic shunt. *Am J Gastroenterol* 1995;90(1):126–130.

197. Mallery S, Freeman ML, Peine CJ, et al. Biliary-shunt fistula following transjugular intrahepatic portosystemic shunt placement. *Gastroenterology* 1996;111(5):1353–1357.

198. Jalan R, Harrison DJ, Redhead DN, et al. Transjugular intrahepatic portosystemic stent-shunt (TIPSS) occlusion and the role of biliary venous fistulae. *J Hepatol* 1996;24(2):169–176.

199. Clark TW, Agarwal R, Haskal ZJ, et al. The effect of initial shunt outflow position on patency of transjugular intrahepatic portosystemic shunts. *J Vasc Interv Radiol* 2004;15(2, pt 1):147–152.

200. Sauer P, Theilmann L, Herrmann S, et al. Phenprocoumon for prevention of shunt occlusion after transjugular intrahepatic portosystemic stent shunt: a randomized trial. *Hepatology* 1996;24(6):1433–1436.

201. Siegerstetter V, Huber M, Ochs A, et al. Platelet aggregation and platelet-derived growth factor inhibition for prevention of insufficiency of the transjugular intrahepatic portosystemic shunt: a randomized study comparing trapidil plus ticlopidine with heparin treatment. *Hepatology* 1999;29(1):33–38.

202. Nishimine K, Saxon RR, Kichikawa K, et al. Improved transjugular intrahepatic portosystemic shunt patency with PTFE-covered stent-grafts: experimental results in swine. *Radiology* 1995;196(2):341–347.

203. Kichikawa K, Saxon RR, Nishimine K, et al. Experimental TIPS with spiral Z-stents in swine with and without induced portal hypertension. *Cardiovasc Intervent Radiol* 1997;20(3):197–203.

204. Pavcnik D, Saxon RR, Kubota Y, et al. Attempted induction of chronic portal venous hypertension with polyvinyl alcohol particles in swine. *J Vasc Interv Radiol* 1997;8(1, pt 1):123–128.

205. Haskal ZJ, Davis A, McAllister A, et al. PTFE-encapsulated endovascular stent-graft for transjugular intrahepatic portosystemic shunts: experimental evaluation. *Radiology* 1997;205(3):682–688.

206. Saxon RR, Timmermans HA, Uchida BT, et al. Stent-grafts for revision of TIPS stenoses and occlusions: a clinical pilot study. *J Vasc Interv Radiol* 1997;8(4):539–548.

207. Ferral H, Alcantara-Peraza A, Kimura Y, et al. Creation of transjugular intrahepatic portosystemic shunts with use of the Cragg Endopro System I. *J Vasc Interv Radiol* 1998;9(2):283–287.

208. Haskal ZJ, Weintraub JL, Susman J. Recurrent TIPS thrombosis after polyethylene stent-graft use and salvage with polytetrafluoroethylene stent-grafts. *J Vasc Interv Radiol* 2002;13(12):1255–1259.

209. Andrews RT, Saxon RR, Bloch RD, et al. Stent-grafts for de novo TIPS: technique and early results. *J Vasc Interv Radiol* 1999;10(10):1371–1378.

210. DiSalle RS, Dolmatch BL. Treatment of TIPS stenosis with ePTFE graft-covered stents. *Cardiovasc Intervent Radiol* 1998;21(2):172–175.

211. Haskal ZJ. Improved patency of transjugular intrahepatic portosystemic shunts in humans: creation and revision with PTFE stent-grafts. *Radiology* 1999;213(3):759–766.

212. Sze DY, Vestring T, Liddell RP, et al. Recurrent TIPS failure associated with biliary fistulae: treatment with PTFE-covered stents. *Cardiovasc Intervent Radiol* 1999;22(4):298–304.

213. LaBerge JM, Kerlan RK. Liver infarction following TIPS with a PTFE-covered stent: is the covering the cause? *Hepatology* 2003;38(3):778–779; author reply 9.

214. Cejna M, Peck-Radosavljevic M, Thurnher SA, et al. Creation of transjugular intrahepatic portosystemic shunts with stent-grafts: initial experiences with a polytetrafluoroethylene-covered nitinol endoprosthesis. *Radiology* 2001;221(2):437–446.

215. Cejna M, Peck-Radosavljevic M, Thurnher S, et al. ePTFE-covered stent-grafts for revision of obstructed transjugular intrahepatic portosystemic shunt. *Cardiovasc Intervent Radiol* 2002;25(5):365–372.

216. Hausegger KA, Portugaller H, Macri NP, et al. Covered stents in transjugular portosystemic shunt: healing response to non-porous ePTFE covered stent grafts with and without intraluminal irradiation. *Eur Radiol* 2003; 13(7):1549–1558.

217. Angeloni S, Merli M, Salvatori FM, et al. Polytetrafluoroethylene-covered stent grafts for TIPS procedure: 1-year patency and clinical results. *Am J Gastroenterol* 2004;99(2):280–285.

218. Hausegger KA, Karnel F, Georgieva B, et al. Transjugular intrahepatic portosystemic shunt creation with the Viatorr expanded polytetrafluoroethylene-covered stent-graft. *J Vasc Interv Radiol* 2004;15(3):239–248.

219. Maleux G, Nevens F, Wilmer A, et al. Early and long-term clinical and radiological follow-up results of expanded-polytetrafluoroethylene-covered stent-grafts for transjugular intrahepatic portosystemic shunt procedures. *Eur Radiol* 2004;14(10):1842–1850.

220. Maleux G, Pirenne J, Vaninbroukx J, et al. Are TIPS stent-grafts a contraindication for future liver transplantation? *Cardiovasc Intervent Radiol* 2004;27(2):140–142.

221. Rossi P, Salvatori FM, Fanelli F, et al. Polytetrafluoroethylene-covered nitinol stent-graft for transjugular intrahepatic portosystemic shunt creation: 3-year experience. *Radiology* 2004;231(3):820–830.

222. Riggio O, Ridola L, Angeloni S, et al. Clinical efficacy of transjugular intrahepatic portosystemic shunt created with covered stents with different diameters: results of a randomized controlled trial. *J Hepatol* 2010; 53(2):267–272.

223. Bureau C, Garcia-Pagan JC, Otal P, et al. Improved clinical outcome using polytetrafluoroethylene-coated stents for TIPS: results of a randomized study. *Gastroenterology* 2004;126(2):469–475.

224. Hernandez-Guerra M, Turnes J, Rubinstein P, et al. PTFE-covered stents improve TIPS patency in Budd-Chiari syndrome. *Hepatology* 2004;40(5):1197–1202.

225. Ockenga J, Kroencke TJ, Schuetz T, et al. Covered transjugular intrahepatic portosystemic stents maintain lower portal pressure and require fewer reinterventions than uncovered stents. *Scand J Gastroenterol* 2004;39(10): 994–999.

226. Barrio J, Ripoll C, Banares R, et al. Comparison of transjugular intrahepatic portosystemic shunt dysfunction in PTFE-covered stent-grafts versus bare stents. *Eur J Radiol* 2005;55(1):120–124.

227. Echenagusia M, Rodriguez-Rosales G, Simo G, et al. Expanded PTFE-covered stent-grafts in the treatment of transjugular intrahepatic portosystemic shunt (TIPS) stenoses and occlusions. *Abdom Imaging* 2005;30(6):750–754.

228. Vignali C, Bargellini I, Grosso M, et al. TIPS with expanded polytetrafluoroethylene-covered stent: results of an Italian multicenter study. *AJR Am J Roentgenol* 2005;185(2):472–480.

229. Bureau C. Covered stents for TIPS: are all problems solved? *Eur J Gastroenterol Hepatol* 2006;18(6):581–583.

230. Tripathi D, Ferguson J, Barkell H, et al. Improved clinical outcome with transjugular intrahepatic portosystemic stent-shunt utilizing polytetrafluoroethylene-covered stents. *Eur J Gastroenterol Hepatol* 2006;18(3):225–232.

231. Fanelli F, Bezzi M, Bruni A, et al. Multidetector-row computed tomography in the evaluation of transjugular intrahepatic portosystemic shunt performed with expanded-polytetrafluoroethylene-covered stent-graft. *Cardiovasc Intervent Radiol* 2011;34(1):100–105.

Transjugular Liver Biopsy

STEVEN J. KROHMER and NIK BHAGAT

HISTORY

Soft-tissue biopsy is the gold standard for evaluating both histology and pathology in the liver.[1,2] Additionally, liver biopsy provides a tool for assessing prognosis, especially in patients with acute liver failure (ALF)[3] and chronic viral hepatitis.[4] Transjugular liver biopsy (TJLB) is an established alternative for obtaining hepatic tissue when there are contraindications to percutaneous liver biopsy (PLB) for diffuse liver disease.[5] Dr. Charles Dotter,[6] in 1964, was the first to report on transvenous liver biopsy performed through the jugular vein in several dogs. Later, Rosch et al.[7] discussed utilizing the transjugular approach to liver biopsy in people, following the previously described use of the same approach for cholangiography.[8] Rosch et al.[7] used the transjugular approach to biopsy 44 patients, yielding adequate tissue for evaluation in 39 of the patients, giving an 89% success rate. Transvenous cholangiography was found to lead more frequently to infectious complications, and, therefore, the percutaneous transhepatic approach is preferred in this and also for portal venography. In contradistinction, however, infectious complications are extremely rare in TJLB.[9]

Since its inception, TJLB was considered an inferior biopsy technique compared to PLB because of concern that the prior provided smaller and more fragmented samples.[4,10,11] Kalambokis et al.[12] reviewed 64 series reporting on 7,649 TJLBs and evaluated the safety of the technique and quality of the specimen obtained. They concluded that TJLB was as safe as PLB and provided specimens that were qualitatively comparable. The quality of the specimen obtained by TJLB improves with the use of a Tru-cut needle compared to an aspiration-type biopsy needle (such as the Menghini needle), likely related to less sample fragmentation with the Tru-cut needle. Further, the quality of the specimen, as characterized by the number of complete portal tracts (CPTs) obtained with TJLB, was comparable with the number obtained by PLB when a mean number of 2.3 passes were obtained.[12]

The development of TJLB was the culmination of years spent in the lab, designing and constructing catheters that could be negotiated from the internal jugular vein (IJV) into a hepatic vein and successfully extract adequate tissue samples that could be used for pathologic evaluation. Routine use of the technique initially involved utilizing a modified Ross transseptal needle.[13] A needle with a reverse bevel was later introduced to overcome the tendency of the needle to perforate the catheter walls as it curves into the vein.[14,15] Further advancement in TJLB needle sets included a variation of the Tru-cut needle (Baxter Healthcare) and the Quick-Core needle system (Cook, Bloomington, IN).

These sets use a semiautomated Tru-cut system for obtaining tissue specimens. Since the initial introduction of the technique, numerous advancements and refinements have been made to provide greater ease and reliability of adequate tissue sampling. This chapter discusses the current state of the technique of TJLB, including indications, contraindications, complications, and use in special circumstances, such as in liver transplant recipients.

QUALITY

Because liver biopsy is an essential tool in working up patients with both acute and chronic liver disease, it is important that the obtained specimens for analysis are of sufficient quality for evaluation. The sample should be of sufficient size, minimizing fragmentation and containing as many CPTs as possible. As defined by Crawford et al.,[16] a CPT needs to be visible in its full circumference or when at least three-quarters of its circumference is visible and contain three luminal structures, namely, portal vein, hepatic artery, and bile duct. Number has been considered the most important criterion for assessing the adequacy of the liver biopsy sample.[12] When evaluating a liver with cirrhosis, advanced fibrosis, and/or massive necrosis, a given mean length of sample may have fewer portal tracts or none compared to a noncirrhotic liver and is therefore an unreliable measure of quality in this situation.[17] In such cases, one must then rely on sample length for evaluation of sample quality. A liver specimen greater than or equal to 15 mm is considered sufficient in diffuse liver disease for diagnostic purposes.[10,18]

In a noncirrhotic patient, an adequate specimen for optimal histologic analysis should consist of a length greater or equal to 15 mm and containing six to eight CPTs.[10,18] Additionally, in assessing chronic liver disease, such as fibrosis from chronic hepatitis and nonalcoholic fatty liver disease, the obtained specimen should have a length of 20 to 25 mm and/or greater than 11 CPTs for reliability in grading and staging and to reduce sampling errors.[19,20] Historically, there has been concern that TJLB provided specimens that were inadequate for diagnostic and prognostic analysis. In a study by Cholongitas et al.,[21] a total of 326 consecutive TJLB specimens obtained using either a 19-gauge Cook or a Kimal Tru-cut needle were compared with 40 consecutive PLB specimens collected with a 15-gauge Menghini needle. No statistically significant difference in mean specimen length or CPTs procured was found, given three passes obtained with the TJLB. Although earlier in the history of TJLB there was concern that the samples obtained were considered inferior to those collected by PLB secondary to smaller size and fragmentation,[1] this concern has largely been alleviated with the introduction of the Tru-cut needles.

Additionally, smaller needle diameter correlates with a larger mean length of the specimen obtained and lesser specimen fragmentation.[12]

▌ TECHNIQUE

As with any interventional radiology procedure, patient evaluation is an important step in the planning process. A history, physical, and a review of routine laboratory studies, such as the CBC, coagulation profile, and basic chemistries, should be performed to assess the patient for adequacy of the procedure and for patient safety. Although the procedure is virtually painless, the use of mild conscious sedation may help to relieve anxiety invoked by the procedure and alleviate any discomfort. Midazolam is a good choice for a sedative because it does not affect hepatic hemodynamics.[22] Typically, no antibiotic coverage is required because complications arising from infectious causes are very unusual.[9] The patient's vital signs must be monitored during the procedure, including continuous electrocardiographic monitoring, because a catheter will proceed through the right atrium and induced arrhythmias need to be detected. For the typical right-side IJV approach, the patient should be positioned supine with the head turned slightly to the left, while maintaining comfortable positioning for the patient. Then after subcutaneously injecting local analgesia, a micropuncture needle is advanced into the IJV under ultrasound guidance. Anatomically, the puncture site is immediately anterior to the sternomastoid muscle, halfway between the mastoid process and the sternal notch.[23] If the IJV is small in caliber, making it difficult to cannalize, placing a wedge beneath the patient to elevate the feet may help distend it.[13] After the vein has been accessed with the micropuncture needle using standard exchange techniques, a 5 French micropuncture sheath is placed. Through this, a guide wire, such as a 3J or Bentson wire, is advanced into the superior vena cava, through the right atrium, and into the inferior vena cava (IVC) (FIGURE 33.1).

Over this wire, the micropuncture sheath is exchanged for the 9 French introducer sheath. The guide wire is then manipulated under fluoroscopic guidance into the right hepatic vein with the use of an angled, steerable catheter, such as a 5 French angled glide catheter, Cobra, or a 5 French multipurpose catheter. Once the wire is appropriately placed within the right hepatic vein, the catheter is advanced over the wire into the vein. The right and middle hepatic veins are the preferred sites to perform the TJLB because of the larger volumes of adjacent liver to do the biopsy, decreasing the risk of capsular perforation.[24] Once there is secure placement of the wire within the hepatic vein, hepatic venography can be performed to demonstrate patency and to further elucidate the relationship and proximity of the hepatic vein to the IVC, planning for the best central location from which to perform the biopsy (FIGURE 33.2).[13]

The wire then may be changed to a stiffer working wire, such as the Rosen or Amplatz Super-Stiff guide wire. The sheath is then advanced and hepatic venography is performed through the catheter to evaluate the hepatic vein anatomy and to assess the position of the tip of the sheath. A stable position of the sheath tip within the proximal portion of the hepatic vein close to the origin from the IVC will usually provide the safest position for performing the transvenous biopsy.[15] The catheter is then removed and the curved metal cannula is advanced through the introducer sheath and into the right hepatic vein. In our institution, a Tru-cut needle is first prepared by pulling back the plunger until there is a definite click. The biopsy needle tip is introduced into the metal cannula and before advancing the tip out into the hepatic vein, the cannula is rotated in an anterior direction (FIGURE 33.3).

If the middle hepatic vein was selected, then the cannula is directed in a lateral/posterior position.[5] One could consider cannulating the left hepatic vein in patients with a decreased right hepatic lobe and hypertrophied left lobe.[5]

The biopsy device is then fired and the device is withdrawn and specimen is obtained. After three sufficient passes, the cannula is removed from the sheath and a hepatic venogram

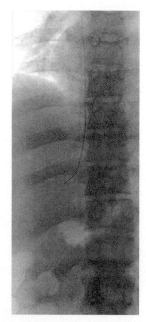

FIGURE 33.1 Right internal jugular venous access with guide wire tip in the IVC.

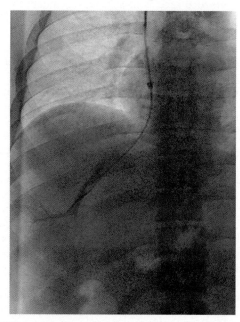

FIGURE 33.2 Hepatic venography via a 5 French catheter.

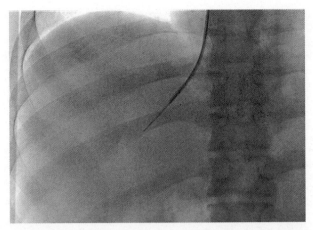

FIGURE 33.3 Biopsy needle advanced across the middle hepatic vein into liver parenchyma after rotating the metal cannula anteriorly.

performed to ensure through the side arm of the introducer sheath to evaluate for possible capsular perforation.

Multiple passes may be needed to obtain an adequate sample. In between passes, the system must be held in place within the hepatic vein to prevent cardiac pulsation and respiratory motion from displacing the system out of the vein.

In a study of 326 consecutive TJLBs in 274 patients, Cholongitas et al.[21] found three passes to be safe and to provide an adequate liver specimen. In the event of capsular perforation, gelfoam pledgets may be used to embolize the needle tract. Embolization of the needle tract immediately after the detection of capsular perforation may decrease the risk of developing hemoperitoneum.[23]

Although the sheath and cannula assembly of the TJLB set is designed for the straight line formed from the right IJV, superior vena cava, right atrium, and IVC, in certain circumstances, a left IJV approach may be used. Indications for a left-side IJV approach include: documented previous difficult catheterization of a target hepatic vein for a right IJV approach, partial or total occlusion of the right IJV, overlying skin infection, or existing tunneled right-side central venous catheters. In the case of an existing tunneled dialysis catheter, typically one could access the IJV above the level of the catheter.[24] Additionally, the right-side IJV approach may not provide the best approach for transvenous biopsy in patients with severe chronic liver disease secondary to distorted anatomy from atrophy or compensatory hypertrophy. Similarly, the anatomy of the hepatic vein origins as well as intrahepatic venous anatomy may be irregular after transplantation.[25] In these circumstances, there may be severe angulation between the IVC and the hepatic veins, making cannulation quite difficult. Having the patient take a deep inspiration may help facilitate a more favorable hepatic vein orientation in relation to the IVC.[5]

Additionally, one could increase the likelihood for a successful transvenous liver biopsy attempt from a right-sided IJV access through modification of the curve on the biopsy cannula or by employing secondary or tertiary curves in the shaft of the cannula. One must remain cognizant, however, that customization of the biopsy cannula may make it difficult to insert the

cannula. Overly acute angles of the curve of the cannula may make it challenging to pass the biopsy needle and furthermore may hinder the normal function of the biopsy needle itself.[24] Conversely, one may try a left-side IJV access for the transvenous biopsy. The left-side access poses an additional technical challenge, namely, crossing the mediastinum through the central veins. Using a stiffer guide wire, such as the Amplatz Super-Stiff or Lunderquist, should improve the safety of passing the potentially traumatic rigid cannula through the central veins and right atrium.[24] Indeed, the anatomy of the hepatic vein origins may be such that the angle with the IVC becomes too acute to approach from a superior venous access and must be approached from below, using the right common femoral vein (FIGURE 33.4).

Transcaval biopsies may also be utilized in cases where cannulation of the hepatic veins is not possible, such as in Budd-Chiari syndrome.[5] To perform a transcaval biopsy, one may utilize both ultrasound and fluoroscopic guidance. First, the operator must properly identify the intrahepatic vena cava. With the tip of the cannula located at the intrahepatic IVC, point the tip of the cannula anteriorly and to the right, wedging it into the liver parenchyma. Use the ultrasound to confirm adequate liver parenchyma anterior to the cannula tip. Advance the biopsy needle into the parenchyma and obtain biopsy specimens.[5] Another alternative for patients with difficult hepatic venous anatomy is the percutaneous or plugged-percutaneous liver biopsy. Free hepatic, wedged hepatic, IVC, and right atrial (RA) pressures may also be obtained during the procedure.[5] To perform reliable pressure measurements, one will need a recorder that can produce a permanent tracing of pressure values, a pressure transducer that can detect changes in venous pressure, and an occlusion balloon catheter (preferable to an end-hole catheter). A balloon-tipped catheter can be used to occlude a larger hepatic branch and therefore can measure a wedged hepatic venous

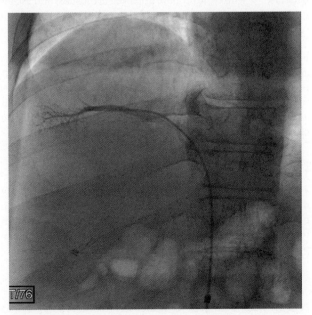

FIGURE 33.4 Hepatic venous cannulation from the right common femoral vein.

pressure (WHVP) over a wider vascular territory of the liver, as compared to that obtained with a straight catheter (which needs to be wedged in a distal hepatic vein to obtain accurate WHVP measurements).[26]

INDICATIONS

TJLB is mostly performed when hepatic tissue is needed for evaluation and PLB is contraindicated. The most common indications for TJLB are severe coagulopathy (platelets <60,000 or INR ≥ 2) and moderate or severe ascites.[12,23,27] Coagulopathy can be considered more of a relative contraindication rather than an absolute contraindication for TJLB. PLB with plugging the needle tract with gelfoam has been previously described.[28,29] Sawyerr et al.[30] investigated 117 patients with impaired blood coagulation who were randomized to either TJLB or plugged-percutaneous liver biopsy. Both methods proved to be very successful with a low incidence of complications. However, the authors did suggest that there may be a higher risk of hemorrhage with the plugged-percutaneous liver biopsy because two of the patients biopsied in that manner required blood transfusion for hemorrhage (platelet count 49 and 134 × 10^9/L, respectively, and INR of 1.2 and 2.1, respectively).[30] Atar et al.[31] retrospectively compared plugged-percutaneous liver biopsy to TJLB, evaluating their own in-hour protocol for method selection. Those patients with platelet counts of less than 60,000/mm^3 or an INR of greater than or equal to 2 received TJLB, whereas those patients with platelet counts of 60,000 to 100,000/mm^3 or an INR of 1.4 to 2 were selected for plugged-percutaneous liver biopsy. They found no statistically significant difference between the two groups in regard to complication rate to technical success.[31] Given that plugged-percutaneous liver biopsy is simpler, with lower cost and less radiation, Atar et al. further believe that the division of patients in this manner is effective and safe.

Other indications for TJLB include post-liver transplant patients,[32–36] who typically have impaired hemostasis and ascites in the early post-transplant period,[35,37] and those patients with fulminant and ALF.[3,5,38] Liver biopsy may be both diagnostic and prognostic in early ALF and congenital clotting disorders.[39–43] Further, patients with renal failure who are undergoing hemodialysis and receiving heparin[5,44] and those with difficult percutaneous biopsy and borderline parameters may also be candidates for TJLB.[5] TJLB also has a role in evaluating liver dysfunction after bone marrow transplant that has been shown to be safe and effective (Table 33.1).[45]

CONTRAINDICATIONS

There are no absolute contraindications to TJLB. In general, any derangements in the coagulation profile should be corrected if possible. The technique should not be used for the biopsy of focal liver lesions. The patient will need to have venous access to perform the procedure.

FOLLOW-UP

Patients were monitored for heart rate, respiratory rate, blood pressure, neck hematoma, and abdominal girth every 2 hours for 6 hours. Diet should be advanced as tolerated (liquid to solid).[5]

Table 33.1

Indications for Transjugular Liver Biopsy^a

Major

Coagulation disorders^b
Ascites^c
Need for concurrent procedures^d

Minor

Massive obesity
Small cirrhotic liver
Suspected vascular tumor or peliosis hepatic

^{a}Reported by McAfee et al.[9]

^{b}Prothrombin time >3 sec over control value and/or platelet count <60,000/cm^3.

^{c} Moderate or severe.

^{d} Hepatic and caval venous pressure measurements, hepatic venography, portography, or transjugular intrahepatic portosystemic shunts.

COMPLICATIONS

Procedural and postprocedural complications are documented according to Society of Interventional Radiology (SIR) guidelines as described in Table 33.2.[46]

In a large review of 64 series reporting on 7,649 TJLBs, complications were reported in 7.1% of cases.[12] Minor complications were reported in 6.5%, 3.2% of which were liver puncture related. Importantly, reported complications involving minor neck complications were significantly less than those performed under ultrasound guidance (1.9% versus 2.8%). In another series of 7,493 TJLBs, the total complication rate was 6.7% with a major complication rate of 0.5%, 0.2% of which were liver puncture related.[12] Death was reported in 0.09% of cases caused by intraperitoneal hemorrhage or ventricular arrhythmia.

In a large series of PLBs, all deaths reported were attributed to hemoperitoneum.[47] Hemoperitoneum is also a significant cause of procedure-related death after TJLB because it occurs

Table 33.2

SIR Classification System for Complications by Outcome

Minor complications

A. No therapy, no consequence
B. Nominal therapy, no consequence; includes overnight admission for observation only

Major complications

C. Require therapy, minor hospitalization (<48 h)
D. Require major therapy, unplanned increase in level of care, prolonged hospitalization (>48 h)
E. Permanent adverse sequelae
F. Death

Reprinted with permission from Sacks D, McClenny T, Cardella J, et al. Society of Interventional Radiology clinical practice guidelines. *J Vasc Interv Radiol* 2003;14:S199–S202.

secondarily to capsular perforation.[15] Performing the TJLB from a stable central position within the hepatic vein close to its origin from the IVC will limit the number of capsular perforations.[15] As the location of the TJLB becomes more peripheral in the hepatic vein, the number of capsular perforations increases.[23,48,49] Corr et al.[23] reported that capsular perforation was the most serious complication encountered in their series of 200 TJLBs (FIGURE 33.5). Immediate embolization of the needle tract with gelfoam makes the development of hemoperitoneum less likely.[23] Gamble et al.[48] reported capsular perforation in 18 of 461 TJLBs (3.9% of patients). The needle tract was treated with gelfoam in 17 of the 18 patients with capsular perforation because it was identified at the time of the biopsy. Of these patients, 14 stabilized with no further evidence of intraperitoneal bleed, whereas 2 of the other patients stabilized with continued conservative management. One of the patients developed further signs of intraperitoneal hemorrhage and died 12 days following the biopsy.[48]

Concerning major hemorrhage and mortality, the complication rates are similar between PLB and TJLB, ranging between 0.16% to 0.32% and 0.01% to 0.12%, respectively.[12] Kalambokis et al.[12] have shown that three passes with TJLB using a Tru-cut needle is relatively safe, without increase in the complication rate, whereas increasing the number of passes from one with PLB does increase the complication rate.[50–53] With TJLB, complications are generally limited to hemorrhage within the liver, within the peritoneal space, and damage to adjacent organs. Limiting the number of passes will limit the risk of complication for hemobilia and arterioportal fistulas.

Cardiac arrhythmia is a complication that is unique to TJLB. In the series of TJLBs reported by Gamble et al.,[48] two procedure-related cardiac arrhythmias occurred. Transient supraventricular tachycardia most commonly resolves with removal of the guide wire or catheter from the right atrium.[23] Kalambokis et al.[12] reported a 0.3% rate of supraventricular arrhythmia and a 0.03% death rate from ventricular arrhythmia in their review of 7,469 TJLBs.

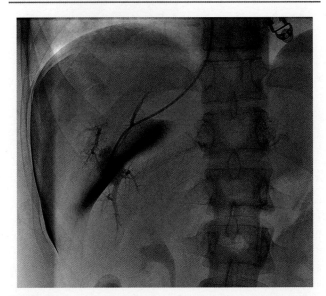

FIGURE 33.5 Capsular perforation after TJLB. The patient was monitored overnight and was stable.

RESULTS

It is uncommon for TJLB to be unsuccessful. Failed attempts at TJLB can usually be attributed to problems with puncture of the IJV, catheterization of the hepatic veins, or retrieval of liver tissue.[9] In a systematic review of 7,526 TJLB samples by Kalambokis et al., inability to catheterize a suitable hepatic vein was the most common reason for technical failure. Failure to cannulate the jugular vein and failure to obtain a liver sample were the number two and three reasons for failure of the TJLB. Improved successful attempts of cannulating the IVC were achieved with ultrasound guidance.[12]

Concerning sample acquisition and sample adequacy, the type of needle and its gauge are important factors. In a study by Choo et al., 18 patients with contraindications to PLB subsequently underwent TJLB. Of these 18 patients, 11 underwent a biopsy using an aspiration technique (modified transseptal needle) and 7 with a Tru-cut needle (Quick-Core biopsy needle); specimen length was significantly longer with less fragmentation using the Tru-cut needle. That being said, 17 of 18 specimens were considered to be adequate with the single exception of a specimen obtained using the aspiration technique.[54] The number of CPTs obtained in a specimen is considered to be superior to sample size when evaluating sample adequacy.[10,20]

The Quick-Core biopsy system (Cook) contains a 49-cm, 7 French transjugular guiding catheter, an 80-cm 5 French multipurpose curve catheter, a 50.5-cm 14-gauge thin-wall stainless steel stiffening cannula, and the Quick-Core biopsy needle.[13] Using the Quick-Core biopsy needle for TJLB, Little et al.[13] reported adequate specimens in 100% of the 42 patients in whom hepatic tissue was sampled. Middlebrook et al.[15] also reported a 100% success rate in a study of 25 consecutive patients. Mammen et al.[5] reported adequate specimens in 97% of patients in whom hepatic tissue was sampled and an overall technical success rate of 98.8% in a series of 601 patients.

ACUTE LIVER FAILURE

Optimum management of the patient with ALF requires early and accurate diagnostic and prognostic evaluation because the eligibility for liver transplant must be quickly decided and because submassive or massive liver necrosis and cirrhosis are predictors of poor long-term prognosis.[3] Severe liver dysfunction, jaundice, coagulopathy, and encephalopathy characterize ALF with symptoms presenting within 8 weeks in a patient without previously known liver disease.[55–57] ALF is associated with a mortality rate of 65% to 85%.[58,59] Medical management alone is associated with a poor prognosis. Donaldson et al.[38] reported retrospectively the results of TJLB in 61 patients with ALF, noting a successful biopsy in 60 of the patients. In another study of 17 patients with the clinical presentation of ALF, Miraglia et al.[3] reported a successful biopsy in 100% without complication with average time of biopsy and frozen section analysis of 80 minutes. Therefore, TJLB is a quick, useful tool in evaluating patients with ALF and selecting those for liver transplantation over conservative management.

TRANSPLANT

Over 106,000 liver transplants were performed in the United States between January 1988 and October 2010.[60] Transplant recipients are surviving longer with improvement in surgical technique, technologic advancements, and immunosuppressive agents.[61] According to the Organ Procurement and Transplantation Network,[60] the 1-, 3-, and 5-year survival rates after liver transplant are 87%, 78%, and 72%, respectively. The interventional radiologist plays an essential role in caring for these patients as a member of a multidisciplinary team along with surgeons and other clinical practitioners. In addition to laboratory analysis, histopathologic analysis is an important element in evaluating post-transplant complications. Liver biopsy remains the gold standard for evaluating acute rejection.[51,62,63] The interventional radiologist may be asked to perform the liver biopsy in such a patient and must decide the safest and most efficacious procedure to obtain hepatic tissue for analysis. Many post-liver transplant patients have indications that would suggest TJLB as a more suitable approach to biopsy over PLB, such as coagulopathy and/or ascites, especially in the first 30 days.[35,64] As noted earlier, however, TJLB is more technically challenging when the hepatic vein to be cannulated forms an acute angle with the IVC, which is common with one type of hepatic venous anastomosis with liver transplant.

There are two main surgical techniques used in orthotopic liver transplantation: the traditional in-line venous anastomosis and the piggyback technique.[64] In the traditional in-line technique, the donor's IVC is anastomosed to the recipient's IVC, leaving intact the anatomic relationship and angulation between the hepatic vein and the IVC (FIGURE 33.6). This is in contradistinction to the piggyback technique, in which the end of the donor IVC is anastomosed to the side of the recipient IVC (FIGURE 33.7).

This may produce acute angulation of the hepatic vein to the native IVC. The hepatic vein is typically more difficult to catheterize because of this acute angulation.[35,65] The decision on which technique to use for orthotopic liver transplantation (from the surgeon's perspective) depends on a number of issues involving the patient. The piggyback technique has several advantages over the traditional in-line technique including: maintenance of caval flow during explantation, improved maintenance of core body temperature, and improved cardiac hemodynamic stability.[66] Therefore, prior to performing TJLB on a post-liver transplant patient, one should be aware of the surgical technique utilized to be prepared for potential challenges.

In a study of 269 consecutive TJLB procedures in 139 patients who had received cadaveric liver transplants, 131 using the in-line technique and 138 using the piggyback technique, Miller et al. found TJLB to be equally safe with acceptable tissue yields. Of note, however, TJLB was less likely to provide diagnostic tissue in patients in which the piggyback technique was employed.[64] As described earlier, there are several techniques one may use to approach the patient with acute angles between the hepatic vein and the IVC, including using stiffer guide wires, reshaping the metal cannula from the biopsy set, and timing catheterization with respiratory effort.[5,67,68] At our institution, we have used a reverse curve catheter, such as a Simmons 1, to catheterize a difficultly angled hepatic vein. More experience with TJLB is likely to improve the success rate in patients with challenging hepatic anatomy.[35] Additionally, the transcaval technique may

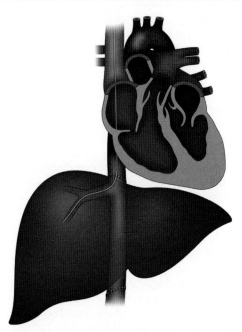

FIGURE 33.6 Inline orthotopic liver transplant. The recipient's IVC is resected and replaced with the donor IVC, retaining anatomic relationships.

Redrawn from Miller M, Smith T, Kuo P, et al. Transjugular liver biopsy results in the transplanted liver: comparison of two surgical hepatic venous anastomotic configurations in 269 consecutive biopsies over a 14-year period. *J Vasc Interv Radiol* 2010;21:508–514.

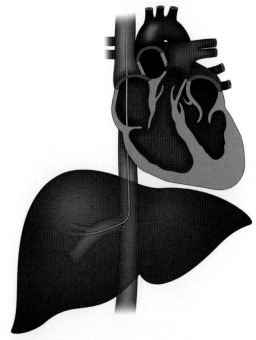

FIGURE 33.7 Piggyback orthotopic liver transplant. The recipient's IVC is retained. The donor's IVC is sutured onto the recipient's IVC in the location of the native hepatic veins.

Redrawn from Miller M, Smith T, Kuo P, et al. Transjugular liver biopsy results in the transplanted liver: comparison of two surgical hepatic venous anastomotic configurations in 269 consecutive biopsies over a 14-year period. *J Vasc Interv Radiol* 2010;21:508–514.

be employed for transvenous liver biopsy in these situations. At our institution, we have also performed transvenous liver biopsy in post-piggyback technique liver transplant patients from a right-side common femoral vein approach. When using this approach, one must be cognizant of the increased risk of pneumothorax when obtaining the biopsy specimen. Additionally, the patient must be of normal-to-smaller stature due to the length of the biopsy cannula and needle provided in the biopsy set.

Although TJLB has been proven to be safe and effective in the post-liver transplant population,[35,64] some transplant centers continue to rely on percutaneous approaches for liver biopsy. The transplant centers using only the percutaneous approach advocate correcting the coagulopathy, draining the ascites,[69] and leaving the fascia of the incision open for easier access.[70] These methods may lead to increased complications from potential leak of ascites, increased risk of infection, and graft thrombosis.

CONCLUSION

TJLB continues to remain instrumental in providing care for patients requiring a liver biopsy but having contraindications to PLB. The evolution of the technique to include the use of the Tru-cut type of biopsy needle with three passes provides adequate samples for analysis with comparable complication and mortality rates as compared to PLB.[12] TJLB is also indicated in the case of ALF and in early post-liver transplant recipients.[12] Additionally, TJLB should be employed when hepatic pressures are also needed for patient evaluation.

Compared to PLB, TJLB is more time consuming and requires operator experience, patient monitoring, and moderate sedation. It is a safe alternative technique, however, for obtaining adequate liver tissue for histopathologic analysis when PLB may be contraindicated.

REFERENCES

1. Lebrec D. Various approaches to obtaining liver tissue—choosing the biopsy technique. *J Hepatol* 1996;25(suppl 1):20–24.
2. Campbell M, Reddy K. Review article: the evolving role of liver biopsy. *Aliment Pharmacol Ther* 2004;20:249–259.
3. Miraglia R, Luca A, Gruttadauria S, et al. Contribution of transjugular liver biopsy in patients with the clinical presentation of acute liver failure. *Cardiovasc Intervent Radiol* 2006;29:1008–1010.
4. Guido M, Rugge M. Liver biopsy sampling in chronic viral hepatitis. *Semin Liver Dis* 2004;24:89–97.
5. Mammen T, Keshava S, Eapen C, et al. Transjugular liver biopsy: a retrospective analysis of 601 cases. *J Vasc Interv Radiol* 2008;19:351–358.
6. Dotter C. Catheter biopsy: experimental technic for transvenous liver biopsy. *Radiology* 1964;82:312–314.
7. Rosch J, Lakin P, Antonovic R, et al. Transjugular approach for liver biopsy and transhepatic cholangiography. *N Engl J Med* 1973;289:227–231.
8. Hanafee W, Weiner M. Transjugular percutaneous cholangiography. *Radiology* 1967;88:35–39.
9. McAfee J, Keeffe E, Lee R, et al. Special article: transjugular liver biopsy. *Hepatology* 1992;15:726–732.
10. Bravo A, Sheth S, Chopra S. Liver biopsy. *N Engl J Med* 2001;344:495–500.
11. Sheela H, Seela S, Caldwell C, et al. Liver biopsy: evolving role in the new millennium. *J Clin Gastroenterol* 2005;39:603–610.
12. Kalambokis G, Manousou P, Vibhakorn S, et al. Transjugular liver biopsy—indications, adequacy, quality of specimens, and complications—a systematic review. *J Hepatol* 2007;47:284–294.
13. Little A, Zajko A, Orons P. Transjugular liver biopsy: a prospective study in 43 patients with the Quick-Core biopsy needle. *J Vasc Interv Radiol* 1996;7:127–131.
14. Colapinto R, Blendis L. Liver biopsy through the transjugular approach. *Radiology* 1983;148:306.
15. Middlebrook M, Cohen A, Wallace M, et al. Improved method for transjugular liver biopsy. *J Vasc Interv Radiol* 1999;10:807–809.
16. Crawford A, Lin X, Crawford J. The normal adult human liver biopsy: a quantitative reference standard. *Hepatology* 1998;28:323–331.
17. Rocken C, Meier H, Klauck S, et al. Large-needle biopsy versus thin-needle biopsy in diagnostic pathology of liver diseases. *Liver Int* 2001;21:391–397.
18. Schlichting P, Holund B, Poulsen H. Liver biopsy in chronic aggressive hepatitis. Diagnostic reproducibility in relation to size of specimen. *Scand J Gastroenterol* 1983;18:27–32.
19. Colloredo G, Guido M, Sonzogni A, et al. Impact of liver biopsy size on histological evaluation of chronic viral hepatitis: the smaller the sample, the milder the disease. *J Hepatol* 2003;39:239–244.
20. Bedossa P, Dargere D, Paradis V. Sampling variability of liver fibrosis in chronic hepatitis C. *Hepatology* 2003;38:1449–1457.
21. Cholongitas E, Quaglia A, Samonakis D, et al. Transjugular liver biopsy: how good is it for accurate histological interpretation? *Gut* 2006;55:1789–1794.
22. Steinlauf A, Garcia-Tsao G, Zakko M, et al. Low-dose midazolam sedation: an option for patients undergoing serial hepatic venous pressure measurements. *Hepatology* 1999;29:1070–1073.
23. Corr P, Beningfield S, Davey N. Transjugular liver biopsy: a review of 200 biopsies. *Clin Radiol* 1992;45:238–239.
24. Yavuz K, Geyik S, Barton R, et al. Transjugular liver biopsy via the left internal jugular vein. *J Vasc Interv Radiol* 2007;18:237–241.
25. Kardache M, Soyer P, Boudiaf M, et al. Transjugular liver biopsy with an automated device. *Radiology* 1997;204:369–372.
26. Groszman R, Wongcharatrawee S. The hepatic venous pressure gradient: anything worth doing should be done right. *Hepatology* 2004;39:280–282.
27. Scotto J, Opolon P, Eteve R, et al. Liver biopsy and prognosis in acute liver failure. *Gut* 1973;14:927–933.
28. Riley S, Ellis W, Irving H, et al. Percutaneous liver biopsy with plugging of needle track: a safe method for use in patients with impaired coagulation. *Lancet* 1984;2:436.
29. Tobin M, Gilmore I. Plugged liver biopsy in patients with impaired coagulation. *Dig Dis Sci* 1989;34:13–15.
30. Sawyerr A, McCormick P, Tennyson G, et al. A comparison of transjugular and plugged-percutaneous liver biopsy in patients with impaired coagulation. *J Hepatol* 1993;17:81–85.
31. Atar E, Ari Z, Bachar G, et al. A comparison of transjugular and plugged-percutaneous liver biopsy in patients with contraindications to ordinary percutaneous liver biopsy and an "in-house" protocol for selecting the procedure of choice. *Cardiovasc Intervent Radiol* 2010;33:560–564.
32. Blasco A, Forns X, Carrion J, et al. Hepatic venous pressure gradient identifies patients at risk for severe hepatitis C recurrence after liver transplantation. *Hepatology* 2006;43:492–499.
33. Abujudeh H, Huggins R, Patel A. Emergency transjugular liver biopsies in post-liver-transplant patients: technical success and utility. *Emerg Radiol* 2004;10:268–269.
34. Romero M, Banares R, Salcedo M, et al. Diagnostic value of transjugular liver biopsy in liver transplant recipients. *Gastroenterol Hepatol* 1999;22:493–496.
35. Azoulay D, Raccuia J, Roche B, et al. The value of early transjugular liver biopsy after liver transplantation. *Transplantation* 1996;61:406–409.
36. Mentha G, Widmann J, Schneider P, et al. Hepatic venography, manometric studies and transjugular liver biopsy in the follow-up of liver transplant patients. *Transplant Proc* 1987;19:3323–3326.
37. Papatheodoridis G, Patch D, Watkinson A, et al. Transjugular liver biopsy in the 1990s: a 2-year audit. *Aliment Pharmacol Ther* 1999;13:603–608.
38. Donaldson B, Gopinath R, Wanless I, et al. The role of transjugular liver biopsy in fulminant liver failure: relation to other prognostic indicators. *Hepatology* 1993;18:1370–1374.
39. Dawson M, McCarthy P, Walsh M, et al. Transjugular liver biopsy is a safe and effective intervention to guide management for patients with a congenital bleeding disorder infected with hepatitis C. *Intern Med J* 2005;35:556–559.
40. Shin J, Teitel J, Swain M, et al. A Canadian multicenter retrospective study evaluating transjugular liver biopsy in patients with congenital bleeding disorders and hepatitis C: is it safe and useful? *Am J Hematol* 2005;78:85–93.
41. Saab S, Cho D, Quon D, et al. Same day outpatient transjugular liver biopsies in haemophilia. *Haemophilia* 2004;10:727–731.
42. Stieltjes N, Ounnoughene N, Save E, et al. Interest of transjugular liver biopsy in adult patients with heamophilia or other congenital bleeding disorders infected with hepatitis C virus. *Br J Haematol* 2004;125:769–776.

43. Dimichele D, Mirani G, Canchis W, et al. Transjugular liver biopsy is safe and diagnostic for patients with congenital bleeding disorders and hepatitis C infection. *Haemophilia* 2003;9:613–618.

44. Pereira B, Levey A. Hepatitis C virus infection in dialysis and renal transplantation. *Kidney Int* 1997;51:981–999.

45. Carreras E, Granena A, Navasa M, et al. Transjugular liver biopsy in BMT. *Bone Marrow Transplant* 1993;11:21–26.

46. Sacks D, McClenny T, Cardella J, et al. Society of Interventional Radiology clinical practice guidelines. *J Vasc Interv Radiol* 2003;14:S199–S202.

47. Piccinino F, Sagnelli E, Pasquale G, et al. Complications following percutaneous liver biopsy: a multicentre retrospective study on 68,276 biopsies. *J Hepatol* 1986;2:165–173.

48. Gamble P, Colapinto R, Colman J, et al. Transjugular liver biopsy: a review of 461 biopsies. *Radiology* 1985;157:589–593.

49. Colapinto R. Transjugular biopsy of the liver. *Clin Gastroenterol* 1985;14:451–467.

50. Grant A, Neuberger J. Guidelines on the use of liver biopsy in clinical practice. British Society of Gastroenterology. *Gut* 1999;45(suppl 4):IV1–IV11.

51. McGill D, Rakela J, Zinmeister A, et al. A 21-year experience with major hemorrhage after percutaneous liver biopsy. *Gastroenterology* 1990;99:1396–1400.

52. Maharaj B, Bhoora I. Complications associated with percutaneous needle biopsy of the liver when one, two or three specimens are taken. *Postgrad Med J* 1992;68:964–967.

53. Cadranel J, Rufat P, Degos F. Practices of liver biopsy in France: results of a prospective nationwide survey. For the Group of Epidemiology of the French Association for the Study of the Liver (AFEF). *Hepatology* 2000;32:477–481.

54. Choo S, Do Y, Park K, et al. Transjugular liver biopsy: modified Ross transseptal needle versus Quick-Core biopsy needle. *Abdom Imaging* 2000;25:483–485.

55. Raham T, Humphrey H. Clinical management of acute hepatic failure. *Intensive Care Med* 27:467–476.

56. Schiodt F, Lee W. Fulminant liver disease. *Clin Liver Dis* 2003;7:331–349.

57. Henegan M, Lara L. Fulminant hepatic failure. *Semin Gastrointest Dis* 2003;14:87–100.

58. Brems J, Hiatt J, Ramming K, et al. Fulminant hepatic failure: the role of liver transplantation as primary therapy. *Am J Surg* 1987;154:137–141.

59. Peleman R, Gavaler J, Van Thiel D, et al. Orthotopic liver transplantation for acute and subacute hepatic failure in adults. *Hepatology* 1987;7:484–489.

60. Organ Procurement and Transplantation network. Available at http://optn.org. Accessed January 14, 2011.

61. Amesur N, Zajko A. Interventional radiology in liver transplantation. *Liver Transpl* 2006;12:330–351.

62. Colonna J, Brems J, Goldstein L, et al. The importance of percutaneous liver biopsy in the management of the liver transplant recipient. *Transplant Proc* 1988;20(suppl 1):682–684.

63. Bubak M, Porayko M, Krom R, et al. Complications of liver biopsy in liver transplant patients: increased sepsis associated with choledochojejunostomy. *Hepatology* 1991;14:1063–1065.

64. Miller M, Smith T, Kuo P, et al. Transjugular liver biopsy results in the transplanted liver: comparison of two surgical hepatic venous anastomotic configurations in 269 consecutive biopsies over a 14-year period. *J Vasc Interv Radiol* 2010;21:508–514.

65. Richard H, Cooper J, Ahn J, et al. Transjugular intrahepatic portosystemic shunts in the management of Budd-Chiari syndrome in the liver transplant patient with intractable ascites: anatomic considerations. *J Vasc Interv Radiol* 1998;9:137–140.

66. Shokouh-Amiri M, Gaber A, Bagous W, et al. Choice of surgical technique influences perioperative outcomes in liver transplantation. *Ann Surg* 2000;231:814–823.

67. Chevallier P, Dausse F, Berthier F, et al. Transjugular liver biopsy: prospective evaluation of the angle formed between the hepatic veins and the vena cava main axis and the modification of a semi-automated biopsy device in cases of an unfavorable angle. *Eur Radiol* 2007;17:169–173.

68. de Hoyos A, Loredo M, Martinez M, et al. Use of a stiff guidewire in transjugular liver biopsy in patients with a pronounced angle of the suprahepatic veins. *Ann Hepatol* 2004;3:72–73.

69. Belghiti J, Panis Y, Sauvanet A, et al. A new technique of side to side caval anastomosis during orthotopic hepatic transplantation without inferior vena cava occlusion. *Surg Gynecol Obstet* 1992;175:270–272.

70. Hadengue A, Lebrec D, Gaudin C, et al. Transvenous biopsy of orthotopic liver grafts—feasible and effective. *Transplantation* 1991;5:915–917.

CHAPTER 34
Retrograde Balloon Occlusion Variceal Ablation

KEIGO OSUGA, HIRO KIYOSUE, and HIROSHI ANAI

INTRODUCTION

Gastric varices are present in 5% to 33% of patients with portal hypertension commonly caused by cirrhosis.[1] Although gastric varices bleed less frequently than esophageal varices, their bleeding can be massive and fatal because of the large size and rapid blood flow of the varices. Thus, gastric variceal bleeding is not sufficiently controlled by medical treatment alone or it is often more difficult to control by endoscopic intervention than bleeding from esophageal varices. Transjugular intrahepatic portosystemic shunt (TIPS) has been a salvage therapy for refractory variceal bleeding; however, TIPS is not always effective because the portal venous pressure can be decreased by the accompanying large gastrorenal (GR) shunt.[2–4] Today, a surgical shunt, despite the definitive therapy, has a limited role for gastric variceal bleeding because of the invasiveness and high mortality, especially in patients with poor liver function. Because gastric variceal bleeding remains a therapeutic challenge, a transcatheter treatment of retrograde approach has been developed. In 1984, Olson et al.[5] first reported a case of gastroesophageal variceal bleeding successfully treated by retrograde ethanol sclerotherapy. In 1996, Kanagawa et al.[6] first published a case series of balloon-occluded retrograde transvenous obliteration (B-RTO) using ethanolamine oleate (EO) for fundal gastric varices. Since then, B-RTO has been rapidly spreading, mainly in Japan, as an effective treatment to control or prevent gastric variceal bleeding.[7–21] The intent of B-RTO is to ablate gastric varices by filling a sclerosing agent retrogradely via the dominant draining vein, thereby reducing the mortality from gastric variceal bleeding.

PATIENT SELECTION

B-RTO is indicated for isolated gastric varices that have bled or are at a bleeding risk. Endoscopic and imaging evaluations are important to select patients with a favorable venous anatomy for B-RTO. The existence of the dominant draining route, usually GR shunt or gastrocaval (GC) shunt, is essential for catheter access. Risk factors for gastric variceal bleeding include the presence of red color sign, enlarging variceal size, and impaired liver function.[22] Gastric varices that are newly developed or aggravated after endoscopic intervention for esophageal varices also have a high bleeding risk.[23] B-RTO should be carefully indicated or avoided in patients with refractory ascites, severely impaired liver function or Child-Pugh grade C, and main portal vein thrombosis.

ANATOMIC CONSIDERATIONS

Gastric varices are anatomically divided into four types: (1) the gastoesophageal varices located at the cardia contiguous with esophageal varices; (2) the isolated gastric varices located in the fundus in the absence of esophageal varices; (3) the combined type of gastroesophageal and isolated gastric varices; and (4) the ectopic varices secondary to the splenic vein thrombosis.[24] Among them, the isolated gastric varices dominantly draining into the GR shunt are most suitable for B-RTO. The isolated gastric varices form in a large portosystemic shunt between the gastric veins and the left inferior phrenic vein in the bare area of the stomach. They are mainly supplied from the left gastric vein and/or the posterior gastric vein but less frequently from the short gastric vein.[25] They drain into the left inferior phrenic vein, which runs inferiorly into the left renal vein (GR shunt) (80% to 85%), and/or directly into the inferior vena cava, forming the GC shunt (10% to 15%).[25] The isolated gastric varices can also drain into the pericardiacophrenic vein, the subcostal and intercostal veins, the right inferior phrenic vein, and the azygos vein (FIGURE 34.1).

DEVICE CONSIDERATIONS

Balloon Catheter

A 10- to 20-mm Simmons-shaped balloon catheter is useful for occlusion of the GR shunt via the transfemoral approach (FIGURE 34.2A). A C-shaped balloon catheter is useful for occlusion of the GC shunt or GR shunt via the transjugular approach (FIGURE 34.2B). Placement of a specific 8 French S-curved sheath (Medikit, Tokyo, Japan) in the GR shunt is also useful to support insertion of a 5 French C- or cobra-shaped balloon catheter. Recently, a 5 French/9 French double coaxial balloon catheter system (Medikit, Tokyo, Japan) has been developed to allow more selective balloon insertion (FIGURE 34.2C).[26] Size 10-mm microballoon catheters (Attendant, Terumo, Tokyo, Japan; Temporally occlusion balloon catheter, Fuji Systems, Tokyo, Japan) are also available for selective occlusion of a small or tortuous shunt. They can be introduced through a 6 French guiding catheter or 4 French sheath over a 0.014-inch microguide wire.

Sclerosing Agent

Five percent ethanolamine oleate-iopamidol (EOI) has been mainly used in B-RTO. It is a viscous agent, consisting of a mixture of 10% EO (Oldamin, Grelan Pharmaceutical, Tokyo, Japan) and the same dose of a nonionic iodinated contrast medium (Iopamidol 300, Bayer Healthcare, Osaka, Japan). Five percent EOI is radiopaque and it is easy to monitor its filling or escape under X-ray fluoroscopy. Recently, sclerosing foams using polidocanol or sodium tetradecyl sulfate have been applied.[27,28] These foams can reduce the net amount of the drug itself and enhance contact with the venous wall. There are potential risks of air embolism, however. Ethanol and 50% glucose also have been supplementary used before injecting 5% EOI.[7,29]

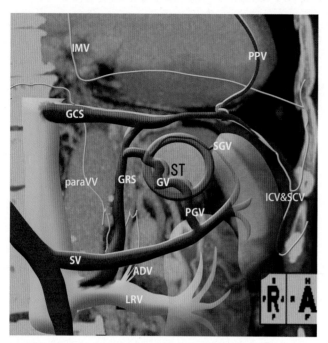

FIGURE 34.1 Diagram of the venous anatomy around gastric varices. ADV, adrenal vein; GCS, gastrocaval shunt; GRS, gastrorenal shunt; GV, gastric varices; ICV, intercostal vein; IMV, internal mammary vein; LRV, left renal vein; paraVV, paravertebral vein; PGV, posterior gastric vein; PPV, pericardiacophrenic vein; SCV, subcostal vein; SGV, short gastric vein; ST, stomach; SV, splenic vein.

TREATMENT SELECTION STRATEGIES

There are three situations for control of gastric variceal bleeding by B-RTO. First is emergent B-RTO to stop acute bleeding from the ruptured varices. Hypovolemic shock should be stabilized first by conservative treatment and balloon tamponade. If the bleeding remains active, direct B-RTO is controversial because balloon occlusion may increase variceal pressure and aggravate bleeding. It is preferable to perform B-RTO once initial hemostasis is obtained. The second situation is elective B-RTO to prevent rebleeding from varices once previously ruptured. If the varices remain unstable and are resistant to endoscopic interventions, B-RTO is indicated if the varices are anatomically feasible. The last is prophylactic B-RTO to prevent bleeding from unruptured varices at a certain bleeding risk. Periodic endoscopic screening is important because the bleeding is not always predictable. B-RTO is indicated when the varices show a red color sign or enlargement over time.

The success of B-RTO can be disturbed by drug escape into collateral drainage veins. Hirota et al.[7] classified the degree of collateral visualization on balloon-occluded venography into four grades: G-1, no collateral drainage; G-2, small and a few collaterals with stagnation of contrast medium in the varices for 3 minutes or more; G-3, medium to large collateral drainage with contrast stagnation in the varices less than 3 minutes; G-4, large and multiple collateral drainages without contrast filling in the varices. For G-1 to G-2 varices, the standard B-RTO is effective in most cases. In contrast, G-3 to G-4 varices are refractory to the standard B-RTO, and the modified techniques are necessary.

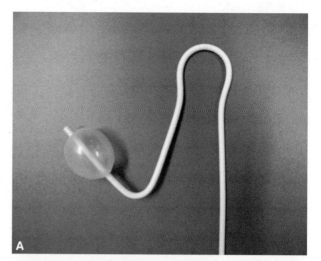
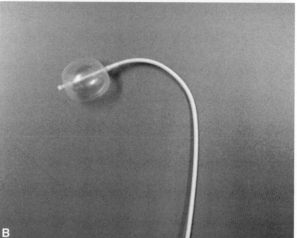
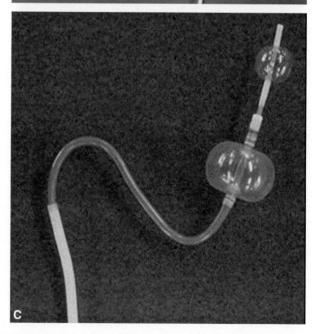

FIGURE 34.2 Balloon catheters for B-RTO. **A.** 5 French Simmons-shaped catheter with a 10-mm balloon. **B.** 5 French C-shaped catheter with a 10-mm balloon. **C.** Double coaxial balloon catheter system: a 9 French guiding catheter with a 20-mm balloon and a 5 French coaxial catheter with a 10-mm balloon.

PLANNING THE INTERVENTIONAL PROCEDURE

Because balloon and coaxial catheters are advanced retrogradely toward the varices, image assessment of the drainage routes from the gastric varices is important. By angiography, the superior mesenteric and celiac arteriograms are useful to grasp the whole portal venous system. Arteriography is not always necessary, however, because such a venous anatomy can be evaluated by the current vascular imaging technique using multidetector row computed tomography (MDCT). Contrast-enhanced CT images of the late arterial or portal venous phase are essential to demonstrate the portal venous system. Image reconstruction with multiplanar reformation, maximum intensity protection, or volume-rendering technique allows three-dimensional analysis.[30] Magnetic resonance (MR) portography is an alternative to MDCT for patients with an allergic history to iodinated contrast media. Size and shape of balloon catheters are determined based on the diameter and configuration of the estimated access route veins. When the GR shunt is not clearly shown, the alternative access routes, such as the GC shunt and the left pericardiacophrenic vein, are sought.

SPECIFIC INTRAPROCEDURAL TECHNIQUES

The standard B-RTO is usually effective for G-1 to G-2 varices according to Hirota's classification. A balloon catheter is placed in the GR or GC shunt via the right femoral or right jugular vein. A transjugular approach may allow deeper balloon insertion and reduce patient discomfort when the balloon inflation is planned until the next day. Balloon-occluded venography is then performed by manual contrast injection to demonstrate the gastric varices (FIGURE 34.3A). A power injector should not be used to avoid variceal rupture caused by forceful pressure. The volume of sclerosing agent is estimated according to the contrast volume to fill the varices. Subsequently, a sclerosing agent is injected intermittently until the variceal cavity is fully filled (FIGURE 34.3B). The balloon is kept inflated until adequate blood flow stasis of the varices is obtained. If there are small collateral veins, stepwise injection of 5% EOI or 50% glucose solution is useful to prevent the escape of sclerosing agent through them.[29]

For G-3 to G-4 varices, where the sclerosing agent easily escapes into collateral veins, several modified techniques are required. First, coil or glue embolization is necessary to occlude large or high-flow collateral veins. A 25% to 33% n-butyl-2-cyanoacrylate (NBCA)-lipiodol mixture is used when the microcatheter position is unstable for coil deployment.[13] Second, if the collateral veins remain or are difficult to embolize, a balloon catheter is advanced distally beyond the collateral veins, or a microcatheter is further inserted as close as possible to the varices (downgrade technique). Gentle manipulation to insert the microcatheter is mandatory to avoid vessel perforation. If the microcatheter reaches the varices, intravariceal glue injection can be performed and coils are deployed in the draining vein to avoid glue migration.[12] When the gastric varices are drained via both the GR and GC shunts, B-RTO is performed under dual balloon occlusion of both shunts (double-balloon technique) (FIGURE 34.4). When the drainage route is available, B-RTO may be performed via the left pericardiacophrenic vein by approaching from the femoral, left brachial, or left jugular vein. B-RTO

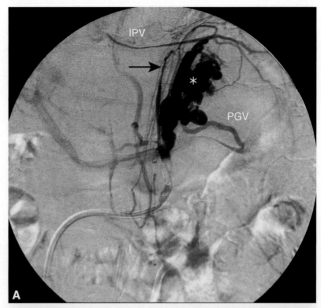

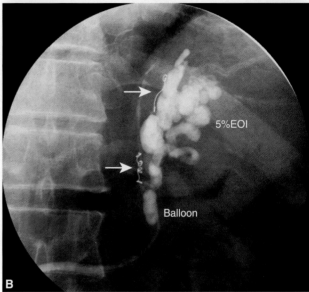

FIGURE 34.3 B-RTO for gastric varices with a small collateral drainage vein. **A.** Balloon-occluded venography shows the gastric varices (*) and their afferent vein, the posterior gastric vein (PGV). There is a collateral vein (*arrow*) draining into the inferior phrenic vein (IPV). **B.** Following microcoil embolization of the collateral vein (*arrows*), the varices were sufficiently filled with 5% EOI under balloon occlusion.

via the azygos vein is usually difficult because of the complex venous network.[31] If the outlet of the GR shunt is too large to occlude by a single balloon catheter, selective insertion of a coaxial balloon catheter may help. If this fails, a combination of percutaneous transhepatic obliteration (PTO) is considered to reduce the flow of the GR shunt.

Even without its escape into the collateral veins, the sclerosing agent does not always stagnate in the entire varices. This may occur when there is pressure gradient among multiple afferent veins, and the sclerosing agent distributes only in the

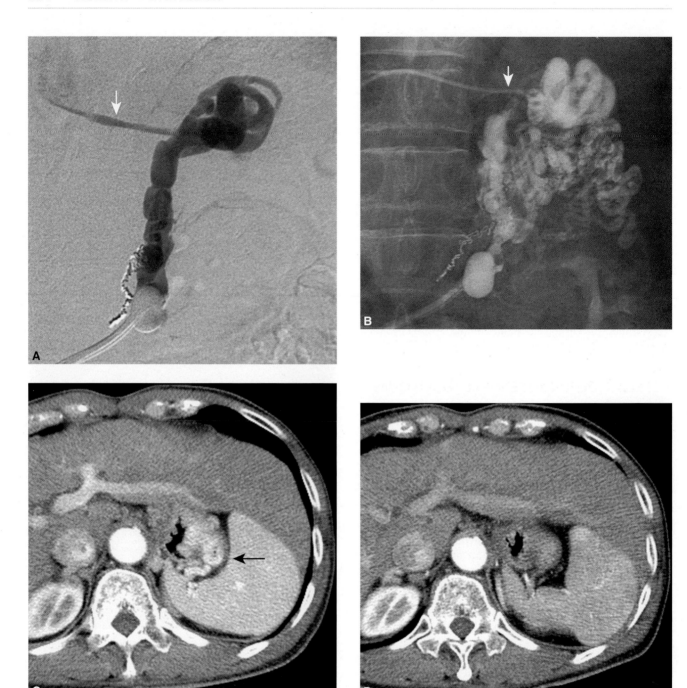

FIGURE 34.4 B-RTO with double balloon technique. **A.** Balloon-occluded venography shows collateral drainage into the inferior phrenic vein (*arrow*) without filling the gastric varices. **B.** With the inferior phrenic vein occluded with another 10-mm balloon catheter (*arrow*), 18 mL of 5% EOI was injected from the balloon catheter in the GR shunt. Sufficient filling of the sclerosing agent was obtained in the entire varices. **C.** Contrast-enhanced CT before B-RTO shows the fundal gastric varices (*arrow*). **D.** On the 3-year follow-up CT, the gastric varices remain disappeared.

lower pressure side in the varices.[13] In this situation, PTO of high-pressure afferent veins using coils or ethanol may aid the filling of sclerosing agent in the entire varices.[13,16] If a microcatheter reaches the varices via the route of PTO, a sclerosing agent or glue can be injected to obliterate the varices themselves. Another method is temporary balloon occlusion of the splenic artery during B-RTO to reduce pressure from the posterior and

short gastric veins (FIGURE 34.5).[32] Partial splenic embolization also can be applied to reduce the flow of the GR shunt.[33] Lastly, inhomogeneous distribution of sclerosing agent may result from the effect of gravity in the supine position. EOI tends to retain in the dorsal part of the varices, whereas foams in the ventral part. Change of body position may help the sclerosing agent to enter into the unfilled part of the varices.

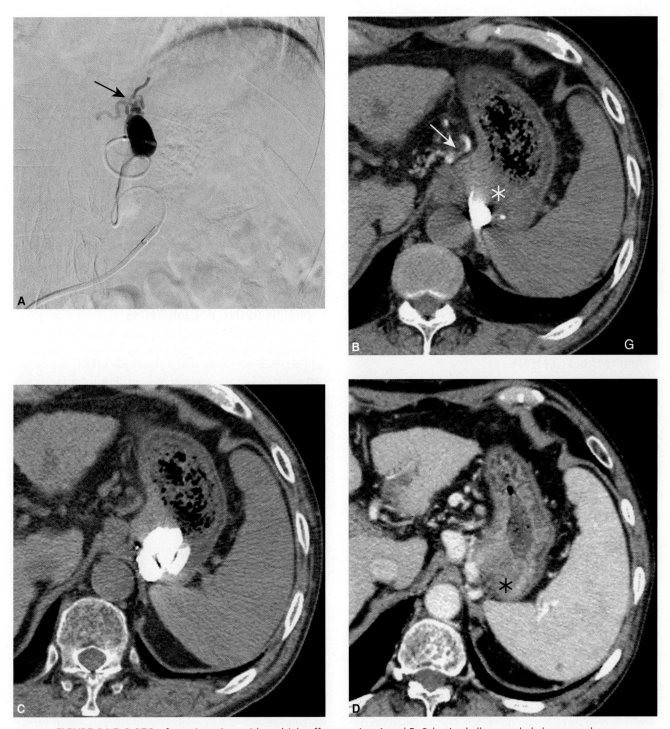

FIGURE 34.5 B-RTO of gastric varices with multiple afferent veins. **A** and **B.** Selective balloon-occluded venography as well as CT during the venography only shows a part of the GR shunt and the left gastric veins (*arrows*). Gastric varices (*) are not opacified because of the pressure gradient between the posterior or short gastric vein and the left gastric vein. **C.** Then CT during the venography under temporary balloon occlusion of the splenic artery shows the contrast media filling the entire varices. B-RTO was performed in this condition. **D.** Contrast-enhanced CT after 1 week confirms complete thrombosis of the varices (*).

ENDPOINT ASSESSMENT OF THE PROCEDURE

The endpoint of the procedure is sufficient stagnation of the sclerosing agent in the entire gastric varices to obtain complete thrombosis. To judge whether the varices are fully filled with the sclerosing agent, a CT or C-arm CT during the procedure is useful to monitor the distribution of 5% EOI (FIGURE 34.5C).[27] The balloon occlusion time to meet the endpoint is often unpredictable, however. In the first report by Kanagawa et al.,[6] the balloon was kept inflated for 30 minutes, but 22% of patients required additional sessions due to incomplete thrombosis. We normally leave the balloon inflated for 30 to 60 minutes, but if a residual flow remains, an additional dose of sclerosing agent is injected. Especially in patients with a large variceal cavity or severe thrombocytopenia, overnight balloon inflation is considered. Practically, shorter occlusion time would minimize the procedure time as well as patient strain but may increase the risk of pulmonary embolism due to the migration of unstable clots. Thrombosis of gastric varices depends on several factors including variceal size, local hemodynamics, and coagulation profiles. Further investigation will be necessary to optimize the balloon occlusion time.

PROCEDURAL COMPLICATIONS AND MANAGEMENT

Procedural complications are mainly related to the use of sclerosing agent. Hemoglobinuria is frequently seen due to hemolysis by 5% EOI. Haptoglobin (Green Cross, Osaka, Japan) 2,000 to 4,000 units is administered intravenously during the procedure to prevent acute renal failure.[34] The residual 5% EOI or hemolytic blood is withdrawn as much as possible before balloon deflation. Pulmonary edema, disseminated intravascular coagulopathy, and anaphylactic shock can also occur after use of EO.[11] The safe dose has been proposed as less than 0.6 mL/kg.[35] To avoid excessive use of 5% EOI, the coaxial balloon catheter or microcatheter is selectively advanced close to the varices, and 50% glucose solution or ethanol is complementarily used.[7,29] Injection of 5% EOI should be carefully monitored under X-ray fluoroscopy because overflow or reflux of the sclerosing agent will cause thrombosis in the adjacent portal or systemic veins.

Other technical complications include retroperitoneal bleeding caused by catheter injury, migration of coils or glues, and dislodgment or rupture of the balloon.[36] Catheters should be manipulated gently in thin and distended veins. Contrast media should be injected carefully by avoiding the catheter wedge to the vein wall. To avoid coil migration, oversized coils should be selected, although vein size may alter with its dilatation or collapse. During balloon inflation, the integrity of the balloon should be checked by X-ray fluoroscopy. If any balloon trouble occurs, because it can lead to serious pulmonary embolism, another balloon catheter should be repositioned immediately. Postprocedural side effects including pyrexia, abdominal pain, hemoglobinuria, nausea, and hypertension are mostly self-limiting or can be managed conservatively.

OUTCOMES AND PROGNOSIS

The clinical outcomes of B-RTO are summarized in Table 34.1. Technical success rates were 90% to 100%, and 78% to 100% of gastric varices showed complete thrombosis. Repeat B-RTO was necessary, however, until complete thrombosis was obtained in some studies. After successful B-RTO, 88% to 100% of the gastric varices were eradicated, and recurrence and rebleeding were seen in 0% to 7% and 0% to 6% of the gastric varices, respectively. Therefore, once the procedural success is achieved, variceal ablation with durable bleeding control can be highly expected. The 1-, 3- and 5-year survival rates ranged from 90% to 98%, 71% to 97%, and 39% to 82%, respectively. Some studies revealed Child-Pugh grade C and the coexistence of hepatocellular carcinoma (HCC) as the significant prognostic factors by multivariate analyses. As the secondary effects of B-RTO, Fukuda et al.[10] reported that the Child-Pugh score was improved in 50% at 6 months after B-RTO, and hepatic encephalopathy was normalized in all patients due to complete occlusion of the GR shunt. The same group also experienced the improvement of refractory ascites due to elevation of serum albumin.[37]

DISEASE SURVEILLANCE AND TREATMENT MONITORING ALGORITHMS

Contrast-enhanced CT 1 week after B-RTO is necessary to confirm complete thrombosis of gastric varices or to detect unintended thrombosis of the portal or systemic venous system. If a part of the varices remain enhanced, additional B-RTO should be considered. Once they show complete thrombosis, patients should be followed up to assess the morphologic change of the varices, hepatic function tests, and clinical symptoms every 1 to 3 months as the condition demands. Endoscopy is essential for assessment of the treatment response of gastric varices and to the aggravation of esophageal varices. At 1 week, the endoscopy typically shows a localized congestive mucosal change of the thrombosed varices resembling portal hypertensive gastropathy.[36]

EARLY AND LATE FAILURES AND MANAGEMENT

B-RTO fails when the balloon catheter cannot be placed in position due to the large size or tortuosity of the GR shunt. Other reasons for failure include incomplete thrombosis caused by the altered hemodynamics in the varices, shorter balloon occlusion time than necessary, and impaired clotting function.[10,15,18] B-RTO should be repeated when the initial follow-up CT reveals the incomplete thrombosis of the gastric varices. Thrombocytopenia or coagulopathy should be corrected prior to the procedure. Once B-RTO is successful, the concerns are mostly worsening of the esophageal varices and refractory ascites. Such adverse effects result from portal venous pressure increase by losing the dominant hepatofugal shunts by B-RTO. The reported incidence of worsening of esophageal varices was 0% to 50% at 3 to 5 years, although they often can be controlled by endoscopic interventions.[15,17] Preexisting esophageal varices, hepatofugal flow of the left gastric vein, and poor liver dysfunction are the significant predictive factors for worsening of esophageal varices.[8,15] Ascites can also increase after B-RTO due to the overload of the portal flow in patients with poor liver function, although they are usually manageable conservatively.[9]

Table 34.1

Clinical Outcomes of B-RTO for Gastric Varices

Author (year)	Indication	Technical success (%)	Complete thrombosis of GV (%)	Eradication of GV (%)	Recurrence of GV (%)	Bleeding of GV (%)	Survival rates	Risk factors
Fukuda et al. (2001)[10]	Bleeding control or prophylaxis	100 (45/45)[a]	100 (43/43)	100 (43/43)	7.0 (3/43)	NA	1 y 97.6%, 2 y 79.3%, 5 y 69%	CP-C
Takuma et al. (2005)[14]	Prophylaxis	100 (17/17)	82.4 (14/17)	88.2 (15/17)	NA	5.9 (1/17)	1 y 94%, 3 y 85%, 5 y 39%	NA
Ninoi et al. (2005)[15]	Bleeding control or prophylaxis	87.2 (82/94)	95 (78/82)	97.4 (76/78)	2.6 (2/78)	1.3 (1/78)	1 y 93%, 3 y 76%, 5 y 54%	HCC, CP-C
Arai et al. (2006)[16]	Bleeding control or prophylaxis	100 (75/75)	90.7 (68/75)	100 (75/75)	4.0 (3/75)	1.3 (1/75)	1 y 92%, 3 y 75%	NA
Hiraga et al. (2007)[17]	Bleeding control	91.2 (31/34)	91.2 (31/34)	96.8 (30/31)	0 (0/31)	0 (0/31)	1 y 90%, 3 y 75%, 5 y 68%, 7 y 55%	NA
Akahoshi et al. (2008)[18]	Bleeding control or prophylaxis	92.6 (63/68)	NA	96.8 (61/63)	NA	3.2 (2/63)	3 y 96.5%, 5 y 81.7%, 8 y 79.0%	HCC
Kasuga et al. (2010)[19]	Bleeding control or prophylaxis	100 (21/21)[a]	100 (21/21)	100 (21/21)	0 (21/21)	0 (21/21)	1 y 90.5%, 3 y 71.1%, 5 y 53.7%	None
Katoh et al. (2010)[20]	Bleeding control or prophylaxis	78.7 (37/47)[a]	78.1 (25/32)	NA	6.3 (2/32)	0 (0/32)	1 y 92%, 3 y 90%, 5 y 73%	NA
Maruyama et al. (2010)[21]	Bleeding control or prophylaxis	96.0 (94/98)	96.0 (94/98)	NA	0 (0/81)	0 (0/81)	1 y 90%, 3 y 74.8%, 5 y 52.7%, 7 y 45.8%	HCC, CP-B/C, GP-R ≥ 1.0

[a]Secondary success after repeating B-RTO.

NA, not applicable; GV, gastric varices; EV, esophageal varices; CP, Child-Pugh; HCC, preexisting hepatocellular carcinoma; GP-R, flow volume ratio of gastric vein and portal vein measured by ultrasound.

▌ PRACTICAL ADVANTAGES AND LIMITATIONS

Because it does not require needle puncture of the liver, B-RTO is less invasive than TIPS and PTO with the risk of liver injury or peritoneal bleeding.[7,10,18] B-RTO is a highly feasible procedure as long as there are dominant draining routes to place a balloon catheter. B-RTO can have secondary effects to improve liver function and hepatic encephalopathy as mentioned before. The technique of B-RTO can be applied not only to treat gastric varices but also bleeding from ectopic varices, such as those in the duodenum,[38] small intestines,[39] large intestines,[40] and around the stoma after a colostomy.[41] B-RTO can be technically difficult, however, when there is no draining route to access or when the GR shunt is too large to occlude by a balloon catheter. B-RTO also requires the use of specific balloon catheters and proper sclerosing agents.

▌ RELATIVE EFFECTIVENESS COMPARED TO OTHER TREATMENTS

There have been few studies comparing B-RTO with other treatments to treat gastric varices. B-RTO is often performed as a prophylactic or elective treatment, whereas endoscopic treatments and TIPS are rather rescue therapies for acute variceal bleeding. Additionally, treatment responses are different between gastroesophageal and isolated gastric varices, which are often mixed in studies. Therefore, treatment effects are difficult to compare among studies as long as indications and types of varices are inhomogeneous. One study of surgery showed a good result of gastric devascularization and splenectomy in well-compensated patients.[42] Eradication of gastric varices was obtained in all patients, and the cumulative recurrence and nonbleeding rates at 5 years were 0% and 100%, respectively. For acute gastric variceal bleeding, endoscopic interventions achieve initial hemostasis in 52% to 100% of patients, but the varices rebled in 23% to 53% of patients.[43–47] TIPS achieves initial hemostasis in 90% to 100% of patients; however, the varices rebleed in 7% to 31% of patients, which is often related to shunt occlusion. TIPS also induces hepatic encephalopathy in 17% to 36% of patients.[48–51] The varices tend to rebleed within the first year after both endoscopic interventions and TIPS. In a small randomized study comparing B-RTO and TIPS for acute gastric variceal bleeding, B-RTO was as effective as TIPS for immediate hemostasis, but the Child-Pugh score was significantly decreased in B-RTO.[52] These results suggest that B-RTO is more effective than TIPS to ablate gastric varices and reduce their rebleeding risk.

▪ THE FUTURE

B-RTO has not yet been popular in Western countries because TIPS has been widely performed instead, the practice guidelines do not yet support B-RTO,[4] there is concern about worsening of portal hypertension after B-RTO, and, finally, appropriate balloons and sclerosing agents are not always available. It might be difficult to conduct a randomized controlled trial comparing B-RTO with other interventions with endpoints of bleeding-free or overall survivals because survivals are also affected by progression of cirrhosis or coexisting HCC. If B-RTO and TIPS could be considered as complementary to each other, it will be necessary to clarify each of their indication and role to optimize treatment selection or even their combination.

▪ CONCLUSION

B-RTO effectively obliterates gastric varices and achieves long-term control or prevention of their bleeding. The success of B-RTO depends on proper patient selection and thorough evaluation of vascular anatomy and local hemodynamics around the varices. According to the change in local hemodynamics after B-RTO, liver function can be improved, whereas portal hypertension can be aggravated. Therefore, the benefits and risks of B-RTO should be carefully weighed based on each individual condition.

▪ REFERENCES

1. Sarin SK, Lahoti D, Saxena SP, et al. Prevalence, classification and natural history of gastric varices: a long-term follow-up study in 568 portal hypertension patients. *Hepatology* 1992;16:1343–1349.
2. Watanabe K, Kimura K, Matsutani S, et al. Portal hemodynamics in patients with gastric varices. A study in 230 patients with esophageal and/or gastric varices using portal vein catheterization. *Gastroenterology* 1988;95:434–440.
3. Sanyal AJ, Freedman AM, Luketic VA, et al. The natural history of portal hypertension after transjugular intrahepatic portosystemic shunts. *Gastroenterology* 1997;112:889–898.
4. Garcia-Tsao G, Sanyal AJ, Grace ND, et al. Prevention and management of gastroesophageal varices and variceal hemorrhage in cirrhosis. *Hepatology* 2007;46:922–938.
5. Olson E, Yune HY, Klatte EC. Transrenal-vein reflux ethanol sclerosis of gastroesophageal varices. *AJR Am J Roentgenol* 1984;143:627–628.
6. Kanagawa H, Mima S, Kouyama H, et al. Treatment of gastric fundal varices by balloon-occluded retrograde transvenous obliteration. *J Gastroenterol Hepatol* 1996;11:51–58.
7. Hirota S, Matsumoto S, Tomita M, et al. Retrograde transvenous obliteration of gastric varices. *Radiology* 1999;211:349–356.
8. Matsumoto A, Hamamoto N, Nomura T, et al. Balloon-occluded retrograde transvenous obliteration of high risk gastric fundal varices. *Am J Gastroenterol* 1999;94:643–649.
9. Kiyosue H, Matsumoto S, Onishi R, et al. Balloon-occluded retrograde transvenous obliteration (B-RTO) for gastric varices: therapeutic results and problems. *Nihon Igaku Hoshasen Gakkai Zasshi* 1999;59:12–19.
10. Fukuda T, Hirota S, Sugiura K, et al. Long-term results of balloon-occluded retrograde transvenous obliteration for the treatment of gastric varices and hepatic encephalopathy. *J Vasc Interv Radiol* 2001;12:327–336.
11. Kitamoto M, Imamura M, Kamada K, et al. Balloon-occluded retrograde transvenous obliteration of gastric fundal varices with hemorrhage. *AJR Am J Roentgenol* 2002;178:1167–1174.
12. Kiyosue H, Mori H, Matsumoto S, et al. Transcatheter obliteration of gastric varices: part 1, anatomic classification. *RadioGraphics* 2003;23:911–920.
13. Kiyosue H, Mori H, Matsumoto S, et al. Transcatheter obliteration of gastric varices: part 2, strategy and techniques based on hemodynamic features. *RadioGraphics* 2003;23:921–937.
14. Takuma Y, Nouso K, Makino Y, et al. Prophylactic balloon-occluded retrograde transvenous obliteration for gastric varices in compensated cirrhosis. *Clin Gastroenterol Hepatol* 2005;3:1245–1252.
15. Ninoi T, Nishida N, Kaminou T, et al. Balloon-occluded retrograde transvenous obliteration of gastric varices with gastrorenal shunt: long-term follow-up in 78 patients. *AJR Am J Roentgenol* 2005;184:1340–1346.
16. Arai H, Abe T, Takagi H, et al. Efficacy of balloon-occluded retrograde transvenous obliteration, percutaneous transhepatic obliteration and combined techniques for the management of gastric fundal varices. *World J Gastroenterol* 2006;12:3866–3873.
17. Hiraga N, Aikata H, Takaki S, et al. The long-term outcome of patients with bleeding gastric varices after balloon-occluded retrograde transvenous obliteration. *J Gastroenterol* 2007;42:663–672.
18. Akahoshi T, Hashizume M, Tomikawa M, et al. Long-term results of balloon-occluded retrograde transvenous obliteration for gastric variceal bleeding and risky gastric varices: a 10-year experience. *J Gastroenterol Hepatol* 2008;23:1702–1709.
19. Kasuga A, Mizumoto H, Matsutani S, et al. Portal hemodynamics and clinical outcomes of patients with gastric varices after balloon-occluded retrograde transvenous obliteration. *J Hepatobiliary Pancreat Sci* 2010;17:898–903.
20. Katoh K, Sone M, Hirose A, et al. Balloon-occluded retrograde transvenous obliteration for gastric varices: the relationship between the clinical outcome and gastrorenal shunt occlusion. *BMC Med Imaging* 2010;10:2.
21. Maruyama H, Okugawa H, Kobayashi S, et al. Pre-treatment hemodynamic features involved with long-term survival of cirrhotic patients after embolization of gastric fundal varices. *Eur J Radiol* 2010;75:e41–e45.
22. Kim T, Shijo H, Kokawa H, et al. Risk factors for hemorrhage from gastric fundal varices. *Hepatology* 1997;25:307–312.
23. Sarin SK, Agarwal SR. Gastric varices and portal hypertensive gastropathy. *Clin Liver Dis* 2001;5:727–767.
24. Sarin SK, Kumar A. Gastric varices: profile, classification, and management. *Am J Gastroenterol* 1989;84:1244–1249.
25. Chikamori F, Kuniyoshi N, Shibuya S, et al. Correlation between endoscopic and angiographic findings in patients with esophageal and isolated gastric varices. *Dig Surg* 2001;18:176–181.
26. Tanoue S, Kiyosue H, Matsumoto S, et al. Development of a new coaxial balloon catheter system for balloon-occluded retrograde transvenous obliteration (B-RTO). *Cardiovasc Intervent Radiol* 2006;29:991–996.
27. Koizumi J, Hashimoto T, Myojin K, et al. C-arm CT-guided foam sclerotherapy for the treatment of gastric varices. *J Vasc Interv Radiol* 2010;21:1583–1587.
28. Sabri SS, Swee W, Turba UC, et al. Bleeding gastric varices obliteration with balloon-occluded retrograde transvenous obliteration using sodium tetradecyl sulfate foam. *J Vasc Interv Radiol* 2011;22:309–316.
29. Yamagami T, Kato T, Hirota T, et al. Infusion of 50% glucose solution before injection of ethanolamine oleate during balloon-occluded retrograde transvenous obliteration. *Australas Radiol* 2007;51:334–338.

30. Willmann JK, Weishaupt D, Böhm T, et al. Detection of submucosal gastric fundal varices with multi-detector row CT angiography. *Gut* 2003;52:886–892.

31. Araki T, Hori M, Motosugi U, et al. Can balloon-occluded retrograde transvenous obliteration be performed for gastric varices without gastrorenal shunts? *J Vasc Interv Radiol* 2010;21:663–670.

32. Kiyosue H, Tanoue S, Kondo Y, et al. Balloon-occluded retrograde transvenous obliteration of complex gastric varices assisted by temporary balloon occlusion of the splenic artery. *J Vasc Interv Radiol* 2011;22:1045–1048.

33. Chikamori F, Kuniyoshi N, Kawashima T, et al. Gastric varices with gastrorenal shunt: combined therapy using transjugular retrograde obliteration and partial splenic embolization. *AJR Am J Roentgenol* 2008;191:555–559.

34. Miyoshi H, Ohshiba S, Matsumoto A, et al. Haptoglobin prevents renal dysfunction associated with intravariceal infusion of ethanolamine oleate. *Am J Gastroenterol* 1991;86:1638–1641.

35. Takase Y, Kikuchi M, Ozaki A, et al. Pathological studies on esophageal varices treated with injection sclerotherapy. *Jpn J Surg* 1985;15:30–35.

36. Shimoda R, Horiuchi K, Hagiwara S, et al. Short-term complications of retrograde transvenous obliteration of gastric varices in patients with portal hypertension: effects of obliteration of major portosystemic shunts. *Abdom Imaging* 2005;30:306–313.

37. Fukuda T, Hirota S, Matsumoto S, et al. Application of balloon-occluded retrograde transvenous obliteration to gastric varices complicating refractory ascites. *Cardiovasc Intervent Radiol* 2004;27:64–67.

38. Zamora CA, Sugimoto K, Tsurusaki M, et al. Endovascular obliteration of bleeding duodenal varices in patients with liver cirrhosis. *Eur Radiol* 2006;16:73–79.

39. Hashimoto N, Akahoshi T, Yoshida D, et al. The efficacy of balloon-occluded retrograde transvenous obliteration on small intestinal variceal bleeding. *Surgery* 2010;148:145–150.

40. Anan A, Irie M, Watanabe H, et al. Colonic varices treated by balloon-occluded retrograde transvenous obliteration in a cirrhotic patient with encephalopathy: a case report. *Gastrointest Endosc* 2006;63:880–884.

41. Minami S, Okada K, Matsuo M, et al. Treatment of bleeding stomal varices by balloon-occluded retrograde transvenous obliteration. *J Gastroenterol* 2007;42:91–95.

42. Tomikawa M, Hashizume M, Saku M, et al. Effectiveness of gastric devascularization and splenectomy for patients with gastric varices. *J Am Coll Surg* 2000;191:498–503.

43. Sarin SK. Long-term follow-up of gastric variceal sclerotherapy: an eleven-year experience. *Gastrointest Endosc* 1997;46:8–14.

44. Ogawa K, Ishikawa S, Naritaka Y, et al. Clinical evaluation of endoscopic injection sclerotherapy using n-butyl-2-cyanoacrylate for gastric variceal bleeding. *J Gastroenterol Hepatol* 1999;14:245–250.

45. Kind R, Guglielmi A, Rodella L, et al. Bucrylate treatment of bleeding gastric varices: 12 years' experience. *Endoscopy* 2000;32:512–519.

46. Huang YH, Yeh HZ, Chen GH, et al. Endoscopic treatment of bleeding gastric varices by N-butyl-2-cyanoacrylate (Histoacryl) injection: long-term efficacy and safety. *Gastrointest Endosc* 2000;52:160–167.

47. Akahoshi T, Hashizume M, Shimabukuro R, et al. Long-term results of endoscopic Histoacryl injection sclerotherapy for gastric variceal bleeding: a 10-year experience. *Surgery* 2002;131(suppl 1):S176–S181.

48. Stanley AJ, Jalan R, Ireland HM, et al. A comparison between gastric and oesophageal variceal haemorrhage treated with transjugular intrahepatic portosystemic stent shunt (TIPSS). *Aliment Pharmacol Ther* 1997;11:171–176.

49. Chau TN, Patch D, Chan YW, et al. "Salvage" transjugular intrahepatic portosystemic shunts: gastric fundal compared with esophageal variceal bleeding. *Gastroenterology* 1998;114:981–987.

50. Barange K, Peron JM, Imani K, et al. Transjugular intrahepatic portosystemic shunt in the treatment of refractory bleeding from ruptured gastric varices. *Hepatology* 1999;30:1139–1143.

51. Rees CJ, Nylander DL, Thompson NP, et al. Do gastric and oesophageal varices bleed at different portal pressures and is TIPS an effective treatment? *Liver* 2000;20:253–256.

52. Choi HY, Yoon CJ, Park JH, et al. Obliteration for gastric variceal bleeding: its feasibility compared with transjugular intrahepatic portosystemic shunt. *Korean J Radiol* 2003;4:109–116.

SECTION V

Arterial Occlusive Disease

Epidemiology, Pathophysiology and Natural History of Atherosclerotic Peripheral Vascular Disease

TODD S. PERLSTEIN and MARK A. CREAGER

The growing general awareness of the effects of cardiovascular diseases in the increasingly older global population is creating a sharper focus on the epidemiology, pathophysiology, and natural history of atherosclerotic peripheral (i.e., noncoronary) vascular disease (APVD). In the context of this chapter, APVD includes peripheral artery disease (PAD) of the extremities, mesenteric artery disease, renal artery disease, and extracranial carotid and vertebral artery disease.

▌ NOMENCLATURE

An American Heart Association Conference Proceedings recommended nomenclature for APVD (Table 35.1).[1] PAD refers to disease that affects the upper or lower extremities. Mesenteric artery disease refers to diseases of the celiac trunk, superior mesenteric artery, or inferior mesenteric artery. Renal artery disease refers to disease of the main renal arteries and extrarenal branches. Cerebral artery disease refers to disease of the extracranial cerebral and intracranial cerebral arteries. Aortic aneurysms are often associated with atherosclerosis but are not caused by atherosclerosis and are not included herewith. Nonatherosclerotic disorders that can cause peripheral vascular disease include dysplastic (fibromuscular dysplasia), inflammatory (arteritis), and thrombotic disorders.

▌ PATHOBIOLOGY OF ATHEROSCLEROSIS

Atherosclerosis is initiated by a qualitative change in the endothelium monolayer of the inner arterial surface (FIGURE 35.1).[2] In response to a physical or chemical stimulus (e.g., oxidized cholesterol, mechanical stress), endothelial cells express adhesion molecules that capture leukocytes on their surfaces. Concomitant changes in endothelial permeability and the extracellular matrix beneath the endothelium promote the entry and retention of cholesterol-containing particles in the artery wall.[3] Modified cholesterol particles undergo endocytosis by monocyte-derived macrophages that become resident foam cells. Other types of leukocytes accumulate in the developing atheroma but in far fewer number than macrophages. Smooth muscle cells migrate into the intima and proliferate. These produce extracellular matrix molecules, such as elastin and collagen, forming a fibrous cap over the atheromatous plaque. Cellular debris and extracellular lipids can accumulate within the plaque secondary to the inefficient clearance of dead cells, a process called efferocytosis.[4] The result is a lipid-rich pool at the core of the plaque.

Clinical manifestations of atherosclerotic vascular disease generally arise as a consequence of stenotic or occlusive lesions. Acute events most commonly occur due to rupture of a thin fibrous cap overlying the lipid-rich core and less commonly due to plaque erosion. The contents of the plaque's core are prothrombotic, and exposure of these to the bloodstream can result in thrombotic occlusion of the vessel or thromboembolism and occlusion of smaller downstream vessels. Chronic syndromes (e.g., intermittent claudication) typically result from progressive growth in the atherosclerotic plaque and the development of a flow-limiting stenosis. This is associated with loss of kinetic energy manifest as a pressure gradient across the stenosis and a fall of downstream perfusion pressure. The relationship between the residual radius of the artery, the pressure gradient, and flow is described by the Poiseuille equation that states:

$$\text{Pressure drop across stenosis} = \text{flow}\,[8L\eta] \div \pi r^4$$

Where L = length of stenosis, r = internal radius, and η = viscosity.[5]

From this equation it can be appreciated that a 50% reduction in vessel diameter results in a 16-fold increase in the pressure drop across a stenosis. The loss of laminar flow at high-flow velocities can exponentially increase the pressure drop across a stenosis. Thus, a 50% stenosis that is not hemodynamically significant at rest might result in significant drop in distal flow or pressure with exercise-induced high-flow velocity.[6]

▌ PERIPHERAL ARTERY DISEASE

Normal Anatomy

The arterial tree of the lower extremities begins with the bifurcation of the aorta into the right and left common iliac arteries. Each common iliac artery bifurcates into internal and external iliac arteries. The internal iliac arteries supply the pelvis. Each external iliac artery gives rise to a common femoral artery that bifurcates into the deep and superficial femoral arteries, the latter traversing the thigh and becoming the popliteal artery at the knee. Below the knee, the popliteal artery first gives off the anterior tibial artery and then the tibioperoneal trunk that bifurcates into the posterior tibial and peroneal arteries. The two tibial arteries continue into the foot, the anterior tibial artery as the dorsalis pedis artery, and communicate via the plantar arch, which then gives rise to the digital arteries.

The arterial tree of the right upper extremity normally begins with the brachiocephalic (innominate) artery arising as the first of the aortic arch branch vessels. This becomes the right subclavian artery after the takeoff of the right common carotid artery (CCA). The left subclavian artery is normally the third of the arch vessels. The right and left subclavian arteries course below the clavicle and continue on to become the axillary and then

Table 35.1

Major Vascular Terms

Recommended	Previous terms	Pathophysiology	Anatomy	Duration and severity	Comments
Vascular diseases		Diseases of arteries, veins, and lymphatics; includes atherosclerosis and nonatherosclerotic diseases	All vessels without anatomic designation	Acute to chronic; asymptomatic to severe	Broadest term to describe all vascular diseases: coronary, cerebral, peripheral, renal, and mesenteric artery occlusive disease, aneurysms, venous and lymphatic diseases
Atherosclerotic vascular diseases		Diseases of arteries caused by atherosclerosis	All vessels without anatomic designation	Acute to chronic; asymptomatic to severe	
Peripheral artery disease	Peripheral vascular disease, peripheral arterial disease, peripheral arterial occlusive disease, arteriosclerosis obliterans	Atherosclerosis, thrombosis, noncardiac emboli, inflammatory, etc.	Stenosis or occlusion of upper- or lower-extremity arteries	Acute to chronic; may be asymptomatic; symptoms and signs range from asymptomatic with functional limitations to intermittent claudication, rest pain, ulcers, and gangrene	Limited to artery disease; excludes renal, coronary cerebral, mesenteric, and aneurysms
Mesenteric artery disease	Visceral or mesenteric ischemia or angina, intestinal ischemia/angina	Atherosclerosis, thrombosis, emboli, extrinsic compression, vasculitis	Celiac trunk, superior mesenteric artery, inferior mesenteric artery	Acute to chronic; most patients are asymptomatic; symptoms include postprandial pain and weight loss	
Renal artery disease	Renal artery stenosis, renovascular disease	Atherosclerosis, thrombosis, emboli, arterial dysplasia	Main renal arteries and extrarenal branches	Acute to chronic, mild to severe	Associated with hypertension and/or renal insufficiency
Cerebral artery disease	Cerebral vascular disease (confused with cardiovascular disease); extracranial arterial occlusive disease	Atherosclerosis and nonatherosclerotic causes such as dissection, arterial dysplasia	Aortic arch to intracranial vessels	Acute and chronic; symptoms and signs of stroke and transient ischemic attack depend on affected territory	May be asymptomatic
Extracranial cerebral artery disease	Cervical carotid disease, vertebralbasilar insufficiency	Atherosclerosis and nonatherosclerotic causes as above	Aortic arch, carotid, vertebral, and extracranial vessels	As above	Excludes intracranial artery diseases
Intracranial cerebral artery disease		Atherosclerosis and nonatherosclerotic causes	Intracerebral vessels	As above	Excludes extracranial artery diseases (although may coexist)

From Hiatt WR, Goldstone J, Smith SC Jr, et al. Atherosclerotic Peripheral Vascular Disease Symposium II: nomenclature for vascular diseases. *Circulation* 2008;118:2826–2829.

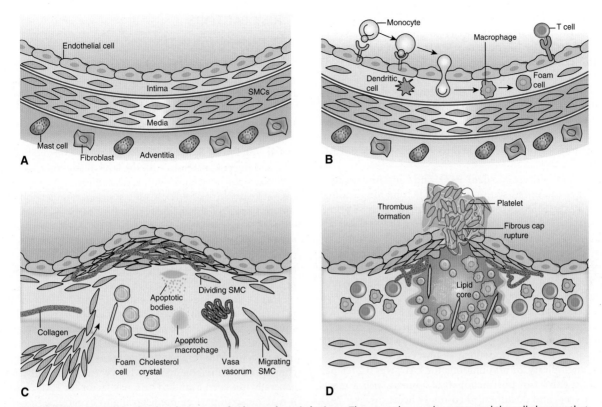

FIGURE 35.1 Stages in the development of atherosclerotic lesions. The normal muscular artery and the cell changes that occur during disease progression to thrombosis are shown. **A.** The normal artery contains three layers. The inner layer, the tunica intima, is lined by a monolayer of endothelial cells that is in contact with blood overlying a basement membrane. In contrast to many animal species used for atherosclerosis experiments, the human intima contains resident smooth muscle cells (SMCs). The middle layer, or tunica media, contains SMCs embedded in a complex extracellular matrix. Arteries affected by obstructive atherosclerosis generally have the structure of muscular arteries. The arteries often studied in experimental atherosclerosis are elastic arteries, which have clearly demarcated laminae in the tunica media, where layers of elastin lie between strata of SMCs. The adventitia, the outer layer of arteries, contains mast cells, nerve endings, and microvessels. **B.** The initial steps of atherosclerosis include adhesion of blood leukocytes to the activated endothelial monolayer, directed migration of the bound leukocytes into the intima, maturation of monocytes (the most numerous of the leukocytes recruited) into macrophages, and their uptake of lipid, yielding foam cells. **C.** Lesion progression involves the migration of SMCs from the media to the intima, the proliferation of resident intimal SMCs and media-derived SMCs, and the heightened synthesis of extracellular matrix macromolecules, such as collagen, elastin, and proteoglycans. Plaque macrophages and SMCs can die in advancing lesions, some by apoptosis. Extracellular lipid derived from dead and dying cells can accumulate in the central region of a plaque, often denoted the lipid or necrotic core. Advancing plaques also contain cholesterol crystals and microvessels. **D.** Thrombosis, the ultimate complication of atherosclerosis, often complicates a physical disruption of the atherosclerotic plaque. Shown is a fracture of the plaque's fibrous cap, which has enabled blood coagulation components to come into contact with tissue factors in the plaque's interior, triggering the thrombus that extends into the vessel lumen, where it can impede blood flow.

From Libby P, Ridker PM, Hansson GK. Progress and challenges in translating the biology of atherosclerosis. *Nature* 2011;473:317–325.

brachial arteries. The brachial artery bifurcates below the elbow into the radial and ulnar arteries. These continue to the hand and are connected by the superficial and deep palmar arches that give rise to the digital arteries.

Prevalence and Incidence of Lower Extremity PAD

Estimates of PAD prevalence come from ankle brachial index (ABI) screening programs. The ABI is calculated by dividing the higher of the posterior tibial and dorsalis pedis artery systolic pressure by the higher of the systolic pressures of the two upper extremities; a value less than or equal to 0.90 indicates a greater than or equal to 50% stenosis of the arterial tree of the affected limb.[7] An ABI less than or equal to 0.90 in either leg is diagnostic of PAD. In a 1999 to 2004 sample from the National Health and Nutrition Examination Survey, a cross-sectional cohort representative of the population of the United States, the estimated prevalence of PAD in those greater than or equal to 40 years was 5.9%, corresponding to approximately 7.1 million U.S. adults with PAD.[8] The prevalence of PAD increases somewhat exponentially with aging. As such, PAD is uncommon in those under 40 years of age, and its prevalence increases to greater than 25% in octogenarians.[9] The likelihood of PAD is also increased in populations at greater risk for atherosclerosis because PAD is most commonly caused by atherosclerotic vascular disease. For example, in a multicenter study conducted in primary care clinics across the United States examining adults considered at risk for PAD based on being either age 70 years or older or being age 50 through 69 years with a history of cigarette smoking or diabetes mellitus, the prevalence of PAD was 29%.[10]

Fewer data address incident PAD, and most prospective studies have examined symptomatic PAD. The longitudinal Limburg PA(O)D Study of 5,201 older (range, 48 to 85 years) adults selected from the general population in the Netherlands found an incidence rate of asymptomatic PAD of approximately 1% per year and symptomatic PAD of approximately 0.1% per year with women having a higher incidence rate than men.[11] In a cohort of Quebec men the incidence rate of symptomatic PAD increased progressively with age, being 0.07% in men ages 35 to 44 years, 0.3% in men ages 45 to 54 years, 0.7% in men ages 55 to 64 years, and 0.9% in men aged 65 years or more.[12] Among Medicare-eligible adults 65 years or older, the rate of incident PAD, defined as lower-extremity bypass surgery, angioplasty, or amputations for PAD, was 0.21% per year.[13] In a cohort of postmenopausal women with a mean age of 67 years and documented coronary heart disease, PAD events defined as revascularization or amputation occurred at a rate of approximately 1.4% per year.[14]

Prevalence and Incidence of Upper Extremity PAD

Upper extremity PAD is clinically less common than lower extremity PAD but may, in fact, have similar prevalence. A systolic blood pressure (SBP) difference of greater than or equal to 15 mm Hg has been considered diagnostic of upper extremity PAD, although differences of 10 and 20 mm Hg have also been used. The interarm SBP gradient will underestimate the prevalence of upper extremity PAD, however, because bilateral disease will not be detected, and the proximity of the cervical vessels allows for collateral circulation that may mask the subclavian disease. A systematic review of population studies only found four studies of sufficient quality to include in the analysis; it estimated the prevalence of an interarm SBP gradient greater than 10 mm Hg to be 19.6% and greater than 20 mm Hg to be 4.2%.[15] English and colleagues found the prevalence of angiographically defined proximal left subclavian stenosis to vary directly with cardiovascular risk factor burden and extent of vascular disease in other arterial beds.[16] For example, the prevalence of proximal left subclavian artery stenosis was 1.5% in persons at low cardiovascular risk, 6.8% in patients with diabetes, and 11.5% when lower extremity PAD was present. Gutierrez et al.[17] found an 18.7% prevalence of angiographically defined subclavian stenosis in a small cohort of patients with peripheral vascular disease referred for coronary angiography. Left-sided disease is approximately five times more common than right-sided disease.[17] To our knowledge, no study has examined incident upper extremity PAD.

■ RISK FACTORS

Risk Factors for PAD

The risk factors for PAD are generally the same as those for coronary heart disease. As such, the strongest risk factor is aging. Age of onset also affects the distribution of lesions in PAD because younger adults (<50 years) have been reported to have more proximal disease than older adults.[18] Among commonly considered cardiovascular risk factors, smoking appears uniquely associated with PAD.[19] Smoking confers a two- to fourfold increased risk, and the risk increases with the level of smoking.[20] Diabetes is also strongly associated with PAD, conferring a two- to fourfold increased risk of PAD. Insulin resistance, understood to be the root cause of the majority of type 2 diabetes, is associated with PAD independent of diabetes itself.[21] High total cholesterol increases the risk of PAD one- to twofold, and low high-density lipoprotein (HDL) cholesterol does the same. The total cholesterol-to-HDL cholesterol ratio may be the strongest lipid predictor of PAD risk.[22]

Hypertension is associated with a 1.5- to 2.2-fold increased risk of PAD. Although the magnitude of increased risk is relatively small, the high prevalence of hypertension makes it a significant contributor to the population burden of PAD. For example, 30% of the risk for symptomatic PAD in the Framingham cohort was considered attributable to stage II hypertension.[23] Obesity has generally not been found to be a risk factor for PAD; however, it may do so in part by predisposing to hypertension and diabetes mellitus. The association between alcohol and protection from PAD is inconsistent because alcohol intake and cigarette smoking are closely correlated, and failure to fully account for the latter might mask the protective effect of the former. Several studies have found that black race is associated with a higher risk for PAD than white race.[24–26] The relative risk for PAD attributed to black race compared with white race has ranged from 1.5 to 3.5. Non-Hispanic whites and Asians may have a lower prevalence of PAD than whites, but data are limited.[27,28] Circulating markers of inflammation including C-reactive protein (CRP) and fibrinogen demonstrate consistent associations with PAD. For example, an elevated CRP is associated with an approximately twofold increased risk of PAD.[29] Chronic kidney disease is a newly recognized risk factor for PAD with some estimates suggesting up to a fivefold increased risk, although the role of confounding from hypertension and diabetes is unclear.[13,30,31] Microalbuminuria alone, absent chronic kidney disease, is associated with a nearly threefold increased risk of PAD.[32] Chronic kidney disease is also associated with medial calcinosis, and the resultant noncompressible vessels might cause the ABI examination to underestimate the prevalence of PAD in patients with renal insufficiency.[33]

Risk Factors for Upper Extremity PAD

Less is known about risk factors for subclavian artery stenosis. In a study of 1,090 Japanese adults, aging, hypertension, obesity, elevated HgbA1c, and the presence of PAD were all associated with an interarm blood pressure gradient.[34] In an U.S.-based community cohort, smoking, higher blood pressure, and lower HDL were associated with subclavian artery stenosis. The presence of lower extremity PAD increased the risk of upper extremity PAD by fivefold.[35]

Lower Extremity PAD Clinical Syndromes and Pathophysiology

Asymptomatic Disease

Most patients with lower extremity PAD are asymptomatic, and the disease is therefore most often unrecognized. In such patients, diminished pulses or a femoral bruit may be noted on physical examination, or an imaging study might identify incidental arterial stenosis.[7] The recognition of PAD in asymptomatic individuals is potentially important because of the prognostic implications (reviewed later). It may be that the application of intensive medical therapy to persons with asymptomatic PAD identified by a screening examination and application of intensive prevention therapies could potentially reduce the risk for cardiovascular morbidity and mortality, but this has not been adequately addressed in clinical trials.[8,36]

Intermittent Claudication

Intermittent claudication is defined as exertional leg muscle discomfort relieved by rest and which does not occur at rest. Claudication can range in severity from mild to severely limiting. Claudication occurs when the metabolic demand of the exercising muscle is not met by the blood perfusion.[5] There are several determinants of the threshold at which symptoms of intermittent claudication occur. As reflected in the Poiseuille equation (discussed previously), the pressure drop across a stenosis is determined by the degree of stenosis (the radius), the length of the stenosis, the velocity of flow across the stenosis, and the blood viscosity. Collateral circulation can partially, but not fully, compensate for loss of native flow, and the adequacy of collateral formation varies widely between individuals. Vascular function, in part mediated by locally synthesized vasoactive factors, such as nitric oxide and prostacyclin, influences the ability to augment flow to the exercising muscle. Nonvascular structural changes in the limb, such as distal axonal denervation and skeletal muscle type II fiber loss, contribute to muscle weakness. Metabolic changes within the skeletal muscle, such as impaired mitochondrial function and reduced skeletal muscle glucose uptake secondary to insulin resistance, influence metabolic demand at a given workload. Finally, ischemia and ischemia-reperfusion injury contribute to excess oxidant production and impaired antioxidant defenses, leading to oxidative stress, which in turn adversely affects vascular, muscle, and metabolic function and propagates tissue injury.[5]

Atypical Leg Pain and Functional Disability

Patients with lower extremity PAD are more likely to have leg pain that is not typical of intermittent claudication than individuals without PAD. Factors that predispose to PAD may also be associated with sources of leg discomfort, such as degenerative arthritis or lumbar radiculopathy. Moreover, patients with PAD typically walk more slowly and for shorter distances before fatiguing, even in the absence of claudication.[37–39]

Critical Limb Ischemia

Critical limb ischemia (CLI) occurs when blood perfusion is inadequate at rest. Symptoms and signs of CLI include rest pain, pallor, paresthesias, poikilothermia (cold), and pulselessness. Dependent rubor, caused by resistance vessel vasodilation, may be evident. The pain of CLI is often improved by placing the limb in a dependent position, such as hanging the leg over the side of the bed. The skin of the affected limb is susceptible to ulceration and infection, and wound healing is greatly impaired. Ultimately tissue loss and gangrene set in.

The development of CLI typically depends on multiple levels of hemodynamically significant stenosis or occlusion. These might occur in series, such as aortoiliac and femoral-popliteal disease, or in parallel, such as superficial and deep femoral artery disease. These combinations of lesions impair the development of effective collateral circulation. When perfusion pressure falls below the level necessary to sustain basal tissue metabolism, tissue ischemia and necrosis result.

Acute Limb Ischemia

Acute limb ischemia (ALI) owing to an abrupt decrease in limb perfusion can be caused by embolism, in situ thrombosis, vasospasm (e.g., ergotism), arterial disruption or compression, or phlegmasia cerulea. The typical presentation is the abrupt onset of limb pain, pallor, and pulselessness. The prognosis of the affected limb is predicted by limb characteristics at presentation (Table 35.2).[40]

Upper Extremity PAD Syndromes and Pathophysiology

Asymptomatic

Atherosclerosis of the upper extremity is usually localized to the region of the subclavian artery.[41] The majority of patients with upper extremity PAD are asymptomatic.

Table 35.2

Clinical Categories of Acute Limb Ischemia

Grade	Category	Sensory loss	Motor deficit	Prognosis
I	Viable	None	None	No immediate threat
IIA	Marginally threatened	None or minimal (toes)	None	Salvageable if promptly treated
IIB	Immediately threatened	More than toes	Mild/moderate	Salvageable if promptly treated
III	Irreversible	Profound, anesthetic	Profound, paralysis (rigor)	Major tissue loss Amputation Permanent nerve damage inevitable

Adapted from Rutherford RB, Baker JD, Ernst C, et al. Recommended standards for reports dealing with lower extremity ischemia: revised version. *J Vasc Surg* 1997;26:517–538.

Arm Claudication/Ischemia

If the degree of stenosis is severe enough such that the affected limb does not maintain adequate perfusion pressure with activity or at rest, arm claudication or rest ischemia will ensue. Subclavian artery stenosis can also provoke or exacerbate preexisting Raynaud's phenomenon due to the decreased perfusion pressure of the hand.[42]

Vertebrobasilar Insufficiency and Subclavian Steal Syndrome

Atherosclerotic stenosis of the innominate/subclavian arteries occurs most commonly at or near their origin and therefore proximal to the takeoff of the vertebral arteries. This can present as dizziness, lightheadedness, imbalance, hearing loss, or tinnitus provoked by use of the arm, which causes reversal of flow in the ipsilateral vertebral artery.[43] Flow reversal in the vertebral artery caused by subclavian artery stenosis is referred to as subclavian steal.

Left Internal Mammary Artery Insufficiency

Stenosis of the left subclavian artery proximal to an "in situ" left internal mammary artery (LIMA) coronary artery bypass graft (CABG) can cause a coronary-subclavian steal syndrome. This has been reported in approximately 2.5% of patients referred for CABG surgery.[44,45] It can present as angina occurring after CABG surgery, which is provoked by left arm exertion.[46] Acute atherosclerotic proximal occlusion of the left subclavian artery has been reported to cause acute myocardial infarction in the setting of a prior "in situ" LIMA graft.[47]

Prognosis and Natural History of PAD

The severity of PAD progresses threefold more rapidly in the first year after diagnosis compared with later years. In an angiographic study of superficial femoral artery disease, 9.1% of patients per year had evidence of disease progression.[48] Several studies have examined the change in ABI among patients with PAD. One of these reported a fall in ABI of greater than 0.15 in 37% of patients over 5 years. A more rapid rate of progression, 50% decline in ABI over 4 years, was found in a group of smokers.[49] In a relatively recent study of patients referred to a vascular laboratory and followed for a mean of 4.6 years, ABI measurements indicated that 30% of limbs progressed to worse disease, but 23% of limbs regressed to less severe disease.[50]

The prognosis of patients with PAD, regardless of symptom status, is characterized by an increased risk of cardiovascular ischemic events compared with persons who do not have PAD. The prevalence of significant coronary artery disease in patients with PAD ranges from 30% to 80%, the higher estimates from coronary angiography.[51–55] An estimated 12% to 25% of patients with PAD have hemodynamically significant carotid artery stenosis, and the severity of PAD is directly correlated with the severity of carotid artery disease.[56–59] Coronary and cerebrovascular events exceed lower extremity ischemic events by approximately two- to fourfold in persons with PAD (FIGURE 35.2).

The burden of coexistent coronary and cerebrovascular disease results in high rates of myocardial infarction, stroke, and cardiovascular death. In a sample of 3,649 adults identified from general practice centers in the Netherlands in whom screening ABI examination was performed, there was an 8% per year

nonfatal cardiovascular event in patients with PAD compared with 1.5% per year in patients without PAD.[11] Cardiovascular mortality rates were 3.5% and 0.2% per year in patients with and without PAD, respectively. A recent report of screening ABI examination performed in community dwelling German adults greater than or equal to 65 years found that individuals with asymptomatic and symptomatic PAD had similarly increased cardiovascular event rates compared with persons without PAD.[60] The combined all-cause mortality and cardiovascular event rates were 2.7%, 6%, and 10% per year in patients without PAD, with asymptomatic PAD, and with symptomatic PAD, respectively. In a meta-analysis including 48,294 men and women from 16 population studies, the 10-year cardiovascular mortality risk in persons with a low ABI (≤0.90) was three to four times that of persons with a normal ABI (1.11 to 1.40).[61]

Prognosis and Natural History of Upper Extremity PAD

Little is known about the natural history and prognosis of upper extremity PAD. The majority of patients with subclavian artery stenosis or occlusion do not develop symptoms of arm ischemia or subclavian steal. In an ultrasound study of 67 patients with either subclavian artery stenosis or occlusion, there were 47 instances of stenosis detected at the baseline examination. Of these, six stenoses were no longer detectable and eight had progressed to occlusion at 2 years. No instances of arm ischemia were reported. One study reported that 54% of patients with symptomatic subclavian steal resolved their symptoms over 2 years without revascularization.[62,63]

Upper extremity PAD is associated with an increased risk of cardiovascular morbidity and mortality. In a cohort of 1,778 patients either from a vascular laboratory (1,248) or from the community (624), an interarm blood pressure gradient of greater than or equal to 15 mm Hg was associated with a 42% and 50% increased risk of all-cause and cardiovascular mortality, respectively, associations that persisted even after accounting for baseline cardiovascular disease or lower extremity PAD.[64] In addition, there was a graded relationship between severity of upper extremity PAD and mortality risk. The prognostic significance of upper extremity PAD was also studied in 423 male patients from a general medical or renal disease clinic. For every 10 mm Hg increase in the difference between arms, mortality increased 24%.[65]

■ CEREBROVASCULAR DISEASE

Normal Arterial Anatomy

The brachiocephalic (innominate), left CCA, and left subclavian arteries usually have separate origins from the aortic arch (FIGURE 35.3).[66] The right CCA most often arises from the brachiocephalic artery. The most common variant of this anatomy is a shared common origin of the brachiocephalic and left CCA. Less frequently the left CCA arises from the brachiocephalic artery. Least frequently, the three branch vessels share a common origin, and a bicarotid trunk gives rise to the carotid arteries. The distal CCA typically bifurcates into the internal and external carotid arteries at the level of the thyroid cartilage. The carotid bulb, a dilated portion at the origin of the internal carotid artery (ICA), usually extends approximately 2 cm; the ICA is more uniform after the bulb. The left vertebral artery normally originates from

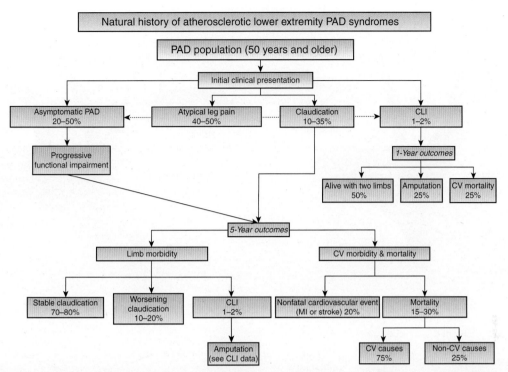

FIGURE 35.2 The natural history of atherosclerotic lower extremity PAD. Individuals with atherosclerotic lower extremity PAD may be: (a) asymptomatic (without identified ischemic leg symptoms, albeit with a functional impairment); (b) present with leg symptoms (classic claudication or atypical leg symptoms); or (c) present with CLI. All individuals with PAD face a risk of progressive limb ischemic symptoms as well as a high short-term cardiovascular ischemic event rate and increased mortality. These event rates are most clearly defined for individuals with claudication or CLI and less well defined for individuals with symptomatic PAD. PAD, peripheral artery disease; CLI, critical limb ischemia; CV, cardiovascular; MI, myocardial infarction.

Adapted from Hirsch AT, Haskal ZJ, Hertzer NR, et al. ACC/AHA 2005 Practice guidelines for the management of patients with peripheral arterial disease (lower extremity, renal, mesenteric, and abdominal aortic): a collaborative report from the American Association for Vascular Surgery/Society for Vascular Surgery, Society for Cardiovascular Angiography and Interventions, Society for Vascular Medicine and Biology, Society of Interventional Radiology, and the ACC/AHA Task Force on Practice Guidelines (Writing Committee to Develop Guidelines for the Management of Patients With Peripheral Arterial Disease): endorsed by the American Association of Cardiovascular and Pulmonary Rehabilitation; National Heart, Lung, and Blood Institute; Society for Vascular Nursing; TransAtlantic Inter-Society Consensus; and Vascular Disease Foundation. *Circulation* 2006;113:e463–e654.

the left subclavian artery, and the right vertebral artery from the right subclavian artery. The ICAs and vertebral arteries each connect to the circle of Willis, providing an extensive network of collateral support to the cerebral circulation. The anatomy of the circle of Willis is highly variable with fewer than 50% of individuals having a complete circle.

Prevalence, Incidence, and Risk Factors

Population surveys utilizing carotid artery duplex ultrasonography have found significant carotid stenosis in 5% to 7% of female and 7% to 9% of male adults aged greater than or equal to 65 years.[67,68] Approximately one-third of patients with an asymptomatic carotid bruit have a greater than or equal to 50% ICA stenosis.[69] The presence of an asymptomatic carotid bruit on physical examination is a weak predictor of cerebrovascular events. The proportion of stroke events attributable to carotid disease is somewhat difficult to define but is estimated to be 10% to 20%. Atherosclerotic plaques often develop at sites of

nonlaminar flow and, as such, there is a predilection for plaque formation at the carotid bifurcation. Stroke as a consequence of carotid artery atherosclerotic disease can result from (1) artery-to-artery embolism of thrombus formed on atherosclerotic plaque, (2) atheroembolism of cholesterol crystals or other atheromatous debris, (3) acute thrombotic occlusion resulting from plaque rupture, (4) structural disintegration of the arterial wall resulting from dissection or subintimal hematoma, and (5) reduced cerebral perfusion resulting from critical stenosis or occlusion.

Clinical Syndromes and Pathophysiology

Stroke is defined as an acute, irreversible neurologic injury caused by a disruption of blood flow. *Cerebral infarction*, analogous to myocardial infarction, has been adopted to reflect a tissue definition of an ischemic event.[70] The defining characteristic of cerebral infarction is imaging evidence of neurologic injury (i.e., brain, spinal cord, retina), similar to how cardiac

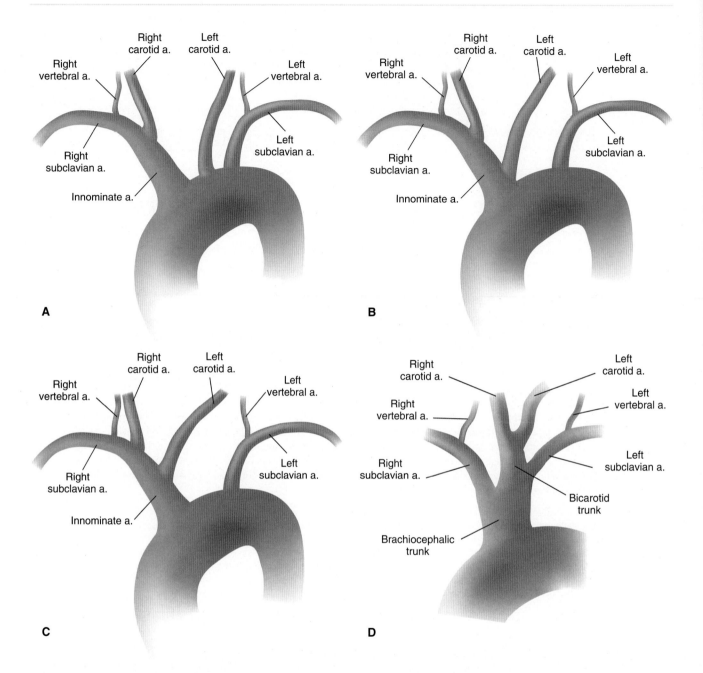

FIGURE 35.3 Aortic arch types. **A.** The most common aortic arch branching pattern found in humans has separate origins for the innominate, left common carotid, and left subclavian arteries. **B.** The second most common pattern of human aortic arch branching has a common origin for the innominate and left common carotid arteries. This pattern has erroneously been referred to as a "bovine arch." **C.** In this variant of aortic arch branching, the left common carotid artery originates separately from the innominate artery. This pattern has also been erroneously referred to as a "bovine arch." **D.** The aortic arch branching pattern found in cattle has a single brachiocephalic trunk originating from the aortic arch that eventually splits into the bilateral subclavian arteries and a bicarotid trunk. ("a" indicates artery.)

Reprinted with permission from Layton KF, Kallmes DF, Cloft HJ, et al. Bovine aortic arch variant in humans: clarification of a common misnomer. *AJNR Am J Neuroradiol* 2006;27:1541–1542.

biomarkers provide evidence of myocardial injury. Thus, a cerebral infarction can be symptomatic or asymptomatic, and a clinical event of transient neurologic symptoms but accompanied by imaging-defined neurologic injury is considered a cerebral infarction. It follows that the appropriate definition of transient ischemic attack (TIA) is a brief episode neurologic dysfunction caused by focal brain, spinal cord, or retinal ischemia without acute infarction.[71]

Acute ischemic cerebral syndrome is used to indicate that an active vascular process (e.g., unstable plaque) likely contributed to an acute ischemic stroke, and that there is a high risk of recurrence of stroke/TIA.[72] Advances in neuroimaging have allowed recognition that time criteria to define stroke events (e.g., TIA lasting <24 hours, reversible ischemic neurologic deficit [RIND] lasting <3 weeks, and completed stroke as lasting ≥3 weeks) are inaccurate in terms of identifying neurologic injury. For example, acute cerebral injury has been identified in 30% to 45% of cases with clinical symptoms lasting less than 24 hours.

ICA stenosis most commonly is recognized to cause acute ischemic events of the anterior circulation. The location and size of the infarct or focus of ischemia determines the specific neurologic deficit.[73] In a stroke affecting the territory of the carotid artery, unilateral signs predominate: weakness (hemiparesis) or paralysis (hemiplegia), loss of sensation (hemiasthenia), bilateral visual field loss (hemianopia), impairment of language (aphasia), and loss of ability to recognize objects, persons, sounds, shapes, or smells while the specific sense is not defective (agnosia) are the usual consequences. ICA disease can also cause retinal ischemia and/or infarction, presenting as amaurosis fugax or monocular blindness.

High-grade ICA stenosis or occlusion can be associated with watershed infarcts, or infarcts of the distal fields of two nonanastomosing arterial systems. Classic neuropathologic studies describe two distinct supratentorial watershed areas: (1) the cortical watershed between the cortical territories of the anterior cerebral artery (ACA), middle cerebral artery (MCA), and posterior cerebral artery (PCA); and (2) the internal watershed in the white matter along and slightly above the lateral ventricle, between the deep and the superficial arterial systems of the MCA, or between the superficial systems of the MCA and ACA.[74] The watershed areas are susceptible to ischemia due to their "distal field" situation, where cerebral perfusion pressure is lowest. Autopsy and imaging studies reveal that microemboli also are important contributors to watershed infarcts, particularly those of the cortical watershed. The typical presentation of watershed infarct includes episodic, fluctuating, or progressive weakness of the hand, occasionally associated with upper limb shaking, sometimes with the occurrence of syncope at the initial presentation, and often in the setting of a cardiac disturbance such as myocardial infarction or arrhythmia.[74–78]

Prognosis and Natural History of Carotid Artery Disease

In a cohort of 465 asymptomatic patients with 60% to 79% ICA stenosis identified by ultrasonography and followed between 1989 and 1994, 5%, 11%, and 20% of patients had progression to 80% to 99% stenosis over 1, 2, and 3 years, respectively.[79] The rate of TIA and stroke associated with asymptomatic significant carotid stenosis has fallen progressively over the last 25 years (FIGURE 35.4).[80] The most recently reported ipsilateral stroke event rates in patients with greater than or equal to 50% asymptomatic carotid stenosis was less than 1% per year.[80,81] Of note, many strokes that occur in the setting of high-grade asymptomatic carotid stenosis are not caused by the carotid disease. For example, in 1,820 patients with asymptomatic carotid artery stenosis of 60% to 99% severity and followed for 5 years, 45% of strokes were attributable to lacunes or cardioembolism.[82]

In contrast, symptomatic ICA stenosis presents a high risk of stroke. A TIA predicts a 13% stroke risk in the first 90 days after the event, a risk that is highest in the first week.[83,84] A reflection

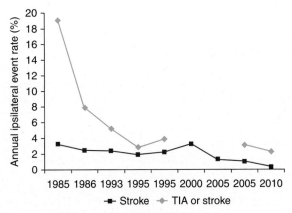

FIGURE 35.4 Risk of stroke attributable to asymptomatic high-grade internal carotid artery stenosis.

Data from Abbott AL. Medical (nonsurgical) intervention alone is now best for prevention of stroke associated with asymptomatic severe carotid stenosis: results of a systematic review and analysis. *Stroke* 2009;40:e573–e583, and Marquardt L, Geraghty OC, Mehta Z, et al. Low risk of ipsilateral stroke in patients with asymptomatic carotid stenosis on best medical treatment: a prospective, population-based study. *Stroke* 2009;41:e11–e17.

of the high early risk is that the benefit of carotid endarterectomy in patients with symptomatic ICA stenosis falls sharply after the first 2 weeks.[85]

The risk of nonstroke cardiovascular events and death in individuals with asymptomatic carotid artery stenosis is two to five times greater than that of stroke attributable to the carotid disease. For example, combining data from the Asymptomatic Carotid Atherosclerosis Study (ACAS) and the Asymptomatic Carotid Surgery Trial (ACST) trials, there were 53 stroke-related deaths and 285 nonstroke deaths in the deferral of carotid endarterectomy arms over 5 years of follow-up. The rate of stroke events is increased with greater degrees of carotid artery stenosis but so does the rate of cardiac ischemic events.[82,86] Progression of carotid artery stenosis on serial examinations also predicts increased risk for cerebral ischemic events, as do echolucency and heterogeneity of the carotid plaque.[79,87]

▌ MESENTERIC VASCULAR DISEASE
Normal Arterial Anatomy

The celiac trunk supplies the foregut, including the lower esophagus, the stomach, and the first two parts of the duodenum. The superior mesenteric artery supplies the third part of the duodenum, the entire small bowel, and the large bowel up to the splenic flexure. The inferior mesenteric artery supplies the descending colon, sigmoid colon, and the rectum. The intestine around the splenic flexure marks a watershed zone between the supply of the superior and inferior mesenteric arteries, an area that is susceptible to ischemia. The marginal artery of Drummond is the anastomotic connection between the colic branches of the superior mesenteric and inferior mesenteric arteries and is of great importance in protecting the colon from ischemia. The rectum also receives blood from branches of the internal iliac artery. Total mesenteric blood flow, regulated by the mesenteric arteriole, increases up to twofold in response to a meal to support digestion.

Epidemiology

The Prevalence and Incidence of Mesenteric Vascular Disease

The prevalence of mesenteric artery disease is not well defined. Autopsy studies have reported a prevalence of mesenteric artery stenosis ranging up to 80%.[88] In a cohort of male military veterans referred for abdominal aortography, 27% had greater than or equal to 50% stenosis in a mesenteric artery, including 50% of those with advanced renal artery stenoses. The only population-based study, utilizing ultrasound to examine the mesenteric vessels in 553 Cardiovascular Health Study participants, found the prevalence of any mesenteric stenosis to be 17.5%; only 1% of the cohort had at least two-vessel stenosis.[89] The mean age at presentation of chronic mesenteric ischemia is 68 years and is equally distributed between men and women.[90] Hypertension, diabetes mellitus, and chronic kidney disease are all associated with chronic mesenteric ischemia. Patients with chronic mesenteric ischemia typically have a history of other vascular disease.

Acute mesenteric ischemia can be caused by thrombosis or embolism of a mesenteric artery, mesenteric venous thrombosis, Nonocclusive mesenteric ischemia (NOMI), or by a variety of other causes. Retrospective studies support that age older than 50 years, congestive heart failure, cardiac arrhythmias, recent myocardial infarction, hypovolemia, hypotension, or sepsis predispose to acute mesenteric ischemia. NOMI is increasingly reported after dialysis and cardiac surgery.[91,92] Vasculitis and hypercoaguable states increase risk for acute mesenteric ischemia. It is important to recognize, however, that acute mesenteric ischemia has been reported in young patients without apparent predisposing factors.[93]

Clinical Syndromes and Pathophysiology

Acute Mesenteric Ischemia

The classic clinical presentation of acute mesenteric ischemia is the sudden onset of severe abdominal pain. Shortly after onset, the pain typically exceeds the physical findings. Within a few hours, however, the complications of perforation and/or peritonitis set in, leading to the examination findings of abdominal guarding, rebound tenderness, distention, and rigidity. Vomiting, diarrhea, and fever are variably present. The presenting symptoms in the elderly may be limited to mental status changes or tachycardia. A high-anion gap metabolic acidosis and leukocytosis are common, particularly later in the course.[94]

Emboli to the mesenteric vessels cause between one-third and one-half of cases of mesenteric ischemia. The most common origin of these emboli is the heart in the setting of arrhythmia, valvular disease, focal severe segmental left ventricular wall motion abnormality following a myocardial infarction, and severe global left ventricular dysfunction. The superior mesenteric artery is more commonly involved than the celiac artery and inferior mesenteric artery because the angle of its origin is least acute. Mesenteric arterial thrombosis accounts for 15% to 30% of cases of acute mesenteric ischemia. These often occur at the site of preexisting atherosclerotic stenosis. As such, most patients with acute mesenteric ischemia caused by arterial thrombosis have a history of chronic mesenteric ischemia. Venous thrombosis accounts for approximately 15% of cases of acute mesenteric ischemia and should be suspected in patients with a history of prior venous thrombosis, a history

of thrombophilia, or recent abdominal surgery. Nonocclusive mesenteric ischemia can occur in low-flow states, such as severe heart failure, and postdialysis, or it can be caused by vasoconstrictor stimuli, such as intravenous vasopressors, cocaine, or triptans.

Chronic Mesenteric Ischemia

Patients with chronic mesenteric ischemia usually present with abdominal angina, a clinical syndrome characterized by painful abdominal cramps and colic typically occurring during the postprandial phase.[95,96] Patients may suffer from ischemic gastropathy and enteropathy, a condition characterized by the fear of food, nausea, vomiting, diarrhea, symptoms of malabsorption, and unintended progressive weight loss (Table 35.3). Chronic mesenteric ischemia is most often considered the result of atherosclerotic disease compromising the blood flow of at least two of the three major mesenteric arteries.[97] That multivessel disease is usually necessary for chronic mesenteric ischemia and is supported by case series describing relief of symptoms by restoring patency of a single mesenteric vessel.[98–100] Single vessel disease, however, is increasingly recognized as a cause of chronic mesenteric ischemia.[101] Nonatherosclerotic causes of chronic mesenteric ischemia are listed in the Table 35.4.

Natural History

Chronic Mesenteric Ischemia

Few data address the natural history of mesenteric artery stenosis. One study reported the incidence of mesenteric ischemia among 60 patients referred for aortography and found to have greater than or equal to 50% stenosis of at least one mesenteric artery but no symptoms of intestinal ischemia.[96] Over a mean 2.6 years of follow-up, mesenteric ischemia developed in 4 of the 15 patients (27%) with significant three-vessel disease, and none of the other patients developed mesenteric ischemia. Wilson and colleagues[102] reported a 6½-year follow-up in a population-based sample of 553 elderly adults screened by duplex ultrasonography for the presence of mesenteric artery stenosis. The mortality rate (20.6%) in the subjects found to have mesenteric artery stenosis was not different from that of those without mesenteric artery stenosis (20.4%). Not all patients with chronic mesenteric ischemia require revascularization. In an analysis of 242 patients with chronic mesenteric ischemia pooled from three case series, 46% of patients did well with conservative management.[90]

Acute Mesenteric Ischemia

Acute mesenteric ischemia is an immediately life-threatening disorder. Acute mesenteric ischemia should be suspected in cases of acute onset severe abdominal pain that persists for more than 2 to 3 hours. In-hospital mortality rates are between 60% and 80%.[93] Outcome in acute mesenteric ischemia declines rapidly with delays in diagnosis, with intestinal viability in 100% of patients if the duration of symptoms is less than 12 hours, 56% if it is between 12 and 24 hours, and only 18% if symptoms are more than 24 hours in duration prior to diagnosis.[103] Several studies have reported improved survival if the diagnosis of acute mesenteric ischemia is made within 24 hours of symptom onset.[93] A strategy of early angiography and catheter-based intervention was found to reduce the mortality rate of NOMI from historical levels of 70% to 90% down to 55%. The recurrence rate of acute mesenteric ischemia is not well described, but patients should be

Table 35.3

Presenting Characteristics of Patients with Chronic Mesenteric Ishcemia

	Moawad et al. *Surg Clin North Am* 1997 $n = 330^a$	Mensink et al. *Br J Surg* 2006 $n = 107$	Silva et al. *J Am Coll Cardiol* 2006 $n = 59$	Kruger et al. *J Vasc Surg* 2007 $n = 39$
Weight loss	78%	78%	68%	95%
Abdominal pain	94%	NR	100%	NR
Postprandial abdominal pain	88%	86%	78%	90%
Exercise-induced abdominal pain	NR	43%	NR	NR
Abdominal bruit	63%	24%	NR	NR
Triad of "abdominal angina"[†]	NR	21%	NR	NR
Nausea/vomiting/fullness	33%	NR	22%	NR
Diarrhea/constipation	36/18%	NR	22%	41%
Hematochezia/lower gastrointestinal bleeding	NR	NR	8%	NR

^{a}A summary of cases reported in the literature up to 1997.
NR, not reported.
[†]abdominal bruit, postprandial pain, and weight loss
Data in table derived form: Moawad, J. and Gewertz BL. "Chronic mesenteric ischemia. Clinical presentation and diagnosis. "Surg Clin North Am, 1997, 77: 357–369; Mensink, P. B., et al. "Clinical significance of splanchnic artery stenosis. "Br J Surg, 2006; 93: 1377–1382; Silva, J. A., et al. "Endovascular therapy for chronic mesenteric ischemia. "J AM Coll Cardiol, 2006; 47: 944–950; Kruger, A. J., et al. "Open surgery for atherosclerotic chronic mesenteric ischemia. "J Vasc Surg, 2007; 46: 941–945.

considered at high risk for occurrence if an underlying condition, such as atrial fibrillation or hypercoaguable state, persists.[93]

RENAL ARTERY DISEASE

Normal Arterial Anatomy

The kidneys are paired, retroperitoneal organs. A single renal artery normally supplies each kidney, but accessory arteries are not uncommon. The main renal artery divides into the anterior and posterior main branches, the former supplying the lower

Table 35.4

Nonatherosclerotic Conditions Associated with Chronic Mesenteric Ischemia

Neurofibromatosis	Polyarteritis nodosa
Middle aortic syndrome	Cogan syndrome
Median arcuate ligament syndrome	Aortic coarctation repair
Visceral artery dissection	Radiation injury
Thromboangiitis obliterans	Thrombosis associated with Thoraco-abdominal aortic aneurysm repair
Connective tissue diseases	Mesenteric arteritis
Cocaine abuse	Congenital afibrinogenemia
Ergot poisoning	

pole, the apex, and upper and middle segments of the anterior surface of the kidney. The segmental arteries of the kidney are end arteries, meaning without collateral circulation, such that occlusion of a segmental artery will lead to occlusion of a focal segment of the kidney. The segmental arteries divide into interlobar arteries, which in turn divide into arcuate arteries at the level of the corticomedullary junction. These branch into interlobular arteries that give rise to the afferent arterioles. The glomeruli are drained by efferent arterioles of two types. Juxtamedullary glomeruli efferent arterioles give rise to capillaries that supply the outer and inner medulla in separate networks. Cortical efferent arterioles from superficial and midcortical glomeruli supply the peritubular capillaries of the cortex.

Epidemiology

Prevalence and Incidence

Renal artery disease is most commonly caused by atherosclerosis. Risk factors for renal artery disease are therefore those for atherosclerosis. Population-based data are scarce. In a series of 5,194 consecutive autopsies, 4.3% had renal artery stenosis. Medical records review revealed that only 7.3% of the cases of renal artery stenosis had been recognized, and only 73% had been diagnosed with hypertension, suggesting that a large proportion of renal artery stenosis is undiagnosed.[104] An analysis of the United States Medicare population suggested that the incidence of renal artery stenosis in the elderly is 3.7 per 1,000 patient years.[105] These same authors reported that the rate of diagnosis of atherosclerotic renal artery disease increased threefold in this population from 1992 to 2004.[106] A population-based study of 834 elderly adults screened by duplex ultrasonography found a prevalence of significant renal artery stenosis of 7%.[107] In a study of 1,554 hypertensive patients referred for renal angiography, a stenosis of greater than 60% was present in 15.1%.[108] In a group of hypertensive patients referred for renal angiography for either treatment-resistant hypertension or a rise in creatinine in response to angiotensin-converting enzyme therapy, renal artery stenosis was found in 41% and 46%, respectively.[109] Renovascular hypertension was diagnosed by angiography and renal vein sampling in 30% of patients with severe hypertension identified as grade III or IV hypertensive retinopathy.[110] Renal artery stenosis was detected by computed tomography in 41% of patients initiating renal replacement therapy.[111] Independent analyses of recent U.S. Renal Data System data found that the rate of atherosclerotic renal artery disease in patients initiating dialysis is increasing, notably increasing at a rate faster than end-stage renal disease (ESRD) caused by diabetes and ESRD overall.[112,113] In a pooled meta-analysis of 40 studies including 15,879 patients reported from 1966 through 2007, renal artery stenosis was found at angiography in 10.5% of patients referred for coronary angiography, 25.3% of patients with PAD, and 54.1% of patients with congestive heart failure.[114]

Clinical Syndromes and Pathophysiology

Asymptomatic

Atherosclerotic renal artery disease is most often identified in individuals with other atherosclerotic vascular disease. Hypertension and chronic kidney disease are highly prevalent among patients with atherosclerotic vascular disease, and it is often unclear whether an identified renal artery stenosis is contributing to or is coincident with those risk factors. Hypertension and renal insufficiency are clinically "silent" until end organ damage or uremia occurs. It is therefore impractical to categorize renal artery disease as asymptomatic or symptomatic. A proposed classification scheme that would help assess the probability that an individual patient is symptomatic from renal artery stenosis is the following[115,116]:

Grade 1: Renal artery stenosis is present, but there are no clinical manifestations (i.e., normotensive with normal renal function).

Grade II: Renal artery stenosis is present, but patients have medically controlled hypertension and normal renal function.

Grade III: Renal artery stenosis is present, and patients have evidence of abnormal renal function, medically refractory hypertension, or evidence of volume overload.

With this scheme, grade I patients would be truly asymptomatic, whereas grade III patients would be highly likely to be symptomatic from their renal artery stenosis. Grade II subjects would fall somewhere in between.

Renovascular Hypertension

Renovascular hypertension should be suspected in three clinical settings related to hypertension (Table 35.5). The first is the sudden onset of hypertension in a previously normotensive individual. This scenario is most likely to occur in younger adults because hypertension is highly prevalent among older adults. In this setting, renal artery stenosis caused by fibromuscular dysplasia is common.[117] The second is the sudden acceleration of preexisting hypertension, more likely to occur in an older hypertensive patient who acquires atherosclerotic renal artery disease. Finally, hypertensive patients who develop azotemia attributable

Table 35.5

Clinical Situations Where the Diagnosis of Renal Artery Disease Should Be Considered

Clinical presentation
- Onset of hypertension before the age of 30 y and after 55 y
- Hypertension with hypokalemia, in particular when receiving thiazide diuretics
- Hypertension and abdominal bruit
- Accelerated hypertension (sudden and persistent worsening of previously controlled hypertension)
- Resistant hypertension (failure of blood-pressure control despite full doses of an appropriate three-drug regimen including a diuretic)
- Malignant hypertension (hypertension with coexistent end-organ damage, i.e., acute renal failure, flash pulmonary edema, hypertensive left ventricular failure, aortic dissection, new visual or neurological disturbance, and/or advanced retinopathy)
- New azotemia or worsening renal function after the administration of an angiotensin-converting enzyme inhibitor or an angiotensin II receptor blocker
- Unexplained hypotrophic kidney
- Unexplained renal failure

From Tendera M, Aboyans V, Bartelink ML, et al. ESC guidelines on the diagnosis and treatment of peripheral artery diseases: document covering atherosclerotic disease of extracranial carotid and vertebral, mesenteric, renal, upper and lower extremity arteries: the Task Force on the Diagnosis and Treatment of Peripheral Artery Diseases of the European Society of Cardiology (ESC). *Eur Heart J* 2011;32(22):2851–2906.

to angiotensin-converting enzyme inhibitor (ACEI) or angiotensin receptor blocker (ARB) therapy have a high probability of bilateral renal artery stenosis or renal artery stenosis to a solitary functioning kidney.[118,119]

Goldblatt and colleagues demonstrated in 1934 that renal artery stenosis is sufficient to cause a persistent rise in blood pressure.[120,121] Their work demonstrated that the mechanism of hypertension in renal artery stenosis depends on whether or not there is an unaffected kidney. The "two-kidney" model—one clipped, the other intact—was the model of renovascular hypertension with renin excess as the driving force. The "one-kidney" model—one kidney clipped, the other removed—modeled renovascular hypertension with volume excess as the primary mechanism.[122,123] The latter model mimics bilateral renal artery stenosis. It is the ability of an unaffected kidney to excrete sodium in response to the excess blood pressure that defines the difference of these two types of renovascular hypertension. Typically, a 65% to 70% luminal stenosis is required before a fall in renal blood flow occurs. It is difficult to predict the hemodynamic consequences of a given renal artery stenosis because: (1) at high degrees of stenosis, small changes in diameter can result in marked changes in perfusion pressure; (2) turbulence, which can increase the pressure gradient across a stenosis, is influenced by the surface of the stenosis and therefore cannot be judged; and (3) the hemodynamic effect of a stenosis depends, in large part, on the peripheral resistance in the kidney.[119,124]

Renal blood flow is maintained over a wide range of perfusion pressure. At high pressures, a myogenic response increases renal vascular resistance. In the setting of low renal perfusion pressures secondary to stenosis, renal neurohormonal activation and tubuloglomerular feedback result in elevated systemic pressure and, therefore, preserved renal perfusion pressure.[125]

Ischemic Nephropathy

Ischemic nephropathy should be suspected in patients with renal dysfunction and (1) asymmetrical kidneys, with the smaller kidney corresponding to the side of stenosis, or (2) otherwise unexplained progressive renal dysfunction, or (3) azotemia during ACEI or ARB therapy.[119] The mechanisms of renal damage in renal artery stenosis are complex and are largely unrelated to renal hypoxia per se.[126] Increased levels of the components of the renin-angiotensin system, endothelin, thromboxane, and oxidative stress, coupled with reduction in nitric oxide and vasodilating prostaglandins, such as PGE$_2$, likely all contribute to the renal injury.[127] Tubulointerstitial injury is the most prominent pathologic feature and the best prognostic indicator in ischemic nephropathy.[127,128]

Recurrent Congestive Heart Failure and Flash Pulmonary Edema

Recurrent congestive heart failure and flash pulmonary edema not attributable to ischemic heart disease can result from bilateral renal artery stenosis or unilateral renal artery stenosis to a single functional kidney.[129] Flash pulmonary edema has been reported in 13% to 19% of patients referred for percutaneous renal artery intervention and responds to successful revascularization of the affected kidney(s).[130,131] The mechanisms underlying renal artery stenosis–associated flash pulmonary edema are unclear but may include activation of the renin-angiotensin system, impairment of renal sodium excretion, and lack of ACEI/ARB therapy caused by intolerance.[129]

Natural History

There are several facets to the natural history of renal artery disease: progression of stenosis, decline in renal function, and cardiovascular morbidity and mortality.[132] The pathophysiology of progressive renal artery stenosis is presented in FIGURE 35.5.

Progression of stenosis has been examined by angiographic and ultrasonographic studies. In a study from 1984, baseline and follow-up angiograms were obtained in 85 patients with renal artery stenosis who did not undergo revascularization; at a mean of 52 months, 37 (44%) had progressive stenosis and 14 (16%) developed occlusion.[133] In a more contemporary series of 1,189 patients who underwent coronary angiography including abdominal aortography and then a repeat procedure approximately 2.6 years later, 133 (11.1%) demonstrated progression of degree of renal artery stenosis.[134] Improvements in medical therapy are likely to account for the apparent reduction in disease progression. In a series of 79 patients with renal artery stenosis who underwent repeat angiography at a mean interval of 27.8 months, treatment with statin therapy was associated with approximately one-third the risk of disease progression (RR 0.28, 95% CI 0.10 to 0.77).[135] Using duplex ultrasound to characterize the renal arteries, a recent study reported a rate of anatomic progression of 9.1% over a mean of 34.4 months in hypertensive patients referred for ultrasonography.[136] A previous study found that the rate of progression from less than 60%

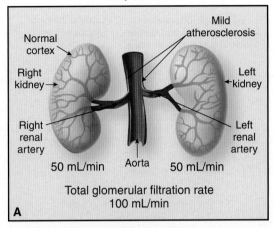

Early disease

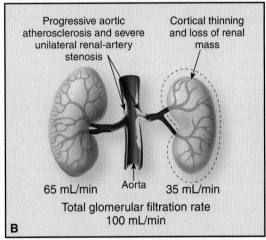

Progressive disease

FIGURE 35.5 Progressive atherosclerosis, renal-artery stenosis, and ischemic nephropathy. In the early phase (**A**), there is mild atherosclerosis of the perirenal abdominal aorta and normal renal function. Renal blood flow, renal mass, and the serum creatinine concentration are normal. The dimensions of the kidneys are normal, and there is no cortical atrophy. The total glomerular filtration rate (100 mL/min) and the glomerular filtration rate in each kidney (50 mL/min) are normal. As the disease progresses (**B**), there is progressive aortic atherosclerosis and severe unilateral renal-artery stenosis. The left kidney is smaller than the right kidney, and there may be cortical thinning and asymmetry in renal blood flow. The serum creatinine concentration remains normal as long as the right kidney is normal, despite the loss of renal mass. The total glomerular filtration rate may be normal (100 mL/min) or only slightly depressed owing to compensatory changes in the right kidney, but renal blood flow is decreased in the left kidney (35 mL/min). In advanced disease (**C**), there is bulky atherosclerotic plaque in the perirenal aorta and severe bilateral renal-artery stenosis. Both kidneys are small, and there is marked cortical thinning and irregularity. Loss of more than 50% of renal mass is usually associated with an elevation in the serum creatinine concentration (ischemic nephropathy), which may not be reversible. The total glomerular filtration rate (30 mL/min) and the glomerular filtration rate in each kidney (15 mL/min) are depressed.

From Safian RD, Textor SC. Renal-artery stenosis. *N Engl J Med* 2001;344: 431–442. *(continued)*

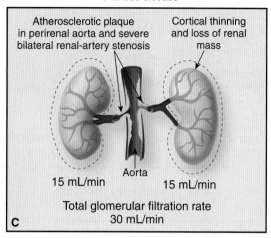

Advanced disease

Atherosclerotic plaque in perirenal aorta and severe bilateral renal-artery stenosis

Cortical thinning and loss of renal mass

Aorta

15 mL/min   15 mL/min

Total glomerular filtration rate
30 mL/min

C

FIGURE 35.5 (Continued)

to greater than or equal to 60% was 48%, and the rate of progression to occlusion from greater than or equal to 60% stenosis was 7% over 2 years.[137] Another duplex scan follow-up study found the 3-year incidence of renal artery disease progression for baseline disease categorized as normal, less than 60%, and greater than 60% was 18%, 28%, and 49%, respectively.[138]

Progression to renal failure over 2 years occurred in 2.7%, 17.6%, and 55.3% of patients with unilateral stenosis, bilateral stenosis, and unilateral occlusion plus contralateral occlusion or stenosis.[139] Over a 2-year period, renal atrophy, defined as a reduction in renal length of greater than 1 cm, occurred in 5.5%, 11.7%, and 20.8% of kidneys with a degree of renal artery stenosis categorized as normal, less than 60%, and greater than or equal to 60%, respectively.[140] In the Angioplasty and Stenting for Renal Artery Lesions (ASTRAL) trial of 806 patients with atherosclerotic renal artery stenosis and an estimated mean glomerular filtration rate of 40 mL/min who were randomized to either percutaneous revascularization plus medical therapy or medical therapy alone, the rate of progression to ESRD was 8% over 5 years in each treatment arm.[141]

Cardiovascular morbidity and mortality occurs at an accelerated rate in patients with atherosclerotic renal artery disease. An analysis of United States Medicare claims data suggests that elderly patients with atherosclerotic renal artery stenosis have a 4-fold increased risk of coronary heart disease, 5-fold increased risk of PAD, 3½-fold increased risk of heart failure, 3-fold increased risk of an acute ischemic cerebral syndrome, and a 2.6-fold increased risk of death compared with the general elderly population.[105] The aforementioned ASTRAL trial provides an estimate of cardiovascular event rates in patients with atherosclerotic renal artery stenosis on optimal medical therapy (e.g., 96% of patients were on statin therapy).[141] Over 5 years of follow-up, 27% of patients in that trial experienced a myocardial infarction, stroke, or death from cardiovascular causes. A combined endpoint of all cardiovascular events accrued a 50% event rate. Of 806 studied patients, 87 died of cardiovascular causes, yielding a 5-year cardiovascular mortality rate of 11%; the 5-year overall mortality rate was 26%. Thus, even with optimal medical therapy, patients with atherosclerotic renal artery stenosis are at high risk of cardiovascular morbidity and mortality.

The Cardiovascular Outcomes in Renal Atherosclerotic Lesions (CORAL) trial randomized patients with hypertension requiring two or more medications or stage 3 or higher chronic kidney disease and found to have one or more severe renal artery stenoses to optimal medical therapy or angioplasty plus stenting of the renal artery. This trial will provide additional information on current cardiovascular event rates in patients with renal artery stenosis and is testing whether percutaneous renal artery revascularization can modify those event rates.[142,143]

■ REFERENCES

1. Hiatt WR, Goldstone J, Smith SC Jr, et al. Atherosclerotic Peripheral Vascular Disease Symposium II: nomenclature for vascular diseases. *Circulation* 2008;118:2826–2829.
2. Libby P, Ridker PM, Hansson GK. Progress and challenges in translating the biology of atherosclerosis. *Nature* 2011;473:317–325.
3. Tabas I, Williams KJ, Boren J. Subendothelial lipoprotein retention as the initiating process in atherosclerosis: update and therapeutic implications. *Circulation* 2007;116:1832–1844.
4. Tabas I. Macrophage death and defective inflammation resolution in atherosclerosis. *Nat Rev Immunol* 2010;10:36–46.
5. Hiatt WR, Brass EP. Pathophysiology of intermittent claudication. In: Creager MA, Dzau V, Loscalzo CE, eds. *Vascular Medicine: A Companion to Braunwald's Heart Disease.* Philadelphia, PA: Saunders Elsevier; 2006.
6. Young DF, Cholvin NR, Kirkeeide RL, et al. Hemodynamics of arterial stenoses at elevated flow rates. *Circ Res* 1977;41:99–107.
7. Brott TG, Halperin JL, Abbara S, et al. 2011 ASA/ACCF/AHA/AANN/ AANS/ACR/ASNR/CNS/SAIP/ SCAI/SIR/SNIS/SVM/SVS guideline on the management of patients with extracranial carotid and vertebral artery disease: executive summary: a report of the American College of Cardiology Foundation/American Heart Association Task Force on Practice Guidelines, and the American Stroke Association, American Association of Neuroscience Nurses, American Association of Neurological Surgeons, American College of Radiology, American Society of Neuroradiology, Congress of Neurological Surgeons, Society of Atherosclerosis Imaging and Prevention, Society for Cardiovascular Angiography and Interventions, Society of Interventional Radiology, Society of NeuroInterventional Surgery, Society for Vascular Medicine, and Society for Vascular Surgery. *Vasc Med* 2011;16:35–77.
8. Pande RL, Perlstein TS, Beckman JA, et al. Secondary prevention and mortality in peripheral artery disease: National Health and Nutrition Examination Study, 1999 to 2004. *Circulation* 2011;124:17–23.
9. Hirsch AT, Haskal ZJ, Hertzer NR, et al. ACC/AHA 2005 Practice Guidelines for the management of patients with peripheral arterial disease (lower extremity, renal, mesenteric, and abdominal aortic): a collaborative report from the American Association for Vascular Surgery/Society for Vascular Surgery, Society for Cardiovascular Angiography and Interventions, Society for Vascular Medicine and Biology, Society of Interventional Radiology, and the ACC/AHA Task Force on Practice Guidelines (Writing Committee to Develop Guidelines for the Management of Patients With Peripheral Arterial Disease): endorsed by the American Association of Cardiovascular and Pulmonary Rehabilitation; National Heart, Lung, and Blood Institute; Society for Vascular Nursing; TransAtlantic Inter-Society Consensus; and Vascular Disease Foundation. *Circulation* 2006;113:e463–e654.
10. Hirsch AT, Criqui MH, Treat-Jacobson D, et al. Peripheral arterial disease detection, awareness, and treatment in primary care. *JAMA* 2001;286:1317–1324.
11. Hooi JD, Stoffers HE, Kester AD, et al. Peripheral arterial occlusive disease: prognostic value of signs, symptoms, and the ankle-brachial pressure index. *Med Decis Making* 2002;22:99–107.
12. Dagenais GR, Maurice S, Robitaille NM, et al. Intermittent claudication in Quebec men from 1974–1986: the Quebec Cardiovascular Study. *Clin Invest Med* 1991;14:93–100.
13. O'Hare AM, Rodriguez RA, Bacchetti P. Low ankle-brachial index associated with rise in creatinine level over time: results from the atherosclerosis risk in communities study. *Arch Intern Med* 2005;165:1481–1485.
14. Hsia J, Simon JA, Lin F, et al. Peripheral arterial disease in randomized trial of estrogen with progestin in women with coronary heart disease: the Heart and Estrogen/Progestin Replacement Study. *Circulation* 2000;102:2228–2232.

15. Clark CE, Campbell JL, Evans PH, et al. Prevalence and clinical implications of the inter-arm blood pressure difference: a systematic review. *J Hum Hypertens* 2006;20:923–931.

16. English JA, Carell ES, Guidera SA, et al. Angiographic prevalence and clinical predictors of left subclavian stenosis in patients undergoing diagnostic cardiac catheterization. *Catheter Cardiovasc Interv* 2001;54:8–11.

17. Gutierrez GR, Mahrer P, Aharonian V, et al. Prevalence of subclavian artery stenosis in patients with peripheral vascular disease. *Angiology* 2001;52:189–194.

18. Hansen ME, Valentine RJ, McIntire DD, et al. Age-related differences in the distribution of peripheral atherosclerosis: when is atherosclerosis truly premature? *Surgery* 1995;118:834–839.

19. Fowkes FG, Housley E, Riemersma RA, et al. Smoking, lipids, glucose intolerance, and blood pressure as risk factors for peripheral atherosclerosis compared with ischemic heart disease in the Edinburgh Artery Study. *Am J Epidemiol* 1992;135:331–340.

20. Kannel WB, Shurtleff D. The Framingham Study. Cigarettes and the development of intermittent claudication. *Geriatrics* 1973;28:61–68.

21. Pande RL, Perlstein TS, Beckman JA, et al. Association of insulin resistance and inflammation with peripheral arterial disease: the National Health and Nutrition Examination Survey, 1999 to 2004. *Circulation* 2008;118:33–41.

22. Pradhan AD, Shrivastava S, Cook NR, et al. Symptomatic peripheral arterial disease in women: nontraditional biomarkers of elevated risk. *Circulation* 2008;117:823–831.

23. Murabito JM, D'Agostino RB, Silbershatz H, et al. Intermittent claudication. A risk profile from The Framingham Heart Study. *Circulation* 1997;96:44–49.

24. Newman AB, Siscovick DS, Manolio TA, et al. Ankle-arm index as a marker of atherosclerosis in the Cardiovascular Health Study. Cardiovascular Heart Study (CHS) Collaborative Research Group. *Circulation* 1993;88:837–845.

25. McDermott MM, Fried L, Simonsick E, et al. Asymptomatic peripheral arterial disease is independently associated with impaired lower extremity functioning: the women's health and aging study. *Circulation* 2000;101:1007–1012.

26. Zheng ZJ, Sharrett AR, Chambless LE, et al. Associations of ankle-brachial index with clinical coronary heart disease, stroke and preclinical carotid and popliteal atherosclerosis: the Atherosclerosis Risk in Communities (ARIC) Study. *Atherosclerosis* 1997;131:115–125.

27. Curb JD, Masaki K, Rodriguez BL, et al. Peripheral artery disease and cardiovascular risk factors in the elderly. The Honolulu Heart Program. *Arterioscler Thromb Vasc Biol* 1996;16:1495–1500.

28. Perlstein TS, Pande RL, Beckman JA, et al. Serum total bilirubin level and prevalent lower-extremity peripheral arterial disease: National Health and Nutrition Examination Survey (NHANES) 1999 to 2004. *Arterioscler Thromb Vasc Biol* 2008;28:166–172.

29. Ridker PM, Stampfer MJ, Rifai N. Novel risk factors for systemic atherosclerosis: a comparison of C-reactive protein, fibrinogen, homocysteine, lipoprotein(a), and standard cholesterol screening as predictors of peripheral arterial disease. *JAMA* 2001;285:2481–2485.

30. Fried LF, Shlipak MG, Crump C, et al. Renal insufficiency as a predictor of cardiovascular outcomes and mortality in elderly individuals. *J Am Coll Cardiol* 2003;41:1364–1372.

31. O'Hare AM, Glidden DV, Fox CS, et al. High prevalence of peripheral arterial disease in persons with renal insufficiency: results from the National Health and Nutrition Examination Survey 1999–2000. *Circulation* 2004;109:320–323.

32. Baber U, Mann D, Shimbo D, et al. Combined role of reduced estimated glomerular filtration rate and microalbuminuria on the prevalence of peripheral arterial disease. *Am J Cardiol* 2009;104:1446–1451.

33. Leskinen Y, Salenius JP, Lehtimaki T, et al. The prevalence of peripheral arterial disease and medial arterial calcification in patients with chronic renal failure: requirements for diagnostics. *Am J Kidney Dis* 2002;40:472–479.

34. Kimura A, Hashimoto J, Watabe D, et al. Patient characteristics and factors associated with inter-arm difference of blood pressure measurements in a general population in Ohasama, Japan. *J Hypertens* 2004;22:2277–2283.

35. Shadman R, Criqui MH, Bundens WP, et al. Subclavian artery stenosis: prevalence, risk factors, and association with cardiovascular diseases. *J Am Coll Cardiol* 2004;44:618–623.

36. Perlstein TS, Creager MA. The ankle-brachial index as a biomarker of cardiovascular risk: it's not just about the legs. *Circulation* 2009;120:2033–2035.

37. McDermott MM, Greenland P, Liu K, et al. Leg symptoms in peripheral arterial disease: associated clinical characteristics and functional impairment. *JAMA* 2001;286:1599–1606.

38. McDermott MM, Mehta S, Liu K, et al. Leg symptoms, the ankle-brachial index, and walking ability in patients with peripheral arterial disease. *J Gen Intern Med* 1999;14:173–181.

39. Wang JC, Criqui MH, Denenberg JO, et al. Exertional leg pain in patients with and without peripheral arterial disease. *Circulation* 2005;112:3501–3508.

40. Rutherford RB, Baker JD, Ernst C, et al. Recommended standards for reports dealing with lower extremity ischemia: revised version. *J Vasc Surg* 1997;26:517–538.

41. Zimmerman NB. Occlusive vascular disorders of the upper extremity. *Hand Clin* 1993;9:139–150.

42. Creager MA, Perlstein TS, Halperin JL. Raynaud's Phenomenon. In: Creager MA, Beckman JA, Loscalzo J. Eds, *Vascular Medicine*, Elsevier, 2013: 587–599.

43. Psillas G, Kekes G, Constantinidis J, et al. Subclavian steal syndrome: neurotological manifestations. *Acta Otorhinolaryngol Ital* 2007;27:33–37.

44. Hwang HY, Kim JH, Lee W, et al. Left subclavian artery stenosis in coronary artery bypass: prevalence and revascularization strategies. *Ann Thorac Surg* 2010;89:1146–1150.

45. Prasad A, Varghese I, Roesle M, et al. Prevalence and treatment of proximal left subclavian artery stenosis in patients referred for coronary artery bypass surgery. *Int J Cardiol* 2009;133:109–111.

46. Angle JF, Matsumoto AH, McGraw JK, et al. Percutaneous angioplasty and stenting of left subclavian artery stenosis in patients with left internal mammary-coronary bypass grafts: clinical experience and long-term follow-up. *Vasc Endovascular Surg* 2003;37:89–97.

47. Barlis P, Brooks M, Hare DL, et al. Subclavian artery occlusion causing acute myocardial infarction in a patient with a left internal mammary artery graft. *Catheter Cardiovasc Interv* 2006;68:326–331.

48. Walsh DB, Gilbertson JJ, Zwolak RM, et al. The natural history of superficial femoral artery stenoses. *J Vasc Surg* 1991;14:299–304.

49. Nicoloff AD, Taylor LM Jr, Sexton GJ, et al. Relationship between site of initial symptoms and subsequent progression of disease in a prospective study of atherosclerosis progression in patients receiving long-term treatment for symptomatic peripheral arterial disease. *J Vasc Surg* 2002;35:38–46; discussion 46–47.

50. Bird CE, Criqui MH, Fronek A, et al. Quantitative and qualitative progression of peripheral arterial disease by non-invasive testing. *Vasc Med* 1999;4:15–21.

51. Mendelson G, Aronow WS, Ahn C. Prevalence of coronary artery disease, atherothrombotic brain infarction, and peripheral arterial disease: associated risk factors in older Hispanics in an academic hospital-based geriatrics practice. *J Am Geriatr Soc* 1998;46:481–483.

52. Dormandy J, Mahir M, Ascady G, et al. Fate of the patient with chronic leg ischaemia. A review article. *J Cardiovasc Surg* (Torino) 1989;30:50–57.

53. Valentine RJ, Grayburn PA, Eichhorn EJ, et al. Coronary artery disease is highly prevalent among patients with premature peripheral vascular disease. *J Vasc Surg* 1994;19:668–674.

54. A randomised, blinded, trial of clopidogrel versus aspirin in patients at risk of ischaemic events (CAPRIE). CAPRIE Steering Committee. *Lancet* 1996;348:1329–1339.

55. Golomb BA, Criqui MH, Budens W. Epidemiology. In: Creager MA, ed. *Management of Peripheral Arterial Disease*. London, UK: ReMEDICA Pub; 2000:1–18.

56. Klop RB, Eikelboom BC, Taks AC. Screening of the internal carotid arteries in patients with peripheral vascular disease by colour-flow duplex scanning. *Eur J Vasc Surg* 1991;5:41–45.

57. Alexandrova NA, Gibson WC, Norris JW, et al. Carotid artery stenosis in peripheral vascular disease. *J Vasc Surg* 1996;23:645–649.

58. Cheng SW, Wu LL, Ting AC, et al. Screening for asymptomatic carotid stenosis in patients with peripheral vascular disease: a prospective study and risk factor analysis. *Cardiovasc Surg* 1999;7:303–309.

59. Long TH, Criqui MH, Vasilevskis EE, et al. The correlation between the severity of peripheral arterial disease and carotid occlusive disease. *Vasc Med* 1999;4:135–142.

60. Diehm C, Allenberg JR, Pittrow D, et al. Mortality and vascular morbidity in older adults with asymptomatic versus symptomatic peripheral artery disease. *Circulation* 2009;120:2053–2061.

61. Fowkes FG, Murray GD, Butcher I, et al. Ankle brachial index combined with Framingham Risk Score to predict cardiovascular events and mortality: a meta-analysis. *JAMA* 2008;300:197–208.

62. Ackermann H, Diener HC, Dichgans J. Stenosis and occlusion of the subclavian artery: ultrasonographic and clinical findings. *J Neurol* 1987;234:396–400.

63. Ackermann H, Diener HC, Seboldt H, et al. Ultrasonographic follow-up of subclavian stenosis and occlusion: natural history and surgical treatment. *Stroke* 1988;19:431–435.

64. Aboyans V, Criqui MH, McDermott MM, et al. The vital prognosis of subclavian stenosis. *J Am Coll Cardiol* 2007;49:1540–1545.

65. Agarwal R, Bunaye Z, Bekele DM. Prognostic significance of between-arm blood pressure differences. *Hypertension* 2008;51:657–662.

66. Layton KF, Kallmes DF, Cloft HJ, et al. Bovine aortic arch variant in humans: clarification of a common misnomer. *AJNR Am J Neuroradiol* 2006;27:1541–1542.

67. Fine-Edelstein JS, Wolf PA, O'Leary DH, et al. Precursors of extracranial carotid atherosclerosis in the Framingham Study. *Neurology* 1994;44:1046–1050.

68. O'Leary DH, Polak JF, Kronmal RA, et al. Distribution and correlates of sonographically detected carotid artery disease in the Cardiovascular Health Study. The CHS Collaborative Research Group. *Stroke* 1992;23:1752–1760.

69. Johansson EP, Wester P. Carotid bruits as predictor for carotid stenoses detected by ultrasonography: an observational study. *BMC Neurol* 2008;8:23.

70. Saver JL. Proposal for a universal definition of cerebral infarction. *Stroke* 2008;39:3110–3115.

71. Easton JD, Saver JL, Albers GW, et al. Definition and evaluation of transient ischemic attack: a scientific statement for healthcare professionals from the American Heart Association/American Stroke Association Stroke Council; Council on Cardiovascular Surgery and Anesthesia; Council on Cardiovascular Radiology and Intervention; Council on Cardiovascular Nursing; and the Interdisciplinary Council on Peripheral Vascular Disease. The American Academy of Neurology affirms the value of this statement as an educational tool for neurologists. *Stroke* 2009;40:2276–2293.

72. Kidwell CS, Warach S. Acute ischemic cerebrovascular syndrome: diagnostic criteria. *Stroke* 2003;34:2995–2998.

73. Ropper AH, Samuels MA. Cerebrovascular diseases. In: Ropper AH, Samuels MA, eds. *Adams & Victor's Principles of Neurology*. 9th ed. New York, NY: McGraw-Hill; 2009.

74. Momjian-Mayor I, Baron JC. The pathophysiology of watershed infarction in internal carotid artery disease: review of cerebral perfusion studies. *Stroke* 2005;36:567–577.

75. Bladin CF, Chambers BR. Clinical features, pathogenesis, and computed tomographic characteristics of internal watershed infarction. *Stroke* 1993;24:1925–1932.

76. Bladin CF, Chambers BR. Frequency and pathogenesis of hemodynamic stroke. *Stroke* 1994;25:2179–2182.

77. Howard R, Trend P, Russell RW. Clinical features of ischemia in cerebral arterial border zones after periods of reduced cerebral blood flow. *Arch Neurol* 1987;44:934–940.

78. Yanagihara T, Sundt TM Jr, Piepgras DG. Weakness of the lower extremity in carotid occlusive disease. *Arch Neurol* 1988;45:297–301.

79. Olin JW, Fonseca C, Childs MB, et al. The natural history of asymptomatic moderate internal carotid artery stenosis by duplex ultrasound. *Vasc Med* 1998;3:101–108.

80. Abbott AL. Medical (nonsurgical) intervention alone is now best for prevention of stroke associated with asymptomatic severe carotid stenosis: results of a systematic review and analysis. *Stroke* 2009;40:e573–e583.

81. Marquardt L, Geraghty OC, Mehta Z, et al. Low risk of ipsilateral stroke in patients with asymptomatic carotid stenosis on best medical treatment: a prospective, population-based study. *Stroke* 2009;41:e11–e17.

82. Inzitari D, Eliasziw M, Gates P, et al. The causes and risk of stroke in patients with asymptomatic internal-carotid-artery stenosis. North American Symptomatic Carotid Endarterectomy Trial Collaborators. *N Engl J Med* 2000;342:1693–1700.

83. Lisabeth LD, Ireland JK, Risser JM, et al. Stroke risk after transient ischemic attack in a population-based setting. *Stroke* 2004;35:1842–1846.

84. Johnston SC, Rothwell PM, Nguyen-Huynh MN, et al. Validation and refinement of scores to predict very early stroke risk after transient ischaemic attack. *Lancet* 2007;369:283–292.

85. Rerkasem K, Rothwell PM. Carotid endarterectomy for symptomatic carotid stenosis. *Cochrane Database Syst Rev* 2011:CD001081.

86. Chambers BR, Norris JW. Outcome in patients with asymptomatic neck bruits. *N Engl J Med* 1986;315:860–865.

87. Coli S, Magnoni M, Sangiorgi G, et al. Contrast-enhanced ultrasound imaging of intraplaque neovascularization in carotid arteries: correlation with histology and plaque echogenicity. *J Am Coll Cardiol* 2008;52:223–230.

88. Reiner L, Rodriguez FL, Jimenez F, et al. Injection studies on mesenteric arterial circulation: III, occlusions without intestinal infarction. *Arch Pathol* 1962;73:461–472.

89. Hansen KJ, Wilson DB, Craven TE, et al. Mesenteric artery disease in the elderly. *J Vasc Surg* 2004;40:45–52.

90. Sreenarasimhaiah J. Diagnosis and management of intestinal ischaemic disorders. *BMJ* 2003;326:1372–1376.

91. Diamond SM, Emmett M, Henrich WL. Bowel infarction as a cause of death in dialysis patients. *JAMA* 1986;256:2545–2547.

92. Gennaro M, Ascer E, Matano R, et al. Acute mesenteric ischemia after cardiopulmonary bypass. *Am J Surg* 1993;166:231–236.

93. Brandt LJ, Boley SJ. AGA technical review on intestinal ischemia. American Gastrointestinal Association. *Gastroenterology* 2000;118:954–968.

94. Herbert GS, Steele SR. Acute and chronic mesenteric ischemia. *Surg Clin North Am* 2007;87:1115–1134, ix.

95. Zeller T, Rastan A, Sixt S. Chronic atherosclerotic mesenteric ischemia (CMI). *Vasc Med* 2010;15:333–338.

96. Thomas JH, Blake K, Pierce GE, et al. The clinical course of asymptomatic mesenteric arterial stenosis. *J Vasc Surg* 1998;27:840–844.

97. White CJ. Chronic mesenteric ischemia: diagnosis and management. *Prog Cardiovasc Dis* 2011;54:36–40.

98. Steinmetz E, Tatou E, Favier-Blavoux C, et al. Endovascular treatment as first choice in chronic intestinal ischemia. *Ann Vasc Surg* 2002;16:693–699.

99. Allen RC, Martin GH, Rees CR, et al. Mesenteric angioplasty in the treatment of chronic intestinal ischemia. *J Vasc Surg* 1996;24:415–421; discussion 21–23.

100. Hollier LH, Bernatz PE, Pairolero PC, et al. Surgical management of chronic intestinal ischemia: a reappraisal. *Surgery* 1981;90:940–946.

101. Mensink PB, Moons LM, Kuipers EJ. Chronic gastrointestinal ischaemia: shifting paradigms. *Gut* 2011;60:722–737.

102. Wilson DB, Mostafavi K, Craven TE, et al. Clinical course of mesenteric artery stenosis in elderly Americans. *Arch Intern Med* 2006;166:2095–2100.

103. Lobo Martinez E, Merono Carvajosa E, Sacco O, et al. Embolectomy in mesenteric ischemia [in Spanish]. *Rev Esp Enferm Dig* 1993;83:351–354.

104. Sawicki PT, Kaiser S, Heinemann L, et al. Prevalence of renal artery stenosis in diabetes mellitus—an autopsy study. *J Intern Med* 1991;229:489–492.

105. Kalra PA, Guo H, Kausz AT, et al. Atherosclerotic renovascular disease in United States patients aged 67 years or older: risk factors, revascularization, and prognosis. *Kidney Int* 2005;68:293–301.

106. Kalra PA, Guo H, Gilbertson DT, et al. Atherosclerotic renovascular disease in the United States. *Kidney Int* 2010;77:37–43.

107. Hansen KJ, Edwards MS, Craven TE, et al. Prevalence of renovascular disease in the elderly: a population-based study. *J Vasc Surg* 2002;36:443–451.

108. Kuczera P, Wloszczynska E, Adamczak M, et al. Frequency of renal artery stenosis and variants of renal vascularization in hypertensive patients: analysis of 1550 angiographies in one centre. *J Hum Hypertens* 2009;23:396–401.

109. van Jaarsveld BC, Krijnen P, Derkx FH, et al. Resistance to antihypertensive medication as predictor of renal artery stenosis: comparison of two drug regimens. *J Hum Hypertens* 2001;15:669–676.

110. Davis BA, Crook JE, Vestal RE, et al. Prevalence of renovascular hypertension in patients with grade III or IV hypertensive retinopathy. *N Engl J Med* 1979;301:1273–1276.

111. van Ampting JM, Penne EL, Beek FJ, et al. Prevalence of atherosclerotic renal artery stenosis in patients starting dialysis. *Nephrol Dial Transplant* 2003;18:1147–1151.

112. Fatica RA, Port FK, Young EW. Incidence trends and mortality in end-stage renal disease attributed to renovascular disease in the United States. *Am J Kidney Dis* 2001;37:1184–1190.

113. Guo H, Kalra PA, Gilbertson DT, et al. Atherosclerotic renovascular disease in older US patients starting dialysis, 1996 to 2001. *Circulation* 2007;115: 50–58.

114. de Mast Q, Beutler JJ. The prevalence of atherosclerotic renal artery stenosis in risk groups: a systematic literature review. *J Hypertens* 2009;27: 1333–1340.

115. Rocha-Singh KJ, Eisenhauer AC, Textor SC, et al. Atherosclerotic Peripheral Vascular Disease Symposium II: intervention for renal artery disease. *Circulation* 2008;118:2873–2778.

116. Creager MA, White CJ, Hiatt WR, et al. Atherosclerotic Peripheral Vascular Disease Symposium II: executive summary. *Circulation* 2008;118: 2811–2825.

117. Slovut DP, Olin JW. Fibromuscular dysplasia. *N Engl J Med* 2004;350: 1862–1871.
118. Textor SC, Tarazi RC, Novick AC, et al. Regulation of renal hemodynamics and glomerular filtration in patients with renovascular hypertension during converting enzyme inhibition with captopril. *Am J Med* 1984;76:29–37.
119. Fisher JEE, Olin JW. Renal artery stenosis: clinical evaluation. In: Creager MA, Dzau VJ, Loscalzo J, eds. *Vascular Medicine: A Companion to Braunwald's Heart Disease.* Philadelphia, PA: Saunders Elsevier; 2005: 335–347.
120. Goldblatt H, Lynch J, Hanzal RF, et al. Studies on experimental hypertension : I. The production of persistent elevation of systolic blood pressure by means of renal ischemia. *J Exp Med* 1934;59:347–379.
121. Gollan F, Richardson E, Goldblatt H. Hypertension in the systemic blood of animals with experimental renal hypertension. *J Exp Med* 1948;88:389–400.
122. Kaplan NM. The Goldblatt memorial lecture. Part II: the role of the kidney in hypertension. *Hypertension* 1979;1:456–461.
123. Goldblatt H. The renal origin of hypertension. *Physiol Rev* 1947;27: 120–165.
124. Pemsel HK, Thermann M. The haemodynamic effects of renal artery stenosis (author's transl) [in German]. *Rofo* 1978;129:189–192.
125. Textor SC, Smith-Powell L. Post-stenotic arterial pressures, renal haemodynamics and sodium excretion during graded pressure reduction in conscious rats with one- and two-kidney coarctation hypertension. *J Hypertens* 1988;6:311–319.
126. Wiecek A, Kokot F, Kuczera M, et al. Plasma erythropoietin concentrations in renal venous blood of patients with unilateral renovascular hypertension. *Nephrol Dial Transplant* 1992;7:221–224.
127. Textor SC, Lerman LO. Renal artery disease: pathophysiology. In: Creager M, Dzau VJ, Loscalzo J, eds. *Vascular Medicine: A Companion to Braunwald's Heart Disease.* Philadelphia, PA: Saunders Elsevier; 2006:323–334.
128. Wright JR, Duggal A, Thomas R, et al. Clinicopathological correlation in biopsy-proven atherosclerotic nephropathy: implications for renal functional outcome in atherosclerotic renovascular disease. *Nephrol Dial Transplant* 2001;16:765–770.
129. Pickering TG, Herman L, Devereux RB, et al. Recurrent pulmonary oedema in hypertension due to bilateral renal artery stenosis: treatment by angioplasty or surgical revascularisation. *Lancet* 1988;2:551–552.
130. Gray BH, Olin JW, Childs MB, et al. Clinical benefit of renal artery angioplasty with stenting for the control of recurrent and refractory congestive heart failure. *Vasc Med* 2002;7:275–279.
131. Pelta A, Andersen UB, Just S, et al. Flash pulmonary edema in patients with renal artery stenosis—the Pickering syndrome. *Blood Press* 2010;20:15–19.
132. Safian RD, Textor SC. Renal-artery stenosis. *N Engl J Med* 2001;344: 431–442.
133. Schreiber MJ, Pohl MA, Novick AC. The natural history of atherosclerotic and fibrous renal artery disease. *Urol Clin North Am* 1984;11:383–392.
134. Crowley JJ, Santos RM, Peter RH, et al. Progression of renal artery stenosis in patients undergoing cardiac catheterization. *Am Heart J* 1998;136: 913–918.
135. Cheung CM, Patel A, Shaheen N, et al. The effects of statins on the progression of atherosclerotic renovascular disease. *Nephron Clin Pract* 2007;107:c35–c42.
136. Davis RP, Pearce JD, Craven TE, et al. Atherosclerotic renovascular disease among hypertensive adults. *J Vasc Surg* 2009;50:564–570, 571.e1–e3; discussion 71.
137. Zierler RE, Bergelin RO, Davidson RC, et al. A prospective study of disease progression in patients with atherosclerotic renal artery stenosis. *Am J Hypertens* 1996;9:1055–1061.
138. Caps MT, Perissinotto C, Zierler RE, et al. Prospective study of atherosclerotic disease progression in the renal artery. *Circulation* 1998;98:2866–2872.
139. Connolly JO, Higgins RM, Walters HL, et al. Presentation, clinical features and outcome in different patterns of atherosclerotic renovascular disease. *Q J Med* 1994;87:413–421.
140. Caps MT, Zierler RE, Polissar NL, et al. Risk of atrophy in kidneys with atherosclerotic renal artery stenosis. *Kidney Int* 1998;53:735–742.
141. Wheatley K, Ives N, Gray R, et al. Revascularization versus medical therapy for renal-artery stenosis. *N Engl J Med* 2009;361:1953–1962.
142. Cooper CJ, Murphy TP, Matsumoto A, et al. Stent revascularization for the prevention of cardiovascular and renal events among patients with renal artery stenosis and systolic hypertension: rationale and design of the CORAL trial. *Am Heart J* 2006;152:59–66.
143. Murphy TP, Cooper CJ, Dworkin LD, et al. The Cardiovascular Outcomes with Renal Atherosclerotic Lesions (CORAL) Study: rationale and methods. *J Vasc Interv Radiol* 2005;16:1295–1300.
144. Tendera M, Aboyans V, Bartelink ML, et al. ESC guidelines on the diagnosis and treatment of peripheral artery diseases: document covering atherosclerotic disease of extracranial carotid and vertebral, mesenteric, renal, upper and lower extremity arteries: the Task Force on the Diagnosis and Treatment of Peripheral Artery Diseases of the European Society of Cardiology (ESC). *Eur Heart J* 2011;32(22):2851–2906.

IDO WEINBERG and MICHAEL R. JAFF

CHAPTER

36 Diagnostic Noninvasive Evaluations: Ultrasound and Hemodynamic Studies

▌ INTRODUCTION

Noninvasive vascular imaging has made giant strides over the past decades. The potential for high-quality imaging without the risk of invasive procedures renders these tests the first line in the diagnostic algorithm for patients with vascular disease. Judicious use of noninvasive vascular imaging, coupled with excellent history taking and comprehensive physical examination, will aid clinicians both in diagnosing and establishing treatment pathways for their patients with noncardiac vascular diseases.

▌ THE BASICS OF ULTRASOUND

Introduction

This section focuses on basic ultrasound principles. Duplex ultrasound offers a combination of two-dimensional gray scale imaging of vascular structures, color-coding of blood flow, and Doppler-derived velocity and direction. Correct clinical interpretation and use of ultrasound technology mandates first understanding its basic principles.

Ultrasound utilizes the reflection of high-frequency sound waves from various structures to create a two-dimensional image of these structures (this is called *B-mode*, or brightness mode). The Doppler effect is used to measure movement in a sampled volume, such as that of blood flow.

Measuring Velocity—The Doppler Effect

When sound waves reflect off a moving object, the frequency of the reflected wave is deferent than that of the transmitted one. This is called a *frequency shift* and is known as the *Doppler effect*. In audible terms, this phenomenon may be encountered while observing a moving car passing by a stationary observer. As the car nears and then passes, the pitch (or rather, frequency) of its engine sound seems to change. This change is known as the *Doppler shift frequency*:

$$f_d = f_t - f_r$$
f_d = Frequency shift; f_t = Transmitted frequency;
f_r = Received frequency

According to the Doppler effect, the frequency shift correlates to the relative movement (or velocity) between two objects:

$$f_d = 2f_t{}^* v/c$$
v = Relative speed between objects; c = Speed of sound

In medical applications, the practical meaning of this formula is that the velocity by which blood flow correlates to changes in the sound frequency. This can be represented as audible sounds or visual outputs that reflect blood velocity.

When measuring velocity of an angular object, such as blood flow through a blood vessel, the angle between the transducer and the direction of flow needs to be incorporated into the formula:

$$f_d = 2f_t{}^* \cos\theta{}^* v/c$$
θ = the angle between the ultrasound beam
and the direction of flow

The measuring angle should be 60 degrees or less due to several factors:

1. At an angle below 60 degrees the ultrasound beam scatter from the vessel walls increases, making it less efficient.
2. Angles above 60 degrees are not recommended because small errors in angle measurement may result in large errors in velocity estimation due to the dependency on the cosine in the equation.

Practically, an angle of 60 degrees is used most often because it is the easiest to accomplish and most reproducible between observers.

Ultrasound Technology

Medical ultrasound transducers emit high-frequency sound waves that are produced by *piezoelectric* materials. When subjected to electric currents, piezoelectric materials (crystals) vibrate at a rate that corresponds to the electric current frequency.

Thus, when subjected to a high-frequency electrical current, high-frequency vibrations take place and these in turn produce high-pitched sound waves emitted from the crystals. Higher-frequency transducers tend to produce a more defined image, whereas lower-frequency transducers penetrate deeper into tissue while sacrificing image quality.

Pulsed wave (PW) Doppler systems transmit ultrasound waves in pulses. The number of such pulses transmitted per second is known as the *pulse repetition frequency (PRF)*. A PRF of 1 KHz would mean 1,000 cycles per second. Sound waves need to travel to the selected tissue and back before a new pulse can be triggered; otherwise two pulses will overlap. That is why the PRF limits the highest velocity that can be measured. If blood flows at a velocity too high for a certain PRF, an artifact known as *aliasing* occurs (FIGURE 36.1).

Spectral waveform analysis—Blood flowing through a blood vessel has a velocity but also a mass. The more the number of blood cells flowing through a measured area, the stronger the signal amplitude picked up by the detector. Modern ultrasound machines analyze these waveforms and conveys the information to the observer in a graphic format, where the velocity is on the *y*-axis, time is on the *x*-axis, and the intensity of shades of gray depict the volume of flowing blood (FIGURE 36.2).

As opposed to spectral waveform analysis, *color flow* is an imaging tool that presents frequency shift estimates (as opposed to accurate measurements) in real time and in color. This allows for an area of flow to be rapidly identified. Flow direction and velocity are depicted as color hue and intensity, typically on a spectrum of red and blue. Modern duplex ultrasound equipment, however, allows the technologist to alter the color "map."

Together with its obvious advantages, duplex ultrasonography (DUS) has some limitations that should be appreciated when interpreting vascular duplex scanning. These are shown in Table 36.1.

To summarize, DUS is a method that combines two-dimensional imaging of structures with color-coding and the ability to sample blood flow velocities with PW Doppler.

PERIPHERAL ARTERY DISEASE OF THE LOWER EXTREMITIES

Peripheral artery disease (PAD) of the lower extremities is a common condition affecting as many as 29% of people age 70 and above, more so in those who smoke and/or have diabetes mellitus.[1] Only half of elderly people with PAD are symptomatic.[2,3] Symptoms may include leg tightness or discomfort, numbness, or heaviness exacerbated by exertion and relieved with rest. Symptoms of PAD may present in classically (intermittent claudication) or, more commonly, with atypical symptoms. Differentiation from other nonvascular causes of limb pain may be difficult to determine. Noninvasive diagnostic testing methods complement careful history taking and physical examination in the diagnosis and evaluation of patients with PAD. Indications for noninvasive lower extremity testing include, but are not limited to, lower extremity discomfort with exertion, lower extremity ischemic rest pain, the presence of ischemic ulcerations or gangrene, absent pulses on physical examination, digital ischemia, and assessment of wound healing potential.

Ankle Brachial Index

The ankle brachial index (ABI) is a simple noninvasive test that is used to quickly and reliably assess artery circulation to the legs. As arterial narrowing progresses, there is a decrease in systolic blood pressure distal to the site of stenosis. The extent by which pressure falls depends on the degree of stenosis. Measurement of the pressure drop will allow assessment of the presence and severity of arterial disease.[3] Although the ABI cannot localize arterial disease to a specific segment, it is easy to obtain and correlates well with PAD. A recent meta-analysis confirmed that the ABI does not only provide information regarding the lower extremities, but is also a marker of systemic atherosclerosis and survival.[4] It is therefore recommended as a screening

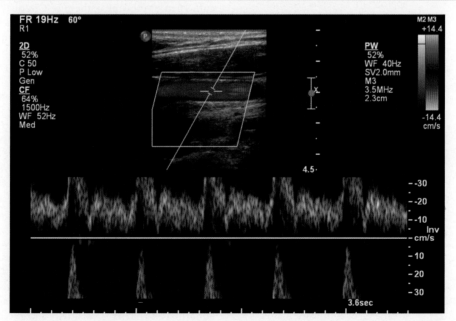

FIGURE 36.1 Duplex showing aliasing evident as wrapping of the waveform (*arrow*) from the top to the bottom of each pulse (+ to +).

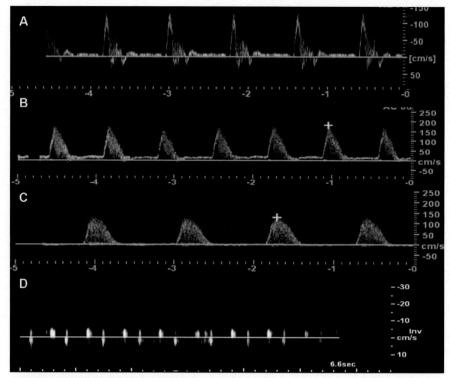

FIGURE 36.2 Doppler waveforms. **A.** Triphasic waveform. **B.** Biphasic waveform with mild spectral broadening. **C.** Monophasic waveform. **D.** Nonpulsatile waveform.

Table 36.1

Technical Limitations and Common Errors in Duplex Ultrasound

Limitation	Solution
Incorrect sample volume size and location	Sample volume should be appropriate to vessel size and placed in the center of flow with a proper Doppler angle
Incorrect angle of insonation provides inaccurate results	The angle of insonation should always be ≤60 degrees
Aliasing	Adjust the pulse repetition frequency
Shadow artifact	When calcification is present, attempt different angles of insonation
Mirror artifact	Suspect when there is lack of correlation between the image and known anatomy and/or lack of displacement or distortion of adjacent objects by the "pseudolesion"
Tortuous vessel may be hard to assess	If increased peak systolic velocity in an area of tortuosity, assess for poststenotic turbulence

tool in asymptomatic individuals by most,[5] but not all, experts.[6] The multispecialty performance measures for adults with PAD suggest ABI measurements in patients at risk for PAD.[7]

The ABI is measured by dividing the systolic blood pressure at the level of the ankle by that in the upper arm. Specifically, ABI measuring technique involves inflating a pneumatic cuff to obliterate blood flow to the limb. A sensing unit (such as a continuous wave Doppler or plethysmograph) is placed distal to the cuff. Then, as pressure in the cuff is gradually deflated, the point at which arterial blood flow is resumed is noted as the systolic blood pressure at that level. The ABI is calculated by dividing the higher of the dorsalis pedis or posterior tibial systolic pressures by the higher of the two brachial pressures.[1] This is repeated for each leg. Within a range, a reduction of the ABI indicates reduced blood flow to the legs. Normal and abnormal ABIs are depicted in Table 36.2. An ABI under 0.9 is 95% sensitive and 99% specific for the diagnosis of PAD.[8] An ABI of 0.9 or less and an ABI greater than 1.4 have been found to be a useful adjunct to the Framingham risk score in determining cardiovascular risk.[4] ABI can also be used for surveillance of PAD. A change of 0.15 or more is considered clinically significant. When measuring the ABI the absolute pressure should be noted as well as the ratio of pressures. An ankle pressure of 50 mm Hg or less suggests critical ischemia.[3]

When an ABI cannot be measured because of undetectable blood pressure or noncompressible arteries, an alternative is the toe brachial index (TBI). This is most often, but not exclusively, the case in elderly patients and those with diabetes mellitus or advanced chronic kidney disease. A TBI under 0.7 is considered abnormal and has 41% sensitivity and 99% specificity for PAD.[9] An absolute toe pressure of 30 mm Hg or less denotes the likelihood of critical limb ischemia (ischemic rest pain, nonhealing

Table 36.2

Normal and Abnormal Values of ABI and TBI

TBI	ABI	Clinical significance
>0.7	>1.0–1.3	Normal
N/A	0.91–1.0	Borderline
0.5–0.7	0.7–0.9	Mild
0.35–0.5 or 30–40 mm Hg	0.4–0.7	Moderate
<0.35 or <30 mm Hg	<0.4 or <50 mm Hg	Severe
—	>1.3	Noncompressible

ischemic ulcerations, or gangrene).[10] Normal and abnormal values for TBI are depicted in Table 36.2.

Segmental Pressure

Although ABI alone cannot localize segments of arterial disease, multiple blood pressure cuffs applied along the lower extremities can offer more information. This procedure is known as segmental limb pressure measurements. Segmental pressures are performed by applying blood pressure cuffs to several locations along the lower extremities (upper thigh, lower thigh, calf, ankle, foot and digit). Each segment is compared to the contralateral segment, the ipsilateral adjacent segments, and the higher of the two brachial pressures. A reduction in pressure greater than 20 mm Hg from one level to the next distal segment, or compared to the contralateral similar segment, is considered significant.[11–13]

Segmental pressures do not reflect the blood flow in specific anatomic arteries but rather the sum of all arterial circulation to the limb—both in named arteries and collateral vessels. It therefore provides more physiologic than anatomic information.[1]

As with the ABI, noncompressible arteries secondary to calcification may be encountered in patients with diabetes mellitus and/or renal failure and may hamper the ability to use segmental pressures for diagnosing and following patients with PAD.

Pulse Volume Recordings

Segmental plethysmographic pulse volume recordings (PVRs) offer additional information regarding the presence, location, and severity of PAD. PVRs are acquired at sites along the lower limbs similar to when performing segmental limb pressure measurements. Blood pressure cuffs are inflated to obliterate venous, but not arterial, flow, commonly to a level of approximately 65 mmHg. Using plethysmographic methods the arterial flow pattern is then recorded.

An advantage of PVR is its ability to demonstrate diminished arterial blood flow in persons with noncompressible arteries, cases in which segmental pressures are not useful. As an example, of 396 patients who were referred to a vascular clinic, 13.6% had noncompressible lower limb arteries. Of these, 24% had abnormal PVR.[14]

A normal PVR has a sharp upstroke, a narrow complex, and a dicrotic notch in the downstroke. Changes to this pattern denote PAD with worsening waveform morphology suggesting more severe PAD (Table 36.3).

Limitations of PVRs include[1]:

- PVRs are less accurate in states of low cardiac output.[15]
- PVR offers a qualitative, *not* a quantitative, measure of perfusion.
- Abnormal PVRs denote physiologic lack of perfusion to a particular limb segment but do not localize the lesion to particular arteries.[11]
- PVRs are less accurate in distal rather than in proximal arterial segments.

Exercise Testing

Exercise prompts an increase in demand for arterial flow to the lower extremities. Healthy people can maintain blood flow to the lower extremities with increasing exercise load, whereas people with PAD cannot. Exercise testing can thus increase the sensitivity of ABI, PVRs, and segmental pressure measurements for detecting PAD and to discern etiologies of exercise-induced limb discomfort.[14,16,17] This is particularly helpful in determining the etiology of exertional limb discomfort in patients with atypical limb symptoms.

A standard protocol for treadmill testing is 5 minutes in duration at a speed of 2 mph and 12% incline. While patients walk they are asked to report onset of symptoms of leg pain, chest pain, shortness of breath, or fatigue. The test is terminated based on patient symptoms. Immediately after the exercise test has been completed, repeat ABI and PVRs are obtained and compared to the resting figures. A postexercise reduction of 20% in the ABI or a recovery time of over 3 minutes denotes PAD.[3]

Plantar flexion ("toe-ups" or "heel raise") exercise may substitute treadmill exercise if a patient cannot walk on a treadmill, or if one is not available.[17] This correlates well with treadmill exercise.[14] Patients should perform up to 50 repetitions or as many as they can. The number of repetitions at the first onset of pain and the total number of repetitions should be recorded. A major limitation of heel-raise exercise in relation to treadmill exercise is lack of reproducibility.

In patients who cannot perform exercise, such as those who cannot stand or walk, and for those patients with other comorbidities, such as congestive heart failure or chronic pulmonary disease, reactive hyperemia testing is an alternative to exercise testing. Limb cuffs are inflated on the thighs at suprasystolic pressure for a maximum of 3 to 5 minutes, resulting in distal ischemia. After releasing the cuffs, reactive hyperemia confers reduced resistance to blood flow with vasodilation of the arteries distal to the occlusive cuff, similar to that achieved with exercise.[18] PVR and segmental pressures are measured immediately after the cuffs are released and every 2 minutes thereafter until blood flow returns to its precuff inflation quality. Reactive hyperemia is considered a difficult test for patients largely because of discomfort.

Duplex Ultrasonography

DUS of the arteries of the lower extremities offers anatomic information together with Doppler waveforms and flow velocities and is accurate in diagnosing stenosis and occlusion of native arteries, arteries with stents, and surgical bypass grafts (FIGURE 36.3). It is used to assess patients with moderate to severe intermittent claudication and to follow patients after surgery and endovascular therapy.

Table 36.3		
Pulse Volume Recording Patterns in Relation to Disease Severity		
Disease severity	PVR pattern	PVR diagram
Sharp upstroke Narrow complex Flat interval between waveforms Possible dicrotic notch	Normal	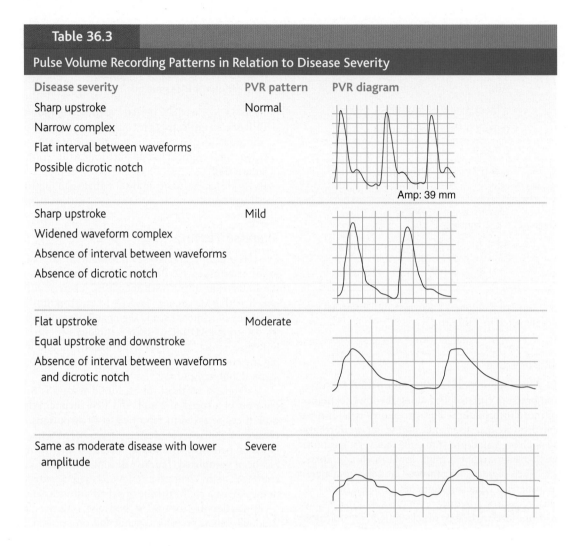 Amp: 39 mm
Sharp upstroke Widened waveform complex Absence of interval between waveforms Absence of dicrotic notch	Mild	
Flat upstroke Equal upstroke and downstroke Absence of interval between waveforms and dicrotic notch	Moderate	
Same as moderate disease with lower amplitude	Severe	

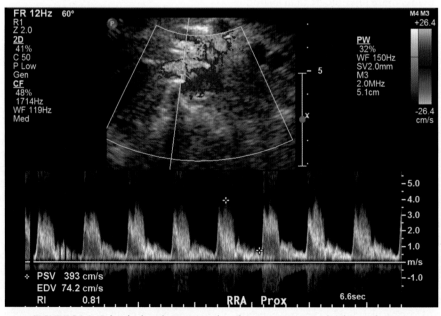

FIGURE 36.3 Color duplex ultrasonography of a stenotic proximal right renal artery.

Doppler Waveforms

Normal Doppler waveforms in the lower extremity arteries are triphasic, but as PAD progresses the signal changes to biphasic and monophasic and eventually is nonpulsatile.[13,16] Normal waveform patterns in the posterior tibial and the dorsalis pedis arteries may be biphasic (FIGURE 36.2).

A hemodynamically significant stenosis may result in (1) an increase in peak systolic velocity (PSV) at the site of narrowing, which may be coupled with a visible obstruction, and in severe cases a "string sign" can be seen with color Doppler; (2) turbulence (termed *poststenotic turbulence*) at and distal to the obstruction; (3) slowed PSV distal to the lesion ("parvus et tardus" waveform pattern); (4) loss of the reverse flow component of the Doppler waveform; and (5) spectral broadening of the Doppler waveform. Although these changes are most commonly recorded by PW Doppler, an initial assessment can be made at the bedside with a continuous wave Doppler by an experienced examiner.

The information that can be obtained from Doppler waveforms has limitations. Dampened signals may be obtained proximal to an obstruction but also distal to it. Collaterals surrounding a total occlusion may resemble flow distal to an occlusion because they are low resistance.

Flow Velocities

Although normal ranges for PSVs in lower extremity arteries have been described,[10] it is not solely the PSV but rather a ratio of PSVs between the area of greatest stenosis and the normal artery proximal to the stenosis.[15,19]

The sensitivity of duplex ultrasound for detecting greater than or equal to 50% stenosis in the lower limb arteries is 80% to 96% and the specificity 89% to 99%. The sensitivity and specificity for detecting occlusion were even higher (90% and 96% to 100%, respectively).[20]

The following criteria may be used to quantify stenosis severity in native arteries of the lower extremities (Table 36.4).[10,11]

Evaluation of Arteries Treated with Endovascular Therapy

Endovascular therapy of the lower extremity arteries has become a widely accepted mode of treatment for patients with symptomatic PAD. Restenosis following percutaneous transluminal angioplasty (PTA) is seen in over 60% of patients, however, and following stent deployment[21] in as many as 40% of patients within 1 year.[22] In general, duplex ultrasound-based surveillance is commonly recommended to determine areas of restenosis prior to arterial thrombosis.[23]

Stenting alters vessel compliance and thus the measured velocities.[23,24] A recent study comparing DUS criteria to angiography in 78 limbs found that combining a PSV greater than 275 cm/second and a velocity ratio above 3.5 to determine greater than 80% in-stent stenosis had 74% sensitivity, 94% specificity, a 88% positive predictive value, and a 85% negative predictive value.[23]

Surgical Bypass Graft Surveillance

In patients who have undergone surgical bypass graft revascularization, graft stenosis is a common problem. Most vein graft restenosis occurs during the first 6 to 12 months postoperatively[25] with an estimated 60% primary patency at 5 years.[26] Salvage procedures for thrombosed autologous vein grafts have far worse outcomes than revision procedures for failing, yet patent, grafts.[27] Vein graft surveillance programs have been shown to improve femoropopliteal and femorotibial graft-assisted primary patency rates in a cost-effective manner.[25] A study of intensive duplex ultrasound-based surveillance compared to symptom onset testing after vein bypass graft surgery in 539 patients demonstrated improved secondary patency (80% versus 67%) and limb salvage (94% versus 73%) for those assigned to intensive duplex ultrasound-based surveillance at 5 years.[28] The use of an intensive surveillance program has been less beneficial in prosthetic grafts when compared to autologous grafts.[27]

Graft surveillance protocols are similar to native vessel DUS. If the ratio of the PSV within a stenotic segment relative to the normal segment proximal to the stenosis is greater than 2, this suggests 50% to 75% diameter reduction. The addition of end-diastolic velocities greater than 100 cm/second suggest greater than 75% stenosis.[29] A PSV of less than 40 cm/second measured in the early postoperative period or during surveillance suggests impending graft thrombosis, as shown in a series of 67 patients (Table 36.5).[30]

Duplex ultrasound of lower extremity arteries has limitations. Although it can locate areas of stenosis, in cases of multiple stenosis it may be difficult to determine the hemodynamically significance of the distal stenosis. Also, DUS is of limited use in patients with heavily calcified arteries because of acoustic shadowing artifact.

Table 36.4
Duplex Ultrasound Grading of Arterial Stenosis in the Lower Extremities

PSV ratio to adjacent segments	Spectral broadening	Waveform	Categories of stenosis severity	Degree of stenosis
1	–	Triphasic	0	Normal
>1.3, <2	+	Triphasic	1–19%	Mild
<2	+	Biphasic	20–49%	Moderate
>2	+	Monophasic	50–99%; String sign may be present	Severe
No flow	No flow	No flow	100%	Occlusion

Table 36.5

Duplex Ultrasound Classification of Graft Stenosis

Velocity ratio (Vr) and velocity spectra	Diameter reduction
Vr < 1.5, mild spectral broadening in systole, PSV < 150 cm/sec	Normal, <20% stenosis
1.5 < Vr < 2.5, spectral broadening throughout systole, no change in waveform configuration across stenosis, PSV > 150 cm/sec	20–50% stenosis
Vr > 2.5, severe spectral broadening in systole with reversed flow components, PSV > 180 cm/sec	50–75% stenosis, moderate
Vr > 3.5, severe lumen reduction and "flow jet" present by color Doppler imaging; PSV > 300 cm/sec, EDV in flow-jet >40 cm/sec, damped velocity waveform in distal arteries	>75% stenosis, severe

Modified from Bandyk DF. Infrainguinal vein bypass graft surveillance: how to do it, when to intervene, and is it cost-effective? *J Am Coll Surg* 2002;194 (suppl 1):S40–S52.

PERIPHERAL ARTERY DISEASE OF THE UPPER EXTREMITIES

Upper extremity arterial disease is rare in comparison to other forms of PAD; however, it is a cause of morbidity and even mortality. Noninvasive imaging plays a central role in the diagnosis of upper extremity PAD and often assists clinicians in making decisions regarding the need for invasive therapy. Segmental pressures and PVRs in the upper extremities are measured in a similar fashion to those in the lower extremities. Cuffs are inflated on the upper arms, forearms, and wrists. The wrist brachial index (WBI) is the upper extremity equivalent of the lower extremity ABI. A WBI under 0.7 denotes obstruction to flow, although no standardization has been published. Some use the digital-brachial index, whereas others claim digital pressures are unreliable.[31]

Digital photo-plethysmography (PPG) offers further information regarding blood flow quality to the fingers. As flow diminishes, the PPG waveform widens and flattens.[32] PPG is used to assess arterial flow to the fingers and also response of the microcirculation to cold, medication, and sympathectomy. The method allows single digit flow quantification, enabling mapping of pathology to the distribution of particular vascular beds, such as in the case of the hypothenar hammer syndrome.

THORACIC OUTLET SYNDROME

The thoracic outlet is a narrow anatomic space between the sternum, the first rib, and the vertebrae. It is bordered by the scalene muscles. The subclavian artery and vein, along with the brachial plexus, traverse through the thoracic outlet. Functional or anatomic abnormalities that narrow this space may impinge on these structures, resulting in thoracic outlet syndrome (TOS), which may result in various upper extremity symptoms. Though neurogenic TOS is the most common type, arterial as well as venous types, although less common, may result in serious limb compromise.[33]

Noninvasive testing for TOS is needed in two scenarios—to aid in diagnosis or to search for arterial complications. PVRs in multiple arm positions may complement the physical examination (i.e., Adson maneuver) in confirming the diagnosis of TOS. DUS may also be used to examine the subclavian artery in neutral, 90-degree, 120-degree, and military positions. A supraclavicular or infraclavicular approach may be used. Absence of flow denotes occlusion. An increased flow velocity with the maneuver denotes significant stenosis. The same criteria that have been described for lower extremity arterial stenosis may be used.

DUS can also be used to look for subclavian thrombi or aneurysms, both complications of arterial TOS.[33,34] Collateral arteries may be evident in cases of chronic obstruction.

Provocative Testing for Vasospasm

Cold challenge testing assesses the ability of the digital vascular bed to respond to cold stimuli and recovery. Digital blood flow is assessed before, during, and after exposure to cold stimuli. There are several protocols described in the literature. Cold challenge test is reproducible and is often used in patients with suspicion of secondary Raynaud phenomenon (i.e., scleroderma, thromboangiitis obliterans, etc.).[31,35]

EXTRACRANIAL CAROTID ARTERY DISEASE

The carotid duplex ultrasound examination (CDUS) can identify plaque, stenoses, occlusions, and direction of flow. It is commonly used to diagnose and follow patients with extracranial internal carotid disease in native arteries as well as after surgery and stent deployment. CDUS can demonstrate carotid artery dissection with variable degrees of sensitivity and is generally recommended when the likelihood that the diagnosis will affect management is low[36,37] and carotid body tumors.[38] Indications for CDUS include a history of transient ischemic attacks, stroke, cervical bruits, surveillance following surgical or endovascular revascularization, and in patients deemed to be at high risk for the presence of carotid stenosis.[11] Furthermore, carotid plaque visualized by CDUS has been linked to increased risk of mortality in the elderly,[39] whereas echolucent plaque morphology is suggested as an increased risk for stroke.[40]

Intima-media thickness (IMT) can be visualized with DUS. It is measured in a straight segment of the distal common carotid artery (CCA) that has no plaque. Measurement acquisition can be performed manually or with automated edge detection software programs while the operator holds the transducer at the correct location. Although increments in the IMT have been linked to cardiovascular risk[41] and IMT has been shown to be an independent risk factor for cardiovascular events,[41,42] current evidence fails to support additional benefit of IMT to traditional risk factors in cardiovascular risk stratification. Serial IMT measurements are currently not recommended.[6]

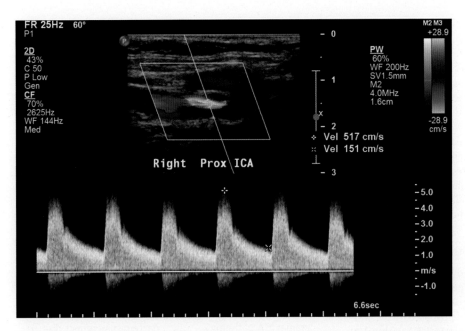

FIGURE 36.4 Color duplex ultrasonography of a stenotic proximal right internal carotid artery in longitudinal view.

Duplex Ultrasonography

By linking both anatomic visualization and Doppler-derived flow measurements, the degree of carotid stenosis can be determined with a high degree of accuracy by CDUS (FIGURE 36.4). With properly developed criteria the sensitivity and specificity of CDUS for detecting internal carotid artery stenosis exceed 90%.[43] Sensitivity and specificity of CDUS increase as the degree of stenosis increases.[43,44] The accuracy of CDUS varies between different vascular laboratories.[43] Individual quality assurance is mandatory, and developing therapeutic strategies based on CDUS results from nonaccredited vascular laboratories should be performed with caution.[45]

Native Arteries

The CDUS examination must include at least views of the common carotid (CCA), internal carotid (ICA), external carotid (ECA), and vertebral arteries (VA). Of note, the origin of the VAs is usually not visualized by DUS.

Specific duplex criteria for diagnosing ICA stenosis have been described by a consensus conference of different specialists (Table 36.6).

Other diagnostic characteristics must be included in the standard CDUS examination. Flow in the VA should be antegrade (toward the brain) and demonstrate a low-resistance pattern. Flow quality in the CCA should also be assessed. Normal CCA

Table 36.6

Duplex Classification of Carotid Artery Stenosis

Comments	B-mode plaque estimate	ICA/CCA ratio	Diastolic velocity (cm/sec)	Peak systolic velocity (cm/sec)	Interpretation
—	No plaque	<2	40>	125>	Normal
Poststenotic mosaic pattern may be evident	50%>	<2	40>	125>	0–49%
—	≥50%	2–4	40–100	125–230	50–69% (moderate)
—	≥50%	>4	>100	>230	70–99% (severe)
"String sign" may be evident	Visible	Variable	Variable	High, low, or undetectable	Near occlusion
No flow	100% occlusion	Not applicable	Not applicable	Undetectable	Occlusion

Modified from Grant EG, Benson CB, Moneta GL, et al. Carotid artery stenosis: gray-scale and Doppler US diagnosis—Society of Radiologists in Ultrasound Consensus Conference. *Radiology* 2003;229:340–346.

Doppler waveforms represent components of the ICA and ECA. If the CCA waveform demonstrates ECA morphology (see later), this suggests an ICA occlusion. A parvus et tardus waveform may suggest proximal CCA stenosis or occlusion. If the Doppler spectral waveform morphology is parvus et tardus bilaterally, this suggests critical aortic stenosis or impaired cardiac output. A recent publication defined duplex-based criteria for determining greater than 50% CCA stenosis. A PSV greater than 182 cm/second had a sensitivity of 64% and a specificity of 88% and an EDV greater than 30 cm/second had a sensitivity of 54% and a specificity of 74%.[46] ECA waveforms are high resistance.[47] An ECA may be further differentiated from the ICA by demonstrating the superior thyroidal artery and oscillations upon temporal tap, although both methods have limited capabilities.[48]

Postcarotid Endarterectomy Surveillance

Although DUS surveillance after carotid endarterectomy may not be cost-effective,[49] it is commonly performed because the prevalence of postendarterectomy restenosis may be as frequent as 20% within 5 years of surgery. A model proposed by the University of South Florida suggests surveillance CDUS within 1 to 2 months after operation and annually thereafter if there is no residual disease. If there is disease on either side, surveillance every 6 months is indicated.[50] Intraoperative duplex may also improve surgical results.

Carotid Artery Stent Surveillance

CDUS is utilized following carotid artery stenting. Carotid stents alter the flow dynamics caused by loss of compliance of the ICA. Therefore, native artery velocity criteria tend to overestimate the degree of stenosis in stented arteries.[24] A recent trial compared stenosis as assessed by duplex velocity criteria to computed tomography angiography (CTA) and invasive angiography measurements in 310 carotid arteries. A high degree of correlation was found; for a stenosis of 50% to 79%, PSV greater than 220 cm/second produced sensitivity of 100% and specificity of 96.2%, and for a stenosis of 80% to 99%, PSV greater than 340 cm/second resulted in sensitivity of 100% and specificity of 98.6%.[51] Ideally, velocities should be documented soon after the procedure and if an increase in PSV, EDV, or ICA/CCA ratio is observed, it may prompt further investigation for in-stent restenosis.

Common Errors with Carotid Duplex Ultrasonography

When performing a CDUS examination, it is important to recognize some common errors that may arise. Operator-dependent and physiologic errors are shown in Table 36.7.

Transcranial Doppler/Duplex

Transcranial Doppler (TCD) is a portable, inexpensive examination used to evaluate the blood flow in the intracerebral arterial system.[52] Uses for TCD include efficacy of thrombolytic therapy, assessment of collateral flow, detection of microemboli as stratification of risk for recurrent stroke, detection of vasospasm after subarachnoid hemorrhage, and assessment of brain death. TCD may be used intraoperatively during carotid endarterectomy to monitor brain perfusion and embolic phenomena

Table 36.7

Common Errors and Pitfalls in Carotid Duplex Ultrasonography

Limitation	Solution
Operator dependent performance and interpretation errors	
Incorrect identification of ICA versus ECA	Identify anatomy, use temporal tap in ECA, assess Doppler spectral waveform pattern
Lack of identification of ostial CCA pathology	Always attempt to visualize the CCA origin
Lack of identification of distal ICA pathology	Scan distally and look for fibromuscular dysplasia pattern
Lack of suspicion for intracranial ICA pathology	High-resistance CCA flow pattern may reflect distal stenosis
Inadequate assessment of central etiologies for inflow stenosis (e.g., innominate stenosis)	Parvus et tardus CCA flow pattern may reflect "inflow" stenosis or poor cardiac output
Physiologic	
High and low cardiac output may affect PSV	In this case, ICA/CCA ratio is more central in estimating stenosis
Overestimation of stenosis in the setting of contralateral occlusion	Always perform bilateral exam
Tandem lesions or long lesions	May diminish ability of standard criteria

(high-intensity transient signals, HITS). TCD is also used to complement CDUS to reveal intracranial hemodynamic consequences of carotid lesions and vertebral reversal of flow in patients with subclavian steal physiology.[53]

TCD utilizes one of three bone windows to detect blood flow in major intracerebral arteries. The bone windows are the transorbital, transtemporal, and transforaminal. Although TCD is a blind examination, knowledge of the insonated blood vessel is gained by combining the window, depth, and direction of flow. TCD is more accurate in the anterior circulation than in the vertebro-basilar (posterior) system.

■ SUBCLAVIAN ARTERIES/INNOMINATE ARTERY

Roughly 2% of the general population and over 7% of patients with vascular disease are estimated to have asymptomatic subclavian artery stenosis. The etiology is most commonly atherosclerosis.[12] Subclavian steal may result from subclavian artery stenosis or occlusion. It is characterized by posterior circulation symptoms of diplopia, ataxia, and vertigo. Physical examination findings include an absent or diminished radial pulse, blood pressure differences between the two brachial arteries, and a supraclavicular bruit.[54] The subclavian artery is usually implicated, yet on the right this may be secondary to the innominate artery in as many as one-third of cases.[12]

ABDOMINAL AORTA

Early detection of abdominal aortic aneurysms (AAA) may be lifesaving, and ultrasound-based screening is effective in reducing AAA-related mortality.[55] A true aneurysm of the abdominal aorta is a localized dilatation of all three arterial layers measuring more than 3 cm in diameter.[56] Because not all AAAs rupture, elective repair is undertaken only when the risk of rupture is high. The diagnosis should be suspected if a pulsatile abdominal mass is palpated or when a family history of an AAA in a first-degree relative is present. Some advocate screening for an AAA in all men over age 55 who have ever smoked, all women over the age 65, or all men over the age 65.[55] A large population-based trial found that duplex ultrasound screening of men over age 65 was both cost-effective and reduced aneurysm-related death after 10 years.[57]

The strongest known predictor of rupture is the maximal diameter of the aneurysm. Thus, if an aneurysm is found, continued surveillance is mandatory because aneurysms grow with time.[58] Aneurysms measuring 3 to 5.9 cm typically grow at a rate of 0.26 to 0.4 cm per year.[59] Growth is more rapid, on average, for larger aneurysms or in patients with collagen disorders (e.g. Ehlers-Danlos syndrome). Therefore, follow-up imaging is recommended at 12-month intervals for patients with an AAA of 3.5 to 4.4 cm in diameter and at 6-month intervals for patients with an AAA diameter between 4.5 and 5.4 cm.[55]

AAA can be reliably diagnosed and followed with DUS. Accuracy of ultrasound for AAA detection approaches 100% as compared with surgical specimens.[56] Prior to the scan, patients fast overnight. The examination is performed in the supine, reverse Trendelenburg position. Using a low frequency (i.e., 3.5 mHz) transducer, the aorta is identified at the level of the diaphragm in the sagittal plane throughout its length. The ultrasound probe is then reoriented in the coronal plane, and transverse measurements are obtained in the suprarenal, juxtarenal, and infrarenal positions. The aorta should be measured in two planes. When reporting an AAA, information regarding size, location, shape, visible thrombus, calcifications, relation to renal arteries, and presence of iliac aneurysms should be noted.

Duplex Ultrasound Following Endovascular Aortic Stent-Graft Repair

Since 1951, the standard therapy for larger AAA has been surgical repair.[60] Despite apparent equality of long-term mortality, and the potential need for reintervention,[60,61] endoluminal repair has become as prevalent as open surgical repair in the United States.[62] A potentially catastrophic complication of endoluminal stent-grafts is an endoleak, which is arterial flow outside the endoluminal graft and into the native aneurysm sac. Endoleaks may occur at the proximal or distal attachment zones (Type I), via patent lumbar or intercostals arteries (Type II), or directly through the fabric of the implant: either due to tears of the fabric (Type III)[63] or due to porosity of the stent itself.[64] If unrecognized or untreated, this persistent flow may result in expansion of the aneurysm and cause it to rupture.

Although traditionally three-dimensional helical computerized tomographic scans have been used to detect endoleaks after endoluminal repair, color DUS has demonstrated accuracy in detecting endoleaks, although quality remains operator dependent.[65] A recent comparison of CTA and duplex surveillance after endovascular repair of aortic aneurysms examined 117 patients for an average of 32 months. Each patient underwent both CTA and ultrasound and 406 examinations were compared. Although the positive predictive value was low (45%), the sensitivity was 86% and the negative predictive value was high (94%) for DUS compared to computed tomography (CT).[65]

RENAL ARTERIES

Atherosclerotic renal artery stenosis (ARAS) may contribute to the development of hypertension and end-stage renal dysfunction. The proper diagnosis of ARAS has practical implications. Indications for renal artery imaging include new-onset hypertension in the young or elderly, difficult to control hypertension, unexplained azotemia (especially if exacerbated following angiotensin-converting enzyme inhibitor administration), recurrent flash pulmonary edema without a proper cardiac explanation, and as surveillance following revascularization.[66]

Duplex Ultrasonography of Native Renal Arteries

Renal artery duplex ultrasonography (RADUS) is an appealing noninvasive option for confiming the diagnosis of renal artery stenosis (FIGURE 36.5). In a prospective series comparing 102 RADUS exams to contrast angiography, the sensitivity of DUS was 98%, specificity 99%, positive predictive value 99%, and negative predictive value 97%.[67]

Renal artery duplex is performed after an overnight fast. Patients may take their medications with a sip of water. Insonation is performed from the anterior and oblique positions at a Doppler angle of less than 60 degrees. All segments of the renal artery need to be visualized. The lateral and posterior approaches may prove to be particularly useful for studying obese patients with excessive overlying bowel gas. ARAS is diagnosed using peak systolic and end-diastolic velocities as well as the ratio of the aortic PSV as measured at the level of the superior mesenteric artery and the PSV in the renal artery, known as the renal/aortic ratio (RAR). The renal artery PSV is obtained by interrogating the entire main renal artery from the ostium to the hilum. Persistent diastolic flow is normal because the renal artery provides circulation to a low-resistance system.

RADUS criteria are categorized as 0% to 59%, 60% to 99% stenosis, or occluded. In a study of 67 renal arteries, comparing RADUS to angiography, the RAR was found to be more accurate than PSV in the renal artery. If the RAR is 3.5 or more, this implies a 60% to 99% stenosis. If the aortic blood flow velocity is less than 40 cm/second or more than 100 cm/second, the RAR is not accurate, and the PSV should be used.[68] In these cases a PSV greater than 200 cm/second and poststenotic turbulence by RADUS denote 60% to 99% stenosis. A recent trial compared RADUS to angiography and pressure gradient measurements in 56 stenosed renal arteries. Using a PSV cutoff of 180 cm/second, false positive rates were 55%, whereas relying on a RAR of 3.5 produced a false positive of 15% for hemodynamically

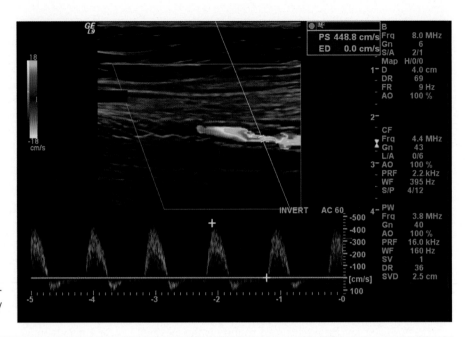

FIGURE 36.5 Color duplex ultrasonography of the superficial femoral artery revealing focal stenosis within a stent.

significant renal artery stenosis. It was suggested that values should be more stringent with a PSV of 318 cm/second and an RAR of 3.74.[69] This may result, however, in a raised false negative rate.

Renal hilar artery insonation may be easier to perform than main renal artery investigation. It is performed by using an oblique approach at a 0-degree Doppler angle. A direct comparison performed in 41 patients proved to be less accurate. Hilar scanning had a sensitivity of 32% with a specificity of 100% as compared to angiography.[70] Other limitations include inability to discriminate between stenosis and occlusion and inadequate determination of accessory renal arteries.

The renal resistive index (RRI) has been suggested as a predictor of success of percutaneous renal revascularization. The RRI is thought to represent intrinsic renovascular resistance and may reflect renal parenchymal disease. It is calculated as the PSV minus the end-diastolic velocity divided by the PSV.[71] It is measured in the renal parenchymal arteries. Severe renal artery stenosis may actually produce a low RRI due to poststenotic flow characteristics.[72]

A prospective study examined the utility of the RRI less than or equal to 0.8 to predict outcomes of renal revascularization. A high preintervention resistive index, especially when combined with impaired renal function, predicted lack of blood pressure response and continued renal function deterioration over time.[71] Because the contralateral RRI may affect measurement, this publication was criticized for not reporting the contralateral RRI. A recent review recommended against use of the RRI as the main predictive tool until further data are gathered.[72]

Renal artery DUS is time consuming and requires skilled technologists and physicians to perform and interpret the results.[66,67] Main renal artery and hilar ultrasonography have been found to miss polar (accessory) renal arteries.[70] Exams deemed technically difficult may be uncommon in some centers and should be interpreted with caution or repeated by a second technologist.[67]

Renal Artery Duplex Ultrasonography of Stented Arteries

DUS is useful in surveillance of stented renal arteries because the entire renal artery can be imaged despite the presence of a metallic endoprosthesis. Restenosis is detected by an increase in the PSV within the stented segment of the renal artery as well as an increase in the RAR. Suggested criteria for detecting RAS greater than 60% include a PSV greater than or equal to 300 cm/second with poststenotic turbulence and/or an RAR greater than or equal to 4.3. A PSV less than 240 cm/second accurately excludes significant stenosis.[73] A comparison was conducted between the duplex findings in 31 stenotic stented renal arteries and 30 native stenotic renal arteries. Stenosis was angiographically proven in both groups.[74] The mean PSV was higher in the stented group (452 versus 360 cm/second, $p = .002$) and the RAR in patients with in-stent stenosis was 6 versus 4 in native renal artery stenosis ($p = .02$). Receiver operating characteristics (ROC) curves were used to calculate the optimal threshold for predicting in-stent restenosis of greater than or equal to 70%. This was found with a PSV of 395 cm/second that yielded a sensitivity of 83%, specificity of 88% and accuracy of 87%, and an RAR of 5.1 that yielded an accuracy of 88%. Using native renal artery stenosis parameters may thus overestimate the finding in stented arteries.

■ MESENTERIC ARTERIES

Chronic mesenteric ischemia manifests as weight loss, abdominal pain, and "fear of food" and is more common in patients with PAD than in the general population.[75] Although CTA and angiography offer a definitive diagnosis, ultrasound has gained favor as a primary diagnostic test. When acute mesenteric ischemia is suspected, on the other hand, prompt imaging, commonly with invasive arteriography or CTA, is performed.

Duplex Ultrasonography

DUS of the mesenteric arteries may be a challenging examination. It involves interrogation of the celiac, superior mesenteric, and inferior mesenteric arteries. Anatomic variants must be readily recognized.[76] Mesenteric artery DUS is performed after a 6-hour fast to avoid overlying bowel gas. In the fasting state, the normal superior mesenteric artery (SMA) Doppler waveform has a high-resistance pattern. First, aortic flow velocities are measured throughout the entire abdominal aorta. Then celiac artery peak systolic and end-diastolic velocities are measured at the ostium and within the artery toward the bifurcation to the hepatic and splenic arteries.[76] Often, particularly when concerns exist regarding celiac artery compression syndrome, Doppler spectral waveforms are obtained during held inspiration and exhalation.[77,78] The superior and inferior mesenteric artery peak systolic and end-diastolic velocities are also measured at the ostium and as far into the arteries as possible.

The normal celiac waveform is biphasic because this is a low-resistance system supplying the liver and spleen. The normal superior mesenteric artery Doppler waveform is high resistant and triphasic in the fasted state, changing to biphasic with a lower resistance pattern after a meal as blood flow to the intestines increases. The inferior mesenteric artery waveform is triphasic as well.

In a prospective study involving 100 patients with and without abdominal symptoms, DUS was compared to angiography. SMA PSV greater than or equal to 275 cm/second and celiac artery PSV greater than or equal to 200 cm/second identified angiographic stenosis of greater than 70% severity with a sensitivity of 92% and 87% and a specificity of 96% and 80%, respectively.[79] In a retrospective validation study an EDV greater than or equal to 45 cm/second or no flow in the SMA had a sensitivity of 90% and a specificity of 91% to stenosis greater than or equal to 50%, as shown by angiography. PSV greater than or equal to 300 cm/second resulted in a low sensitivity of 60% but a specificity of 100%. Differences between various thresholds may be secondary to gender preponderance, instrumentation, and pretest probability as drawn from patient selection method.[76]

A normal response to a meal includes increased PSV and loss of reversed diastolic flow in the superior mesenteric artery. In mesenteric ischemia, the artery cannot dilate further, and flow does not rise.[80] Some authorities claim a meal challenge is not necessary in light of the excellent results of fasting studies.[76]

There are no duplex criteria for stenosis of stented mesenteric arteries. Mitchell et al. retrospectively examined mesenteric artery PSVs before and after stenting in 18 and 13 patients, respectively. Pre-stent average PSV was 450 cm/second and post-stent average PSV was 336 cm/second; both were higher than the traditional native artery cutoff of 275 cm/second, although most patients demonstrated long-term symptomatic relief. The authors concluded that native artery criteria could not be applied to stented arteries for detection of restenosis.[81]

Mesenteric artery bypass graft surgery is an established treatment for mesenteric ischemia. A retrospective analysis of the natural history of 34 mesenteric bypass grafts in 22 patients showed that symptom-based assessment of graft patency was only 33% accurate compared to duplex and angiographic follow-up.[82] Another retrospective analysis of duplex ultrasound surveillance of 43 bypass graft operations showed that although the inflow artery PSV varied between grafts of various types,

midgraft and perianastomotic velocities were similar. Only three graft events presented during the trial period, but in normal grafts velocities remained consistent throughout follow-up. Most measured PSV values ranged from 140 to 200 cm/second.[83]

Limitations of mesenteric artery DUS include overlying bowel gas, abdominal wall scars, and medications that affect mesenteric blood flow (such as vasopressin or adrenaline). Obesity is often cited as an obstacle for abdominal ultrasound; however, in the case of mesenteric ischemia it may challenge the diagnosis because these patients are usually underweight.

PSEUDOANEURYSMS AND ARTERIOVENOUS FISTULAE

Iatrogenic complications of arterial catheterization include pseudoaneurysm and arteriovenous fistulae. Pseudoaneurysm prevalence is as high as 6% of punctures performed for coronary or peripheral artery interventions.[84] DUS can detect a pseudoaneurysm by demonstrating an extravascular blood collection (sac) with "to and fro" arterial flow in the "neck" between it and the "feeding" artery. Blood flow inside the collection may demonstrate the classic "yin-yang" pattern as bidirectional blood flow is detected. Ultrasound-guided compression or direct thrombin injection may be successful in 91% to 100% of cases; otherwise surgical repair is needed.[84,85] An arteriovenous fistula, on the other hand, is diagnosed by demonstrating the connection between the artery and the vein and by demonstrating arterialization of flow in the vein. This arterial flow pattern decreases with increasing distance from the vessel wall defect but may persist well into the vena cava.

CONCLUSION

Noninvasive testing and technologic advances in particular have improved, and standardization over the past decades has resulted in great value in the management of many vascular disorders. Physiologic testing for PAD offers reliable, simple, and painless options to confirm the presence of PAD, the severity of the disorder at rest and with exercise, and can be used to follow the outcomes of patients treated for PAD. DUS provides accurate identification of pathology, assists in treatment planning, and, in certain situations, surveillance after interventions, particularly in the lower extremities, carotid arteries, abdominal visceral arteries, and the abdominal aorta. These modalities are expected to continue to play a vital role for the foreseeable future.

REFERENCES

1. Olin JW, Sealove BA. Peripheral artery disease: current insight into the disease and its diagnosis and management. *Mayo Clin Proc* 2010;85(7):678–692.
2. Aronow WS. Office management of peripheral arterial disease. *Am J Med* 2010;123(9):790–792.
3. Weitz JI, Byrne J, Clagett GP, et al. Diagnosis and treatment of chronic arterial insufficiency of the lower extremities: a critical review. *Circulation* 1996;94(11):3026–3049.
4. Ankle Brachial Index Collaboration; Fowkes FG, Murray GD, et al. Ankle brachial index combined with Framingham risk score to predict cardiovascular events and mortality: a meta-analysis. *JAMA.* 2008;300(2):197–208.
5. Executive summary: standards of medical care in diabetes—2010. *Diabetes Care* 2010;33(suppl 1):S4–S10.
6. U.S. Preventive Services Task Force. Using nontraditional risk factors in coronary heart disease risk assessment: U.S. Preventive Services Task Force recommendation statement. *Ann Intern Med* 2009;151(7):474–482.

7. Olin JW, Allie DE, Belkin M, et al. ACCF/AHA/ACR/SCAI/SIR/SVM/SVN/ SVS 2010 performance measures for adults with peripheral artery disease: a report of the American College of Cardiology Foundation/American Heart Association Task Force on Performance Measures, the American College of Radiology, the Society for Cardiac Angiography and Interventions, the Society for Interventional Radiology, the Society for Vascular Medicine, the Society for Vascular Nursing, and the Society for Vascular Surgery (writing committee to develop clinical performance measures for peripheral artery disease). *Circulation* 2010;122(24):2583–2618.
8. McDermott MM, Greenland P, Liu K, et al. The ankle brachial index is associated with leg function and physical activity: the Walking and Leg Circulation Study. *Ann Intern Med* 2002;136(12):873–883.
9. Feigelson HS, Criqui MH, Fronek A, et al. Screening for peripheral arterial disease: the sensitivity, specificity, and predictive value of noninvasive tests in a defined population. *Am J Epidemiol* 1994;140(6):526–534.
10. Hirsch AT, Haskal ZJ, Hertzer NR, et al. ACC/AHA 2005 practice guidelines for the management of patients with peripheral arterial disease (lower extremity, renal, mesenteric, and abdominal aortic): a collaborative report from the American Association for Vascular Surgery/Society for Vascular Surgery, Society for Cardiovascular Angiography and Interventions, Society for Vascular Medicine and Biology, Society of Interventional Radiology, and the ACC/AHA Task Force on Practice Guidelines (writing committee to develop guidelines for the management of patients with peripheral arterial disease): endorsed by the American Association of Cardiovascular and Pulmonary Rehabilitation; National Heart, Lung, and Blood Institute; Society for Vascular Nursing; TransAtlantic Inter-society Consensus; and Vascular Disease Foundation. *Circulation* 2006;113(11):e463–e654.
11. Gerhard-Herman M, Gardin JM, Jaff M, et al. Guidelines for noninvasive vascular laboratory testing: a report from the American Society of Echocardiography and the Society for Vascular Medicine and Biology. *Vasc Med* 2006;11(3):183–200.
12. Shadman R, Criqui MH, Bundens WP, et al. Subclavian artery stenosis: prevalence, risk factors, and association with cardiovascular diseases. *J Am Coll Cardiol* 2004;44(3):618–623.
13. Andersen CA. Noninvasive assessment of lower extremity hemodynamics in individuals with diabetes mellitus. *J Vasc Surg* 2010;52(suppl 3):76S–80S.
14. Stein R, Hriljac I, Halperin JL, et al. Limitation of the resting ankle-brachial index in symptomatic patients with peripheral arterial disease. *Vasc Med* 2006;11(1):29–33.
15. Allard L, Cloutier G, Guo Z, et al. Review of the assessment of single level and multilevel arterial occlusive disease in lower limbs by duplex ultrasound. *Ultrasound Med Biol* 1999;25(4):495–502.
16. Marinelli MR, Beach KW, Glass MJ, et al. Noninvasive testing vs clinical evaluation of arterial disease. A prospective study. *JAMA* 1979;241(19):2031–2034.
17. Carter SA. Response of ankle systolic pressure to leg exercise in mild or questionable arterial disease. *N Engl J Med* 1972;287(12):578–582.
18. Fronek A, Johansen K, Dilley RB, et al. Ultrasonographically monitored postocclusive reactive hyperemia in the diagnosis of peripheral arterial occlusive disease. *Circulation* 1973;48(1):149–152.
19. Kohler TR, Nance DR, Cramer MM, et al. Duplex scanning for diagnosis of aortoiliac and femoropopliteal disease: a prospective study. *Circulation* 1987;76(5):1074–1080.
20. Collins R, Cranny G, Burch J, et al. A systematic review of duplex ultrasound, magnetic resonance angiography and computed tomography angiography for the diagnosis and assessment of symptomatic, lower limb peripheral arterial disease. *Health Technol Assess* 2007;11(20):iii, iv, xi–xiii, 1–184.
21. Rocha-Singh KJ, Jaff MR, Crabtree TR, et al. Performance goals and endpoint assessments for clinical trials of femoropopliteal bare nitinol stents in patients with symptomatic peripheral arterial disease. *Catheter Cardiovasc Interv* 2007;69(6):910–919.
22. Schillinger M, Sabeti S, Loewe C, et al. Balloon angioplasty versus implantation of nitinol stents in the superficial femoral artery. *N Engl J Med* 2006;354(18):1879–1888.
23. Baril DT, Rhee RY, Kim J, et al. Duplex criteria for determination of in-stent stenosis after angioplasty and stenting of the superficial femoral artery. *J Vasc Surg* 2009;49(1):133, 138; discussion 139.
24. Ringer AJ, German JW, Guterman LR, et al. Follow-up of stented carotid arteries by Doppler ultrasound. *Neurosurgery* 2002;51(3):639, 643; discussion 643.
25. Bandyk DF. Infrainguinal vein bypass graft surveillance: how to do it, when to intervene, and is it cost-effective? *J Am Coll Surg* 2002;194(suppl 1):S40–S52.
26. Berceli SA, Hevelone ND, Lipsitz SR, et al. Surgical and endovascular revision of infrainguinal vein bypass grafts: analysis of midterm outcomes from the PREVENT III trial. *J Vasc Surg* 2007;46(6):1173–1179.
27. Carter A, Murphy MO, Halka AT, et al. The natural history of stenoses within lower limb arterial bypass grafts using a graft surveillance program. *Ann Vasc Surg* 2007;21(6):695–703.
28. Bergamini TM, George SM Jr, Massey HT, et al. Intensive surveillance of femoropopliteal-tibial autogenous vein bypasses improves long-term graft patency and limb salvage. *Ann Surg* 1995;221(5):507, 515; discussion 515–516.
29. Bandyk DF. Postoperative surveillance of infrainguinal bypass. *Surg Clin North Am* 1990;70(1):71–85.
30. Bandyk DF, Cato RF, Towne JB. A low flow velocity predicts failure of femoropopliteal and femorotibial bypass grafts. *Surgery* 1985;98(4):799–809.
31. Chloros GD, Smerlis NN, Li Z, et al. Noninvasive evaluation of upper-extremity vascular perfusion. *J Hand Surg Am* 2008;33(4):591–600.
32. Allen J. Photoplethysmography and its application in clinical physiological measurement. *Physiol Meas* 2007;28(3):R1–R39.
33. Sanders RJ, Hammond SL, Rao NM. Diagnosis of thoracic outlet syndrome. *J Vasc Surg* 2007;46(3):601–604.
34. Urschel HC, Kourlis H. Thoracic outlet syndrome: a 50-year experience at Baylor University Medical Center. *Proc (Bayl Univ Med Cent)* 2007;20(2):125–135.
35. Maricq HR, Valter I, Maricq JG. An objective method to estimate the severity of Raynaud phenomenon: digital blood pressure response to cooling. *Vasc Med* 1998;3(2):109–113.
36. Arnold M, Baumgartner RW, Stapf C, et al. Ultrasound diagnosis of spontaneous carotid dissection with isolated horner syndrome. *Stroke* 2008;39(1):82–86.
37. Goyal MS, Derdeyn CP. The diagnosis and management of supraaortic arterial dissections. *Curr Opin Neurol* 2009;22(1):80–89.
38. Sajid MS, Hamilton G, Baker DM, et al. A multicenter review of carotid body tumour management. *Eur J Vasc Endovasc Surg* 2007;34(2):127–130.
39. Stork S, Feelders RA, van den Beld AW, et al. Prediction of mortality risk in the elderly. *Am J Med* 2006;119(6):519–525.
40. Mathiesen EB, Bonaa KH, Joakimsen O. Echolucent plaques are associated with high risk of ischemic cerebrovascular events in carotid stenosis: the Tromso Study. *Circulation* 2001;103(17):2171–2175.
41. O'Leary DH, Bots ML. Imaging of atherosclerosis: carotid intima-media thickness. *Eur Heart J* 2010;31(14):1682–1689.
42. Touboul PJ, Labreuche J, Vicaut E, et al. Carotid intima-media thickness, plaques, and Framingham risk score as independent determinants of stroke risk. *Stroke* 2005;36(8):1741–1745.
43. Jahromi AS, Cina CS, Liu Y, et al. Sensitivity and specificity of color duplex ultrasound measurement in the estimation of internal carotid artery stenosis: a systematic review and meta-analysis. *J Vasc Surg* 2005;41(6):962–972.
44. Grant EG, Duerinckx AJ, El Saden SM, et al. Ability to use duplex US to quantify internal carotid arterial stenoses: fact or fiction? *Radiology* 2000;214(1):247–252.
45. Brown OW, Bendick PJ, Bove PG, et al. Reliability of extracranial carotid artery duplex ultrasound scanning: value of vascular laboratory accreditation. *J Vasc Surg* 2004;39(2):366, 371; discussion 371.
46. Slovut DP, Romero JM, Hannon KM, et al. Detection of common carotid artery stenosis using duplex ultrasonography: a validation study with computed tomographic angiography. *J Vasc Surg* 2010;51(1):65–70.
47. Garth KE, Carroll BA, Sommer FG, et al. Duplex ultrasound scanning of the carotid arteries with velocity spectrum analysis. *Radiology* 1983;147(3):823–827.
48. Kliewer MA, Freed KS, Hertzberg BS, et al. Temporal artery tap: usefulness and limitations in carotid sonography. *Radiology* 1996;201(2):481–484.
49. Post PN, Kievit J, van Baalen JM, et al. Routine duplex surveillance does not improve the outcome after carotid endarterectomy: a decision and cost utility analysis. *Stroke* 2002;33(3):749–755.
50. Roth SM, Back MR, Bandyk DF, et al. A rational algorithm for duplex scan surveillance after carotid endarterectomy. *J Vasc Surg* 1999;30(3):453–460.
51. Lal BK, Hobson RW 2nd, Tofighi B, et al. Duplex ultrasound velocity criteria for the stented carotid artery. *J Vasc Surg* 2008;47(1):63–73.
52. Sarkar S, Ghosh S, Ghosh SK, et al. Role of transcranial Doppler ultrasonography in stroke. *Postgrad Med J* 2007;83(985):683–689.
53. Harper C, Cardullo PA, Weyman AK, et al. Transcranial Doppler ultrasonography of the basilar artery in patients with retrograde vertebral artery flow. *J Vasc Surg* 2008;48(4):859–864.
54. Berguer R, Higgins R, Nelson R. Noninvasive diagnosis of reversal of vertebral-artery blood flow. *N Engl J Med* 1980;302(24):1349–1351.

55. Chaikof EL, Brewster DC, Dalman RL, et al. SVS practice guidelines for the care of patients with an abdominal aortic aneurysm: executive summary. *J Vasc Surg* 2009;50(4):880–896.
56. LaRoy LL, Cormier PJ, Matalon TA, et al. Imaging of abdominal aortic aneurysms. *AJR Am J Roentgenol* 1989;152(4):785–792.
57. Thompson SG, Ashton HA, Gao L, et al. Screening men for abdominal aortic aneurysm: 10 year mortality and cost effectiveness results from the Randomised Multicentre Aneurysm Screening Study. *BMJ* 2009;338:b2307.
58. Lederle FA, Wilson SE, Johnson GR, et al. Immediate repair compared with surveillance of small abdominal aortic aneurysms. *N Engl J Med* 2002;346(19):1437–1444.
59. Brady AR, Thompson SG, Fowkes FG, et al. Abdominal aortic aneurysm expansion: risk factors and time intervals for surveillance. *Circulation* 2004;110(1):16–21.
60. De Bruin JL, Baas AF, Buth J, et al. Long-term outcome of open or endovascular repair of abdominal aortic aneurysm. *N Engl J Med* 2010;362(20):1881–1889.
61. United Kingdom EVAR Trial Investigators; Greenhalgh RM, Brown LC, et al. Endovascular versus open repair of abdominal aortic aneurysm. *N Engl J Med* 2010;362(20):1863–1871.
62. Kent KC. Endovascular aneurysm repair—is it durable? *N Engl J Med.* 2010;362(20):1930–1931.
63. Sato DT, Goff CD, Gregory RT, et al. Endoleak after aortic stent graft repair: diagnosis by color duplex ultrasound scan versus computed tomography scan. *J Vasc Surg* 1998;28(4):657–663.
64. White GH, May J, Waugh RC, et al. Type III and type IV endoleak: toward a complete definition of blood flow in the sac after endoluminal AAA repair. *J Endovasc Surg* 1998;5(4):305–309.
65. Manning BJ, O'Neill SM, Haider SN, et al. Duplex ultrasound in aneurysm surveillance following endovascular aneurysm repair: a comparison with computed tomography aortography. *J Vasc Surg* 2009;49(1):60–65.
66. Dworkin LD, Cooper CJ. Clinical practice. Renal-artery stenosis. *N Engl J Med* 2009;361(20):1972–1978.
67. Olin JW, Piedmonte MR, Young JR, et al. The utility of duplex ultrasound scanning of the renal arteries for diagnosing significant renal artery stenosis. *Ann Intern Med* 1995;122(11):833–838.
68. Soares GM, Murphy TP, Singha MS, et al. Renal artery duplex ultrasonography as a screening and surveillance tool to detect renal artery stenosis: a comparison with current reference standard imaging. *J Ultrasound Med* 2006;25(3):293–298.
69. Drieghe B, Madaric J, Sarno G, et al. Assessment of renal artery stenosis: side-by-side comparison of angiography and duplex ultrasound with pressure gradient measurements. *Eur Heart J* 2008;29(4):517–524.
70. Motew SJ, Cherr GS, Craven TE, et al. Renal duplex sonography: main renal artery versus hilar analysis. *J Vasc Surg* 2000;32(3):462, 469; 469–471.
71. Radermacher J, Chavan A, Bleck J, et al. Use of Doppler ultrasonography to predict the outcome of therapy for renal-artery stenosis. *N Engl J Med* 2001;344(6):410–417.
72. Krumme B, Hollenbeck M. Doppler sonography in renal artery stenosis—does the resistive index predict the success of intervention? *Nephrol Dial Transplant* 2007;22(3):692–696.
73. Galin I, Trost B, Kang J, et al. In: *Validation of Renal Duplex Ultrasound in Detecting Renal Artery Stenosis Post Stenting.* American College of Cardiology Annual Scientific Sessions; March 2008; Chicago, Illinois.
74. Chi YW, White CJ, Thornton S, et al. Ultrasound velocity criteria for renal in-stent restenosis. *J Vasc Surg* 2009;50(1):119–123.
75. Sanders BM, Dalsing MC. Mesenteric ischemia affects young adults with predisposition. *Ann Vasc Surg* 2003;17(3):270–276.
76. Zwolak RM, Fillinger MF, Walsh DB, et al. Mesenteric and celiac duplex scanning: a validation study. *J Vasc Surg* 1998;27(6):1078, 1087; discussion 1088.
77. Erden A, Yurdakul M, Cumhur T. Marked increase in flow velocities during deep expiration: a duplex Doppler sign of celiac artery compression syndrome. *Cardiovasc Intervent Radiol* 1999;22(4):331–332.
78. Baccari P, Civilini E, Dordoni L, et al. Celiac artery compression syndrome managed by laparoscopy. *J Vasc Surg* 2009;50(1):134–139.
79. Moneta GL, Lee RW, Yeager RA, et al. Mesenteric duplex scanning: a blinded prospective study. *J Vasc Surg* 1993;17(1):79, 84; discussion 85–86.
80. Lilly MP, Harward TR, Flinn WR, et al. Duplex ultrasound measurement of changes in mesenteric flow velocity with pharmacologic and physiologic alteration of intestinal blood flow in man. *J Vasc Surg* 1989;9(1):18–25.
81. Mitchell EL, Chang EY, Landry GJ, et al. Duplex criteria for native superior mesenteric artery stenosis overestimate stenosis in stented superior mesenteric arteries. *J Vasc Surg* 2009;50(2):335–340.
82. McMillan WD, McCarthy WJ, Bresticker MR, et al. Mesenteric artery bypass: objective patency determination. *J Vasc Surg* 1995;21(5):729, 740; discussion 740–741.
83. Liem TK, Segall JA, Wei W, et al. Duplex scan characteristics of bypass grafts to mesenteric arteries. *J Vasc Surg* 2007;45(5):922, 927; discussion 927–928.
84. Webber GW, Jang J, Gustavson S, et al. Contemporary management of postcatheterization pseudoaneurysms. *Circulation* 2007;115(20):2666–2674.
85. Paulson EK, Sheafor DH, Kliewer MA, et al. Treatment of iatrogenic femoral arterial pseudoaneurysms: comparison of US-guided thrombin injection with compression repair. *Radiology* 2000;215(2):403–408.

Diagnostic Noninvasive Evaluations: CT

JONATHAN K. WEST, PATRICK T. NORTON, and KLAUS D. HAGSPIEL

INTRODUCTION

Computed tomography angiography (CTA) and magnetic resonance angiography (MRA) are highly accurate cross-sectional vascular imaging tools that have completely replaced diagnostic catheter angiography.[1,2] This chapter reviews the role of CTA for the evaluation and follow-up of patients with occlusive arterial disease involving the upper and lower extremities as well as the visceral aortic branches. CTA requires the acquisition of a three-dimensional (3D) volume during the peak enhancement phase of the vessels of interest following intravenous injection of iodinated contrast material. Helical (or spiral) CT is a method of CT scanning with continuous gantry rotation and data acquisition during table movement along the z-axis.[3,4] The advent of multidetector-row CT (MDCT) scanners in conjunction with powerful computer workstations rendered CTA the powerful vascular imaging tool it is today.[5,6] MDCT uses multiple detector rows for helical scanning that are switched together to allow scanning a number of slices or channels simultaneously. MDCT scanners achieve large anatomic coverage and allow scanning with isotropic collimation (submillimeter voxels, typically 0.5 to 0.6 mm).[7,8] At the time of this writing, systems were available with gantry rotation times of 300 msec or less and between 16 and 320 active detector rows, in addition to dual-source CT scanners. The more detectors a system has, the greater the coverage speed with fully comparable or better image quality.[9,10] This also translates into reduced contrast doses. Shorter scan times also mean better breath-hold compatibility, which improves the diagnostic accuracy for some applications. CT scan parameters and contrast administration have to be custom tailored to the anatomic area of interest as well as the CT scanner used for a particular exam.[11]

CTA requires the use of intravenous contrast media with the scan delay chosen such that the peak enhancement of the target vessel occurs during the actual data acquisition. We use automated bolus timing techniques like Smart Prep (General Electric Medical Systems, Milwaukee, PA) or Carebolus (Siemens Medical Systems, Malvern, PA) for all of our extracardiac CTA scans.

Table 37.1 gives typical scan parameters for CTA protocols used at our institution. We perform initial image analysis using the axial source data. Due to the large data sets, however, the use of 3D techniques is necessary for efficient image interpretation, specifically multiplanar reformation (MPR), maximum intensity projection (MIP), and volume rendering (VR). MPR techniques allow the acquisition of planar images in sagittal, coronal, or oblique orientations and are particularly useful for the evaluation of stent patency or vessels with eccentric calcifications.[12] Curved MPRs are particularly suitable to display tortuous vessels, such as iliac arteries. The creation of two perpendicular longitudinal cross-sections along the median center line of the target vessel aids in stenosis quantification. The MIP algorithm creates images that are most like a conventional angiogram, but the algorithm has several limitations. Although MIPs facilitate detection of calcium and stents, they do not allow imaging of the vascular lumen within a stent or calcified plaque. Also, MIP requires bone removal, which can, despite the availability of automated bone removal algorithms, be a time-consuming task. Multiple overlapping vessels can make MIP images difficult to interpret, but this can be overcome by using only a subvolume of the data (thin-slab MIP).[2]

Unlike MIP techniques, VR allows the simultaneous display of structures with differing attenuation levels. Depending on the chosen opacity parameters, all voxels can contribute to the final image, which makes VR techniques more computing intensive than MIP and MPR. VR allows quick review of large datasets, however, because bone removal is generally not necessary. VR techniques also allow virtual angioscopy, a fly-through simulation.

LOWER EXTREMITY ARTERIAL SYSTEM

Imaging assessment of patients with peripheral arterial disease (PAD) requires coverage of the abdominal aorta, inflow, outflow, and runoff vessels. Such an extensive scan range became feasible with the advent of 4-channel MDCTA technology. In 2001, a study of 24 consecutive patients with symptomatic lower extremity arterial disease who underwent both 4-channel MDCT and digital subtraction arteriography (DSA), a mean scanning time of 66 seconds was required to cover a mean of 1,233 mm, producing a mean of 908 reconstructed transverse images (1.6-mm reconstructed slice thickness). All 504 arterial segments imaged were of diagnostic quality, using now 10-year-old technology.[13] With current 64-channel MDCT technology, acquisition time is reduced, resulting in the acquisition of 2,000 slices of 0.6-mm thickness in approximately 30 seconds or less.[14] The achieved spatial resolution outperforms the best MRA techniques. For analysis of runoff studies, we primarily interactively review coronal thin-slab MIPs in conjunction with the axial slices. MPRs, curved MPRs, and VR reconstructions are used as an adjunct. Oblique MPRs and thin slab MIPs are particularly useful for analysis of bifurcations, such as the aortic, iliac, and femoral bifurcations. They are also very useful for evaluation of the proximal runoff vessels because they do not require bone removal. We only use curved planar reconstruction (CPR) for stenosis quantification if an exact value is critical; otherwise we report a vessel as patent, mildly (<50%), moderately (50% to 70%) or severely (>70%) stenosed, or occluded. We also report the length of the stenotic or occluded segment.

Table 37.1

CTA Protocol Scan Parameters

	Scan range	16-Sector collimation	64-Sector collimation	16-Sector pitch	64-Sector pitch	kV
Renal CTA	Diaphragm to iliac crest	0.6–1.0	0.6–1.0	1.375	1.375	120
Mesenteric CTA (a) Arterial phase	Diaphragm to ischial tuberosity	0.6–1.0	0.6–1.0	1.375	1.375	120
(b) Portal venous phase	Same	1.0–1.5	1.0–1.5	1.375	1.375	120
Lower extremity CTA	Diaphragm to knee joint	0.6–1.0	0.6–1.0	1.75	1.375	120
	Knee joint to toes	0.6–1.0	0.6–1.0	1.75	1.0	100
Upper extremity CTA	Arch to elbow	0.6–1.0	0.6–1.0	1.75	1.0	120
	Elbow to fingertips	0.6–1.0	0.6–1.0	1.75	1.0	100

MIPs and thin-slab MIPs are particularly useful for the display of embolic disease because abrupt cutoffs and asymmetries of small vessels can become more apparent.[15]

The postprocessing of MDCTA data of the peripheral vascular system has been significantly facilitated by automated and semiautomated bone segmentation algorithms. A remaining significant limitation of CTA as compared to MRA is the impaired visualization of small vessel lumens in the presence of arterial wall calcification, particularly circumferential wall calcifications. Because these occur more frequently in patients with tissue loss or rest pain and diabetes, we usually perform MRA in these patients. One "problem" with 64-row MDCT and its inherently high-scan speeds is the possibility of outrunning the arterial bolus, resulting in nonopacification of distal vessels, particularly in patients who have severe upstream disease with poor collateralization. A reduction of table speed (decrease of pitch) or the use of two station protocols (which require extra time to switch kilovoltage) generally alleviate this problem (Table 37.1). Alternatively, a two-timing bolus technique can be used (one in the proximal abdominal aorta, one at the popliteal level), and the table speed and injection rate are then custom tailored to the individual patient's cardiac output and lower extremity flow. In reality, we find this approach rarely necessary.

Atherosclerotic Disease of the Lower Extremities

The vast majority of lower extremity steno-occlusive PAD is caused by atherosclerosis. It is estimated that the prevalence of atherosclerotic PAD is 2.5% in individuals 50 to 59 years of age and 14.5% in those over the age of 70. Of PAD patients, 40% to 60% have concomitant coronary artery disease and a significantly increased prevalence of cerebrovascular disease.[14]

Atherosclerotic plaques in the aortoiliac inflow vessels and femoropopliteal outflow vessels can be readily evaluated by

CTA, as can plaque composition, that is, calcific versus fibrofatty plaque. CTA allows evaluation of the length and severity of a stenosis or occlusion, and lesions can be categorized using the TASC II classification, which is used to guide management of aortoiliac and femoropopliteal occlusive disease.[16]

Because of the large size of the aorta, CTA allows excellent evaluation of distal abdominal aortic occlusive disease (FIGURE 37.1). Leriche syndrome is defined as atherosclerotic occlusive disease involving the abdominal aorta and, often, the iliac arteries. Classic symptoms include buttock, thigh, and leg claudication with erectile dysfunction in males. Therapy depends on the extent of disease, and CTA allows assessment of this as well as evaluating the presence of collateral pathways and level of arterial reconstitution, thus allowing accurate treatment planning.

A study comparing contrast enhanced MRA (ceMRA) and 4-channel MDCT to DSA in the evaluation of hemodynamically significant arterial stenosis of the aortoiliac system reported sensitivities greater than 90% and specificities greater than 98% for both modalities with excellent interobserver and intermodality agreement (kappa 0.88 to 0.90). Three-dimensional data postprocessing was significantly more time consuming for CTA ($p < .001$). Patients preferred CTA over ceMRA ($p = .016$).[17] The same group also compared the accuracy of 16-channel MDCTA with conventional DSA in the assessment of aortoiliac and lower extremity arteries in 39 patients with PAD. MDCTA demonstrated a sensitivity of 96% and a specificity of 97% with excellent interobserver agreement (kappa 0.84 to 1.00). The presence of anteroposteriorly located luminal narrowing and extensive vascular calcifications were the main factors leading to disparate results between the two modalities.[10] A meta-analysis of studies published between January 2000 and April 2006 analyzing the performance of MDCTA for the detection of stenoses greater than 50% in the lower extremity arterial system as compared to DSA included 12 studies. These included 9,551 arterial segments in 436 patients, resulting in a

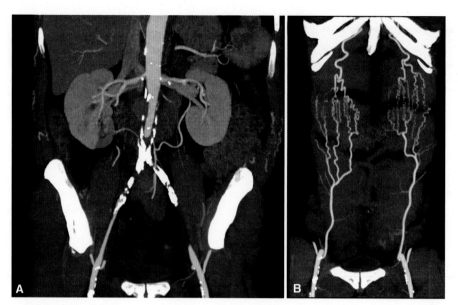

FIGURE 37.1 Leriche syndrome. **A**. Coronal subvolume MIP reconstruction from aortoiliac CTA demonstrates occlusion of the abdominal aorta just distal to the origin of the inferior mesenteric artery. The right common iliac artery and left common and external iliac arteries are also occluded. The lower pole of the right kidney is infarcted due to occlusion of an inferior right accessory renal artery. **B**. Coronal subvolume MIP reconstruction of the abdominal wall in the same patient reveals dense collateral formation between the mammillary arteries (superiorly) and the inferior epigastic arteries.

combined sensitivity and specificity of 92% (95% confidence interval: 89%, 95%) and 93% (95% confidence interval: 91%, 95%), respectively.[18]

Another meta-analysis included 20 studies performed between 2002 and 2008 and demonstrated that 94% of occlusions and 87% of stenoses greater than 50% identified by DSA were correctly identified by CTA. This study also showed superior performance of 16- and 64-channel CT scanners (sensitivity 97%, specificity 98%) compared to 2- and 4-channel models (sensitivity 92%, specificity 93%).[19] A retrospective Italian study comparing 64-channel MDCTA and DSA obtained in individuals with PAD found a 97.2% sensitivity, 97% specificity, 97.1% diagnostic accuracy, and 95.4% concordance with DSA on degree of stenosis.[20] Shareghi et al. showed a sensitivity of 99% and specificity of 98% for the detection of stenoses in the inflow, outflow, and runoff vessels using 64-row MDCTA with DSA as the "gold standard." In this study, MDCTA visualized more segments of the vascular tree than DSA, suggesting MDCTA to be as good as or better than DSA.[21] In the most recent prospective nonrandomized study comparing CTA and DSA in 212 patients for diagnosis of stenoses greater than 70%, CTA had an accuracy of 98%, Positive Predictive Value (PPV) of 96%, and Negative Predictive Value (NPV) of 99% with excellent interobserver agreement (kappa ≥ 0.928). Additionally, CTA was faster (12 versus 58 minutes on average) and better tolerated by patients.[22]

MDCTA is constantly evolving and improving. In an effort to reduce radiation and iodinated contrast doses, a group from Japan compared 120 and 80 kVp scan protocols in 80 patients with suspected PAD. This prospective randomized trial showed a 30% reduction in contrast dose and radiation dose (mean dose length product) for the 80 kVp arm without significant difference in image quality or vascular enhancement.[23] The high average body mass index (BMI) in our patient population precludes us from using a 80 kVp protocol routinely, but we use a two-station runoff protocol with the upper station (diaphragm to knee joint) acquired at 120/100 kVp and the lower station at 100/80 kVp.

Dual energy CTA holds promise for improving the accuracy of CTA, even in the setting of significant vascular calcifications. The technology allows the differentiation of calcium and iodine based on attenuation differences at different peak kilovoltage levels, thus making it possible to subtract mural calcifications and osseous structures automatically from the images (FIGURE 37.2). Kau et al.[24] found good agreement between stenosis grading using 3D MIPs after automated dual energy CTA plaque and bone removal and DSA above the knee, moderate agreement in the calf, and insufficient agreement in the pedal arteries (overall sensitivity 84%, specificity 67%). Time-resolved CTA has also been studied in the form of a 12-phase scan of the runoff vessels. A significant decrease in venous contamination and improved diagnostic confidence was found at the expense of higher radiation and contrast dose.[25]

CTA provides an excellent roadmap to plan treatment, be it medical, open surgical, or endovascular. It allows choice of the appropriate vascular access as well as determination of the optimal angulation of the X-ray tube during interventions. The TASC guidelines use catheter angiography–based measurements of location, degree, and length of steno-occlusions. MDCTA provides much of the same information and one study found

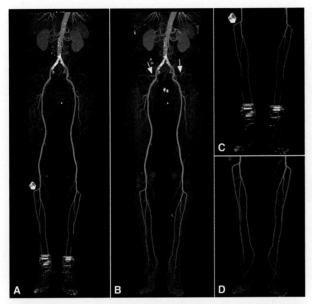

FIGURE 37.2 Postprocessing bone removal. When displaying full-volume CTA data, it is useful to remove bones so that arteries can be displayed without obscuration. Bone removal is typically performed using density threshold and continuity algorithms on 3D workstations (**A, C**). This process can be improved utilizing material separation properties of dual energy CT (**B, D**). In **A**, there is incomplete removal of the right patella as well as incomplete removal of bone within the ankles and feet. Additionally, there has been errant removal of portions of the anterior tibial arteries (**C**). In **B**, material separation based on dual energy provides improved retention of small vessels (*arrows*) as compared to **A** as well as complete bone removal. Additionally, the anterior tibial artery, with its close proximity to bone, was preserved (**D**).

that an MDCTA-based treatment plan was identical to a DSA-based plan in 190 of 191 patients.[22] A retrospective study evaluating the appropriateness of CTA-based treatment decisions for Fontaine Stage IIb PAD concluded that CTA-based decisions were highly reliable and accurate for treatment planning.[26] The same group performed a similar retrospective analysis in patients with Fontaine Stage IV PAD (critical limb ischemia) and again demonstrated that MDCTA was accurate in assigning TASC classification and management planning. All endovascular and surgical treatments in this series were performed as indicated by findings on CTA.[27]

Embolic Disease

Arterial embolic disease of the lower extremities can be easily diagnosed with CTA. Emboli often originate in the heart, particularly in individuals with atrial fibrillation or heart failure, or from aortic atheromas or thrombus within aneurysms. Embolic disease can be bilateral or unilateral (especially if the source is an iliac lesion or popliteal aneurysm) (FIGURE 37.3). CTA shows the presence and location of embolic occlusion and identifies the source in many cases. Use of prospective ECG-gating for the thoracic portion of the CTA can aid in detection of cardiac thrombus. Unexpected emboli are frequently present in internal

iliac and deep femoral branches. CTA offers a good roadmap to guide surgical or catheter-based embolectomy and vascular reconstruction (FIGURE 37.3).

Aortic Dissection

Abdominal aortic dissections are usually extensions of thoracic dissections but can rarely be isolated. The dissection can extend into the iliofemoral arteries, occasionally resulting in flow limitation. The main task for the assessment of dissections of the abdominal aorta is to determine involvement of the renal and visceral branches as well as the iliofemoral arteries, demonstrating whether the arteries arise from the true or false lumen. The high spatial resolution of CTA allows the detailed assessment of the aortic dissection flap as well as its relationship with the side branches. If surgical or endovascular intervention is required, CTA is an excellent planning tool to determine stent graft sizing and positioning of fenestration sites. CTA is often used for follow-up of dissections to detect aneurysmal dilatation and to evaluate for extension of the dissection flap.

Arterial Endofibrosis

Cyclists are the athletes most commonly affected by arterial endofibrosis, a disease that manifests mainly in the external iliac artery (EIA). Intimal fibrotic thickening results in stenosis caused by repetitive vessel damage from hemodynamic and mechanical stress in highly trained athletes. Symptoms are unilateral (85% of cases) claudication-like pain, feeling of loss of power, and leg cramps after supramaximal effort. DSA is the reference standard and requires multiple projections and dynamic examination in different hip positions simulating cycling. Angiographic findings are frequently subtle and consist of smooth or irregular eccentric stenoses without calcifications. CTA (and MRA) allows acquisition of images in different hip positions (extended and flexed) and can show luminal narrowing, wall thickening, and kinking during hip flexion as well as excessive vessel length. CTA has been shown to assist with the diagnosis and is also useful for surgical planning and treatment monitoring.[28] Treatment is surgical; endofibrosectomy with vein patch angioplasty, bypass placement, shortening of the artery, and release from the psoas muscle or inguinal ligament are the main therapeutic options.[28]

Cystic Adventitial Disease

Cystic adventitial disease is a rare cause of nonatherosclerotic popliteal artery stenosis. Other vessels can be involved, but 85% of these lesions are found in the popliteal artery. The disease is characterized by a mucus-containing cyst between the arterial adventitia and media, which leads to compression and even occlusion of the artery. The classic angiographic finding is an abrupt but smooth narrowing of the vessel. If the lesion is circumferential it can have an "hourglass" appearance, and if it is eccentric it presents with the "scimitar sign." On CTA, a low-density cystic lesion is seen intimately associated with the artery, causing stenosis of the lumen by mass effect on the artery. MRI is generally considered superior to CTA for this disease.[29]

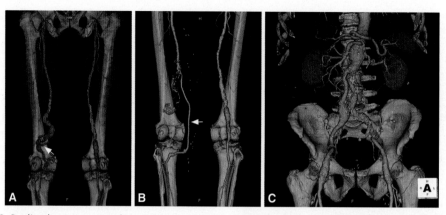

FIGURE 37.3 Popliteal aneurysms and intervention. **A**. Volume-rendered posterior reconstruction from CTA in a patient with bilateral popliteal artery aneurysm. The larger left aneurysm is bound by calcification (*arrow*) surrounding the lumen, and the mural thrombus is not visualized. **B**. CTA after surgical ligation of the aneurysm sac and vein bypass (*arrow*) from left superficial femoral artery to distal popliteal artery. **C**. The same patient also had undergone surgical repair of an infrarenal abdominal aortic aneurysm using a bifurcated aortoiliac graft. There is also aneurysmal dilatation of the juxtarenal abdominal aorta, the common iliac, and the common femoral arteries. About one-third of patients with a unilateral popliteal and two-thirds of those with bilateral popliteal artery aneurysm will have an abdominal aortic aneurysm.

Popliteal Entrapment Syndrome

Popliteal entrapment syndrome is characterized by calf pain and intermittent claudication most commonly encountered in young, active men. The etiology is an anomalous relationship between the gastrocnemius muscle, its tendons, and the popliteal vessels, which results in compression and symptomatic stenosis of the artery or vein.[30] Six types of popliteal entrapment have been described. Type I entrapment involves an abnormal course of the popliteal artery medial to the medial head of the gastrocnemius muscle. Type II entrapment is a result of an abnormally lateral distal femur insertion of the medial head of the gastrocnemius displacing the popliteal artery medially. Type III is caused by an accessory slip from the medial head of the gastrocnemius wrapping around a normally positioned popliteal artery. Type IV entrapment is caused by a fibrous band or popliteal muscle. Type V entrapment involves the vein. Type VI is more of a functional type with normal positional anatomy but hypertrophy of the gastrocnemius.[31] Repetitive trauma caused by these anatomic variants can result in abnormalities of the vessel itself, such as early atherosclerosis, aneurysm formation, and intrinsic stenosis. Both CTA and magnetic resonance imaging/magnetic resonance angiography (MRI/MRA) are useful noninvasive modalities to make the diagnosis (FIGURE 37.4).[32]

Stents and Bypass Grafts

Peripheral arterial bypass grafts of the lower extremities are periodically monitored, most commonly with duplex ultrasound, to detect abnormalities early and intervene before progression to graft failure. MDCTA demonstrates excellent performance in the evaluation of peripheral arterial bypass grafts and is useful for triaging patients with bypass complications and planning for either endovascular or open surgical repair (FIGURE 37.3). Common problems with bypass grafts include occlusion, anastomotic stenoses, and poor inflow or outflow caused by native disease progression. Other problems include vein graft injury, retained valves, kinks, graft infection (indicated by presence

of air, perigraft fluid, or soft tissue), pseudoaneurysms, arteriovenous fistulae, as well as extravascular complications.[33] Willmann et al. studied 99 arterial bypass graft segments in 27 patients to evaluate for hemodynamically significant stenoses

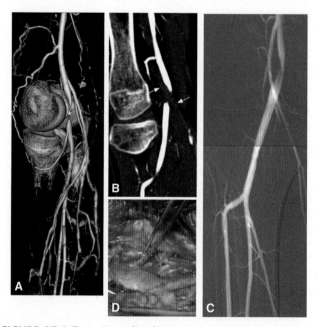

FIGURE 37.4 Type III popliteal artery entrapment. **A**. Volume-rendered imaging from a CTA of the lower extremity performed during forced plantar flexion. There is complete occlusion (*) of the popliteal artery, near the level of the insertion of the medial head of the gastrocnemius. **B**. Sagittal MIP reconstruction reveals the accessory muscle slip (*arrows*) from the gastrocnemius compressing the popliteal artery (type III entrapment). **C**. AP projection catheter angiogram demonstrating medial displacement and compression of the popliteal artery typical of entrapment. **D**. Intraoperative photo of the accessory muscle slip (*forceps*).

using MDCTA and duplex ultrasound, comparing the findings to DSA as the reference standard. Twenty-nine significant stenoses were detected at DSA out of 99 bypass graft segments yielding sensitivities and specificities for MDCTA of 97% to 100% and 100%, respectively, and for duplex ultrasound of 100% and 96%, respectively.[17] CTA is useful to follow stented arterial segments when duplex ultrasound is inconclusive. Using reduced field of view and medium or sharp kernels in concert with coronal, oblique MPR, or CPR views improves evaluation of in-stent stenosis.[34] Li et al. performed a prospective comparison of 64-slice MDCTA and DSA for evaluation of 81 peripheral stents in 41 patients. The overall sensitivity and specificity for in-stent stenosis of MDCTA were 85.7% and 71.7%, respectively, for all stents. Excluding the 23.5% of stents that were not assessable on MDCTA due to metal and motion artifact resulted in 95.4% and 96.4%, respectively.[35] CTA can also demonstrate other stent complications such as migration, fracture, and infection (FIGURE 37.5).

Nonatherosclerotic Causes of Lower Extremity Occlusive Disease

Fibromuscular dysplasia (FMD) can rarely manifest in the iliac, femoral, popliteal, and anterior tibial arteries, with the EIA most commonly affected.[36] Vasculitides can cause occlusive disease of the aortoiliac and peripheral arterial system. The more common vasculitides affecting the lower extremities are TA, Buerger disease, and giant cell arteritis. Takayasu arteritis

(TA) is an idiopathic, large-vessel vasculitis most commonly found in young Asian women that typically involves the thoracoabdominal aorta and its branches as well as the pulmonary arteries. Steno-occlusive disease involving the abdominal aorta and proximal iliac arteries with normal distal iliac and outflow/runoff vessels in the appropriate patient population should raise the question of TA.[37] CTA may demonstrate thickening of the vessel wall or mural enhancement with more progressive disease showing areas of stenosis, occlusion, or aneurysm. Planning for intervention or follow-up with CTA may be necessary if significant stenosis or aneurysm is present because these features can worsen despite corticosteroid treatment (FIGURE 37.6).[14] Giant cell arteritis more commonly affects the upper extremities and is discussed in more depth in that section. Buerger disease, an occlusive vasculitis of medium-sized arteries, presents in smokers in the fifth decade of life with rest pain and tissue loss. There is a characteristic lack of atherosclerotic disease with specific location of lesions in the distal femoral, popliteal, and proximal tibioperoneal arteries associated with significant collateral vessel formation. CTA or DSA demonstrate high-grade focal, concentric stenosis with collateral formation resulting in a "corkscrew appearance."[14]

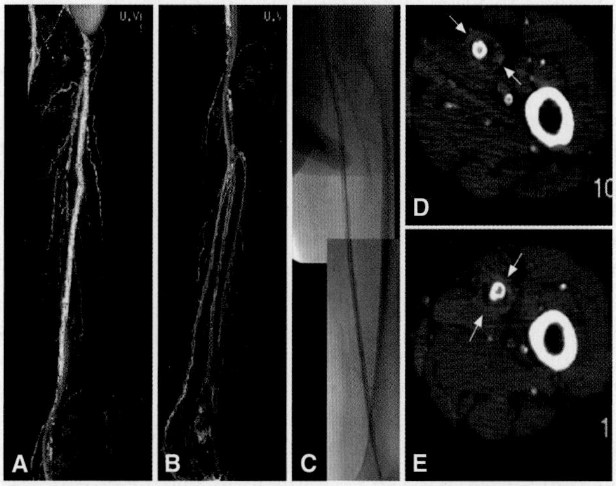

FIGURE 37.5 Infected stents. A 62-year-old man presented with fevers and tenderness of the upper thigh after subintimal recanalization and stenting of the left superficial femoral artery (SFA). CTA revealed infection of the SFA stents. VR reconstruction of the left thigh (**A**) and below knee runoff vessels (**B**) after bone removal demonstrates the extent of stenting within the SFA and venous contamination in the calf vessels (**B**) and, to a lesser extent, in the popliteal vein (**A**). Venous contamination is more often encountered in infected extremities caused by hyperemia. **C**. Completion catheter angiogram demonstrates patency of the SFA stents. Infected fluid collection surrounds the stent in the upper (**D**) and lower (**E**) thigh. The fluid collections are lower density centrally and have a thick, enhancing rim (*arrows*).

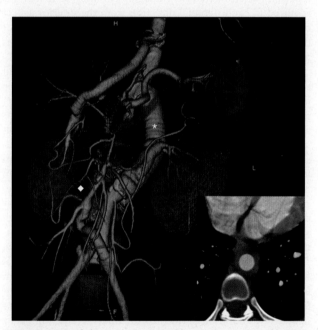

FIGURE 37.6 Abdominal aortic and visceral reconstruction in a woman with Takayasu vasculitis. A young woman developed severe occlusive disease of the abdominal aorta with involvement of the visceral vessels. She underwent surgical reconstruction of the abdominal aorta (*) from just superior to the celiac artery to above the origin of the inferior mesenteric artery. A graft was placed to reconnect the left renal artery with the aortic graft. The right renal artery was revascularized with a supraceliac graft. The superior mesenteric artery was supplied via a graft from the left common iliac artery. An occluded celiac bypass graft is seen originating from the right common iliac artery (υ). (*Inset*) Axial image from the same CTA demonstrates descending thoracic aortic wall thickening typical for Takayasu vasculitis.

Abdominal coarctation is extremely rare and can be acquired or congenital. Neurofibromatosis (NF 1) can lead to stenoses of the abdominal aorta and its branches.

UPPER EXTREMITY ARTERIAL SYSTEM

Occlusive arterial disease is less frequent in the upper than in the lower extremity. Imaging of the upper extremity (UE) arterial system is necessary in trauma for the diagnosis of atherosclerotic/embolic events, vasculitis, and the preoperative planning of complex UE reconstructions or endovascular procedures. DSA has been the main imaging modality for evaluation of UE arterial disease due to its high spatial and temporal resolution. MDCTA has become a noninvasive alternative to DSA, however, and it is now the initial diagnostic test of choice for the evaluation of UE vascular pathology at our institution. MDCTA demonstrates excellent diagnostic performance from the aortic arch and the arm vessels to the level of the deep and superficial palmar arches. The distal vessels of the hand still remain the realm of DSA. The scan is performed with the extremity of interest over the head and fingers extended. If necessary, patients can be imaged with the arms at the side; however, this results in significantly degraded image quality. Intravenous access is obtained in the contralateral arm.[38] Alternatively, central lines or femoral access can be used, especially when bilateral UE imaging is required. Imaging is acquired in caudo-cranial direction from the inferior aspect of the aortic arch to the tips of the fingers with the center of the field of view weighted toward the extremity of interest as much as possible.

Vascular injuries of the UE account for up to 50% of all peripheral vascular injuries, and CTA has been shown to be invaluable in this setting. Traumatic lesions of peripheral arteries occur mainly as a result of penetrating injuries (such as gunshot wounds) and motor vehicle accidents. Trauma can result in vasospasm, extrinsic vascular compression, dissection, occlusion, arteriovenous fistula (AVF) formation, pseudoaneurysm formation, and rupture or transection. Imaging is employed in hemodynamically stable patients if clinical findings suggest arterial injury, including diminished distal pulses or neuromuscular dysfunction. As early as 1999 spiral CTA was found to have high sensitivity (95.1%) and specificity (98.7%) for detection of traumatic arterial injuries, including partial and complete occlusion, pseudoaneurysm formation, and presence of AVFs and intimal flaps.[39] Seamon et al. prospectively studied 22 patients with less than 0.9 ankle brachial index (ABI) or evidence of extremity injury after trauma who went on to have CTA and DSA or operative exploration performed for injury evaluation. They reported 100% sensitivity and specificity of CTA for the diagnosis of traumatic injury with only one nondiagnostic study. Seven of these studies were of the UE.[40] Inaba et al. performed a similar prospective study of adults who sustained extremity trauma. MDCTA was compared to DSA, operative findings, or clinical follow-up. The authors concluded that CTA was 100% sensitive and specific in identifying clinically significant vascular injuries of the extremities, although 7 of the 89 studies (9.6%) in their series were not diagnostic due to metallic artifact or reformatting errors.[41]

Atherosclerotic disease affects the UE less often than the lower extremity. In our experience, the accuracy for detecting occlusion is greater than that for grading stenosis, especially in small-caliber vessels. Similar to CTA for the lower extremity, UE CTA effectively evaluates for stenosis, occlusion, aneurysm, and embolic events, especially when they affect vessels proximal to the wrist.

The imaging appearance of thrombembolic disease in the UE is similar to that of other vascular territories with emboli appearing as filling defects within larger arteries, typically with a meniscus sign. Emboli can be occlusive or nonocclusive. In smaller arteries, filling defects are not typically appreciated and abrupt occlusion is the dominant finding. Most emboli originate from the heart. There are several sources of emboli that are unique to the UE, however, including thoracic outlet compression, hypothenar hammer syndrome (HHS), the circumflex humeri artery in baseball pitchers, and occluded axillary-femoral bypass grafts. Thoracic outlet syndrome (TOS) occurs when the neurovascular bundle is compressed by the structures of the thoracic outlet. The neurovascular bundle exits the thorax at the thoracic outlet between the scalene muscles and the first rib and clavicle. It is classified into arterial, venous, or neurogenic TOS based on the compressed structure with neurogenic TOS accounting for 85% to 98% of cases. Neurogenic TOS generally presents with pain, numbness, and paresthesia radiating from the shoulder down the arm, especially with overhead activity. Arterial TOS (<1% of cases) presents with claudication of the arm with activity and can result in subclavian artery aneurysm formation with thrombus formation and distal embolization to the fingers. Venous TOS results in swelling and pain of the affected extremity and symptoms associated with venous thrombosis. The diagnosis of arterial TOS on CTA is made with the arm in hyperabduction. Subtle dilatation or aneurysm formation distal to a stenosis with or without wall adherent thrombus or distal embolization can be present (FIGURE 37.7). A search for osseous abnormalities that can cause thoracic outlet compression, such as cervical ribs or fractures of the clavicle or first rib, should be performed. Arterial TOS is not a commonly encountered clinical entity.[42] CTA may also be helpful in diagnosing the more common neurogenic TOS.[43] It is important to realize that CTA can be false negative in the evaluation of TOS, primarily due to problems of positioning the arm in the gantry in the position that causes the symptoms. In cases with abnormal stress Doppler examination and negative CTA, we usually perform catheter angiography.

HHS is a result of repetitive trauma to the distal ulnar artery and superficial palmar arch caused by entrapment between an external force and the hamulus. This results in arterial wall damage and stenosis, thrombosis, or aneurysm formation with distal embolic disease. Symptoms are that of ischemia in the second to the fifth digits. HHS can occasionally be diagnosed with CTA, which demonstrates occlusion of the distal ulnar artery near the hypothenar eminence.[44]

MDCTA is suitable to diagnose vasculitis of the proximal UE arterial system. Takayasu arteritis, giant cell arteritis, and thromboangiitis obliterans are also the most common types of vasculitides affecting the UE vessels. Acute vasculitis can be differentiated from atherosclerotic disease by the presence of constitutional symptoms including fevers, malaise, myalgias, and arthralgias. Laboratory values, such as elevated inflammatory markers, provide supporting evidence for the diagnosis. On CTA, vasculitis tends to present as long, segmental stenoses with gentle tapering, as opposed to the focal stenosis and abrupt occlusion of atherosclerosis. Vessel wall thickening

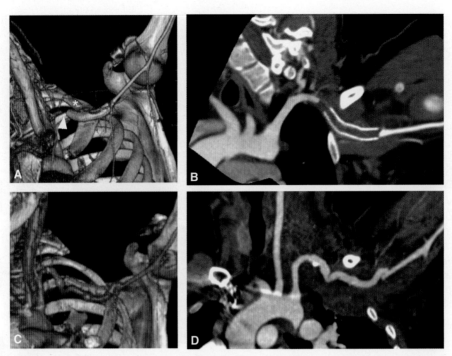

FIGURE 37.7 Thoracic outlet syndrome. A 17-year-old woman underwent placement of a covered stent for occlusive disease at an outside institution. Several months after the procedure, the patient presented with heaviness and coolness of the left arm and hand. **A.** VR image demonstrates the occluded subclavian artery and stent (*arrowhead*) and the presence of a left cervical rib (*). The clavicle was removed on the workstation for clarity. **B.** Curved MPR of the left subclavian artery demonstrates a completely thrombosed stent. The patient underwent surgical revision with subclavian artery bypass with vein graft and resection of the left cervical and first ribs, shown on this VR image (**C**). Curved MPR confirms patency of the subclavian bypass (**D**).

and enhancement are also characteristic signs. Thickening of the arterial wall in vasculitis is typically isodense to muscle, as opposed to hypodense noncalcific atherosclerotic plaque. A delayed phase scan can be helpful to demonstrate wall enhancement, although MRI would be the better test in our opinion if vasculitis is suspected. Skip lesions in the axillary and brachial arteries are typical for giant cell vasculitis. As in other vascular beds, CTA is helpful for both treatment planning and evaluation of bypass grafts or stents (FIGURE 37.7).

Renal Arteries

CTA displays the normal arterial and venous anatomy and its normal variants in exquisite detail.[45] Modern 64-slice scanners allow coverage of the aorta, the renal arteries, and the kidneys with isotropic resolution in as little as 5 seconds.[9,46] The main renal arteries typically originate from the aorta below the superior mesenteric artery at the L1 to L2 vertebral level before dividing into segmental arteries near the renal hilum.[47] RA variations are divided into arteries with early division (proximal segmental artery branching) and extrarenal arteries. Extrarenal arteries can be hilar (accessory) arteries that enter the kidney in the hilum or polar (aberrant) arteries (which enter outside the hilum).[48,49]

The main clinical uses of CTA of the renal arteries are the detection of renal artery stenosis (RAS) and, less frequently, the evaluation of kidney donors, kidney trauma, renal aneurysms, or hematuria of unknown origin.

The most common indication for imaging of the renal artery (RA) in our center is the evaluation of patients with suspected renovascular hypertension (RVH) and or insufficiency. RVH is the leading cause of secondary hypertension and is thought to occur in 3% to 5% of all hypertensive patients. Because it is theoretically curable with revascularization, detection is important.[50] Most RVH patients have atherosclerotic RAS (estimated to occur in 70% to 90% of cases), followed by FMD. Atherosclerotic RAS is typically ostial (within 10 mm of the aortic wall) or truncal (in the proximal to mid-RA more than 10 mm from the ostium). DSA is considered the gold standard for the diagnosis of RAS due to high spatial and temporal resolution and the ability to perform intra-arterial pressure measurements. CTA has been shown to have relatively high sensitivities (>90%) and specificities (83% to 98%), however, for the detection of atherosclerotic RAS in a number of single center series.[17,50–61] It was shown to be superior to Doppler sonography for the detection of RAS.[53] As in other vascular territories, lesion quantification can be difficult due to small vessel size or calcifications of the aorta or renal arteries, generally resulting in overestimation. The latter has been improved with the advent of dual energy CT-based calcific plaque subtraction (FIGURE 37.8). We consider 64-detector MDCTA the modality of choice for elderly patients with normal renal function, whereas we perform contrast-enhanced or noncontrast MRA in children, younger patients, and patients with renal insufficiency.

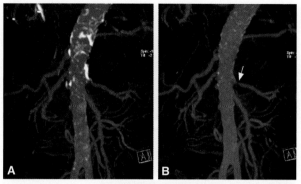

FIGURE 37.8 Dual energy plaque subtraction. Using dual energy CT, calcified atherosclerotic plaques can be subtracted from CTA datasets using separation based on difference in atomic properties between calcium and iodine. **A**. Full-thickness MIP from a dual energy CTA of the renal arteries with calcified plaques included. **B**. Same MIP reconstruction after calcified plaques have been removed reveals the presence of a high-grade left renal artery stenosis (*arrow*) that is difficult to visualize in **A**.

Nonatherosclerotic Occlusive Renal Artery Disease

FMD is a nonatherosclerotic, noninflammatory vascular disease of unclear etiology and the most common cause of RVH in young patients.[62,63] It is estimated to account for 30% to 40% of RAS and predominantly affects young and middle-aged females.[62] The FMD classification is based on the involved arterial wall layer and the histopathologic findings (FIGURE 37.9).[62] Medial fibroplasia (60% to 70%) is the most common type in adults. It tends to affect the mid-to-distal portion of the main RA but can extend into the proximal segmental branches and has the classic "string of beads" appearance. Perimedial fibroplasia (10% to 25%) presents with focal and, occasionally, multiple stenoses. The beads are less numerous and smaller than in medial fibroplasias due to lack of aneurysm formation. Medial hyperplasia (5% to 15%) and intimal fibroplasia (1% to 2%) manifest as smooth band-like stenoses in the proximal or distal main renal arteries. Adventitial fibroplasia (<1%) presents as localized tubular stenosis. Complications of FMD include aneurysm formation, dissection, and RA occlusion. The detection of moderate-to-severe FMD is generally possible on a high-quality CTA scan, although the determination of the hemodynamic impact and the detection of subtle FMD or FMD in small side branches require DSA. The differentiation of atherosclerosis from FMD is straightforward, with the former affecting the ostial and proximal RA in older patients, and the latter the mid-to-distal arterial segments in younger patients. Segmental arterial mediolysis (SAM) is a rare condition whose cause is not known.[64] CTA findings described are arterial dilation, dissection, occlusion and fusiform aneurysm formation, perivascular stranding, and hemorrhage. It resembles FMD but SAM predominantly affects the visceral and renal arteries of elderly patients, whereas FMD tends to affect a younger age group.[65]

TA can affect the renal arteries.[37,48] CTA findings are renal arterial wall thickening with or without luminal narrowing, occlusion, and aneurysm formation.[66]

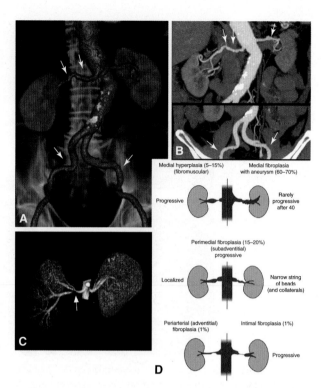

FIGURE 37.9 Fibromuscular dysplasia. **A**. VR reconstruction of CTA from a patient with medial fibroplasia type of fibromuscular dysplasia (FMD) involving the renal arteries and external iliac arteries. FMD involves the renal arteries most commonly, followed by the carotid arteries and then iliac arteries (*arrows*). **B**. MIP reconstruction from the same dataset demonstrates the regions of alternating web-like stenosis and aneurysms that are typical of this type of FMD (*arrows*). Note the involvement of the mid and distal renal arteries. **C**. Intimal fibroplasia-type FMD in a 3-month-old boy with persistent hypertension despite multiple medications. There is a long segment high-grade stenosis (*arrow*) in the branch supplying the anterior segment, resulting in decrease perfusion of the majority of the right kidney. **D**. Illustrations show the manifestations and relative incidences of various subtypes of FMD that involve the renal arteries.

Polyarteritis nodosa (PAN) is a medium and small artery vasculitis and frequently involves the kidneys.[48] Catheter angiographic findings include vessel irregularity, microaneurysms, dissection, stenosis, and occlusion. Microaneurysms tend to be multiple and intraparenchymal and CTA is not well suited for their diagnosis due to the small size and the fact that they are usually obliterated by parenchymal background enhancement. CT scans can show renal infarcts or perirenal and subcapsular hematomas in cases of arterial occlusion or aneurysm rupture. The evaluation of small or medium artery vasculitides remains the realm of angiography. Radiation vasculitis can involve the renal arteries and can cause stenoses or occlusions with a latency of months to years.

Renal Artery Dissection.   Most renal artery (RA) dissections are an extension of aortic dissection. Isolated RA dissections are rare and usually iatrogenic due to catheter manipulation or balloon dilation. RA dissection can compromise renal perfusion and require revascularization. RA dissections can also be seen in FMD and SAM.[48]

RA embolism is the most common cause of acute renal infarction in the elderly with the heart being the most common source. The diagnosis is often delayed because the clinical symptoms of renal infarction are vague and ambiguous. CTA can show both the filling defects in the renal arteries, the renal infarct, as well as intracardiac thrombus.[48]

Retroperitoneal fibrosis (RPF) can involve and obstruct the renal arteries and veins. CTA findings are periaortic and perirenal soft tissue as well as encasement of arteries, veins, and ureters.[48]

Neurofibromatosis syndrome type I (NF-1) is associated with a wide spectrum of vascular abnormalities, most notably aneurysms or stenoses of the aortic, renal, and mesenteric circulation.[11] The RA is the most frequent site of involvement.[48]

Median arcuate ligament compression of the renal arteries is a recognized, although rare, entity. Cases of RA stents fractured or compressed by the median arcuate ligament have been described in the literature.[48]

CTA is well suited to plan renal revascularization procedures and for follow-up of these procedures (FIGURE 37.6).[67]

MESENTERIC ARTERIAL SYSTEM

The blood supply to the intestinal tract is derived from the three major anterior branches of the abdominal aorta: the celiac artery (CA), the superior mesenteric artery (SMA), and the inferior mesenteric artery (IMA).

MDCTA has become the initial technique of choice for the diagnosis of mesenteric ischemia.[68,69] It allows for the assessment of vascular abnormalities as well as evaluation of secondary signs of bowel ischemia, such as bowel wall thickening, submucosal hemorrhage, abnormal enhancement, mesenteric stranding, or pneumatosis.

Acute Mesenteric Ischemia

Acute interruption of the blood supply to the small bowel and/or colon is a catastrophic event and carries a morbidity and mortality rate exceeding 60%. The four major causes of acute mesenteric ischemia (AMI) are SMA embolus, SMA thrombosis, mesenteric venous thrombosis (MVT), and nonocclusive mesenteric vasoconstriction (NOMI).[23] Aortic dissections have also been reported to cause AMI on rare occasions.[23]

Acute emboli to the SMA account for approximately 40% to 50% of all episodes of AMI with the typical patient having a history of cardiovascular disease. The majority of emboli in the SMA lodge just beyond the origin of the middle colic artery. Acute mesenteric arterial thrombosis is associated with a preexisting atherosclerotic lesion and consequently a history of intestinal angina is present in up to 50% of cases.[23] In contrast to the abrupt catastrophic onset of symptoms associated with an embolus to the SMA, the abdominal pain and symptoms associated with acute mesenteric arterial thrombosis may be more insidious due to the development of collateral circulation. Thrombotic occlusion of the SMA occurs typically near the ostium, unlike embolic occlusion. CTA demonstrates calcified and noncalcified ostial plaque, thrombus, and collateral vessels.[68]

MVT accounts for approximately 5% to 15% of all cases of AMI and occurs most commonly in patients with associated risk factors, such as portal hypertension, hypercoagulable states, trauma, intraabdominal inflammatory diseases, the use of oral contraceptives, and recent surgery affecting the portomesenteric venous system, especially splenectomy. Portal venous phase CT (70-second scan delay) has been demonstrated to be highly accurate for the evaluation of SMV and PV thrombosis.[68,69]

NOMI is thought to be responsible for approximately 25% of cases of AMI with a mortality rate as high as 70%.[68] NOMI usually develops during an episode of cardiogenic shock or a state of hypoperfusion in which excessive sympathetic activity results in secondary splanchnic vasoconstriction. The response to intraarterial papaverine during DSA is both diagnostic and therapeutic, but the diagnosis can occasionally be made with CTA if there is lack of mesenteric venous enhancement on the portal phase scan in conjunction attenuated SMA branches (FIGURE 37.10).[70]

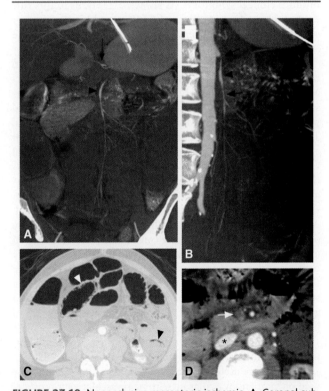

FIGURE 37.10 Nonocclusive mesenteric ischemia. **A.** Coronal subvolume MIP reconstruction of the mesenteric vasculature shows attenuation of the branches of the celiac artery (*arrow*) and superior mesenteric artery (*arrowhead*). **B.** Sagittal MIP reconstruction of the abdominal aorta and mesenteric vessels. Vasospasm, which is the key finding in NOMI, is suggested by alternating segments of smooth stenosis (*arrows*) and normal caliber vessels (*arrowhead*) as present in the superior mesenteric artery. **C.** The presence of gas with the bowel wall is diagnostic of pneumatosis and suggests bowel necrosis (*arowheads*). **D.** Lack of enhancement of the superior mesenteric vein (*arrow*) on portal venous phase is probably the most sensitive sign for NOMI in the appropriate clinical setting. Note strong enhancement of the infrarenal IVC (*) and absent enhancement in the SMV, a highly abnormal finding.

Approximately 5% of patients with aortic dissection develop mesenteric ischemia as a complication of the dissection process.[23] Isolated dissections of the SMA either in association with cystic degeneration or as a complication of catheter angiography are extremely rare but readily diagnosed on CTA. In acute cases, perivascular stranding is typical in isolated SMA dissections.[68]

Chronic Mesenteric Ischemia

Chronic mesenteric ischemia (CMI) is almost always caused by severe atherosclerotic disease and characterized by a classical clinical triad of postprandial abdominal pain, weight loss, and food avoidance. Although atherosclerosis of the mesenteric branches is frequent in the elderly, CMI is relatively uncommon, primarily due to the abundant mesenteric collateral circulation. This mesenteric collateral network makes it difficult to estimate the degree of mesenteric vascular stenosis necessary to cause intestinal angina.[68] It is generally accepted that at least two of the three main vessels have to be affected by occlusive or significant stenotic disease to produce clinical symptoms. As always, exceptions to this rule exist and we have seen cases of CMI caused by proximal or segmental mesenteric artery stenosis or occlusion in only one artery.

A number of nonatherosclerotic vascular pathologies can cause CMI. FMD is a rare but well-recognized cause of CMI.[71] Median arcuate ligament syndrome is caused by extrinsic compression of the celiac trunk and/or the celiac neural plexus by the central tendon of the crura of the diaphragm. The classic finding on a lateral view of the aorta consists of a smooth indentation of the superior aspect of the proximal CA, which is more marked on expiration than on inspiration.[71] Median arcuate ligament compression can occasionally involve the proximal SMA and even renal arteries. CTA scans should be done in expiration if this entity is suspected. Aortic dissections can cause both acute and CMI, usually by one of three mechanisms: there can be complete obliteration of the true lumen by the false lumen at the visceral artery ostia, resulting in the intimal flap covering the visceral ostia; the dissection flap may extend into a visceral artery, causing stenosis or occlusion; or the visceral artery may arise from a poorly perfused true or false lumen, resulting in visceral hypoperfusion.[71]

CMI has also been described as one of the many manifestations of vasculitides, especially TA.[71]

MDCTA is a useful tool to follow patients after all currently used open or endovascular mesenteric revascularization procedures, including surgical embolectomy, thrombectomy, bypass graft placement, endarterectomy, surgical release of the median arcuate ligament, mechanical thrombectomy, angioplasty, catheter-directed thrombolysis, fenestration of the dissection membrane, stenting, and endoluminal stent-graft placement (FIGURE 37.11).[71]

Early postoperative graft occlusion is almost always caused by surgical or technical problems, such as twisting, kinking, or inadequate anastomoses. A rare immediate complication of successful revascularization is the development of reperfusion syndrome, where massive bowel and visceral organ hyperemia can lead to liver failure, ascites, pancreatitis, and food intolerance. CTA demonstrates massive hyperemia of the visceral organs and

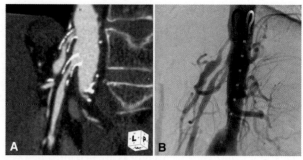

FIGURE 37.11 In-stent intimal hyperplasia. **A**. Oblique MPR reconstruction from CTA with 0.6-mm isotropic voxels shows severe stenosis of stents in the ostium of the celiac and superior mesenteric arteries. CTA is an excellent modality for the evaluation of in-stent stenosis caused by intimal hyperplasia when Doppler ultrasound is inconclusive. **B**. Comparison imaging with digital subtraction angiography.

the bowel, evidenced by early filling of the mesenteric veins on arterial phase imaging.[71]

CTA has also an important role in the preoperative evaluation of liver and kidney transplant donors as well as the postoperative evaluation of liver, kidney, and pancreas transplant recipients (FIGURE 37.12).[72,73]

■ THE FUTURE

One of the major concerns in CT scanning is radiation exposure. All vendors actively pursue ways to reduce patient radiation dose while maintaining image quality. The standard CT reconstruction process, filtered back projection (FBP), is a rapid and reliable reconstruction technique but not optimized for low-dose scans. Newer image reconstruction techniques, so called iterative reconstruction techniques, have recently been introduced and are under clinical investigation. They are based on maximum likelihood algorithms that can be applied to the raw data or the slice data, or both. Although more computing intensive, their use has shown to allow significant dose reductions while maintaining image quality in both neurologic and body CT scanning. These techniques will likely become mainstream in cardiovascular CT in the near future.[74] Flat-panel volume CT is a technologic approach aimed at increasing the spatial resolution of CT. Rather than using multirow detectors, a flat-panel area detector is used in these systems. Whereas spatial resolution on current CT systems is limited to 0.4 mm (in-plane) and 0.5 mm (z-axis), one such flat-panel CT prototype achieved a maximum resolution of 150 μm.[75] Technical disadvantages of these systems are currently inferior contrast resolution, higher radiation dose, and longer scan times. New flat-panel detector technology might, however, change this in the future. Dual energy computed tomography (DECT) is a recently commercially available CT technique using two acquisitions at different energy levels that are performed simultaneously. Single-source CT units using sandwich detectors or rapid kilovolt switching as well as dual-source scanners allow the acquisition of DE studies. The differentiation of material in CT is based on quantifiable differences in X-ray attenuation.[76] The use of different energy levels results in different degrees of X-ray attenuation, measured

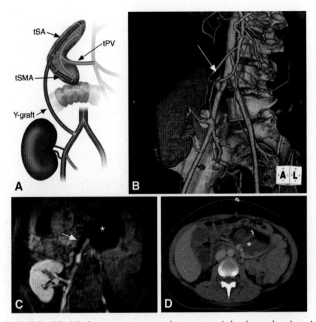

FIGURE 37.12 Pancreas transplant arterial thrombosis. A 47-year-old man developed abdominal pain, elevated lipase, and poor glucose control in the immediate postoperative period following combined kidney-pancreas transplantation. **A.** The patient underwent porto-enteric drainage-type pancreas allograft transplantation. Dual transplant renal arteries were anastomosed to the right common and external iliac arteries. The pancreas transplant arterial supply is from the recipient common iliac artery via a donor Y-graft to the allograft splenic artery (tSA) and superior mesenteric artery (tSMA). Venous drainage of the transplant pancreas is via the transplant portal vein (tPV) that was anastomosed to the native superior mesenteric vein into the recipient portal system. **B.** VR image demonstrates patency of the transplant renal arteries and homogenous enhancement of the transplant kidney. The Y-graft to the pancreas is completely thrombosed (*arrow*) with only a stump remaining. Comparison MRA demonstrates thrombosis of the Y-graft (*arrow*) and the infarcted pancreas allograft (*) (**C**), as does the portal venous phase CT (**D**).

in Hounsfield units (HU), for different materials. The variation in the HU is minimal for soft tissues but significant for materials with large atomic numbers.[76] DECT thus allows the characterization of iodine, calcium, and other materials within tissues by their different absorptiometric characteristics at low and high kilovoltages. DECT-based automated bone removal and calcified plaque removal are of potential benefit for CTA of occlusive disease and undergo active investigation.

CONCLUSION

CTA is a highly advanced noninvasive vascular imaging modality. It allows accurate diagnosis of virtually all vascular occlusive disease in the aorta and its branches and facilitates treatment planning and follow-up. Its main disadvantages are radiation exposure and the need to use potentially nephrotoxic iodinated contrast agents. Current technologic developments aim at increasing spatial resolution and reducing radiation and contrast doses.

REFERENCES

1. Rubin GD, Shiau MC, Schmidt AJ, et al. Computed tomographic angiography: historical perspective and new state-of-the-art using multi detector-row helical computed tomography. *J Comput Assist Tomogr* 1999;23(suppl 1):S83–S90.
2. Prokop M. Multislice CT angiography. *Eur J Radiol* 2000;36:86–96.
3. Kalender WA, Seissler W, Klotz E, et al. Spiral volumetric CT with single-breath-hold technique, continuous transport, and continuous scanner rotation. *Radiology* 1990;176:181–183.
4. Kalender WA, Polacin A. Physical performance characteristics of spiral CT scanning. *Med Phys* 1991;18:910–915.
5. Rubin GD, Walker PJ, Dake MD, et al. Three-dimensional spiral computed tomographic angiography: an alternative imaging modality for the abdominal aorta and its branches. *J Vasc Surg* 1993;18:656–664; discussion 665.
6. Liang Y, Kruger RA. Dual-slice spiral versus single-slice spiral scanning: comparison of the physical performance of two computed tomography scanners. *Med Phys* 1996;23:205–220.
7. Hu H, He HD, Foley WD, et al. Four multidetector-row helical CT: image quality and volume coverage speed. *Radiology* 2000;215:55–62.
8. Klingenbeck-Regn K, Schaller S, Flohr T, et al. Subsecond multi-slice computed tomography: basics and applications. *Eur J Radiol* 1999;31:110–124.
9. Fleischmann D. MDCT of renal and mesenteric vessels. *Eur Radiol* 2003;13(suppl 5):M94–M101.
10. Willmann JK, Baumert B, Schertler T, et al. Aortoiliac and lower extremity arteries assessed with 16-detector row CT angiography: prospective comparison with digital subtraction angiography. *Radiology* 2005;236:1083–1093.
11. Zeman RK, Silverman PM, Vieco PT, et al. CT angiography. *AJR Am J Roentgenol* 1995;165:1079–1088.
12. Rubin GD, Dake MD, Napel S, et al. Spiral CT of renal artery stenosis: comparison of three-dimensional rendering techniques. *Radiology* 1994;190:181–189.
13. Rubin GD, Schmidt AJ, Logan LJ, et al. Multi-detector row CT angiography of lower extremity arterial inflow and runoff: initial experience. *Radiology* 2001;221:146–158.
14. Foley WD, Stonely T. CT angiography of the lower extremities. *Radiol Clin North Am* 2010;48:367–396.
15. Fleischmann D, Hellinger J, Napoli A. Multidetector-row CT angiography of peripheral arteries: imaging upper-extremity and lower-extremity vascular disease. In: Anonymous. *Multidetector-Row CT Angiography.* New York, NY: Springer; 2005:187–198.
16. Norgren L, Hiatt WR, Dormandy JA, et al. Inter-society consensus for the management of peripheral arterial disease (TASC II). *J Vasc Surg* 2007;45(suppl S):S5–S67.
17. Willmann JK, Wildermuth S, Pfammatter T, et al. Aortoiliac and renal arteries: prospective intraindividual comparison of contrast-enhanced three-dimensional MR angiography and multi-detector row CT angiography. *Radiology* 2003;226:798–811.
18. Heijenbrok-Kal MH, Kock MCJM, Hunink MGM. Lower extremity arterial disease: multidetector CT angiography—a meta-analysis. *Radiology* 2007;245:433–439.
19. Met R, Bipat S, Legemate DA, et al. Diagnostic performance of computed tomography angiography in peripheral arterial disease: a systematic review and meta-analysis. *JAMA* 2009;301:415–424.
20. Cernic S, Pozzi Mucelli F, Pellegrin A, et al. Comparison between 64-row CT angiography and digital subtraction angiography in the study of lower extremities: personal experience. *Radiol Med* 2009;114:1115–1129.
21. Shareghi S, Gopal A, Gul K, et al. Diagnostic accuracy of 64 multidetector computed tomographic angiography in peripheral vascular disease. *Catheter Cardiovasc Interv* 2009;75(1):23–31.
22. Napoli A, Anzidei M, Zaccagna F, et al. Peripheral arterial occlusive disease: diagnostic performance and effect on therapeutic management of 64-section CT angiography. *Radiology* 2011;261:976–986.
23. Utsunomiya D, Oda S, Funama Y, et al. Comparison of standard- and low-tube voltage MDCT angiography in patients with peripheral arterial disease. *Eur Radiol* 2010;20:2758–2765.
24. Kau T, Eicher W, Reiterer C, et al. Dual-energy CT angiography in peripheral arterial occlusive disease—accuracy of maximum intensity projections in clinical routine and subgroup analysis. *Eur Radiol* 2011;21:1677–1686.
25. Sommer WH, Helck A, Bamberg F, et al. Diagnostic value of time-resolved CT angiography for the lower leg. *Eur Radiol* 2010;20:2876–2881.
26. Schernthaner R, Stadler A, Lomoschitz F, et al. Multidetector CT angiography in the assessment of peripheral arterial occlusive disease: accuracy

in detecting the severity, number, and length of stenoses. *Eur Radiol* 2007;18:665–671.

27. Schernthaner R, Fleischmann D, Stadler A, et al. Value of MDCT angiography in developing treatment strategies for critical limb ischemia. *Am J Roentgenol* 2009;192:1416–1424.

28. Flors L, Leiva-Salinas C, Bozlar U, et al. Imaging evaluation of flow limitations in the iliac arteries in endurance athletes: diagnosis and treatment follow-up. *AJR Am J Roentgenol* 2011;197:W948–W955.

29. Maged IM, Turba UC, Housseini AM, et al. High spatial resolution magnetic resonance imaging of cystic adventitial disease of the popliteal artery. *J Vasc Surg* 2010;51:471–474.

30. Housseini AM, Maged IM, Abdel-Gawad EA, et al. Popliteal artery entrapment syndrome. *J Vasc Surg* 2009;49:1056.

31. Rich NM, Collins GJ Jr, McDonald PT, et al. Popliteal vascular entrapment. Its increasing interest. *Arch Surg* 1979;114:1377–1384.

32. Zhong H, Gan J, Zhao Y, et al. Role of CT angiography in the diagnosis and treatment of popliteal vascular entrapment syndrome. *Am J Roentgenol* 2011;197:W1147–W1154.

33. Lopera JE, Trimmer CK, Josephs SG, et al. Multidetector CT angiography of infrainguinal arterial bypass. *Radiographics* 2008;28:529–548.

34. Heuschmid M, Wiesinger B, Tepe G, et al. Evaluation of various image reconstruction parameters in lower extremity stents using multidetector-row CT angiography: initial findings. *Eur Radiol* 2006;17:265–271.

35. Li XM, Li YH, Tian JM, et al. Evaluation of peripheral artery stent with 64-slice multi-detector row CT angiography: prospective comparison with digital subtraction angiography. *Eur J Radiol* 2010;75:98–103.

36. Rastogi N, Kabutey NK, Kim D, et al. Symptomatic fibromuscular dysplasia of the external iliac artery. *Ann Vasc Surg* 2012;26:574.e9–574.e13.

37. Abdel-Gawad EA, Housseini AM, Maged IM, et al. Computed tomography angiography of type III Takayasu arteritis. *J Rheumatol* 2009;36:652–653.

38. Pieroni S, Foster BR, Anderson SW, et al. Use of 64-row multidetector CT angiography in blunt and penetrating trauma of the upper and lower extremities. *Radiographics* 2009;29:863–876.

39. Soto JA, Munera F, Cardoso N, et al. Diagnostic performance of helical CT angiography in trauma to large arteries of the extremities. *J Comput Assist Tomogr* 1999;23:188–196.

40. Seamon MJ, Smoger D, Torres DM, et al. A prospective validation of a current practice: the detection of extremity vascular injury with CT angiography. *J Trauma* 2009;67:238–244.

41. Inaba K, Branco BC, Reddy S, et al. Prospective evaluation of multidetector computed tomography for extremity vascular trauma. *J Trauma* 2011;70:808–815.

42. Criado E, Berguer R, Greenfield L. The spectrum of arterial compression at the thoracic outlet. *J Vasc Surg* 2010;52:406–411.

43. Hasanadka R, Towne JB, Seabrook GR, et al. Computed tomography angiography to evaluate thoracic outlet neurovascular compression. *Vasc Endovascular Surg* 2007;41:316–321.

44. Abdel-Gawad EA, Bonatti H, Housseini AM, et al. Hypothenar hammer syndrome in a computer programmer: CTA diagnosis and surgical and endovascular treatment. *Vasc Endovascular Surg* 2009;43:509–512.

45. Turkvatan A, Ozdemir M, Cumhur T, et al. Multidetector CT angiography of renal vasculature: normal anatomy and variants. *Eur Radiol* 2009;19:236–244.

46. Brink JA, Lim JT, Wang G, et al. Technical optimization of spiral CT for depiction of renal artery stenosis: in vitro analysis. *Radiology* 1995;194:157–163.

47. Turba UC, Uflacker R, Bozlar U, et al. Normal renal arterial anatomy assessed by multidetector CT angiography: are there differences between men and women? *Clin Anat* 2009;22:236–242.

48. Flors L, Leiva-Salinas C, Ahmad EA, et al. MD CT angiography and MR angiography of nonatherosclerotic renal artery disease. *Cardiovasc Intervent Radiol* 2011;34:1151–1164.

49. Oz M, Hazirolan T, Turkbey B, et al. CT angiography evaluation of the renal vascular pathologies: a pictorial review. *JBR-BTR* 2010;93:252–257.

50. Rountas C, Vlychou M, Vassiou K, et al. Imaging modalities for renal artery stenosis in suspected renovascular hypertension: prospective intraindividual comparison of color Doppler US, CT angiography, GD-enhanced MR angiography, and digital substraction angiography. *Ren Fail* 2007;29:295–302.

51. Galanski M, Prokop M, Chavan A, et al. Renal arterial stenoses: spiral CT angiography. *Radiology* 1993;189:185–192.

52. Berg MH, Manninen HI, Vanninen RL, et al. Assessment of renal artery stenosis with CT angiography: usefulness of multiplanar reformation, quantitative stenosis measurements, and densitometric analysis of renal parenchymal enhancement as adjuncts to MIP film reading. *J Comput Assist Tomogr* 1998;22:533–540.

53. Halpern EJ, Rutter CM, Gardiner GA Jr, et al. Comparison of Doppler US and CT angiography for evaluation of renal artery stenosis. *Acad Radiol* 1998;5:524–532.

54. Kim TS, Chung JW, Park JH, et al. Renal artery evaluation: comparison of spiral CT angiography to intra-arterial DSA. *J Vasc Interv Radiol* 1998;9:553–559.

55. Rubin GD, Napel S. Helical CT angiography of renal artery stenosis. *AJR Am J Roentgenol* 1997;168:1109–1111.

56. Van Hoe L, Gryspeerdt S. Helical CT angiography of renal artery stenosis. *AJR Am J Roentgenol* 1997;168:1380–1381.

57. Beregi JP, Elkohen M, Deklunder G, et al. Helical CT angiography compared with arteriography in the detection of renal artery stenosis. *AJR Am J Roentgenol* 1996;167:495–501.

58. Farres MT, Lammer J, Schima W, et al. Spiral computed tomographic angiography of the renal arteries: a prospective comparison with intravenous and intraarterial digital subtraction angiography. *Cardiovasc Intervent Radiol* 1996;19:101–106.

59. Elkohen M, Beregi JP, Deklunder G, et al. Evaluation of spiral computed tomography of the renal arteries alone or combined with Doppler ultrasonography in the detection of renal artery stenosis. Prospective study of 114 renal arteries. *Arch Mal Coeur Vaiss* 1995;88:1159–1164.

60. Wittenberg G, Kenn W, Tschammler A, et al. Spiral CT angiography of renal arteries: comparison with angiography. *Eur Radiol* 1999;9:546–551.

61. Fraioli F, Catalano C, Bertoletti L, et al. Multidetector-row CT angiography of renal artery stenosis in 50 consecutive patients: prospective interobserver comparison with DSA. *Radiol Med* 2006;111:459–468.

62. Luscher TF, Lie JT, Stanson AW, et al. Arterial fibromuscular dysplasia. *Mayo Clin Proc* 1987;62:931–952.

63. Slovut DP, Olin JW. Fibromuscular dysplasia. *N Engl J Med* 2004;350:1862–1871.

64. Slavin RE, Cafferty L, Cartwright J Jr. Segmental mediolytic arteritis. A clinicopathologic and ultrastructural study of two cases. *Am J Surg Pathol* 1989;13:558–568.

65. Kalva SP, Somarouthu B, Jaff MR, et al. Segmental arterial mediolysis: clinical and imaging features at presentation and during follow-up. *J Vasc Interv Radiol* 2011;22:1380–1387.

66. Gotway MB, Araoz PA, Macedo TA, et al. Imaging findings in Takayasu's arteritis. *AJR Am J Roentgenol* 2005;184:1945–1950.

67. Behar JV, Nelson RC, Zidar JP, et al. Thin-section multidetector CT angiography of renal artery stents. *AJR Am J Roentgenol* 2002;178:1155–1159.

68. Shih MC, Hagspiel KD. CTA and MRA in mesenteric ischemia: part 1, role in diagnosis and differential diagnosis. *AJR Am J Roentgenol* 2007;188:452–461.

69. Barmase M, Kang M, Wig J, et al. Role of multidetector CT angiography in the evaluation of suspected mesenteric ischemia. *Eur J Radiol* 2011;80:e582–e587.

70. Bozlar U, Turba UC, Hagspiel KD. Nonocclusive mesenteric ischemia: findings at multidetector CT angiography. *J Vasc Interv Radiol* 2007;18:1331–1333.

71. Shih MC, Angle JF, Leung DA, et al. CTA and MRA in mesenteric ischemia: part 2, normal findings and complications after surgical and endovascular treatment. *AJR Am J Roentgenol* 2007;188:462–471.

72. Bhatti AA, Chugtai A, Haslam P, et al. Prospective study comparing three-dimensional computed tomography and magnetic resonance imaging for evaluating the renal vascular anatomy in potential living renal donors. *BJU Int* 2005;96:1105–1108.

73. Byun JH, Kim TK, Lee SS, et al. Evaluation of the hepatic artery in potential donors for living donor liver transplantation by computed tomography angiography using multidetector-row computed tomography: comparison of volume rendering and maximum intensity projection techniques. *J Comput Assist Tomogr* 2003;27:125–131.

74. Nelson RC, Feuerlein S, Boll DT. New iterative reconstruction techniques for cardiovascular computed tomography: how do they work, and what are the advantages and disadvantages? *J Cardiovasc Comput Tomogr* 2011;5:286–292.

75. Gupta R, Cheung AC, Bartling SH, et al. Flat-panel volume CT: fundamental principles, technology, and applications. *Radiographics* 2008;28:2009–2022.

76. Johnson TR, Krauss B, Sedlmair M, et al. Material differentiation by dual energy CT: initial experience. *Eur Radiol* 2007;17:1510–1517.

CHAPTER

38

Diagnostic Noninvasive Evaluations: MRI

MOAZZEM KAZI and MARTIN R. PRINCE

INTRODUCTION

Magnetic resonance (MR) has transformed imaging the human body using magnetic relaxation phenomena to produce images with unique soft-tissue contrast different from conventional X-ray and computed tomography (CT) scans. Magnetic fields and radiofrequency (RF) energy used in MR scanning avoid the radiation exposure risks of X-ray-based methods. Gadolinium-based contrast agents used in magnetic resonance angiography (MRA) are typically safer than iodinated contrast agents and noninvasively visualize arteries and veins throughout the body. MRA has also been revolutionized with new imaging sequences that do not even require contrast agent injection.

PREPROCEDURE ASSESSMENT

Safety Screening

Safety is paramount for anyone entering an MR scanner room. Patients undergoing an MR scan need to be thoroughly screened for objects incompatible with the magnetic field. Loose objects that contain iron or other magnetic material are subject to the attractive forces of the magnetic field and can become dangerous projectiles when they are brought into the MR scanner room.[1] MR-incompatible objects may also create artifacts in the image. The most severe consequence for an MR-incompatible object is lethal bodily harm if the object becomes a projectile or an implant moves from its imbedded location within the body when subject to the strong magnetic force of modern MR magnets.

The following is a list of everyday objects that need to be removed before entering an MR scanner room: cellular phones, beepers, watches, credit cards (or any card with a magnetic strip), hearing aids, eyeglasses, keys, pens, money clips, coins, safety pins, paperclips, nail clippers, scissors, pocket knives, or any metallic tools. Articles of clothing that patients need to remove include belts, steel-tipped shoes/boots, hairpins, metallic jewelry (including body-piercing jewelry), clothing that contain magnetic threading, zippers, and snaps (e.g., bras).[2,3] Nonmetallic jewelry (e.g., gold wedding rings) can be worn but preferably should not be located within the area being scanned. If unsure of the magnetic properties of an object, a small handheld magnet can be used to determine if the object has risk.[3] When in doubt, the object should be kept safely outside the scanner room and control room with at least two doors between the unsafe object and MR scanner. Because the list of objects prohibited in the MR scanner room can be extensive, patients are instructed to remove all clothing and wear a hospital gown before being scanned.[2]

Before an MR scan is ordered and certainly before a patient enters the scanner room, he or she needs to be evaluated for medically implanted devices that are contraindicated for MR scanning. The short list of contraindicated devices include brain aneurysm clips, cardiac pacemakers, implantable cardioverter defibrillators (ICD), cochlear implants or implanted hearing aids, electronic implants or devices (including those that are magnetically activated), and neurostimulation systems (e.g., spinal cord stimulators).[2] Nonferromagnetic vena cava filters, especially if not in close proximity to the scanning site, do not generally pose a safety hazard.[3] With the increasing popularity of MR scanning, many manufacturers are developing MR-compatible devices, so it is advisable to contact the manufacturer directly to determine if its device is safe for MR scanning.

Intravenous Access

Because most conventional MRA involves the use of contrast (e.g., gadolinium), intravenous (IV) access is obtained prior to scanning. Right arm IV access is ideal because it directly leads to the central circulation. A small-gauge (e.g., 20 or 22 gauge) angiocatheter access line in the right antecubital fossa, hand, or wrist is preferred. If the IV access is delicate or tenuous, using a low-osmolar, nonionic gadolinium solution is suggested because it has lower viscosity and can minimize pain caused by extravasation, when compared to high-osmolar, ionic gadolinium solutions.[3] It also may be helpful to warm the gadolinium to body temperature prior to injection to reduce its viscosity and resistance to flow, especially when using a small-caliber IV.[4]

Although MR-compatible power injector devices are available for contrast infusion, hand injection devices offer multiple advantages. Hand injection is required for pediatric patients, IV access from central lines or peripherally inserted central catheter (PICC) lines, or delicate IV access in the hand or wrist.[5] Hand injection allows for quicker detection of problems with the IV access or contrast extravasation because the operator can sense changes in the resistance of infusion. It also allows for ideal breath-holding because the operator is beside the patient and directly observing the patient breathing. Finally, hand injection allows for earlier detection of contrast reactions compared to power injection because the operator is closer to the patient.

IV access should be maintained for at least 5 to 10 minutes after injection of contrast because most allergic reactions occur during this time.[5] The IV access line may become necessary for the administration of medication to stabilize a patient in the event of an allergic reaction.

Contrast Agents

Contrast agents accentuate signal intensity differences between adjacent regions that are imaged together. This is accomplished through the shortening of the T1 (spin-lattice) relaxation times of protons within tissues. Gadolinium-based, iron-containing, and manganese-containing compounds are currently approved by the U.S. Food and Drug Administration (FDA) for use as contrast agents.[6]

Extracellular Contrast

Gadolinium is toxic to tissues in its ionic-free form. Therefore, it is chelated to an organic ligand, like diethylenetriamine pentaacetic acid (DTPA), to eliminate its toxicity, limit its interaction with tissues, and promote its excretion from the body.[7] Gadolinium complexes primarily shorten T1, so areas where the contrast accumulates appear bright on T1-weighted scans. These are referred to as positive or paramagnetic contrast media.[8]

Gadolinium-based contrast agents were among the first approved for clinical use in patients. These complexes can be linear in structure, such as gadopentetate dimeglumine (Gd-DTPA).[8] They can also have a macrocyclic structure, such as gadoteridol (Gd-HP-DO3A) or gadobutrol (Gd-DO3A-butrol), which are usually more stable than linear structures. These agents are rapidly excreted through the kidneys with an elimination half-life of 15 to 90 minutes in patients with normal renal function.

After injection into a vein, most gadolinium-based contrast agents travel to the arterial circulation, leak through capillaries, and finally redistribute into extracellular spaces.[5] Imaging must be timed appropriately to capture the contrast in the arterial phase, ideally during its first pass through circulation, before there has been any appreciable extracellular redistribution.

Blood-Pool Contrast

In addition to extracellular distribution, some gadolinium-based contrast agents can have blood-pool (intravascular), tissue-specific, or intracellular distributions.[7] Blood-pool agents have been developed that reversibly bind serum albumin, prolonging plasma half-life, so they tend to remain primarily in the intravascular space. This enables better visualization of veins, smaller vessels, and vessels with slow or complex flow. Blood-pool agents have the potential for perfusion imaging, detection of gastrointestinal bleeding and stent graft leaks, and tumor imaging by way of demonstrating angiogenesis.[9]

Gadofosveset trisodium is designed as a blood-pool agent and is currently FDA approved for MRA. It binds noncovalently to plasma albumin, enabling the visualization of blood vessels.[9] The reversible nature of its bond with albumin enhances its effectiveness, allowing for lower doses to achieve the same degree of contrast than other gadolinium-based agents, yet still permitting removal by the kidneys.

Tissue-Specific Contrast

Tissue-specific and intracellular contrast agents currently have a limited role in MRA. An example of a tissue-specific agent with a potential role in MRA is gadobenate dimeglumine (Gd-BOPTA).[8] It is used to visualize the hepatobiliary system and has a delayed entry into hepatocytes after administration. Also, it transiently binds to albumin, which enables it to function as a conventional extracellular agent.

Nongadolinium Contrast Agents

Ferumoxide and mangafodipir trisodium (Mn-DPDP) are nongadolinium-containing complexes with FDA approval for contrast imaging.[6] They are both tissue-specific contrast agents used for evaluating liver lesions. Mangafodipir trisodium is a positive contrast agent, like the gadolinium-based agents, but with less enhancement at clinical doses.[8] Ferumoxide, an iron oxide superparamagnetic molecule, is a negative contrast agent that mainly shortens T2 (spin-spin) relaxation times, so areas where the contrast accumulates appear darker on T2-weighted scans. Their use in patients is primarily for hepatic visualization and they currently have limited MRA applications. Ferumoxytol is another iron oxide agent that can be a positive or negative contrast agent and has been used effectively for blood-pool MRA.[10,11]

Nephrogenic Systemic Fibrosis

A rare entity seen with the widespread use of gadolinium contrast in patients with severe renal failure is nephrogenic systemic fibrosis (NSF).[12] The first cases thought to be NSF can be traced back to 1997.[13] NSF has been observed in patients with acute or severe chronic kidney disease who have received gadolinium contrast, usually at high doses. Symptoms commonly occur a month after exposure to the contrast. Clinical features of the disease are fibrosis of skin and connective tissue throughout the body. Movement becomes restricted as skin becomes rigid and firm. Fibrosis may occur in internal organs, such as the heart, lungs, and esophagus, and may disrupt their normal function. Death can occur in severe cases.

A proposed pathophysiology of NSF is gadolinium transmetallation, whereby other cations (e.g., Ca^{2+} and Zn^{2+}) displace gadolinium from its chelator into its free ionic form (Gd^{3+}).[7] Free Gd^{3+} may precipitate with phosphates, deposit in cells, and provoke an inflammatory response with subsequent fibrosis.[12] Free Gd^{3+} also interferes with calcium-ion passage through muscle and nerve cells, disrupting proper tissue function. In addition, gadolinium has been detected in biopsy samples from NSF lesions.[14]

With improvements in renal function, there have been reports documenting a slowing of NSF progression, symptom reversal,[12] or even cure.[15] Despite this, NSF tends to be a progressive condition and there is no effective medical treatment available. Since 2006, the FDA has requested manufacturers of gadolinium-based contrast agents to include a boxed warning on labels of their products.[16] This includes the suggestion to weigh the risks and benefits of gadolinium contrast use in any patient with a glomerular filtration rate (GFR) less than 30 mL/min/1.73 m^2. Noncontrast MRA remains a viable option in those at risk for NSF.

Despite the risk of NSF (i.e., decreased renal function), gadolinium-based contrast agents have an acceptable safety profile for patients with GFR greater than 30 mL/min/1.73 m^2.[7] In these individuals, most of the gadolinium is excreted from the body in its chelated form and not enough, if any, free Gd^{3+} accumulates to cause an appreciable disruption of normal bodily function.

Sedation

An intrinsic part of obtaining clear MR images is the requirement for the patient to be motionless while being scanned. This can be difficult for patients with claustrophobia or who are otherwise anxious about being in an unfamiliar environment with noises (e.g., Lorentz forces from gradient switching), motions (e.g., the moving table), and the solitude of the scanner room. These patients will probably be able to cooperate with the scan if premedicated with benzodiazepines, such as diazepam or alprazolam. An effective dose for a typical adult patient is 5 to 10 mg of diazepam or 1 to 2 mg of alprazolam taken orally approximately 30 minutes before scanning.[3] Patients that require oral sedation need to be accompanied from the scanning facility by another responsible adult.

Suspending Respiration

Imaging vasculature in the chest or abdomen also requires patient cooperation with breath-holding. Even slight respiratory motions can obscure images of the intricate vasculature in these regions. It is possible to observe a patient breathing at baseline to estimate how long he or she will be able to hold his or her breath.[5] For instance, if a patient is breathing at a rate of 20 breaths per minute with long pauses between breaths, he or she may be able to easily suspend breathing for approximately 30 to 40 seconds on inspiration when coached to hyperventilate just before breath-holding. If a patient is breathing at a rate of over 30 breaths per minute with little or no pauses between breaths, he or she may not be able to suspend breathing at all.

Even though most patients find it easiest to hold their breath at maximum inhalation, it is sometimes preferred for them to hold their breath at end exhalation. This increases reproducibility in terms of anatomic positioning, especially when multiple, successive breath-holds are required.[5] Additionally, end-exhalation breath-holds are particularly advantageous for electrocardiogram (ECG)-gated acquisitions because the heart is brought closer to the skin, which produces larger ECG signals.

▌ MAGNETIC RESONANCE ANGIOGRAPHY TECHNIQUES

Contrast-Enhanced Magnetic Resonance Angiography

Contrast agent injection for MRA increases the signal-to-noise ratio (SNR) over noncontrast techniques and can increase image resolution while eliminating many artifacts. In addition to the type of contrast agent used, the rate of injection and concentration of the contrast agent can be altered to increase SNR.[17] The current recommended dose for most gadolinium-based contrast agents is 0.1 mmol/kg body weight and the recommended injection rate is 2 mL/second.[18] Generally, higher SNR images can be obtained by increasing the rate of contrast injection, although T2* effects can degrade image quality at very high injection rates (e.g., >4 mL/second). There is a physiologic limit for how fast the veins will allow contrast to be injected. For a typical peripheral IV line, the tolerable rate of contrast injection is 3 to 4 mL/

second.[5] Alternatively, using higher concentrations of contrast agents effectively increases the injection rate. Using a double-concentrated solution (e.g., gadobutrol) with a constant injection rate would be the same as doubling the injection rate of a single-concentrated solution. With these strategies, SNR can be optimized for MRA imaging.

Three-dimensional (3D) MRA has replaced the use of two-dimensional (2D) MRA techniques.[5] This is largely caused by multiple advantages 3D imaging offers over 2D imaging, including higher spatial resolution, increased SNR, reduced motion artifacts, image reconstruction at oblique angles, and an added dimension for volume perception.

Contrast-Timing Methods

Three-dimensional contrast-enhanced MRA is one of the most widely used imaging techniques in MRA. It offers high spatial resolution with a minimum of artifacts to accurately diagnose numerous vascular conditions.[4] Accurate timing of contrast injection to synchronize the bolus with periods of optimal data gathering is necessary. Multiple methods have been developed that estimate when the contrast is expected to arrive at the imaging site.

The "best guess" technique is one method for estimating the arrival of contrast at the imaging site.[4] In this method, equations have been developed for the imaging delay using factors, such as estimated contrast travel time, injection time, imaging time, and rise time:

$$\text{Imaging delay} = (\text{estimated contrast agent travel time}) \\ + (\text{injection time}/2) - (\text{imaging time}/2) \tag{1}$$

$$\text{Imaging delay} = (\text{estimated contrast agent travel time}) \\ - (\text{imaging time}/2) + (\text{rise time}) \tag{2}$$

Imaging delay is the time from starting the injection to starting the scan, and rise time is the length of time contrast takes from arterial arrival to arterial peak concentration. As its name suggests, this method can be inaccurate at times. This is partly caused by the variability of equation parameters in different disease states, location of the IV site (e.g., hand, upper arm), and the patient's level of conditioning.

Another method for estimating the arrival of contrast at the imaging site is the "test-bolus" technique. In this method, a small bolus (e.g., 2 mL) of contrast followed by 20 mL of saline is injected and rapidly imaged at fixed time intervals, usually every 1 to 2 seconds, to determine when the contrast arrives in the region of interest.[4] Contrast arrival can be detected by visual inspection or by sequential signal intensity measurements at the imaging site. Image acquisition times can then be adjusted with this information with a few more seconds added because the full contrast volume is normally larger than the test bolus. Limitations of this method include an error from early signal peaking due to the small, short-duration test bolus. The test bolus can add to background signal during the actual scanning because it has enough time to spread to the extracellular space.

Automatic triggering and fluoroscopic triggering are other methods for timing the contrast with image acquisition.[5]

Automatic triggering uses a pulse sequence that automatically detects contrast arrival in the aorta to synchronize data acquisition with the arterial phase of the contrast. In fluoroscopic triggering, multiple, rapid 2D MR images of the aorta are taken, and the operator switches to 3D MRA with centric or recessed elliptical centric k-space ordering when contrast is seen arriving in the aorta.

Time-resolved 3D contrast-enhanced MRA has been developed to remove the effect of contrast timing on image quality.[4] In this technique, multiple 3D image datasets are quickly acquired in succession and independent of contrast injection timing. The operator then selects the image set that shows the best detail. Fast scanning is needed for proper image detail in the appropriate phase for time-resolved techniques.[5] To separate the arterial and venous phase, scanners must gather data at a rate of 2 to 3 seconds per dataset. Recent technologic advances in MRA now allow 4 to 5 3D volumes per second to be acquired using radial or spiral acquisitions that over-sample central k-space and share peripheral k-space data. More primitive commercially available implementations include 3D time-resolved imaging of contrast kinetics (TRICKS).[19]

Comparison of 1.5 and 3.0 T Magnets

The 3.0 Tesla (T) magnets increase SNR in MRA, albeit with more imaging artifacts, compared to 1.5 T magnets. This is caused by twice as many protons aligning with the magnetic field at 3.0 T compared to 1.5 T and prolonged T1 relaxation times at 3.0 T compared to 1.5 T.[20] SNR increases can translate into increased spatial resolution in a 3.0 T scan for the same scan duration and amount of gadolinium contrast as a 1.5 T scan. Less gadolinium contrast can also be used at 3.0 T without an appreciable decrease in image quality compared to scans at 1.5 T. Lower gadolinium doses at 3.0 T may be particularly beneficial for scanning patients with poor renal function who are at risk for NSF because NSF occurs primarily with high doses of gadolinium contrast.

Despite the advantages of 3.0 T magnets in 3D MRA, there are concerns of over incomplete imaging, artifacts, and patient safety.[20] In a 3.0 T magnet, the RF wavelength is 26 cm (compared to 52 cm at 1.5 T) because the resonance frequency of water protons is 128 MHz (compared to 64 MHz at 1.5 T). The decreased RF wavelength has implications on anatomic accuracy and artifacts in the resulting image. Smaller RF wavelengths are more likely to produce constructive interference as they interact within the imaging field and appear as areas that are artificially brighter. Conversely, they can produce destructive interference and appear artificially darker with the possible loss of anatomic detail. New coil designs and pulse sequences are being developed that minimize these effects of 3.0 T magnets.

Another concern of 3.0 T magnets is patient safety due to the specific absorption rate (SAR) of RF energy. SAR is the normalized rate per kilogram body mass that RF power is coupled with biologic tissue.[21] It is an estimate of the energy that enters tissues from an RF pulse and the current accepted SAR limit is 4 W/kg for the entire body over 15 minutes.[20] Higher resonance frequency at 3.0 T leads to an increase in SAR, compared to 1.5 T. The increase in energy, which ultimately becomes heat, can potentially have adverse health effects. New pulse sequences, which decrease scan time and thereby reduce RF and SAR, can minimize these effects of 3.0 T magnets.

Noncontrast Magnetic Resonance Angiography

Time-of-Flight

Noncontrast techniques, such as time-of-flight (TOF), rely on the motion of flowing blood to image vasculature.[22] The principle behind TOF is that stationary protons become increasingly saturated when exposed to repeated excitations and produce low signal intensities. Protons that flow into the imaging volume are not saturated by RF pulses until entering the imaging volume, however, and produce high signal intensities. The differences in behavior of in-plane stationary protons and the protons in flowing blood when exposed to RF pulses are utilized in TOF to create an image (FIGURE 38.1B).

TOF-MRA imaging can be 2D or 3D, depending on the area to be imaged.[22] The intracranial vessels are typically imaged using 3D techniques at low flip angles to prevent excessive saturation of in-plane flow around the Circle of Willis. Three-dimensional methods yield higher spatial resolution with no slice misregistration and work well with low-resistance flow. For peripheral imaging, however, 2D methods are used because they work better with slower, high-resistance, pulsatile flow.

Another consideration in TOF-MRA is synchronization with the cardiac cycle.[22] For imaging the lower extremities, TOF-MRA requires ECG-gating to synchronize image acquisition with systole. This increases image contrast because there is more consistently reliable blood in flow.

A limitation of TOF-MRA is the unintended saturation of protons in flowing blood because the blood vessel was oriented parallel to the imaging plane.[22] This leads to difficulty in distinguishing signal intensity differences between blood and stationary tissues. Sequences to minimize this effect have been developed, such as tilt optimized nonsaturated excitation (TONE). In this sequence, increasing amounts of RF are used to overcome the saturation of protons in intracranial blood vessels. Another limitation of TOF-MRA is clear visualization of vessel walls because slow blood flow along the wall may not be visualized, especially in the presence of an ulcerated plaque.

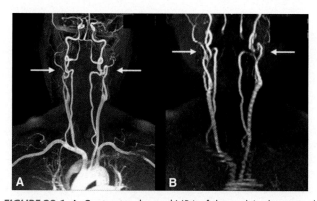

FIGURE 38.1 **A.** Contrast-enhanced MRA of the neck in the coronal plane. The internal carotid arteries are tortuous at the midcervical level (*arrows*). **B.** Time-of-flight MRA of the neck acquired axially and reformatted in the coronal plane. In this noncontrast image, there are multiple artifacts along the carotid arteries bilaterally, especially where the carotid artery is tortuous and subject to in-flow saturation (*arrows*). Clinical information: 78-year-old woman with a history of lightheadedness.

Phase Contrast

Phase contrast is another noncontrast technique that utilizes the motion of flowing blood to visualize blood vessels.[5] In this technique, a phase shift that is proportional to flow rate is produced, and then the phase images are reconstructed with the signal being proportional to velocity.[3] A velocity encoding value (Venc) can be set, which allows the estimation of blood flow velocity in a blood vessel of interest.

Uses of phase contrast MRA include finding the direction of blood flow and calculating hemodynamic information, such as its velocity. Phase contrast MRA also has better background suppression than TOF.[20] Low spatial resolution phase contrast techniques are commonly used as a scout sequence (e.g., for carotid MRA).[22] An exciting recent advance is the use of phase contrast to estimate pressure gradients across stenoses.[23]

Phase contrast MRA is limited, however, by long image acquisition times. Also, it is sensitive to eddy currents, partial volume averaging, and changes in the velocity and amount of blood flow, such as with variations in cardiac output.[20]

Balanced Steady-State Free Precession

In balanced steady-state free precession (SSFP) sequences, image contrast is determined by the ratio of T2/T1 and results in blood appearing bright, independent of inflow.[20] Arteries and veins both produce a bright signal in balanced SSFP (FIGURE 38.2). This is useful in imaging the thoracic area because visualizing both arteries and veins is important for evaluating conditions, such as congenital heart disease. Venous suppression techniques can also be used to isolate only the arterial signal if purely arterial imaging is needed, like in renal angiography.

A common use of balanced SSFP is for coronary imaging.[22] Three-dimensional techniques using thin slab breath-holding and free-breathing whole-heart acquisitions have been developed. These techniques use T2 effects to suppress signal from the myocardium and fat. Because cardiac motion negatively affects balanced SSFP image quality, acquisitions are usually timed to diastole, when cardiac motion is minimal.

Another application of balanced SSFP is for thoracic imaging.[22] The minimal need for fat and venous signal suppression and fast blood flow in thoracic imaging are ideal for balanced SSFP, especially when combined with ECG-gating and local shimming. Measurements of the thoracic aorta and evaluations of aortic disease comparable to contrast-enhanced MRA techniques are possible, albeit at a smaller field-of-view (FOV) due to shimming limitations.[20]

Balance SSFP is limited by magnetic field inhomogeneities, such as air-tissue interfaces and metallic implants.[22] Also, special suppression techniques are needed to minimize visualization of veins to produce purely arterial images.

Arterial Spin Labeling in Steady-State Free Precession

Arterial spin labeling (ASL) can be used in conjunction with SSFP to produce greater visualization of arteries.[20] In this technique, protons in blood vessels upstream to the area being imaged are tagged with an RF pulse. Suppression of background tissue is achieved by digitally subtracting the untagged image from the tagged image, leaving an arterial image with a high SNR.

The renal and carotid arteries are imaged well using ASL with SSFP, particularly due to the limitation of flow artifacts because of multidirectional flow in these areas.[22] ASL can also be used to provide hemodynamic information, such as blood velocity, because the time between application of the tag and imaging and the distance between these two areas is known. Additionally, by varying the time delay between tagging and imaging, perfusion-like images of the kidneys, lungs, and liver can be produced without the use of contrast.

A limitation of ASL is a reduction in signal caused by slow blood velocity.[20] Tagged blood flowing into the area to be imaged is essential in ASL. If blood is moving slowly (e.g., in peripheral arteries), the time needed to replace blood in the imaged area can approach the T1 of tagged blood, which reduces the tagging effect. This limitation can be minimized by using multiple thin-slab acquisitions. There may be a subsequent increase in imaging time. Another limitation of ASL is the potential for motion artifact.[22] This is caused by motion occurring between tagged and untagged acquisitions, which interfere with quality of image subtraction.

Time-Spatial Labeling Inversion Pulse

Time-spatial labeling inversion pulse (Time-SLIP) is an imaging technique where venous blood signal is eliminated with an inversion pulse and arteries are imaged with 3D SSFP readout.[24] An additional spectro-spatial inversion pulse eliminates fat signal and respiratory gating minimizes motion artifact. It has been utilized to evaluate the renal artery and can be used to diagnose renal artery stenosis. A limitation of this technique is signal interference from the intestines and fatty tissue as well as long acquisition times and poor gating in some patients.

Systolic-Diastolic subtraction

Single-shot fast spin echo (FSE) is a method that utilizes digital subtraction techniques and T2 properties to make a 3D image.[22] Because there is low signal caused by the fast flow during systole, arteries appear dark during this time. Alternatively, there is high signal caused by the slow flow during diastole, making arteries appear bright. Digital subtraction of datasets gathered during systolic acquisitions from datasets gathered during diastolic acquisitions produce contrast in the image. Venous blood signal subtracts away because of slow flow during both systole and diastole. ECG-gating is employed to time acquisitions appropriately with the cardiac cycle.

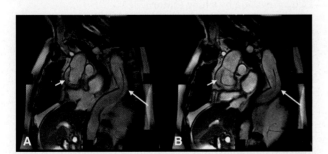

FIGURE 38.2 Balanced steady-state free precession MRA of the chest in the sagittal plane (**A** and **B**). There is an ascending aortic dissection (*short arrow*) and a descending thoracic aortic dissection (*long arrow*) with blood flowing in the true and false lumen. Clinical information: 70-year-old man with a Stanford type A dissection.

Double Inversion Recovery

Double inversion recovery (DIR) is an MRA sequence in which blood appears black because of T1 effects.[3] Acquisitions are done with ECG-gating and breath-holding. Two sequential RF pulses are applied to different areas in the imaging region. The first 180-degree pulse is applied to the entire region. The second 180-degree pulse is applied to a specific slice, such that all spins outside the plane of imaging are inverted, whereas spins within the image plane rotate 360 degrees and are unaffected. The read-out is performed after waiting for blood to reach the null point. DIR imaging creates fine resolution between the boundary of the lumen and vessel wall (FIGURE 38.3A). This can be used to identify areas of subtle dissection flaps within a blood vessel.

DIR can be used to evaluate the carotid arteries for atherosclerotic plaque.[25] ECG-gating reduces artifact from carotid artery pulsation and breath-holding reduces overall motion artifact. Black-blood techniques such as this are not affected by turbulent flow, so the degree of stenosis in a vessel is not overestimated. Plaque components, such as calcification and fibrosis, can also be evaluated using DIR.

STANDARD MAGNETIC RESONANCE ANGIOGRAPHY SCANS

Radiologists, physicists, biomedical engineers, and other specialists have been programming sequences encoding specific parameters and commands to acquire and display MR images since the advent of this technology. Over time, protocols using specific sequences have been developed and refined for accurately imaging specific regions of the body and disease states. Parameters such as FOV, slice thickness and spacing, frequency and phase encoding, repetition time (TR), echo time (TE), and flip angle need to be adjusted according to the anatomy being imaged to optimize image resolution and contrast. Appropriate coils (devices that send an RF pulse and/or receive a signal) and body landmarks also need to be used.

Carotid Arteries and Aortic Arch

Three-dimensional contrast-enhanced MRA is typically used to evaluate the carotid arteries and aortic arch.[26] Primary clinical indications for this exam include stroke, transient ischemic attack (TIA), confirming carotid ultrasound findings, and

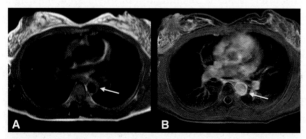

FIGURE 38.3 (A) Double inversion recovery (DIR) and **(B)** liver accelerated volume acquisition (LAVA) of the chest in the axial plane. In both DIR and LAVA images, there is circumferential enhancement and wall thickening of the descending thoracic aorta (*arrow*). No thoracic aortic aneurysm is seen. Clinical information: 26-year-old woman with Takayasu arteritis.

preoperative evaluation for carotid endarterectomy. The aortic arch, great-vessel origins, and surrounding vasculature are also the location of certain disease states, such as atherosclerosis, vasculitis, aneurysms, as well as anatomic variations (FIGURE 38.1).[5]

A neurovascular coil that extends to the chest overlying the aortic arch is needed for simultaneous imaging of the origins and bifurcation of the carotid arteries using a single injection of contrast.[3] If this coil is not available, a torso array coil can be used with its components placed from the upper chest to above the chin. The conventional landmark for neck imaging is just below the angle of the mandible.[26] The series of carotid arteries and aortic arch images starts with a three-plane localizer and calibration scan. This is followed by axial 2D TOF of the neck and coronal 3D pre- and postcontrast MRA. Axial 3D TOF of the carotid bifurcation and axial DIR black-blood imaging may be done precontrast to assess carotid plaque.

Fluoroscopic triggering is used to detect the arrival of contrast for 3D acquisitions.[26] When contrast is seen arriving in the carotid arteries, an operator can activate 3D scanning. Two-dimensional projection imaging can be shifted down to the chest because it may be difficult to detect exactly when contrast arrives in the carotid arteries. With this strategy, contrast can be seen in the venous system, traveling through the right heart, pulmonary vasculature, and left heart, and then the operator can begin scanning when the contrast arrives in the aortic arch. It may be beneficial to utilize centric ordering of k-space acquisition with the absolute center of k-space recessed in from the very beginning of the scan by a few seconds to avoid ringing artifacts.

Pulmonary Vessels

Three-dimensional contrast-enhanced MRA is normally used to evaluate the pulmonary vasculature. Clinical indications for this exam include suspicion of a pulmonary embolism, evaluation of pulmonary hypertension, arteriovenous malformations (AVM), congenital heart disease, and even lung tumors.[5] MRA offers the advantage of scanning the lungs for pulmonary embolism and also scanning the lower extremities for a source of the embolus, such as deep venous thrombosis (DVT), in a single exam. Pulmonary MRA can be used to detect chronic thromboembolism as a cause of pulmonary hypertension or for preoperative evaluation prior to their removal and for mapping pulmonary veins prior to RF ablation. Although CT is routinely used for lung tumor staging, MRA is an alternative in patients who cannot be given iodinated contrast. MRA is also capable of detecting vascular invasion by a lung tumor.

The series of pulmonary MRA imaging begins with a three-plane localizer and calibration scan using a cardiac coil.[27] Two-dimensional imaging is done using DIR in oblique planes. This is followed by 3D contrast-enhanced imaging in the axial and coronal planes, imaging both lungs with a single injection of a blood-pool contrast agent (e.g., gadofosveset trisodium).

Thoracic Aorta

Similar to pulmonary MRA, 3D contrast-enhanced MRA is also utilized to evaluate the thoracic aorta. Indications for imaging the thoracic aorta include suspected aortic dissection, aortic aneurysm, coarctation, aortitis, and great-vessel anomalies.[5] MRA scans for aortic dissection can display the extent of the dissection, entry and reentry locations, and side-branch involvement

(FIGURE 38.2). Three-dimensional contrast-enhanced MRA for the evaluation of aortic aneurysm shows the relationship of the aneurysm to origins of branch vessels, the morphology of the aortic wall, and distinguishes areas of thrombus from flowing blood. In coarctation of the aorta, MRA evaluation can show the location of the stenosis and the exact luminal size. For the assessment of aortitis, both the aortic wall and surrounding tissues need to be examined for inflammation (FIGURE 38.3). The degree of enhancement from imaging can serve as a marker for disease activity. Great-vessel anomalies, such as double aortic arch, right-sided aortic arch, and patent ductus arteriosus, are clearly displayed on 3D contrast-enhanced MRA.

A body coil is normally used for imaging the thoracic aorta.[28] A torso coil can also be used. The conventional landmark is the midsternum. The MRA sequences for the thoracic aorta are essentially the same as those for pulmonary MRA. ECG-gating can be used to remove artifact from cardiac motion. This is particularly important for the visualization of dissection flaps near the aortic root.

Abdominal Aorta

Three-dimensional contrast-enhanced MRA is used to visualize the abdominal aorta. Primary clinical indications for imaging the abdominal aorta include evaluating abdominal aortic aneurysms (AAA), aortic dissections, and aortic occlusion.[5] Characteristics of the AAA, such as maximum diameter, proximal-distal extent, relationship to nearby major arteries, and inflammatory changes, are well-visualized in 3D contrast-enhanced MRA. Also, monitoring for disease progression, preoperative, and stent graft assessments can be done for MR-compatible stents (FIGURE 38.4). Similar to thoracic aorta dissections, those in the abdominal aorta need to be assessed for extent, entry and reentry locations, and involvement of side vessels. Also, extension of the dissection flap to block flow in side vessels, such as the renal arteries, can be visualized using contrast. Three-dimensional contrast-enhanced MRA can be used to visualize stenosis in the abdominal aorta from diseases like atherosclerosis and also show wall irregularities and collateral vessels.

A body coil is used for imaging the abdominal aorta, mainly due to the large field of view, which enables viewing from the diaphragm to the femoral heads (FIGURE 38.5).[29] The standard landmark is the lower anterior rib margin or upper margin of the iliac crest. Scanning begins with a three-plane localizer and calibration scan. Two-dimensional coronal and axial images are then obtained using single-shot FSE. Then coronal 3D contrast MRA is acquired. Next, 3D postcontrast liver accelerated volume acquisition (LAVA) images are obtained in the axial and coronal planes. Two-dimensional balanced SSFP images of the aorta and aneurysm can also be acquired in the oblique plane.

Mesenteric Vessels

Clinical indications for performing 3D MRA of the mesenteric vessels include postprandial abdominal pain, preoperative mapping of mesenteric arterial anatomy and postoperative evaluation, and pre- and post-liver transplantation.[30] Three-dimensional contrast-enhanced MRA can be used to visualize mesenteric vessels for stenosis in the diagnosis of mesenteric ischemia. These can serve as preoperative images prior to surgical revascularization and can also serve as a comparison for

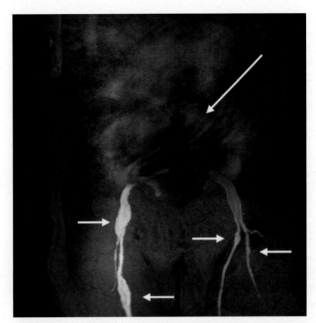

FIGURE 38.4 Contrast-enhanced MRA of the pelvis in the coronal plane. There is stent graft artifact in the middle of the abdomen (*long arrow*) caused by an aortic endograft. There are multiple aneurysms in the common, internal, and external iliac arteries bilaterally (*short arrows*). Clinical information: 73-year-old man with a history of femoral artery aneurysm and an abdominal aortic endograft.

patients with persisting symptoms. Three-dimensional contrast-enhanced MRA can be used to visualize aneurysms in the mesenteric system, such as in the proximal celiac artery, which is commonly associated with AAA.

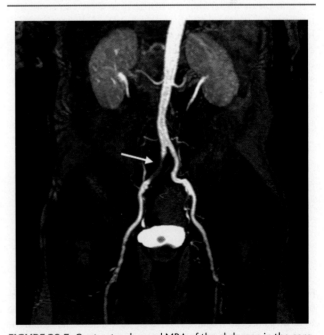

FIGURE 38.5 Contrast-enhanced MRA of the abdomen in the coronal plane. There is a stent in the right common iliac artery (*arrow*) with associated stent artifact. Clinical information: 61-year-old man being evaluated for claudication.

FIGURE 38.6 Contrast-enhanced MRA of the abdomen in the coronal plane. **A.** Thin maximum intensity projection (MIP) showing narrowing and dilatation of the left renal artery (*arrow*). **B.** Thicker MIP showing the entire left renal artery (*arrow*). Clinical information: 49-year-old woman being evaluated for vasculitis. Differential diagnosis includes fibromuscular dysplasia, Ehlers-Danlos syndrome, and polyarteritis nodosa.

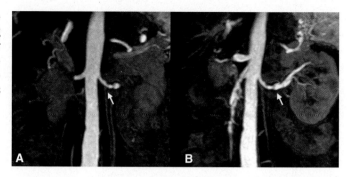

A body coil is used in MRA scans of the mesenteric arteries.[30] The xyphoid process serves as a standard landmark. Scanning begins with a three-plane localizer and calibration scan. Then images are acquired using 2D coronal and axial single-shot FSE. Next, 3D contrast-enhanced MRA and postcontrast 3D axial and coronal LAVA are performed.

Renal Arteries

Difficult-to-control hypertension, renal failure, preoperative arterial mapping, and renal transplantation are some indications for performing an MRA of the renal arteries.[5] Atherosclerosis and fibromuscular dysplasia, both implicated in difficult-to-control hypertension, can be visualized on MRA of the renal arteries (FIGURE 38.6). Limiting iodinated contrast, which can promote further nephropathy, makes MRA advantageous in the evaluation of renal failure (FIGURE 38.7). Imaging the vasculature in both the donor and recipient before and after renal transplantation is another utility of renal MRA.

A body array coil is used in renal MRA. The lower anterior rib margin or upper margin of the iliac crest can serve as a landmark.[31] Protocols with and without gadolinium contrast have been developed for renal MRA. Noncontrast scanning can be particularly useful if there is a concern for NSF in individuals with poor renal function. Noncontrast protocols start with a three-plane localizer and calibration scan. The

majority of scanning is done with 2D single-shot FSE, 2D and 3D balanced SSFP sequences. Phase contrast imaging can help assess the hemodynamic significance of any stenosis found.

Peripheral Arteries

Imaging the peripheral arteries can be done for the evaluation of claudication, rest pain, nonhealing ulcers, and to assess bypass graft patency.[3] Some medical conditions where 3D contrast-enhanced MRA techniques are commonly used include peripheral vascular disease (PVD) and AVM.[5] This technique enables the visualization of the length of the occlusion in the aortoiliac or femoropopliteal vessel segments in PVD (FIGURE 38.8). It is also used to find AVM or fistulas in the upper and lower extremities, and multiphase acquisitions can be done that show venous drainage from these areas (FIGURE 38.9).

Total body coil arrays, torso, extremity, or knee coils can be used.[5] Alternatively, the extremity being imaged can be placed inside a head coil. Imaging can be done at multiple anatomic stations and a single injection of contrast can be followed as it circulates to distal parts of the extremity. This is referred to as the "bolus-chase" or "floating table" technique.

Lower extremity imaging begins with axial TOF scout images at multiple spots along the extremity.[5] These are for locating the arteries for upcoming precontrast 3D mask images that will be used for digital subtraction. After contrast injection, 3D contrast-enhanced MRA images are acquired at three imaging

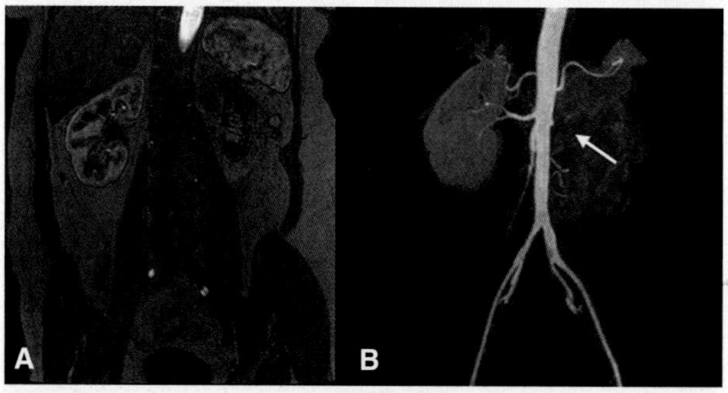

FIGURE 38.7 Contrast-enhanced MRA of the abdomen in the coronal plane (**A**) and reconstructed image (**B**). The left kidney was found to be atrophic with a delayed perfusion, so it is not visualized in the reconstructed imaged. The left renal artery is completely occluded versus high-grade narrowing near its origin (*arrow*). Clinical information: 40-year-old woman with a history of uncontrolled hypertension and chronic myelogenous leukemia.

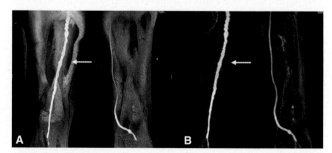

FIGURE 38.8 Contrast-enhanced MRA of the lower extremities in the coronal plane (**A**) with digital subtraction (**B**). There are multiple superficial femoral artery aneurysms (*arrow*) in the right lower extremity and a femoral-to-below-the-knee bypass graft in the left lower extremity. Clinical information: 73-year-old man with a femoral artery aneurysm found on prior ultrasound.

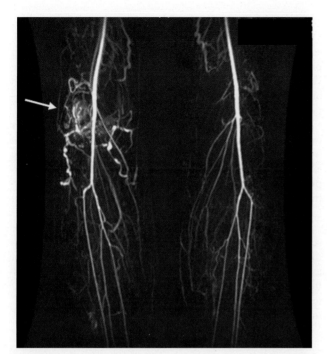

FIGURE 38.9 Contrast-enhanced MRA of the lower extremities in the coronal plane. Early increased pattern of enhancement is seen (*arrow*) at the level of the knee in the right lower extremity, indicating an arteriovenous malformation (AVM) because only arteries should enhance with contrast during the arterial phase. This shows normal appearance of left lower extremity vasculature. Clinical information: 42-year-old woman with a history of an AVM.

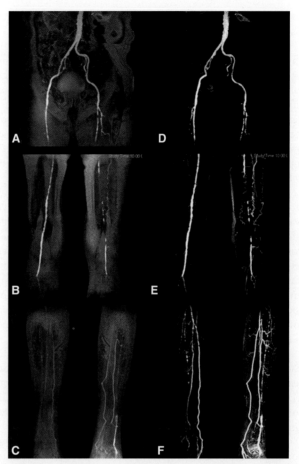

FIGURE 38.10 "Bolus chase" MRA of the lower extremities in the coronal plane. After contrast injection, images were acquired at three stations: pelvis (**A**), thigh (**B**), and calf (**C**) as the table moved to track the bolus as it flowed down the legs. Improved contrast is created with digital subtraction of a precontrast mask (**D–F**). This study clearly details segmental occlusions of the left superficial femoral artery. Clinical information: 85-year-old man being evaluated for claudication.

stations (e.g., pelvis, thigh, and calf) as the table moves to track the bolus as it flows down the legs (FIGURE 38.10). Bolus chase is difficult to perform if the circulation is too fast compared to the time needed for table movement and image acquisitions. In these cases, a second injection of contrast can be used. Alternatively, blood pressure cuffs placed on the thighs inflated to 50 to 60 mm Hg can help to delay venous enhancement.

Portal Venous System

Portal hypertension, liver transplantation, and hepatic and portal vein thrombosis can be imaged using 3D contrast-enhanced MRA.[5] Imaging can help plan where to place a portosystemic shunt and also assess shunt-flow volume. It can also be used to visualize the patency of the hepatic artery, hepatic veins, and portal veins before and after transplantation, especially in the case of posttransplant elevation of liver function tests. Flow limitations due to thrombus in the hepatic and portal veins can also be seen on 3D contrast-enhanced MRA.

A body coil is used to image the portal venous system, which can be imaged during MRI examinations of the abdomen, renal, or mesenteric vessels, so routine scanning protocols for those regions can include the portal veins.[5] Acquisitions can be done using 2D phase contrast, TOF, and postcontrast gradient echo sequences. Precontrast T1 and T2 spin echo imaging can be done to visualize liver parenchymal disease. Imaging in the coronal plane can simultaneously visualize the superior and inferior

mesenteric arteries along with the portal venous system. Alternatively, imaging in the axial plane can result in higher spatial resolution because the portal vein courses along this plane.

Contrast dilution must be taken into consideration when imaging the portal venous system.[5] A large amount of contrast may be needed (e.g., 10 mL gadofosveset trisodium or at least 0.1 mmol/kg of an extracellular agent) due to contrast traveling into the extracellular space and starting to be excreted by the liver before reaching the portal vein.

Peripheral Venography

Two approaches can be used for visualization of the peripheral veins: indirect and direct.[5] The indirect approach images during the equilibrium phase of contrast after it is injected through a peripheral IV site. This has the advantage of avoiding cannulation of veins in the affected extremity. This approach requires a large amount of contrast, however, to compensate for the extracellular distribution of contrast before it reaches the veins of the affected extremity. Image quality can be improved by obtaining images that have been digitally subtracted from precontrast datasets.

The direct approach involves injecting contrast at an upstream site on the affected extremity. This has the advantage of using less contrast than the indirect approach. A large volume of dilute contrast is needed, however, for continuous infusion during the scanning. Also, if imaging central veins, contrast infusions from both arms may need to be used because of the physiologic dilution of contrast from the systemic venous system as it enters the central veins. Similar to the indirect approach, digital subtraction is used to enhance image quality in the direct approach.

Clinical indications for visualizing upper extremity veins include arm swelling, prepacemaker placement, preoperative evaluation prior to dialysis fistula, and a poorly functioning dialysis fistula.[32] Axillary, subclavian, innominate veins, and superior vena cava can be visualized by contrast magnetic resonance venography (MRV) (FIGURE 38.11).[5] The middle of the sternum is the standard landmark.[32] A torso coil can be used for visualizing one arm or a body coil can be used for visualization of both arms and central veins. The arms may need to be elevated anteriorly to the level of the subclavian vein to be easily included in the FOV.

Imaging at multiple anatomic stations may be needed to visualize the entire upper extremity.[32] Imaging at each station begins with a three-plane localizer. Two-dimensional inversion recovery with fat saturation, 3D TOF with contrast, and 2D TOF postcontrast acquisitions are normally utilized for visualizing upper extremity veins.

Indications for lower extremity MRV include leg swelling, nondiagnostic ultrasound for DVT, to rule out pelvic DVT, to determine the proximal extension of a known DVT, to evaluate for a free-floating thrombus, and preoperative evaluation for

venous reconstructive surgery (FIGURE 38.12).[33] Two-dimensional TOF acquisitions without contrast can image the iliac, femoral, and popliteal veins for diagnosing a DVT.[5] Using contrast can provide higher-resolution images. Also, methods to increase venous flow may be utilized, such as keeping the legs warm with blankets, elevating the legs,[3] or using tourniquets at certain locations (e.g., ankle, thigh).[5]

The pubic symphysis is the conventional landmark for lower extremity imaging and a body coil is typically used because of its large FOV.[33] Similar to upper extremity venography, imaging is done at multiple anatomic stations and begins with a three-plane localizer. Two-dimensional TOF and 2D phase contrast images are usually acquired during scanning. Postcontrast LAVA acquisitions can be used to image small DVTs.[3]

An area with a filling defect may be reimaged using 2D phase contrast with superior-to-inferior flow encoding.[3] This can help distinguish a true filling defect from a flow artifact. Postcontrast axial T1 and T2 acquisitions can help distinguish an acute DVT from a chronic DVT because acute ones appear bright on T2 images and enhance with contrast due to a perivenous inflammatory response.

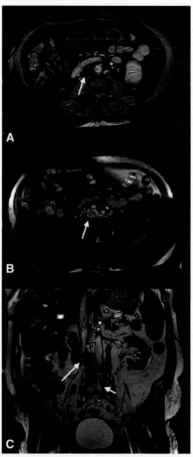

FIGURE 38.12 Balanced steady-state free precession MRV of the abdomen in the axial plane (**A** and **B**) and coronal plane (**C**). An inferior vena cava (IVC) filter is seen (image **A**, *arrow*) with a thrombus distal to it (image **B**, *arrow*). The IVC filter (*long arrow*) and distal thrombus (*short arrow*) can be seen in a single coronal image **C**. Clinical information: 58-year-old man with leg swelling.

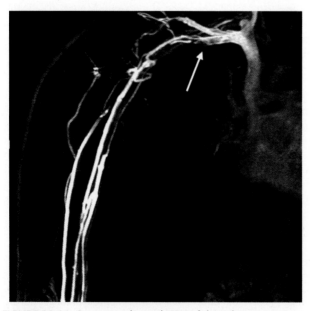

FIGURE 38.11 Contrast-enhanced MRV of the right upper extremity in the coronal plane using gadolinium diluted 20:1 with normal saline. A filling defect (*arrow*) occludes the subclavian vein where it enters the thoracic cage. Clinical information: 31-year-old woman with right arm swelling.

ACKNOWLEDGMENTS

We wish to thank Keigo Kawaji, MS, for his assistance with MR physics and image preparation, and Nanda Thimmappa, MD, for her assistance with image preparation.

REFERENCES

1. McRobbie DW, Moore EA, Graves MJ, et al. *MRI from Picture to Proton.* 2nd ed. Cambridge, UK: Cambridge University Press; 2007.
2. Shellock FG, Spinazzi A. MRI safety update 2008: part 2, screening patients for MRI. *Am J Roentgenol* 2008;191(4):1140–1149.
3. Winchester PA, Prince MR. Magnetic resonance angiography. In: Kandarpa K, Machan L, eds. *Handbook of Interventional Radiologic Procedures.* 4th ed. Philadelphia, PA: Lippincott Williams & Wilkins; 2011.
4. Zhang H, Maki JH, Prince MR. 3D contrast-enhanced MR angiography. *J Magn Reson Imaging* 2007;25(1):13–25.
5. Prince MR, Grist TM, Debatin JF. *3D Contrast MR Angiography.* 3rd ed. Berlin, Germany: Springer; 2003.
6. U.S. Food and Drug Administration. Questions and answers on gadolinium-based contrast agents. August 13, 2009. Available at: http://www.fda.gov/Drugs/DrugSafety/DrugSafetyNewsletter/ucm142889.htm.
7. Ersoy H, Rybicki FJ. Biochemical safety profiles of gadolinium-based extracellular contrast agents and nephrogenic systemic fibrosis. *J Magn Reson Imaging* 2007;26(5):1190–1197.
8. Burtea C, Laurent S, Vander Elst L, et al. Contrast agents: magnetic resonance. *Handb Exp Pharmacol* 2008;185(pt 1):135–165.
9. Bremerich J, Bilecen D, Reimer P. MR angiography with blood pool contrast agents. *Eur Radiol* 2007;17:3017–3024.
10. Ersoy H, Jacobs P, Kent CK, et al. Blood pool MR angiography of aortic stent-graft endoleak. *Am J Roentgenol* 2004;182(5):1181–1186.
11. Anzai Y, Prince MR, Chenevert TL, et al. MR angiography with an ultrasmall superparamagnetic iron oxide blood pool agent. *J Magn Reson Imaging* 1997;7(1):209–214.
12. Saxena SK, Sharma M, Patel M, et al. Nephrogenic systemic fibrosis: an emerging entity. *Int Urol Nephrol* 2008;40(3):715–724.
13. Cowper SE, Robin HS, Steinberg SM, et al. Scleromyxoedema-like cutaneous diseases in renal-dialysis patients. *Lancet* 2000;356:1000–1001.
14. High WA, Ayers RA, Chandler J, et al. Gadolinium is detectable within the tissue of patients with nephrogenic systemic fibrosis. *J Am Acad Dermatol* 2007;56(1):21–26.
15. Prince MR, Zhang HL, Roditi GH, et al. Risk factors for NSF: a literature review. *J Magn Reson Imaging* 2009;30(6):1298–1308.
16. U.S. Food and Drug Administration. Information for healthcare professionals: gadolinium-based contrast agents for magnetic resonance imaging (marketed as Magnevist, MultiHance, Omniscan, OptiMARK, ProHance). December 23, 2010. Available at: http://www.fda.gov/Drugs/DrugSafety/PostmarketDrugSafetyInformationforPatientsandProviders/ucm142884.htm.
17. Waugh SA, Ramkumar PG, Gandy SJ, et al. Optimization of the contrast dose and injection rates in whole-body MR angiography at 3.0T. *J Magn Reson Imaging* 2009;30(5):1059–1067.
18. Bellin MF, Van Der Molen AJ. Extracellular gadolinium-based contrast media: an overview. *Eur J Radiol* 2008;66(2):160–167.
19. Korosec FR, Frayne R, Grist TM, et al. Time-resolved contrast-enhanced 3D MR angiography. *Magn Reson Med* 1996;36(3):345–351.
20. Hartung MP, Grist TM, Francois CJ. Magnetic resonance angiography: current status and future directions. *J Cardiovasc Magn Reson* 2011;13:19.
21. Shellock FG, Crues JV. MR procedures: biologic effects, safety, and patient care. *Radiology* 2004;232(3):635–652.
22. Miyazaki M, Lee VS. Nonenhanced MR angiography. *Radiology* 2008;248(1):20–43.
23. Bley TA, Johnson KM, Francois CJ, et al. Noninvasive assessment of transstenotic pressure gradients in porcine renal artery stenoses by using vastly undersampled phase-contrast MR angiography. *Radiology* 2011;261:266–273.
24. Shonai T, Takahashi T, Ikeguchi H, et al. Improved arterial visibility using short-tau inversion-recovery (STIR) fat suppression in non-contrast-enhanced time-spatial labeling inversion pulse (Time-SLIP) renal MR angiography (MRA). *J Magn Reson Imaging* 2009;29(6):1471–1477.
25. Chen J, Di YJ, Bu CQ, et al. A comparative analysis of double inversion recovery TFE and TSE sequences on carotid artery wall imaging. *Eur J Radiol.* 2012;81(2):223–225. doi:10.1016/j.ejrad.2010.12.048.
26. Arch and carotids. In: MRprotocols.com [database online]. May 19, 2010. Available at: http://www.mrprotocols.com/?p=538.
27. Pulmonary MRA. In: MRprotocols.com [database online]. May 25, 2010. Available at: http://www.mrprotocols.com/?p=641.
28. Thoracic MRA. In: MRprotocols.com [database online]. May 25, 2010. Available at: http://www.mrprotocols.com/?p=644.
29. Abdominal aortic aneurysm. In: MRprotocols.com [database online]. May 24, 2010. Available at: http://www.mrprotocols.com/?p=630.
30. Mesenteric-portal. In: MRprotocols.com [database online]. May 24, 2010. Available at: http://www.mrprotocols.com/?p=632.
31. Renal artery without contrast. In: MRprotocols.com [database online]. May 26, 2010. Available at: http://www.mrprotocols.com/?p=670.
32. Subclavian venography. In: MRprotocols.com [database online]. May 25, 2010. Available at: http://www.mrprotocols.com/?p=647.
33. Deep venous thrombosis. In: MRprotocols.com [database online]. May 24, 2010. Available at: http://www.mrprotocols.com/?p=634.

Diagnostic Catheter-Based Evaluations

JOHN H. RUNDBACK, DANIEL ANGHELESCU, and ROBERT A. LOOKSTEIN

INTRODUCTION

The angiographic diagnosis of vascular diseases was first defined in the 1940s[1] and further refined in the early 1950s.[2,3] Although cross-sectional imaging and duplex sonography have facilitated the noninvasive diagnosis of peripheral arterial disease (PAD), diagnostic catheter-based angiography remains the gold standard for intervention. Although the fundamental technique for percutaneous access, formulated in the 1950s by Ivan Seldinger, remains the same,[4,5] advances in sheaths, catheters, needles, and wires have optimized subselective catheterization capability, improving diagnostic accuracy that makes targeted therapy possible by allowing for consistent selective and subselective catheterization. Advances in flat-panel imaging equipment also allow for more improved spatial and contrast resolution, leading to more accurate delineation of pathology while minimizing risks associated with intervention.[6] The recent availability of rotational angiography with multidimensional reconstructions further enhances diagnostic capability, particularly for the imaging of cerebrovascular and visceral arterial segments.[7,8]

DIAGNOSTIC EVALUATION STRATEGIES AND RECOMMENDATIONS

Generally, patients being evaluated for symptomatic PAD undergo noninvasive testing utilizing flow studies (ankle brachial indices [ABIs], segmental limb pressures, pulse volume recordings) for physiologic data, and imaging (computed tomography angiography, CTA; magnetic resonance angiography, MRA; or duplex sonography) for anatomic information. These tests have shown excellent concordance when compared with catheter-based angiography.[9,10] As noted in earlier chapters, however, noninvasive imaging has several limitations, particularly for accurate diagnosis in patients with complex multisegmental patterns of occlusive disease, extensive vascular calcification, and prior interventions. Whether performed in a separate setting or concurrently with interventional management, catheter-based angiography remains the gold standard for disease mapping and treatment planning. To ensure the most favorable imaging and interventional planning, a full knowledge of optimal angiographic techniques is necessary (FIGURES 39.1 to 39.5). Further, specific interventional strategies and interventional device selection is predicated on contrast angiographic features of lesion extent (length and severity), eccentricity, calcification, and patterns of reconstitution. Hence, a diagnostic algorithm in symptomatic patients being considered for endovascular therapy invariably and ultimately relies on catheter-based angiography.

GENERAL PRINCIPLES AND SPECIFIC TECHNIQUES

Diagnostic angiography and intervention are performed in dedicated suites compliant with existing standards for safety, sterility, and monitoring. Regular and planned testing and maintenance of equipment is mandatory. Both mobile C-arm imaging equipment and fixed-ceiling or wall-mounted dedicated angiographic equipment can be utilized; the latter has additional acquisition and processing capabilities and usually provides for better quality imaging. Features, such as pixel shifting, are generally available on all modern angiographic equipment and can help compensate for image degradation caused by patient motion (FIGURE 39.2).

Diagnostic catheters and wires come in multiple configurations and types of construction and consist of nonselective (i.e., pigtail type) as well as selective (consisting of preformed distal curves and tip shapes) catheters, sheaths, and guides. Typical catheter shapes for diagnostic catheterization are shown in Table 39.1. Most diagnostic studies are initially performed using 4 or 5 French catheters placed via the femoral artery using arterial puncture and Seldinger technique. In selective cases, alternate access routes, such as radial or brachial puncture sites, are used. Larger-bore catheters and sheaths, as well as coaxially introduced 3 French or smaller microcatheters, are often used for intervention but may be necessary for diagnostic purposes alone, either to stabilize selective catheter placement (larger sheaths) or to allow diagnostic assessment of smaller second- and third-order vascular branches (microcatheters). To ensure better torque control, most modern selective catheters are formed with a strong shaft that incorporates braided metals, such as steel, into the catheter polymer to provide reinforcement and facilitate the 1:1 rotational control of the tip during manipulations of the catheter outside the puncture site. Microcatheters allow deeper penetration into arterial segments to be studied for detailed selective and subselective arteriography and transcatheter treatments (Table 39.2).

Catheter tips are selected to match the expected shape and tortuosity of the artery to be accessed. Appropriate selection maximizes pushability while minimizing damage to the catheterized vessel. To optimally function, all of the elements of the system (often a sheath, catheter, microcatheter, and wires) need to fit together. For example, most microcatheter systems fit into 5 French catheter, although 4 French hydrophilic catheters accommodate many microcatheter systems. Consideration of the ideal combination of sheath, catheter, microcatheter, and wires to optimize entry into the desired vessel should be thought of in advance so that all tools will be ready prior to starting catheterization.

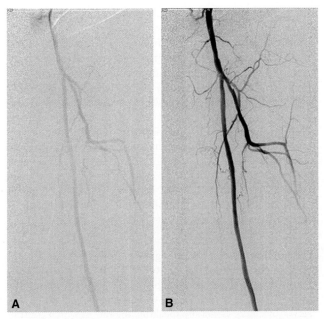

FIGURE 39.1 The importance of adequate opacification. Angiography of the leg obtained with insufficient contrast volume does not show adequate vascular detail (**A**). Repeat image with appropriate contrast rates and volumes clearly depicts vascular anatomy (**B**).

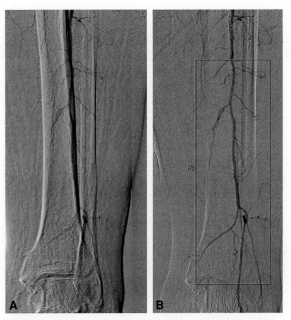

FIGURE 39.2 Pixel shifting. An initial tibial arteriogram (**A**) does not adequately depict the course of the distal vessels due to overlapping bone artifact. After pixel shifting (**B**) the bone artifact is largely eliminated and the arterial structures are well seen.

Standard Arterial Puncture

The standard puncture site for most therapeutic percutaneous interventions is the right common femoral artery. Although looking for landmarks, such as the lateral inguinal crease, is

helpful, confirmation of the puncture site such that the site of arterial entry is overlying the lower to middle third of the femoral head with fluoroscopy is recommended. With the beveled tip up, using an angle of entry between 45 and 85 degrees, the

Table 39.1		
Examples of Selective Catheter Configurations		
Catheter	Uses	Shape
Flush (e.g., pigtail, flush, tennis racket)	Aortography	
Angled (e.g., cobra, multipurpose, Berenstein)	Selective visceral angiography, extremity catheterization	
Shepherds crook (e.g., reverse curve, Sos, Simmons)	Selective visceral	

Table 39.2			
Examples of Peripheral Microcatheters			
Name	Company	Distal tip size (Fr)	Wire (inches)
Renegade	Boston Scientific (Nadick, MA)	2.4–2.7	0.018
ProGreat	Terumo (Somerset, NJ)	2.4–2.8	0.018–0.025
Miraflex	Cook (Bloomington, IN)	2.5–2.8	0.018
ProTrack	Baylis (Montreal, CA)	2.7, 2.9	0.021, 0.024
Marksman	ev3 (Minneapolis, MN)	2.8	0.023
Courier	Micrus Endovascular (San Jose, CA)	1.8, 1.9	0.014

vessel wall is punctured with an 18- or 19-gauge needle either between or below fingers palpating the pulse. When necessary, pulseless groins can be punctured using the femoral vein as an indicator of position and then redirecting the needle more laterally, or by using ultrasound guidance, often with 21-gauge micropuncture needles. A single puncture technique, where the needle is slowly advanced until blood return is observed, is now almost exclusively used for arterial access, especially in the coagulopathic patient or if a closure device is to be used. A floppy tipped straight or "J"-tipped wire is then passed into the artery and exchange made over the wire for a diagnostic catheter or low-profile introducer sheath. Although pulsatile flow suggests entry into the arterial lumen, a minor adjustment (medial, lateral, superficial, or deep) may be necessary if a wire does not travel easily through the vessel lumen, especially in patients with severe atherosclerotic disease or with tortuous arteries. The 19-gauge needle allows for direct access with a 0.035-inch diameter wire, most often a Benson wire, which incorporates a relatively long floppy tip with a minimally stiff main wire. Micropuncture sets uses a thinner 0.018-inch diameter wire, which can be switched out for a 0.035-inch wire after the inner stylet of the micropuncture sheath is removed. Minimizing the impedance of overlying tissues with a dermatotomy at least 2 mm larger in diameter than the largest sheath helps with sheath insertion; similarly, applying manual pressure over the arterial puncture while inserting catheters and sheaths stabilizes the artery and eases insertion.

Superselective Catheterization (FIGURE 39.3)

Catheterization of tortuous second- and third-order branches often requires the use of coaxial catheter systems, utilizing a catheter or guide at the ostium of the parent vessel, and the placement of smaller catheters in a telescoped fashion through the ostial catheter for subselective positioning (Table 39.2).

Size 3 French and smaller microcatheters can be advanced through 4 to 5 French catheters over 0.014- to 0.018-inch specialty wires. These wires often have shapeable tips and excellent torque control, thereby facilitating access to distal vessels for secure catheter advancement. Continuous fluoroscopy while advancing using the coaxial technique will ensure that the tension in the coaxial system does not push the guide catheter out of the first-order vessel. If too much tension develops in the system, the microcatheter/wire system is slowly retracted over the wire until the guide catheter is reengaged in the ostia.

■ OPTIMIZING ANGIOGRAPHIC TECHNIQUE

Careful preprocedure planning, meticulous basic technique, and appropriate catheter selection are the initial steps toward successful catheter-based angiography. To further enhance diagnostic performance, several other technical factors should be considered, as shown in Table 39.3. Adequate volumes of contrast need to be injected to opacify the desired target vessels (FIGURE 39.1). Generally speaking, the rate at which contrast is injected is determined by the anticipated rate of flow in the catheterized vessel to allow cross-sectional arterial filling and avoid artifacts that may be caused by contrast layering. When the catheter is well upstream from the vascular bed being imaged, somewhat lower contrast rates may be sufficient to allow mixing with blood and ensure complete vessel filling. The total volume of contrast injected depends on the volume of distribution to be imaged. For example, if an operator is performing magnification arteriography over a small vascular region, minimal amounts of contrast may be needed; on the contrary, for visceral angiography in which the entire splanchnic arterial bed and portal venous return is to be studied, considerably larger volumes of contrast are needed. Sample contrast rates and volumes are shown in Table 39.4. The use of power injectors ensures uniform contrast delivery at prespecified pressures, injection rates, and volumes, thereby improving vascular opacification. Injection pressures of 1,000 to 1,200 psi (pounds per square inch) are used for larger lumen catheters and catheters with sideholes. Microcatheters require injection pressures of 300 to 350 psi.

■ POTENTIAL ERRORS

Angiography remains the gold standard for diagnosis of vascular lesions; however, even with the most advanced equipment, there are potential pitfalls that can result in poor image resolution or clinically irrelevant information if optimal technique is not used (Table 39.3). Other potential causes of error are listed in Table 39.5. Patient positioning should lead to a full profile of the desired vessel; this is particularly important to see the origins of branching vessels and avoid misinterpretation caused by vascular overlap (FIGURE 39.4). As an example, the best imaging obliquity to visualize the iliac bifurcation is the 30-degree contralateral anterior oblique, and the femoral bifurcation is best seen in the 30-degree ipsilateral anterior oblique. Inadequate blood flow may require use of vasodilatation with an agent, such as nitroglycerin, administered intra-arterially 20 to 30 seconds before the acquisition of angiographic images. Poor collimation leads to flare ("burnout"), incorrect exposure, and gray

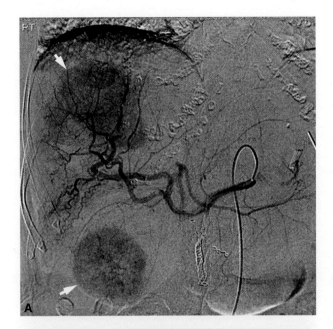

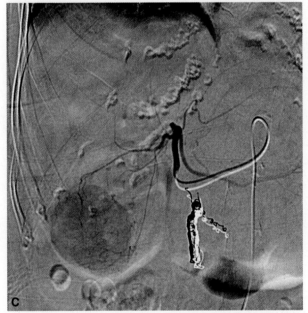

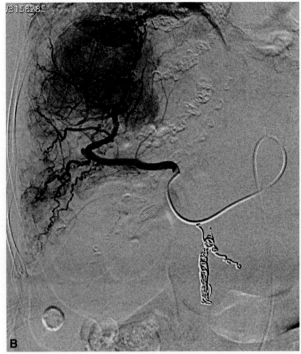

FIGURE 39.3 Value of selective catheterization. Celiac arteriography (**A**) prior yttrium-90 radioembolization shows two hypervascular right hepatic tumors (*arrowheads*) as previously demonstrated on CT. Selective right hepatic arteriography (**B**) does not show the segment 5 lesion. Subsequently, selective left hepatic arteriography (**C**) shows anomalous supply to the segment 5 tumor from a left hepatic artery branch. This finding resulted in a change in the radioembolization treatment plan.

Table 39.3
Keys to Optimizing Catheter-Based Angiography

1. Digital subtraction angiography when possible
2. Selective injections for distal arterial evaluation
3. Inject sufficient contrast volumes to avoid underfilling
4. Tight collimation and filters
5. Proper patient position
6. Restraints or cushions to avoid motion artifact
7. Oblique views to characterize lesions and treatment response
8. Remasking/pixel shifting to reduce motion artifacts
9. Vasodilators if needed to enhance peripheral vessel filling

scale compression. Excessive distance between patient and film or detector enhances the penumbra effects and causes magnification unsharpness as well as higher radiation exposure to the operator. Patient movement may be minimized with restraints or cushions.

COMPLICATIONS

Catheter angiography with modern technique is extremely safe with major complications occurring in less than 3% to 5% of cases. The Society of Interventional Radiology has defined thresholds for complications based on extensive literature review and expert consensus,[11] and this document provides an excellent and detailed resource regarding potential complications of angiographic procedures. In a large series of 999 patients

Table 39.4

Sample Rates and Volumes of Contrast Injection for Diagnostic Angiography

Vascular bed	Contrast rate (cc/sec)	Contrast volume (cc)
Aortogram	10–20	20–40
Pelvic angiography and lower extremity runoff	6–10	15–20
Selective extremity	4–6	10–15
Carotid	4–6	6–12
Celiac, SMA	4–6	6–12 (proximal evaluation)
		25–30 (include portal phase)
IMA	3–5	12–20
Microcatheter injection	1–3 cc (lower psi)	6–15

SMA, superior mesenteric artery; IMA, inferior mesenteric artery.

Table 39.5

Causes of Error During Diagnostic Arteriography

1. Inadequate dose and density of injected contrast medium
2. Nonselective or proximal injection, causing poor opacification
3. Incorrect patient positioning, resulting in failure to profile lesions
4. Patient restraints compressing vessels, leading to pseudo-occlusion
5. Plantar flexion, leading to pseudo-occlusion of the dorsalis pedis artery
6. Inadequate blood flow (requiring vasodilation)
7. Poor collimation, leading to flare ("burnout"), incorrect exposure, and gray scale compression
8. Anatomy preventing adequate collimation due to angulation of the area of interest (e.g., lateral view of ankle)
9. Excessive distance between patient and film or detector (magnification unsharpness)
10. Poor contrast resolution from screen-film arteriography
11. Poor contrast and spatial resolution from old DSA equipment
12. Patient movement
13. Improper timing between injection of contrast material and imaging

DSA, digital subtraction arteriography.

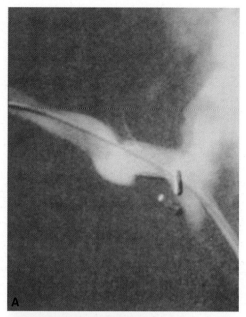

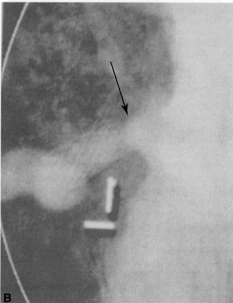

FIGURE 39.4 Utilization of proper oblique imaging. **A.** Selective renal arteriography in the left anterior oblique view shows a stent that appears to extend to the aortic lumen. **B.** Repeat angiography in the 10-degree right anterior oblique projection shows that the stent does not cover an ostial renal artery stenosis (*arrow*). The patient had recurrent hypertension and was treated with additional stent placement.

Reprinted with permission from Rundback JH, Weintraub JL. Renal vascular interventions. *Semin Roentgenol* 2002;37:312–326.

undergoing diagnostic angiography,[12] renal insufficiency was the most important risk and affected patient care in 1.5%. Major complications were described in 1.6%. The risk of major complication correlates with the experience of the operator. In a report evaluating outcomes in inexperienced physicians compared with practiced physicians, major complication rates for

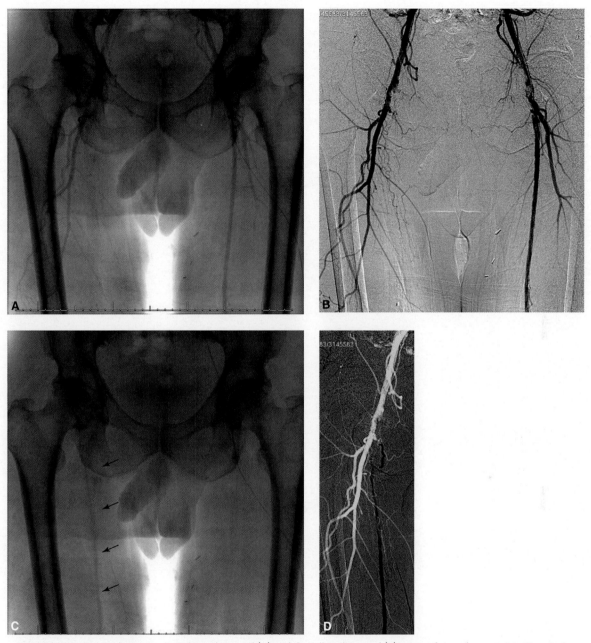

FIGURE 39.5 Delayed imaging. Initial unsubtracted (**A**) and digitally subtracted (**B**) images from a lower extremity arteriogram show apparent long segment occlusion of the right superficial femoral artery (SFA). Delayed imaging allows collateral reconstitution and retrograde filling of most of the SFA (**C**, *arrows*). A subtracted remasked image (**D**) using a late mask shows that the SFA occlusion is relatively short (*bracketed segment*). Using a late mask, early opacified vessels appear in white, and later filling vessels are black. Utilization of "stacking" software would also produce a picture of the entire patent vessel but can be limited if there is patient movement.

the initial 25 procedures was 8% but was reduced for the final 119 procedures to 0.8%.[13]

Lesser complications including puncture site ecchymosis, small hematomas, minor and self-limited arterial injury due to wire or catheter manipulation, asymptomatic microemboli, vasovagal reactions, and transient deteriorations in renal function are likely more common but not well characterized. Only a minority of these require specific therapy. Prevention of contrast-induced nephropathy may be improved by using low- or iso-osmolar contrast, limiting contrast volume, and making sure the patient is well hydrated.[14]

▌ CONCLUSION

Catheter angiography remains the gold standard for vascular diagnosis and affords an opportunity for simultaneous endovascular interventions. Using modern equipment and adherence to state-of-the-art technique, successful diagnostic studies can be obtained with minimal risk. Although the accuracy of alternative vascular imaging techniques will continue to improve, catheter-based angiography is likely to remain integral to the care of vascular patients for many years to come.

▌REFERENCES

1. Stuhlberg NM, Chechikian GM. Angiography in diseases of the peripheral vascular system. *Vestn Rentgenol Radiol* 1946;26(4):12.
2. Dotter CT, Steinber I, Ball RP. Angiography. *Circulation* 1951;3(4):606.
3. Dotter CT, Steinber I. Rapid serial contrast angiography. *Angiology* 1951;2(3):173–183.
4. Seldinger SI. Catheter replacement of the needle in percutaneous arteriography; a new technique. *Acta Radiol* 1953;39(5):368.
5. Hawkins IF. Carbon dioxide digital subtraction arteriography. *AJR Am J Roentgenol* 1982;139(1):19.
6. Chida K, Inaba Y, Saito H, et al. Radiation dose of interventional radiology system using a flat-panel detector. *AJR Am J Roentgenol* 2009;193(6):1680–1685.
7. Katoh M, Opitz A, Minko P, et al. 2D rotational angiography for fast and standardized evaluation of peripheral and visceral artery stenoses. *Cardiovasc Intervent Radiol* 2011;34(3):474–480.
8. Louie JD, Kothary N, Kuo WT, et al. Incorporating cone-beam CT into the treatment planning for yttrium-90 radioembolization. *J Vasc Interv Radiol* 2009;20(5):606–613.
9. Fleischmann D, Lammer J. Peripheral CT angiography for interventional treatment planning. *Eur Radiol* 2006;16(suppl 7):M58–M64.
10. Leiner T. Magnetic resonance angiography of abdominal and lower extremity vasculature. *Top Magn Reson Imaging* 2005;16(1):21–66.
11. Singh H, Cardella JF, Cole PE, et al. Quality improvement guidelines for diagnostic arteriography. *J Vasc Interv Radiol* 2003;14:S283–S288.
12. Gates J, Hartnell GG. Optimized diagnostic angiography in high-risk patients with severe peripheral vascular disease. *Radiographics* 2000;20(1):121.
13. Balduf LM, Langsfeld M, Marek JM, et al. Complication rates of diagnostic angiography performed by vascular surgeons. *Vasc Endovascular Surg* 2002;36(6):439–445.
14. Rundback JH, Weintraub JL. Renal vascular interventions. *Semin Roentgenol* 2002;37:312–326.

Medical Management of Peripheral Artery Disease

NEIL J. WIMMER and JOSHUA A. BECKMAN

INTRODUCTION

Peripheral artery disease (PAD) is a condition caused by atherosclerosis of the abdominal aorta, iliacs, and lower extremity arteries leading to stenoses or occlusions. In primary care practices across the United States, 29% of patients older than 70 or 50 years with a history of smoking or diabetes have PAD.[1] The severity of PAD is closely associated with the risk of myocardial infarction, ischemic stroke, and death from vascular causes. Multiple studies have demonstrated that the lower (or worse) the ankle brachial index (ABI), a measure of the severity of PAD, the greater the risk of cardiovascular events (FIGURE 40.1).[2,3]

PAD is most commonly asymptomatic on presentation but often presents with either a history of intermittent claudication or atypical leg pain. Classic claudication is pain or discomfort (aching, heaviness, tiredness, tightness, cramping, or burning) that is (1) reproducible with a similar level of walking from day to day, (2) disappears after predictable period of rest, and (3) occurs at the same distance once walking has resumed. There are other, less common symptomatic presentations of PAD, such as critical limb ischemia, but classic claudication and atypical pain are the most common. Patient outcomes with PAD are also variable. Clinical outcomes occur in two distinct categories: (1) limb specific morbidity and (2) cardiovascular morbidity and mortality including myocardial infarction, stroke, and cardiovascular-related death.

Once the diagnosis is established, the patient should always be treated medically with a risk factor modification and exercise program to reduce subsequent risk. Symptoms can be managed with exercise, symptom-targeted medications, or with revascularization by percutaneous intervention or surgery. The medical management of PAD, excluding antiplatelet therapy, is presented here. A discussion of antiplatelet agents, percutaneous interventional approaches, and surgery is presented in other chapters.

TREATMENT OBJECTIVES AND APPROACHES

The two primary treatment goals in individuals with PAD are to decrease cardiovascular morbidity and mortality and to improve limb-related symptoms and quality of life. These two goals should be addressed simultaneously in every patient.

LOWERING CARDIOVASCULAR MORBIDITY AND MORTALITY

The risk factors for PAD are identical to those for other forms of atherosclerotic vascular disease, and PAD is similarly associated with an increased risk of coronary, cerebrovascular, and

renovascular disease. As a result, PAD is considered a coronary heart disease equivalent, elevating it to the highest category of cardiovascular risk.[4] The 2005 American College of Cardiology/American Heart Association (ACC/AHA) practice guidelines and the 2007 TASC II consensus document on the management of PAD recommend smoking cessation, lipid-lowering therapy with statins, and the treatment of diabetes and hypertension.[5,6] Data from a Dutch prospective cohort study of 2,420 patients with PAD (ABI ≤ 0.90) support these conclusions and demonstrate that a comprehensive approach to risk factor modification can have additive benefits.[7] In this study, Feringa et al. demonstrated that after adjustment for risk factors and propensity scores, statins (hazard ratio [HR], 0.46; 95% confidence interval [CI], 0.36 to 0.58), beta blockers (HR, 0.68; 95% CI, 0.58 to 0.80), aspirin (HR, 0.72; 95% CI, 0.61 to 0.84), and angiotensin-converting enzyme (ACE) inhibitors (HR, 0.80; 95% CI, 0.69 to 0.94) were significantly associated with a reduced risk of long-term mortality in this cohort. The benefits of these therapies appear additive, and these data support the universal nature of atherosclerotic vascular disease, whether in the form of PAD or elsewhere.

Hyperlipidemia

Several cholesterol-lowering trials in patients with hyperlipidemia and coronary artery disease and/or PAD have evaluated the effects of lipid lowering on PAD. Initial studies, performed before the availability of statins, showed either regression or less progression of femoral atherosclerosis with lipid-lowering therapy.[8–10]

Studies in the statin era confirm these initial results. For instance, in the Heart Protection Study, which randomized 20,536 high-risk participants to 40 mg/day of simvastatin or placebo, a 24% relative risk reduction was observed in first-time cardiovascular events in the patients who received simvastatin. The subgroup of patients with PAD had similar cardiovascular benefits regardless of history of myocardial infarction or coronary artery disease. Even the subgroup population who had LDL-C levels less than 100 mg/dL at baseline benefited from statin therapy.[11] A post-hoc analysis of the Scandinavian Simvastatin Survival Study (4S), which included 4,444 patients with angina or previous myocardial infarction and a baseline total cholesterol between 212 and 309 mg/dL, found that treatment with 20 to 40 mg/day of simvastatin reduced the incidence of new or worsening claudication by 38% (2.3% vs. 3.6% with placebo).[12]

Independent of cholesterol-lowering effects, statin use improves pain-free walking distance and walking speed in patients with PAD and claudication.[13] Two studies randomized patients with claudication to simvastatin 40 mg daily or placebo.

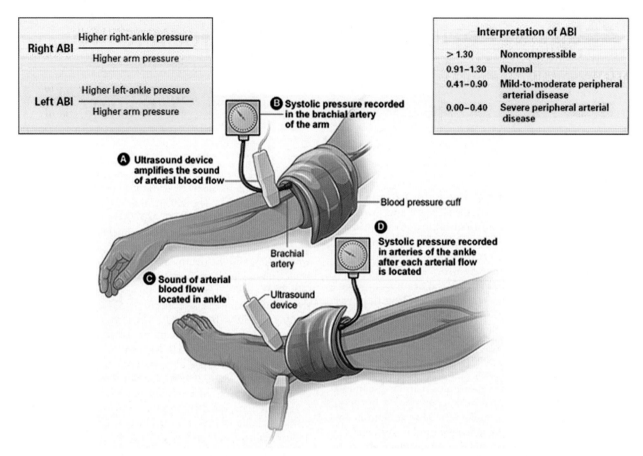

FIGURE 40.1 Ankle brachial index (ABI) examination. A blood pressure cuff is applied to the patient's arm and inflated. A Doppler ultrasound placed at the radial artery is used to record the first sound as the cuff is deflated. The cuff is then applied to the other arm and the procedure is repeated. The highest of the two arm blood pressures is accepted as the "baseline" upper extremity reading. The cuff is then applied to the midcalf on one leg and inflated. The Doppler ultrasound is placed at the dorsalis pedis (DP) and the posterior tibial (PT) arteries to record the first sound as the cuff is deflated. The cuff is then placed on the opposite leg, and the procedure is repeated. The highest ankle pressure for each leg is used as the lower extremity "baseline" reading. The ratio of each ankle-to-brachial pressure is determined by dividing the ankle pressure by the highest brachial pressure. An equal ratio implies no blockage of blood flow into the lower extremities. If the ratio of blood flow into the ankles is less than 0.9, PAD is likely to exist. A ratio of less than 0.8 correlates with symptomatic exercise-induced claudication. Patients with a ratio of less than 0.4 are likely to experience pain at rest in their legs. Severe, limb-threatening PAD is diagnosed when the ratio is less than 0.25.

Reprinted with permission from Unger J. *Diabetes Management in Primary Care*. Philadelphia, PA: Lippincott Williams & Wilkins; 2013.

Aronow et al.[14] reported an improvement in pain-free walking distance of 24% increase at 6 months and of 42% increase at 1 year after imitation of treatment. Interestingly, total walking distance and ABI did not improve. In contrast, Mondillo et al.[15] reported increases in the ABI, total walking distance, and pain-free survival in patients randomized to simvastatin. Mohler et al.[16] randomized 354 subjects with claudication to atorvastatin 10 mg, 80 mg, or placebo. Patients receiving atorvastatin had an increased pain-free walking distance but not total walking distance or ABI. Patients with PAD who take statins have been shown to have less annual decline in lower extremity performance than those who do not.[17] Overall, the aggregate data suggest that statin use may increase the walking distance

until the onset of pain, but statin use does not clearly impact total walking time or change lower extremity blood flow as measured by ABI.

The current recommendations advocate a goal LDL-C less than 100 mg/dL for patients with PAD; for very high-risk patients, the goal is an LDL-C less than 70 mg/dL. All patients with PAD should be treated with statins as first-line lipid-lowering therapy, if tolerable.[5]

There is also a role for fibrate therapy in the treatment of PAD. The Fenofibrate Intervention and Event Lowering in Diabetes (FIELD) study randomized 9,795 patients aged 50 to 75 years with type 2 diabetes to either fenofibrate 200 mg/day or placebo for 5 years' duration. The risks of first amputation

(45 vs. 70 events; HR, 0.64; 95% CI, 0.44–0.94; p = .02) and minor amputation events without known large-vessel disease (18 vs. 34 events; 0.53, 0.30 to 0.94; p = .027) were lower for patients assigned to fenofibrate than for patients assigned to placebo with no difference between groups in risk of major amputations.[18] A reduction in amputation events has not been similarly shown with statin therapy.

Smoking Cessation

Several nonrandomized studies have shown that patients who successfully quit smoking have decreased rates of PAD progression, critical limb ischemia, amputation, myocardial infarction, and stroke and have increased survival.[19,20] Unfortunately, the spontaneous cessation rates without intervention range from 2% to 5% in the United States, despite nearly 75% of smokers expressing a desire to stop. Given the importance of smoking cessation, it is important for health care providers to consistently convey to patients that discontinuation of tobacco products is extremely important to overall survival, well-being, and limb preservation.[21,22] Behavioral interventions can improve cessation rates but only modestly. Only 5% of patients who receive physician advice, follow-up correspondence, phone calls, and supplementary visits will quit smoking.[23] Randomized trial evidence, however, has demonstrated that a 10-week intervention that results just a 21.7% smoking cessation rate at 5 years significantly improves survival in patients with chronic lung disease compared to those treated with usual care.[24] Thus, efforts at cessation should be made.

Henrikus et al. have specifically demonstrated that individuals with PAD respond to intensive counseling and education in a randomized trial of 124 subjects. They compared an intensive tobacco cessation counseling program with a minimal educational program over 6 months. Study participants assigned to the intensive intervention group were significantly more likely to be abstinent of tobacco at 6-month follow-up: 21.3% versus 6.8% in the minimal intervention group (p = .023).[25]

Smoking cessation can be aided in many ways including the use of pharmacotherapy, such as short-term nicotine replacement products including gums, long-acting nicotine replacement patches, buproprion, or varenicline. Pharmacologic interventions are more effective than medical advice alone. In controlled studies, the rates of stopping smoking using pharmacologic treatment interventions has varied from 17% to 48% at 6 months and between 11% and 34% at 1 year.[26] Buproprion, via a poorly understood mechanism, diminishes the desire for smoking. It is associated with cessation rates of 27% to 35% at 6 months and 23% to 30% at 1 year.[27] Varenicline, a partial agonist selective for the alpha-4, beta-2 nicotinic acetylcholine receptor, is a newer agent than buproprion. Two large randomized trials have suggested that varenicline performs better when the two are compared directly. In a study of 1,025 smokers where subjects were randomized to placebo, sustained-release buproprion, or varenicline, abstinence rates from weeks 9 to 52 were significantly elevated in the two drug arms compared to placebo. Cessation rates were 8.4%, 16.1%, and 21.9%, respectively, for individuals taking placebo, buproprion, and varenicline.[28] In a second large randomized trial, Jorenby et al.[29] found similar abstinence rates

in individuals treated with placebo, buproprion, or varenicline as well.

The United States Public Health Services task force smoking cessation guidelines do not recommend any one of the first-line agents over another.[30] Instead, they recommend that patient preference and previous experience with the medications guide the choice among the first-line therapy (nicotine replacement, bupropion, and varenicline). Meta-analyses done for the guideline update addressed the question of whether any drug was more effective than the nicotine patch. In this analysis, there was no statistically significant difference between the patch and other nicotine replacement products or bupropion, but varenicline had a higher efficacy than the nicotine patch (OR, 1.6; 95% CI, 1.3 to 2.0). The analysis also compared the nicotine patch to combinations of drugs. The combination of nicotine patch and short-acting nicotine replacement products, used for an extended period, was more effective than the patch alone (OR, 1.9; 95% CI, 1.3 to 2.7), as was the combination of nicotine patch and sustained-release buproprion (OR, 1.3; 95% CI, 1.0 to 1.8).

Until further trials are performed, varenicline and the combination of long-acting patch plus short-acting nicotine replacement therapies appear to be roughly equivalent first-line choices. Patients treated with varenicline should be monitored for possible adverse neuropsychiatric events.

Despite multiple options for the approach to tobacco cessation in individuals with PAD, there appears to be continued risk in individuals who successfully become abstinent. Recently published data from the Women's Health Study demonstrate that although smoking cessation substantially reduces risk for PAD events in women, there remains an increased occurrence of PAD events in former smokers compared to individuals who never smoked.[31]

Hypertension

In a large number of clinical trials involving thousands of patients, antihypertensive drug therapy has been associated with a 35% to 40% mean reduction in the rate of stroke, 20% to 25% reduction in myocardial infarction, greater than 50% reduction in heart failure, and a significant reduction in the development of chronic kidney disease.[32] Although treating hypertension has been studied in many contexts, there are limited data available to determine whether treatment of hypertension will prevent the development of claudication or alter the course of PAD itself.

The Treatment of Mild Hypertension Study (TOMHS) showed that drug treatment in addition to nutritional interventions was superior to nutritional interventions alone in preventing the development of intermittent claudication and PAD over an average follow-up of 4.4 years.[33]

Reports on the effect of blood pressure lowering on the ability to walk in patients with intermittent claudication are mixed.[34–36] These small studies have demonstrated that the ACE inhibitor captopril maintains and may increase walking distance in patients with claudication. Alpha-adrenergic blockers, beta blockers, and calcium-channel blockers may adversely affect walking distance, particularly if there is a substantial decrease in systolic blood pressure. In a 6-month crossover trial of 20 hypertensive patients with PAD randomized to atenolol, labetalol, pindolol, captopril, or placebo, only individuals treated with captopril maintained walking distance.[36] This appears to be a class effect because enalapril and ramipril seem to improve lower extremity blood flow in patients with claudication as well.[37,38]

Antihypertensive therapy should be administered to hypertensive patients with PAD to achieve a goal of less than 140/90 mm Hg for nondiabetic patients or to less than 130/80 mm Hg for patients with diabetes or chronic kidney disease to reduce the risk of myocardial infarction, stroke, heart failure, and cardiovascular death.[5]

In PAD patients with diabetes, the Appropriate Blood Pressure Control in Diabetes (ABCD) study supports intensive management of hypertension.[39] The ABCD study randomized 480 normotensive subjects (baseline diastolic blood pressure of 80 to 89 mm Hg) with type 2 diabetes to either an intensive blood pressure regimen with enalapril or nisoldipine or placebo. Individuals were followed for 5 years. Of the subjects, 53 had PAD as defined by an ABI less than 0.90. In patients with PAD, there were 3 cardiovascular events (13.6%) on intensive treatment compared with 12 events (38.7%) on placebo ($p = .046$). After adjustment for multiple cardiovascular risk factors, an inverse relationship between ABI and cardiovascular events was observed with placebo ($p = .009$) but not with intensive treatment ($p = .91$). Thus, with intensive blood pressure control, the risk of an event was not increased, even at the lowest ABI values, and was the same as in patients without PAD. The conclusion from the trial was that intensive blood pressure lowering to a mean of 128/75 mm Hg resulted in a marked reduction in cardiovascular events.

Additional Benefits of Renin-Angiotensin System Antagonism

Although the achievement of goal blood pressure level outweighs a specific class of antihypertensive agents, the use of renin-angiotensin system antagonists should be considered an initial drug class of choice.

Both ACE inhibitors and angiotensin receptor blockers (ARBs) have favorable effects on the cardiovascular system beyond their ability to lower blood pressure. Based on the Heart Outcomes Prevention Evaluation (HOPE) study, patients with diabetes or evidence of vascular disease plus one other cardiovascular risk factor who received ramipril had a 22% relative risk reduction of the combined endpoint of stroke, myocardial infarction, and death compared with patients who received placebo, despite a baseline blood pressure considered at goal for most subjects. These outcomes were seen despite a relatively modest overall blood pressure reduction of 3/2 mm Hg.[40] Overall, 17.8% of patients in the placebo group reached the primary study endpoint of myocardial infarction, stroke, or cardiovascular death. The rate was 22% for the 4,051 patients with PAD compared to 14.3% for the 5,246 patients without PAD.

In the European trial on Reduction of cardiac events with Perindopril in patients with stable coronary Artery disease (EUROPA), 12,218 patients with stable coronary artery disease were randomly assigned to perindopril or placebo. After a mean follow-up of 4.2 years, cardiovascular events were significantly decreased in patients treated with perindopril. All predefined subgroups, including the 883 patients who had documented PAD, benefited from perindopril.[41] These data concurred with the HOPE trial.

Thus, based on two studies of subjects with normal blood pressure at rest and only modest changes in blood pressure with therapy, ACE inhibitors decrease cardiovascular morbidity and mortality more than expected with the observed blood pressure lowering.

Similar to ACE inhibitors, ARBs have documented cardiovascular benefits beyond their antihypertensive properties. In particular, ARBs have been shown to improve endothelial function through decreased vascular inflammation.[42] Patients with high cardiovascular risk, including those with PAD, are likely to benefit from ARBs. ARBs, such as losartan and candesartan, have shown morbidity and mortality benefits either alone or in combination with ACE inhibitors, as demonstrated in the Losartan Intervention for Endpoint (LIFE) and the Candesartan in Heart Failure Assessment of Reduction in Mortality and Morbidity (CHARM) studies.[43,44] In the LIFE study, losartan was compared to atenolol in hypertensive patients with electrocardiographic evidence of left ventricular hypertrophy. Overall, losartan significantly lowered the incidence of cardiovascular events, particularly stroke, despite similar decreases in blood pressure. Thus, similar to ACE inhibitors, ARBs should be thought of as having cardiovascular benefits beyond blood pressure reduction. Interestingly, in Swedish National Registry Data, patients treated with candesartan were less likely to develop PAD compared to patients treated with losartan despite similar blood pressure lowering.[45]

Beta Blockers in Peripheral Artery Disease

The commonly held belief that beta-blocking agents worsen claudication and shorten the amount of exercise required to bring on discomfort in the legs has been challenged. In a carefully performed meta-analysis of 11 randomized controlled trials, Radack and Deck[46] demonstrated that beta-adrenergic blocker therapy does not worsen claudication symptoms in people with PAD. Only 1 of 11 studies in this meta-analysis showed that pain-free and maximal treadmill walking distances were decreased by atenolol, labetalol, or pindolol, but not captopril.

Beta blockers should not be considered a first-line agent in the treatment of hypertension and PAD, however, given the beneficial effects of ACE-I and ARBs already discussed. If there are clear indications for beta-blocker use, such as congestive heart failure, post-myocardial infarction, angina pectoris, arrhythmias, or for perioperative cardiovascular protection, then beta blockers can and should be used.[47]

Diabetes Mellitus

To date, no prospective trials have been performed to assess whether improved glycemic control decreases the cardiovascular risk associated with PAD, walking distance of patients with claudication, or frequency of amputation. In a retrospective review of the Diabetes Control and Complications Trial of subjects with type 1 diabetes mellitus, there was a 22% risk reduction in the development of PAD in the group that received intensive insulin therapy.[48] Epidemiologic studies also support the benefit of tight glycemic control. The prospective Belfast Diet Study of type 2 diabetic subjects demonstrated an increasing risk for myocardial infarction of 1.04/mmol increase in fasting plasma glucose.[49] In the UK Prospective Diabetes Study of 2,693 subjects followed for nearly 8 years, subjects in the highest tertile of glycosylated hemoglobin had a 1.5-fold greater risk for myocardial infarction compared to those in the lowest tertile.[50] Although no prospective trial has demonstrated the benefits of improved glycemic control, it is nevertheless recommended. The American Diabetes Association recommends that all patients with diabetes and PAD should be aggressively treated to reduce their glycosylated hemoglobin levels to less than 7%.[51] Further reduction in goal glycosylated hemoglobin levels have been tested in several recent trials.[52–54] Although intensive glycemic control reduced the incidence of microvascular events, there were no significant reductions in macrovascular outcomes between standard and intensive glycemic control. The ACCORD trial, for instance, randomized 10,251 subjects with a history of a cardiovascular event or significant cardiovascular risk to intensive glycemic control (target HbA_{1c}, <6.0%) or standard glycemic control (target HbA_{1c}, 7.0% to 7.9%). Within 12 months of randomization, the intensive glycemic group reached a median HbA_{1c} of 6.4% (from a baseline median of 8.1%) compared with a median HbA_{1c} of 7.5% in the standard glycemic group. The glycemic control arm was stopped, however, owing to an increased mortality rate in the intensive glycemic control group.[52] At this time, the optimal HbA_{1c} goal for individuals with PAD remains less than 7%.

Despite a paucity of clinical trial evidence, meticulous foot care is also recommended in patients with diabetes and PAD to reduce the risk of skin ulceration, necrosis, and subsequent amputation. This includes the use of appropriate footwear to avoid pressure injury, daily inspection and cleansing by the patient, and the use of moisturizing cream to prevent dryness and fissuring. Frequent foot inspection by patients and health care providers is thought to enable early identification of foot lesions and ulcerations and facilitate prompt referral for treatment.[51]

Obesity and Weight Reduction

An association between obesity and PAD has been observed in some studies but not others. For instance, in the Framingham cohort of 5,209 subjects, relative weight was only a weak risk factor for claudication.[55] In contrast, obesity, as determined by a body mass index greater than 30, was not a risk factor for PAD or intermittent claudication in the Edinburgh Artery Study, Whitehall Study, or Lipid Research Clinics Study.[56–58] Despite the mixed evidence for a direct relationship between obesity and PAD, obesity may heighten the risk for PAD by increasing the prevalence of other previously established risk factors. For instance, in a study of 8,688 men followed for 5 years, being overweight was the most significant predictor of who was going to develop type 2 diabetes mellitus.[59] McDermott et al.[60] have shown that over 4 years of follow-up, subjects with intermittent claudication and a body mass index greater than 30 kg/m² had significantly more functional decline. Thus it reasons that any decrease in weight will decrease the work required for walking and will improve exercise capacity. Therefore, weight reduction is recommended for patients with PAD.

THERAPY FOR THE TREATMENT OF CLAUDICATION

Aside from modifying risk factors to improve overall cardiovascular morbidity and mortality, there are noninterventional strategies available to treat the mobility limitations caused by symptomatic PAD. Only two medications carry approval by the Food and Drug Administration (FDA) for the improvement of walking distance in PAD, pentoxifylline and cilostazol.

Pentoxifylline

Pentoxifylline is a rheologic modifier approved by the FDA for symptomatic relief of claudication. It is thought to act by improving red blood cell and leukocyte flexibility, inhibiting neutrophil activation and adhesion, decreasing fibrinogen concentrations, and reducing blood viscosity, thus permitting improved muscular perfusion.

Studies investigating the efficacy of pentoxifylline have yielded conflicting results. A meta-analysis found that pentoxifylline improved walking distance by 29 m compared with placebo.[61] The improvement was approximately 50% in the placebo group, whereas pentoxifylline added an additional 30%. The benefit was substantially less, however, than that achieved with a supervised exercised program.[62]

The beneficial response to pentoxifylline is small in most patients, and the overall data are insufficient to support its widespread use in patients with claudication. Pentoxifylline may be considered for patients who cannot take cilostazol, have not responded adequately to an exercise program, and/or are not candidates for revascularization, either with percutaneous or surgical approaches.

Cilostazol

Cilostazol is a phosphodiesterase-III inhibitor that suppresses platelet aggregation and is a direct arterial dilator.[63] The efficacy of cilostazol has been demonstrated in several studies[64–66] and in a meta-analysis[67] of eight randomized, placebo-controlled trials that included 2,702 patients with stable moderate-to-severe claudication. In the meta-analysis, treatment with 100 mg twice daily for 12 to 24 weeks increased maximal and pain-free walking distances by 50% and 67%, respectively. Because cilostazol is a phosphodiesterase inhibitor similar to milrinone, it is contraindicated in patients with symptomatic congestive heart failure or patients with a left ventricular ejection fraction less than 40%.

Cilostazol is more effective than pentoxifylline when compared directly. Superiority was illustrated in a trial of 698 patients randomized to cilostazol, pentoxifylline, or placebo for 24 weeks. The increase in mean walking distance over baseline with pentoxifylline and placebo was the same (30% and 34%, respectively), but the increase with cilostazol was significantly greater (54%).[68]

The most common adverse effects with cilostazol are headache, palpitations, and diarrhea. The optimal dose of cilostazol is 100 mg twice daily. The medication should be given on an empty stomach. Because of the inhibitory effects of cilostazol on drug metabolism, the dose should be halved in patients taking medications that inhibit the cytochrome P450 isoenzymes CYP3A4 and CYP2C19 (erythromycin, diltiazem, omeprazole, etc.).[69]

Other Pharmacologic Agents

Multiple other agents have been used in the treatment of claudication. Naftidrofuryl, a 5-hydroxytryptamine serotonin receptor inhibitor, has been available in Europe for a number of years. The mechanism of action of this drug is not clear, but it is thought to promote glucose uptake and increase adenosine triphosphate levels. A meta-analysis of four trials showed an increase in the time to initial pain development with treadmill walking over a 3- to 6-month period.[70]

Buflomedil is an alpha-adrenolytic agent available in Europe, but not the United States, that has been used in the treatment of claudication. The LIMB trial evaluated the efficacy and safety of buflomedil in 2,078 patients with claudication and an ABI between 0.3 and 0.8, in a randomized, placebo-controlled trial. At a median follow-up of 2.8 years, the rate of a composite endpoint of cardiovascular death, nonfatal myocardial infarction, nonfatal stroke, symptomatic deterioration in PAD, or leg amputation was significantly lower in patients who received buflomedil (9.1% vs. 12.4%). The benefit was largely driven by a reduction in symptoms of PAD.[71]

Ginkgo biloba has also been studied in the treatment of claudication with some modest success. Ginkgo is thought to act via an antioxidant mechanism that inhibits vascular injury. It is also thought to have some antithrombotic effects. The effect of ginkgo has been reviewed in a meta-analysis that showed that patients receiving ginkgo extract significantly increased pain-free walking of approximately 34 m compared to placebo.[72]

Many other agents have been tried in the treatment of symptomatic claudication. These include estrogen replacement therapy, chelation therapy with intravenous ethylenediaminetetra-acetic acid (EDTA), and vitamin E supplementation. None have been shown to have significant benefit, and none are recommended by current therapy guidelines.

Exercise

Many prospective trials have demonstrated that supervised exercise is an effective method of treating patients with claudication.[73] The magnitude of the effect from a supervised exercise program exceeds that achieved with any of the pharmacologic agents available. A meta-analysis of 21 studies by Gardner and Poehlman,[74] which included both randomized and nonrandomized trials, showed that pain-free walking time improved by an average of 180% and maximal walking time by 120% in patients with claudication who underwent supervised exercise training. Furthermore, a meta-analysis from the Cochrane Collaboration that included only randomized, controlled trials showed that exercise improved maximal walking ability by an average of 150% (range 74% to 230%).[75]

There are several mechanisms by which exercise training may improve claudication, although the available data are not sufficient to render firm conclusions regarding their relative importance. These mechanisms include improved endothelial function via increases in nitric oxide synthase and prostacyclin; reduction of local inflammation; increased exercise pain tolerance; induction of vascular angiogenesis; improved muscle metabolism by favorable effects on muscle carnitine metabolism; and reductions in blood viscosity and red cell aggregation.[76]

Although less well studied, exercise may also improve survival in PAD. This idea was addressed in a prospective, observational study of 225 men with PAD evaluated in whom physical activity was measured with a vertical accelerometer. Patients were followed for a mean duration of 57 months over which time 33% of patients died. Individuals in the highest quartile of accelerometer-measured activity had a significantly lower mortality than those in the lowest quartile (HR, 0.29; 95% CI, 0.10 to 0.83).[77]

The current PAD guidelines state that a program of supervised exercise training is recommended as an initial treatment modality for patients with claudication (class I, level of evidence A) and that supervised exercise training should be performed for a minimum of 30 to 45 minutes in sessions performed at least three times per week for a minimum of 12 weeks (class I, level of evidence A).[5]

Exercise programs have several important limitations. First, patients must be motivated, which is often difficult when they experience claudication-related pain whenever they walk. Second, the best results occur when patients enroll in a supervised program as with cardiac rehabilitation ensuring compliance. Unfortunately, there is often a lack of financial reimbursement for supervised programs and patients instructed by health care providers to exercise on their own do not achieve the same improvement as those in structured programs.[78]

THE FUTURE IN THE TREATMENT OF CLAUDICATION

There are several promising agents being evaluated for the treatment of symptoms of PAD.

In general vasodilators have not been effective in treating PAD symptoms. A randomized, double-blind, placebo-controlled crossover trial of 44 patients with stable claudication demonstrated, however, that patients treated with verapamil for 4 weeks increased mean pain-free walking distance by 29% and maximal walking distances by 49% compared with placebo. In the study, verapamil had minimal effect on systolic ankle pressure, ABI, peripheral leg temperature, or systolic blood pressure, all arguing against its effects being mediated by improved peripheral hemodynamics.[79]

Several members of the prostaglandin family of compounds, such as prostaglandin E_1 (PGE_1), have also been studied. In a study of 80 patients with intermittent claudication, intravenous administration of a PGE_1 prodrug produced a dose-related improvement in walking distance in walking distance and quality of life at 4 and 8 weeks.[80] A Cochrane review of five small studies comparing different forms of PGE_1 with placebo found that significant increases in walking distances were attained with PGE_1, which persisted even after termination of treatment.[81] Similarly, beraprost is an orally active prostaglandin I_2 (prostacyclin) analog that has also been studied in the BERCI-2 trial. In the study, 549 patients were shown to increase their pain-free walking distance by 82% and the incidence of critical cardiovascular events was lower but not statistically significant (4.8% vs. 8.9% for placebo).[82] A similarly designed trial found no difference in walking distance or quality of life in patients treated with beraprost compared with placebo.[83] In the aggregate, the ACC/AHA guidelines concluded that oral vasodilation therapy with prostaglandins was not effective in the treatment of intermittent claudication.

INTEGRATED APPROACH

An overall approach to the patient with claudication is presented in FIGURE 40.2.[84]

As we have stressed, while symptomatic claudication is being addressed, all attempts must be made to enact plans for smoking cessation and for the control of hypertension, dyslipidemia, and diabetes. The most up-to-date societal guidelines for the

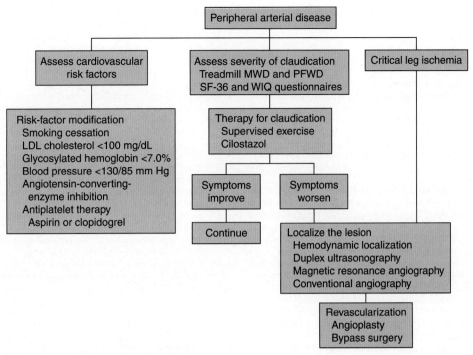

FIGURE 40.2 Assessment and treatment of PAD.

Adapted from Hiatt WR. Medical management of peripheral arterial disease and claudication. *N Engl J Med* 2001;344:1608.

treatment of PAD were published in *Circulation* in 2006.[5] A summary of the recommendations is in FIGURE 40.3.

CONCLUSION

Patients with PAD range from the asymptomatic to those who experience intermittent claudication to those with critical limb ischemia. Both symptomatic and asymptomatic patients with

PAD have markedly increased rates of myocardial infarction, stroke, and cardiovascular events. There are two major strategies that should be undertaken for the treatment of PAD at the same time. These include strategies to improve symptoms and quality of life with medical therapy alone or with revascularization (surgical or percutaneous) and strategies to prevent cardiovascular events with a comprehensive program that addresses patient specific high-risk features including tobacco use,

ACC/AHA recommendations	Aspirin	Clopidogrel as an alternative to aspirin	Pentoxifylline	Cilostazol	Supervised exercise program	Smoking cessation	Target BP <140/90 mm Hg	Target BP <130/80 mm Hg with DM or CKD	Statin for all patients for LDL goal <100 mg/dL	Statin for all patients for LDL goal < 70 mg/dL	in DM HbA1C goal of <7%
Class I	A	B		A	A	B	A	A	B		
Class IIa										B	C
Class IIb			A								
Class III											

Class I Procedure/Treatment SHOULD be performed/administered	Class IIa IT IS REASONABLE to perform procedure/administer treatment	Class IIb Procedure/Treatment MAY BE CONSIDERED	Class III Procedure/Treatment should NOT be performed/administered SINCE IT IS NOT HELPFUL AND MAY BE HARMFUL

Level A	Multiple (3–5) population risk strata evaluated. General consistency of direction and magnitude of effect
Level B	Limited (2–3) population risk strata evaluated
Level C	Very limited (1–2) population risk strata evaluated

FIGURE 40.3 Summary of the American College of Cardiology/American Heart Association recommendations for medical therapy of PAD.

Adapted from Goei AD, Findeiss LK, Slim AM. Medical management in peripheral arterial disease: a systematic approach to medical therapy. *J Vasc Interv Radiol* 2010;21:603.

sedentary lifestyle, hypertension, dyslipidemia, and the control of diabetes.

■ REFERENCES

1. Hirsch AT, Criqui MH, Treat-Jacobson D, et al. Peripheral arterial disease detection, awareness, and treatment in primary care. *JAMA* 2001;286(11):1317–1324.
2. McKenna M, Wolfson S, Kuller L. The ratio of ankle and arm arterial pressure as an independent predictor of mortality. *Atherosclerosis* 1991;87(2–3):119–128.
3. Vogt MT, McKenna M, Anderson SJ, et al. The relationship between ankle-arm index and mortality in older men and women. *J Am Geriatr Soc* 1993;41(5):523–530.
4. Third Report of the National Cholesterol Education Program (NCEP) Expert Panel on Detection, Evaluation, and Treatment of High Blood Cholesterol in Adults (Adult Treatment Panel III) final report. *Circulation* 2002;106(25):3143–3421.
5. Hirsch AT, Haskal ZJ, Hertzer NR, et al. ACC/AHA 2005 Practice Guidelines for the management of patients with peripheral arterial disease (lower extremity, renal, mesenteric, and abdominal aortic): a collaborative report from the American Association for Vascular Surgery/Society for Vascular Surgery, Society for Cardiovascular Angiography and Interventions, Society for Vascular Medicine and Biology, Society of Interventional Radiology, and the ACC/AHA Task Force on Practice Guidelines (Writing Committee to Develop Guidelines for the Management of Patients with Peripheral Arterial Disease): endorsed by the American Association of Cardiovascular and Pulmonary Rehabilitation; National Heart, Lung, and Blood Institute; Society for Vascular Nursing; TransAtlantic Inter-Society Consensus; and Vascular Disease Foundation. *Circulation* 2006;113(11):e463–e654.
6. Norgren L, Hiatt WR, Dormandy JA, et al. Inter-Society Consensus for the Management of Peripheral Arterial Disease (TASC II). *J Vasc Surg* 2007;45(suppl S):S5–S67.
7. Feringa HH, van Waning VH, Bax JJ, et al. Cardioprotective medication is associated with improved survival in patients with peripheral arterial disease. *J Am Coll Cardiol* 2006;47(6):1182–1187.
8. Barndt R Jr, Blankenhorn DH, Crawford DW, et al. Regression and progression of early femoral atherosclerosis in treated hyperlipoproteinemic patients. *Ann Intern Med* 1977;86(2):139–146.
9. Duffield RG, Lewis B, Miller NE, et al. Treatment of hyperlipidaemia retards progression of symptomatic femoral atherosclerosis. A randomised controlled trial. *Lancet* 1983;2(8351):639–642.
10. Blankenhorn DH, Azen SP, Crawford DW, et al. Effects of colestipol-niacin therapy on human femoral atherosclerosis. *Circulation* 1991;83(2):438–447.
11. MRC/BHF Heart Protection Study of cholesterol lowering with simvastatin in 20,536 high-risk individuals: a randomised placebo-controlled trial. *Lancet* 2002;360(9326):7–22.
12. Pedersen TR, Kjekshus J, Pyörälä K, et al. Effect of simvastatin on ischemic signs and symptoms in the Scandinavian simvastatin survival study (4S). *Am J Cardiol* 1998;81(3):333–335.
13. McDermott MM, Guralnik JM, Greenland P, et al. Statin use and leg functioning in patients with and without lower-extremity peripheral arterial disease. *Circulation* 2003;107(5):757–761.
14. Aronow WS, Nayak D, Woodworth S, et al. Effect of simvastatin versus placebo on treadmill exercise time until the onset of intermittent claudication in older patients with peripheral arterial disease at six months and at one year after treatment. *Am J Cardiol* 2003;92(6):711–712.
15. Mondillo S, Ballo P, Barbati R, et al. Effects of simvastatin on walking performance and symptoms of intermittent claudication in hypercholesterolemic patients with peripheral vascular disease. *Am J Med* 2003;114(5):359–364.
16. Mohler ER III, Hiatt WR, Creager MA. Cholesterol reduction with atorvastatin improves walking distance in patients with peripheral arterial disease. *Circulation* 2003;108(12):1481–1486.
17. Giri J, McDermott MM, Greenland P, et al. Statin use and functional decline in patients with and without peripheral arterial disease. *J Am Coll Cardiol* 2006;47(5):998–1004.
18. Rajamani K, Colman PG, Li LP, et al. Effect of fenofibrate on amputation events in people with type 2 diabetes mellitus (FIELD study): a prespecified analysis of a randomised controlled trial. *Lancet* 2009;373(9677):1780–1788.
19. Jonason T, Bergstrom R. Cessation of smoking in patients with intermittent claudication. Effects on the risk of peripheral vascular complications, myocardial infarction and mortality. *Acta Med Scand* 1987;221(3):253–260.
20. Quick CR, Cotton LT. The measured effect of stopping smoking on intermittent claudication. *Br J Surg* 1982;69(suppl):S24–S26.
21. Hobbs SD, Wilmink AB, Adam DJ, et al. Assessment of smoking status in patients with peripheral arterial disease. *J Vasc Surg* 2005;41(3):451–456.
22. Hobbs SD, Bradbury AW. Smoking cessation strategies in patients with peripheral arterial disease: an evidence-based approach. *Eur J Vasc Endovasc Surg* 2003;26(4):341–347.
23. Law M, Tang JL. An analysis of the effectiveness of interventions intended to help people stop smoking. *Arch Intern Med* 1995;155(18):1933–1941.
24. Anthonisen NR, Skeans MA, Wise RA, et al. The effects of a smoking cessation intervention on 14.5-year mortality: a randomized clinical trial. *Ann Intern Med* 2005;142(4):233–239.
25. Hennrikus D, Joseph AM, Lando HA, et al. Effectiveness of a smoking cessation program for peripheral artery disease patients: a randomized controlled trial. *J Am Coll Cardiol* 2010;56(25):2105–2112.
26. Okuyemi KS, Ahluwalia JS, Harris KJ. Pharmacotherapy of smoking cessation. *Arch Fam Med* 2000;9(3):270–281.
27. Dalsgareth OJ, Hansen NC, Søes-Petersen U, et al. A multicenter, randomized, double-blind, placebo-controlled, 6-month trial of bupropion hydrochloride sustained-release tablets as an aid to smoking cessation in hospital employees. *Nicotine Tob Res* 2004;6(1):55–61.
28. Gonzales D, Rennard SI, Nides M, et al. Varenicline, an alpha4beta2 nicotinic acetylcholine receptor partial agonist, vs sustained-release bupropion and placebo for smoking cessation: a randomized controlled trial. *JAMA* 2006;296(1):47–55.
29. Jorenby DE, Hays JT, Rigotti NA, et al. Efficacy of varenicline, an alpha4beta2 nicotinic acetylcholine receptor partial agonist, vs placebo or sustained-release bupropion for smoking cessation: a randomized controlled trial. *JAMA* 2006;296(1):56–63.
30. Fiore MC, Jaen CR. A clinical blueprint to accelerate the elimination of tobacco use. *JAMA* 2008;299(17):2083–2085.
31. Conen D, Everett BM, Kurth T, et al. Smoking, smoking status, and risk for symptomatic peripheral artery disease in women: a cohort study. *Ann Intern Med* 2011;154(11):719–726.
32. Chobanian AV, Bakris GL, Black HR, et al. The Seventh Report of the Joint National Committee on Prevention, Detection, Evaluation, and Treatment of High Blood Pressure: the JNC 7 report. *JAMA* 2003;289(19):2560–2572.
33. The treatment of mild hypertension study. A randomized, placebo-controlled trial of a nutritional-hygienic regimen along with various drug monotherapies. The Treatment of Mild Hypertension Research Group. *Arch Intern Med* 1991;151(7):1413–1423.
34. Novo S, Abrignani MG, Pavone G, et al. Effects of captopril and ticlopidine, alone or in combination, in hypertensive patients with intermittent claudication. *Int Angiol* 1996;15(2):169–174.
35. Solomon SA, Ramsay LE, Yeo WW, et al. Beta blockade and intermittent claudication: placebo controlled trial of atenolol and nifedipine and their combination. *BMJ* 1991;303(6810):1100–1104.
36. Roberts DH, Tsao Y, McLoughlin GA, et al. Placebo-controlled comparison of captopril, atenolol, labetalol, and pindolol in hypertension complicated by intermittent claudication. *Lancet* 1987;2(8560):650–653.
37. Sonecha TN, Nicolaides AN, Kyprianou P, et al. The effect of enalapril on leg muscle blood flow in patients with claudication. *Int Angiol* 1990;9(1):22–24.
38. Ahimastos AA, Lawler A, Reid CM, et al. Brief communication: ramipril markedly improves walking ability in patients with peripheral arterial disease: a randomized trial. *Ann Intern Med* 2006;144(9):660–664.
39. Mehler PS, Coll JR, Estacio R, et al. Intensive blood pressure control reduces the risk of cardiovascular events in patients with peripheral arterial disease and type 2 diabetes. *Circulation* 2003;107(5):753–756.
40. Yusuf S, Sleight P, Pogue J, et al. Effects of an angiotensin-converting-enzyme inhibitor, ramipril, on cardiovascular events in high-risk patients. The Heart Outcomes Prevention Evaluation Study Investigators. *N Engl J Med* 2000;342(3):145–153.
41. Fox KM. Efficacy of perindopril in reduction of cardiovascular events among patients with stable coronary artery disease: randomised, double-blind, placebo-controlled, multicentre trial (the EUROPA study). *Lancet* 2003;362(9386):782–788.
42. Navalkar S, Parthasarathy S, Santanam N, et al. Irbesartan, an angiotensin type 1 receptor inhibitor, regulates markers of inflammation in patients with premature atherosclerosis. *J Am Coll Cardiol* 2001;37(2):440–444.
43. Dahlof B, Devereux RB, Kjeldsen SE, et al. Cardiovascular morbidity and mortality in the Losartan Intervention For Endpoint reduction in hypertension study (LIFE): a randomised trial against atenolol. *Lancet* 2002;359(9311):995–1003.

44. Pfeffer MA, Swedberg K, Granger CB, et al. Effects of candesartan on mortality and morbidity in patients with chronic heart failure: the CHARM-Overall programme. *Lancet* 2003;362(9386):759–766.

45. Kjeldsen SE, Stålhammar J, Hasvold P, et al. Effects of losartan vs candesartan in reducing cardiovascular events in the primary treatment of hypertension. *J Hum Hypertens* 2010;24(4):263–273.

46. Radack K, Deck C. Beta-adrenergic blocker therapy does not worsen intermittent claudication in subjects with peripheral arterial disease. A meta-analysis of randomized controlled trials. *Arch Intern Med* 1991;151(9):1769–1776.

47. Olin JW. Hypertension and peripheral arterial disease. *Vasc Med* 2005;10(3):241–246.

48. Effect of intensive diabetes management on macrovascular events and risk factors in the Diabetes Control and Complications Trial. *Am J Cardiol* 1995;75(14):894–903.

49. Hadden DR, Patterson CC, Atkinson AB, et al. Macrovascular disease and hyperglycaemia: 10-year survival analysis in type 2 diabetes mellitus: the Belfast Diet Study. *Diabet Med* 1997;14(8):663–672.

50. The effect of intensive treatment of diabetes on the development and progression of long-term complications in insulin-dependent diabetes mellitus. The Diabetes Control and Complications Trial Research Group. *N Engl J Med* 1993;329(14):977–986.

51. Standards of medical care for patients with diabetes mellitus. *Diabetes Care* 2003;26(suppl 1):S33–S50.

52. Gerstein HC, Miller ME, Byington RP, et al. Effects of intensive glucose lowering in type 2 diabetes. *N Engl J Med* 2008;358(24):2545–2559.

53. Patel A, MacMahon S, Chalmers J, et al. Intensive blood glucose control and vascular outcomes in patients with type 2 diabetes. *N Engl J Med* 2008;358(24):2560–2572.

54. Duckworth W, Abraira C, Moritz T, et al. Glucose control and vascular complications in veterans with type 2 diabetes. *N Engl J Med* 2009;360(2):129–139.

55. Kannel WB, McGee DL Update on some epidemiologic features of intermittent claudication: the Framingham Study. *J Am Geriatr Soc* 1985;33(1):13–18.

56. Fowkes FG, Housley E, Riemersma RA, et al. Smoking, lipids, glucose intolerance, and blood pressure as risk factors for peripheral atherosclerosis compared with ischemic heart disease in the Edinburgh Artery Study. *Am J Epidemiol* 1992;135(4):331–340.

57. Smith GD, Shipley MJ, Rose G. Intermittent claudication, heart disease risk factors, and mortality. The Whitehall Study. *Circulation* 1990;82(6):1925–1931.

58. Criqui MH, Browner D, Fronek A, et al. Peripheral arterial disease in large vessels is epidemiologically distinct from small vessel disease. An analysis of risk factors. *Am J Epidemiol* 1989;129(6):1110–1119.

59. Medalie JH, Papier CM, Goldbourt U, et al. Major factors in the development of diabetes mellitus in 10,000 men. *Arch Intern Med* 1975;135(6):811–817.

60. McDermott MM, Criqui MH, Ferrucci L, et al. Obesity, weight change, and functional decline in peripheral arterial disease. *J Vasc Surg* 2006;43(6):1198–1204.

61. Hood SC, Moher D, Barber GG. Management of intermittent claudication with pentoxifylline: meta-analysis of randomized controlled trials. *Can Med Assoc J* 1996;155(8):1053–1059.

62. Hiatt WR, Regensteiner JG, Hargarten ME, et al. Benefit of exercise conditioning for patients with peripheral arterial disease. *Circulation* 1990;81(2):602–609.

63. Reilly MP, Mohler ER III. Cilostazol: treatment of intermittent claudication. *Ann Pharmacother* 2001;35(1):48–56.

64. Dawson DL, Cutler BS, Meissner MH, et al. Cilostazol has beneficial effects in treatment of intermittent claudication: results from a multicenter, randomized, prospective, double-blind trial. *Circulation* 1998;98(7):678–686.

65. Money SR, Herd JA, Isaacsohn JL, et al. Effect of cilostazol on walking distances in patients with intermittent claudication caused by peripheral vascular disease. *J Vasc Surg* 1998;27(2):267–274; discussion 274–275.

66. Beebe HG, Dawson DL, Cutler BS, et al. A new pharmacological treatment for intermittent claudication: results of a randomized, multicenter trial. *Arch Intern Med* 1999;159(17):2041–2050.

67. Thompson PD, Zimet R, Forbes WP, et al. Meta-analysis of results from eight randomized, placebo-controlled trials on the effect of cilostazol on patients with intermittent claudication. *Am J Cardiol* 2002;90(12):1314–1319.

68. Dawson DL, Cutler BS, Hiatt WR, et al. A comparison of cilostazol and pentoxifylline for treating intermittent claudication. *Am J Med* 2000;109(7):523–530.

69. Dobesh PP, Stacy ZA, Persson EL. Pharmacologic therapy for intermittent claudication. *Pharmacotherapy* 2009;29(5):526–553.

70. Girolami B, Bernardi E, Prins MH, et al. Treatment of intermittent claudication with physical training, smoking cessation, pentoxifylline, or nafronyl: a meta-analysis. *Arch Intern Med* 1999;159(4):337–345.

71. Leizorovicz A, Becker F. Oral buflomedil in the prevention of cardiovascular events in patients with peripheral arterial obstructive disease: a randomized, placebo-controlled, 4-year study. *Circulation* 2008;117(6):816–822.

72. Pittler MH, Ernst E. Ginkgo biloba extract for the treatment of intermittent claudication: a meta-analysis of randomized trials. *Am J Med* 2000;108(4):276–281.

73. Regensteiner JG, Gardner A, Hiatt WR. Exercise testing and exercise rehabilitation for patients with peripheral arterial disease: status in 1997. *Vasc Med* 1997;2(2):147–155.

74. Gardner AW, Poehlman ET. Exercise rehabilitation programs for the treatment of claudication pain. A meta-analysis. *JAMA* 1995;274(12):975–980.

75. Watson L, Ellis B, Leng GC. Exercise for intermittent claudication. *Cochrane Database Syst Rev* 2008;(4):CD000990.

76. Hamburg NM, Balady GJ. Exercise rehabilitation in peripheral artery disease: functional impact and mechanisms of benefits. *Circulation* 2011;123(1):87–97.

77. Garg PK, Tian L, Criqui MH, et al. Physical activity during daily life and mortality in patients with peripheral arterial disease. *Circulation* 2006;114(3):242–248.

78. Bendermacher BL, Willigendael EM, Teijink JA, et al. Supervised exercise therapy versus non-supervised exercise therapy for intermittent claudication. *Cochrane Database Syst Rev* 2006;(2):CD005263.

79. Bagger JP, Helligsoe P, Randsbaek F, et al. Effect of verapamil in intermittent claudication A randomized, double-blind, placebo-controlled, cross-over study after individual dose-response assessment. *Circulation* 1997;95(2):411–414.

80. Belch JJ, Bell PR, Creissen D, et al. Randomized, double-blind, placebo-controlled study evaluating the efficacy and safety of AS-013, a prostaglandin E1 prodrug, in patients with intermittent claudication. *Circulation* 1997;95(9):2298–2302.

81. Reiter M, Bucek RA, Stümpflen A, et al. Prostanoids for intermittent claudication. *Cochrane Database Syst Rev* 2004;(1):CD000986.

82. Lievre M, Morand S, Besse B, et al. Oral Beraprost sodium, a prostaglandin I(2) analogue, for intermittent claudication: a double-blind, randomized, multicenter controlled trial. Beraprost et Claudication Intermittente (BERCI) Research Group. *Circulation* 2000;102(4):426–431.

83. Mohler ER III, Hiatt WR, Olin JW, et al. Treatment of intermittent claudication with beraprost sodium, an orally active prostaglandin I2 analogue: a double-blinded, randomized, controlled trial. *J Am Coll Cardiol* 2003;41(10):1679–1686.

84. Hiatt WR. Medical treatment of peripheral arterial disease and claudication. *N Engl J Med* 2001;344(21):1608–1621.

CHAPTER
41

Endovascular Interventions: Upper Extremity

STEPHEN T. KEE and JOHN M. MORIARTY

INTRODUCTION

Endovascular interventions in the veins of the upper extremity have increased greatly in recent years, primarily driven by the expansion of the endovascular options for the management of dialysis graft or fistula complications, the ever expanding need for stable chronic venous access, and the increasingly common diagnosis of, and hence call for management of, upper limb deep venous thrombosis.[1-3] Within the arteries, however, with the exception of acute trauma, endovascular interventions are relatively rare with upper limb arterial disease being estimated to be one-sixth as common as in the leg.[4] This is caused by a combination of differences in the muscle bulk of the arms, and hence arterial oxygen supply requirements, decreased sheer stress on the vessels of the arm compared to the ambulating legs, and the degree of collateralization between large transport vessels, such as the brachial artery and radial artery, and nutrient vessels such as the interosseous artery.[5]

Arterial occlusive disease of the upper extremity can be classified as either acute or chronic. Thromboembolism, most commonly from cardiac sources in the setting of valvular heart disease or atrial fibrillation, is the most common cause of acute arterial occlusion, although it frequently presents in an "acute-on-chronic" fashion on a background of atherosclerotic large-vessel stenosis or occlusion. It should be noted that although acute critical ischemia of the upper limb is rare even in diabetes, there is a significantly increased risk of digital ischemia in patients with end-stage renal disease.[6]

The causes of chronic arterial occlusion are numerous (Table 41.1); however, atherosclerosis is the most common cause with 80% occurring in males.[7] Similarly symptomatology will vary widely depending on the etiology, ranging from arm claudication, rest pain, ulceration, and muscle wasting to Raynaud phenomenon. Furthermore, clinical presentation is often complicated by the fact that the presenting symptoms are frequently the result of the arm "stealing" blood from another area, such as the brain in vertebral-subclavian steal, and the heart in the presence of a previous internal mammary coronary bypass graft, and coronary-subclavian steal.[8,9]

PATIENT SELECTION

Indications for investigation includes patients presenting with symptomatic upper extremity ischemia, claudication, rest pain, ulceration, symptomatic vertebral-subclavian steal syndrome,

and symptomatic coronary-subclavian steal syndrome. Catheter angiography has been superseded mostly by noninvasive modalities, such as ultrasound, multidetector computed tomography angiography (CTA) and magnetic resonance angiography (MRA). Advances in CTA, such as dual energy acquisition, allows submillimeter resolution of digital vessels,[10] whereas time-resolved MRA can be of great benefit in evaluating flow patterns and collateral channels in the arterial tree with minimal contrast dose and scan time.[11,12] Both CTA and MRA provide highly detailed images of the peripheral vascular tree with the added bonus of visualizing beyond the vessel lumen to surrounding anatomic structures (FIGURE 41.1). With high-field strength MRA and the newest MDCTA systems isotropic voxel sizes of $0.4 \times 0.4 \times 0.4$ mm are possible, allowing truly three-dimensional datasets with reconstructions that can be viewed as analogous to conventional catheter angiography but in an infinity of perspectives.

With increasing awareness of the level of renal impairment in the community and the identification of some gadolinium-based agents as cofactors in the development of nephrogenic systemic fibrosis (NSF), interest in noncontrast imaging techniques has risen. Although newer techniques, such as balanced steady-state free precession (bSSFP) and half-Fourier fast spin echo MRA have been evaluated in the lower limb, their use in the upper limb is unproven. Noncontrast techniques have centered around the use of time-of-flight MRA (TOF-MRA) and phase contrast MRA (PC-MRA). Both suffer from limitations. With TOF-MRA the acquisition times are long with difficulties in orientation of the saturation pulses to the tortuous path of the upper limb vasculature and inherent artifacts that lead to overestimation of the degree and length of stenoses.[13] PC-MRA meanwhile is mainly used in a limited fashion to assess directionality of flow, such as in cases of subclavian steal, although there is ongoing research into its use to assess flow velocities in failing dialysis grafts.[14]

There remains some controversy with regard to treatment of incidentally identified, asymptomatic lesions in the upper limb arteries. Standard of care is to avoid intervention in asymptomatic lesions with the possible exception of asymptomatic subclavian stenosis or occlusion where the internal mammary artery is to be harvested for coronary artery bypass grafting (CABG).[15]

Relative contraindications, such as severe atherosclerosis of the aortic arch, renal insufficiency, and concurrent infection, must be balanced against the clinical indication and urgency of intervention. It is generally accepted that signs of irreversible

Table 41.1	
Etiologic Causes of Upper Limb Arterial Occlusion	

Inflammatory disorders

    Atherosclerosis

    Radiation arteriopathy

Vasculitis

    Takayasu's Arthritis

    Rheumatoid Arthritis

    Giant cell arteritis

    SLE

    Polyarteritis nodosa

    Scleroderma

Immunologic

    Cryoglobulinaeima

    Multiple myeloma

Embolic

    Valvular heart disease

    Atrial fibrillation

    Atherosclerotic plaques

Iatrogenic

Traumatic

limb ischemia with severe sensorimotor deficits and muscle rigor are a contraindication to endovascular therapy, and these patients should have urgent surgical intervention.

ENDOVASCULAR TREATMENT OPTIONS AND TECHNICAL/DEVICE CONSIDERATIONS

The full range of endovascular treatment options commonly applied for management of lower extremity arterial occlusive disease is also available for use in the upper limb. These include transcatheter thrombolysis, either mechanical or pharmacologic, angioplasty, and stenting.

The variety of devices available for use in the upper limb depends somewhat on the need for devices with long shaft lengths that can reach from the femoral arteriotomy access point to the arm and even to the hand. Long access sheaths of between 45 and 90 cm and angioplasty balloons with 110-cm shaft lengths are standard. Maneuverability, pushability, and torqueability of devices at this remove from the access point can be suboptimal and, hence, the use of triaxial techniques with a long sheath or brachial/radial access can be of benefit.

Equipment:

- 4 to 5 French micropuncture access sets for arterial access
- 5 to 9 French 90-cm long vascular sheaths
- Straight and angled-tip hydrophilic guide wires
- Pigtail, Simmons, Headhunter, angled-glide, straight flush catheters
- Microcatheter system, for example, Renegade HI-FLO (Boston Scientific, Natick, MA) or Progreat (Terumo, Somerset, NJ) microcatheters

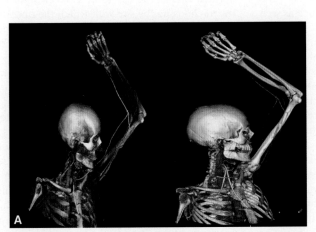
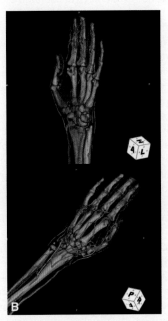

FIGURE 41.1 Multidetector row CT angiography allows rapid, noninvasive evaluation of the upper limb vessels. With near isotropic voxel sizes, true 3D imaging of the entire arm (**A**) or high-fidelity imaging of the small vessels in the hand (**B**) is possible.

Courtesy of C. Arellano, MD, Diagnostic Cardiovascular Imaging, UCLA Medical Center.

- 0.035 Angioplasty balloons, typically 4 to 80 mm in diameter, 2 to 4 cm in length with elongated 110- to 135-cm shaft lengths, for example, OptaPro (Cordis, Miami Lakes, FL) or Synergy (Boston Scientific, Natick, MA)
- 0.018 Angioplasty balloons, for example, Sterling (Boston Scientific, Natick, MA)
- Fogarty embolectomy balloon (Edwards Life Sciences, Irving, CA)
- Balloon-expandable stents, for example, Omnilink 0.018 and 0.035 (Guidant, Santa Clara, CA), and self-expanding stents, for example, Precise (Cordis Endovascular, Warren, NJ) and Zilver (Cook, Bloomington, IN)
- Stent-grafts, particularly for use with emergent complications, such as vessel rupture restenosis, for example, ViaBahn (Gore, Flagstaff, AZ) and Fluency (Bard, Covington, GA)
- Thrombectomy devices, such as aspiration thrombectomy catheters, for example, Pronto Extraction Catheter (Vascular Solutions, Minneapolis, MN), fluid jet devices, for example, AngioJet (Possis, Minneapolis, MN), or mechanical fragmentation devices, for example, Arrow-Trerotola (Arrow International, Reading, PA)

ANATOMIC CONSIDERATIONS

The arterial supply of the upper limb originates in the subclavian artery, which in the majority of cases (70%)[16] comes directly off the aortic arch on the left-hand side, and off the brachiocephalic trunk on the right. Variation in arch and great-vessel anatomy is common. The branches of the subclavian artery include the vertebral, internal thoracic, cervical trunk, costocervical trunk, and supreme intercostal arteries. It should be noted that symptomatic disease of the left subclavian artery is eight times more frequent than the right subclavian,[17] which is fortunate because intervention in the right subclavian artery typically involves crossing the arch and working in close concert with the right common carotid artery.

The axillary artery commences at the lateral border of the clavicle and extends to the lateral margin of teres minor where it becomes the brachial artery. Its branches include the lateral and superior thoracic arteries, the thoracoacromial trunk, and the subscapular and the circumflex humeral arteries. Aneurysms of these branch vessels and the axillary artery itself have been associated with repetitive rotatory motion injuries, such as seen with baseball pitchers and tennis players.[18]

The brachial artery runs inferiorly on the ventral surface of the arm, closely applied to the medial aspect of the median nerve. Proximally it gives off the profunda brachialis branch to the posterolateral muscles of the arm before terminating in the radial, ulnar, and interosseous arteries in the antecubital fossa. Anomalous early takeoff of the radial or ulnar artery from the brachial or axillary artery is present in 15% and 3% of patients, respectively.[19]

The radial and ulnar arteries continue along the lateral and medial aspects of the forearm respectively to the hand where they form the palmar arches. There is considerable variation in the supply of the arches, and either vessel may dominate; however, typically the more proximal deep arch is mainly supplied by the radial artery and the distal superficial arch by the ulnar. Of note in 2% of people the interosseous artery may continue to the hand as the median artery.

Within the hand the paired common metacarpal and digital arteries originate in the arches and join at the web spaces to form the palmar digital arteries that supply the fingers. The priceps pollicis artery arises from the radial artery as it turns medially into the palm and is the major blood supply to the thumb.

TREATMENT SELECTION STRATEGIES AND PLANNING THE INTERVENTIONAL PROCEDURE

Proper technique and successful outcomes begin with good clinical evaluation. Before performing endovascular therapy in the upper limb vessels, evaluation and documentation of the presence or absence of the axillary, brachial, radial, and ulnar pulses should be performed. Preprocedure assessment of digital capillary refill and measurement of bilateral brachial artery blood pressure may also be of benefit.

Patients with chronic occlusive arterial disease are generally excellent candidates for noninvasive imaging with CTA or MRA. Acute ischemia may require urgent endoluminal evaluation and management, and noninvasive imaging may be skipped to save time and contrast dose. Although there is sparse literature on when and where CTA or MRA should be used in the acute setting, advances in the speed of acquisition of MRA, utilizing techniques, such as parallel imaging and repetitive centric k-space filling techniques, and CTA, with the newest generation multidetector scanners (e.g., Siemens Definition Flash, Erlangen, Germany) able to scan a 70-cm upper extremity field of view in 3 seconds, may increase their use in the acute scenario. Furthermore as fusion software improves and previously obtained cross-sectional images are mated to angiographic systems, allowing noncontrast and virtual roadmapping, overall contrast dose savings may be accomplished.[20]

Review of any preprocedure imaging, such as CTA or MRA, is essential, being careful to note the degree of systemic atherosclerosis, prominent collaterals, and the presence of anatomic variants that could alter catheter selection or approach. Long occlusions, tight ostial stenoses, extensive mural thrombus, and proximity of target vessels to the vertebral or carotid arteries are all "warning signs" that should be noted on preprocedure imaging.

Following review of the indications and potential contraindications of the procedure the interventionist must select the optimal vascular access point. A balance must be reached between choosing the site with which the operator has the most experience, the greatest chance of success, the lowest risk of complication, the ease of passage to the target lesion, and the ability to deploy devices safely. In general this is the common femoral artery; however, the axillary artery, brachial artery, or radial artery may all be selected.

Previous literature reported unacceptably high rates of complication with brachial artery access (up to 36%)[21]; however, with modern micropuncture access techniques and ultrasound guidance, complication rates equivalent to femoral access can be expected (5%).[22] Similarly the radial artery has been shown, primarily through the interventional cardiology literature, to be a safe and acceptable site for arterial access, although typically the sheath access size is limited to 4 to 6 French.[23-25]

Axillary arterial access is considered high risk due to the proximity of the vessel to the brachial plexus and the relatively noncompressible site in the axilla. Furthermore although it has been shown to be a relatively safe site for retrograde insertion of large-caliber sheaths,[26,27] there is little evidence for its use for antegrade access down the arm.

▌SPECIFIC INTRAPROCEDURAL TECHNIQUES

Once safe and secure vascular access has been obtained, diagnostic angiography of the area in question should be performed. Evaluation of the ostia of the great vessels is best performed with an arch aortogram. Counterpoint oblique views, right anterior oblique to visualize the bifurcation of the brachiocephalic artery and left anterior oblique to visualize the ostia of the left common carotid and left subclavian arteries, are performed with a 5 French pigtail catheter situated in the ascending aorta.

From a femoral access selective catheterization of the subclavian arteries can be made with a 5 French angled catheter, such as an angled glide-catheter, although often a backward seeking catheter, such as a Simmons-1 or Simmons-2 catheter, is necessary when selecting great vessels arising with an acute angle from the arch.

It is important to ensure overlap of images to confirm that the vessels are seen in their entirety. The catheter tip should be positioned just distal to the vertebral arteries when imaging the subclavian or axillary arteries, and images should be obtained down to the digital vessels. Care must be made not to place the diagnostic catheter too distal, for example, into the brachial artery, to ensure that a high arising radial or ulnar artery is not missed. In cases of digital artery vasculitis or spasm, intra-arterial vasoactive agents, such as nitroglycerin (100 mcg bolus) or verapamil (2.5 to 5 mg bolus), and warming of the hands with warm towels may be of benefit.

Acute Upper Extremity Ischemia

In a series of 36 patients with acute ischemia of the upper limb,[28] 17 (47.2%) had embolic occlusion, 9 (25%) had iatrogenic thrombosis of the brachial artery, and 10 (27.8%) had primary arterial thrombosis, presumably on the background of a chronic atherosclerotic lesion. Most of the acute emboli to the upper limb originate in the heart in patients with atrial fibrillation (70%) with further sources, such as proximal aneurysms, endocarditic vegetations, and paradoxical emboli, being less common.[29,30]

Although there is copious published literature concerning the efficacy of catheter-directed thrombolysis in the lower limb,[31,32] similar data are lacking in the upper limb. Furthermore early reports, primarily using streptokinase or urokinase, showed poor outcomes when compared to surgical thrombectomy/embolectomy in the upper limb.[33–35] More recent data have shown that catheter-directed administration of second-generation thrombolytic agents, such as tissue plasminogen activator (tPA, e.g., Altepelase) or Reteplase, has greater efficacy and results that approach or surpass surgical embolectomy.[36,37]

Protocols differ and the selection of aspiration thrombectomy, mechanical thrombectomy, cathether-directed pharmacologic thrombectomy, and novel ultrasound-based devices depends mostly on local availability and operator experience.[38–40] In general, for thrombolysis of occlusions proximal to the brachial artery, excellent (95% to 100% limb salvage) angiographic and symptomatic results can be expected with infusion of thrombolysis through a catheter, for example, Cragg-McNamara 4 or 5 French infusion catheter (ev3, Plymouth, MN) positioned abutting the proximal aspect of the occlusion[36] (FIGURE 41.2). Lysis protocols and angiographic follow-up vary from institution to institution; however, the patient typically will return for a lysis check at 12 and 24 hours with manipulation of the catheter distally if applicable.

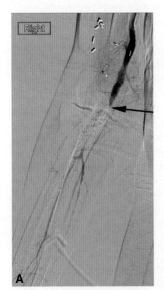 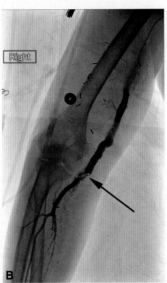 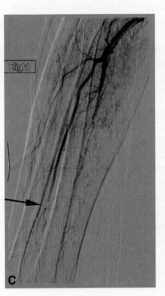 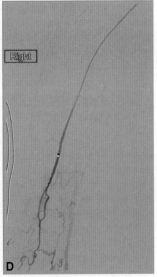

FIGURE 41.2 A. Acute right arm ischemia in a man with dialysis dependent chronic renal failure and severe systemic arterial calcification. Angiography of the cold right arm demonstrated an acute occlusion in the brachial artery (*arrow*). Catheter-directed TpA thrombolysis was commenced. **B.** Repeat angiogram performed after 24 hours of TpA lysis demonstrates resumption of antegrade flow. This was associated with symptomatic relief. However, a markedly irregular area of calcific stenosis in the brachial artery persisted. This was balloon angioplastied. **C.** Angiography of the forearm following balloon angioplasty of the brachial artery lesion demonstrated a focal filling defect in the interosseous artery, consistent with an iatrogenic embolus. **D.** The embolus was directly retrieved with the reperfusion catheter of the Penumbra system (Penumbra Inc., Alameda, CA) with good inline flow in the interosseous artery demonstrated on completion angiography.

Catheter-directed thrombolysis is less successful in the treatment of distal forearm or hand emboli. Typically a 5 French sheath is positioned in the distal brachial artery with thrombolysis performed through either a small-lumen microcatheter or an infusion wire (e.g., Cragg, Boston Scientific, Natick, MA). Angiographic success, typically defined as restoration of blood flow with at least one patent forearm vessel, is less common than with above elbow interventions (33% to 50%).[36,41,42] It should be noted, however, that clinical improvement, that is, relief of ischemia symptoms and prevention of amputation, occurs despite lack of angiographic recanalization.

Chronic Upper Extremity Ischemia

Chronic occlusions will typically be crossed using a hydrophilic straight or angled wire; however, care must be taken to prevent iatrogenic dissection. Although commonly used in lower limb vessels, such as the SFA, due to the risk of propagating the false lumen plane proximally into the vertebral artery or aorta, subintimal approaches are discouraged in the upper limb.[43] Once the guide wire is free in the distal lumen it is advisable to pass a hydrophilic diagnostic catheter through the occlusion and do a hand injection to confirm luminal placement prior to insertion of an exchange wire.

Once the lesion is crossed angioplasty with or without stenting is generally performed. There is little evidence to suggest that stenting offers greater primary patency or improved time to revascularization in the upper limb,[23,44,45] and indeed it is common practice to perform balloon angioplasty and only stent if the postdilatation angiogram demonstrates inadequate inline flow.

Predilatation prior to stenting has several advantages including better visualization of landing points, proof of calcific lesion distensibility, and physiologic sizing of the vessel lumen. The main disadvantages are the possibility of creating or propagating a dissection and vessel rupture, necessitating covered stent-graft insertion.[46] Stent migration prior to deployment has also been recorded,[47] and careful positioning regarding branch and collateral vessels, especially the vertebral and internal mammary vessels, is required.

ENDPOINT ASSESSMENT OF THE PROCEDURE

After either angioplasty or stenting, repeat angiography to assess for luminal patency and both site and downstream complications should be performed. Postdilatation with no more than a 1:1 balloon size-to-vessel ratio can be undertaken, if necessary, with postdilatation angiography to evaluate the distal flow. Embolic material in the distal vessels should be removed, primarily using aspiration, although novel techniques initially used in clot retrieval in the brain may also be of use, for example, the Merci Retriever (Concentric Medical, Inc., Mountain View, CA).

COMPLICATIONS, OUTCOMES, AND PROGNOSIS

Potential complications include those associated with angiography in general, such as access site trauma, contrast reactions, and nephrotoxicity. If the brachial artery is used for access then vasospasm or acute thrombosis should be evaluated prior to sheath removal with palpation of radial pulses and a limited angiogram. Acute brachial thrombosis can be dealt with endovascularly; however, when caused by access site injury it is frequently preferable to undergo a surgical procedure to repair the vessel and extract the thrombus rather than obtaining secondary access.[48]

Lesion-specific complication rates vary greatly depending on the site, chronicity, and calcification of the lesion; however, major complication rates for noncarotid arch and upper extremity vessel intervention are low, estimated at 1%.[45,49–52] As described previously, operators should be familiar with endovascular mechanisms of embolism retrieval or dissolution. Most emboli occur secondary to either a cardiac source or vessel trauma at the time of intervention; however, if the source of embolization is a proximal atherosclerotic plaque then this lesion should also be addressed with either angioplasty or stenting.

Management of vessel rupture is as elsewhere in the body, initially with balloon tamponade, reversal of anticoagulation, and, if necessary, stent-graft placement[53] (FIGURE 41.3).

Outcomes of upper extremity occlusive disease treated with endovascular approaches are good. Initial clinical success ranges from between 60% and 100% for occlusive lesions to 100% for stenoses.[51,54,55] Reported long-term outcomes largely relate to subclavian and innominate artery intervention with 1-year patency rates of 91% to 100%, falling to 85% at 3 years and 75% at 5 years.[17,56–58] One exception to this rule of good outcomes seems to be in the subgroup of patients with radiation-induced vasculopathy and stenosis, who may respond better to surgical than endovascular reconstruction.[59]

As with occlusive disease in the lower limbs, upper limb occlusive disease is a sign of systemic atherosclerosis and, hence, risk factor modification is required in all patients. This includes blood sugar and lipid control, smoking cessation, antiplatelet therapy, and investigation for other sites of atherosclerotic occlusion, such as the coronaries, carotids, and lower limbs.

THE FUTURE

As risk factors for systemic atherosclerosis increase in prevalence, particularly in patients with chronic renal disease with its frequent need for upper limb vascular intervention, the incidence of chronic occlusions in the upper limb will doubtless increase as well. With the advent of volumetric fast CT angiographic acquisition and high-resolution MRA with dedicated limb coils, accurate, timely noninvasive diagnosis is possible. It is highly likely that there will be an increased need for dedicated upper limb equipment, whether low-profile balloons on long shafts or flexible stents capable of withstanding the repetitive motion of the forearm and elbow hinge points.

CONCLUSION

Upper extremity arterial insufficiency is common in vascular practice and likely to become more so. Acute symptoms typically present in the affected limb, whereas chronic occlusive disease of the great vessels may present with cerebral or coronary symptoms due to steal phenomenon. Although most acute lesions are cardioembolic and chronic lesions are caused by atherosclerosis, other etiologies including vasculitis, radiation, and spontaneous dissection can also cause vascular occlusion. Noninvasive imaging is sensitive and specific, and endovascular methods akin to those used in the lower limb can be safely used.

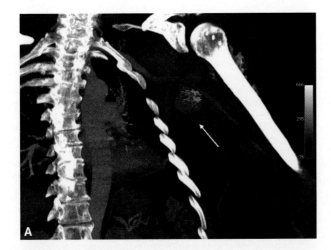

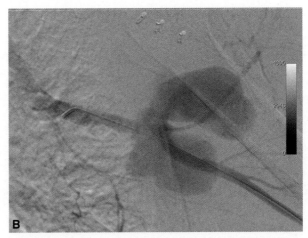

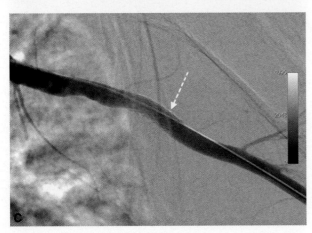

FIGURE 41.3 Contrast-enhanced CTA following a road traffic accident demonstrated a large pseudoaneurysm arising from the left axillary artery (**A**, *solid arrow*). The bilobed pseudoaneurysm was confirmed on selective angiography (**B**) with endovascular exclusion of the lesion with a covered stent-graft (**C**, *dashed arrow*).

Courtesy of L. Lawler, MD, Mater Misericordieae Hospital, Dublin, Ireland.

▌ REFERENCES

1. Bent CL, Sahni VA, Matson MB. The radiological management of the thrombosed arteriovenous dialysis fistula. *Clin Radiol* 2011;66:1–12.
2. Anaya-Ayala JE, Younes HK, Kaiser CL, et al. Prevalence of variant brachial-basilic vein anatomy and implications for vascular access planning. *J Vasc Surg* 2011;53(3):720–724.
3. Nemcek AA Jr. Upper extremity deep venous thrombosis: interventional management. *Tech Vasc Interv Radiol* 2004;7:86–90.
4. Sotta RP. Vascular problems in the proximal upper extremity. *Clin Sports Med* 1990;9:379–388.
5. Ciccone M, Di Noia D, Di Michele L, et al. The incidence of asymptomatic extracoronary atherosclerosis in patients with coronary atherosclerosis. *Int Angiol* 1993;12:25–28.
6. Chang BB, Roddy SP, Darling RC 3rd, et al. Upper extremity bypass grafting for limb salvage in end-stage renal failure. *J Vasc Surg* 2003;38:1313–1315.
7. Fields WS, Lemak NA. Joint study of extracranial arterial occlusion: VII, subclavian steal—a review of 168 cases. *JAMA* 1972;222:1139–1143.
8. Ferrara F, Meli F, Raimondi F, et al. Subclavian stenosis/occlusion in patients with subclavian steal and previous bypass of internal mammary interventricular anterior artery: medical or surgical treatment? *Ann Vasc Surg* 2004;18:566–571.
9. Mulvihill NT, Loutfi M, Salengro E, et al. Percutaneous treatment of coronary subclavian steal syndrome. *J Invasive Cardiol* 2003;15:390–392.
10. Pieroni S, Foster BR, Anderson SW, et al. Use of 64-row multidetector CT angiography in blunt and penetrating trauma of the upper and lower extremities. *Radiographics* 2009;29:863–876.
11. Brauck K, Maderwald S, Vogt FM, et al. Time-resolved contrast-enhanced magnetic resonance angiography of the hand with parallel imaging and view sharing: initial experience. *Eur Radiol* 2007;17:183–192.
12. Reisinger C, Gluecker T, Jacob AL, et al. Dynamic magnetic resonance angiography of the arteries of the hand. A comparison between an extracellular and an intravascular contrast agent. *Eur Radiol* 2009;19:495–502.
13. Cavagna E, D'Andrea P, Schiavon F, et al. Failing hemodialysis arteriovenous fistula and percutaneous treatment: imaging with CT, MRI and digital subtraction angiography. *Cardiovasc Intervent Radiol* 2000;23:262–265.
14. Misra S, Fu AA, Misra KD, et al. Wall shear stress measurement using phase contrast magnetic resonance imaging with phase contrast magnetic resonance angiography in arteriovenous polytetrafluoroethylene grafts. *Angiology* 2009;60:441–447.
15. Prasad A, Varghese I, Roesle M, et al. Prevalence and treatment of proximal left subclavian artery stenosis in patients referred for coronary artery bypass surgery. *Int J Cardiol* 2009;133:109–111.
16. Layton KF, Kallmes DF, Cloft HJ, et al. Bovine aortic arch variant in humans: clarification of a common misnomer. *AJNR Am J Neuroradiol* 2006;27:1541–1542.
17. De Vries JP, Jager LC, Van den Berg JC, et al. Durability of percutaneous transluminal angioplasty for obstructive lesions of proximal subclavian artery: long-term results. *J Vasc Surg* 2005;41:19–23.
18. Kee ST, Dake MD, Wolfe-Johnson B, et al. Ischemia of the throwing hand in major league baseball pitchers: embolic occlusion from aneurysms of axillary artery branches. *J Vasc Interv Radiol* 1995;6:979–982.
19. Panagouli E, Tsaraklis A, Gazouli I, et al. A rare variation of the axillary artery combined contralaterally with an unusual high origin of a superficial ulnar artery: description, review of the literature and embryological analysis. *Ital J Anat Embryol* 2009;114:145–156.
20. Duckett SG, Ginks MR, Knowles BR, et al. Advanced image fusion to overlay coronary sinus anatomy with real-time fluoroscopy to facilitate left ventricular lead implantation in CRT. *Pacing Clin Electrophysiol* 2011;34(2):226–234.

21. Hildick-Smith DJ, Khan ZI, Shapiro LM, et al. Occasional-operator percutaneous brachial coronary angiography: first, do no arm. *Catheter Cardiovasc Interv* 2002;57:161–165; discussion 166.
22. Gan HW, Yip HK, Wu CJ. Brachial approach for coronary angiography and intervention: totally obsolete, or a feasible alternative when radial access is not possible? *Ann Acad Med Singapore* 2010;39:368–373.
23. Kawarada O, Yokoi Y, Higashimori A. Angioplasty of ulnar or radial arteries to treat critical hand ischemia: use of 3- and 4-French systems. *Catheter Cardiovasc Interv* 2010;76:345–350.
24. Bertrand OF, Rao SV, Pancholy S, et al. Transradial approach for coronary angiography and interventions: results of the first international transradial practice survey. *JACC Cardiovasc Interv* 2010;3:1022–1031.
25. Rao SV, Cohen MG, Kandzari DE, et al. The transradial approach to percutaneous coronary intervention: historical perspective, current concepts, and future directions. *J Am Coll Cardiol* 2010;55:2187–2195.
26. Kucuker A, Sener E. Safety of axillary artery cannulation. *J Thorac Cardiovasc Surg* 2010;139:797; author reply 797–798.
27. Rescigno G, Aratari C, Matteucci ML. Axillary artery cannulation pitfalls. *J Thorac Cardiovasc Surg* 2009;138:251; author reply 251–252.
28. James EC, Khuri NT, Fedde CW, et al. Upper limb ischemia resulting from arterial thromboembolism. *Am J Surg* 1979;137:739–744.
29. Widlus DM, Venbrux AC, Benenati JF, et al. Fibrinolytic therapy for upper-extremity arterial occlusions. *Radiology* 1990;175:393–399.
30. Banis JC Jr, Rich N, Whelan TJ Jr. Ischemia of the upper extremity due to noncardiac emboli. *Am J Surg* 1977;134:131–139.
31. Results of a prospective randomized trial evaluating surgery versus thrombolysis for ischemia of the lower extremity. The STILE trial. *Ann Surg* 1994;220:251–266; discussion 266–268.
32. Ouriel K, Veith FJ, Sasahara AA. A comparison of recombinant urokinase with vascular surgery as initial treatment for acute arterial occlusion of the legs. Thrombolysis or Peripheral Arterial Surgery (TOPAS) Investigators. *N Engl J Med* 1998;338:1105–1111.
33. Michaels JA, Torrie EP, Galland RB. The treatment of upper limb vascular occlusions using intraarterial thrombolysis. *Eur J Vasc Surg* 1993;7:744–746.
34. Tisnado J, Bartol DT, Cho SR, et al. Low-dose fibrinolytic therapy in hand ischemia. *Radiology* 1984;150:375–382.
35. Katz SG, Kohl RD. Direct revascularization for the treatment of forearm and hand ischemia. *Am J Surg* 1993;165:312–316.
36. Cejna M, Salomonowitz E, Wohlschlager H, et al. rt-PA thrombolysis in acute thromboembolic upper-extremity arterial occlusion. *Cardiovasc Intervent Radiol* 2001;24:218–223.
37. Saemi AM, Johnson JM, Morris CS. Treatment of bilateral hand frostbite using transcatheter arterial thrombolysis after papaverine infusion. *Cardiovasc Intervent Radiol* 2009;32:1280–1283.
38. Sharafuddin MJ, Hicks ME. Current status of percutaneous mechanical thrombectomy: part III, present and future applications. *J Vasc Interv Radiol* 1998;9:209–224.
39. Sharafuddin MJ, Hicks ME. Current status of percutaneous mechanical thrombectomy: part II, devices and mechanisms of action. *J Vasc Interv Radiol* 1998;9:15–31.
40. Magishi K, Izumi Y, Shimizu N. Short- and long-term outcomes of acute upper extremity arterial thromboembolism. *Ann Thorac Cardiovasc Surg* 2010;16:31–34.
41. Wheatley MJ, Marx MV. The use of intra-arterial urokinase in the management of hand ischemia secondary to palmar and digital arterial occlusion. *Ann Plast Surg* 1996;37:356–362; discussion 362–363.
42. Pfyffer M, Schneider E, Jager K, et al. Local thrombolysis of acute and subacute forearm, hand and finger artery occlusions. Early and late results [in German]. *Vasa* 1989;18:128–135.
43. Bolia A, Nasim A, Bell PR. Percutaneous extraluminal (subintimal) recanalization of a brachial artery occlusion following cardiac catheterization. *Cardiovasc Intervent Radiol* 1996;19:184–186.
44. Rhyne D, Mann T. Hand ischemia resulting from a transradial intervention: successful management with radial artery angioplasty. *Catheter Cardiovasc Interv* 2010;76:383–386.
45. Dineen S, Smith S, Arko FR. Successful percutaneous angioplasty and stenting of the radial artery in a patient with chronic upper extremity ischemia and digital gangrene. *J Endovasc Ther* 2007;14:426–428.
46. Kurimoto Y, Tsuchida Y, Saito J, et al. Emergency endovascular stent-grafting for infected pseudoaneurysm of brachial artery. *Infection* 2003;31:186–188.
47. Woo EY, Fairman RM, Velazquez OC, et al. Endovascular therapy of symptomatic innominate-subclavian arterial occlusive lesions. *Vasc Endovascular Surg* 2006;40:27–33.
48. Alvarez-Tostado JA, Moise MA, Bena JF, et al. The brachial artery: a critical access for endovascular procedures. *J Vasc Surg* 2009;49:378–385; discussion 385.
49. Bates MC, Broce M, Lavigne PS, et al. Subclavian artery stenting: factors influencing long-term outcome. *Catheter Cardiovasc Interv* 2004;61:5–11.
50. Queral LA, Criado FJ. Endovascular treatment of aortic arch occlusive disease. *Semin Vasc Surg* 1996;9:156–163.
51. Criado FJ, Queral LA. The role of angioplasty and stenting in the treatment of occlusive lesions of supra-aortic trunks. *J Mal Vasc* 1996;21(suppl A):132–138.
52. Carrafiello G, Lagana D, Mangini M, et al. Percutaneous treatment of traumatic upper-extremity arterial injuries: a single-center experience. *J Vasc Interv Radiol* 2011;22:34–39.
53. Patel T, Shah S, Sanghavi K, et al. Management of radial and brachial artery perforations during transradial procedures—a practical approach. *J Invasive Cardiol* 2009;21:544–547.
54. Queral LA, Criado FJ. The treatment of focal aortic arch branch lesions with Palmaz stents. *J Vasc Surg* 1996;23:368–375.
55. Amor M, Eid-Lidt G, Chati Z, et al. Endovascular treatment of the subclavian artery: stent implantation with or without predilatation. *Catheter Cardiovasc Interv* 2004;63:364–370.
56. Farina C, Mingoli A, Schultz RD, et al. Percutaneous transluminal angioplasty versus surgery for subclavian artery occlusive disease. *Am J Surg* 1989;158:511–514.
57. Stone PA, Srivastiva M, Campbell JE, et al. Diagnosis and treatment of subclavian artery occlusive disease. *Expert Rev Cardiovasc Ther* 2010;8:1275–1282.
58. Longo GM, Pipinos II. Endovascular techniques for arch vessel reconstruction. *J Vasc Surg* 2010;52:77S–81S.
59. Atabek U, Spence RK, Alexander JB, et al. Upper extremity occlusive arterial disease after radiotherapy for breast cancer. *J Surg Oncol* 1992;49:205–207.

CHAPTER 42

Endovascular Therapies: Proximal Great Vessels

ANDREW S. FERRELL and TONY P. SMITH

INTRODUCTION

Diseases of the aortic arch and proximal great vessels primarily consist of atherosclerotic disease, trauma, and various uncommon arteriopathies. The indications for treating these abnormalities are incompletely clear. The relative infrequency of these entities has led to a relative inexperience in dealing with them in large numbers and, thus, a lack of evidence-based studies to guide decision making. Most of the available literature is composed of case series, leaving the operator with little sound science to guide clinical decisions. Treatment choice is individualized not only to the capabilities of the center but also to the patient him/herself, including general medical condition, presence or absence of symptoms, as well as anatomic considerations. This chapter summarizes the available information and attempt to define a reasonable approach to endovascular therapies of the great vessels.

ANATOMIC CONSIDERATIONS

Conventional Configuration Thoracic Aorta

The thoracic aorta extends proximally from the aortic annulus to the diaphragmatic crura distally and can be divided into ascending, transverse, isthmus, and descending segments.[1,2] The transverse aorta, commonly referred to as the aortic arch, extends from the brachiocephalic trunk to the origin of the left subclavian artery. The branches of the transverse aorta in typical order of origin are the brachiocephalic trunk (innominate), left common carotid, and left subclavian arteries (FIGURE 42.1). The brachiocephalic trunk is the first and largest branch ascending posterolateral to the trachea and bifurcating at the level of the sternoclavicular joint into the right subclavian and right common carotid arteries.[1] The left common carotid artery passes initially in front of the trachea and then ascends along its left posterolateral aspect, bifurcating into the left internal and external carotid arteries at the level of the thyroid cartilage.[1] The left subclavian artery is typically the final branch of the ascending aorta, coursing superior and lateral to the level of the scalene muscles where it becomes the axillary artery.[1]

Variants and Anomalies

The classic three-vessel configuration of the aortic arch is seen in 80% or less of the adult population.[3,4] The largest autopsy series described by Liechty et al.[4] in 1,000 adult cadavers noted this configuration in only 65% of cases. More recently two large series of arch variants and configurations have been described using multidetector computed tomographic angiography

(CTA).[5,6] In the larger of these studies (1,000 patients), variants were identified in 32.4%.[6] Although these variants usually have little physiologic consequence, knowledge of these variations is important to ensure proper endovascular therapeutic planning.

The most common branching pattern variant is a common origin of the brachiocephalic and left common carotid arteries, commonly referred to as a bovine configuration and is seen in 27.4%[6] (FIGURE 42.2A). Although this is a common term ingrained in the medical literature, the bovine arch is a misnomer; cows actually have a single brachiocephalic trunk that splits into the bilateral subclavian arteries and a bicarotid trunk.[2,7] The second most common variant is a direct origin of the left vertebral artery from the aortic arch (6.6%). Other, less common variants include the left common carotid artery arising from the brachiocephalic trunk

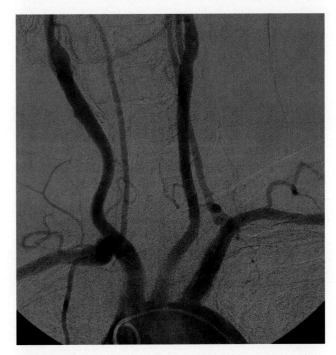

FIGURE 42.1 Normal arch. Note the typical three-vessel configuration consisting of the right brachiocephalic, left common carotid, and left subclavian arteries. In this patient, both vertebral arteries are well visualized originating from their respective subclavian artery. In this patient, the left vertebral artery is only slightly larger than the right.

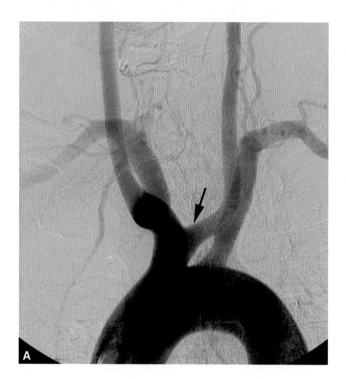

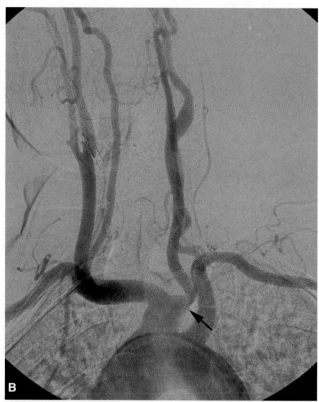

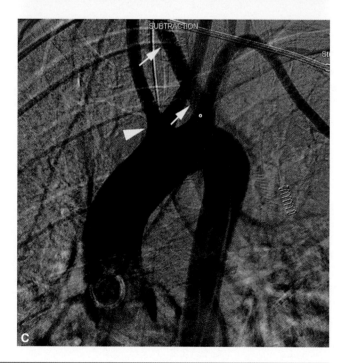

FIGURE 42.2 Great vessel branching patterns from the arch. **A.** Common origin (*arrow*) of the right brachiocephalic and left common carotid arteries, the so-called bovine configuration. **B.** Left common carotid appears as a branch of the right brachiocephalic artery (*arrow*). Many would still refer to this as a bovine configuration. **C.** Right subclavian artery (*arrows*) originates distal to the left subclavian artery. This configuration is referred to as an aberrant right subclavian artery. Note also the common origin of the right brachiocephalic and left common carotid arteries (bovine configuration) (*arrowhead*).

(7%) (FIGURE 42.2B) and the left common carotid and left subclavian arteries from a left-sided brachiocephalic trunk (1% to 2%).[1,3,6,8,9]

Often considered an anomaly rather than a true variant, a left aortic arch with aberrant right subclavian artery occurs in approximately 0.9%[10] (FIGURE 42.2C). In this situation the subclavian originates from the descending aorta distal to the left subclavian artery, often with an associated diverticular orifice (Kommerall), and courses posterior to the esophagus toward the right arm.[11] Recognizing this variant is important to ensure

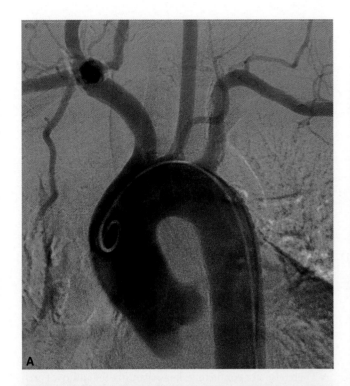

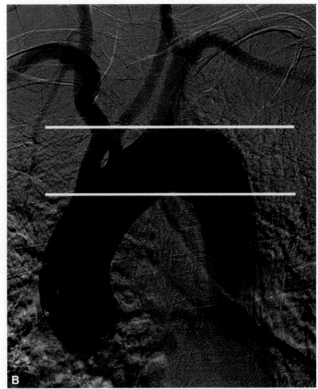

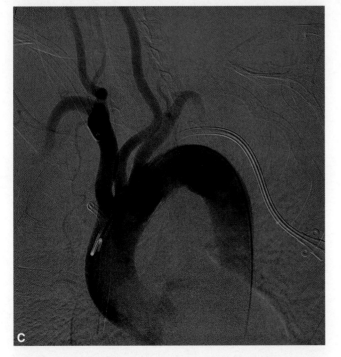

FIGURE 42.3 Aortic arch classification. Moving from arch I to arch III classes usually corresponds with increasing difficulty of vessel catheterization. **A.** Class I, where great vessels originate from the top of the arch. **B.** Class II, where great vessels originate between parallel lines (*drawn in white*) along the outer and inner curves of the arch. **C.** Class III, where great vessels originate caudal to the inner surface of the arch or off the ascending aorta.

that complete angiographic studies are performed including visualization of the right vertebral artery.

Arch Classification

With advanced age, hypertension, and atherosclerotic changes, the arch sinks deeper into the thoracic cavity, drawing the great vessel origins with it, resulting in arch elongation and a more caudal position of the great vessel origins with respect to the top of the arch.[12] A classification has been developed for this change in configuration that is felt to correspond with increasing difficulty of vessel cannulation with class I vessels originating from the top of the arch, class II between parallel lines drawn along the outer and inner curves of the arch, and type III caudal to the inner surface of the arch or off the ascending aorta[13] (FIGURE 42.3). In theory moving from arch I to arch III corresponds with increasing difficulty of catheterization and often requiring reformed backward-facing catheters (e.g., Simmons).

DIAGNOSTIC ANGIOGRAPHY

Anatomy and diseases of the thoracic aorta and the great vessels can be studied with catheter-based angiography, CTA, magnetic resonance angiography (MRA), and ultrasound. Each of these modalities has specific strengths and limitations that are the subject of other chapters within this text. Assessment of aortic arch anatomy and disease is initially evaluated by one or more of these noninvasive methods; however, conventional aortic arch angiography and selective branch injection may be imperative in procedural planning and is, of course, an integral part of endovascular therapy.[14]

Arch aortography is typically performed with a pigtail catheter placed in the ascending aorta just above the aortic valve.[11] The left anterior oblique (LAO) projection will typically remove overlap of the branch vessels and provide adequate anatomic detail[11] (FIGURE 42.4A). Craniocaudal views may be necessary to "open up" torturous origins occurring in the anterior-posterior (AP) plane. In the LAO projection the right subclavian and right common carotid arteries often overlap, which can be overcome with a variable right anterior oblique (RAO) projection[14] (FIGURE 42.4B). Selective catheterization of the proximal great vessels is usually performed with a 4 or 5 French angled catheter. For steep (type III) arches use of a reformed backward-facing catheter is often needed as noted earlier.[14]

Catheter-based studies of the aortic arch and great vessels are often performed in conjunction with cerebral angiography and there has long been debate regarding the need for performance of arch injections with these evaluations. Many consider the time, effort, and difficulty as well as contrast load involved with injections of the ascending aorta to be of little benefit considering potential risks.[15] Akers et al. reported on 100 consecutive patients with arch and cerebral four-vessel angiography studies, finding that only 0.6% had hemodynamically significant stenosis of the intrathoracic vessels.[15,16] Another study of 129 patients undergoing evaluation for carotid endarterectomy compared arch aortography to noninvasive testing including clinical recording of upper limb pulses, blood pressure, supraclavicular bruits, and duplex examinations to evaluate proximal inflow to the carotid arteries. They identified 19 (14.7%) patients with angiographic evidence of aortic branch disease of whom 7 (5.4%) underwent additional surgery. All of these lesions were detected by a combination of noninvasive tests, leading the authors to conclude that arch injections are unnecessary in the absence of clinical or noninvasive findings.[17] In yet another study the utility of arch injections was evaluated prospectively in 100 patients undergoing evaluation for carotid distribution ischemic events. All patients underwent selective carotid angiography followed by arch aortography and in only two cases (2%) did the arch injection affect patient management. In 69 patients the study provided no useful information and 29 demonstrated abnormalities that did not affect patient care.[18]

There also are conflicting data regarding the utility of arch evaluation in the modern era of CTA. In a study of three-dimensional CT angiographic assessment prior to carotid stenting in 59 patients, CTA significantly influenced the plan for carotid artery stenting in 37%.[19] Theoretically, CTA evaluation of the arch provides the same anatomic and pathologic information as traditional catheter-based angiography and

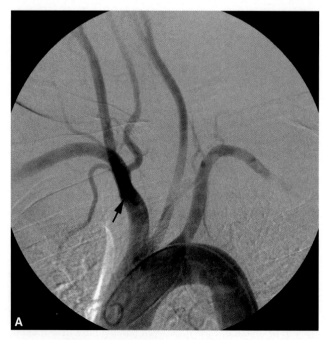
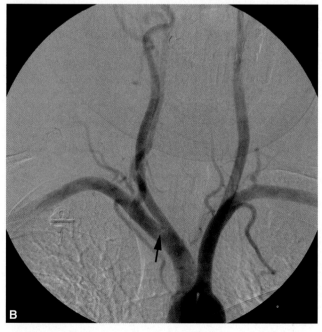

FIGURE 42.4 Obliquities of aortic arch. **A.** The left anterior oblique projection lessens any overlap of the great vessels but tends to accentuate overlap of the right subclavian and common carotid arteries (*arrow*) at the bifurcation of the brachiocephalic artery. **B.** The right anterior oblique projection lessens the overlap of the proximal right subclavian and right common carotid arteries (*arrow*) as they originate from the right brachiocephalic artery.

any discrepancy in the conclusions drawn between this study and catheter-based ones again suggests variability in what is considered significant given the lack of standardization. Arch aortography certainly does provide useful information in the setting of proximal great vessel stenosis, tortuosity, or anatomic variation. If there is clinical or imaging concern for supra-aortic trunk vessel stenosis then adequate delineation of the origins of these vessels is imperative for both diagnostic purposes as well as facilitating safe selective catheterization. If there is no reasonable concern for the possibility of atherosclerotic disease (such as in the workup of ischemic stroke) then arch aortography may be unnecessary.

TREATMENT OF ATHEROSCLEROTIC STENOSES OF THE SUPRA-AORTIC TRUNK VESSELS

The supra-aortic trunk vessels specifically refer to the direct branches of the aortic arch, namely, the brachiocephalic, left common carotid, and left subclavian arteries. This section also considers the proximal right common carotid and subclavian arteries in the same discussion. Although these branches do not directly arise from the arch, disease processes and treatment options are essentially the same and the available literature often includes them, making separation of these vessels for this discussion counterintuitive. A separate section is devoted to intervention of the proximal vertebral artery as well.

Surgical Therapy

The first surgical report for the treatment of proximal carotid artery disease was published in 1951 by Shimizu and Sano who described treatment of two common carotid occlusions, one by retrograde thrombectomy and the other by venous interposition graft.[20,21] As with lesions of the common carotid artery (CCA), surgical therapy has traditionally been the mainstay of treatment for brachiocephalic and subclavian stenosis. Transthoracic brachiocephalic endarterectomy was described by Davis et al.[22] in 1956 and, subsequently, prosthetic bypass grafting of the great vessels by De Bakey et al.[23] in 1958. Parot and coworkers introduced carotid subclavian transposition in 1964 and Diethrich and coworkers carotid subclavian bypass in 1967.[24] Crawford et al. confirmed the efficacy of carotid-subclavian bypass and demonstrated a reduced mortality rate of 5.6% as compared to 22% with transthoracic procedures.[21,25]

The patency of surgical procedures remains excellent with 5-year rates of 90% for bypasses and 96% for transpositions.[24] More recently Fry et al.[26] demonstrated a 100% 4-year patency rate for carotid-subclavian bypass, and Perler and Williams[27] showed 92% and 83% primary patency rates at 5 and 8 years, respectively. These, along with other studies, have clearly demonstrated the efficacy and durability of surgical approaches to lesions of the supra-aortic trunk vessels.

Although well defined with regard to its efficacy and durability,[28,29] open surgical treatment has become increasingly avoided because of the morbidity of the approaches as well as their technical difficulty given the relatively uncommon occurrence. The combined stroke/death rate associated with surgical revascularization of proximal CCA and other supra-aortic trunk lesions with a transthoracic approach can be as high as 16%.[28,29] Although reduced significantly with the introduction

of extra-anatomic repairs, this remains approximately 4%,[28] resulting in continued desire for less invasive endovascular solutions.

GENERAL ENDOVASCULAR TECHNIQUE

Prior to intervention, antiplatelet therapy is essential to reduce the risk of subacute stent thrombosis and thromboembolic complications. Dual antiplatelet therapy with aspirin (81 to 325 mg daily) and clopidogrel (75 mg daily) or ticlopidine (250 mg twice daily) is initiated 3 to 5 days prior to the procedure. In urgent situations one-time loading doses of aspirin 650 mg and clopidogrel 300 to 600 mg can be given followed by daily standard dose therapy although this is less than desirable. Following femoral access and routine diagnostic aortography, heparin anticoagulation of 60 units/kg of body weight is given with target activated clotting time (ACT) greater than or equal to 250 or twice baseline. Alternatively, agents are available for use in patients with heparin allergies.

The femoral approach is preferable because of long-term experience and low rate of complications compared to other approaches. Alternatively, brachial or retrograde cervical (open or percutaneous) approaches have been reported to be particularly useful in the setting of tight ostial stenosis or occlusions, aorto-iliac-femoral occlusive disease, or aortic arch tortuosity preventing a femoral approach.[14] The axillary approach is avoided due to the potential for brachial plexus injury if an expanding hematoma is to occur. In fact, brachial and axillary approaches have been limited or largely replaced in selected centers by the radial artery approach, now an option because of lower-profile angioplasty and stent delivery platforms.

Following anticoagulation a sheath or guide catheter with large enough inner diameter to accommodate appropriate angioplasty balloons and stent delivery systems (usually 6 French sheath or 7 French guide catheter) is placed in the aortic arch for an ostial lesion or within the proximal target vessel for more distal lesions. If stability of the sheath within the aorta becomes an issue it can be supported by passage of a 0.035-inch buddy wire into the axillary or external carotid arteries.

The use of embolic protection devices (EPDs) is currently unclear. Although embolic potential appears to be low with supra-aortic trunk lesions, it is logical to think that distal filter protection will enhance the safety of the procedure and this approach has been adopted in most centers, although there is no consensus evidence supporting their use.[14] Because EPDs are typically designed for use within the internal carotid artery, sizing becomes an issue. If an EPD is to be used, it should be deployed within a nondiseased segment of the target vessel several centimeters distal to the lesion (FIGURE 42.5). Close attention must be made to ensure that the vessel size is appropriate for the size of the EPD. If the vessel is too large, the EPD will have limited efficacy. The device can be deployed within the more appropriate-sized internal carotid artery if the target lesion is within the CCA. At times trouble will be encountered crossing the lesion itself and/or the angulated arch origins with the filter wire; in these situations the procedure may have to be performed without embolic protection.[14]

The technique for treating supra-aortic trunk vessel stenosis is similar to that for treating carotid bifurcation lesions with slight modifications due to the working position in the arch or proximal great vessels. Balloon angioplasty alone has had reported success as noted later. As with many atherosclerotic

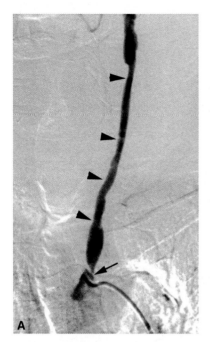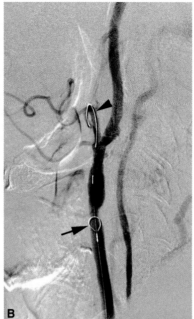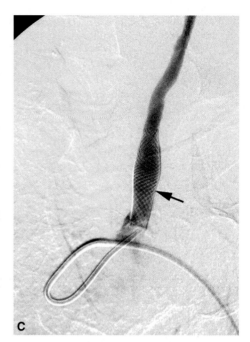

FIGURE 42.5 Angioplasty and stenting of the left common carotid artery (LCCA) origin. **A.** High-grade stenosis (*arrow*) of the origin of the LCCA from the aortic arch. There is disease more superiorly in the vessel (*arrowheads*) that was not thought to be significant. **B.** Distal protection device (*arrow*) placed in the distal LCCA with the wire (*arrowhead*) extending into the left external carotid artery. **C.** Post-balloon angioplasty and stenting with an acceptable angiographic result. Note that a self-expanding stent (*arrow*) was used based on study protocol at the time. Most often a lesion in this location would be treated with a balloon-expandable stent.

lesions today, however, stents are typically preferred for truly ostial or extremely calcified lesions and in the endovascular treatment of total occlusions. Balloon-expandable stents are usually preferred in this location because they allow more precise, controlled deployment; have a greater hoop strength; are within the thoracic cage, preventing crushing by external forces; and are less prone to misplacement in high-grade lesions (watermelon-seed) compared to self-expanding stents[14,30] (FIGURE 42.6). Self-expanding stents are reserved for extrathoracic long segment nonostial disease in which differential vessel size, vessel tortuosity, or compression by external anatomic structures/forces favors use of a self-expanding stent (FIGURE 42.5). Within the mid- or distal subclavian, for example, self-expandable stents are preferred, limiting the potential for external compression by the clavicle or first rib.[24] In general, as with other sites, balloon-expandable stents should be sized as close to the exact size of the vessel as possible, whereas self-expandable stents are typically slightly oversized.[14]

VESSEL-SPECIFIC CONSIDERATIONS AND OUTCOMES

Common Carotid Artery

Although the carotid bifurcation remains the primary area of interest with regard to therapy for cerebrovascular disease, the origin and proximal CCA is the second most common location for extracranial carotid stenosis, accounting for 1% to 2% of ischemic cerebral events[31] (FIGURE 42.6). Despite this, however,

the natural history of these lesions is poorly understood, as are the indications, efficacy, and durability of various therapies.

There are only two notable studies specifically regarding endovascular treatment of proximal CCA lesions. In 2003 Chio et al.[32] reported prospective experience in 37 patients undergoing elective stenting of lesions of greater than 50% stenosis of the origin and proximal CCA. They reported a technical success rate of 95% with a 30-day all-death/stroke rate of 7.1% with mean follow-up of 24 months.[32] They also observed a restenosis rate of 5.1%. A larger retrospective study by Paukovits et al.[31] in 2008 reported their experience with 147 patients undergoing angioplasty alone (45) or angioplasty with stenting (108) with an inclusion criteria of at least 70% stenosis in symptomatic (31.2%) or 85% stenosis in asymptomatic patients (68.7%). The neurologic complication rate in this study was lower with a 2.8% 30-day all-stroke/death rate with a similarly high-technical success rate of 98.6%. There have been a number of series that describe synchronous bifurcation carotid endarterectomy coupled with retrograde endovascular treatment of proximal common carotid stenoses. These reports, however, are all small cohorts ranging from 6 to 23 patients with variable indications and inclusion criteria, limiting useful conclusion.[31]

With these limitations, evidence-based clinical decisions regarding treatment of these lesions is difficult and has classically been left to the discretion of the treating physician. Typically, operators presume with reasonable assumption that these lesions will behave similarly to those seen at the carotid bifurcation. Typical indications include symptomatic disease, such as amaurosis fugax, transient ischemic attacks (TIAs), and

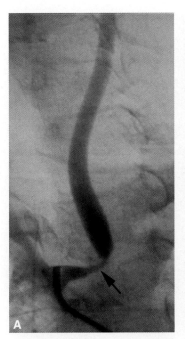
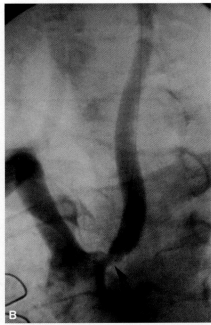
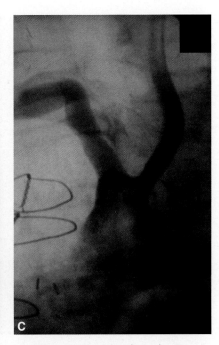

FIGURE 42.6 Angioplasty and stenting of left common carotid artery (LCCA) lesion. **A.** Proximal LCCA lesion (*arrow*). Note the common origin of the right brachiocephalic artery and LCCA. Such anatomy necessitates very accurate positioning of the proximal end of the stent. **B.** Post-balloon angioplasty demonstrates a residual stenosis (*arrow*). Intervention is being performed using a distal protection device, which is in the distal LCCA (off the images). **C.** Poststent angioplasty and stent placement (*arrow*) demonstrating an excellent radiographic result.

nondevastating stroke with good recovery, as well as at least 50% stenosis, or asymptomatic stenosis of at least 75% to 80%.[14] A lesion may be in isolation or in tandem with a more distal plaque for which treatment is planned.

Subclavian Artery

The left subclavian artery is the most common site of atherosclerotic disease of the supra-aortic trunk vessels, being affected three to four times more frequently than its counterpart on the right.[33,34] Subclavian and brachiocephalic disease considered together account for 17% of symptomatic extracranial cerebrovascular disease.[34,35] Although the presence of subclavian atherosclerotic disease is common, related symptoms are relatively rare. In a study of 1,114 patients with disease involving the brachiocephalic and subclavian arteries, only 168 (15%) demonstrated clinical signs of subclavian stenosis.[24,36] In another study of 6,534 patients by Perler and Williams, only 17% were noted to have a stenosis of 30% or more and, of those, only 24% had clinical and angiographic evidence of steal phenomena.[24,27] Additionally, disease progression is limited. Ackerman and coworkers found disease progression in only 17% of 67 patients over a 2-year interval and, ultimately, only 4 of 55 asymptomatic patients developed vertebrobasilar symptoms within 4 years.[24,37]

Although most subclavian lesions are asymptomatic, if symptoms are present they are primarily arm claudication and/or neurologic events. One of the most notable conditions related to subclavian atherosclerosis is subclavian steal (FIGURE 42.7). First described in 1961 by Reivich and coworkers,[35,38] this syndrome arises in the setting of subclavian artery stenosis or occlusion proximal to the vertebral artery origin. The stenosis leads to decreased distal subclavian perfusion and, thus, a progressive decrease and ultimately reversal of flow in the ipsilateral vertebral artery to restore blood flow toward the arm. This results in shunting of blood away from the brain toward the arm and clinical symptoms of vertebrobasilar insufficiency including ataxia, vertigo, dizziness, syncope, diplopia, nausea, and vomiting. Additional collaterals that may provide flow to the ipsilateral arm but are of less clinical importance include the external carotid artery, ascending cervical artery, and thyrocervical trunk.

Upper extremity ischemic symptoms may also occur due to flow restriction or embolic events and may result in arm claudication, paresis, or atheroembolic digital ischemia.[24] Along the same lines, the coronary subclavian steal may develop where a proximal subclavian stenosis causes reversal of flow within a mammary artery graft. At times endovascular techniques may be used to maintain patency of the proximal subclavian to preserve supply to the inferior mesenteric artery (IMA) for coronary bypass procedures. Treatment of lesions is also indicated to maintain subclavian patency for patients undergoing or in expected need of future hemodialysis grafts.[24] Patients who are to receive axillofemoral bypass procedures with proximal subclavian stenosis may also be candidates for revascularization techniques.

Typically patients will present with evidence of arm ischemia or vertebrobasilar insufficiency and on examination show upper extremity pressure gradients of 20 mm Hg or more between the affected and nonaffected sides.[24] Initial diagnosis typically is performed with Doppler sonography.[39] MRA and CTA are

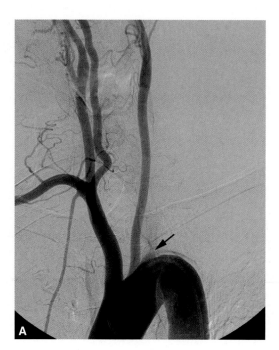

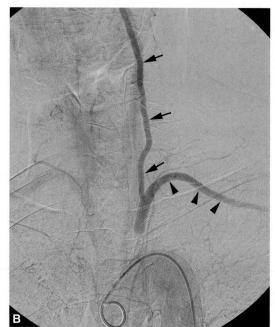

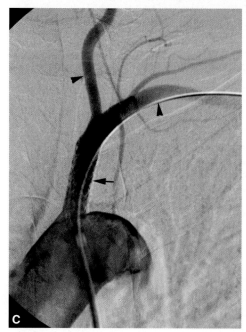

FIGURE 42.7 Patient with symptoms referable to the posterior fossa and arch aortogram confirming subclavian steal. **A.** Image from an arch aortogram early in the sequence showing occlusion of the left subclavian artery (*arrow*). **B.** Image from an arch aortogram later in the sequence showing retrograde flow in the left vertebral artery (*arrows*) filling the left subclavian artery (*arrowheads*). **C.** Left subclavian angiogram following angioplasty and stenting of the proximal left subclavian artery. Note the excellent radiographic result (*arrow*) with antegrade flow in the left vertebral and left subclavian arteries (*arrowheads*).

acceptable screening studies as well and may be useful to confirm or refute Doppler findings; however, angiography remains the gold standard for definitive diagnosis and treatment planning.

As with other great vessel lesions, surgical therapy has traditionally been the mainstay of treatment for subclavian stenosis. Angioplasty for subclavian artery stenosis was first described in 1980[40]; however, due to uncertainty over long-term patency as well as potential for distal embolism and stroke, the procedure was not fully adopted until well over a decade later. By the mid-1990s several reports of successful endovascular treatment of subclavian stenosis emerged with initial technical success rates of 92% to 100% in selected patients and 85% to 100% patency rates at a mean follow-up of 27 months.[21,41–44]

Both carotid-subclavian bypass and endovascular stenting are safe, effective, and durable; however, bypass procedures are more durable in the long term.[45] Patients tend to have focal lesions in large vessels relatively early in disease progression, which leads to early presentation and promotes favorable outcome. In general, relief of ischemic symptoms is excellent, whereas results for improving dizziness are poor (only 20%).[24] Neurologic complications are surprisingly low, possibly caused by the protective effect of flow reversal within the vertebral artery, which is not restored until 20 seconds to 4 minutes following angioplasty and stent placement.[24] Patency rates have drastically improved with the advent of lower-profile balloons, improved wire technology, and stent design, decreasing to 0% to 18% for 2- to 4-year follow-up periods.[24]

A unique consideration when stenting the subclavian artery is the proximity of the lesion with respect to the vertebral artery origin. Angioplasty performed over the origin can cause plaque disruption and distal emboli or dissection. Techniques to prevent this include undersizing of balloons, dilatation proximal or distal to the vertebral origin, and, if necessary, placement of an indwelling 0.014-inch guide wire following selective catheterization for troubleshooting after the angioplasty.[14] Fortunately, the stent cell size will typically allow for adequate inflow to preserve vessel patency and rarely results in occlusion. In cases of high-grade stenosis or concern for distal embolism, a distal protection device can be deployed into the vertebral artery, although this represents an off-label indication.

Angioplasty and stenting of the right subclavian artery is often more difficult than its counterpart on the left due to the proximity of the right common carotid and vertebral artery origins as well as difficulty in displaying the anatomy accurately given the overlap of the above-mentioned structures (FIGURE 42.8). An RAO projection with slight craniocaudal tilt is often best for removing overlay of the common carotid and vertebral arteries as well as adequately demonstrating the origins from the brachiocephalic and subclavian arteries, respectively.[14] Because of the close proximity of these branch vessels, precise angioplasty and stent placement is critical, often necessitating use of balloon-mounted stents.[14]

Brachiocephalic Artery

Compared to the proximal common carotid and subclavian arteries, brachiocephalic stenosis is relatively uncommon. Symptoms related to brachiocephalic stenosis, however, may be severe and result in retrograde flow from the vertebral artery into both the right common carotid and subclavian arteries. Patients will generally present with symptoms of vertebrobasilar insufficiency or upper extremity claudication (FIGURE 42.8).

Technique for intervening upon brachiocephalic lesions is similar to that for the left subclavian or left CCA origins (FIGURE 42.9). Intervention of brachiocephalic lesions is often problematic because of the propensity of these lesions to be very short within a large-diameter vessel, which makes stability and precise placement of angioplasty balloons and stents difficult.[14] For accurate placement, balloon-mounted stents are preferred. If the lesion closely approximates the CCA origin, then kissing stents may be necessary.[24] At times a combined femoral and brachial approach can be helpful to provide stability during wire access.[14]

OUTCOMES OF ENDOVASCULAR THERAPY FOR SUPRA-AORTIC VESSEL STENOSIS

Determining effectiveness of therapies for supra-aortic trunk vessels is difficult given that some reports are specific to these branches, whereas others include distal branches, such as the

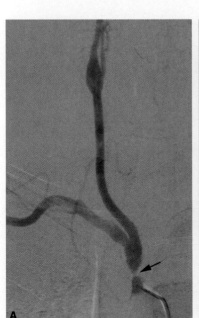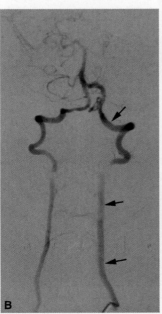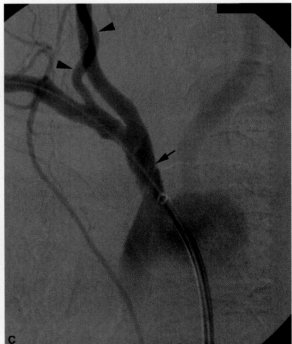

FIGURE 42.8 Distal right brachiocephalic stenosis resulting in retrograde flow in the right vertebral artery. Patient presented with right arm claudication. **A.** Angiogram of the right brachiocephalic artery shows high-grade stenosis just proximal to the bifurcation (*arrow*). Note no filling of the right vertebral artery. **B.** Selective angiogram of the left vertebral artery shows some filling of the posterior intracranial vessels as well as retrograde flow in the right vertebral artery (*arrows*). **C.** Right brachiocephalic angiogram following angioplasty and stenting. Excellent radiographic result (*arrow*) with antegrade filling of the right vertebral artery (*arrowheads*).

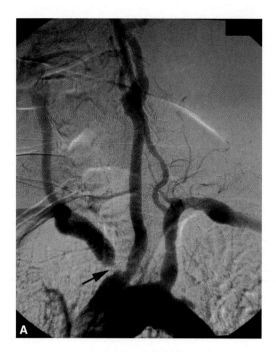

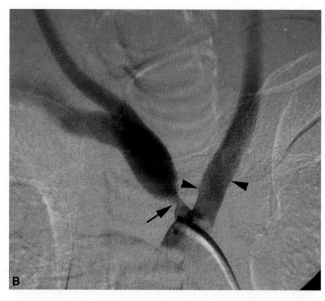

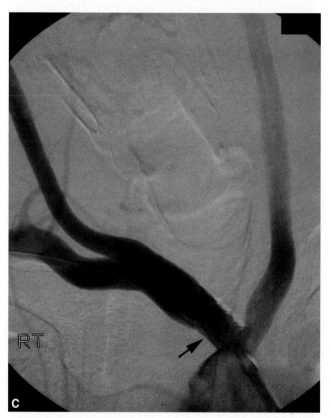

FIGURE 42.9 Right brachiocephalic angioplasty and stent placement. **A.** Aortic arch angiogram shows a high-grade stenosis of the right brachiocephalic artery (*arrow*). Note there is a common origin of the right brachiocephalic and left common carotid arteries. **B.** Selective injection of the right brachiocephalic artery showing the stenosis (*arrow*) in very close proximity to the left common carotid artery (*arrowheads*). **C.** Post-angioplasty and stenting of the right brachiocephalic artery with a balloon-expandable stent. There is an excellent radiographic result (*arrow*) with very minimal stent exposure to the left common carotid artery.

vertebral origin or right CCA. There is also difficulty interpreting literature because inclusion criteria, patient selection, follow-up, and various technical factors, such as stent type, are not standardized. Some series only included patients considered poor surgical candidates, whereas in others endovascular therapy was the first-line treatment. Some authors performed procedures under general anesthesia, whereas others under conscious sedation.

In general primary technical success rates are high with variable rates of restenosis. Primary technical success rates

of 88% to 100% have been reported for balloon angioplasty alone, although recurrence rates as high as 22% have also been reported.[46–51] Cumulative patency rates at 3 years range from 86% to 98%, although one report showed a clinical success rate of only 56%, including nine occlusions.[52,53]

As stent placement was added to angioplasty during the 1990s the technical success rates remained high, ranging from 83% to 100%[21,33,35,41,43–46,52,54–67] (Table 42.1). Primary patency rates overall were improved with stenting, ranging from 83% to 100%

Table 42.1

Available Literature Related to Stenting of Supra-Aortic Trunk Vessels

Author	Year	Patients/ lesions	Subclav artery	Innom artery	Common carotid	Stents	Tech success	Minor compl	Major compl	30-day	Mean F/U	Restenosis	1% patent	2% patent
Kumar et al.[44]	1995	27/31	28	3	—	100%	100%	7.4%	0%	0%	NA	NA	NA	NA
Queral and Criado[41]	1996	22/26	12	8	6	100%	92.3%	0%	0%	0%	27 mo	15%	85% @ 27 mo	NA
Sueoka[43]	1996	7/7	7	—	—	100%	100.0%	0%	0%	0%	12 mo	NA	NA	NA
Sullivan et al.[21]	1998	66/66	66	7	—	100%	93.9%	4.5%	4.5%	0%	14.3 mo	4.5%	84% @ 35 mo	NA
Rodriguez-Lopez et al.[33]	1999	69/70	70	—	—	100%	96%	11.40%	4.3%	1.4%	13 mo	10%	92% @ 18 mo	96% @ 18 mo
Al-Mubarak et al.[54]	1999	38/38	38	—	—	100%	92.1%	0%	0%	0%	20 mo	6%	91% @ 20 mo	NA
Henry et al.[55]	1999	113/113	113	—	—	41%	91.2%	2.6%	2.6%	0.9%	4.3 y	15.5%	83% @ 8 y	90% @ 8 y
Hadjipetrou et al.[35]	1999	18/18	15	3	—	100%	100%	11.1%	0%	0%	17 mo	0%	100% @ 17 mo	NA
Schillinger et al.[56]	2001	115/115	115	—	—	23%	85%	NA	NA	NA	NA	NA	59% @ 4 y	NA
Huttl et al.[46]	2002	89/89	—	89	—	1.1%	96.4%	6%	2%	NA	NA	3.4%	93% @ 117 mo	98% @ 117 mo
Bates et al.[65]	2004	91/101	96	—	—	100%	97%	14.3%	0%	1.1%	36.1 mo	14.6%	89% @ 40 mo	NA
Brountzos et al.[66]	2004	39/39	39	10	—	100%	94.9%	5.1%	0%	5.1%	12.3 mo	10.8%	77% @ 24 mo	92% @ 24 mo
Amor et al.[60]	2004	86/89	89	—	—	100%	93.3%	16.2%	4.5%	2.3%	3.51 y	19.5%	85% @ 3 y	98% @ 3 y
Allie et al.[57]	2004	11/11	—	11	—	100%	97%	NA	NA	NA	34 mo	0%	100% @ 34 mo	NA
De Vries et al.[58]	2005	110/110	110	—	—	58%	93%	7%	1.1%	2%	34 mo	7.80%	89% @ 5 y	NA
Przewlocki et al.[67]	2006	75/76	73	2	—	87%	93.3%	9.3%	0%	0%	24.4 mo	15.6%	77% @ 5 y	95% @ 3 y
Peterson et al.[59]	2006	20/18	3	8	9	100%	100%	0%	0%	0%	12 mo	0%	100% @ 12 mo	NA
Woo et al.[146]	2006	25/27	—	—	—	81.5%	89%	0%	0%	0%	18 mo	12%	88% @ 18 mo	NA
Patel et al.[61]	2008	170/177	166	11	—	100%	98.3%	1.8%	4.1%	0.6%	35.2 mo	15.9%	83% @ 66 mo	96% @ 54 mo
AbuRahma et al.[45]	2007	121/121	121	—	—	100%	98%	9.2%	5.9%	0.8%	3.4 y	NA	97% @ 30 d	70% @ 5 y
Van Noord et al.[64]	2007	43/43	40	3	—	88.4%	97.7%	NA	NA	0%	12 mo	NA	NA	NA
Van Hattum et al.[63]	2007	30/30	—	30	—	66.7%	83%	13.3%	6.7%	3.3%	24 mo	50%	50% @ 24 mo	NA
Bakken et al.[52]	2008	44/45	26	8	11	93%	98%	11.0%	2.0%	0%	NA	23%	77% @ 3 y	88% @ 3 y
Sixt et al.[62]	2009	107/108	—	—	—	87%	97%	1.9%	0%	0%	29 mo	12%	88% @ 1 y	97% @ 1 y

Tech, technical; Compl, complication; Patent, patency; F/U, follow-up; S, subclavian artery; IA, innominate artery; CC, common carotid artery; NA, not applicable.

at a mean follow-up of 23.8 months, with acceptable 30-day cumulative rates of stroke and all-cause death ranging from 0% to 3.3% (Table 42.1).[21,33,35,41,43–45,54,57–64]

A 2007 report compared 121 patients undergoing stenting versus 51 carotid-subclavian bypasses for subclavian stenoses and showed technical success rates of 98% and 100%, respectively, with a major complication rate of 5.8% in the percutaneous transluminal angioplasty (PTA)/stent group and 5.9% in the surgical group. The overall periprocedural complication rate including minor complications was lower in the surgical (5.9%) versus the endovascular (15.1%) group; however, the increase in minor complications in the PTA/stent group was primarily related to access site complications. Primary patency was 100% at 1 year and 96% at 5 years for surgery, whereas the endovascular group showed patency rates of 93% at 1 year and 70% at 5 years.[45]

These results suggest that endoluminal stenting for ostial disease of the supra-aortic trunk vessels provides excellent primary results and adequate long-term patency rates with low morbidity, mortality, and secondary intervention rates.[52]

PROXIMAL VERTEBRAL ARTERY

Background, Indications, and Patient Selection

The pathophysiologic methods of ischemia involving the vertebrobasilar system have improved in recent years with advanced imaging modalities as well as data from characterized groups of patients possessing definitive signs and symptoms of posterior circulation ischemia.[68] The pathology is twice as frequent in men as in women, typically developing after age 60.[69] Embolism is the most common mechanism accounting for approximately 40% of cases. Embolic material may originate in the heart, aorta, or proximal great vessels but the vertebral origin is the most common site.[70,71] Embolic events present with sudden maximum onset of neurologic symptoms and may resolve quickly if spontaneous thrombolysis occurs.[72] The second most common mechanism is hemodynamic compromise from focal stenosis or local thrombosis without embolism. Vertebral artery atherosclerotic stenosis accounts for approximately 32% of cases.[70] In either setting, symptoms will typically develop slowly and may have a fluctuating course occurring over hours to days.[72] Flow-limiting lesions may be particularly susceptible to presentation during the setting of even a moderate decrease in mean arterial pressure seen in situations of cardiac failure, myocardial infarction, or subclavian steal. This may also be positional in nature, associated with a stereotypical movement, such as extension or rotation of the head or neck.[72]

The vertebral artery typically arises along the superior or posterior portion of the subclavian artery and is usually the first branch. The vertebral artery arises directly from the arch in about 6% of people and rarely may arise from the CCA. The first segment of the vertebral artery (V1) extends from the subclavian origin to its entrance into the transverse foramina, typically at the sixth cervical vertebra and is the subject of discussion here. Muscular branches arise from the vertebral artery and share a collateral circulation with the external carotid artery and thyrocervical trunk, providing collateral supply to the vertebral artery beyond a proximal occlusion.[71,72]

Atherosclerotic disease has a predilection to involve the origin or proximal section of the vertebral artery, although there is also significant incidence of disease within the intracranial

segment.[73] Although extracranial vertebral artery stenoses has traditionally been considered to have a benign course compared to its intracranial counterpart, evidence has shown extracranial vertebra artery disease to be the primary cause of ischemia in a significant portion of patients.[70] Based on registry data, disease in the proximal vertebral artery is present in 20% of patients presenting with symptoms of vertebrobasilar insufficiency and is thought to be the primary cause of ischemia in 9%.[74] In the setting of disease of the proximal vertebral artery, 50% will present initially with stroke alone with 26% experiencing TIA rapidly followed by stroke.[71,72]

Symptoms of vertebrobasilar insufficiency are often nonspecific, typically occurring in the elderly population with overlapping signs of other common diseases, particularly those of cardiac origin.[75] Often, dizziness is the dominant symptom and accompanied by other signs of posterior circulation ischemia including diplopia, vertigo, blurred vision, tinnitus, ataxia, bilateral weakness or sensory deficits, and syncope.

Initial diagnosis often begins with noninvasive imaging studies including ultrasonography, MRA, and CTA. In a review of 11 studies comparing noninvasive imaging with catheter-based angiography for the detection of vertebral artery disease, CTA and contrast-enhanced MRA were associated with higher sensitivity (94%) and specificity (95%) than ultrasonography (sensitivity 70%); however, neither CTA nor MRA reliably defined vertebral origin stenosis; therefore, if clinically necessary, catheter-based angiography remains essential to confirm or dispute initial findings of noninvasive imaging studies in this region.[75,76]

The safety and efficacy of invasive treatments are uncertain with only one small randomized trial comparing the efficacy of endovascular intervention to medical therapy alone, and no randomized trials exist comparing surgery to medical therapy or endovascular treatment. In the international, multicenter Carotid And Vertebral Artery Transluminal Angioplasty Study (CAVATAS), 16 patients with symptomatic vertebral artery stenosis were randomized in equal proportions to receive endovascular (angioplasty and/or stenting) or best medical therapy and were followed neurologically for as long as 8 years.[77] Although this trial failed to show a benefit of intervention over best medical therapy, the study was severely underpowered with only 16 patients and, therefore, little definitive conclusions can been drawn from the data.

For these reasons physicians have been conservative with decisions to intervene and, until recently, most patients with vertebral artery stenosis have been treated with medical therapy alone. In the setting of posterior circulation ischemia and imaging evidence of thrombus within the extracranial vertebral artery, anticoagulant therapy is generally recommended for at least 3 months.[75,78–81]

Indication for intervention on proximal vertebral artery lesions is generally reserved only for symptomatic patients with high grade (>70%) stenosis refractory to medical therapy.[77] Subjective factors that may influence decisions include severity of symptoms, angiographic appearance of stenosis, adequacy of collaterals, and the age of the patient.[70] Asymptomatic patients generally do not warrant therapy given that one must consider the vertebrobasilar circulation as a confluence of two vessels, either of which may adequately perfuse the posterior circulation. Significant numbers of patients remain asymptomatic with occlusion of one vertebral artery. Patients with extracranial vertebral artery disease may often present with severe stroke and no preceding TIA. For this reason many operators will treat asymptomatic high-grade (≥70%) stenosis in the setting of a dominant or singular vertebral artery.[72]

Surgical therapy for vertebral ostial stenosis includes transsubclavian endarterectomy, transposition of the vertebral to the ipsilateral common carotid, and reimplantation of the vertebral artery with vein graft extension to the subclavian artery, all rarely performed today.[75] Reports of surgical endarterectomy and vessel reconstruction are challenging and complications are not infrequent with morbidity and mortality rates as high as 20%.[70,77,82,83] For proximal vertebral artery reconstruction, early complication rates have been reported from 2.5% to 25% with perioperative mortality rates of 0% to 4%.[75,84,85]

Multiple nonrandomized case series reporting outcomes of endovascular treatment for vertebral artery stenosis exist.[12,77,86–103] Most of these series are for primary stenting reporting good technical success rates with mean 30-day major stroke or death rates of 3.2%.[77,104] One series specific to ostial lesions showed periprocedural stroke risks of 5% in 58 patients, whereas another series showed an overall stroke risk of 8% over 25 months.[105–107] In a 2006 literature review of 300 interventions for proximal vertebral artery stenosis, the mortality rate was 0.3%, with a 5.5% rate for periprocedural neurologic complications, and 0.7% rate of future posterior circulation stroke with a mean follow-up of 14.2 months. After a mean period of 12 months, a 26% restenosis rate was observed but the range was large (0% to 43%) and was not consistently correlated with recurrent symptoms.[107,108]

Based on available data, stenting of the proximal vertebral artery has been deemed safe with a low risk of periprocedural and future ischemic events. The procedure appears efficacious given that it is performed in symptomatic patients with high-grade stenosis who are refractory to medical management; however, patient selection as well as proficiency and experience with interventional technique remains important in reproducing similar results. Restenosis does appear to be a potential problem, although it does not always correlate with recurrent symptoms.[107]

Technique

Preprocedural diagnostic angiography including cervicocerebral arch and intracranial injections should be performed to adequately plan the procedure. Intracranial views serve to identify collateral flow including the contralateral vertebral artery and adequacy of the posterior communicating arteries (FIGURE 42.10). As with other great-vessel interventions, antiplatelet therapy is essential and the femoral approach is preferred. A 6 French guide catheter or equivalent sheath will typically accommodate most stents appropriate for vertebral artery lesions.[72]

Although some success has been shown with angioplasty alone, recurrence rates are high, occurring in up to 10% in one series[92] and 75% in another,[91] and, in general, primary stenting is indicated to prevent elastic recoil and restenosis.[100] Vertebral origin lesions are usually managed with balloon-expandable stents (3.5 to 6 mm) for reasons of precise placement as previously discussed as well as the advantage of immediate protection if dissection is to occur given the potential stroke risk (FIGURE 42.11). The vertebral artery origin typically has a well-developed muscularis, and plaque burden often extends into the subclavian artery, requiring a stent with high radial force.[72] In proximal lesions it is important that the stent completely covers the ostium of the vessel, which usually requires leaving

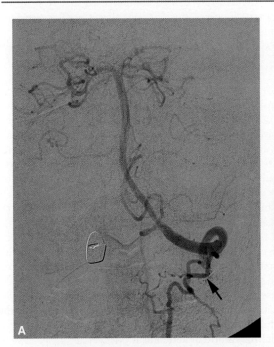
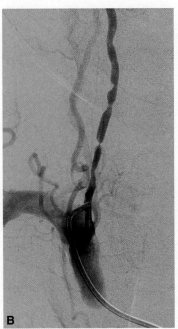
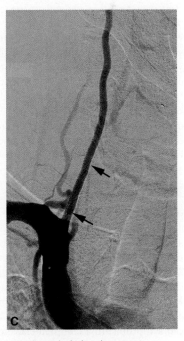

FIGURE 42.10 Right vertebral angioplasty and stent placement. **A.** Proximal left vertebral artery is occluded and reconstitutes via collaterals distally (*arrow*). **B.** Multiple stenosis along the proximal right vertebral artery. Distally the right vertebral is widely patent. **C.** Post-angioplasty and stenting of the proximal right vertebral artery with a self-expanding stent shows an excellent radiographic result (*arrows*).

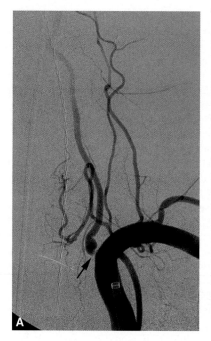
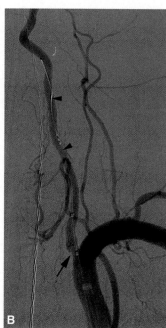

FIGURE 42.11 Left vertebral angioplasty and stent placement. **A.** High-grade stenosis (*arrow*) of the proximal left vertebral artery. Right vertebral artery (not shown) is stenotic as well. **B.** Post-angioplasty and stenting of the proximal left vertebral artery with a balloon-expandable stent shows an acceptable radiographic result (*arrow*); performed without distal embolic protection over a conventional guide wire (*arrowheads*).

1 to 2 mm of stent extending into the subclavian artery. This allows for adequate coverage of plaque within the subclavian artery contributing to the vertebral artery origin lesion, decreasing the likelihood of restenosis. Typically no further angioplasty will be necessary, although poststent dilatation may be required to achieve an adequate angiographic result.

The use of EPDs is unclear. Although one may assume that embolic protection may be of benefit, this has not been definitively shown, and, in general, its use largely depends on the size of the vertebral lumen and ability to accommodate the device, which is usually 4 mm.[70] The small size of the vertebral artery as well as difficulty in identifying a straight segment of the vessel in which to deploy the EPD may preclude routine use. One must also consider possible difficulties in retrieving the device including unfavorable angles of the vertebral artery origin subsequent to stent placement. Complications from proximal vertebral artery intervention include posterior distribution stroke and TIAs, which are generally embolic and occur in approximately 5% of interventions.

Outcomes

Multiple retrospective case series have been reported on the efficacy of angioplasty and stenting for the treatment of extracranial vertebral artery disease (Table 42.2). In general the technical success rate is high, ranging from 93% to 100% with 30-day rates of stroke and all-cause death ranging from 0% to 6.3%.[12,77,86,88–90,93,96,97,100,107,109–111] Regarding long-term patency, restenosis rates have been somewhat high, ranging from 3% to 50%, although restenosis does not always correlate with recurrent symptoms. In a comprehensive review of all available literature until 2005, 300 interventions for proximal vertebral artery stenosis were identified with a mortality rate of 0.3%, a 5.5% rate of periprocedural neurologic complications, and a 0.7% rate of future posterior circulation stroke with a mean

follow-up of 14.2 months. After a mean period of 12 months, a 26% recurrent stenosis rate was observed but the range was large (0% to 43%) and was not consistently correlated with recurrent symptoms.[107,108]

In summary proximal vertebral artery endovascular intervention is safe and feasible with high primary success rates and a low risk of periprocedural neurologic complications. The recurrent stenosis rate is high compared to that seen in the carotid artery; however, this does not always predict recurrent symptoms.

Proximal Great-Vessel Dissection

Dissection involving the supra-aortic trunk vessels is most often an extension of dissection of the aortic arch. Traumatic dissection occurs in approximately 1% of all patients with blunt injury mechanisms and is often initially unrecognized.[112] Focal, isolated dissections involving the great vessels may occur from trauma but will most commonly be iatrogenic, often resulting from inadvertent wire or line placement or as a complication of endovascular procedures (FIGURE 42.12).

The annual incidence of spontaneous carotid artery dissection is 2.5 to 3 per 100,000 (most of which occur in the ICA), whereas the incidence of spontaneous vertebral artery dissection is 1 to 1.5 per 100,000.[112] Carotid dissection accounts for approximately 2% of ischemic strokes and for 15% to 20% of ischemic strokes in patients younger than 45.[112] The incidence and consequences of vertebral artery dissections are less well-defined.[113] Spontaneous dissections of the proximal great vessels do occur; however, the incidence is minor compared to that seen in the internal carotid or vertebral arteries.

Carotid dissection typically presents with pain on one side of the head or neck accompanied by a sudden onset of neurologic symptoms including possible cerebral or retinal ischemia and Horner syndrome. Vertebral artery dissection may

Table 42.2

Available Literature Related to Stenting of the Proximal Vertebral Artery

Author	Year	Patients/ lesions	Vertebral artery	Subclav artery	Stents	Tech success	Minor compl	Major compl	30-day	Mean F/U	Restenosis	1% patent	2% patent
Chastain et al.[88]	1999	50/55	—	—	100%	98%	0%	0%	4%	25 mo	10%	90% @ 25 mo	NA
Malek et al.[97]	1999	21/21	13	8	100%	100%	9.5%	9.5%	4.8%	20.7 mo	50%	NA	NA
Piotin et al.[100]	2000	7/7	7	—	100%	100%	0%	0%	0%	15 mo	0%	100%	NA
Jenkins et al.[93]	2001	32/37	—	—	100%	100%	NA	NA	3%	10.6 mo	3%	97% @ 10.6 mo	100% @ 10.6 mo
Mukherjee et al.[12]	2001	12/12	12	—	100%	100%	NA	NA	NA	NA	NA	NA	NA
Chiras et al.[89]	2002	11/11	11	—	100%	100%	NA	0%	NA	NA	NA	NA	NA
Albuquerque et al.[86]	2003	33/33	33	—	100%	97%	6.1%	0%	3%	16.2 mo	43% (>50%)	67% @ 16.2 mo	NA
Cloud et al.[90]	2003	14/14	14	—	71.4%	100%	0%	0%	0%	33.6%	10% stents	90% stents	NA
Lutsep et al.[96]	2004	18/18	—	—	100%	100%	NA	NA	0%	6 mo	42.9% @ 6 mo	67	NA
Hauth et al.[109]	2004	16/16	16	—	31.3%	87%	18.8%	6.3%	6.3%	NA	NA	NA	NA
Dabus et al.[110]	2006	25/28	—	—	82.1%	92.8%	NA	0%	0%	24 mo	NA	NA	NA
Eberhardt et al.[107]	2006	11/11	11	—	100%	100%	NA	NA	0%	6–36 mo	50%	NA	NA
Coward et al.[77]	2007	8/8	8	—	33%	100%	25%	0%	0%	4.5 y	50% @ 9.6 mo	50% @ 9.6 mo	NA
Zavala-Alarcon et al.[111]	2008	28/35	25	10	100%	96%	3.5%	0%	0%	14.2 mo	NA	NA	NA

Tech, technical; Compl, complication; Patent, patency; F/U, follow-up; S, subclavian artery; V, vertebral artery; NA, not applicable.

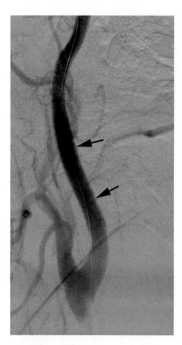

FIGURE 42.12 Dissection of the left internal carotid artery by the guiding catheter during an intracranial embolization procedure. Dissection successfully treated by self-expanding stent placement (*arrows*).

be propagated by sudden or excessive neck movement and may present with headache, neck pain, vertigo, nausea, visual disturbances, or syncope.[75] Diagnosis usually begins with noninvasive imaging, such as CTA or MRA; however, catheter-based angiographic evaluation may be necessary to confirm or dispute findings of noninvasive imaging methods prior to initiating potential medical or interventional therapies.

Treatment for asymptomatic dissection is debatable with both anticoagulation and antiplatelet agents advocated as treatment methods; however, there is limited evidence on which to base recommendations with no randomized trials comparing anticoagulant and antiplatelet therapy to each other or placebo.[112,114–116] Arterial dissections typically heal within 3 to 6 months, with resolution of stenosis in 90%, and recanalization of occlusions in approximately 50%.[112] For symptomatic patients anticoagulant therapy is typically recommended with antiplatelet therapy replacing it once symptoms have resolved and imaging demonstrates healing of the dissection flap.[75] There is no clear length of time for which antiplatelet therapy should be continued.

Surgical or endovascular therapy is generally reserved for patients who have persistent or recurrent symptoms and have failed to respond to anticoagulation or for flow-limiting dissections. Urgent intervention is recommended by some operators for all symptomatic patients to stabilize the dissection flap and reduce risks of additional thrombotic events and to restore cerebral perfusion provided that irreversible infarction has not already occurred. If intervention is deemed necessary, the specific technique is the same as that described for atherosclerotic disease. Use of self-expanding stents is more plausible because they may extend into areas subject to external compression (FIGURE 42.12).

Inadvertent Brachiocephalic Arterial Catheter Placement

Insertion of central venous catheters is performed millions of times per year, most of which are successful and uncomplicated even when performed without imaging guidance. Arterial complications are reported between 0.5% and 3.7%, although the true incidence is likely unknown due to underreporting.[117–119] Typically these are simple access needle punctures with an estimated inadvertent arterial large-caliber catheter placement occurring in some 0.1% to 0.8% of attempted central line placements.[120] Risk factors contributing to this include obesity, prior surgery or radiation therapy to the neck or upper chest, multiple prior central venous catheter insertions, multiple needle passes, and inexperience.[117] Although inadvertent arterial puncture with a small needle is usually benign, arterial cannulation with larger dilators, sheaths, or catheters will result in arteriotomy sites, which will often lead to significant hemorrhage, pseudoaneurysm formation, arteriovenous fistula formation, hemothorax, ischemic stroke, and potential airway obstruction from expanding hematoma and thus requiring therapy.[117,120–122] These complications may lead to significant morbidity and mortality as well as litigation.[123]

In patients with normal clotting factors, puncture of the subclavian artery with an 18- to 25-gauge access needle is unlikely to result in significant complication and the needle can simply be withdrawn and pressure held if the site is accessible.[124,125] The same is true for inadvertent needle placement within the carotid artery. If large-bore inadvertent catheter placement does occur, the treatment options will depend on the size of the catheter, presence or absence of symptoms, artery canalized, and length of time before recognition. Depending on these factors there are several treatment options available including removal and external compression, off-label use of percutaneous closure devices, endovascular intervention with stent-graft placement, or surgical repair.[126]

Usually for catheters of 7 French size or larger, removal with manual pressure is not recommended. With catheters of this size, manual pressure control may be associated with significant morbidity including pseudoaneurysm, expanding hematoma with airway compromise, and stroke rates as high as 5.6%.[125] Adequate pressure in the cervical area may not be possible without inducing at least some degree of cerebral hypoperfusion. With regard to inadvertent subclavian artery catheterization, the clavicle and first rib typically prevent adequate manual pressure. Prolonged arterial canalization is worrisome because thrombus formation at the site of arterial injury may result in vascular occlusion or thromboembolism and stroke. If immediate treatment is not possible, anticoagulation should be initiated.[125] If inadvertent placement occurs in an anesthetized patient, then elective surgery should be postponed and the catheter dealt with first. Several cases of unrecognized stroke in the anesthetized patient following the pull/pressure method have been reported in this setting even in light of normal carotid sonography.[125,127] If the pull/pressure method is used, it is imperative to be aware that pseudoaneurysm or arteriovenous fistula formation may be observed as late as 2 weeks after the event and, therefore, follow-up imaging is indicated.[125]

If inadvertent subclavian arterial catheterization is recognized promptly before the catheter is removed, the access site may be successfully controlled with one of several available percutaneous closure devices.[117,128] These closure devices are generally not recommended for the carotid artery because any inadvertent arterial narrowing, occlusion, or thrombus may result in carotid ischemia. Arteriotomy closure can be augmented with arterial balloon catheterization of the injured vessel to provide balloon tamponade as an adjunct for manual pressure hemostasis of inadvertent arterial punctures (FIGURE 42.13).

If the preceding removal measures are not possible, then additional options are placement of a covered stent or surgical exploration. Surgery for inadvertent subclavian, proximal carotid, or vertebral catheter placement presents significant morbidity, requiring partial removal of the first rib or thoracotomy. Surgery

typically is reserved if stent grafting is not a viable option. Percutaneous stent grafting of iatrogenic and noniatrogenic bleeding, arterial injury, and pseudoaneurysm formation is a recognized successful treatment with low complication rates when compared to surgery.[117]

ENDOVASCULAR THERAPY FOR ARTERIOPATHIES

The two forms of arteriopathies that affect the great vessels are Takayasu arteritis and temporal arteritis (see also Section 6: Vasculitides). Both are forms of giant cell arteritis but with

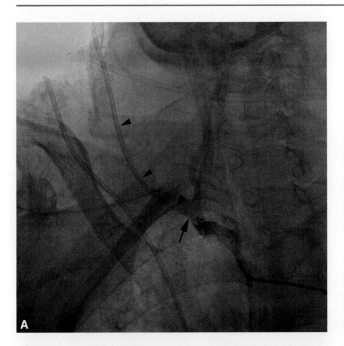

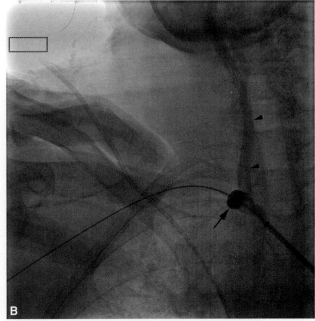

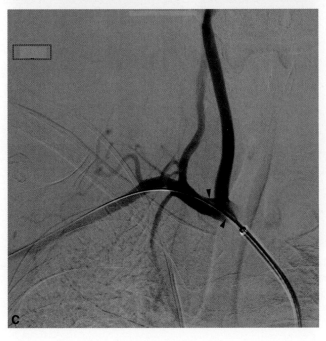

FIGURE 42.13 Central venous catheter inadvertently placed into the left subclavian artery. **A.** Brachiocephalic angiography shows central venous catheter (*arrowheads*) coursing into the proximal left subclavian artery (*arrow*). **B.** Removal of central venous catheter was undertaken using a combination of external manual compression (hand in image) and internally using an occlusion balloon (*arrow*). Injection via the introducer sheath in the right brachiocephalic artery shows flow into the right carotid artery (*arrowheads*) but no flow into the subclavian artery. **C.** Subclavian angiogram following manual compression and balloon occlusion for 10 minutes shows an excellent radiographic result without contrast extravasation. Filling defect in the contrast column extending into the right subclavian artery (*arrowheads*) is the deflated balloon catheter, which is left in place in the event hemorrhage is noted. If hemorrhage is noted, treatment options at this stage include additional balloon inflation (balloon still in place) or placing a covered stent over the bleeding site via an existing guide wire and through the introducer sheath in place in the right brachiocephalic artery. However, the stent may have to cover the right vertebral artery. Fortunately, the left vertebral artery is the dominate vertebral in this patient, allowing covered stent placement to be an acceptable option if necessary.

different clinical presentations. Temporal arteritis involves the medium and large branches of the great vessels but will typically spare the supra-aortic trunk vessels themselves. The condition is usually seen in females and 95% of patients are over age 50.[1] Headache and scalp tenderness are typically associated with a nodular superficial temporal artery. Biopsy is usually required to make the diagnosis. Angiography may be normal or show smooth areas of stenosis with more severe cases demonstrating vascular occlusion.[1]

Takayasu arteritis is a primary panarteritis of unknown etiology primarily affecting females ages 15 to 45. The pathology involves medium and large vessels producing stenosis, occlusions, segmental dilation, or aneurysm formation including the aorta and its branches.[1,129] Although more common in Asia, the disease is seen worldwide.[129] For Takayasu-related stenoses there are several treatment options including steroid therapy, PTA with or without stenting, and surgery.[130,131]

Glucocorticoids may help improve symptoms in the active stage of the disease.[132] Steroids however, require high doses and long-term administration with variable effects on the degree of stenosis.[131,133] Steroid therapy is usually given in the setting of acute inflammation, this being the most likely time that anti-inflammatory agents will have an effect on improving both symptoms and reducing degree of stenosis. Chronic inactive stenosis may respond less favorably or not at all to medical therapy, leaving endovascular or surgical therapy as the only reasonable option for symptomatic lesions.

Surgery, as with atherosclerotic disease, is rather morbid given the thoracic exposures required. Surgery has also been shown to have a higher morbidity in the setting of revascularization for arteritis than in atherosclerosis due to an increased incidence of graft occlusion, suture failure, or aneurysm formation, especially in the active phase of the disease.[134–137] The progressive inflammatory nature of the disease also precludes use of reconstructive surgery because multiple procedures may be needed at various points in time.

Interventional therapy in the setting of acute inflammatory disease should be avoided if possible. Chronic stenotic lesions of Takayasu arteritis tend to be firm, fibrotic, and nonulcerated without superimposed thrombus formation.[132] PTA alone has been used to treat Takayasu-related stenoses of the renal, carotid, subclavian, and superior mesenteric arteries with relatively high success rates.[134,138–145] Unfortunately, with PTA alone there tends to be persistent lesional pressure gradients, which can be improved with stent placement (FIGURE 42.14).

In 2009[147] reported results of angioplasty alone ($n = 18$) or angioplasty and stenting ($n = 17$) in 24 patients with 35 chronic, inactive lesions of the renal, subclavian/innominate, and carotid arteries as well as abdominal aorta. They achieved target lesion revascularization with no residual or minimal residual stenosis in 26 of 35 lesions. Thirty lesions achieved satisfactory hemodynamic correction. Restenosis was observed in eight lesions treated with angioplasty alone and in three lesions treated with angioplasty and stenting with all recurrent stenoses undergoing successful reintervention without significant complication.

Endovascular therapy of chronic, inactive stenotic lesions related to Takayasu arteritis also seems to result in clinical improvement in most patients and appears to be a relatively durable treatment option. Long-term follow-up studies are needed to

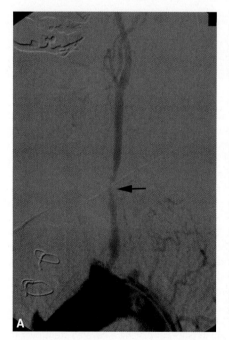 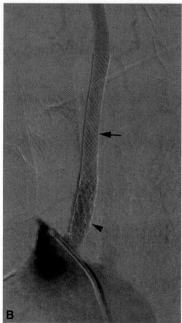 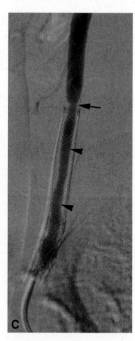

FIGURE 42.14 Angioplasty and stenting of chronic stage of Takayasu arteritis. **A.** Arch aortogram shows stenosis of the proximal left common carotid artery (*arrow*) with occlusion of the right brachiocephalic and left subclavian arteries. **B.** Angiogram following angioplasty and stenting of the proximal left common carotid artery with a self-expanding stent distally (*arrow*) and a balloon-expandable stent proximally (*arrowhead*). There is a good radiographic result. **C.** Six-month follow-up angiogram of the left common carotid artery shows stenosis within the stent (*arrowheads*) and at its distal end (*arrow*).

determine the exact rates of restenosis and other delayed complications (FIGURE 42.14C). The effectiveness of therapy for long-segment disease and occlusions is yet to be defined.

▌ REFERENCES

1. Osborn AG, Jacobs JM, Osborn AG. *Diagnostic Cerebral Angiography.* 2nd ed. Philadelphia, PA: Lippincott Willims & Wilkins; 1999.
2. Chung JH, Ghoshhajra BB, Rojas CA, et al. CT angiography of the thoracic aorta. *Radiol Clin North Am* 2010;48:249–264, vii.
3. Ochkurenko AM. Variants of the aortic arch branches [in Russian]. *Klin Khir* 1966;12:17–18.
4. Liechty JD, Shields TW, Anson BJ. Variations pertaining to the aortic arches and their branches; with comments on surgically important types. *Q Bull Northwest Univ Med Sch* 1957;31:136–143.
5. Jakanani GC, Adair W. Frequency of variations in aortic arch anatomy depicted on multidetector CT. *Clin Radiol* 2010;65:481–487.
6. Berko NS, Jain VR, Godelman A, et al. Variants and anomalies of thoracic vasculature on computed tomographic angiography in adults. *J Comput Assist Tomogr* 2009;33:523–528.
7. Layton KF, Kallmes DF, Cloft HJ, et al. Bovine aortic arch variant in humans: clarification of a common misnomer. *AJNR Am J Neuroradiol* 2006;27:1541–1542.
8. Pavlova-Poliakova MM. On anatomical variants of the aortic arch and its branches [in Russian]. *Khirurgiia (Mosk)* 1962;38:51–55.
9. Terentev GV. Variants of aortic arch branches [in Russian]. *Grudn Khir* 1964;6:55–57.
10. Tsutsumi M, Ueno Y, Kazekawa K, et al. Aberrant right subclavian artery—three case reports. *Neurol Med Chir (Tokyo)* 2002;42:396–398.
11. Morris P. *Practical Neuroangiography.* 2nd ed. Philadelphia, PA: Lippincott Williams & Wilkins; 2007.
12. Mukherjee D, Roffi M, Kapadia SR, et al. Percutaneous intervention for symptomatic vertebral artery stenosis using coronary stents. *J Invasive Cardiol* 2001;13:363–366.
13. Lin SC, Trocciola SM, Rhee J, et al. Analysis of anatomic factors and age in patients undergoing carotid angioplasty and stenting. *Ann Vasc Surg* 2005;19:798–804.
14. Criado FJ. Endovascular techniques for supra-aortic trunk intervention. *Perspect Vasc Surg Endovasc Ther* 2007;19:231–237.
15. Caplan LR, Wolpert SM. Angiography in patients with occlusive cerebrovascular disease: views of a stroke neurologist and neuroradiologist. *AJNR Am J Neuroradiol* 1991;12:593–601.
16. Akers DL, Markowitz IA, Kerstein MD. The value of aortic arch study in the evaluation of cerebrovascular insufficiency. *Am J Surg* 1987;154:230–232.
17. Kadwa AM, Robbs JV, Abdool-Carrim AT. Aortic arch angiography prior to carotid endarterectomy. Is its continued use justified? *Eur J Vasc Endovasc Surg* 1997;13:527–530.
18. Goldstein SJ, Fried AM, Young B, et al. Limited usefulness of aortic arch angiography in the evaluation of carotid occlusive disease. *AJR Am J Roentgenol* 1982;138:103–108.
19. Wyers MC, Powell RJ, Fillinger MF, et al. The value of 3D-CT angiographic assessment prior to carotid stenting. *J Vasc Surg* 2009;49:614–622.
20. Shimizu A, Matsuzaki M. Pulseless disease, Takayasu' disease [in Japanese]. *Ryoikibetsu Shokogun Shirizu* 1996;(14):415–416.
21. Sullivan TM, Gray BH, Bacharach JM, et al. Angioplasty and primary stenting of the subclavian, innominate, and common carotid arteries in 83 patients. *J Vasc Surg* 1998;28:1059–1065.
22. Davis JB, Grove WJ, Julian OC. Thrombic occlusion of the branches of the aortic arch, Martorell's syndrome: report of a case treated surgically. *Ann Surg* 1956;144:124–126.
23. De Bakey ME, Morris GC Jr, Jordan GL Jr, et al. Segmental thromboobliterative disease of branches of aortic arch; successful surgical treatment. *J Am Med Assoc* 1958;166:998–1003.
24. Wholey MH. The supraaortic and vertebral endovascular interventions. *Tech Vasc Interv Radiol* 2004;7:215–225.
25. Crawford ES, De Bakey ME, Morris GC Jr, et al. Surgical treatment of occlusion of the innominate, common carotid, and subclavian arteries: a 10 year experience. *Surgery* 1969;65:17–31.
26. Fry WR, Martin JD, Clagett GP, et al. Extrathoracic carotid reconstruction: the subclavian-carotid artery bypass. *J Vasc Surg* 1992;15:83–88; discussion 8–9.
27. Perler BA, Williams GM. Carotid-subclavian bypass—a decade of experience. *J Vasc Surg* 1990;12:716–722; discussion 22–23.
28. Berguer R, Morasch MD, Kline RA, et al. Cervical reconstruction of the supra-aortic trunks: a 16-year experience. *J Vasc Surg* 1999;29:239–246; discussion 46–48.
29. Berguer R, Morasch MD, Kline RA. Transthoracic repair of innominate and common carotid artery disease: immediate and long-term outcome for 100 consecutive surgical reconstructions. *J Vasc Surg* 1998;27:34–41; discussion 2.
30. Harrigan MR, Deveikis JP. *Handbook of Cerebrovascular Disease and Neurointerventional Technique.* Dordecht, The Netherlands: Humana Press; 2009.
31. Paukovits TM, Haasz J, Molnar A, et al. Transfemoral endovascular treatment of proximal common carotid artery lesions: a single-center experience on 153 lesions. *J Vasc Surg* 2008;48:80–87.
32. Chio FL Jr, Liu MW, Khan MA, et al. Effectiveness of elective stenting of common carotid artery lesions in preventing stroke. *Am J Cardiol* 2003;92:1135–1137.
33. Rodriguez-Lopez JA, Werner A, Martinez R, et al. Stenting for atherosclerotic occlusive disease of the subclavian artery. *Ann Vasc Surg* 1999;13:254–260.
34. Hass WK, Fields WS, North RR, et al. Joint study of extracranial arterial occlusion: II, arteriography, techniques, sites, and complications. *JAMA* 1968;203:961–968.
35. Hadjipetrou P, Cox S, Piemonte T, et al. Percutaneous revascularization of atherosclerotic obstruction of aortic arch vessels. *J Am Coll Cardiol* 1999;33:1238–1245.
36. Fields WS, Lemak NA. Joint study of extracranial arterial occlusion: VII, subclavian steal—a review of 168 cases. *JAMA* 1972;222:1139–1143.
37. Ackermann H, Diener HC, Seboldt H, et al. Ultrasonographic follow-up of subclavian stenosis and occlusion: natural history and surgical treatment. *Stroke* 1988;19:431–435.
38. Reivich M, Holling HE, Roberts B, et al. Reversal of blood flow through the vertebral artery and its effect on cerebral circulation. *N Engl J Med* 1961;265:878–885.
39. Kliewer MA, Hertzberg BS, Kim DH, et al. Vertebral artery Doppler waveform changes indicating subclavian steal physiology. *AJR Am J Roentgenol* 2000;174:815–819.
40. Bachman DM, Kim RM. Transluminal dilatation for subclavian steal syndrome. *AJR Am J Roentgenol* 1980;135:995–996.
41. Queral LA, Criado FJ. The treatment of focal aortic arch branch lesions with Palmaz stents. *J Vasc Surg* 1996;23:368–375.
42. Lyon RD, Shonnard KM, McCarter DL, et al. Supra-aortic arterial stenoses: management with Palmaz balloon-expandable intraluminal stents. *J Vasc Interv Radiol* 1996;7:825–835.
43. Sueoka BL. Percutaneous transluminal stent placement to treat subclavian steal syndrome. *J Vasc Interv Radiol* 1996;7:351–356.
44. Kumar K, Dorros G, Bates MC, et al. Primary stent deployment in occlusive subclavian artery disease. *Cathet Cardiovasc Diagn* 1995;34:281–285.
45. AbuRahma AF, Bates MC, Stone PA, et al. Angioplasty and stenting versus carotid-subclavian bypass for the treatment of isolated subclavian artery disease. *J Endovasc Ther* 2007;14:698–704.
46. Huttl K, Nemes B, Simonffy A, et al. Angioplasty of the innominate artery in 89 patients: experience over 19 years. *Cardiovasc Intervent Radiol* 2002;25:109–114.
47. Millaire A, Trinca M, Marache P, et al. Subclavian angioplasty: immediate and late results in 50 patients. *Cathet Cardiovasc Diagn* 1993;29:8–17.
48. Mathias KD, Luth I, Haarmann P. Percutaneous transluminal angioplasty of proximal subclavian artery occlusions. *Cardiovasc Intervent Radiol* 1993;16:214–218.
49. Duber C, Klose KJ, Kopp H, et al. Percutaneous transluminal angioplasty for occlusion of the subclavian artery: short- and long-term results. *Cardiovasc Intervent Radiol* 1992;15:205–210.
50. Selby JB Jr, Matsumoto AH, Tegtmeyer CJ, et al. Balloon angioplasty above the aortic arch: immediate and long-term results. *AJR Am J Roentgenol* 1993;160:631–635.
51. Dorros G, Lewin RF, Jamnadas P, et al. Peripheral transluminal angioplasty of the subclavian and innominate arteries utilizing the brachial approach: acute outcome and follow-up. *Cathet Cardiovasc Diagn* 1990;19:71–76.
52. Bakken AM, Palchik E, Saad WE, et al. Outcomes of endoluminal therapy for ostial disease of the major branches of the aortic arch. *Ann Vasc Surg* 2008;22:388–394.
53. Hebrang A, Maskovic J, Tomac B. Percutaneous transluminal angioplasty of the subclavian arteries: long-term results in 52 patients. *AJR Am J Roentgenol* 1991;156:1091–1094.
54. Al-Mubarak N, Liu MW, Dean LS, et al. Immediate and late outcomes of subclavian artery stenting. *Catheter Cardiovasc Interv* 1999;46:169–172.

55. Henry M, Amor M, Henry I, et al. Percutaneous transluminal angioplasty of the subclavian arteries. *J Endovasc Surg* 1999;6:33–41.
56. Schillinger M, Haumer M, Schillinger S, et al. Risk stratification for subclavian artery angioplasty: is there an increased rate of restenosis after stent implantation? *J Endovasc Ther* 2001;8:550–557.
57. Allie DE, Hebert CJ, Lirtzman MD, et al. Intraoperative innominate and common carotid intervention combined with carotid endarterectomy: a "true" endovascular surgical approach. *J Endovasc Ther* 2004;11:258–262.
58. De Vries JP, Jager LC, Van den Berg JC, et al. Durability of percutaneous transluminal angioplasty for obstructive lesions of proximal subclavian artery: long-term results. *J Vasc Surg* 2005;41:19–23.
59. Peterson BG, Resnick SA, Morasch MD, et al. Aortic arch vessel stenting: a single-center experience using cerebral protection. *Arch Surg* 2006;141:560–563; discussion 3–4.
60. Amor M, Eid-Lidt G, Chati Z, et al. Endovascular treatment of the subclavian artery: stent implantation with or without predilatation. *Catheter Cardiovasc Interv* 2004;63:364–370.
61. Patel SN, White CJ, Collins TJ, et al. Catheter-based treatment of the subclavian and innominate arteries. *Catheter Cardiovasc Interv* 2008;71:963–968.
62. Sixt S, Rastan A, Schwarzwalder U, et al. Results after balloon angioplasty or stenting of atherosclerotic subclavian artery obstruction. *Catheter Cardiovasc Interv* 2009;73:395–403.
63. van Hattum ES, de Vries JP, Lalezari F, et al. Angioplasty with or without stent placement in the brachiocephalic artery: feasible and durable? A retrospective cohort study. *J Vasc Interv Radiol* 2007;18:1088–1093.
64. Van Noord BA, Lin AH, Cavendish JJ. Rates of symptom reoccurrence after endovascular therapy in subclavian artery stenosis and prevalence of subclavian artery stenosis prior to coronary artery bypass grafting. *Vasc Health Risk Manag* 2007;3:759–762.
65. Bates MC, Broce M, Lavigne PS, et al. Subclavian artery stenting: factors influencing long-term outcome. *Catheter Cardiovasc Interv* 2004;61:5–11.
66. Brountzos EN, Petersen B, Binkert C, et al. Primary stenting of subclavian and innominate artery occlusive disease: a single center's experience. *Cardiovasc Intervent Radiol* 2004;27:616–623.
67. Przewlocki T, Kablak-Ziembicka A, Pieniazek P, et al. Determinants of immediate and long-term results of subclavian and innominate artery angioplasty. *Catheter Cardiovasc Interv* 2006;67:519–526.
68. Caplan L. Posterior circulation ischemia: then, now, and tomorrow. The Thomas Willis Lecture-2000. *Stroke* 2000;31:2011–2023.
69. Zaytsev AY, Stoyda AY, Smirnov VE, et al. Endovascular treatment of supra-aortic extracranial stenoses in patients with vertebrobasilar insufficiency symptoms. *Cardiovasc Intervent Radiol* 2006;29:731–738.
70. Mukherjee D, Pineda G. Extracranial vertebral artery intervention. *J Interv Cardiol* 2007;20:409–416.
71. Wityk RJ, Chang HM, Rosengart A, et al. Proximal extracranial vertebral artery disease in the New England Medical Center Posterior Circulation Registry. *Arch Neurol* 1998;55:470–478.
72. Wehman JC, Hanel RA, Guidot CA, et al. Atherosclerotic occlusive extracranial vertebral artery disease: indications for intervention, endovascular techniques, short-term and long-term results. *J Interv Cardiol* 2004;17:219–232.
73. Schwartz CJ, Mitchell JR. Atheroma of the carotid and vertebral arterial systems. *Br Med J* 1961;2:1057–1063.
74. Caplan LR, Wityk RJ, Glass TA, et al. New England Medical Center Posterior Circulation registry. *Ann Neurol* 2004;56:389–398.
75. Brott TG, Halperin JL, Abbara S, et al. 2011 ASA/ACCF/AHA/AANN/AANS/ACR/ASNR/CNS/SAIP/SCAI/SIR/SNIS/SVM/SVS Guideline on the management of patients with extracranial carotid and vertebral artery disease: executive summary. *J Am Coll Cardiol* 2011 Feb 22;57(8):1002–44.
76. Long A, Lepoutre A, Corbillon E, et al. Critical review of non- or minimally invasive methods (duplex ultrasonography, MR- and CT-angiography) for evaluating stenosis of the proximal internal carotid artery. *Eur J Vasc Endovasc Surg* 2002;24:43–52.
77. Coward LJ, McCabe DJ, Ederle J, et al. Long-term outcome after angioplasty and stenting for symptomatic vertebral artery stenosis compared with medical treatment in the Carotid And Vertebral Artery Transluminal Angioplasty Study (CAVATAS): a randomized trial. *Stroke* 2007;38:1526–1530.
78. Savitz SI, Caplan LR. Vertebrobasilar disease. *N Engl J Med* 2005;352:2618–2626.
79. Caplan LR. Atherosclerotic vertebral artery disease in the neck. *Curr Treat Options Cardiovasc Med* 2003;5:251–256.
80. Canyigit M, Arat A, Cil BE, et al. Management of vertebral stenosis complicated by presence of acute thrombus. *Cardiovasc Intervent Radiol* 2007;30:317–320.
81. Eckert B. Acute vertebrobasilar occlusion: current treatment strategies. *Neurol Res* 2005;27(suppl 1):S36–S41.
82. Ausman JI, Diaz FG, Sadasivan B, et al. Intracranial vertebral endarterectomy. *Neurosurgery* 1990;26:465–471.
83. Blacker DJ, Flemming KD, Wijdicks EF. Risk of ischemic stroke in patients with symptomatic vertebrobasilar stenosis undergoing surgical procedures. *Stroke* 2003;34:2659–2663.
84. Berguer R. Suboccipital approach to the distal vertebral artery. *J Vasc Surg* 1999;30:344–349.
85. Berguer R, Morasch MD, Kline RA. A review of 100 consecutive reconstructions of the distal vertebral artery for embolic and hemodynamic disease. *J Vasc Surg* 1998;27:852–859.
86. Albuquerque FC, Fiorella D, Han P, et al. A reappraisal of angioplasty and stenting for the treatment of vertebral origin stenosis. *Neurosurgery* 2003;53:607–614; discussion 14–16.
87. Barakate MS, Snook KL, Harrington TJ, et al. Angioplasty and stenting in the posterior cerebral circulation. *J Endovasc Ther* 2001;8:558–565.
88. Chastain HD II, Campbell MS, Iyer S, et al. Extracranial vertebral artery stent placement: in-hospital and follow-up results. *J Neurosurg* 1999;91:547–552.
89. Chiras J, Vallee JN, Spelle L, et al. Endoluminal dilatations and stenosis of symptomatic vertebral arteries [in French]. *Rev Neurol (Paris)* 2002;158:51–57.
90. Cloud GC, Crawley F, Clifton A, et al. Vertebral artery origin angioplasty and primary stenting: safety and restenosis rates in a prospective series. *J Neurol Neurosurg Psychiatry* 2003;74:586–590.
91. Crawley F, Brown MM, Clifton AG. Angioplasty and stenting in the carotid and vertebral arteries. *Postgrad Med J* 1998;74:7–10.
92. Higashida RT, Tsai FY, Halbach VV, et al. Transluminal angioplasty for atherosclerotic disease of the vertebral and basilar arteries. *J Neurosurg* 1993;78:192–198.
93. Jenkins JS, White CJ, Ramee SR, et al. Vertebral artery stenting. *Catheter Cardiovasc Interv* 2001;54:1–5.
94. Kachel R, Basche S, Heerklotz I, et al. Percutaneous transluminal angioplasty (PTA) of supra-aortic arteries especially the internal carotid artery. *Neuroradiology* 1991;33:191–194.
95. Levy EI, Hanel RA, Bendok BR, et al. Staged stent-assisted angioplasty for symptomatic intracranial vertebrobasilar artery stenosis. *J Neurosurg* 2002;97:1294–1301.
96. Stenting of Symptomatic Atherosclerotic Lesions in the Vertebral or Intracranial Arteries (SSYLVIA): study results. *Stroke* 2004;35:1388–1392.
97. Malek AM, Higashida RT, Phatouros CC, et al. Treatment of posterior circulation ischemia with extracranial percutaneous balloon angioplasty and stent placement. *Stroke* 1999;30:2073–2085.
98. Motarjeme A, Keifer JW, Zuska AJ. Percutaneous transluminal angioplasty of the brachiocephalic arteries. *AJR Am J Roentgenol* 1982;138:457–462.
99. Nahser HC, Henkes H, Weber W, et al. Intracranial vertebrobasilar stenosis: angioplasty and follow-up. *AJNR Am J Neuroradiol* 2000;21:1293–1301.
100. Piotin M, Spelle L, Martin JB, et al. Percutaneous transluminal angioplasty and stenting of the proximal vertebral artery for symptomatic stenosis. *AJNR Am J Neuroradiol* 2000;21:727–731.
101. Qureshi AI, Suri MF, Khan J, et al. Abciximab as an adjunct to high-risk carotid or vertebrobasilar angioplasty: preliminary experience. *Neurosurgery* 2000;46:1316–1324; discussion 24–25.
102. Rasmussen PA, Perl J II, Barr JD, et al. Stent-assisted angioplasty of intracranial vertebrobasilar atherosclerosis: an initial experience. *J Neurosurg* 2000;92:771–778.
103. Sampei K, Hashimoto N, Kazekawa K, et al. Autoperfusion balloon catheter for treatment of vertebral artery stenosis. *Neuroradiology* 1995;37:561–563.
104. Coward LJ, Featherstone RL, Brown MM. Percutaneous transluminal angioplasty and stenting for vertebral artery stenosis. *Cochrane Database Syst Rev* 2005;(2):CD000516.
105. Lin YH, Juang JM, Jeng JS, et al. Symptomatic ostial vertebral artery stenosis treated with tubular coronary stents: clinical results and restenosis analysis. *J Endovasc Ther* 2004;11:719–726.
106. Ko YG, Park S, Kim JY, et al. Percutaneous interventional treatment of extracranial vertebral artery stenosis with coronary stents. *Yonsei Med J* 2004;45:629–634.
107. Eberhardt O, Naegele T, Raygrotzki S, et al. Stenting of vertebrobasilar arteries in symptomatic atherosclerotic disease and acute occlusion: case series and review of the literature. *J Vasc Surg* 2006;43:1145–1154.
108. Brott TG, Halperin JL, Abbara S, et al. 2011 ASA/ACCF/AHA/AANN/AANS/ACR/ASNR/CNS/SAIP/SCAI/SIR/SNIS/SVM/SVS Guideline on the management of patients with extracranial carotid and vertebral artery disease. *J Am Coll Cardiol* 2011 Feb 22;57(8):e16–94.

109. Hauth EA, Gissler HM, Drescher R, et al. Angioplasty or stenting of extra- and intracranial vertebral artery stenoses. *Cardiovasc Intervent Radiol* 2004;27:51–57.

110. Dabus G, Gerstle RJ, Derdeyn CP, et al. Endovascular treatment of the vertebral artery origin in patients with symptoms of vertebrobasilar ischemia. *Neuroradiology* 2006;48:917–923.

111. Zavala-Alarcon E, Emmans L, Little R, et al. Percutaneous intervention for posterior fossa ischemia. A single center experience and review of the literature. *Int J Cardiol* 2008;127:70–77.

112. Redekop GJ. Extracranial carotid and vertebral artery dissection: a review. *Can J Neurol Sci* 2008;35:146–152.

113. Schievink WI. Spontaneous dissection of the carotid and vertebral arteries. *N Engl J Med* 2001;344:898–906.

114. Lyrer P, Engelter S. Antithrombotic drugs for carotid artery dissection. *Stroke* 2004;35:613–614.

115. Lyrer P, Engelter S. Antithrombotic drugs for carotid artery dissection. *Cochrane Database Syst Rev* 2000;(4):CD000255.

116. Lyrer P, Engelter S. Antithrombotic drugs for carotid artery dissection. *Cochrane Database Syst Rev* 2003;(3):CD000255.

117. Nicholson T, Ettles D, Robinson G. Managing inadvertent arterial catheterization during central venous access procedures. *Cardiovasc Intervent Radiol* 2004;27:21–25.

118. Mansfield PF, Hohn DC, Fornage BD, et al. Complications and failures of subclavian-vein catheterization. *N Engl J Med* 1994;331:1735–1738.

119. Mercer-Jones MA, Wenstone R, Hershman MJ. Fatal subclavian artery haemorrhage. A complication of subclavian vein catheterisation. *Anaesthesia* 1995;50:639–640.

120. Reuber M, Dunkley LA, Turton EP, et al. Stroke after internal jugular venous cannulation. *Acta Neurol Scand* 2002;105:235–239.

121. Shah PM, Babu SC, Goyal A, et al. Arterial misplacement of large-caliber cannulas during jugular vein catheterization: case for surgical management. *J Am Coll Surg* 2004;198:939–944.

122. Eckhardt WF, Iaconetti J, Kwon JS, et al. Inadvertent carotid artery cannulation during pulmonary artery catheter insertion. *J Cardiothorac Vasc Anesth* 1996;10:283–290.

123. Domino KB, Bowdle TA, Posner KL, et al. Injuries and liability related to central vascular catheters: a closed claims analysis. *Anesthesiology* 2004;100:1411–1418.

124. Sznajder JI, Zveibil FR, Bitterman H, et al. Central vein catheterization. Failure and complication rates by three percutaneous approaches. *Arch Intern Med* 1986;146:259–261.

125. Guilbert MC, Elkouri S, Bracco D, et al. Arterial trauma during central venous catheter insertion: case series, review and proposed algorithm. *J Vasc Surg* 2008;48:918–925; discussion 25.

126. Powers CJ, Zomorodi AR, Britz GW, et al. Endovascular management of inadvertent brachiocephalic arterial catheterization. *J Neurosurg* 2011;114:146–152.

127. Kron IL, Joob AW, Lake CL, et al. Arch vessel injury during pulmonary artery catheter placement. *Ann Thorac Surg* 1985;39:223–224.

128. Berlet MH, Steffen D, Shaughness G, et al. Closure using a surgical closure device of inadvertent subclavian artery punctures during central venous catheter placement. *Cardiovasc Intervent Radiol* 2001;24:122–124.

129. Yamato M, Lecky JW, Hiramatsu K, et al. Takayasu arteritis: radiographic and angiographic findings in 59 patients. *Radiology* 1986;161:329–334.

130. Shelhamer JH, Volkman DJ, Parrillo JE, et al. Takayasu's arteritis and its therapy. *Ann Intern Med* 1985;103:121–126.

131. Li D, Ma S, Li G, et al. Endovascular stent implantation for isolated pulmonary arterial stenosis caused by Takayasu's arteritis. *Clin Res Cardiol* 2010;99:573–575.

132. Sharma BK, Jain S, Bali HK, et al. A follow-up study of balloon angioplasty and de-novo stenting in Takayasu arteritis. *Int J Cardiol* 2000;75(suppl 1):S147–S152.

133. Fukuda Y, Shirai K, Takamiya Y, et al. Isolated pulmonary arterial stenosis caused by Takayasu's arteritis in an elderly male. *J Cardiol* 2008;51:196–200.

134. Kumar S, Mandalam KR, Rao VR, et al. Percutaneous transluminal angioplasty in nonspecific aortoarteritis (Takayasu's disease): experience of 16 cases. *Cardiovasc Intervent Radiol* 1989;12:321–325.

135. Inada K, Katsumura T, Hirai J, et al. Surgical treatment in the aortitis syndrome. *Arch Surg* 1970;100:220–224.

136. Ishikawa K. Survival and morbidity after diagnosis of occlusive thromboaortopathy (Takayasu's disease). *Am J Cardiol* 1981;47:1026–1032.

137. Kimoto S. The history and present status of aortic surgery in Japan, particularly for aortitis syndrome. *J Cardiovasc Surg (Torino)* 1979;20:107–126.

138. Park JH, Han MC, Kim SH, et al. Takayasu arteritis: angiographic findings and results of angioplasty. *AJR Am J Roentgenol* 1989;153:1069–1074.

139. Srur MF, Sos TA, Saddekni S, et al. Intimal fibromuscular dysplasia and Takayasu arteritis: delayed response to percutaneous transluminal renal angioplasty. *Radiology* 1985;157:657–660.

140. Hodgins GW, Dutton JW. Transluminal dilatation for Takayasu's arteritis. *Can J Surg* 1984;27:355–357.

141. Yagura M, Sano I, Akioka H, et al. Usefulness of percutaneous transluminal angioplasty for aortitis syndrome. *Arch Intern Med* 1984;144:1465–1468.

142. Theron J, Tyler JL. Takayasu's arteritis of the aortic arch: endovascular treatment and correlation with positron emission tomography. *AJNR Am J Neuroradiol* 1987;8:621–626.

143. Tyagi S, Gambhir DS, Kaul UA, et al. A decade of subclavian angioplasty: aortoarteritis versus atherosclerosis. *Indian Heart J* 1996;48:667–671.

144. Tyagi S, Verma PK, Gambhir DS, et al. Early and long-term results of subclavian angioplasty in aortoarteritis (Takayasu disease): comparison with atherosclerosis. *Cardiovasc Intervent Radiol* 1998;21:219–224.

145. Joseph S, Mandalam KR, Rao VR, et al. Percutaneous transluminal angioplasty of the subclavian artery in nonspecific aortoarteritis: results of long-term follow-up. *J Vasc Interv Radiol* 1994;5:573–580.

146. Woo EY, Fairman RM, Velazquez OC, Golden MA, Karmacharya J, Carpenter JP. Endovascular therapy of symptomatic innominate-subclavian arterial occlusive lesions. *Vasc Endovascular Surg.* 2006 Jan–Feb; 40(1):27–33.

147. Lee BB, Laredo J, Neville R, and Villavicencio JL. Endovascular management of takayasu arteritis: is it a durable option? *Vascular* 2009 May–June; 17: 138–46.

Endovascular Therapies: Carotid Bifurcation

WILLIAM A. GRAY

▌ INTRODUCTION

Prior to describing the genesis of carotid artery stenting (CAS) and its early history, it is worthwhile to point out that carotid artery bifurcation stenosis is unique among arterial stenoses causing symptoms; therefore, carotid intervention has different objectives and sensitivities. In all other arterial atherosclerotic stenoses, clinical symptoms and end-organ failure are caused by restriction of flow and ischemia that result in the distal circulatory bed (lower limb, mesenteric, renal, subclavian, etc.). The primary goal of intervention in those lesions is to restore distal flow by relieving the stenosis (endovascular intervention) or bypassing the offending lesion (surgical revascularization), thus relieving symptoms. In carotid bifurcation disease, ongoing symptoms caused by distal cerebral ischemia due to flow restriction are the exception and not the rule as a result of both intra- (circle of Willis) and extracranial collateral supplies. Therefore, most mischief arising from carotid stenosis is related to rupture of the stenotic atherosclerotic plaque and the embolization of the ensuing thrombus and/or atheromatous debris into the distal cerebral circulation, which is exquisitely sensitive to such an assault—this susceptibility to even minor emboli also makes this circulation unique among revascularization targets—surgical or endovascular. The goal of intervention in the carotid lesion, therefore, is not primarily to reduce the stenosis, restore flow, and eliminate ongoing symptoms but to eliminate its future potential to embolize, either by removing it altogether (carotid endarterectomy [CEA]) or covering it and allowing the resulting neointima to "seal" and passivize the lesion (CAS). Thus, in most cases, CEA and CAS are prophylactic interventions meant to avert future symptoms and disability and not to relieve current symptoms.

The current thresholds for justification to intervene on a bifurcation carotid lesion are detailed in a recent multidisciplinary guidelines document, which gives a Class I indication for both CEA and CAS for symptomatic patients (transient ischemic attack [TIA] or nondisabling stroke within the past 6 months) with stenosis greater than 50% by angiography, and a Class IIa and IIb indication for CEA and CAS, respectively, in asymptomatic patients with lesions greater than 70%.[1]

The origins of endovascular therapy for carotid bifurcation disease date back over 30 years with simple balloon angioplasty first being performed in patients with fibromuscular dysplasia.[2] Extending the concept to patients with atherosclerotic internal carotid artery disease, Mathias then performed carotid angioplasty (there being no stents available for the first dozen or so years of percutaneous therapy) in patients with severe stenosis and poor surgical options.[3] In that first experience, three patients were treated and one neurologic event occurred. The subsequent practice of carotid angioplasty was sporadic and primarily in

Europe.[4] In the mid-1990s, Theron reported 259 carotid angioplasties, a minority of which were accompanied by stenting and 188 of which were atherosclerotic. Importantly, roughly half of these cases were performed with a triple coaxial cerebral protection distal occlusion catheter that had previously been proposed by the same author.[5,6] This was the first series of any size that employed an emboli protection device (EPD) and its use was truly prescient. Although it was a nonrandomized experience, Theron found a differential advantage in outcomes among the cases in which the cerebral protection was used. At approximately the same time in the United States, Diethrich published a smaller series of 117 procedures, all with carotid balloon-expandable stents but no embolic protection in patients at high surgical risk, with acceptable results in that early experience.[7] Rounding out the largely pre-EPD and pre-self-expanding stent era is the only multicenter study performed, the Carotid and Vertebral Artery Transluminal Angioplasty Study (CAVATAS) trial, which randomized 504 recently symptomatic patients to either angioplasty of the carotid artery (only ~25% of patients in the trial received stents when they became available) or CEA.[8] Although this trial found no early or late differences in outcomes for stroke and death between CEA and carotid angioplasty, the event rates for both groups were, by today's standards, unacceptably high with a 30-day death and major stroke rate of approximately 6% and death and all stroke rate of approximately 10%. Not surprisingly, there was a greater incidence of late restenosis among the unscaffolded lesions in the angioplasty group.

The outcomes of CAS in the dedicated device era are detailed later in this chapter.

▌ PATIENT SELECTION

Patient selection for CAS has only recently come into sharper focus with increasing experience with outcomes associated with different clinical, comorbid, and anatomic patient types. This relatively late appreciation of selection criteria is not surprising given that, in the United States at least, CAS was initially positioned as the alternative to most of the anatomic and medical comorbidities that actually served as exclusion criteria in previous landmark CEA trials; thus patients with significant comorbidities were intentionally included in the majority of early US CAS studies. Additionally, given the lack of broad experience with the procedure, there were few well understood exclusions for CAS during its early practice.

A gathering experience demonstrates that it is now very clear patient selection in CAS is as important as for CEA (or any intervention), and several analyses of large multicenter CAS databases from the serve to inform regarding the selection considerations in both high and standard surgical risk patients.[9–15]

Patients who have been recently symptomatic (defined as non-disabling stroke or TIA in the past 180 days) undergoing CAS are at roughly twofold increased risk for death/stroke compared with asymptomatic patients, much in the same proportion as with CEA. Those CAS patients over the age of 80 years (and likely increasing continuously through the age ranges) have a greater risk for death/stroke/myocardial infarction (MI) with CAS as well. In the only randomized trial to compare CEA to CAS in the standard surgical risk octogenarian, the per-protocol analysis performed by the Food and Drug Administration (FDA)[12] demonstrated no difference in outcomes between the two therapies by age, albeit with worse outcomes than in the patient under age 80 for both CEA and CAS. CAS in the octogenarian has also been confirmed as safe in high-volume centers without an apparent differential compared with the nonoctogenarian and emphasizes the need for expert and experienced operators, especially in such at-risk patients.[16] Interestingly, and somewhat counter-intuitively, CAS outcomes in both Stent-Protected Angioplasty Versus Carotid Endarterectomy (SPACE) and Carotid Revascularization Endarterectomy Versus Stent Trial (CREST) trials were better in the younger patient under the age of 68 and 60 years, respectively.[13,17]

Prospective, multicenter independent core lab analyses of outcomes by anatomy are limited, but most experienced operators agree, and analyses previously referenced confirm, that lesions with excessive distortion of arch access anatomy, proximal/distal carotid or lesion tortuosity, circumferential lesion calcification, thrombus in situ, lengthy lesions, occluded external carotid artery (ECA), low bifurcations, and total occlusions are to be taken on with caution. Macdonald et al.[18] used a Delphi-style expert consensus document to confirm some of these and other qualities as being high-risk features, especially for the novice carotid stenter. These have not only been subsequently validated using a patient-specific simulation model, but it also appears that a multiplicity of these factors is additive in increasing risk of CAS.[19,20] Patients with severe aortic stenosis and/or severe triple vessel/left main coronary artery disease, especially when accompanied by significant left ventricular dysfunction, need to be approached with care given the possibility of carotid sinus stimulation and the accompanying bradycardia and hypotension that can compromise myocardial perfusion. Additionally, patients with renal failure have demonstrated worse outcomes with CAS in some series.[21] Table 43.1 outlines the various features that have been associated with worse outcomes in CAS and/or make the procedure more technically demanding.

ENDOVASCULAR TREATMENT OPTIONS

CAS is generally a procedure in four parts: access, embolic protection (deployment and retrieval), balloon angioplasty, and stent implantation. Options to vary the endovascular procedure itself, therefore, are quite limited because each part is considered essential to a properly performed intervention although there may be variability among these elements, as discussed later.

ANATOMIC AND LESION CONSIDERATIONS

When planning for a CAS procedure, anatomic and lesion-specific considerations are paramount in achieving not only an uncomplicated outcome but also streamlining the procedure for the patient and operator alike.

Table 43.1

Anatomic and Clinical Features Associated with Worse Outcomes or More Technically Demanding Procedures in CAS

Type III or bovine aortic arch	Age >80 years
Circumferential lesion calcification	Symptoms in the past 6 months
Low carotid bifurcation	Atrial fibrillation
Angulated ICA origin	End-stage renal disease
Severe arch atheroma	Impending major surgery
Occluded ECA	

Anatomic considerations begin with femoral access, which is the typical access point for CAS. Excessive iliac tortuosity can limit the ability to maneuver catheters in the more proximal aorta or carotid vessels. If iliac access is unavailable altogether, then radial or brachial approaches to the procedure can be performed safely but will require some experience and special technical considerations.[22] When upper extremity access is used, it is generally considered easier to work from the contralateral upper extremity from the index lesion because this allows for a simpler, less abrupt and less tortuous entry into the target common carotid artery (CCA) with the guide or sheath, although this will always be dictated primarily by the patient-specific anatomy.

The next anatomic consideration is the aortic arch, a critical feature that can make difficult or prevent the performance of the CAS procedure altogether and may lead to neurologic complication. Data from the CAPTURE postmarket registry demonstrate that roughly 20% of all periprocedural strokes that occur in CAS are in a nonipsilateral territory from the lesion being treated. This presumes an etiology arising from the aortic arch during access, and, therefore, since an equal distribution to the ipsilateral carotid can also be assumed, the rate of stroke related to access may be as high as 35%–40%.[23] Accordingly, attention has been focused on minimizing or eliminating the arch as a source of this complication. Specifically, new device approaches (to be detailed) have been developed and the more routine use of cross-sectional imaging of the aortic arch to facilitate patient selection and planning is now advocated, especially for less experienced operators.

The aforementioned differential outcomes noted with the octogenarian patients with CAS are thought to be at least partially linked to age-related changes in the aorta, making establishing safe access more challenging because as patients age, the aorta can become elongated, redundant, and rotated. There are three general types of arches, each with increasing complexity and difficulty of catheterization (FIGURE 43.1). Because within the thorax the aorta is "fixed" between the sternum and spine, not only are the great vessel origins displaced proximally toward the heart, there is significant worsening of the acuity of their angle of origin when approaching from femoral access, but the distal arch can also become "humpbacked." This latter feature results in an even greater acuity in the angle of entry because now the

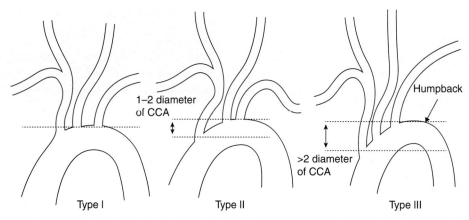

FIGURE 43.1 Variability of aortic arch types increasing in catheterization difficulty as described by Madhwal S, Rajagopal V, Bhatt DL, et al. Predictors of difficult carotid stenting as determined by aortic arch angiography. *Cath Lab Digest* 2008;20:5.

catheter path does not travel directly retrograde from the aorta to the CCA entry in the cranial direction, but rather ultimately travels caudal from the apex formed by the elongated distal aorta and then back to cranial as it enters the CCA. Additionally, the ability to advance catheters cranially is reduced because their forward motion is stored in the deformed distal arch. Adding to the anatomic considerations of arch complexity is the presence of atherosclerotic disease, especially when calcification involves the origins of the great vessels, which can independently cause difficulty with catheter passage.

Following the aortic arch, the anatomy of the carotid artery—common, bifurcation, and internal segments—additionally factors into the ability to perform CAS and, potentially, what form of EPD is chosen. It will also be evident to the reader that complexity of the arch married to a convoluted carotid artery anatomy additively impedes procedural planning and performance. Regarding CCA considerations, a bovine origin of the left CCA that originates not from the aorta but from the proximal innominate artery and typically is accompanied by retroflexion of the proximal CCA can result in a difficult-to-establish 180-degree course of the catheter from the aorta to the distal CCA (FIGURE 43.2A). An elongated and horizontal segment of the proximal right CCA after the bifurcation of the innominate artery can cause problems establishing a vertical/coaxial sheath position, which can lead to loss of guide/sheath position intraprocedurally and/or trauma to the proximal CCA (FIGURE 43.2B). Lastly, any proximal tortuosity in the CCA will generally be translated into the more distal carotid vasculature once straightened by the placement of a guide catheter or sheath and will exaggerate any circuitous anatomy already present there (FIGURE 43.2C).

Regarding carotid bifurcation considerations, the occlusion of the ECA will necessitate that the operator must gain guide/sheath access into the CCA over a guide wire that will not be able to be anchored in the ECA as is common practice (FIGURE 43.2D). This will create a challenge, especially if the CCA is short or access routes are tortuous, or both, because the length of supportive wire may be inadequate to allow catheter transit. Separate from access issues, the bifurcation anatomy can also be made complex by the presence of a large distal CCA (i.e., nontapered) combined with a 90-degree or more entry angle into the internal

carotid artery (ICA) because wires will typically prolapse into the ongoing ECA. This is especially true with fixed-wire filter systems that will not easily track the angulated entry of the distal flexible part of the wire into the ICA. Severe ICA entry angulation can be further exacerbated by an ostial/proximal location of the stenosis and/or proximal (not ostial) severe angulation of the ICA. Lastly, distal ICA tortuosity, loops, or disease (FIGURE 43.2E) can preclude the use of distal EPD and require the consideration of proximal protection or therapy alternative to CAS altogether.

Lesion-specific considerations for CAS include the following:

- Severity: In the United States, the standard for the determination of stenosis severity is based on the North American Symptomatic Carotid Endarterectomy Trial (NASCET) method.[24] As is seen in FIGURE 43.3, the minimum lumen diameter on the tightest angiographic view of the stenosis ("A") is divided by the reference segment ("C"), which is defined as the portion of the ICA where the walls of the vessel become parallel. The European Carotid Surgery Trial (ECST) method utilizes the assumed diameter of the proximal ICA ("B"), which uses the larger carotid bulb as the denominator, so that for every ECST stenosis, the NASCET percent stenosis will be less severe.

- Calcification: Severe, circumferential calcification can result in the underexpansion/nonexpansion of the lesion and, subsequently, the implanted stent. It may also lead to more profound carotid sinus-mediated hypotension and bradycardia as a result of the required aggressive dilations combined with a "knuckle" effect of the calcium pushing into the sinus. Lastly, in rare instances dissection, perforation or rupture of the carotid artery has been reported in calcified lesions due to the high pressures or adjunctive therapies (e.g., cutting or scoring balloons) employed.[25]

- Thrombus: Classically the presence of thrombus was a strict contraindication to CAS due to the concern of distal embolization and stroke. With the advent of proximal protection, however, such lesions are now being considered possible targets, although without large-scale proof of safety.

- Prior CEA with patch angioplasty: Depending on the location of the lesion and the degree of carotid expansion and vessel mismatch created by the patch angioplasty at the time of the

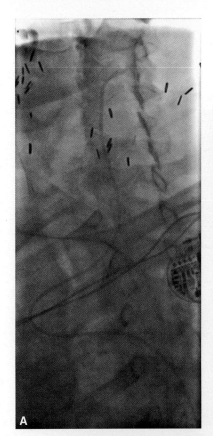
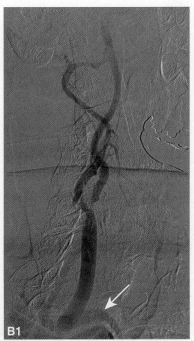
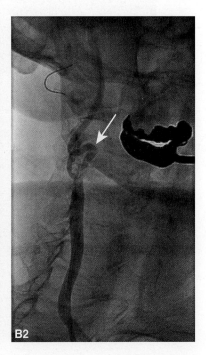
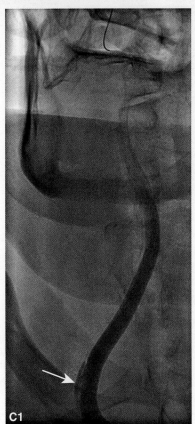
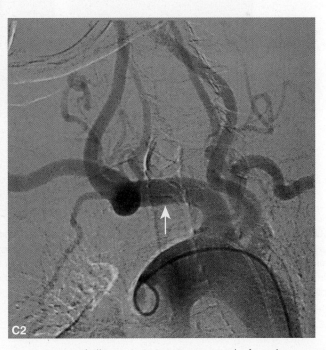

FIGURE 43.2 Angiographic demonstrations of various anatomic challenges in CAS. **A.** Tortuous path of a catheter engaged in a bovine left CCA. **B1.** Bifurcation lesion demonstrated with angiographic catheter. Note the proximal ICA tortuosity. **B2.** Severe kinking in the proximal ICA after establishing sheath access for CAS. Patient was referred for CEA. **C1.** Traumatic catheter-induced dissection of the right CCA (*arrow*). **C2.** The horizontal orientation of the innominate artery (*arrow*) led to catheter malorientation and dissection even in a favorable arch. *(continued)*

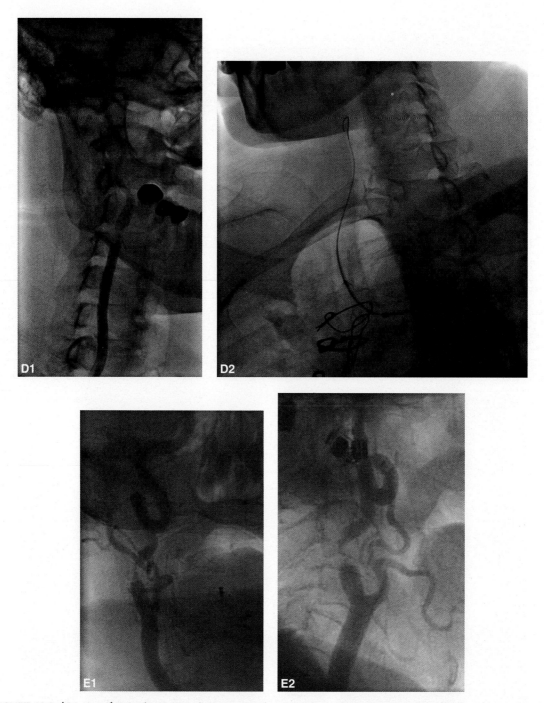

FIGURE 43.2 (*Continued*) **D1.** Absent ECA eliminates usual access wire anchoring position. **D2.** Pigtail curl in access wire allows for catheter passage while safely maintaining position below the lesion. **E1** and **E2.** Angiographic demonstration of severe distal ICA tortuosity/loop in oblique and lateral projections. **F.** Prior CEA with patch angioplasty and complex stenosis in the proximal and distal patch. Late recurrent stenosis after remote CEA demonstrating complex neoatherosclerosis on Duplex imaging (**G1**), and difficult-to-visualize angiographic lesion (**G1** and **G2**). Another complex late neoatherosclerotic lesion post-CEA in a different patient (**G4**).

original CEA, there may be significant difficulty in appropriate stent sizing and placement. Specifically, self-expanding stents require early vessel engagement to stabilize their position; otherwise they will "spring" forward into a potentially undesirable distal position (FIGURE 43.2G).

- "String-sign": Although, strictly speaking, there is no uniform definition of this term, it is generally considered to be present when the lesion is relatively long (greater than ~2 cm); the antegrade passage of contrast is within a serpiginous channel that amounts to a 99% stenosis; and the distal ICA is

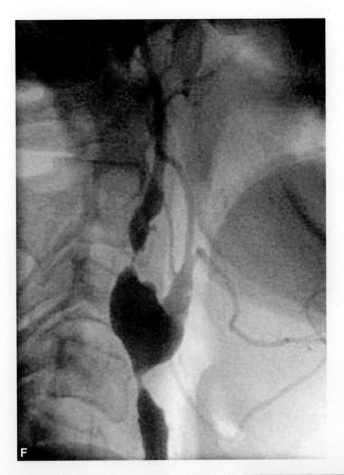

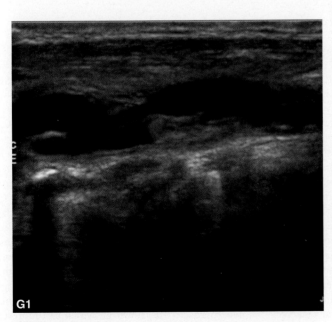

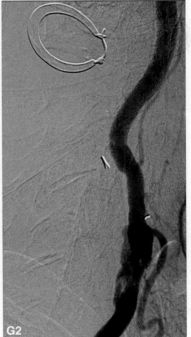

FIGURE 43.2 (*Continued*)

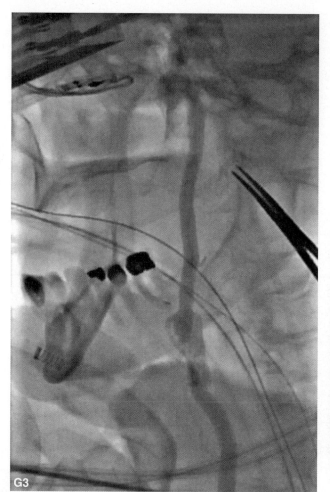

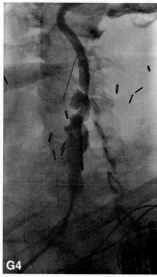

FIGURE 43.2 (*Continued*)

"collapsed," that is, it is undersized and underfilled. In most cases, filling of the distal intracranial circulation will be delayed and slower than filling of the distal ECA. Many of these lesions are generally believed to be recanalized total occlusions and to have a low-risk natural history and, therefore, not in need of revascularization by any method. From an interventional perspective, the bulky, potentially thrombotic nature of the lesion was felt to be, in combination with the expected benign natural history, a relative contraindication to intervention. This viewpoint may be in flux given certain considerations regarding selected patient natural history and newer interventional methods and tools. This is addressed in combination with chronic total occlusions (CTOs) next.

- Chronic total occlusion: Because the stroke potential from carotid bifurcation CTOs was felt to be benign, revascularization by any method was generally not pursued. In patients with recurrent events or in whom cerebrovascular reserve was abnormal, rates of neurologic complication on medical therapy at 2 years were similar to that seen in symptomatic stenoses in NASCET.[24] This has prompted two multicenter studies[26,27] to assess the possible benefit of external carotid-to-intracranial bypass in such patients. In neither study was there a benefit observed compared to the medical arm, at

least in part due to the inadequacy of both donor and recipient vessels as well as to perioperative morbidity. There has not been a randomized evaluation of either surgical or endovascular revascularization of such lesions. An interesting recent report from Taiwan described a single-center experience in patients with carotid bifurcation CTO with reported rates of death/stroke at 3 months of 4%.[28] This compares favorably with the perioperative rate of complication seen in the Carotid Occlusion Surgery Study (COSS) (>10%) and opens the possibility to study CAS as a potential benefit to such patients.

- Restenosis of prior CEA: Typically these lesions are felt to have a low emboligenic potential because they comprise neointimal tissue and they are usually stented with a very low rate of complication. Post-CEA lesions developing greater than 2 years after the surgical procedure can be caused by neoatherosclerosis, however, which can represent some of the most complex lesions in this anatomic location and are characterized by multiple, septated components that may be difficult to visualize angiographically and are best understood via Duplex evaluation (FIGURE 43.3). In these infrequent lesions, many operators will favor a proximal protection approach.

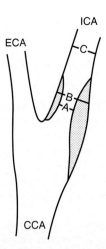

FIGURE 43.3 Schematic of carotid stenosis and various points of measurement as described by Wael E. Shaalan, et al. Reappraisal of velocity criteria for carotid bulb/internal carotid artery stenosis utilizing high-resolution B-mode ultrasound validated with computed tomography angiography. *J Vasc Surg* 2008;48(1):104–113.

CCA: Common carotid artery ICA: Internal carotid artery ECA: External carotid artery.

PLANNING THE INTERVENTIONAL PROCEDURE

Once the decision to proceed with CAS is made, procedural planning and preparation are straightforward. Typically, pretreatment with aspirin and clopidogrel are initiated at least 3 days prior to the procedure, or a loading dose of 300 to 600 mg clopidogrel is given several hours before intervention. Antihypertension medications are held on the day of the procedure to allow for a margin of blood pressure during carotid body stimulation. Because the patient will be NPO for at least 6 hours prior to the procedure, and considerably longer on occasion, either continuous saline or bolus hydration to maintain euvolemia will help mitigate carotid body-mediated hypotension should it occur, the management of which is discussed in a later section.

Preprocedural imaging (Duplex, computed tomography angiography [CTA], magnetic resonance angiography [MRA], or digital subtraction angiography [DSA]) should be used to define the extent of the lesion and its severity, calcification, tortuosity, thrombus or other plaque CAS characteristics, any associated proximal or distal lesions, and arch access issues. Based on the experience and comfort level of the operator, assessment of the aortic arch may be reserved for the procedural angiography itself. In the symptomatic patient, intracranial imaging should be performed to exclude other potential pathology that may be primarily responsible for the clinical presentation or which might modify the decision or approach to revascularization. In the asymptomatic patient, transcranial Doppler (TCD) physiologic assessment of cerebrovascular reserve[29] or silent high-intensity transients representing microemboli[30] have been proposed as useful in stratifying both natural history and procedural risk and therefore in patient selection, but as yet without randomized data to support their routine use. Other modalities, such as plaque characterization using close-field high-resolution MRA,[31] intravascular ultrasound virtual histology,[32] and other

techniques are also not yet clinically mature enough to predict either natural history or procedural outcomes. Even earlier phase investigations assessing plaque activity using measures of adventitial neovascularization[33] and matrix metalloproteinase concentration as a marker of inflammation are as yet speculative.[34]

ACCESS

Femoral artery access made difficult secondary to iliac tortuosity may be mitigated by a long sheath (45 to 65 cm), which helps straighten the path and limits the primary interventional sheath involvement with the iliac, therefore allowing easier catheter transit/manipulation. Femoral artery access that is altogether absent will require access from alternative routes. These typically include percutaneous approaches from the radial or brachial artery but can also involve surgical access points from the subclavian/axillary and the proximal CCA. However, some of these alternate access points may impose a considerably more circuitous path for the operator to negotiate.

Difficult arch anatomy as previously described may be approached using a variety of methods, which are generally variations on the "standard" method of CCA access. This is usually accomplished, in straightforward cases, by first intubating the target CCA with a diagnostic catheter. Diagnostic catheters generally can be divided into two broad categories: simple and complex shapes. The former (vertebral, Berenstein, etc.) is useful in uncomplicated anatomy where selection of the vessel is not at issues and have the advantage of being easily advanced over nonsupportive wires into the CCA. The complex shape catheters (Vitek, Simmons, etc.) are useful for engaging challenging anatomy where the necessary torqueing or wire passage is encumbered with simple catheter shapes. These catheters may require forming in the body and therefore a greater expertise on the part of the operator. Moreover, they are not as easily advanced into the CCA and beyond over nonsupportive wires due to their preshape and will generally require a stiffer jacketed wire.

Regardless of the catheter chosen, once the target CCA/innominate is intubated and scout angiography performed, a wire is advanced into the ECA as a point of anchorage for either advancement of the diagnostic catheter into the external artery or removal of the diagnostic catheter and exchange for the guide sheath. In the former method, once the diagnostic catheter is in the ECA the nonsupportive wire is exchanged for a supportive wire over which the guide sheath will be advanced. The latter method depends on the ability of the operator to steer a supportive wire into the ECA, and the wire of choice here is the TAD II wire (Covidien, Mansfield, MA), which has a 0.018" distal tip that gradually tapers to a 0.035" supportive shaft. Stiffer 0.035" to 0.038" wires are not steerable and should not be used to access the ECA unless a catheter has already been placed there. A stiff jacketed hydrophilic wire (0.035" to 0.038") is steerable enough to be maneuvered into the ECA safely but can be difficult to perform exchanges over, resulting in loss of access position.

Generally a 6 French 90-cm sheath is preferred for CAS. Although some CAS systems will allow use of a 5 French sheath, the operator gives up a measure of stability and support with the smaller caliber system, and some operators actually prefer 7 French sheaths for their stability. Lastly, proximal occlusion catheters are currently 9 French due to the need for both an ECA balloon/port and a channel to inflate the CCA balloon. But because they are meant to be used with a sheath (i.e., the dilator and distal aspects are not required to pierce/traverse the soft tissue tract in at the access site), their more flexible construction allows for greater trackability in tortuous arch anatomy, thus offsetting the greater French size.

Although planning for CCA access can be significantly enhanced by the use of preprocedural imaging, such as CTA or MRA, occasionally the anatomy identified on axial imaging can be misleading, both to the positive and negative, and until the operator "engages" the anatomy it may be difficult to predict how demanding the task of access will be.

In cases of difficult arch anatomy it may not be possible to advance the catheter or even a nonsupportive wire into the CCA. Alternative methods of procedural access include the following:

- The sheath can be "loaded" onto the diagnostic catheter, typically complex shaped, instead of its dilator. This creates two advantages. First, the dilator is generally too short and stiff to negotiate difficult turns in the vasculature owing to its mandate to also provide entry through the skin, and the diagnostic catheter will be more supportive of the required course. Second, this ad hoc system may provide a bit more support for wire passage because the sheath now closely backs up the catheter. Once this system has engaged the artery, a supportive wire can be advanced partway into the CCA, and over the diagnostic catheter the sheath can gradually be advanced. Specific systems have been created for this approach that incorporate longer (125 cm), more supportive (6.5 French) diagnostic catheters meant to minimize the inherent gap that would otherwise exist between the inner diameter of a sheath and a standard diagnostic catheter.

- Preshaped 8 French coronary guide catheters (internal mammary, extra-backup, Amplatz shapes) can be used as an alternative to a 6 French sheath. This has the advantage of not requiring deep intubation of a sheath into the CCA because if the correct shape is chosen, a reasonably stable position in the ostium of the CCA/innominate can be obtained. The obvious disadvantage is that the operator is then necessarily working on the lesion at a distance, and contrast visualization (especially in the right CCA given the nonselective method), wire steerage, and platform stability are compromised. To address the latter issue, a supportive 0.014" buddy wire can be advanced into the ECA (for left carotid intervention) or into the subclavian/axillary artery (or snared and externalized through a 4 French brachial sheath) for right carotid intervention. The operator should be cautious in gaining initial access using this method because the preformed catheters can be more traumatic to the arch and can liberate particulates in a diseased aorta. A "no-touch" technique using a second wire in the aorta can be useful in this regard.

- Although not yet available in the United States, there two other catheter systems that enable access in difficult anatomy. The first is the SAAD (Cordis/Johnson and Johnson, Warren, NJ) and other lines of guide catheters with shapes specifically designed for carotid access and stable positioning. The second is the Piton catheter (Medtronic, Santa Rosa, CA), which has two wire ports and a preformed tip designed to easily engage the carotid/innominate ostium on rotation. A supportive wire is placed in the central lumen of the catheter that has an exit through a side hole at the bend point of the distal catheter and positioned in the aortic root. Using this wire as a stabilizing platform, the catheter can be turned in an atraumatic fashion

to engage the target vessel and then a second, less supportive, wire can be advanced to engage the CCA. The supportive wire is then withdrawn from the aortic root and redirected into the CCA. Access with the interventional sheath/guide of choice is then performed over the supportive wire.

Once the arch access issues are overcome, there still may be CCA tortuosity to manage. As mentioned previously this can lead to loss of access during the procedure, trauma to the CCA, or the transmission of the proximal tortuosity to the ICA segment, causing kinking. These issues can be at least partly mitigated by the use of an 8 French coronary multipurpose guide that can generally be situated to achieve a more coaxial position in the vessel.

In an effort to eliminate the arch both as an obstacle to carotid access but also as a source of emboli and clinical events, a system is being trialed in the United States that accesses the proximal CCA directly via a small incision just above the clavicle (detailed further on). Initial results have been encouraging.[35]

■ LESION

The nature of the lesion, both clinical and anatomic, will have a bearing on the operator's choice of equipment and method of CAS. Regarding the choice of embolic protection, in difficult ICA anatomy, including entry angle, lesion stenosis severity, or distal tortuosity, a bare wire filter system (Emboshield, Abbott Vascular, Santa Clara, CA, or Spider Rx Covidien, Mansfield, MA) will generally be preferred over fixed-wire systems because they allow a greater degree of independent wire tip control. For these and other difficult anatomic scenarios, as well as the at-risk populations of symptomatic patients and octogenarians, there are some data suggesting that proximal occlusion with flow cessation (Mo.Ma, Medtronic, Santa Rosa, CA) or flow reversal (Neuroprotection System [NPS], WL Gore, Flagstaff, AZ) may afford a greater degree of embolic protection for stroke and death in these subgroups.[36,37]

Although there are operators who prefer not to predilate most of their lesions, this, in fact, is considered one of the least risky steps of the CAS procedure, as evidenced by TCD monitoring and confirmed by clinical experience. Most will predilate with a 3- to 4-mm balloon, which can allow for less traumatic stent placement and better contrast visualization.[38] Consideration is occasionally given to high-pressure cutting or scoring balloon angioplasty in cases where the lesion is resistant due to calcium, but this should be undertaken with caution because perforation can ensue when predilation is pursued too aggressively. Predilation balloon length is typically longer (30 to 40 mm) inasmuch as there will be no balloon trauma imparted at the nonlesion site (because the balloon is subnominally sized and atraumatic in these segments) and the longer length affords stability and prevents balloon dislocation during inflation.

A lesion-specific choice of stents is discussed next. Once the stent is implanted, the option to postdilate is available but increasingly not being performed. When it is, balloon sizing for bifurcation/ICA lesions should not exceed 5 mm because this will result, in almost every instance, in nominal sizing for the NASCET reference mid/distal ICA vessel, and remembering that the goal of CAS is to cover the lesion and allow neointimal stabilization of the plaque, with stenosis relief a secondary aim (usually just enough that stent flow is not compromised, usually <30% residual NASCET stenosis).

CHOICE OF STENT

Stents used in CAS have various qualities that may distinguish them from each other, such as conformability (to the vessel wall), scaffolding, visibility, deliverability, and radial strength. In the early CAS experience, balloon-expandable stents were used for their radial strength and exactness of placement. Because the carotid bifurcation is exposed to the potential of extrinsic forces, a minority of these stents was noted on follow-up to be crushed and deformed, leading to stenosis, and their use was abandoned in favor of self-expanding varieties. But this example highlights, in the extreme, the various tradeoffs that are made between the desirable qualities in stent design. All stents, save one, used for CAS are nitinol (nickel-titanium alloys). The non-nitinol stent is made from an Elgiloy stainless steel and is a woven mesh design, whereas the nitinol stents are laser-cut from a nitinol tube.

There has been much debate as to the potential for the stents themselves to act as EPDs inasmuch as the size of their cells theoretically could be a determinant of the ability of freshly disrupted plaque—either by the adjunctive balloon angioplasty or the inherent instability of a recently symptomatic plaque to embolize through the stent. Advocates of this view point to data from prospective registries that demonstrate that approximately one-third of stroke events occur postdischarge following CAS,[23] and the speculative causal etiology is the late embolization from the plaque protruding through the cells. There have been retrospective analyses with the typical selection biases inherent that suggest an advantage of closed-cell stents over open-cell stents for stroke outcomes.[40] Skeptics point out that the late events are in the main minor strokes, most of which are potentially a late manifestation of an intraprocedural event that does not come to light until anticoagulation is reversed (allowing for thrombus formation at a small, distally located thrombo- or athero-embolism), and the usual permissive hypertension (allowed to counter carotid body stimulation) is reversed, which then allows the expression of the neurologic findings resulting from reduced collateralization of the affected area. There are also equally compelling retrospective data suggesting no difference between stent types for outcomes.[41] The most voluminous and convincing data actually exist in a pair of prospective studies run contemporaneously and which can be used to assess the impact of stent design on outcomes. These high surgical risk postmarket approval surveillance (PMS) studies had very similar inclusion and exclusion criteria with independent assessment of both neurologic outcomes on site and adjudication of neurologic events by an independent Clinical Events Committee.[42] In several thousand patients with similar demographic characteristics there was no difference in outcomes for open-cell and closed-cell stents (5.7% vs. 5.1% S/D, respectively). In addition, several of the later trials in the United States designed to gain FDA clearance for EPD systems allowed the use of any approved stent, and although the number available for analysis is small, there were no observed differences in outcomes by stent design.[36,37] Of note, there are reports of closed-cell stent fracture in CAS application, although no significant clinical sequelae have been associated with this phenomenon, and this has not been similarly seen in open-cell designs.[39]

Incorporating the benefits of both design features, operators outside the United States have the option of a hybrid stent (Cristallo, Medtronic, Santa Rosa, CA), which has open cells at each end for greater flexibility and closed cells in the midportion for greater lesion coverage, although there are no compelling data supporting a difference in outcomes. In the United States, an Investigational Device Exemption (IDE) approval trial of a mesh-covered open-cell stent is nearing initiation but will not be powered to detect a difference in outcomes, noting that a 1% reduction in stroke rates in CAS would require a trial of several thousand patients. It is possible that some surrogate, such as postprocedural TCD or diffusion-weighted magnetic resonance imaging (DWMRI), could discern a difference but would likely be confounded by factors having to do with EPD, operator experience, and patient and lesion subtypes.

So although there is a theoretical advantage to suggest that closed-cell stents are preferable, in fact there is no empirical evidence to support this contention. Therefore, because the choice of stent to use in any given patient cannot be programmatically determined according to outcome data, it is typically made based on operator ease of use and lesion characteristics. Specifically, many operators will prefer a tapered stent for bifurcation disease (which accounts for most CAS performed) given the size disparity between the ICA and CCA, an open-cell design when there is a concern about deliverability or conformability to the vessel once deployed, closed-cell for calcified or symptomatic lesions, and so on—all of which is without a basis in data. Most operators will choose to use a 4-cm stent because it has the best chance of not missing the lesion coverage and because there does not appear to be a "penalty" in terms of restenosis associated with stent length in the carotid circulation. The delivery systems of the various stents may drive choice as well with several systems having a triaxial sheath catheter, which stabilizes the device during stent delivery and allows for exacting placement. In cases where a proximal embolic protection system is chosen, many operators will prefer a closed-cell stent to minimize snagging the ECA balloon during its withdrawal from behind the stent. Lastly, the woven mesh stents will, by their very nature, shorten to fit the vessel they are placed into, so the final length of stent cannot be accurately predetermined. In this case, operators are required to make their best estimate shortening and ensuring to cover the target zone.

Although covered stents have been used in carotid intervention for carotid blowouts (traumatic, oncologic, etc.) and pseudoaneurysm treatment, they have not been routinely advocated for obstructive atherosclerotic treatment due to the larger size of their delivery systems and the concern over the possibility of stent thrombosis, an exceedingly rare event in CAS with current stents.

CHOOSING AN EMBOLIC PROTECTION DEVICE

Although there are those who would argue that embolic protection has no randomized data with differentiated clinical outcomes to support its use, and in fact that there may be objective, albeit subclinical, evidence of increased high-intensity transients signals (HITS) on TCD and increased white matter findings on DWMRI,[43] meta-analyses suggest that the advent of EPDs has been associated with a reduction in overall death and stroke rates, although it is admittedly difficult to separate other possible influences of improved outcomes, such as operator experience, dedicated carotid stents, and patient selection.[44] Further supportive data for the use of EPD come from the CREST study, which showed a fourfold increase in the death and stroke rates for those procedures performed without EPD, albeit with a clearly "selected" population in whom it could not be placed for anatomic or operator reasons.[13] Most operators who have practiced in the eras with and without EPD believe that there is, in fact, a protective effect worth incorporating as a standard component for all CAS. In the United States, CAS performed without EPD is not considered standard of care by Medicare and therefore does not meet coverage requirements.

In point of fact the current controversy around EPDs centers more on the type of device that is necessary to achieve optimal outcomes. The current options include distal, primarily filter, devices (distal balloon occlusion not used in practice significantly), and proximal balloon occlusion devices with either flow cessation or flow reversal.

Distal filter EPDs come in various designs, the differences generally meant to address some of the challenges with distal filter placement and embolic capture efficiency, especially on bends. Table 43.2 gives some of the elements of the various filters currently available.

Bare wire systems are meant to be advantageous when there is a significant degree of angulation or tortuosity in the access to or in the ICA proper because the wire can be placed through the difficult anatomy first and the filter can follow once distal wire position has been established. Remote deployment filters allow for one less step in the procedure and potentially a smaller crossing profile absent the usual covering sheath that releases a nitinol-based filter frame. Partial frame filters are more flexible in tortuous segments but may have the disadvantage of less robust wall apposition than a fully framed filter might have and therefore less capture efficiency. It should be noted that the particulate capture efficiency of most filters will be reduced if they are situated in the bend point of a vessel, and this is to be avoided whenever possible. Lastly, the porous membranes allow for an infinite variety of pore sizes, distribution and density, the possibility of surface coatings (e.g., heparin), and, typically, good flow. The filament type filter actually may partially/completely interrupt flow, which may in fact be its mechanism of protective action. Lastly, a nitinol-woven basket filter allows good flow and filter volume but has variability in its "pore" size.

Whichever filter is chosen, it should ideally be placed as atraumatically through the lesion as possible and distally in the ICA just below the petrous segment where the vessel is generally straight and the bony turn will stabilize the device somewhat. Occasionally, a lesion will be so tight and/or calcified that the filter will not pass easily and should not be forced. Instead the nonocclusive platinum tip should be left across the lesion, and a second 0.014" wire passed into the distal vessel and used to predilate the lesion with a small (2 mm) diameter balloon, which will then allow passage of the filter. Occasionally, a buddy wire is required to straighten a vessel so that a filter can pass, but in both instances strong consideration for a proximal protection device should be given because predilation prior to filter placement has been associated with poorer outcomes.[9]

Proximal embolic protection comes in three varieties, all with the same basic principle founded on the surgical approach to protection; that is, a clamp placed on the CCA and ECA to prevent forward flow in the ICA while the lesion is being removed. In the endovascular version, a balloon-tipped catheter is positioned proximally in the CCA and when inflated serves as a "vascular clamp" to occlude antegrade flow. In two of the three proximal protection systems, a small balloon is placed in the ECA to block retrograde flow into the ICA circulation and represents the second "clamp." This ECA balloon should be placed as proximally in the vessel as possible to occlude flow from early branches (e.g., superior thyroidal). In one system, flow is stopped after the "clamps" are inflated (these are elastomeric volume-based balloons and therefore largely atraumatic) and when the procedure is completed, active aspiration is performed until the aspirant is clear. In the other two versions, flow is reversed after balloon inflation via a conduit to the femoral vein throughout the entire procedure. The system that does not employ an ECA balloon has been designed with a switch to permit both high flow (which reverses flow out of both the ECA and ICA) and low flow, which can be used in between the embaligenic parts of the procedure. This system has an additional "protection" feature, namely, it is placed directly into the proximal CCA (currently with a small surgical exposure and repair), which eliminates the risk of liberating emboli from traversing/manipulating catheters in the aorta.

In a following section, the outcomes for both types of protection are detailed, and operators' choices for EPD are, at least in

Table 43.2

Various Design Features of Distal Filter EPD

Wire		Deployment mechanism		Frame element		Filter element	
Bare (independent of filter)	Fixed (attached to filter)	Sheath	Remote actuation	Full frame	Partial/no frame	Porous membrane	Filament/ woven
Emboshield	All	All	Fibernet	All	Emboshield	All	Fibernet
Spider Rx	All				Filterwire		Spider Rx
	All				Gore Filter		
					Fibernet		

part, influenced by these data. Other factors include anatomy that favors a particular system, such as excessive ICA looping or tortuosity that favors a proximal system; a difficult arch access, which may favor the filters (because they only require a 6 French sheath rather than the 9 French proximal systems); and the patient with a truly isolated intracranial circulation distal to the lesion who would have a high probability of intolerance to flow cessation or reversal. This last point bears further comment: it is very difficult, a priori, to accurately predict intolerance to proximal CCA flow interruption simply by an examination of cerebral angiography and many an operator has been surprised in both directions. Therefore, the decision to use proximal protection is typically made with factors other than intolerance in mind. The management of intolerance is discussed in the following section.

PROCEDURAL COMPLICATIONS AND HOW TO MANAGE THEM SUCCESSFULLY

CAS intraprocedural complications occur in several broad categories: neurologic, hemodynamic, device related, and access related. The last of these is generic, its management well described, and is not addressed here.

Neurologic complications are distinctly unusual, as discussed in the outcomes section of this chapter, but important to know how to diagnose and manage when they occur. They can be manifest as either focal or generalized, and major or minor. Focal neurologic syndromes are largely caused by either a distal

(intracranial circulation) embolization or reduction of flow that is planned (proximal occlusion EPD, which is termed *intolerance*) or unplanned (dilating balloon inflation, or slow flow in a distal filter device, or acute vessel closure—a rare event). There can also be focal neurologic deficits following a seizure caused by marked intolerance to flow interruption and a resulting Todd paralysis.

Depending on the procedural scenario, distal embolization should be ruled out in most cases of focal neurologic disturbance. Additionally, it is important to characterize the event as associated with either a major or minor deficit by neurologic exam because the combination of emboli location and severity will drive decision making. If an embolus is noted in a distal intracranial vessel and the deficit is limited/minor (NIHSS <3 or 4) then conservative management (permissive hypertension, hydration, etc.) is generally recommended because most minor strokes resolve and leave little or no deficit,[13,44] whereas endovascular manipulation of these small distal branch carries an increased risk of larger and more permanent complication. If the embolism is proximal there is usually a major deficit and immediate intervention is warranted. Intracranial intervention is described in another chapter and the reader is referred there for detail.

The proximal cause of embolization should also be investigated. In most cases it will not be evident by angiography, but stent thrombosis rarely will be present (FIGURE 43.4). The distinction between this entity and plaque protrusion can be difficult, although plaque protrusion usually appears more distinctly, whereas stent thrombosis tends to be more diffuse. Stent thrombosis, when it occurs, is a biologic problem in that there is an exuberant platelet activation and aggregation response to the tissue factors and other

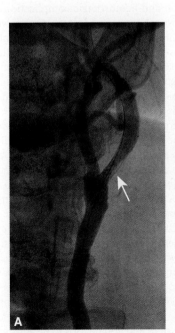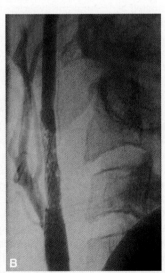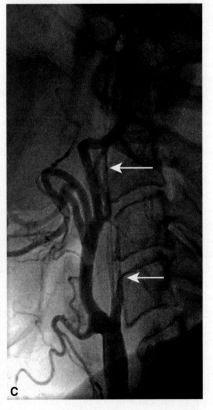

FIGURE 43.4 A. Stent thrombosis (*arrow*). **B.** Massive stent thrombosis causing a "moth-eaten" appearance. **C.** No flow caused by filter occlusion following successful stent implantation, arrows define previous course of carotid artery.

material of the carotid plaque core, which has been exposed to the bloodstream during the procedure. For this reason, aggressive postdilation with balloons is to be avoided after stent placement given that the aim in CAS is to displace, but not to further rupture, the underlying plaque, which is different from most other arterial intervention for obstructive disease. Given the pathogenesis of this entity, the operator should check that the activated clotting time is adequate and consider 2b3a platelet inhibitors. Both thrombosis and plaque protrusion may be treated with catheter aspiration or relining the stent with another stent. In either scenario, maneuvers should be carried out with the EPD in place.

When a neurologic syndrome is caused by intolerance, the patient will likely have no long-term sequelae due to it alone, so the primary focus should always be on completing the procedure at hand safely. Intolerance can be generalized and subtle, presenting as yawning, inattention, agitation/movement, or it can be more definitively focal. It is the rare case where intolerance is generated by the short balloon inflations used during the CAS procedure, and today almost always related to proximal balloon occlusion EPD, or to a lesser extent to slowed flow in a distal filter (which is usually an asymptomatic event but its management is covered here). For the proximal occlusion EPD, there are several methods of managing intolerance. The primary one is to make certain that systolic blood pressure is adequate, usually over 160 mm Hg, because this will enhance collateral flow into the affected cortex and significantly reduce the clinical intolerance. Many patients also can be conditioned to tolerance by intermittent occlusion such that progressively longer periods of occlusion can be sustained. Intermittent balloon inflation during lesion manipulation and deflation between steps, making certain to clear the column of blood by aspiration before releasing the "clamp," can be used in the persistently intolerant patient. Ensuring that all necessary equipment is available and prepared before the CAS procedure should be standard practice but especially important when minimizing time of occlusion is critical. Lastly, a distal EPD can be used in many cases when intolerance cannot be otherwise managed.

Distal filter EPDs may occasionally become partially or completely occluded, resulting in slow or no flow (FIGURE 43.4). The appearance of slow flow can also be caused by vessel spasm, dissection, and pseudostenosis/kinking and these should be eliminated as possibilities or treated with vasodilators (e.g., intra-arterial nitroglycerin), additional stenting, or wire removal, respectively. Filters may become occluded due to captured material or fibrin deposits; the latter is especially true if the time of dwell is excessive (most procedures should be completed in well under 10 minutes of filter dwell or proximal occlusion time). If this occurs, they should be treated as occlusion devices, meaning that the column of blood below the filter is stagnant and therefore has the potential to contain significant amounts of debris from the lesion, and therefore should be aspirated until the aspirant is free of debris. The filter can then be removed, typically restoring flow quickly.

Hemodynamic perturbations during CAS are common but only rarely lead to clinical sequelae. During CAS, excepting in the previously operated/deenervated vessel (e.g., prior CEA), the carotid sinus will be stimulated by not only the balloon angioplasty but also the continued outward force of the stent after implantation, especially in calcified lesions where there is no compression of the calcium but rather just displacement and transmission of the dilating forces into the carotid sinus. This reflex is modulated through medullary pathways in the brain:

the resulting parasympathetic outflow in primarily bradycardia/asystole with some associated hypotension and is typically transient after balloon depressurization, or easily treated with belladonna alkaloids (e.g., atropine) and very rarely with a pacemaker, whereas the resulting sympathetic response causes significant venodilation and precipitous, profound (e.g., 100 mm Hg) drops in blood pressure, which can be prolonged. In anticipation of this hypotensive response, antihypertensive medications are typically withheld on the morning of the procedure and it is not unusual for preprocedural systolic blood pressure to range over 180 mm Hg as a result. In addition, most patients should be given at least 500 cc of saline before the procedure, and preparations should be made to rapidly administer alpha agonists (e.g., phenylephrine 100 to 200 mcg IV) and atropine as needed. Occasionally, a vasopressor drip will be needed if the blood pressure continues to sag postprocedure. If persistent, other causes of hypotension should not be overlooked, principally access site bleeding. In a real sense, the patient with persistent hypotension caused by carotid sinus stimulation has an "acquired" autonomic dysfunction, the treatment for which is pressor support, continued aggressive hydration as tolerated, and early/frequent ambulation, which favors the use of access closure devices. Although counterintuitive to most, ambulating the patient while on pressor support can significantly limit the time spent on pressors and should be encouraged where possible.

A couple of caveats regarding carotid sinus stimulation: First, in patients with critical aortic stenosis or severe multivessel coronary disease associated with marked left ventricular dysfunction, there is little, if any, tolerance for hypotension and bradycardia and in these instances a prophylactic temporary pacemaker should be considered. Second, in deciding whether to postdilate a stented lesion, the degree of residual lesion as well as the patient's hemodynamic response to predilation and stent implantation should be considered.

Equally important as hypotension following CAS is controlling hypertension, which has been thought to be associated with both hyperperfusion and hemorrhagic complication postprocedure (these syndromes are covered later). Aggressive control of hypertension is important and can be achieved with various intravenous pharmacologic agents (until the reinstitution of oral antihypertensives), such as beta blockers, calcium-channel blockers, and nitroglycerin, although the latter can lead to headache, and confusion (i.e. intracranial hemorrhage vs. medication effect) as to its etiology.

Device-related complications have largely to do with exquisite attention to procedural detail and avoidance: avoiding losing sheath/guide access in the CCA (and into the aorta), especially while a distal filter is in place; avoiding snagging a framed filter on an open-cell stent (which can require an operation to remove); avoiding CCA dissection by a catheter placed in a bend, and so on. There is one scenario that cannot always be avoided: difficulty passing the filter EPD retrieval device through the stent owing to it snagging the stent. This is an issue that relates to the bias of the wire across the stent struts. Any maneuver that changes this bias will be helpful in getting the retrieval device across the stent: bowing the wire by pushing it distally, turning the neck, swallowing, dorsiflexion of the head, and so on. In the event these do not work, a shaped catheter (e.g., multipurpose, JR4, etc.) can be steered through the stent and also be used to recapture the filter.

A loss of consciousness in or immediately following a CAS procedure is an ominous event usually signaling an acute intracerebral hemorrhage, which is almost uniformly fatal. This is fortunately a rare event, occurring well less than 1% of the time, and has been associated with aggressive procedural anticoagulation/antiplatelet therapy (e.g., 2b3a inhibitors).[45,46]

Late complications following CAS are numerically unusual given the overall low rates of events, but on a proportionate basis they can be significant.[23] These complications consist of a late stroke, hyperperfusion syndrome, and cerebral hemorrhage. As discussed previously under the stent section, late stroke may in fact be a misnomer because many of these events may have occurred intraprocedurally and only clinically manifest after blood pressure is controlled, and so on. Therefore, although it is certain that late embolic events occur after CAS, it is not clear what proportion of the neurologic deficits that come to attention late (after 24 hours) they actually represent. Fortunately, these events are generally minor and do not result in significant deficit. Hyperperfusion syndrome is an autoregulatory failure of cerebral blood flow and may present as headache, seizure, and altered mental status. It can occur in up to 5% of patients after CEA or CAS in the hours that follow the revascularization. Patients who develop this syndrome are more likely to have had a recent TIA (but not stroke) and uncontrolled blood pressure following the procedure, will have characteristic CT evidence of sulcal effacement (FIGURE 43.5) confirming the etiology of their clinical presentation, and will recover completely from the syndrome. At the end of the spectrum of autoregulatory failure is postprocedural intracranial hemorrhage, considered a form of hyperperfusion syndrome. It is distinguished from the intraprocedural hemorrhage largely by its timing (usually presenting more than a day after the procedure) and by its generally more favorable prognosis because most patients will both survive and recover.

RECURRENCE OF STENOSIS FOLLOWING SUCCESSFUL CAROTID ARTERY STENTING

Unlike most of the endovascular procedures performed for obstructive atherosclerotic disease where the durability of the intervention is the major determinant of its utility (the acute procedural outcomes generally being significantly less morbid than the surgical alternatives), in CAS the opposite holds true. The durability of the stent, once implanted, is exceptional (~1% per year need for revascularization) and compares favorably with CEA durability,[13] such that the acute procedural/30-day safety has been the principal focus of CAS utility versus CEA.

Determining whether restenosis after CAS has occurred can be challenging by noninvasive means. Cross-sectional imaging can be encumbered by stent artifact, and Duplex velocity measurements, although easily acquired, are elevated due to the

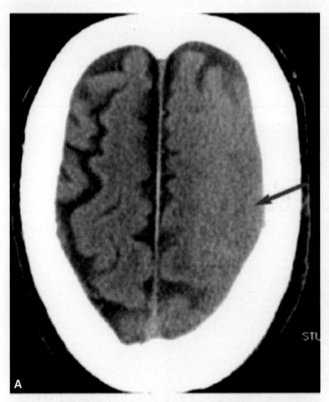
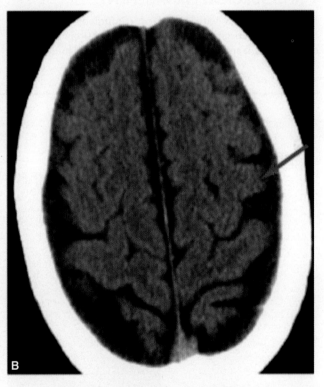

4 hours post procedure   24 hours post procedure

FIGURE 43.5 A. Sulcal effacement in a patient with hyperperfusion syndrome following successful CAS. **B.** Normalization of CT findings.

From Brantley HP, Kiessling JL, Milteer HB, et al. Hyperperfusion syndrome following carotid artery stenting: the largest single-operator series to date. *J Invasive Cardiol* 2009;21:27–30.

presence of the stent alone when there is little or no significant lesion. There has been speculation as to the cause of this stent artifact, such as a stiffening of the vessel and disruption of normal flow dynamics. Several authors have suggested, based on correlation with angiography, that only when the systolic velocity is greater than 250 to 300 cm/second is there a significant in-stent restenosis (ISR).[47,48] Once confirmed by angiography, the management of CAS ISR is relatively straightforward, although there are little systematic outcome data to drive interventional approach because it is infrequent. Most operators will deploy a distal EPD; cutting or scoring balloon inflation will result in an angiographically attractive reduction in stenosis severity. If the stent appears underexpanded it is reasonable to try to achieve a greater expansion. It is advisable after a successful procedure to obtain an early (<30 days) Duplex velocity measurement: the stent velocity will not likely ever achieve a normal value, so having an early assessment can allow subsequent comparisons of elevated velocities to assess for any changes. If there is a re-recurrence, then it is reasonable to reline the stent with another, which can trap exuberant material and lead to further vessel expansion, both of which will lead to greater luminal dimensions (FIGURE 43.6). For repeated failures caused by ISR, it is reasonable to consider a surgical explant of the stent by a skilled surgeon.

OUTCOMES AND RELATIVE THERAPEUTIC EFFECTIVENESS COMPARED TO MEDICAL AND SURGICAL MANAGEMENT

Multicenter trials with dedicated equipment—stents and EPDs—did not begin until the early 2000s. In Europe, where access to the stent and EPD technology preceded the United States,

three major trials randomizing CAS and CEA were initiated during the early and midpart of the decade in standard surgical risk patients who had sustained a nondisabling ischemic neurologic event—TIA or stroke—in the previous 6 months: Endarterectomy Versus Stenting in patients with Symptomatic Severe Carotid Stenosis (EVA-3S, ~500 subjects), Stent-Protected Angioplasty Versus Carotid Endarterectomy (SPACE, ~1,200 subjects), and International Carotid Stenting Study (ICSS, ~1,700 subjects).[49–51] In contradistinction, the U.S. path for CAS was more measured, involved several FDA IDE multicenter trials throughout the decade, and was initiated primarily in patients at high surgical risk for CEA (Table 43.3).[36,37,44,52–56] All U.S. IDE studies mandated EPD use (in several cases this was the device being primarily assessed), prospective neurologic assessment of outcomes, core lab-controlled angiographic assessment, routine ascertainment of MI (postprocedure electrocardiogram [ECG] and enzyme determination) with its inclusion as a primary endpoint, and independent adjudication of outcome events. In every case, the device being tested met its prespecified endpoint, usually an objective performance goal determined by the historical outcomes in these patients with CEA, and received approval or clearance from the FDA as safe and effective for the patient at medical or anatomic high surgical risk for CEA.

In contradistinction, only one of the European trials was completed (ICSS); EVA-3S stopped for futility and safety, and SPACE because the sponsors would not support the remaining 1,000 or so patients mandated by a prespecified interim analysis of the data. These trials were further problematic from several trial construct and conduct perspectives. First, none mandated EPD as part of their initial trial design and as a result its use was as low as 27% (SPACE), and thus did not represent "modern" CAS. Second, MI was not part of the primary endpoint or

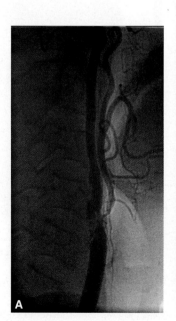
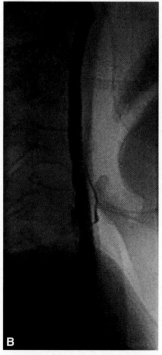

FIGURE 43.6 A. Recurrent in-stent restenosis. **B.** Result following restenting and further balloon expansion of original stent.

Table 43.3	
Criteria for the Designation of a High Surgical Risk CEA Patient	
Ejection fraction <30%	NYHA class III or IV
Dialysis-dependent renal failure	Restenosis following previous CEA
FEV_1 <30% of predicted	Surgically inaccessible lesion
Prior neck irradiation	Prior radical neck surgery
Spinal immobility	Tracheostomy stoma
Contralateral laryngeal nerve palsy	Contralateral ICA occlusion
Unstable angina	MI in past 30 days
Two or more diseased (>70%) coronary arteries	Requirement for open-heart surgery within 30 days

FEV_1, forced expiratory volume in 1 second.

even routinely assessed, and this event was routinely underreported: in SPACE not a single myocardial infarct was reported in 1,200 patients undergoing CEA and CAS. Finally, operator training and experience in the two treatment arms (CEA and CAS) of EVA-3S and ICSS was not equivalent, the CAS operators being significantly less expert than not only the surgical investigators, but also to many of the extant CAS standards.[57] As a result, these trials are considered by some to be fatally flawed in terms of the ability to glean meaningful comparative data between the two therapies.[58]

CREST studying symptomatic and asymptomatic patients at standard surgical risk started at roughly the same time as the aforementioned European trials but took the longest to enroll (~8 years).[12,13] It was completed last owing to its size of approximately 2,500 subjects (the largest trial of any carotid intervention to date), along with its mandate that its CAS operators be suitably experienced, to at least a comparable level to the surgeons performing CEA in the trial.[56] This proved to be difficult in the early going because the procedure was not widely practiced in the United States at the onset of the trial and for some years after because of limited FDA approval and Medicare coverage and had the effect of slowing enrollment and completion of the study.

In fact, a significant experience in CAS in the United States did not occur until the FDA and Centers for Medicare and Medicaid Services (CMS) approvals, albeit limited, and the initiation of several postmarket surveillance studies. This dramatically increased the ability of operators to treat patients and gain experience, both technical and in patient selection. As a manifestation of this volume increase, the stroke and death rates from the IDE trials, performed largely in the same high surgical risk population and by many of the same operators, was reduced by more than half from the beginning of the decade to the end, independent of devices being tested. Further, it is likely that this experience outside the CREST trial translated into improved outcomes within the trial as well, as was demonstrated in an analysis presented to the FDA panel reviewing the data.[13]

CREST demonstrated no difference in the primary composite endpoint of death, stroke, and MI in the first 30 days plus ipsilateral stroke out to 4 years.[12] Within the composite, there were some differences noted: patients experienced roughly twice the number of minor strokes in the CAS group, but no long-term differences between groups for neurologic sequelae, and roughly twice the number of MIs in the CEA group, which were associated with a significant worsening in mortality at 4 years. It should be noted that event rates in both groups were very low, both procedures proving quite safe, so that the absolute differences being discussed are in the 1% to 1.5% range. Beyond the primary outcome measures, CAS had significantly fewer access-related complications than CEA and no cranial nerve injury, whereas CEA had approximately 5% 30-day incidence. Based on these data, the FDA granted an extension of indication to standard risk symptomatic and asymptomatic patients for the devices tested. At this time, however, Medicare coverage to match the U.S. FDA approvals is still not forthcoming and is only present for symptomatic patients at high surgical risk.

The postmarket surveillance registries have produced voluminous data on CAS in high surgical risk patients.[9–11,42] In fact, there are over 50,000 high surgical risk patients studied in these multicenter prospective trials and postmarket single-arm studies in the past decade, and outcomes have achieved stroke and death guidelines of the American Heart Association (AHA) for CEA for both symptomatic (3%) and asymptomatic (6%) patients.[42] Because many of these risk factors were exclusion criteria for the landmark surgical trials, there are no comparable data for CEA in the same population and therefore has not been shown to satisfy the same AHA guidelines. Accordingly, for those patients with severe carotid stenosis requiring revascularization who are at risk for CEA, CAS is arguably the treatment of choice based on the available data.

It should be noted that there are no direct comparisons of CAS with medical therapy either for symptomatic or asymptomatic patients. This is because prior studies established CEA as the standard of care for symptomatic (NASCET)[24] and asymptomatic patients (Asymptomatic Carotid Atherosclerosis Study [ACAS] and Asymptomatic Carotid Surgery Trial [ACST]),[59,60] and CAS was compared to that standard of care—it would have been unethical to do otherwise. There is now a question as to the best management of the asymptomatic patient with severe carotid bifurcation stenosis given improvements in medical therapy for atherosclerosis. Unfortunately, prior studies are either too old (ACAS) or did not programmatically institute medical therapy with targeted goals (ACST) to adequately address this issue definitively. The data available for CEA for the proportion of patients on medical therapy in the ACST trial demonstrates that the proportional benefit of CEA is not diminished. A well-designed trial in this area will be filled with questions as to the severity of stenosis that should be studied, the proper medical therapeutic approach (e.g., which class of drugs, what targets for blood pressure, lipids, etc.), and figures to be a ripe area of research in the years to come. Similarly, the question as to the significance of clinically silent microembolization manifesting as DWMRI abnormalities will be an important one. Currently it appears that although CEA creates fewer abnormalities than filter-protected CAS, the volume of the abnormalities is similar. Furthermore, proximal protection CAS is now beginning to approach CEA in this objective measure of microembolization.[61]

CONCLUSION

In the short decade since the advent of dedicated devices for CAS there has been rapid outcome improvement, which is now on par with the much older practice of CEA in most measures. The remaining opportunity in this field is to continue to lower rates of minor stroke by a combination of operator improvement, better patient selection, and evolution in the tools sets—including small-pore stents, proximal protection, and so on. This will likely almost certainly lead to continued reductions in not only the clinical event rates, which are already very low, but also the objective measures of microembolization. And this will merge seamlessly with the goal of providing the lowest revascularization risk possible to the asymptomatic patient, for whom medical therapy alternative remains to be proven, but will likely be tested in the years to come.

REFERENCES

1. Brott TG, Halperin JL, Abbara S, et al. 2011 ASA/ACCF/AHA/AANN/AANS/ACR/ASNR/CNS/SAIP/SCAI/SIR/SNIS/SVM/SVS guideline on the management of patients with extracranial carotid and vertebral artery disease: executive summary. *Stroke* 2011;42(8):e420–e463.
2. Mathias K, Bockenheimer S, von Reutern G, et al. Catheter dilatation of arteries supplying the brain [in German]. *Radiologe* 1983;23(5):208–214.
3. Bockenheimer SA, Mathias K. Percutaneous transluminal angioplasty in arteriosclerotic internal carotid artery stenosis. *AJNR Am J Neuroradiol* 1983;4(3):791–792.
4. Courtheoux P, Theron J, Tournade A, et al. Percutaneous endoluminal angioplasty of post endarterectomy carotid stenoses. *Neuroradiology* 1987;29(2):186–189.
5. Theron J. Protected carotid angioplasty and carotid stents [in French]. *J Mal Vasc* 1996;21(suppl A):113–122.
6. Theron J, Courtheoux P, Alachkar F, et al. New triple coaxial catheter system for carotid angioplasty with cerebral protection. *AJNR Am J Neuroradiol* 1990;11(5):869–874.
7. Diethrich EB, Ndiaye M, Reid DB. Stenting in the carotid artery: initial experience in 110 patients. *J Endovasc Surg* 1996;3(1):42–62.
8. CAVATAS Investigators. Endovascular versus surgical treatment in patients with carotid stenosis in the Carotid and Vertebral Artery Transluminal Angioplasty Study (CAVATAS): a randomised trial. *Lancet* 2001;357(9270):1729–1737.
9. Gray WA, Yadav JS, Verta P, et al. The CAPTURE registry: predictors of outcomes in carotid artery stenting with embolic protection for high surgical risk patients in the early post-approval setting. *Catheter Cardiovasc Interv* 2007;70(7):1025–1033.
10. Massop D, Dave R, Metzger C, et al. Stenting and angioplasty with protection in patients at high-risk for endarterectomy: SAPPHIRE Worldwide Registry first 2,001 patients. *Catheter Cardiovasc Interv* 2009;73(2):129–136.
11. Aronow HD, Gray WA, Ramee SR, et al. Predictors of neurological events associated with carotid artery stenting in high-surgical-risk patients:

12. insights from the Cordis Carotid Stent Collaborative. *Circ Cardiovasc Interv* 2010;3(6):577–584.
12. Brott TG, Hobson RW II, Howard G, et al. Stenting versus endarterectomy for treatment of carotid-artery stenosis. *N Engl J Med* 2010;363(1):11–23.
13. Gray WA, Simonton CA, Verta P. Overview of the 2011 Food and Drug Administration Circulatory System Devices Panel meeting on the ACCU-LINK and ACCUNET Carotid Artery Stent System. *Circulation* 2012;125(18):2256–2264.
14. Werner M, Bausback Y, Bräunlich S, et al. Anatomic variables contributing to a higher periprocedural incidence of stroke and TIA in carotid artery stenting: single center experience of 833 consecutive cases. *Catheter Cardiovasc Interv* 2012;80(2):321–328.
15. Hawkins BM, Kennedy KF, Giri J, et al. Pre-procedural risk quantification for carotid stenting using the CAS score: a report from the NCDR CARE Registry. *J Am Coll Cardiol* 2012;60(17):1617–1622.
16. Grant A, White C, Ansel G, et al. Safety and efficacy of carotid stenting in the very elderly. *Catheter Cardiovasc Interv* 2010;75(5):651–655.
17. Stingele R, Berger J, Alfke K, et al. Clinical and angiographic risk factors for stroke and death within 30 days after carotid endarterectomy and stent-protected angioplasty: a subanalysis of the SPACE study. *Lancet Neurol* 2008;7(3):216–222.
18. Macdonald S, Lee R, Williams R, et al. Towards safer carotid artery stenting: a scoring system for anatomic suitability. *Stroke* 2009;40(5):1698–1703.
19. Willaert WI, Cheshire NJ, Aggarwal R, et al. Improving results for carotid artery stenting by validation of the anatomic scoring system for carotid artery stenting with patient-specific simulated rehearsal. *J Vasc Surg* 2012;56(6):1763–1770.
20. Hawkins BM, Kennedy KF, Giri J, et al. Pre-procedural risk quantification for carotid stenting using the CAS score: a report from the NCDR CARE Registry. *J Am Coll Cardiol* 2012;60(17):1617–1622.
21. Wimmer NJ, Yeh RW, Cutlip DE, et al. Risk prediction for adverse events after carotid artery stenting in higher surgical risk patients. *Stroke* 2012;43(12):3218–3224.
22. Etxegoien N, Rhyne D, Kedev S, et al. The transradial approach for carotid artery stenting. *Catheter Cardiovasc Interv* 2012;80(7):1081–1087.
23. Fairman R, Gray WA, Scicli AP, et al. The CAPTURE registry: analysis of strokes resulting from carotid artery stenting in the post approval setting: timing, location, severity, and type. *Ann Surg* 2007;246(4):551–556.
24. North American Symptomatic Carotid Endarterectomy Trial Collaborators. Beneficial effect of carotid endarterectomy in symptomatic patients with high-grade carotid stenosis. *N Engl J Med* 1991;325(7):445–453.
25. Dieter RS, Ikram S, Satler LF, et al. Perforation complicating carotid artery stenting: the use of a covered stent. *Catheter Cardiovasc Interv* 2006;67(6):972–975.
26. The EC/IC Bypass Study Group. Failure of extracranial-intracranial arterial bypass to reduce the risk of ischemic stroke. Results of an international randomized trial. *N Engl J Med* 1985;313:1191–1200.
27. Powers WJ, Clarke WR, Grubb RL, et al. Results of the carotid occlusion surgery study [abstract]. Presented at: American Heart Association 2011 International Stroke Conference; Los Angeles, CA.
28. Lin MS, Lin LC, Li HY, et al. Procedural safety and potential vascular complication of endovascular recanalization for chronic cervical internal carotid artery occlusion. *Circ Cardiovasc Interv* 2008;1(2):119–125.
29. Gur AY, Bova I, Bornstein NM. Is impaired cerebral vasomotor reactivity a predictive factor of stroke in asymptomatic patients? *Stroke* 1996;27:2188–2190.
30. Spence JD, Tamayo A, Lownie SP, et al. Absence of microemboli on transcranial Doppler identifies low-risk patients with asymptomatic carotid stenosis. *Stroke* 2005;36(11):2373–2378.
31. Watanabe Y, Nagayama M. MR plaque imaging of the carotid artery. *Neuroradiology* 2010;52(4):253–274.
32. Inglese L, Fantoni C, Sardana V. Can IVUS-virtual histology improve outcomes of percutaneous carotid treatment? *J Cardiovasc Surg (Torino)* 2009;50(6):735–744.
33. Hoogi A, Akkus Z, van den Oord SC, et al. Quantitative analysis of ultrasound contrast flow behavior in carotid plaque neovasculature. *Ultrasound Med Biol* 2012;38(12):2072–2083.
34. Hermus L, van Dam GM, Zeebregts CJ. Advanced carotid plaque imaging. *Eur J Vasc Endovasc Surg* 2010;39(2):125–133.
35. Criado E, Fontcuberta J, Orgaz A, et al. Transcervical carotid stenting with carotid artery flow reversal: 3-year follow-up of 103 stents. *J Vasc Surg* 2007;46(5):864–869.
36. Clair DG, Hopkins LN, Mehta M, et al. Neuroprotection during carotid artery stenting using the GORE flow reversal system: 30-day outcomes in the EMPiRE Clinical Study. *Catheter Cardiovasc Interv* 2011;77(3):420–429.

37. Ansel GM, Hopkins LN, Jaff MR, et al. Safety and effectiveness of the IN-VATEC MO.MA proximal cerebral protection device during carotid artery stenting: results from the ARMOUR pivotal trial. *Catheter Cardiovasc Interv* 2010;76(1):1–8.

38. Orlandi G, Fanucchi S, Fioretti C, et al. Characteristics of cerebral microembolism during carotid stenting and angioplasty alone. *Arch Neurol* 2001;58(9):1410–1413.

39. Ling AJ, Mwipatayi P, Gandhi T, et al. Stenting for carotid artery stenosis: fractures, proposed etiology and the need for surveillance. *J Vasc Surg* 2008;47(6):1220–1226.

40. Bosiers M, de Donato G, Deloose K, et al. Does free cell area influence the outcome in carotid artery stenting? *Eur J Vasc Endovasc Surg* 2007;33(2):135–141; discussion 142–143.

41. Grunwald IQ, Reith W, Karp K, et al. Comparison of stent free cell area and cerebral lesions after unprotected carotid artery stent placement. *Eur J Vasc Endovasc Surg* 2012;43(1):10–14.

42. Gray WA, Chaturvedi S, Verta P, et al. Thirty-day outcomes for carotid artery stenting in 6320 patients from 2 prospective, multicenter, high-surgical-risk registries. *Circ Cardiovasc Interv* 2009;2(3):159–166.

43. Macdonald S, Evans DH, Griffiths PD, et al. Filter-protected versus unprotected carotid artery stenting: a randomised trial. *Cerebrovasc Dis* 2010;29(3):282–289.

44. Gray WA, Hopkins LN, Yadav S, et al. Protected carotid stenting in high-surgical-risk patients: the ARCHeR results. *J Vasc Surg* 2006;44(2):258–268.

45. Qureshi AI, Saad M, Zaidat OO, et al. Intracerebral hemorrhages associated with neurointerventional procedures using a combination of antithrombotic agents including abciximab. *Stroke* 2002;33(7):1916–1919.

46. Chan AW, Yadav JS, Bhatt DL, et al. Comparison of the safety and efficacy of emboli protection devices versus platelet glycoprotein IIb/IIIa inhibition during carotid stenting. *Am J Cardiol* 2005;95:791–795.

47. Gray WA, White HJ Jr, Barrett DM, et al. Carotid stenting and endarterectomy: a clinical and cost comparison of revascularization strategies. *Stroke* 2002;33(4):1063–1070.

48. Yan BP, Clark DJ, Jaff MR, et al. Carotid duplex ultrasound velocity measurements versus intravascular ultrasound in detecting carotid in-stent restenosis. *Circ Cardiovasc Interv* 2009;2(5):438–443.

49. Ringleb PA, Allenberg J, Bruckmann H, et al. 30 day results from the SPACE trial of stent-protected angioplasty versus carotid endarterectomy in symptomatic patients: a randomised non-inferiority trial. *Lancet* 2006;368(9543):1239–1247.

50. Mas JL, Chatellier G, Beyssen B, et al. Endarterectomy versus stenting in patients with symptomatic severe carotid stenosis. *N Engl J Med* 2006;355(16):1660–1671.

51. Ederle J, Dobson J, Featherstone RL, et al. Carotid artery stenting compared with endarterectomy in patients with symptomatic carotid stenosis (International Carotid Stenting Study): an interim analysis of a randomised controlled trial. *Lancet* 2010;375(9719):985–997.

52. Yadav JS, Wholey MH, Kuntz RE, et al. Protected carotid-artery stenting versus endarterectomy in high-risk patients. *N Engl J Med* 2004;351(15):1493–1501.

53. Safian RD, Bresnahan JF, Jaff MR, et al. Protected carotid stenting in high-risk patients with severe carotid artery stenosis. *J Am Coll Cardiol* 2006;47(12):2384–2389.

54. Iyer SS, White CJ, Hopkins LN, et al. Carotid artery revascularization in high-surgical-risk patients using the Carotid WALLSTENT and FilterWire EX/EZ: 1-year outcomes in the BEACH Pivotal Group. *J Am Coll Cardiol* 2008;51(4):427–434.

55. Higashida RT, Popma JJ, Apruzzese P, et al. Evaluation of the Medtronic exponent self-expanding carotid stent system with the Medtronic guardwire temporary occlusion and aspiration system in the treatment of carotid stenosis: combined from the MAVErIC (Medtronic AVE Self-expanding CaRotid Stent System with distal protection In the treatment of Carotid stenosis) I and MAVErIC II trials. *Stroke* 2010;41(2):e102–e109.

56. Hopkins LN, Myla S, Grube E, et al. Carotid artery revascularization in high surgical risk patients with the NexStent and the Filterwire EX/EZ: 1-year results in the CABERNET trial. *Catheter Cardiovasc Interv* 2008;71(7):950–960.

57. Hopkins LN, Roubin GS, Chakhtoura EY, et al. The Carotid Revascularization Endarterectomy versus Stenting Trial: credentialing of interventionalists and final results of lead-in phase. *J Stroke Cerebrovasc Dis* 2010;19(2):153–162.

58. Gensicke H, Zumbrunn T, Jongen LM, et al. Characteristics of ischemic brain lesions after stenting or endarterectomy for symptomatic carotid artery stenosis: results from the international carotid stenting study-magnetic resonance imaging substudy. *Stroke* 2013;44(1):80–86.

59. Endarterectomy for asymptomatic carotid artery stenosis. Executive Committee for the Asymptomatic Carotid Atherosclerosis Study. *JAMA* 1995;273(18):1421–1428.

60. Halliday A, Harrison M, Hayter E, et al.10-year stroke prevention after successful carotid endarterectomy for asymptomatic stenosis (ACST-1): a multicentre randomized trial. *Lancet* 2010;376(9746):1074–1084.

61. Bijuklic K, Wandler A, Hazizi F, et al. The PROFI study (Prevention of Cerebral Embolization by Proximal Balloon Occlusion Compared to Filter Protection During Carotid Artery Stenting): a prospective randomized trial. *J Am Coll Cardiol* 2012;59(15):1383–1389.

Diagnosis and Management of Mesenteric Ischemia

JAMES R. STONE, ULKU CENK TURBA, SAHER S. SABRI, WAEL E. SAAD, JOHN F. ANGLE, and ALAN H. MATSUMOTO

Acute Mesenteric Ischemia

OVERVIEW

Acute mesenteric ischemia is a serious and life-threatening condition that occurs when blood flow cannot sustain the functional demands of the intestines, leading to bowel infarction. Primary etiologies include mesenteric arterial embolus, mesenteric arterial thrombosis, mesenteric venous thrombosis, and nonocclusive mesenteric ischemia (NOMI). Less common causes include vasculitides, trauma, aortic dissections, volvulus, intussusceptions, hernias, adhesions, drugs (cocaine), cholesterol emboli, and intestinal obstruction.[1,2] Once bowel infarction occurs, mortality rates increase significantly and can approach 90%.[3] As such, an important goal with this disease process is to establish an early diagnosis, allowing for the provision of aggressive treatment prior to the onset of bowel infarction.

The classic clinical presentation of acute mesenteric ischemia is an abrupt onset of severe abdominal pain that is out of proportion to the physical examination. Diagnosis of this condition may be aided by a high index of clinical suspicion, history of cardiovascular disease, presence of hypotension requiring vasopressor support, and diagnostic imaging evaluation.

In the diagnostic imaging assessment of mesenteric ischemia, catheter-based angiography remains the gold standard given its superior resolution, accuracy in detection of both large- and small-vessel disease, and ability to dynamically follow a delivered contrast bolus from arterial through venous phases. With advancements in noninvasive imaging techniques, catheter-based angiography is now generally employed in anticipation of endovascular therapy, to clarify findings of an equivocal noninvasive imaging study, or to further define vascular anatomy prior to surgery. With its widespread availability, multidetector helical computed tomographic angiography (CTA) has assumed the primary role as the initial diagnostic examination for patients in whom acute mesenteric ischemia is a consideration.[4,5] CTA can be performed very rapidly and can be used to identify the presence of a critical stenosis or occlusion of the superior mesenteric artery (SMA) or thrombosis of the superior mesenteric vein (SMV) while also providing information concerning the presence of bowel infarction or other ancillary findings, such as an abdominal aortic aneurysm, an aortic dissection, or an internal hernia. Its sensitivity is limited for detection of very small emboli or a subtle vasculitis, however, and its use may be contraindicated in patients with severe renal insufficiency.

Magnetic resonance angiography (MRA) can provide insight into the location of stenotic or occlusive disease. Additionally, newer sequences can track a contrast bolus from the arterial through venous phases, allowing for the detection of both arterial lesions and mesenteric vein thrombosis. Its utility in small-vessel disease and in the assessment of bowel integrity is limited, however. Lack of widespread availability of a good cardiovascular magnetic resonance imaging (MRI) unit, limited technical staffing during "off hours," and difficulty in patient monitoring makes MRA less useful than CTA. MRA can be used in patients in whom the estimated glomerular filtration rate (eGFR) is greater than 30 mL/min. Below an eGFR of 30, concern for the development of nephrogenic systemic fibrosis (NSF) may limit the use of contrast-enhanced MRA in this patient population.[6,7] Plain films of the abdomen may demonstrate bowel wall thickening or thumbprinting, bowel dilatation, intramural gas, or portal venous gas, all of which would be secondary signs of end-organ damage resulting from acute mesenteric ischemia.

Treatment has traditionally involved aggressive surgical management. Endovascular management, however, has played an increasing role with multiple case series and reports describing success with initial endovascular therapy or in combination with open surgical intervention.[8–10] Factors that may affect treatment decisions include the acuity of presentation, presence or absence of bowel infarction, extent of occlusive disease, risk factors, etiology of the ischemia, and availability of technical expertise for a planned treatment approach.

ETIOLOGY AND TREATMENT OF ACUTE MESENTERIC ISCHEMIA

Arterial Occlusive Disease

Embolization of thrombotic material to the mesenteric arterial vasculature is responsible for 40% to 50% of cases of acute mesenteric ischemia with a cardiac source being the most common etiology. A frequent association with atrial fibrillation or prior myocardial infarction is seen and approximately 20% of individuals will have a concurrent peripheral arterial embolus. About 33% of individuals presenting with acute mesenteric ischemia from an embolic source will have had a history of a prior embolic event. The clinical presentation of embolic acute mesenteric ischemia typically involves an abrupt onset of severe abdominal pain, diarrhea, and/or hematochezia. Imaging features generally involve a filling defect, outlined by contrast with a convex meniscus in a location that is typically at least 3 cm beyond the origin of the SMA. Generally there are no apparent collaterals and there is poor distal flow given the abrupt onset of this flow-limiting event (FIGURE 44.1).

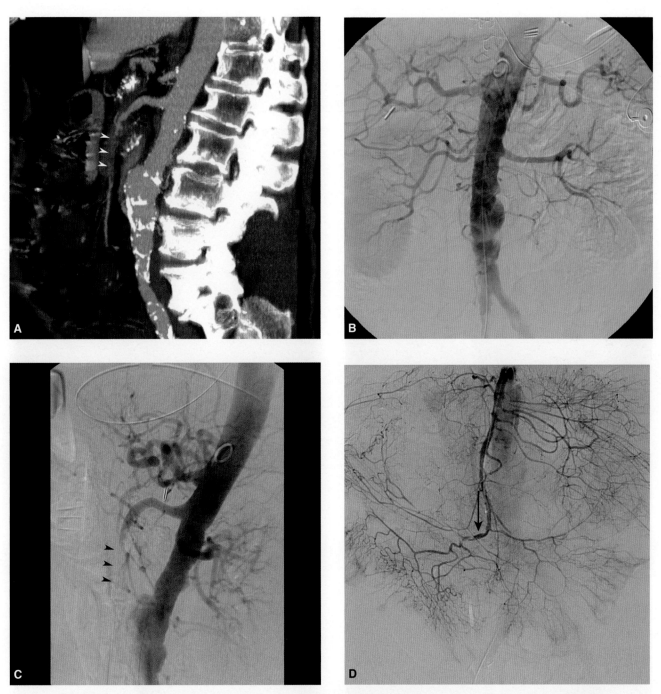

FIGURE 44.1 A 72-year-old patient with ischemic cardiomyopathy and previous ventricular tachycardia arrest requiring automatic implantable cardioverter defibrillator placement, referred for evaluation of acute abdominal pain. **A.** Maximum intensity projection reconstruction of a CTA in a sagittal plane demonstrates acute-appearing embolus (*arrowheads*) within the SMA, approximately 5 cm from the origin of this vessel. **B.** AP nonselective aortogram demonstrates only minimal filling of proximal SMA branches. **C.** Lateral nonselective aortogram again shows the location of embolus (*arrowheads*) within the proximal SMA. **D.** AP arteriogram following 24 hours of SMA catheter-directed thrombolysis demonstrates significant improved flow with patchy areas of end-organ perfusion and some residual clot (*arrow*).

Formation of thrombus directly within the mesenteric arterial vasculature occurs in about 25% of cases of acute mesenteric ischemia. It is typically seen in patients with underlying atherosclerotic lesions and is associated with previous reports of intestinal angina in up to 50% of cases. In contrast to acute embolic mesenteric ischemia, acute thrombotic mesenteric ischemia generally has a less abrupt, more insidious onset. Imaging evaluation reveal occlusive lesions generally located 1 to 2 cm from the origin of the SMA. Collateral vessels may be present, consistent with a more chronic condition in which an acute on chronic process has developed. Findings of bowel ischemia and/or infarction may be observed on a CTA.

An aortic dissection that involves the abdominal aorta or the SMA accounts for less than 5% of all cases of acute mesenteric ischemia. The mesenteric arterial vasculature can be supplied by either the true or the false lumen in these patients (FIGURE 44.2). Inadequate flow results when blood flow fails to

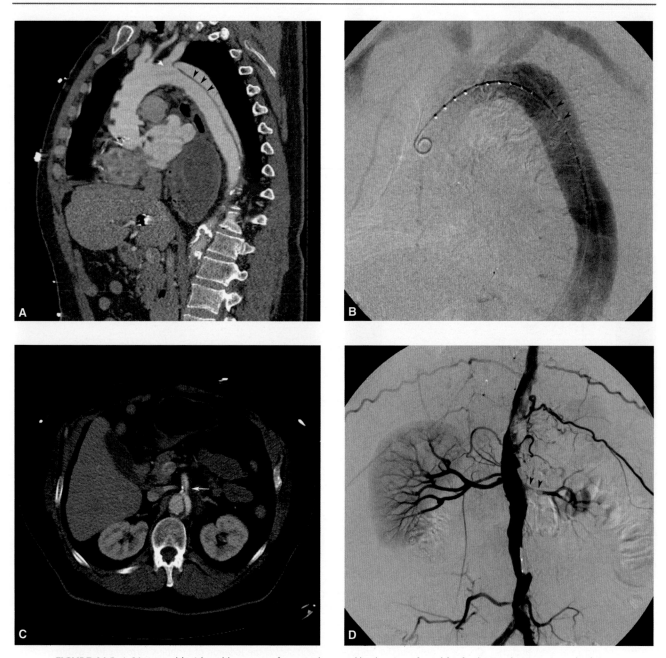

FIGURE 44.2 A 61-year-old with sudden onset of severe chest and back pain, referred for further evaluation. **A.** Multiplanar reformation of CTA in oblique plane demonstrates a dissection septum (*arrowheads*) arising just distal to the left subclavian artery. **B.** Nonselective thoracic aortogram again demonstrates dissection (*arrowheads*). **C.** Axial CTA of the abdomen demonstrates dissection flap extending into the SMA (*arrow*). **D.** Nonselective abdominal aortogram reveals dissection extending through the abdominal aorta. Dissection flap involves the left renal artery (*arrowheads*), resulting in marked reduction in flow to the left kidney. No appreciable filling of the SMA branches is appreciated. **E.** Thoracic aortogram demonstrates positioning of TAG thoracic endograft (W.L. Gore & Associates, Flagstaff, AZ) with the proximal aspect of the prosthesis located at the aortic isthmus. **F.** Abdominal aortogram following thoracic endograft deployment demonstrates marked improvement in flow to both the SMA (*arrowheads*) and left renal artery (*arrow*).

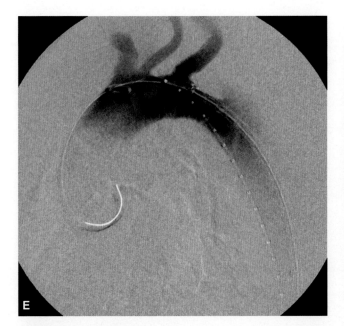 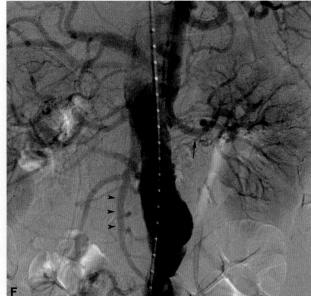

FIGURE 44.2 *(Continued)*

meet the metabolic needs of the bowel due to absence of a distal reentry site, insufficient fenestrations between the true and false lumens, or compression of the main vascular lumen by the other lumen with resultant decreased perfusion in the SMA vascular bed. CTA is typically the best imaging modality to identify the true and false lumens while defining the nature and anatomic relationship of the dissection flap and the adequacy of perfusion to the mesenteric arterial vascular bed. Findings of bowel ischemia or infarction may be seen as well on the CTA study.

Historically, treatment of arterial occlusive acute mesenteric ischemia has involved primary surgical exploration, revascularization, and resection of infarcted bowel.[11–13] Recent reports suggest, however, that endovascular revascularization is associated with relatively favorable outcomes as compared with a more traditional open approach. In a report by Acosta et al.,[8] 10 patients with acute embolic occlusion of the SMA underwent endovascular therapy using percutaneous embolectomy techniques followed by stenting as needed. Embolic protection devices were not used. Satisfactory results were observed in seven patients with two of these requiring adjunctive local thrombolysis. Bowel resection was required in only 1 of the 10 patients. Two deaths were observed in this group with one in-hospital death and one delayed death secondary to a long SMA dissection that led to bowel infarction. In the same report, a separate group of 11 patients were studied who presented with acute SMA occlusion secondary to atherosclerotic disease. In this group, endovascular therapy was performed with all patients undergoing stent or stent-graft placement. Additionally, one patient received open surgical thrombectomy, one received suction thrombectomy, and one underwent local thrombolysis. Four of these patients also underwent subsequent bowel resection. Two deaths were seen in this group and were felt to be secondary to chronic

obstructive pulmonary disease (COPD) and bowel infarction, respectively. Distal emboli that occurred due to the aggressive endovascular interventions were relatively well tolerated[8] (FIGURE 44.3).

In a separate study performed by Bjornsson et al.,[9] the utility of local arterial thrombolytic therapy for acute SMA occlusion was studied in 34 patients. Most patients included in this study (82%) had embolic occlusion. No patients with acute peritonitis received arterial thrombolysis. In 10 of these patients, aspiration thromboembolectomy was performed. Thirteen patients underwent exploratory laparotomies and eight underwent bowel resection. An in-hospital survival rate of 74% was observed with successful thrombolysis being associated with a decrease in mortality.

The management of acute arterial occlusive mesenteric ischemia is evolving to include more aggressive application of endovascular therapy as an initial approach, even in the presence of bowel infarction. With imaging-verified mesenteric arterial occlusion or with a high level of clinical suspicion, the management of each patient depends heavily on the presence of bowel infarction versus bowel ischemia. If bowel infarction is present, revascularization with embolectomy/ bypass or endovascular revascularization approaches should be performed as soon as possible, followed by an exploratory laparotomy to remove infarcted bowel. As an adjunct to treatment, the potent vasodilator papaverine should be administered directly within the SMA to relieve the associated mesenteric arterial vasoconstriction. Papaverine is given as a 45- to 60-mg bolus directly within the SMA, followed by a papaverine infusion at a rate of 1 mg/min directly into the SMA. The intra-arterial papaverine is administered during the surgical procedure and in the postoperative period to optimize intestinal perfusion.

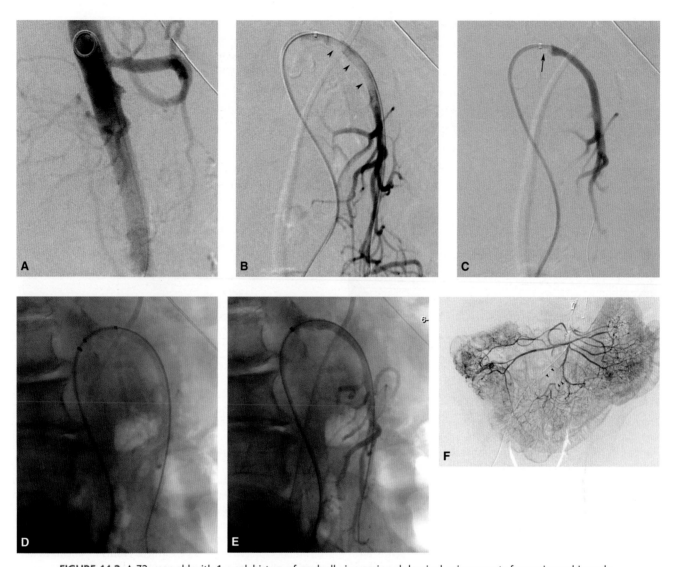

FIGURE 44.3 A 73-year-old with 1-week history of gradually increasing abdominal pain presents for angiographic evaluation. **A.** Nonselective lateral aortogram demonstrates occlusion of the SMA near the ostium of this vessel. **B.** Occlusion was crossed with a hydrophilic guide wire and catheter, after which a sheath was placed. Contrast injection into the SMA demonstrates thrombus extending through the proximal portion of this vessel (*arrowheads*). **C.** After 4 mg of tPA administration into the SMA and suction thrombectomy, significant clearance of thrombus is noted. Persistent focal occlusion (*arrow*) is still seen at the proximal aspect of this vessel, likely secondary to atherosclerotic disease. **D.** A 6 × 18 mm balloon-expandable bare metal stent is positioned within the proximal SMA. **E.** Poststent deployment, the SMA is patent with good flow as seen on the lateral view. **F.** Completion AP SMA arteriogram demonstrates dramatic improved flow into the SMA. Persistent occlusions of secondary and tertiary branches are seen (*arrowheads*). However, continuous perfusion of bowel is supplied through abundant mesenteric collaterals.

In the absence of bowel infarction, occlusions can be recanalized and treated with percutaneous transluminal angioplasty (PTA)/stents. Lysis of an acute embolus/thrombus can be performed with the use of mechanical thrombectomy and embolic protection devices. Intra-arterial papaverine can also be added to the treatment regimen to maximize intestinal perfusion. Anticoagulation should be initiated and continued in all patients who present with an arterial embolus.

In the setting of an aortic dissection causing acute mesenteric ischemia, operative repair is associated with a mortality rate that approaches 90%. Early intervention with endograft and endovascular therapy may reduce mortality rates. Endografts can be used to cover the primary aortic fenestration to depressurize the false lumen and enhance true lumen flow into the SMA. Dilatation of an existing fenestration(s) or creation of de novo fenestrations using percutaneous techniques can be performed to more closely equilibrate flow within the true and false lumens to enhance intestinal perfusion.[14] Use of stents to approximate an occlusive, fixed dissection flap within the SMA to reestablish flow can be performed as well (FIGURE 44.2).

Nonocclusive Mesenteric Ischemia

NOMI is responsible for approximately 20% to 30% of acute mesenteric ischemia cases and commonly results from prolonged hypotension. The presentation of NOMI has been associated with a variety of vasopressors and other pharmaceuticals, such as digitalis and dopamine. Clinically, this condition can present with an ileus, increasing pain, use of vasopressors, an episode of profound hypotension, and/or increasing transaminases. Catheter-based angiography, CTA, or MRA demonstrates diffuse arterial vasospasm with segmental, sausage-like narrowings or diffuse narrowing of the arterial circulation. These findings are most commonly seen near vessel branch points. Delayed filling of distal branches, asymmetric bowel perfusion, and/or delayed venous filling are commonly seen. Additionally, reflux of contrast from the SMA into the aorta during catheter-based angiography secondary to high pressure in the mesenteric vascular bed is often observed (FIGURE 44.4).

Treatment of NOMI should first attempt to reverse the existing causes of hypotension to prevent further end-organ injury. A mainstay of therapy for NOMI is intra-arterial infusion of papaverine directly into the SMA. Treatment is generally

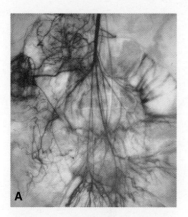
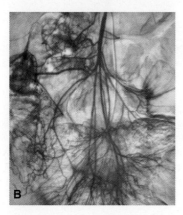

FIGURE 44.4 Patient with nonocclusive mesenteric ischemia. A. Pretreatment, diffuse reduction in caliber of the mesenteric vessels are noted with overall reduction in end-organ perfusion. B. Intra-arterial papaverine was administered directly into the SMA to promote vasodilation. After intra-arterial papaverine administration, marked increase in vessel caliber is noted. Significantly improved end-organ perfusion is seen as well.

continued until symptoms resolve (usually 1 to 2 days). If peritoneal signs develop or serum lactate levels continue to rise, exploratory laparotomy should be performed to assess for and resect nonviable bowel.

Superior Mesenteric Vein Thrombosis

Thrombosis of the SMV accounts for less than 5% of all cases of acute mesenteric ischemia. Predisposing factors for SMV thrombosis include portal hypertension, abdominal inflammatory disease, oral contraceptives, prior surgery involving the portal venous system, trauma, and a hypercoagulable state. Thrombosis of the SMV generally leads to intestinal venous congestion, mucosal edema, and arterial hypoperfusion. SMV thrombosis is typically diagnosed with a CTA or MRA during venous phase imaging. The imaging studies will often reveal a filling defect or no flow in the mesenteric veins and associated mucosal edema of the small bowel.

Catheter-based angiographic evaluation of a patient with concern for SMV thrombosis will demonstrate high resistance to arterial flow with diffuse arterial vasospasm seen, persistence of the arterial phase and prolonged mucosal enhancement, lack of opacification of the mesenteric veins, prolonged opacification of venules or larger regional veins, and a fixed intraluminal filling defect within the mesenteric veins on venous phase. Mucosal edema might also be identified.

Treatment includes stabilizing the cardiovascular status and correcting any predisposing factors with appropriate hydration and antibiotics. Patients who present with mesenteric venous thrombosis can often be managed conservatively with supportive care and anticoagulation.[15] In a study conducted by Turnes et al.,[16] mesenteric vein recanalization rates were 69% when anticoagulation therapy was instituted within 1 week but dropped to 25% if therapy was administered later than 1 week after symptom onset.

Surgical intervention should be performed when peritoneal signs are present or with rapidly increasing serum lactic acid levels. The primary goal of surgery is to resect nonviable bowel but, on occasion, surgical thrombectomy is performed. Surgical thrombectomy does not appear to benefit venous patency in the long term, however.[17,18] Preoperative and postoperative anticoagulation is employed because up to one-third of patients experience recurrent thrombosis of uninvolved segments. If coexistent mesenteric arterial vasoconstriction is present, intra-arterial (SMA) papaverine can be used.

In the presence of persistent abdominal pain, peritoneal signs, or elevated lactic acid levels, endovascular options include transarterial, systemic, or direct transhepatic or transjugular infusion of thrombolytics[18–23] (FIGURE 44.5). Adjunctive mechanical thrombectomy, angioplasty, and stent placement can be used if direct access into the mesenteric venous system is obtained. A study performed by Liu et al.,[24] explored the efficacy of direct access to the portal system with mechanical thrombectomy and thrombolysis versus indirect thrombolysis through placement of a catheter in the SMA and infusion thrombolytic therapy from the arterial side of the mesenteric vascular bed. In this study, complete clearance of thrombus from the portal vein (PV) and SMV was seen in 81% of patients with partial clearance from the remaining 19% treated with this approach. The indirect thrombolysis group showed partial clearance of clot in 14% of patients that was accompanied by complete

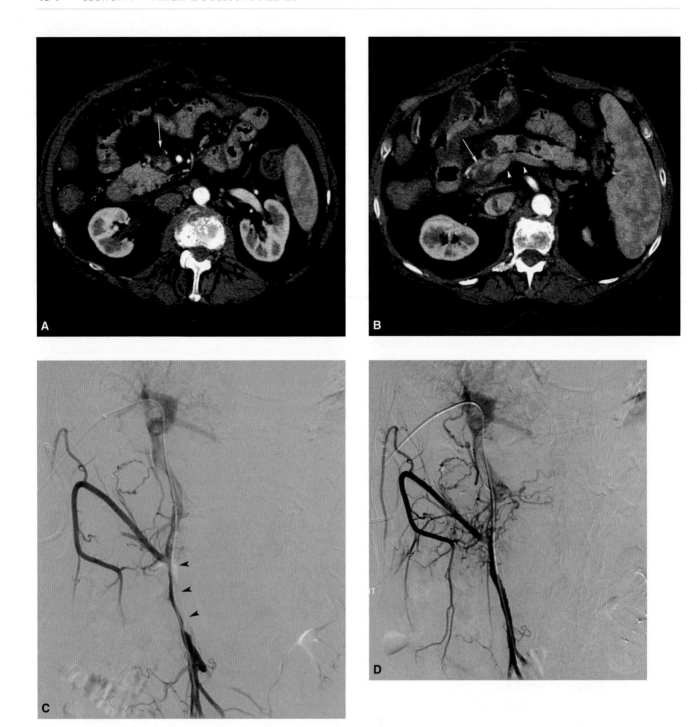

FIGURE 44.5 Acute abdominal pain and elevated lactate seen in the setting of SMV thrombosis. **A.** Axial CTA demonstrates an enlarged SMV containing partially occlusive thrombus (*arrow*). **B.** Axial CTA shows thrombus extending within the SMV (*arrow*) to the confluence of the splenic vein (*arrowheads*). **C.** Transhepatic access to the portal system has been obtained and catheterization of the SMV performed. Venogram demonstrates partially occlusive clot within the SMV (*arrowheads*). **D.** Following mechanical thrombectomy and thrombolysis, clearance of thrombus within the SMV is seen, accompanied by marked improvement in flow.

symptom relief. The remaining 86% showed no gross change in thrombus burden. Lateral branch angiogenesis and dramatic improvement in symptoms was seen in 92% of patients showing no bulk change in thrombus burden. A study by Wang et al.[25] explored the utility of prolonged transradial SMA infusion for treatment of SMV thrombosis. In these patients, 5 French Cobra catheters were introduced into the SMA and infusions were performed ranging from 5 to 11 days. All patients demonstrated significant clinical improvement. Near-complete clearance of PV-SMV thrombosis was seen in 56% of the patients, whereas partial recanalization of the PV-SMV was seen in the remaining 44%. Another study performed by Hollingshead et al.[19] evaluated the utility of transcatheter thrombolytic therapy in patients with portal and/or mesenteric vein thrombosis. Twenty patients were included in the analysis. Overall, 15 of the 20 patients (75%) achieved lysis with 3 patients experiencing complete lysis (15%) and 12 patients (60%) experiencing partial lysis. Symptom improvement was seen in 17 of the 20 patients (85%). Twelve patients (60%) developed major complications, which included one death and bleeding requiring transfusion. After completion of thrombolytic therapy, no patients developed further portal or mesenteric vein thromboses during follow-up. This study underscores observations that direct transhepatic or transjugular approaches to mesenteric venous thrombosis are associated with risks for intraperitoneal bleeding or liver injury associated with the direct access of the mesenteric circulation and is particularly hazardous in the presence of ascites.

In general, the treatment of SMV thrombosis should be guided by clinical presentation and distribution of thrombus burden. Conservative management with early anticoagulation and supportive care is often an effective approach. In patients with persistent abdominal pain, peritoneal signs, and/or elevated lactic acid, endovascular therapy may provide benefit. Transhepatic access to the portal system with retrograde catheterization of the SMV may provide the greatest benefit to those patients with the bulk of clot located in the main trunk of the SMV and PV. When clot is primarily distributed peripherally within small venules and/or capillaries, however, thrombolysis through the SMA may provide sufficient small-vessel clearance to afford symptom relief. When bowel infarction is present, surgical exploration should be performed to resect nonviable bowel.

Systemic Effects of Bowel Infarction

Although acute mesenteric ischemia may result from a spectrum of etiologies, a final common pathway of this disease process can involve bowel infarction, systemic inflammatory response syndrome (SIRS), refractory shock, and multiorgan dysfunction syndrome (MODS).[26] Clinical criteria for SIRS is met by observing two or more of the following: (1) temperature greater than 38°C or less than 36°C, (2) heart rate greater than 90 beats/min, (3) respiratory rate greater than 20 breaths/min or partial pressure of arterial carbon dioxide ($PaCO_2$) less than 32 mm Hg, (4) white blood cell (WBC) count greater than 12,000/mm³, less than 4,000/mm³, or greater than 10% immature (band) cells.[27] With even brief interruptions in blood flow, intestinal mucosal integrity may begin to fail and become permeable to gut flora. More prolonged interruption of blood flow can cause a shift from aerobic to anaerobic metabolism with resultant accumulation of lactic acid. Failure of anaerobic energy production to keep up with metabolic demands can result in loss of ability to maintain cellular homeostasis, necrotic cell death, and release of intracellular contents into the extracellular space leading to an inflammatory response. With widespread intestinal necrosis, a robust inflammatory response may overwhelm normal immune inhibitory feedback loops, resulting in a self-enforcing cytokine storm, which may manifest as the clinical sequelae of SIRS. If unchecked, SIRS can be associated with profound hypotension, multiorgan failure, and death.

Although a primary goal of treatment for acute mesenteric ischemia includes restoration of mesenteric blood flow, reperfusion injury may occur following therapy secondary to formation of reactive oxygen species (ROS) from interactions between oxygen-rich blood and free radicals locally produced during the inflammatory response.[28] ROS may lead to further cell death through direct injury to the plasma membrane, proteins, and DNA. Reperfusion injury should be considered in the posttreatment period for all patients receiving successful treatment for acute mesenteric ischemia.

Summary

Acute mesenteric ischemia is a serious and life-threatening condition. Rapid diagnosis and restoration of blood flow is of paramount importance in decreasing the morbidity and mortality associated with this condition. Given the profound systemic effects of bowel infarction, the key to successful treatment of acute mesenteric ischemia involves early intervention to correct the underlying abnormality. Although surgical exploration may be required for resection of nonviable bowel, an increasing body of evidence suggests that aggressive endovascular approaches are associated with reductions in the high morbidity and mortality associated with this disease process. When clinical concern exists for acute mesenteric ischemia, patients should be seen as soon as possible and stat diagnostics should be obtained to guide therapy. Once a diagnosis is confirmed, therapy should be instituted without delay and cannot wait until the next morning or following day.

Chronic Mesenteric Ischemia

▌ OVERVIEW

Chronic mesenteric ischemia is a relatively rare clinical phenomenon, largely due to the rich collateral intestinal circulation. Although classic descriptions of chronic mesenteric ischemia describe a requisite for narrowing or occlusion of two or more main visceral arteries prior to symptom development, it is increasingly believed that compromise of one or more of the celiac, superior mesenteric, or inferior mesenteric arteries, in any configuration, may lead to symptoms.

Patients with chronic mesenteric ischemia typically present with postprandial pain and weight loss. Postprandial pain generally begins shortly after eating and lasts 1 to 2 hours and can lead to the patient developing a fear of food given the association between food intake and pain. Differential considerations for this symptom complex include functional bowel disorders, atrophic gastritis, gallbladder disease, chronic pancreatitis, hernias, surgical adhesions, median arcuate ligament compression syndrome, and malignancy.[29,30] Nonspecific symptoms can also be seen and include nausea, diarrhea, and vomiting. Chronic mesenteric ischemia most often occurs secondary to atherosclerotic narrowing of one or more mesenteric arteries. In contrast to most other atherosclerotic diseases, chronic mesenteric ischemia is seen more frequently in females.[29] Gender-related differences are seen in the orientation of the mesenteric vessels to the aorta with the mesenteric vessels possessing a more acute angle to the aorta than in males. Specifically, in a study conducted by Oderich et al.,[31] females with a body mass index (BMI) of 25 to 29.9 were noted to possess a mean angle between the aorta and SMA of 49.5, whereas males in this BMI range were noted to possess a mean aortomesenteric angle of 63.8. It has been suggested that this difference in anatomic configuration may affect flow dynamics and predispose females to atherosclerotic disease of the mesenteric vessels. Occlusive or stenotic lesions of the SMA may also occur secondary to fibromuscular dysplasia (FMD), vasculitides, and intimal hyperplasia after a surgical procedure involving the SMA.

The natural history and factors affecting progression of mesenteric artery stenoses is not well defined. Therefore, it is difficult to predict disease progression. Although progression from chronic to acute mesenteric ischemia is associated with greater than 50% mortality, controversy exists concerning if and when to treat asymptomatic mesenteric arterial lesions given the risks associated with both open surgical and minimally invasive endovascular approaches to correct asymptomatic lesions. At present, there exists no laboratory test to assess for the physiologic significance of a given mesenteric arterial lesion.

▌ DIAGNOSIS

Assessments of chronic mesenteric ischemia can be performed with catheter-based angiography, ultrasound, CTA, and MRA. Catheter-based angiography remains the gold standard for the diagnosis of occlusive mesenteric arterial disease, although its role is now limited to cases determined to be equivocal by other noninvasive imaging modalities or as part of a planned endovascular intervention. Angiography typically involves an initial aortogram in anteroposterior (AP) and lateral projections. The AP aortogram allows for the identification of distal arterial disease while providing an overview of the mesenteric vascular anatomy and dynamic flow from one territory to another. The lateral aortogram will allow for the detection of ostial disease of the celiac artery, SMA, and inferior mesenteric artery (IMA). This initial diagnostic information may be supplemented by selective catheter-directed angiography and translesional pressure measurements. Lesions with a greater than 60% diameter narrowing or with a 70% to 80% reduction in cross-sectional area, in combination with at least a 20 mm Hg systolic translesion pressure gradients at rest, without provocative maneuvers, are generally considered significant. These criteria have largely been adapted from the renovascular hypertension literature.[32–34]

Although catheter-based methods provide superb diagnostic information, advances in noninvasive methods for assessing the visceral vasculature have led to the adoption of ultrasound, CTA, or MRA as the initial diagnostic tests to evaluate for the presence or extent of mesenteric arterial disease prior to proceeding to angiography.

Duplex ultrasound (US) is an inexpensive and readily available imaging modality to screen for chronic mesenteric ischemia. This noninvasive imaging option provides physiologic flow data. Some interventionists have advocated that duplex US can be performed in the fasting and postprandial states to detect physiologically significant stenoses.[35] In the fasting state, the celiac and SMA differ in waveform with the celiac artery, demonstrating higher end diastolic velocities (EDV) with flow throughout the cardiac cycle caused by the low resistance within the liver and spleen. In contrast, the SMA possesses a high-resistance waveform characteristic of the splanchnic circulation. In the postprandial state, a marked increase in EDV will be seen in the SMA with a less dramatic increase seen in the celiac circulation. Physiologically, significant stenoses will

be characterized by increases in the peak systolic velocity (PSV) and EDV during duplex US interrogation. Retrograde flow in the hepatic artery may be seen with a severe stenosis or occlusion of the celiac artery. Additionally, loss of diastolic flow or flow reversal may be seen with a significant stenosis of the SMA. Despite its low cost and ready availability, duplex US may be limited by the presence of overlying bowel gas, normal variant arterial anatomy, patient body habitus, operator training, and lack of uniform criteria for interpretation of the duplex US findings.[35] Additionally, multivessel disease can lead to the overestimation of stenotic lesions secondary to the development of rich collateral arterial flow. Contrast-enhanced ultrasound using commercially available gas-containing microbubbles when compared with nonenhanced US demonstrated improved sensitivity (94.1% enhanced vs. 80% nonenhanced) and equivalent specificity (100% with both enhanced and nonenhanced) for the diagnosis of mesenteric ischemia.[36]

With the advent of multidetector helical scanners, CTA has become increasingly used to aid in the diagnosis of chronic mesenteric ischemia. Using present-day equipment, the temporal and spatial resolution afforded by CTA is almost as good as catheter-based angiography.[37] In addition to localizing sites of occlusive lesions, CTA allows for the assessment of tissue structural findings that may provide insight into lesion etiology while allowing for assessment of secondary findings that may detect an occult pancreatic malignancy or the presence of bowel ischemia/infarction. In the setting of previous endovascular or surgical treatment, CTA can allow for assessment of stent or graft patency, respectively.[38] In the utilization of CTA for the diagnosis of chronic mesenteric ischemia, an initial noncontrast study can be performed to gather information on the presence of calcifications, extravascular blood, surgical clips, stents, or foreign bodies. Arterial phase contrast-enhanced acquisitions are then performed to allow evaluation of the arterial anatomy. A delayed phase can then be acquired 70 seconds after contrast bolus administration to gain additional information on the mucosal surface of the bowel, mesentric venous patency and the anatomy of other end organs. Negative oral contrast may be administered to increase the sensitivity and specificity for detecting bowel-related findings. Positive oral contrast should not be used during a CTA study because the presence of high-density material within the intestines can decrease the overall quality of postprocessed images and create streak artifacts caused by the density differences between the positive contrast and the adjacent air interface in the intestines.

Much progress has been made in recent years with the display of acquired CT data. Multiplanar reformation (MPR), maximum intensity projection (MIP), volume rendering (VR), and surface shaded display have been used to project 3D data sets on a 2D display to optimally demonstrate anatomically significant relationships.[39] Utilization of these postprocessing algorithms has had a significant impact on the amount of meaningful information that can be extracted from a given CTA examination. Postprocessing can be performed by a technologist following acquisition of the data sets and sent to the computer workstation along with the source axial images. Alternatively, with the increased availability of faster, more powerful computer processors, thin-slice isovoxel axial images can be processed at the workstation by the clinician to optimize the direct examination of the clinically significant findings.

MRA represents another noninvasive methodology for the assessment of chronic mesenteric ischemia. Although phase contrast (PC) and time-of-flight (TOF) techniques have been historically used for characterization of mesenteric vascular anatomy, the use of fast, contrast-enhanced techniques provide superior imaging secondary to minimization of motion artifact and flow effects. Three-dimensional (3D) contrast-enhanced acquisitions can provide insight into anatomic relationships while providing an overview of the abdominal arterial and venous vascular supply. Overall, the spatial resolution of MRA is inferior to catheter-based angiography and CTA, although its sensitivity and specificity for evaluation of proximal stenotic or occlusive lesions within the renal arteries exceeds 90%.[40] In addition to the acquisition of anatomic information, MRA can be used to perform functional assessment of intestinal perfusion. Using cine PC, flow rates may be assessed to compare flow within the SMA and SMV following a meal. A significant increase in flow through the SMV as compared to the SMA has been found to be a good predictor of mesenteric ischemia.[41] In addition to flow assessment, in vivo oximetry has also been previously performed using heavily T2-weighted images and relying on the strong paramagnetic properties of deoxyhemoglobin to determine oxygen extraction. Although the previously described functional techniques may provide physiologically meaningful data in the setting of chronic mesenteric ischemia, they are rarely used in routine clinical practice.[42]

TREATMENT

The primary goal of treatment of chronic mesenteric ischemia is to provide adequate revascularization of the mesenteric arterial bed. Surgery has classically been performed for the treatment of chronic mesenteric ischemia and has typically involved either transaortic endarterectomy or mesenteric artery bypass grafting.[43]

Endovascular management has taken on an increasing role in the treatment of chronic mesenteric ischemia caused by atherosclerotic occlusive lesions or FMD.[44] Hemodynamically significant stenoses or frank occlusions can be crossed with a guide wire and a reverse curve catheter, facilitating PTA and stent placement. Median arcuate ligament compression of either the celiac artery or SMA is generally a contraindication to endovascular management given the tendency for stents to be crushed or fractured by extrinsic forces associated with diaphragmatic compression. These cases are generally better managed with surgical decompression of the affected arteries because surgical decompression also alleviates compression of the celiac ganglion and the neural plexus.[45–47] In the setting of mesenteric arterial occlusion, a stump of an occluded vessel arising from the aorta is generally required to allow engagement of the occluded artery for traversing the lesion. If no such stump exists, then surgical intervention will likely be necessary to reestablish vascular patency.

Over the past 20 years, a marked increase in the number of procedures for mesenteric revascularization has been performed. Much of this increase is secondary to an escalated utilization of endovascular techniques.[44] A number of case series have been published assessing the efficacy of endovascular therapy in chronic mesenteric ischemia. In a study performed by Razavi and Chung, 70 symptomatic patients underwent stent placement for treatment of this disease. Technical success was seen in 97%. A mean follow-up of 3 years was achieved and a recurrence rate of 10.5% was observed. Risks for recurrence included occlusions,

lesions greater than 3 cm in length, and stent diameter less than 5 mm[48] (FIGURE 44.6). In a separate study of chronic mesenteric ischemia endovascular therapy, a clinical success rate of 87.9% was seen in a cohort of 33 patients. A mean period of clinical follow-up of 38 months demonstrated a 17% rate of recurrent symptoms with a primary assisted long-term clinical success rate of 96.6%. Of note in this study, isolated IMA treatment was associated with durable results[49] (Table 44.1, FIGURE 44.7).

In the comparison of open surgical versus endovascular techniques, Oderich et al.[31] performed a 14-year retrospective review of outcomes in 229 patients receiving open surgical versus PTA/stent placement for treatment of chronic mesenteric ischemia. Morbidity was 36% in the open surgical group versus 18% in the endovascular group ($p < .001$). However, 5-year recurrence-free survival was 55% in the endovascular group versus 89% in the open surgical group ($p < .05$). Additionally, open surgical repair was associated with improved primary (88% vs. 41%, $p < .05$) and secondary rates (97% vs. 88%, $p < .05$) when compared with endovascular repair (Table 44.2).

ENDOVASCULAR APPROACH

A variety of disease processes can compromise the mesenteric arterial vasculature, leading to acute, acute on chronic, or chronic mesenteric ischemia. Endovascular approaches for treatment of most causes of mesenteric ischemia share common tools and techniques and are similar to those used for the treatment of renal artery disease.

Arterial access through a femoral approach is generally preferred. Brachial artery access may be utilized in the setting of aortoiliac occlusive disease or with an acute downward angle of the mesenteric arterial branches in relation to the aorta. When brachial artery access is used, care should be taken to minimize the profile of catheters and sheaths to prevent brachial artery thrombosis or formation of an arterial hematoma that may compromise the arterial supply to the extremity and/or result in compressive injury to the median nerve. An SOS Omni 2, RC 1, or Simmons 1 catheter (AngioDynamics, Glen Falls, NY; Cook, Inc., Bloomington, IN; Boston Scientific, Natick, MA; Cordis Endovascular, Warrenton, NJ) may be used for catheterization of the celiac artery or SMA. Catheterization of the IMA may be achieved through use of an SOS Omni 2 or an RIM catheter (AngioDynamics or Cook, Inc., respectively). In the setting of arterial occlusion or critical stenosis, a hydrophilic steerable guide wire may be used to cross the lesion. This guide wire may be exchanged for a stiff exchange wire once the lesion is traversed, over which a guiding sheath or catheter may be used to perform PTA or stent placement. In the celiac or SMA branches, a 0.035″ system is preferred for the treatment of heavily calcified lesions, given the increased durability of balloons and stents on a 0.035″ platform as compared with those available for use with 0.018″ or 0.014″ wires. Treatment of IMA lesions may require 0.018″ or 0.014″ wires given the relatively small caliber of this vessel.

A decision whether to intervene can be guided by translesional pressure measurements. In general, systolic peak-to-peak pressure gradient greater than 20 or 10 mm Hg arterial mean pressure is considered an indication for treatment. A systolic peak measurement of less than 10 mm Hg is considered not significant, whereas 10 to 20 mm Hg is considered borderline with treatment guided by the presence and nature of clinical symptoms.

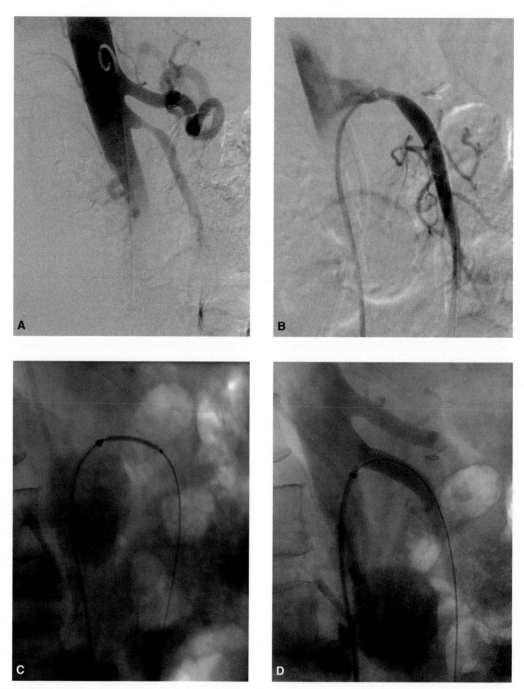

FIGURE 44.6 A 72-year-old patient presents with history of postprandial pain and weight loss, gradually worsening over the past several months. **A.** Nonselective lateral abdominal aortogram demonstrates stenosis within the proximal portion of the SMA. **B.** Selective arteriogram demonstrates proximal stenosis of the SMA. Translesional pressure measurements demonstrate systolic gradient of 28 mm Hg. **C.** Balloon-expandable stent positioned across this lesion. **D.** Poststent deployment, the SMA is widely patent.

When stent placement is required, the choice of stent is generally dictated by the location and type of lesion. For ostial lesions, balloon-expandable stents are generally preferred. Lesions within the trunk of the mesenteric arteries may be treated with either balloon-expandable or self-expanding stents. Although bare metal stents are often used, covered stents may be employed in the setting of soft plaque, in arteries less than 6 mm in diameter (to reduce the risk for in-stent restenosis), or for the treatment of in-stent restenosis secondary to intimal hyperplasia. Balloon or stent advancement may be hindered by tortuosity of the iliac vessels, acute angle of the artery to be treated, and/or the presence of a tight or occlusive lesion. In these settings, an 8 French Morph catheter (Biocardia, San Carlos, CA) may be of some use given the ability to steer the tip of the catheter and provide additional

Table 44.1

Chronic Mesenteric Ischemia: Endovascular Study Results

Study (2000–2011)	Number of patients	Technical success (%)	Early symptom relief (%)	Long-term symptom relief (%)	Mean follow-up (months)
Kasirajan et al.[52]	28	100	NA	66	36
Matsumoto et al.[49]	33	88	88	84	38
Razavi and Chung[48]	70	97	98.5	90	36
Landis et al.[53]	29	97	90	79	28
Silva et al.[54]	59	96	88	83	38
Lee et al.[55]	31	98	70	56	6
Sarac et al.[56]	65	NA	85	75	31
Peck et al.[57]	49	88	90	61	37
Malgor et al.[58]	101	98	98	91	41
Fioole et al.[59]	51	93	78	67	25
Schoch et al.[60]	107	100	100	53	16

NA, not available.

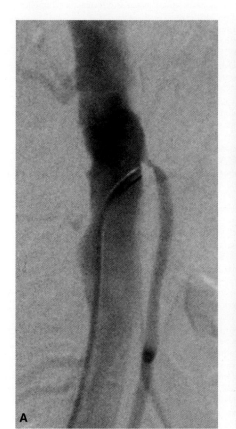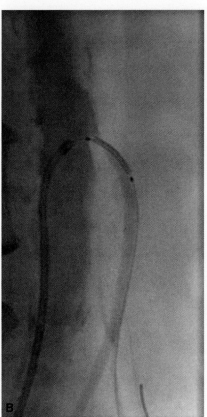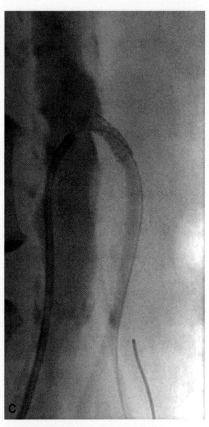

FIGURE 44.7 Patient referred for evaluation of postprandial pain and weight loss. **A.** Lateral aortogram demonstrates isolated high-grade stenosis of the IMA. **B.** Balloon-expandable stent positioned at the IMA. **C.** Poststent deployment, the IMA is widely patent.

Table 44.2					
Chronic Mesenteric Ischemia: Endovascular Treatment Versus Open Surgery					
Study (2000–2011)	Number of patients ET/OS	Technical success ET/OS (%)	Early symptom relief ET/OS (%)	Long-term symptom relief ET/OS (%)	Mean follow-up ET/OS (months)
Kasirajan et al.[52]	28/85	100/100	NA/NA	66/87	60/24
Brown et al.[61]	14/33	NA/93	NA/NA	NA/NA	13/34
Sivamurthy et al.[62]	19/41	95/100	33/71	22/59	19/25
Biebl et al.[63]	23/26	NA/NA	79/100	75/89	10/25
Atkins et al.[50]	31/49	97/100	87/90	74/91	15/42
Zerbib et al.[64]	14/15	93/100	NA/NA	71/93	15/21
Davies et al.[51]	15/17	93/100	86/100	73/100	34/34
Oderich et al.[31]	83/146	95/100	93/95	69/94	30/36
Rawat and Gibbons[65]	36/40	NA/NA	83/90	70/82	22/41

ET, endovascular treatment; OS, open surgery; NA, not available.

support. Treatment of tight or occlusive lesions may also be aided by predilation of the lesion with a low-profile balloon.

Pharmacologic adjuncts to acute arterial occlusive mesenteric ischemia or chronic mesenteric ischemia include the use of intravenous heparin of 3,000 to 5,000 international units with a target activated clotting time of greater than 220 seconds. Intra-arterial nitroglycerin in 100 to 200 mcg boluses may be administered to prevent or minimize spasm. When a stent is deployed, 325 mg of aspirin and 300 mg of clopidogrel may be administered in the recovery room. Aspirin 81 to 325 mg should then be continued for life and 75 mg of clopidogrel should be administered for at least 30 days.

Summary

Chronic mesenteric ischemia is a relatively uncommon clinical phenomenon due to the rich collateral circulation of the gastrointestinal tract. When strong clinical suspicion for this disease process is present, assessments can be performed with US, CTA, or MRA to confirm a diagnosis. Catheter-directed angiography can be performed in patients with equivocal findings on noninvasive imaging or when intervention is anticipated. The primary goal of treatment is to improve blood flow to the mesenteric vascular bed. Endovascular therapy has taken on an increasing role in the primary management of chronic mesenteric ischemia in recent years. Although prospective comparisons of endovascular and open surgical approaches remain lacking, retrospective studies comparing these two approaches suggest that surgical bypass is associated with a more durable result. Open surgery, however, is associated with increased periprocedural morbidity and mortality when compared with endovascular approaches.[31,50,51] As such, current recommendations for treatment involve endovascular management with stent placement as a first-line approach, particularly in patients who are poor surgical candidates secondary to nutrition status, comorbidities, or those who have undergone previous abdominal surgery. In those patients who are surgical candidates and fail endovascular therapy, bypass generally remains an option.

■ REFERENCES

1. Wyers MC. Acute mesenteric ischemia: diagnostic approach and surgical treatment. *Semin Vasc Surg* 2010;23:9–20.
2. Acosta S. Epidemiology of mesenteric vascular disease: clinical implications. *Semin Vasc Surg* 2010;23:4–8.
3. Stamatakos M, Stefanaki C, Mastrokalos D, et al. Mesenteric ischemia: still a deadly puzzle for the medical community. *Tohoku J Exp Med* 2008;216:197–204.
4. Shih MC, Hagspiel KD. CTA and MRA in mesenteric ischemia: part 1, role in diagnosis and differential diagnosis. *AJR Am J Roentgenol* 2007;188:452–461.
5. Ofer A, Abadi S, Nitecki S, et al. Multidetector CT angiography in the evaluation of acute mesenteric ischemia. *Eur Radiol* 2009;19:24–30.
6. Abujudeh HH, Rolls H, Kaewlai R, et al. Retrospective assessment of prevalence of nephrogenic systemic fibrosis (NSF) after implementation of a new guideline for the use of gadobenate dimeglumine as a sole contrast agent for magnetic resonance examination in renally impaired patients. *J Magn Reson Imaging* 2009;30:1335–1340.
7. Lauenstein TC, Salman K, Morreira R, et al. Nephrogenic systemic fibrosis: center case review. *J Magn Reson Imaging* 2007;26:1198–1203.
8. Acosta S, Sonesson B, Resch T. Endovascular therapeutic approaches for acute superior mesenteric artery occlusion. *Cardiovasc Intervent Radiol* 2009;32:896–905.
9. Bjornsson S, Bjorck M, Block T, et al. Thrombolysis for acute occlusion of the superior mesenteric artery. *J Vasc Surg* 2011;54:1734–1742.
10. Resch TA, Acosta S, Sonesson B. Endovascular techniques in acute arterial mesenteric ischemia. *Semin Vasc Surg* 2010;23:29–35.
11. Rogers DM, Thompson JE, Garrett WV, et al. Mesenteric vascular problems. A 26-year experience. *Ann Surg* 1982;195:554–565.
12. Boley SJ, Sprayregen S, Veith FJ, et al. An aggressive roentgenologic and surgical approach to acute mesenteric ischemia. *Surg Annu* 1973;5:355–378.
13. Krausz MM, Manny J. Acute superior mesenteric arterial occlusion: a plea for early diagnosis. *Surgery* 1978;83:482–485.
14. Williams DM, Brothers TE, Messina LM. Relief of mesenteric ischemia in type III aortic dissection with percutaneous fenestration of the aortic septum. *Radiology* 1990;174:450–452.
15. Condat B, Pessione F, Helene Denninger M, et al. Recent portal or mesenteric venous thrombosis: increased recognition and frequent recanalization on anticoagulant therapy. *Hepatology* 2000;32:466–470.
16. Turnes J, Garcia-Pagan JC, Gonzalez M, et al. Portal hypertension-related complications after acute portal vein thrombosis: impact of early anticoagulation. *Clin Gastroenterol Hepatol* 2008;6:1412–1417.
17. Friedenberg MJ, Polk HC Jr, McAlister WH, et al. Superior mesenteric arteriography in experimental mesenteric venous thrombosis. *Radiology* 1965;85:38–45.
18. Abdu RA, Zakhour BJ, Dallis DJ. Mesenteric venous thrombosis—1911 to 1984. *Surgery* 1987;101:383–388.

19. Hollingshead M, Burke CT, Mauro MA, et al. Transcatheter thrombolytic therapy for acute mesenteric and portal vein thrombosis. *J Vasc Interv Radiol* 2005;16:651–661.

20. Di Minno MN, Milone F, Milone M, et al. Endovascular thrombolysis in acute mesenteric vein thrombosis: a 3-year follow-up with the rate of short and long-term sequaelae in 32 patients. *Thromb Res* 2010;126:295–298.

21. Antoch G, Taleb N, Hansen O, et al. Transarterial thrombolysis of portal and mesenteric vein thrombosis: a promising alternative to common therapy. *Eur J Vasc Endovasc Surg* 2001;21:471–472.

22. Yankes JR, Uglietta JP, Grant J, et al. Percutaneous transhepatic recanalization and thrombolysis of the superior mesenteric vein. *AJR Am J Roentgenol* 1988;151:289–290.

23. Rivitz SM, Geller SC, Hahn C, et al. Treatment of acute mesenteric venous thrombosis with transjugular intramesenteric urokinase infusion. *J Vasc Interv Radiol* 1995;6:219–223; discussion 224–228.

24. Liu FY, Wang MQ, Fan QS, et al. Interventional treatment for symptomatic acute-subacute portal and superior mesenteric vein thrombosis. *World J Gastroenterol* 2009;15:5028–5034.

25. Wang MQ, Guo LP, Lin HY, et al. Transradial approach for transcatheter selective superior mesenteric artery urokinase infusion therapy in patients with acute extensive portal and superior mesenteric vein thrombosis. *Cardiovasc Intervent Radiol* 2010;33:80–89.

26. Yasuhara H, Niwa H, Takenoue T, et al. Factors influencing mortality of acute intestinal infarction associated with SIRS. *Hepatogastroenterology* 2005;52:1474–1478.

27. Rangel-Frausto MS, Pittet D, Costigan M, et al. The natural history of the systemic inflammatory response syndrome (SIRS). A prospective study. *JAMA* 1995;273:117–123.

28. Cerqueira NF, Hussni CA, Yoshida WB. Pathophysiology of mesenteric ischemia/reperfusion: a review. *Acta Cir Bras* 2005;20:336–343.

29. White CJ. Chronic mesenteric ischemia: diagnosis and management. *Prog Cardiovasc Dis* 2011;54:36–40.

30. Yamamoto W, Kono H, Maekawa M, et al. The relationship between abdominal pain regions and specific diseases: an epidemiologic approach to clinical practice. *J Epidemiol* 1997;7:27–32.

31. Oderich GS, Bower TC, Sullivan TM, et al. Open versus endovascular revascularization for chronic mesenteric ischemia: risk-stratified outcomes. *J Vasc Surg* 2009;49:1472–1479; e1473.

32. Mangiacapra F, Trana C, Sarno G, et al. Translesional pressure gradients to predict blood pressure response after renal artery stenting in patients with renovascular hypertension. *Circ Cardiovasc Interv* 2010;3:537–542.

33. Corriere MA, Pearce JD, Edwards MS, et al. Endovascular management of atherosclerotic renovascular disease: early results following primary intervention. *J Vasc Surg* 2008;48:580–587; discussion 587–588.

34. Drieghe B, Madaric J, Sarno G, et al. Assessment of renal artery stenosis: side-by-side comparison of angiography and duplex ultrasound with pressure gradient measurements. *Eur Heart J* 2008;29:517–524.

35. Armstrong PA. Visceral duplex scanning: evaluation before and after artery intervention for chronic mesenteric ischemia. *Perspect Vasc Surg Endovasc Ther* 2007;19:386–392; discussion 393–394.

36. Hamada T, Yamauchi M, Tanaka M, et al. Prospective evaluation of contrast-enhanced ultrasonography with advanced dynamic flow for the diagnosis of intestinal ischaemia. *Br J Radiol* 2007;80:603–608.

37. Hellinger JC. Evaluating mesenteric ischemia with multidetector-row CT angiography. *Tech Vasc Interv Radiol* 2004;7:160–166.

38. Shih MC, Angle JF, Leung DA, et al. CTA and MRA in mesenteric ischemia: part 2, normal findings and complications after surgical and endovascular treatment. *AJR Am J Roentgenol* 2007;188:462–471.

39. Calhoun PS, Kuszyk BS, Heath DG, et al. Three-dimensional volume rendering of spiral CT data: theory and method. *Radiographics* 1999;19:745–764.

40. Bhatti AA, Chugtai A, Haslam P, et al. Prospective study comparing three-dimensional computed tomography and magnetic resonance imaging for evaluating the renal vascular anatomy in potential living renal donors. *BJU Int* 2005;96:1105–1108.

41. Burkart DJ, Johnson CD, Ehman RL. Correlation of arterial and venous blood flow in the mesenteric system based on MR findings.

1993 ARRS Executive Council Award. *AJR Am J Roentgenol* 1993;161: 1279–1282.

42. Heiss SG, Li KC. Magnetic resonance angiography of mesenteric arteries. A review. *Invest Radiol* 1998;33:670–681.

43. Shanley CJ, Ozaki CK, Zelenock GB. Bypass grafting for chronic mesenteric ischemia. *Surg Clin North Am* 1997;77:381–395.

44. Schermerhorn ML, Giles KA, Hamdan AD, et al. Mesenteric revascularization: management and outcomes in the United States, 1988–2006. *J Vasc Surg* 2009;50:341–348; e341.

45. Kohn GP, Bitar RS, Farber MA, et al. Treatment options and outcomes for celiac artery compression syndrome. *Surg Innov* 2011;18:338–343.

46. Roseborough GS. Laparoscopic management of celiac artery compression syndrome. *J Vasc Surg* 2009;50:124–133.

47. Grotemeyer D, Duran M, Iskandar F, et al. Median arcuate ligament syndrome: vascular surgical therapy and follow-up of 18 patients. *Langenbecks Arch Surg* 2009;394:1085–1092.

48. Razavi M, Chung HH. Endovascular management of chronic mesenteric ischemia. *Tech Vasc Interv Radiol* 2004;7:155–159.

49. Matsumoto AH, Angle JF, Spinosa DJ, et al. Percutaneous transluminal angioplasty and stenting in the treatment of chronic mesenteric ischemia: results and longterm followup. *J Am Coll Surg* 2002;194:S22–S31.

50. Atkins MD, Kwolek CJ, LaMuraglia GM, et al. Surgical revascularization versus endovascular therapy for chronic mesenteric ischemia: a comparative experience. *J Vasc Surg* 2007;45:1162–1171.

51. Davies RS, Wall ML, Silverman SH, et al. Surgical versus endovascular reconstruction for chronic mesenteric ischemia: a contemporary UK series. *Vasc Endovascular Surg* 2009;43:157–164.

52. Kasirajan K, O'Hara PJ, Gray BH, et al. Chronic mesenteric ischemia: open surgery versus percutaneous angioplasty and stenting. *J Vasc Surg* 2001;33:63–71.

53. Landis MS, Rajan DK, Simons ME, et al. Percutaneous management of chronic mesenteric ischemia: outcomes after intervention. *J Vasc Interv Radiol* 2005;16:1319–1325.

54. Silva JA, White CJ, Collins TJ, et al. Endovascular therapy for chronic mesenteric ischemia. *J Am Coll Cardiol* 2006;47:944–950.

55. Lee RW, Bakken AM, Palchik E, et al. Long-term outcomes of endoluminal therapy for chronic atherosclerotic occlusive mesenteric disease. *Ann Vasc Surg* 2008;22:541–546.

56. Sarac TP, Altinel O, Kashyap V, et al. Endovascular treatment of stenotic and occluded visceral arteries for chronic mesenteric ischemia. *J Vasc Surg* 2008;47:485–491.

57. Peck MA, Conrad MF, Kwolek CJ, et al. Intermediate-term outcomes of endovascular treatment for symptomatic chronic mesenteric ischemia. *J Vasc Surg* 2010;51:140–147; e141–142.

58. Malgor RD, Oderich GS, McKusick MA, et al. Results of single- and two-vessel mesenteric artery stents for chronic mesenteric ischemia. *Ann Vasc Surg* 2010;24:1094–1101.

59. Fioole B, van de Rest HJ, Meijer JR, et al. Percutaneous transluminal angioplasty and stenting as first-choice treatment in patients with chronic mesenteric ischemia. *J Vasc Surg* 2010;51:386–391.

60. Schoch DM, LeSar CJ, Joels CS, et al. Management of chronic mesenteric vascular insufficiency: an endovascular approach. *J Am Coll Surg* 2011;212:668–675; discussion 675–667.

61. Brown DJ, Schermerhorn ML, Powell RJ, et al. Mesenteric stenting for chronic mesenteric ischemia. *J Vasc Surg* 2005;42:268–274.

62. Sivamurthy N, Rhodes JM, Lee D, et al. Endovascular versus open mesenteric revascularization: immediate benefits do not equate with short-term functional outcomes. *J Am Coll Surg* 2006;202:859–867.

63. Biebl M, Oldenburg WA, Paz-Fumagalli R, et al. Surgical and interventional visceral revascularization for the treatment of chronic mesenteric ischemia—when to prefer which? *World J Surg* 2007;31:562–568.

64. Zerbib P, Lebuffe G, Sergent-Baudson G, et al. Endovascular versus open revascularization for chronic mesenteric ischemia: a comparative study. *Langenbecks Arch Surg* 2008;393:865–870.

65. Rawat N, Gibbons CP. Surgical or endovascular treatment for chronic mesenteric ischemia: a multicenter study. *Ann Vasc Surg* 2010;24: 935–945.

Endovascular Therapies: Renal

LOUIS G. MARTIN

INTRODUCTION

It has been over 75 years since Harry Goldblatt and his coworkers reported their seminal experiment that established the association of renal artery stenosis (RAS) and hypertension.[1] Since then we have seen the invasive treatment for renovascular hypertension (RVH) evolve from surgical nephrectomy to surgical atherectomy and bypass to percutaneous angioplasty and stenting. The first percutaneous renal angioplasty (percutaneous transluminal renal angioplasty [PTRA]) was reported by Eberhard Zeitler in 1971 who used the Dotter coaxial catheter technique.[2] This technique, which involved pushing the intraluminal plaque aside by coaxially placing progressively larger catheters over their predecessor, worked fairly well in a straight line but was limited by the acute angle from which the renal artery arises from the aorta; therefore, most renal artery stenoses were excluded from treatment. Percutaneous renal angioplasty did not become a serious competitor to surgical atherectomy and bypass until the development of the angioplasty balloon by Andreas Grüntzig, a German cardiologist.[3] Grüntzig was the first to report the use of this new balloon angioplasty catheter for renal artery dilatation in 1978.[4] As they say, "The rest is history," or is it? Renal artery angioplasty and stenting have become the standard procedure for the treatment of a hemodynamically significant renal artery stenoses associated with fibromuscular dysplasia (FMD) and for cardiac decompensation associated with flash pulmonary edema; however, its role is less clear for the treatment of hypertension and renal insufficiency in the adult atherosclerotic patient with RAS.

On a recent PubMed.gov literature search for renal artery angioplasty and stenting, 3,125 publications were available. The overwhelming reported experience is that hypertension associated with a hemodynamically significant atherosclerotic RAS is better controlled on fewer medications following renal angioplasty and stenting. This generalization is supported by studies included in three meta-analyses of clinical series and a meta-analysis of randomized controlled trials. A meta-analysis of small series indicated that renal function is improved in about 40%, unchanged in 30%, and worsened in 30% of patients with severe functional impairment (mean serum creatinine 3.0 mg/dL).[5–8] Despite this experience, PTRA is under serious attack. It has failed to show convincing benefit over optimal medical therapy in four randomized trials.[9–12] There are serious flaws in the design, administration, and interpretations of all of these trials; however, the evidence seems to be growing against the benefit of renal angioplasty and stenting. Many physicians specializing in the treatment of patients with hypertension are reluctant to submit them to interventional therapy, which is an invasive procedure associated with potential complications, high costs, and possibly has no benefit over optimal medical control.[13,14] The major issue is whether PTRA/stenting significantly prolongs survival compared with optimal medical management. This is presently being addressed in the Cardiovascular Outcomes in Renal Atherosclerotic Lesions (CORAL) study (NCT00081731), which is a large, multicenter, randomized, controlled trial funded by the National Institutes of Health scheduled to be completed in 2012. This study comparing the effects of optimal medical therapy plus stent revascularization with medical therapy alone has a composite endpoint of cardiovascular and renal events: cardiovascular or renal death, myocardial infarction, hospitalization for congestive heart failure, stroke, doubling of serum creatinine, and need for renal replacement therapy.[15] Pending the results of the study, the best treatment for RAS and even whether to evaluate patients for this disease remain uncertain.

Blood pressure (BP) control has important survival attributes. Data from observational studies involving more than 1 million individuals have indicated that death from both ischemic heart disease and stroke increases progressively and linearly from BP levels as low as 115 mm Hg systolic and 75 mm Hg diastolic upward. The increased risks are present in all age groups, ranging from 40 to 89 years old. For every 20 mm Hg systolic or 10 mm Hg diastolic increase in BP, there is a doubling of mortality from both ischemic heart disease and stroke[16]; therefore, it is very important to search for patients in whom interventional treatment can be beneficial. Adult RVH is most often due to hemodynamically significant atherosclerotic narrowing of the main renal artery. In many, if not the majority of patients, it is best managed by medical therapy. The role of percutaneous renal artery angioplasty in this population is for medical treatment failures. Failure may manifest as poorly controlled hypertension, loss of renal function or mass, or episodes of unexplained flash pulmonary edema. Because loss of renal function or mass is less obvious and may occur even in well-controlled hypertension it is important to establish baseline parameters to be followed; generally, these are the serum creatinine value and the renal size. In the past renal size was measured on an abdominal X-ray; now it is more accurately measured by an ultrasound examination, which has the added bonus of eliminating the risk of radiation exposure. Ideally the ultrasound examination should include a Doppler flow study of the renal arteries to rule out stenosis and to establish baseline velocities. Table 45.1 lists clinical signs that should prompt noninvasive screening for RAS. As we know all "noninvasive

Table 45.1

Clinical Signs of Renovascular Hypertension Which Should Prompt Noninvasive Screening for Renal Artery Stenosis

1. History, or recent onset of significant hypertension after the age of 55 years

2. An abdominal bruit, particularly if it continues into diastole and is lateralized

3. Accelerated or resistant hypertension

4. Recurrent (i.e., flash) pulmonary edema

5. Renal failure of uncertain cause, especially with a normal urinary sediment and <1 g of protein per daily urinary output

6. Coexisting, diffuse atherosclerotic vascular disease, especially in heavy smokers

7. Acute renal failure precipitated by antihypertensive therapy, particularly angiotensin-converting enzyme inhibitors or angiotensin II receptor blockers

8. Malignant hypertension, defined as hypertension with end organ damage including left ventricular hypertrophy, congestive heart failure, visual or neurologic disturbance, or advanced retinopathy

9. Hypertension with a unilateral small kidney

10. Hypertension associated with medication intolerance

11. Unstable angina in the setting of suspected renal artery stenosis

Society of Interventional Radiology. *Quality improvement guidelines for angiography, angioplasty, and stent placement for the diagnosis and treatment of renal artery stenosis in adults.*[24]

studies" do not have equal sensitivity and specificity; therefore, if the signs of RVH are clinically severe or the ultrasound examination suggests a hemodynamically significant stenosis or a small kidney, a computed tomography angiography (CTA) or magnetic resonance angiography (MRA) should be performed. Catheter-directed angiography should be reserved for cases where treatment will be performed if a hemodynamically significant stenosis is confirmed or when performing angiography in another organ system in a patient with clinical signs strongly suggestive of RAS. Forty-seven percent of 851 consecutive patients undergoing coronary catheterization who exhibited at least one of four predefined selection criteria (severe hypertension, unexplained renal dysfunction, acute pulmonary edema with hypertension, or severe atherosclerosis) were found to have greater than 50% RAS. Multivariate analysis found that severe RAS was associated with age, female gender, reduced creatinine clearance, increased systolic BP, and peripheral or carotid artery disease.[17] Table 45.2 lists the indications for catheter angiography. Care must be taken not to misinterpret the preceding statements. Catheter-based renal angiography should not be performed in "all" procedures primarily performed for evaluation of another organ system, but only on those having strong clinical signs of RAS. In a loose sense I am suggesting "drive-by angiography" on this patient set; however, I am not recommending "drive-by angioplasty or stenting." These patients must be carefully evaluated to ensure that they are receiving "optimal medical care" for their hypertension and that the loss of renal function or mass is progressive and secondary to the RAS. Indications for intervention that are accepted by the Society of Interventional Radiology, the American College of Cardiology, and the American Heart Association are listed in Table 45.3.

PATIENT SELECTION, DEMOGRAPHIC CONSIDERATIONS

Demographic information, such as age at presentation, etiology, and location of disease were addressed by the Cooperative Study of Renovascular Hypertension. The analysis indicates that the age distribution of patients with atherosclerotic lesions of the renal arteries was almost identical in males and females, the mean age being 52.1 for males and 51.2 for females. This was not the

Table 45.2

Indications for Catheter-Directed Diagnostic Angiography[17,24]

1. Noninvasive vascular imaging suggests that a significant RAS is present (>50%)

2. Noninvasive imaging is not likely to have adequate sensitivity and specificity

3. Onset of hypertension occurs in a patient under the age of 30 years, or older than age 30 years but with FMD suspected as the etiology of RAS

4. There are appropriate indications for screening and a very high clinical suspicion of RAS, in which case noninvasive screening can be bypassed

5. In patients with strong clinical signs of RAS while evaluating another organ system; i.e., cerebral, coronary, or peripheral

Table 45.3

Indications for Renal Artery Angioplasty or Stenting in the Presence of a Hemodynamically Significant Stenosis[23,24]

1. Uncontrolled hypertension on three medications
2. Loss of renal function or mass while on antihypertensive treatment
3. Hypertension with unexplained unilateral small kidney
4. Unexplained recurrent congestive heart failure or flash pulmonary edema
5. Hypertension with intolerance to medicine

case, however, for fibromuscular hyperplasia of the renal arteries. For females with fibromuscular hyperplasia the shape of the curve parallels that of subjects with atherosclerosis, but a decade earlier. Although the mean ages for males and females (38.6 vs. 40.2, respectively) were similar, there were a larger proportion of males with fibromuscular hyperplasia occurring prior to the age of 30. Seventy-five percent of the atherosclerotic lesions were on the left side. Thus, there is a significant difference of unilateral lesions with respect to etiology. Of the atherosclerotic lesions, 30.6% were bilateral and 25% of the fibromuscular lesions were bilateral. Thus, atherosclerotic lesions predominate in males and are more prevalent on the left side, whereas fibromuscular hyperplasia shows a striking predilection for the right renal artery and for female patients.[18] Severe RAS was associated with age, female gender, reduced creatinine clearance, increased systolic BP, and peripheral or carotid artery disease in a multivariate model of patients undergoing cardiac catheterization who were deemed at risk for RAS based on clinical or laboratory criteria for study entry, but who had not previously been suspected of having RAS.[17]

Is race an issue in the incidence of RAS? Thirty percent of the 2,442 patients in the Cooperative Study of Renovascular Hypertension were nonwhite. The age distribution and incidence of RVH of the white and nonwhite groups were similar. The nonwhites had a higher representation in the FMD group (10%) than in the atherosclerotic disease group (7%).[18,19] When correction is made for age, smoking, and hyperlipidemia, there is no significant difference in the incidence of RAS or RVH in the white and nonwhite populations.[20–22]

PATIENT SELECTION, FUNCTIONAL CONSIDERATIONS

An interventional procedure resulting in normal BP on no medications is possible in children and young adults who are treated for FMD. Cure is extremely rare in older patients with atherosclerotic RAS, presumably because of concurrent essential hypertension. Therefore, the goal in the atherosclerotic patients must be control of BP on as few medications as possible and preservation of renal function and renal tissue. Unexplained renal dysfunction (creatinine clearance ≤50 mL/min) without a clearly established cause and especially with a normal urinary sediment containing less than 1 g of urinary

protein daily, acute renal dysfunction attributable to angiotensin-converting enzyme inhibitor or angiotensin receptor blocking medications, unexplained loss of renal mass, and episodes of congestive heart failure with "flash pulmonary edema" should prompt evaluation and treatment of a hemodynamically significant RAS.[23,24]

PATIENT SELECTION, PHYSIOLOGIC CONSIDERATIONS

Although a stenosis is the result of an abnormal process in the arterial wall, it is not usually of hemodynamic significance until the luminal cross-sectional area is reduced by 75%, which usually occurs when the vessel diameter is narrowed by 50% or more. These numbers vary depending on characteristics of the stenosis, such as its length, irregularity, multiplicity, the resistance of the distal vascular bed, and the available collateral blood supply.[25] Although mild stenoses are of no hemodynamic significance, a stenosis that narrows the luminal diameter by 75% (>90% of cross-sectional area) almost certainly is significant.[26] The physiologic significance of degrees of diameter stenosis between 50% and 75% may depend on the resistance of the peripheral renal vasculature or the condition of the renal autoregulatory system.[27] Because it is not possible to record orthogonal views of a renal artery, it is frequently more accurate to evaluate the physiologic significance of a stenosis by measuring a pressure gradient across the lesion. Difficulty measuring the pressure without affecting it, and the physiologic variations that occur during its measurement, make pressure gradient thresholds problematic. Ten percent of the peak systolic pressure and an absolute gradient of 10 or 20 mm Hg have been proposed by many interventionists as a measure of hemodynamic significance. Others have proposed using mean rather than peak systolic gradients. There is emerging science regarding the best method for determining the hemodynamic relevance of RAS, including the routine use of low-profile pressure-sensing wires instead of catheters positioned across the stenosis and determinations of renal fractional flow reserve following the intra-arterial administration of vasodilator medications.[28–30] Various measurements using the 0.014-inch pressure wire were compared by Leesar et al., who concluded that a systolic gradient greater than or equal to 21 mm Hg following hyperemic stimulation provided the highest accuracy in predicting hypertension improvement after stenting of RAS.[31] Therefore, it is the interventionist's responsibility to adopt a method of measurement and pressure threshold that he or she considers reliable and objectively use this to confirm that a stenosis is hemodynamically significant before treating it. It is worthwhile to note that it is extremely difficult, if not impossible, to visually determine whether a stenosis caused by the medial hyperplastic form of FMD is hemodynamically significant. Use of a pressure wire is recommended to determine a significant gradient both before and after angioplasty in these lesions.

PLANNING THE PROCEDURE

Planning the procedure begins with a review of noninvasive imaging. Does it suggest the presence of a hemodynamically significant RAS? If not, the procedure is over; if you cannot tell, additional noninvasive tests or catheter-directed angiography may be necessary. A medical history and chart review is required to confirm that the patient has received optimal medical therapy and that intervention is appropriate. You should not proceed if the patient is normotensive on two medications, has normal renal function, and has no sign of renal atrophy. This patient has already achieved the goal of your proposed therapy. Review laboratory tests, especially serum creatinine, platelets, and international normalized ratio (INR). Then it is time to have an honest discussion with the patient and family. They need to know the treatment options and which you consider to be the best. *Pretend it is your mother.* They need to be told the risks involved, the goal of therapy, the likelihood of reaching it, and the effect it will have on the patient's health and life expectancy. If you are not sure, tell them.

ENDOVASCULAR TREATMENT OPTIONS

Although endovascular treatment options for RAS theoretically includes the entire armamentarium available for use in peripheral, coronary, and cerebral interventions, in reality, in 99% of de novo cases the decision is between plain old balloon angioplasty (POBA) and stenting (PTRAS). The choices are more difficult and numerous for the treatment of restenosis, especially in-stent restenosis. Most pediatric and FMD cases can be treated by POBA as can most truncal atherosclerotic stenoses. There is no evidence that primary stenting is of any benefit in these cases. Pediatric and adult intimal fibroplastic FMD may rarely need the assistance of a cutting balloon. Most adult ostial atherosclerotic lesions will require a bare metal stent. There is no demonstrated benefit to primary use of drug-eluting stents (DESs), cryoplasty, self-expanding stents, or covered stents (CS), although there may be a use for each in specific cases or in treatment of complications. Brachytherapy has been safely used by a few investigators to increase primary patency and to treat restenosis with modest benefit. In-stent restenosis is a difficult and frequent problem following treatment of RAS, occurring in 10% to 30% of cases. Acceptable patency rates have been reported following placement of covered and DES within the restenosis. Cryoplasty, cutting balloon angioplasty (CBA), and POBA have been of little benefit.[32–39]

The operator is working in a hostile environment. It is imperative that the interventionist plans to avoid complications as carefully as he or she plans for success. The etiology of the stenosis is most commonly atherosclerotic disease. Plaques lining the aorta and renal arteries have the potential for renal or distal embolization. It is important to identify obstacles to successful and safe catheter manipulation and to be able to react to technical problems that become apparent during the procedure; however, some decisions need to be addressed preoperatively. Are you going to use a straight sheath, guide sheath, or guide catheter? Do you plan to use a 0.014- or 0.035-inch catheter system? The equipment that you need should be readily available in the room before the procedure is started. The most common complication associated with renal angioplasty involves the access puncture site. A pseudoaneurysm or hematoma at the puncture site is the most common complication; a retroperitoneal hematoma may be fatal. The femoral artery must be punctured below the inguinal ligament. A femoral artery puncture guided by ultrasound has the advantage that it can evaluate plaque or a high femoral artery bifurcation that might complicate the puncture. It has a demonstrated

superiority in obese patients and those with a weak arterial pulse[40] but has the disadvantage that a high (retroperitoneal) puncture may be undetected unless the puncture site is evaluated fluoroscopically. As is frequently the case, a multifaceted approach is best. Palpate the femoral artery to ensure that the pulse is strong and ultrasound it to exclude plaque and high bifurcation of the common femoral artery (CFA). Fluoroscope the groin to locate the midpoint of the femoral head and mark it. Plan to puncture the skin 1 to 3 cm below this mark at a 45-degree cephalad angulation. Guide the needle into the CFA under ultrasound. Fluoroscope the result to make sure puncture has been made correctly; if not, remove the needle and guide wire and try again.

Make sure that every patient is well hydrated before the procedure. Use low-osmolar, isotonic contrast in as low a volume as possible or substitute CO_2. Adequate intravenous volume expansion with isotonic crystalloid (1.0 to 1.5 mL/kg/hour) for 3 to 12 hours before the procedure and continued for 6 to 24 hours afterward can lessen the probability of contrast-induced nephropathy (CIN) in patients at risk; no other adjunctive medical or mechanical treatment has been proved to be efficacious in reducing risk for CIN. Prophylactic hemodialysis and hemofiltration have not been validated as effective strategies. A multidisciplinary CIN Consensus Working Panel reported that, of the pharmacologic agents that have been evaluated, theophylline, 3-hydroxy-3-methylglutaryl coenzyme A reductase inhibitors (statins), ascorbic acid, and prostaglandin E_1 deserve further evaluation. N-acetylcysteine is not consistently effective in reducing the risk for CIN. Fenoldopam, dopamine, calcium channel blockers, atrial natriuretic peptide, and L-arginine have not been shown to be effective. Use of furosemide, mannitol, or an endothelin receptor antagonist is potentially detrimental. Nephrotoxic drugs should be withdrawn before contrast administration in patients at risk for CIN.[41]

ANATOMIC OR LESION CONSIDERATIONS

Clinical and technical success is to a great extent dependent on the anatomic characteristics of the stenosis. What part of the renal artery is involved? Is the stenosis focal or multifocal? Are there tandem stenoses? Does the stenosis affect the main renal artery, an accessory renal artery, or branch vessels? Each feature will affect the way we approach endovascular treatment and the prognosis. Over 95% of the RAS treated in the United States are caused by atherosclerotic plaque narrowing the arterial lumen. Most of these involve the renal artery ostium, which is the junction between the renal artery and the aorta. These stenoses are thought to be caused by aortic thickening and plaque that narrows the renal artery lumen like a curtain. Stents are commonly used to treat these lesions to prevent the curtain from reoccluding the ostium following balloon angioplasty. The truncal or nonostial portion of the main renal artery responds to balloon angioplasty in a manner similar to stenoses in other peripheral arteries of similar size.

The beneficial role of percutaneous transluminal angioplasty (PTA) for the treatment of FMD, in particular its medial fibroplastic form, is well established in children and adults in whom 25% to 75% may be cured and typically over 85% improved in most reported series. There are three distinct types of FMD based on pathologic findings: medial dysplasia, intimal fibroplasias, and adventitial (periarterial) fibroplasia. There are three subcategories of medial dysplasia all of which primarily affect the distal two-thirds of the main renal artery and its secondary and tertiary branches: (1) *medial fibroplasia* the most common, about 75% to 80%, has a string of beads appearance in which the bead diameters are larger than the parent artery; (2) *perimedial fibroplasia*, about 10% to 15%, has beads that are smaller than the affected artery; (3) *medial hyperplasia*, about 1% to 3%, has a concentric smooth stenosis (FIGURE 45.1). Intimal fibroplasias, about 10%, which may occur in an ostial location presents as a focal or long smooth narrowing caused by replacement of adventitial fibrous tissue with dense collagen that is difficult to treat effectively by balloon angioplasty and may require the use of a cutting balloon or stent. In medial and perimedial fibroplasia it is impossible to tell whether the stenosis is hemodynamically significant by its angiographic appearance; the interventionist must rely on intravascular pressure measurements because of the beaded, irregular appearance of most cases of FMD.[42,43]

There is existing important information on noninvasive imaging procedures that are available in a majority of patients. It is imperative that the interventionist reviews and uses this information to plan and implement the procedure. Is the renal artery oriented at a right angle from the aorta or in a cephalad or caudad direction? Is the aortorenal artery angle so acute that an approach from the arm might be better? Most renal arteries do not arise at a horizontal angle from the axial plane of the aorta; in fact 93% of right renal arteries arise anterior-lateral and the 52% of left renal arteries posterior-lateral to this plane.[44] Prior knowledge of the anatomic orientation may influence the choice of vascular access, guide catheter, sheath, or aid in crossing a tight stenosis. Most interventionists prefer to work from a right femoral artery access, but this is not always the optimal approach. In general, a catheter and guide wire introduced from a femoral puncture will rest along the contralateral side of the aorta (FIGURE 45.2). Advancing a balloon or stent into a renal artery with an acute inferior angulation can be very difficult from a contralateral femoral puncture. I prefer to perform a renal intervention from an ipsilateral femoral puncture so that my guide catheter is stabilized against the contralateral aortic wall. You may feel differently; however, the approach should be planned preoperatively.

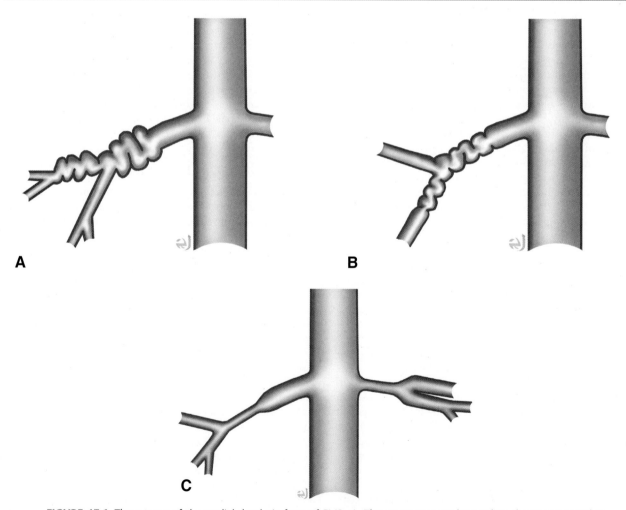

A   **B**   **C**

FIGURE 45.1 Three types of the medial dysplasia form of FMD: **A**. The aneurysms are larger than the parent vessel in *medial fibroplasia*. **B**. The aneurysms are smaller than the parent vessel in *perimedial fibroplasia*. **C**. Concentric smooth stenoses are observed in *medial hyperplasia*.

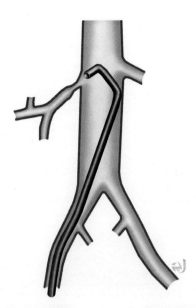

FIGURE 45.2 The curvature of the guide catheter is usually supported by the contralateral aortic wall when introduced from a femoral puncture ipsilateral to the lesion being treated.

TECHNICAL/DEVICE CONSIDERATIONS

Hundreds of articles have been published over the years claiming that a recent innovation was much better than its predecessors: that the 0.014-inch system is better than the 0.018-inch system and is better than the 0.035-inch-based catheter system; that the rapid exchange (monorail) system is better than the over-the-wire system; that it is better to use a guide catheter than a guide sheath, which is better than a straight sheath, and so on. It really does not make much difference in most cases. It is more important for the interventionist to be able to use one system safely and effectively, to know when he or she has reached the limits of his or her ability, and to avoid major complications—especially those caused by neglect and stupidity.

TREATMENT SELECTION STRATEGIES

Our goal in the treatment of RVH is to provide the patient with a safe and effective method to prolong life and to avoid the adverse effects of his or her disease. This involves much more than dilating and stenting an RAS. It includes a program of weight control, lipid control, cessation of smoking, preservation of renal function, preservation of renal tissue, and optimal medical management of the patient's BP. Cure, that is, normal BP on no antihypertensive medications, is only a realistic goal in children and adults with FMD. All others are likely to require ancillary medical therapy for life. Therefore, our strategy is to control BP medically on two or less medications before considering an intervention (FIGURE 45.3).

Once we have decided *who* to treat we must decide *how* to treat the stenosis. Our present treatment options include: POBA, CBA, non–drug-eluting stent (n-DES), DES, and CS. Our choice is affected by the location (ostial, truncal, branch, or mixed), whether it is the primary treatment or treatment

of a restenosis, or complication, that is, flow-limiting dissection or rupture. Almost all ostial stenoses will require stenting. Stents should be avoided in nonostial stenoses and in arteries less than 5 mm in diameter. The use of DES has been disappointing for both primary and restenotic lesions.[45] CBA has been used successfully in a small number of cases of in-stent restenosis, children with resistant stenoses, and transplant stenosis.[46,47] The use of the CS has primarily been limited to treatment of renal artery rupture and RAS associated with renal artery aneurysm.

PLANNING THE INTERVENTIONAL PROCEDURE

1. Prior to the procedure
   - Perform patient evaluation and consent.
   - Perform preprocedure tests: electrocardiogram (ECG), basic metabolic panel, hemoglobin, hematocrit, platelets, INR.
   - Discontinue warfarin at least 4 days prior to the procedure. Substitute enoxaparin if necessary.
   - Discontinue nephrotoxic medications.
   - Start clopidogrel, aspirin, and a statin at least 2 days prior to the procedure.

2. The day of the procedure
   - Diabetics
     - On insulin eat a small breakfast and take one-half dose of insulin. Schedule the procedure for 6 hours later.
     - Insulin-dependent diabetics on oral medication should withhold medication and fast for 6 hours. If the procedure is scheduled in the afternoon, they may eat a light breakfast.
     - Diabetics on diet control should fast for 6 hours. If the procedure is scheduled in the afternoon, they may eat a light breakfast.
   - Nondiabetics should fast for 6 hours and take their normal medications with a small sip of water.

3. The procedure
   - Determine what the risks are to using iodinated contrast. Substitute CO_2 or gadolinium if necessary.
   - Make sure that all the catheters and other devices that you plan to use and those that you may need in case of a complication are readily available in the procedure room.

SPECIFIC INTRAPROCEDURAL TECHNIQUES

1. It does not make any difference how good a job you do if you put the patient's life at risk because of a retroperitoneal hematoma. Make sure that the access puncture site is below the inguinal ligament.
2. Always keep the tip of the guide wire in the fluoroscopic field and pay attention to it. If the end of the wire begins to buckle (accordion), it means that the tip is wedged against a plaque, beneath the intima or in a small branch vessel, and that a perforation or intimal dissection is in the near future. This goes double for glide wires! "J"-shaped guide wires are not immune to causing dissections. The configuration of

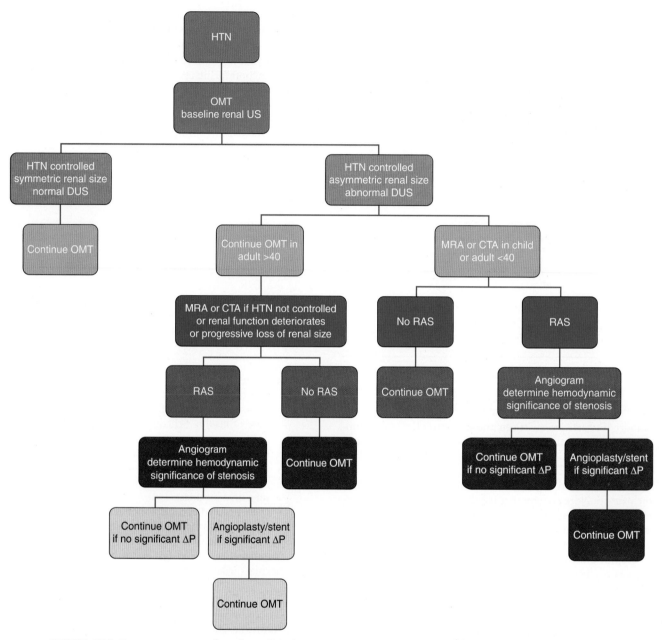

FIGURE 45.3 Treatment strategy flow chart. HTN, hypertension; OMT, optimal medical therapy; US, ultrasound; DUS, Doppler ultrasound; MRA, magnetic resonance angiogram; CTA, computed tomographic angiogram; RAS, renal artery stenosis; ΔP, pressure gradient.

the "J" changes to an "O" as the wire is pushed further into a narrowing vessel. The "O-sign" predicts intimal injury (FIGURE 45.4).

3. The arterial access site should be planned after review of all available noninvasive imaging procedures (see the above discussion).

4. Take measures to cross the stenosis safely. This means that you should cross the lumen of the stenosis parallel to its axis with a soft guide wire. Think of it as trying to advance the guide wire through the stenosis without touching its walls. To do this you would have to have the axis of the catheter guiding the wire in perfect alignment with the stenosis.

5. Stay within safe limits of contrast dosage and accept the fact that the safe dose is frequently less than you would suspect. A serum creatinine of 1.1 mg/dL may fall within normal limits in your laboratory, but it is not normal in an 80-year-old female with very little muscle mass. Make sure every patient is well hydrated before the procedure. Use low-osmolar, isotonic contrast in as low a volume as possible or substitute CO_2. Small volumes of a gadolinium-based contrast agent (GBCA) are substituted in patients with a history of severe or life-threatening contrast allergy in whom CO_2 angiography is inadequate.* The Food and Drug Administration's (FDA) review of the safety of the most widely used

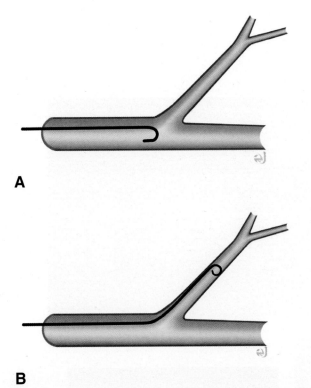

A

B

FIGURE 45.4 The "J" shape of the guide wire (**A**) is compressed into an "O" as it is advanced into a vessel too small to accommodate it (**B**).

GBCAs determined that Magnevist, Omniscan, and Optimark are associated with a greater risk than other GBCAs for nephrogenic systemic fibrosis (NSF) in certain patients with kidney disease. Data suggest that NSF may follow the administration of any GBCA and the FDA continues to assess the safety of each GBCA to better estimate its NSF risks.*

6. Make sure that you are attempting to treat a hemodynamically significant stenosis; otherwise you will be exposing the patient to risk without the chance of reward. Pressure measurements are required on stenoses narrowing the lumen diameter by 50% to 75%; most of us can accurately judge a greater degree of stenosis and pressure measurements are not required in these lesions, although they are useful compared to completion pressures to determine benefit. This said, I have had one case in which there was no gradient across a 75% in-stent stenosis that was being treated for a second time. I assume this was because of adequate retroperitoneal collateral blood supply or high resistance in the distal vascular bed, possibly related to atheroembolism. We did not re-treat the lesion.

7. Be on the look out for soft atheromatous plaque! Symptomatic embolization has been reported in 1% to 3% of renal angioplasties.[24] Most often this is related to relatively hard plaque being dislodged by guide wire or catheter manipulation. Soft plaque can be recognized as intraluminal vegetations in the aorta or renal artery during an intravascular ultrasound (IVUS) examination or during the fluoroscopic procedure when the contrast fails to wash away

*http://www.fda.gov/NewsEvents/Newsroom/PressAnnouncements/ucm225286.htm. Accessed January 15, 2011.

from the vessel wall following a small test injection. This is an extremely dangerous situation and almost always ends in disaster. My advice is to terminate the procedure and seek medical or surgical consultation for alternative therapy.

8. Heparinize after the arterial puncture. Goal should be an ACT (activated coagulation time) between 350 and 375.[48]

9. Be liberal with the use of a vasodilator during the procedure. I infuse 50 to 100 mcg of nitroglycerine (TNG) into the renal artery each time I have the opportunity, that is, during catheter and guide wire exchanges. This is especially important during procedures on pediatric patients and young females.

10. Perform an aortogram only if information is needed that is not available from the noninvasive images. Optimize the information by placing the image tube at a 15-degree left anterior oblique (LAO) position, place the sideholes of the aortic catheter at the level of the L_{1-2} disc space, and inject 15 mL of the contrast agent at 1,000 to 1,200 psi with no rate rise. Record images as rapidly as possible on your equipment; frequently, view of the origin of the renal artery is obstructed by aortic branches after the first several frames. Alter the angulation or catheter position if necessary to observe the renal artery origin in profile.

11. Form reverse curve catheters below the aortic arch, that is, in the contralateral iliac, celiac, or mesenteric arteries or in the aorta using the Cope technique.[49,50]

12. Avoid scraping the aortic endothelium as much as possible. Introduce the catheter or guiding system chosen to cross the stenosis over a soft, straight guide wire (usually a Benson guide wire). Advance 2 to 3 cm of the guide wire beyond the catheter tip so that it prevents the tip from scoring the endothelium as it moves along the aortic wall; that is, position the tip of the reverse curve catheter about 1 cm below the expected origin of the renal artery and remove the guide wire. Push the catheter superiorly, expecting the tip to make a quick lateral movement as it enters the renal artery ostium. If blood can be aspirated, confirm the catheter tip position by injecting a small amount of contrast.

13. When treating ostial stenoses, the stent should protrude at least 2 mm into the aorta. It is not necessary to flare its aortic margin, but it may make it easier to re-catheterize in the event of in-stent restenosis. Special care must be taken not to damage branch vessels when treating an adjacent truncal stenosis; the branch can be ruptured or dissected if too large a balloon is used. This situation is most commonly encountered when treating FMD or arteritis. Consider using "kissing balloons" to treat these lesions. The balloons must be sized to safely dilate the branch vessels and not over-dilate their parent artery (FIGURE 45.5). Consider that the effect on the parent artery of dilating with two equally sized balloons is not the sum of their diameters, but it is 82% of the sum (FIGURE 45.6). The geometry of more than two unequally sized balloons can be calculated using the Gaylord algorithm.[51]

14. Arterial access closure devices are optional. I feel that they are of special benefit in the obese, the elderly, and patients with chronic back pain who are unlikely to keep their leg straight during recovery. I use a closure device on almost every patient.

15. For a 0.035-inch-based system
   • When using a reverse curve catheter, the Bentson guide wire is advanced beyond the stenosis and the shaft of the catheter pulled inferiorly, causing the tip to cross the stenosis. Note that the guide wire may need to be retracted

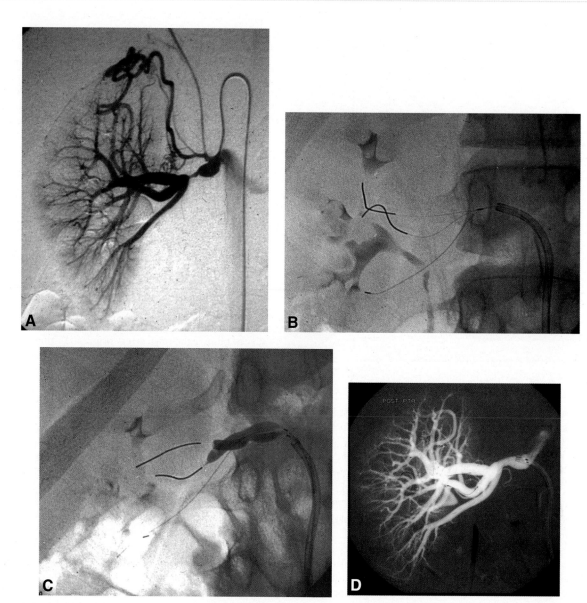

FIGURE 45.5 Teenage female with malignant hypertension caused by stenosis of the trifurcation of the right main renal artery: **A.** Diagnostic arteriogram. **B.** Placement of guide wires into the branches. **C.** Balloon angioplasty. **D.** Completion angiogram.

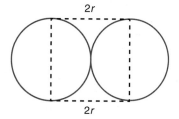

Circumference of two adjacent equally sized balloons is equal to $2\pi r + 4r$, which equals 82% of their added diameters

FIGURE 45.6 The circumference (C_{1+2}) of two equally sized balloons inflated simultaneously equals the circumference (C_1) of one balloon plus two times the balloon's diameter.

as the catheter tip is pulled forward to prevent it from damaging branch vessels.

- The guide wire is then removed and the catheter tip position confirmed by injecting a small amount of contrast. A stiffer guide wire, such as a Rosen or TAD wire, is then placed beyond the stenosis and the catheter removed. A guide catheter or guide sheath is then advanced to the renal artery ostium and a magnified angiogram recorded to determine vessel size and the degree of stenosis.

- If the stenosis is greater than 75% of the renal artery diameter or a significant gradient is present across a lesser stenosis, the lesion is predilated with a 4- or 5-mm angioplasty balloon and then stented if: it is an ostial stenosis, there is a flow-limiting dissection, or there is greater than 30% residual stenosis.

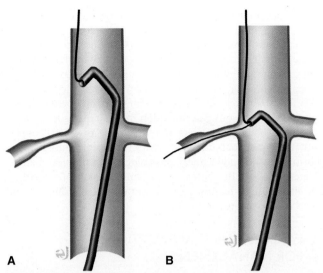

FIGURE 45.7 "No touch" technique: **A.** Guide catheter with a Bentson guide wire placed in the aorta above the renal artery. **B.** The guide catheter is pulled inferiorly until the renal orifice is located and the stenosis crossed with a guide wire.

- Some prefer to advance the guide sheath across the stenosis, "Dottering" it rather than predilating it with a balloon and then positioning the stent through the stenosis for deployment and unsheathing it as you would an inferior vena cava (IVC) filter.

16. For a 0.014-inch-based system
   - Select the properly shaped guide catheter based on preoperative information or from an aortogram as discussed above.
   - The guide catheters are rather stiff and likely to injure or scrape plaque off the aortic wall if moved without protection. The "no touch" technique accomplishes this by placing a soft guide wire cephalad through the catheter tip, which reduces its wall contact. Contrast injected through a Touhey-Borst adapter will confirm that the tip is adjacent to the renal artery lumen after which a 0.014-inch pressure wire or guide wire is directed across the stenosis before the safety wire is removed (FIGURE 45.7).[52]

ENDPOINT ASSESSMENT OF THE PROCEDURE

The immediate postprocedural evaluation begins with an angiogram. This is performed prior to relinquishing access across the stenosis. Let me be clear! Never remove the guide wire before you are absolutely sure that the stenosis has been completely and optimally treated. It would be foolish to remove the guide wire from the renal artery to use it to place a pigtail catheter in the aorta for a flush aortogram and then discover that the stenosis has not been adequately treated or that a flow-limiting dissection has occurred. I recommend performing the completion arteriogram through the guide catheter or guide sheath with the image tube angled to view the vessel origin in tangent. All of the renal branches must be included in the examination. Because of vessel curvature, more

than one projection may be necessary to completely evaluate your result. Pay attention to rate of flow through the peripheral vessels. The normal renal circulation is a low-resistance system with very rapid flow. Delayed washout or stasis of contrast indicates inadequate treatment of the stenosis, dissection, or peripheral embolization. Completion pressure measurements are usually not needed for a stented ostial stenosis but are definitely needed for nonstented truncal lesions, especially for FMD. Pressure measurements should be recorded postoperatively across most lesions being evaluated by CO_2 angiography; because of its buoyancy and rapid flow, the CO_2 angiogram rarely provides the physical information available on an iodinated study.

PROCEDURAL COMPLICATIONS AND HOW TO MANAGE THEM SUCCESSFULLY

A meta-analysis of complications reported in the Society of Interventional Radiology Quality improvement guidelines for angiography, angioplasty, and stent placement in the diagnosis and treatment of RAS in adults indicates that access site complications are by far the most common, occurring in over 5% of cases; next were symptomatic embolization in 3% followed by acute renal failure, worsening of chronic renal failure, main renal artery occlusions, and branch renal artery occlusions occurring in about 2% each.[24] These complications are best avoided by meticulous attention to preventive measures. Acute renal failure and worsening of chronic renal failure are most often related to contrast agents. Their treatment is detailed in an excellent review in emedicine and will not be repeated here.[53]

Arterial access site bleeding is rarely a major complication unless it results in a retroperitoneal hemorrhage or causes a compartment syndrome; the latter is usually associated with a brachial or axillary artery puncture in which case it is a surgical emergency.[54] Much has been written about the treatment of the pseudo-aneurysm and will not be repeated here.[55]

Cholesterol emboli to the peripheral renal vessels have a dismal outlook. Treatment associated with combined therapy consisting of plasma exchange and low-to-intermediate-dose corticosteroid therapy has been shown to be effective in some cases of renal cholesterol embolism. Prostanoid drugs and cholchicine are also possible adjuvant treatments. The medical treatment is mostly symptomatic: rest, warm conditions, appropriate dressing, antiplatelet drugs, hydration, and hemodialysis when necessary to ensure renal function.[56,57]

Occlusions of the main renal artery and its branches are usually caused by thrombus or dissection. The cause must be quickly identified and treated because of the short warm ischemic time of the kidney. The occlusions are usually related to either inadequate anticoagulation and/or flow-limiting subintimal dissection. Acute thrombosis is almost always successfully treated by intra-arterial infusion of a combination of t-PA and a glycoprotein IIb/IIIa receptor antagonist, such as abciximab. The latter is given at a loading dose of 0.25 mg/kg over 1 minute, which can be followed by a drip at 21 mL/hour (0.125 mcg/kg/minute) for 12 hours if necessary. Treatment of the dissection by stenting should be avoided if possible because of their high restenosis rate. If they are necessary, I recommend a DES, which has an unproven but theoretical advantage. Crossing a dissection is very hazardous and frequently results in occlusion. Surgical consultation is advised before attempting it in most situations. Dissections that do not completely occlude flow can often be treated by extended anticoagulation and observation.

Hemorrhage secondary to renal arterial perforation or rupture is a serious threat to the patient's life as well as the kidney; therefore, it must be controlled at all costs. The first measure is to reinflate the angioplasty balloon to tamponade the site of rupture. Anticoagulation must be reversed: 1 to 1.5 mg of protamine sulfate must be given for every 100 units of active heparin; therefore, the dose depends on the calculated amount of circulating heparin. Approximately one-half of the heparin is metabolized every hour—if 6,000 units had been given 1 hour earlier, 30 to 45 mg of protamine would be necessary to neutralize it. The BP must be supported by crystalloid infusion until matched blood is available for transfusion. You must be prepared to evaluate and reevaluate the effects of the tamponade by interval balloon deflation without losing access across the rupture; therefore, a second arterial puncture may be necessary from which to evaluate renal flow and measure arterial pressure during resuscitation. Because the warm ischemic time of the kidney is fairly short (30 to 120 minutes), cold saline should be infused if prolonged treatment is necessary. A small rupture or perforation will frequently seal following heparin reversal and tamponade; if not, a covered stent should be placed to cover the rupture. The basic steps of heparin reversal and crystalloid infusion are appropriate for treatment of a peripheral arterial perforation. If the perforation can be located, it should be occluded by supraselective embolization or a more central embolization if tamponade of the main artery has failed.

OUTCOMES/PROGNOSIS

The goals of renal artery angioplasty are control of hypertension and prevention of the progression of ischemic nephropathy. A meta-analysis of small series indicated that renal function is improved in about 40%, unchanged in 30%, and worsened in 30% of patients with severe functional impairment (mean serum creatinine 3.0 mg/dL).[57] This benefit has not been substantiated in recent prospectively randomized trials, which are under attack for biased patient recruitment and poor design. Although a distinguishing advantage for revascularization compared with medical therapy alone is the potential for a hypertension cure, only 1% to 3% of patients with atherosclerotic RAS are reported as cured following revascularization. The clinical profile of the patient most likely to be cured has not been defined for the patient with atherosclerotic RVH, but it is clear that cure and benefit are over 75% in patients with FMD. The mean cure rate for renal revascularization for stenoses secondary to FMD was 44% in a meta-analysis.[58] No attempt was made to separate the results of treatment of the various types of FMD in this document. It seems reasonable to assume that the majority of those treated had the "medial fibroplastic" type of FMD, which is the most common variety. This type affects 60% to 70% of patients with FMD and most likely a higher percentage of the adult population.

DISEASE SURVEILLANCE AND TREATMENT MONITORING ALGORITHMS

Our therapy is not directed at a stenosis but at its clinical sequelae; therefore, surveillance must be multifocal: directed at maintaining optimal medical therapy, limiting the progression of coronary and cerebral vascular disease, controlling BP, preserving renal function and mass, as well as detecting restenosis,

which occurs in approximately 15% of stented renal arteries. Most of us will rely on a nephrologist or internist to optimize medical therapy; however, it is our responsibility also, and many patients "fall through the cracks" between the interests of their subspecialized physicians. Poor BP control, accelerated loss of renal function, or reduction of renal size should alert us to the possibility of restenosis. It is important to obtain a baseline postprocedural ultrasound examination from a reliable laboratory. It should include measurement of renal size as well as Doppler flow assessment of both renal arteries.[59,60] Postprocedural monitoring must include clinical, physiologic, and physical metrics. Deterioration of BP control or renal function, loss of renal mass, or alteration of the flow patterns in the treated kidney should alert us to evaluate for restenosis.

EARLY FAILURES AND OPTIONS FOR MANAGEMENT

Early failure, that is, within the first 30 days following PTRA and stenting, is associated with contrast nephropathy, cholesterol embolization, intimal dissection, thrombosis, and vessel rupture or perforation. As is the case with most complications, they are best treated by prevention. These have been discussed earlier under procedural techniques and procedural complications.

LATE FAILURES AND OPTIONS FOR MANAGEMENT

Late failures are almost always associated with restenosis. In the case of FMD, more aggressive re-treatment with a larger balloon should be considered. A stent should be your last option. In cases treated for atherosclerotic stenoses, in-stent restenosis can be very difficult to treat. Reexpansion or overdilatation of the existing stent, possibly preceded by CBA and placement of a second noncovered, covered, or DES can be attempted. The latter has limited value at present because of its small diameter. Brachytherapy has been reported to have success but the experience is so limited that it cannot be recommended with any confidence. Surgical bypass should always be considered as an option, both as an initial treatment and for treatment of restenosis.

PRACTICAL ADVANTAGES AND LIMITATIONS

The obvious practical advantage of percutaneous angioplasty and stenting are that they are much less invasive and associated with less postprocedural morbidity than surgery. Limitations of the above advantage include the expertise of the interventionist, the availability of optimal equipment, and that the procedure is being performed in a potentially hostile environment with equipment that can be harmful to the vessel, organ, and patient, not to mention that technical and clinical success are far from guaranteed.

RELATIVE THERAPEUTIC EFFECTIVENESS COMPARED TO MEDICAL AND SURGICAL MANAGEMENT

The therapeutic effect of renal revascularization has been centered on control of BP and improvement of renal function; however, RAS is independently associated with mortality in patients with coronary artery disease. There is an incremental effect on mortality according to the severity of RAS at baseline. Four-year adjusted survival for patients with 50%, 75%, or greater than or equal to 95% stenosis was 70%, 68%, and 48%, respectively. Bilateral disease was associated with 4-year survival of 47% as compared with 59% for patients with unilateral disease ($p < .001$).[61] There is no compelling evidence to suggest that renal angioplasty has a significant benefit for treatment in patients responding to medical control or that it preserves normal function or prolongs survival. Neither percutaneous nor surgical intervention for treatment of RAS has any role in the patient with medically controlled hypertension, stable renal function, or no evidence of loss of renal mass. Therefore, any improvement in these parameters seen following interventional correction of RAS in the poorly controlled patient, albeit percutaneous or surgical, is testimony to their effectiveness over failed medical treatment. There are two prospectively randomized trials comparing percutaneous renal intervention and surgical revascularization. The evidence from direct comparisons of these interventions is vague, contradictory, and does not support one treatment approach over another for atherosclerotic renal artery stenosis; therefore, the choice between percutaneous and surgical treatment of RAS must be left to the patient and his physician to decide.[62,63]

THE FUTURE?

There are many competitors in the foot race to the future of RAS. Clarification of the risk factors for RVH and genetic profiling are in the forefront. We can expect new medications with fewer side effects—medications directed at the underlying risk factors of atherosclerosis, diabetes, obesity, and others. Technologic advances on the horizon, such as atherectomy and embolic protection devices optimized for renal use, should be expected. Control of myointimal hyperplasia and stents covered with biologically engineered tissue will be available for the renal arteries as for other parts of the body.

CONCLUSION

Our predecessors have supplied us with the hammer; despite the proven efficacy of surgical revascularization, endovascular therapy is increasingly being performed using PTRA and endoluminal stenting. Yet, the value of PTRA remains the source of considerable debate.

In summary, percutaneous renal revascularization with stentingis usually effective in improving (but rarely in curing) hypertension, in stabilizing renal failure in a substantial percentage of patients, and in eliminating recurrent cardiac events (i.e., flash pulmonary edema) in patients with atherosclerotic RAS. Current guidelines suggest that revascularization may benefit specific subgroups of patients, including those with hemodynamically significant RAS and recurrent, unexplained congestive heart failure or unexplained, sudden-onset or "flash" pulmonary edema (class I recommendation). Percutaneous revascularization is reasonable (class IIa) for patients with hemodynamically significant RAS and unstable angina or accelerated hypertension, resistant hypertension, and malignant hypertension. It is also reasonable for patients with RAS and progressive chronic kidney disease with bilateral RAS, or RAS to a solitary functioning kidney, and for patients with RAS and chronic renal insufficiency with global renal ischemia.

REFERENCES

1. Goldblatt H, et al. Studies on experimental hypertension: 1, the production of persistant elevation of systolic blood pressure by means of renal ischemia. *J Exp Med* 1934;59:347–379.
2. Zeitler E. Angiographic problems in the diagnosis and therapy of renovascular hypertension [in German]. *Radiologe* 1971;11(2):43–49.
3. Grüntzig A, Hopff H. Percutaneous recanalization after chronic arterial occlusion with a new dilator-catheter (modification of the Dotter technique) (author's transl) [in German]. *Dtsch Med Wochenschr* 1974;99(49):2502–2510.
4. Grüntzig A, et al. Treatment of renovascular hypertension with percutaneous transluminal dilatation of a renal-artery stenosis. *Lancet* 1978;311(8068):801–802.
5. Martin LG, Rees CR, O'Bryant T. Percutaneous angioplasty of the renal arteries. In: Strandness DE Jr, van Breda A, eds. *Vascular Diseases: Surgical and Interventional Therapy*. New York, NY: Churchill Livingstone; 1994:721–741.
6. Isles CG, Robertson S, Hill D. Management of renovascular disease: a review of renal artery stenting in ten studies. *QJM* 1999;92(3):159–167.
7. Leertouwer TC, et al. Stent placement for renal arterial stenosis: where do we stand? A meta-analysis. *Radiology* 2000;216(1):78–85.
8. Nordmann AJ, et al. Balloon angioplasty or medical therapy for hypertensive patients with atherosclerotic renal artery stenosis? A meta-analysis of randomized controlled trials. *Am J Med* 2003;114(1):44–50.
9. Webster J, et al., Randomised comparison of percutaneous angioplasty vs continued medical therapy for hypertensive patients with atheromatous renal artery stenosis. Scottish and Newcastle Renal Artery Stenosis Collaborative Group. *J Hum Hypertens* 1998;12(5):329–335.
10. Plouin PF, et al. Blood pressure outcome of angioplasty in atherosclerotic renal artery stenosis: a randomized trial. Essai Multicentrique Medicaments vs Angioplastie (EMMA) Study Group. *Hypertension* 1998;31(3):823–829.
11. Van Jaarsveld BC, et al. The effect of balloon angioplasty on hypertension in atherosclerotic renal-artery stenosis. Dutch Renal Artery Stenosis Intervention Cooperative Study Group. *N Engl J Med* 2000;342(14):1007–1014.
12. Astral-Investigators, et al. Revascularization versus medical therapy for renal-artery stenosis. *N Engl J Med* 2009;361(20):1953–1962.
13. Sacks D, Rundback JH, Martin LG. Renal angioplasty/stent placement and hypertension in the year 2000. *J Vasc Interv Radiol* 2000;11(8):949–953.
14. White CJ. Kiss my astral: one seriously flawed study of renal stenting after another. *Catheter Cardiovasc Interv* 2010;75(2):305–307.
15. Cooper CJ, et al. Stent revascularization for the prevention of cardiovascular and renal events among patients with renal artery stenosis and systolic hypertension: rationale and design of the CORAL trial. *Am Heart J* 2006;152(1):59–66.
16. Lewington S, et al. Age-specific relevance of usual blood pressure to vascular mortality: a meta-analysis of individual data for one million adults in 61 prospective studies.[Erratum appears in *Lancet* 2003;361(9362):1060]. *Lancet* 2002;360(9349):1903–1913.
17. Buller CE. The profile of cardiac patients with renal artery stenosis. *J Am Coll Cardiol* 2004;43(9):1606–1613.
18. Maxwell MH, et al. Cooperative study of renovascular hypertension. Demographic analysis of the study. *JAMA* 1972;220(9):1195–1204.
19. Simon N, et al. Clinical characteristics of renovascular hypertension. *JAMA* 1972;220(9):1209–1218.
20. Alhaddad IA, et al. Renal artery stenosis in minority patients undergoing diagnostic cardiac catheterization: prevalence and risk factors. *J Cardiovasc Pharmacol Ther* 2001;6(2):147–153.
21. Hansen KJ, et al. Prevalence of renovascular disease in the elderly: a population-based study. *J Vasc Surg* 2002;36(3):443–451.
22. Jazrawi A, et al. Is race a risk factor for the development of renal artery stenosis? *Cardiol Res Pract* 2009;2009:817–987.
23. Hirsch AT, et al. ACC/AHA 2005 guidelines for the management of patients with peripheral arterial disease (lower extremity, renal, mesenteric, and abdominal aortic): executive summary a collaborative report from the American Association for Vascular Surgery/Society for Vascular Surgery, Society for Cardiovascular Angiography and Interventions, Society for Vascular Medicine and Biology, Society of Interventional Radiology, and the ACC/AHA Task Force on Practice Guidelines (Writing Committee to Develop Guidelines for the Management of Patients With Peripheral Arterial Disease) endorsed by the American Association of Cardiovascular and Pulmonary Rehabilitation; National Heart, Lung, and Blood Institute; Society for Vascular Nursing; TransAtlantic Inter-Society Consensus; and Vascular Disease Foundation. *J Am Coll Cardiol* 2006;47(6):1239–1312.

24. Martin LG, et al. Quality improvement guidelines for angiography, angioplasty, and stent placement for the diagnosis and treatment of renal artery stenosis in adults. *J Vasc Interv Radiol* 2010;21(4):421–430; quiz 230.

25. Kohler TR. Hemodynamics of arterial occlusive disease. In: Strandness DE Jr, van Breda A, eds. *Vascular Diseases: Surgical and Interventional Therapy.* New York, NY: Churchill Livingstone; 1994:65–71.

26. Simon G. What is critical renal artery stenosis? Implications for treatment. *Am J Hypertens* 2000;13(11):1189–1193.

27. May AG, et al. Critical arterial stenosis. *Surgery* 1963;54:250–259.

28. Gross CM, et al. Determination of renal arterial stenosis severity: comparison of pressure gradient and vessel diameter. *Radiology* 2001;220(3):751–756.

29. Subramanian R, et al. Renal fractional flow reserve: a hemodynamic evaluation of moderate renal artery stenoses. *Catheter Cardiovasc Interv* 2005;64(4):480–486.

30. Mitchell JA, et al. Predicting blood pressure improvement in hypertensive patients after renal artery stent placement: renal fractional flow reserve. *Catheter Cardiovasc Interv* 2007;69(5):685–689.

31. Leesar MA, et al. Prediction of hypertension improvement after stenting of renal artery stenosis: comparative accuracy of translesional pressure gradients, intravascular ultrasound, and angiography. *J Am Coll Cardiol* 2009;53(25):2363–2371.

32. Zeller T, et al. Treatment of reoccurring instent restenosis following reintervention after stent-supported renal artery angioplasty. *Catheter Cardiovasc Interv* 2007;70(2):296–300.

33. Giles H, et al. Balloon-expandable covered stent therapy of complex endovascular pathology. *Ann Vasc Surg* 2008;22(6):762–768.

34. Hendricks DE, Hagspiel KD. Cryoplasty for the treatment of in-stent renal artery restenosis? *Tex Heart Inst J* 2008;35(4):489–491; author reply 491.

35. Stoeteknuel-Friedli S, et al. Endovascular brachytherapy for prevention of recurrent renal in-stent restenosis. *J Endovasc Ther* 2002;9(3):350–353.

36. Zahringer M, et al. Sirolimus-eluting versus bare-metal low-profile stent for renal artery treatment (GREAT Trial): angiographic follow-up after 6 months and clinical outcome up to 2 years. *J Endovasc Ther* 2007;14(4):460–468.

37. Jefferies JL, Dougherty K, Krajcer Z. First use of cryoplasty to treat in-stent renal artery restenosis. *Tex Heart Inst J* 2008;35(3):352–355.

38. Gupta R, Zoghbi G, Aqel R. Brachytherapy for rental artery in-stent restenosis [Erratum appears in *J Invasive Cardiol* 2007;19(7):A16]. *J Invasive Cardiol* 2006;18(8):E227–E229.

39. Lekston A, et al. Comparison of early and late efficacy of percutaneous transluminal renal angioplasty with or without subsequent brachytherapy: the effect on blood pressure in patients with renovascular hypertension. *Cardiol J* 2009;16(6):514–520.

40. Dudeck O, et al. A randomized trial assessing the value of ultrasound-guided puncture of the femoral artery for interventional investigations. *Int J Cardiovasc Imaging* 2004;20(5):363–368.

41. Stacul F, et al. Strategies to reduce the risk of contrast-induced nephropathy. *Am J Cardiol* 2006;98(6A):59K–77K.

42. Begelman SM, Olin JW. Fibromuscular dysplasia. *Curr Opin Rheumatol* 2000;12(1):41–47.

43. Das CJ, et al. Fibromuscular dysplasia of the renal arteries: a radiological review. *Int Urol Nephrol* 2007;39(1):233–238.

44. Verschuyl EJ, et al. Renal artery origins: location and distribution in the transverse plane at CT. *Radiology* 1997;203(1):71–75.

45. Kiernan TJ, et al. Treatment of renal artery in-stent restenosis with sirolimus-eluting stents. *Vasc Med* 2010;15(1):3–7.

46. Towbin RB, et al. Cutting balloon angioplasty in children with resistant renal artery stenosis. *J Vasc Interv Radiol* 2007;18(5):663–669.

47. Tanemoto M, et al. Cutting balloon angioplasty of resistant renal artery stenosis caused by fibromuscular dysplasia. *J Vasc Surg* 2005;41(5):898–901.

48. Chew DP, et al. Defining the optimal activated clotting time during percutaneous coronary intervention: aggregate results from 6 randomized, controlled trials. *Circulation* 2001;103(7):961–966.

49. Cope C. Suture technique to reshape the "Sidewinder" catheter curve. *J Interv Radiol* 1986;1:63–64.

50. Silberstein M, Tress BM, Hennessy O. Selecting the right technique to reform a reverse curve catheter (Simmons style): critical review. *Cardiovasc Intervent Radiol* 1992;15(3):171–176.

51. Gaylord GM, et al. The geometry of triple-balloon dilation. *Radiology* 1988;166(2):541–545.

52. Feldman RL, Wargovich TJ, Bittl JA. No-touch technique for reducing aortic wall trauma during renal artery stenting. *Catheter Cardiovasc Interv* 1999;46(2):245–248.

53. Siddiqi NH. Contrast medium reactions, recognition and treatment. 2010. Available at: http://emedicine.medscape.com/article/422855-overview

54. Tsao BE, Wilbourn AJ. The medial brachial fascial compartment syndrome following axillary arteriography. *Neurology* 2003;61(8):1037–1041.

55. Tisi PV, Callam MJ. Treatment for femoral pseudoaneurysms. *Cochrane Database Syst Rev* 2009(2):CD004981.

56. Hasegawa M, et al. The evaluation of corticosteroid therapy in conjunction with plasma exchange in the treatment of renal cholesterol embolic disease. A report of 5 cases. *Am J Nephrol* 2000;20(4):263–267.

57. Scolari F, et al. The challenge of diagnosing atheroembolic renal disease: clinical features and prognostic factors. *Circulation* 2007;116(3):298–304.

58. Martin LG, Rees CR, O'Bryant T. Percutaneous angioplasty of the renal arteries. In: Strandness DE Jr, van Breda A, eds. *Vascular Diseases: Surgical and Interventional Therapy.* New York, NY: Churchill Livingstone; 1994:721–742.

59. Sharafuddin MJ, et al. Renal artery stenosis: duplex US after angioplasty and stent placement. *Radiology* 2001;220(1):168–173.

60. Rocha-Singh K, Jaff MR, Lynne Kelley E. Renal artery stenting with noninvasive duplex ultrasound follow-up: 3-year results from the RENAISSANCE renal stent trial. *Catheter Cardiovasc Interv* 2008;72(6):853–862.

61. Conlon PJ, et al. Severity of renal vascular disease predicts mortality in patients undergoing coronary angiography. *Kidney Int* 2001;60(4):1490–1497.

62. Weibull H, et al. Percutaneous transluminal renal angioplasty versus surgical reconstruction of atherosclerotic renal artery stenosis: a prospective randomized study. *J Vasc Surg* 1993;18(5):841–850; discussion 850–852.

63. Balzer KM, et al. Prospective randomized trial of operative vs interventional treatment for renal artery ostial occlusive disease (RAOOD). *J Vasc Surg* 2009;49(3):667–674; discussion 674–675.

Endovascular Therapies: Aortoiliac

SUN HO AHN and TIMOTHY P. MURPHY

INTRODUCTION

Charles Dotter performed the first successful percutaneous dilation of a superficial femoral artery (SFA) in 1963,[1] giving birth to a new field of image-guided minimally invasive therapy. What ensued is a paradigm shift in preferred treatment of vascular disease, best exemplified by aortoiliac occlusive disease (AIOD). The first endovascular dilations of iliac arteries were reported in 1966, also by Dotter and his colleagues.[2] Other groundbreaking advances included the development of percutaneous angioplasty balloons and stents. Dr. Gruntzig is largely credited for developing the first clinically applicable percutaneous transluminal angioplasty (PTA) balloon in 1974, allowing rapid advancement in endovascular therapy. Subsequent development of stents allowed endovascular treatment of more complex vascular diseases, including chronic occlusions. A myriad of angioplasty balloons and stents are now available. With refinement of technique and modern equipment, endovascular revascularization has become the preferred modality of AIOD treatment.

Although femoropopliteal disease may be three to five times more common than aortoiliac disease,[3] aortoiliac insufficiency is a very common cause of peripheral artery disease (PAD). Approximately 10 million of the U.S. population is affected by PAD, and the prevalence rate increases with age.[4] It has been reported that over 20% of patients older than 75 years may have PAD.[5] Screening questionnaires aimed mainly at detection of symptoms have underestimated the prevalence due to those patients who have PAD but are without symptoms or have atypical symptoms. Compared with noninvasive physiologic tests (segmental blood pressures, flow velocity, postocclusive reactive hyperemia, and pulse reappearance half-time), the Rose questionnaire failed to identify 80% of patients with PAD.[5] The Edinburgh artery study also reported the underestimation of PAD with the WHO questionnaire compared to physiologic test.[6] Accurate identification of patients with asymptomatic or symptomatic PAD may prove to be crucial for secondary prevention of cardiovascular disease because recent studies have identified PAD as an independent risk factor for future cardiovascular events.[7,8]

Intermittent claudication (IC) is the most common presentation of PAD; however, some patients may present with critical limb ischemia (CLI)—that is, rest pain or tissue loss. Asymptomatic patients are not subject to revascularization. It is important to note that most patients with IC may not admit to having classic symptoms. As a result, patients may erroneously attribute symptoms of claudication to other causes of leg pain.

Most claudicants will have stable symptoms over a 5-year period. Approximately 20% of patient will suffer progression of disease with 6% requiring an amputation and 9.5% requiring bypass surgery over the same 5-year period.[9] Major amputation rate has been shown to be less than 4%.[10] Therefore, open surgical treatments were reserved for those with CLI or severe symptoms, and patients with IC were typically managed nonoperatively—that is, smoking cessation and exercise. With the emergence of safer minimally invasive techniques, additional options for endovascular revascularization are available, but still should be used judiciously. Moreover, studies have shown significant improvements in quality of life (QOL) after endovascular treatment.[11,12]

All patients with PAD, regardless of symptoms, should be assessed for cardiovascular risk factors and secondary cardiovascular disease prevention; for example, hypertension, lipid levels, blood glucose level, smoking, and so on. Appropriate measures should be taken for risk factor modification (please refer to Adult Treatment Panel III and ACC/AHA guidelines).[13,14]

PATIENT SELECTION

Treatment of symptomatic AIOD comprises medical, endovascular, and surgical therapies. Cilastazol and supervised exercise program (SEP) are the mainstays of medical management. A 3-month trial of cilastazol (50 or 100 mg twice a day) is recommended in those with claudication, which has shown improvements in maximum walking distance (MWD) as well as QOL.[15] Cilastazol has also shown to be more effective than pentoxyphylline.[16] Potential side effects include diarrhea and headache. Cilastazol is contraindicated in patients with congestive heart failure because of the potential risk of mortality. SEP therapy also has demonstrated improvements in MWD and QOL.[17] For maximum benefit, programs with 35- to 50-minute sessions three to five times a week are recommended.[18] SEP utilization is hindered by patient noncompliance, access limitations, and lack of reimbursement. The benefits of unsupervised programs are controversial.

For patients who fail medical management or present with CLI, invasive management is indicated. Endovascular interventions may be contraindicated in those with uncorrectable coagulopathy, severe nondialysis-dependent renal insufficiency, and systemic or access site infections. These contraindications are shared with open surgical procedures, however, and may be addressed with appropriate corrective measures.

The debate of endovascular versus surgical management for AIOD is more of a historical one in the current medical practice. From 1996 to 2000, an 850% increase in endovascular treatment, a 15.5% decrease in aortofemoral bypass surgery, and a 34% increase in overall procedures were reported in one U.S. study.[19] Endovascular technique has become the first-line invasive treatment for AIOD; however, open bypass surgery remains as an alternative option in situations where endovascular may be undesirable or unsuccessful.

ENDOVASCULAR TREATMENT OPTIONS

AIOD endovascular treatment options are mainly PTA and stenting. Prior to the introduction of stents, PTA was performed with reasonable success but was limited to only focal stenoses. Because of high complication rates, occlusions and lengthy lesions were felt to be best treated with open bypass.[20] As a result, PTA was only applicable in 60% of AIOD.[3] Stents have effectively removed this limitation and have allowed treatment of the most complex AIOD, including total occlusions (FIGURE 46.1). The interventionalist now has the option of primary PTA with secondary stenting or primary stenting. Stent options include balloon expandable (BE) or self-expandable (SE) types as well as bare metal or covered stent-grafts. Covered stents also provide definitive endovascular treatment of arterial ruptures, which, although rare, may occur during iliac interventions.

ANATOMIC OR LESION CONSIDERATION

AIOD management algorithm is one that is fluid and continues to evolve. Past and current guidelines have been predominantly based on lesion morphology and distribution.[14,21–23] Although recommendations, such as the TransAtlantic Inter-Society Consensus (TASC) I and II exist, suffice it to say that almost all patients with aortoiliac insufficiency can be treated interventionally.

TECHNICAL AND DEVICE CONSIDERATIONS

Single plane digital subtraction fluoroscopy unit with a moving table and a power contrast injector is sufficient for AIOD interventions. The angiography rooms should be equipped with continuous hemodynamic and oxygenation monitoring and advanced cardiac life support (ACLS) emergency equipment. The treating physician and staff should be ACLS-certified and possess commanding knowledge of conscious sedation medications and their reversal agents.

Diagnostic arteriogram equipment consists of access needles (18, 19, or 22 gauge), 4 or 5 French catheters (multiple side holed catheters are required for distal aortic injections), standard length spring coiled or hydrophilic guide wires, and a 5 French vascular sheath. For interventions, larger and longer length sheaths—that is, 6 to 9 French and 45 cm, respectively—may be required. Stiffer spring coiled guide wires will facilitate passage of sheaths through complex lesions and occlusions. PTA balloons and stents are manufactured in various delivery lengths. For common femoral artery (CFA) access, 75-cm length PTA and stent systems are preferred. Arm access

will require longer catheters, sheaths, and delivery systems for obvious reasons.

For iliac artery interventions, 6- to 10-mm diameter PTA balloons and stents are sufficient. For distal aorta purposes, balloon and stents up to 15 mm in diameter may be needed. Inflation device with a pressure gauge is useful. Because most arterial dilations are generally successful with less than 10 atmospheres of pressure, high-pressure balloons are not necessary. Arterial pressure transducer capability should be available to measure pressure gradients.

A large number of stents are available today.[24] Stents can be divided into BE or SE types. The Palmaz stent was the original BE stent composed of rigid stainless steel and required manual mounting on a balloon. The early designs required ipsilateral access, and contralateral delivery over the aortic bifurcation was challenging, if not prohibited. The modern BE stents, however, are premounted and have much improved trackability. In general, BE stents consist of stainless steel and possess greater hoop strength and radial force than SE. A major advantage of BE stents is the ability for precise placement. Examples of BE stents include Palmaz (Cordis Endovascular/Johnson & Johnson, Warren, NJ), Palmaz Genesis (Cordis Endovascular/Johnson & Johnson, Warren, NJ), Express (Boston Scientific, Natick, MA), and Bridge Assurant (Medtronic, Minneapolis, MN). The Wallstent was the first SE stent. SE stents are more flexible, allowing better trackability and conformity to the vessel wall. SE stents are made of nitinol (except the Wallstent, which is made from Elgiloy), tend to be more crush resistant, and are manufactured in longer lengths, which may avoid the need for multiple overlapping stents. Examples of SE stents are Wallstent (Boston Scientific, Natick, MA), Absolute (Guidant, Santa Clara, CA), Luminexx (C.R. Bard, Covington, GA), SMART (Cordis Endovascular/Johnson & Johnson, Warren, NJ), and Zilver (Cook, Bloomington, IN). Covered stents are now commercially available and are composed of synthetic material, which covers or lines a metal stent. Examples of covered stents include Fluency (SE) (C.R. Bard, Covington, GA), ViaBahn (SE) (W.L. Gore, Flagstaff, AZ), Wallgraft (SE) (Boston Scientific, Natick, MA), and iCast (BE) (Atrium Medical, Hudson, NH). The lists of stents are selective and not meant to be exhaustive. FIGURE 46.2 shows selective examples.

TREATMENT SELECTION STRATEGIES

Primary PTA with secondary stenting or primary stenting may be performed. Direct comparative data are limited and consist of one randomized trial and a meta-analysis.[25,26] The Dutch Iliac Stent Trial Study (DIST), which randomized patients to either PTA with selective stenting group or primary stenting group, did not show any statistically significant patency outcomes in early or long-term follow-up.[25,27] The reader should be aware, however, that 43% of patients required secondary stent placement. In addition, if 5 mm Hg mean translesional gradient was used to define technical success (TS), rather than 10 mm Hg mean used in the study, a higher number of cases would have likely required stents. Also, complication rate for the PTA group was nearly twice that of the primary stent group.[25] In a meta-analysis comparing PTA and stenting (six PTA and eight stent studies), stenting had higher TS (96% vs. 91%) and higher primary patency rates (77% vs. 64%).

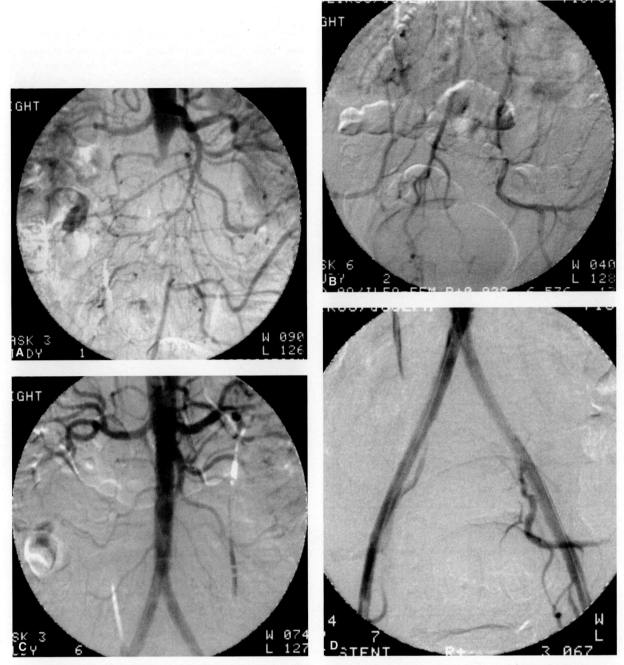

FIGURE 46.1 Total infrarenal aortoiliac occlusion treated with catheter-directed thrombolysis and stent placement. Abdominal aortogram shows infrarenal aortic and iliac artery occlusions (**A**, **B**). Catheter-directed short-term thrombolysis was performed followed by stent placements. Palmaz stents were used in the aorta and Wallstents were used in the iliac arteries. Postendovascular revascularization angiogram (**C**, **D**).

The superiority of stents was further demonstrated by a 39% reduction in long-term failure rate.[26] The authors' preference is primary stent placement for most AIOD. If PTA is desired, it should be reserved for short, focal, noncalcified stenoses. Early limited data for utility of covered stents have arisen for complex lesions[28] and for common iliac artery (CIA) origin disease[29] with promising outcomes.

PLANNING THE INTERVENTIONAL PROCEDURE

As in any intervention, the treating physician should perform an appropriate history and physical examination. Prior revascularization treatment(s) should be noted. If an iodinated contrast allergy is present, appropriate premedications should

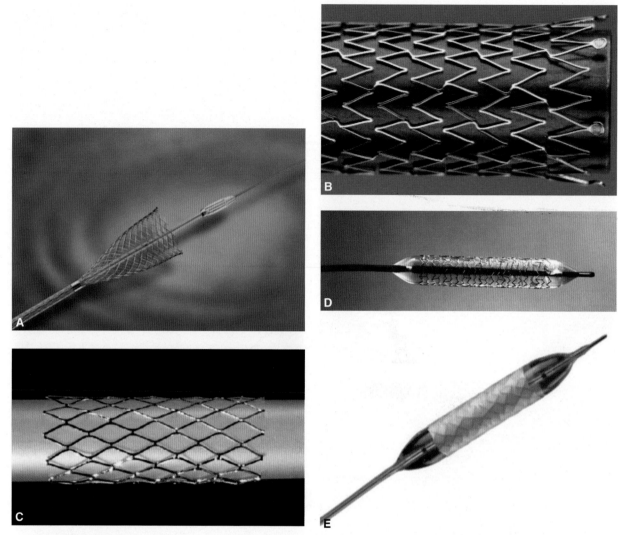

FIGURE 46.2 Selective examples of various stents. Photographs of (**A**) partially expanded Wallstent, (**B**) expanded SMART stent, (**C**) Palmaz stent, (**D**) Express LD stent, and (**E**) iCAST. (**A** and **B** are self-expanding, **C** and **D** are balloon expandable, and **E** is balloon expandable covered stent).

Images are courtesy of Boston Scientific (**A**, **D**), Cordis Endovascular/Johnson & Johnson (**B**, **C**), and Atrium Medical (**E**).

be prescribed (e.g., 32 mg methylprednisolone 12 and 2 hours prior to contrast exposure). In the presence of AIOD, CFA pulse may be diminished and should be noted. Pertinent laboratory evaluations include complete blood count, blood urea nitrogen, serum creatinine, and coagulation profile. A severe baseline renal insufficiency may preclude use of iodinated contrast. Renal protection maneuvers should be taken in the presence of mild or moderate renal insufficiency. The literature for prevention of contrast-induced nephropathy (CIN) is confusing and contradictory. Minimizing contrast volume and hydration with 0.9% saline at 1 mL/kg/hour for 24 hours starting 2 to 12 hours prior to contrast exposure may help prevent CIN.[30] Efficacy of sodium bicarbonate and n-acetyl-cysteine is debated because the data are equivocal.[30,31] Use of an alternative contrast agent, namely, carbon dioxide, may help to decrease the contrast volume. For insulin-dependent diabetics, the morning dose of insulin should be reduced in half. For patients on metformin or its derivates, a

serum creatinine should be checked 48 hours after contrast exposure prior to reinitiation of therapy. Warfarin therapy should be withheld prior to the procedure. In cases where anticoagulation cannot be interrupted, Lovenox and unfractionated heparin may be required to minimize cessation of anticoagulation. If an intervention is anticipated, antiplatelet therapy should be initiated prior to it. Preprocedure cardiac clearance and electrocardiogram are not routinely recommended. Any prior diagnostic examinations or interventions (endovascular and surgical), if present, should be reviewed. Pulse volume recordings, segmental blood pressures, computed tomography angiograms (CTA), and magnetic resonance angiograms (MRA) can provide critical information for access planning, device selection, and risk stratification (FIGURE 46.3).

Patients are instructed to have a clear liquid diet for a minimum of 6 hours prior to the procedure. Daily medications, with the exception of warfarin and insulin (see preceding discussion),

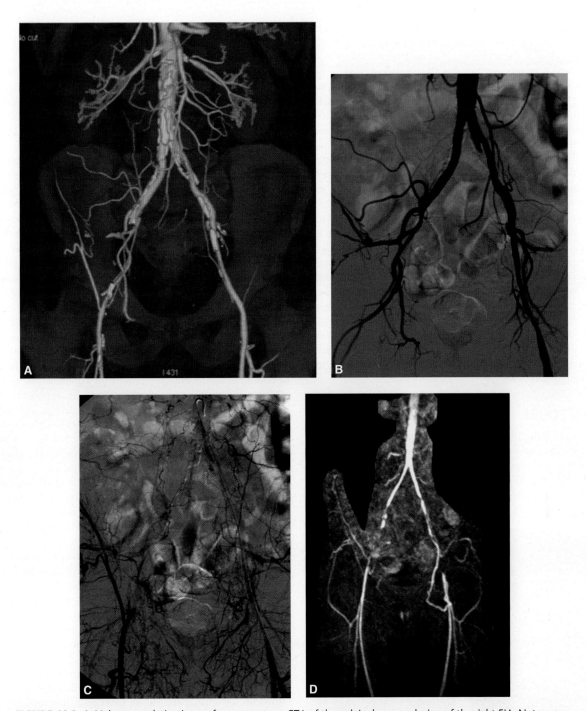

FIGURE 46.3 **A**. Volume rendering image from a contrast CTA of the pelvis shows occlusion of the right EIA. Note reconstitution of flow in the distal EIA. **B**. Digital subtraction angiogram correlation at time of treatment. Early image shows right EIA occlusion, and delayed image (**C**) shows reconstitution of the distal EIA. **D**. MRA of the pelvis with gadolinium (different patient) demonstrates right external iliac occlusion with reconstitution at the level of CFA, left CIA stenosis, and EIA occlusion with reconstitution at the level of the mid-CFA.

should be taken with a small amount of water. American Society of Anesthesiologists classification and conscious sedation risk should be assessed. Bilateral inguinal regions should be prepared with a shave. If left brachial arterial access is anticipated, the left arm should be additionally prepped. A bladder catheter should be placed if an intervention is planned.

Laterality of access should be considered in advance. In general, access contralateral to the symptomatic leg may be preferred in situations where no preceding diagnostic imaging is available. With wider application of preprocedure CTA and MRA, however, access can be tailored to the anticipated intervention(s). Ipsilateral access is most appropriate for CIA origin disease. Conversely, external iliac artery (EIA) lesions are best treated from a contralateral approach because the lesion may be too close to the access site if an ipsilateral access is used. With advances in modern braided sheath designs and stents, contralateral treatment is quite viable. When CFA access is not possible, brachial artery (BA) access may be required. Left BA is preferred to the right BA to avoid crossing of the right vertebral and both common carotid arteries. Reported complications include BA thrombosis and pseudoaneurysms, which are more frequently observed in women and often require surgical intervention.[32,33] Although BA access is an option, impractical length issues and reported higher complication rates limit its use as a primary option.

A recently published SIR practice guideline does not recommend routine antibiotic prophylaxis for AIOD procedures including angiography, PTA, thrombolysis, arterial access closures, and stenting. Decisions should be individualized and considered in those who are high risk—that is, repeated accesses within 7 days, long-term indwelling arterial catheters, or long procedure duration. Cefazolin (1 g intravenously) is the suggested first-line agent with vancomycin and clindamycin as alternatives in patients with penicillin allergy. Antibiotic should be administered at least 1 hour prior to the procedure. Prophylactic antibiotics are recommended for routine peripheral endograft placement.[34]

▌ PROCEDURE

If a pulse is palpable, CFA can be targeted at midfemoral head level. In cases of an absent pulse, one or more of the following techniques may be useful. Fluoroscopic guidance can be used if the CFA is calcified (FIGURE 46.4). Typically the

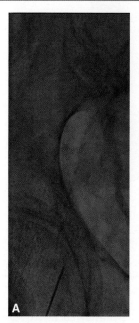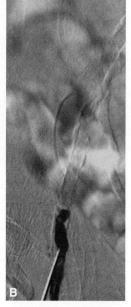

FIGURE 46.4 Fluoroscopic-guided access of a nonpalpable artery. **A.** Fluoroscopic image shows calcification of the CFA wall used as a guide for access needle placement. **B.** Digital subtraction angiogram confirms successful access.

calcification involves the posterior and medial walls of the CFA. Alternatively, ultrasound (US) can be used and may be preferred for routine accesses, but in the authors' opinion, US is rarely required. If the common femoral vein is inadvertently accessed, the course of the wire can be used to localize the artery immediately lateral to the vein. In thin patients, a calcified artery may be able to be palpated for access despite an absent pulse. If CFA access is not possible, then BA access can be used. Authors prefer an 18 gauge access needle, but 19 or 22 gauge needles are reasonable alternatives. With smaller gauged needles, determination of adequate arterial access may be more challenging due to slower blood return in patients with proximal occlusions.

After successful arterial access, a tailored diagnostic arteriogram and pressure gradients, if needed, should be obtained. With increased utilization and accuracy of peripheral CTA and MRA, the need for complete diagnostic arteriogram has been reduced. Rather, confirmation of suspected disease may be performed. Oblique imaging may reveal stenoses, which may be obscured by overlapping branches of the internal iliac artery (IIA). For nonocclusive stenoses, hemodynamic significance should be determined. Pressure gradient measurement is the most accurate determinant of hemodynamic significance. Although there is a lack of complete consensus, a resting gradient greater than 5 mm Hg (mean pressure) or 10 mm Hg (systolic pressure) is felt to be significant. When resting pressures are equivocal, pharmacologic provocation (e.g., IA nitroglycerin) and a resultant gradient greater than 10 mm Hg (mean) or 20 mm Hg (systolic) denote significance. Simultaneous measurement above and below the lesion via separate accesses is the most accurate technique. This avoids a false pressure gradient, which may be created when a catheter is across the lesion. If a single access, coaxial measurement is used, a 2 French sized difference between the inner catheter and outer sheath is usually required, or a pressure-sensing guide wire can be used. Pullback pressure measurement is unreliable because of temporal variations in blood pressure and should be avoided if possible. Diameter reduction can also be used to determine hemodynamic significance. Although a threshold of greater than 50% diameter reduction is routinely used, sole reliance on anatomic measurement may lead to inaccuracies. Pressure gradients should be used to ascertain the presence of a significant stenosis for marginal or equivocal stenoses.[35]

Once the decision to treat is made, intravenous heparin is usually administered, although it can be avoided when interventions are anticipated to be brief and uncomplicated and when the patient is not hypercoagulable. Activated clotting time (ACT) between 250 and 300 seconds is sufficient. The lesion should be crossed carefully to avoid dissections or plaque dislodgment and embolization. Steps should be planned to minimize the number of lesion traversals. After the lesion is crossed with a wire and catheter, the wire should be exchanged for one with greater stiffness. An appropriately sized sheath should be advanced across the lesion. Bareback placement of BE stents should be avoided because traversal of severe stenosis or occlusions without a sheath may lead to stent dislodgment from the balloon (FIGURE 46.5). Once the stent is properly positioned, the sheath is retracted to allow stent deployment. Contrast can be injected via the sidearm of the sheath to confirm

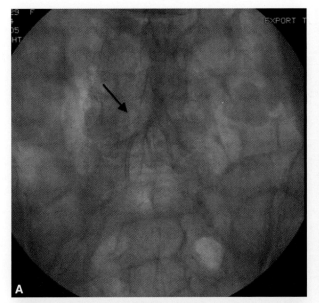

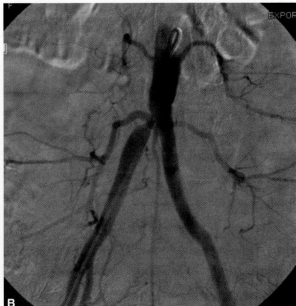

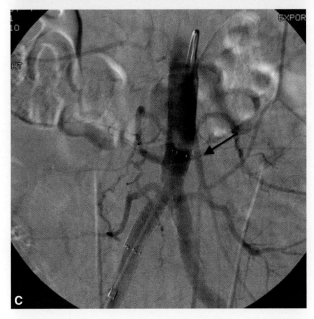

FIGURE 46.5 Stent mishaps. **A**. Fluoroscopic image demonstrates a balloon expandable stent (*arrow*) in the distal aortic bifurcation. The stent fell off the balloon as it was advanced over the bifurcation in a bareback manner (without a guiding sheath). The stent was successfully removed using an intravascular snare. **B**. Digital subtraction angiogram demonstrates a hemodynamically significant stenosis of the right CIA. **C**. A self-expanding stent was placed; however, note the inadvertent placement extending into the distal aorta (*arrow*).

proper positioning and, subsequently, the stent is deployed (FIGURE 46.6). Stent length should be sufficiently long enough to completely cover the lesion. SE stents typically require dilation with a balloon to fully expand to the intended diameter and to achieve wall apposition, especially in calcified stenoses. In addition, there is a learning curve for delivery of SE stents due to foreshortening and unjacketing technique (FIGURE 46.5). With experience, however, precise placement can also be obtained with SE stents. Balloon and stent diameters should be oversized to the vessel by 1 mm to account for intimal hyperplasia. If more than one stent is required, a 1-cm overlap is sufficient. Although arterial ruptures have occurred at low inflation pressures, greater than 10 to 12 atmospheres should be avoided for PTA or stent deployment in the aorta and iliac arteries, if

possible, and symptoms should be monitored. Severe pain can herald arterial rupture. If the patient has pain despite balloon deflation, it may be a signal that an arterial rupture has taken place. Maintenance of guide wire access across the lesion is mandatory until a completion angiogram is performed to determine TS and exclude vessel rupture or dissection.

Once the procedure is completed, hemostasis is obtained after anticoagulation is waned (ACT below 160). Manual compression for 15 to 20 minutes or use of percutaneous closure devices is effective for hemostasis. Bed rest for 6 hours is recommended for manual compression patients. Serial vascular exams, postintervention ankle brachial indices (ABI), and overnight observation should be performed. Antiplatelet therapy should be initiated if not already begun. Patient with renal insufficiency

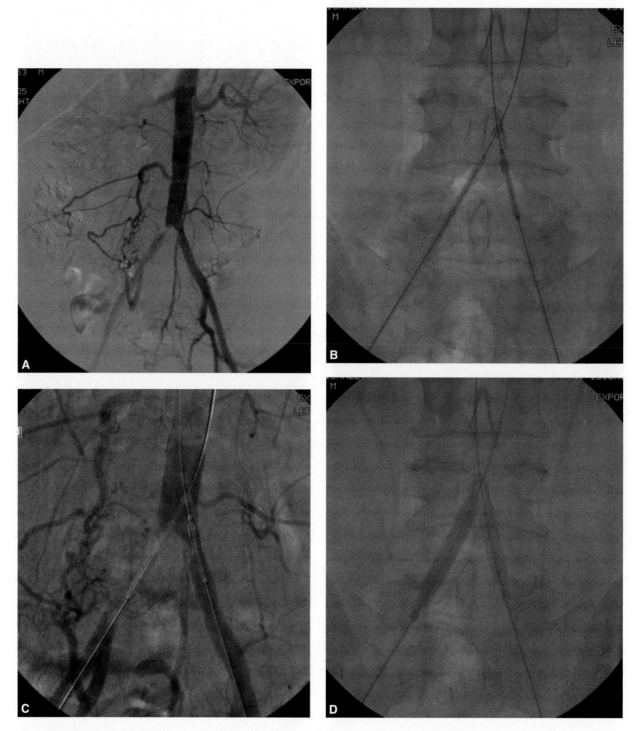

FIGURE 46.6 Stent placement—step-by-step guide. **A**. Digital subtraction angiogram shows a near occlusive right CIA stenosis and hemodynamically significant left CIA stenosis. **B**. After the guide wires are negotiated into the distal aorta, appropriately sized sheaths are advanced above the stenosis and the stents are advanced to the approximate location of expected placement. **C**. Stents are positioned as guided by contrast injected via either vascular sheath. **D**. The sheaths are then retracted to fully expose the balloon expandable stent and subsequently bilateral stents are deployed simultaneously.

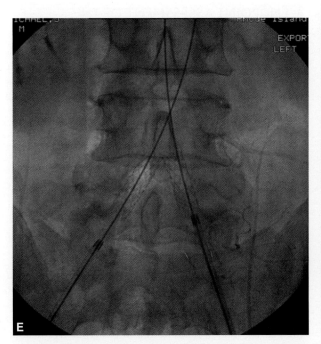
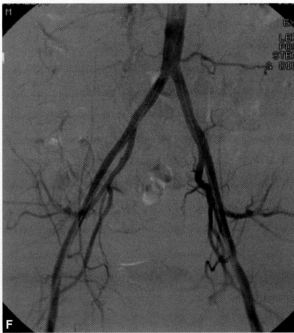

FIGURE 46.6 (*Continued*) **E**. Digital fluoroscopic image of the deployed stents. **F**. Completion angiogram shows technically successful stent placements.

should continue with hydration therapy. Diet can be reinitiated with clear liquids and advanced as tolerated. Routine creatinine checks are not recommended.

Special consideration should be given in certain situations in AIOD interventions. CIA origin disease may require what has been described as "kissing stents." To preserve the luminal patency of the contralateral CIA, stents may need to be placed simultaneously, even if the other side does not have a significant stenosis. Stents may be placed 1 to 2 mm into the distal aorta. Extending the stent too high into the aorta may preclude future interventions from a contralateral approach. If the stenosis begins in the distal aorta and extends into the CIA, then an aortic stent can be placed and CIA stents can be deployed overlapping into the aortic stent. Hypogastric or IIA disease can lead to buttock claudication and/or impotence. As such, preservation of IIA patency should be maintained if possible. Although stenting across the IIA origin should be avoided, small series have shown patency of IIA in nearly all patients despite stent placement over the ostium of the IIA.[36,37] Stent placement across the inguinal ligament is not recommended. External compressive forces may lead to stent deformation and subsequent vessel occlusion. Moreover, stents extending into the CFA may preclude future CFA bypass options. If stent placement across the inguinal ligament is not avoidable, then an SE stent is recommended.

Chronic occlusions represent the most technically challenging of cases in AIOD interventions. Despite potential difficulties in traversal, chronic occlusions can be successfully treated with endovascular technique. The decision to treat is predicated on the presence of relatively normal artery proximal and distal to the occlusion. In the early endovascular experience, some have suggested a trial of thrombolysis in patients whose symptoms

can be dated to less than 1 year in duration or increase in severity. Thrombolysis may (1) reduce an occlusion to a stenosis or (2) reduce the length of the occlusions by lysing the acute or subacute thrombus often found in chronic occlusions. Motarjeme and his group reported overall success of 88% and 5-year symptom-free rate of 80% in a retrospective analysis of 99 chronic occlusions managed with thrombolysis and subsequent PTA.[38] Some of the limitations of thrombolysis include increased procedure times, risk of hemorrhage, distal embolization, and prolonged hospitalization stays. As such and with emergence of primary stenting,[39,40] thrombolysis for chronic occlusions has become antiquated except in cases of total distal aortic occlusions.

For traversal of chronic occlusions, a directable catheter and a hydrophilic guide wire should be the initial tools of choice. Contrast injected directly at the occlusion (above and below) may reveal a hint of the occluded true lumen. Wire should be aimed directly at the true lumen assisted by a directable catheter. Although a retrograde approach typically provides the best mechanical advantage, in certain situations, both retrograde and anterograde attempts are required. A "modified wire loop technique" as described by McLean et al.,[41] which modified the initial technique by Gaines and Cumberland,[42] utilizes a gooseneck snare to pull the guide wire from a contralateral approach into the ipsilateral access, forming a wire loop. Then two catheters can be placed over both ends of the guide wire and be advanced into the distal aorta, allowing access for stent placement after true lumen location is confirmed.

Careful guide wire manipulation affords the highest chance for true lumen passage. Although early interventionalists purported the use of long, tapered spring coiled wires, the authors prefer 0.035-inch hydrophilic wire. Although true lumen recanalization is optimal, subintimal passage may not be avoidable and hence may be perfectly acceptable as long as true lumen reentry is gained prior to stent placement. If the combination of the guide wire and directable catheter is not successful, then multiple options exist for true lumen reentry. For very short distances, the back end of the guide wire can be used to dissect into the true lumen. If unsuccessful, then sharp needle recanalization may be required. As described by Murphy et al.,[43] several steps should be taken to ensure safe traversal. The distance of needle traversal should be minimized. Then a compliant balloon should be placed from the contralateral access as a target. Prior to unsheathing the needle, multiple projections should be obtained for triangulation. Correct trajectory should be confirmed with indentation on the balloon with the outer cannula. The needle is then advanced into the balloon. The balloon should immediately deflate, and then a wire is advanced through the lumen of the cannula. True lumen reentry should be confirmed prior to advancement of the sheath. Finally, prior to stent deployment, the sheath should be retracted while contrast is injected to ensure that passage is not external to the artery (FIGURE 46.7).[43] In a recent report of 112 limbs with chronic occlusions, sharp needle recanalization was successful in 9 of 11 cases, which had failed both conventional methods and the back end of the guide wire attempts.[44] Some interventionalists may favor the use of alternative devices designed specifically for true lumen reentry. These include the Frontrunner (Cordis, Warren, NJ), the Outback (Cordis, Warren, NJ), and the Pioneer (Medtronic, Minneapolis, MN). Positive early experiences with reentry devices have been recently reported for chronic iliac occlusions.[45,46]

ENDPOINT ASSESSMENT OF THE PROCEDURE

Determination of TS and exclusion of complications is obtained by a mandatory postintervention arteriogram. Published reporting standards have defined criteria for TS based on anatomic, hemodynamic, and clinical means. Less than 30% residual stenosis and reduction of the pressure gradient to less than 5 mm Hg mean or less than 10 mm Hg systolic are considered successful. Restoration of a 2+ CFA or dorsalis pedis and posterior tibial pulses provides added reassurance of success. Postintervention ABI should demonstrate greater than 0.10 improvement in technically successful procedures.[47]

PROCEDURAL COMPLICATIONS AND HOW TO MANAGE THEM SUCCESSFULLY

Endovascular AIOD revascularization can be performed safely with low morbidity and mortality rates. The aforementioned meta-analysis of over 2,116 patients treated endovascularly showed an overall 30-day mortality rate of 1% for PTA and 0.8% for stenting. Major complication rates between 4.3% and 7% for PTA and 4% and 5.2% for stenting have been reported.[25,26] A more recent large retrospective study of 505 arterial segments demonstrated a 30-day overall mortality and major complication rates of 0.5% and 7%, respectively.[48] Stratified to lesion complexity, complication rates tend to be higher with treatment of more complex disease.[26,49] Potential complications include arterial rupture, dissection, distal embolization, stent

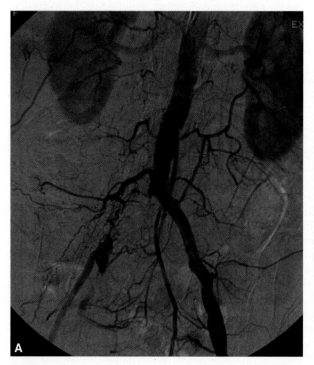
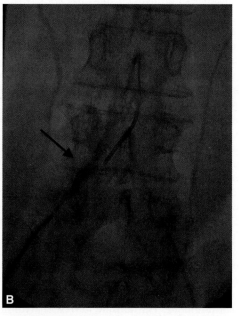

FIGURE 46.7 Sharp needle recanalization. **A.** Digital subtraction angiogram shows right CIA chronic total occlusion. **B.** Anterograde and retrograde true lumen recanalization attempts were unsuccessful. Note the subintimal contrast along the right lateral aspect of the right CIA (*arrow*).

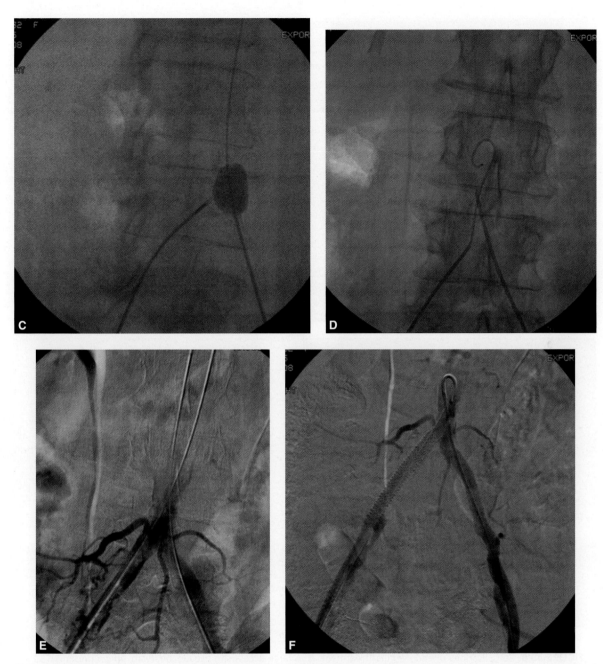

FIGURE 46.7 (*Continued*) **C.** A compliant balloon is placed from the contralateral access to serve as the target. A sheathed curved needle is positioned directly adjacent to the balloon and confirmed by multiple projections. **D.** After the balloon is burst (not shown), a guide wire is advanced into the true lumen. **E.** Prior to stent placement, subintimal tract passage is confirmed, and not extravascular tract, by retracting the sheath while injecting contrast with the wire across the occlusion. **F.** Completion angiogram shows successful endovascular revascularization with primary stent placement.

thrombosis, stent infection, access-related hematoma and pseudoaneurysm, renal failure, gastrointestinal bleeding, septicemia, and myocardial infarction (FIGURE 46.8).[26,48,49]

Arterial ruptures of the distal aorta or iliac arteries can result in catastrophic outcomes. Fortunately, the reported incidence is low, between 0.8% and 0.9%.[50,51] Intraprocedural and delayed presentations have been both described in the literature.[50,52] Patients may complain of persistent pain despite balloon

deflation and postintervention arteriogram may reveal free or contained extravasation of contrast. Medial displacement of the bladder may be present. Alternatively, hemodynamic collapse may precede the radiographic findings. Once the arterial rupture is confirmed, several steps need to be performed immediately and in concert to avert an undesired outcome. Appropriate resuscitation including oxygenation and pressure support should be started. Intravascular volume support—that is, intravenous

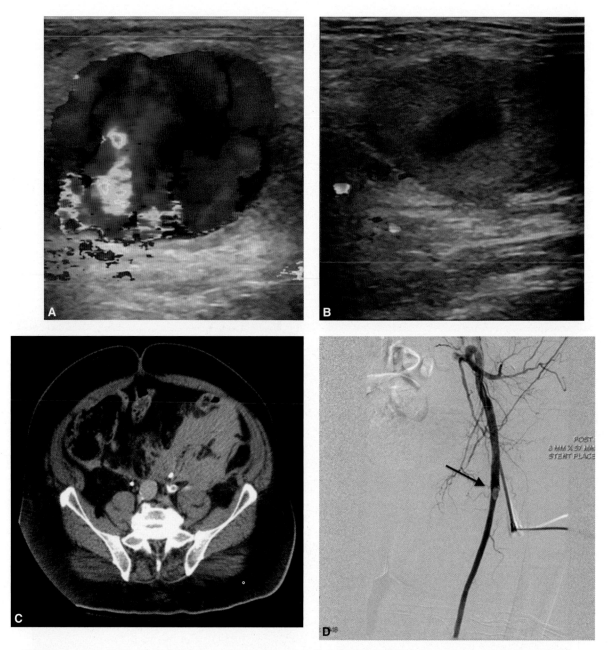

FIGURE 46.8 Complications of endovascular treatment. **A.** A large access site pseudoaneurysm, which presented as a painful pulsatile mass on initial outpatient follow-up visit. Note the characteristic yin-yang flow pattern on color Doppler US image. Given its size, percutaneous thrombin injection was performed. **B.** After successful embolization, no flow is seen in the thrombosed pseudoaneurysm. **C.** CT scan image of the pelvis after left external iliac artery rupture during recanalization shows a large hematoma. The rupture was successfully managed with percutaneous covered stent placement at the time of intervention. **D.** Intraprocedure arteriogram shows embolus (*arrow*) in the left common femoral artery bifurcation after successful recanalization of a chronic total occlusion of the left CIA. The embolus has occluded the profunda femoris artery origin.

saline bolus infusion or blood transfusion, should be initiated. A balloon catheter should be advanced quickly and inflated at the site of the extravasation to tamponade the bleeding. Contrast should be injected from above and below to confirm adequate exclusion. Anticoagulation should be reversed with protamine sulfate infusion. Although successful treatment with prolonged balloon tamponade has been reported,[53] availability of covered

stents allow more definitive treatment. Proposed risk factors for rupture include calcified high-grade stenosis, inappropriately sized balloon catheter, inflation without a manometric control, diabetes, corticosteroids, and recent endarterectomy.[50] In a small series of five patients with postintervention ruptures, patients (three) treated with covered stents had good outcome, whereas those treated with surgery (one) or conservative management (one) resulted in fatalities.[50] Once hemostasis is accomplished with a covered stent, the patient should be monitored in critical care. CT scan of the abdomen and pelvis may be considered.

PTA or stenting may be complicated by arterial dissection. If a dissection is present, occurrence of blood flow limitation and loss of branch arteries should be assessed. Typically, focal, retrograde, and non–flow-limiting dissections are self-limiting and do not require intervention. If distal blood flow is compromised, a stent should be placed to tack down the flap. Stent placement can also result in a dissection, typically at the proximal or distal margin(s) of the stent. In such instances, additional stents may need to be extended.

AIOD intervention may be complicated by distal embolization. A completion angiogram should include imaging of the arteries distal to the intervention, especially at major branching points; that is, CFA bifurcation and popliteal trifurcation. Depending on embolus location and burden, suction embolectomy, percutanous mechanical thrombectomy, thrombolysis, or, rarely, open surgical thrombectomy may be required.

Stent infections are rare events. As a result, data are drawn from few single case reports. Although Darcy[54] reported that only eight published cases as of year 2000 were found, the authors agree with his suggestion that stent infections may be underdiagnosed and likely more common given the increased utilization of stents. Patients may present with fever, leukocytosis, pain, bacteremia, sepsis, or pseudoaneurysm formation. *Staphylococcus aureus* infection has been most commonly associated with stent infections.[55,56] High index suspicion and prompt therapy with intravenous antibiotics or surgical resection may help to avert poor outcomes. As mentioned previously, prophylactic antibiotics are not recommended for routine arterial stent placement.

▌ OUTCOMES/PROGNOSIS

Numerous studies have been published regarding outcomes of endovascular treatment of AIOD. Despite recommended reporting standards, studies vary in patient characteristics, indication for treatment (claudication vs. CLI), severity of disease (TASC classification), presence of concomitant CFA or distal occlusive disease, technique (primary stent vs. selective stent placement), follow-up intervals, and measures of patency (ABI, US velocity, arteriography, etc.). As a result, direct comparative analysis is challenging.

Before the advent of stents, PTA performed reasonably well. Most PTA data are from earlier experiences in endovascular technique. TS rates have been reported between 91% and 95%,[22,26] and not surprisingly, TS rate for stenoses are higher than for occlusions. Bosch and Hunink[26] reported an average of 96% TS rate for stenosis and 80% TS rates for occlusion. Overall patency rate of 75% at 5-year follow-up was reported by Becker's group,[57] in their review of 2,697 noncoronary PTA. Subsequent review by Pentecost et al.[22] showed slight higher patency rate of 80% at 4 years. In the aforementioned meta-analysis that included over 1,300 patients treated with PTA, a 4-year primary patency rate of 64% and secondary patency rate of 80% were reported.[26] Because stent placement has become more popular, outcome discussion of PTA alone is more of a historical interest.

Palmaz et al.[58] published the first large series (171 procedures) of stent placement for AIOD after failure of PTA in 1990. Subsequent reports have shown high TS, primary patency, and secondary patency rates. In a meta-analysis of 816 patients with stent placement published in 1997, 4-year primary and secondary patency rates were 74% and 88%, respectively.[26] Table 46.1 is a list of selective published studies on endovascular AIOD intervention outcomes chosen by the authors for their larger sample size and long-term follow-up data. TS, primary patency, and secondary patency rates are enumerated for provided follow-up intervals. The largest series of 496 limbs treated by Murphy's group showed a TS rate of 98% with 8-year primary and secondary patency rates of 74% and 84%, respectively.[48]

DIST compared primary PTA and selective stenting with primary stenting and found no difference in outcome at 2 years.[25] Interestingly, subsequently long-term follow-up results showed better symptomatic outcome (Fontaine classification) for the PTA and selective stent group despite no difference in ABI, iliac patency, and QOL between the two treatment arms.[27] The reader should note that a large number of the primary PTA with selective stenting group received stents (43%) and that TS was defined as residual gradient less than 10 mm Hg mean.[25] If a gradient less than 5 mm Hg mean was applied instead, it is likely that a larger number of patients would have required selective stenting. Nevertheless, DIST is the only randomized trial comparing selective stenting and primary stenting for AIOD to the authors' knowledge.

Numerous studies have tried to identify markers for successful endovascular intervention for AIOD but the proposed predictors of favorable outcome have not been able to be consistently validated. The studies of earlier experiences in general were consistent with TASC recommendations. In the previously mentioned meta-analysis, stenoses showed higher patency rates compared to occlusions, regardless of treatment technique (PTA or stent) and indication (claudication or CLI).[26] In contrast, more recent publications have demonstrated improved outcomes for the lesions with higher complexity including occlusions, challenging open surgical management. Balzer et al.[59] showed 3-year primary and secondary patency rates of 89.9% and 95.5%, respectively, in 89 patients with TASC C and D lesions, emphasizing the lack of utility of that system for patient selection. In another study of 103 patients with chronic iliac artery occlusions, the reported 4-year primary and secondary patency rates were 78% and 88%, respectively.[39] A recent review of studies on TASC C and D lesions published between years 2000 and 2009 revealed 5-year primary patency rates between 60% and 86%, respectively, and secondary patency rates between 80% and 98%, respectively.[60] Many studies have found no significant association of between TASC classification and patency rates.[49,61,62] Not surprisingly, the recent 2007 TASC II classification has expanded the role of endovascular treatment.

Longer lesion lengths, EIA disease, younger age, female sex, poor runoff vessel patency, presence of comorbid diseases, and smoking have been implicated in one or more studies as predictors of poor outcome. Longer lesion lengths have been associated with decreased patency rates in two recent large series,[48,49] contradicting earlier results from Galaria and Davies[62] who did not find longer lesion length to be a significant indicator of decreased patency. EIA involvement has been a source of much controversy and confusion. Timaran et al.[63] reported higher loss of patency in EIA disease; however, when adjusted for gender, only women with EIA disease but not men had worse outcome. Interestingly, Lee et al.[64] showed a nonstatistically significant trend in which EIA had higher patency compared to CIA.

Table 46.1

Studies Published after Year 2000 Selected for Endovascular Treatment of AIOD, Sample Size, and Long-Term Follow-Up

Study	Year	N	TS	PPR (%)						SPR (%)					
				1 y	2 y	3 y	4 y	5 y	10 y	1 y	2 y	3 y	4 y	5 y	10 y
Pulli et al.[86]	2011	212 PT	98.9												
		114 stenosis	99.2					77.7						92.8	
		109 CTO	99.1					82.4						93.1	
Ichihashi et al.[49]	2011	288 TASC A/B PT	99	95		91		88	83	99		99		97	97
		125 TASC C/D PT	99	90		88		83	71	99		98		98	98
Koizumi et al.[87]	2009	487 lesions	95.7												
		177 PTA				67		54	50						
		212 SSP				88		82	75						
Park et al.[88]	2005	88 TASC A PT	98	96		84		81		98 PAP		88 PAP		88 PAP	
		92 TASC B PT		95		85		85		98 PAP		91 PAP		91 PAP	
		32 TASC C PT		94		94		78		97 PAP		97 PAP		74 PAP	
		16 TASC D PT		93		74		74		94 PAP		85 PAP		85 PAP	
Kudo et al.[69]	2005	151 lesions	99.3	76		59		49						99 (7 y)	
Galaria and Davies[62]	2005	394 lesions	98					53	27					79	72
		TASC A/B													
Murphy et al.[48]	2004	505 limbs	98	89	86	83	78	75	74 (8 y)	95	93	91	87	86	84 (8 y)
Reyes et al.[66]	2004	303 limbs	99	87	82	76	71	70	57	96	95	94	93	92	87
Timaran et al.[67]	2003	188 PT	97	85		72		64							
Reekers et al.[89]	2002	143 limbs	94	89						86 PAP					
Schurmann et al.[90]	2002	126 limbs		92	81	76	71	66	46	96	91	87	83	79	55
Scheinert et al.[91]	2001	212 CTO PT	90	84	81	78	76	66		88	88	86	85	80	
Powell et al.[92]	2000	210 lesions	97	61		43				87 PAP		72 PAP			

TS, technical success; PPR, primary patency rate; SPR, secondary patency rate; PT, patients; CTO, chronic total occlusion; PTA, percutaneous transluminal angioplasty; SSP, selective stent placement; PAP, primary assisted patency; TASC, transAtlantic inter-society consensus.

Younger age[48,65] and female gender[63,66] also have been found to be risk factors for loss of patency. Presence of patent runoff vessels (i.e., femoral and tibial) has been associated with higher patency rates after AIOD intervention.[62,65,67,68] Reyes et al.[66] did not find that association to be true. Coexisting diseases including diabetes, hypertension, hypercholesterolemia, chronic renal failure, and smoking all have been also associated with less patency.[61,62,65,69] Despite these statistical associations, outcomes for all lesions and with all comorbid conditions are satisfactory; there are no patients or lesion types that should be routinely excluded from interventional therapy for aortoiliac insufficiency because of them.

DISEASE SURVEILLANCE AND TREATMENT MONITORING ALGORITHMS

Longitudinal office follow-up is required for all patients regardless of medical or endovascular therapy. At the initial postprocedural follow-up, specific evaluation of the access site(s) and the lower extremities should be performed. Improvement in clinical symptoms and hemodynamics (ABI) should be documented. Antiplatelet therapy should be confirmed. If no clinical improvement is noted despite improvement in ABI (>0.10), other etiologies for leg symptoms should be investigated. Subsequent follow-up with clinical examinations and ABI are recommended at regular intervals (e.g., 6 months then yearly or as required). Along with lower extremity evaluations, patients should be monitored for continued cardiovascular risk factor reductions—that is, blood pressure, serum cholesterol, blood sugar control for diabetics (hemoglobin A1c), smoking cessation, physical activity, and proper diet.

Patients on cilastazol therapy or SEP should be reassessed at 3 to 6 months for improvements in symptoms. For those with no clinical improvement on medical or exercise therapy, endovascular revascularization should be offered depending on severity of symptoms. If recurrence of disease or loss of patency is suspected (symptom worsening or decrease in ABI >0.10) corroboration with noninvasive imaging (e.g., CTA or MRA) may be helpful for confirmation and treatment planning. Endovascular reintervention is recommended as appropriate.

EARLY FAILURE

Early loss of patency may be secondary to acute thrombosis of the treated segment or early restenosis. With increased utilization of stents, acute thrombosis is a rare event. Patients may present with no improvement or worsening symptoms and ABI, diminished femoral pulse(s), or acute limb ischemia. If acute stent thrombosis is suspected then a repeat arteriogram is recommended. Contralateral access is recommended for diagnostic purposes. Once confirmed, percutaneous mechanical thrombectomy or short-term catheter-directed thrombolysis may alleviate the occlusion and/or unmask the etiology. Repeat PTA or stent placement may be necessary. Restenosis is a complex process involving neointimal hyperplasia, remodeling, and thrombosis. Restenosis may occur within the stent or at the proximal or distal edges of the stent. If restenosis is encountered, repeat PTA or restenting will suffice. Preliminary experience with cutting balloon and cryoplasty for iliac restenosis is encouraging but limited.[70,71]

LATE FAILURES AND OPTIONS FOR MANAGEMENT

Similar to early loss of patency, late failures of AIOD treatment include recurrence of disease (stent restenosis or occlusion) and de novo stenosis. Regardless of etiology, surveillance may show return of symptoms, abnormal femoral pulses, and decreased ABI. Similar to the initial diagnostic algorithm, a CTA or MRA (less helpful because of metal artifact) should help to confirm the presence of disease and aid in treatment planning. Most in-stent restenosis can be effectively ameliorated by balloon angioplasty. A second stent may be required in some cases. Occasionally, new occlusive disease remote to the site of prior intervention may be present rather than restenosis and should be treated as appropriate. In the rare patient, who requires frequent repeated treatments, open surgical bypass remains an option.

PRACTICAL ADVANTAGES AND LIMITATIONS

The practical benefits of endovascular revascularization compared to open bypass surgery lies in the inherent minimally invasive nature. Because endovascular therapy only requires conscious sedation, the risks related to general anesthesia are averted. As such, patients with comorbid diseases who are poor surgical candidates can be treated with reduced risk. Several studies have shown less major complications and 30-day mortality rates. A Cochrane Database review of direct anatomic open surgical repair of AIOD encompassing 5,738 patients in 29 published studies from 1970 to 2007 showed a 4.1% perioperative death rate and 16.0% systemic morbidity rate.[72] As mentioned earlier, the endovascular 30-day all-inclusive mortality rates for PTA and stenting were 1% and 0.8%, respectively, and major complication rates ranged from 4% to 7%.[26,48] These figures are more impressive if one considers that endovascular patients tend to have more comorbid disease.[73] Aside from less morbidity and mortality and wider applicability to patients with comorbid diseases, endovascular technique does not preclude future surgical bypass options. Thus, open surgical bypass remains a viable option for patients who fail endovascular therapy. Other practical advantages include shorter length of hospital stay and less hospital cost with endovascular revascularization.[73–75] Finally, reintervention for recurrent disease does not present added technical challenges in contrast to open aortofemoral bypass surgery. Repeat access, PTA, or stenting can be performed without the risks associated with open revision of aortofemoral bypass surgery.

Limitations of endovascular treatment are few. Heavily calcified lesions may not be able to be fully expanded despite placement of a stent and balloon dilation. In such rare instances, surgical bypass may be prudent if clinical benefit is not realized. A second limitation is seen in patients with concomitant CFA disease who may require a CFA endarterectomy in combination with inflow intervention to provide optimal AIOD patency.

RELATIVE THERAPEUTIC EFFECTIVENESS COMPARED TO MEDICAL AND SURGICAL MANAGEMENT

Direct comparison studies of endovascular treatment with medical or open surgical therapy are lacking. To the authors' knowledge, there are only five published randomized, controlled trials that have compared endovascular treatment (none involving stents) to either medical or surgical treatments.[76–82] The Mild to Moderate Intermittent Claudication trial participants prospectively compared best medical management with best medical management with PTA for AIOD and femoropopliteal disease.[78] Although the study population was small (34 for the AIOD limb of the trial), significant increases in outcomes measures—that is, absolute walking distance (AWD) and initial claudication distance—were observed at 24 months for the best medical management and PTA compared to best medical management alone. In fact, AWD was 78% greater for the PTA group.[78] The treatment regimen for exercise therapy in this study was low, however, as was the response to exercise.[77] Two earlier studies with a small number of patients with iliac or femoropopliteal occlusive disease compared PTA with exercise and found short-term benefits in symptom relief and walking distance in the PTA groups; however, at long-term follow-up, the PTA advantages were no longer observed.[76,79–81] The CLEVER (Claudication: Exercise Vs. Endoluminal Revascularization) trial is a randomized study evaluating efficacy, safety, and health economic impact for treatment options: (1) optimal medical care, (2) primary stenting, and (3) SEP, and showed superior treadmill outcomes (MWD) for SEP compared with stents.[17]

In general, aortoiliac bypass surgery tends to have higher primary patency rates but similar rates of primary assisted or secondary patency rates compared to endovascular treatment. In the only randomized, controlled study comparing endovascular treatment with surgery, Wolf et al. randomized 263 patients with iliac, femoral, or popliteal occlusive disease to either PTA or bypass surgery. They found a nonsignificant trend favoring surgery for primary success and PTA for limb salvage, and concluded that there was no difference in outcomes at 4-year follow-up.[77] A recent retrospective study of 169 patients (288 limbs) with greater than TASC B disease compared open bypass to endovascular revascularization. The aortobifemoral bypass surgery group showed 93% primary patency, 97% secondary patency rate, 98% limb salvage rate. and 80% long-term survival at 3 years. The endovascular group had 74% primary patency, 95% secondary patency, 98% limb salvage, and 80% long-term survival.[83] In a smaller series, aortoiliac bypass surgery showed higher primary patency rate at 4 years compared to stenting (93% vs. 69%).[74] The abovementioned Cochrane Database review of direct anatomic open surgical repair of AIOD revealed an 86.3% 5-year primary patency rate for aortofemoral bypass surgery.[72] In an earlier meta-analysis, surgical 5- and 10-year patency rates were reported to be 87.5% to 91.0% and 81.8% to 86.8%, respectively.[84] These numbers are nearly comparable to those of endovascular treatment (Table 46.1). Although the surgical data tend to have better primary patency rates, perhaps the more relevant comparison would be to secondary patency rates because endovascular techniques are minimally invasive and repeat interventions can be performed without the added risk associated with repeat open surgical procedure. It is unlikely that a randomized controlled trial comparing stenting to surgery would ever be performed given the positive endovascular results and greater invasive nature of open bypass surgery.

THE FUTURE

An ideal vascular intervention would have high TS, primary patency, and be minimally invasive as possible. Medical and technical advances may lead to regression of already present plaque and prevent restenosis. Coronary atherosclerosis regression with intensive statin therapy, as measured by intravascular US, has shown encouraging preliminary results.[85] No specific data for AIOD atherosclerosis are available, however. Prevention of restenosis has been the holy grail of revascularization. In other vascular beds, atherectomy, cryoplasty, drug-eluting stents, and drug-eluting balloons have been proposed in an effort to reduce restenosis. Future studies would be required to demonstrate consistent superiority to the current PTA and stenting therapy.

CONCLUSION

Technologic advances have allowed endovascular management to become the first-line invasive treatment for AIOD. PTA and stenting can effectively manage AIOD with high TS and patency rates and low complication rates. Longitudinal follow-up care and secondary prevention of cardiovascular events by risk factor reduction are recommended.

REFERENCES

1. Dotter CT, Judkins MP. Transluminal treatment of arteriosclerotic obstruction. Description of a new technic and a preliminary report of its application. *Circulation* 1964;30:654–670.
2. Dotter CT, Frische LH, Judkins MP, et al. The "nonsurgical" treatment of iliofemoral arteriosclerotic obstruction. *Radiology* 1966;86(5):871–875.
3. Martin EC. The impact of angioplasty: a perspective. *J Vasc Interv Radiol* 1992;3(3):511–514.
4. Criqui MH. Peripheral arterial disease—epidemiological aspects. *Vasc Med* 2001;6(3 suppl):3–7.
5. Criqui MH, Fronek A, Barrett-Connor E, et al. The prevalence of peripheral arterial disease in a defined population. *Circulation* 1985;71(3):510–515.
6. Fowkes FG, Housley E, Cawood EH, et al. Edinburgh Artery Study: prevalence of asymptomatic and symptomatic peripheral arterial disease in the general population. *Int J Epidemiol* 1991;20(2):384–392.
7. Hirsch AT, Criqui MH, Treat-Jacobson D, et al. Peripheral arterial disease detection, awareness, and treatment in primary care. *JAMA* 2001;286(11):1317–1324.
8. Steg PG, Bhatt DL, Wilson PW, et al. One-year cardiovascular event rates in outpatients with atherothrombosis. *JAMA* 2007;297(11):1197–1206.
9. Jelnes R, Gaardsting O, Hougaard Jensen K, et al. Fate in intermittent claudication: outcome and risk factors. *Br Med J (Clin Res Ed)* 1986;293(6555):1137–1140.
10. McDaniel MD, Cronenwett JL. Basic data related to the natural history of intermittent claudication. *Ann Vasc Surg* 1989;3(3):273–277.
11. Murphy TP, Soares GM, Kim HM, et al. Quality of life and exercise performance after aortoiliac stent placement for claudication. *J Vasc Interv Radiol* 2005;16(7):947–953; quiz 954.
12. Kalbaugh CA, Taylor SM, Blackhurst DW, et al. One-year prospective quality-of-life outcomes in patients treated with angioplasty for symptomatic peripheral arterial disease. *J Vasc Surg* 2006;44(2):296–302; discussion 302–303.
13. Third Report of the National Cholesterol Education Program (NCEP) Expert Panel on Detection, Evaluation, and Treatment of High Blood Cholesterol in Adults (Adult Treatment Panel III) final report. *Circulation* 2002;106(25):3143–3421.
14. Hirsch AT, Haskal ZJ, Hertzer NR, et al. ACC/AHA Guidelines for the Management of Patients with Peripheral Arterial Disease (lower extremity, renal, mesenteric, and abdominal aortic): a collaborative report from the American Associations for Vascular Surgery/Society for Vascular Surgery, Society for Cardiovascular Angiography and Interventions, Society for Vascular Medicine and Biology, Society of Interventional Radiology, and the ACC/AHA Task Force on Practice Guidelines (writing committee to develop guidelines for the management of patients with peripheral arterial disease)—summary of recommendations. *J Vasc Interv Radiol* 2006;17(9):1383–1397; quiz 1398.
15. Regensteiner JG, Ware JE Jr, McCarthy WJ, et al. Effect of cilostazol on treadmill walking, community-based walking ability, and health-related quality of life in patients with intermittent claudication due to peripheral arterial disease: meta-analysis of six randomized controlled trials. *J Am Geriatr Soc* 2002;50(12):1939–1946.

16. Dawson DL, Cutler BS, Hiatt WR, et al. A comparison of cilostazol and pentoxifylline for treating intermittent claudication. *Am J Med* 2000;109(7):523–530.

17. Murphy TP, Cutlip De, Regensteiner, JG, et al. Supervised exercise versus primary stenting for claudication resulting from aortoiliac peripheral artery disease: six-month outcomes from the claudication: exercise versus endoluminal revascularization (CLEVER) study. *Circulation* 2012 Jan 3; 125(1): 130–139.

18. Stewart KJ, Hiatt WR, Regensteiner JG, et al. Exercise training for claudication. *N Engl J Med* 2002;347(24):1941–1951.

19. Upchurch GR, Dimick JB, Wainess RM, et al. Diffusion of new technology in health care: the case of aorto-iliac occlusive disease. *Surgery* 2004;136(4):812–818.

20. Ring EJ, Freiman DB, McLean GK, et al. Percutaneous recanalization of common iliac artery occlusions: an unacceptable complication rate? *AJR Am J Roentgenol* 1982;139(3):587–589.

21. Dormandy JA, Rutherford RB. Management of peripheral arterial disease (PAD). TASC Working Group. TransAtlantic Inter-Society Concensus (TASC). *J Vasc Surg* 2000;31(1, pt 2):S1–S296.

22. Pentecost MJ, Criqui MH, Dorros G, et al. Guidelines for peripheral percutaneous transluminal angioplasty of the abdominal aorta and lower extremity vessels. A statement for health professionals from a Special Writing Group of the Councils on Cardiovascular Radiology, Arteriosclerosis, Cardio-Thoracic and Vascular Surgery, Clinical Cardiology, and Epidemiology and Prevention, the American Heart Association. *J Vasc Interv Radiol* 2003;14(9, pt 2):S495–S515.

23. Norgren L, Hiatt WR, Dormandy JA, et al. Inter-society consensus for the management of peripheral arterial disease (TASC II). *J Vasc Surg* 2007;45(suppl S):S5–67.

24. Leung DA, Spinosa DJ, Hagspiel KD, et al. Selection of stents for treating iliac arterial occlusive disease. *J Vasc Interv Radiol* 2003;14(2, pt 1): 137–152.

25. Tetteroo E, van der Graaf Y, Bosch JL, et al. Randomised comparison of primary stent placement versus primary angioplasty followed by selective stent placement in patients with iliac-artery occlusive disease. Dutch Iliac Stent Trial Study Group. *Lancet* 1998;351(9110):1153–1159.

26. Bosch JL, Hunink MG. Meta-analysis of the results of percutaneous transluminal angioplasty and stent placement for aortoiliac occlusive disease. *Radiology* 1997;204(1):87–96.

27. Klein WM, van der Graaf Y, Seegers J, et al. Dutch iliac stent trial: long-term results in patients randomized for primary or selective stent placement. *Radiology* 2006;238(2):734–744.

28. Rzucidlo EM, Powell RJ, Zwolak RM, et al. Early results of stent-grafting to treat diffuse aortoiliac occlusive disease. *J Vasc Surg* 2003;37(6):1175–1180.

29. Sabri SS, Choudhri A, Orgera G, et al. Outcomes of covered kissing stent placement compared with bare metal stent placement in the treatment of atherosclerotic occlusive disease at the aortic bifurcation. *J Vasc Interv Radiol* 2010;21(7):995–1003.

30. Barrett BJ, Parfrey PS. Clinical practice. Preventing nephropathy induced by contrast medium. *N Engl J Med* 2006;354(4):379–386.

31. Kagan A, Sheikh-Hamad D. Contrast-induced kidney injury: focus on modifiable risk factors and prophylactic strategies. *Clin Cardiol* 2010;33(2):62–66.

32. Armstrong PJ, Han DC, Baxter JA, et al. Complication rates of percutaneous brachial artery access in peripheral vascular angiography. *Ann Vasc Surg* 2003;17(1):107–110.

33. Alvarez-Tostado JA, Moise MA, Bena JF, et al. The brachial artery: a critical access for endovascular procedures. *J Vasc Surg* 2009;49(2):378–385; discussion 385.

34. Venkatesan AM, Kundu S, Sacks D, et al. Practice guideline for adult antibiotic prophylaxis during vascular and interventional radiology procedures. *J Vasc Interv Radiol* 2010;21(11):1611–1630; quiz 1631.

35. Bonn J. Percutaneous vascular intervention: value of hemodynamic measurements. *Radiology* 1996;201(1):18–20.

36. Long AL, Page PE, Raynaud AC, et al. Percutaneous iliac artery stent: angiographic long-term follow-up. *Radiology* 1991;180(3):771–778.

37. Gunther RW, Vorwerk D, Bohndorf K, et al. Iliac and femoral artery stenoses and occlusions: treatment with intravascular stents. *Radiology* 1989;172(3):725–730.

38. Motarjeme A, Gordon GI, Bodenhagen K. Thrombolysis and angioplasty of chronic iliac artery occlusions. *J Vasc Interv Radiol* 1995;6(6, pt 2 suppl):66S–72S.

39. Vorwerk D, Guenther RW, Schurmann K, et al. Primary stent placement for chronic iliac artery occlusions: follow-up results in 103 patients. *Radiology* 1995;194(3):745–749.

40. Dyet JF, Gaines PA, Nicholson AA, et al. Treatment of chronic iliac artery occlusions by means of percutaneous endovascular stent placement. *J Vasc Interv Radiol* 1997;8(3):349–353.

41. McLean GK, Cekirge S, Weiss JP, et al. Stent placement for iliac artery occlusions: modified "wire-loop" technique with use of the goose neck loop snare. *J Vasc Interv Radiol* 1994;5(5):701–703.

42. Gaines PA, Cumberland DC. Wire-loop technique for angioplasty of total iliac artery occlusions. *Radiology* 1988;168(1):275–276.

43. Murphy TP, Marks MJ, Webb MS. Use of a curved needle for true lumen re-entry during subintimal iliac artery revascularization. *J Vasc Interv Radiol* 1997;8(4):633–636.

44. Sharafuddin MJ, Hoballah JJ, Kresowik TF, et al. Impact of aggressive endovascular recanalization techniques on success rate in chronic total arterial occlusions (CTOs). *Vasc Endovascular Surg* 2010;44(6):460–467.

45. Etezadi V, Benenati JF, Patel PJ, et al. The reentry catheter: a second chance for endoluminal reentry at difficult lower extremity subintimal arterial recanalizations. *J Vasc Interv Radiol* 2010;21(5):730–734.

46. Jacobs DL, Motaganahalli RL, Cox DE, et al. True lumen re-entry devices facilitate subintimal angioplasty and stenting of total chronic occlusions: initial report. *J Vasc Surg* 2006;43(6):1291–1296.

47. Sacks D, Marinelli DL, Martin LG, et al. Reporting standards for clinical evaluation of new peripheral arterial revascularization devices. *J Vasc Interv Radiol* 2003;14(9, pt 2):S395–S404.

48. Murphy TP, Ariaratnam NS, Carney WI Jr, et al. Aortoiliac insufficiency: long-term experience with stent placement for treatment. *Radiology* 2004;231(1):243–249.

49. Ichihashi S, Higashiura W, Itoh H, et al. Long-term outcomes for systematic primary stent placement in complex iliac artery occlusive disease classified according to Trans-Atlantic Inter-Society Consensus (TASC)-II. *J Vasc Surg* 2011;53(4):992–999.

50. Allaire E, Melliere D, Poussier B, et al. Iliac artery rupture during balloon dilatation: what treatment? *Ann Vasc Surg* 2003;17(3):306–314.

51. Palmaz JC, Laborde JC, Rivera FJ, et al. Stenting of the iliac arteries with the Palmaz stent: experience from a multicenter trial. *Cardiovasc Intervent Radiol* 1992;15(5):291–297.

52. Sobrinho G, Albino JP. Delayed rupture of the external iliac artery after balloon angioplasty and stent placement. *J Vasc Interv Radiol* 2008;19(3):460–462.

53. Cooper SG, Sofocleous CT. Percutaneous management of angioplasty-related iliac artery rupture with preservation of luminal patency by prolonged balloon tamponade. *J Vasc Interv Radiol* 1998;9(1, pt 1):81–83.

54. Darcy M. Complications of iliac angioplasty and stenting. *Tech Vasc Interv Radiol* 2000;3(4):226–239.

55. Hoffman AI, Murphy TP. Septic arteritis causing iliac artery rupture and aneurysmal transformation of the distal aorta after iliac artery stent placement. *J Vasc Interv Radiol* 1997;8(2):215–219.

56. Bunt TJ, Gill HK, Smith DC, et al. Infection of a chronically implanted iliac artery stent. *Ann Vasc Surg* 1997;11(5):529–532.

57. Becker GJ, Katzen BT, Dake MD. Noncoronary angioplasty. *Radiology* 1989;170(3, pt 2):921–940.

58. Palmaz JC, Garcia OJ, Schatz RA, et al. Placement of balloon-expandable intraluminal stents in iliac arteries: first 171 procedures. *Radiology* 1990;174(3, pt 2):969–975.

59. Balzer JO, Gastinger V, Ritter R, et al. Percutaneous interventional reconstruction of the iliac arteries: primary and long-term success rate in selected TASC C and D lesions. *Eur Radiol* 2006;16(1):124–131.

60. Jongkind V, Akkersdijk GJ, Yeung KK, et al. A systematic review of endovascular treatment of extensive aortoiliac occlusive disease. *J Vasc Surg* 2010;52(5):1376–1383.

61. Leville CD, Kashyap VS, Clair DG, et al. Endovascular management of iliac artery occlusions: extending treatment to TransAtlantic Inter-Society Consensus class C and D patients. *J Vasc Surg* 2006;43(1):32–39.

62. Galaria, II, Davies MG. Percutaneous transluminal revascularization for iliac occlusive disease: long–term outcomes in TransAtlantic Inter-Society Consensus A and B lesions. *Ann Vasc Surg* 2005;19(3):352–360.

63. Timaran CH, Stevens SL, Freeman MB, et al. External iliac and common iliac artery angioplasty and stenting in men and women. *J Vasc Surg* 2001;34(3):440–446.

64. Lee ES, Steenson CC, Trimble KE, et al. Comparing patency rates between external iliac and common iliac artery stents. *J Vasc Surg* 2000;31(5):889–894.

65. Yasuhara H, Shigematsu H, Muto T. Risk factors for restenosis after balloon angioplasty in focal iliac stenosis. *Surgery* 1998;123(6):658–665.

66. Reyes R, Carreira JM, Gude F, et al. Long-term follow-up of iliac wallstents. *Cardiovasc Intervent Radiol* 2004;27(6):624–631.

67. Timaran CH, Prault TL, Stevens SL, et al. Iliac artery stenting versus surgical reconstruction for TASC (TransAtlantic Inter-Society Consensus) type B and type C iliac lesions. *J Vasc Surg* 2003;38(2):272–278.

68. Funovics MA, Lackner B, Cejna M, et al. Predictors of long-term results after treatment of iliac artery obliteration by transluminal angioplasty and stent deployment. *Cardiovasc Intervent Radiol* 2002;25(5):397–402.

69. Kudo T, Chandra FA, Ahn SS. Long-term outcomes and predictors of iliac angioplasty with selective stenting. *J Vasc Surg* 2005;42(3):466–475.

70. McCaslin JE, Macdonald S, Stansby G. Cryoplasty for peripheral vascular disease. *Cochrane Database Syst Rev* 2007;(4):CD005507.

71. Tsetis D, Belli AM, Morgan R, et al. Preliminary experience with cutting balloon angioplasty for iliac artery in-stent restenosis. *J Endovasc Ther* 2008;15(2):193–202.

72. Chiu KW, Davies RS, Nightingale PG, et al. Review of direct anatomical open surgical management of atherosclerotic aorto-iliac occlusive disease. *Eur J Vasc Endovasc Surg* 2010;39(4):460–471.

73. Indes JE, Mandawat A, Tuggle CT, et al. Endovascular procedures for aorto-iliac occlusive disease are associated with superior short-term clinical and economic outcomes compared with open surgery in the inpatient population. *J Vasc Surg* 2010;52(5):1173–1179, 1179.e1.

74. Hans SS, DeSantis D, Siddiqui R, et al. Results of endovascular therapy and aortobifemoral grafting for Transatlantic Inter-Society type C and D aortoiliac occlusive disease. *Surgery* 2008;144(4):583–589; discussion 589–590.

75. Indes JE, Tuggle CT, Mandawat A, et al. Age-stratified outcomes in elderly patients undergoing open and endovascular procedures for aortoiliac occlusive disease. *Surgery* 2010;148(2):420–428.

76. Whyman MR, Fowkes FG, Kerracher EM, et al. Randomised controlled trial of percutaneous transluminal angioplasty for intermittent claudication. *Eur J Vasc Endovasc Surg* 1996;12(2):167–172.

77. Wolf GL, Wilson SE, Cross AP, et al. Surgery or balloon angioplasty for peripheral vascular disease: a randomized clinical trial. Principal investigators and their Associates of Veterans Administration Cooperative Study Number 199. *J Vasc Interv Radiol* 1993;4(5):639–648.

78. Greenhalgh RM, Belch JJ, Brown LC, et al. The adjuvant benefit of angioplasty in patients with mild to moderate intermittent claudication (MIMIC) managed by supervised exercise, smoking cessation advice and best medical therapy: results from two randomised trials for stenotic femoropopliteal and aortoiliac arterial disease. *Eur J Vasc Endovasc Surg* 2008;36(6):680–688.

79. Whyman MR, Fowkes FG, Kerracher EM, et al. Is intermittent claudication improved by percutaneous transluminal angioplasty? A randomized controlled trial. *J Vasc Surg* 1997;26(4):551–557.

80. Perkins JM, Collin J, Creasy TS, et al. Exercise training versus angioplasty for stable claudication. Long and medium term results of a prospective, randomised trial. *Eur J Vasc Endovasc Surg* 1996;11(4):409–413.

81. Creasy TS, McMillan PJ, Fletcher EW, et al. Is percutaneous transluminal angioplasty better than exercise for claudication? Preliminary results from a prospective randomised trial. *Eur J Vasc Endovasc Surg* 1990;4(2):135–140.

82. Holm J, Arfvidsson B, Jivegard L, et al. Chronic lower limb ischaemia. A prospective randomised controlled study comparing the 1-year results of vascular surgery and percutaneous transluminal angioplasty (PTA). *Eur J Vasc Surg* 1991;5(5):517–522.

83. Kashyap VS, Pavkov ML, Bena JF, et al. The management of severe aortoiliac occlusive disease: endovascular therapy rivals open reconstruction. *J Vasc Surg* 2008;48(6):1451–1457, 1457.e1–1457.e3.

84. de Vries SO, Hunink MG. Results of aortic bifurcation grafts for aortoiliac occlusive disease: a meta-analysis. *J Vasc Surg* 1997;26(4):558–569.

85. Nissen SE, Nicholls SJ, Sipahi I, et al. Effect of very high-intensity statin therapy on regression of coronary atherosclerosis: the ASTEROID trial. *JAMA* 2006;295(13):1556–1565.

86. Pulli R, Dorigo W, Fargion A, et al. Early and long-term comparison of endovascular treatment of iliac artery occlusions and stenosis. *J Vasc Surg* 2011;53(1):92–98.

87. Koizumi A, Kumakura H, Kanai H, et al. Ten-year patency and factors causing restenosis after endovascular treatment of iliac artery lesions. *Circ J* 2009;73(5):860–866.

88. Park KB, Do YS, Kim JH, et al. Stent placement for chronic iliac arterial occlusive disease: the results of 10 years experience in a single institution. *Korean J Radiol* 2005;6(4):256–266.

89. Reekers JA, Vorwerk D, Rousseau H, et al. Results of a European multicentre iliac stent trial with a flexible balloon expandable stent. *Eur J Vasc Endovasc Surg* 2002;24(6):511–515.

90. Schurmann K, Mahnken A, Meyer J, et al. Long-term results 10 years after iliac arterial stent placement. *Radiology* 2002;224(3):731–738.

91. Scheinert D, Schroder M, Ludwig J, et al. Stent-supported recanalization of chronic iliac artery occlusions. *Am J Med* 2001;110(9):708–715.

92. Powell RJ, Fillinger M, Bettmann M, et al. The durability of endovascular treatment of multisegment iliac occlusive disease. *J Vasc Surg* 2000;31(6):1178–1184.

Endovascular Therapies: Femoropopliteal

GARY M. ANSEL and JOHN A. PHILLIPS

INTRODUCTION

The prevalence of peripheral arterial disease continues to increase in the United States due to an aging population and increasing incidence of diabetes. Data from participants in the Framingham Study found that symptomatic disease onset, as manifest by intermittent claudication, increases 10-fold in men and 20-fold in women by the seventh decade of life.[1] Femoropopliteal disease is the most common cause of claudication and typically presents with diffuse atherosclerotic degeneration even when only focal disease is angiographically apparent. The femoropopliteal disease process is often bilateral and progressive: At 3-year follow-up, one out of three stenoses progress and one out of seven stenoses will occlude.[2] The prevalence of diabetes is upward of 16% of the population and has become a major challenge in providing health care.[3] The development of critical limb ischemia (CLI) is often associated with multilevel vascular obstruction of which the femoropopliteal bed is commonly involved.

FEMOROPOPLITEAL ANATOMY

As the common femoral artery continues in the femoral triangle, it divides into the profunda femoral and superficial femoral arteries (SFA). The profunda femoral artery most commonly arises from the posterolateral side of the common femoral artery fairly high in the femoral triangle. As the main supply of the muscles of the thigh, the profundus femoral artery is the true "lifeline of the leg." The common femoral artery may occasionally give off small, muscular branches. The SFA lies anterior, and medial, to the profundus femoral artery. A large muscle (adductor longus) separates the SFA branches from the profunda femoral branches. Distally the SFA traverses the adductor canal through the tendinous opening in the adductor magnus muscle to reach the popliteal fossa. As the SFA exits the adductor canal into the popliteal fossa, the SFA changes its title to the popliteal artery. Atherosclerotic degeneration of the SFA often arises at the adductor canal tendinous as a result of trauma to the vessel wall by the tendons that surround this area. The popliteal artery extends distally until the takeoff of the anterior tibial and tibioperoneal trunk arteries.

IMPORTANT COLLATERAL CIRCULATION

The integrity of the profundus femoral artery should always be a priority during any treatment planning because it is the most important collateral source vessel to the lower extremity. This is extremely important, especially when evaluating endovascular treatment options that may occur near the ostium of the SFA. The two largest branches of the profundus femoral artery are the medial and lateral femoral circumflex vessels (FIGURE 47.1). The medial femoral circumflex artery typically arises from the medial or posteromedial side of the profundus femoral artery and turns posteriorly between the iliopsoas and pectineus muscles. The lateral femoral circumflex artery may arise from the common femoral artery itself but typically arises from the lateral side of the upper end of the profunda. A very important collateral pathway occurs proximally, where the medial and lateral circumflex branches have collateral connections to the internal iliac artery. In the distal aspect of the profunda femoral artery, perforating muscular branches provide perfusion to the muscles of the thigh. Also distally, the lateral circumflex artery has connections to the collateral circulation at the knee joint, which may provide an important collateral to the popliteal and tibial arteries. The descending genicular branch, which typically arises in the arterial segment proximal to the adductor canal, provides an important collateral channel to the infrapopliteal vessels from the distal SFA (FIGURE 47.2).

FEMOROPOPLITEAL DISEASE CHARACTERIZATION

The femoropopliteal bed is unique in its disease process due to the multiple external forces as well as the presence of few side branches. The disease process is frequently diffuse in nature. With the relative paucity of significant sized side branches, total occlusions tend to be relatively long compared to stenoses. Often the occlusion will progress proximally to near the bifurcation of the profunda femoral artery. Involvement of the ostium may lead to complex considerations for endovascular treatment. Femoropopliteal arterial occlusive obstructions are also often associated with significant calcification and thrombus.

Although less frequently involved with vascular obstruction, the profunda femoral should be adequately imaged to ensure that any stenoses are noted. Ostial profunda femoral disease can often easily be treated with improvement in symptoms in patients with diffuse superficial femoral disease.

PATIENT SELECTION FOR TREATMENT CONSIDERATION

There is no indication for treatment of asymptomatic femoropopliteal disease unless the patency of a previous surgical venous bypass graft is threatened. Currently there are little data about whether asymptomatic restenosis of other endovascular procedures is prolonged with reintervention.

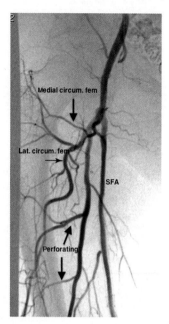

FIGURE 47.1 Angiogram demonstrating the typical anatomy of the femoral bifurcation.

Although feared by patients with symptomatic peripheral arterial disease, the progression to amputation in the nondiabetic is a relatively rare outcome. Typically only 1% to 3% of nondiabetic claudicants will require a major amputation over a 5-year period. In a study by Cox et al.[4] that included patients with SFA disease, the risk for patients requiring invasive treatment was 11% at 5 years and only progressed to 14% at 5 years. In contrast the

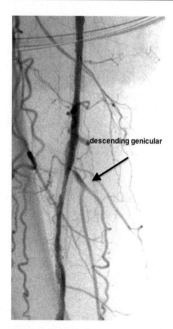

FIGURE 47.2 Angiogram demonstrating the genicular branches of the distal superficial femoral artery.

diabetic patient with intermittent claudication does not have such a benign prognosis. Jonason and Ringquist[5] studied nondiabetic and diabetic patients over a 6-year period. Gangrene occurred in 31% of diabetics as opposed to only 5% of patients without diabetes, and rest pain and/or gangrene occurred in 40% of patients with diabetes mellitus and only in 18% of those without. Interestingly, progression in symptoms is most common during the first year after diagnosis. Evaluating the benefit of treatment based solely on the development of CLI is not appropriate. Claudication significantly affects a patient's quality of life and as more effective and durable technologies are developed the number of patients treated is expected to increase.

Femoropopliteal intervention should always be preceded by investigation of aortoiliac disease. Any hemodynamically significant obstructive disease should be treated prior to femoropopliteal disease for claudicants or concomitantly to provide straight-line flow to the foot in the case of patients with limb-threatening ischemia.

Before undertaking any therapeutic option the patient's risk benefit should be weighed. Certainly medical risk factor modification should play a role in all patients even when more aggressive surgical or endovascular procedures are considered. This effort is important to try and decrease the associated cardiac and cerebrovascular mortality. Supervised walking programs and pharmacologic treatment have been met with some success in patients with claudication symptoms. In appropriate settings both approaches may be desirable before more aggressive intervention. In cases where doubling of the walking distance will not lead to an acceptable ambulation status, invasive treatment may be an appropriate first-line therapy. Historically, patients with diffuse symptomatic femoropopliteal artery disease have been treated surgically. For patients with an available venous bypass conduit, fempop venous bypass continues to be associated with the highest patency rates of any invasive treatment option. The indications for infrainguinal surgical bypass have not changed over the last several years and continue to include vocation-limiting claudication and limb-threatening ischemia. Broadening of the classic surgical indications would be difficult due to the associated surgical morbidities, such as infection (15% to 25%) and mortality (1% to 2%).[6] Keeping the traditional surgical indications in mind is important. With the broadening of endovascular indications and the significant femoropopliteal restenosis rate many patients could be faced with being offered surgical repair for failed endovascular treatment without the development of the classic level of symptoms or meeting traditional indications.

In the hands of skilled interventionists and properly selected patients, femoropopliteal endovascular procedures offer inherently lower-risk, repeatable techniques compared to the risks associated with open surgical bypass procedures. Thus indications for endovascular treatment of symptomatic peripheral vascular disease are often liberalized to also include patients with more function-limiting symptoms. Two groups of patients are relatively contraindicated for endovascular treatment: those with significant renal insufficiency and may not tolerate the use of contrast, and those who cannot be placed on antiplatelet therapy. The TASC II (Inter-Society Consensus for the Management of PAD) guidelines are a relative guide that assists in patient selection.[7] Because endovascular procedure outcome data have improved, these guidelines continue to be liberalized, resulting in an endovascular-first approach. Currently the strongest anatomic and lesion characteristics leading to relative contraindications for endovascular procedures in the femoropopliteal area include severe calcification and total occlusion of the common femoral artery or mid- to distal popliteal artery.

TECHNOLOGY REVIEW

The typical percutaneous endovascular procedure may utilize one or several techniques, including different types of angioplasty, stents, stent-grafts, laser, and atherectomy. Only recently has the controversy over the actual indications that have existed due to the paucity of reliable controlled and comparable outcome data started to be replaced by randomized trial data. The optimization of any technology in the femoropopliteal arterial segment has been complex, however, because this arterial bed experiences many unique forces, such as torque, compression, elongation, and bending. Furthermore, there are lesion and patient variables that may affect outcome durability including lesion length, vessel diameter, diabetes, renal insufficiency, smoking, and quality of distal runoff.[8,9]

PERCUTANEOUS BALLOON ANGIOPLASTY (PLAIN, SUBINTIMAL, CUTTING/SCORING, CRYOPLASTY)

Plain Balloon Angioplasty

Balloon angioplasty continues to be the cornerstone of endovascular treatment. Most other technologies also utilized balloon angioplasty to some degree during the treatment process. Technical advances in balloon design and technique have been made with improved durability at even high inflation pressures (upward of 30 atmospheres) and increased balloon lengths (up to 300 cm). No improvement in primary patency rates after percutaneous transluminal angioplasty (PTA) has been documented however. A recent publication utilizing controlled data and literature with hard endpoints has demonstrated very low primary patency of 33% in the common mid-length lesions of 4 to 15 cm.[10] Examining previous controlled endovascular trials can assist in defining the durability for balloon angioplasty in shorter and longer atherosclerotic lesions. For shorter lesion lengths the multicenter, randomized, Intracoil stent versus balloon angioplasty femoropopliteal trial allows for some insight into restenosis rates. Although this trial allowed for lesion lengths up to 16 cm, investigators typically enrolled patients with focal disease, leading to a short average lesion length of only 3.3 cm. The 9-month angiographic restenosis (≥50%) rate for the PTA control arm was 33.7%.[11] Another randomized trial evaluated the use of PTA versus balloon expandable stents for lesions less than 5 cm. The 1-year angiographic restenosis rate for the balloon arm was 47%.[12] Even more unsatisfactory results of PTA would be expected in long femoropopliteal lesions. Utilization in patients with claudication would appear to be suboptimal due to the high recurrence rate. In patients with tissue breakdown, however, patency appears to be less of an issue as long as an acceptable result is obtained at the time of the angioplasty.

Subintimal Angioplasty

Some authors have espoused the technique of subintimal angioplasty. Typically utilized for patients with total vessel occlusion, this technique establishes a channel between the intima and media with wire reentry into the native vessel lumen beyond the distal edge of the occlusion. A meta-analysis of 23 studies including over 1,500 patients resulted in technical success of 80% to 90% and primary patency at 1 year of only 50% with procedural complication rates between 8% and 17%.[13] During this type of procedure, which by its very nature creates a dissection, stents are typically utilized only for compromised flow.

Cutting/Scoring Balloon Angioplasty

The theory of providing controlled dissection during balloon angioplasty leading to a lower restenosis rate has long been sought. In a large randomized coronary trial no difference was found in restenosis.[14] Beyond restenosis, however, cutting or scoring balloons may play a role by improving the acute result in lesions that are in a location where stenting may be suboptimal, difficult to dilate, such as calcified lesions, or where uncontrolled dissection may compromise a side branch, as in a bifurcation lesion.[15,16] In the femoropopliteal segment this technology is typically reserved for the common femoral, ostial SFA, midpopliteal, and calcified lesions.

Cryoplasty

Registry data evaluating the use of near-freezing balloon technology (cryoplasty) have been published. This system has been shown in laboratory data to bring about apoptosis (planned cell death), which is hoped to limit intimal hyperplasia. This registry allowed for up to 10-cm lesions (mean enrolled lesion length 4.7 cm) and showed the 9-month, duplex-controlled restenosis rate to be similar to that of plain balloon angioplasty of short lesions, that is, 30%.[17] A more recent single-center randomized evaluation has not demonstrated any evidence of advantage in patency or dissection rate.[18] With these data it appears that cryoplasty should have a limited role until more extensive randomized data are completed.

ATHERECTOMY AND LASER

Mechanical atherectomy devices are typically available in two types: rotational spinning and directional cutting. Both mechanical atherectomy and excimer laser continue to undergo evolutionary changes with improvement in the ability to treat vessel locations unfavorable for stenting, larger vessel diameters, as well as an improved effect on calcification (FIGURES 47.3 and 47.4). Unfortunately to date only excimer laser has been evaluated in a randomized trial to PTA. No mechanical type of atherectomy has shown any improved patency over balloon angioplasty in a randomized trial.[19–22]

The role of these devices is yet to be fully defined, but certainly they may play a role in areas where current technology options are limited, such as the common femoral, ostial superficial femoral, and popliteal vessels. The role of debulking (especially in calcified vessels) is attractive but still has no supporting data.

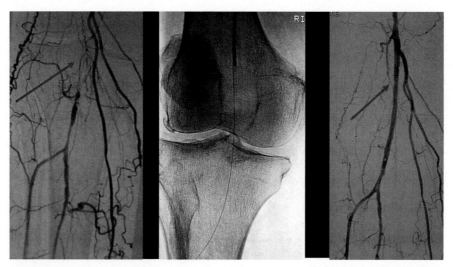

FIGURE 47.3 Angiograms demonstrating a total occlusion of the midpopliteal artery (**far left**), directional atherectomy atherotome (**middle**) and angiographic result postatherectomy (**far right**).

The efficacy of atherectomy prior to other complementary technology to increase the maximal luminal gain is not currently known. Broader application of atherectomy may be affected by the risk of embolization and perforation inherent in the procedure.[23,24] Further broadening of atherectomy use may depend on the interaction between the atherectomized artery drug-coated balloon technologies that are in an early developmental evaluation.

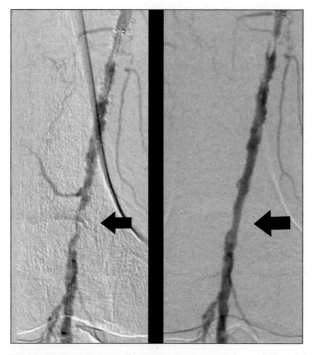

FIGURE 47.4 Angiogram demonstrating a severely stenotic calcified popliteal stenosis (**right**) and standalone rotational atherectomy result (**left**).

■ BARE METAL STENTS

Bare metal stents have been utilized in an effort to decrease clinically significant dissection and restenosis by increasing the postprocedural vessel luminal diameter. Early stainless steel stents did not show much clinical utility for a multitude of reasons, including poor study design.[25,26] Early attempts at balloon expandable stents were compromised by stent crush primarily at the adductor canal region.[27] The first stent approved by the Food and Drug Administration (FDA) for the femoropopliteal arterial bed was a nitinol coil stent. This stent in a randomized study against balloon angioplasty in short lesions did not show a restenosis benefit but did demonstrate that a primary stent approach was associated with a lower complication rate (1.8% vs. 8.7%).[11] Tubular nitinol stents with improved luminal coverage have since displaced this coiled stent (FIGURE 47.5). It has become evident that not all tubular nitinol stents appear to react the same to the forces present in the femoropopliteal bed. Although some have demonstrated excellent durability, other nitinol stents have demonstrated a clinically relevant higher rate and complexity of stent fracture that may, in fact, affect patency if the stent fractures are complex (FIGURE 47.6).[28,29] A randomized study evaluated a tubular nitinol stent designed for iliac usage (particularly prone to fracture) compared to PTA in relatively short lesions (mean lesion length 4.5 cm). There was no improvement in patency at 1 year in the stent-treated patients.[30] Whether this demonstrated poor stent design or truly a lack of stent efficacy in short lesions is debatable. A grading scheme for stent fractures has been reported.[31] Soon these schemes may be outdated, however, because newer stent designs appear to be significantly reducing the incidence of stent fracture.

Superior results compared to PTA at 1-year follow-up has been demonstrated in two randomized trials of tubular nitinol stents for mid-length femoropopliteal lesions.[32,33] In further follow-up, at 2 years, the patency advantage of nitinol stents was preserved, but the exercise improvement was no longer statistically significant.[34] Insight into the need for intravenous

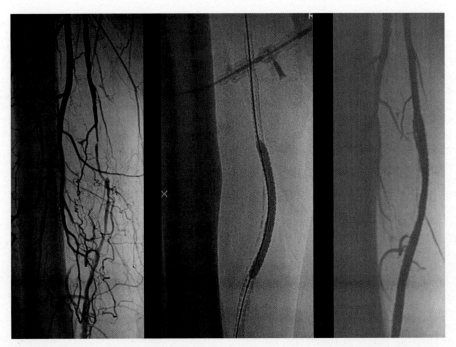

FIGURE 47.5 Angiogram demonstrating an occlusion of the superficial femoral artery (**right**), balloon angioplasty and stenting (**middle**), and final angiogram (**left**).

antiplatelet therapy was evaluated in the multicenter, randomized, and blinded "Bilateral Lower Arterial Stenting Employing Reopro (BLASTER) study" of complex superficial femoral disease. At 9-month follow-up no superiority was demonstrated in the group treated with abciximab. The combined study groups demonstrated a duplex restenosis rate of 24% with a mean lesion length of over 10 cm. Both groups experienced functional outcome improvement as well with significantly improved treadmill study in 88% of patients.[35] Prospective longer-term data on these nitinol tubular stents have been lacking. A retrospective study of mid-length lesions (mean >10 cm) with duplex follow-up appears to show an approximately 40% restenosis rate at 2 years.[36]

COVERED STENTS

Interest in covered stent exclusion of atherosclerotic disease emerged in an effort to improve longer-term restenosis rates. This potential use stemmed from the successful utilization of these devices for the treatment of aneurysmal disease.[37,38] Earlier versions of covered stents included devices, such as the Cragg system (Min Tec) and Wallgraft (Boston Scientific), for the treatment of atherosclerotic disease. Early clinical efficacy in the femoropopliteal arterial bed was suboptimal. The early covering materials, such as Dacron, seem to elicit a significant inflammatory response with associated poor patency and high thrombosis rates.[39–41]

Subsequently, most industry attention has been directed to the use of stents covered with polytetrafluoroethylene (PTFE). The efficacy of PTFE in surgical bypass is well documented, and this material has shown favorable tissue interaction. Complete neointimal formation has been documented although for long-segment disease, this process may take many months.[42]

An international feasibility trial of the earlier version of the currently approved femoral stent-graft was associated with very high technical success and a 79% primary patency at 1 year.[43] There are three small published series that have evaluated the

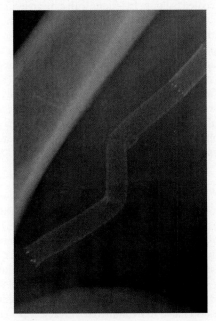

FIGURE 47.6 X-ray demonstrating bare metal stent fracture.

PTFE-covered stent in patient populations with primarily CLI. Railo et al.,[44] in a small series of 15 patients (73% with CLI) with relatively short lesions (4 to 10 cm), reported a primary patency at 1 and 2 years of 93% and 84%, respectively. The only randomized comparison of claudicants versus CLI reported similar 1-year primary patencies of 81.3% and 88.9%, respectively. The average lesion lengths were similar at 9.8 and 11.7 cm, respectively. The tibial outflow status and treatment were significantly different between these two groups. Poor runoff defined as 0 to 1 patent tibial vessel was present in only 18.7% of the claudicants, whereas 88.9% of the CLI group had poor runoff. Outflow treatment was completed in only 6.3% of the claudicants versus 66.7% of the CLI cohort.[45]

Stent-grafts have the ability to easily exclude both occlusive and ecstatic disease (FIGURE 47.7). A single center randomized trial comparing stent grafting to PTFE surgical bypass demonstrated equivalent results at 1-year follow-up.[46] The randomized VIBRANT trial (VIaBahn [Endoprosthesis] veRsus bAre Nitinol stenT for the treatment of long lesion [≥8 cm] SFA occlusive disease) comparing stent-graft to tubular nitinol stenting has completed enrollment and as hypothesized has no significant difference in patency. Interestingly, even with the concern of covering potential collaterals, no difference was seen at 1 or 3-year follow-up. For lesions over 15 cm stent fractures were common in the bare nitinol stent groups whereas rare in the stent-graft group.[47] Restenosis patterns were different, however with primarily focal stenoses at the stent-graft edge versus diffuse restenosis in the bare metal group (FIGURE 47.8). The VIPER registry (Gore Viabahn Endoprosthesis with Heparin Bioactive Surface in the Treatment of Superficial Femoral Artery Obstructive Disease) demonstrated a primary patency of 79% in long femoral lesions with a mean length of 19 cm.[48]

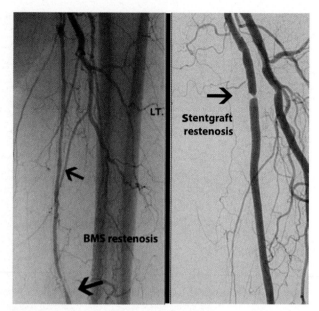

FIGURE 47.8 Angiograms demonstrating diffuse restenosis in bare metal stenting (**right**) and focal edge restenosis with stent grafting (**left**).

DRUG-COATED BALLOONS

With concern for stent fracture and restenosis, there has been recent increasing enthusiasm for the use of PTA with balloons coated with antirestenosis agents. Two randomized trial publications using balloon catheters coated with paclitaxel demonstrated encouraging results when compared to uncoated balloons.[49,50] In the Local Taxan with Short Time Exposure for Reduction of Restenosis in Distal Arteries (THUNDER) trial, 154 patients were randomly assigned to one of three strategies: bare balloon, bare balloon with paclitaxel dissolved in contrast media, and a paclitaxel-coated balloon. In lesions with a mean lesion length of 7.5 cm the late lumen loss was significantly lower in the segments treated with the coated balloon, 92 (FIGURE 47.9). In a second study, 87 patients were randomized to bare balloon versus paclitaxel-coated balloon, and in mean lesion lengths ranging from 5.7 to 6.1 cm, late lumen loss and target lesion revascularization were significantly lower in the coated balloon-treated segments.

Many trials using different drug and coating technologies are currently being planned. These investigations may result in a significant alteration in treatment strategies for patients with femoropopliteal artery disease.

DRUG-COATED STENTS

The addition of drug elution to peripheral metal stents appears to be more complex than in the coronary vasculature. In the first trial the addition of the sirolimus to a self-expanding nitinol stent using a polymer base demonstrated early but not sustained significant benefit possibly due to problematic drug elution rates and better-than-expected results with bare nitinol stents.[51,52] The second trial of a polymer-based drug-eluting stent utilizing everolimus also failed to demonstrate efficacy.[53] Presentation of data from the Zilver PTX European registry, which utilized a

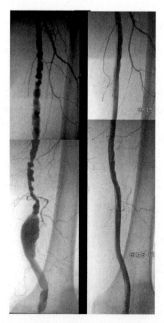

FIGURE 47.7 Angiograms demonstrating stenotic and ecstatic femoral artery disease before (**right**) and after placement of stent grafts (**left**).

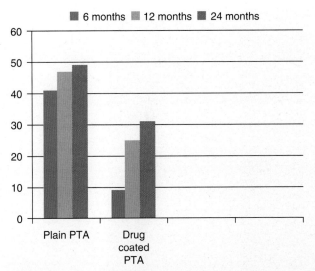

FIGURE 47.9 Patency rates at various time intervals for the Thunder Trial.

non–polymer-based, paclitaxel-coated nitinol stent has demonstrated improved clinical effect both early and in 2-year follow-up in a wide spectrum of infrainguinal disease (Table 47.1).[54] These data were further supported by the Randomized Zilver PTX trial. This large, randomized, multicenter, international trial demonstrated 1- and 2-year primary patency rates of over 80% as well as a 3-year freedom from repeat revascularization rate of 83%. This represents a 50% reduction in restenosis over both balloon angioplasty and bare metal stents. The 1-year stent fracture rate was very low at 0.9% and the pattern of recurrent obstruction appears to be typically very focal in nature (FIGURE 47.10).[55]

Table 47.1

Rates of Freedom from Target Lesion Revascularization from the Zilver PTX European Registry Study

Subgroup	12 months	24 months
Overall	89% (n = 818)	82% (n = 427)
De novo (all)	91%	88%
≤7 cm lesions	94%	91%
>7 to 15 cm lesions	92%	86%
>15 cm lesions	84%	80%
Occlusions	86%	77%
Stenosis	90%	85%
Restenosis (all)	81%	70%
Restenosis (not ISR)	87%	73%
In-stent restenosis (ISR)	78%	69%

RESTENOSIS AND PATENCY FAILURES

The etiology of endovascular procedure failure is related to the amount of time that has lapsed since the procedure. Early procedural failure may be related to lack of periprocedural anticoagulation or patient-specific coagulation abnormalities. Early technical issues that may lead to failure include suboptimal lesion dilation, stent-graft oversizing leading to material redundancy, and unrecognized proximal or distal dissection. Appropriate sizing of balloons, stents, and stent-grafts and covering all dilated areas with stents or stent-grafts may minimize these failures. Although no data exist, pressure gradient measurement may be utilized to assess adequacy of lesion treatment after PTA, atherectomy, or stent (graft) placement.

An intermediate time for procedural failure (6 to 24 months) is most commonly caused by excessive intimal hyperplasia at the site of intervention. Bare metal stents typically restenoses diffusely, whereas stent-grafts more commonly restenosed at the leading edge. Late failure is most often secondary to progression of proximal or distal vascular occlusive disease.

Treatment of restenosis has been problematic. Although some profess that the main reason to refrain from stenting is the ease of re-treatment after angioplasty or atherectomy, one must remember that restenosis is a multifaceted process. This process includes recoil, intimal hyperplasia, and, most importantly, vascular atresia. Thus all restenoses may be problematic. In-stent restenosis can be especially difficult to treat, however, because of the dense nature of the intimal hyperplasia. To date treatment of in-stent restenosis with plain balloon angioplasty, cutting balloon angioplasty, and cryoplasty have not demonstrated efficacy.[56,57] Atherectomy may have of some benefit,[58] but one must be careful not to entrap the stent in the atherotome because it can lead to serious results. Stent grafting has limited data of efficacy as well.[59] It appears that restenosis will continue to challenge the interventionist in the longer-term care of the vascular patient. It is hoped that drug-coated balloons or drug-coated stents may improve the current results. Further in the future bioabsorbable stents have started to demonstrate early efficacy in the coronary vascular bed.[60]

TECHNICAL CONSIDERATIONS

Vascular Access

Retrograde femoral access is by far the most common vascular access utilized for endovascular procedures. Today's angiographic suites are uniformly designed for this access site for procedures that are cephalad to this site. The common femoral artery is typically large enough for even the larger sheaths available and usually offers a readily compressible site for postprocedure homeostasis. Care should be taken that the true common femoral artery is entered. With the prevalence of obesity the potential for a low puncture is increased. When too low of a puncture is utilized the risk of pseudoaneursym increases (FIGURE 47.11). When utilizing retrograde vascular access for contralateral procedures the choice of sheath is important. Non-kinkable, typically braided sheaths should be utilized. Previous aortobi-iliac or bifemoral bypass may make it difficult or impossible to utilize the contralateral femoral access due to the severity of the bifurcation angulation.

Antegrade femoral access is utilized for complex femoropopliteal procedures. One important benefit that this

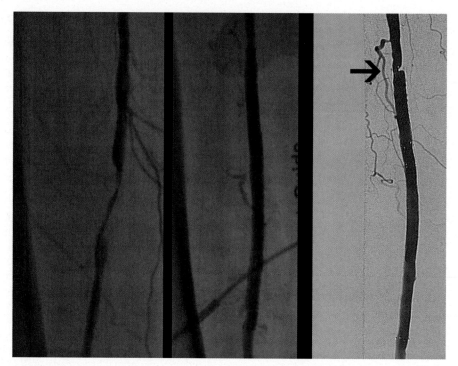

FIGURE 47.10 Angiogram demonstrating a severe stenosis of the superficial femoral artery prior to treatment (**right**), post nonpolymer drug-coated stenting (**middle**), and at 1-year follow-up with focal edge restenosis (**left**).

technique offers is lowered physician operator radiation exposure.[61,62] Because the cutaneous entry site is above the inguinal ligament great care must be taken to ensure that the common femoral artery is entered and not the external iliac, where compression for homeostasis will be very difficult, thereby increasing the risk of retroperitoneal hemorrhage. Too low of

a puncture may also lead to needle entry into the profunda femoral artery, which would prevent access into the SFA. Utilization of Plexiglas protection, placed over the head of the patient, may allow for a simplified working field. Antegrade access may be very problematic and occasionally unfeasible in the obese patient.

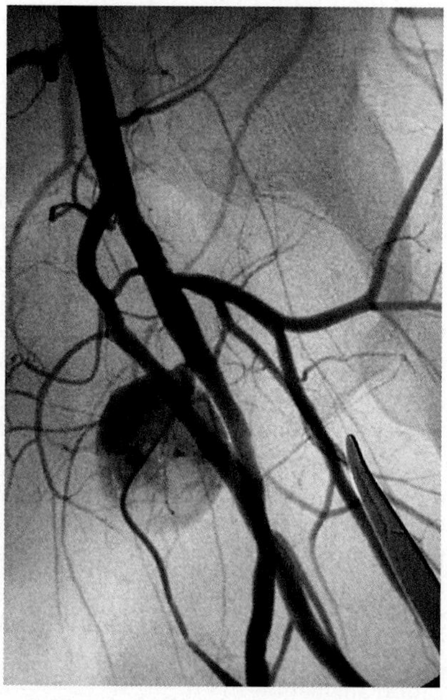

The popliteal artery offers a "backdoor" approach to the superficial artery. This approach is usually reserved for total occlusions that have not been able to be traversed from a more cephalad approach. The popliteal artery lies deep in the popliteal space with a vein that lies posterior and slightly lateral. The tibial nerve lies directly posterior. The artery should be entered above the joint line to decrease the chance of bleeding into the joint space. Popliteal hematomas are often very symptomatic and the development of compartment syndrome is a significant consideration. After definition of the anatomic landmarks on fluoroscopy, the vessel is effectively located for needle entry by utilizing duplex ultrasound or a Doppler probe. If a more cephalad sheath is in place, angiography or "road mapping" may also define the vessel. Micropuncture tools may theoretically allow for less chance of complication. With the recent development of effective reentry type and total occlusion devices, the need for popliteal access has diminished considerably.

Although possibly more important for stent-grafts, inflow is important for any endovascular femoropopliteal procedure. Iliac disease should be treated before undertaking the femoropopliteal segment. Status of distal runoff vessels has been shown to affect the durability of endovascular procedures. Intervention with 2- to 3-vessel distal runoff is associated with significant improvement in patency compared to patients with 0- to 1-vessel runoff.[63,64] Both surgical and endovascular procedures appear to be more durable in claudicants. This is in contrast to patients

FIGURE 47.11 Angiogram demonstrating a pseudoaneurysm of the profunda femoral artery.

with CLI where tibial patency is typically reduced, as is procedure durability.[65–67] However, whether treatment of outflow lesions at the time of femoropopliteal intervention affects patency has not been demonstrated.[68,69]

Although not currently studied in the occlusive disease population, studies evaluating covered stent grafting of popliteal aneurysms have seen stent-graft occlusion in 16% to 22% (1 year).[70–72] One must weigh the risk/benefit of crossing a diseased but potential collateral source to end the stent-graft in a less-diseased, more distal vessel. Special attention to oral antiplatelet therapy may be beneficial, although comparative data are lacking.

CHRONIC TOTAL OCCLUSION TRAVERSAL

When treating chronic total occlusions (CTO) of the femoropopliteal bed the operator should first reevaluate the indication for the procedure because treatment of total occlusions is typically more complex and associated with increased complications, such as distal embolization. Before deciding on the optimal invasive approach, the etiology of the femoropopliteal occlusion should be evaluated. The differential diagnosis most commonly includes atherosclerotic thrombosis, embolization, aneurysmal thrombosis, and, more rarely, arterial entrapment, adventitial cystic disease, and traumatic dissection. Atherosclerotic occlusions typically include an eccentric plaque that generally starts on the back wall. The occlusion will also typically extend side branch to side branch. Collateral flow around the occlusion may lead the operator to overestimate the occlusion length. Prior to gaining vascular access the operator should evaluate which major side branches or collaterals should optimally not be compromised. The preferable access and wire direction as well as evaluating the extent of disease at the reentry segment should then be completed. If the arterial vessel at the site of reconstitution has little disease then the wire will typically reenter spontaneously; however, if there is significant disease then reentry will be more problematic.

At times the operator may prefer to utilize subintimal angioplasty. The objective is to create a subintimal dissection plane proximal to occlusion, through the subintimal space, and then reenter into the true lumen at the distal portion of the lesion. The theory behind utilizing the subintimal channel is that it is free from endothelium and atheroma that can invite thrombus and neointimal hyperplasia to accumulate. To date the data are not clear that this is beneficial.[73,74]

CHRONIC TOTAL OCCLUSION TECHNOLOGY

When the physician operator contemplates utilizing a CTO device, several issues are important, including procedural and physician time. Any worthwhile CTO device should increase success in crossing a CTO while also decreasing complications. Devices that assist in crossing CTOs are generally classified into two categories. The first category of devices is designed to stay in the true vessel lumen, whereas the second category of devices is generally thought of as reentry devices. Use of the reentry devices allows for successful crossing of all but the most heavily calcified lesions. The reentry type of devices allows for precise reentry and should lead to reduced occlusion extension as well as less side branch occlusion (FIGURE 47.12).

SUMMARY

Endovascular revascularization techniques continue to evolve and offer patients a low-risk alternative to open surgical bypass. Angioplasty has been the cornerstone of therapy but randomized trials have demonstrated superiority of both stents and stent-grafts. However, patency of bare metal stents and stent-grafts is still suboptimal and techniques of successfully treating restenosis have yet to be defined. Other, more niche techniques have been successfully utilized but currently there are no randomized data to allow us to compare to angioplasty or stents. Drug-eluting

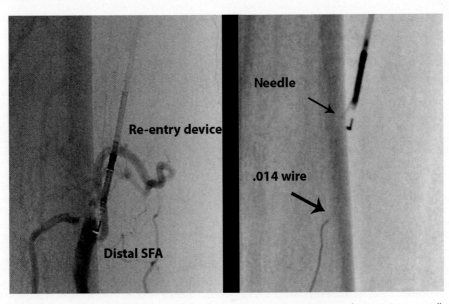

FIGURE 47.12 Angiogram demonstrating the use of a chronic total occlusion reentry device prior to needle deployment (**right**) and after needle advancement and wire placement into arterial lumen (**left**).

balloons and non–polymer-based stents have demonstrated superior results and appear to make up the cornerstone of future therapy. CTO devices appear to be expanding the interventionists' ability to safely traverse long total occlusions.

▌ REFERENCES

1. Kannel W, Skinner JJ, Schwartz M, et al. Intermittent claudications: incidence in the Framingham Study. *Circulation* 1970;41:875–883.
2. Walsh DB, Gilbertson JJ, Zwolak RM, et al. The natural history of superficial femoral artery stenoses. *J Vasc Surg* 1991;14:299–304.
3. Steinbrook R. Facing the diabetes epidemic—mandatory reporting of glycosylated hemoglobin values in New York City. *N Engl J Med* 2006; 354:545–548.
4. Cox GS, Hertzer NR, Young JR, et al. Non-operative treatment of superficial femoral artery disease: long term follow-up. *J Vasc Surg* 1993;17:172–182.
5. Jonason T, Ringquist I. Diabetes mellitus and intermittent claudication. Relation between peripheral vascular complications and location of occlusive atherosclerosis in the legs. *Acta Med Scand* 1985;218:217–221.
6. Conte MM, Belkin M, Upchurch GR, et al. Impact of increasing comorbidity on infrainguinal reconstruction: a 20-year perspective. *Ann Surg* 2001;233:445–452.
7. Norgren L, Hiatt WR; TASC II Working Group. Inter-society consensus for the management of peripheral arterial disease (TASC II). *J Vasc Surg* 2007;45(suppl S):S5–67.
8. Johnson KW. Femoral and popliteal arteries: reanalysis of results of balloon angioplasty. *Radiology* 1992;183:767–771.
9. Muradin G, Bosch J, Stijnen T, et al. Balloon dilation and stent implantation for treatment of femoropopliteal arterial disease: meta-analysis. *Radiology* 2001;221:137–145.
10. Rocha-Singh KJ, Jaff MR, Crabtree TR, et al. Performance goals and endpoint assessments for clinical trials of femoropopliteal bare nitinol stents in patients with symptomatic peripheral arterial disease. *Catheter Cardiovasc Interv* 2007;69:910–919.
11. Food and Drug Administration: Cardiovascular and Radiologic Health Advisory Board. *FDA Intracoil Data*. Silver Spring, MD: U.S. Food and Drug Administration; 2001.
12. Cejna M, Thurnher S, Illiasch H, et al. PTA versus Palmaz stent placement in femoropopliteal artery obstructions: a multicenter prospective randomized study. *J Vasc Interv Radiol* 2001;12:23–31.
13. Met R, Van Lieden KP, Koelemay MJW, et al. Subintimal angioplasty for peripheral arterial occlusive disease: a systematic review. *Cardiovasc Intervent Radiol* 2008;31:687–697.
14. Mauri L, Bonan R, Weiner BH, et al. Cutting balloon angioplasty for the prevention of restenosis: results of the Cutting Balloon Global Randomized Trial. *Am J Cardiol* 2002;90:1079–1083.
15. Cotroneo AR, Pascali D, Iezzi R. Cutting balloon versus conventional balloon angioplasty in short femoropopliteal arterial stenoses. *J Endovasc Ther* 2008;15:283–291.
16. Ansel GM, Sample NS, Botti III CF Jr, et al. Cutting balloon angioplasty of the popliteal and infrapopliteal vessels for symptomatic limb ischemia. *Catheter Cardiovasc Interv* 2004;61:1–4.
17. Laird J, Jaff MR, Biamino G, et al. Cryoplasty for the treatment of femoropopliteal arterial disease: results of a prospective, multicenter registry. *J Vasc Interv Radiol* 2005;16:1067–1073.
18. Jahnke T, Mueller-Huelsbeck S, Charalambous et al. Prospective, randomized single-center trial to compare cryoplasty versus conventional angioplasty in the popliteal artery: midterm results of the COLD study. *J Vasc Interv Radiol* 2010;21:186–194.
19. Scheinert D, Laird J, Schroeder M, et al. Excimer laser-assisted recanalization of long, chronic superficial femoral artery occlusions. *J Endovasc Ther* 2001;8:156–166.
20. Tielbeek AV, Vroegindeweij D, Bluth J, et al. Comparison of balloon angioplasty and Simpson atherectomy for lesions in the femoropopliteal artery: angiographic and clinical results of a prospective randomized trial. *J Vasc Interv Radiol* 1996;7:837–844.
21. Zeller T, Rastan A, Schwarzwalder U, et al. Percutaneous peripheral atherectomy of femoropopliteal stenoses using a new-generation device: six-month results from a single-center experience. *J Endovasc Ther* 2004;11:676–685.
22. Nguyen MC, Garcia LA. Recent advances in atherectomy and devices for treatment of infra-inguinal arterial occlusive disease. *J Cardiovasc Surg (Torino)* 2008;49:167–177.
23. Kaid KA, Gopinathapillai R, Qian F, et al. Analysis of particulate debris after superficial femoral artery atherectomy. *J Invasive Cardiol* 2009;21:7–10.
24. Shrikhande GV, Khan SZ, Hussain HG, et al. Lesion types and device characteristics that predict distal embolization during percutaneous lower extremity interventions. *J Vasc Surg* 2011;53:347–352.
25. Martin EC, Katzen BT, Benenati JF, et al. Multicenter trial of the wallstent in the iliac and femoral arteries. *J Vasc Interv Radiol* 1995;6:843–849.
26. Gray BH, Sullivan TM, Childs MB, et al. High incidence of restenosis/reocclusion of stents in the percutaneous treatment of long-segment superficial femoral artery disease after suboptimal angioplasty. *J Vasc Surg* 1997;25:74–83.
27. Rosenfield K, Schainfeld R, Pieczek A, et al. Restenosis of endovascular stents from stent compression. *J Am Coll Cardiol* 1997;29:328–338.
28. Scheinert D, Scheinert S, Sax J, et al. Prevalence and clinical impact of stent fractures after femoropopliteal stenting. *J Am Coll Cardiol* 2005;45:312–315.
29. Iida O, Nanto S, Uematsu M, et al. Influence of stent fracture on the long-term patency in the femoro-popliteal artery. *J Am Coll Cardiol Interv* 2009;2:665–671.
30. Krankenburg H, Schluter M, Steinkamp HJ, et al. Nitinol stent implantation versus percutaneous transluminal angioplasty in superficial femoral artery lesions up to 10 cm in length. *Circulation* 2007;116:285–292.
31. Jaff M, Dake M, Pompa J, et al. Standardized evaluation and reporting of stent fractures in clinical trials of noncoronary devices. *Catheter Cardiovasc Interv* 2007;70:460–462.
32. Schillinger M, Sabeti S, Loewe C, et al. Balloon angioplasty versus implantation of nitinol stents in the superficial femoral artery. *N Engl J Med* 2006;354:1879–1888.
33. Laird JR, Katzen BT; for the RESILIENT Investigators. Nitinol stent implantation versus balloon angioplasty for lesions in the superficial femoral artery and proximal popliteal artery: twelve-month results from the RESILIENT randomized trial. *Circ Cardiovasc Interv* 2010;3:267–276.
34. Schillinger M, Sabeti S, Dick P, et al. Sustained benefit at 2 years of primary femoropopliteal stenting compared with balloon angioplasty with optional stenting. *Circulation* 2007;115:2745–2749.
35. Ansel GM, Silver MJ, Botti CF Jr, et al. Functional and clinical outcomes of nitinol stenting with and without abciximab for complex superficial femoral artery disease: a randomized trial. *Catheter Cardiovasc Interv* 2006;67:288–297.
36. Mewissen MW. Self-expanding nitinol stents in the femoropopliteal segment: technique and mid-term results. *Tech Vasc Interv Radiol* 2004;7:2–5.
37. Marin ML, Veith FJ, Panetta TF, et al. Transfemoral endoluminal stented graft repair of a popliteal artery aneurysm. *J Vasc Surg* 1994;19:754–757.
38. Dorros G, Bates M, Kumar K. Percutaneous deployment of a polytetrafluoroethylene (PTFE) graft to repair a pseudoaneurysm produced by a graft to graft anastomotic dehiscence. *Cathet Cardiovasc Diagn* 1994;32:372–375.
39. Cragg AH, Dake MD. Treatment of peripheral vascular disease with stent-grafts. *Radiology* 1997;205:307–314.
40. Henry M, Amor M, Cragg A, et al. Occlusive and aneurysmal peripheral arterial disease: assessment of a stent-graft system. *Radiology* 1996;201:717–724.
41. Ahmadi R, Schillinger M, Maca T, et al. Femoropopliteal arteries: immediate and long-term results with a Dacron-covered stent-graft. *Radiology* 2002;223:345–350.
42. Marin J, Veith F, Cynamon J, et al. Human transluminal placed endovascular stented grafts: preliminary histopathologic analysis of healing grafts in aortoiliac and femoral artery occlusive disease. *J Vasc Surg* 1995;21:595–604.
43. Lammer J, Dake MD, Bleyn J, et al. Peripheral arterial obstruction: prospective study of treatment with a transluminally placed self-expanding stent-graft. International Trial Study Group. *Radiology* 2000;217:95–104.
44. Railo M, Roth WD, Edgren J, et al. Preliminary results with endoluminal femoropopliteal thrupass. *Ann Chir Gynaecol* 2001;90:15–18.
45. Hartung O, Otero M, Dubuc M, et al. Efficacy of Hemobahn in the treatment of superficial femoral artery lesions in patients with acute or critical ischemia: a comparative study with claudicants. *Eur J Vasc Endovasc Surg* 2005;30:300–306.
46. Kedora J, Hohmann S, Garrett W, et al. Randomized comparison of percutaneous Viabahn stent grafts vs prosthetic femoral-popliteal bypass in the treatment of superficial femoral arterial occlusive disease. *J Vasc Surg* 2007;45:10–16.
47. Ansel GM. VIBRANT trial 1-year interim results. Presented at the VIVA meeting; October 2011; Las Vegas, NV.
48. Saxson R. VIPER trial. Presented at the VIVA meeting; October 2011; Las Vegas, NV.

49. Tepe G, Zeller T, Albrecht T, et al. Local delivery of paclitaxel to inhibit restenosis during angioplasty of the leg. *N Engl J Med* 2008;358:689–699.

50. Werk M, Langner S, Reinkensmeier B, et al. Inhibition of restenosis in femoropopliteal arteries: paclitaxel-coated versus uncoated balloons: femoral paclitaxel randomized pilot trial. *Circulation* 2008;118:1358–1365.

51. Duda SH, Pusich B, Richter G, et al. Sirolimus-eluting stents for the treatment of obstructive superficial femoral artery disease: six-month results. *Circulation* 2002;106:1505–1509.

52. Duda SH, Bosiers M, Lammer J, et al. Sirolimus-eluting versus bare nitinol stent for obstructive superficial femoral artery disease: the SIROCCO II trial. *J Vasc Interv Radiol* 2005;16:331–338.

53. Lammer J. The STRIDES trial results. Presented at the CIRSE meeting; September 2009; Lisbon, Portugal.

54. Dake M. The ZILVER REGISTRY-2-year results. Presented at the CIRSE meeting; September 2009; Lisbon, Portugal.

55. Dake M. ZILVER PTX randomized trial results. Presented at the TCT meeting; September 2010; Washington, DC.

56. Dick P, Sabeti S, Mlekusch W, et al. Conventional balloon angioplasty versus peripheral cutting balloon angioplasty for treatment of femoropopliteal artery in-stent restenosis. *Radiology* 2008;248:297–302.

57. Karthik S, Tuite DJ, Nicholson AA, et al. Cryoplasty for arterial restenosis. *Eur J Vasc Endovasc Surg* 2007;33:40–43.

58. Zeller T, Rastan A, Schwarzwälder U, et al. Percutaneous peripheral atherectomy of femoropopliteal stenoses using a new-generation device: six-month results from a single-center experience. *J Endovasc Ther* 2004;11:676–685.

59. Kwa AT, Yeo KK, Laird JR. The role of stent-grafts for prevention and treatment of restenosis. *J Cardiovasc Surg* (Torino) 2010;51:579–589.

60. Serruys PW, Ormiston JA, Onuma Y, et al. A bioabsorbable everolimus-eluting coronary stent system (ABSORB): 2-year outcomes and results from multiple imaging methods. *Lancet* 2009;373:897–910.

61. Nice C, Timmons G, Bartholemew KH, et al. Retrograde vs antegrade puncture for infra-inguinal angioplasty. *Radiology* 2003;26:370–374.

62. Khoury M, Batra S, Berg R, et al. Influence of arterial access sites and interventional procedures on vascular complications after cardiac catheterizations. *Am J Surg* 1992;164:205–209.

63. Gallino A, Mahler F, Probst P, et al. Percutaneous transluminal angioplasty of the arteries of the lower limbs: a 5 year follow-up. *Circulation* 1984;70:619–623.

64. Jeans WD, Armstrong S, Cole SEA, et al. Fate of patients undergoing transluminal angioplasty for lower-limb ischemia. *Radiology* 1990;177:559–564.

65. Vainio E, Salenius JP, Lepäntalo M, et al. Endovascular surgery for chronic limb ischaemia. Factors predicting immediate outcome on the basis of a nationwide vascular registry. *Ann Chir Gynaecol* 2001;90:86–91.

66. Trocciola SM, Chaer R, Dayal R, et al. Comparison of results in endovascular interventions for infrainguinal lesions: claudication versus critical limb ischemia. *Am Surg* 2005;71:474–479.

67. Hunink MG, Wong JB, Donaldson MC, et al. Revascularization for femoropopliteal disease. A decision and cost-effectiveness analysis. *JAMA* 1995;274:165–171.

68. Ihnat DM, Duong ST, Taylor ZC, et al. Contemporary outcomes after superficial femoral artery angioplasty and stenting: the influence of TASC classification and runoff score. *J Vasc Surg* 2008;47:967–974.

69. Davies MG, Saad WE, Peden EK, et al. Impact of runoff on superficial femoral artery endoluminal interventions for rest pain and tissue loss. *J Vasc Surg* 2008;48:619–625.

70. Midy D, Berard X, Ferdani M, et al. A retrospective multicenter study of endovascular treatment of popliteal artery aneurysm. *J Vasc Surg* 2010;51:850–856.

71. Tielliu IF, Verhoeven EL, Prins TR, et al. Treatment of popliteal artery aneurysms with the Hemobahn stent-graft. *J Endovasc Ther* 2003;10:111–116.

72. Tielliu IF, Verhoeven EL, Zeebregts CJ, et al. Endovascular treatment of popliteal artery aneurysms: results of a prospective cohort study. *J Vasc Surg* 2005;41:561–567.

73. Markose G, Miller FN, Bolia A. Subintimal angioplasty for femoro-popliteal occlusive disease. *J Vasc Surg* 2010;52:1410–1416.

74. Met R, Van Lienden KP, Koelemay MJ, et al. Subintimal angioplasty for peripheral arterial occlusive disease: a systematic review. *Cardiovasc Intervent Radiol* 2008;31:687–697.

Endovascular Therapies: Tibial/Pedal

THOMAS ZELLER, ALJOSCHA RASTAN, and ANDREJ SCHMIDT

INTRODUCTION

Interventional treatment of patients with peripheral arterial disease (PAD) has become the treatment of choice in the aortoiliac and in the femoropopliteal region.[1-7] Compared to these regions, however, the number of interventional procedures in below the knee (BTK) arteries is still low and focused on experienced centers.[8-13] The TASC 2000 recommendations[1] considered BTK lesions longer than 2 cm as indication for surgical revascularization, and the TASC II paper published in 2007[7] offers no clear recommendations regarding the choice of treatment method relative to the complexity of the lesion.

Treatment indications BTK are either an adjunct to iliac or femoropopliteal inflow procedures with the intention to improve patency of those proximal interventions or endovascular procedures in isolated infrapopliteal disease. Isolated focal proximal lesions can result in disabling claudication or—more frequently—in critical limb ischemia (CLI). CLI represents the most advanced stage of PAD and is associated with a high risk of limb loss, demanding for revascularization, either by surgical or endovascular means.[7,14-19]

CLINICAL ASPECTS OF CRITICAL LIMB ISCHEMIA BELOW THE KNEE

An estimated 10 million people in the United States suffer from symptomatic PAD—20 to 30 million from asymptomatic PAD.[20] The prevalence of PAD increases with age, affecting approximately 20% of patients over 65 years.[21,22] Risk factors that are linked to the development of CLI are diabetes mellitus, tobacco abuse, lipid abnormalities, age over 65 years, male gender, and reduced ankle brachial index (ABI). Surveys suggest that approximately half the patients with CLI will undergo some kind of revascularization. After revascularization, ulcer healing may require adjunctive treatments that may be best achieved in dedicated foot centers with a multidisciplinary team. After revascularization, local wound care and, possibly, surgical foot salvage procedures, must be considered. Limb salvage after revascularization is defined as preservation of a part or the total foot.

Patients with chronic CLI have 20% mortality in the first year after presentation, and long-term data suggest that mortality continues at the same rate. Coronary artery disease is by far the most common cause of death among patients with PAD (40% to 60%) with cerebral artery disease accounting for 10% to 20% of deaths. Only 20% to 30% of patients with PAD die of noncardiovascular causes. The presence of PAD indicates an extensive and severe degree of systemic atherosclerosis that is responsible for mortality, independent of the presence of risk factors.[7,23]

Patients presenting with CLI and complex BTK lesions represent an increasing patient population due to the increasing prevalence of diabetes and end-stage renal failure.[23] The primary aims of the treatment of CLI are to relieve ischemic pain, to heal (neuro) ischemic ulcers, to prevent limb loss, and to improve quality of life. Secondary aim is prolongation survival. The most important outcome for the patients is amputation-free survival. To obtain these outcomes, most patients will need revascularization procedures requiring referral to a vascular specialist. Additionally, the patients should have aggressive modification of their cardiovascular risk factors and should be prescribed antiplatelet drugs.[7,24]

PATIENT SELECTION

1. *Patients with infrapopliteal disease and intermittent claudication:* Indication for intervention depends on the individual lifestyle limitation and the lesion morphology. In more focal lesions with a good chance of long-term patency following the revascularization procedure, the indication for an endovascular intervention is more liberal, whereas all conservative options must have failed before long diffuse infrapopliteal lesions should be approached due to the limited chance for a durable postprocedural outcome.

2. *Patients with infrapopliteal disease and CLI:* The natural history of CLI is such that intervention is indicated to salvage a useful and pain-free extremity.[25] The selected treatment depends on the premorbid condition of the patient and the extremity as well as estimating the risk of intervention based on comorbid conditions and the expected patency and durability of the reconstruction.[26] As shown in the BASIL trial,[27] percutaneous revascularization is as effective as surgical reconstruction in terms of limb salvage (FIGURE 48.1). It is noteworthy that temporary restoration of blood flow leads to pain relief and wound healing in simple ulcerations; however, in infected wounds or in large wounds requiring extensive wound debridement (FIGURE 48.2), long-term durability of sufficient blood supply to the foot is crucial.[28]

For some CLI patients with severe comorbidities where ambulation is unlikely or impossible and for patients with a very limited chance of successful revascularization, primary amputation following appropriate imaging and

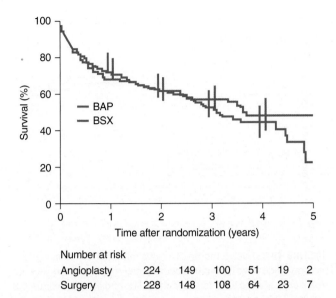

FIGURE 48.1 Amputation-free survival of CLI patients following surgical or endovascular revascularization according to the BASIL trial data.

Data from Adam DJ, Beard JD, Cleveland T, et al. Bypass versus angioplasty in severe ischaemia of the leg (BASIL): multicentre, randomised controlled trial. *Lancet* 2005;366(9501):1925–1934.

determination of the correct level of amputation may still be the most appropriate treatment.[7]

Recanalization is not indicated in asymptomatic BTK obstructions because there is currently no evidence of prognostic benefit. There are, generally, reservations about performing BTK angioplasty on patients who are in an active stage of thrombangiitis obliterans even if some single-center reports indicated favorable outcomes of endovascular treatment.

ENDOVASCULAR TREATMENT OPTIONS

Balloon Angioplasty

With the introduction of low-profile catheters and dedicated guide wires, percutaneous transluminal balloon angioplasty (PTA) of the lower limbs was increasingly performed over the past 10 years.[1,7,29,30] Using plain balloon angioplasty (POBA) limb salvage rates were reported in 80% to 90%.[31] In case of a failed revascularization attempt, however, limb loss was 40% to 50% and the mortality approximately 20%.[7] Even using long low-profile balloon catheters, BTK interventions are limited by a considerable number of restenosis or reocclusion, especially in long and severely calcified lesions.[13,16,23,32] There is need for endovascular techniques, resulting in more durable procedural success.

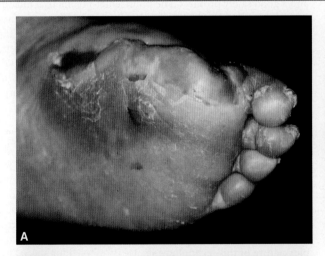

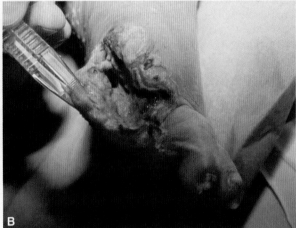

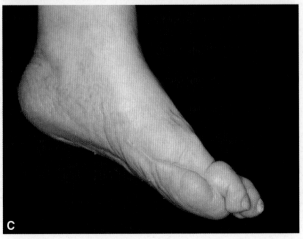

FIGURE 48.2 Infected wound after amputation of the left first toe (**A**), during debridement and before revascularization (**B**), and healed wound 6 months after angioplasty (**C**).

Plaque Modulation Techniques

So-called focal force devices, such as Cutting Balloon (Boston Scientific, Natick, MA), scoring balloon (Angiosculpt, Biotronik, Berlin, Germany), and VascuTrac (Bard PV, Tempe, AZ), are balloon catheters with additional arteriotoms or nitinol wires fixed on or around the balloon with the goal to focally increase the dilatation pressure to create controlled dissections that should improve vessel compliance and, thus, reduce balloon pressures necessary to fully expand the balloon. Aim is the reduction of the so-called barotrauma including flow-limiting dissections. Single-center experiences report fair acute outcomes,[33,34] but no comparative studies exist evaluating the longer-term technical and clinical impact of these devices.

Plaque Excision/Atherectomy

Atherectomy may be an alternative tool to improve procedural success, to avoid stent placement, and to potentially reduce the restenosis rate compared to conventional balloon angioplasty.[6,35–37]

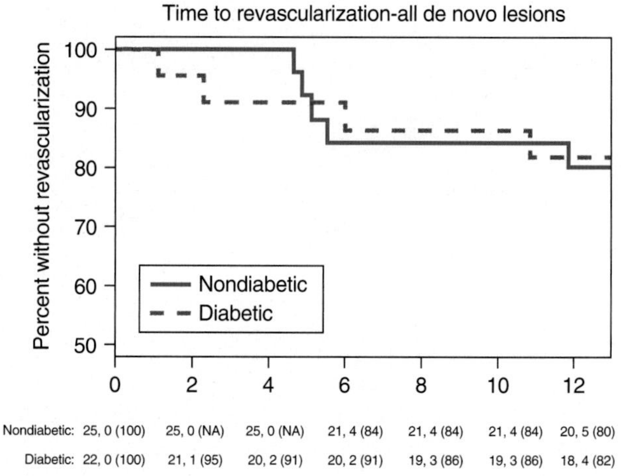

Excimer Laser-Assisted Angioplasty

The LACI trial[38] was the first trial investigating the impact of using a debulking tool to facilitate angioplasty in CLI patients. In this international multicenter registry including 127 patients with 155 threatened limbs, a mean of 2.4 lesions were treated per intervention. The 6-month limb salvage rate following laser-assisted angioplasty (Spectranetics, Colorado Springs, CO) among the survivors was 93%.

Directional Atherectomy

The Silverhawk technology (Covedian-ev3, Paris, France) represents a directional plaque excision technique.[6,35,39–41] A U.S. multicenter registry including 69 CLI patients demonstrated efficacy of directional plaque excision in avoiding amputation.[41] At 6-month follow-up, no unplanned major amputation had to be performed following successful debulking procedure with a 6-month target lesion revascularization rate (TLR) of only 4%. In a small single-center study,[35] 1- and 2-year primary patency rates were 67% and 60%, respectively, and the according secondary patency rates were 91% and 80%, respectively. An inverse correlation of lesion length and vessel patency was found. The TALON registry suggests equivalent TLR rates for above- and below-the-knee lesions for diabetic and nondiabetic patients,[40] a result that was confirmed by own data (FIGURE 48.3).

Rotational Aspiration Atherectomy

The Jetstream Atherectomy System (Pathway Medical, Redmond, WA) is a rotating, aspirating, expandable catheter for active removal of atherosclerotic debris and thrombus from peripheral vasculature. The Pathway PV System uses a fluted differentially cutting catheter tip to preferentially remove both hard and soft diseased tissue from peripheral arteries. Additionally, the removed material is aspirated at the treatment site, via

Time to revascularization-all de novo lesions

Nondiabetic:	25, 0 (100)	25, 0 (NA)	25, 0 (NA)	21, 4 (84)	21, 4 (84)	21, 4 (84)	20, 5 (80)
Diabetic:	22, 0 (100)	21, 1 (95)	20, 2 (91)	20, 2 (91)	19, 3 (86)	19, 3 (86)	18, 4 (82)

FIGURE 48.3 Twelve-month TLR rates following directional atherectomy of de novo lesions in diabetics (*green line*) and nondiabetics (*blue line*). Hazard ratio for 12 months TLR of diabetes mellitus: 0.8 (95% CI: 0.25 to 2.6).

ports in the fluted tip, into the catheter lumen, and transported to a collection bag. A first published safety and feasibility study on 15 patients resulted in a remarkable 0% 6-month TLR rate and a good safety profile.[42] The multicenter pivotal trial including only a minority of BTK lesions resulted in fair 1-year patency and TLR rates.[36] A subgroup analysis confirmed the data of the plaque excision studies with equivalent TLR rates for diabetic and nondiabetic patients following Jetstream atherectomy.[43] Because of the diameter of 2.1 to 3 mm of the current device generation, the application of the device is limited to large proximal BTK arteries (FIGURE 48.4).

High-Speed Rotational Atherectomy

Highly calcified atherosclerotic plaque has created the need for the development of high-speed rotational devices aimed specifically toward lesions where POBA has been shown to be suboptimal. The Rotablator system (Boston Scientific) is the oldest technology utilizing plaque ablation to achieve larger lumens. The device is a high-speed "rotary sander." Because of the complex nature of this technology, its use is reserved for special indications, such as when balloon catheters cannot cross or dilate BTK lesions (FIGURE 48.5). No larger series on Rotablator use in CLI patients in BTK lesions exists.

Orbital Atherectomy

The Diamondback 360° Orbital Atherectomy device (Cardiovascular Systems Inc., St. Paul, MN) represents a modified Rotablator technology featuring a drive shaft with an eccentrically mounted diamond-coated abrasive crown. This eccentric position of the abrasive crown creates an orbital spin that increases with rising rotational speed. This should lead to lumen gain up to 100% larger than the crown size.[44,45] In our own experience, the best indication for the device is diffuse calcified BTK arterial disease equivalent to the indication for

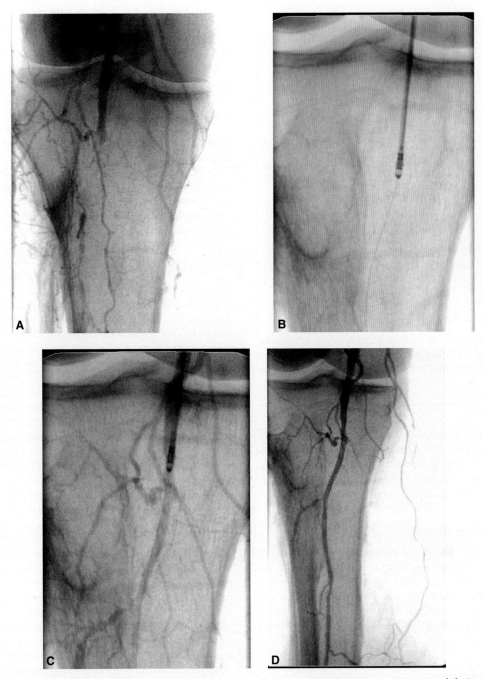

FIGURE 48.4 Distal occlusion of the right popliteal artery involving the infrapopliteal bifurcation before (**A**), during (**B, C**), and after Jetstream atherectomy (**D**).

the Rotablator. Larger series in CLI patients, however, are still missing.

Bare Metal Stents

In CLI patients, implantation of carbon-coated stents showed superior patency rates compared to conventional balloon angioplasty in focal lesions (6-month primary patency rate 86% vs. 45%[46]). Even in limited lesion length up to 10 cm, 1-year restenosis rates for bare metal balloon-expandable stents exceed 50%.[47–51] Currently, only one balloon-expandable stent device is dedicated to infrapopliteal use, the cobalt-chromium Chromis Deep stent (Medtronic-Invatec Corp., Concesio Brescia, Italy), with a length up to 8 cm. Initial single-center experiences are promising.[52]

Dedicated BTK self-expanding nitinol stents, such as Expert (Abbott Vascular, Diegem, Belgium), Astron pulsar (Biotronik), or Maris deep (Medtronic-Invatec), may be indicated in bended proximal vessel segments, such as the anterior tibial artery, and distally at the level of the ankle where balloon-expandable stents

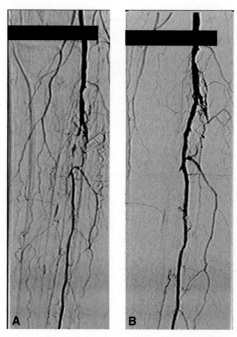

FIGURE 48.5 Highly calcified subtotal occlusion of the left tibioperoneal trunk (could not be engaged with a 1-mm coronary balloon catheter) before (**A**) and after 2-mm high-speed rotational atherectomy (Rotablator) (**B**).

might potentially be crushed by external compression forces. First registry reports were promising in terms of midterm patency.[53,54] The randomized controlled XXS trial comparing the Expert stent with PTA only in lesions with a length of up to 18 cm just recently closed enrollment.

Bioabsorbable Stents

The AMS INSIGHT study,[55,56] designed to evaluate the safety and performance of the first-generation absorbable metal stent (AMS) for the treatment of infrapopliteal lesions in patients with CLI, resulted in inferior patency outcomes compared with PTA alone. A first in man trial evaluating a new-generation bioabsorbable drug-eluting stent will start enrollment soon (ABSORB trial).

Drug-Eluting Stents

Data from small monocenter studies[49–51,57] reported 6-month restenosis rates ranging from 0% for focal lesions with full lesion coverage[51] to 8% for spot stenting in long diffusely diseased arteries using the sirolimus-eluting Cypher select stent device (Cordis J&J), the currently only CE marked DES for the indication of CLI. In larger series, 1-year restenosis rates more realistically are in the range of 15% to 20%.[58,59] Three randomized multicenter trials (YUKON-BTK, ACHILLES, DESTINY) have finished the follow-up program. YUKON-BTK and DESTINY data had been presented recently with superior patency rates for the DES compared to the bare metal stent platform. In the YUKON-BTK double-blind controlled trial using a polymer-free sirolimus-eluting stent (Yukon, Translumina, Hechingen, Germany), the 1-year primary patency rates were 80.6% and

55.6% ($p = .004$) for DES and bare metal stents, respectively. In the DESTINY trial comparing the everolimus-eluting Xience V stent (Abbott Vascular) with the bare metal Multilink Vision stent (Abbott Vascular), the primary 1-year patency rates were 85.2% and 54.4% ($p < .001$), respectively. The ACHILLES trial comparing the performance of the Cypher select stent (Cordis J&J) with plain balloon angioplasty confirmed the results of the 2 former trials with a significant patency benefit for the DES cohort (80.6% vs. 58.1%, $p < 0.0001$). Interestingly, the performance of the balloon cohort in the ACHILLES trial was as good as the one of the bare metal stent cohorts in the other two trials. As a result of these three proof-of-concept trials, DES might become the treatment of choice in BTK lesions of short and moderate length even if none of the three trials resulted in superior limb salvage rates due to their limited sample size. DES in sufficient length for infrapopliteal use is still lacking, however.

Drug-Eluting Balloons

Encouraged by the results with paclitaxel-coated balloons in the superficial femoral artery, the Leipzig Below-the-Knee registry was initiated comparing two registry cohorts treated either with plain balloons[32] or with IN.PACT Amphirion balloons in lesions with a mean length of 17 and 18 cm, respectively. Angiographic restenosis rate (>50%) after 3 months was significantly lower in the DEB BTK group compared to the standard PTA group (27% vs. 69%, and restenosis of the whole treated segment: 11% vs. 56% [FIGURE 48.6]). Two randomized, single-blinded, two-arm, multicenter studies are currently investigating the impact of DEBs in BTK lesions in patients presenting with CLI. The German **PICCOLO** trial assesses the efficacy of Paccocath balloons versus uncoated conventional balloons for prevention of restenosis in 114 patients with one or two lesions 15 to 200 mm in length. Follow-up includes control angiography after 6 and 18 months and clinical follow-up examinations up to 18 months. The primary endpoint is late lumen loss at 6 months. Eighteen months follow-up of the trial had been finished in 2010. However, due to consistent protocol violations, final data release is still pending. A case of a patient with a long occlusion in the anterior tibial artery treated with a Paccocath balloon in the PICCOLO study is presented in FIGURE 48.7. In the European **IN.PACT-DEEP** trial, 357 patients with BTK CLI (Rutherford Class 4-6) will be treated with either an IN.PACT Amphirion drug-coated balloon (Invatec S.p.A., Italy) or a standard Amphirion PTA balloon (2:1 randomization). The primary endpoints are late lumen loss at 12 months as assessed by quantitative angiography in a subcohort of 168 patients with lesions up to 10 cm in length and the clinically driven TLR rate of the target lesion in the amputation-free surviving patients at 12 months. This study has a long-term follow-up schedule up to 5 years. Until October 2010, 104 patients had been enrolled in the trial.

▌ ANATOMIC OR LESION CONSIDERATIONS

CLI is considered to be the result of multilevel arterial occlusive disease in most cases resulting in significant management problems because proximal revascularizations may not remain patent due to lack of arterial outflow without additional infrainguinal procedures. In patients with diabetes mellitus, arteries proximal to the knee joint are often spared or moderately diseased—except the deep femoral artery—and the majority of

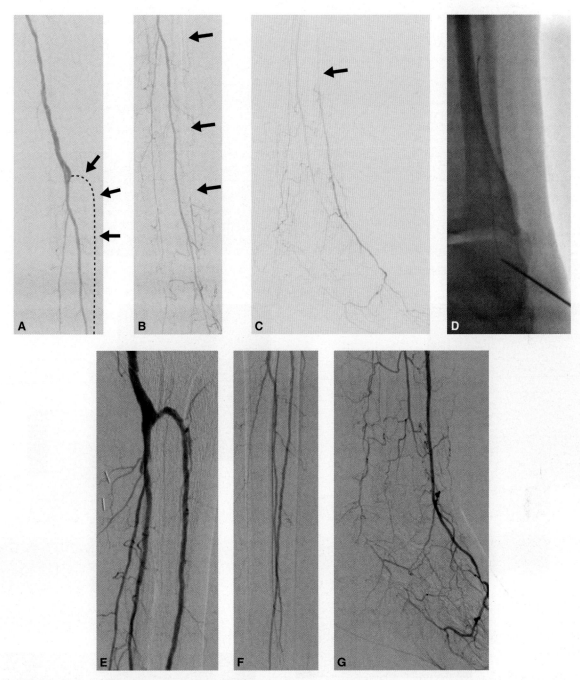

FIGURE 48.6 Occlusion of the left anterior tibial artery (**A–C**) (*arrows*), retrograde puncture (**D**), result after balloon angioplasty with DEB (**E–G**), and 3-month angiographic result with focal restenosis (**H–J**). *(continued)*

occlusions occur at the tibial peroneal trunk and distally. Often, the peroneal artery and the dorsalis pedis artery are patent beyond these occlusions and serve as potential distal targets for a bypass or retrograde endovascular revascularization.[7,8] Recently endovascular tools used for infrapopliteal interventions had been adapted from coronary interventions because of similar vessel diameters. Compared to coronary artery disease, however, tibial artery occlusions are frequently much longer and less bended, demanding different recanalization techniques, as compared to coronary interventions, such as intentional subintimal wire recanalization using soft 0.035-inch hydrophilic-coated

guide wires (Radiofocus, Terumo, AquaTrack, Cordis J&J). Most patients presenting with significant infrapopliteal disease have diabetes mellitus or are in end-stage renal insufficiency. Concentric calcification of the medial vessel wall layers is a typical appearance in these patients, resulting in difficulties to reenter the true lumen distal to the occlusion in case of subintimal wire position. Distal vessel reconstitutions can be used for retrograde, mostly sheathless recanalization attempts if the antegrade attempt failed. Alternatively, similar to retrograde coronary recanalization procedures, the plantar arch can serve as a retrograde approach to an occluded tibial artery.

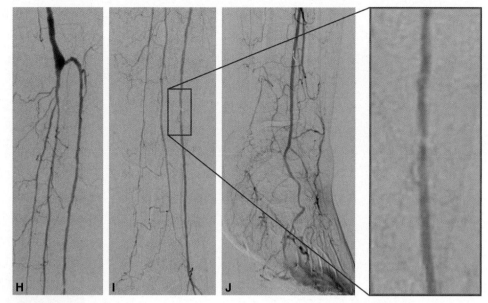

FIGURE 48.6 (Continued)

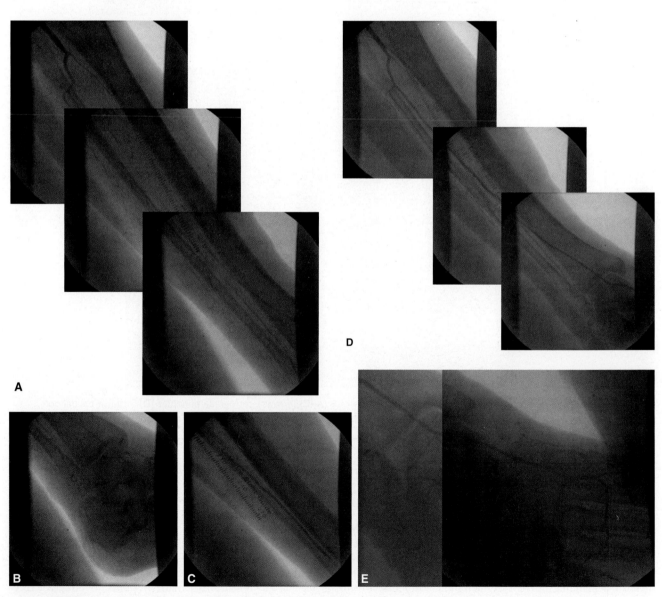

FIGURE 48.7 Proximal occlusion of a right anterior tibial artery (**A, B**), balloon angioplasty with a 3-mm diameter, 120-mm-long paclitaxel-coated balloon (**C**), and final result (**D, E**).

▌TECHNICAL AND DEVICE CONSIDERATIONS

Access Routes

Key for a successful interventional procedure is the selection of the appropriate access route. If anatomically feasible, the antegrade access via the ipsilateral common femoral artery should be the preferred approach due to the short and straight access to the target area, resulting in more precise steerability of interventional devices, particularly guide wires (FIGURE 48.8). Downsizing of interventional devices allows the use of 4 French or 5 French sheaths, either dedicated for infrapopliteal access with various lengths of 35 to 55 cm or in standard length combined with a 100-cm-long guiding catheter. Both techniques, long sheath or guiding catheter, reduce the amount of contrast medium needed due to the local administration and increase pushability of the devices. In obese patients, contralateral crossover access may be necessary. Marked tortuosity or severe calcification of the pelvic arteries may lead to significant loss of maneuverability in the guide wires, demanding either the use of a 90-cm-long sheath or a 100-cm-long guiding catheter. In case an occlusion cannot be passed via an antegrade access, retrograde recanalization techniques, such as transpedal access or transcollateral access, may be successful.

Guide Wires

Whether a stenosis or an occlusion is present is the major factor involved in deciding on the choice of the guide wire. Although shorter stenoses are most easily crossed with coronary 0.014-inch floppy guide wires, hydrophilic-coated 0.014-inch guide wires (Pilot wire series, Abbott Vascular; Choice wire series, Boston Scientific) are more suitable to cross longer occlusions. In severely calcified lesions, dedicated stiff coronary 0.014-inch guide wires (Miracle, Confienza; Asahi, Abbott Vascular) may be helpful but involves the risk of perforation, in particular in longer lesions with a bended course. Alternatively, hydrophilic-coated 0.018-inch guide wires provide a greater firmness (V18 Control

Wire, Boston Scientific). In occlusions difficult to cross, standard stiff straight hydrophilic-coated 0.035-inch guide wires (Radiofocus, Terumo; AquaTrack, Cordis J&J) can be used with the expense of an increased risk of perforation. Sometimes a loop technique for intentional subintimal wire recanalization is successful, preferably by using a dedicated 0.035-inch half-stiff 180-degree-angled guide wire (Radiofocus, Terumo [FIGURE 48.9]).

Support Catheter

Long obstructions, in particular, require the guide wire to be stabilized with a dedicated support catheter (e.g., Quick-Cross, Spectranetics; Diver, Medtronic-Invatec; or CXI-Support-catheter, Cook). The cheapest and probably most effective support catheter, however, is still simply a balloon catheter offering the best possible profile, a hydrophilic coating on the balloon surface and the advantage of—if getting stuck in a rigid plaque—being able to stepwise predilate the lesion by following the guide wire. Additional support provides the telescoping technique, the combined use of wire, balloon catheter, and guiding catheter that can be stepwise advanced into the lesion following predilatation with the balloon catheter.

Crossing Devices

The oldest crossing device for chronic total occlusions (CTOs) is the excimer laser (Spectranetics). Using the "step-by-step" technique by stepwise, advancing the recanalization wire followed by the 0.9-mm laser probe, is one of the techniques used for intentional intraluminal crossing of a CTO. Even using this technique, in longer lesions, the wire frequently enters the subintimal vessel layers at least partially. Photoablation with the excimer laser is very effective in long diffuse stenotic lesions even as a stand-alone intervention. More recent devices that should facilitate the passage of a CTO are the Frontrunner XP (Cordis J&J) and the Crosser (Bard PV/FlowCardia Inc., Sunnyvale, CA).[60,61]

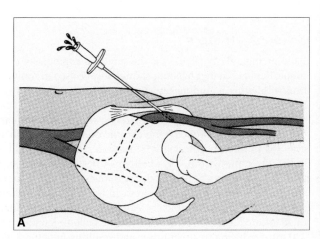
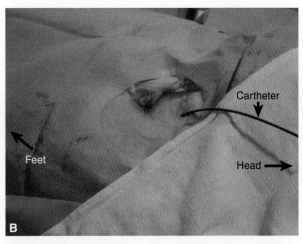

FIGURE 48.8 Schematic drawing showing proper needle position for right antegrade access (**A**) and photographic image of left antegrade access (**B**).

A: Reprinted with permission from Kandarpa K, Machan L. *Handbook of Interventional Radiologic Procedures*. Philadelphia, PA: Lippincott Williams & Wilkins; 2011.

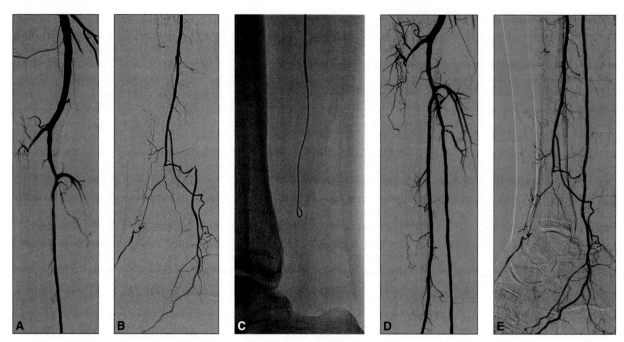

FIGURE 48.9 Total occlusion of the posterior tibial artery right leg with distal reconstitution (**A, B**); subintimal passage using the wire loop of a half-stiff-type 0.035-inch Terumo guide wire (**C**); result after subintimal recanalization of the posterior tibial artery with final 3-mm balloon angioplasty (**D, E**).

The *Frontrunner XP* CTO catheter is a wireless device using blunt microdissection to create a channel through the occlusion for easier guide wire placement.[60] First, the Frontrunner XP catheter is delivered to the proximal cap of the CTO, using a microguide catheter as support. The blunt tip engages the CTO, penetrating its proximal cap. The actuating jaws of the Frontrunner XP catheter delivers enough force to microdissect the plaque. With support from the microguide catheter, the Frontrunner XP catheter continues separating plaque to create a channel through the occlusion. Once a channel has been established, the microguide catheter facilitates the placement of a conventional guide wire across the CTO.

The *Crosser device* consists of reusable electronics (generator and transducer) and the single-use rapid exchange Crosser catheter, which is delivered over standard 0.014-inch guide wires.[61] High-frequency mechanical vibration is transmitted to the tip of the Crosser catheter. The high-frequency mechanical vibration should facilitate guide wire passage of the CTO and should allow for subsequent balloon angioplasty, debulking, and/or stent placement.

Both devices, the Frontrunner XP and the Crosser, are CE marked and approved by the Food and Drug Administration (FDA) for peripheral use. Both tools have not yet proven superiority in acute success crossing CTOs, however, compared to a traditional guide wire. Moreover, because of their axial stiffness their use is limited to straight occluded vessel sections.

Reentry Devices

Recanalization success of CTOs, regardless of the location and occlusion length, is limited to approximately 90%.[7] Main reasons for crossing failure are either a failed crossing attempt caused by extensive calcification of all vessel wall layers or the failed reentry into the true lumen distal to the lesion after crossing the CTO subintimally.[62]

Currently, two reentry devices are available primarily for femoropopliteal use: the intravascular ultrasound (IVUS)-guided Pioneer device (Medtronic, Santa Rosa, CA) and the fluoroscopically oriented Outback LTD device (Cordis J&J). In experienced hands, these devices can also be used in infrapopliteal interventions depending on the target vessel size.[63] Antegrade recanalization attempts may fail in small and severely calcified vessels in which reentry devices cannot be applied.

Balloon Catheters

Balloon angioplasty (POBA) is the standard angioplasty technique. Rapid exchange balloons should only be used in conjunction with either a guiding catheter or a long sheath; otherwise the axial support may be insufficient, particularly in CTOs. With the support of a guiding catheter, lowest-profile coronary balloons can be helpful crossing chronic calcified CTOs where even the profile of dedicated BTK balloon catheters is still too bulky. Over-the-wire (OTW) balloons offer better axial support and the advantage of local dye administration via the guide wire lumen. Moreover, guide wires can be exchanged without removing the balloon catheter. Various companies are offering dedicated low-profile balloons with a balloon length up to 220 mm, reducing treatment time and resulting in better acute angioplasty results with less edge dissections following long balloon inflations of 2 to 5 minutes.[32]

Focal force balloons, such as the Cutting Balloon, Angio-Sculpt, or Vascutrak, are recommended for rigid lesions that cannot be completely dilated even with high-pressure balloons.[33,34] Their use is limited by the relatively large crossing profile, however, in particular, of the Cutting Balloon. A valuable alternative to those balloon devices are high-speed rotational atherectomy systems, such as the Diamondback or the Rotablator.

Debulking Devices

Even having not yet proven superior longer-term performance compared to POBA, atherectomy devices are a valuable alternative or additive to POBA. Directional plaque excision with the Silverhawk catheter is mainly indicated in proximal, more focal, and eccentric fibrotic lesions.[35,41] The main limitation of this device is the bulky nosecone that prevents the catheter in crossing severely calcified lesions. For this purpose, front-cutting devices, such as excimer laser, Rotablator, and Diamondback, are more effective. The main indications for laser angioplasty are long diffuse lesions with limited degree of calcification. The laser is the only device that can be applied without having already passed the lesion successfully with a guide wire (step-by-step technique).[38] Provided the lesion could be crossed with a dedicated guide wire, high-speed rotational atherectomy devices are indicated in calcified lesions (FIGURE 48.5).

Stents

It has not yet been investigated whether systematic stenting is clinically superior to balloon angioplasty. Main indication for stenting is still an inadequate balloon angioplasty result, such as flow-limiting dissection, early elastic recoil, and significant residual stenosis (FIGURE 48.10). It is not yet investigated whether self-expanding or balloon-expandable stents result in different outcomes. Balloon-expandable stents should be favored for the treatment of significant residual stenosis; elastic recoil and dissections can be treated with both kinds of stents. Due to their flexibility, self-expanding nitinol stents should be preferred if the distal segment of the popliteal artery and the origin of the anterior tibial artery are involved (FIGURE 48.11). Balloon-expandable stents and self-expanding stents can be applied by either a 5 French guiding catheter or a 4 French sheath and are available in a length up to 8 and 10 cm, respectively. Evidence is increasing that DES offer superior patency rates in lesions up to 10 cm in length compared to bare metal stents or POBA (YUKON-BTK, DESTINY, ACHILLES). Thus, it can be expected that DES may play an important future role in the treatment of claudicants with isolated infrapopliteal disease or with CLI and complex wounds, both representing clinical situations where long-term patency is mandatory, to either consistently improve quality of life or to guarantee wound healing and with this limb salvage.[64]

Drug-Coated Balloons

Based on the initial Leipzig experience, the main indication for DEB in the future might become long lesions and lesions in vessel segments where stents are contraindicated, such as near the ankle and the foot arteries (FIGURE 48.12). Prior to the use of a DEB the lesion must be predilated with an undersized standard balloon for two reasons:

- In DEB, the hydrophilic balloon coating is replaced by the active drug and a spacer, resulting in higher friction when engaging the lesion, which makes the direct treatment of tight lesions, severely calcified lesions, and CTOs impossible.

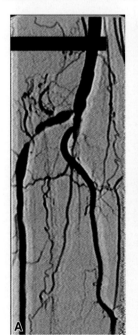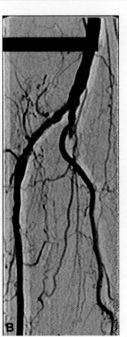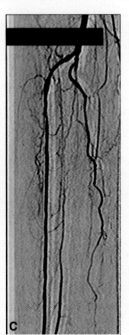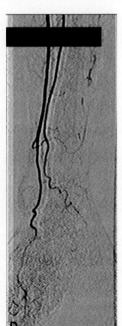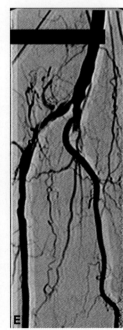

FIGURE 48.10 Tandem lesion of the right anterior tibial artery involving the origin and total occlusion of the tibioperoneal trunk (**A**); result after 3-mm balloon angioplasty with residual stenosis and dissection (**B**); result after implantation of a 3.5-mm diameter, 18-mm-long coronary stent (**C–E**).

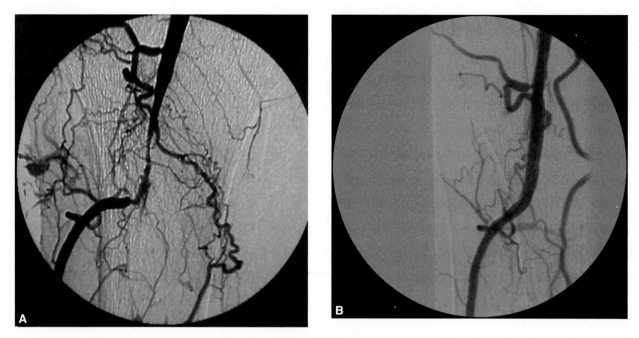

FIGURE 48.11 High-grade stenosis of a right popliteal artery and anterior tibial artery and total occlusion of the tibioperoneal trunk (**A**); result after implantation of a self-expanding Expert stent (**B**).

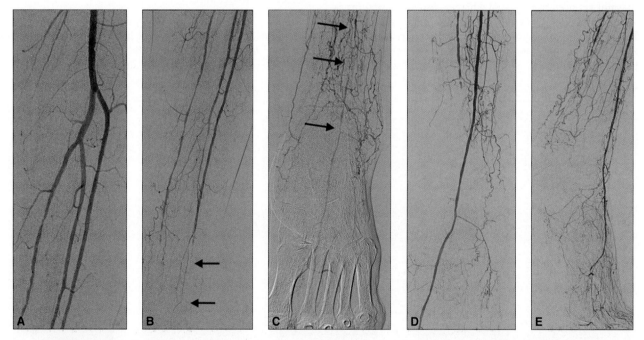

FIGURE 48.12 Occlusion of a left distal anterior tibial artery/dorsalis pedis artery (**A–C**); acute paclitaxel-eluting balloon result after treatment with an In.Pact Amphirion 2.5-mm diameter, 120-mm long (Medtronic-Invatec, Santa Rose, CA) (**D, E**); 3-month angiography without restenosis (**F, G**). The arrows in **B** & **C** mark the target lesion before the treatment.

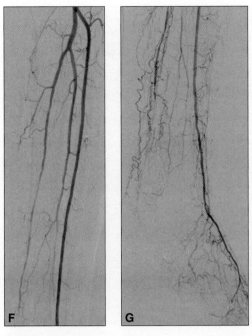

FIGURE 48.12 *(Continued)*

- In tight lesions, a significant amount of the drug could be lost at the proximal edge of the lesion, resulting in inhomogeneous drug distribution with higher drug concentration in the proximal lesion segment and lower concentration distal.

An interesting not yet investigated concept might become debulking first with atherectomy devices followed by DEB application.

Aspiration Devices

Embolic events result most frequently in an obstruction of the bifurcation into the tibioperoneal trunk and the anterior tibial artery. Those emboli can be easily aspirated with either dedicated end-hole aspiration catheters or simply with guiding catheters of appropriate lumen diameter. More difficult is the retrieval of more distal emboli. For this purpose the wire lumen of a 3-mm 5 French shaft balloon catheter can be used for aspiration (FIGURE 48.13) or dedicated coronary aspiration devices that run over a 0.014-inch guide wire, such as Export, Medtronic, Diver CE, Medtronic-Invatec, and Quickcath, Spectranetics (FIGURE 48.14). Before aspiration, locally applied lytic agents or GP IIb/IIIa receptor antagonists can facilitate the aspiration procedure. Aspiration is carried out with a 20-mL, or in proximal occlusions an even better 50-mL, syringe, and the catheter is withdrawn slowly while maintaining aspiration. Because the aspirate is sometimes lost in the hemostatic valve of the sheath during catheter withdrawal, sheaths with removable valves are preferred.

▌ TREATMENT SELECTION STRATEGIES

Focal Lesion

In focal lesions the treatment selection strategy depends on the clinical presentation of the patient. Claudicants—suffering from a lifestyle-limiting disease—should be treated with the most durable interventional technique, currently DES and probably DEB; however, for the latter treatment strategy, controlled data are still lacking. Alternatively, atherectomy techniques seem to provide also acceptable patency results. The same treatment strategy should be applied in patients with CLI and complex wounds.

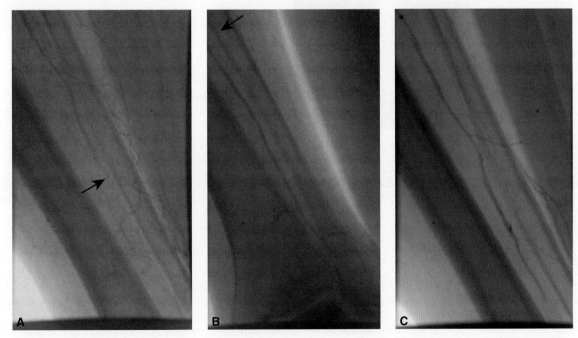

FIGURE 48.13 Embolic occlusion of left distal peroneal artery the arrow marks the beginning of the lesion (**A**); result after aspiration using a 3-mm diameter, 20-mm long Admiral extreme balloon catheter (*arrow*, **B, C**).

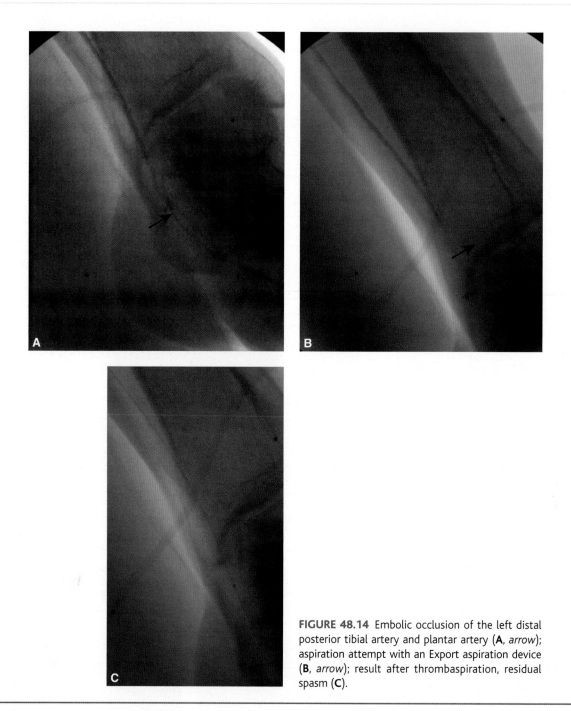

FIGURE 48.14 Embolic occlusion of the left distal posterior tibial artery and plantar artery (**A**, *arrow*); aspiration attempt with an Export aspiration device (**B**, *arrow*); result after thrombaspiration, residual spasm (**C**).

Patients presenting with CLI and simple focal wounds without a previous history of claudication can be treated with a less durable technique, such as plain balloon angioplasty or bare metal stenting (FIGURE 48.15).

Complex Lesions

For patients with CLI and simple wounds, plain balloon angioplasty might be sufficient for wound healing and symptom relief. For claudicants and CLI patients with complex wounds, a potentially more durable treatment technique should be selected, such as atherectomy (high-speed rotational atherectomy, such as Diamondback or Rotablator, Silverhawk, and excimer

laser [FIGURE 48.16]) or DEB. Full lesion coverage with DES in lesion lengths more than 10 cm is rarely cost effective and not yet investigated (FIGURE 48.17).

Embolic Lesions

Treatment strategy of embolic lesions depends on the acuity of the symptoms: If acute ischemia is clinically compensated, simply local lysis can be established for several hours, mostly overnight. If the clinical symptoms are urgent in terms of neurologic and muscular deficits, acute thrombectomy is indicated, usually started after a bolus application of a lytic agent and/or a GP IIb/IIIa receptor antagonist. For this purpose, dedicated aspiration

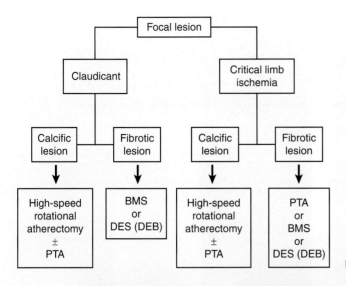

FIGURE 48.15 Treatment selection strategy for focal lesions.

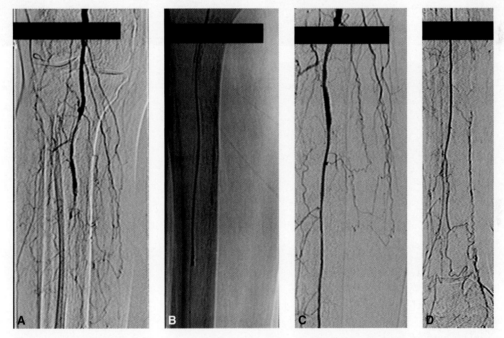

FIGURE 48.16 Subtotal occlusion of the right peroneal artery and total occlusion of the anterior and posterior tibial artery (**A**); small vessel Silverhawk atherectomy device in the peroneal artery (**B**); result after plain atherectomy (**C, D**).

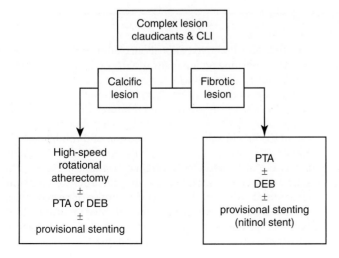

FIGURE 48.17 Treatment selection strategy complex lesions.

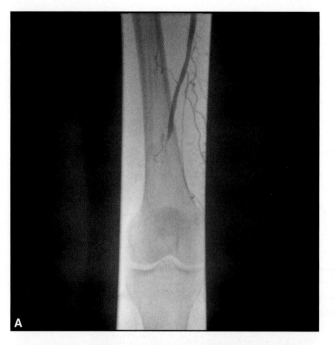

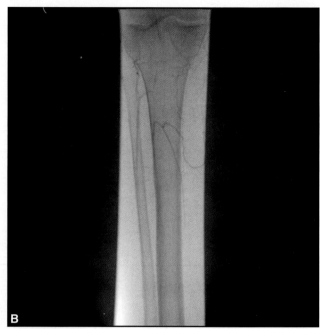

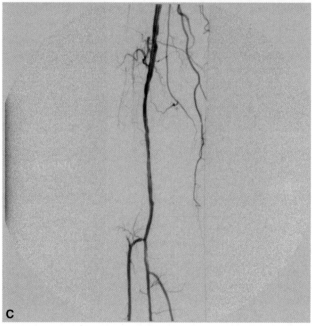

FIGURE 48.18 Thrombotic occlusion of the right popliteal artery and tibioperoneal trunk (**A, B**); result after 6 French Straub Rotarex thrombectomy (**C**).

catheters, guiding catheters, or mechanical thrombectomy devices (Angiojet, Straub Aspirex, and Rotarex, etc. [FIGURE 48.18]) can be used to reestablish some direct flow to the foot, followed by additional local lysis in the presence of residual thrombi after mechanical thrombus removal (FIGURE 48.19).

PLANNING THE INTERVENTIONAL PROCEDURE

Preinterventional Patient Examination

Basis for a successful infrapopliteal angioplasty is a proper preinterventional patient examination. This includes patient examination with pulse palpation and auscultation of potential puncture sites. Preinterventional calculation of the ABI is essential (1) for documentation of the severity of the perfusion deficit and (2) for comparison with the postprocedural measurement. Duplex ultrasound is essential for planning the correct access (puncture site calcification, femoral bifurcation abnormalities) and the interventional strategy. Duplex offers the option of analysis of lesion morphology, determination of thrombus burden, and exact measurement of vessel diameter even BTK. Duplex is very useful to detect even minimal postocclusive flow in the main foot arteries, such as the dorsalis pedis artery or the plantar artery distal, to long occlusions of the anterior or posterior tibial arteries. Based on this information, dedicated procedural tools, such as thrombectomy or atherectomy devices, and potential retrograde access sites can be predetermined.

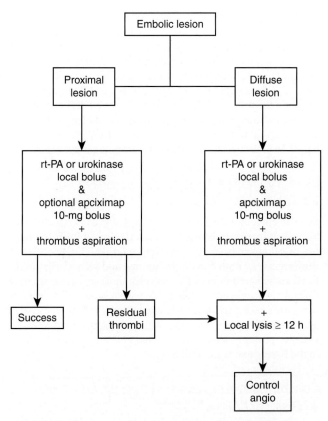

FIGURE 48.19 Treatment selection strategy for embolic lesions.

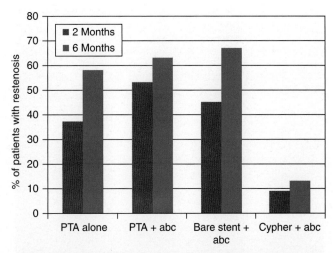

FIGURE 48.20 Two- and six-month angiographic outcome of the BELOW trial[65] stratified to the four treatment cohorts. No significant impact of ReoPro administration; significantly reduced restenosis rate with Cypher select drug-eluting stent.

abc, abciximab.

Magnetic resonance (MRA) and computed tomography angiograms (CTA) can provide a good anatomic overview about the infrapopliteal vessels. Lesion length and distal landing zones can be identified as well as anatomic variations of access site arteries. In diabetic patients and in patients with end-stage renal failure, in particular, it can become hard to differentiate between a contrast medium–filled vessel lumen and a severely calcified occluded vessel segment.

Medication

No controlled trials are available comparing different peri- and postprocedural anticoagulation and antiplatelet regimens in peripheral interventions. In infrapopliteal interventions in particular, where frequently long sheaths or guiding catheters are used with the potential risk of thrombus formation. Thus, most recommendations are adapted to standards of coronary interventional procedures. Thus, it is common sense that periprocedural anticoagulation should be at least 5,000 international units of unfractionated heparin. Measurement of activated clotting time (ACT, at least 250 seconds) is recommended but not international standard of care. Alternative anticoagulation regimens, such as bivalirudin, are not investigated in peripheral procedures. Postprocedural prolongation of anticoagulation is only indicated in thrombotic occlusive disease with residual thrombi following the intervention.

Antiplatelet therapy usually consists at least of aspirin 100 mg once a day and clopidogrel 75 mg once a day for 30 days following bare metal stent placement or for 6 months following

DES placement. In our institutions, patients are preloaded with 500 mg of aspirin and 600 mg of clopidogrel in every procedure. The adjunctive administration of a glycoprotein IIb/IIIa receptor antagonist (ReoPro) had been tested in a small randomized controlled trial[65] and did not result in a significant technical or clinical benefit (FIGURE 48.20). In our institution, ReoPro is given as a bolus dose of 10 mg in complex interventions with prolonged low- or no-flow periods.

Intra-arterial administration of vasodilators plays an important role in infrapopliteal recanalization procedures. Particularly in younger and female patients, there is a strong tendency for vasospasm to develop during the dilatation process, which is exacerbated by the injection of contrast medium. Before or directly after balloon dilatation or other recanalization maneuvers, administration of nitroglycerin 0.2 to 0.3 mg (1 mg nitroglycerin diluted in 10 mL NaCl, stepwise administration of 2 to 3 mL), 30 to 60 mg papaverine, calcium antagonists (e.g., up to 5 mg verapamil), or adenosine is carried out. The guide wire sometimes promotes spasm and consequently has to be withdrawn to assess the result of the angioplasty.

❙ SPECIFIC INTRAPROCEDURAL TECHNIQUES

Intraluminal Recanalization Technique

The most effective technique of staying in the true lumen is the coaxial technique. A low-profile balloon catheter or support catheter is used together with a dedicated 0.014-inch recanalization wire (either hydrophilic coated, e.g., Pilot or Choice series, or uncoated with a progressively stiffened tapered tip, Miracle series, Confienza series, Asahi, all Abbott Vascular). In our institution, we use a "dual coaxial" technique: A straight 5 French guiding-catheter (STR, Cordis J&J) is selectively introduced into the affected tibial artery and positioned close to the occlusion. The guide wire and a coronary balloon catheter (low-profile, monorail, 2 to 2.5 mm diameter, 2 to 4 cm in length) are stepwise introduced into the CTO, advancing the

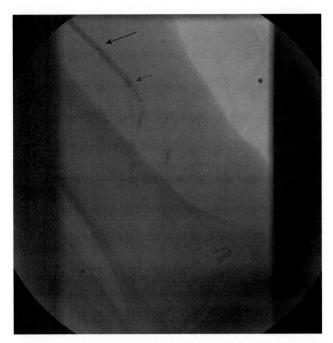

FIGURE 48.21 "Double coaxial" technique: 5 French straight guiding catheter advanced into an occluded posterior tibial artery following stepwise predilatation (*red arrow*), 0.014-inch guide wire stepwise advanced, a 2.5-mm diameter, 40-mm-long balloon catheter (distal marker band inside tip of the guiding catheter, *black arrow*) supports the wire.

guide wire only 1 to 2 cm followed by the balloon catheter (FIGURE 48.21). If friction is increasing, the already traversed CTO segment is predilated with the balloon catheter. During balloon catheter deflation, the guiding catheter is further advanced into the CTO. These procedural steps are repeated as many times as necessary until the lesion is crossed in total. After the completed crossing attempt, the CTO wire can be exchanged against a more floppy guide wire; the guiding catheter is once again pulled back to the beginning of the former occlusion and the lesion is dilated with a second balloon catheter of at least appropriate diameter and length. The success rate of intraluminal crossing attempts is inversely correlated with lesion length. In some cases, double wire techniques can result in a crossing success if the first recanalization wire got stuck in a dissection plane.

Subintimal Recanalization Technique[66]

The first step of the recanalization procedure is to engage the occlusion with a 0.014-inch guide wire for at least 1 or 2 cm and to predilate this occlusion segment with a low-profile balloon (2.5 to 3 mm in diameter). Thereafter, a 5 French shaft 3-mm balloon catheter (length 4 to 8 cm) is introduced over the 0.014-inch guide wire, which is then exchanged against a soft 0.035-inch guide wire (e.g., Radiofocus standard J tip, Terumo). This wire has to be shaped into a small loop primal or inside the predilated vessel segment, which is then pushed through the occlusion followed by the OTW balloon catheter. Alternatively a dedicated 0.035-inch half-stiff-angled Terumo wire can be used with a preshaped loop for subintimal wire passage (FIGURE 48.9).

The balloon catheter can be stepwise inflated if the friction is becoming too high. In most cases, distal to the CTO, the wire loop pops into the true lumen without additional wire manipulation. In rare cases, it can become necessary to straighten the tip of the wire and to perforate the intima plane with the straightened wire tip. If this does not succeed, a stiff 0.014-inch CTO can be used to probe the true vessel lumen. After successful lesion crossing, a balloon catheter of appropriate diameter and length has to be used for a final prolonged balloon dilatation. In experienced hands, overall success rate with this technique is 80% to 90%.

Reentry Device Application After Failed Subintimal Recanalization[63]

Even if current reentry devices (Outback LTD, Cordis J&J, Pioneer, Medtronic-Invatec) are not dedicated for infrapopliteal use, they can be applied to infrapopliteal CTOs. FIGURE 48.22 shows a case of both failed intraluminal and secondarily subintimal crossing attempts of a relatively short proximal anterior tibial artery occlusion. After guide wire passage failed initially using the straight and slightly bended tip of a hydrophilic-coated coronary CTO wire (Pilot 150, Abbott Vascular) due to extravascular position, a loop was created and the occlusion passed in the subintimal vessel wall layer.

Combined Antegrade and Retrograde Tibial Access Technique[63,67–69]

This technique is usually applied after a failed intraluminal or subintimal antegrade crossing attempt. Injecting contrast medium via the antegrade access makes it possible to identify the reconstituted vessel segment distal to the occlusion (FIGURE 48.23). Some operators just mark the course of the artery on the skin; others use fluoroscopy to either detect the calcified native artery or to guide the puncture attempt of the vessel by serial small contrast medium injections. As soon as lumen access is established with a micropuncture needle, a 0.014- or 0.18-inch wire is introduced for the "sheathless" approach or a 4 to even 6 French sheath is introduced. In almost all cases, it is relatively easy to pass the remaining occluded segment retrograde with the 0.014- or 0.018-inch wire, which is usually supported by an OTW balloon catheter, because a recanalization channel has been left behind after the failed antegrade recanalization attempt. After retrograde wire passage, there are two options to proceed with the intervention: (1) in easy cases, the lesion can be dilated from below with a balloon catheter of appropriate dimensions (according to lesion length and reference vessel diameter); (2) in more complex cases, the retrograde wire can be externalized through the femoral sheath (FIGURE 48.24); thereafter, an OTW balloon catheter is pushed over the externalized wire distal to the occlusion and the wire is turned with the flexible tip oriented distally. In the meantime, the tibial access site can be compressed manually by a second operator.

In rare cases, it can be impossible even from retrograde to reconnect with the true lumen proximal to the occlusion. Two potential solutions exist to overcome this problem: (1) Forming a guide wire loop from antegrade and retrograde (0.035-inch Radiofocus soft tip guide wires) and to pass the lesion with both wires from each end. This frequently results in a perforation of the separating membrane. (2) Placing two balloons (2.5 or

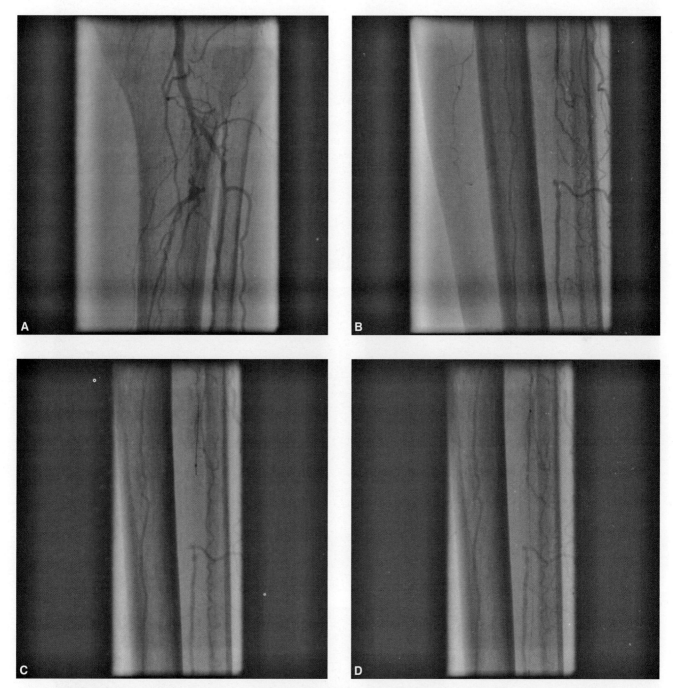

FIGURE 48.22 A–K. Recanalization of a proximal anterior tibial occlusion using the Outback LTD reentry device. After failed intraluminal crossing of a short proximal left anterior tibial artery occlusion, a guide wire loop was created and the occlusion passed subintimally. Because of media calcification, however, the wire could not be repositioned in the true lumen distal to the occlusion. Thus, the subintimal lumen was predilated with a 2.5-mm balloon to create a lumen large enough to accept the Outback LTD reentry device. Then the Outback system was positioned distal to the occlusion and lateral to the true lumen of the reconstituted vessel segment. By only advancing the puncture needle 1 to 2 mm toward the vessel lumen, which had a diameter of about 2 mm, the puncture needle could be positioned into the true lumen and a 0.014-inch guide wire was inserted down to the distal segment of the anterior tibial artery. The next procedural steps were the balloon dilatation of the reentry site followed by the placement of a single low-profile Chromis Deep stent (3.5 mm diameter, and 75 mm long, Medtronic-Invatec). *(continued)*

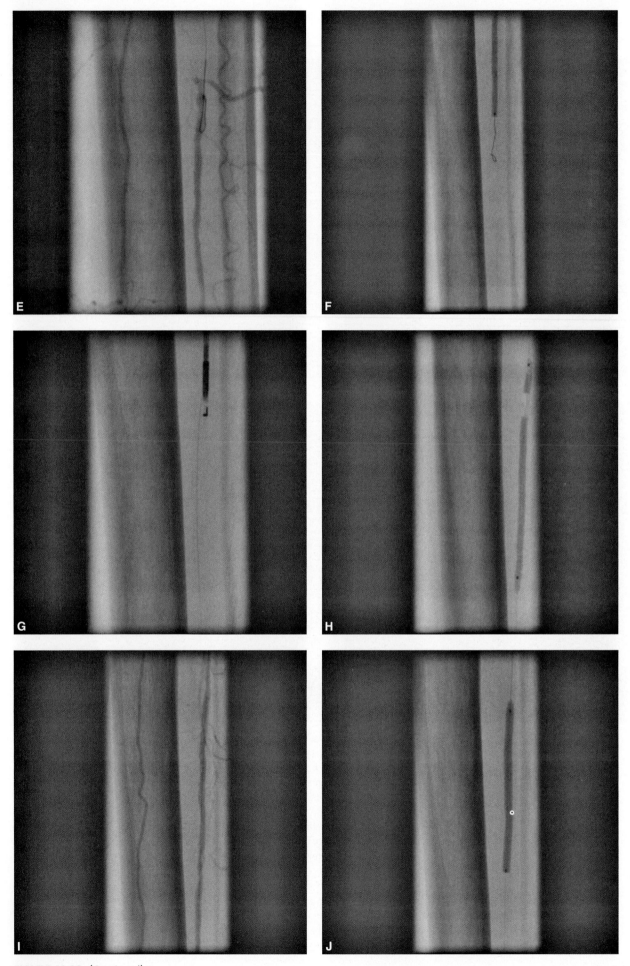

FIGURE 48.22 *(Continued)*

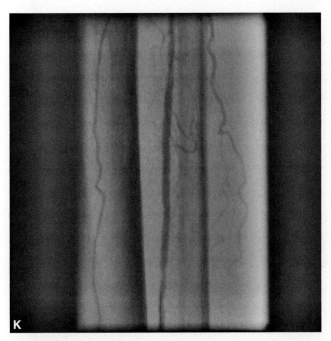

FIGURE 48.22 *(Continued)*

3 mm in diameter), one each introduced from antegrade and retrograde, in a fashion that the distal balloon shoulders just meet when the balloons are inflated (CART technique[68]). This maneuver also results in disrupting the intimal membrane connecting both channels with the option to orient one of the wires into the corresponding lumen. Most of these interventions end in stent placement to fix the resulting dissection planes.

Retrograde Collateral Access Technique[63,70]

It is a frequently seen pathoanatomic situation that the anterior and posterior tibial arteries are occluded with reperfusion of the distal vessel segments or at least the dorsalis pedis artery or plantar artery via collaterals originating from the peroneal artery (anterior and posterior perforating arteries). Such collateral vessel connections can be used as retrograde access to tibial occlusions following a failed antegrade recanalization attempt. FIGURE 48.25 demonstrates a case example where a recanalization attempt of a long posterior tibial artery occlusion failed due to subintimal wire position distal to the occlusion following predilatation of the whole occlusion length. In this case a retrograde recanalization was performed via the posterior perforating artery originating from the peroneal artery. For this purpose, a 5 French STR guiding catheter was advanced into the distal peroneal artery. A hydrophilic-coated 0.014-inch guide wire (Pilot 50, Abbott Vascular) was maneuvered retrograde into the occlusion via the posterior perforating artery (a dummy wire had to be used because the wire unintentionally went into a small side branch). After entering the occlusion from retrograde, the distal occlusion segment was dilated with a 2.5-/40-mm balloon catheter and finally a second wire could be passed through the lesion from above, connecting with the true lumen of the distal posterior tibial artery. The intervention was finished with balloon angioplasty of the entire lesion length including the distal connection to the true lumen with a 3-/120-mm balloon catheter (Amphirion deep, Medtronic-Invatec).

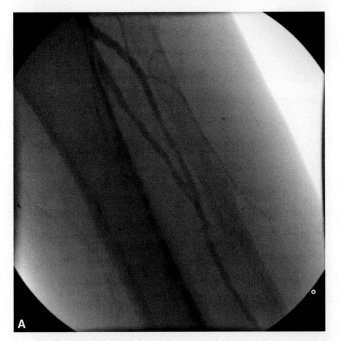
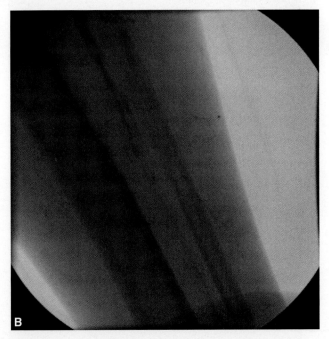

FIGURE 48.23 Calcified total occlusion of a left anterior tibial artery (**A–C**); antegrade recanalization attempt, dummy wire technique (**D, E**); retrograde puncture of the dorsalis pedis artery (*arrow*, **F, G**); one 0.014-inch wire each introduced antegradely and retrogradely (**H**); 2-mm balloon angioplasty after connecting the retrograde lumen with the antegrade lumen (**I**); implantation of a Chromis Deep stent via the antegrade access (**J, K**); angiographic result 6 months postprocedure (**L–N**). *(continued)*

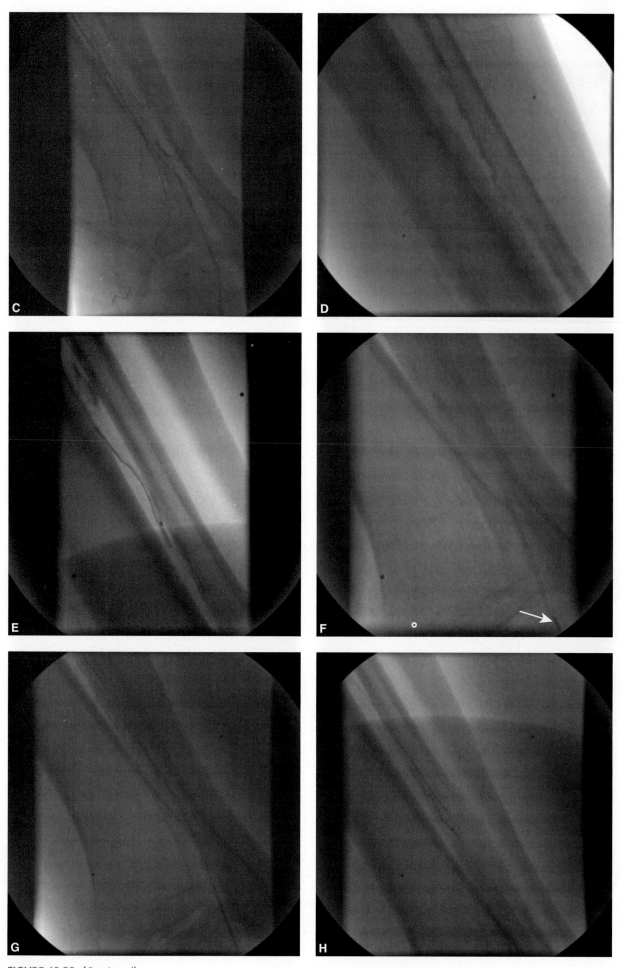

FIGURE 48.23 (Continued)

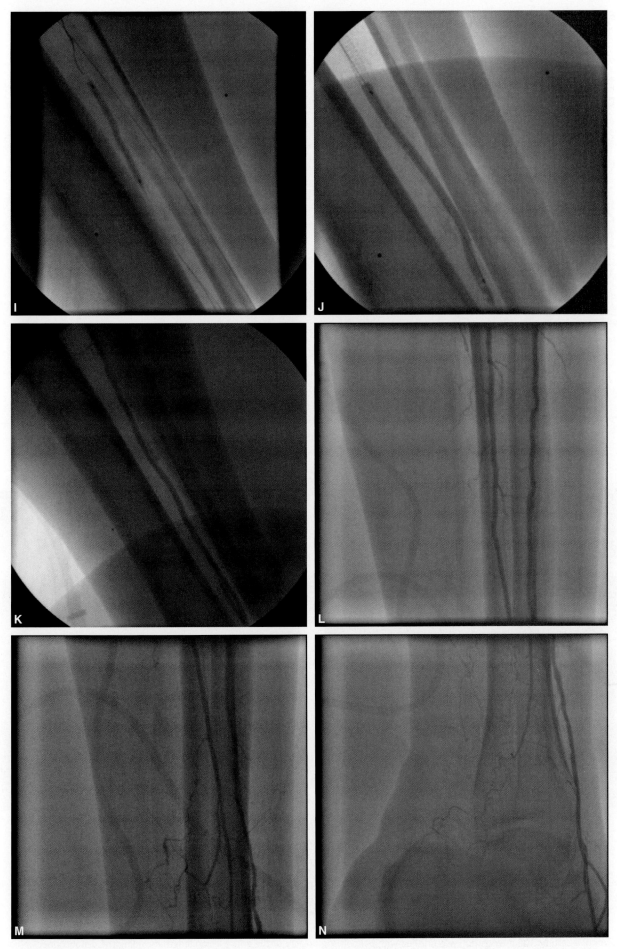

FIGURE 48.23 *(Continued)*

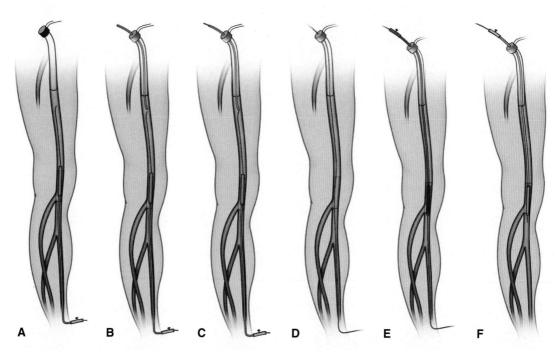

FIGURE 48.24 Technique of femoral externalization of a retrograde-introduced guide wire: The wire crossed the occlusion via tibial access (**A**); an angled diagnostic catheter (vertebral or Judkins right configuration) is introduced via the femoral sheath and the lumen of the catheter is oriented to the vessel wall. Thereafter, the wire is introduced into the diagnostic catheter (**B**) and pushed into the diagnostic catheter until the hemostatic valve of the femoral sheath is passed (**C, D**); an over-the-wire balloon catheter is now introduced via the femoral sheath to antegradely cross the lesion (**E**) and to exchange the wire with external compression of the tibial puncture site (**F**).

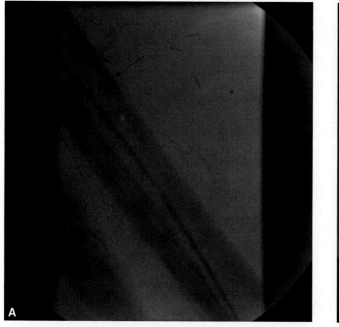

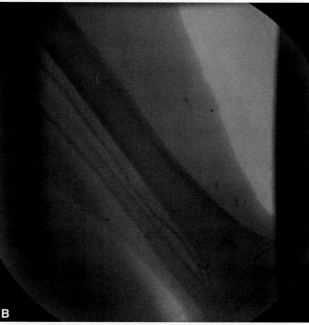

FIGURE 48.25 Occlusion of the right proximal posterior tibial artery (**A**) (*arrow*) with distal reconstitution (**B**); stepwise crossing attempt with a hydrophilic-coated 0.014-inch guide wire (Pilot 150 [**C**]) supported by a 2-mm coronary monorail balloon (**D**); 5 French guiding catheter advanced to the distal occlusion segment (**E**); two wires in subintimal planes (**F**). Retrograde wire recanalization attempt via the posterior perforating artery originating from the peroneal artery advancing a flexible hydrophilic-coated 0.014-inch guide wire (Pilot 50, *red arrow*) into the occlusion (a dummy wire had to be used because this first wire unintentionally went into the collateral branch, *black arrow* [**G, H**]). After complete passage of the occlusion from retrograde (**I, J**), the distal occlusion segment was dilated with a 2.5-mm diameter, 40-mm-long balloon catheter (**K**) and, finally, a second wire could be passed through the lesion from above connecting with the true lumen of the distal posterior tibial artery. The intervention was finished with balloon angioplasty of the entire lesion length including the distal connection to the true lumen with a 3-mm diameter, 120-mm-long balloon catheter (Amphirion Deep, Medtronic-Invatec [**L, M**]).

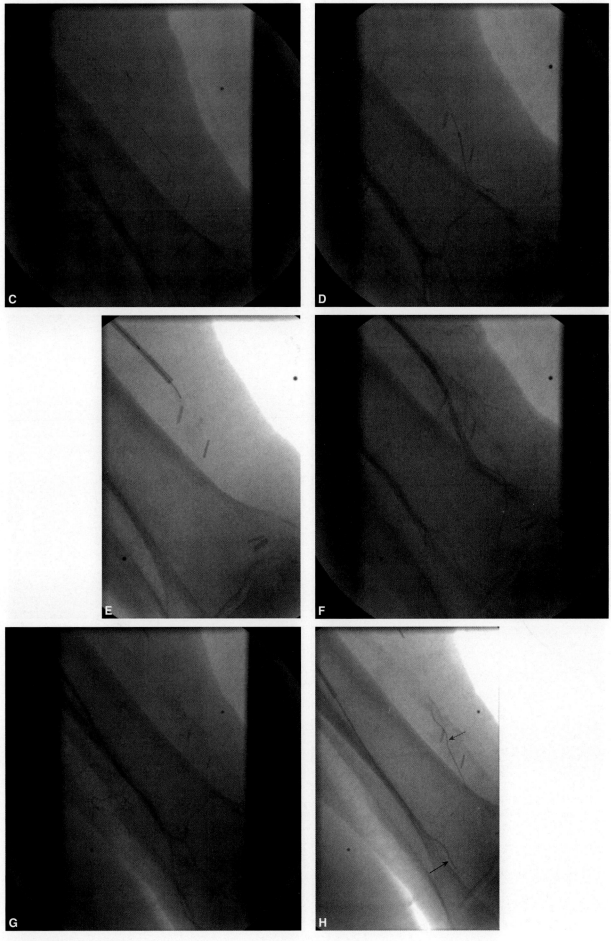

FIGURE 48.25 *(Continued)*

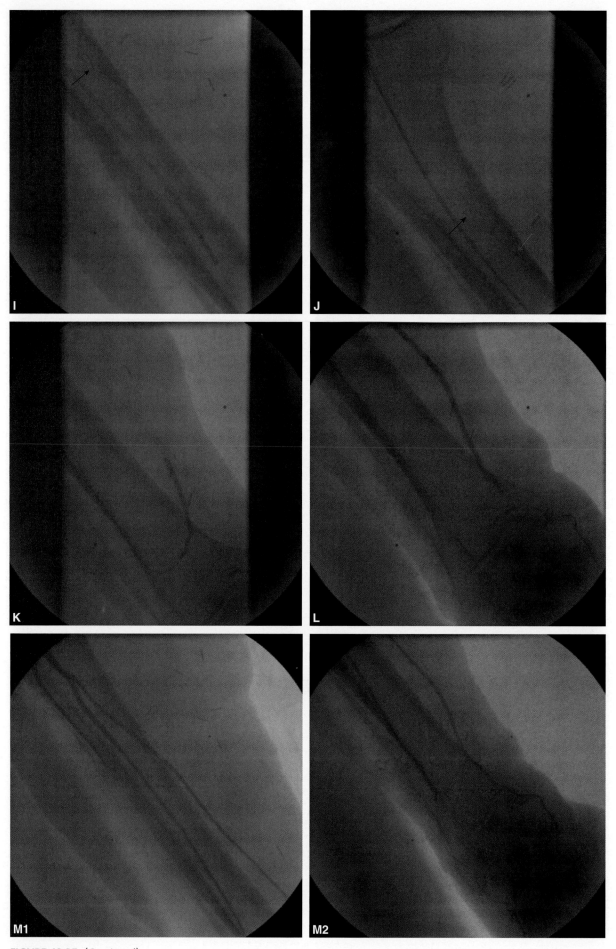

FIGURE 48.25 *(Continued)*

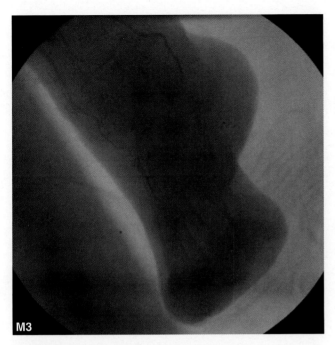

FIGURE 48.25 *(Continued)*

Plantar Arch/Pedal-Plantar Loop Technique

Manzi et al.[71] reported the largest series of 135 patients suffering from CLI, which were treated with a pedal-plantar loop technique to recanalize the foot arteries. The tibial artery was involved in most cases. The tibial artery could be approached

for PTA in 100% of the cases, whereas acute success for the pedal-plantar loop technique was 85%. The background of this technique is to reconnect the foot arch and to establish at least a sufficient retrograde perfusion of one branch of the arch that is not directly provided by an antegrade flow due to occlusion of the providing tibial artery (anterior tibial artery in case of the dorsalis pedis artery and posterior tibial artery in case of the plantar artery). The first step of the procedure is to establish a straight line flow through one of the tibial arteries. Next, the foot artery circulation has to be analyzed and a collateral branch of sufficient diameter (at least 1 mm) needs to be identified connecting the dorsalis pedis artery with the plantar artery. In case of a CTO of the posterior tibial artery, a 0.014-inch hydrophilic-coated floppy guide wire (e.g., Pilot 50, Abbott Vascular) has to be advanced through the dorsalis pedis artery into a plantar artery branch and further upstream until the distal end of the posterior tibial artery occlusion. The entire foot arch is dilated with a long 2-mm low-profile balloon catheter, establishing with this a retrograde flow into the plantar artery and their side branches. The technique to retrogradely recanalize a distal artery occlusion via the foot loop is also helpful in cases where a patent tibial artery does not provide sufficient blood supply to the ischemic area of the foot and another occluded tibial artery cannot be recanalized from antegrade (FIGURE 48.26).

Duplex-Guided Angioplasty

Ascher et al.[72,73] reported their experience with duplex-guided endovascular treatment of occlusive and stenotic lesions. The rationale for this technique was to avoid the nephrotoxic effect of the contrast agent and to eliminate or minimize radiation exposure. In a subgroup of infrapopliteal angioplasties (15% of all cases),

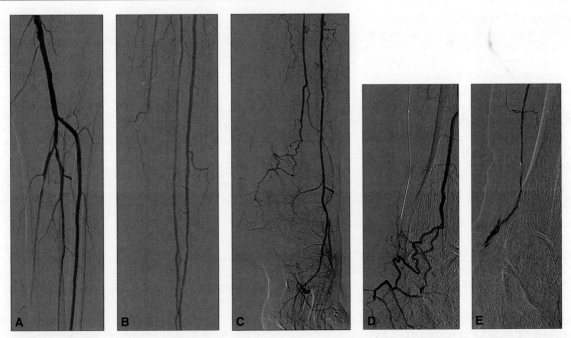

FIGURE 48.26 Distal occlusion of the right posterior tibial artery in a patient with a nonhealing ischemic heel ulcer (**A–C**); failure of antegrade guide wire passage with perforation, successful retrograde wire passage via the foot loop (**D–F**); result after balloon dilatation of the posterior tibial artery (**G–I**). *(continued)*

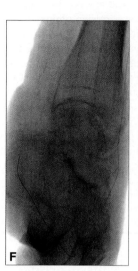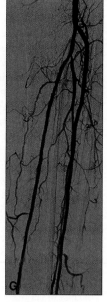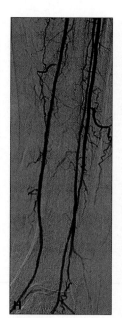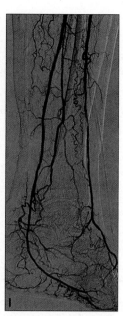

FIGURE 48.26 *(Continued)*

technical success was achieved in 77 of their 80 cases with an overall success rate of 96%.[73] In our institutions we usually prefer the fluoroscopic-guided puncture and intervention techniques.

ENDPOINT ASSESSMENT OF THE PROCEDURE

Acute Technical Success

Technical success is usually defined as restoration of antegrade flow to the foot without a residual stenosis of more than 30% in the postprocedural completion angiogram. This angiogram should be done selectively if no substracted imaging technique is used. Due to the overlay with the bones and the superposition of the peroneal and anterior tibial arteries, completion angiograms should be performed in two different planes.

Angiographic interventional success should be confirmed by postprocedural clinical examination (pulse palpation, skin temperature), calculation of the ABI, and in dedicated patients (prior to planned amputation) the measurement of skin oxygenation. Pre- and postprocedural photographic wound documentation is recommended.

Clinical Success

Clinical success is defined as either relief or improvement of disabling claudication documented in an improved treadmill test or walking impairment questionnaire or relief of rest pain and improved wound healing, finally resulting in limb preservation or distalization of a planned amputation level.

PROCEDURAL COMPLICATIONS AND HOW TO MANAGE THEM SUCCESSFULLY

Complications of endovascular treatment of infrapopliteal arteries are rare but can become limb threatening.

Guide wire perforations are rare but are probably the most frequent complication, although they do not always make it necessary to stop the intervention and rarely require treatment. Angiographically visible bleeding must always be stopped before the end of the intervention, however, because there is otherwise a substantial risk of compartment syndrome development. If external compression, for example, using a blood pressure cuff and/or heparin antagonization using protamine is not sufficient, coil embolization or implantation of a stent graft (Graft-Master, Abbott Vascular) should be performed.

Peripheral embolization during a selective infrapopliteal intervention is a rarity due to the relatively low plaque burden. Exceptions are (1) the treatment of proximal embolic occlusions with the risk of distal thrombus movement during aspiration maneuvers sometimes resulting in the need for prolonged local lysis if the thrombi are occluding small distal branches, such as collateral branches of the distal peroneal artery to the dorsalis pedis artery or plantar artery, which cannot be removed even using dedicated coronary aspiration catheters, and (2) atherectomy procedures, particularly using the Silverhawk device.

The frequency of *flow-limiting dissections* has been remarkably reduced since the availability of dedicated long low-profile balloons for infrapopliteal intervention. If such a dissection persists despite prolonged balloon inflation, dedicated low-profile stents can be placed—preferably self-expanding nitinol stents (e.g., Expert, Abbott Vascular) due to their wider range in available stent lengths.

Vasospasm is a frequent event, particularly in younger patients. If low blood pressure does not prevent its use, prophylactic selective administration of nitroglycerin prior to the start of the intervention might be helpful. In severe cases of vasospasm not responding to nitroglycerin administration, prostanoides (1 to 10 μg as intra-arterial bolus) can solve the problem. If not, prolonged inflation—at least 5 minutes—of a long balloon can result in a satisfying result.

Reperfusion syndrome is a dreaded limb and—in particular circumstances—even life-threatening complication requiring intensive care supervision. It develops mostly in cases of prolonged acute limb ischemia following restoration of blood supply to the calf and foot muscles but in rare cases also in patients suffering from chronic CLI. Reperfusion syndrome is characterized by a local response, which follows reperfusion, and consists of limb swelling with its potential for aggravating tissue injury and the systemic response, resulting in multiple-organ failure and death. It is apparent that skeletal muscle is the predominant tissue in the limb but also the tissue that is most vulnerable to ischemia. Physiologic and anatomic studies show that irreversible muscle cell damage starts after 3 hours of ischemia and is nearly complete at 6 hours. These muscle changes are paralleled by progressive microvascular damage. Microvascular changes appear to follow, rather than precede, skeletal muscle damage because the tolerance of capillaries to ischemia vary with the tissue being reperfused. The more severe the cellular damage, the greater the microvascular changes and with death of tissue, microvascular flow ceases within a few hours—the no-reflow phenomenon. At this point tissue swelling ceases. The inflammatory responses following reperfusion varies greatly. When muscle tissue death is uniform, as would follow tourniquet ischemia or limb replantation, little inflammatory response results. In most instances of reperfusion, which follows thrombotic or embolic occlusion, there will be a variable degree of ischemic damage in the zone where collateral blood flow is possible. The extent of this region will determine the magnitude of the inflammatory response, whether local or systemic.[74]

The systemic release of myoglobine can result in acute renal failure, and the release of potassium in life-threatening arrhythmias and, finally, heart arrest. In such emergency cases, acute hemodialysis is the only lifesaving treatment option. Compartment syndrome requires urgent surgical fasciotomy to prevent compression of microcirculation, resulting in complete necrosis of the calf muscle. Moreover, surgical decompression prevents irreversible nerve compression.

OUTCOMES/PROGNOSIS

Depending on clinical presentation, treatment modality, and severity of infra-popliteal disease overall prognosis following infrapopliteal intervention is good for claudicants. For those patients, life style modification and guidelines conform adjustment of risk factor treatment is an essential part of the treatment strategy.

CLI patients however have a poor survival prognosis with a cardiovascular mortality up to 50% after 2 years.[7] Thus, patient care is not only limited to treatment of peripheral artery disease and wound care but needs in addition close surveillance by a cardiologist.

Claudication

In patients suffering from disabling claudication and exclusive infrapopliteal artery disease, lesion distribution and extension is more focal and mostly affects the proximal vessel segments (FIGURES 48.10 and 48.11). These focal lesions have an excellent long-term prognosis if treated with DES (Yukon-BTK and DESTINY) or atherectomy[34] with durable symptom relief.

Critical Limb Ischemia

Limb salvage rates following infrapopliteal intervention are exceeding 90% in most publications irrespective of the treatment modality used. In patients with chronic wounds, the clinical impact of revascularization in preventing amputation is hard to predict. These patients require a multidisciplinary approach including wound care specialists, podiatrists, plastic surgeons, and diabetologists.[75] Focal superficial skin lesions can heal even if a vessel reoccludes within a few weeks following plain balloon angioplasty. Restenosis and reocclusion rates of more than 60% are reported 3 months after balloon angioplasty of long diffuse lesions.[32] Complex wounds definitely require a prolonged restored skin perfusion. Stents are not useful for the treatment of long lesions; whether DEB will increase the duration of revascularization success is still under investigation. No controlled data exist about the effect of high-speed rotational atherectomy in long diffuse lesions. Thus, CLI patients with long diffuse lesions and complex wounds need close supervision by a vascular specialist including serial control angiograms and, if clinically indicated, multiple redo procedures.[76]

DISEASE SURVEILLANCE AND TREATMENT MONITORING ALGORITHMS

Claudicants with Isolated Infrapopliteal Disease

In general, follow-up visits every 6 months are recommended including clinical examination, ABI measurement, and, if appropriate, duplex ultrasound. A treadmill test might be helpful in case of uncertain symptoms. Appropriate cardiologic tests are recommended at least once a year to exclude significant coronary artery disease.

Critical Limb Ischemia

Appropriate wound care is essential following the revascularization procedure. Follow-up visits by the vascular specialist are recommended after 1, 3, 6, and 12 months depending on the progress of wound healing and the patient's general condition. Cardiologic supervision is essentially the same as in claudicants.

EARLY FAILURES AND OPTIONS FOR MANAGEMENT

Early interventional failure is usually defined as recurrence of symptoms or restenosis/reocclusion within 30 days. In situations suspicious for restenosis, early reangiography is indicated. Early restenosis following balloon angioplasty is usually a result of early recoil or dissection and can be treated by a repeat balloon angioplasty, atherectomy, or stenting procedure. In early reocclusion, thrombus aspiration followed by balloon angioplasty might be indicated; atherectomy could result in distal thrombus migration. If angiography does not result in an early failure of the previous intervention but no progress in wound healing was noted, revascularization of an additional infrapopliteal artery should be considered.

LATE FAILURES AND OPTIONS FOR MANAGEMENT

Late interventional failure is defined as revascularization failure later than 1 month and usually represents typical neointimal growth-induced restenosis or natural disease progression. For disease progression, the standard interventional tools can be applied. Typical restenosis requires, in most cases, more advanced techniques than a simple repeat balloon angioplasty. In lesions shorter than 10 cm, bare metal stents or even better DES are viable treatment options to guarantee a more durable treatment success. Atherectomy, or, if available, DEB are indicated in longer lesions. DEB seems to offer durable results irrespective of their use in de novo lesions or restenotic lesions. The final treatment option, if endovascular strategies repeatedly failed and if a distal vessel segment would be available for anastomosis, might be distal crural or pedal bypass surgery.

PRACTICAL ADVANTAGES AND LIMITATIONS

The obvious *advantage* of endovascular revascularization of infrapopliteal arteries is the limited invasiveness of the procedure and the option for redo procedures if clinically indicated. A stepwise approach oriented on the clinical benefit of a first procedure is possible. Moreover, complete infrapopliteal revascularization procedures including the foot arteries are possible with endovascular approach, whereas a bypass reconstruction is mostly limited to one infrapopliteal vessel. If distal landing zones for bypass anastomosis are not affected by endovascular procedures, the option for surgical revascularization is still preserved in case of acute or late endovascular revascularization failure.

Currently, only a few *limitations* exist for endovascular infrapopliteal interventions: The major limitation is the dependency on operator experience and the limited access to interventional tools in some institutions. Technically, major limitations are (1) missing outflow distal to an occluded vessel segment and (2) severe vessel calcification.

RELATIVE THERAPEUTIC EFFECTIVENESS COMPARED TO MEDICAL AND SURGICAL MANAGEMENT (INCLUDING CLINICAL, PATHOPHYSIOLOGIC, AND ANATOMIC MEASURES)

Compared to conservative treatment only, adding revascularization procedures to the management of critical limb or diabetic foot management resulted in a significant reduction of amputation rates.[77–79] Even if the BASIL trial[27] was not limited to infrapopliteal disease, the trial resulted in equivalent limb salvage rates for open surgical reconstruction and endovascular therapy of CLI patients. Noteworthy is that the only endovascular treatment tool used in this trial was the balloon catheter, resulting in higher restenosis and TLR rates for the endovascular cohort.

Currently, no dedicated trial results are available comparing the clinical efficacy of medical therapy, endovascular therapy, and surgical therapy of infrapopliteal disease.

THE FUTURE

Even if isolated infrapopliteal disease as the cause of disabling claudication is a relatively rare condition, advances in the durability of endovascular therapy as a result of DES and DEB availability will make interventional therapy the treatment of choice in this particular patient cohort. Moreover, improvement of infrapopliteal outflow in conjunction with femoropopliteal inflow procedures might become standard of care if these procedures will result in sustained patency of both inflow and outflow procedures.

In patients with CLI, endovascular treatment has already become the first-line treatment where available. Further improvement of endovascular tools, such as the availability of dedicated crossing devices, long focal force balloons, longer DES, and the combined approach of atherectomy and DEB application might result in further improvement of acute success and durability of the endovascular procedure. The most relevant predictor for treatment success is still the operator experience. Thus, technically challenging interventions should be focused on experienced centers of excellence. In parallel, individual physician training in such experienced centers should be offered more frequently.

CONCLUSION

Improvements in interventional tools and operator skills have made infrapopliteal interventions safe and technically effective. Durability of the procedures is still a matter of concern; however, drug-eluting solutions might become a breakthrough in the near future. Whether these technical improvements can be translated in improved patient outcomes has still to be proven.

REFERENCES

1. Dormandy JA, Rutherford RB. Management of peripheral arterial disease (PAD). TASC Working Group. TransAtlantic Inter-Society Consensus (TASC). *J Vasc Surg* 2000;31:S1–S296.
2. Rutherford RB, Baker JD, Ernst C, et al. Recommended standards for reports dealing with lower extremity ischemia: revised version. *J Vasc Surg* 1997;26:517–538. Erratum in: *J Vasc Surg* 2001;33:805.
3. Schillinger M, Sabeti S, Loewe C, et al. Balloon angioplasty versus implantation of nitinol stents in the superficial femoral artery. *N Engl J Med* 2006;354:1879–1888.
4. Krankenberg H, Schluter M, Steinkamp HJ, et al. Nitinol stent implantation vs. percutaneous transluminal angioplasty in superficial femoral artery lesions up to 10 cm in length: the Femoral Artery Stenting Trial (FAST). *Circulation* 2007;116:285–292.
5. Zeller T, Tiefenbacher C, Steinkamp HJ, et al. Nitinol stent implantation in TASC A and B superficial femoral artery lesions: the Femoral Artery Conformexx Trial (FACT). *J Endovasc Ther* 2008;15(4):390–398.
6. Zeller T, Rastan A, Schwarzwalder U, et al. Long-term results after directional atherectomy of femoro-popliteal lesions. *J Am Coll Cardiol* 2006;48(8):1573–1578.
7. Norgren L, Hiatt WR, Dormandy JA, et al. Intersociety consensus for the management of peripheral arterial disease. *Int Angiol* 2007;26(2):81–157.
8. Buckenham TM, Loh A, Dormandy JA, et al. Infrapopliteal angioplasty for limb salvage. *Eur J Vasc Surg* 1993;7:21–25.
9. Brown K, Moore ED, Getrajdman G, et al. Infrapopliteal angioplasty: long-term follow-up. *J Vasc Interv Radiol* 1993;4:139–144.
10. Hanna GP, Fujise K, Kjellgren O, et al. Infrapopliteal transcatheter interventions for limb salvage in diabetic patients: importance of aggressive interventional approach and role of transcutaneous oximetry. *J Am Coll Cardiol* 1997;30:664–669.
11. Häuser H, Bohndorf K, Wack C, et al. Percutaneous transluminal angioplasty (PTA) of isolated crural arterial stenoses in critical arterial occlusive disease [in German]. *Rofo* 1996;164:238–243.

12. Saab MH, Smith DC, Aka PK, et al. Percutaneous transluminal angioplasty of tibial arteries for limb salvage. *Cardiovasc Intervent Radiol* 1992;15:211–216.

13. Soder HK, Manninen HI, Jaakkola P, et al. Prospective trial of infrapopliteal artery balloon angioplasty for critical limb ischemia: angiographic and clinical results. *J Vasc Interv Radiol* 2000;11:1021–1031.

14. Bakal CW, Cynamon J, Sprayregen S. Infrapopliteal percutaneous transluminal angioplasty: what we know. *Radiology* 1996;200:36–43.

15. Bates MC, Aburahma AF. An update on endovascular therapy of the lower extremities. *J Endovasc Ther* 2004;11(suppl 2):II107–II127.

16. Boyer L, Therre T, Garcier JM, et al. Infrapopliteal percutaneous transluminal angioplasty for limb salvage. *Acta Radiol* 2000;41:73–77.

17. Dormandy J, Belcher G, Broos P, et al. Prospective study of 713 below-knee amputations for ischaemia and the effect of a prostacyclin analogue on healing. Hawaii Study Group. *Br J Surg* 1994;81(1):33–37.

18. Ouriel K, Fiore WM, Geary JE. Limb-threatening ischemia in the medically compromised patient: amputation or revascularization? *Surgery* 1988;104:667–672.

19. Tunis SR, Bass EB, Steinberg EP. The use of angioplasty, bypass surgery, and amputation in the management of peripheral vascular disease. *N Engl J Med* 1991;325(8):556–562.

20. Allagaband S, Solis J, Kazemi S, et al. Endovascular treatment of peripheral vascular disease. *Curr Probl Cardiol* 2006;31(11):711–760.

21. Diehm C, Schuster A, Allenberg H, et al. High prevalence of peripheral arterial disease and comorbidity in 6,880 primary care patients: cross sectional study. *Atherosclerosis* 2004;172:95–105.

22. Alberts MJ, Bhatt DL, Mas JL, et al. Three-year follow-up and event rates in the international REduction of Atherothrombosis for Continued Health Registry. *Eur Heart J* 2009;30(19):2318–2326.

23. DeRubertis BG, Pierce M, Ryer EJ, et al. Reduced primary patency rate in diabetic patients after percutaneous intervention results from more frequent presentation with limb-threatening ischemia. *J Vasc Surg* 2008; 47(1):101–108.

24. Hirsch AT, Haskal Z, Hertzer N, et al. ACC/AHA guidelines for the management of patients with peripheral arterial disease (lower extremity, renal, mesenteric, and abdominal aortic). *Circulation* 2006; 113:463–654.

25. Bosiers M, Hart JP, Deloose K, et al. Endovascular therapy as the primary approach for limb salvage in patients with critical limb ischemia: experience with 443 infrapopliteal procedures. *Vascular* 2006;14:63–69.

26. Abdelsalam H, Markose G, Bolia A. Revascularisation strategies in below the knee interventions. *J Cardiovasc Surg (Torino)* 2008;49(2):187–191.

27. Adam DJ, Beard JD, Cleveland T, et al. Bypass versus angioplasty in severe ischaemia of the leg (BASIL): multicentre, randomised controlled trial. *Lancet* 2005;366(9501):1925–1934.

28. Arain SA, White CJ. Endovascular therapy for critical limb ischemia. *Vasc Med* 2008;13(3):267–279.

29. Krankenberg H, Sorge I, Zeller T, et al. Percutaneous transluminal angioplasty of infrapopliteal arteries with intermittent claudication: acute and 1-year results. *Catheter Cardiovasc Interv* 2005;64:12–17.

30. Mousa A, Rhee JY, Trocciola SM, et al. Percutaneous endovascular treatment for chronic limb ischemia. *Ann Vasc Surg* 2005;19:186–191.

31. Zeller T, Sixt S, Rastan A. New techniques for endovascular treatment of peripheral artery disease with focus on chronic critical limb ischemia. *Vasa* 2009;38(1):3–12.

32. Schmidt A, Ulrich M, Winkler B, et al. Angiographic patency and clinical outcome after balloon-angioplasty for extensive infrapopliteal arterial disease. *Catheter Cardiovasc Interv* 2010;76(7):1047–1054.

33. Ansel GM, Sample NS, Botti CF III Jr, et al. Cutting balloon angioplasty of the popliteal and infrapopliteal vessels for symptomatic limb ischemia. *Catheter Cardiovasc Interv* 2004;61(1):1–4.

34. Bosiers M, Deloose K, Cagiannos C, et al. Use of the AngioSculpt scoring balloon for infrapopliteal lesions in patients with critical limb ischemia: 1-year outcome. *Vascular* 2009;17(1):29–35.

35. Zeller T, Sixt S, Schwarzwalder U, et al. Two-year results after directional atherectomy of infrapopliteal arteries with the SilverHawk device. *J Endovasc Ther* 2007;14:232–240.

36. Zeller T, Krankenberg H, Steinkamp HJ, et al. One-year outcome of percutaneous rotational and aspiration atherectomy in infrainguinal peripheral arterial occlusive disease: the Multi-Centre Pathway PVD Trial. *J Endovasc Ther* 2009;16:653–662.

37. Rastan A, Sixt S, Schwarzwälder U, et al. Initial experience with laser directed atherectomy using the CLiRpath photoablation atherectomy system and Bias Sheath in superficial femoral artery lesions. *J Endovasc Ther* 2007;14:365–373.

38. Laird JR, Zeller T, Gray BH, et al. Limb salvage following laser-assisted angioplasty for critical limb ischemia: results of the LACI Multicenter Trial. *J Endovasc Ther* 2006;13:1–9.

39. McKinsey JF, Goldstein L, Khan HU, et al. Novel treatment of patients with lower extremity ischemia: use of percutaneous atherectomy in 579 lesions. *Ann Surg* 2008;248(4):519–528.

40. Ramaiah V, Gammon R, Kiesz SJ, et al. Midterm outcomes from the TALON registry: treating peripherals with Silverhawk: outcome collection. *J Endovasc Ther* 2006;13:592–602.

41. Kandzari DE, Kiesz RS, Allie D, et al. Procedural and clinical outcomes with catheter-based plaque excision in critical limb ischemia. *J Endovasc Ther* 2006;13(1):12–22.

42. Zeller T, Krankenberg H, Rastan A, et al. Percutaneous rotational and aspiration atherectomy in infrainguinal peripheral arterial occlusive disease: a multi-centre pilot study. *J Endovasc Ther* 2007;14:357–364.

43. Sixt S, Scheinert D, Rastan A, et al. One-year outcome after percutaneous rotational and aspiration atherectomy in infrainguinal arteries in patient with and without diabetes mellitus type 2. *Ann Vasc Surg* 2011;25(4):520–529.

44. Weinstock B, Dulas D. A new treatment option for treating peripheral vascular stenosis: orbital atherectomy. *Vasc Dis Manage* 2008;5:88–92.

45. Safian RD, Niazi K, Runyon JP, et al. Orbital atherectomy for infrapopliteal disease: device concept and outcome data for the OASIS trial. *Catheter Cardiovasc Interv* 2009;73(3):406–412.

46. Rand T, Basile A, Cejna M, et al. PTA versus carbofilm-coated stents in infrapopliteal arteries: pilot study. *Cardiovasc Intervent Radiol* 2006;29: 29–38.

47. Feiring AJ, Wesolowski AA, Lade S. Primary stent-supported angioplasty for treatment of below-knee critical limb ischemia and severe claudication: early and one-year outcomes. *J Am Coll Cardiol* 2004;44:2307–2314.

48. Schmehl J, Tepe G. Current status of bare and drug-eluting stents in infrainguinal peripheral vascular disease. *Expert Rev Cardiovasc Ther* 2008; 6(4):531–538.

49. Siablis D, Kraniotis P, Karnabatidis D, et al. Sirolimus-eluting versus bare stents for bailout after suboptimal infrapopliteal angioplasty for critical limb ischemia: 6-month angiographic results from a nonrandomized prospective single-center study. *J Endovasc Ther* 2005;12:685–695.

50. Siablis D, Karnabatidis D, Katsanos K, et al. Sirolimus-eluting versus bare stents for after suboptimal infrapopliteal angioplasty for critical limb ischemia: enduring 1-year angiographic and clinical benefit. *J Endovasc Ther* 2007;14:241–250.

51. Scheinert D, Ulrich M, Scheinert S, et al. Comparison of sirolimus-eluting vs. bare-metal stents for the treatment of infrapopliteal obstructions. *EuroIntervention* 2006;2:169–174.

52. Deloose K, Bosiers M, Peeters P. One year outcome after primary stenting of infrapopliteal lesions with the Chromis Deep stent in the management of critical limb ischaemia. *EuroIntervention* 2009;5(3):318–324.

53. Tepe G, Zeller T, Heller S, et al. Acute and mid-term results of 4 French sheath compatible self-expanding nitinol stents for treatment of infragenicular arteries following unsuccessful balloon angioplasty. *Eur Radiol* 2007;17(8):2088–2095.

54. Bosiers M, Deloose K, Verbist J, et al. Nitinol stenting for treatment of "below-the-knee" critical limb ischemia: 1-year angiographic outcome after Xpert stent implantation. *J Cardiovasc Surg (Torino)* 2007;48:455–461.

55. Peeters P, Bosiers M, Verbist J, et al. Preliminary results after application of absorbable metal stents in patient with critical limb ischemia. *J Endovasc Ther* 2005;12:1–5.

56. Bosiers M, Peeters P, D'Archambeau O, et al. AMS INSIGHT—absorbable metal stent implantation for treatment of below-the-knee critical limb ischemia: 6-month analysis. *Cardiovasc Intervent Radiol* 2009;32:424–435.

57. Commeau P, Barragan P, Roquebert PO. Sirolimus for below the knee lesions: mid-term results of SiroBTK study. *Catheter Cardiovasc Interv* 2006;68:793–798.

58. Balzer JO, Zeller T, Rastan A, et al. Percutaneous interventions below the knee in patients with critical limb ischemia using drug eluting stents. *J Cardiovasc Surg* 2010;51:183–191.

59. Rastan A, Schwarzwälder U, Noory E, et al. Primary use of sirolimus-eluting stents for angioplasty of infrapopliteal arteries. *J Endovasc Ther* 2010;17:480–487.

60. Charalambous N, Schäfer PJ, Trentmann J, et al. Percutaneous intraluminal recanalization of long, chronic superficial femoral and popliteal occlusions using the Frontrunner XP CTO device: a single-center experience. *Cardiovasc Intervent Radiol* 2010;33(1):25–33.

61. Gandini R, Volpi T, Pipitone V, et al. Intraluminal recanalization of long infrainguinal chronic total occlusions using the Crosser system. *J Endovasc Ther* 2009;16(1):23–27.

62. Beschorner U, Sixt S, Schwarzwälder U, et al. Recanalization of chronic occlusions of the superficial femoral artery using the Outback™ re-entry catheter: a single centre experience. *Catheter Cardiovasc Interv* 2009; 74:934–938.

63. Schwarzwälder U, Zeller T. Debulking procedures: potential device specific indications. *Tech Vasc Interv Radiol* 2010;13:43–53.

64. Feiring AJ, Krahn M, Nelson L, et al. Preventing leg amputations in critical limb ischemia with below-the-knee drug-eluting stents: the PaRADISE (PReventing Amputations using Drug eluting StEnts) trial. *J Am Coll Cardiol* 2010;55(15):1580–1589.

65. Tepe G, Schmehl J, Heller S, et al. Drug eluting stents versus PTA with GP IIb/IIIa blockade below the knee in patients with current ulcers—The BELOW Study. *J Cardiovasc Surg (Torino)* 2010;51(2):203–212.

66. Met R, Van Lienden KP, Koelemay MJ, et al. Subintimal angioplasty for peripheral arterial occlusive disease: a symptomatic review. *Cardiovasc Intervent Radiol* 2008;31(4):687–697.

67. Fusaro M, Dalla Paola L, Biondi-Zoccai GG. Retrograde posterior tibial artery access for below-the-knee percutaneous revascularisation by means of sheathless approach and double wire technique. *Minerva Cardioangiol* 2006;54(6):773–777.

68. Kimura M, Katoh O, Tsuchikane E, et al. The efficacy of a bilateral approach for treating lesions with chronic total occlusions the CART (controlled antegrade and retrograde subintimal tracking) registry. *JACC Cardiovasc Interv* 2009;2(11):1135–1141.

69. Montero-Baker M, Schmidt A, Bräunlich S, et al. Retrograde approach for complex popliteal and tibioperoneal occlusions. *J Endovasc Ther* 2008;15:594–604.

70. Fusaro M, Agostani P, Biondi-Zoccai GG. "Trans-collateral" angioplasty for a challenging chronic total occlusion of the tibial vessels: a novel approach tor percutaneous revascularisation in critical lower limb ischemia. *Catheter Cardiovasc Interv* 2008;71(2):268–272.

71. Manzi M, Fusaro M, Ceccacci T, et al. Clinical result of below-the-knee intervention using pedal-plantar loop technique for the revascularisation of foot arteries. *J Cardiovasc Surg (Torino)* 2009;50(3):331–337.

72. Ascher E, Hingorani AP, Marks N. Duplex-guided balloon angioplasty of lower extremity arteries. *Perspect Vasc Surg Endovasc Ther* 2007;19(1):23–31.

73. Ascher E, Marks NA, Hingorani AP, et al. Duplex-guided endovascular treatment for occlusive and stenotic lesions of the femoro-popliteal arterial segment: a comparative study in the first 253 cases. *J Vasc Surg* 2006;44(6):1230–1237; discussion 1237–1238.

74. Blaisdell FW. The pathophysiology of skeletal muscle ischemia and the reperfusion syndrome: a review. *Cardiovasc Surg* 2002;10(6):620–630.

75. Zayed H, Halawa M, Maillardet L, et al. Improving limb salvage rate in diabetic patients with critical leg ischaemia using a multidisciplinary approach. *Int J Clin Pract* 2009;63(6):855–858. Epub 2008 Feb 1.

76. Fernandez N, McEnaney R, Marone LK, et al. Predictors of failure and success of tibial interventions for critical limb ischemia. *J Vasc Surg* 2010;52:834–842.

77. McCaslin JE, Hafez HM, Stansby G. Lower-limb revascularization and major amputation rates in England. *Br J Surg* 2007;94(7):835–839.

78. Abou-Zamzam AM Jr, Gomez NR, Molkara A, et al. A prospective analysis of critical limb ischemia: factors leading to major primary amputation versus revascularization. *Ann Vasc Surg* 2007;21(4):458–463. Epub 2007 May 17.

79. Faglia E, Clerici G, Clerissi J, et al. When is a technically successful peripheral angioplasty effective in preventing above-the-ankle amputation in diabetic patients with critical limb ischaemia? *Diabet Med* 2007;24(8): 823–829. Epub 2007 Jun 8.

Endovascular Management of Multilevel Lower Extremity Disease

AMARDEEP JOHAR and BOB R. SMOUSE

INTRODUCTION

Lower extremity peripheral arterial disease (PAD) commonly affects the entire arterial tree in a tandem pattern and so isolated lesions are less common and usually are diagnosed and treated at an earlier stage of the disease process. Endovascular management of single-level occlusive disease has been discussed elsewhere, so in this chapter we focus on the management of more complex, multilevel PAD. Patients with multilevel disease, which include both inflow and outflow occlusions, represent a more advanced stage of PAD and have historically been treated with surgical bypass. With the advancement of percutaneous devices and endovascular techniques the nonsurgical treatment options for multilevel disease have expanded as represented by the evolution of the TransAtlantic Inter-Societal Consensus (TASC) guidelines for endovascular management of lower extremity arterial vascular disease.[1]

In January 2000, the TASC work group printed the first set of guidelines recommending which lower extremity vascular lesions should be treated by endovascular means (TASC A) or surgical means (TASC D).[1] Also contained in the guidelines were two additional classifications for lesions in the gray area that may be treated with either endovascular or surgical means. Those lesion subsets include TASC B lesions, which may be better treated with endovascular therapy, and TASC C lesions, which may be better treated with open surgery. These so-called gray areas allow the operator to stratify patients on a case-by-case basis, taking into account patient comorbidities, anatomic concerns, and the operator's experience and skill level. In 2007, those guidelines were updated and the indications within each group were changed based on data collected from centers treating peripheral vascular disease.[2] As a whole, the treatment recommendations for more complex lesions have shifted downward, favoring endovascular methodologies.

The TASC guidelines demonstrate the limited success of endovascular therapy in multilevel, diffuse disease. Surgery may also be challenging in these patients because they tend to have comorbidities and advanced atherosclerosis affecting other vascular territories, such as coronary, renal, visceral, and cerebrovascular systems that may make them poor surgical and anesthesia candidates. Although surgery remains the gold standard, the endovascular approach may be the best option available to salvage limbs and reestablish distal perfusion without causing considerable morbidity.

PATIENT DEMOGRAPHICS

PAD affects approximately 10 million Americans.[3] Multilevel atherosclerotic disease in the lower extremity is usually seen in an older male patient with limited functional capacity and symptomatic ischemia of one or both legs, presenting as either severe intermittent claudication or critical limb-threatening ischemia with rest pain, to nonhealing ulcers. With multilevel disease the process has been long-standing with associated ischemic dermatopathic changes, hair loss and, in some cases, peripheral neuropathy of chronic vascular ischemia and/or diabetes. There is a strong association with diabetes, hypertension, dyslipidemia, smoking, and symptomatic cerebral, coronary, or other visceral arterial disease.[4] Due to the natural history of the disease, these patients present late in the course of their illness and as the U.S. population survives longer, this subset of patients will continue to grow.

There are two ways to clinically categorize PAD: Fontaine's stages or Rutherford categories.[5] The Fontaine stages were introduced by Rene Fontaine in 1954 for ischemia and are primarily based on clinical symptomatology. Stage 1 is no pain when walking (asymptomatic), incomplete blood vessel obstruction. Stage 2 is pain when walking relatively short distances (intermittent claudication); 2a is pain triggered by walking after a distance of greater than 200 m, and 2b after less than 200 m. Stage 3 is pain while resting (rest pain), mostly in the feet, increasing when the limb is raised. Stage 4 is biologic tissue loss (gangrene) and difficulty walking. A more recent classification by Rutherford consists of three grades and six categories: stage 1 is mild claudication, stage 2 is moderate claudication, stage 3 is severe claudication, stage 4 is ischemic pain at rest, stage 5 is minor tissue loss, and stage 6 is major tissue loss (Table 49.1).

The location and extent of arterial occlusive disease found on angiography or cross-sectional imaging (computer tomography angiography [CTA] or magnetic resonance angiography [MRA]) can be further categorized into one of the TASC classifications. As mentioned earlier, these range from TASC A to TASC D, depending on the extent of the vascular disease process and whether the limb is treated best with an endovascular or a surgical approach. Once the clinical, comorbid, and anatomic data have been determined, patient stratification is performed for appropriate invasive management. This will run the gambit from doing nothing, endovascular treatment, open surgery, or a combination of both. This applies to patients with intermittent claudication to critical limb-threatening ischemia and possible limb loss. One subset of patients, those with diabetes, is particularly challenging when it comes to management. Many present

Table 49.1

Fontaine Stages & Rutherford Categories

Fontaine		Rutherford		
Stage	Clinical	Grade	Category	Clinical
I	Asymptomatic	0	0	Asymptomatic
IIa	Mild claudication	I	1	Mild claudication
IIb	Moderate to severe claudication	I	2	Moderate claudication
		I	3	Severe claudication
III	Ischemic rest pain	II	4	Ischemic rest pain
IV	Ulceration or gangrene	III	5	Minor tissue loss
		III	6	Major tissue loss

with soft-tissue infections and chronic ulcers that interfere with surgery and wound healing. Venous insufficiency is not uncommon as is chronic pedal edema. Dermatopathic changes of chronic venous stasis and concomitant venous ulcer disease complicate potential surgical options. In this context there is patient self-selection toward endovascular techniques. The conventional surgical management of these lesions is lengthy and requires extensive revascularization, adequate vein, long wound healing, and higher perioperative risks. Therefore, the need for less-invasive, shorter, and better-tolerated procedures has driven the rapid adoption of endovascular management in this patient subset.

When determining the aggressiveness of the treatment plan it is useful to divide patients into (1) those presenting with claudication (Rutherford stages 1–3) and (2) those presenting with critical limb ischemia (CLI) (Rutherford stages 4–6). The distinction is pragmatic because the endovascular goals and risk benefit ratios for treatment are different between the two. A patient with claudication will benefit more with a low-risk intervention with focus on treatment durability. This usually involves treating suprapopliteal lesions. A patient with critical limb-threatening ischemia, however, will do better with a more complex and inherently riskier endovascular procedure that includes treating the infrapopliteal circulation. Shorter patency durability is acceptable as long as there is wound healing. CLI patients are on the verge of limb loss due to their limited vascular capacity and plethora of medical comorbidities. Therefore, short-term improvement in quality of life and limb preservation are considered acceptable outcomes even in the absence of long-term vessel patency. Primary patency rates of 8 to 12 weeks usually suffice for wound healing, and, if done properly, endovascular interventions may be able to revitalize a pulseless or infected limb without precluding subsequent surgical procedures.

DRAWING UP THE TREATMENT PLAN

Achieving successful reperfusion of a limb with multisegment disease begins with making this assessment: whether inflow revascularization alone or both inflow and outflow procedures are necessary. Furthermore, in patients who require both inflow and outflow revascularizations, the interventionist must

decide if these procedures are to be done in a staged or a combined fashion.[6] In staged management, performing therapy in the large proximal arteries first improves inflow immediately and also allows time for clinical reassessment for wound healing before proceeding to more complex infrainguinal or infrapopliteal therapies, such as long recanalizations. Staged procedures may come at the cost of increased operating room time, with double bookings, and interim tissue loss. Simultaneous intervention for both inflow and outflow lesions avoid potential tissue loss, but it may subject some patients to riskier outflow procedures that could be avoided. Furthermore, multisegment revascularizations also test the endurance of the operator and patient because they tend to be much more time-intensive.

A newer emerging option is the hybrid procedure: combining endovascular and surgical approaches at the same setting. Technical and hemodynamic success rates have been as high as 95% and 100%, respectively, and long-term durability of suprapopliteal artery revascularizations have been reported. Hybrid procedures involve endarterectomy and/or bypass grafting combined with endovascular therapy, such as stenting or subintimal recanalization, of the proximal or distal vascular territory. An example of such a procedure would be common femoral artery endarterectomy combined with superficial femoral artery recanalization and stenting. Hybrid procedures are promising but more long-term investigation is needed before this approach can be recommended in most cases.[7–11] With hybrid procedures general anesthesia can be minimized in high-risk patients with the use of epidural or local anesthesia.

ANATOMIC CONSIDERATIONS IN MULTILEVEL PERIPHERAL ARTERY DISEASE

The anatomic course of the arteries in the leg and the forces on them during ambulation affect outcome of treatment. Cadaver models and three-dimensional in vivo imaging have demonstrated significant femoropopliteal artery deflection and distortion with hip flexion and knee bending. There is axial compression, bending, torsion, and some elongation of the femoral and popliteal arteries.[12] The common femoral artery (CFA)

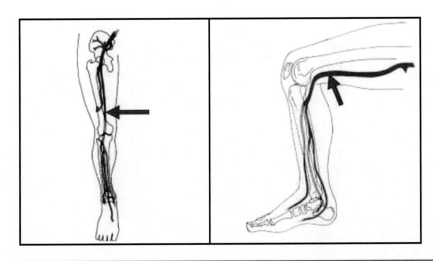

FIGURE 49.1 Upper popliteal a. segment (*red arrow*).

is relatively fixed between the inguinal ligament superiorly and the sartorius muscle inferiorly; however, at the margins of the CFA, bending occurs with hip flexion.

The superficial femoral artery (SFA) is relatively mobile and undergoes axial compression to absorb arterial slack with hip flexion and knee bending. Some sinusoidal bending will occur along the course of the artery but this is relatively minor in the normal artery. With arterial stenting axial compression is restricted and additional bending will occur to absorb the arterial slack. Furthermore, the SFA is externally supported by the adductor ring as it exits the adductor hiatus, and the ring acts as a fulcrum, resulting in arterial bending.

The popliteal artery begins after the takeoff of the supreme geniculate artery from the SFA and can be divided into three segments: the superior, middle, and inferior popliteal arterial segments.

1. The superior popliteal artery extends from adductor ring to superior border of the femoral condyle (FIGURE 49.1). The abundant areolar tissue around the neurovascular trunk allows for enlargement of the popliteal triangle with knee bending. During ambulation slack occurs within the popliteal artery that must be taken up and this arterial

redundancy is absorbed by a series of bends within the popliteal triangle. These bends can result in stent deformation, kinking, and strut fracture with ambulation.

2. The middle popliteal artery lies behind the femoral condyles opposite the intercondylar notch and this region is anatomically narrowed and restricts popliteal artery (PA) movement (FIGURE 49.2). During knee bending there is axial compression or foreshortening of the artery along with bending behind the knee. With maximal knee bend more axially rigid stents may kink and repetitive deformation of the stent can result in stent fracture.[13] Impedance matching is another concept to be cognizant of when stenting the compliant muscular inflow arteries because doing so can result in turbulent blood flow, leading to abnormal wall shear and intimal hyperplasia.[14] With the development of more flexible stents, strut fracture and intimal hyperplasia should improve.

3. The inferior popliteal artery extends from the joint line to the soleus arcade (FIGURE 49.3). The neurovascular bundle is deeply inserted in the ventrally concave gutter, marking the position of the medial and lateral heads of the gastrocnemius muscles. The course of the inferior popliteal artery is in a narrow canal that restricts popliteal artery movement;

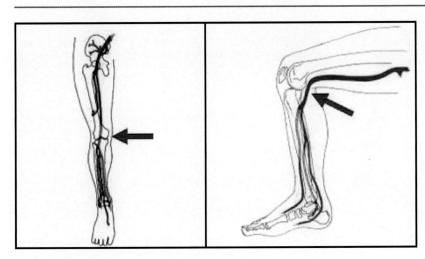

FIGURE 49.2 Middle popliteal a. segment (*red arrow*).

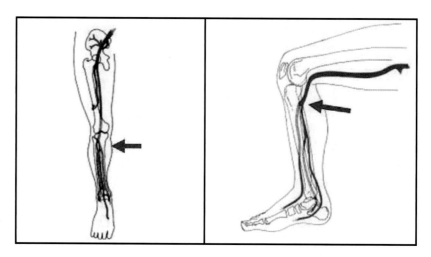

FIGURE 49.3 Lower popliteal a. segment (*red arrow*).

however, with knee bending the inferior popliteal artery will pull away from the tibial arteries, which are fixed, forming a 90-degree angle. This severe angulation can result in stent kinking and vessel occlusion. This hostile arterial environment is one leading theory on why endovascular repair and long-term vessel patency tends to be wanting in the femoropopliteal segment.

In contradistinction, the small tibial arteries are relatively fixed with little deflection and bending during ambulation and stair climbing. The small caliber of the arteries, their frequent occlusions, slow blood flow, and remote location present different challenges for endovascular management of the distal limb, however.

ACCESS AND DEVICE CONSIDERATIONS

Multilevel disease treatment can potentially involve the endovascular management of the aorta, iliac, femoropopliteal, and infrageniculate arteries during the same session.

In the inflow tract, the muscular arteries are relatively large and readily accessible by either an ipsilateral or a contralateral groin approach or by either a brachial or an axillary approach. A contralateral groin approach is commonly chosen because this will allow a "stem-to-stern" approach for vessel access and treatment (FIGURES 49.4–49.7). By accessing the groin contralateral to the symptomatic leg, the abdominal aorta and iliac and contralateral leg arteries are accessible for endovascular treatment with a single arterial puncture. If both legs are to be treated during the

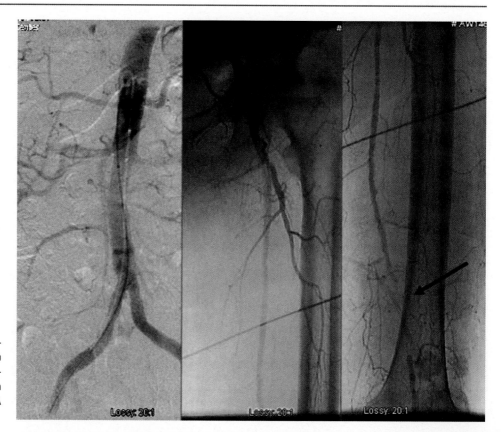

FIGURE 49.4 Contralateral common femoral artery approach with digital subtraction angiography showing distal SFA occlusion (*arrow*). This corresponds to CTA in figure 8.

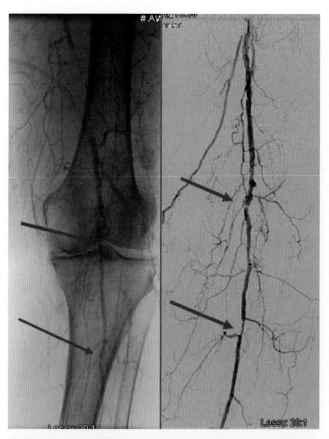

FIGURE 49.5 Standard angiography (unsubtracted and digitally subtracted) demonstrating focal stenoses of the popliteal and peroneal arteries (*arrows*). This corresponds to CTA in figure 9.

same session, then bilateral CFA punctures can be performed for bilateral up-and-over sheath placements to allow treatment of both legs. If the disease is bilateral and proximal (above the knee) then a brachial or axillary approach can be used to give appropriate access to the diseased arteries of both legs, usually using the left arm to avoid crossing the origin of the carotid arteries.

A common strategy is to start with a short 4 or 5 French vascular sheath placed into the contralateral CFA followed by pigtail diagnostic arteriography. Once a plan for treatment has been decided then the diagnostic sheath is exchanged for a larger diameter and longer working sheath. A pigtail or reverse-curve catheter is used to select the contralateral iliac artery, allowing for guide wire placement into the contralateral limb followed by sheath exchange over the aortoiliac bifurcation. This will allow treatment of most or the entirety of the contralateral leg vessels. A common working sheath has an internal diameter from 6 to 8 French and is 45 cm in length. Additionally, some sheaths have a hydrophilic coating on the leading half to ease with placement through the atherosclerotic arteries. Once sheath access has been accomplished wire crossing is performed to allow treatment. This step is straightforward with the exception of chronic total occlusions (CTOs), which can be challenging.

In the infrapopliteal segment, the arteries are much smaller and have numerous collaterals with slower flow. Catheter access and wire crossing can be difficult because of the long distance from the usual contralateral groin approach and their high rate of chronic occlusions. Once guide wire access has been gained care must be taken to prevent vasospasm, preserve distal runoff, and prevent emboli.[15] Stenting in this region is also hindered by the small arterial caliber, diffuse long-segment disease, and numerous vital collaterals, which should not be blocked. Given the distance of the vessels from the contralateral groin, an ipsilateral

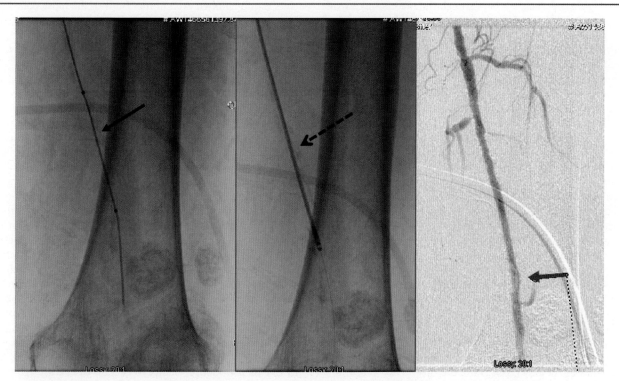

FIGURE 49.6 Treatment of the distal SFA occlusion seen in figures 4 & 8. The occlusion is crossed using a Quick Cross catheter (Spectranetics, Colorado Springs, CO) over a 0.035 guidewire (Cook Medical, Bloomington, IN) (*black arrow*). Atherectomy is performed using the Jetstream rotational atherectomy device (Bayer HealthCare, Warrendale, PA) (*dashed arrow*). Digital subtraction angiography demonstrating patent SFA after atherectomy (*red arrow*).

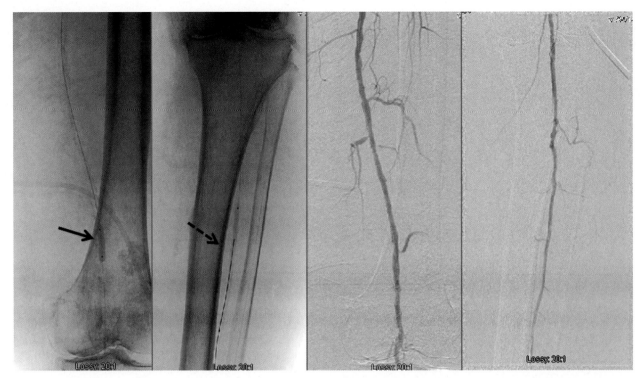

FIGURE 49.7 Treatment of the popliteal and peroneal artery stenoses seen in figures 5 & 9. Simple angioplasty of the popliteal (*black arrow*) and peroneal (*dashed arrow*) arteries and follow-up digital subtraction angiography demonstrating widely patent vessels.

approach can be used to reach the vessels for treatment. The ipsilateral groin approach will allow straight-line access and provide a mechanical advantage to crossing CTOs that the contralateral groin approach does not offer. With the recent introduction of long-shaft angioplasty balloons dedicated to tibial vessel treatment, the contralateral groin approach is feasible in most cases and is gaining in popularity.

Improved sheaths and catheters borrowed from neurovascular and coronary work have made it possible to access smaller and more distal arteries in the leg and their small collaterals. New low-profile catheters are constantly being developed to help treat the infrageniculate vascular bed, including specifically designed crossing catheters and wires for long-segment distal recanalizations. Low-profile balloons have also been developed to cope with the anatomic challenges of this circulation, specifically long chronic occlusions, which can be navigated when used in tandem with crossing wires. Stents of various sizes and flexibilities are available and in development for treating large- to small-diameter proximal and distal arteries. Hydrophilic coated and uncoated wires, available in 0.014-, 0.018-, and 0.035-inch diameters, have been developed with stiffer tips that can be used in combination with support catheters, for crossing of tight stenosis, and CTOs. Reentry catheters, such as the Outback LTD (Cordis, Bridgewater, NJ) and the Pioneer (Medtronic, Minneapolis, MN), allow successful reentry into the true lumen during endovascular subintimal recanalization of long CTOs above the knee.

Unfortunately, given the small diameter of the tibial arteries, guide wire crossing of tibial CTOs usually requires an intraluminal approach and the successful use of reentry catheters is quite limited even in the hands of the most skilled and experienced operator. Current devices for intraluminal crossing include the Frontrunner XP (Cordis), the Crosser (Bard), Wildcat (Avinger, Redwood City, CA), and, most recently, the TruePath catheter (Boston Scientific Corp, Boston, MA).

The complexity including length of lesions are considered when planning for therapy because surgery remains the gold standard for long-segment multilevel disease and should be implemented in treatment when appropriate. Severe medical comorbidities, lack of adequate vein, and absence of a nondiseased target vessel can stymie traditional distal bypass surgeries, however. When bypass is not desirable, the overall clinical picture can aid in the selection of an appropriate treatment strategy. For example, in early ischemic foot damage, only a small improvement in inflow perfusion using angioplasty with or without stenting may be sufficient to help heal the lesion. This procedure should be conducted first and the clinical effect observed before a second more distal procedure is planned. In a patient with intermittent claudication who desires complete ambulation, improving both inflow and the outflow will yield the best results and provide the greatest increase in exercise tolerance.

Unfortunately, most patients present in the late stages of the disease process with more complex and challenging lesions. Diabetics, for example, often have diffuse disease and present with digital or leg ulceration that requires complete revascularization to give their wounds a chance to heal. In cases with significant forefoot or heel gangrene that is caused by the compounding of moderate proximal disease and severe outflow obstruction, the best treatment is simultaneous inflow and outflow treatment to give the wound its best chance to heal. And in these cases, revascularization of at least one tibial artery, giving straight-line flow from the abdominal aorta into the foot, is the minimum requirement for most wound healing.

When the need for a combined procedure is less clear, certain preangiographic measurements can be utilized to aid in the decision-making process. Many people with multilevel disease have moderate proximal disease of unclear clinical consequence. Their pulses are normal but angiography later reveals stenosis. To assess the hemodynamics before angiography any one or more of the following can be used: noninvasive testing that measures Doppler-derived high thigh pressure, femoral artery pulsatility index, power spectrum analysis, femoral artery pulse volume recording, and color flow duplex scanning.[4,16,17] The duplex scan and Doppler-derived high thigh pressure have proved to be the most clinically useful due to their high sensitivity and specificity and, thus, are most often used.[17–19] When used in conjunction with preprocedure cross-sectional imaging (CTA and MRA), these tests can clarify the nature of multisegmental PAD.

PLANNING THE INTERVENTIONAL PROCEDURE

Before embarking on any endovascular therapy, a complete vascular assessment is paramount. In addition to a complete investigation of the target occlusion, it is important to have knowledge of any prior endovascular or surgical procedures. History of aortic bypass graft, kissing iliac stent placements, or other procedures that may preclude the contralateral approach will necessitate an ipsilateral or brachial/axillary approach. Proper history taking can thus prevent major access site complications and eliminate any unforeseen surprises.

To fully visualize, the target vasculature CTA or MRA should be scheduled prior to all procedures if possible. The exception is for those with severe chronic kidney disease (FIGURE 49.8 and FIGURE 49.9). In reviewing the imaging results, the operator should pay particular attention to the presence of calcium, location of collateral vessels, and the morphology of the lead-in vessels. This information can then be used to plan the wire approach to the target lesion and give some idea as to the therapy that may be needed, whether it is balloon angioplasty alone, stenting, percutaneous atherectomy, other endovascular therapy, open surgery, or a hybrid procedure. The distal runoff vessels should also be noted because improper distal flow is a factor known to compromise primary patency. Patients with two to three patent tibial vessels have significantly better long-term patency than those with no or one patent vessel.[20–24] In the case of poor distal flow, additional interventions may need to be planned to address limited distal patency.

Another important consideration in the treatment planning for outflow problems or infrageniculate vessels, especially in the case of diabetics with infected vascular ulcers, is the concept of angiosomes. First described by Taylor and Palmer in 1992, angiosomes are the vascular equivalent of dermatomes.[25] An angiosome is an anatomic unit of tissue (which has skin, subcutaneous tissue, fascia, muscle, and bone) fed by a source artery. There are six distinct angiosomes in the leg that originate from the anterior tibial, posterior tibial, and peroneal arteries. The artery that directly supplies the ischemic angiosome should be preferentially revascularized. The dorsal foot is fed by the anterior tibial artery, the plantar foot by the posterior tibial artery, the lateral foot by

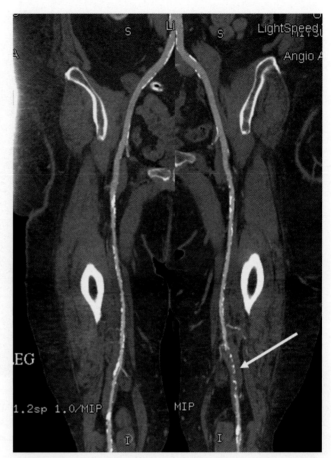

FIGURE 49.8 CTA of the pelvis and upper legs demonstrating 7 cm occlusion lower left SFA (*arrow*).

the peroneal artery, and the calcaneal region is fed from both the posterior tibial and peroneal arteries. A case where a progressive calcaneal ulcer leads to an amputation despite an excellent dorsalis pedis pulse demonstrates the importance of this concept. Simply reestablishing distal flow seems to be insufficient. Understanding the angiosome principle allows the interventionist to plan for a revascularization that directly optimizes the perfusion to the region of a particular wound for maximal healing.[26]

SPECIFIC INTRAPROCEDURAL TECHNIQUES

Like all other interventional procedures the approach to intraluminal recanalization in multilevel disease involves the classic CFA approach with a guide wire and catheter. The difference is that there are multiple lesions to traverse during the course of the procedure. Nonetheless, the methodology is the same and begins with pretreatment with clopidogrel and the use of 70 to 100 mg/kg of heparin during the procedure to maintain an activated clotting time greater than 250 seconds. A 0.014-, 0.018-, or 0.035-inch guide wire or hydrophilic guide wire is implemented to traverse the plaque-filled arterial lumen with the support of a catheter, hydrophilic glide catheter, or low-profile angioplasty balloon. The catheter becomes important when using the floppy guide wire to approach the hard cap that is usually present on the proximal end of an occlusive atherosclerotic lesion. The combination of a glide wire and glide catheters along with

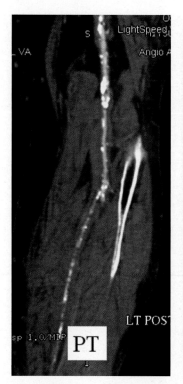
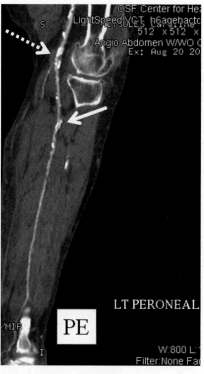
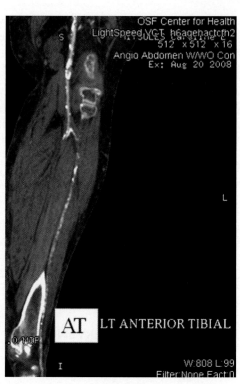

FIGURE 49.9 CTA of the popliteal and tibial arteries showing multilevel disease. The posterior tibial (PT) and anterior tibial (AT) arteries are diffusely calcified and occluded. The peroneal artery (PE) is patent with proximal calcified stenosis (*solid arrow*). The middle popliteal artery has a focal stenosis secondary to arteriosclerosis (*dashed arrow*).

the use of a twisting motion while advancing can result in the successful transversal of up to 95% of tight lesions.[27–29]

Once the proximal cap is penetrated, the catheter is advanced into the occlusion to give more support to the wire as it is used to completely cross the lesion. The wire will start to loop at this point but if the size of the loop exceeds the diameter of the vessel, it is signifying a subintimal dissection. The wire should be immediately drawn back into the catheter and the wire and catheter redirected and slowly readvanced. The tactile response from the wire and catheter helps the interventionist continue until the target lesion is crossed. Endovascular therapy can then be performed whether with low-profile monorail or coaxial balloons, percutaneous stenting, atherectomy, or other endovascular procedure. Care should be taken not to overdilate the artery and cause dissection and barotrauma.

Sometimes this classic approach is not successful and a subintimal route has to be used to cross a lesion. In 1990, Bolia et al.[30] first described the percutaneous intentional extraluminal recanalization (PIER) technique to cross difficult or chronically occluded vessels. The subintimal space is a potential space that provides little resistance to the wire as it is advanced and can be much easier than crossing a tight stenosis intraluminally, especially when they are longer than 5 cm.[31] This technique involves intentionally dissecting into the subintimal space, extending the dissection along the full length of the lesion in question, and then gaining reentry into the true lumen before using balloon angioplasty to tack open the newly created lumen. If the true lumen cannot be gained distal to the lesion, the wire is left in place and a direct attempt to access the lesion from its distal aspect in a retrograde fashion can be attempted.

Direct retrograde access from the dorsalis pedis, tibial, and popliteal arteries has been described as the "back door" access. Sometimes this approach can be advantageous and lead to traversal of an otherwise impassable lesion. Recently, sharp puncture into the true lumen has been made possible with the use of reentry catheters. There are several reentry catheters that are designed specifically to gain access from the subintimal space into the true lumen with use of an angled needle that accepts a 0.014-inch wire. These are the Outback LTD (Cordis Johnson & Johnson, Miami Lakes, FL) and the Pioneer (Medtronic, Minneapolis, MN) catheters. The Outback catheter has indicator marks on the device to allow fluoroscopic-guided steering of the needle toward the reconstituted true lumen. The Pioneer catheter uses an attached intravascular ultrasound probe to direct the needle toward the pulsatile reconstituted true lumen. With both devices, the angled needle allows placement of an exchange length 0.014-inch wire into the reconstituted true lumen of the artery, allowing treatment of the occluded segment. Antispasmodics are commonly used with approaches from distal arteries because these arteries are sensitive to manipulation. In cases where femoral access is not possible but a proximal lesion exists, the brachial or axillary approach can be utilized.

How does one treat calcaneal ulcers in patients with diffuse infrageniculate arterial disease? When there is only one patent artery but it is not in the appropriate angiosome distribution for wound healing, the plantar loop technique may be a last resort.[32] This involves advancing a microwire (0.014 inch) from the patent tibial artery anterior tibial (AT) or posterior tibial (PT), around the plantar arch, and into the occluded tibial artery supplying the angiosome in question. The wire will travel retrograde through the occluded artery and exit into the lower popliteal artery at which point the wire is snared or advanced through an indwelling catheter. This will allow wire exchange and treatment of the occluded tibial artery (AT or PT).

In sensitive areas where stenting is not desirable, such as behind the knee or in the smaller infrapatellar arteries, endovascular thrombectomy can be used to debulk the lesion before angioplasty is performed. This method has seen high technical success, and as a result numerous new atherectomy devices have infiltrated the market. Long-term primary patency has yet to be demonstrated, however. Four devices are available and are classified based on their mechanism of action. The SilverHawk (Covidien, Mansfield, MA) is a directional atherectomy device with a rotating cutter mounted in an angled catheter. As plaque is shaved off the arterial wall, it is packed into the nose cone of the catheter and then removed from the nose cone once the catheter is withdrawn from the patient. The catheter can then be reused as necessary until adequate luminal diameter is obtained. The Jetstream (Pathway, Redmond, WA) is a rotational atherectomy device with a spinning catheter with articulated tip-mounted cutting blades. The device rides over a guide wire and when spinning clockwise the cutting diameter is 2.1 mm, whereas when spinning counterclockwise the articulated blades project outward, cutting a diameter of 3 mm. There are aspiration ports proximal to the cutting blades to remove atherosclerotic particulates. The device is approved by the Food and Drug Administration (FDA) for atheroma and thrombus removal. The Diamondback (CSI, St. Paul, MN) is an orbital atherectomy device that runs over a wire with an eccentrically mounted cutter on a wire that is pneumatically spun at high revolutions per minute (RPM). The faster the spin, the greater the wobble or perturbation and the greater the diameter of the atherectomized channel. The high rate of spin breaks down the debris to sub-red blood cell size. With rotational and orbital devices the use of an intra-arterial vasodilator is desirable to prevent distal runoff vessel occlusion. The last available atherectomy device is the CVX-300 Excimer laser (Spectranetics, Colorado Springs, CO) and is a so-called cold-tipped laser. This device is approved for crossing CTOs in which guide wire access is not possible. The device exposes a xenon-chloride gas mixture to 15,000 volts generating extremely short high-energy bursts of photochemical, photothermal, and photomechanical energy that disrupt plaque, calcium, and thrombus, creating a channel in a previously narrowed or occluded vessel. It is important to advance the catheter very slowly (no faster than 0.5 to 1 mm per second) to prevent embolization. It is also important to use a laser catheter that is no greater than two-thirds the reference vessel in diameter to prevent vessel perforation.

ENDPOINT ASSESSMENT OF THE PROCEDURE

Assessing the effectiveness of a vascular procedure includes evaluation of vessel patency and patient-based assessments of changes in functional status and quality of life. Markers of success generally accepted by most interventionists include clinical improvement, hemodynamic improvement, patency, and freedom from amputation, stroke, death, myocardial infarction, and other accepted major adverse events. Although vessel patency and limb salvage are essential for proper evaluation, the

patient's improvement in functional status and quality of life must be considered equally when determining whether or not the appropriate treatment outcome has occurred.[33] If there has been no significant improvement in functional status, further objective assessment should be performed to determine whether additional intervention is warranted.

How to judge patency? A reconstructed arterial segment may be considered patent when any of the following criteria are met: demonstrated patent on conventional angiography, contrast-enhanced CTA, or MRA; maintenance of the achieved improvement in the appropriate segmental pressure index with no more than 0.10 drop from the highest postoperative index; maintenance of plethysmographic tracing distal to the reconstitution that is significantly greater in value than the preoperative value. This criterion is the weakest and only used when segmental pressures cannot be accurately obtained. In most cases, direct imaging is preferable; the presence of a palpable pulse or the recording of a biphasic or triphasic Doppler waveform at two points along the course of the artery or graft; direct observation of patency at operation or postmortem examination.[34]

With multisegment revascularizations close patient surveillance is indicated to appropriately reintervene when needed at the earliest possible point. This is achieved in part based on Doppler and imaging studies as well as regular monitoring of symptoms.

PROCEDURAL COMPLICATIONS AND THEIR MANAGEMENT

Major complications are limited to approximately 6% of cases and mostly consist of puncture site hematomas and acute occlusions, both of which can be particularly dangerous in older patients undergoing multilevel revascularization.[1,35] Because anticoagulation is a necessary component of these procedures, caution should be taken postoperatively and patients should be monitored closely for early signs of retroperitoneal or groin site hemorrhage.[36] Acute puncture site and treated vessel occlusions may need reintervention with suction embolectomy or thrombolysis, and symptomatic or expanding hematomas may need operative repair. Other complications include intracranial bleeding, embolization, and access-site infections.[37] Embolization can be particularly damaging if there is already downstream ischemic tissue damage present, so suction embolectomy is commonly implemented to chase any visualized emboli at the end of these procedures. Aspiration catheters range from 6 to 10 French devices with maximal distal end diameters from 1.3 to 3.25 mm and catheter lengths from 40 cm (dialysis graft use) to 145 cm. Most require a 0.014-inch exchange-length guide wire, and the 10 French device works over a 0.035-inch exchange-length guide wire. Infections are not very common, but when procedures are lengthy or infections are already present in any ulcers or wounds distally, antibiotics should be given preoperatively and continued postoperatively. Diabetic patients with calcified vessels are prone to arterial perforation, which may sometimes require coil embolization or balloon tamponade.[38] With commercially available covered stents, such as the Viabahn stent-graft (Gore Medical, Flagstaff, AZ), ICast (Atrium, Hudson, NH), and Wallgraft (Boston Scientific Corp, Boston, MA), large-vessel perforations can often be managed with an endovascular approach without surgical intervention. All of these complications are usually correctable but are associated with added costs.

■ AFTERMATH POST-TREATMENT

Currently no level I data evaluate the treatment of complex multilevel PAD using endovascular or hybrid therapies. Most patients with CLI have multilevel infrainguinal PAD. One-third of CLI patients will have isolated tibial disease. After revascularization for CLI, isolated tibial disease carries a worse prognosis (amputation-free survival, limb salvage, survival, maintenance of ambulation, and independent living status) compared with patients with multilevel infrainguinal PAD, despite the "greater" disease burden in these patients and despite no difference in primary patency rates out to 2 years after revascularization. Isolated tibial disease patients are more likely to have confounding factors, such as diabetes mellitus, renal disease, and worse ischemia at presentation than those with multilevel PAD. The recognition of isolated tibial disease may be helpful in identifying high-risk patients but is not an independent risk factor for poor outcomes.[39]

Technical success for percutaneous transluminal angioplasty (PTA) in the infrapopliteal circulation ranges from 78% to 100%, and primary patency at 1 year ranges from 13% to 81% and at 2 years from 48% to 78%.[24,31,40–47] The same studies have reported limb salvage rates at 1 year of 77% to 89%, a discrepancy that highlights that there is no direct correlation between long-term patency and clinical success. This means that patients continue to avoid amputation and feel no pain despite restenosis in their vessels, either due to collateralization or decreased tissue oxygen demand. It is known that an open ulcer has a higher oxygen demand than that required by the same tissue once the ulcer has healed, a fact that likely plays a part in the discrepancy between long-term patency and clinical success.[48]

Diabetics have a lower limb salvage rate by PTA than other groups of patients.[49–51] This may be caused by any number of factors that are important to wound healing and that are impaired in diabetic patients, including renal insufficiency, elevated lipoprotein levels, and the presence of gangrene.[40,52] These patients also have the heaviest and most diffuse atherosclerotic disease burden, which itself has a negative outcome on the procedure.[42]

Hybrid vascular procedures, combining open surgery and endovascular treatment of multilevel PAD during the same treating session, usually involve CFA endarterectomy combined with iliac and or infrainguinal angioplasty or recanalization. Single-center technical success of 98% and 5-year primary, primary-assisted, and secondary patencies of 60%, 97%, and 98%, respectively, have been reported.[53]

Because most patients with long-standing multilevel PAD live on the edge of inadequate blood flow for tissue maintenance, an acute technical success with improved blood flow without long-term durability allows for wound healing and downgrading on the Rutherford scale. Vascular reinterventions are common and can be complex but when performed judiciously will not preclude future endovascular or surgical treatment, as needed.

■ DISEASE SURVEILLANCE AND TREATMENT MONITORING

Patients with multilevel PAD have recurrent stenoses, occlusions, and disease progression despite early technical success. Close patient monitoring must be performed for adequate treatment response (wound healing, improved ambulation, resolution of ischemic rest pain). This usually involves serial office visits and noninvasive vascular testing. There is no consistent approach to long-term follow-up, however. After revascularization a baseline duplex ultrasound study with ankle brachial index (ABI) should be obtained within 30 days. The initial response to revascularization will be monitored by symptomatic improvement and improvement in hemodynamic testing. A persistent increase in ABI greater than 0.1 is considered significant. The timing of scheduled follow-ups will depend on the extent and complexity of the vascular procedures performed and the clinical presentation. Patients with CLI should be scheduled for short interval office follow-up with duplex and ABI testing to ensure adequate response to the revascularization procedure and appropriate wound healing. Patients treated for intermittent claudication are scheduled for office visits and noninvasive vascular testing at extended time periods. Duplex ultrasound imaging is obtained for patients who have been stented or who have undergone bypass surgeries to evaluate for the development of hemodynamically significant neointimal hyperplasia within the stents or at the proximal and distal anastomoses of the bypass graft. Patients with long femoropopliteal stent-grafts are monitored closely to discern hemodynamically significant edge stenosis before stent-graft thrombosis occurs, which can present as acute limb-threatening ischemia. At the author's institution all vascular patients are initially seen in the office within 1 to 3 months, depending on the complexity of the procedure, and then followed at 6-month intervals for at least 2 years. Although arguable, at each office visit the patient undergoes evaluation of the ABI with treadmill exercise testing when possible, and the results are compared to baseline postoperative values. Duplex ultrasound imaging of all implanted stents is performed, as mentioned earlier. Patients with implanted bare metal stents and short-length stent-grafts are intervened upon when the patient becomes symptomatic. Recurrent stenosis is considered hemodynamically significant (>50% stenosis) when the peak systolic velocity is 2.5 times greater than the reference vessel peak systolic velocity. Patients with implanted long-length stent-grafts are placed into graft surveillance for serial duplex ultrasound imaging. When duplex imaging indicates greater than 50% stenosis at the proximal or distal margins of the stent-graft, further evaluation is performed with CTA or MRA for confirmation prior to intervening. Intervention is performed when there is greater than 50% diameter stenosis because longer stent-grafts may fail in the absence of clinical deterioration. The failure mode of stent-grafts is similar to bypass grafts with acute in situ thrombosis and limb-threatening ischemia.

■ EARLY FAILURES AND THEIR MANAGEMENT

Early treatment failures of complex recanalizations are similar to single-level revascularizations but occur more frequently due to the extensive nature of tandem repairs.

With angioplasty early failures are related to barotrauma, vascular recoil, vessel rupture, and discontinuation of the internal elastic lamina, resulting in flow-limiting dissection. Bare metal stenting has largely resolved vessel recoil and dissection, and covered stents can repair large vessel perforation. However, stenting leaves a foreign body in place with the downstream risk of neointimal hyperplasia and recurrent stenosis or occlusion, including the risk of stent fracture, especially in the femoropopliteal segment.

Atherectomy has the risk of embolization with tibial vessel occlusion. Kaid et al.[54] treated 15 consecutive patients with directional atherectomy and found debris within the embolic protection device in 14 of the 15 cases (93%) and large debris in 7 of the 15 cases (47%).

The liberal use of intra-arterial antispasmodics, such as nitroglycerin and verapamil, and the judicious use of filter wires, can reduce tibial occlusions.

Early failures with stenting include subacute in-stent thrombosis and persistent stenosis. Subacute in-stent thrombosis is usually seen in long-segment stenting and can be prevented with the use of an oral antiplatelet regimen postrevascularization. Persistent stenosis after stenting is found in lesions with dense circumferential fibrocalcific plaque, resulting in recoil. In cases of inappropriate stent selection incomplete vessel wall apposition of the stent to the wall of the artery will reduce primary patency. Balloon-expandable stents are recommended for origin stenoses because they tend to be heavily calcified, and self-expanding stents are recommended for nonostial and femoropopliteal stenoses.

Unrecognized hemodynamically significant lesions are another cause of early treatment failure. Adequate imaging during treatment with digital subtraction angiography and orthogonal views is vital to identifying and appropriately assessing stenoses. Post-treatment subtraction angiography will also identify acute treatment failures, allowing for immediate repair. Angiographic borderline lesions can be assessed for hemodynamic significance with pullback pressure gradient evaluation, and a mean pressure drop of 5-mm mercury is considered hemodynamically significant. Pullback pressure measures in smaller arteries may not be attainable due to the pressure gradient introduced by the catheter itself. A PressureWire (St. Jude Medical) has a diameter of 0.014 inch and is better for obtaining pressure gradient measurements in smaller vessels.

Because hybrid procedures use endovascular and surgical therapies, early failures can be a result of operative and endovascular causes. Surgical reexploration may be warranted depending on etiology of failure.

Infection is a rare cause of treatment failure but needs to be investigated in the appropriate clinical setting of fever, leukocytosis, elevated c-reactive protein, erythrocyte sedimentation rate, access site erythema, swelling, exquisite tenderness, and presence of foreign body, including arterial closure device, bypass graft, or stent.

If failure is suspected, hemodynamic evaluation with ABI and duplex ultrasound imaging is performed. Abnormal results can be followed up with cross-sectional imaging with CTA and MRA, as needed. This will help in determining the location and extent of treatment failure and assist in operative planning.

LATE FAILURES AND THEIR MANAGEMENT

Late failures are usually caused by neointimal hyperplasia, progression of atherosclerotic disease, or a combination of the two. Close clinical surveillance with hemodynamic monitoring will often pick up stenoses and disease progression before graft or vessel occlusion occurs. Once stenosis of a bypass graft, stent, or treated artery is suspected, cross-sectional imaging with CTA or MRA can be obtained to better evaluate the underlying pathology. Based on clinical and anatomic findings, close surveillance monitoring or reintervention can be planned.

PRACTICAL ADVANTAGES AND LIMITATIONS

Endovascular therapies are considered low-risk procedures that rarely compromise later surgical procedures and preserve the saphenous vein for future coronary or lower extremity

bypass should the need arise.[55] They also avoid general anesthesia, which is hazardous to many of the patients who need treatment for multilevel PAD. The hospital stays associated with endovascular procedures are considerably shorter than those associated with open bypass surgery.[56] Additionally, endovascular treatment can be easily repeated when needed, whereas surgical reintervention is more difficult. These reasons make a compelling argument to disregard surgical therapy and proceed only with the endovascular approach. However, the fact remains that surgical management can achieve greater long-term patency and remains the gold standard for treatment of diffusely diseased vessels.

RELATIVE THERAPEUTIC EFFECTIVENESS COMPARED TO SURGERY

There have been no direct head-to-head trial between endovascular and surgical procedures in multilevel lower extremity disease but success rates from both types of therapy can be compared. Limb salvage rates at 1 year are very comparable between the two approaches, 81% to 88% for surgery and 77% to 89% for PTA.[47,57,58] After 1 year, bypass grafting is clearly more successful than PTA; however, up to one-third of these grafts have to be intervened on to maintain patency.[59]

PTA has a lower mortality rate, which is estimated to be near 1.7% at 30 days, compared with bypass surgery, which ranges from 1.8% to 6%.[60–63] This group of patients is at high risk of mortality from cardiovascular disease. Of this group of patients, 25% end up with amputations despite surgical attempts at revascularization, possibly caused by a lack of attention to angiosomes.[64] Studies have shown that patients that have successful revascularization of their diseased arteries go on to survive longer however, and with a higher quality of life than those who get amputations.[59,65] For this reason alone, tailored endovascular therapy should be attempted whenever possible to try to reestablish blood flow to the proper vascular territory in the ischemic legs of every one of these patients. When there are numerous comorbidities, no distal vessels available for bypass, or superficial leg infections present that prohibit surgery, endovascular management is the only therapeutic option available for these patients. And even in cases where amputation cannot be avoided, lesser amputations may be possible if partial revascularization can be achieved.

Hybrid procedures are an exciting, emerging tactic in treating complex multilevel disease. They are a viable alternative to more invasive open procedures both in terms of decreasing perioperative complications and increasing long-term patency. Early data suggest that primary patency rates may be lower than open surgical procedures; however, many patients enjoy continued patency with only percutaneous reintervention. Overall, the hybrid procedure is well tolerated. Additionally, many of these patients would not be candidates for abdominal revascularization procedures and would benefit from the shortened hospital stay and overall decreased trauma of a limited groin exposure.[53]

THE FUTURE

The next generation of interventionists will be able to rely on newer technology that was developed to deal with the challenges being faced today. There are already some hints at what the future may hold as innovative new devices are being released. For example, there are currently two reentry devices on the market in the United States for the subintimal recanalization technique. When initially described, reentry into the true lumen of the vessel after subintimal dissection relied on angled catheters and wires, but now an ultrasound-guided catheter, Pioneer (Medtronic, Santa Rosa, CA), and a fluoroscopically oriented catheter, Outback (Cordis Johnson & Johnson), are both available to aid in the process by providing better visualization.

As mentioned earlier, debulking or atherectomy devices are being developed to decrease the plaque burden before PTA or stenting. This has the benefit of preventing barotrauma from overdilation and also can lessen the risk of acute recoil or excessive neointimal formation after stent implantation. Device manufacturers have taken new and unique approaches to creating these tools with rotational aspiration, high speed, orbital, and laser atherectomy mechanism of actions.[66] Each of these devices will remove plaque but studies need to be conducted on their long-term effectiveness. So-called plaque modification with atherectomy devices, that is, to prep the vessel, may assist with adjuvant therapies with drug-coated balloons, drug-eluting stents (DES), and simple low-pressure angioplasty.

The potential advantage that DES may have over bare metal stents was not validated by the SIROCCO I and II trials.[67,68] Recent data from the Zilver PTX randomized trial was shown to reduce SFA restenosis rate by 50%, however. Zilver PTX combines mechanical and drug therapies using the Zilver nitinol stent (Cook Medical) with a polymer-free paclitaxel coating.[69] Drug-eluting balloons (DEB) are very exciting technologies that have become available in recent years, and based on the early randomized experience from the THUNDER study[70] and the FemPac study,[71] there is a lot of interest and promise for this technology. In fact, both studies have shown a significant reduction in neointimal proliferation for the paclitaxel/iopromide-coated balloon as compared to standard balloon dilatation, measured by late lumen loss at 6 months. Moreover, standard efficacy parameters, such as binary restenosis and target lesion revascularization (TLR) rates, showed a significant and sustained improvement with this new technology up to 2 years. Nevertheless, because the efficacy of a DEB may largely depend on the dose and formulation of the active coating, no general conclusions can be made for different DEB devices. It will be mandatory in the future that efficacy and safety data are provided for each commercially available product. Their use in complex multilevel PAD is strongly anticipated.

Lastly, hybrid procedures combining the "best of both" open and endovascular therapies are exciting, and preliminary studies have shown high technical success rates and good long-term durability. As techniques develop and devices are made specifically for this niche market, we should anticipate that more patients will be treated in a hybrid fashion.

CONCLUSION

As the population ages and the prevalence of obesity and diabetes in the population rises, the number of patients with multilevel complex PAD will increase as well. This will necessitate the continued improvement of endovascular and hybrid techniques for the management of complex multilevel lower extremity arterial disease.

REFERENCES

1. Dormandy JA, Rutherford RB. Management of peripheral arterial disease (PAD). TASC working group. TransAtlantic inter-society consensus (TASC). J Vasc Surg 2000;31(1, pt 2):S1–S296.
2. Norgren L, Hiatt WR, Dormandy JA, et al. Inter-society consensus for the management of peripheral arterial disease (TASC II). J Vasc Surg 2007;45(suppl S):S5–S67.
3. Stoyioglou A, Jaff MR. Medical treatment of peripheral arterial disease: a comprehensive review. J Vasc Interv Radiol 2004;15(11):1197–1207.
4. Moneta GL, Yeager RA, Taylor LM Jr, et al. Hemodynamic assessment of combined aortoiliac/femoropopliteal occlusive disease and selection of single or multilevel revascularization. Semin Vasc Surg 1994;7(1):3–10.
5. Bernstein EF, Fronek A. Current status of noninvasive tests in the diagnosis of peripheral arterial disease. Surg Clin North Am 1982;62(3):473–487.
6. Collins GJ Jr, Rich NM, Andersen CA, et al. Staged aortofemoropopliteal revascularization. Arch Surg 1978;113(2):149–152.
7. Antoniou GA, Sfyroeras GS, Karathanos C, et al. Hybrid endovascular and open treatment of severe multilevel lower extremity arterial disease. Eur J Vasc Endovasc Surg 2009;38(5):616–622.
8. Chang RW, Goodney PP, Baek JH, et al. Long-term results of combined common femoral endarterectomy and iliac stenting/stent grafting for occlusive disease. J Vasc Surg 2008;48(2):362–367.
9. Lantis J, Jensen M, Benvenisty A, et al. Outcomes of combined superficial femoral endovascular revascularization and popliteal to distal bypass for patients with tissue loss. Ann Vasc Surg 2008;22(3):366–371.
10. Timaran CH, Ohki T, Gargiulo NJ, III, et al. Iliac artery stenting in patients with poor distal runoff: influence of concomitant infrainguinal arterial reconstruction. J Vasc Surg 2003;38(3):479–484; discussion 484–485.
11. Cotroneo AR, Iezzi R, Marano G, et al. Hybrid therapy in patients with complex peripheral multifocal steno-obstructive vascular disease: two-year results. Cardiovasc Intervent Radiol 2007;30(3):355–361.
12. Smouse HB, Nikanorov A, LaFlash D. Biomechanical forces in the femoropopliteal arterial segment. Endovasc Today 2005;(6):60–66.
13. Arena FJ. Arterial kink and damage in normal segments of the superficial femoral and popliteal arteries abutting nitinol stents—a common cause of late occlusion and restenosis? A single-center experience. J Invasive Cardiol 2005;17(9):482–486.
14. Schajer GS, Green SI, Davis AP, et al. Influence of elastic nonlinearity on arterial anastomotic compliance. J Biomech Eng 1996;118(4):445–451.
15. Blevins WA Jr, Schneider PA. Endovascular management of critical limb ischemia. Eur J Vasc Endovasc Surg 2010;39(6):756–761.
16. O'Donnell TF Jr, Lahey SJ, Kelly JJ, et al. A prospective study of Doppler pressures and segmental plethysmography before and following aortofemoral bypass. Implications for predicting success and for adopting a uniform method of classifying arterial disease. Surgery 1979;86(1):120–129.
17. Kohler TR, Nance DR, Cramer MM, et al. Duplex scanning for diagnosis of aortoiliac and femoropopliteal disease: a prospective study. Circulation 1987;76(5):1074–1080.
18. Legemate DA, Teeuwen C, Hoeneveld H, et al. How can the assessment of the hemodynamic significance of aortoiliac arterial stenosis by duplex scanning be improved? A comparative study with intraarterial pressure measurement. J Vasc Surg 1993;17(4):676–684.
19. Langsfeld M, Nepute J, Hershey FB, et al. The use of deep duplex scanning to predict hemodynamically significant aortoiliac stenoses. J Vasc Surg 1988;7(3):395–399.
20. Gallino A, Mahler F, Probst P, et al. Percutaneous transluminal angioplasty of the arteries of the lower limbs: a 5 year follow-up. Circulation 1984;70(4):619–623.
21. Darling RC, Linton RR. Durability of femoropopliteal reconstructions. endarterectomy versus vein bypass grafts. Am J Surg 1972;123(4):472–479.
22. Jeans WD, Armstrong S, Cole SE, et al. Fate of patients undergoing transluminal angioplasty for lower-limb ischemia. Radiology 1990;177(2):559–564.
23. Hunink MG, Wong JB, Donaldson MC, et al. Patency results of percutaneous and surgical revascularization for femoropopliteal arterial disease. Med Decis Making 1994;14(1):71–81.
24. Varty K, Bolia A, Naylor AR, et al. Infrapopliteal percutaneous transluminal angioplasty: a safe and successful procedure. Eur J Vasc Endovasc Surg 1995;9(3):341–345.
25. Taylor GI, Palmer JH. Angiosome theory. Br J Plast Surg 1992;45(4):327–328.
26. Neville RF, Attinger CE, Bulan EJ, et al. Revascularization of a specific angiosome for limb salvage: does the target artery matter? Ann Vasc Surg 2009;23(3):367–373.

27. Leville CD, Kashyap VS, Clair DG, et al. Endovascular management of iliac artery occlusions: extending treatment to TransAtlantic Inter-society Consensus class C and D patients. *J Vasc Surg* 2006;43(1):32–39.

28. Giles KA, Pomposelli FB, Spence TL, et al. Infrapopliteal angioplasty for critical limb ischemia: relation of TransAtlantic InterSociety Consensus class to outcome in 176 limbs. *J Vasc Surg* 2008;48(1):128–136.

29. Dosluoglu HH, Cherr GS, Harris LM, et al. Rheolytic thrombectomy, angioplasty, and selective stenting for subacute isolated popliteal artery occlusions. *J Vasc Surg* 2007;46(4):717–723.

30. Bolia A, Miles KA, Brennan J, et al. Percutaneous transluminal angioplasty of occlusions of the femoral and popliteal arteries by subintimal dissection. *Cardiovasc Intervent Radiol* 1990;13(6):357–363.

31. Bolia A, Sayers RD, Thompson MM, et al. Subintimal and intraluminal recanalisation of occluded crural arteries by percutaneous balloon angioplasty. *Eur J Vasc Surg* 1994;8(2):214–219.

32. Fusaro M, Dalla Paola L, Biondi-Zoccai G. Pedal-plantar loop technique for a challenging below-the-knee chronic total occlusion: a novel approach to percutaneous revascularization in critical lower limb ischemia. *J Invasive Cardiol* 2007;19(2):E34–E37.

33. Rutherford RB. Essential considerations in evaluating the results of treatment. In: Rutherford RB, ed. *Vascular Surgery.* 6th ed. Philadelphia, PA: Elsevier Saunders; 2005:21–30.

34. Dayal R, Kent KC. Standardized reporting practices. In: Rutherford RB, ed. *Vascular Surgery.* 6th ed. Philadelphia, PA: Elsevier Saunders; 2005:41–52.

35. Heintzen MP, Strauer BE. Peripheral arterial complications after heart catheterization [in German]. *Herz* 1998;23(1):4–20.

36. Michalis LK, Rees MR, Patsouras D, et al. A prospective randomized trial comparing the safety and efficacy of three commercially available closure devices (angioseal, vasoseal and duett). *Cardiovasc Intervent Radiol* 2002;25(5):423–429.

37. Dosluoglu HH, Harris LM. Endovascular management of subacute lower extremity ischemia. *Semin Vasc Surg* 2008;21(4):167–179.

38. Hayes PD, Chokkalingam A, Jones R, et al. Arterial perforation during infrainguinal lower limb angioplasty does not worsen outcome: results from 1409 patients. *J Endovasc Ther* 2002;9(4):422–427.

39. Gray BH, Grant AA, Kalbaugh CA, et al. The impact of isolated tibial disease on outcomes in the critical limb ischemic population. *Ann Vasc Surg* 2010;24(3):349–359. Epub 2010 Jan 4.

40. Soder HK, Manninen HI, Jaakkola P, et al. Prospective trial of infrapopliteal artery balloon angioplasty for critical limb ischemia: angiographic and clinical results. *J Vasc Interv Radiol* 2000;11(8):1021–1031.

41. Dorros G, Jaff MR, Murphy KJ, et al. The acute outcome of tibioperoneal vessel angioplasty in 417 cases with claudication and critical limb ischemia. *Cathet Cardiovasc Diagn* 1998;45(3):251–256.

42. Bull PG, Mendel H, Hold M, et al. Distal popliteal and tibioperoneal transluminal angioplasty: long-term follow-up. *J Vasc Interv Radiol* 1992;3(1):45–53.

43. Buckenham TM, Loh A, Dormandy JA, et al. Infrapopliteal angioplasty for limb salvage. *Eur J Vasc Surg* 1993;7(1):21–25.

44. Matsi PJ, Manninen HI, Suhonen MT, et al. Chronic critical lower-limb ischemia: prospective trial of angioplasty with 1–36 months follow-up. *Radiology* 1993;188(2):381–387.

45. Lofberg AM, Lorelius LE, Karacagil S, et al. The use of below-knee percutaneous transluminal angioplasty in arterial occlusive disease causing chronic critical limb ischemia. *Cardiovasc Intervent Radiol* 1996;19(5):317–322.

46. Parsons RE, Suggs WD, Lee JJ, et al. Percutaneous transluminal angioplasty for the treatment of limb threatening ischemia: do the results justify an attempt before bypass grafting? *J Vasc Surg* 1998;28(6):1066–1071.

47. London NJ, Varty K, Sayers RD, et al. Percutaneous transluminal angioplasty for lower-limb critical ischaemia. *Br J Surg* 1995;82(9):1232–1235.

48. Reekers JA. Percutaneous intentional extraluminal (subintimal) revascularization (PIER) for critical lower limb ischemia: too good to be true? *J Endovasc Ther* 2002;9(4):419–421.

49. Vainio E, Salenius JP, Lepantalo M, et al. Endovascular surgery for chronic limb ischaemia. Factors predicting immediate outcome on the basis of a nationwide vascular registry. *Ann Chir Gynaecol* 2001;90(2):86–91.

50. Danielsson G, Albrechtsson U, Norgren L, et al. Percutaneous transluminal angioplasty of crural arteries: diabetes and other factors influencing outcome. *Eur J Vasc Endovasc Surg* 2001;21(5):432–436.

51. Mlekusch W, Schillinger M, Sabeti S, et al. Clinical outcome and prognostic factors for ischaemic ulcers treated with PTA in lower limbs. *Eur J Vasc Endovasc Surg* 2002;24(2):176–181.

52. Brillu C, Picquet J, Villapadierna F, et al. Percutaneous transluminal angioplasty for management of critical ischemia in arteries below the knee. *Ann Vasc Surg* 2001;15(2):175–181.

53. Chang RW, Goodney PP, Baek JH, et al. Long-term results of combined common femoral endarterectomy and iliac stenting/stent grafting for occlusive disease. *J Vasc Surg* 2008;48(2):362–367.

54. Kaid KA, Gopinathapillai R, Qian F, et al. Analysis of particulate debris after superficial femoral artery atherectomy. *J Invasive Cardiol* 2009;21(1):7–10.

55. Isner JM, Rosenfield K. Redefining the treatment of peripheral artery disease. Role of percutaneous revascularization. *Circulation* 1993;88(4, pt 1):1534–1557.

56. Holm J, Arfvidsson B, Jivegard L, et al. Chronic lower limb ischaemia. A prospective randomised controlled study comparing the 1-year results of vascular surgery and percutaneous transluminal angioplasty (PTA). *Eur J Vasc Surg* 1991;5(5):517–522.

57. Ballard JL, Killeen JD, Smith LL. Popliteal-tibial bypass grafts in the management of limb-threatening ischemia. *Arch Surg* 1993;128(9):976–980; discussion 980–981.

58. Biancari F, Kantonen I, Alback A, et al. Popliteal-to-distal bypass grafts for critical leg ischaemia. *J Cardiovasc Surg (Torino)* 2000;41(2):281–286.

59. Kalra M, Gloviczki P, Bower TC, et al. Limb salvage after successful pedal bypass grafting is associated with improved long-term survival. *J Vasc Surg* 2001;33(1):6–16.

60. Nehler MR, Moneta GL, Edwards JM, et al. Surgery for chronic lower extremity ischemia in patients eighty or more years of age: operative results and assessment of postoperative independence. *J Vasc Surg* 1993;18(4):618–624; discussion 624–626.

61. Pomposelli FB Jr, Marcaccio EJ, Gibbons GW, et al. Dorsalis pedis arterial bypass: durable limb salvage for foot ischemia in patients with diabetes mellitus. *J Vasc Surg* 1995;21(3):375–384.

62. Belli AM, Cumberland DC, Knox AM, et al. The complication rate of percutaneous peripheral balloon angioplasty. *Clin Radiol* 1990;41(6):380–383.

63. Wengerter KR, Veith FJ, Gupta SK, et al. Prospective randomized multicenter comparison of in situ and reversed vein infrapopliteal bypasses. *J Vasc Surg* 1991;13(2):189–197; discussion 197–199.

64. Dormandy JA. Rationale for antiplatelet therapy in patients with atherothrombotic disease. *Vasc Med* 1998;3(3):253–255.

65. Klevsgard R, Risberg BO, Thomsen MB, et al. A 1-year follow-up quality of life study after hemodynamically successful or unsuccessful surgical revascularization of lower limb ischemia. *J Vasc Surg* 2001;33(1):114–122.

66. Laird JR Jr, Reiser C, Biamino G, et al. Excimer laser assisted angioplasty for the treatment of critical limb ischemia. *J Cardiovasc Surg (Torino)* 2004;45(3):239–248.

67. Duda SH, Bosiers M, Lammer J, et al. Drug-eluting and bare nitinol stents for the treatment of atherosclerotic lesions in the superficial femoral artery: long-term results from the SIROCCO trial. *J Endovasc Ther* 2006; 13(6):701–710.

68. Duda SH, Bosiers M, Lammer J, et al. Sirolimus-eluting versus bare nitinol stent for obstructive superficial femoral artery disease: the SIROCCO II trial. *J Vasc Interv Radiol* 2005;16(3):331–338.

69. Dake M. The Zilver PTX randomized trial of paclitaxel-eluting stents for femoropopliteal disease: 24-month update. Presented at: 7th edition of the Leipzig Interventional Course (LINC) 2011; January 19–22, 2011; Leipzig, Germany.

70. Werk M, Langner S, Reinkensmeier B, et al. Inhibition of restenosis in femoropopliteal arteries: paclitaxel-coated versus uncoated balloon: femoral paclitaxel randomized pilot trial. *Circulation* 2008;118:1358–1365.

71. Tepe G, Zeller T, Albrecht T, et al. Local delivery of paclitaxel to inhibit restenosis during angioplasty of the left leg. *N Engl J Med* 2008;358: 689–699.

Management of Acute Thromboembolic Events in Lower Extremity Interventions

MAHMOOD K. RAZAVI

INTRODUCTION

The number of patients with symptomatic peripheral arterial disease is on the rise due to factors, such as the changing demographics of the populations and increasing prevalence of metabolic disorders. With progressive improvement in techniques and outcome, endovascular approaches are now the dominant mode of treatment for these patients. As the number of endovascular procedures increases, so does the number of procedural complications. As such, acute thromboembolic events (ATE), an uncommon but well-recognized complication of peripheral endovascular interventions, are also on the rise and considered to be an emerging challenge.

The clinical significance of ATE in terms of worsening of symptoms or the outcome of intervention, however, is not well studied in the lower limbs. Although showering of emboli with occlusion of the terminal arterial branches in the foot is considered a poor outcome, the significance of the loss of a tibial artery in a patient with more than one-vessel runoff is not as clear. Similarly, embolic occlusion of a severely stenotic and well-collateralized segment of a vessel during or after an intervention may not produce immediate additional symptoms. Good interventional technique, however, mandates searching for and treating angiographically visible distal embolization.

The risk factors, detection, prevention, and treatment strategies for ATE are reviewed in this chapter. The technical details of treating patients with ATE are beyond the scope of this writing and readers are referred to previous publications on the subject.[1,2]

INCIDENCE AND SIGNIFICANCE OF ACUTE THROMBOEMBOLIC EVENTS

ATE is an uncommon complication of endovascular techniques. The incidence of ATE rises with the increasing complexity of the lesion and intervention. The expected clinical outcome of thromboembolic complications is also poorer in patients with more advanced disease. Although the overall risk of ATE is low, the number of events is expected to grow. Factors contributing to this trend include interventional management of more complicated lesions, such as chronic total occlusions (CTOs) of native and stented vessels, and increasing use of complex tools, such as atherectomy devices.

In a single center registry, the severity of lesions, presence of thrombus, and prior amputation, all indicators of advanced disease, were predictors of distal embolization in peripheral

interventions.[3] Lam et al.[4] studied the rate of ATE during superficial femoral artery (SFA) interventions in a relatively small number of patients. Ipsilateral popliteal arteries were continuously monitored using 4-MHz Doppler probes during the procedures. Although they observed embolic signals during all phases of the interventions, they reported only one case of angiographically and clinically significant distal embolization.[4] In a larger retrospective analysis from the same institution, an overall distal embolization rate of 1.6% was observed after SFA interventions.[5] Rotational atherectomy had a higher risk of distal embolization as compared to angioplasty and stenting (22% vs. 0.7%). Anatomic features associated with ATE in this study included CTOs, in-stent restenosis, and TASC-II C and D lesions. Measures of outcome reported included primary and secondary patency as well as limb salvage rates. Interestingly, the clinical outcome of patients with and without distal embolization was not significantly different in this study.[5] It should be noted that 34 patients with distal emboli were treated using various techniques and flow was reestablished in 32 of them.

Conversely, Davies and colleagues[6] in a retrospective analysis of their experience reported that distal embolization during SFA interventions resulted in a significantly lower limb salvage and freedom from recurrent symptoms. They observed an overall distal embolization rate of 3.8% and in situ thrombosis rate of 3.5% with female gender being a risk factor for both. In situ thrombosis was associated with lower patency rates in the same study.[6]

All publications specifically studying ATE show that it is a complication associated with lower limb arterial interventions. The rate is widely variable depending on the definition of distal embolization used in the study, the methods employed to diagnose it, and the technique and technologies utilized for revascularization. The clinical significance of procedural ATE, however, is not well studied or reported in the literature. Prudence dictates to search for and treat all such events when detected.

PREDISPOSING FACTORS TO ACUTE THROMBOEMBOLIC EVENTS

Interventions for Acute Limb Ischemia

Catheter-based interventions for acute limb ischemia are one of the most common causes of distal embolization. During catheter-directed thrombolytic therapy (CDT) partial flow may be established as a result of the therapy with residual clot migrating downstream. This phenomenon can temporarily occlude either the collateral flow or the previously patent runoff vessels into the foot causing exacerbation of symptoms. No specific additional therapy is necessary unless profound ischemia is noted. Flow is usually reestablished with continuation of thrombolytic therapy. The incidence of permanent embolization with angiographic loss of runoff vessels during CDT is reported to be between 7% and 12%.[7,8] This is likely an underestimate because asymptomatic distal emboli occur during the management of an acute clot but the data are neither captured nor reported due to the asymptomatic nature of the events. Similarly, distal embolization with segmental or total loss of a tibial vessel may remain initially asymptomatic due to the presence of other runoff vessels. It should be noted, however, that asymptomatic distal embolization is not a benign event. Lower rates of limb salvage, primary and secondary patency, and freedom from recurrent symptoms have been reported in association with procedure-related ATE as discussed previously.[6]

Another common cause of distal embolization in patients who have undergone CDT for acute limb ischemia is angioplasty or debulking of underlying lesions "uncovered" after thrombolysis. Angiographic stenoses after CDT may contain or entirely comprise organized thrombus and angioplasty could dislodge and cause its migration downstream. Treatment of such lesions can be performed using an embolic capture device to prevent ATE. In case it occurs, it can be retrieved by aspiration embolectomy or further CDT (see next).

Crossing and Treatment of Chronic Total Occlusions

Crossing CTOs in iliac and superficial femoral arteries has also been associated with ATE. In occluded arterial segments there is usually organized athrothrombotic debris that may not be adherent to vessel wall. Studies have shown that these particles consist of platelet and fibrin aggregates with or without trapped erythrocytes and inflammatory cells, cholesterol crystals, and extracellular matrix. Reestablishment of flow through channels filled with such unattached debris could release them into the distal circulation.

Older studies on recanalization of occluded iliac arteries reported high rates of ATE but more contemporary publications indicate rates as low as 2.5% to 4.1%.[9,10] As might be expected, however, studies using embolic protection device (EPD) report a much higher rate of embolic detection in filters during aortoiliac interventions. Karnabatidis et al.[11] reported the capture of particles greater than 1 mm in 58% and greater than 3 mm in 12% of their infraaortic interventions using distal protection devices. Similar to other studies, CTOs, acute thrombosis interventions, and long lesions all correlated with increased ATE.

In the SFA the reported rates of ATE are widely varied, ranging from 1.6% to 90%.[4,12] As discussed earlier, this variability stems from inconsistent definitions of embolization and nonstandard thresholds for treating it. Some authors suggest that any Doppler signal during continuous sonographic monitoring or capture of any debris in an EPD constitutes "distal embolization." Others consider the development of clinical symptoms or angiographic loss of a runoff vessel as the only indication of significant embolization. In the study by Müller-Hülsbeck et al.[12] using EPDs, 90% of devices contained debris ranging from 90 to

2,000 microns after SFA interventions. Although larger particles as reported by Karnabatidis have a high likelihood of occluding runoff vessels, it is unclear if microscopic debris generated during routine interventions have any clinical sequelae in lower extremities.

Recanalization of Occluded Stents and Stent-Grafts

The most common cause of stent failure in lower extremities is neointimal tissue ingrowth or stent-adjacent lesions. As such, presence of material with embolic potential is typically discounted during interventions for occluded stents. Clot at various stages of organization, however, could exist, especially in totally occluded stent-grafts or recently occluded stents of any kind. Time of onset of symptoms and the tactile feeling during the passage of wire through a previously stented segment should provide clues as to the likelihood of presence of mobile thrombus. Acute and subacute clot are usually softer and more easily crossed. In such cases recanalization without preventive measures may lead to macroscopic thromboembolism. Use of aspiration devices, EPDs, or pharmacomechanical thrombolysis should be considered prior to maneuvers, such as angioplasty or atherectomy.

Atherectomy and Debulking Devices

Use of some atherectomy or debulking devices may also increase the risk of distal embolization during lower extremity revascularization.[4,5,13–16] These studies report capture of macroscopic debris in a large number of EPDs with all of the currently available devices including the SilverHawk atherectomy (ev3/Covidien, Minneapolis, MN), excimer laser ablation (Spectranetics, Colorado Springs, CO), Jetstream (Pathway Medical, Kirkland, WA), and Diamondback orbital atherectomy (Cardiovascular Systems Inc., St. Paul, MN). In studies not using EPD, the reported rates of distal embolization range from 0% to 22%.[4,17,18] This variability may be indicative of the learning curve associated with each individual device as well as other factors alluded to earlier. Centers with more experience with one device tend to report lower embolization rates than others. Although bias toward a center's or operator's "favorite" device cannot be excluded in these publications, device experience is clearly beneficial in reducing the complication rates.

In addition to device experience, it appears that the length and complexity of the lesion increases the risk of ATE during debulking procedures as well. This can be minimized by careful attention to appropriate patient selection, use of EPDs, and overcoming the learning curve for these technologies.

DETECTION OF PROCEDURAL THROMBOEMBOLIC EVENTS

The diagnostic method used to detect ATE has a significant impact on its reported incidence. Using continuous Doppler ultrasound, Lam et al.[4] observed embolic signals in 100% of their patients undergoing lower extremity arterial interventions. Embolic signals were detected during every stage of the procedures including wire passage, balloon angioplasty, stenting, atherectomy, and so on. The number of signals was proportionally higher during plaque excision and debulking. Despite this finding, only 1 of 60 patients in this analysis suffered from what was considered "clinically significant" distal embolization by the authors. Studies using EPDs report a similarly high percentage of captured debris and particulate material.[12–16] The clinical relevance of distal embolization, however, has only been partially validated when the loss of antegrade flow is detected by contrast angiography.[6] It should be noted that in studies reporting angiographic loss of a named distal vessel, successful attempts at reestablishment of flow were made in the majority of cases.

Similar to other vascular territories, loss of flow in a named artery or major collateral branch of the lower extremity will likely harbor a poorer prognosis. Without a better understanding of the long-term consequences of emboli detected by Doppler or EPD, however, conclusive statements regarding their clinical impact cannot be made. It is therefore prudent to perform complete arteriography before and after any upstream interventions, especially in patients and interventions considered high risk for distal emboli. Deteriorations in antegrade flow should be treated aggressively.

PREVENTION OF ACUTE THROMBOEMBOLIC EVENTS

Recognition of at-risk patients or lesions is the first step in preventing procedure-related thromboembolic events. Appropriate measures could then be taken to minimize such risks. Most patients undergoing peripheral interventions do not require special measures except appropriate anticoagulation and standard good practices, such as routine flushing of sheaths and catheters. In general, careful manipulation of devices across stenotic lesions, utilization of lower profile devices, minimization of the number of steps (such as catheter exchanges and balloon inflations), use of long balloons matching lesion lengths, and so on, all reduce the risk of distal emboli. In addition, familiarity with various specialty devices, such as atherectomy catheters, stent-grafts, recanalization tools, and drug-coated balloons as well as understanding their performance characteristics and limitations is paramount to good immediate and long-term outcome.

ANTICOAGULATION AND ANTIPLATELET THERAPY

In patients at higher relative risks of in situ thrombosis or atheroembolization, sufficient anticoagulants should be administered to keep the activated clotting time (ACT) above 250 seconds during the intervention. Proper anticoagulation will reduce the risk of in situ clotting as well as acute thrombosis of the vascular beds distal to an embolic occlusion, allowing the operator to treat the offending embolus. Although our preferred anticoagulant of choice during such cases is bivalirudin, use of heparin would also be adequate provided ACT is measured at regular intervals and maintained above 250 seconds. There has been no randomized study comparing unfractionated heparin with bivalirudin in peripheral interventions but reported experience with the latter reveals safety and efficacy equivalent to or better than heparin. The main advantage of bivalirudin during peripheral procedures is that it avoids the inconsistency of dose-response relationship that

is common with the use of unfractionated heparin and the need for multiple ACT measurements during prolonged interventions. Use of anticoagulants after routine endovascular interventions has not been shown to prevent recurrence.

Use of dual antiplatelet therapy has gained more acceptance and popularity before and after lower extremity arterial interventions. This may be caused by an extrapolation of the beneficial data from the coronary circuit to the carotid and peripheral arterial disease territories. There is currently no evidence that dual therapy is superior to monoantiplatelet therapy in the prevention of secondary peripheral arterial disease after endovascular interventions.[19] Monotherapy with either aspirin or clopidogrel before and after interventions in patients with peripheral arterial disease should be routine. Although the role of antiplatelet therapy in preventing procedural ATE in the peripheral circulation has not been rigorously studied, the evidence supporting its use in this patient population is strong.[19,20]

▌ EMBOLIC PROTECTION DEVICES

Despite the recommendation of some authors in favor of the routine use of EPDs during peripheral interventions,[16,21] their use is not common and cannot be justified in most cases. The benefits of EPDs during peripheral interventions should be carefully weighed against their complications and costs. Although distal embolization or acute thrombosis could occur during the routine treatment of even simple lesions, the risk is low enough that the use of EPDs during such interventions is not likely to prove beneficial or cost-effective. High-risk interventions, however, may warrant the use of EPDs.[13–15]

Embolic Protection Devices and Thrombolytic Therapy

A patient presenting with acute limb ischemia may undergo CDT as the initial step. Once the clot is removed and an underlying lesion exposed, care must be exercised in treating that lesion. Stenoses in freshly lysed arterial segments may harbor acute or organized residual clot, which could be released after angioplasty or debulking procedures. An unusual stenosis, such as a lesion in the middle of a synthetic graft or the angiographic appearance of any "filling defect," should raise the suspicion of adherent clot. Deployment of an EPD may be prudent prior to catheter manipulation of these lesions. For this purpose, the use of any one of the available distal protection devices would be adequate as long as the length of its wire matches the shaft length of the planned balloon or stent to be used. Most EPDs are designed for carotid and coronary circulation where all devices used are on a 0.014-inch rapid-exchange platform. The short wires of rapid-exchange platforms are frequently incompatible with the required devices for lower limb interventions. For this reason EPDs on longer exchange lengths should be deployed.

Following the intervention, repeat angiography is done and if a large amount of embolic material is seen in the EPD, care should be exercised during its retrieval. An overloaded basket could release some of its content during recapture maneuvers, causing more distal embolization. A commonly used technique is to advance a guiding or aspiration catheter to the basket and apply suction to partially empty it before recapture. We routinely aspirate the sheath vigorously once the basket reaches its tip during removal.

Embolic Protection Device and Atherectomy

Although the distal embolization potential of all debulking devices is well recognized, the routine use of EPDs during these procedures is controversial. The existing scant data on the subject are further confused by the marketing efforts and pseudo-scientific literature on ATE and the use of atherectomy. It is commonly accepted, however, that debulking of long lesions may be associated with sufficient atheroemboli to justify the use of EPDs. Hence, compatibility of debulking devices with the wire of the distal protection devices should be considered before their application. The use of the current generations of Diamondback and Predator 360 atherectomy systems (CSI, St. Paul, MN), for example, is not recommended over the EPDs. Diamondback has its own dedicated wire (ViperWire) designed to prevent the advancement of the crown of the device beyond the wire tip. Similarly, Jetstream (Pathway Medical, Kirkland, WA) may shear the covering of some 0.014 wires of EPDs and lead to excessive friction between the wire and the device. SilverHawk atherectomy (ev3/Covidien, Minneapolis, MN) and TurboElite laser (Spectranetics, Colorado Springs, CO) catheters are compatible with most EPD wires.

Embolic Protection Device and Chronic Total Occlusion

Most available EPDs in current use can be negotiated across stenotic lesions in the lower extremity arteries but the current generations of basket-type devices are not designed for primary crossing of a CTO. Successful deployment prior to the treatment of a CTO can therefore be problematic. Their placement distal to an occluded segment first requires the passage of a guide catheter with a large enough inner diameter to accommodate the basket across the occlusion. This maneuver could prove difficult in severely calcified or fibrotic lesions without prior angioplasty. Furthermore, the passage of a large guide catheter itself can cause distal embolization by "plowing" embolic material downstream. The use of the Spider (ev3, Minneapolis, MN) or Emboshield/NAV-6 (Abbott Vascular, Snata Clara, CA) can avoid these problems. The BareWire of the Emboshield device is not attached to the basket and can move independent of it. Hence an exchange length BareWire can be advanced through the support catheter used to cross the CTO and the catheter exchanged for the cartridge containing the constrained NAV 6 basket without the need for larger guide catheters or preangioplasty. The Spider embolic protection system can be advanced through its own microcatheter and hence does not require a guide catheter.

Other Preventive Technologies

A new and novel method of preventing distal emboli during lower extremity interventions includes the use of the Proteous embolic capture angioplasty balloon (Angioslide, Ltd., Caesarea, Israel). This device provides the operators with a balloon angioplasty catheter and the option of embolic capture in one device.[22] The long-term efficacy as well as cost-effectiveness of this device, however, is not known at this time. Experience with the use of proximal protection devices in the periphery is limited and hence cannot be recommended at present time.

TREATMENT OF ACUTE THROMBOEMBOLIC EVENTS

As mentioned previoulsy, prevention is the best strategy in dealing with patients at high risk of ATE who require endovascular interventions. Applying good catheter techniques, using adequate pharmacologic adjuncts, and employing protection devices when indicated are common examples. Despite these measures distal embolization and/or in situ thrombosis can occur. The following is a brief description of approaches that have been shown to be effective in treating ATE.

Aspiration Embolectomy

In case of distal embolization and loss of runoff vessels, the simplest and fastest approach is aspiration embolectomy using either a large lumen guide catheter or one of several specialty devices designed for this purpose. Examples of various aspiration/extraction catheters include the Pronto (Vascular Solutions, Minneapolis, MN), Diver (Invatec/Medtronic, Brescia, Italy), Export (Medtronic, Minneapolis, MN), Rescue (Boston Scientific, Natick, MA), QuickCat (Spectranetics, Colorado Springs, CO), Xtract (Lumen Biomedical, Maple Grove, MN), and Fetch (Medrad Interventional, Minneapolis, MN).

These are all manual aspiration catheters with variable performance characteristics. Familiarity with their specific dimensions and aspiration capabilities is critical to the success of rescue maneuvers.

Long segment occlusions of previously stented vessels may contain a nonadherent organized clot that could embolize once partial flow is reestablished. This is particularly true of arteries treated by stent-grafts. Stent-adjacent stenoses were the most common cause of loss of patency in the VIBRANT trial.[23] As such, the interior of a recently occluded stent-graft may contain thrombus. If such is suspected, prophylactic application of suction thrombectomy with or without EPD prior to any intervention can remove a nonadherent clot, preventing distal embolization.

Adjunctive Pharmacotherapy

The applications and dosing of thrombolytic therapies in acute limb ischemia is described elsewhere in this text. The following discussion is related to patients with acute procedural thromboembolic complications. Pharmacomechanical thrombolysis using automated mechanical thrombectomy devices with thrombolytic drugs in the treatment of procedural complications is reserved for in situ thrombosis. This is an uncommon occurrence at the site of intervention. One retrospective study reported an incidence of 3.5% in situ thrombosis in their patients undergoing SFA interventions.[6] In our own analysis of 102 consecutive patients we observed only one in situ thrombosis of the femoropopliteal segment. This patient was undergoing atherectomy and sustained an injury to the vessel wall, causing acute thrombosis. The incidence of true in situ thrombosis in adequately anticoagulated patients is likely to be significantly less than 3.5%, as reported by Davies et al.[6] Many acute closures at the sites of intervention are likely caused by recoil, dissection, or focal rupture and spasm rather than thrombosis. These are usually treated by placement of stents rather than declotting maneuvers.

Thrombosis of the vascular bed distal to an acute embolic occlusion can occur in patients with suboptimal anticoagulation and/or antiplatelet therapy and could be addressed by either pharmacomechanical or catheter-directed thrombolysis. Angioject (Medrad Interventional/Possis, Minneapolis, MN) is currently the most commonly used device for this purpose. The Trellis-6 catheter (Covidien, Mansfield, MA) may be used in longer occlusions of the SFA or bypass grafts. It is currently too large for more distal vessels.

It should be emphasized that the only role for pharmacomechanical thrombectomy in ATE is to remove the hyperacute clot and not the atheroembolic loads. Neither the lytic agents nor the mechanical thrombectomy devices are suited for atherosclerotic debris. The latter should be removed by aspiration using one of a variety of aspiration catheters as discussed earlier.

Use of glycoprotein IIb/IIIa inhibitors in peripheral ATE is not well studied. Based on the mechanism of action of these agents and the experience in other vascular beds it is safe to assume that they are effective in reducing the risk of procedural thrombosis during peripheral interventions but may increase the risk of bleeding complications. As with the coronary circulation, GP IIb/IIIa inhibition could be utilized in situations where there is massive distal embolization into the small vessels or the microcirculation causing slow flow or trashed foot.[24]

CONCLUSION

The procedural ATE are uncommon in peripheral interventions but their incidence is rising due to the increasing number and complexity of endovascular procedures. Our understanding of their risk factors and clinical significance is improving, leading to better preventive strategies and treatment approaches.

REFERENCES

1. Razavi MK. Detection and treatment of acute thromboembolic events in lower extremities. *Tech Vasc Interv Radiol* 2011;14:80–85.
2. Lookstein RA, Lewis S. Distal embolic protection for infrainguinal interventions: how to and when? *Tech Vasc Interv Radiol* 2010;13:54–58.
3. Shammas NW, Shammas GA, Dippel EJ, et al. Predictors of distal embolization in peripheral percutaneous interventions: a report from a large peripheral vascular registry. *J Invasive Cardiol* 2009;21(12):628–631.
4. Lam RC, Shah S, Faries PL, et al. Incidence and clinical significance of distal embolization during percutaneous interventions involving the superficial femoral artery. *J Vasc Surg* 2007;46(6):1155–1159.
5. Shrikhande GV, Khn SZ, Hussain HG, et al. Lesion types and device characteristics that predict distal embolization during percutaneous lower extremity interventions. *J Vasc Surg* 2011;53:347–352.
6. Davies MG, Bismuth J, Saad WE, et al. Implications of in situ thrombosis and distal embolization during superficial femoral artery endoluminal intervention. *Ann Vasc Surg* 2010;24(1):14–22.
7. Ouriel K, Kandarpa K, Schuerr DM, et al. Prourokinase versus urokinase for recanalization of peripheral occlusions, safety and efficacy: the PURPOSE trial. *J Vasc Interv Radiol* 1999;10(8):1083–1091.
8. Razavi MK, Lee DS, Hofmann L *J Vasc Interv Radiol*. 2004 Jan;15:13-23.
9. Kondo Y, Dardik A, Muto A, et al. Primary stent placement for iliac artery chronic total occlusions. *Surg Today* 2010;40(5):433–439.
10. Lupattelli L, Maselli A, Barzi F, et al. Chronic iliac artery occlusion: treatment with the Strecker stent after PTA. *Eur J Radiol* 1998;28(1):80–85.
11. Karnabatidis D, Katsanos K, Kagadis GC, et al. Distal embolism during percutaneous revascularization of infra-aortic arterial occlusive disease: an underestimated phenomenon. *J Endovasc Ther* 2006;13(3):269–280.
12. Müller-Hülsbeck S, Hümme TH, Philipp Schäfer J, et al. Final results of the protected superficial femoral artery trial using the FilterWire EZ system. *Cardiovasc Intervent Radiol* 2010;33(6):1120–1127.
13. Hellinger JC, Hergret E, Frisoli J, et al. Peripheral arterial endovascular interventions: early results using distal protection. *J Vasc Interv Radiol* 2005;16:S100.
14. Shammas NW, Dippel EJ, Coiner D, et al. Preventing lower extremity distal embolization using embolic filter protection: results of the PROTECT registry. *J Endovasc Ther* 2008;15(3):270–276.
15. Shammas NW, Coiner D, Shammas GA, et al. Distal embolic event protection using excimer laser ablation in peripheral vascular interventions: results of the DEEP EMBOLI registry. *J Endovasc Ther* 2009;16(2):197–202.
16. Siablis D. Atheroembolization and peripheral vascular interventions: the evidence is mounting. *J Endovasc Ther* 2009;16(2):203–205.
17. Kandzari DE, Kiesz RS, Allie DE, et al. Procedural and clinical outcomes with catheter-based plaque excision in critical limb ischemia. *J Endovasc Ther* 2006;13:12–22.
18. Rastan A, Sixt S, Schwarzwälder U, et al. Initial experience with directed laser atherectomy using the CLiRpath photoablation atherectomy system and bias sheath in superficial femoral artery lesions. *J Endovasc Ther* 2007;14(3):365–373.
19. Alonso-Coello P, Bellmunt S, McGorrian C, et al. Antithrombotic therapy in peripheral artery disease: antithrombotic therapy and prevention of thrombosis, 9th ed: American College of Chest Physicians Evidence-Based Clinical Practice Guidelines. *Chest* 2012;141(2 suppl):e669S–e690S.
20. Hayden M, Pignone M, Phillips C, et al. Aspirin for the primary prevention of cardiovascular events: a summary of the evidence for the U.S. Preventive Services Task Force. *Ann Intern Med* 2002;136(2):161–172.
21. Allie DE. To PROTECT or not to PROTECT? In lower extremity angioplasty procedures, "why not?" is the question! *J Endovasc Ther* 2008;15(3):277–282.
22. Zankar A, Brilakis ES, Banerjee S. Use of embolic capture angioplasty for the treatment of occluded superficial femoral artery segments. *J Invasive Cardiol* 2011;23(11):480–484.
23. Ansel G. Initial results of the VIBRANT Trial. Presented at: Vascular Interventional Advances (VIVA); 2009; Las Vegas, Nevada.
24. Shammas NW, Dippel EJ, Shammas GA, et al. Utilization of GP IIb/IIIa inhibitors in peripheral percutaneous interventions: current applications and in-hospital outcomes at a tertiary referral center. *J Invasive Cardiol* 2008;20:266–269.

Classification, Diagnosis, Natural History, and Medical Management of Vaculitides

KENNETH J. WARRINGTON, TANAZ A. KERMANI, and THOM W. ROOKE

OVERVIEW AND CLASSIFICATION OF VASCULITIS

Vasculitis encompasses a group of heterogeneous autoimmune disorders that are characterized by inflammation of blood vessels. The most commonly used classification system for these diseases is based on the size of the vessel involved and is divided into large-, medium-, and small-sized-vessel vasculitis (Table 51.1).[1] Giant cell arteritis (GCA) and Takayasu arteritis (TAK) are both large-vessel vasculitides that affect the aorta and its primary and secondary branches. Polyarteritis nodosa (PAN) involves medium-sized and, occasionally, small muscular arteries. Small-vessel vasculitides include Wegener granulomatosis (WG), microscopic polyangiitis (MPA) and Churg-Strauss syndrome (CSS), often referred to collectively as antineutrophil cytoplasmic antibody (ANCA)-associated vasculitis (AAV). Cryoglobulinemic vasculitis, Henoch-Schönlein purpura, leukocytoclastic vasculitis, and other forms of vasculitis associated with connective tissue diseases, such as systemic lupus erythematosus, also predominantly affect the small vessels. In this chapter, we review the epidemiology, clinical manifestations, diagnosis, and medical management of the major forms of vasculitis based on the classification system outlined previously. In particular, we will focus on large- and medium-sized-vessel vasculitis because patients with these conditions most often require angiographic imaging studies for diagnosis and/or disease monitoring.

LARGE-VESSEL VASCULITIS

Giant Cell Arteritis

GCA, also known as temporal arteritis, is a granulomatous vasculitis of medium- and large-sized arteries. Although GCA primarily involves the extracranial branches of the carotid artery, it can also affect the aorta and its major branches. GCA can cause vision loss through ischemic optic neuropathy, a dreaded and typically irreversible consequence of this arteritis. Extracranial complications may include stenosis of the great vessels with resultant ischemic complications or aortic disease with aneurysm formation and possible rupture.[2]

Epidemiology

GCA is the most common form of systemic vasculitis in adults over the age of 50 years. Its incidence varies by race and geographic location. The highest incidence rates have been reported among people of Northern European descent, whereas GCA is rare in African Americans and Asians.[3] The estimated annual incidence in Olmsted County, Minnesota, is 18.9 per 100,000 people aged 50 years and above.[4] GCA appears to have an age restriction and almost never affects people under the age of 50 years. Indeed, the incidence of GCA increases with age and the mean age at diagnosis is approximately 74 years.[4] Women are affected two to three times more often than men.

Although the vasculitic process in GCA preferentially involves the extracranial branches of the carotid artery, involvement of the aorta and its primary and secondary branches is commonly seen on radiographic imaging studies. In a population-based study, 27% of patients with GCA developed clinically significant large-vessel involvement (aortic aneurysm/dissection or large-artery stenosis).[5]

Etiology and Pathogenesis

Genetic and environmental factors are thought to play a role in disease pathogenesis. Genetic polymorphisms of the human leukocyte antigen (HLA) class II region, specifically HLA-DRB1*04

Table 51.1
Classification of Vasculitis by Size of Vessel Involvement
Large vessel
Takayasu arteritis
Giant cell arteritis
Medium vessel
Kawasaki disease
Polyarteritis nodosa
Small vessel
Wegener's granulomatosis
Microscopic polyangiitis
Churg-Strauss syndrome
Henoch-Schönlein purpura
Cryoglobulinemic vasculitis
Cutaneous leukocytoclastic vasculitis

Adapted from Jennette JC, et al. Nomenclature of systemic vasculitides. Proposal of an international consensus conference. *Arthritis Rheum* 1994; 37(2):187–192.

and DRB1*01 alleles, are associated with susceptibility to GCA.[6] A number of genetic polymorphisms in "immune function" genes have also been implicated in disease pathogenesis. The exact cause of GCA, however, remains unknown. Although several bacterial and viral organisms have been evaluated as potential etiologic agents, to date the inciting trigger remains elusive.[2]

GCA is a T-cell–dependent disease.[7] The inflammatory process begins in the adventitial layer of the arterial wall where resident vascular dendritic cells (DC) are activated via toll-like receptors.[8] DCs appear to be the predominant antigen-presenting cell in GCA. Activated DCs recruit CD4+ T cells by providing the necessary costimulatory signals for T-cell activation. T cells produce cytokines, particularly interferon-gamma (IFN-γ), which activates macrophages and results in the formation of multinucleated giant cells. Recently, T cells producing interleukin-17 have also been implicated in disease pathogenesis.[9] Macrophages in the arterial wall amplify inflammation and release matrix metalloproteinases and reactive oxygen species that cause tissue damage.

In response to immunologic injury, the artery releases growth and angiogenic factors that induce migration and proliferation of myofibroblasts, neoangiogenesis, and intimal proliferation.[7] The neointimal proliferation can result in narrowing or occlusion of the arterial lumen.

The hallmark histopathologic feature of GCA is transmural (intimal, medial, and adventitial) inflammation. This inflammatory process is frequently segmental. Macrophages tend to concentrate around the internal elastic lamina and fragmentation of this elastic layer often occurs. Although most macrophages are singly distributed, they may coalesce to form multinucleated giant cells. The absence of giant cells may be noted in up to one-third of biopsies and does not exclude the diagnosis.

Clinical Features and Diagnosis

Patients with GCA often present with new temporal or occipital headaches that may be accompanied by scalp tenderness. Occasionally, thickening and nodularity of the temporal arteries may be observed clinically. Jaw claudication from involvement of the facial and internal maxillary arteries supplying the muscles of mastication is present in only one-third of patients but is highly specific for this diagnosis.[10] Approximately 20% of patients experience partial or complete vision loss and can progress to blindness. Other visual symptoms related to ischemia may include amaurosis fugax and diplopia. Symptoms of polymyalgia rheumatica with aching and prolonged morning stiffness of the shoulder and hip-girdle are present in 40% to 60% of patients with GCA. Constitutional symptoms, such as fatigue, fever, or weight loss, can also be present at diagnosis.

A subset of GCA patients present with constitutional symptoms in the absence of more typical cranial symptoms. Vasculitis, particularly GCA, should be in the differential diagnosis for an elderly person who presents with fever of unknown origin or unexplained constitutional symptoms. Another subset of GCA patients present with symptoms of vascular insufficiency affecting the extremities, especially the arms. These patients tend to be younger and do not have typical cranial manifestations, often resulting in a delayed diagnosis.[5,11] Other less common presenting symptoms include upper respiratory symptoms, such as dry cough, sore throat, and hoarseness. Neurologic manifestations are less common and may include stroke, transient ischemic attack, or neuropathy.

Physical examination of patients suspected of having GCA should include a careful assessment of the temporal arteries and a detailed cardiovascular examination. Abnormalities of the temporal artery (nodularity, swelling, diminished pulse, or tenderness to palpation) are predictive of a positive temporal artery biopsy.[10] Subclavian bruits, asymmetry in upper extremity blood pressure, or absent radial pulses may suggest extracranial involvement of the proximal upper extremity arteries. An aortic insufficiency murmur could indicate the presence of aortic root dilatation caused by involvement of the thoracic aorta.

Laboratory findings are nonspecific in GCA. Complete blood counts often show a normocytic anemia and reactive thrombocytosis secondary to the inflammatory process. Erythrocyte sedimentation rate (ESR) and C-reactive protein (CRP) are usually elevated, although some patients may have a normal ESR. Autoantibodies including antinuclear antibody (ANA) and rheumatoid factor are typically negative.

The American College of Rheumatology 1990 has developed classification criteria for GCA, which are listed in Table 51.2.[12] The classification criteria are useful in distinguishing GCA from other forms of vasculitis and are not diagnostic criteria. Temporal artery biopsy and careful histologic examination of the arterial sample remains the gold standard for the diagnosis of GCA. Temporal artery biopsy may be negative for arteritis in 10% of cases.[13] Ultrasonographic examination of the temporal arteries has been used for diagnosis and in GCA may show a characteristic "halo" caused by vessel wall edema.[14] This technique is highly operator dependent, however, and is not routinely employed in clinical practice.

It is important to note that a greater proportion of GCA patients with upper extremity arterial involvement may have a negative biopsy compared to patients with cranial symptoms. In one study, 42% of GCA patients with subclavian, axillary, or brachial artery involvement had a negative temporal artery biopsy.[11] These patients also tend to have fewer cranial symptoms,[11] and imaging studies are often helpful in establishing the diagnosis. Computed tomography angiography (CTA) and magnetic resonance angiography (MRA) may demonstrate arterial wall thickening suggestive of inflammation or smooth,

Table 51.2

1990 American College of Rheumatology Classification Criteria for Giant Cell Arteritis[a]

Age ≥50 y

New localized headache

Temporal artery abnormality (tenderness to palpation, decreased or absent pulses)

Erythrocyte sedimentation rate ≥50 mm/hr by Westergren method

Abnormal temporal artery biopsy showing vasculitis with predominance of mononuclear cell infiltration or granulomatous inflammation

[a]Presence of three or more of the criteria listed above indicates a sensitivity of 94% and specificity of 91% for diagnosis of GCA.

From Hunder GG, et al. The American College of Rheumatology 1990 criteria for the classification of giant cell arteritis. *Arthritis Rheum* 1990;33(8):1122–1128.

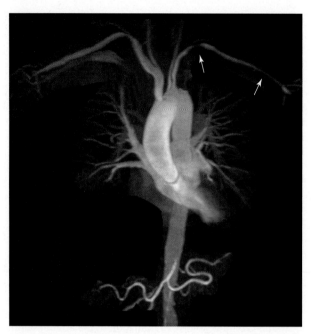

FIGURE 51.1 MR angiogram (chest) in a patient with giant cell arteritis. The 3D reconstruction images demonstrate long segments of smooth and tapered stenoses of the left subclavian/axillary artery (*arrows*) characteristic of vasculitis.

tapered, long-segment vascular stenoses characteristic of vasculitis (FIGURE 51.1).[15] Thickening of the wall of the aorta indicative of aortitis may also be observed (FIGURE 51.2). In recent years, positron emission tomography (PET) scanning has become useful in the evaluation of large-vessel vasculitis (FIGURE 51.3). Increased diffuse 18-fluorodeoxyglucose (FDG) uptake in the aorta and large vessels has been found in up to 83% of patients with GCA at diagnosis.[16] Although PET appears to be a sensitive imaging modality for the diagnosis of large-vessel vasculitis, its role in follow-up evaluations is unclear. Persistent vascular uptake is often present on serial imaging studies even when the patient is clinically in remission.[16]

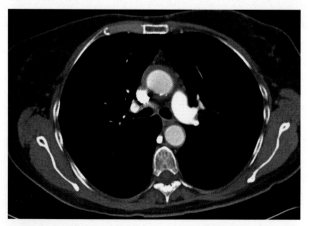

FIGURE 51.2 CT scan (chest) with contrast in a patient with giant cell arteritis demonstrates soft tissue thickening of the ascending and descending thoracic aorta indicative of aortitis.

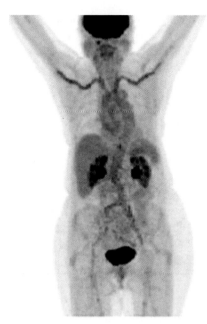

FIGURE 51.3 FDG-PET scan in a patient with giant cell arteritis demonstrates avid FDG uptake in the aorta, bilateral subclavian, and proximal lower extremity arteries.

Treatment

Glucocorticoids remain the mainstay for treatment of GCA. A typical starting dose is between 40 and 60 mg of prednisone for 4 weeks followed by a gradual taper over several months.[2] In cases where clinical suspicion is high, treatment should be initiated promptly and should not be delayed while awaiting temporal artery biopsy. Studies have shown that the temporal artery biopsy can be diagnostic even after several weeks of corticosteroid therapy.[17] In cases of impending vision loss, high-dose intravenous methylprednisolone (1 g daily for 3 days) is often used. Prednisone therapy for GCA has been shown in clinical practice over decades to be a very effective treatment modality. In an early retrospective study comparing treated patients to a precorticosteroid-era group, it was demonstrated that cortisone significantly lowered the risk of visual loss. After 4 weeks of treatment, the daily prednisone dose should be tapered gradually by about 10% every 2 to 4 weeks. Disease relapses are common during prednisone taper and require an increase in the corticosteroid dosage. The typical total duration of treatment is 1 to 2 years.[2] Corticosteroid therapy use is associated with serious adverse events in up to 86% of patients.[18] These may include infection, osteoporosis and fractures, avascular necrosis, cataracts, diabetes mellitus, and gastrointestinal bleeding.[18] In cases where frequent relapses require increases in glucocorticoid doses, methotrexate may be a useful adjunctive therapeutic agent. Prospective, randomized clinical trials evaluating the efficacy of methotrexate in GCA have yielded conflicting results. A recent meta-analysis found that treatment with methotrexate lowers the risk of relapse and reduces corticosteroid exposure.[19] Overall, the steroid-sparing effect of methotrexate is modest at best and this medication is reserved for use as an adjunct in GCA patients in whom corticosteroid taper is complicated by frequent relapses. Finally, addition of low-dose aspirin may be beneficial in reducing the risk of ischemic complications. In retrospective studies GCA patients on aspirin had a lower risk of cranial ischemic events including vision loss.[20,21]

Prognosis

Vision loss from ischemic optic neuropathy caused by GCA is often irreversible even after initiation of treatment. The probability of vision loss after initiation of treatment is estimated at 1% over 5 years in patients without visual manifestations at diagnosis and 13% at 5 years in patients with a visual deficit at disease onset.[22]

GCA patients are at increased risk of aortic aneurysm formation compared to the general population (FIGURE 51.4).[5,23] In contrast to atherosclerosis, which more commonly affects the abdominal aorta, GCA has a predilection for the thoracic aorta. In a population-based study, GCA was associated with a 17.3-fold increased risk of developing thoracic aortic aneurysm and a 2.4-fold increased risk of developing an isolated abdominal aortic aneurysm compared to the general population.[23] Because of the increased risk of aortic aneurysmal disease in GCA, long-term surveillance with periodic imaging of the aorta is recommended.[24]

The overall mortality is not increased in patients with GCA compared with the general population. Mortality, however, is increased in the subset of patients who develop aortic dissection (FIGURE 51.5).[25]

■ TAKAYASU ARTERITIS

TAK is a chronic granulomatous vasculitis that primarily affects the aorta and its major branches. TAK typically affects young females below the age of 40 years. The clinical presentation can

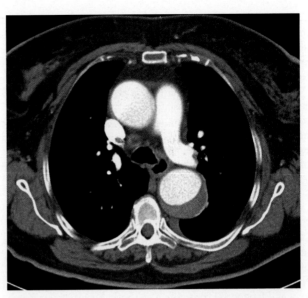

FIGURE 51.5 CT scan of the chest of an acute dissection of the descending thoracic aorta with thrombosed false lunch in a 77-year-old woman with giant cell arteritis. A prior CT scan 3 months earlier demonstrated dilatation of the descending thoracic aorta measuring 43 mm.

be variable and depends on the pattern of vascular involvement. Vascular inflammation in TAK may lead to major vessel stenoses, occlusion, or aneurysm formation. Although patients often have an accompanying systemic inflammatory syndrome, this is not always present. Most patients with TAK have a chronic relapsing course and require long-term immunosuppression.

Epidemiology

TAK is an uncommon disease and the reported incidence in the United States is 2.6 cases per million population per year.[26] A more recent population-based study from the United Kingdom reported an incidence of 0.8 cases per million population.[27] In Asian countries, the incidence is higher; autopsy studies from Japan report that evidence of TAK is found in 1 of every 3,000 cases. The majority (80% to 90%) of cases occur in women and the peak incidence is in the third decade of life. TAK causes different aortic lesions in different countries. TAK in the Far East tends to affect mainly the aortic arch, whereas in Southern Asia the disease frequently affects the abdominal aorta.[28]

Etiology and Pathogenesis

TAK is considered to be an autoimmune disease. However, the exact cause remains unknown. Environmental factors, such as infection, may be an important trigger of TAK. In addition, genetic factors that determine host response are thought to play a role in disease pathogenesis.

Histologic examination of arterial specimens from patients with TAK in the inflammatory phase reveals granulomatous inflammation and mononuclear cell infiltrates. Cell-mediated immune mechanisms have been implicated in disease pathogenesis. The vascular inflammatory process in TAK is very similar to that observed in the large arteries of patients with GCA.[7]

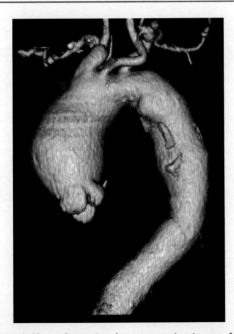

FIGURE 51.4 Three-dimensional reconstruction images from a CT angiogram of the aorta showing a large ascending thoracic aortic aneurysm and diffuse dilatation of the descending thoracic aorta in a patient with giant cell arteritis.

T lymphocytes are prominent in the initial cellular response and macrophage activation is also seen. Antiendothelial cell antibodies have been described in TAK, although the exact significance is unclear. Elevated levels of proinflammatory cytokines are often present in patients with active disease.

The intimal lining of the vessels affected by TAK demonstrates profound hyperplasia and may result in luminal narrowing. The medial layer of the vessel often undergoes laminar necrosis and the adventitial layer increases in thickness caused by fibrosis. In the later stages of the disease, vascular damage is often accompanied by atherosclerotic plaques and calcification (FIGURE 51.6).[28]

Clinical Features and Diagnosis

Claudication of the extremities is a common presenting feature in TAK. Similarly, patients may present because of the finding of absent pulse or blood pressure in one extremity (FIGURE 51.7). Nonspecific constitutional symptoms including fever, weight loss, and fatigue are common. New-onset hypertension may be present in up to a third of cases and is often related to renal artery stenosis (FIGURE 51.8). Aortic valvular regurgitation secondary to aortic root dilatation is the most common cardiac finding. Angina pectoris, pericarditis, and congestive heart failure are uncommon presentations. Pulmonary artery involvement may result in chest pain, dyspnea, or hemoptysis. Involvement of cervical or cranial arteries can cause headache, transient ischemic attack, or stroke. Visual symptoms can include blurring, scotoma, diplopia, and amaurosis fugax. Mesenteric artery involvement can produce abdominal pain, intestinal angina, or gastrointestinal hemorrhage. Cutaneous involvement is uncommon and may include the presence of erythema nodosum. Development of collateral circulation patterns can lead to variety of other findings, particularly the subclavian steal syndrome caused by a stenotic lesion proximal to the origin of the vertebral artery, resulting in lightheadedness with exercise of the upper limb. The physical examination of patients with TAK should include an evaluation of all peripheral pulses and auscultation for bruits.[26,29]

The diagnosis of TAK should be considered in patients under the age of 40 years with symptoms of ischemia, especially when risk factors for atherosclerosis are absent. The American College of Rheumatology classification criteria for TAK are listed in

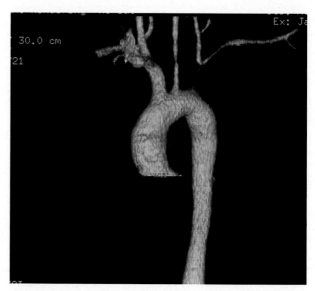

FIGURE 51.7 Three-dimensional reconstruction images from a CT angiogram of the aortic arch in a patient with Takayasu arteritis demonstrates occlusion of the left subclavian artery with reconstitution from the vertebral artery.

Table 51.3.[30] Classification of the types of TAK according to site of involvement is shown in Table 51.4.[31]

The diagnosis of TAK may be delayed due to the nonspecific nature of clinical symptoms and laboratory findings. Acute phase markers including the ESR and CRP are usually elevated in patients with TAK but may occasionally be normal. Other nonspecific markers of inflammation, such as normocytic anemia and thrombocytosis, may be found. No laboratory tests are

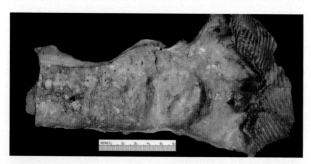

FIGURE 51.6 Autopsy specimen of the aorta from a patient with Takayasu arteritis who had undergone previous graft repair. There is "cobblestoning" of the intima with white patches and intervening normal intima.

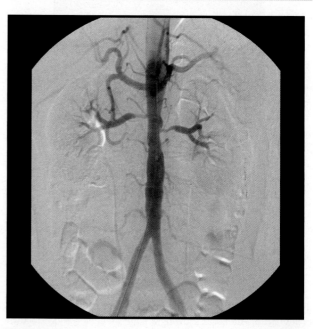

FIGURE 51.8 Catheter-based renal arteriogram demonstrates bilateral renal artery stenosis in a patient with Takayasu arteritis.

Table 51.3
American College of Rheumatology Classification Criteria for Takayasu Arteritis[a]

1. Age at disease onset <40 y

   Development of symptoms or findings related to Takayasu arteritis at age <40 y

2. Claudication of extremities

   Development and worsening of fatigue and discomfort in muscles of one or more extremity while in use, especially the upper extremities

3. Decreased brachial artery pulse

   Decreased pulsation of one or both brachial arteries

4. BP difference >10 mm Hg

   Difference of >10 mm Hg in systolic blood pressure between arms

5. Bruit over subclavian arteries or aorta

   Bruit audible on auscultation over one or both subclavian arteries or abdominal aorta

6. Arteriogram abnormality

   Arteriographic narrowing or occlusion of the entire aorta, its primary branches, or large arteries in the proximal upper or lower extremities, not due to arteriosclerosis, fibromuscular dysplasia, or similar causes; changes usually focal or segmental

[a]Presence of three or more of the above criteria indicates a sensitivity of 90.5% and specificity of 97.8% for the diagnosis of Takayasu arteritis. BP, blood pressure.
From Arend WP, et al. The American College of Rheumatology 1990 criteria for the classification of Takayasu arteritis. *Arthritis Rheum* 1990;33(8):1129–1134.

specific for the diagnosis of TAK and testing for autoantibodies, such as ANA, is typically unrevealing. Imaging studies including computed tomography (CT) and MRA imaging, as well as conventional angiography, are currently the most important modalities for establishing the diagnosis of TAK and can be helpful for monitoring disease activity.[15] MRA imaging is used most often because it is a radiation-free and noninvasive means of assessing the large vessels. MRA imaging may reveal structural lesions, such as arterial stenoses and/or occlusions, but also provides useful information regarding the vessel wall (particularly the presence of edema that may suggest active vascular inflammation). In one study, 94% of patients with clinically active disease had

vessel wall edema seen on MR. Vessel wall edema was also encountered in patients who were judged to be clinically inactive. Overall, the presence of vessel wall edema did not consistently correlate with the occurrence of new anatomic changes found on subsequent studies.[32] PET has been suggested as a means for identifying inflammation in the large arteries, although the sensitivity and specificity of the method are not well established. Noninvasive vascular ultrasonography can also be a useful tool for the initial evaluation of patients with suspected TAK. Arterial biopsy from an affected vessel is usually not feasible. Biopsy specimens from patients requiring revascularization procedures may show active inflammation and/or sequelae of vasculitis, depending on disease activity at the time of surgery, but biopsy is not the usual approach to the diagnosis of TAK.

Treatment

The goal of treatment for TAK is not only to improve symptoms but also to suppress vascular inflammation to prevent progressive damage to blood vessels. Corticosteroids are the mainstay of treatment, and most patients require additional immunosuppressive agents. Surgical or percutaneous revascularization procedures may be required to improve blood flow or to prevent rupture of aneurysms.

For newly diagnosed, active TAK, oral prednisone is typically started at about 1 mg/kg/day in a single daily dose and this dose is maintained for 4 weeks. Once the symptoms of active disease have resolved and acute phase markers have normalized, prednisone is then gradually tapered. A common tapering regimen is to reduce prednisone by 5 mg/week until reaching a dose of 20 mg daily. Thereafter, the prednisone dose is tapered by 2.5 mg each week until reaching a dose of 10 mg daily. Below 10 mg, the daily dose is typically lowered by 1 mg each week until prednisone is discontinued or a relapse occurs. No studies

Table 51.4	
Classification of Takayasu Arteritis	
Type	**Site of involvement**
I	Branches of the aortic arch
IIa	Ascending aorta, aortic arch and its branches
IIb	Ascending aorta, aortic arch and its branches, and thoracic descending aorta
III	Thoracic descending aorta, abdominal aorta, and/or renal arteries
IV	Abdominal aorta and/or renal arteries
V	Combination of types IIb and IV

The involvement of coronary or pulmonary arteries should be indicated as C (+) or P (+), respectively.

From Hata A, et al. Angiographic findings of Takayasu arteritis: new classification. *Int J Cardiol* 1996;54(suppl):S155–S163.

have established the optimal way to lower prednisone, and this has to be tailored according to clinical progress and inflammatory markers.

More than 90% of patients will go into remission with corticosteroid therapy. Disease relapses occurs in the majority of patients during steroid taper, however, and about three-fourths of patients will require additional immunosuppressive therapy. Immunosuppressive agents, such as methotrexate, azathioprine, or mycophenolate mofetil, are often used for treatment of TAK.[29] In an open-label study of 18 patients with active TAK, methotrexate was effective as steroid-sparing therapy for a subset of patients.[33] Azathioprine and mycophenolate mofetil have been studied in small open label trials with promising results and can therefore be considered for patients who are intolerant to, or relapse, while on methotrexate. In patients with severe, refractory and life-threatening disease, use of cyclophosphamide may be indicated. Anti-tumor necrosis factor (TNF) therapy should be considered for patients with TAK who have relapsing disease despite treatment with corticosteroids and immunosuppressive agents.

In an open-label study of 15 patients with relapsing TAK, anti-TNF therapy resulted in improvement in 93% of patients and sustained remission in 67%. Most patients in this study were treated with infliximab and were able to successfully reduce their corticosteroid dose.[34] In a follow-up study of refractory cases from the Cleveland Clinic, 60% of patients achieved complete remission and 28% achieved partial remission with anti-TNF therapy. Relapses also occurred in patients on anti-TNF therapy, however, often requiring an increase in the dose of infliximab. In this study, serious adverse effects were uncommon but included opportunistic infections and one case of malignancy.[35]

In addition to immunosuppressive therapy, low-dose aspirin should be recommended for patients with TAK. A recent retrospective study demonstrated that antiplatelet therapy with aspirin reduces the risk of acute ischemic events, in particular cerebrovascular and cardiovascular, in patients with TAK. On the other hand, anticoagulant therapy had no effect on the risk of ischemic events.[36]

Disease relapses occur frequently and it may be difficult to determine whether the disease is active or not. Kerr et al.[37] have proposed that TAK should be considered active if a patient has new or worsening of two or more of the following disease features: (1) signs or symptoms of vascular ischemia or inflammation, (2) elevated ESR, (3) angiographic findings, (4) systemic symptoms not attributable to another cause. Symptoms and inflammatory markers, however, may not correlate well with disease activity. Indeed, new vascular lesions may develop even when no other signs, symptoms, or laboratory features of disease activity are present. In such circumstances, the disease has to be viewed as being active. Conversely, acute phase markers may be elevated from other causes and do not always imply active disease.

Patients with TAK should be routinely evaluated by clinical examination and serial measurement of inflammatory markers. Vascular imaging studies should be performed at least yearly to identify any new vascular lesions and more frequent imaging may be required depending on the patient's symptoms.

Immunosuppressive therapy can lead to significant treatment-related morbidity and, therefore, strategies to reduce treatment toxicity should be implemented. Particularly, prevention of corticosteroid-induced bone loss with calcium/ vitamin D supplements, and bisphosphonates when indicated, is important. Other complications, such as steroid-related diabetes and hypertension, should be sought and treated appropriately. Immunosuppressive agents, such as methotrexate, azathioprine, and mycophenolate mofetil, require regular laboratory monitoring including complete blood count and liver enzymes. Appropriate vaccinations, such as influenza and pneumococcal vaccines, should be recommended. Live vaccines, such as the herpes zoster vaccine, are contraindicated for patients on immunosuppressive therapy. Prior to receiving anti-TNF therapy, patients should be screened for latent tuberculosis (TB) because TB reactivation can occur with these agents. Patients receiving intense immunosuppressive therapy, particularly high-dose corticosteroids, should be given prophylaxis for *Pneumocystis jiroveci* pneumonia. This typically consists of trimethoprim-sulfamethoxazole, one single-strength tablet once daily, and for patients with a sulfonamide allergy, alternatives include dapsone or atovaquone.

Surgical intervention may be required in patients with severe complications of TAK. Vascular lesions are usually not reversible with immunosuppression alone, and thus patients with symptomatic vascular insufficiency may require surgical intervention. Percutaneous angioplasty with stenting can be effective in the short term, but restenosis is common. Good long-term outcomes have been reported with vascular bypass surgery. Indications for bypass surgery may include symptomatic carotid artery stenoses, coronary artery disease, renovascular hypertension, and limb claudication. Patients with aortic insufficiency and aortic aneurysms may require aneurysm repair. Long-term complications of bypass surgery may include anastomotic aneurysms, congestive heart failure, cerebrovascular accident, renal failure, and graft failure. Surgical outcomes are better among the patients who undergo revascularization when the disease is in an inactive state. Indeed, patients with active inflammatory disease who undergo vascular surgery are more likely to require revision procedures. Therefore, control of inflammation prior to vascular surgery is important to improve outcomes.[38]

Prognosis

Most patients with TAK have a chronic, progressive, and relapsing course requiring long-term immunosuppression. Serial angiographic studies have shown that new lesions can be found in a significant proportion of patients even when the disease is thought to be clinically quiescent.[37] In one series, sustained remission, lasting for at least 6 months while on less than 10 mg of prednisone daily, was attained by only 28% of patients, and only 17% remained in remission after prednisone was discontinued.[29] Still, some patients may have a monophasic disease course and this has been described in up to 20% of cases.

Long-term morbidity is related primarily to complications from ischemia and patients with frequent relapses are more likely to become disabled. Mortality rates for patients with TAK vary from 3% to 15%. The causes of death described have included congestive heart failure, cerebrovascular events, postoperative complications, and myocardial infarction.[29] Systemic hypertension and presence of cardiovascular disease were significant mortality predictors in a series of Mexican patients with TAK.[39]

▌MEDIUM-VESSEL VASCULITIS

Polyarteritis Nodosa

PAN is a systemic necrotizing vasculitis that predominantly involves medium-sized and small arteries without involvement of arterioles, venules, or capillaries.[1] Most cases of PAN are idiopathic and ANCA are typically absent. There is an association between PAN and hepatitis B virus (HBV) infection.[40] Commonly affected organs in PAN are the kidneys, skin, joints, and gastrointestinal tract. Although PAN is a systemic vasculitis, there are organ-limited forms, particularly cutaneous PAN (cPAN), which appears to be a separate entity.[41]

Epidemiology

PAN is a rare disease with an annual incidence ranging from 4.6 to 9.7 per million cases.[42] In a study from France, the prevalence was estimated at approximately 30 per million.[43] The frequency of HBV-associated PAN has been declining since the early 1990s, likely coincident with vaccination against HBV and increased safety of transfusion-related products.[44] The peak age at onset of PAN is in the fifth and sixth decades with a male preponderance in most cases.[44]

Etiology and Pathogenesis

Most cases of PAN are idiopathic. Approximately one-third of patients are carriers of HBV.[45] Other less commonly associated infections include human immunodeficiency virus (HIV) and Epstein-Barr virus (EBV).[46,47] A well-documented association also exists with hairy cell leukemia, a rare B-cell lymphoproliferative disorder that can cause paraneoplastic PAN.[48] Although the exact mechanism by which this occurs is unclear, there has been direct evidence linking the two conditions with cases of histopathology showing direct invasion of the vessel wall by leukemic cells.[48]

The pathogenesis of PAN is also not well understood. In HBV-associated cases, circulating viral antigen-antibody complexes can lead to immune activation with recruitment and activation of neutrophils.[49,50] The exact mechanism by which this activation results in medium-sized blood vessel inflammation is unknown. T cells, particularly CD8+ T cells, may also be involved in disease pathogenesis.[51] In other cases, immune complexes may play a less central role. Thickening of the vessel wall and intimal proliferation can cause luminal narrowing and ischemia. On the other hand, inflammation can also result in weakening of the vessel wall and aneurysm formation.

Histologically, PAN is characterized by segmental, transmural, necrotizing inflammation of the muscular arteries. According to the Chapel Hill Nomenclature, involvement of arterioles, venules, or capillaries should suggest an alternate diagnosis, such as MPA.[1] The inflammatory infiltrate in PAN consists mainly of neutrophils and mononuclear cells. Leukocytoclasis (fragmentation of white blood cells) may be observed. Disruption of the internal elastic lamina and external elastic lamina can lead to aneurysm formation. Although circulating immune complexes have been implicated in the pathogenesis of this process, typical immune complex deposits (as demonstrated by immunofluorescence and/or electron microscopy) are absent in PAN.

Clinical Features and Diagnosis

Nonspecific symptoms, such as fever, weight loss, myalgias, and arthralgias, may occur in up to 93% of patients at diagnosis.[52] Although any organ system can be involved, the skin, kidneys, peripheral nerves, joints, and gastrointestinal tract are most often involved. Neurologic manifestations, such as mononeuritis multiplex or sensorimotor peripheral neuropathy, may occur in up to 79% of individuals.[52] Cutaneous lesions may include livedo reticularis, subcutaneous nodules, purpura, and skin ulcerations (FIGURE 51.9).[52] Peripheral arterial occlusions can result in digital ischemia and infarction. Abdominal pain is a common presenting feature, which suggests gastrointestinal involvement. Mesenteric ischemia, bowel infarction, or hemorrhage as well as pancreatitis may occur.[52] Severe gastrointestinal involvement often requires surgery and is associated with a worse prognosis.[53,54] Renal involvement often leads to arterial hypertension and ischemic nephropathy with renal insufficiency. Imaging studies may show renal parenchymal infarcts with stenoses and microaneurysms, which can rupture and cause hematomas.[55] Testicular pain from testicular artery ischemia is a characteristic disease manifestation but only occurs in about 17% of patients.[52] Vasculitis-related cardiomyopathy or coronary vasculitis is rare but is associated with a poor prognosis.[54,56] Compared to patients with idiopathic PAN, patients with HBV-PAN tend to have more frequent peripheral neuropathy, abdominal pain, cardiomyopathy, orchitis, and hypertension.[52] Localized PAN involving a single organ (e.g., appendix, gallbladder) is occasionally identified on histopathologic examination of surgical specimens and is frequently cured by surgical resection alone.

Laboratory studies in PAN are often nonspecific and include elevated markers of inflammation, such as ESR and CRP. Other laboratory abnormalities may include anemia and leukocytosis. Evaluation should include assessment of renal function, liver enzymes, and hepatitis serologies. There is no diagnostic

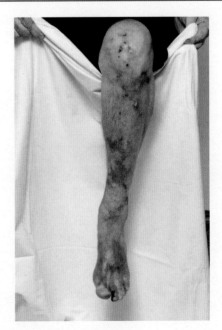

FIGURE 51.9 Livedoid skin changes, leg ulcers, and ischemic toes in a patient with polyarteritis nodosa.

laboratory test for PAN. ANCA serologies are typically negative in PAN and their presence should suggest an AAV. Urinalysis may show proteinuria and hematuria but active urinary sediment is usually absent.

In cases with cutaneous or peripheral nerve involvement, biopsy of the affected area should be obtained to confirm the diagnosis. A deep skin biopsy is usually required rather than a punch biopsy given the size of cutaneous vessels involved in PAN. In the absence of a site for biopsy, the diagnosis depends on imaging findings. CT of the abdomen may show vessel stenoses, intra-abdominal organ infarcts, and/or bowel thickening but findings are often nonspecific. Conventional angiogram may show characteristic finding, such as multiple microaneurysms of the celiac, mesenteric, and renal artery branches (FIGURE 51.10).[57] Surgical specimens from patients with visceral involvement (e.g., small intestine) can also provide the diagnosis.

The 1990 American College of Rheumatology has established 10 criteria to distinguish PAN from other forms of vasculitis (Table 51.5).[58] Presence of 3 of the 10 criteria has sensitivity of 82% and specificity of 87% for PAN in a patient with vasculitis.

Treatment

The treatment of PAN should be tailored according to disease severity. Mild disease can be treated with glucocorticoids alone. The typical starting dose of prednisone is 1 mg/kg/day for 4 weeks with subsequent taper for total treatment duration of 9 to 12 months.[59] Patients with major organ involvement, such as renal insufficiency, gastrointestinal, or cardiac or neurologic disease, are treated with cyclophosphamide in addition to glucocorticoids.[59] Cyclophosphamide is usually given orally as a single daily dose or by monthly intravenous infusion.[59] Treatment with cyclophosphamide is typically continued for no longer than 6 months, after which it is replaced with a remission

Table 51.5
1990 American College of Rheumatology Classification Criteria for Polyarteritis Nodosa[a]
Weight loss ≥4 kg
Livedo reticularis
Testicular pain or tenderness
Myalgias, weakness or leg tenderness
Mononeuropathy or polyneuropathy
Diastolic blood pressure >90 mm Hg
Elevated blood urea nitrogen (>40 mg/dL) or creatinine (>1.5 mg/dL)
Evidence of hepatitis B virus infection (serum antibody or hepatitis B surface antigen)
Arteriographic abnormality with aneurysms or occlusions of the visceral arteries not secondary to atherosclerosis, fibromuscular dysplasia, or other noninflammatory causes
Biopsy of small- or medium-sized artery with polymorphonuclear infiltrates

[a]Presence of three or more of the criteria indicates a sensitivity of 82.2% and specificity of 86.6% for polyarteritis nodosa.
Adapted from Lightfoot RW Jr, et al. The American College of Rheumatology 1990 criteria for the classification of polyarteritis nodosa. *Arthritis Rheum* 1990;33(8):1088–1093.

maintenance agent, such as methotrexate or azathioprine, for total treatment duration of 12 to 18 months.

In HBV-related PAN, plasma exchange may be helpful for removal of the antigen-antibody immune complexes.[44] In this subset of patients, treatment with corticosteroids, antiviral agents, and plasma exchange has been used successfully.[44] Treatment in these patients is aimed at stopping viral replication and clearing the viral infection.[44] Cyclophosphamide is typically avoided in these patients.

Prognosis

Involvement of the cardiac, gastrointestinal, renal, or central nervous system is associated with a poor prognosis in PAN.[56] The overall 5-year survival is estimated at 75%.[52] The major contributor to mortality is uncontrolled newly diagnosed vasculitis or relapsing vasculitis.[52] Other causes of death include sepsis, cardiac causes, or stroke.

ANTINEUTROPHIL CYTOPLASMIC ANTIBODY-ASSOCIATED VASCULITIS: WEGENER GRANULOMATOSIS, MICROSCOPIC POLYANGIITIS, AND CHURG-STRAUSS SYNDROME

WG, MPA, and CSS are systemic vasculitides that primarily involve small-sized vessels, such as arterioles, venules, and capillaries. These three conditions are often associated with the

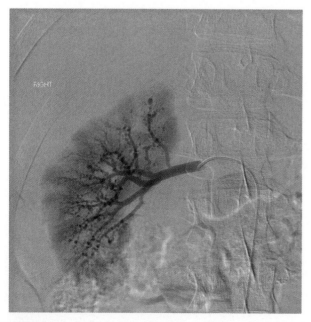

FIGURE 51.10 Right renal arteriogram in a patient with polyarteritis nodosa demonstrates innumerable microaneurysms.

presence of circulating ANCA and, therefore, WG, MPA, and CSS are also collectively known as the AAV.

Epidemiology

The incidence of AAV is approximately 10 to 20 per million population per year. WG is the most common form of AAV (incidence of 8 to 10/million/year), followed by MPA (2 to 6/million) and CSS (1 to 4/million). These conditions occur more frequently in older adults with a peak onset in the 65- to 70-year-old age group and they affect men and women equally.[42,60]

Pathogenesis

The etiology of AAV remains unknown, but these are considered autoimmune conditions. As with other forms of vasculitis, genetic and environmental factors are thought to be important in disease pathogenesis. A number of candidate gene association studies have identified variants associated with an increased incidence of AAV. Most of the genes so far described encode proteins involved in the immune response. Environmental triggers may include toxins (e.g., silica), drugs (e.g., propylthiouracil), and infectious agents (e.g., *Staphylococcus aureus*). ANCA are present in most patients with small-vessel vasculitis and are specific for antigens in neutrophil granules and monocyte lysosomes. These antibodies can be detected by immunofluorescent techniques, which produce two major staining patterns: cytoplasmic ANCA (c-ANCA) and perinuclear ANCA (p-ANCA). Most patients with WG are c-ANCA positive and the target antigen is typically proteinase-3 (PR-3). On the other hand, most patients with MPA and CSS have a positive p-ANCA due to reactivity with myeloperoxidase (MPO). Antibodies to PR-3 and MPO can be measured directly in the peripheral blood using enzyme-linked immunosorbent assays (ELISAs) and these are often used for clinical diagnosis. ANCA appear to have an important pathogenic role in the development of AAV; however, the exact mechanism remains controversial. The current hypothesis is that ANCA interact with their target antigens on neutrophils, causing neutrophil activation with subsequent endothelial and tissue damage. Histologically, WG is characterized by a necrotizing granulomatous vasculitis. Necrotizing granulomatous inflammation is also seen in CSS, typically with eosinophilic tissue infiltration. MPA is characterized by necrotizing small-vessel vasculitis without pathologic evidence of granulomatous inflammation.[61–64]

Clinical Features and Diagnosis

For a patient with multiorgan dysfunction and a systemic inflammatory process, small-vessel vasculitis should be included in the differential diagnosis. Constitutional symptoms including fever and weight loss, as well as arthralgias and myalgias, are present in most patients with AAV. WG classically involves the kidney along with the upper and lower respiratory tract. Clinical manifestations may include epistaxis, sinusitis, and/or otitis in addition to oral and nasal ulcers. Tracheal inflammation can present with stridor and respiratory distress. Pulmonary involvement may vary from asymptomatic pulmonary nodules/masses to alveolar capillaritis presenting with hemoptysis and respiratory distress (FIGURE 51.11). Most patients with WG will develop glomerulonephritis, which can lead to rapidly progressive renal failure. Other disease manifestations may include

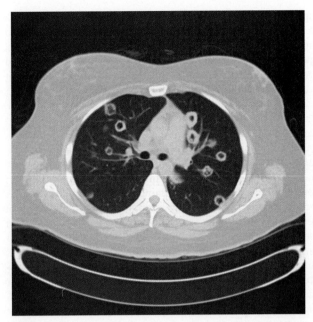

FIGURE 51.11 CT scan of the chest shows bilateral thick-walled cavitary pulmonary nodules consistent with Wegener granulomatosis.

ocular inflammation (scleritis, proptosis), cutaneous vasculitis (purpuric rash, leg ulcers) (FIGURE 51.12), mononeuritis multiplex, and gastrointestinal vasculitis.

The clinical features of MPA can be very similar to those encountered in WG. Rapidly progressive glomerulonephritis and alveolar hemorrhage are the most common clinical manifestations. Cutaneous vasculitis, peripheral neuropathy, and vasculitis of the gastrointestinal tract can also be part of the clinical

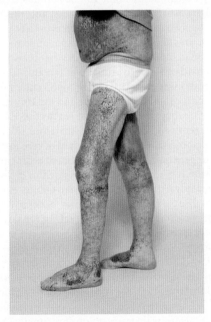

FIGURE 51.12 Extensive purpuric rash caused by cutaneous leukocytoclastic vasculitis.

spectrum in MPA. CSS typically has three main features: allergic rhinitis and asthma; eosinophilic infiltrative disease; and systemic small-vessel vasculitis. CSS often involves the lungs, peripheral nerves, and skin but less frequently the heart and gastrointestinal tract. Cardiac involvement can be a significant cause of morbidity and mortality in patients with CSS.[65,66]

The diagnosis of AAV requires an integration of clinical, laboratory, and histopathologic findings. Laboratory assessment for inflammatory markers (ESR, CRP), liver and renal function, ANCA, antinuclear antibodies, complement, cryoglobulins, hepatitis serologies, rheumatoid factor, and urinalysis should be obtained. ANCA testing is helpful in reaching a diagnosis of AAV, but false-positive as well as false-negative tests can be encountered. Patients should undergo chest imaging for assessment of pulmonary involvement and when indicated, nerve-conduction studies to evaluate for peripheral nerve changes. Pathologic examination of involved tissue, such as the skin, muscle, nerve, lung, or kidney, is often desirable to document small-vessel vasculitis. Given the toxicity associated with treatment, histologic confirmation of a vasculitic process is preferable. A prompt diagnosis of AAV, however, is essential because end-organ damage may progress rapidly in the absence of appropriate therapy.[63,64]

Treatment

The prognosis of untreated AAV is very poor; however, in the past few decades much progress has been made in the treatment of this disease. Although AAV is rare, several multicenter randomized clinical trials have been conducted to evaluate optimal treatment strategies. The treatment of AAV can be divided into three phases: induction of remission, maintenance of remission, and treatment of relapses. Because of the severity of AAV, most patients require induction therapy with cyclophosphamide for 3 to 6 months in combination with high-dose corticosteroids. A typical initial treatment regimen includes oral cyclophosphamide 2 mg/kg/day combined with oral prednisone 1 mg/kg/day. Alternatively, cyclophosphamide can be administered as intravenous pulses, usually every 3 to 4 weeks, and this treatment route may be associated with less adverse effects. Induction therapy with prednisone and cyclophosphamide results in disease remission in most patients with AAV but is associated with significant toxicity. Recently, rituximab (an anti-CD20 monoclonal antibody) was evaluated in two multicenter randomized controlled trials conducted in Europe and the United States. In these trials, rituximab was shown to be as effective as cyclophosphamide for remission induction and, therefore, this agent may replace cyclophosphamide as the standard of care for remission induction in generalized AAV.[67] Treatment with rituximab is associated with less adverse events compared to cyclophosphamide, particularly leukopenia and ovarian failure. Patients with severe renal disease related to AAV may benefit from plasma exchange because this can increase the rate of renal recovery.

Once disease remission is achieved, prednisone is usually tapered over a 6- to 9-month period, although some patients require long-term low-dose prednisone. Maintenance immunosuppressive therapy usually consists of either azathioprine or methotrexate and these medications should be continued for at least 18 months. A European randomized clinical trial confirmed that maintenance therapy with oral azathioprine (2 mg/kg/day) avoids prolonged cyclophosphamide exposure without increasing the rate of relapse.[68] Methotrexate can also be used as an alternative to azathioprine for remission maintenance but it is contraindicated in patients with renal insufficiency. Another option for remission maintenance is mycophenolate mofetil, although this was recently shown to be associated with increased relapses when compared to azathioprine. Anti-TNF agents do not appear to have a role in the management of AAV and may be associated with an increased malignancy risk. As for other types of vasculitis, the morbidity associated with therapy is significant and preventive measures to minimize risk of fractures and infections are essential. In particular, patients should receive *Pneumocystis jiroveci* prophylaxis with trimethoprim/sulfamethoxazole (either one single-strength tablet daily or one double-strength tablet three times per week). For patients with limited forms of AAV and no vital organ failure, methotrexate in combination with prednisone can be effective for inducing disease remission. High-dose corticosteroid treatment alone may be adequate for CSS, although most patients require additional immunosuppressive agents.

In summary, prednisone and cyclophosphamide remain the mainstay of induction therapy for most patients with AAV, although rituximab has recently been shown to be equally effective as cyclophosphamide. For maintenance therapy, azathioprine and methotrexate are the preferred medications.[69,70]

■ CONCLUSION

Vasculitis refers to a group of autoimmune disorders characterized by inflammation of blood vessel walls. The classification of vasculitis takes into consideration the predominant vessel size affected by the inflammatory process. The clinical manifestations of individual vasculitic diseases are highly variable but often reflect involvement of multiple organ systems. A systemic inflammatory process characterized by immune activation occurs in most patients. The diagnosis of vasculitis often requires radiographic imaging studies and histologic examination of the affected tissues. The treatment of vasculitis varies according to the severity of disease manifestations but typically includes prolonged immunosuppression. Patients with vasculitis warrant close long-term monitoring for disease- and treatment-related complications.

■ REFERENCES

1. Jennette JC, et al. Nomenclature of systemic vasculitides. Proposal of an international consensus conference. *Arthritis Rheum* 1994;37(2):187–192.
2. Salvarani C, Cantini F, Hunder GG. Polymyalgia rheumatica and giant-cell arteritis. *Lancet* 2008;372(9634):234–245.
3. Gonzalez-Gay MA, et al. Epidemiology of giant cell arteritis and polymyalgia rheumatica. *Arthritis Rheum* 2009;61(10):1454–1461.
4. Kermani TA, et al. Increase in age at onset of giant cell arteritis: a population-based study. *Ann Rheum Dis* 2010;69(4):780–781.
5. Nuenninghoff DM, et al. Incidence and predictors of large-artery complication (aortic aneurysm, aortic dissection, and/or large-artery stenosis) in patients with giant cell arteritis: a population-based study over 50 years. *Arthritis Rheum* 2003;48(12):3522–3531.
6. Weyand CM, et al. The HLA-DRB1 locus as a genetic component in giant cell arteritis. Mapping of a disease-linked sequence motif to the antigen binding site of the HLA-DR molecule. *J Clin Invest* 1992;90(6):2355–2361.
7. Weyand CM, Goronzy JJ. Medium- and large-vessel vasculitis. *N Engl J Med* 2003;349(2):160–169.
8. Weyand CM, et al. Vascular dendritic cells in giant cell arteritis. *Ann N Y Acad Sci* 2005;1062:195–208.
9. Deng J, et al. Th17 and Th1 T-cell responses in giant cell arteritis. *Circulation* 2010;121(7):906–915.
10. Smetana GW, Shmerling RH. Does this patient have temporal arteritis? *JAMA* 2002;287(1):92–101.
11. Brack A, et al. Disease pattern in cranial and large-vessel giant cell arteritis. *Arthritis Rheum* 1999;42(2):311–317.

12. Hunder GG, et al. The American College of Rheumatology 1990 criteria for the classification of giant cell arteritis. *Arthritis Rheum* 1990;33(8):1122–1128.

13. Salvarani C, et al. Reappraisal of the epidemiology of giant cell arteritis in Olmsted County, Minnesota, over a fifty-year period. *Arthritis Rheum* 2004;51(2):264–268.

14. Schmidt WA, et al. Do temporal artery duplex ultrasound findings correlate with ophthalmic complications in giant cell arteritis? *Rheumatology (Oxford)* 2009;48(4):383–385.

15. Pipitone N, Versari A, Salvarani C. Role of imaging studies in the diagnosis and follow-up of large-vessel vasculitis: an update. *Rheumatology (Oxford)* 2008;47(4):403–408.

16. Blockmans D, et al. Repetitive 18F-fluorodeoxyglucose positron emission tomography in giant cell arteritis: a prospective study of 35 patients. *Arthritis Rheum* 2006;55(1):131–137.

17. Achkar AA, et al. How does previous corticosteroid treatment affect the biopsy findings in giant cell (temporal) arteritis? *Ann Intern Med* 1994;120(12):987–992.

18. Proven A, et al. Glucocorticoid therapy in giant cell arteritis: duration and adverse outcomes. *Arthritis Rheum* 2003;49(5):703–708.

19. Mahr AD, et al. Adjunctive methotrexate for treatment of giant cell arteritis: an individual patient data meta-analysis. *Arthritis Rheum* 2007;56(8):2789–2797.

20. Nesher G, et al. Low-dose aspirin and prevention of cranial ischemic complications in giant cell arteritis. *Arthritis Rheum* 2004;50(4):1332–1337.

21. Lee MS, et al. Antiplatelet and anticoagulant therapy in patients with giant cell arteritis. *Arthritis Rheum* 2006;54(10):3306–3309.

22. Aiello PD, et al. Visual prognosis in giant cell arteritis. *Ophthalmology* 1993;100(4):550–555.

23. Evans JM, O'Fallon WM, Hunder GG. Increased incidence of aortic aneurysm and dissection in giant cell (temporal) arteritis. A population-based study. *Ann Intern Med* 1995;122(7):502–507.

24. Bongartz T, Matteson EL. Large-vessel involvement in giant cell arteritis. *Curr Opin Rheumatol* 2006;18(1):10–17.

25. Nuenninghoff DM, et al. Mortality of large-artery complication (aortic aneurysm, aortic dissection, and/or large-artery stenosis) in patients with giant cell arteritis: a population-based study over 50 years. *Arthritis Rheum* 2003;48(12):3532–3537.

26. Hall S, et al. Takayasu arteritis. A study of 32 North American patients. *Medicine (Baltimore)* 1985;64(2):89–99.

27. Watts R, et al. The epidemiology of Takayasu arteritis in the UK. *Rheumatology (Oxford)* 2009;48(8):1008–1011.

28. Kobayashi Y. Takayasu's arteritis. In: Ball GV, Bridges SL, eds. *Vasculitis.* Oxford, UK: Oxford University Press; 2008:323–334.

29. Maksimowicz-McKinnon K, Clark TM, Hoffman GS. Limitations of therapy and a guarded prognosis in an American cohort of Takayasu arteritis patients. *Arthritis Rheum* 2007;56(3):1000–1009.

30. Arend WP, et al. The American College of Rheumatology 1990 criteria for the classification of Takayasu arteritis. *Arthritis Rheum* 1990;33(8):1129–1134.

31. Hata A, et al. Angiographic findings of Takayasu arteritis: new classification. *Int J Cardiol* 1996;54(suppl):S155–S163.

32. Tso E, et al. Takayasu arteritis: utility and limitations of magnetic resonance imaging in diagnosis and treatment. *Arthritis Rheum* 2002;46(6):1634–1642.

33. Hoffman GS, et al. Treatment of glucocorticoid-resistant or relapsing Takayasu arteritis with methotrexate. *Arthritis Rheum* 1994;37(4):578–582.

34. Hoffman GS, et al. Anti-tumor necrosis factor therapy in patients with difficult to treat Takayasu arteritis. *Arthritis Rheum* 2004;50(7):2296–2304.

35. Molloy ES, et al. Anti-tumour necrosis factor therapy in patients with refractory Takayasu arteritis: long-term follow-up. *Ann Rheum Dis* 2008;67(11):1567–1569.

36. de Souza AW, et al. Antiplatelet therapy for the prevention of arterial ischemic events in Takayasu arteritis. *Circ J* 2010;74(6):1236–1241.

37. Kerr GS, et al. Takayasu arteritis. *Ann Intern Med* 1994;120(11):919–929.

38. Fields CE, et al. Takayasu's arteritis: operative results and influence of disease activity. *J Vasc Surg* 2006;43(1):64–71.

39. Soto ME, et al. Takayasu arteritis: clinical features in 110 Mexican Mestizo patients and cardiovascular impact on survival and prognosis. *Clin Exp Rheumatol* 2008;26(3 suppl 49):S9–S15.

40. Hughes LB, Bridges SL Jr. Polyarteritis nodosa and microscopic polyangiitis: etiologic and diagnostic considerations. *Curr Rheumatol Rep* 2002;4(1):75–82.

41. Segelmark M, Selga D. The challenge of managing patients with polyarteritis nodosa. *Curr Opin Rheumatol* 2007;19(1):33–38.

42. Watts RA, et al. Epidemiology of vasculitis in Europe. *Ann Rheum Dis* 2001;60(12):1156–1157.

43. Mahr A, et al. Prevalences of polyarteritis nodosa, microscopic polyangiitis, Wegener's granulomatosis, and Churg-Strauss syndrome in a French urban multiethnic population in 2000: a capture-recapture estimate. *Arthritis Rheum* 2004;51(1):92–99.

44. Guillevin L, et al. Hepatitis B virus-associated polyarteritis nodosa: clinical characteristics, outcome, and impact of treatment in 115 patients. *Medicine (Baltimore)* 2005;84(5):313–322.

45. Guillevin L, et al. Polyarteritis nodosa related to hepatitis B virus. A prospective study with long-term observation of 41 patients. *Medicine (Baltimore)* 1995;74(5):238–253.

46. Massari M, et al. Polyarteritis nodosa and HIV infection: no evidence of a direct pathogenic role of HIV. *Infection* 1996;24(2):159–161.

47. Calabrese LH. Vasculitis and infection with the human immunodeficiency virus. *Rheum Dis Clin North Am* 1991;17(1):131–147.

48. Hasler P, Kistler H, Gerber H. Vasculitides in hairy cell leukemia. *Semin Arthritis Rheum* 1995;25(2):134–142.

49. Zuckerman AJ. Proceedings: hepatitis B, immune complexes, and the pathogenesis of polyarteritis nodosa. *J Clin Pathol* 1976;29(1):84–85.

50. Pernice W, et al. Antigen-specific detection of HBsAG-containing immune complexes in the course of hepatitis B virus infection. *Clin Exp Immunol* 1979;37(2):376–380.

51. Panegyres PK, et al. Vasculitis of peripheral nerve and skeletal muscle: clinicopathological correlation and immunopathic mechanisms. *J Neurol Sci* 1990;100(1–2):193–202.

52. Pagnoux C, et al. Clinical features and outcomes in 348 patients with polyarteritis nodosa: a systematic retrospective study of patients diagnosed between 1963 and 2005 and entered into the French Vasculitis Study Group Database. *Arthritis Rheum* 2010;62(2):616–626.

53. Levine SM, Hellmann DB, Stone JH. Gastrointestinal involvement in polyarteritis nodosa (1986–2000): presentation and outcomes in 24 patients. *Am J Med* 2002;112(5):386–391.

54. Bourgarit A, et al. Deaths occurring during the first year after treatment onset for polyarteritis nodosa, microscopic polyangiitis, and Churg-Strauss syndrome: a retrospective analysis of causes and factors predictive of mortality based on 595 patients. *Medicine (Baltimore)* 2005;84(5):323–330.

55. Hachulla E, et al. Embolization of two bleeding aneurysms with platinum coils in a patient with polyarteritis nodosa. *J Rheumatol* 1993;20(1):158–161.

56. Guillevin L, et al. Prognostic factors in polyarteritis nodosa and Churg-Strauss syndrome. A prospective study in 342 patients. *Medicine (Baltimore)* 1996;75(1):17–28.

57. Jee KN, et al. Radiologic findings of abdominal polyarteritis nodosa. *AJR Am J Roentgenol* 2000;174(6):1675–1679.

58. Lightfoot RW Jr, et al. The American College of Rheumatology 1990 criteria for the classification of polyarteritis nodosa. *Arthritis Rheum* 1990;33(8):1088–1093.

59. Guillevin L, Lhote F. Treatment of polyarteritis nodosa and microscopic polyangiitis. *Arthritis Rheum* 1998;41(12):2100–2105.

60. Lane SE, Watts R, Scott DG. Epidemiology of systemic vasculitis. *Curr Rheumatol Rep* 2005;7(4):270–275.

61. Chen M, Kallenberg CG. New advances in the pathogenesis of ANCA-associated vasculitides. *Clin Exp Rheumatol* 2009;27(1 suppl 52):S108–S114.

62. Jennette JC, Falk RJ. New insight into the pathogenesis of vasculitis associated with antineutrophil cytoplasmic autoantibodies. *Curr Opin Rheumatol* 2008;20(1):55–60.

63. Guillevin L, Pagnoux C, Teixeira L. Microscopic polyangiitis. In: Ball GV, Bridges SL, eds. *Vasculitis.* Oxford, UK: Oxford University Press; 2008: 355–364.

64. Gross W, Csernok E. Wegener's granulomatosis:clinical and immunodiagnostic aspects. In: Ball GV, Bridges SL, eds. *Vasculitis.* Oxford, UK: Oxford University Press; 2008:403–413.

65. Keogh KA, Specks U. Churg-Strauss syndrome: update on clinical, laboratory and therapeutic aspects. *Sarcoidosis Vasc Diffuse Lung Dis* 2006;23(1):3–12.

66. Abril A, Calamia KT, Cohen MD. The Churg Strauss syndrome (allergic granulomatous angiitis): review and update. *Semin Arthritis Rheum* 2003;33(2):106–114.

67. Stone JH, et al. Rituximab versus cyclophosphamide for ANCA-associated vasculitis. *N Engl J Med* 2010;363(3):221–232.

68. Jayne D, et al. A randomized trial of maintenance therapy for vasculitis associated with antineutrophil cytoplasmic autoantibodies. *N Engl J Med* 2003;349(1):36–44.

69. Langford CA. Small-vessel vasculitis: therapeutic management. *Curr Rheumatol Rep* 2007;9(4):328–335.

70. Mukhtyar C, et al. EULAR recommendations for the management of primary small and medium vessel vasculitis. *Ann Rheum Dis* 2009;68(3):310–317.

Endovascular Management of Vasculitides

ANDREW HOLDEN, SANJIV SHARMA, BRENDAN BUCKLEY, BRIGID N. CONNOR, and PRIYA JAGIA

▍ INTRODUCTION

Vasculitis, or inflammation of the blood vessels, includes infective and noninfective inflammatory conditions. Noninfective inflammatory conditions include a heterogeneous group of autoimmune systemic vasculitides that are usually classified according to the size of the vessel involved. Large-vessel arteritis involves the aorta and its proximal branches and includes Takayasu arteritis. In addition to the systemic vasculitides, localized vasculitis may be seen after irradiation and in conditions, such as Buerger disease.

This chapter reviews the evidence for endovascular treatment in a number of vasculitides. Treatment techniques and outcomes are covered. First, intervention in infective arteritis is discussed. The role of endovascular intervention in systemic vasculitis is largely limited to large-vessel arteritis and is the focus of much of the chapter. Intervention in localized vasculitis is reviewed last.

▍ ENDOVASCULAR MANAGEMENT OF INFECTIVE ARTERITIS

Infective arteritides are uncommon. Although they can affect any artery in the body, different sites have different pathogenesis. The aorta is the most commonly infected artery and can be involved via contiguous spread from a vertebral body, intervertebral disk, or paravertebral infection.[1] Alternatively, an existing aneurysm or ulcerated plaque can be colonized via circulating bloodstream organisms. Cerebral and visceral arteries are less commonly affected.[2] Peripheral arteries may be infected by direct trauma including penetrating trauma, surgery, and, in particular, intravenous drug users.

Arterial infection may result in the formation of an aneurysm—often called a "mycotic aneurysm." The term *mycotic* was first used in 1885 in relation to endocarditis[3] and does not imply the presence of fungi. Infective aneurysms may be true or false aneurysms and are often a combination of both. Most infected aneurysms are caused by *Staphylococcus*, *Streptococcus*, or *Salmonella*.[1,2]

Patients with aortic infection usually present with nonspecific symptoms including fevers, malaise, and weight loss. Back pain may also be present and an abdominal aortic mycotic aneurysm may be tender to palpation. The insidious nature of the symptoms often leads to a delayed diagnosis. Imaging plays an important role with computed tomography (CT) and magnetic resonance imaging (MRI) being the most important modalities.[4] The key findings on cross-sectional imaging of an infected aneurysm include a saccular morphology, a ring of enhancing periaortic soft tissue, and an adjacent inflammatory change (FIGURE 52.1). A source of contiguous infection may also be

demonstrated. Peripheral infected aneurysms, by virtue of their location, are generally more clinically apparent.

The treatment of mycotic aneurysm traditionally involves both medical and surgical management. Appropriate antibiotics are the mainstay of medical treatment and it may be possible to treat asymptomatic, unruptured, infected aneurysms with antibiotics alone.[2,5] It is important to culture a specific organism from blood cultures so that antibiotic sensitivities can be assessed and appropriate antibiotic regimens commenced. This may be problematic in patients who have been arbitrarily commenced on antibiotics. In this regard, the polymerase chain reaction (PCR) laboratory test is useful because it detects dead or alive bacterial DNA.[6] Tissue specimens (surgical or percutaneous biopsy), however, are required.

The surgical treatment of infected aneurysms involves excision of infected tissue followed by arterial reconstruction. The reconstruction is often extra-anatomic to avoid the infected surgical bed, particularly if synthetic material is required for the arterial bypass. For example, an infected infrarenal abdominal aortic aneurysm may be managed with excision and axillofemoral bypass grafting. In situ grafts may also be used. In such cases, synthetic grafts may be soaked in antibiotics or vein grafts may be used (FIGURE 52.2).

In recent years, endovascular options for managing infected aortic pathologies have been explored.[7–9] The minimally invasive nature of these interventions is obviously appealing, particularly where extra-anatomic bypass is technically challenging, such as the thoracic aorta.[10] There is controversy regarding the placement of foreign material in an infected field, particularly because there are no large published series reporting this technique. The literature is confined to small series and single case reports. Some authors have suggested that, rather than a definitive treatment, endovascular treatment may be used as a bridge to surgery.[8] This allows the patient to be medically stabilized before the infected artery is resected without the risk of aneurysm rupture. In particular, thoracic aortic pathologies may be complicated by aortoesophageal or aortotracheal fistula, and a bridging strategy with a thoracic aortic endograft may allow fistula control prior to surgical resection (FIGURE 52.3). In some patients, such as those with significant comorbidities, a combination of antibiotics and endograft may be used as a palliative approach. Occasional reports have documented apparent complete resolution of the infective episode with no clinical or imaging evidence of active infection on long-term follow-up.

The endovascular technique for mycotic aortic aneurysm is similar to other endovascular techniques for aneurysmal disease. Endografts are sized and planned to extend from the noninfected aorta proximal to the aneurysm to the noninfected aorta or iliac arteries distally. Guide wire and catheter manipulation is minimized to avoid the risk of perforation through the infected

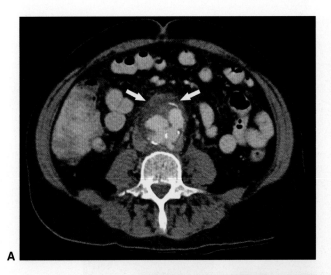

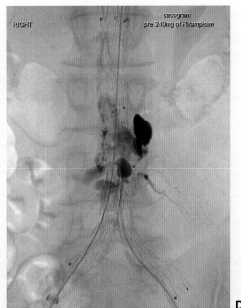

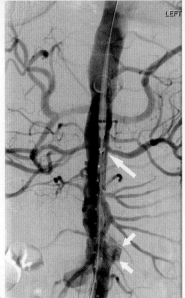

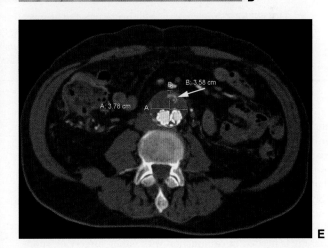

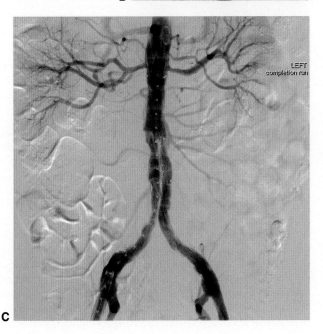

FIGURE 52.1 Mycotic abdominal aortic aneurysm in an 82-year-old man caused by *Staphylococcus aureus* sepsis from an infected, thrombosed brachial vein. Because of significant patient comorbidities, the patient was not considered fit for open surgical repair so endoluminal repair was undertaken. **A.** Contrast-enhanced CT at the time of acute presentation. Note the irregular, ulcerated blood lumen within an abdominal aortic aneurysm with surrounding periaortic inflammatory tissue (*arrows*). **B.** Aortogram during endoluminal repair. The top of the graft (*long arrow*) is positioned immediately below the renal arteries. Note the irregular blood lumen within the aneurysm (*short arrows*). **C.** Completion angiogram after endoluminal repair. A Medtronic Endurant (Medtronic, Minneapolis, MN) endograft was used. **D.** Contrast injected via a catheter within the aneurysm sac but outside the deployed endograft ("sacogram"). Subsequently, antibiotic (rifampicin, 240 mg) was injected into the excluded aneurysm sac. **E.** Contrast-enhanced CT 6 months after endoluminal repair. Note the dramatic aneurysm shrinkage and resolution of the periaortic inflammatory tissue. Calcification is present with mural thrombus (*arrow*).

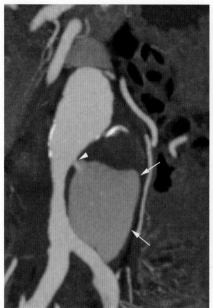 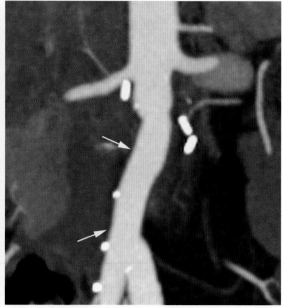

FIGURE 52.2 Aortic false aneurysm presumed to be mycotic in etiology, although an organism was not identified because the patient had been on antibiotics for unexplained fevers. **A.** Contrast-enhanced CT. Coronal reconstruction demonstrates an aortic false aneurysm (*arrows*). Note the discrete aortic wall defect (*arrowhead*). **B.** Coronal reconstruction of contrast-enhanced CT after surgical excision of the infected aorta and replacement with superficial femoral vein as a conduit (*arrows*).

and weakened aortic wall. Some authors have reported adding antibiotic to the preprocedural flushing of the graft while it is loaded in its delivery system in an attempt to deliver a high dose of the antibiotic locally to the aneurysm. There is no evidence that the antibiotic adheres to the graft, however, so this is probably unhelpful. An alternative is to leave a catheter within the aneurysm but outside the endograft and inject antibiotic into the isolated aneurysm sac (FIGURE 52.1). Prolonged antibiotic therapy is needed in conjunction with either surgery or endovascular therapy, but the optimal duration of treatment has not been established.[7,10]

The management of infected surgical grafts or endografts within the aorta primarily involves resection or explantation, debridement, and bypass, usually with an extra-anatomic bypass graft.[11] The incidence of endograft infection is estimated at 0.5% to 3% with *Staphylococcus*, the most common organism.[11] Endograft infection may present with rupture or endoleak but also on unexplained aneurysm sac expansion or "endotension." In these cases, image-guided percutaneous sac pressure measurements and aspiration of the sac contents allow differentiation from noninfective causes of endotension (such as occult endoleak and sac hygroma) and diagnosing a specific infective etiology (FIGURE 52.4).

ENDOVASCULAR MANAGEMENT OF SYSTEMIC ARTERITIS

Endovascular intervention in systemic vasculitis is largely limited to large-vessel arteritis, known as nonspecific aortoarteritis (NSAA) or Takayasu disease. This is an uncommon idiopathic, chronic vasculitis involving the aorta, its major branches, and the pulmonary arteries.[12] Cell-mediated vessel inflammation

results in thickening of the wall, fibrosis, stenosis, and thrombus formation in the involved vessels. The inflammation can also destroy the arterial media and lead to dilatation or aneurysm formation in some patients (FIGURE 52.5). Heterogeneous angiographic manifestations have been reported from different geographical areas with predilection for stenotic versus dilative and thoracic versus abdominal aortic involvement in different locations.[13,14]

The diagnosis of NSAA requires correlation of clinical, radiologic, and biochemical findings. The criteria for the diagnosis include the presence of:

- Ischemic symptoms of the central nervous system, upper extremities, or kidneys
- Fever, absent or decreased pulses, bruits, and fundoscopic findings
- Increased erythrocyte sedimentation rate (ESR) and presence of C-reactive protein

Angiographic findings considered diagnostic of NSAA include a spectrum of changes ranging from minimal intimal irregularity to typical rat-tail narrowing, complete obstruction, or aneurysm formation in the involved vessels. Involvement of the aorta and/or at least two medium-sized branches is considered essential for the diagnosis (FIGURE 52.6).

The disease is characterized by an early phase marked by nonspecific constitutional symptoms and signs, such as arthralgia, fever, fatigue, headaches rashes, and weight loss. In the late occlusive phase, ischemic symptoms in the involved vascular territories predominate. Signs of active vascular inflammation include aggravation of clinical features, the appearance of new vascular lesions, worsening of existing vascular lesions, or the presence of abnormal serologic tests showing increased levels

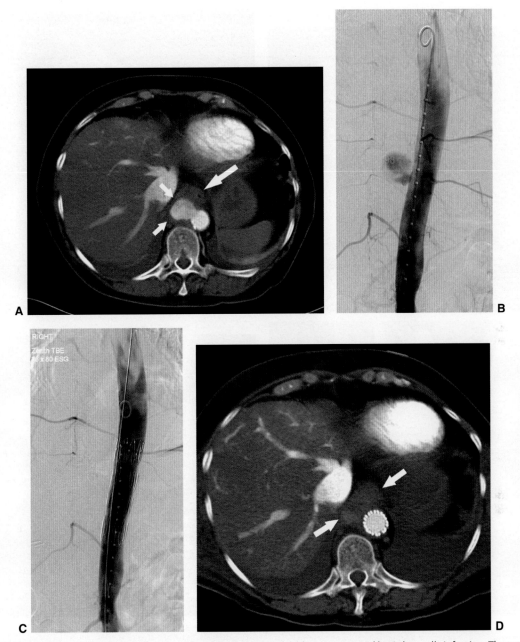

FIGURE 52.3 Mycotic distal thoracic aortic aneurysm in a 78-year-old woman caused by *Salmonella* infection. The patient presented with massive hematemesis caused by an aortoesophageal fistula. Endoluminal repair was planned as a bridge to possible surgery. **A.** Contrast-enhanced CT. Note the saccular false aneurysm of the distal thoracic aorta (*short arrows*) with the esophagus adjacent (*long arrow*). **B.** Catheter aortogram showing a false aneurysm. **C.** Arteriogram following endolumi-nal repair using a Cook TX2 (Cook Medical, Bloomington, IN) endograft. **D.** Contrast-enhanced CT 7 days after endoluminal repair showing exclusion and thrombosis of the false aneurysm (*arrows*).

of acute phase reactants, such as ESR and C-reactive protein ti-ters. Active vascular lesions often produce long diffuse concen-tric stenosis in the involved vessel (FIGURE 52.7). The presence of an active disease has important therapeutic implications. The outcome of various revascularization techniques is adversely af-fected by the presence of active disease. It is therefore important to identify clinical remission before advocating endovascular or surgical revascularization to treat the complications of vascular inflammation.

Clinical and biochemical markers are relatively poor predic-tors of clinical activity. Surgical biopsy may be the most sensitive method of assessing disease activity. Noninvasive imaging tech-niques, including duplex sonography, CT, and MRI, have been used for detecting active disease. Unenhanced CT may show a high-density arterial wall of variable thickness in the aorta or its branches occasionally with calcification. CT angiography may show enhancement of the thickened aortic wall in the presence of an active inflammation (FIGURE 52.8) with low attenuation ring

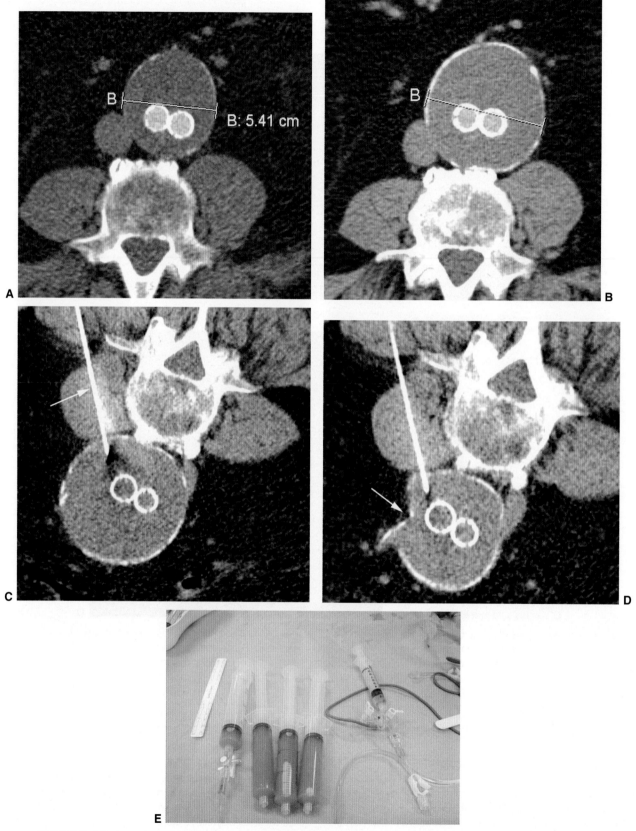

FIGURE 52.4 Endotension managed by aneurysm sac aspiration. **A.** Contrast-enhanced CT 1 month after endoluminal repair. **B.** Contrast-enhanced CT 2 years after endoluminal repair shows aneurysm sac expansion without evidence of an endoleak. There were no clinical features of infection. **C.** CT-guided needle aspiration (*arrow*) of the aneurysm sac with the patient positioned prone. **D.** Following sac aspiration, there is partial collapse of the aneurysm sac (*arrow*). **E.** Discolored fluid aspirated from the aneurysm sac. Culture showed no evidence of an infective etiology.

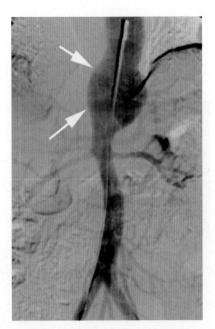

FIGURE 52.5 NSAA in a 28-year-old woman who presents with uncontrolled hypertension. Catheter angiography of the abdominal aorta shows a thoracoabdominal aortic aneurysm (*arrows*).

on delayed scans.[15] These mural changes correlate with disease activity and have been shown to decrease in the follow-up after clinical remission.[16] MRI can show subtle wall thickening in early cases. T2-weighted images may show a bright signal caused

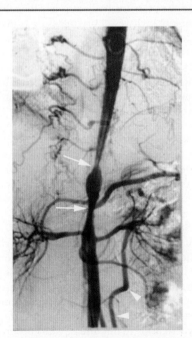

FIGURE 52.6 NSAA in a 25-year-old woman with uncontrolled hypertension. A catheter angiogram shows focal stenoses in the distal thoracic and suprarenal aorta (*arrows*). Both renal arteries show mild ostial and proximal stenosis. In addition, a large marginal artery of Drummond arising from the inferior mesenteric artery (*arrowheads*) is seen. This was supplying the superior mesenteric artery (SMA) caused by an ostial occlusion of the SMA.

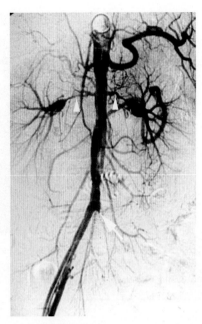

FIGURE 52.7 NSAA in a 16-year-old girl with uncontrolled hypertension. Catheter angiography shows a long diffuse severe stenosis of both the renal arteries beginning at their origin and extending up to their bifurcation (*arrowheads*). Such lesions are usually associated with active disease. In addition, there is an ostial occlusion of the left common iliac artery (*arrow*).

by edema in and around the inflamed vessel (FIGURE 52.9). During the acute phase, enhancement of the aortic wall and periadventitious soft tissues can also be observed. These MR criteria are not highly sensitive but are specific of disease activity.[17] Aortic wall thickness by itself may reflect activity of the disease.[18] Most patients with inactive disease have a wall thickness

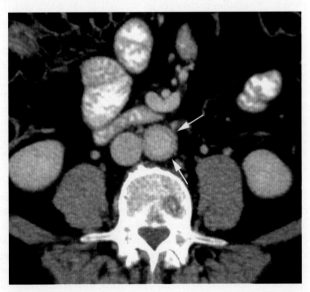

FIGURE 52.8 NSAA in a 32-year-old man with uncontrolled hypertension. Axial CT image of the abdominal aorta shows circumferential mural thickening (*arrows*) with enhancement.

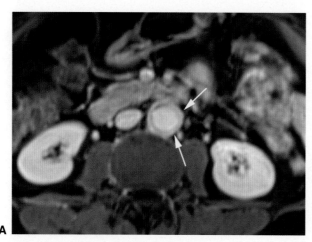
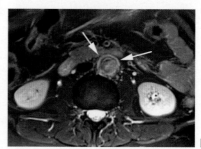

FIGURE 52.9 MRI evaluation of NSAA in the same patient shown in FIGURE 52.8 with uncontrolled hypertension. **A.** Axial T1-weighted MR image postcontrast shows concentric aortic wall enhancement (*arrows*). **B.** Axial T2-weighted MR image shows concentric wall brightening (*arrows*).

of less than 4 mm and most of those with an acute or chronic active disease have a wall thickness of 5 to 7 mm.[18] Imaging with 18-fluorodeoxyglucose and positron emission tomography (FDG PET) also demonstrates the distribution and inflammatory activity of involved vessels and may show response to therapy.[19]

The goals of therapy include the control of clinical activity by pharmacologic treatment with steroids and/or immunosuppressive therapy, restoration of blood flow to the stenosed vessel by surgical or endovascular techniques, pharmacologic control of blood pressure (BP), and supportive management. Some form of revascularization is necessary to relieve ischemia secondary to a hemodynamically significant stenosis. Surgical revascularization can be performed in the form of a bypass graft, excision of segment and in situ graft, patch angioplasty, and end-arterectomy. Surgical repair should be undertaken in the "burnt-out" phase of the disease when further progression is unlikely.[20] The complexity of pathologic changes in the wall of the aorta and its branches, widespread nature of this involvement, and long length of steno-occlusive lesions with diffuse adjacent disease make surgical revascularization technically difficult. Patients are often young and tend to outgrow the bypass grafts over time. There is a significant prevalence of graft occlusion, aneurysm formation at the surgical anastomoses, and progressive symptomatic disease at other sites.[21] Patients with active disease are more likely to require revision or develop progressive symptomatic disease at another site. Given the limitations of open surgery, nonsurgical revascularization techniques have been increasingly used in the treatment of this disease.

Renovascular hypertension (RVH) is the most common treatable clinical presentation of this disease. RVH is typically caused by obstructing lesions involving the aorta and/or the renal arteries. Indications for endovascular treatment include poorly controlled hypertension, flash pulmonary edema, or severe left ventricular dysfunction in the presence of a significant stenosis in the renal artery or adjacent aorta with angiographic evidence of at least 70% stenosis. In hypertensive patients, intervention should be performed in the setting of clinically inactive disease. Patients presenting with flash pulmonary edema or severe left ventricular dysfunction may undergo endovascular revascularization even

in the presence of an active disease as an emergency salvage. Where the severity of the arterial stenosis is uncertain, a pressure gradient across the stenosis should be measured (a peak systolic gradient of >20 mm Hg is considered significant).

Angioplasty is the primary technique used for renal artery revascularization (FIGURE 52.10). A femoral, brachial, or radial approach may be used. Angioplasty is considered technically successful if the arterial lumen has less than 30% residual stenosis, the arterial lumen is at least 50% larger than its pretreatment diameter, and the pressure gradient is less than 20 mm Hg. In lesions where a branch vessel originates or is involved in the stenosis, a kissing balloon technique is employed using a coaxial approach (FIGURE 52.11). Most patients experience an intense, transient backache during balloon inflation, often accompanied by a transient fall in BP. This subsides soon after balloon deflation. After angioplasty, patients are considered cured if normal BP is achieved without antihypertensive drug therapy, improved if there is at least a 15% reduction in diastolic pressure or the diastolic pressure is less than 90 mm Hg with the patient taking less antihypertensive medication than before the procedure, and failed if there is no change in BP after the procedure.

The results of renal angioplasty have been reported in many small case series but one of the largest series involved 193 patients and reported a technical success rate of 96%, clinical benefit of 91%, and complication rate of 5.8%.[22] The restenosis rate was 17% and the cumulative 5-year patency rate was 67%. Factors predicting restenosis included an ostial location of the stenosis, residual stenosis of greater than 30%, residual pressure gradient of greater than 10 mm Hg after angioplasty, coexisting juxtadiaphragmatic aortic stenosis, and reactivation of the underlying disease.[22] Overall, renal angioplasty is safe and effective in treating hypertension in this disease with encouraging follow-up results and a low complication rate. Follow-up angiograms are performed in patients with recurrence of hypertension, and angioplasty is usually repeated if restenosis is detected.

Primary stenting of renal artery stenoses is not advised. The patients are often young and still growing, the anatomy is often complex involving the aorto-ostial region and extending to the renal artery bifurcation, and the risk of in-stent restenosis is

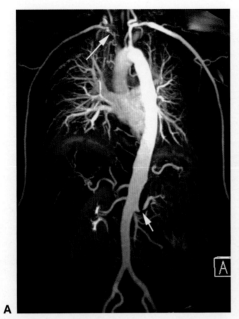
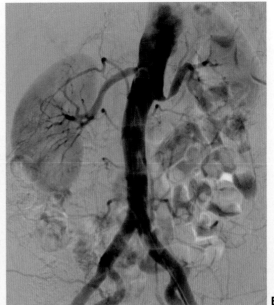
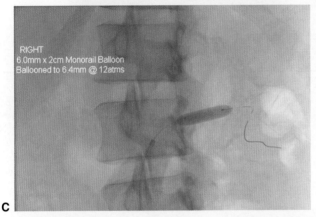
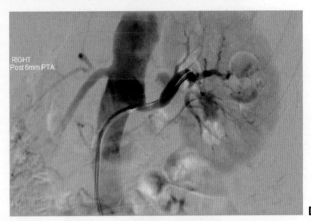

FIGURE 52.10 A 24-year-old man with NSAA presents with severe hypertension. **A.** Contrast-enhanced MR angiogram. Note the brachiocephalic artery occlusion (*long arrow*) and critical left renal artery stenosis (*short arrow*). **B.** Catheter arteriogram confirms the left renal artery stenosis. **C.** Balloon angioplasty of the left renal artery stenosis. **D.** Postangioplasty angiography shows improved vessel caliber.

high. Exacerbation of disease activity, small caliber of arteries in young patients, and aggressive neointimal hyperplasia contribute to the high risk of in-stent restenosis. Stenting should be reserved as a bailout option for complications of angioplasty, including flow-limiting dissection. Balloon-mounted stents are preferred in the renal arteries, whereas self-expanding stents are more often used in the aorta. In patients with significant residual stenosis after angioplasty, repeat angioplasty with a cutting or scoring balloon can be considered.[23]

The outcomes of endovascular interventions in the mesenteric arteries are less rewarding. Due to the presence of diffuse lesions and increased wall thickness, the stenosis responds less well to balloon angioplasty. Even after initial successful angioplasty, the restenosis rate is high. Although mesenteric lesions are frequently present, they are rarely symptomatic, presumably due to the extensive collateral pathways of the visceral circulation. Endovascular treatment is therefore much less common.

The use of angioplasty for the treatment of aortic stenoses has been infrequently reported. Patients with short segment (<4 cm long) stenosis showed better overall results than those with long segment (>4 cm long) stenosis (FIGURE 52.12). Adverse angiographic features include eccentric and diffuse stenoses, location in juxtadiaphragmatic segment of the aorta, and presence of calcification.[24] In these patients, angioplasty is often complicated by dissection (FIGURE 52.13) and stenting is required.

Endovascular reconstruction is rarely performed for aneurysmal disease in NSAA. The aneurysm typically involves the perirenal segment of the aorta including the visceral arteries, making endovascular reconstruction with standard endografts impossible. Mural inflammatory involvement in angiographically normal segments contributes to the unsuitability for endograft placement because adequate landing zones free of disease are rarely available. The aortic segment above the aortic bifurcation is also usually not large enough to accommodate the graft limbs. For these reasons, patients with aneurysmal disease are usually managed by reconstructive surgery.

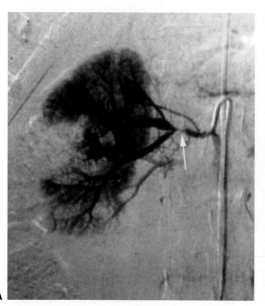
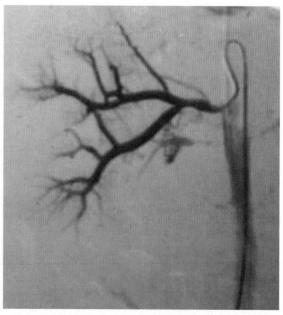

FIGURE 52.11 A 16-year-old girl with NSAA and uncontrolled hypertension. **A.** Selective right renal artery catheter arteriogram. There is a critical nonostial stenosis of the main renal artery extending to and involving its bifurcation (*arrow*). The patchy nephrogram was caused by nonopacification of an additional renal artery in this patient. **B.** Selective angiography after kissing balloon angioplasty shows no significant residual stenosis and brisk antegrade flow into lobar branches.

Symptomatic carotid artery stenoses are usually best treated with surgical bypass as are coronary and long lower limb arterial lesions. Focal limb arterial stenoses in claudicants may respond well to angioplasty.

Overall, endovascular techniques, including angioplasty and stenting, are useful in the management of selected patients with NSAA. Judicious case selection and a proper understanding of the technical complexity of the procedures are essential for their optimal utilization. Disease activity should be assessed before accepting patients for revascularization treatment. The natural history of this disease is better understood today, advances in imaging have made some impact in detecting clinical activity,

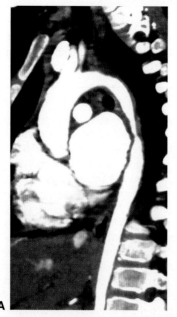
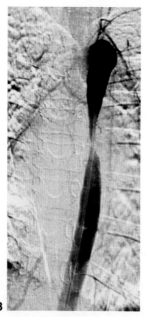
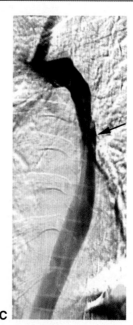

FIGURE 52.12 A 24-year-old man with uncontrolled hypertension and severe left ventricular dysfunction. **A.** Sagittal reconstruction of CT angiogram shows an eccentric severe stenosis in the upper thoracic aorta with mural thickening. **B.** Catheter angiography demonstrates the same stenosis. There was a 90 mm Hg pressure gradient across the stenosis. **C.** Angiography after angioplasty shows improvement in the luminal caliber with no significant residual stenosis or gradient. There is a small nonobstructive dissection flap at the angioplasty site (*arrow*).

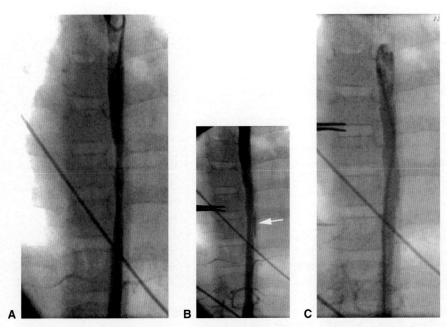

FIGURE 52.13 A 9-year-old boy with NSAA, hypertension, and severe left ventricular dysfunction. **A.** Catheter angiogram shows a long diffuse up to 70% diameter stenosis in the lower thoracic aorta associated with a 60 mm Hg trans-stenotic pressure gradient. **B.** Catheter angiography after balloon angioplasty shows a 50% residual stenosis and an obstructive dissection flap (*arrow*) at the angioplasty site with a residual gradient of 40 mm Hg. **C.** This resolved after self-expanding stent placement with no residual pressure gradient.

the drug treatment of active disease is evolving, and long-term outcomes of surgical and nonsurgical revascularization have validated an aggressive management of these patients. Despite these developments, this disease remains an enigma because the etiopathogenesis is still not established, the course of the disease is unpredictable, reliable markers of activity remain elusive, and the optimal treatment strategy is, as yet, not defined.

Endovascular intervention in other systemic arteritides is much less common. Giant cell arteritis (GCA) is another granulomatous arteritis but it involves medium and small arteries, especially the extracranial branches of the carotid artery. Although aortic involvement is relatively uncommon, the thoracic aorta is most commonly affected,[25] resulting in aneurysmal dilatation. Surgical biopsies of extracranial carotid branches (such as the superficial temporal artery) are often performed to confirm the diagnosis but endovascular treatment is rare. Polyarteritis nodosa (PAN) involves medium- and small-sized arteries. The transmural necrotizing pathologic process seen in PAN can result in arterial thrombosis and aneurysm formation. Thrombosis results in ischemia and infarction involving the skin, digits, and mesenteric circulation. The renal circulation is often involved with a combination of arterial stenoses and micro- and macroaneurysm formation. Catheter angiography of the renal circulation may be used to confirm the diagnosis, demonstrating pathonomic microaneurysms. Endovascular intervention is rarely indicated in PAN and even less common in small-vessel arteritides, such as rheumatoid arthritis and systemic lupus erythematosus. Kawasaki arteritis is an acute illness of infants and young children usually presenting with fever, lymphadenopathy, and oral erythema.[26] Medium-vessel arteritis is an occasional complication, presenting with aneurysm formation and thrombosis. The coronary arteries are most commonly involved by

aneurysms with the subclavian, axillary, brachial, iliac, or femoral arteries occasionally involved (FIGURE 52.14). Surgical revascularization in the form of bypass grafting is the preferred method of intervention when necessary.[26]

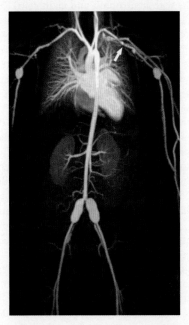

FIGURE 52.14 Magnetic resonance angiogram in a 4-year-old girl with Kawasaki disease. Note the focal aneurysms of the common iliac and axillary arteries. There are also stenoses in the left subclavian artery (*arrow*).

ENDOVASCULAR MANAGEMENT OF LOCALIZED ARTERITIS

Localized arteritides include Buerger disease and radiation arteritis. Thromboangiitis obliterans (TAO) (Buerger disease) is an inflammatory vasculitis of limb vessels. The original description of Buerger disease as a nonatheromatous segmental obliterating thrombosis involving arteries, veins, and adjacent nerve bundles remains valid after over a century.[27] Classically presenting in young men with a history of tobacco use, patients present with symptoms of claudication, Raynaud phenomenon, or critical ischemia (rest pain, ulceration, and gangrene). Ulceration and gangrene typically occur much earlier in the presentation than with atherosclerosis.[28,29] Nerve pain and thrombophlebitis are also recognized presenting symptoms.[30]

TAO affects small- and medium-sized arteries and veins with occlusive inflammatory thrombus. Although predominantly occurring in young men, more recent reports describe patients in their 40s and an increasing number of women diagnosed with TAO, likely as a result of the increased prevalence of smoking in women.[31,32] Lower limb involvement occurs in all patients with the upper limbs affected in 30% to 50%.[33] Disease progression typically involves acute exacerbations and remissions.

Disease prevalence varies around the world, being more common in Asia and the Middle East and Eastern Europe and uncommon in Western Europe; however, over the past two decades the prevalence of TAO has been decreasing worldwide.[34]

The diagnosis of TAO can be challenging with no specific test available. Patients usually require investigations to exclude other causes of peripheral arterial disease, including atherosclerosis and atheroembolic disease, and the more classical vasculitides. Various diagnostic criteria have been proposed to improve specificity for TAO, although none have been validated prospectively.[29,34,35]

In the acute phase, TAO shows a highly cellular inflammatory thrombus with neutrophils and giant cells. Relative sparing of the vessel wall and preservation of the internal elastic lamina are seen as key features by many authors[27,29,34] and is thought to distinguish TAO from GCA and atherosclerosis. Some studies describe involvement of the entire vessel wall more in keeping with a typical vasculitis.[31] In the subacute and chronic phases the thrombus organizes and then progresses to vascular fibrosis.

Over a century after first being described by Buerger, the etiology remains unclear. Although the etiology may be multifactorial, smoking is accepted as the initiating factor. Allergic-immune, autoimmune, or possibly hereditary factors have all been postulated as playing a role.[28] There is evidence for an immune-type response to factors such as type I and III collagen[36] and endothelial cells.[37] There are increased circulating levels of $CD3^+$ T cells[38] that may suggest an immune or autoimmune reaction to an antigen in the intimal layer of the vessel, but to date no single antigen has been identified.

On angiography, proximal arteries are most often normal in appearance; tapering occlusive disease progresses from small- to medium-sized vessels with "corkscrew" vessels (FIGURE 52.15) classically providing collateral supply.[39] Some studies have demonstrated an increased likelihood of ischemic ulcers when small-caliber corkscrew collaterals are shown.[40] Superficial venous occlusive disease and thrombophlebitis are present in up to 50% of limbs.[30]

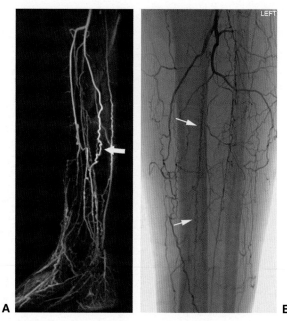

FIGURE 52.15 A 36-year-old man patient with a past history of nicotine abuse and, more recently, symptoms of right foot critical ischemia. **A.** Magnetic resonance angiogram shows occluded tibial and pedal arteries distally with corkscrew collaterals (*arrow*). **B.** Catheter angiogram confirms the MR findings (*arrows*).

Cessation from use of all tobacco products has the most significant impact on slowing the progression of the disease,[33,41] although patients are still more likely to progress to amputation than those with atherosclerosis or other vasculitides. Vascular reconstruction and bypass has a limited role in treatment because arterial bypass surgery has poor long-term patency, likely secondary to inadequate runoff and disease involving superficial veins that would be used as graft vessels.[34] Sympathectomy can be used in conjunction with cessation of smoking but its contribution to reducing disease progression is uncertain.[42]

There have been few reports of endovascular treatment in patients with TAO. The distal extent of tibial and pedal artery disease provides challenges for endovascular as well as surgical bypass techniques. Patients considered for endovascular therapy usually present with lower limb critical ischemia. Catheter-directed thrombolysis has been associated with reasonable amputation-free survival,[43] but it has not been widely used. Recently, angioplasty using low-profile, long balloons in the tibial and pedal arteries has been performed with high technical success and high limb salvage rates.[44]

Recent reports on the use of distraction osteogenesis (Ilizarov technique) to stimulate angioneogenesis and collateral formation suggest this has some benefit.[45] Use of autologous bone marrow mononuclear cells (BM-MNC) implantation shows promise with improvement in symptoms following injection to the affected limb. Several studies have shown a reduction in rest pain and improved ulcer healing.[46] The mechanism of action appears to involve increased angiogenesis and vasculogenesis.

Although rare, Buerger disease should be considered in any young patient presenting with critical limb ischemia and a history of tobacco use. Early intervention by cessation of all tobacco use can avoid progression to limb amputation. Newer treatments aimed at stimulating angiogenesis may also reduce progression to amputation.

The pathogenesis of radiation-induced arteritis is not fully understood. Changes in medium and large arteries exposed to radiation are initially limited to the intima, but eventually there is fibrosis of the internal elastic lamina and media, resulting in fibrosis.[47] These changes are thought to be caused by injury to the vasa vasorum. The medial fibrosis and intimal thickening narrows the arterial lumen, eventually causing thrombus formation and occlusion. Accelerated atherosclerotic changes are also common.

The diagnosis of radiation arteritis should be suspected in a patient presenting with arterial occlusive disease with a past history of irradiation to the relevant anatomic region. The lesions are often in atypical locations for atherosclerosis and may be unilateral with sparing of adjacent arteries (FIGURE 52.16). The most common sites are the extracranial carotid arteries (following irradiation for head and neck malignancy) and the aortoiliac arteries (following irradiation for pelvic malignancy). Historically, radiation injury to the axillary and subclavian arteries frequently complicated treatment for breast carcinoma but this is now rare.

Treatment options for patients who present with symptoms from radiation arteritis include medical therapy, surgical repair (anatomic revascularization or extra-anatomic bypass), and endovascular techniques including angioplasty, stenting, and covered stenting. Operating in a surgical field with radiation-damaged tissues is often problematic so extra-anatomic bypass and endovascular techniques hold appeal.[48]

Hemodynamically significant carotid artery lesions are much more prevalent than age and sex match controls in patients following head and neck irradiation.[49] The pattern of arterial disease may resemble atherosclerosis, being largely confined to the carotid bifurcation and proximal internal carotid artery. An atypical pattern is not uncommon, however, often with long stenoses of the common carotid artery (FIGURE 52.16) and sparing of the internal carotid artery.[50]

Because the carotid artery lesions are often extensive in radiation arteritis, extra-anatomic bypass with vein graft is often undertaken. Carotid endarterectomy in patients with radiation arteritis is associated with a higher incidence of cranial nerve palsy, wound complications, and restenosis when compared with nonirradiated patients.[51] Carotid artery stenting offers an attractive alternative to surgery in patients with hemodynamically significant radiation arteritis of the carotid arteries. Authors have reported high rates of technical success with short- and medium-term results comparable to open surgery.[52,53] There have been concerns, however, regarding apparent reduced long-term patency after carotid artery stenting in the setting of radiation arteritis when compared to surgical bypass with a higher rate of late, asymptomatic stent occlusion.[54] The technique of carotid artery stenting in radiation arteritis is generally the same as that of atherosclerotic stenoses with the use of dedicated nitinol self-expanding stents being most common (FIGURE 52.17). Embolic protection devices are usually used although their benefit in this condition is unclear.[54]

Radiation arteritis involving the aortoiliac arteries usually presents with occlusive lesions that correlate in distribution to the radiation field. These lesions are often indistinguishable

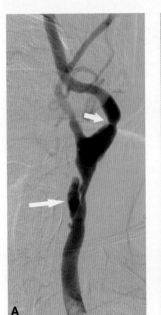
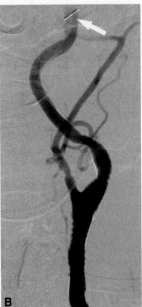

FIGURE 52.17 Radiation arteritis involving the right distal common and proximal internal carotid arteries in an 80-year-old male who presented with a small right cerebral hemispheric ischemic stroke. **A.** Digital subtraction angiography of the right carotid artery demonstrates an ulcerated lesion in the distal common carotid artery (*long arrow*) as well as a proximal internal carotid stenosis (*short arrow*). **B.** Lesion after treatment with a nitinol self-expanding stent (Precise, Cordis, Johnson & Johnson, Miami, FL). Note the distal embolic filter (Filterwire, Boston Scientific, Natick, MA) in the internal carotid artery (*arrow*).

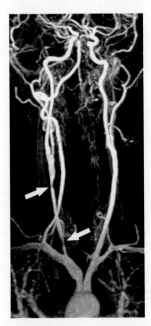

FIGURE 52.16 Magnetic resonance angiogram in a 72-year-old woman with right cerebral hemispheric transient ischemic attacks. The patient underwent radiotherapy for pharyngeal carcinoma 12 years previously. Note the stenoses in the proximal and distal right common carotid artery (*arrows*).

from atherosclerotic lesions. Localized stenoses or occlusions often respond well to angioplasty and stenting with both self-expanding and balloon expandable stents used.[55] For more extensive lesions, covered stent-grafts may be used, particularly if there is evidence of penetrating ulceration or rupture after angioplasty. Occasionally, frank aneurysmal change may occur, often representing a false or mycotic aneurysm.[56] These are best managed surgically, although endografts may be used in a bridging or palliative context.

▌CONCLUSION

Endovascular management of vasculitides is limited to medium- and large-artery arteritis. The most common application of endovascular techniques is seen in NSAA (Takayasu disease). There are expanding endovascular options in other arterial inflammatory conditions, however, including mycotic aneurysm and radiation arteritis.

▌REFERENCES

1. Leon LR, Mills JL. Diagnosis and management of aortic mycotic aneurysms. *Vasc Endovascular Surg* 2010;44(1):5–13.
2. Lee W-K, Mossop PJ, Little AF, et al. Infected (mycotic) aneurysms: spectrum of imaging appearances and management. *Radiographics* 2008;28(7):1853–1868.
3. Osler W. The Gustonian lectures on malignant endocarditis. *Br Med J* 1885;1:467–470.
4. Macedo TA, Stanson AW, Oderich GS, et al. Infected aortic aneurysms: imaging findings. *Radiology* 2004;232(1):250–257.
5. Chapot R, Houdart E, Saint-Maurice JP, et al. Endovascular treatment of cerebral mycotic aneurysms. *Radiology* 2002;222(2):389–396.
6. Marques da Silva R, Caugant DA, Eribe ER, et al. Bacterial diversity in aortic aneurysms determined by 16S ribosomal RNA gene analysis. *J Vasc Surg* 2006;44(5):1055–1060.
7. Kan CD, Lee HL, Yang YJ. Outcome after endovascular stent graft treatment for mycotic aortic aneurysm: a systematic review. *J Vasc Surg* 2007;46(5):906–912.
8. Liu WC, Kwak BK, Kim KN, et al. Tuberculous aneurysm of the abdominal aorta: endovascular repair using stent grafts in two cases. *Korean J Radiol* 2000;1(4):215–218.
9. Forbes TL, Harding GEJ. Endovascular repair of *Salmonella*-infected abdominal aortic aneurysms: a word of caution. *J Vasc Surg* 2006;44(1):198–200.
10. Vaughan-Huxley E, Hamady MS, Metcalfe MJ, et al. Endovascular repair of an acute, mycotic, ascending aortic pseudoaneurysm. *Eur J Vasc Endovasc Surg* 2011;41:488–491.
11. Setacci C, De Donato G, Setacci F, et al. Management of abdominal endograft infection. *J Cardiovasc Surg* 2010;51:33–41.
12. Numano F, Okawara M, Inomata H, et al. Takayasu's arteritis. *Lancet* 2000;356:1023–1025.
13. Kerr GS, Hallahan CW, Giordano J, et al. Takayasu arteritis. *Ann Intern Med* 1994;120(11):919–929.
14. Sharma S, Rajani M. Regional differences in the angiographic morphology in nonspecific aorto-arteritis (Takayasu's disease) in the Indian subcontinent. *Indian J Radiol Imaging* 1994;4:23–26.
15. Park JH, Chung JW, Im JG, et al. Takayasu arteritis: evaluation of mural changes in the aorta and pulmonary artery with CT angiography. *Radiology* 1995;196(1):89–93.
16. Kim SY, Park JH, Chung JW, et al. Follow-up CT evaluation of the mural changes in active Takayasu arteritis. *Korean J Radiol* 2007;8(4):286–294.
17. Choe YH, Han BK, Koh EM, et al. Takayasu's arteritis: assessment of disease activity with contrast-enhanced MR imaging. *AJR Am J Roentgenol* 2000;175(2):505–511.
18. Matsunaga N, Hayashi K, Sakamoto I, et al. Takayasu arteritis: MR manifestations and diagnosis of acute and chronic phase. *J Magn Reson Imaging* 1998;8(2):406–414.
19. Kobayashi Y, Ishii K, Oda K, et al. Aortic wall inflammation due to Takayasu arteritis imaged with 18F-FDG PET co-registered with enhanced CT. *J Nucl Med* 2005;46(6):917–922.
20. Scott D, Awang H, Sulieman B, et al. Surgical repair of visceral artery occlusions in Takayasu's disease. *J Vasc Surg* 1986;3(6):904–910.
21. Fields CE, Bower TC, Cooper LT, et al. Takayasu's arteritis: operative results and influence of disease activity. *J Vasc Surg* 2006;43(1):64–71.
22. Sharma S, Gupta A. Visceral artery interventions in Takayasu's arteritis. *Semin Intervent Radiol* 2009;26(3):230–241.
23. Tanaka R, Higashi M, Naito H. Angioplasty for non-arteriosclerotic renal artery stenosis: the efficacy of cutting balloon angioplasty versus conventional angioplasty. *Cardiovasc Intervent Radiol* 2007;30(4):601–606.
24. Sharma S, Jagia P. Endovascular management of nonspecific aortoarteritis. In: Kandarpa K, ed. *Peripheral Vascular Interventions.* Philadelphia, PA: Lippincott Williams & Wilkins; 2008:277–286.
25. Evans JM, O'Fallon WM, Hunder GG. Increased incidence of aortic aneurysm and dissection in giant cell (temporal) arteritis. A population-based study. *Ann Intern Med* 1995;122(7):502–507.
26. Newburger JW, Takahashi M, Gerber MA, et al. Diagnosis, treatment and long-term management of Kawasaki disease. *Circulation* 2004;110:2747–2771.
27. Buerger L. Thrombo-angiitis obliterans: a study of the vascular lesions leading to presenile spontaneous gangrene. *Am J Med Sci* 1908;136:567–580.
28. Malecki R, Zdrojowy K, Adamiec R. Thromboangiitis obliterans in the 21st century—a new face of disease. *Atherosclerosis* 2009;206:328–334.
29. Olin JW. Thromboangiitis obliterans (Buerger's disease). *N Engl J Med* 2000;343:864–869.
30. Olin JW, Shih A. Thromboangiitis obliterans (Buerger's disease). *Curr Opin Rheumatol* 2006;18:18–24.
31. Lie JT. The rise and fall and resurgence of thromboangiitis obliterans (Buerger's disease). *Acta Pathol Jpn* 1989;39:153–158.
32. Yorukoglu Y, Ilgit E, Zengin M, et al. Thromboangiitis obliterans (Buerger's disease) in women (a re-evaluation). *Angiology* 1993;44:527–532.
33. Olin JW, Young JR, Graor RA, et al. The changing clinical spectrum of thromboangiitis obliterans (Buerger's disease). *Circulation* 1990;82:3–8.
34. Mills JL. Buerger's disease in the 21st century: diagnosis, clinical features, and therapy. *Semin Vasc Surg* 2003;16:179–189.
35. Papa MZ, Rabi I, Adar R. A point scoring system for the clinical diagnosis of Buerger's disease. *Eur J Vasc Endovasc Surg* 1996;11:335–339.
36. Adar R, Papa MZ, Halpern Z, et al. Cellular sensitivity to collagen in thromboangiitis obliterans. *N Engl J Med* 1983;308:1113–1116.
37. Eichhorn J, Sima D, Lindschau C, et al. Antiendothelial cell antibodies in thromboangiitis obliterans. *Am J Med Sci* 1998;315:17–23.
38. Kobayashi M, Ito M, Nakagawa A, et al. Immunohistochemical analysis of arterial wall cellular infiltration in Buerger's disease (endarteritis obliterans). *J Vasc Surg* 1999;29:451–458.
39. Suzuki S, Mine H, Umehara I, et al. Buerger's disease (thromboangiitis obliterans): an analysis of the arteriograms of 119 cases. *Clin Radiol* 1982;33:235–240.
40. Fujii Y, Soga J, Nakamura S, et al. Classification of corkscrew collaterals in thromboangiitis obliterans (Buerger's disease): relationship between corkscrew type and prevalence of ischemic ulcers. *Circ J* 2010;74:1684–1688.
41. Ohta T, Shionoya S. Fate of the ischemic limb in Buerger's disease. *Br J Surg* 1988;75:259–262.
42. Roncon-Albuquerque R, Serrao P, Vale-Pereira R, et al. Plasma catecholamines in Buerger's disease: effects of cigarette smoking and surgical sympathectomy. *Eur J Vasc Endovasc Surg* 2002;24:338–343.
43. Hussein EA, el Dorri A. Intra-arterial streptokinase as adjuvant therapy for complicated Buerger's disease: early trials. *Int Surg* 1993;78:54–58.
44. Graziani L, Morelli L, Parini F, et al. Clinical outcome after extended endovascular recanalization in Buerger's disease in 20 consecutive cases. *Ann Vasc Surg* 2012;26(3):387–395.
45. Patwa JJ, Krishnan A. Buerger's disease (thromboangiitis obliterans)—management by Ilizarov's technique of horizontal distraction. A retrospective study of 60 cases. *Indian J Surg* 2011;73(1):40–47.
46. Durdu S, Akar AR, Arat M, et al. Autologous bone-marrow mononuclear cell implantation for patients with Rutherford grade II-III thromboangiitis obliterans. *J Vasc Surg* 2006;44:732–739.
47. Butler MJ, Lane RHS, Webster JHH. Irradiation injury to large arteries. *Br J Surg* 1980;67:341–343.
48. Modrall G, Sadjadi J. Early and late presentations of radiation arteritis. *Semin Vasc Surg* 2003;16(3):209–214.

49. Carmody BJ, Arora S, Avena R, et al. Accelerated carotid artery disease after high-dose head and neck radiotherapy: is there a role for routine carotid duplex surveillance? *J Vasc Surg* 1999;30:1045–1051.

50. Silverberg GD, Britt RH, Goffinet DR. Radiation-induced carotid artery disease. *Cancer* 1978;41:130–137.

51. Hassen-Khodja R, Sala F, Declemy S, et al. Surgical management of atherosclerotic carotid artery stenosis after cervical radiation therapy. *Ann Vasc Surg* 2000;14:608–611.

52. Ting AC, Cheng SW, Yeung KM, et al. Carotid stenting for radiation-induced extracranial carotid artery occlusive disease: efficacy and midterm outcomes. *J Endovasc Ther* 2004;11:53–59.

53. Harrod-Kim P, Kadkhodayan Y, Derdeyn CP, et al. Outcomes of carotid angioplasty and stenting for radiation-associated stenosis. *AJNR Am J Neuroradiol* 2005;26:1781–1788.

54. Protack CD, Bakken AM, Saad WA, et al. Radiation arteritis: a contraindication to carotid stenting? *J Vasc Surg* 2007;45:110–117.

55. Baerlocher MO, Rajan DK, Ing DJ, et al. Primary stenting of bilateral radiation-induced external iliac stenoses. *J Vasc Surg* 2004;40:1028–1031.

56. Ross HB, Sales JEL. Post-irradiation femoral aneurysm treated by iliopopliteal by-pass via the obturator foramen. *Br J Surg* 1972;59:400–405.

SECTION VII

Arteriopathies

Diagnosis and Role of Interventional Techniques

RYAN M. HICKEY and ALBERT A. NEMCEK, Jr.

▌ FIBROMUSCULAR DYSPLASIA

Introduction

Fibromuscular dysplasia (FMD) is a nonatherosclerotic, non-inflammatory arteriopathy that causes narrowing of small- and medium-sized vessels. FMD affects the renal arteries in 60% to 75% of cases, of which 35% have bilateral renal artery involvement. The extracranial carotid and vertebral arteries are affected in 25% to 30% of cases. Although intracranial FMD itself is rare, there is an association with intracranial aneurysms in 7% to 51% of cases of carotid or vertebral artery FMD.[1] Mesenteric arterial FMD is also rare and usually coexists with renal artery FMD.[2]

Renal artery FMD is the second leading cause of renal artery stenosis after atherosclerosis and is the cause of 10% of cases of renovascular hypertension.[1] Women are more commonly affected than men (M:F 1:3), typically presenting with hypertension between the ages of 15 and 50 years, and less commonly presenting with acute flank pain caused by arterial dissection or renal infarction. In contrast to atherosclerotic renal artery stenosis, which typically affects the ostial and proximal renal artery, FMD affects the mid- and distal renal artery. Because FMD is not an inflammatory condition, there should be no evidence of active inflammation, such as elevated acute phase reactants, as is typically seen with vasculitis.[1]

The five subtypes of FMD include medial fibroplasia (75% to 80%), perimedial fibroplasia (<10%), intimal fibroplasia (<10%), medial hyperplasia (<1%), and adventitial fibroplasia (<1%).[2] Medial fibroplasia is characterized by a "string-of-beads" appearance of the mid- to distal renal artery with the "beads" being larger than the normal vessel and pathologically proven to be true aneurysms (FIGURE 53.1). Perimedial fibrosis causes focal stenoses and arterial beading in which the "beads" are smaller than the normal vessel. Medial hyperplasia and intimal fibroplasia are angiographically indistinguishable and result in long segments of smoothly narrowed stenoses, similar to those seen in larger vessels affected by Takayasu or giant cell arteritis.[3] Finally, adventitial fibroplasia is characterized by sharply demarcated tubular areas of stenosis.

Diagnosis

Duplex ultrasonography has a high sensitivity and specificity for diagnosing main renal artery stenosis. Because FMD typically involves the mid- and distal main renal artery, it is critical that the entire renal artery be evaluated. Furthermore, patients should be scanned via an oblique or flank approach, additionally to the traditional anterior approach, to accurately insonate the distal renal arteries.[2] A renal-to-aortic peak systolic velocity greater than or equal to 3.5 suggests a stenosis of 60% to 99%. An end-diastolic velocity greater than or equal to 150 cm/second

in the renal artery corresponds to a severe stenosis ranging from 80% to 99%.[2]

Catheter angiography is the gold standard for diagnosing FMD of both the main renal arteries as well as branch vessels.[2] Although the sensitivities and specificities of both multidetector computed tomography angiography (CTA) and magnetic resonance angiography (MRA) exceed 90% for diagnosing main renal artery stenosis, spatial resolution of the distal and branch vessels remains insufficient to adequately diagnose or exclude FMD using these modalities.[4]

Treatment

Pharmacologic management of hypertension is the first line of therapy for patients with hypertension and renal artery FMD. For patients whose blood pressure cannot be controlled with medication, are noncompliant with or intolerant to blood pressure medication, or for those with evidence of ischemic nephropathy, endovascular or surgical revascularization is recommended. Percutaneous transluminal angioplasty (PTA) is considered the first-line therapy in young patients with new-onset hypertension due to the high cure rates in this population.[5] Primary stent placement is not recommended in the treatment of FMD and should be reserved for cases of suboptimal luminal gain following PTA (residual stenosis >30%) or dissection. Successful exclusion of renal artery aneurysms with covered stents has been described.[6]

Outcomes

A recent meta-analysis of published angioplasty and surgical revision studies involving more than 2,600 patients reports a success rate of 88.2% for PTA. Hypertension cure (i.e., blood pressure <140/90 mm Hg without pharmacologic therapy) was achieved in 35.8% of patients. Hypertension was cured or improved in 86.4% of patients. Cure rates in exclusively pediatric series ranged from 67% to 100%. There was no significant difference in the cure rate of patients with unilateral compared to bilateral disease, and no significant difference in cure rates between patients with branch stenosis compared to stenosis of other locations. The probability of curing hypertension with PTA was significantly lower in medial fibroplasia ("string-of-beads") compared to nonmedial fibroplasia ("unifocal" or "tubular"), however, and significantly decreased with increasing patient age and longer duration of hypertension.[7]

Restenosis rates following PTA ranged from 11% to 25% during 3- to 25-month follow-up. The complication rates for PTA compared to surgery were 12% and 17%, respectively, with major complications occurring in 6% of endovascular cases compared to 15% of surgical revascularization cases.[7]

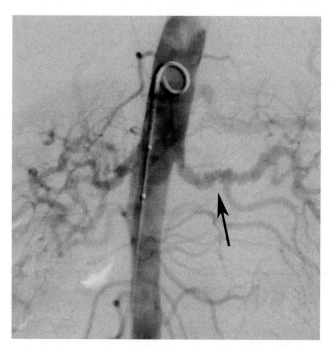

FIGURE 53.1 Digital subtraction abdominal aortogram in a 41-year-old woman with drug-resistant hypertension. The left renal artery (*arrow*) shows typical findings of medial fibroplasia with a "string-of-beads" appearance. The right renal artery is also involved, although less severely.

Surveillance and Follow-Up

The natural history of FMD includes progressive angiographic disease as evidenced by new lesions, worsening stenosis, and enlarging aneurysms in approximately 40% of cases.[8,9] Intimal and perimedial fibroplasia in particular are associated with progressive decline in renal function, although renal failure is rare. Medial fibroplasia generally remains stable with a relatively favorable prognosis.[5] Affected kidneys typically show a loss of renal mass, specifically caused by loss of cortical thickness and renal length, whereas the unaffected kidney also often loses cortical thickness but maintains renal length.[10]

Patients treated with PTA should undergo regular surveillance duplex ultrasonography to evaluate for restenosis, disease progression, or loss of renal volume.[5] Surveillance should begin immediately following treatment to assess treatment response at 6 and 12 months post-treatment and then annually.

◼ COMPRESSIVE ARTERIOPATHIES
Popliteal Entrapment Syndrome
Introduction

Popliteal artery entrapment syndrome is an uncommon cause of intermittent claudication in young adults resulting from a congenitally anomalous relationship between the popliteal artery and the medial head of the gastrocnemius muscle, its musculotendinous junction, or, rarely, the popliteus muscle. As a result, the popliteal artery is subjected to compression against bony structures in the popliteal fossa, particularly in certain provocative positions. In the classic type, delayed migration of the medial head of the gastrocnemius results in displacement of the popliteal artery such that it travels medial to that muscle,[11,12] resulting in intermittent compression and claudication with muscular activity.[13] Five additional types of entrapment have been described, including compression by fibrous or tendinous bands (type III), compression by the popliteus muscle (type IV), vein entrapment (type V), and functional entrapment without aberrant anatomy.[14] In most instances, the artery deviates from its normal course to lie medial to a normally inserting medial head of the gastrocnemius, or the popliteal artery course is normal but it is compressed by atypically inserting muscles, fibers, or tendons.

Popliteal entrapment syndrome is the cause of 60% of cases of ischemic leg pain in young patients (with the bulk of other cases resulting from adventitial cystic disease, see later). The syndrome is more commonly seen in men than women, although whether this is a difference in the prevalence of the anatomic predilection to entrapment or the result of muscular hypertrophy causing this predilection to become clinically manifest is uncertain. Bilateral entrapment occurs in 22% to 67% of cases although symptoms tend to predominate on one side.[15] The degree of arterial wall degeneration depends on the severity and duration of compression. Repetitive trauma and intimal damage cause popliteal artery narrowing, fibrosis, and thrombosis, often with distal embolization.[16] In just under 15% of cases, poststenotic dilatation and true aneurysm formation occur, increasing the risk for distal embolization.[17]

Diagnosis

CTA and MRI/MRA have replaced digital subtraction arteriography (DSA) as the modality of choice for diagnosing and evaluating popliteal entrapment syndrome. CTA very rapidly provides high-spatial-resolution images of the relationship between the popliteal artery and soft-tissue structures within the popliteal fossa. On cross-sectional imaging, for most of the cases, the anatomic substrate for entrapment is readily recognized: normally, the popliteal artery and vein course through the popliteal fossa in close proximity, separated by, if anything, small amounts of fat. In typical entrapment, a soft-tissue band (usually the medial head of the gastrocnemius or a slip of this muscle) separates the artery and vein (FIGURE 53.2). Note that this will not apply if the artery and vein are entrapped together, in which case a "sling" of muscle surrounds both structures, attached at both ends to the distal femur (FIGURE 53.3). Multiplanar reformatted images and maximum intensity projection images can also be used to further characterize vessel stenosis, poststenotic aneurysm formation, thrombosis, and collateralization.

On lower extremity arteriography or projectional reconstructions, the popliteal artery may be deviated medially in its midportion, or it may appear normal if entrapped only by a slip or tendon of the muscle. In either instance, provocative maneuvers—passive dorsiflexion or, preferably, active plantar flexion—may accentuate narrowing or cause occlusion of the artery (FIGURE 53.4). These maneuvers are not specific; however, some narrowing may be produced with normal popliteal fossa anatomy, especially in heavily muscled individuals ("functional" entrapment).

MRI provides better soft-tissue detail than CT and may aid in identifying surgically relevant anatomy. Adding MRA to MRI further increases diagnostic accuracy. The accuracy of MRA has

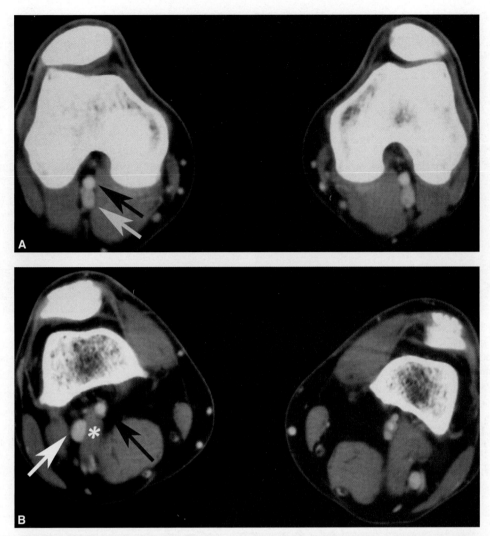

FIGURE 53.2 A. Contrast-enhanced CT of the popliteal fossa in an anatomically normal individual. Note that the artery (*black arrow*) and vein (*white arrow*) run together in the popliteal fossa with no separation. **B.** Contrast-enhanced CT of the popliteal fossa in bilateral entrapment. Note that the artery (*black arrow*) and vein (*white arrow*) are separated on each side by a muscular band (*asterisk*).

been reported to be comparable to DSA with an absolute agreement between the modalities of 95%. Additionally, MRI simultaneously diagnoses or excludes the presence of cystic adventitial disease, the leading differential diagnosis in a young patient presenting with intermittent claudication.[18] Note that confirmation of the anatomic abnormalities requires careful review of the anatomic relationship of the popliteal fossa musculature and vasculature on source images. If analysis is confined to projectional three-dimensional reconstructions, the anomalous anatomy will not be appreciated.

Treatment

Endovascular management of popliteal artery entrapment syndrome is limited to the use of catheter-directed thrombolysis and catheter thromboembolectomy for cases of acute limb-threatening ischemia.[19–21] Definitive treatment for popliteal artery entrapment requires surgical decompression of the popliteal fossa and interposition vein grafting if the underlying artery is severely damaged.

Celiac Artery Compression

Introduction

Celiac artery compression syndrome, also known as median arcuate ligament syndrome or Dunbar syndrome, is characterized by extrinsic compression of the celiac trunk (and less often of the superior mesenteric artery) by the median arcuate ligament or celiac ganglionic tissue. Compression occurs during expiration and is relieved upon inspiration due to anterior and inferior movement of the celiac axis during inspiration (FIGURE 53.5). Chronic compression of the celiac axis can result in irreversible arterial damage, including intimal hyperplasia, medial elastic fiber proliferation, and adventitial disorganization.[22] Over time, progressive fixed, hemodynamically significant narrowing of the celiac artery and development of pancreaticoduodenal collaterals may result.

It is controversial whether or not celiac artery compression can result in symptoms of abdominal pain.[23] Many individuals with clear evidence of celiac compression are asymptomatic. Further, it is difficult to posit that ischemic pain can result from

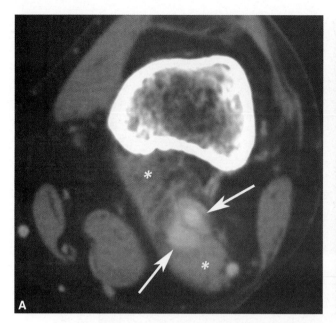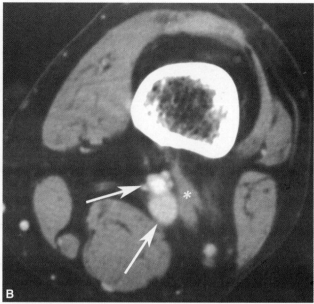

FIGURE 53.3 A. Contrast-enhanced CT of combined popliteal arterial and venous entrapment; the patient presented with lower extremity ischemic symptoms and leg swelling. At the level of the intercondylar notch the artery and vein (*arrows*) are surrounded by a sling of gastrocnemius musculature (*asterisks*). **B.** At a slightly more cephalad level, the sling (*asterisk*) surrounding the vessels is completed.

isolated narrowing of the celiac artery with patent superior and inferior mesenteric arteries that can provide collateral supply to the celiac territory. It may be that if pain can result, it is caused by neural compression in the region of the celiac plexus rather than being related to alterations in blood flow. It has been emphasized that in patients with celiac compression and abdominal pain, a careful search should be made for other causes of abdominal pain.

Regardless of the potential role of celiac compression in abdominal pain, there are two situations in which this condition

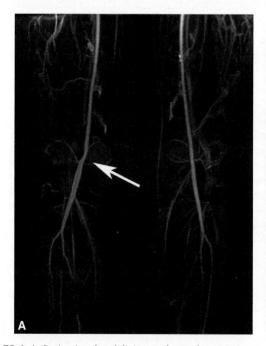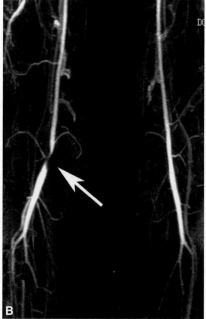

FIGURE 53.4 A. Projectional gadolinium-enhanced magnetic resonance arteriogram in a young man with right calf claudication. Without provocative maneuvers, there is mild narrowing of the mid-popliteal artery (*arrow*). **B.** Same patient as in (**A**), now with passive dorsiflexion of the right foot. Marked narrowing of the popliteal artery results (*arrow*).

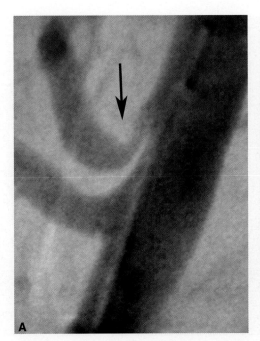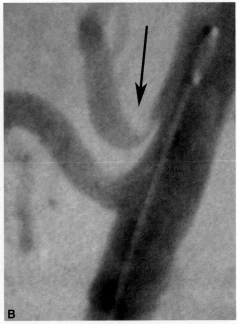

FIGURE 53.5 A. Typical angiographic appearance of celiac artery compression syndrome with eccentric stenosis and caudal displacement of the celiac artery (*arrow*). Lateral digital subtraction aortogram obtained in full inspiration. **B.** Same patient as in (**A**), lateral digital subtraction arteriogram obtained in full expiration. Note the increased severity of the proximal celiac stenosis (*arrow*).

can become clinically important. It has been recognized that pancreaticoduodenal arcade collateralization can result in true aneurysms in patients with celiac compression (as well as other causes of celiac stenosis). These aneurysms may rupture, even at small sizes, typically into the extraenteric mesentery rather than into the lumen of the small bowel (FIGURE 53.6). The other situation in which celiac compression may become clinically significant is in cases of liver transplantation, when the dearth of hepatic artery collaterals can cause a previously clinically silent stenosis to manifest as ischemic cholangiopathy.

Diagnosis

Lateral aortography demonstrates focal, asymmetric, and classically hook-shaped narrowing of the proximal celiac axis with poststenotic dilatation.[23,24] Celiac axis narrowing varies throughout the respiratory cycle and is most severe on expiration.[23]

CTA with volume rendering and three-dimensional reconstruction may replace catheter angiography as the diagnostic modality of choice for celiac artery compression syndrome. Sagittal reconstruction images provide optimal visualization of the celiac axis and often allow visualization of the median arcuate ligament. Because CTA image acquisition typically occurs during inspiration, when celiac artery compression should be minimized, focal narrowing seen at CTA may correlate with clinically significant compression. Poststenotic dilatation and marked collateralization support the diagnosis.[24]

Treatment

Standard treatment of celiac artery compression syndrome includes division of the median arcuate ligament by open or laparoscopic surgery. In one of the largest published series of surgical repair, long-term results suggested that division of the median arcuate ligament alone was insufficient and celiac dilatation or reconstruction was necessary to achieve clinical improvement.[25] Again, it should be noted that there is some support for the idea that the true benefit of surgery is in achieving neurolysis rather than improved mesenteric flow.

Endovascular therapy alone has a poor success rate in the treatment of celiac artery compression syndrome due to the extrinsic compressive forces of the median arcuate ligament.[26,27] However, PTA with or without stent placement, following surgical release, may be beneficial in addressing severe celiac stenosis in place of or prior to undertaking more extensive surgery, such as celiac reconstruction or bypass.[23]

Because of high rates of rupture and secondary mortality associated with pancreaticoduodenal arcade aneurysms, embolization of these aneurysms is recommended. Effective embolization includes packing the aneurysm sac with coils, or excluding the aneurysm from circulation by embolizing the parent artery distal and proximal to the aneurysm.[28,29]

Arterial Thoracic Outlet Syndrome

Introduction

Thoracic outlet syndrome refers to compression of subclavian-axillary neurovascular structures at the thoracic outlet, resulting in a spectrum of clinical signs and symptoms ranging from pain and paresthesias to ischemia of the affected limb. Neurogenic thoracic outlet syndrome is by far the most common cause of compression-induced paresthesias with arterial thoracic outlet syndrome representing less than 1% of cases.[30]

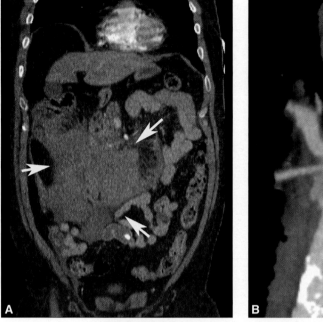
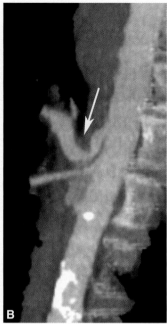
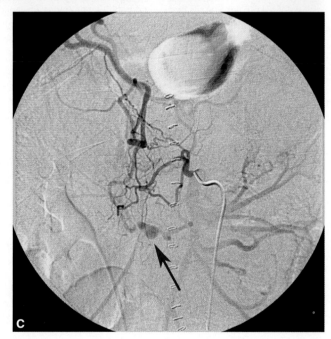

FIGURE 53.6 A 58-year-old man presenting with acute abdominal pain. **A.** Coronal reconstruction, contrast-enhanced abdominal CT. The scan shows a large accumulation of soft-tissue density in the mesentery (*arrows*) consistent with a hematoma. **B.** Sagittal reconstruction, contrast-enhanced abdominal CT. Note the typical configuration of celiac artery compression syndrome (*arrow*). **C.** Superior mesenteric branch digital subtraction arteriography performed following exploratory laparotomy. The laparotomy did not reveal a source for mesenteric bleeding. An aneurysm of the pancreaticoduodenal territory is present (*arrow*). This was subsequently embolized with detachable coils.

Arterial thoracic outlet syndrome most frequently results from compression by an osseus abnormality, such as a cervical rib or anomalous first rib, or by compression from tendons extending from these structures. Rarely, hypertrophy of the scalene muscle can cause compression of the subclavian artery. Repetitive compression causes arterial damage, leading to stenosis or aneurysm formation. Arterial damage may manifest as claudication, pallor, coolness, or paresthesia of the arm and hand with sparing of the neck and shoulder. Arterial thrombosis and distal embolization can cause extensive hand and digital ischemia.[30,31] Retrograde embolization from proximal

subclavian artery aneurysms resulting in cerebral infarcts has also been reported.[32,33]

Diagnosis

Because arterial thoracic outlet syndrome is often associated with rib anomalies, chest radiography is an important screening modality. Duplex ultrasonography reliably detects aneurysms and stenoses of the subclavian artery. Arteriography performed in the neutral, hyperabducted, and hyperextended positions remains an important component of the evaluation of suspected arterial thoracic outlet syndrome and assists with

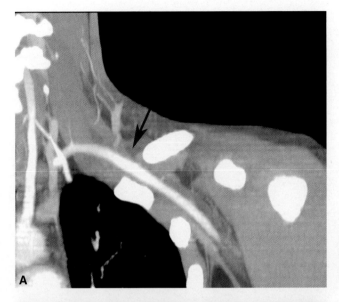

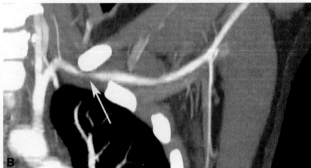

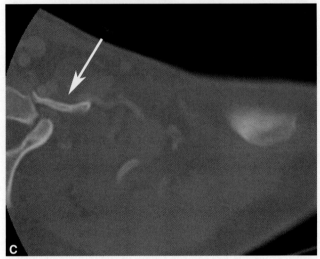

FIGURE 53.7 Contrast-enhanced CT arteriography imaging in a 13-year-old with bilateral upper extremity tingling and numbness. **A.** Coronal maximum intensity projection reconstruction with the left arm in the neutral position. Note a widely patent subclavian artery (*arrow*). **B.** Coronal maximum intensity projection with the left arm hyperabducted and extended. Severe narrowing of the subclavian artery is present. **C.** Axial CT shows a short left-sided cervical rib (*arrow*).

surgical planning.[30,31] CT arteriography and three-dimensional reconstructions can also show compression as well as the musculoskeletal anatomy relevant to the compression (FIGURE 53.7).

Treatment

Treatment of arterial thoracic outlet syndrome requires surgical excision or release of the compressive structure. The presence of intimal damage or aneurysm formation necessitates excision of the affected arterial segment and replacement with interposition graft or reversed saphenous vein.[31] A small series of subclavian artery aneurysms associated with thoracic outlet syndrome successfully treated with stent-grafts, in conjunction with first rib resection, has been reported.[34]

DRUG-INDUCED ARTERIOPATHY

Introduction

Ergotism refers to peripheral vasoconstriction resulting in burning pain and ischemia caused by ingestion of ergot alkaloids. Known as St. Anthony's fire, ergotism was historically caused by alkaloids produced by the fungus *Claviceps purpura* that had infected rye and grain.[35] In modern times, ergotism may result from medications containing ergot alkaloids, such as certain migraine medications, as well as from recreational drug use, such as lysergic acid diethylamide (LSD), synthetically derived from ergot alkaloids.[36]

Although exceedingly rare, patients with acute ergotism may present with convulsions or acute peripheral ischemia, even gangrene. Agonistic effects of the ergot alkaloid on alpha-adrenergic receptors and prostaglandin activity trigger vasoconstriction, most markedly affecting the distal extremities.[37] Catheter angiography remains the standard for diagnosis, demonstrating generalized and symmetric smooth tapering of the peripheral vasculature (FIGURE 53.8) with focal vasospasm being less common.[38]

Treatment

Treatment of ergotism generally consists of therapeutic intravenous anticoagulation with intra-arterial vasodilators and sympatholytics. Raval et al. describe successful PTA of nearly the entire

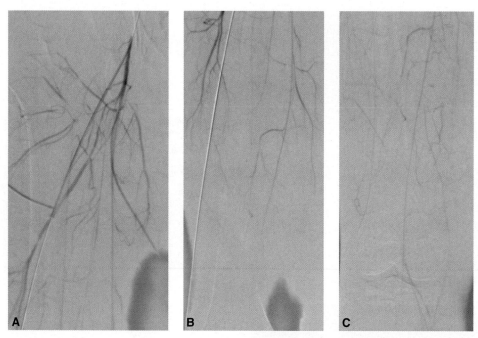

FIGURE 53.8 Ergotism. Images from digital subtraction arteriography on a 19-year-old woman with rapid onset of lower extremity pain, loss of sensation, weakness, and purple discoloration. She was found to have a history of lysergic acid diethylamide (LSD) use 3 days before presentation. Images obtained in the proximal (**A**), mid (**B**), and distal (**C**) thigh show diffuse narrowing of the superficial femoral, profunda femoris, and popliteal arteries consistent with vasospasm.

lower limb vasculature, in combination with oral antiplatelet medication and intra-arterial vasodilators, for a case of extensive bilateral lower extremity ergotism and severe peripheral ischemia related to LSD use. PTA presumably caused interruption of sustained smooth muscle contraction by muscle stretching, resulting in luminal gain and lower extremity reperfusion, sparing the patient major amputation.[36]

CONGENITAL AND HERITABLE ARTERIOPATHIES

Persistent Sciatic Artery

Introduction

Persistent sciatic artery is a rare embryologic anomaly resulting from incomplete regression of the vascular supply to the lower extremity, 20% to 25% of which occur bilaterally. Men and women are affected equally; there may be associated disorders, such as hemihypertrophy, limb hypoplasia, varicosities, and others. The sciatic artery, a branch of the internal iliac artery, persists as the dominant vascular supply to the lower extremity with associated hypoplasia or aplasia of the iliofemoral system. The sciatic artery passes through the sciatic foramen adjacent to the sciatic nerve and continues posteriorly in the thigh along the adductor magnus muscle to reach the popliteal fossa (FIGURE 53.9). Forty percent to 60% of persistent sciatic arteries develop aneurysms that occur adjacent to the greater trochanter of the femur, likely as the result of repetitive trauma. Approximately half of these aneurysms are complicated by thrombosis, thromboembolism, or compressive symptoms.[39,40] Persistent sciatic arteries are also prone to atherosclerotic degeneration

and generalized arteriomegaly. On physical examination, there may be a unique combination of poor femoral pulses and good distal pulses (Cowie sign).

Persistent sciatic artery typically presents in the fifth to sixth decade with sciatic nerve pain caused by compressive effects of an adjacent aneurysm or acute onset of lower extremity ischemia due to thrombosis or embolism. Physical examination may reveal a pulsatile mass in the region of the buttock or greater trochanter. Frank aneurysmal rupture is less common. Aneurysmal degeneration may occur due to chronic trauma at the sciatic foramen and gluteus musculature with a component of congenital dysplasia of the vessel wall.[41] Angiographic imaging, including CTA and MRA, will adequately demonstrate the presence of a persistent sciatic artery and secondary complications (FIGURES 53.10 to 53.12). On these studies, the internal iliac artery is often larger than the external. The profunda femoris artery is usually present but the superficial artery is often hypoplastic, ending in a typical "forked" configuration in the distal thigh. The persistent sciatic artery may be tortuous, irregular, and sometimes diffusely ectatic. Two classification systems for persistent sciatic artery are described by Pillet et al. and Paris et al., both of which reflect the degree of continuity of the sciatic artery and iliofemoral system through the lower extremity.[42] A complete persistent sciatic artery is most common, in which this vessel is continuous from the pelvis (as the continuation of the inferior gluteal artery) to the popliteal artery. An incomplete persistent sciatic artery may also occur, in which there is discontinuity between the persistent sciatic artery and the internal iliac or popliteal artery, and small collaterals may be present. In such cases, the superficial femoral artery may be continuous to the popliteal artery.

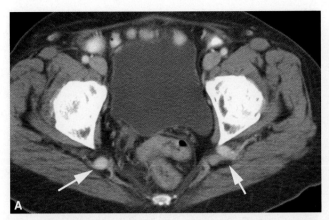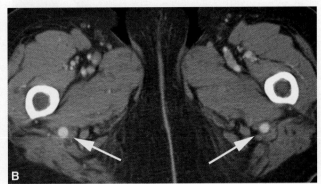

FIGURE 53.9 Asymptomatic persistent sciatic arteries in an 81-year-old woman. Note the arteries (*arrows*) exiting the sciatic notch (**A**) and coursing caudally in the posterior thigh (**B**).

Treatment

For individuals with an incidentally discovered persistent sciatic artery and no aneurysmal degeneration, regular duplex ultrasonographic evaluation is recommended due to the high incidence of developing an aneurysm and its associated complications.

Symptomatic individuals are at high risk for thromboembolic complications and limb loss. In the presence of a normal superficial femoral artery, or sufficient collateral flow to the lower leg in the setting of an incomplete iliofemoral system, the persistent sciatic artery can be ligated, resected, or embolized.[43,44]

Most persistent sciatic arteries are associated with a hypoplastic or aplastic superficial femoral artery, which requires femoropopliteal or iliopopliteal bypass prior to exclusion of the sciatic artery from circulation. The use of vascular plugs to obliterate the sciatic artery, in place of dense coils packing, has been described.[42,43] Interposition grafts in place of resected areas of aneurysmal degeneration are contraindicated due to high rates of thrombosis from compression, sciatic nerve injury, and aneurysmal degeneration of the remaining sciatic artery. The same contraindications would similarly apply to the use of covered stents.[45]

Ehlers-Danlos Syndrome Type IV

Introduction

Ehlers-Danlos syndrome type IV is an autosomal dominant connective tissue disorder of type III collagen, which is predominantly found in skin, blood vessel walls, and hollow viscera, rendering affected individuals prone to spontaneous arterial, intestinal, or uterine rupture.[46] Clinical features of Ehlers-Danlos type IV include a slender facial structure with periorbital pigmentation, thin translucent skin, excessive bruising, and poor wound healing.[47]

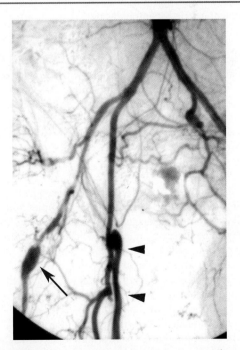

FIGURE 53.11 Digital subtraction arteriogram, right anterior oblique projection, showing a focal aneurysm of a persistent sciatic artery (*arrow*). The patient has had a femoral-popliteal bypass graft (*arrowheads*) needed because of occlusion related to emboli from the aneurysm.

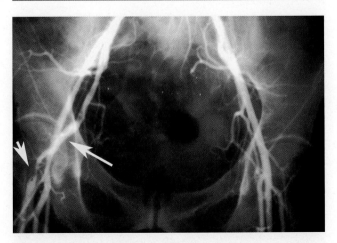

FIGURE 53.10 Conventional arteriogram showing typical appearance of persistent sciatic artery (*arrows*), representing a continuation of the inferior gluteal artery out the sciatic notch, behind the greater trochanter. Note atherosclerotic irregularity of the artery.

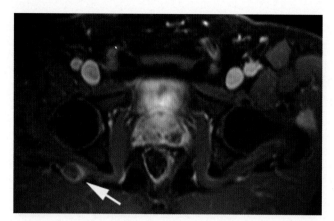

FIGURE 53.12 Axial source images from a gadolinium-enhanced magnetic resonance arteriogram in a 53-year-old man with right lower extremity ischemia. A partially thrombosed persistent sciatic aneurysm (*arrow*) is present. Distally, persistent sciatic artery thrombosis extended to the popliteal artery.

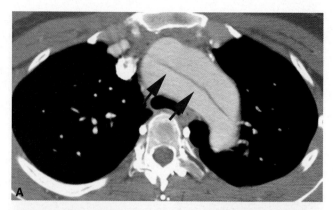

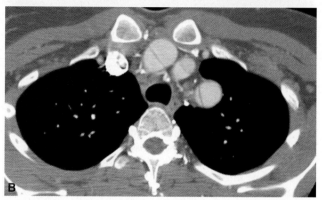

FIGURE 53.13 Axial contrast-enhanced CT scans on a 36-year-old woman with Ehlers-Danlos syndrome type IV. Aortic dissection is present (**A**, *arrows*) extending into the brachiocephalic artery, left common carotid artery, and left subclavian artery (**B**), each of which demonstrates aneurysm formation.

Nearly a quarter of individuals with Ehlers-Danlos IV present with a complication before age 20 with approximately 80% having a related complication by the age of 40.[46] Vascular complications are the leading cause of death and include dissections, aneurysms, and arteriovenous fistulas, often occurring spontaneously and with a predilection for large- and middle-sized arteries, particularly the aorta and its branch vessels.[46] There is a high risk of uterine rupture in pregnancy, particularly during the third trimester and in the puerperal period. Varicose veins are also common in Ehlers-Danlos IV, but surgical management is strictly contraindicated.[47]

Diagnosis

The diagnosis of Ehlers-Danlos type IV should be considered in any young patient presenting with sequelae of spontaneous vascular injury, including intracranial hemorrhage or stroke, or with a combination of vascular complications as noted previously (FIGURES 53.13 to 53.15). Genetic studies would reveal a heterozygous mutation of the COL3A1 gene on chromosome 2.[47]

Management and Treatment

No specific treatments exist for Ehlers-Danlos type IV, and interventions are limited to symptomatic therapies and genetic counseling. All invasive diagnostic modalities, including arteriography and endoscopy, must be avoided or performed with extreme caution, and operative treatments should be limited to life-threatening circumstances.

With relation specifically to arteriography, given the excessively high rates of puncture site pseudoaneurysms and rupture, and a propensity for dissection of selected or catheterized vessels, endovascular therapy is typically reserved for coil embolization of ruptured arteries. Mortality rates associated with arteriography have previously been reported as high as 17% with major complication rates reaching almost 70%; however, lower-profile endovascular systems have likely lowered these rates. Nonetheless, open repair of arterial access sites is recommended.[46,48] Consensus documents recommend avoidance of stent-graft therapy in Ehlers-Danlos IV patients due to high rates of perforation and erosion at landing points as well as very high rates of secondary intervention.[48,49]

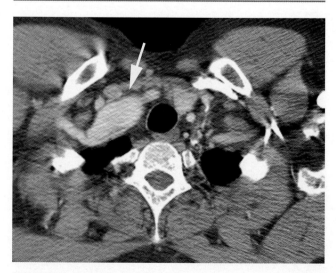

FIGURE 53.14 Brachiocephalic artery aneurysm in a 31-year-old man with Ehlers-Danlos syndrome type IV (*arrow*).

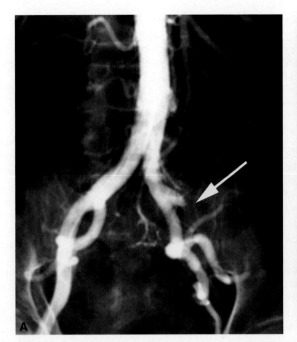
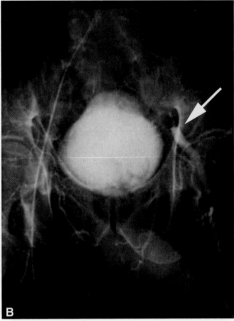

FIGURE 53.15 Endofibrosis of the external iliac artery. A 49-year-old man presenting with left lower extremity ischemia of acute onset. Conventional arteriography shows occlusion of the common iliac artery (**A**, *arrow*) with reconstitution of the external iliac artery (**B**, *arrow*). Thrombolytic therapy uncovered a focal external iliac stenosis. The patient was a vigorous bicycle rider.

Neurofibromatosis Type I

Introduction

Neurofibromatosis (NF) type I is an autosomal dominant disorder or neural crest cells resulting from mutation of the NF1 gene on chromosome 17 and manifesting with diffuse neurofibromas as well as benign and malignant tumors. NF type I-related arteriopathy causes occlusive and aneurysmal disease, most commonly affecting the renal arteries with the abdominal aorta, mesenteric, cerebral, and peripheral arteries being less frequently involved.[50] Most patients with NF arteriopathy have multivessel involvement but remain asymptomatic until late childhood or early adulthood. Renal artery hypertension is the most common clinical manifestation.[51]

Intrinsic arterial wall lesions are present in both the arterial stenoses and aneurysms of NF type I, resulting from enlarging adventitial neurofibromas in medium and large arteries as well as spindle cell proliferation in the walls of smaller arteries. Arterial stenoses or aneurysms may also form due to cell proliferation, degeneration, healing, smooth muscle loss, and fibrosis.[50,51] Four distinct histopathologic subtypes have been described. The purely intimal subtype demonstrates intimal proliferation with thinning of the media in the presence of a normal adventitia, resulting in vessel stenosis. The aneurysmal intimal subtype tends to affect larger vessels and causes hyaline intimal thickening, disruption of the elastic lamina, loss or thinning of the media, and aneurysmal degeneration of the vessel. In the nodular periarterial subtype, nodules develop between the media and adventitia, impinging on the intima and resulting in stenosis. Finally, in the epithelioid subtype, proliferation of fusiform cells causes vessel stenosis.[50]

A review of the published literature by Oderich et al. reports renal artery lesions as the most common manifestation, present in 41% of NF type I patients with vasculopathy, of which 68% were unilateral. Renal artery stenoses were more common than aneurysms.[51] Renal artery stenoses tend to involve the renal artery ostium, whereas aneurysms are more frequently intrarenal.[50,51] Carotid, vertebral, and cerebral artery lesions occurred in 19% of patients and were more often aneurysmal and affected women (72%) more often than men. Abdominal aortic coarctation or aneurysm occurred in 12% of patients.[51]

Treatment

Endovascular therapy with PTA is an option for treatment of clinically relevant renal artery stenoses. Because it has no adverse effects on subsequent surgical management, it may be considered the first-line therapy when medical management has failed. In a review of 10 NF type I patients treated with renal artery PTA, Booth et al.[52] report successful PTA in 33% of the lesions treated and blood pressure control in another 33%. In their comprehensive review, however, Oderich et al. report restenosis requiring intervention occurring in 44% of patients treated with PTA. In general, control of renovascular hypertension in NF type I patients requires a combination of medical, endovascular, and open surgical management.[50,51]

Visceral aneurysms associated with NF type I have been successfully treated with coil embolization.[51,53] Successful use of covered stents has been reported for the treatment of a ruptured subclavian artery aneurysm as well as contained rupture of two superior mesenteric artery aneurysms in a single patient.[54,55] One of these two aneurysms subsequently filled due to an endoleak and was subsequently treated with coil embolization.[56] Despite lack of data on the use of stent-grafts in the treatment of NF-associated aneurysms, no definite contraindications exist and indications for treatment should be the same as for the general population. No data are available regarding endovascular management of aortic coarctation in individuals with NF type I.

Pseudoxanthoma Elasticum

Pseudoxanthoma elasticum is an inherited disorder of connective tissue leading to progressive calcification of the elastic tissues of the skin, eyes, and vasculature.[57] The disorder results from an abnormality of the ABCC6 gene on chromosome 16, of which more than 40 mutations have been discovered.[58] Affected individuals present with premature cardiovascular disease, particularly claudication, in the setting of characteristic yellow skin plaques.[57] Calcium deposition in the elastic laminae of arteries leads to vessel remodeling, stenosis, and, ultimately, ischemia.[59]

Diagnosis relies on skin biopsy. Fundoscopic examination reveals angioid streaks even in the absence of overt skin manifestations.

Treatment of pseudoxanthoma elasticum is limited to addressing vascular lesions that become symptomatic because lifestyle modification and medications appear to have no effect on progression of the vascular disease. Revascularization of affected vascular territories is difficult due to the diffuse and often distal distribution of the disease. PTA of focal stenoses has been reported with favorable outcomes.[59]

Homocystinuria

Homocystinuria refers to urinary excretion of the oxidized form of plasma homocysteine, an intermediate product in the conversion of the amino acid methionine into cysteine. Elevated plasma levels of homocysteine can result from inherited impairment of enzymes of this metabolic pathway or deficiencies in required cofactors, and predispose to intra-arterial thrombosis, arterial dissection, as well as an arteriopathy than can appear similar to FMD due to a combination of endothelial dysfunction, effects on coagulation factors, and platelet activation. Widespread atherosclerosis may develop besides hypercoagulopathy.[60] Classic homocystinuria is an autosomal recessive disorder caused by mutation of nearly 100 alleles that code for the enzyme cystathionine-beta-synthase (CBS).[61]

In a cohort of over 600 patients with homocystinuria reviewed by Mudd et al., 25% presented with thromboembolic events. Peripheral venous thrombosis caused 51% of ischemic events, cerebrovascular infarcts represented 32%, peripheral arterial occlusions 11%, and myocardial infarctions 4%. The risk of a vascular event in this cohort was 25% by age 16 and 50% by age 29.[62]

The diagnosis of homocystinuria relies on measurement of plasma homocysteine levels and should be considered in the diagnostic workup of children or young adults with arterial thrombotic events, as part of all hypercoagulability workups, as well as in the evaluation of patients presenting with atherosclerosis before the age of 40.

Treatment of homocystinuria aims to reduce or normalize plasma levels of homocysteine through dietary regulation and supplementation with vitamin B_6, folate, betaine, and vitamin B_{12}, depending on the precise metabolic abnormality.[60] Patients

with arterial occlusive disease may fail endovascular management until plasma homocysteine levels are normalized. Additionally, given the effects on both the coagulation cascade and platelet activation, patients should be treated with antiplatelet medication as well as anticoagulation.[63]

Tuberous Sclerosis

Tuberous sclerosis is an autosomal dominant disorder with a classic clinical triad of seizures, mental retardation, and facial adenomas. Although vascular manifestations of tuberous sclerosis are rare, their clinical implications are significant. Aneurysms have been reported more often than arterial stenoses or occlusions, and most aneurysms affect the abdominal aorta. Arterial stenoses tend to affect medium and large arteries, most commonly as abdominal aortic coarctation or renal artery stenosis, either in isolation or concomitantly.[64]

Patients with tuberous sclerosis and any signs or symptoms that may be attributable to arterial aneurysms or stenosis should receive either targeted or whole-body vascular screening with CTA or MRA. MRA is preferred in children due to the lack of ionizing radiation. Exam times are longer, however, often necessitating sedation. Because of its better spatial resolution, CTA is preferred for evaluation of the small- and medium-sized vessels, such as the intrarenal arterial branches. Follow-up surveillance can be performed with duplex ultrasonography, MRA, or CTA, depending on the vessel involved.[64]

■ OTHER ARTERIOPATHIES

Endofibrosis of the Iliofemoral Arteries

Endofibrosis of the iliofemoral arteries refers to intimal hyperplasia most often involving the external iliac artery, followed by the common iliac and superficial femoral arteries, in athletically active individuals. The finding has been described most commonly among cyclists, including professional and recreational cyclists, resulting in decreased arterial flow to one or both of the lower extremities during vigorous activity. Affected individuals rarely present with overt claudication, but rather report rapid fatigue, deteriorated performance, loss of power, or weakness.[65]

Endofibrosis has been attributed to several mechanisms, including repeated stretching with prolonged hip flexion, possibly exacerbated by psoas muscle hypertrophy, external compression by the inguinal ligament or hypertrophied abdominal musculature, prolonged high flow through the iliofemoral vessels, and kinking of the vessel due to tethering by external iliac artery branches (Ford).

Diagnosis of endofibrosis may be difficult because clinical findings are absent at rest. Angiographic findings include beaded or smooth stenosis of the affected iliac vessel over 5 to 6 cm, occasionally requiring comparison to the contralateral side to detect subtle stenoses. Pressure gradients across the stenoses are typically normal at rest but may become abnormal following intra-arterial vasodilator administration. MRA and CTA can be helpful in the diagnosis because the images can be acquired with the patient in a variety of positions and then reconstructed in three dimensions.[66,67]

Endofibrosis lesions tend to be resistant to PTA with significant elastic recoil or even dissection in the short-term.[67,68] Stent placement is generally contraindicated due to mechanical compression, migration, and aggressive intimal hyperplasia at the stent margins.[69] Surgical options depend on the underlying cause of endofibrosis and include arterial release, arterial shortening in the setting of vessel kinking, resection of the affected segment with interposition vein graft, or endarterectomy with vein patch angioplasty. Report of a long-term follow-up of endofibrosis suggests that lesions will stabilize once intensive activity has stopped.[65]

Cystic Adventitial Disease

Cystic adventitial disease is an uncommon cause of focal vascular stenoses, in which cysts containing mucinous material are found in the outer media and adventitia of the popliteal artery. The cyst contents are generally clear and gelatinous in consistency but can have a "currant jelly" appearance if hemorrhage has occurred. Although most often involving the popliteal arteries, it has been described in arteries of the forearm (radial and ulnar arteries, external iliac/common femoral arteries), tending to occur near joints and involve nonaxial arteries (i.e., arteries that form at a later stage embryologically than axial arteries). There are rare reports of venous cysts. Men are affected 15 times more frequently than women, and the lesions are nearly always unilateral. Theories as to the etiology of adventitial cysts include chronic trauma, implantation of ganglionic cysts within the adventitia, as well as incorporation of mesenchymal cells into the vessel wall from nearby joints during embryogenesis that secrete mucin later in life.[70] Patients may present with the sudden onset of claudication, and because the cysts are space-occupying, sharp knee flexion may cause the loss of distal pulses. This entity should be considered, along with popliteal entrapment syndrome, in younger individuals presenting with claudication.

Angiographic studies show eccentric, concentric, or spiral stenoses or segmental occlusion of the involved artery. The artery above and below the lesion is normal in caliber, and when involving the popliteal artery the course of the artery is normal. On cross-sectional imaging biconvex, ovoid, or round, often multilocular collections are demonstrated (FIGURES 53.16 and 53.17); at times the lesion may mimic an intraluminal filling defect. MRI and MRA are excellent diagnostic modalities, demonstrating not only the cyst within the vessel wall, but also a connection to the adjacent joint as well as the degree of vessel stenosis.[71]

Treatment of adventitial cysts includes cyst excision with preservation of the vessel or excision of the affected segment with vein graft interposition. PTA as well as stent placement have been shown to be ineffective in treating cystic adventitial disease.[72–74] Although percutaneous aspiration of cyst contents has been described, its effectiveness may be limited by the viscosity of the cyst contents, by the multilocular nature of the cysts, and by recurrence following successful aspiration.

Hypothenar Hammer Syndrome

Hypothenar hammer syndrome (HHS) refers to characteristic injury to the palmar ulnar artery from repetitive blunt trauma to the hypothenar region of the hand, leading to digital ischemia from thromboembolism (FIGURE 53.18). Repetitive trauma to the palmar ulnar artery, typically at the hamate, results in arterial thrombosis or aneurysm formation with distal embolization. The superficial palmar arch, supplied by the ulnar artery, is the dominant source of blood to the digits, particularly the third through fifth digits. Underlying FMD of the palmar ulnar artery has been proposed as a predisposing factor for development of the syndrome.[75]

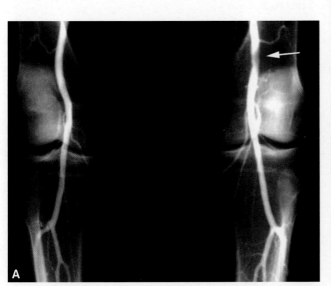
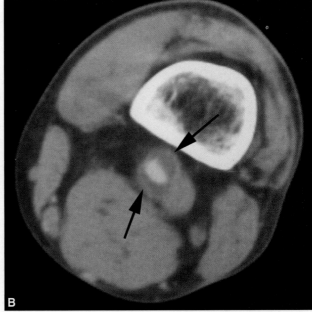

FIGURE 53.16 Adventitial cystic disease of the popliteal artery. A 35-year-old man presenting with left calf claudication. Conventional arteriography (**A**) shows a subtle lucency of the proximal popliteal artery (*arrow*). Contrast-enhanced CT (**B**) shows low-density material within the wall of the popliteal artery with luminal compression (*arrows*).

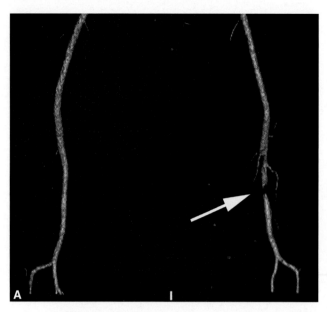
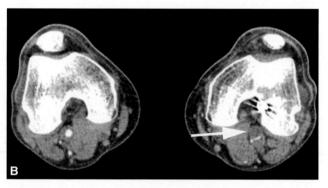

FIGURE 53.17 Adventitial cystic disease of the popliteal artery. A 46-year-old man with left leg pain. CT angiography (**A**) suggests a short focal occlusion of the popliteal artery (*arrow*). Source images (**B**) show low-density material flattening and nearly occluding the popliteal artery lumen (*arrow*).

Catheter angiography of both upper extremities and hands remains the gold standard for diagnosis, although MRA with a 3.0T magnet has been shown to offer excellent depiction of the digital arteries and stenoses.[76,77] Angiographic findings of HHS include

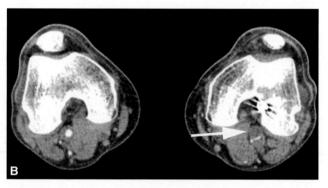

FIGURE 53.18 Hypothenar hammer syndrome. A 33-year-old man who pounded material into place with the heel of his left hand and developed ischemic changes in several digits. Conventional subtraction angiography shows segmental occlusion of the ulnar artery in the palm (*arrow*); multiple proper digital artery occlusions are present consistent with emboli.

segmental occlusion of the ulnar artery or patent ulnar artery with elongation and a corkscrew appearance. These same findings are often present in the contralateral, asymptomatic hand.[76]

Treatment of hypothenar syndrome includes avoidance of blunt trauma, anticoagulation and antiplatelet medication, calcium channel blockers, and smoking cessation. Endovascular therapy is limited to delivery of intra-arterial vasodilators or thrombolytic, often prior to surgical repair. Open surgical repair includes resection of the involved arterial segment with interposition vein graft.[78]

Thermal Injury

Severe tissue freezing and subsequent thawing can cause severe ischemia of the distal extremities, requiring amputation. Tissue freezing induces crystal formation, but more severe injury occurs during the thawing phase, at which point local inflammation and coagulation cause microvascular thrombosis and cell death.[79]

Although treatment has traditionally consisted of rewarming followed by delayed amputation, local thrombolytic and anticoagulation early in the rewarming phase have been shown to reduce rates of amputation, likely due to restoration of perfusion before the onset of tissue necrosis from microvascular thrombosis.[80,81] Bruen et al. reported significant reduction in digital amputation rates and complete avoidance of proximal amputations in patients presenting with circulatory compromise when treated with continuous infusion of intra-arterial tissue plasminogen activator (tPA) within 24 hours of exposure. Infusion was continued until perfusion was restored angiographically or up to a limit of 48 hours.[80] Twomey et al.[80] reported that intra-arterial or intravenous tPA administration were both effective at reducing digital amputations due to frostbite. Intra-arterial vasodilators prior to tPA infusion may also improve outcomes by reducing concomitant vasospasm.[82]

Treatment criteria include severe frostbite with full-thickness involvement or the presence of abnormal perfusion at angiography with therapy initiation within 24 hours of rewarming. Patients who failed endovascular therapy included those with more than 24 hours of cold exposure, warm ischemia times greater than 6 hours, and multiple freeze-thaw cycles.[80,81]

REFERENCES

1. Slovut DP, Olin JW. Fibromuscular dysplasia. *N Engl J Med* 2004;350: 1862–1871.
2. Olin JW. Recognizing and managing fibromuscular dysplasia. *Cleve Clin J Med* 2007;74:273–274, 277–282.
3. Begelman SM, Olin JW. Fibromuscular dysplasia. *Curr Opin Rheumatol* 2000;12:41–47.
4. Slalina M, Zizka J, Klzo L, et al. Contrast-enhanced MR angiography utilizing parallel acquisition techniques in renal artery stenosis detection. *Eur J Radiol* 2010;75:e46–e50.
5. Olin JW, Pierce M. Contemporary management of fibromuscular dysplasia. *Curr Opin Cardiol* 2008;23:527–536.
6. Sciacca L, Ciocca RG, Eslami MH, et al. Endovascular treatment of renal artery aneurysm secondary to fibromuscular dysplasia: a case report. *Ann Vasc Surg* 2009;23:536.e9–536.e12.
7. Trinquart L, Mounier-Vehier C, Sapoval M, et al. Efficacy of revascularization for renal artery stenosis caused by fibromuscular dysplasia: a systematic review and meta-analysis. *Hypertension* 2010;56:525–532.
8. Kincaid OW, Davis GD, Hallerman FJ, et al. Fibromuscular dysplasia of the renal arteries. Arteriographic features, classification, and observations on natural history of the disease. *Am J Roentgenol Radium Ther Nucl Med* 1968;104:271–282.
9. Schreiber MJ, Pohl MA, Novick AC. The natural history of atherosclerotic and fibrous renal artery disease. *Urol Clin North Am* 1984;11:383–392.
10. Goncharenko V, Gerlock AJ Jr, Shaff MI, et al. Progression of renal artery fibromuscular dysplasia in 42 patients as seen on angiography. *Radiology* 1981;139:45–51.
11. Insua JA, Young JR, Humphries AW. Popliteal artery entrapment syndrome. *Arch Surg* 1970;101:771–775.
12. Darling RC, Buckley CJ, Abbott WM, et al. Intermittent claudication in young athletes: popliteal artery entrapment syndrome. *J Trauma* 1974;14:543–552.
13. Rich NM, Collins GJ Jr, McDonald PT, et al. Popliteal vascular entrapment. Its increasing interest. *Arch Surg* 1979;114:1377–1384.
14. Levien LJ. Popliteal artery entrapment syndrome. *Semin Vasc Surg* 2003;16: 223–231.
15. Collins PS, McDonald PT, Lim RC. Popliteal artery entrapment: an evolving syndrome. *J Vasc Surg* 1989;10:484–489; discussion 489–490.
16. Fong H, Downs AR. Popliteal artery entrapment syndrome with distal embolization. A report of two cases. *J Cardiovasc Surg (Torino)* 1989; 30:85–88.
17. Gyftokostas D, Koutsoumbelis C, Mattheou T, et al. Post stenotic aneurysm in popliteal artery entrapment syndrome. *J Cardiovasc Surg (Torino)* 1991;32:350–352.
18. Hai Z, Guangrui S, Yuan Z, et al. CT angiography and MRI in patients with popliteal artery entrapment syndrome. *AJR Am J Roentgenol* 2008;191:1760–1766.
19. Steurer J, Hoffman U, Schneider E, et al. A new therapeutic approach to popliteal artery entrapment syndrome (PAES). *Eur J Vasc Endovasc Surg* 1995;10:243–247.
20. Ring EH Jr, Haines GA, Miller DL. Popliteal artery entrapment syndrome: arteriographic findings and thrombolytic therapy. *J Vasc Interv Radiol* 1999;10:713–721.
21. Shen J, Abu-Hamad G, Makaroun MS, et al. Bilateral asymmetric popliteal entrapment syndrome treated with successful surgical decompression and adjunctive thrombolysis. *Vasc Endovascular Surg* 2009;43:395–398.
22. Duffy AJ, Panait L, Eisenberg D, et al. Management of median arcuate ligament syndrome: a new paradigm. *Ann Vasc Surg* 2009;23:778–784.
23. Glovickzi P, Duncan AA. Treatment of celiac artery compression syndrome: does it really exist? *Perspect Vasc Surg Endovasc Ther* 2007;19:259–263
24. Horton KM, Talamini MA, Fishman EK. Median arcuate ligament syndrome: evaluation with CT angiography. *Radiographics* 2005; 25:177–182.
25. Reilly LM, Ammar AD, Stoney RJ, et al. Late results following operative repair for celiac artery compression syndrome. *J Vasc Surg* 1985;2:79–91.
26. Delis KT, Glovickzi P, Althwaijri M, et al. Median arcuate ligament syndrome: open celiac artery reconstruction and ligament division after endovascular failure. *J Vasc Surg* 2007;46:799–802.
27. Matsumoto AH, Angle JF, Spinosa DJ, et al. Percutaneous transluminal angioplasty and stenting in the treatment of chronic mesenteric ischemia: results and longterm followup. *J Am Coll Surg* 2002;194:S22–S31.
28. Ikeda O, Tamura Y, Nakasone Y, et al. Coil embolization of pancreaticoduodenal artery aneurysms associated with celiac artery stenosis: report of three cases. *Cardiovasc Intervent Radiol* 2007;30:504–507.
29. Ogino H, Sato Y, Banno T, et al. Embolization in a patient with ruptured anterior inferior pancreaticoduodenal arterial aneurysm with median arcuate ligament syndrome. *Cardiovasc Intervent Radiol* 2002;25:318–319.
30. Sanders RJ, Hammond SL, Rao NM. Diagnosis of thoracic outlet syndrome. *J Vasc Surg* 2007;46:601–604.
31. Durham JR, Yao JS, Pearce WH, et al. Arterial injuries in the thoracic outlet syndrome. *J Vasc Surg* 1995;21:57–70.
32. Matsen SL, Messina LM, Laberge JM, et al. SIR 2003 film panel case 7: arterial thoracic outlet syndrome presenting with upper extremity emboli and posterior circulation stroke. *J Vasc Interv Radiol* 2003;14:807–812.
33. Lee TS, Hines GL. Cerebral embolic stroke and arm ischemia in a teenager with arterial thoracic outlet syndrome: a case report. *Vasc Endovascular Surg* 2007;41:254–257.
34. Malliet C, Fourneau I, Daenens K, et al. Endovascular stent-graft and first rib resection for thoracic outlet syndrome complicated by an aneurysm of the subclavian artery. *Acta Chir Belg* 2005;105:194–197.
35. De Costa C. St Anthony's fire and living ligatures: a short history of ergometrine. *Lancet* 2002;359(9319):1768–1770.
36. Raval MV, Gaba RC, Brown K, et al. Percutaneous transluminal angioplasty in the treatment of extensive LSD-induced lower extremity vasospasm refractory to pharmacologic therapy. *J Vasc Interv Radiol* 2008; 19:1227–1230.
37. Ausband SC, Goodman PE. An unusual case of clarithromycin associated ergotism. *J Emerg Med* 2001;21:411–413.
38. Bagby RJ, Cooper RD. Angiography in ergotism. Report of two cases and review of the literature. *Am J Roentgenol Radium Ther Nucl Med* 1972;116:179–186.
39. Chapman EM, Shaw RS, Kubik CS. Sciatic pain from arteriosclerotic aneurysm of pelvic arteries. *N Engl J Med* 1964;271:410–411.
40. Mandell VS, Jacques PF, Delany DJ, et al. Persistent sciatic artery: clinical, embryologic, and angiographic features. *AJR Am J Roentgenol* 1985;44: 245–249.
41. Brantley SK, Rigdon EE, Raju S. Persistent sciatic artery: embryology, pathology, and treatment. *J Vasc Surg* 1993;18:242–248.
42. Santaolalla V, Bernabe MH, Jipola Ulecia JM, et al. Persistent sciatic artery. *Ann Vasc Surg* 2010;24:691.e7–691.e10.
43. Mousa A, Rapp Parker A, Emmett MK, et al. Endovascular treatment of symptomatic persistent sciatic artery aneurysm: a case report and review of literature. *Vasc Endovascular Surg* 2010;44:312–314.
44. Sultan SA, Pacainowski JP, Madhavan P, et al. Endovascular management of rare sciatic artery aneurysm. *J Endovasc Ther* 2000;7:415–422.
45. Rezayat C, Sambol E, Goldstein L, et al. Ruptured persistent sciatic artery aneurysm managed by endovascular embolization. *Ann Vasc Surg* 2010;24:115.e5–115.e9.
46. Oderich GS, Panneton JM, Bower TC. The spectrum, management and clinical outcome of Ehlers-Danlos syndrome type IV: a 30-year experience. *J Vasc Surg* 2005;42:98–106.
47. Germin DP. Clinical and genetic features of vascular Ehlers-Danlos syndrome. *Ann Vasc Surg* 2002;16:391–397.
48. Brooke BS, Arnaoutakis G, McDonnell NB, et al. Contemporary management of vascular complications associated with Ehlers-Danlos syndrome. *J Vasc Surg* 2010;51:131–138; discussion 138–139.
49. Svensson LG, Kouchoukos NT, Miller DC, et al. Expert consensus document on the treatment of descending thoracic aortic disease using endovascular stent-grafts. *Ann Thorac Surg* 2008;85(suppl 1):S1–S41.
50. Delis KT, Glovickzi P. Neurofibromatosis type 1: from presentation and diagnosis to vascular and endovascular therapy. *Perspect Vasc Surg Endovasc Ther* 2006;18:226–237.
51. Oderich GS, Sullivan TM, Bower TC, et al. Vascular abnormalities in patients with neurofibromatosis syndrome type I: clinical spectrum, management, and results. *J Vasc Surg* 2007;46:475–484.
52. Booth C, Preston R, Clark G, et al. Management of renal vascular disease in neurofibromatosis type 1 and the role of percutaneous transluminal angioplasty. *Nephrol Dial Transplant* 2002;17:1235–1240.
53. Hassen-Khodja R, Declemy S, Batt M, et al. Visceral artery aneurysms in Von Recklinghausen's neurofibromatosis. *J Vasc Surg* 1997;25:572–575.

636 SECTION VII ■ ARTERIOPATHIES

54. Santin BJ, Guy GE, Bourekas EC, et al. Endovascular therapy for subclavian artery rupture in von Recklinghausen disease. *Vasc Endovascular Surg* 2010;44:714–717.

55. Mendonca CT, Weingartner J, de Carvalho CA, et al. Endovascular treatment of contained rupture of a superior mesenteric artery aneurysm resulting from neurofibromatosis type I. *J Vasc Surg* 2010;51:461–464.

56. Mendonca CT. Regarding "Endovascular treatment of contained rupture of a superior mesenteric artery aneurysm resulting from neurofibromatosis type I". *J Vasc Surg* 2010;52:1425.

57. Lebwohl M, Halperin J, Phelps RG. Brief report: occult pseudoxanthoma elasticum in patients with premature cardiovascular disease. *N Engl J Med* 1993;329:1237–1239.

58. Ohtani T, Furukawa F. Pseudoxanthoma elasticum. *J Dermatol* 2002;9:615–620.

59. Donas KP, Schulte S, Horsch S. Balloon angioplasty in the treatment of vascular lesions in pseudoxanthoma elasticum. *J Vasc Interv Radiol* 2007;18:457–459.

60. Testai FD, Gorelick PB. Inherited metabolic disorders and stroke part 2: homocystinuria, organic acidurias, and urea cycle disorders. *Arch Neurol* 2010;67:148–153.

61. Scriver CR. *The Metabolic and Molecular Bases of Inherited Disease.* 7th ed. 3 Vols. New York, NY: McGraw-Hill, Health Professions Division; 1995:(xxxvi, 4605, Chapter 88).

62. Mudd SH, Skovby F, Levy HL, et al. The natural history of homocystinuria due to cystathionine beta-synthase deficiency. *Am J Hum Genet* 1985;37:1–31.

63. Lobo CA, Millward SF. Homocystinuria: a cause of hypercoagulability that may be unrecognized. *J Vasc Interv Radiol* 1998;9:971–975.

64. Salerno AE, Marsenic O, Meyers KE, et al. Vascular involvement in tuberous sclerosis. *Pediatr Nephrol* 2010;25:1555–1561.

65. Abraham P, Chevalier M, Saumet JL. External iliac artery endofibrosis: a 40-year course. *J Sports Med Phys Fitness* 1997;37:297–300.

66. Schep G, Bender MH, Kaandorp D, et al. Flow limitations in the iliac arteries in endurance athletes. Current knowledge and directions for the future. *Int J Sports Med* 1999;20:421–428.

67. Wijesinghe LD, Coughlin PA, Robertson I, et al. Cyclist's iliac syndrome: temporary relief by balloon angioplasty. *Br J Sports Med* 2001;35:70–71.

68. Giannoukas AD, Berczi V, Anoop U, et al. Endofibrosis of iliac arteries in high-performance athletes: diagnostic approach and minimally invasive endovascular treatment. *Cardiovasc Intervent Radiol* 2006;29:866–869.

69. Ford SJ, Rehman A, Bradbury AW. External iliac endofibrosis in endurance athletes: a novel case in an endurance runner and a review of the literature. *Eur J Vasc Endovasc Surg* 2003;26:629–634.

70. Levien LJ, Benn CA. Adventitial cystic disease: a unifying hypothesis. *J Vasc Surg* 1998;28:193–205.

71. Maged IM, Turba UC, Housseini AM, et al. High spatial resolution magnetic resonance imaging of cystic adventitial disease of the popliteal artery. *J Vasc Surg* 2010;51:471–474.

72. Fox RL, Kahn M, Adler J, et al. Adventitial cystic disease of the popliteal artery: failure of percutaneous transluminal angioplasty as a therapeutic modality. *J Vasc Surg* 1985;2:464–467.

73. Rai S, Davies RS, Vohra RK. Failure of endovascular stenting for popliteal cystic disease. *Ann Vasc Surg* 2009;23:410.e1–410.e5.

74. Khoury M. Failed angioplasty of a popliteal artery stenosis secondary to cystic adventitial disease—a case report. *Vasc Endovascular Surg* 2004;38:277–280.

75. Ferris BL, Taylor LM Jr, Oyama K, et al. Hypothenar hammer syndrome: proposed etiology. *J Vasc Surg* 2000;31:104–113.

76. Lim RP, Storey P, Atanasova IP, et al. Three-dimensional electrocardiographically gated variable flip angle FSE imaging for MR angiography of the hands at 3.0 T: initial experience. *Radiology* 2009;252:874–881.

77. Winterer JT, Moske-Eick O, Marki M, et al. Bilateral ce-MR angiography of the hands at 3.0 T and 1.5 T: intraindividual comparison of quantitative and qualitative image parameters in healthy volunteers. *Eur Radiol* 2008;18:658–664.

78. McCready RA, Bryant MA, Divelbiss JL. Combined thenar and hypothenar hammer syndromes: case report and review of the literature. *J Vasc Surg* 2008;48:741–744.

79. Murphy JV, Banwell PE, Roberts AH, et al. Frostbite: pathogenesis and treatment. *J Trauma* 2000;48:171–178.

80. Twomey JA, Peltier GL, Zera RT. An open-label study to evaluate the safety and efficacy of tissue plasminogen activator in treatment of severe frostbite. *J Trauma* 2005;59:1350–1354; discussion 1354–1355.

81. Bruen KJ, Ballard JR, Morris SE, et al. Reduction of the incidence of amputation in frostbite injury with thrombolytic therapy. *Arch Surg* 2007;142:546–553.

82. Saemi A, Johnson J, Morris C. Treatment of bilateral hand frostbite using transcatheter arterial thrombolysis after papaverine infusion. *Cardiovasc Intervent Radiol* 2009;32:1280–1283.

83. E. Pàris, E. Fadel, P. Jue-Denis et al. Artère sciatique persistante. In E. Kieffer, P. Godeau (Eds.), Actualités de Chirurgie Vasculaire, Maladies Artérielles Non Athéromateuses de L'Adulte, AERCV, Paris (1994), pp. 67–80

84. J. Pillet, P. Albaret, J.L. Toulemonde et al. Tronc artériel ischopoplité, persistence de l'artère axiale. Bull Assoc Anat, 65 (1980), pp. 97–110.

SECTION VIII

Aneurysmal Disease

Diagnostic Noninvasive Evaluations: CT

RICHARD L. HALLETT and DOMINIK D. FLEISCHMANN

Over the past decade, multidetector-row computed tomography (CT) has become a first-line tool in the evaluation of the thoracic and abdominal aorta. Excellent spatial resolution, short exam times, flexibility of acquisition protocols, and the ubiquity of CT technology have made rapid evaluation of a wide spectrum of aortic disease a reality. To maximize the diagnostic evaluation of aortic disease, adequate knowledge of contrast medium dynamics, CT acquisition parameters, and image postprocessing techniques are necessary. This chapter reviews basic contrast medium kinetics, explores options for aortic computed tomography angiogram (CTA) acquisition and injection protocols, and reviews image postprocessing and interpretation strategies. Imaging considerations for specific aortic diseases and states are reviewed last.

CONTRAST MEDIUM CONSIDERATIONS

Contrast Medium Physiology

Accurate diagnosis during CTA evaluation depends on adequate enhancement of the aorta and its branches by intravenous (IV) contrast media (CM). This requires the selection of injection parameters to achieve the desired degree of enhancement and appropriate synchronization between CM injection and CTA scan acquisition. As the speed of multidetector-row CT (MDCT) acquisitions have increased, the importance of understanding CM dynamics has become more crucial to the design of CTA protocols.

Almost all CTA acquisitions involve IV administration of iodinated CM, of which multiple formulations and concentrations are available. These CM share a primary chemical structure as derivatives of a symmetrically tri-iodinated benzene ring. Iodinated CM absorbs X-ray photons and therefore contributes to the visual enhancement of vascular structures (and organ parenchyma) during CTA. Physiologic effects of CM are typically undesired and attempts are made toward mitigation. The amount of vascular and tissue enhancement is directly proportional to local iodine concentration.[1] Therefore, by controlling CM selection and administration parameters, one can optimize vascular enhancement.

The relatively high IV injection rates of CM require attention to the physicochemical properties of the CM. Viscosity plays a role in determining the maximal flow rates and pressures generated during IV administration and depends on the iodine concentration, chemical structure, and ambient temperature of the CM. Viscosity rises exponentially with increasing iodine concentration. Chemical monomers, being typically smaller molecules, have lower viscosity than dimers. It has been shown that viscosity decreases by approximately 50% when CM is warmed from room temperature (~20°C) to body temperature (37°C).[2]

Administration of CM also carries risks of adverse reactions with unintended physiologic consequences. These risks fall into several categories: idiosyncratic reactions, nonidiosyncratic (dose-dependent) reactions, CM extravasation, drug–drug interactions, and interactions with endocrine function. These effects are summarized in Table 54.1. Although a full discussion of all adverse events is beyond the scope of this chapter, and available elsewhere,[3,4] a few important points are stressed.

Adverse effects occur in approximately 3% of iodinated CM administrations; however, severe reactions occur in only 0.04%.[5] Reactions to CM may be idiosyncratic (acute, allergic-like) or nonidiosyncratic (dose dependent) in nature. In general, idiosyncratic reaction rates can be decreased by appropriate screening of patients for history of previous reactions and drug allergies, by effective premedication protocols for selected patients, and by appropriate personnel training and equipment for treatment of these reactions when they occur. Nonidiosyncratic reactions, especially CM-induced nephropathy (CIN), can be mitigated by careful screening for history and risk factors for renal disease and by evaluation of estimated glomerular filtration rates (eGFR) in those patients with risk factors.[6,7] A protocol for prevention of CIN in appropriate patients is therefore also important (Table 54.2).

Contrast Medium Pharmacokinetics

Pharmacokinetically all iodinated radiographic CM are extracellular fluid markers and rapidly become distributed between intravascular and extravascular interstitial spaces when administered IV.[8] Unlike solid organ enhancement, which is primarily influenced by total iodine dose per unit of extracellular space (approximated by body weight [BW] in kilograms), vascular enhancement in the arterial phase is determined by the iodine flow rate (flux) per unit time relative to total blood flow per unit time (i.e., cardiac output [CO]). Therefore, *iodine CM flow rate is the most important controllable parameter in arterial phase CTA, whereas iodine dose is most important for parenchymal (equilibrium) phase imaging.*

A basic understanding of early CM dynamics is important for optimization of injection protocols for CTA. The time-attenuation curve for IV bolus CM administration is depicted in FIGURE 54.1. Following the bolus, there is an early "first-pass" peak, followed by a second, smaller peak, which occurs secondary to bolus broadening through the heart and lungs, as well as recirculation of CM through highly perfused organs, such as the brain and kidneys.

For any given patient and vascular territory, the time-attenuation response to CM administration is directly proportional to the iodine flow rate (iodine flux). For a given iodine concentration the iodine flux (in mg I/s) is simply

Table 54.1		
Contrast Media Adverse Events, Risks, and Preventive Measures[3]		
Adverse event	**Known (or suspected) risk factors**	**Prevention/actions**
Idiosyncratic reactions	**Acute allergy-like**	Screen for prior reactions and drug history
	Hx prior moderate to severe CM reaction	
	Hx significant allergy requiring Tx	Premedication protocol for at-risk patients
	Asthma	
	Drugs (β-blockers, interleukin-2)	Appropriate equipment and protocols for acute CM reaction treatment
	Delayed (cutaneous) reactions	
	History of prior reaction to specific agent	
	Interleukin-2	
	Hydralazine (acute cutaneous vasculitis)	
Dose-dependent (nonidiosyncratic) reactions	**Cardiovascular effects**	Avoid high flow rates/volumes in very sick, elderly patients
	Very high flow rates/volumes can cause decompensation in elderly	
		Screen for Hx and risk factors for renal disease
	CM-induced nephropathy (CIN)	Obtain serum creatinine when risk factors are present
	Hx renal disease	
	Previous kidney surgery	Calculate eGFR:
	Diabetes	http://www.nephron.com/MDRD_GFR.cgi
	Proteinuria	
	Hypertension	Have protocol for prevention of CIN (Table 54.2)
	Gout	
	Multiple myeloma	
	eGFR <60 mL/min/1.73 m^2	
CM extravasation injury	Unconscious/elderly/noncommunicating patients at increased risk	Manual test injection with NS prior to CM bolus
		Monitor injection site
		Extravasation detectors
		Protocol for Tx and plastic/hand surgery consults
Drug–drug interactions	Metformin	Obtain thorough drug history
	Nephrotoxic drugs (e.g., aminoglycosides)	Stop nephrotoxic agents
	Interleukin-2 (increased risk of both acute urticarial and delayed cutaneous reactions)	After 48 hr, may resume metformin if renal function is found to be normal
	β-blockers	
	Hydralazine	
Endocrinopathy	CM contraindicated in patients with clinical hyperthyroidism syndromes	Screen for manifest thyroid disease
	Thyrotoxicosis in Graves and autonomous multinodular goiter patients	
	CM limits utility of radionuclide thyroid scintigraphy and efficacy of radioiodine Tx for thyroid cancer for 2 mo	Endocrinology consult and follow-up

Table 54.2

Preventive Measures for CIN[3,6,7]

Screening serum creatinine level (S_{cr})	Outpatients >70 y
	ALL inpatients
	Questionnaire to determine need for serum creatinine in outpatients <70 y
Estimate eGFR	http://www.nephron.com/MDRD_GFR.cgi
	Or
	eGFR (mL/min/1.73 m²) = 186(S_{cr} × 0.11)$^{-1.154}$ × (age)$^{-0.203}$ × (1.21, if African American) × (0.742 if female)
Estimate risk for CIN	eGFR ≤60 mL/min/173 m²
Renal protective measures	Consider alternate imaging techniques (ultrasound, MRI)
	Stop nephrotoxic drugs/diuretics × 24 hr or more
	Use low- or iso-osmolar CM
	Use smallest CM dose necessary to answer clinical question
	N-acetyl cysteine (NAC) may be helpful
	600–1,200 mg po b.i.d. 24 hr before and 48 hr after CM
	Hydration protocols:
	NS at 1.0–1.5 mL/kg/hr for 3–12 hr before and 4–24 hr after CM
	Screen for CHF, revise infusion rate if needed
	Or
	150 mEq bicarbonate in 1 L 5% dextrose, infused at:
	3.5 mL/kg BW/hr × 1 hr before CM then 1.18 mL/kg BW/hr × 6 hr
Monitor patient outcomes	Perform follow-up on patients at risk for CIN to document outcomes after CM administration

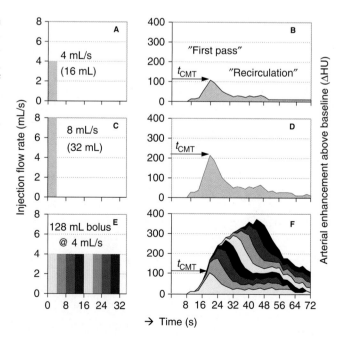

FIGURE 54.1 Basic contrast medium physiology. When injecting a small test bolus (**A, B**), one observes a sharp upstroke of the time-activity curve ("first pass"), followed by rapid decline. There is a second, lower-amplitude, broader peak secondary to recirculation of CM. Injecting at a higher rate (**C, D**) results in an approximate doubling of the observed peaks. **E, F.** Longer injections can be thought of as multiple consecutive test boluses. As shown in (**F**), observed time-attenuation curve reflects an integral function of the individual curves. Note that the composite curve is continuously rising as long as injection continues. Cessation of injection causes rapid decline in the curve.

Note: t_{CMT}, contrast media transit time.

From Fleischmann D. Present and future trends in multiple detector-row CT applications: CT angiography. *Eur Radiol* 2002;12:S11–S16.

controlled by the injection rate (mL/s). Doubling the injection rate thus results in approximately twice the magnitude of vascular enhancement. Although this relationship between injection flow rate and strength of enhancement is intuitive, the effects of changes in injection duration are not as straightforward (FIGURE 54.1). These effects of increasing the injection duration can be best explained by an additive model, where the time-attenuation curve of longer injections is regarded as the summation (integral area function) of smaller "test boluses."[9]

Patient-specific parameters also play a role in early CM dynamics (FIGURE 54.2). Arterial enhancement is inversely proportional to CO; that is, as CO decreases, arterial enhancement increases. CO also correlates with BW. Appropriate increase (or decrease) in injection rates for larger (>90 kg) or smaller (<60 kg) patients is therefore recommended.[10] Central blood volume (CBV) is also inversely proportional to arterial enhancement; thus larger patients require, on average, greater flow rates and volumes to achieve similar degrees of arterial enhancement.

Finally, the introduction of scanners with very short acquisition times (from subseconds to a few seconds) remind us of the fact that the arterial opacification of a given vascular territory is not instantaneous. This is well known for lower extremity arteries in patients with peripheral artery disease but also applies to the aorta—notably in large-diameter, ectatic vessels and in the presence of aneurysms. Additionally, from catheterization data, we know that complete contrast filling of the normal coronary arterial tree by intra-arterial injection takes a few heartbeats. The physiologic time needed to opacify an arterial territory also must be taken into account when scan times are much shorter than territorial filling times.

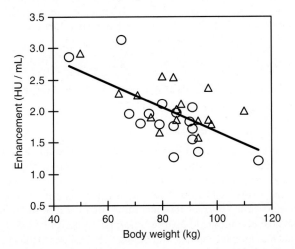

FIGURE 54.2 Arterial enhancement versus body weight. Significant correlation (rPearson = −0.64, *p* < .001) between arterial enhancement and body weight in 32 patients who underwent abdominal CTA. Patients represented as triangles were injected 120 mL of CM at a flow rate of 4 mL/s. Patients represented as circles received individualized volumes and injection rates. Enhancement is given in Hounsfield units (HU) per milliliter of CM injected, correcting for differences in injected volumes in group 2.

Data from Bae KT, Tran HQ, Heiken JP. Multiphasic injection method for uniform prolonged vascular enhancement at CT angiography: pharmacokinetic analysis and experimental porcine model. *Radiology* 2000;216(3):872–880.

Accordingly, the principle rules of early CM dynamics can be summarized as follows (Table 54.3):

1. Arterial enhancement is proportional to iodine flow rate (flux).
2. Arterial enhancement increases over time in a cumulative manner.
3. Arterial enhancement is variable between individuals and depends on CO and CBV.
4. Arterial filling times may be delayed physiologically and/or pathologically.

Athough physiologic parameters, such as CO and CBV, are not modifiable, several CM injection parameters may be modified such that arterial enhancement can be optimized.

The *iodine administration rate* (iodine flux, in mg I/s) has a direct, proportional effect on arterial enhancement. This rate depends on the concentration of iodine molecules (mg I/mL) and the rate at which CM is injected (mL/s). Increasing either the iodine concentration of the CM or the flow rate will increase the arterial enhancement. Increasing both parameters (within practical limits to 370 to 400 mg I/mL CM and 6 to 8 mL/s injection rate) will maximize arterial enhancement.

The *injection duration* also increases arterial enhancement but in a cumulative fashion. As seen in FIGURE 54.1, increasing the injection duration allows additive enhancement relating to recirculation effects. Note that there is also a *minimum* injection duration to allow adequate arterial enhancement and filling of a particular arterial tree: for example, approximately 10 to 15 seconds is necessary for filling of the entire aorta in patients with cardiovascular disease and up to 40 seconds or longer for severely diseased peripheral arterial trees.

The *injection profile* also impacts the magnitude and shape of the enhancement curve. Biphasic or triphasic injection profiles, consisting of initial high flow rates followed by lower flow rates, will produce more uniform enhancement.[10,11] These injection profiles are useful in particular during long injections and acquisitions, such as seen with older CT scanners, large *z*-axis coverage (e.g., lower extremity CTA), and studies utilizing retrospective electrocardiogram (ECG) gating.

The type and quality of IV access can also impact the quality of the CTA. Adequate IV access is important: preferably in a large cubital or antecubital vein and at least 20 gauge in size. We advocate forward flushing (testing) of the IV cannula with normal saline (NS) at the same injection flow rate as the CM protocol. This should be done with the patient's arm in scanning position (typically above his or her head) to truly evaluate IV suitability before CM injection commences and decrease extravasation risk. Placement of the IV cannula in the right arm will reduce streak artifacts across the aortic arch, which is important for maximal evaluation of the thoracic aorta. The injector pressure limit is typically set to 300 psi. Recently, use of power-injectable peripherally inserted central catheters (PICCs) and ports has become possible,[12,13] adding another route for high flow rate CM injection and potentially allowing more compact bolus geometry.[14] Local policy regarding use of such devices, flow rates and pressure limitations, and periprocedural catheter care should be established.

Attention to other injection considerations will further ensure high-quality CTA studies. Warming of CM substantially reduces viscosity,[15] which translates to lower injection pressures and may improve bolus geometry.[16] Therefore, prewarming of

Table 54.3
Key Rules for Early Contrast Medium Dynamics[3,4]

- **Arterial enhancement is proportional to iodine flow rate (flux)**
  - Increasing the injection flow rate and/or iodine concentration of CM will increase the arterial opacification.
    - Increasing from 300 to 370 mg I/mL increases flux by 23%
    - Increasing injection flow rate from 4 to 5 mL/s increases flux by 25%
    - Combination of both increases flux by 54% (1.20 vs. 1.85 g I/s)
- **Arterial enhancement increases over time as a cumulative effect**
  - Arterial enhancement increases with increasing injection duration
  - Minimum injection duration of ~10 s is needed to achieve adequate arterial enhancement
  - Biphasic or multiphasic CM injections result in more uniform enhancement if longer scan times and injection durations are necessary
- **Arterial enhancement is highly variable between individuals**
  - Cardiac output (CO) is inversely proportional to arterial enhancement
    - CO correlates proportionally to body weight/body surface area (BSA)
    - Revising the injection rate and CM volume upward for larger (>90 kg) and downward for smaller (<60 kg) patients will reduce interindividual variability
- **Arterial filling may be delayed physiologically and/or pathologically**
    - Even normal coronary arteries need several heartbeats to fully opacify
    - Mixing of opacified and unopacified blood in aneurysms delays peak enhancement
    - Severe peripheral obstructive atherosclerotic disease can cause substantial delay in bolus propagation

CM and use of a warming cuff on the injector is beneficial. We also advocate use of a NS flush ("chaser") after CM injection, which helps clear residual CM in the arm veins (allowing some CM dose savings), reduce perivenous artifacts in the chest, and promote more compact bolus geometry.[17,18]

Once the CM flow rate and the injection duration for a given scan have been established, the CTA acquisition needs to be synchronized with the expected maximum arterial CM enhancement for a given patient. For arterial CTA, an empiric fixed delay for image acquisition is not recommended. Transit time of CM to the region of interest (ROI) can be reliably determined by utilizing either a test bolus or bolus-triggering software. The test bolus technique utilizes a small bolus of CM injected rapidly with serial, nonincremental image acquisition. The time to peak ROI enhancement can then be calculated; this value is considered the contrast media transit time (t_{CMT}). The t_{CMT} is then used to individualize the scanning delay before image acquisition for CTA. A scan can be initiated at any time relative to the t_{CMT}. For fast scanners this is typically chosen a few seconds after the t_{CMT}. Bolus triggering involves real-time sequential, nonincremental imaging at the ROI, and once an appropriate enhancement level is reached (e.g., increase by 100 HU), the CTA acquisition is automatically or manually commenced. It is important to note that when using bolus-triggering techniques, the monitoring images may require approximately 3 seconds for acquisition, reconstruction, and display. Further, an additional 2 to 4 seconds is required for table movement to scan start position and for breath-hold instructions to be given. It must be realized that bolus triggering—notably with older CT systems—may

result in image acquisition at t_{CMT} plus 8 seconds. Although this may be advantageous given the CM dynamics discussed earlier, the injection duration must be lengthened such that one does not "run out" of CM at the end of the acquisition.

COMPUTED TOMOGRAPHY ACQUISITION PROTOCOLS FOR AORTIC DISEASES

General Considerations

For most examinations of the aorta, the patient should be positioned supine in the gantry, as close to isocenter as possible, with the arms extended comfortably (without extreme abduction) over the head. Correct patient centering is particularly important when automated tube current modulation is used because the tube amperage is computed based on information derived from the digital radiographs ("scout," "topogram"). Exceptions to this rule include simultaneous evaluation of the chest and upper extremity (in which case the contralateral arm can be placed at the side and injection performed from that arm) and desired evaluation of both the chest and carotid/vertebral vessels, where both arms can be placed at the side and automated exposure controls utilized.

Once the patient and CT suite have been prepared, several decisions are then necessary to ensure selection of the most appropriate CTA protocol:

1. Anatomic *range to be imaged:* Inclusion of the appropriate volume of tissue in the scan acquisition will ensure that maximal diagnostic information for a particular disease

process will be available. For example, when evaluating the aorta for dissection, thromboembolic disease, vasculitis, or thoracic aneurysms, evaluation of the entire aorta and iliac arteries (CTA of the chest, abdomen, and pelvis) is recommended. Thoracic aneurysms have a high incidence of coexistent abdominal aortic aneurysms (AAAs), and acute aortic syndromes often involve more than just the thoracic aorta. Further, branch vessel involvement by aortic dissection is a significant cause of morbidity and mortality, and knowledge of iliac vessel size, patency, and tortuosity is important for both staging disease and planning endovascular or surgical treatment.

2. *Noncontrast series:* Depending on the clinical question, nonenhanced CT (NECT) images may be essential for proper interpretation (see below). Given ALARA principles, however, NECT series should only be obtained when they are likely to provide important, additional information.

3. *ECG-synchronized versus nongated CTA:* The use of ECG-triggered or ECG-gated exams (detailed below) is beneficial when evaluating valvular and cardiac function and when vascular pulsation or cardiac motion is expected to interfere with visualization of the anatomy and pathology of interest.[19]

Once the acquisition protocol has been selected, an appropriate CM injection protocol should also be applied. The goal of such an integrated injection/acquisition protocol is to synchronize well-enhanced arteries with data acquisition. In the past, with slower CT scanners, this typically meant that one should scan as fast as possible (within the confines of a breath-hold) and then adjust the injection protocol to provide opacification throughout the duration of image acquisition. For example, for a 25-second scan time, one would inject for 25 to 30 seconds at a flow rate of 4 to 6 mL/s, depending on weight. With the newer (≥64 channel) MDCT scanners, this protocol has changed

because scanning at fast (~10 seconds) or very fast (≤5 seconds) speeds not always ensures good opacification. We use a strategy of fixing the scan time and injection duration for all patients while customizing CM flow rate depending on patient size. Also integrated is an appropriate delay in image acquisition, which allows the bolus a bit of a "head start" to improve vessel filling in the setting of ectatic and/or aneurysmal vessels. The result is an integrated acquisition and injection protocol, which should provide consistently robust CTA imaging across a wide variety of patients and conditions. An example of such an integrated protocol for CTA of the aorta is detailed in Table 54.4.

Scan Acquisition and Reconstruction Considerations

Scan acquisition protocols can be influenced by the patient's clinical condition, size and body habitus, previous or planned interventions, and disease state. The selected CTA protocol should answer the pertinent clinical questions and should be obtained with the lowest necessary radiation dose. Patient size must be factored into the protocol selected. Recent advances, such as dual energy CT, may allow improved diagnosis and radiation dose reduction. Selected acquisition of a noncontrast CT series, utilization of ECG-synchronized ("gated") CT, and implementation of multiple available dose-reduction strategies for aortic CTA will facilitate optimum patient management.

Patient Size Considerations

Image quality, contrast-to-noise ratio (CNR), and signal-to-noise ratio (SNR) are inversely proportional to the patient size.[20,21] Higher levels of image noise in larger patients contribute to a decrease in SNR. It has been shown that for the same

---

Table 54.4

Integrated 64-Channel CT Acquisition and Injection Protocol for CTA of the Thoracic/Abdominal Aorta

Acquisition	64 × 0.6 mm (channels × channel width); automated tube current modulation (250 mAs reference mAs)
Pitch	Variable (depends on volume coverage, usually <1.0)
Scan time	Fixed to 10 s (all patients)
Injection duration	Fixed to 18 s (all patients)
Scanning delay	t_{CMT} + 8 s (scan starts 8 s after CM arrival, as established by automated bolus triggering)
Contrast medium	High concentration (350–370 mg I/mL)
Injection flow rates and volumes	**Individualized to body weight**

Body weight (kg)	CM flow rate (mL/s)	CM volume (mL)
≤55	4.0	72
56–65	4.5	81
66–85	5.0	90
86–95	5.5	99
>95	6.0	108

CM dose and injection rate, larger patients also have lower levels of vascular enhancement. This phenomenon is related to several patient factors. Relative dilution of CM is seen in larger patients, who have correspondingly larger CBV. These patients, in general, also have proportionally higher CO than smaller patients.[20,22] Schindera et al.[23] also showed in both experimental models and with clinical patient data that "hardening" of the polychromatic X-ray beam in larger patients leads to a decrease in arterial enhancement of approximately 10% to 24%, independent of CM concerns. All three of these factors are related to BW as well as body surface area (BSA).[20,24] Conversely, smaller patients benefit from utilization of lower tube potential imaging, for example, 100 kVp. Decreasing tube potential decreases patient radiation dose, even accounting for an increase in tube current (mAs) that may be necessary to offset increased image noise. Given the nearer position of 100 kVp to the k edge of iodine (33.2 keV), iodine-based CM will exhibit greater vascular enhancement as well (FIGURE 54.3).

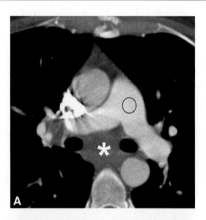

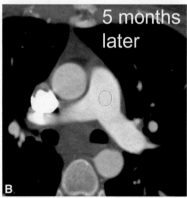

FIGURE 54.3 Effect of lower tube voltage. A 37-year-old female patient weighing 50 kg with pulmonary emboli in the setting of proven histoplasmosis. Injection parameters for both exams were 100 mL CM (370 mg I/mL) injected at 4 mL/s. **A.** Original CTA obtained with 120 kVp tube voltage shows enhancement in the main pulmonary artery (*ellipse*) of 384 ± 15 HU. **B.** Follow-up exam obtained 5 months later using 100 kVp protocol shows enhancement of 528 ± 12 HU. As tube voltage becomes closer to the k edge of iodine, more photons are absorbed, and observed enhancement increases. Note also subcarinal adenopathy (* in figure **A**) related to acute histoplasmosis.

Dual Energy Computed Tomography

In recent years, introduction of new CT scanner technology has also expanded imaging options for vascular disease. Specifically, the use of dual-source CT (DSCT) and gemstone spectral imaging (GSI) allow simultaneous acquisition of different tube potential datasets, which can be utilized in several ways. With DSCT, two X-ray tubes positioned at approximately a 90-degree angle rotate together but function independently, allowing acquisition of two independent datasets (e.g., 80, 140 kVp) at the same location. Alternatively, applications of GSI with rapid kilovolt peak switching during image acquisition also allow generation of dual energy data.

Leveraging the inherent spectral differences between iodine, fat, and soft tissue allows decomposition of different tissues.[25–27] The iodine peak data can then be displayed on the CT image; this iodine (present in CM) within an endoleak can be detected on color-coded dual energy CT images.[28] Dual energy techniques also allow segmentation/removal of bone and calcium from iodine from high-contrast datasets without misregistration artifacts inherent in separate "mask" series acquisition.[26] This ability to discriminate (and remove) calcium and iodine from datasets seem to work best when both materials are very dense and not as well when the materials are less dense, as can be experienced when imaging bone marrow and with partial volume averaging of calcified lesions in smaller vessels.[26] Additionally, gradient-based segmentation techniques are already robust when densities of calcium and iodine are high, thus dual energy imaging at present may not add a large benefit for mask image formation and calcium/iodine identification. Ongoing research may provide additional clarification of value in the near future.

Alternately, by subtracting the iodine data from the average of the CT image, "virtual noncontrast" datasets can be generated, which may obviate the need (and radiation exposure) for a noncontrast series (FIGURE 54.4). This is particularly important in patients who, because of their disease states (e.g., aortic dissection, endovascular aortic stent-grafts), will require frequent or lifelong follow-up CT exams. These virtual image sets have been shown to be of reasonable diagnostic quality and to be effective for the detection and characterization of endoleaks.[29]

Nonenhanced Computed Tomography Acquisitions

Although most abnormalities present on NECT can be visualized as well (if not better) on contrast-enhanced CTA, NECT is important for the optimum evaluation of several cardiovascular processes (FIGURE 54.5). In particular, intramural hematoma (IMH), which is seen in acute aortic syndromes, can only be reliably visualized on NECT. A "hyperdense crescent" within a layer of chronic thrombus of an AAA visualized on NECT may reflect fresh blood burrowing into a thrombus fracture or fissure due to sac increase and can thus be a sign of high risk of an impending rupture. Likewise, periaortic hemorrhage (such as from AAA rupture) is also well demonstrated on NECT. Vascular wall enhancement, as can be seen with vasculitides, is also better assessed when comparison with the nonenhanced data is available. Further, NECT can be beneficial for endograft evaluation because subtle calcifications within the vessel wall or thrombus can be easily detected on NECT but can mimic endoleaks on CTA. Surgical graft material, bioglue, and Teflon felt may also be difficult or

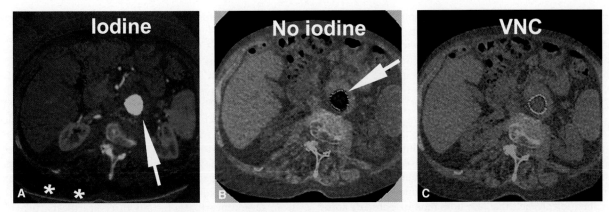

FIGURE 54.4 Applications of dual energy imaging stent-graft evaluation. **A.** Using dual energy techniques, an image can be reconstructed, which displays iodine distribution. Note the inconspicuity of subcutaneous fat (******) in the image, whereas iodinated contrast in the endograft lumen is well displayed (*arrow*). **B.** Conversely, a dataset can be produced by subtracting iodine content. Note lack of displayed signal from the lumen of the endograft (*arrow*). **C.** "Virtual noncontrast" (VNC) image can be produced by deconstructing the added effect of iodine on the composite CT image, allowing radiation dose savings because a dedicated NECT acquisition is not required.

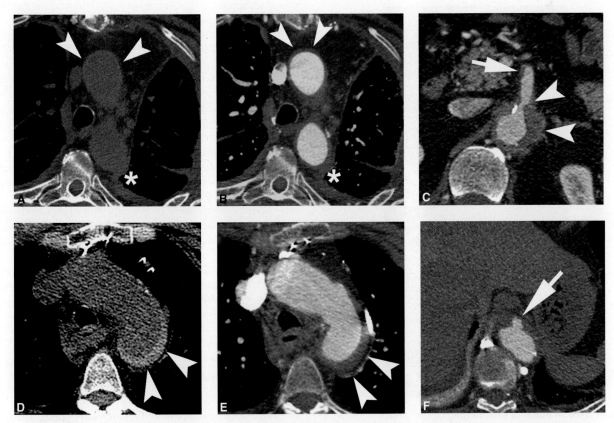

FIGURE 54.5 Importance of nonenhanced CT (NECT) and contrast-enhanced CTA (CECT) images for evaluation of vasculitis and intramural hematoma (IMH). **A–C.** Vasculitis. NECT (**A**) and CECT (**B**) in a 69-year-old with chest and abdominal pain. Note significant mural thickening throughout the proximal (*arrowheads*) and distal (***) transverse thoracic aorta, best visualized on CECT. Density of the mural abnormality (measured at ***) was 37 HU on NECT and increased to 65 HU on CECT. The findings are most consistent with large-vessel vasculitis because IMH does not show enhancement after CM administration. Axial CTA image at the level of the superior mesenteric artery (SMA) shows marked mural thickening (*arrowheads*), which narrows the origin of the SMA and extends along the proximal portions of the vessel (*arrow*). **D–F.** IMH. A 67-year-old female with severe back pain. NECT (**D**) shows hyperdense crescentic mural hematoma (*arrowheads*) with density of 57 HU and no increase in density after contrast administration (**E**). Axial image near diaphragmatic hiatus shows the etiologic agent, a penetrating atherosclerotic ulcer (*arrow*).

impossible to recognize following CM administration but are easily detected by NECT. With the advent of dual energy scanning techniques, it is now possible to reconstruct "virtual noncontrast" CT datasets from the CM-enhanced CTA dataset; this ability may further lessen the need for, and radiation exposure associated with, a dedicated NECT series.

Use of Electrocardiogram Synchronization

The use of ECG-synchronized acquisition can improve evaluation of the aorta, particularly the aortic valve, aortic root, and ascending thoracic aorta.[19] The main benefit of ECG synchronization for aortic imaging comes from the reduction of the notorious pulsation artifacts that may both mimic or obscure aortic pathology. ECG synchronization also can provide additional dynamic information and depict motion of dissection flaps, valves, and leaks, allow analysis of cardiac function and proximal coronary artery segments can be acquired during the diagnostic evaluation of the aorta (FIGURE 54.6). Available techniques

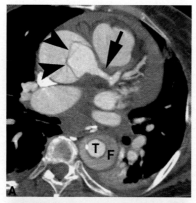

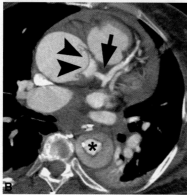

FIGURE 54.6 Importance of ECG synchronization in aortic CTA. A 71-year-old female with Stanford type A aortic dissection, evaluated by retrospectively ECG-gated CTA. **A.** Axial CTA image through aortic root in diastole (70% R-R interval) shows position of dissection flap in the aortic root (*arrowheads*). The left main coronary artery (*arrow*) is also visualized. Note the tubular appearance of the true lumen (*T*) in the descending thoracic aorta, surrounded by the false lumen (*F*). **B.** Systolic image (20% R-R interval) shows movement of the flap (*arrowheads*) over the left coronary ostium (*arrow*). Note also the change in luminal configuration of the true lumen in the descending thoracic aorta (***), secondary to pressurized false lumen.

for ECG synchronization include *prospective ECG triggering* and *retrospective ECG gating.*

Prospective ECG triggering is utilized in a "step and shoot" manner, whereby the CT scanner waits for a user-specified portion of the ECG (typically between 40% and 80% of R-R interval), acquires data, and then moves to the next location, where this process is repeated. The z-axis width of data acquired per heartbeat corresponds to the sum of the active detector widths, which is typically between 2 cm and up to 16 cm on current 64-channel systems. Advantages of prospective triggering include relative lower radiation exposure compared to retrospective gating. The overall scan time to cover the thoracic aorta depends on the detector bank width and may range from several heartbeats to only three heartbeats (two 16-cm scans with interleaved heartbeat for table travel). At least a 4-cm detector bank, or preferably an 8-cm or a 16-cm detector bank is necessary for prospective scanning of the entire thorax. Disadvantages include its limited ability to correct for arrhythmias (ECG editing) and limited ability of valvular and cardiac chamber functional analysis. Because elimination of pulsation artifacts is the main benefit of ECG gating in the setting of acute aortic syndromes, prospective gating is the preferred technique in this setting, provided the scanner has wide enough detector banks.

Retrospective ECG gating, on the other hand, acquires helical data with slow pitch (approximately 0.2 to 0.4) while simultaneously recording the patient's ECG. The data are then retrospectively "binned" into datasets corresponding to the various portions of the R-R interval (for example, 0% to 90% at 10% increments). Reconstruction of retrospective data in this way allows not only freezing of cardiac motion, but also the "cine" review of cardiac and valvular motion and calculation of cardiac functional parameters (ejection fraction, chamber volumes, etc.). Further, because some coronary artery segments are better visualized at different portions of the R-R interval, the review of multiple cardiac phases may allow better assessment of coronary arteries, particularly in patients with higher heart rates. The main drawback of retrospective ECG triggering has been the higher radiation dose owing to the fact that the beam is on during the entire cardiac cycle, pitch is low, and temporal dose efficiency is limited. Latest ECG-based tube current modulation eliminates this disadvantage by exposing the patient only during a desirable (typically diastolic) phase of the cardiac cycle (e.g., 60% to 70% or the R-R interval) while down-modulating the tube current for nondiagnostic phases of the cardiac cycle to only 4% of the full dose.

PROSPECTIVELY TRIGGERED HELICAL COMPUTED TOMOGRAPHY

Although both prospective and retrospective gating were conceptually conceived in the 1970s, prospective triggering of a very fast helical acquisition has been introduced only very recently. This technique takes advantage of the specific dual-source geometry to increase the helical pitch up to 3, which translates in a scan time of 0.6 second for the entire thorax and approximately 2 seconds for the entire chest abdomen and pelvis.[30] Even without ECG synchronization, such a fast acquisition is expected to eliminate or at least substantially reduce cardiac motion artifacts at doses that are equivalent of a standard helical CT.

The selection of ECG synchronization technique for aortic CTA depends on both the scanner capabilities and the clinical question. In the setting of acute aortic syndromes, the main benefit of using ECG synchronization is elimination of cardiac pulsation artifacts in the ascending aorta. Functional information is interesting to visualize, but it (flap motion, etc.) can usually be inferred from high-quality static images as well. Therefore, in the setting of acute aortic syndromes, prospective triggering (for 4- to 16-cm detector banks) or retrospective gating with a narrow, diastolic pulsing window only (for 2- to 4-cm detector banks) is appropriate.

For preoperative planning of valve sparing aortic root surgical repair, transcatheter aortic valve repair, evaluation of postoperative leaks, and other complications, we use retrospective gating with a wider pulsing window that allows both systolic and diastolic assessment of anatomy and pathology.

Of note, we do not use ECG synchronization in the setting of trauma, but instead use nongated CTA of the thorax with portal venous phase abdomen and pelvis CT. The rationale is that traumatic ascending aortic injuries, which would benefit from ECG synchronization, are exceedingly rare in surviving trauma victims. If in doubt—the typical situation is excessive pulsation artifacts in young individuals—an additional scan covering just the ascending aorta can still be obtained to avoid an unnecessary sternotomy.

Dose Reduction Strategies

Some techniques are available to help reduce overall patient dose in CTA, including automated dose modulation, automated exposure control, and ECG-gated tube modulation. *Automated dose modulation* can occur in both the *xy*- and *z*-axis directions. Essentially, the specific X-ray tube current is varied during image acquisition to account for regions of greater thickness and absorption in both angular (*xy*) and longitudinal (*z*) directions, allowing lower exposure for areas of smaller diameter and/or absorption. The result can be an up to 50% reduction in dose in low-absorption areas with preserved image quality throughout the remainder of the scan.[31–36] *Automated exposure control* further adapts the *general* X-ray tube settings to differing patient sizes, which allows consistent image quality across various patient sizes and body thicknesses. This may be accomplished by changing exposure settings to keep a constant "noise index" or adaption of exposure by comparing to a standard patient size or to a known exam template.[32] *ECG-gated tube modulation* ("ECG pulsing") decreases the tube current (by up to 80%) during the retrospective ECG-gated CTA, specifically within the portions of the cardiac cycle where full diagnostic quality is not required. This technique, especially when coupled with lower kilovoltage imaging, can decrease dose up to 50% to 60%,[37,38] albeit at the expense of increased image noise during affected portions of the cardiac cycle. Image quality remains sufficient for calculation of functional data and assessment of cardiac motion. Particularly in smaller patients (<70 kg), routine utilization of 100 kVp tube voltage is recommended; potential dose reduction is significant (up to 25%).[39] Utilization of these techniques should be considered when evaluating patients before, during, and after aortic endograft repair. Given the necessity of multiple follow-up studies for endovascular aneurysm repair (EVAR) or thoracic endovascular aneurysm repair (TEVAR) management, longitudinal dose reduction is quite important.

Raw Data Reconstruction Techniques

For many years, nearly all CT raw data reconstruction has been performed by *filtered back projection* (FBP) techniques, whereby projectional data from multiple angles are mathematically "reversed" to form patient images. The main advantage of FBP is reconstruction speed, which was particularly important in the days of single-slice CT and early MDCT, where computing power was a limiting factor in CT data reconstruction. The FBP algorithm makes several assumptions regarding the CT focal spot, detector configuration, voxel size, and photon statistics that do not represent the reality of CT acquisition. As such, FBP images are prone to high image noise and artifacts. As CT volume coverage and patient size have increased and reconstructed slice thicknesses have decreased, image noise considerations have become more important. As a result, the utility of FBP as a primary reconstruction technique has been questioned. Recently, several vendors have leveraged increases in computational power to allow the reconstruction of CT data with less image noise.

Iterative reconstruction (IR) techniques rely on mathematical modeling of raw CT data without making the assumptions needed for FBP reconstruction. An initial forward projection of image data is formed and then modeled ("iterated") multiple times using a more precise model of CT system optics, photon statistics, and electronic noise until a "final" output image is obtained. Given this computational intensity, the necessary computing power is much greater, and reconstruction times may still be too long for routine clinical use. To make reconstruction times reasonable for routine use, an FBP image can be used as a "starting block" for modeling and iteration of system noise and photon statistics alone (without system optics modeling) can be performed. The result is still a significant reduction in overall image noise at the same acquisition parameters with acceptable reconstruction times. These IR datasets have improved SNR relative to typical FBP images alone. Alternatively, acquisition exposure parameters can be decreased, resulting in image noise levels similar to routine clinical images. Use of IR in this way provides significant reduction in imparted radiation dose while maintaining diagnostic image quality. Much of the advantage of IR techniques is seen in parenchymal organ imaging, where relatively low image contrast predominates. Recent work in higher contrast organ systems, such as coronary, chest, and abdominal aortic regions, has shown that the use of "blended" IR-FBP reconstruction (e.g., 30% to 60% IR) can yield diagnostic quality images at 40% to 50% less radiation dose (FIGURE 54.7).[40–42]

▌ IMAGE POSTPROCESSING CONSIDERATIONS

Once high-quality CTA images are acquired and reconstructed, optimal interpretation of vascular CTA requires knowledge of various postprocessing techniques and development of a consistent workflow for interpretation of increasingly large volumetric datasets.

The transverse "source images" of a volumetric CTA dataset are typically reconstructed with a nominal slice thickness of 1 mm (range 0.5 to 1.5 mm, depending on scanner capabilities and anatomy of interest) and with 0% to 50% overlap in the *z*-direction. Isotropic datasets refer to datasets where voxel dimensions are equivalent in the *x*-, *y*-, and *z*-axes.[43,44] Thicker (but not thinner) images relative to the detector element width in

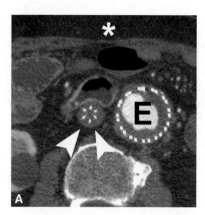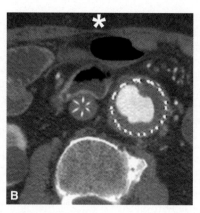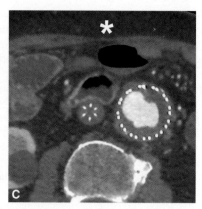

FIGURE 54.7 Effect of iterative reconstruction technique. Axial images obtained with 100% filtered back projection (**A**) and 100% adaptive statistical iterative reconstruction (ASiR) (**C**). Note pronounced decrease in image noise (*) on image (**C**). This marked decrease in image noise may be unpleasant for some viewers, seeming somewhat "plastic" or artificial. On the noncontrast series reconstructed with the clinically typical 40% ASiR blend (**B**), a good balance between noise reduction and visible image changes is struck. Noise levels (measured at *) were 15.8 HU in (**A**), 8.2 HU in (**C**), and 11.0 HU in (**B**). Note also portion of an IVC filter (*arrowheads*) and aortic endograft (*E*) with intraluminal thrombus.

the z-direction can also be reconstructed (e.g., 5 mm). The source images have the highest spatial resolution and often serve as the initial data to establish a diagnosis, notably in the acute setting. Source data viewing is often limited by the sheer number of slices and prominent image noise and may be regarded as a "secondary raw dataset" that is interactively manipulated on a workstation for interpretation. Multiple reconstruction techniques are available for viewing the thin slice source data (FIGURE 54.8).

Multiplanar reconstruction (MPR) is a slice of nominal (1 pixel) thickness, which can be reconstructed in any plane. A stack of MPR images allows quick review of vascular structures. Oriented perpendicular to a vessel, MPRs allow precise calculation of luminal dimensions and any degree of associated stenosis.[45,46] Given the inherent curved course of most vessels, MPR does not allow display of the entire vessel on a single image. Stack review of oblique MPR images enhances the ability to follow curved vascular motion.[45–47]

Curved planar reconstruction (CPR) is generated by propagating a (curved) centerline through a structure of interest, then displaying the associated plane corresponding to the centerline path. CPR has the advantage of display of an entire vessel or vascular territory on one image. Relationships of thrombi, stenoses, aneurysms, and branch vessels can be displayed easily. A secondary set of "slice through" MPR images can be generated perpendicular to the CPR dataset, which can provide more efficient analysis of stenoses.[48] Although recent automated techniques have improved CPR generation accuracy and speed, it remains an operator-dependent technique. Further imitations of CPR technique include unusual artifact generation inherent in the CPR technique and nonvisualization or distortion of surrounding anatomy on the CPR images. For these reasons, review of the centerline traces and source image datasets is mandatory.[46,48]

Maximum intensity projection (MIP) images are a versatile method for the review and display of vascular CTA. A ray-casting technique (which creates 2D images from 3D datasets) was initially developed for the display of vascular magnetic resonance angiogram (MRA) data,[49] MIP displays only the highest (maximum) attenuation voxel within the specified ray. This is advantageous for the review of high-attenuation structures, such as enhanced vessels. Small and/or poorly enhancing vessels are well depicted. Sliding thin-slab (STS) MIP image review is an efficient method for the evaluation of many vascular territories and also has been shown to increase detection of small lung nodules compared to axial images alone.[50,51]

Minimum intensity projection (MINIP), a related technique, displays the minimum attenuation within a ray. Although not as widely applicable to vascular imaging, MINIP is useful for the display of delicate structures, such as cardiac valves. A slab thickness of less than or equal to 5 mm allows optimum depiction. Airways and diffuse lung disease can also be well depicted by the slab MINIP technique.

MIP (and MINIP) images suffer from several limitations, which must be borne in mind when reviewing MIP datasets. Perhaps most importantly, high-density structures (such as calcium or metal) that are adjacent to objects of interest will be preferentially displayed, limiting visualization of the CM-enhanced flow lumen and adjacent anatomy.[44–47,52] Utilizing thinner-slab MIP images, reviewing MPR images in the same plane, and correlating MIP findings to the source image data can minimize this limitation. Also, given the nature of ray casting, the resultant MIP images lack summation of overlapping 3D data and, therefore, spatial relationships can be obscured.[44,46] Additionally, background image noise is additive with MIP/MINIP reconstruction, and this increase in noise can lead to overestimation of stenoses when calculated using MIP data. By the same method, very small vessels can disappear in noisy MIP datasets.

Average intensity projection (AIP), also called "raysum" or "thick MPR," is another ray-casting technique where the averaged voxel value is displayed. Given that this technique averages along the slab, fine detail is limited and image contrast is reduced. This fact limits the utility of AIP for routine vascular review. Image noise is decreased with AIP, however, unlike MIP and MINIP. This factor makes AIP useful as a problem-solving tool for noisy datasets when a trade-off in image contrast and partial volume effects can be tolerated.[46,53]

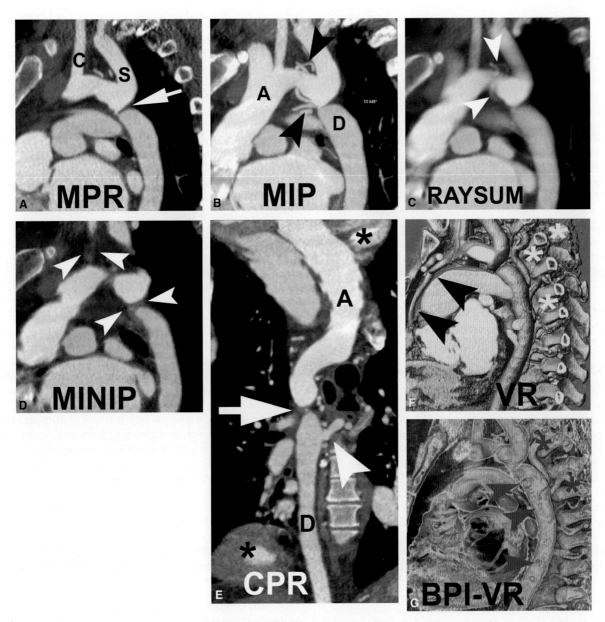

FIGURE 54.8 Basic reconstruction techniques for CTA. A 37-year-old male evaluated for suspected aortic coarctation. **A.** Oblique multiplanar reconstruction (**MPR**) shows a high-grade juxta-ductal coarctation (*arrow*) distal to the left subclavian artery (*S*) and left common carotid artery (*C*). **B.** Oblique sagittal 10-mm maximum intensity projection (**MIP**) image provides a better overview of the entire thoracic aorta and demonstrates a contrast density gradient between the ascending (*A*) and descending (*D*) thoracic aorta, secondary to high-grade obstruction at the coarctation and inflow from collateral blood vessels (*arrowheads*). **C.** A 10-mm raysum (average intensity projection) at the same obliquity as (**B**) shows decreased image noise, but at the expense of low-contrast resolution, demonstrated on the image by poor visualization of the same juxta-ductal collaterals from panel (**B**) (*arrowheads*). **D.** A 10-mm MINIP image at the same obliquity shows limited visualization of vessels, such as the left common carotid artery and coarctation itself (*arrowheads*). Because with MINIP technique only the minimum intensity pixel within the ray is displayed, as slab thickness increases, larger and larger vascular structures may not be well depicted. MINIP is best utilized for valvular or lung imaging. **E.** Curved planar reconstruction (**CPR**) of the entire thoracic aorta. The site of coarctation (*arrow*) and adjacent large intercostal collateral (*arrowhead*) are well depicted. CPR technique can produce odd relationships of structures outside the vessel centerline, as shown by duplication artifact of the left ventricle, displayed at both ends of the image (*). (A, ascending aorta; D, descending aorta.) **F.** Thick-slab volume-rendered (**VR**) image in the same obliquity as (**A**). Note the dilated internal mammary arteries (*arrowheads*), which serve as additional collateral pathways. Multiple intercostal collaterals (*) adjacent to the coarctation are also depicted. Unlike MIP and MINIP, multiple voxels contribute to the output image, and depth information is maintained. The ability of VR to clearly convey complex anatomic relationships is valued by interventionists, surgeons, and referring clinicians. **G.** Blood-pool inversion volume rendering (**BPI-VR**). By reversing the opacity ramp for specific VR opacity transfer functions, one can render the contrast-enhanced lumen transparent. Relationships of the ostia (*arrowheads*) of multiple dilated collateral vessels (*) can be clearly displayed. BPI-VR is also useful for endoluminal viewing of the aortic root.

Volume rendering (VR) is a 3D display technique that developed from the motion picture industry. Unlike MIP and MINIP, VR images allow the display of multiple different voxel attenuations in one image. Individual attenuation ranges can be displayed at varying degrees of opacity. Light sources of varying intensity and perspective are added. These characteristic components of VR images are controlled by "opacity transfer functions," which can be iteratively modified to display tissues and organs of interest. The result is a very flexible method for displaying complex vascular relationships. VR provides an effective overview of complex CTA cases and directs more detailed assessment of lumen and aneurysmal disease by other techniques. Unlike MIP, little to no bone editing is required with VR.[52] VR is effective for the review of endograft integrity and allows communication of complex pathology in only a few images. VR is an interactive technique, and image quality depends on the selection of appropriate opacity transfer functions.[52,54,55] Therefore, the effectiveness of VR display varies with the experience and skill of the operator.

SPECIFIC CLINICAL CONSIDERATIONS FOR COMPUTED TOMOGRAPHY ANGIOGRAM OF THE AORTA

Endovascular Aortic Aneurysm Repair

Technical aspects of placement and management of aortic endografts is addressed elsewhere in this book. CT imaging is important in preoperative, postoperative, and longitudinal follow-up of patients with abdominal and/or thoracic aortic aneurysms. As such, a few technical considerations deserve mention here. CTA is valuable for preprocedural planning for both open and endovascular repair. After endovascular repair of the abdominal aorta (EVAR) or thoracic aorta (TEVAR), follow-up imaging is necessary to detect and classify potential endoleaks and to longitudinally assess the residual aneurysm sac size/volume. Device-related issues, such as endograft fracture, migration, and "bird-beak" proximal apposition of TEVAR devices, which can contribute to endoleak and persistent sac pressurization, can also be well demonstrated by CTA.[56,57]

Preoperative planning benefits from high-resolution CT angiographic depiction of three-dimensional vascular anatomy and CTA have become the gold standard for deriving measurements for EVAR/TEVAR.

Surgically treated thoracic or AAAs typically do not require continued surveillance, unless complications are clinically suspected. EVAR/TEVAR requires lifetime follow-up, however. The traditional CTA protocol for EVAR/TEVAR follow-up is to employ triphasic technique including noncontrast, arterial phase, and delayed (1 to 3 minutes) CT series.[58] Although this is still a prudent approach in the early posttherapeutic phase to assess for early complications and leaks, and in the setting of suspected or known complications, the follow-up strategy for mid- and long-term surveillance may change, notably with newer technology. In the chronic setting, stent-graft integrity and migration are an increasing concern, which can be adequately assessed with noncontrast scans, which also allow assessment of aneurysm sac size. Recent work also suggests that the arterial phase acquisition may not add additional benefit for the detection of endoleaks over the delayed series alone.[59,60] Further, if one obtains the delayed series with dual energy technique (discussed above), a "virtual noncontrast" series can be generated, which may obviate the need for a separate nonenhanced acquisition, thereby decreasing imparted radiation dose by up to 44%.[28,29,61–63] Single-phase CTA acquisition with an intermediate delay (e.g., 40 to 70 seconds) could then be employed to balance the optimum early-phase detection of types I, II, and IV endoleaks with adequate evaluation of type II endoleaks, which may enhance slowly or be better demonstrated later.[28,59] Note, however, that radiation dose may not be as clinically relevant in an older population with advanced atherosclerotic burden who are not surgical candidates for aneurysm repair, but target populations may shift with advances in technology and subsequent clinical use.

Imaging of abdominal aortic aneurysms/thoracoabdominal aortic aneurysms (AAAs/TAAAs) before and after endovascular therapy also requires special attention to image postprocessing. Prior to EVAR selection and placement, accurate length of the infrarenal aneurysm neck (if any), aneurysm neck shape and angulation, orthogonal aneurysmal diameter, aneurysmal sac volume, and status of proposed distal fixation site vessels (e.g., common iliac arteries) must be determined. In addition, for TAAA, the relationship of the aneurysm to the left subclavian artery and the celiac axis, as well as the aortic radius of curvature, must also be determined prior to TEVAR. Given the inherent tortuosity of many aneurysms, the accuracy of measurements made from axial or coronal images alone may be limited.[64,65] Use of a 3D workstation simplifies and standardizes AAA/TAAA evaluation and allows better inter- and intraobserver correlation when compared to catheter angiography.[66,67] CPR and automated centerline tracking images allow accurate measurement of orthogonal vessel diameters and longitudinal vascular landmark relationships at each level. After EVAR or TEVAR, in addition to access site complications and endoleak detection, the size of the residual aneurysm sac must be assessed. Calculation of residual aneurysm sac volume using the segmented aorta has been shown to be accurate and reproducible compared with axial measurements alone. Recently, duplex ultrasound (US) evaluation of EVAR patients has gained popularity given the lack of ionizing radiation and high diagnostic performance in some reports.[68,69] US is operator- and patient dependent, however; thus further work is needed to further clarify the role for US in follow-up of EVAR patients.

Technical Considerations for Imaging of Aortic Dissection

Optimal imaging of aortic dissection requires attention to several specific technical variables. Noncontrast images are acquired because evaluation of IMH may be best detected on NECT. Secondly, given that evaluation of the aortic arch can be limited by streak artifact from contrast medium in the left subclavian and innominate veins, right-sided IV cannula placement is preferred. Placing the arm over the head with the palm against the gantry face will decrease potential venous constriction at the thoracic inlet, which could delay or limit the CM bolus to the SVC and right heart. If there is clinical question of Stanford type A dissection (involving the ascending thoracic aorta), we perform CTA with ECG synchronization to limit artifact from aortic motion. In most instances, we perform retrospective ECG gating (discussed above). Retrospective gating allows assessment of aortic valve morphology and motion and cardiac functional assessment. Also, because side-branch ischemia syndromes from dissection may be the result of static obstruction or dynamic luminal compromise, retrospective ECG gating is valuable to clearly depict the extent of dissection flaps and changes during dynamic obstruction (FIGURE 54.9).[70] Follow-up exams where

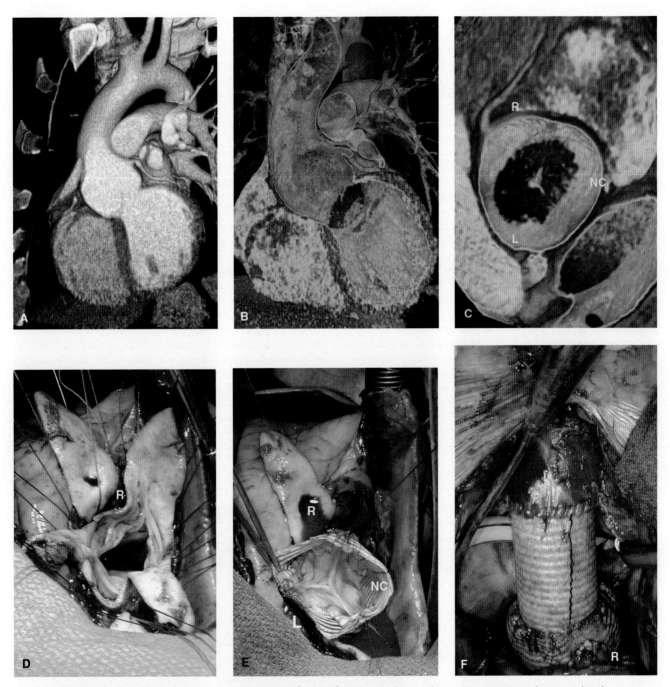

FIGURE 54.9 Valve-sparing aortic root replacement (V-SARR) in the Marfan syndrome. Preoperative volume-rendered image (**A**) of the thoracic aorta in a 27-year-old man with the Marfan syndrome shows aortic root aneurysmal dilatation. Transparent-blood rendering (**B**) and a view from above the valve ("anesthesiologist's perspective") (**C**) illustrate considerable dilatation of the sinuses of Valsalva. Intraoperative photographs demonstrate (**D**) the aortic valve and the residual sinus tissue surrounding the commissures after resection of the sinuses of Valsalva. Note the sutures through the ventriculoaortic junction in the left ventricular outflow tract, which will be used to anchor the graft. The excised right coronary artery button (*R*) with the ostium is seen. In (**E**), the aortic valve is seen resuspended within the proximal graft that has been anchored to the ventriculoaortic junction (not shown). An anterior view of the completed reconstruction (**F**) of the aortic root with the Dacron neosinuses and the reimplanted right coronary artery (*R*), and the second tube graft replacing the tubular portion of the ascending aorta, which re-creates a smaller, new sinotubular junction.

Reprinted, with permission, from Fleischmann D, Liang DH, Mitchell RS, Miller DC. Pre- and postoperative imaging of the aortic root for valve-sparing aortic root repair (V-SARR). *Semin Thorac Cardiovasc Surg*. 2008; 20(4):365–73.

known disease is to be serially monitored can be assessed by prospective ECG-triggered (or even nongated datasets), which provide motion-free datasets with less radiation dose.[70] Recently, time-resolved CTA (TR-CTA) of the aorta has been described, where flow-related information can be acquired utilizing multiple low-dose acquisitions while the CT table moves back and forth, allowing excellent delineation of vascular flow in dissection channels and in endograft imaging.[71] The clinical benefit of this technique remains to be shown.

Technical Considerations for Imaging the Aortic Root and Valve

ECG-synchronized CTA is also very useful in imaging of patients before and after valve-sparing aortic root reconstruction (V-SARR) (FIGURE 54.9) and transcatheter aortic valve implantation (TAVI).[72,73] Retrospective ECG gating is useful for the precise measurement of necessary root and valvular dimensions before these procedures and allows cine evaluation of valvular function and dynamic changes in the root throughout the cardiac cycle. Preoperatively, V-SARR patients are assessed for chest wall/surgical access issues (e.g., pectus deformities), the type and extent of the aortic root aneurysm, coronary artery anatomy and anomalies, and aortic valvular measurements, morphology, and function. Data obtained by MDCT in surgical aortic valve patients have been shown to compare favorably with operative sizing, whereas echocardiographic measurements tend to underestimate true annular dimensions.[74] In postoperative V-SARR patients, we typically obtain a predischarge retrospectively gated CTA as a baseline for further (nongated) follow-up, and, most importantly, to detect complications of the procedure, such as

hematoma or leaks, which may be difficult to assess by echocardiography. We obtain a NECT series in these patients because implanted surgical graft material, felt pledgets, and bioglue are identified as slightly hyperintense at NECT but may be confusing or difficult to characterize without nonenhanced imaging.

Accurate device sizing is essential for procedural success during TAVI. When TAVI is considered, we obtain a retrospectively gated CTA of the chest, followed immediately by switching the scanner acquisition to acquire a nongated CTA of the abdomen and pelvis for evaluation of access vessel suitability and any additional vascular pathology. Accurate preprocedural measurements of the aortic annulus and sinuses of Valsalva (height and diameters), valvular morphologic information, and positions and any anatomic variations of coronary artery origins are obtained by interacting with the 4D dataset on a workstation (FIGURE 54.10).[75] Measurement of aortic root dimensions during both systole and diastole is recommended, given the potentially significant (and somewhat unpredictable) dynamic variability in annular size throughout the cardiac cycle in some patients.[76] Route of access for TAVI also depends on access vessel caliber (≥6 mm), given the size (18 to 19 French) of delivery devices needed for the delivery of the implant. Therefore, assessment of the minimum luminal diameter, calcification, and vessel tortuosity along the planned route of access—either transfemoral or transsubclavian—is important. Other factors, such as extensive bulky atherosclerotic disease, porcelain aorta, and transverse course of the ascending aorta, may preclude transfemoral access secondary to increased risk of cerebrovascular thromboembolic events.[73] In the absence of suitable access vessels, a transapical approach via the left ventricular apex can be performed. Finally,

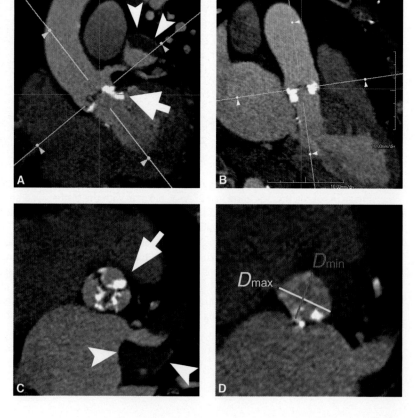

FIGURE 54.10 Utility of ECG-synchronized CTA for preprocedural planning of transcatheter aortic valve implantation (TAVI). A 92-year-old female considered high risk for traditional aortic valve replacement surgery. By placing the imaging plane parallel to the anatomic structure of interest, such as the aortic valve, on both coronal oblique (**A**) and sagittal oblique (**B**) images, an orthogonal image through the aortic valve (*arrow* in **C**) can be obtained. Similar technique will produce an orthogonal image of the aortic annulus (**D**). In figure (**A**), note the extension of aortic valvular calcification along the base of the anterior leaflet of the mitral valve (*arrow*). Extensive, bulky calcification in the implant "landing zone" can predispose to difficulty of sealing the implant with subsequent risks of paravalvular leak and valvular regurgitation. In figures (**A**) and (**C**), a contraindication to TAVI is also demonstrated—thrombus in the left atrium and atrial appendage (*arrowheads*). The maximum (D_{max}) and minimum (D_{min}) diameters can be obtained. The mean diameter (D_{mean}) can then be calculated by $D_{mean} = (D_{max} + D_{min})/2$. The annular perimeter and area can also be calculated from this image.

other structural findings that impact patient eligibility for TAVI, such as LV morphology and function, severe proximal coronary artery stenosis, and cardiac thrombi,[73] can also be visualized by CTA (FIGURE 54.10).

Inflammatory and Infectious Aortic Disease

Vasculitides Affecting the Aorta

CTA is valuable for detecting the presence and extent of large-vessel vasculitis. Hallmarks of large-vessel vasculitis include circumferential mural thickening, intimal low-attenuation ring, absence of calcified atherosclerotic plaque, ectasia/aneurysm formation, and mural enhancement. NECT can demonstrate high density within affected vascular walls and occasional punctate or curvilinear calcification.[77] Arterial phase imaging is useful to show mural thickening, circumferential low-attenuation ring within the mural thickening, and to assess the degree of flow-lumen compromise.[77,78] Delayed-phase imaging (e.g., at 1 to 10 minutes postinjection) is useful to detect areas of enhancement, which correlate to active vasculitis.[78] After steroid therapy, CTA demonstrates decrease or resolution of mural thickening in patients with clinical response.[78,79] Given that many large-vessel vasculitides affect a younger population (who also may better tolerate the longer MR procedure time) and because larger-diameter vessel involvement is common, these patients are also well assessed by contrast-enhanced MRI, where similar imaging findings may be seen.

A recent advance in imaging of vascular inflammation involves the application of 18-fluorodeoxyglucose positron emission tomography/computed tomography (18-FDG PET/CT) to image vascular inflammation. In areas of active infection and inflammation 18-FDG uptake increases, and the use of CT coregistration allows excellent spatial correlation to precise areas of active disease. The amount of tracer accumulation increases with increasing plaque severity. The mechanism of tracer accumulation in plaques and inflammatory lesions is related to the accumulation of metabolically active macrophages.[80,81] Response to therapy can also be assessed by PET/CT.[82–84] PET/CT evaluation of acute aortic syndromes may also have prognostic and therapeutic significance: patients with positive PET/CT have been shown to be at high risk (~80%) for progression of their acute aortic syndrome, whereas most PET-negative patients showed stability or regression of their disease.[85] Likewise, there is strong correlation between 18-FDG avidity and aneurysmal wall stress, progression of size, and rupture.[86–88]

Infections Involving the Aorta

Imaging of infectious (mycotic) aortic aneurysms requires special imaging consideration and clinical correlation. CTA is an excellent modality for depicting mycotic aneurysms and associated complications, including pseudoaneurysm formation, spread of infection to adjacent structures, aortoenteric fistulae, urinary tract obstruction, and rupture.[89] NECT should be obtained as part of the workup and may demonstrate bubbles of gas, which are diagnostic of infection, or evidence of rupture, and therefore should be treated expeditiously. In contrast to atherosclerotic aneurysms, extensive calcification may be conspicuously absent on NECT. NECT may also show adjacent vertebral osteomyelitis, which can be both diagnostic and a causative source.[89] Early in the course of the disease, asymmetric periaortic fat tissue stranding or soft-tissue density may

be present, although this finding is not specific. Irregularity of the adjacent aortic wall may also be seen, and enhancement of the periaortic tissue may occur.[89] Later, saccular aneurysm/pseudoaneurysm formation can occur. A delayed (venous phase) CTA series should also be considered because rim enhancement of perivascular abscesses can be seen, and visualization of a thin mural hypodensity (thought to represent mural edema or necrosis) is often best depicted.[89,90] Rapid appearance of an aneurysm should also suggest mycotic origin; therefore, close follow-up CT may be needed. CTA can also show communication of the mycotic lesion to hollow organs, such as the duodenum, which is diagnostic of an aortoenteric fistula. The protocol for evaluation of such suspected fistulae should include NECT, arterial-phase, and delayed (e.g., 80 seconds) imaging to detect slow-flowing leaks from the aorta.[91] Given the potential for rapid enlargement, serial CT imaging follow-up can be useful.[92] Response to therapy can also be assessed on serial CT examinations. Current therapeutic choices include open surgical resection with in situ or extra-anatomic graft placement or endovascular stent-graft repair.[93–96] Long-term antibiotics are also warranted.[93]

Postoperative Complications

A related application of vascular CT is in the detection of surgical or endovascular graft infection. The incidence of graft and endograft infection is approximately 0.5% to 5%. Early detection is important because graft infection can be life threatening and there is high morbidity from complications, such as rupture, perivascular abscess, aortic fistulae, thrombosis, and embolic disease.[97,98] CT may show bubbles of gas around the graft, which are highly sensitive but nonspecific because bubbles of gas may persist for weeks to months after surgery.[98] Perigraft fluid or soft-tissue thickening is likewise nonspecific; hematoma, lymphocele, seroma, and phlegmon/abscess may all have a similar appearance on CT. Abscess may show rim enhancement, but this is not always seen and likewise not completely specific. CT may also fail to show significant abnormalities in the setting of chronic or low-grade infection. Recently, functional imaging by 18-FDG PET/CT has shown excellent results for the detection, localization, and characterization of suspected graft infection. Focal high-grade tracer accumulation around the graft carries high specificity,[99–102] whereas low-grade linear tracer accumulation is more likely related to aseptic inflammation related to the synthetic graft itself.[98] Inhomogeneous distribution of tracer accumulation should be regarded as nondiagnostic for the presence of infection. Radiolabeled 99-technetium-leukocyte single-photon emission computed tomography/computed tomography (^{99}Tc-WBC SPECT/CT) imaging has also been shown to be effective in detecting graft infections (FIGURE 54.11) and may be of particular value when PET/CT is not readily available, or in the first 2 months after surgery when healing and inflammation (granulation tissue) may produce 18-FDG PET uptake, leading to false positives.[103–105] Using hepatic tracer uptake as an internal control for comparison may allow highest accuracy.[105]

▋ FUTURE DIRECTIONS

Recent introduction of wide-area (volume) CT detector configurations make possible additional techniques for CT imaging of the aorta. Previously, TR-CTA imaging was not practical given that the imaging volume was limited to the width of the

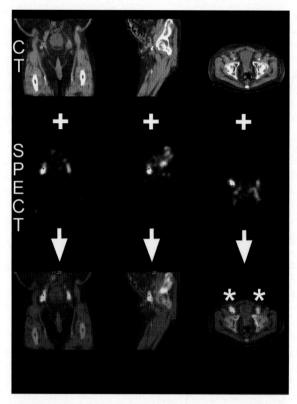

FIGURE 54.11 Technique of SPECT/CT fusion imaging. Infection of the aorto-bifemoral graft. CT images are obtained for anatomic localization (**top row**). The ^{99}Tc-labeled white blood cell (WBC) SPECT datasets in the corresponding projections are acquired (**middle row**). The two datasets are combined into fusion images (**bottom row**), which provide clear localization of abnormal WBC accumulation along the distal portions of both limbs of an aorto-bifemoral graft.

CONCLUSION

CT is a mainstay of aortic imaging over a wide spectrum of disease states. Evolution in CT scanner technology have facilitated tremendous advances in CT evaluation of the aorta, notably the aortic root valve and ascending aorta. Taking advantage of technology requires understanding of the technical principles and fundamentals of contrast dynamics and familiarization with postprocessing tools. In the future, ongoing refinement of these techniques and improved knowledge of the pathophysiology of aortic diseases and new treatments will expand the role of CT as a first-line imaging tool for imaging of the aorta.

detector bank, which was insufficient for coverage of the thoracic or abdominal aorta. Development of large-area detector (volume) CT scanners allow volume acquisition up to 16 cm per rotation, and the introduction of rapid bidirectional table motion (shuttle) techniques allow acquisition of time-resolved data. The ability to evaluate changes in vascular perfusion and flow over time represents a significant advancement in CTA assessment of the aorta and its branches.

Promising preliminary results for TR-CTA have been reported for imaging of aortic dissection, endografts, and peripheral arterial segments.[71] In the setting of dissection, TR-CTA can provide the ability to quantify time and direction of false lumen filling, organ perfusion, and hemodynamic relevance of the dissection flap. In aortic endograft patients, time delay between aortic and endoleak filling can be calculated, and better assessment of the direction and flow (high flow versus low flow) of endoleaks demonstrated. Improved detection of subtle endoleaks (versus traditional CTA) and classification of endoleak type may be expected.[71,106] Assessment of collateral vessel flow in both clinical scenarios should also be improved. In preliminary work in the peripheral circulation, TR-CTA has shown higher contrast enhancement and less venous overlap, and increased diagnostic confidence has been demonstrated compared to standard CTA for calf vessels.[106]

REFERENCES

1. Dawson P, Blomley MJ. Contrast media as extracellular fluid space markers: adaptation of the central volume theorem. *Br J Radiol* 1996;69(824):717–722.
2. Knopp M, Kauczor HU, Knopp MA, et al. Effects of viscosity, cannula size and temperature in mechanical contrast media administration in CT and magnetic resonance tomography [in German]. *Rofo* 1995;163(3):259–264.
3. Fleischmann D. Contrast medium administration in computed tomographic angiography. In: Rubin GD, Rofsky NM, eds. *CT and MR Angiography: Comprehensive Vascular Assessment*. Philadelphia, PA: Lippincott Williams & Wilkins; 2009:128–154.
4. Fleischmann D. CT angiography: injection and acquisition technique. *Radiol Clin North Am* 2010;48(2):237–247, vii.
5. Katayama H, Yamaguchi K, Kozuka T, et al. Adverse reactions to ionic and nonionic contrast media. A report from the Japanese Committee on the Safety of Contrast Media. *Radiology* 1990;175(3):621–628.
6. Choyke PL, Cady J, DePollar SL, et al. Determination of serum creatinine prior to iodinated contrast media: is it necessary in all patients? *Tech Urol* 1998;4(2):65–69.
7. Goldfarb S, McCullough PA, McDermott J, et al. Contrast-induced acute kidney injury: specialty-specific protocols for interventional radiology, diagnostic computed tomography radiology, and interventional cardiology. *Mayo Clin Proc* 2009;84(2):170–179.
8. Dawson P, Blomley MJ. Contrast agent pharmacokinetics revisited: I, reformulation. *Acad Radiol* 1996;3(suppl 2):S261–S263.
9. Fleischmann D. Present and future trends in multiple detector-row CT applications: CT angiography. *Eur Radiol* 2002;12(suppl 2):S11–S15.
10. Fleischmann D, Rubin GD, Bankier AA, et al. Improved uniformity of aortic enhancement with customized contrast medium injection protocols at CT angiography. *Radiology* 2000;214(2):363–371.
11. Bae KT, Tran HQ, Heiken JP. Multiphasic injection method for uniform prolonged vascular enhancement at CT angiography: pharmacokinetic analysis and experimental porcine model. *Radiology* 2000;216(3):872–880.
12. Di Giacomo M. Comparison of three peripherally-inserted central catheters: pilot study. *Br J Nurs* 2009;18(1):8–16.
13. Wieners G, Redlich U, Dudeck O, et al. First experiences with intravenous port systems authorized for high pressure injection of contrast agent in multiphasic computed tomography [in German]. *Rofo* 2009;181(7):664–668.
14. Hittmair K, Fleischmann D. Accuracy of predicting and controlling time-dependent aortic enhancement from a test bolus injection. *J Comput Assist Tomogr* 2001;25(2):287–294.
15. Brunette J, Mongrain R, Rodes-Cabau J, et al. Comparative rheology of low- and iso-osmolarity contrast agents at different temperatures. *Catheter Cardiovasc Interv* 2008;71(1):78–83.
16. Hazirolan T, Turkbey B, Akpinar E, et al. The impact of warmed intravenous contrast material on the bolus geometry of coronary CT angiography applications. *Korean J Radiol* 2009;10(2):150–155.
17. Haage P, Schmitz-Rode T, Hubner D, et al. Reduction of contrast material dose and artifacts by a saline flush using a double power injector in helical CT of the thorax. *AJR Am J Roentgenol* 2000;174(4):1049–1053.
18. Bae KT. Intravenous contrast medium administration and scan timing at CT: considerations and approaches. *Radiology* 2010;256(1):32–61.
19. Roos JE, Willmann JK, Weishaupt D, et al. Thoracic aorta: motion artifact reduction with retrospective and prospective electrocardiography-assisted multi-detector row CT. *Radiology* 2002;222(1):271–277.
20. Bae KT, Seeck BA, Hildebolt CF, et al. Contrast enhancement in cardiovascular MDCT: effect of body weight, height, body surface area, body mass index, and obesity. *AJR Am J Roentgenol* 2008;190(3):777–784.

21. Kubo S, Tadamura E, Yamamuro M, et al. Thoracoabdominal-aortoiliac MDCT angiography using reduced dose of contrast material. *AJR Am J Roentgenol* 2006;187(2):548–554.

22. Nakaura T, Awai K, Yauaga Y, et al. Contrast injection protocols for coronary computed tomography angiography using a 64-detector scanner: comparison between patient weight-adjusted- and fixed iodine-dose protocols. *Invest Radiol* 2008;43(7):512–519.

23. Schindera ST, Tock I, Marin D, et al. Effect of beam hardening on arterial enhancement in thoracoabdominal CT angiography with increasing patient size: an in vitro and in vivo study. *Radiology* 2010;256(2):528–535.

24. Szucs-Farkas Z, Strautz T, Patak MA, et al. Is body weight the most appropriate criterion to select patients eligible for low-dose pulmonary CT angiography? Analysis of objective and subjective image quality at 80 kVp in 100 patients. *Eur Radiol* 2009;19(8):1914–1922.

25. Liu X, Yu L, Primak AN, et al. Quantitative imaging of element composition and mass fraction using dual-energy CT: three-material decomposition. *Med Phys* 2009;36(5):1602–1609.

26. Tran DN, Straka M, Roos JE, et al. Dual-energy CT discrimination of iodine and calcium: experimental results and implications for lower extremity CT angiography. *Acad Radiol* 2009;16(2):160–171.

27. Johnson TR, Krauss B, Sedlmair M, et al. Material differentiation by dual energy CT: initial experience. *Eur Radiol* 2007;17(6):1510–1517.

28. Stolzmann P, Frauenfelder T, Pfammatter T, et al. Endoleaks after endovascular abdominal aortic aneurysm repair: detection with dual-energy dual-source CT. *Radiology* 2008;249(2):682–691.

29. Sommer WH, Graser A, Becker CR, et al. Image quality of virtual noncontrast images derived from dual-energy CT angiography after endovascular aneurysm repair. *J Vasc Interv Radiol* 2010;21(3):315–321.

30. Flohr TG, Leng S, Yu L, et al. Dual-source spiral CT with pitch up to 3.2 and 75 ms temporal resolution: image reconstruction and assessment of image quality. *Med Phys* 2009;36(12):5641–5653.

31. Mastora I, Remy-Jardin M, Delannoy V, et al. Multi-detector row spiral CT angiography of the thoracic outlet: dose reduction with anatomically adapted online tube current modulation and preset dose savings. *Radiology* 2004;230(1):116–124.

32. Greess H, Lutze J, Nomayr A, et al. Dose reduction in subsecond multislice spiral CT examination of children by online tube current modulation. *Eur Radiol* 2004;14(6):995–999.

33. Kalra MK, Rizzo S, Maher MM, et al. Chest CT performed with z-axis modulation: scanning protocol and radiation dose. *Radiology* 2005;237(1):303–308.

34. Kalra MK, Maher MM, D'Souza RV, et al. Detection of urinary tract stones at low-radiation-dose CT with z-axis automatic tube current modulation: phantom and clinical studies. *Radiology* 2005;235(2):523–529.

35. McCollough CH, Bruesewitz MR, Kofler JM Jr. CT dose reduction and dose management tools: overview of available options. *Radiographics* 2006;26(2):503–512.

36. Lee CH, Goo JM, Ye HJ, et al. Radiation dose modulation techniques in the multidetector CT era: from basics to practice. *Radiographics* 2008;28(5):1451–1459.

37. Jakobs TF, Becker CR, Ohnesorge B, et al. Multislice helical CT of the heart with retrospective ECG gating: reduction of radiation exposure by ECG-controlled tube current modulation. *Eur Radiol* 2002;12(5):1081–1086.

38. Hausleiter J, Meyer T, Hadamitzky M, et al. Radiation dose estimates from cardiac multislice computed tomography in daily practice: impact of different scanning protocols on effective dose estimates. *Circulation* 2006;113(10):1305–1310.

39. Nakayama Y, Awai K, Funama Y, et al. Lower tube voltage reduces contrast material and radiation doses on 16-MDCT aortography. *AJR Am J Roentgenol* 2006;187(5):W490–W497.

40. Leipsic J, Nguyen G, Brown J, et al. A prospective evaluation of dose reduction and image quality in chest CT using adaptive statistical iterative reconstruction. *AJR Am J Roentgenol* 2010;195(5):1095–1099.

41. Leipsic J, Labounty TM, Heilbron B, et al. Adaptive statistical iterative reconstruction: assessment of image noise and image quality in coronary CT angiography. *AJR Am J Roentgenol* 2010;195(3):649–654.

42. Singh S, Kalra MK, Hsieh J, et al. Abdominal CT: comparison of adaptive statistical iterative and filtered back projection reconstruction techniques. *Radiology* 2010;257(2):373–383.

43. Cody DD. AAPM/RSNA physics tutorial for residents: topics in CT. Image processing in CT. *Radiographics* 2002;22(5):1255–1268.

44. Rubin GD. 3-D imaging with MDCT. *Eur J Radiol* 2003;45(suppl 1):S37–S41.

45. Salgado R, Mulkens T, Ozsarlak O, et al. CT angiography: basic principles and post-processing applications. *JBR-BTR* 2003;86(6):336–340.

46. Dalrymple NC, Prasad SR, Freckleton MW, et al. Informatics in radiology (infoRAD): introduction to the language of three-dimensional imaging with multidetector CT. *Radiographics* 2005;25(5):1409–1428.

47. Fishman EK, Lawler LP. CT angiography: principles, techniques and study optimization using 16-slice multidetector CT with isotropic datasets and 3D volume visualization. *Crit Rev Comput Tomogr* 2004;45(5–6):355–388.

48. Raman R, Napel S, Beaulieu CF, et al. Automated generation of curved planar reformations from volume data: method and evaluation. *Radiology* 2002;223(1):275–280.

49. Price RR, Creasy JL, Lorenz CH, et al. Magnetic resonance angiography techniques. *Invest Radiol* 1992;27(suppl 2):S27–S32.

50. Napel S, Rubin GD, Jeffrey RB Jr. STS-MIP: a new reconstruction technique for CT of the chest. *J Comput Assist Tomogr* 1993;17(5):832–838.

51. Kim JK, Kim JH, Bae SJ, et al. CT angiography for evaluation of living renal donors: comparison of four reconstruction methods. *AJR Am J Roentgenol* 2004;183(2):471–477.

52. Fishman EK, Ney DR, Heath DG, et al. Volume rendering versus maximum intensity projection in CT angiography: what works best, when, and why. *Radiographics* 2006;26(3):905–922.

53. Philipp MO, Kubin K, Mang T, et al. Three-dimensional volume rendering of multidetector-row CT data: applicable for emergency radiology. *Eur J Radiol* 2003;48(1):33–38.

54. van Ooijen PM, Ho KY, Dorgelo J, et al. Coronary artery imaging with multidetector CT: visualization issues. *Radiographics* 2003;23(6):e16.

55. Baek SY, Sheafor DH, Keogan MT, et al. Two-dimensional multiplanar and three-dimensional volume-rendered vascular CT in pancreatic carcinoma: interobserver agreement and comparison with standard helical techniques. *AJR Am J Roentgenol* 2001;176(6):1467–1473.

56. Roos JE, Hellinger JC, Hallet R, et al. Detection of endograft fractures with multidetector row computed tomography. *J Vasc Surg* 2005;42(5):1002–1006.

57. Ueda T, Fleischmann D, Dake MD, et al. Incomplete endograft apposition to the aortic arch: bird-beak configuration increases risk of endoleak formation after thoracic endovascular aortic repair. *Radiology* 2010;255(2):645–652.

58. Rozenblit AM, Patlas M, Rosenbaum AT, et al. Detection of endoleaks after endovascular repair of abdominal aortic aneurysm: value of unenhanced and delayed helical CT acquisitions. *Radiology* 2003;227(2):426–433.

59. Macari M, Chandarana H, Schmidt B, et al. Abdominal aortic aneurysm: can the arterial phase at CT evaluation after endovascular repair be eliminated to reduce radiation dose? *Radiology* 2006;241(3):908–914.

60. Iezzi R, Cotroneo AR, Filippone A, et al. Multidetector CT in abdominal aortic aneurysm treated with endovascular repair: are unenhanced and delayed phase enhanced images effective for endoleak detection? *Radiology* 2006;241(3):915–921.

61. Chandarana H, Godoy MC, Vlahos I, et al. Abdominal aorta: evaluation with dual-source dual-energy multidetector CT after endovascular repair of aneurysms—initial observations. *Radiology* 2008;249(2):692–700.

62. Numburi UD, Schoenhagen P, Flamm SD, et al. Feasibility of dual-energy CT in the arterial phase: imaging after endovascular aortic repair. *AJR Am J Roentgenol* 2010;195(2):486–493.

63. Karçaaltincaba M, Aktaş A. Dual-energy CT revisited with multidetector CT: review of principles and clinical applications. *Diagn Interv Radiol* 2011;17(3):181–194. Epub 2010 Nov 14.

64. Tillich M, Hill BB, Paik DS, et al. Prediction of aortoiliac stent-graft length: comparison of measurement methods. *Radiology* 2001;220(2):475–483.

65. Broeders IA, Blankensteijn JD, Olree M, et al. Preoperative sizing of grafts for transfemoral endovascular aneurysm management: a prospective comparative study of spiral CT angiography, arteriography, and conventional CT imaging. *J Endovasc Surg* 1997;4(3):252–261.

66. Diehm N, Herrmann P, Dinkel HP. Multidetector CT angiography versus digital subtraction angiography for aortoiliac length measurements prior to endovascular AAA repair. *J Endovasc Ther* 2004;11(5):527–534.

67. Higashiura W, Sakaguchi S, Tabayashi N, et al. Impact of 3-dimensional-computed tomography workstation for precise planning of endovascular aneurysm repair. *Circ J* 2008;72(12):2028–2034.

68. Manning BJ, O'Neill SM, Haider SN, et al. Duplex ultrasound in aneurysm surveillance following endovascular aneurysm repair: a comparison with computed tomography aortography. *J Vasc Surg* 2009;49(1):60–65.

69. Schmieder GC, Stout CL, Stokes GK, et al. Endoleak after endovascular aneurysm repair: duplex ultrasound imaging is better than computed tomography at determining the need for intervention. *J Vasc Surg* 2009;50(5):1012–1017; discussion 7–8.

70. McMahon MA, Squirrell CA. Multidetector CT of aortic dissection: a pictorial review. *Radiographics* 2010;30(2):445–460.

71. Sommer WH, Clevert DA, Bamberg F, et al. Time-resolved computed tomography imaging of the aorta: a feasibility study. *J Thorac Imaging* 2010;25(2):161–167.

72. Fleischmann D, Liang DH, Mitchell RS, et al. Pre- and postoperative imaging of the aortic root for valve-sparing aortic root repair (V-SARR). *Semin Thorac Cardiovasc Surg* 2008;20(4):365–373.

73. Vahanian A, Alfieri O, Al-Attar N, et al. Transcatheter valve implantation for patients with aortic stenosis: a position statement from the European Association of Cardio-Thoracic Surgery (EACTS) and the European Society of Cardiology (ESC), in collaboration with the European Association of Percutaneous Cardiovascular Interventions (EAPCI). *Eur Heart J* 2008;29(11):1463–1470.

74. Dashkevich A, Blanke P, Siepe M, et al. Preoperative assessment of aortic annulus dimensions: comparison of noninvasive and intraoperative measurement. *Ann Thorac Surg* 2011;91(3):709–714.

75. Ewe SH, Klautz RJ, Schalij MJ, et al. Role of computed tomography imaging for transcatheter valvular repair/insertion. *Int J Cardiovasc Imaging* 2011;27(8):1179–1193.

76. de Heer LM, Budde RP, Mali WP, et al. Aortic root dimension changes during systole and diastole: evaluation with ECG-gated multidetector row computed tomography. *Int J Cardiovasc Imaging* 2011;27(8):1195–1204.

77. Park JH, Chung JW, Im JG, et al. Takayasu arteritis: evaluation of mural changes in the aorta and pulmonary artery with CT angiography. *Radiology* 1995;196(1):89–93.

78. Kim SY, Park JH, Chung JW, et al. Follow-up CT evaluation of the mural changes in active Takayasu arteritis. *Korean J Radiol* 2007;8(4):286–294.

79. Marie I, Proux A, Duhaut P, et al. Long-term follow-up of aortic involvement in giant cell arteritis: a series of 48 patients. *Medicine (Baltimore)* 2009;88(3):182–192.

80. Ogawa M, Ishino S, Mukai T, et al. (18)F-FDG accumulation in atherosclerotic plaques: immunohistochemical and PET imaging study. *J Nucl Med* 2004;45(7):1245–1250.

81. Rudd JH, Warburton EA, Fryer TD, et al. Imaging atherosclerotic plaque inflammation with [18F]-fluorodeoxyglucose positron emission tomography. *Circulation* 2002;105(23):2708–2711.

82. Webb M, Chambers A, Al-Nahhas A, et al. The role of 18F-FDG PET in characterising disease activity in Takayasu arteritis. *Eur J Nucl Med Mol Imaging* 2004;31(5):627–634.

83. Kobayashi Y, Ishii K, Oda K, et al. Aortic wall inflammation due to Takayasu arteritis imaged with 18F-FDG PET coregistered with enhanced CT. *J Nucl Med* 2005;46(6):917–922.

84. Tahara N, Kai H, Ishibashi M, et al. Simvastatin attenuates plaque inflammation: evaluation by fluorodeoxyglucose positron emission tomography. *J Am Coll Cardiol* 2006;48(9):1825–1831.

85. Kuehl H, Eggebrecht H, Boes T, et al. Detection of inflammation in patients with acute aortic syndrome: comparison of FDG-PET/CT imaging and serological markers of inflammation. *Heart* 2008;94(11):1472–1477.

86. Sakalihasan N, Van Damme H, Gomez P, et al. Positron emission tomography (PET) evaluation of abdominal aortic aneurysm (AAA). *Eur J Vasc Endovasc Surg* 2002;23(5):431–436.

87. Reeps C, Essler M, Pelisek J, et al. Increased 18F-fluorodeoxyglucose uptake in abdominal aortic aneurysms in positron emission/computed tomography is associated with inflammation, aortic wall instability, and acute symptoms. *J Vasc Surg* 2008;48(2):417–423; discussion 24.

88. Xu XY, Borghi A, Nchimi A, et al. High levels of 18F-FDG uptake in aortic aneurysm wall are associated with high wall stress. *Eur J Vasc Endovasc Surg* 2010;39(3):295–301.

89. Azizi L, Henon A, Belkacem A, et al. Infected aortic aneurysms: CT features. *Abdom Imaging* 2004;29(6):716–720.

90. Rozenblit A, Bennett J, Suggs W. Evolution of the infected abdominal aortic aneurysm: CT observation of early aortitis. *Abdom Imaging* 1996;21(6):512–514.

91. Vu QD, Menias CO, Bhalla S, et al. Aortoenteric fistulas: CT features and potential mimics. *Radiographics* 2009;29(1):197–209.

92. Iimori A, Kanzaki Y, Ito S, et al. Rapidly progressing aneurysm of infected thoracic aorta with pseudoaneurysm formation. *Intern Med* 2010;49(22):2461–2465.

93. Zhou T, Guo D, Chen B, et al. Endovascular stent-graft repair of mycotic aneurysms of the aorta: a case series with a 22-month follow-up. *World J Surg* 2009;33(8):1772–1778.

94. Koeppel TA, Gahlen J, Diehl S, et al. Mycotic aneurysm of the abdominal aorta with retroperitoneal abscess: successful endovascular repair. *J Vasc Surg* 2004;40(1):164–166.

95. Stanley BM, Semmens JB, Lawrence-Brown MM, et al. Endoluminal repair of mycotic thoracic aneurysms. *J Endovasc Ther* 2003;10(3):511–515.

96. Berchtold C, Eibl C, Seelig MH, et al. Endovascular treatment and complete regression of an infected abdominal aortic aneurysm. *J Endovasc Ther* 2002;9(4):543–548.

97. Chang JK, Calligaro KD, Ryan S, et al. Risk factors associated with infection of lower extremity revascularization: analysis of 365 procedures performed at a teaching hospital. *Ann Vasc Surg* 2003;17(1):91–96.

98. Keidar Z, Nitecki S. FDG-PET for the detection of infected vascular grafts. *Q J Nucl Med Mol Imaging* 2009;53(1):35–40.

99. Fukuchi K, Ishida Y, Higashi M, et al. Detection of aortic graft infection by fluorodeoxyglucose positron emission tomography: comparison with computed tomographic findings. *J Vasc Surg* 2005;42(5):919–925.

100. Keidar Z, Engel A, Hoffman A, et al. Prosthetic vascular graft infection: the role of 18F-FDG PET/CT. *J Nucl Med* 2007;48(8):1230–1236.

101. Spacek M, Belohlavek O, Votrubova J, et al. Diagnostics of "non-acute" vascular prosthesis infection using 18F-FDG PET/CT: our experience with 96 prostheses. *Eur J Nucl Med Mol Imaging* 2009;36(5):850–858.

102. Lauwers P, Van den Broeck S, Carp L, et al. The use of positron emission tomography with (18)F-fluorodeoxyglucose for the diagnosis of vascular graft infection. *Angiology* 2007;58(6):717–724.

103. Gardet E, Addas R, Monteil J, et al. Comparison of detection of F-18 fluorodeoxyglucose positron emission tomography and 99mTc-hexamethylpropylene amine oxime labelled leukocyte scintigraphy for an aortic graft infection. *Interact Cardiovasc Thorac Surg* 2010;10(1):142–143.

104. Lee A, Biggs H, Chen S, et al. SPECT/CT of axillofemoral graft infection. *Clin Nucl Med* 2008;33(5):333–334.

105. Lou L, Alibhai KN, Winkelaar GB, et al. 99mTc-WBC scintigraphy with SPECT/CT in the evaluation of arterial graft infection. *Nucl Med Commun* 2010;31(5):411–416.

106. Sommer WH, Helck A, Bamberg F, et al. Diagnostic value of time-resolved CT angiography for the lower leg. *Eur Radiol* 2010;20(12):2876–2881.

Magnetic Resonance Angiography of the Aorta

PHILLIP M. YOUNG and ROBERT J. HERFKENS

INTRODUCTION

Since magnetic resonance (MR) imaging of the cardiovascular system was first described in the early 1980s,[1,2] numerous MR techniques have evolved and been implemented in clinical practice. With the introduction of contrast-enhanced MR angiography (CE-MRA) techniques for imaging the aorta in the mid-1990s,[3,4] use of the technology rapidly increased, taking advantage of the high image contrast, spatial resolution, and diagnostic accuracy such techniques can enable. Although practice patterns have altered in recent years because of increased awareness of the potential association between administration of some gadolinium contrast agents and development of nephrogenic systemic fibrosis (NSF) in patients with renal insufficiency,[5,6] MR techniques continue to advance, and the technology offers an unparalleled array of techniques to noninvasively investigate vessel anatomy, vascular pathology, and hemodynamics. This chapter presents an overview of current strategies for imaging the aorta with MR, including contrast-enhanced and noncontrast techniques, protocol optimization, clinical indications, and current developments with the potential impact in the future of aortic imaging with MR.

SPECIFIC TECHNIQUES

Contrast-Enhanced Magnetic Resonance Angiography

Although use of gadolinium for CE-MRA remains off-label for most of the agents approved for use by the United States Food and Drug Administration, the practice is well established for over 15 years and is commonly employed. State-of-the art imaging can be performed on a 1.5T or 3T magnet with the use of a multichannel-phased array coil. Imaging with a 3T scanner has significant potential advantages for CE-MRA because of higher signal and longer T1s (causing a greater effect of T1 shortening from intravascular gadolinium). To fully exploit these advantages, one must have adequate receiver coils to cover the anatomic region of interest and appropriate pulse sequences. In practice, excellent quality images can be obtained with proper technique at either field strength.

From the perspective of scan technique, CE-MRA employs high spatial resolution 3D spoiled gradient echo images following the intravenous injection of a gadolinium contrast agent. These T1-weighted sequences, which intrinsically lack image contrast and have relatively low signal-to-noise ratios (SNR), exploit the pronounced T1 shortening of intravascular gadolinium to generate image contrast against a low-signal background. There are inherent trade-offs that must be made between scan time, anatomic coverage, and spatial resolution. In general, breath-holding is required for imaging of the thoracic

and abdominal aorta,[7] and the scan should be tailored by the technologist to maximize the patient's breath-holding capacity. This will allow maximum spatial resolution achievable for the anatomic coverage required to answer the clinical question. These sequences are optimized with a high bandwidth (±62.5 to 125 kHz), which allows rapid gradient switches and facilitates use of the minimum repetition time (TR) and echo time (TE) achievable on the system.

To further maximize the spatial resolution achieved in a given scan time, undersampling techniques, such as partial-Fourier acquisition[8,9] and parallel imaging[10,11] are often employed. The former exploits k-space symmetry, whereas the latter exploits spatially varying sensitivities of different coil elements. These techniques, which can be used simultaneously, can allow shorter scan times for a given scan prescription, or alternatively allow acquisition of greater anatomic coverage or higher resolution datasets for a given same scan time. Potential limitations of these techniques include noise-like artifacts related to undersampling and potentially discrete artifacts in the case of parallel imaging.

When performing MRA, the rate and timing of gadolinium contrast injection is critical[12,13] and must be appropriate for the readout method employed. Briefly, data acquired by the MR scanner are placed into k-space—a visual representation of spatial frequencies—before a Fourier transform is employed to convert these data into clinical images. Data in the center of k-space corresponds to low spatial frequencies (the bright-dark contrast of structures in the image). Data at the periphery of k-space, on the other hand, contribute the edge information. Ideally, the peak intravascular gadolinium concentration in the vessel of interest should occur during the acquisition of the center of k-space, but it is also important that the bolus's duration is long enough to maintain signal during acquisition of peripheral k-space to maximize edge definition. Proper timing can be achieved through use of a timing run with a small "test bolus," or alternatively through real-time triggering.[14] Our preference is for the former because it allows more precise determination of the optimal scan time and is less susceptible to mistiming because of patient factors or judgment errors by the MR technologist.

Most MRA acquisitions of the aorta employ either centric or sequential readout. In the case of centric encoding, the center of k-space is obtained at the beginning of the scan, and k-space is filled outward from the center in circular or elliptic fashion for the duration of the scan. This is the most commonly employed technique worldwide. Advantages of this approach include high image contrast and the ability to maximize arterial opacification while minimizing venous contamination.[15,16] This approach employs a high injection rate (2-3 cc/second) to maximize the intravascular concentration of gadolinium at the beginning of the scan. A potential disadvantage of this technique is blurring caused by relative washout of gadolinium from the vessel of interest by the time peripheral k-space is acquired, particularly with long scans or short duration injections (FIGURE 55.1). Additionally, many patients continue to have subtle movement or "settling" of the diaphragm and viscera in the first few seconds after arresting inspiration, causing artifacts related to shifts in the position of structures between the acquisition of the center and periphery of k-space. If the patient fails to maintain the breath-hold at the end of the scan, the edge information in the resulting image can be significantly corrupted. Also, the chance of missing or mistiming the bolus is higher with elliptic techniques than with sequential techniques (especially if using "single dose" 0.1-mmol/kg dosing) because of the short bolus duration. Finally, the rapid injection of contrast can result in a bolus that is too tight to image vessels with different peak enhancement times (for example, simultaneous evaluation of the pulmonary arteries and thoracic aorta). The scan delay after injection for an elliptic centric acquisition is the "peak time" obtained with bolus timing plus an addition of the contrast bolus volume divided by the injection rate—a factor that corrects for the difference in volume between the test bolus and the actual injection for the diagnostic scan. In practice, many technologists simplify this by adding a standard delay of 4 or 5 seconds to the peak time calculated by the timing bolus.

In sequential readout, which we typically employ for aortic imaging, k-space is filled from top to bottom with acquisition of the center of k-space occurring in the middle of the

acquisition. With this technique, a slower injection rate (usually 1 or 1.5 cc/second) is employed than with centric techniques (FIGURE 55.2). Although this causes a lower peak concentration of gadolinium during acquisition of the center of k-space, it "stretches out" the bolus, which has several advantages. Among these is a higher concentration of gadolinium during acquisition of peripheral k-space with resultant improvement in edge definition. Because the bolus has a longer duration, it is possible to push patients to longer breath-holds (sometimes 35 or even 40 seconds in our practices) than can be employed with centric methods, allowing scans with higher resolution, greater anatomic coverage, and/or higher SNR. The longer bolus duration means in practice that the scan is less likely to be corrupted by patient factors, such as loss of breath-hold at the end of the scan or by a technologist making an error in calculation of the scan delay from injection. The timing algorithm for a sequential scan is peak time − (scan time/2) + (contrast volume/injection rate). The addition of the second factor moves the peak of the contrast bolus to the middle of the acquisition when the center of k-space is acquired. Potential disadvantages of this technique include venous contamination, but this is rarely a diagnostically limiting factor when imaging the aorta.

Noncontrast Techniques

Although largely supplanted by CE-MRA, noncontrast MRA techniques for imaging the aorta were employed before CE-MRA became widespread,[17,18] and there is renewed interest worldwide in noncontrast techniques because of the potential risk of NSF with administration of gadolinium contrast to patients with certain risk factors. In addition to "lumenographic" gradient echo "bright-blood" techniques, which offer similar information to

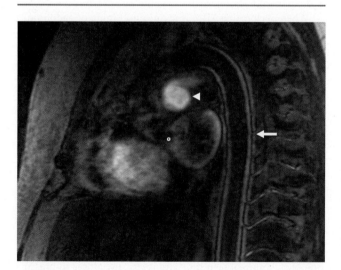

FIGURE 55.1 Short bolus duration and mistiming causing blurring and edge enhancement during centric Magnetic Resonance Angiography. In this sagittal thoracic aortic MRA, the bolus of 11 cc was injected at 3 cc/second with a resulting bolus duration of less than 4 seconds. The bolus was mis-timed. Gadolinium is seen in the right ventricle and pulmonary artery at the time the center of k-space was acquired (the beginning of the acquisition), but the edges are blurred (*arrowhead*) because the contrast had washed out of these areas by the time the peripheral k-space information was acquired (at the end of the scan). By the end of the acquisition contrast had reached the aorta with the result that there is "edge enhancement" (*arrow*) caused by high gadolinium concentration during acquisition of high spatial frequencies at the end of the scan, which was not present when the center of k-space was acquired.

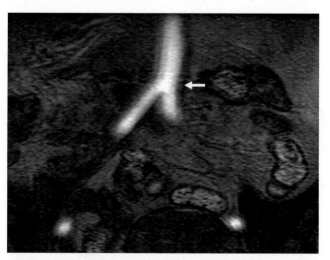

FIGURE 55.2 Blurring and loss of edge information caused by rapid contrast injection and short bolus duration with long scan time. In this case, the scan duration was 35 seconds and a bolus of 10 cc of contrast was administered at 3 cc/second. The rapidly injected bolus (3-second injection), timed to arrive at the center of k-space acquisition during a sequential readout, also washed out very quickly. Consequently, little edge information was acquired during the MRA at the beginning and end of the scan because of the lack of intravascular gadolinium, and there is resultant blurring (*arrow*).

contrast-enhanced MRA, spin echo "dark-blood" techniques offer the potential to directly image the vascular wall, which can be valuable for investigating activity of atherosclerosis disease as well as vasculitis.[19–21]

Gradient echo sequences can achieve "bright-blood" contrast, similar to CE-MRA, and technical improvements have made noncontrast options sometimes rival CE-MRA in spatial resolution and diagnostic utility. Older "time of flight" and phase contrast sequences have the potential advantage of relying on inflow for signal and providing flow-related information as a result. Newer techniques typically rely on balanced steady-state gradient echo imaging and usually employ gating techniques to correct for cardiac and respiratory motion. Diagnostic results can be equal or even superior to CE-MRA (FIGURE 55.3)[22] and may provide additional information when added to a conventional CE-MRA exam.[23] We often use these sequences, employing ECG-gating, to obtain a targeted set of motion-free images of the aortic root and sinuses of Valsalva and complement the CE-MRA of the entire chest. The motion-free images allow more precise and accurate measurement of the sinuses, sinotubular junction, and low ascending aorta, and also can allow assessment of aortic valve abnormalities (such as bicuspid valve or aortic insufficiency) that may be associated with aneurysm formation.

Spin echo sequences, with "black-blood" contrast, are typically used for imaging vessel walls. Although these sequences are rarely used in isolation, they can provide additional information and characterization of vascular pathology when combined with other MR techniques.[24] This approach may be useful to image atherosclerotic plaque or alternatively to assess for inflammation in a number of vasculitic disorders.[25] As discussed later, inclusion of sequences which image vessel wall is critically important when imaging suspected acute aortic pathology, as intramural hematoma may not be easily appreciated on CE-MRA sequences.

ROLE IN INTERVENTIONAL PLANNING

There are little data prospectively comparing current MRA, computed tomography angiography (CTA), and conventional angiographic techniques for planning interventional procedures on the aorta. Earlier studies, many of which do not employ the full capabilities of current technology, demonstrated high accuracy of MRA compared to digital subtraction arteriography (DSA) in evaluating aortoiliac disease.[26] As early as 1994, a blinded evaluation of MRA and DSA images in 47 patients revealed a sensitivity of 99.6% and specificity of 100% for occlusion or hemodynamically significant stenosis.[27] In this series, there was no difference in treatment plan if using MRA data or DSA data independently. There is similarly good evidence supporting the reliability of MRA diameter measurements compared to conventional angiography in patients with great vessel stenoses[28] and congenital heart disease[29]; both studies showed highly accurate results of MRA. With proper technique, interobserver variability is also low[30] and may actually be superior in this regard to DSA.[31] Preprocedural MRA may also decrease the morbidity of thoracic aortic surgery or intervention by mapping the artery of Adamkiewicz.[32,33]

MRA has been shown to be useful to depict preoperative aortic aneurysm morphology[34] and aortoiliac and infrainguinal anatomy for therapeutic planning in patients for whom transfemoral arteriography is not feasible,[35] such as in Leriche syndrome.[36] A preoperative evaluation of 20 patients with abdominal aortic aneurysms performed in 2003 demonstrated equivalent performance between CTA and MRA.[37] In addition to providing a highly accurate analysis without ionizing radiation, the images can be postprocessed much like CT images to provide a three-dimensional method for visualization with maximum intensity projection (MIP) or volume-rendered images (FIGURE 55.4). Although rarely important for diagnostic purposes, these postprocessing tools are important for communicating findings to nonradiologists and may be useful for surgical or interventional planning.

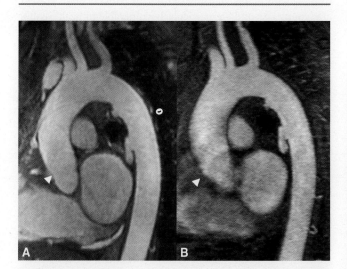

FIGURE 55.3 Noncontrast MRA (**A**) and contrast-enhanced MRA (**B**) in a patient with traumatic pseudoaneurysms of the descending thoracic aorta. Notice the preservation of vessel wall definition in the noncontrast image (*arrowheads*). Because the noncontrast MRA is ECG-gated, it acquires only information from one phase of the cardiac cycle. This area is blurred by motion during the acquisition of the contrast-enhanced MRA.

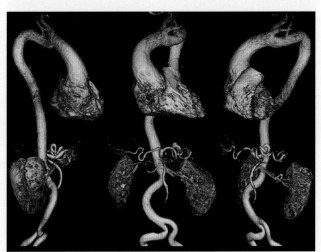

FIGURE 55.4 Multiple-angle volume-rendered contrast-enhanced MRA images in a 29-year-old man with Marfan's syndrome demonstrates extensive tortuosity of the thoracic and abdominal aorta and common iliac arteries.

MRA may also detect additional subclinical lesions requiring treatment in some patients undergoing imaging for another vascular disorder.[38] Because of the ability to perform time-resolved imaging, CE-MRA is also the test of choice if information regarding dynamic transit of contrast is important, or if bolus timing is difficult, such as in an infant.

ROLE IN SURVEILLANCE

CE-MRA has been shown to be highly accurate in detecting and characterizing anastomotic stenoses following complex aortoiliac and aortovisceral reconstruction.[39] Following AAA repair with an endograft, endoleak with continued pressurization of the sac is a significant problem that can lead to continued aneurysm growth and eventual rupture. In these cases, detection of the endoleak and characterization of the source of inflow are critical to planning treatment. Although numerous approaches, including conventional angiography, CTA, contrast-enhanced ultrasound, and color flow ultrasound have been proposed for the diagnosis and characterization of endoleaks, there are growing data to support MRA as the diagnostic method of choice (FIGURE 55.5).[40–46] Blood-pool contrast agents may be particularly useful for this application.[47] Early data support the use of MRA to evaluate for thoracic aortic endoleak as well.[48,49]

For imaging of vasculitis, MR offers some unique potential to assess disease activity through assessment of the vessel wall. Although MRA has been long established as a reliable method to assess for aneurysm, stenosis, or occlusion (FIGURE 55.6), edema-sensitive or postcontrast vessel wall imaging may serve as a useful biomarker of disease activity (FIGURE 55.7). This is accomplished through precontrast T2-weighted imaging and pre- and post-contrast T1-weighted imaging using spin echo or fast spin echo sequences, which can demonstrate both vascular wall thickening and inflammation in the setting of Takayasu arteritis.[25,50] These findings may help to guide medical therapy, although the

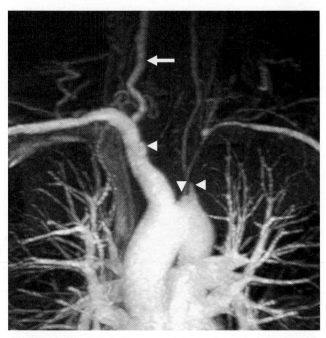

FIGURE 55.6 Coronal maximum intensity projection image of a 34-year-old woman with Takayasu arteritis. Both the left and right common carotid arteries and the left subclavian artery are occluded (*arrowheads*). Only a hypertrophied right vertebral artery (*arrow*) supplies the intracranial circulation.

findings should be interpreted with caution because they have not yet been shown to correlate with subsequent development of new lesions[51] and may not be a reliable indicator of disease activity during therapy.[52]

MRA is also particularly useful for assessing aortic coarctation. As with many congenital problems patients often present at a young age, and are particularly vulnerable to health issues from radiation exposure. These patients typically may need

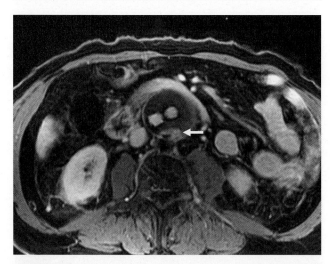

FIGURE 55.5 Post-contrast MRA image in a 78-year-old man with prior endovascular aortic aneurysm repair and a type II endoleak (*arrow*) supplied by lumbar arteries. A CTA had been performed prior to the MRA, and failed to show the leak, leading to referral for CE-MRA.

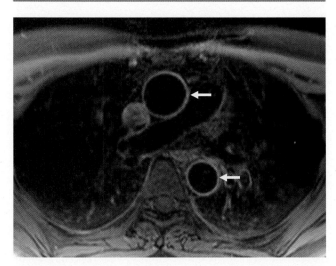

FIGURE 55.7 Delayed enhancement of the aortic wall in a patient with giant cell arteritis on post-gadolinium fat-suppressed ECG-gated T1 weighted spin echo image (*arrows*).

fluoroscopically-guided interventions, and almost certainly will require serial imaging followup over a long period of time. Because of this, MRA should be considered the test of choice for most patients. MRA can clearly depict the coarctation and may also demonstrate extensive intercostal collateral formation, indicating the hemodynamic significance of the coarctation (FIGURE 55.8). In addition to depicting the anatomy of the coarctation and of the collateral arteries, phase contrast techniques can be used to demonstrate the direction of flow in the collateral arteries with retrograde flow in the intercostal arteries indicating hemodynamic significance.[53]

Similarly, although CTA has largely replaced MRA for detection of acute aortic dissection because of faster scan time and more rapid availability in the acute setting, MRA is probably the most appropriate test for long-term followup of known, medically managed aortic dissections because of concerns regarding radiation exposure with serial CT exams. MRA is still a first-line test in some acute clinical situations, such as patients with prior allergic reaction to iodinated contrast (FIGURE 55.9). When imaging patients with suspected acute aortic syndrome, it is important to perform sequences which allow characterization of the aortic wall, usually with "black blood" ECG-gated fast spin echo sequences, as intramural hematoma may be very subtle on CE-MRA (FIGURE 55.10) and invisible on subtracted CE-MRA images.

PRACTICAL ADVANTAGES AND LIMITATIONS

Compared to CT, MRA has the disadvantages of higher cost, often slightly lower spatial resolution, and longer scan time. The availability of CT in the acute setting is usually much more rapid and the scan times are generally much shorter, making CTA the method of choice for emergent evaluation of suspected vascular trauma or dissection. CTA is also superior if evaluation of coronary arteries is required as part of the exam (such as for preoperative evaluation in a low-risk patient). Pregnancy is

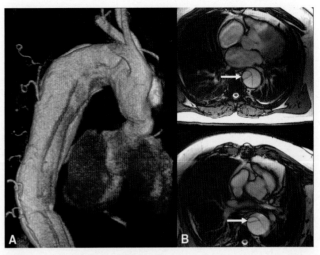

FIGURE 55.9 Volume rendered image from a contrast-enhanced MRA (**A**) in a 50-year-old man with prior Stanford A dissection repair and new sudden onset tearing chest and back pain demonstrates postop changes of previous graft repair of the ascending aorta and hemi-arch, and two distinct dissection flaps in the descending aorta. Balanced steady state free precession images obtained in systole (**A**) and diastole (**B**) demonstrate the two distinct dissection flaps. The true lumen is identified by greater systolic expansion and diastolic collapse (*arrows*).

a contraindication to an MR exam and should be avoided in most cases, and gadolinium should never be administered to a pregnant patient. Some patients have implanted devices, such as pacemakers, which are not safe in the MR environment and

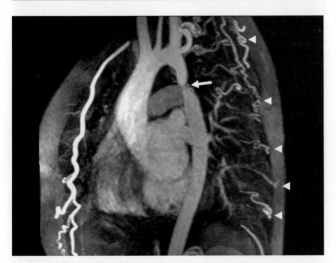

FIGURE 55.8 Sagittal oblique thin maximum intensity projection image of a 33-year-old man with a previously undiagnosed aortic coarctation (*arrow*) who presented with signs of left ventricular failure related to the long-standing coarctation. Dilated and tortuous intercostal arteries (*arrowheads*) and prominent internal mammary artery confirm the hemodynamic significance of the coarctation.

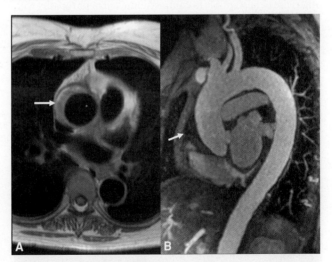

FIGURE 55.10 Aortic intramural hematoma in a 65-year-old female with borderline renal insufficiency who developed a right coronary artery dissection during coronary angiography. The patient was hemodynamically stable, and MRA was performed to assess for extension of the dissection into the aorta. Axial double inversion recovery fast spin echo image (**A**) clearly demonstrates the intramural hematoma (*arrow*) against the flow void in the aortic lumen. The intramural hematoma is visible but subtle on contrast-enhanced MR angiography (**B**, *arrow*).

should be considered an absolute contraindication to the exam. Metallic implants, such as vascular stents, can cause significant artifacts on both MR and CT exams, but with proper technique, the results with MR can be equivalent to CT or conventional angiography.[54]

Although gadolinium-based contrast agents generally have an excellent safety profile, certain agents have been linked with the potential for development of NSF when administered to patients with severe or acute renal insufficiency. Use of these agents should be avoided in patients with a creatinine clearance less than 30 mg/dL or an acute kidney injury unless the potential risks are outweighed by potential benefits, and there are no alternative strategies available providing equivalent information without greater risk to the patient. As knowledge about the risk of NSF continues to evolve, guidelines may continue to change. Helpful guidelines on administration of gadolinium to patients can be obtained from the American College of Radiology, the International Society for Magnetic Resonance in Medicine, and other organizations.

As noted earlier, when serial follow-up is required for nearly any disorder of the aorta, MRA should be considered the first choice for anatomic imaging. This is particularly true for young patients,[55] or those with connective tissue diseases (including Marfan syndrome, Loeys-Dietz syndrome, Ehlers-Danlos type IV, and others), bicuspid valve aortopathy vasculitis, or aortic dissection (FIGURE 55.11). Given the high radiation dose that can be accumulated with serial CT imaging as well as angiographic procedures, all of which are frequently repeated multiple times in young patients, MRA has the potential to significantly reduce the likelihood of radiation-induced complications including iatrogenic carcinogenesis.

Noncontrast MRA techniques are continuing to develop rapidly and often provide the lowest risk option to patients with severe renal insufficiency (but not on hemodialysis), who would otherwise be susceptible to contrast-inducted nephropathy with CTA or NSF with MRA. Such techniques often provide similar

image quality and diagnostic utility to CE-MRA and may obviate the need for gadolinium.[56–58]

THE FUTURE

Already, parallel imaging techniques have allowed dramatic advances in expanding anatomic coverage with maintained spatial resolution. Further advances in parallel imaging techniques, as well as in coil design and reconstruction algorithms, such as compressed sensing,[59] are likely to enable further increases in spatial and temporal resolution of MRA. These techniques also may enable further advances in noninvasive flow quantification such as have been recently demonstrated with the "4d flow" technique. Although to date this application has been limited by long acquisition times and respiratory motion,[60,61] the potential exists for parallel imaging and compressed sensing to reduce acquisition times to within 5 to 15 minutes, which can be clinically feasible. Such techniques may allow an entirely new way to assess vascular flow patterns and hemodynamics and new parameters, such as wall shear stress.[62,63] Early investigations into this technique in disease, such as aortic coarctation,[64] aortic endoleaks[65] and potential sources of embolic plaque in cryptogenic stroke,[66] have all had promising early results. Although post-processing and quantification of the data remains a major challenge, simply visualizing flow patterns may help to understand hemodynamics in diseases such as aortic dissection, and potentially plan interventional therapy (FIGURE 55.12).

Noncontrast MRA techniques already can rival CE-MRA in resolution and image quality, and as they continue to develop, they may become the standard of care, particularly in patients with renal insufficiency or other contraindications to the administration of gadolinium- or iodine-based contrast agents.

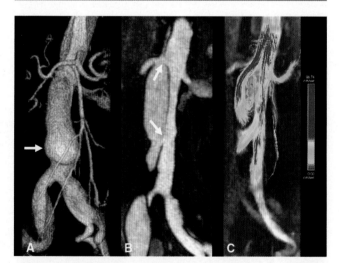

FIGURE 55.12 Comprehensive MRA examination of aortic dissection with increasing aneurysm formation in the abdominal aorta. Coronal volume rendered CE-MRA image (**A**) demonstrates a saccular aneurysm forming above the aortic bifurcation (*arrow*). Coronal oblique multiplanar reformat image demonstrates defects in the intimal-medial flap (*arrows* in **B**) which are confirmed as major entry tears for flow to cross from the true to the false lumen on 4D flow imaging with seed points for streamlines placed in the true lumen above the level of the renal arteries (**C**).

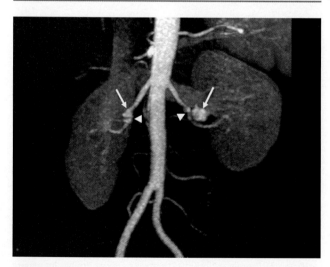

FIGURE 55.11 Coronal maximum intensity projection image in a 54-year-old woman with Type IV Ehlers Danlos syndrome undergoing MRA screening of the aorta demonstrates bilateral renal artery dissections (*arrowheads*) and aneurysms (*arrows*).

CONCLUSION

MRA remains unmatched in offering a variety of tools for the investigation of vascular disease. By offering a combination of techniques that can delineate anatomy, flow physiology, and vascular pathology in a single noninvasive and comprehensive exam, MRA will remain a powerful clinical tool for vascular assessment for the foreseeable future. As further technical developments enable faster scan times, improved spatial and temporal resolution, and better delineation of flow patterns, MR is likely to see increased utilization for all of the indications listed previously. Because MR offers increasing opportunities for vascular imaging without administration of intravascular contrast, it is the preferred modality for many patients with chronic medical conditions. Additionally, because it does not involve use of ionizing radiation, MR should be the preferred noninvasive imaging modality for patients who require serial follow-up for nearly any vascular disorder.

REFERENCES

1. Kaufman L, Crooks L, Sheldon P, et al. The potential impact of nuclear magnetic resonance imaging on cardiovascular diagnosis. *Circulation* 1982; 67:251.
2. Higgins CB, Stark D, MeNamara M, et al. Multiplane magnetic resonance imaging of the heart and major vessels: studies in normal volunteers. *Am J Radiol* 1984;142:558.
3. Prince MR, Narasimham DL, Stanley JC, et al. Breath-hold gadolinium-enhanced MR angiography of the abdominal aorta and its major branches. *Radiology* 1995;197(3):785–792.
4. Prince MR, Narasimham DL, Jacoby WT, et al. Arterial-phase three-dimensional contrast-enhanced MR angiography of the carotid arteries. *AJR Am J Roentgenol* 1996;167(1):211–215.
5. Grobner T. Gadolinium—a specific trigger for the development of nephrogenic fibrosing dermopathy and nephrogenic systemic fibrosis? *Nephrol Dial Transplant* 2006;21:1104–1108.
6. Yang L., Krefting I., Gorovets A., et al. Nephrogenic systemic fibrosis and class labeling of gadolinium–based contrast agents by the Food and Drug Administration. *Radiology* 2012; 265(1):248–53.
7. Maki JH, Chenevert TL, Prince MR. The effects of incomplete breath-holding on 3D MR image quality. *J Magn Reson Imaging* 1997;7(6):1132–1139.
8. MacFall JR, Pelc NJ, Vavrek RM. Correction of spatially dependent phase shifts for partial Fourier imaging. *Magn Reson Imaging* 1988;6:143–155.
9. Noll DC, Nishimura DG, Macovski A. Homodyne detection in magnetic resonance imaging. *IEEE Trans Med Imaging* 1991;10:154–163.
10. Golay X, Brown SJ, Itoh R, et al. Time-resolved contrast-enhanced carotid MR angiography using sensitivity encoding (SENSE). *AJNR Am J Neuroradiol* 2001;22:1615–1619.
11. Maki JH, Wilson GJ, Eubank WB, et al. Utilizing SENSE to achieve lower station sub-millimeter isotropic resolution and minimal venous enhancement in peripheral MR angiography. *J Magn Reson Imaging* 2002;15:484–491.
12. Strouse PJ, Prince MR, Chenevert TL. Effect of the rate of gadopentetate dimeglumine administration on abdominal vascular and soft-tissue MR imaging enhancement patterns. *Radiology* 1996;201(3):809–816.
13. Kreitner KF, Kunz RP, Kalden P, et al. Contrast-enhanced three-dimensional MR angiography of the thoracic aorta: experiences after 118 examinations with a standard dose contrast administration and different injection protocols. *Eur Radiol* 2001;11(8):1355–1363.
14. Prince MR, Chenevert TL, Foo TK, et al. Contrast-enhanced abdominal MR angiography: optimization of imaging delay time by automating the detection of contrast material arrival in the aorta. *Radiology* 1997;203(1):109–114.
15. Wilman AH, Riederer SJ. Improved centric phase encoding orders for three-dimensional magnetization-prepared MR angiography. *Magn Reson Med* 1996;36:384–392.
16. Wilman AH, Riederer SJ, King BF, et al. Fluoroscopically triggered contrast-enhanced three-dimensional MR angiography with elliptical centric view order: application to the renal arteries. *Radiology* 1997;205: 137–146.
17. Kaufman JA, Yucel EK, Waltman AC, et al. MR angiography in the preoperative evaluation of abdominal aortic aneurysms: a preliminary study. *J Vasc Interv Radiol* 1994;5(3):489–496.
18. Kaufman JA, Geller SC, Petersen MJ, et al. MR imaging (including MR angiography) of abdominal aortic aneurysms: comparison with conventional angiography. *AJR Am J Roentgenol* 1994;163(1):203–210.
19. Herfkens RJ, Higgins CB, Hricak H, et al. Nuclear magnetic resonance imaging of atherosclerotic disease. *Radiology* 1983;148(1):161–166.
20. Gold GE, Pauly JM, Glover GH, et al. Characterization of atherosclerosis with a 1.5-T imaging system. *J Magn Reson Imaging* 1993;3(2):399–407.
21. Narvaez J, Narvaez JA, Nolla JM, et al. Giant cell arteritis and polymyalgia rheumatica: usefulness of vascular magnetic resonance imaging studies in the diagnosis of aortitis. *Rheumatology (Oxford)* 2005;44:479–483.
22. Potthast S, Mitsumori L, Stanescu LA, et al. Measuring aortic diameter with different MR techniques: comparison of three-dimensional (3D) navigated steady-state free-precession (SSFP), 3D contrast-enhanced magnetic resonance angiography (CE-MRA), 2D T2 black blood, and 2D cine SSFP. *J Magn Reson Imaging* 2010;31(1):177–184.
23. Iozzelli A, D'Orta G, Aliprandi A, et al. The value of true-FISP sequence added to conventional gadolinium-enhanced MRA of abdominal aorta and its major branches. *Eur J Radiol* 2009;72(3):489–493.
24. Gebker R, Gomaa O, Schnackenburg B, et al. Comparison of different MRI techniques for the assessment of thoracic aortic pathology: 3D contrast-enhanced MR angiography, turbo spin echo and balanced steady state free precession. *Int J Cardiovasc Imaging* 2007;23(6):747–756.
25. Jiang L, Li D, Yan F, et al. Evaluation of Takayasu arteritis activity by delayed contrast-enhanced magnetic resonance imaging. *Int J Cardiol* 2012;155(2):262–267.
26. Venkataraman S, Semelka RC, Weeks S, et al. Assessment of aorto-iliac disease with magnetic resonance angiography using arterial phase 3-D gradient-echo and interstitial phase 2-D fat-suppressed spoiled gradient-echo sequences. *J Magn Reson Imaging* 2003;17(1):43–53.
27. Carpenter JP, Owen RS, Holland GA, et al. Magnetic resonance angiography of the aorta, iliac, and femoral arteries. *Surgery* 1994;116(1):17–23.
28. Loewe C, Schillinger M, Haumer M, et al. MRA versus DSA in the assessment of occlusive disease in the aortic arch vessels: accuracy in detecting the severity, number, and length of stenoses. *J Endovasc Ther* 2004; 11(2):152–160.
29. Valsangioacomo Buechel ER, DiBernardo S, Bauersfeld U, et al. Contrast-enhanced magnetic resonance angiography of the great arteries in patients with congenital heart disease: an accurate tool for planning catheter-guided interventions. *Int J Cardiovasc Imaging* 2005;21(2–3):313–322.
30. Billaud Y, Beuf O, Desjeux G, et al. 3D contrast-enhanced MR angiography of the abdominal aorta and its distal branches: interobserver agreement of radiologists in a routine examination. *Acad Radiol* 2005;12: (2):155–163.
31. Schoenberg SO, Essig M, Hallscheidt P, et al. Multiphase magnetic resonance angiography of the abdominal and pelvic arteries: results of a bicenter multireader analysis. *Invest Radiol* 2002;37(1):20–28.
32. Kawaharada N, Morishita K, Fukada J, et al. Thoracoabdominal or descending aortic aneurysm repair after preoperative demonstration of the Adamkiewicz artery by magnetic resonance angiography. *Eur J Cardiothorac Surg* 2002;21(6):970–974.
33. Yamada N, Okita Y, Minatoya K, et al. Preoperative demonstration of the Adamkiewicz artery by magnetic resonance angiography in patients with descending or thoracoabdominal aortic aneurysms. *Eur J Cardiothorac Surg* 2000;18(1):104–111.
34. Nasim A, Thompson MM, Sayers RD, et al. Role of magnetic resonance angiography for assessment of abdominal aortic aneurysm before endoluminal repair. *Br J Surg* 1998;85(5):641–644.
35. Fenchel S, Wisianowsky C, Schams S, et al. Contrast-enhanced 3D MRA of the aortoiliac and infrainguinal arteries when conventional transfemoral arteriography is not feasible. *J Endovasc Ther* 2002;9(4):511–519.
36. Ruehm SG, Weishaupt D, Debatin JF. Contrast-enhanced MR angiography in patients with aortic occlusion (Leriche syndrome). *J Magn Reson Imaging* 2000;11(4):401–410.
37. Lutz AM, Willman JK, Pfammatter T, et al. Evaluation of aortoiliac aneurysm before endovascular repair: comparison of contrast-enhanced magnetic resonance angiography with multidetector row computed tomographic angiography with an automated analysis software tool. *J Vasc Surg* 2003;37(3):619–627.
38. Napoli A, Anzidei M, Marincola BC, et al. Optimisation of a high-resolution whole-body MR angiography protocol with parallel imaging and biphasic administration of a single bolus of Gd-BOPTA: preliminary experience in

the systemic evaluation of atherosclerotic burden in patients referred for endovascular procedures. *Radiol Med* 2009;114(4):538–552.

39. Fidelman N, Wilson MW, Boddington S, et al. Postoperative evaluation of complex aortovisceral and aortorenal reconstructions by magnetic resonance angiography. *Acad Radiol* 2004;11(9):1055–1058.
40. Alerci M, Oberson M, Fogliata A, et al. Prospective, intraindividual comparison of MRI versus MDCT for endoleak detection after endovascular repair of abdominal aortic aneurysms. *Eur Radiol* 2009;19(5):1223–1231.
41. Cohen EI, Weinreb DB, Siegelbaum RH, et al. Time-resolved MR angiography for the classification of endoleaks after endovascular aneurysm repair. *J Magn Reson Imaging* 2008;27:500–503.
42. Lookstein RA, Goldman J, Pukin L, et al. Time-resolved magnetic resonance angiography as a noninvasive method to characterize endoleaks: initial results compared with conventional angiography. *J Vasc Surg* 2004;39(1):27–33.
43. van der Laan MJ, Bartels LW, Viergever MA, et al. Computed tomography versus magnetic resonance imaging of endoleaks after EVAR. *Eur J Vasc Endovasc Surg* 2006;32:361–365.
44. Pitton MB, Schweitzer H, Herber S, et al. MRI versus helical CT for endoleak detection after endovascular aneurysm repair. *Am J Roentgenol* 2005;185:1275–1281.
45. Wicky S, Fan CM, Geller SC, et al. MR angiography of endoleak with inconclusive concomitant CT angiography. *Am J Roentgenol* 2003;181:736–738.
46. Haulon S, Lions C, McFadden EP, et al. Prospective evaluation of magnetic resonance imaging after endovascular treatment of infrarenal aortic aneurysms. *Eur J Vasc Endovasc Surg* 2001;22:62–69.
47. Wieners G, Meyer F, Halloul Z, et al. Detection of type II endoleak after endovascular aortic repair: comparison between magnetic resonance angiography and blood-pool contrast agent and dual-phased computed tomographic angiography. *Cardiovasc Intervent Radiol* 2010;33(6):1135–1142.
48. Farhat F, Attia C, Boussel L, et al. Endovascular repair of the descending thoracic aorta: mid-term results and evaluation of magnetic resonance angiography. *J Cardiovasc Surg (Torino)* 2007;48(1):1–6.
49. Attia C, Villard J, Boussel L, et al. Endovascular repair of localized pathological lesions of the descending thoracic aorta: midterm results. *Cardiovasc Intervent Radiol* 2007;30(4):628–637.
50. Desai MY, Stone JH, Hellmann DB, et al. Delayed contrast-enhanced MRI of the aortic wall in Takayasu's arteritis: initial experience. *AJR Am J Roentgenol* 2005;184(5):1427–1431.
51. Tso E, Flamm SD, White RD, et al. Utility and limitations of magnetic resonance imaging in diagnosis and treatment. *Arthritis Rheum* 2002;46(6):1634–1642.
52. Both M, Ahmadi-Simab K, Reuter M, et al. MRI and FDG-PET in the assessment of inflammatory aortic arch syndrome in complicated courses of giant cell arteritis. *Ann Rheum Dis* 2008;67:1030–1033.

53. Julsrud PR, Breen JF, Warnes CA, et al. Coarctation of the aorta: collateral flow assessment with phase-contrast MR angiography. *AJR Am J Roentgenol* 1007;169(6):1735–1742.
54. Nordmeyer J, Gaudin R, Tann OR, et al. MRI may be sufficient for non-invasive assessment of great vessel stents: an in vitro comparison of MRI, CT, and conventional angiography. *AJR Am J Roentgenol* 2010;195(4):865–871.
55. Ley-Zaporozhan J, Kreitner KF, Unterhinninghofen R, et al. Assessment of thoracic aortic dimensions in an experimental setting: comparison of different unenhanced magnetic resonance angiography techniques with electrocardiogram-gated computed tomography angiography for possible application in the pediatric population. *Invest Radiol* 2008;43(3):179–186.
56. Srichai MB, Kim S, Axel L, et al. Non-gadolinium–enhanced 3-dimensional magnetic resonance angiography for the evaluation of thoracic aortic disease: a preliminary experience. *Tex Heart Inst J* 2010;37(1):58–65.
57. Francois CJ, Tuite D, Deshpande V, et al. Unenhanced MR angiography of the thoracic aorta: initial clinical evaluation. *AJR Am J Roentgenol* 2008;190(4):902–906.
58. Amano Y, Takahama K, Kumita S. Noncontrast-enhanced MR angiography of the thoracic aorta using cardiac and navigator-gated magnetization-prepared three-dimensional steady-state free precession. *J Magn Reson Imaging* 2008;27(3):504–509.
59. Mistretta CA. Undersampled radial MR acquisition and highly constrained back projection (HYPR) reconstruction: potential medical imaging applications in the post-Nyquist era. *J Magn Reson Imaging* 2009;29(3):501–516.
60. Vock P, Terrier F, Wegmüller H, et al. Magnetic resonance angiography of abdominal vessels: early experience using the three-dimensional phase-contrast technique. *Br J Radiol* 1991;64(757):10–16.
61. Werner R, Ehrhardt J, Frenzel T, et al. Motion artifact reducing reconstruction of 4D CT image data for the analysis of respiratory dynamics. *Methods Inf Med* 2007;46(3):254–260.
62. Harloff A, Nussbaumer A, Bauer S, et al. In vivo assessment of wall shear stress in the atherosclerotic aorta using flow-sensitive 4D MRI. *Magn Reson Med* 2010;62(6):1529–1536.
63. Frydrychowicz A, Stalder AF, Russe MF, et al. Three-dimensional analysis of segmental wall shear stress in the aorta by flow-sensitive four-dimensional-MRI. *J Magn Reson Imaging* 2009;30(1):77–84.
64. Hope MD, Meadows AK, Hope TA, et al. Clinical evaluation of aortic coarctation with 4D flow MR imaging. *J Magn Reson Imaging* 2010;31(3):711–718.
65. Hope TA, Zarins CK, Herfkens RJ. Initial experience characterizing a type I endoleak from velocity profiles using time-resolved three-dimensional phase-contrast MRI. *J Vasc Surg* 2009;49(6):1580–1584.
66. Harloff A, Strecker C, Frydrychowicz AP, et al. Plaques in the descending aorta: a new risk factor for stroke? Visualization of potential embolization pathways by 4D MRI. *J Magn Reson Imaging* 2007;26(6):1651–1655.

CHAPTER

56

Thoracic Aortic Aneurysms

JOSHUA D. ADAMS and ALAN H. MATSUMOTO

INTRODUCTION

Since first reported over 50 years ago, surgical repair of the descending thoracic aorta with resection and graft interposition has become the standard treatment strategy for patients with aneurysmal disease.[1] Despite significant clinical advances, which have allowed operative mortality to decrease to as low as 3% in specialized centers,[2] open surgical repair is generally associated with substantial morbidity and mortality in this patient population that often has multiple medical comorbidities.

Endovascular exclusion of thoracic aortic aneurysms (TAAs) with covered stent-grafts represents a less invasive therapy as compared to open surgical repair. The goal of this chapter is to provide information on the three thoracic endografts that have been approved by the Food and Drug Administration (FDA) and are commercially available; to detail the preoperative evaluation of patients with TAAs including imaging, device selection, and sizing; to elaborate on certain anatomic considerations that guide therapy; and, finally, to review the outcomes and the potential complications specific to thoracic endovascular aneurysm repair (TEVAR).

HISTORY

In the early 1990s, treatment of TAAs entered the era of TEVAR. The principle of complete aneurysm sac exclusion and depressurization using covered stent-grafts for abdominal aortic aneurysms was first reported by Parodi et al.[3] and was subsequently applied to descending TAAs in a high-risk population by Dake et al.[4] in 1994. These first-generation thoracic endograft devices were handmade and consisted of self-expanding stainless steel Z-stents (Cook, Inc., Bloomington, IN) covered with woven polyester graft material, which was hand sewn to the stent body with 5-0 polypropylene sutures.[5] With the development of multiple commercially manufactured endografts and ancillary tools (guide wires, sheaths, molding balloons), the deliverability, flexibility, profile, stability, conformability, and durability of these devices have significantly improved, and complication rates associated with their use have decreased.

In the new millennium, TEVAR results have steadily improved as device and delivery system designs have evolved, strict inclusion and exclusion criteria were employed to guide patient selection, and operator experience increased.[6-9] Currently, three endograft devices are FDA approved and commercially available in the United States for the treatment of descending TAAs. Many groups have reported superior short-term and midterm major perioperative adverse events, 30-day mortality rates, blood loss, and hospital and ICU stay rates when compared with conventional open surgical repair of TAAs.[10-14]

AVAILABLE DEVICES

In March 2005, the first FDA-approved device became available commercially to treat descending TAAs (TAG endoprosthesis, W. L. Gore, Flagstaff, AZ). Subsequently, in 2008, the Zenith TX2 TAA endovascular graft device (Cook, Inc., Bloomington, IN) and the Talent Thoracic Stent Graft System (Medtronic Vascular, Santa Rosa, CA) received FDA approval for both descending thoracic aneurysms and penetrating aortic ulcers. See Table 56.1 for a summary of the individual characteristics of the FDA-approved devices.

TAG Device

The TAG endoprosthesis is a tube composed of expanded polytetrafluoroethylene (ePTFE) externally reinforced with an additional layer of ePTFE and fluorinated ethylene propylene (FEP) and supported by a flexible nitinol exoskeleton (FIGURE 56.1A). The TAG device is available in diameters of 26 to 45 mm and in lengths of 10, 15, and 20 cm. The exoskeleton is commercially bonded to the graft material without sutures and is constrained by an ePTFE-FEP sleeve. ePTFE-covered scalloped flares are present on both ends of the device to aid in its fixation. A circumferential ePTFE sealing cuff is located on the external surface of the endoprosthesis at the base of each flared end to enhance sealing of the endoprosthesis to the wall of the aorta. The device profile depends on the size of the graft and requires a 20 to 24 French sheath for delivery. Deployment is extremely rapid and occurs with the release of the constraining sleeve in a rip-cord fashion. The expansion of the TAG device initiates from the middle of the endograft and simultaneously extends toward both ends to avoid the "windsock effect" from the high arterial flow that would occur in a standard proximal-to-distal deployment mechanism (FIGURE 56.1B). The device is then molded with a specially designed trilobed balloon that allows flow to continue during balloon inflation (FIGURE 56.1C).

Multiple clinical trials were conducted, leading to FDA approval of the TAG endograft. The pivotal trial, which enrolled patients from September 1999 through May 2001, was a nonrandomized multicenter study comparing open surgical repair (n = 94) to endovascular repair (n = 140) in patients with descending TAAs. The primary endpoint of the study was a comparison of the incidence of major adverse events (MAEs) between the two groups at 1 year of follow-up. The study was temporarily interrupted secondary to a high rate of fracture of the longitudinal spine of the TAG device. Following a device modification that included removing the longitudinal spine and adding a low permeability film layer to provide longitudinal stiffness, a nonrandomized multicenter confirmatory study was

665

Table 56.1

Individual Characteristics of the FDA-Approved Thoracic Aortic Devices

	TAG	cTAG	Zenith TX2	Talent thoracic
FDA-approved indication	Descending thoracic aneurysm	Descending thoracic aneurysm	Descending thoracic aneurysm and PAU	Descending thoracic aneurysm and PAU
Stent design and material	Continuous nitinol frame	Continuous nitinol frame (heavier wire)	Individual stainless steel "Z-stents"	Individual nitinol "M-stents"
Graft material	ePTFE	ePTFE	Polyester	Polyester
Active fixation	No	Proximal bare metal	Proximal barbs and distal bare metal	Proximal and distal bare metal
Available diameters	26–45 mm	21–45 mm	28–42 mm (tapered)	22–46 mm (tapered)

PAU, penetrating aortic ulcer.

conducted from January 2004 through June 2004, and compared 51 patients treated with the modified TAG device to the original pivotal study control group. From July 2004 through April 2005, while the device was awaiting FDA approval, an additional 80 patients as part of an ongoing treatment Investigational Device Exemption (IDE) underwent TEVAR utilizing the modified device and using enrollment criteria that were identical to the pivotal and confirmatory studies. For these 80 patients, however, follow-up was performed per the investigators' standard of care.

Results from the three studies, including follow-up through 5 years for the pivotal study, 3 years for the confirmatory study, and 2 years for the ongoing treatment IDE, showed that at 5 years, patients undergoing TEVAR had significantly improved aneurysm-related survival (97% freedom from aneurysm-related death among TEVAR patients versus 88% for open surgical controls; $p = .008$) and a lower incidence of MAEs (42% freedom from MAE among TEVAR patients versus 21% for open surgical controls; $p = .001$).[15] At 1 month, the difference in freedom from MAE was even more impressive (71% freedom from MAE among TEVAR patients versus 21% for open surgical controls; $p < .001$). Pooled data from the three studies demonstrate a rupture incidence of 1.1% ($n = 3$), an incidence of open conversion of 1.1% ($n = 3$), and the need for an additional device implantation of 1.8% ($n = 5$). Comparison of the pivotal study data to the confirmatory data also validates the previously described device modification because there have been no device fractures since the longitudinal spine was removed. Interestingly, since the additional low permeability film layer was added, the percentage of patients demonstrating greater than or equal to 5 mm decrease in aneurysm diameter is increased, 64% in the

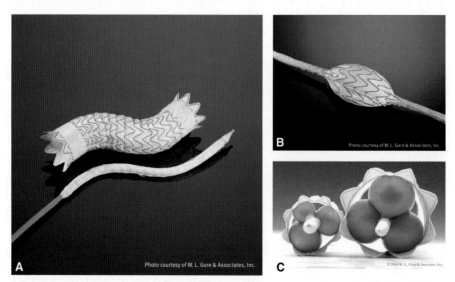

FIGURE 56.1 The TAG endoprosthesis. **A.** The mounted and fully expanded endoprosthesis. **B.** Endograft deployment from the middle of the device to prevent windsocking. **C.** The newly designed trilobed balloon that permits aortic flow during inflation.

Courtesy of WL Gore & Associates, Inc.

confirmatory patients versus 52.7% in the pivotal study patients ($p = .11$), whereas the incidence of aneurysm sac diameter increase ($\geq$5 mm) in the confirmatory and pivotal study patients at 3 years was 6.5% and 16.4% ($p = .0548$), respectively.

Zenith TX2

The Zenith TX2 is designed as a two-piece modular system with a designated proximal and distal device, although one device or the combination of multiple proximal devices may be used depending on the length and characteristics of the treated aorta (FIGURE 56.2). Both components are constructed from stainless steel modified Gianturco Z-stents, which are sutured to full-thickness woven polyester fabric. The small gaps between the individual Z-stents allow the device to conform to the aorta. The fabric is on the outside of the stents at the proximal and distal ends of the device to maximize fabric-to-aortic apposition and on the inside of the stents in the midportion to allow fabric-to-fabric overlap zones. A mechanism of active fixation to the aorta is present in both components with multiple 5-mm staggered external barbs oriented in opposing directions at the most proximal and distal ends of the devices. The device is designed to prevent migration in either direction (FIGURE 56.2A, B). The proximal components are available in straight or tapered configurations and in diameters ranging from 28 to 42 mm and lengths from 120 to 216 mm. The distal component is available in a nontapered configuration only and the diameters range between 28 and 42 mm with lengths from 127 to 207 mm.

The Zenith TX2 is delivered through either the 20 or 22 French H&L-B One-Shot Introduction System (Cook, Inc.), depending on device diameter (FIGURE 56.2C). All 28- to 34-mm diameter components are deployed using a 20 French delivery sheath system, and all 36- to 42-mm diameter components are deployed using a 22 French system. The delivery system features the Flexor braided sheath with hydrophilic coating. The sheath is designed to resist kinking and improve trackability through the iliac arteries to the thoracic aorta. The trigger wire release mechanisms of the delivery system work in tandem to deliver sequential, controlled release of the graft during deployment. Once the sheath is withdrawn, the proximal end of all main body components remain attached to the delivery system via the three trigger wires, which keep the proximal end of the graft in a "trifold" configuration, thus preventing the "windsock effect" by allowing for blood flow around the graft (FIGURE 56.2D). The most recent iteration, the Zenith TX2 TAA Endovascular Graft with Pro-Form and the Z-Trak Plus introduction system (Cook, Inc.) has further improved on proximal stent-graft conformability with trigger wires that hold the entire proximal stent in a position parallel to the inner curvature of the aortic arch until its final deployment. This advancement allows the proximal stent to telescope/invaginate inside the second stent segment, especially along the inner/inferior curvature of the aortic arch, to provide for improved wall apposition in a relatively tight radius of aortic arch curvature (FIGURE 56.3). The stainless steel in this endograft does not obviate the patient's ability to undergo a magnetic resonance imaging (MRI) exam, but it will create

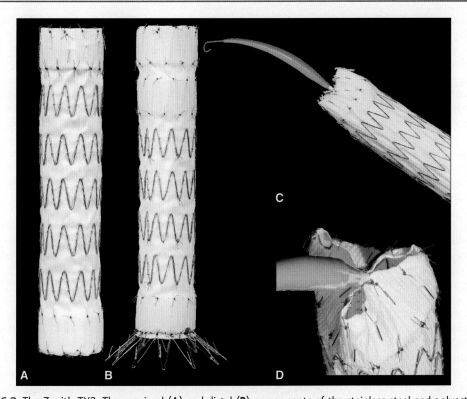

FIGURE 56.2 The Zenith TX2. The proximal (**A**) and distal (**B**) components of the stainless steel and polyester device. **C.** The partially deployed endograft on the H&L-B One-Shot Introduction System. **D.** The trifold configuration prior to release of the proximal trigger wire, therefore allowing flow around the graft and preventing distal migration due to windsock effect.

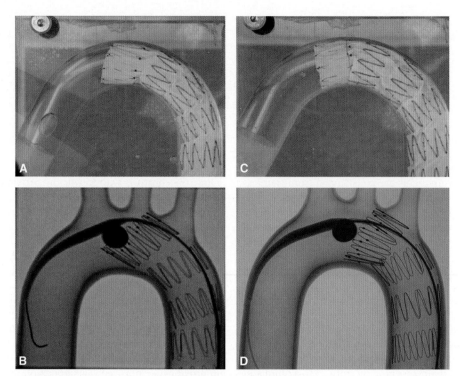

FIGURE 56.3 Comparison of the TX2 without and with the Pro-Form and the Z-Trak Plus introduction system. Photographs and corresponding radiographs comparing deployed TX2 endografts without (**A, B**) and with (**C, D**) the Pro-Form introduction system, which allows the proximal stent to telescope/invaginate inside the second stent segment to improve wall apposition in a relatively tight radius of aortic arch curvature.

local MR susceptibility artifacts. Therefore, MR angiography techniques for imaging the descending thoracic aorta in the presence of this device are limited.

Most of U.S. experience with the Zenith TX2 device has been provided by two clinical trials.[16,17] Greenberg and colleagues first reported their intermediate-term results of TEVAR in their first 100 consecutive patients using the TX1 and TX2 thoracic endografts as part of a site-sponsored investigational device exemption ($n = 97$) or on a compassionate-use basis ($n = 3$). The inclusion of patients considered to be at high risk for conventional surgery was similar to other pivotal TEVAR studies, except that only a 10-mm proximal and distal landing zone neck (seal zone) was required (as compared to 15 mm in the other trials). The indication for treatment was a TAA in 96 patients, including 15 patients with an underlying chronic dissection component. Adjunctive debranching procedures were required to create adequate landing zones in 29% of the patients, including 14 elephant trunk/arch reconstructions, 18 carotid-to-subclavian bypasses, and 4 visceral arterial bypasses. At 1 year, the overall and aneurysm-related mortalities were 17% and 14%, respectively. Secondary interventions were required in 15 patients, 6 of which consisted of successful endovascular treatments of various endoleaks.

The pivotal STARZ-TX2 clinical trial was a nonrandomized, controlled, multicenter, international study designed to evaluate the safety and efficacy of the Zenith TX2 by comparing 30-day survival and 30-day rupture-free survival to contemporary and prospective open surgical controls. Important secondary endpoints included morbidity, clinical utility measures, and freedom from device-related events. In this clinical trial, 160 patients with descending TAAs or penetrating ulcers underwent TEVAR with the Cook device and were compared to 70 open surgical control patients. Follow-up remains ongoing. The 30-day survival rate for TEVAR patients was noninferior to that of open surgical patients, 98.1% versus 94.3%, respectively. At 1 year, freedom from aneurysm-related mortality was 94% in the TEVAR group versus 88% in the open surgical group. TEVAR patients also had significantly lower markers of morbidity than open surgical patients, including severe composite morbidity index, cumulative major morbidity scores, and fewer cardiovascular, pulmonary, and vascular events. All measures of clinical utility were superior in the TEVAR group ($p < .01$), including the duration of intubation and ICU stay, days to ambulation, days to oral intake, and days to hospital discharge. Freedom from any device event, defined as technical failure, secondary intervention, conversion, type I or type III endoleak, or migration, was 90.1% at 1 year and there was no difference in the need for reintervention between the two groups.

Talent Thoracic

The Talent Thoracic Stent Graft System is composed of a polyester woven graft fabric sewn to a series of individual self-expanding, M-shaped nitinol springs (FIGURE 56.4). Between the individual stents is an area of unsupported graft to allow for device conformability. The device has a longitudinal support bar throughout the length of the endograft, which provides columnar strength while maintaining device flexibility as long as the longitudinal bar is oriented along the greater curve of the aorta. This device is also designed in a two-component, modular fashion with slightly different proximal and distal components

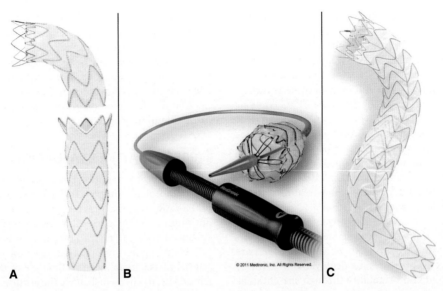

FIGURE 56.4 The Talent and Valiant Thoracic Stent Graft Systems. The proximal and distal components of the Talent (**A**) and the Valiant (**C**) both deployed on the Xcelerant with Captivia Delivery System (**B**) with a tip capture mechanism, which allows for more controlled deployment and precise placement of the Talent Thoracic Stent Graft and has virtually eliminated the problem of device inversion during its initial deployment.

Courtesy of Medtronic, Inc.

(FIGURE 56.4A). The proximal component possesses an uncovered (open web design) nitinol spring and a minisupport spring proximally to allow for implantation across the origin of the left common carotid artery or the left subclavian artery (LSCA) while maintaining patency of the covered branch. These components are available in diameters ranging from 22 to 46 mm and lengths from 112 to 116 mm. The distal component has a "closed web" design in which the most proximal spring is covered with fabric, creating a "tulip" appearance, which helps to ensure fixation within the region of overlap with the proximal endograft component. The distal components are available in straight and tapered configurations with diameters ranging from 26 to 46 mm and lengths from 110 to 114 mm. All devices are deployed through the self-contained Xcelerant delivery system (FIGURE 56.4B), which allows for controlled, ratcheted, and precise deployment of the most proximal portion of the endograft initially with a fast "zip" deployment to prevent "windsock effect" or proximal graft collapse while deploying the remainder of the more distal portion of the endograft. With the initial partial deployment of the endograft device, the stent-graft is usually positioned a few centimeters proximal to its final intended proximal landing zone and then repositioned caudally into its desired position. This deployment technique reduces the occurrence of the unintentional bare spring inversion (folding under itself along the lesser curve), which has been reported with this device deployment system. A recently FDA-approved modification to the delivery system, the Captivia delivery system (Medtronic, Inc.), which features a tip capture mechanism that allows for more controlled deployment and precise placement of the Talent Thoracic Stent Graft, has virtually eliminated the problem of device inversion during its initial deployment (FIGURE 56.4B). In addition to the new tip capture feature, longer proximal main endograft components were made available up

to 200 mm in length (FIGURE 56.4C). The delivery system for the Talent with or without Captivia is between 22 and 25 French, depending on endograft diameters used.

Despite extensive experience with the Talent Thoracic Stent Graft internationally,[18,19] the device did not receive FDA approval until 2008, following submission of the pivotal results of the VALOR trial.[20] The study, which enrolled patients from December 2003 to June 2005, was a prospective, nonrandomized, multicenter trial conducted at 38 sites. This study compared TEVAR in low surgical risk patients to retrospective open surgical data from three centers of excellence: 195 patients underwent TEVAR and were compared to 189 open surgical patients. Vessel access and successful deployment of the device was accomplished in all but one patient (99.5%), who did not receive a device secondary to access failure. Iliac conduits were required in 21.1% of the patients, and preemptive left subclavian revascularization was performed in 5.2% of the patients. The TEVAR group demonstrated significantly better outcomes than the open surgery group, including a 30-day mortality rate of 2% versus 8% ($p < .010$), 30-day MAE of 41% versus 84.4% ($p < .001$), and aneurysm-related mortality at 1 year of 3.1% versus 11.6% ($p < .002$). All measures of clinical utility were significantly better in the TEVAR group. Furthermore, at 1 year, the rate of conversion to open surgery was 0.5%, device migration was 3.9%, endoleak rate was 12.2%, and a stable or decreasing aneurysm sac diameter was noted in 91.5% of patients.

FUTURE DEVICE DEVELOPMENT AND EXTENDED INDICATIONS

More than 15 years after the first relatively primitive handmade endograft was used to repair the thoracic aorta, devices have undergone extensive and rapid evolution. In addition to the three previously discussed FDA-approved devices, several other devices have entered clinical trials and may be FDA approved by the time this text comes to print. Significant modifications have been made to the current TAG device, and this new conformable cTAG endoprosthesis (W. L. Gore) has just received FDA approval to treat TAAs and will soon become commercially available. In comparison to the TAG, the cTAG contains an increased diameter of the nitinol wire with an additional stent apex (9 versus 8) to maximize radial force and prevent endograft collapse. The proximal and distal crowns of the TAG have been removed and replaced with a short, uncovered nitinol stent proximally. The addition of smaller and larger device diameters (21 to 45 mm) and tapered devices will allow treatment to extend to a larger number of patients (FIGURE 56.5).

Recently, Medtronic has received approval for its next generation device, Valiant Captivia Thoracic Stent Graft. In comparison to the Talent, the Valiant features an eight-peak bare metal crown that effectively secures the deployed device inside the aorta and increased conformability through the elimination of the longitudinal connecting bar present on the Talent (FIGURE 56.4C).

As of April 2010, the Relay Plus and Relay NBS (Non Bare Stent) Thoracic Stent Graft (Bolton Medical, Sunrise, FL) had been used extensively in Europe with more than 3,000 devices implanted worldwide. A pivotal clinical trial is currently underway in the United States. This device consists of a polished nitinol exoskeleton of individual stent segments and a unique spiral support strut covered with surgical grade woven polyester and is available in lengths from 100 to 250 mm, diameters from 22 to 46 mm, and both straight and tapered configurations (FIGURE 56.6).

Some anatomic characteristics continue to limit the suitability of patients for TEVAR with currently available devices.

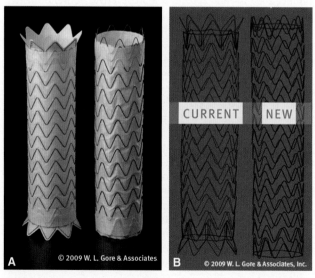

FIGURE 56.5 Comparison of the TAG and the cTAG endoprostheses. Photograph (**A**) and corresponding radiograph (**B**) highlighting the differences between the original device and the newest generation device including the removal of the crowns and the increased gauge nitinol exoskeleton.

Courtesy of WL Gore & Associates, Inc.

Future device designs will continue to increase the range of available device sizes, decrease the profile of the delivery systems, improve device trackability and conformability, allow for more controlled and precise deployment, and eventually include fenestrated and branched endografts. All of these enhancements will continue to expand the applicability of TEVAR to more patients and reduce the rate of complications associated with implantation of the devices.

▌ PREOPERATIVE EVALUATION

There are few interventional procedures where the proverb "if you fail to plan, you plan to fail" rings truer than in the case of TEVAR, and the planning for such a repair begins with optimum imaging assessment. Most centers utilize contrast-enhanced, thin-cut, helical computed tomography angiography (CTA) or magnetic resonance angiography (MRA) timed to the arterial phase, imaging from the base of the neck through the femoral heads (from just above the aortic arch to the level of the common femoral arteries). Additionally, in patients who may require coverage of the LSCA, a CTA or MRA of the head and neck is obtained to establish the presence of a patent circle of Willis, a nondominant left vertebral artery, or other anatomic variants (a vertebral artery ending in the posterior inferior cerebellar artery) that may result in a compromised vascular bed with coverage of the LSCA by the endograft. Imaging software that allows for the creation of multiplanar and three-dimensional reconstructions as well as centerline measurements are critical to establishing the presence of suitable anatomy for endovascular repair and for proper device selection and sizing. This evaluation and planning process includes not only evaluation of the thoracic aorta, but also the size and characteristics of the femoral and iliac arteries, which serve as the access vessels. From a planning standpoint, this preprocedural imaging evaluation also helps determine the optimum projection of the C-arm to show the aortic arch and profile the origins of the great vessels during the fluoroscopically guided placement of the endograft. Cross-sectional imaging also provides useful clinical information, such as degree of atheromatous burden within the aorta, which may allow estimation of a patient's risk for embolic complications and the adequacy of creating a "seal" at the proximal and distal landing zones, the tortuosity of the aorta that may predict the need to use adjunctive techniques for device delivery or alter the exact site of device deployment, and the presence of large intercostal branches that may need to be preserved to reduce the risk for spinal ischemia.

General Sizing and Anatomic Requirements

Although the vascular anatomy required for use of each commercial device may vary depending on the instructions for use (IFU) as detailed in the device-specific descriptions, the general principles for planning and anatomic considerations are the same. Proximal and distal landing zones of relatively normal aortic segments of appropriate length and "quality" must be present to allow for adequate exclusion of the aneurysm by the endograft. Equally important are the characteristics (tortuosity, calcification, and diameter) of the access vessels to allow for safe delivery and deployment of the endograft device into the thoracic aorta. Depending on the device manufacturer and the size and stiffness of the specific device, the variations in access vessel

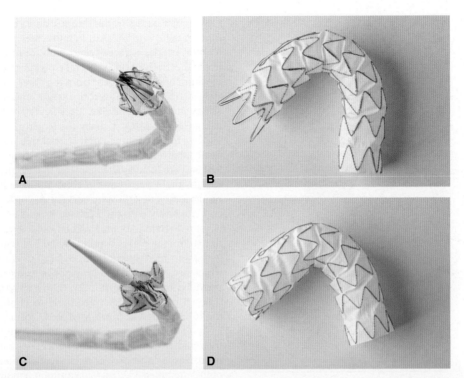

FIGURE 56.6 The Relay Plus and Relay NBS (Non Bare Stent) Thoracic Stent Graft. Photographs of the constrained (**A**) and fully deployed (**B**) Relay Plus demonstrating proximal bare metal stent in contrast to the Relay NBS in constrained (**C**) and fully deployed (**D**) configurations.

tolerance must be considered in the preprocedural planning. Oversizing the diameter of the endograft device relative to the aortic segment landing zones by 10% to 15% aids in both device fixation and the creation of a good seal to exclude flow around the endograft device. Table 56.2 details the specific anatomic requirements and sizing recommendations of the three FDA-approved thoracic endograft devices.

Specific Technical Considerations

TEVAR may still be a viable treatment option in patients who do not meet some of the anatomic requirements as defined in the IFU descriptions. Careful planning in the off-label applications of these endograft devices requires meticulous planning, contingency planning, and open discussions with the patients and referring physicians. For example, the supraaortic vessels may be covered to gain additional proximal landing zone length. Landing zones of the proximal aortic endograft, as defined by Criado et al.,[21] are depicted in FIGURE 56.7. If deployment of the stent-graft will extend into zone 0 or 1, a debranching procedure (i.e., carotid-to-subclavian bypass, ascending aorta-to-bilateral common carotid artery bypasses) must be performed prior to endograft placement. The need for revascularization prior to planned coverage of the LSCA (zone 2), however, has been debated. Some authors have advocated preprocedural revascularization for all of these patients.[22,23] At our institution, we employ

Table 56.2

Anatomic Requirements and Sizing Recommendations of the FDA-Approved Thoracic Aortic Devices

	TAG	Zenith TX2	Talent thoracic
Length of proximal and distal landing zones	≥20 mm	≥25 mm	≥20 mm
Range of treatable aortic diameters	23–42 mm	24–38 mm	18–42 mm
Percentage of oversizing to aorta	6–19% [a]	10–20%	12–22%
Required delivery sheath size	20 French, 22 French, 24 French	20 French or 22 French	22 French, 24 French, 25 French
Outside diameter of delivery system	7.6–9.2 mm (sheath)	7.5–8.5 mm (sheath)	7.3–8.3 mm ("bareback")

[a] TAG device IFU recommends inner-wall to inner-wall measurement of aortic diameter.

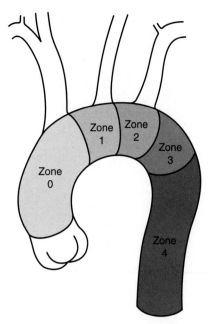

FIGURE 56.7 The zones of proximal aortic stent graft placement sites.

a policy of selective revascularization. Following thorough evaluation of the cerebrovascular blood supply using cross-sectional imaging, LSCA revascularization is performed prior to TEVAR in the presence of an incomplete posterior circulation (i.e., a vertebral artery terminating as the posterior inferior cerebellar artery), a left dominant vertebral artery, a stenosed or occluded right vertebral artery, a patent left internal mammary artery (LIMA) to left anterior descending (LAD) coronary bypass graft, or an aberrant origin of the right subclavian artery. Additionally, in recognizing that branches of the LSCA may contribute to spinal cord perfusion,[24] revascularization of the LSCA is performed when exclusion of a long length of descending thoracic aorta is planned, especially if the patient has undergone prior abdominal aortic repair. LSCA revascularization is most commonly accomplished by left carotid-to-LSCA bypass, although transposition of the LSCA to the left carotid artery has been performed. Bypass techniques and staged embolization of the LSCA origin at time of TEVAR as described by Woo et al.[25] obviates the need for dissection and clamping of the LSCA proximal to the origins of the LIMA and left vertebral artery, thereby minimizing operative ischemic and bleeding risks. Postprocedural LSCA revascularization is performed for patients who develop post-TEVAR ischemic symptoms, such as left arm claudication or symptomatic vertebral-basilar insufficiency. This delayed repair algorithm does not appear to have any untoward consequences, although patients must be specifically queried for these symptoms at follow-up visits post-TEVAR.[26]

Insertion of a lumbar catheter for cerebral spinal fluid (CSF) drainage is performed preoperatively at the discretion of the operator based on assessment of risk factors for spinal ischemia, including the region of planned aortic exclusion, length of planned aortic exclusion, and history of a prior aortic procedure. Spinal drains are managed per protocol in the ICU setting and are discontinued in 48 to 72 hours prior to transferring the patient from the ICU.

Vascular access to the thoracic aorta continues to be a significant issue with TEVAR. In most cases, the bilateral common femoral arteries are accessed to allow for introduction of the delivery sheath from one side and a pigtail catheter for diagnostic injection of contrast agent from the other access site. The diameter, degree of atherosclerotic disease, and the tortuosity of the access site vessels and iliac arteries are assessed preoperatively using CTA or MRA. Usually the larger diameter, less calcified, and less tortuous iliofemoral arterial tree is selected as the main device delivery route. If femoral vessels are not heavily calcified and are of adequate diameter to accommodate the delivery sheath, totally percutaneous access utilizing the "Preclose" technique, as first described by Lee et al. in 2007,[27] can be used safely and effectively with the Perclose Proglide 6F Suture-Mediated Closure System (Abbott Vascular, Redwood City, CA). Briefly, this technique places two individual 3-0 polypropylene sutures with preformed slipknots through the anterior wall of the artery, which are cinched down at the conclusion of the case with the provided knot pusher (FIGURE 56.8). This is a modification of the original technique described by Haas et al. in 1999, in which the 10F Prostar XL Suture-Mediated Closure System was used.[28]

In a follow-up review published 1 year later, Lee et al. reported their midterm outcomes of 292 patients who underwent percutaneous aortic endovascular repairs with successful closure of 408 of the attempted 432 (94.4%) common femoral arterial puncture sites.[29] One hundred of those patients had a CTA at least 6 months postprocedure to assess the 156 preclosed puncture sites and revealed a late complication rate of only 1.92% (3/156), including one asymptomatic femoral artery dissection and two femoral pseudoaneurysms requiring surgical repair. In our institutional experience with percutaneous endografting on 42 AAA and 19 TAA patients with sheath sizes ranging from 12 to 25 French, the success rate in these 61 patients was 100% for effective closure of the arteriotomies. There were no immediate or delayed complications related to the percutaneous closures at clinical follow-up.[30]

Ultrasound (US) guidance for arterial percutaneous access has been reported to significantly reduce access-related complications, especially in patients requiring the use of larger sheath sizes.[31] With US guidance, a technical success rate of 98% was achieved, as compared with a success rate of 94% with manual palpation for arterial access. Complications were 0% in the US guidance group and 7% in the palpation group. With sheath sizes of 20 French or less, both groups had a 97% technical success rate; however, with sheath sizes larger than 20 French, the US group experienced a 100% technical success rate ($n = 24$) as compared with an 82% success rate ($n = 18$) in the manual palpation group ($p < .05$).

Operative surgical control and exposure of the common femoral arteries should be performed in the setting of heavily calcified vessels or if the operating physician has not had adequate training in the "Preclose" technique. If the common femoral or external iliac arteries are not of a size that will accommodate the insertion and advancement of the device delivery system, a surgical conduit, most commonly a 10-mm diameter polyester tube graft, may be sewn to the iliac artery, or less commonly the lower abdominal aorta through a retroperitoneal approach (FIGURE 56.9). The iliac conduit can then be tunneled through a separate stab incision and accessed either through a small "graftotomy" or a direct puncture of the graft (FIGURE 56.10). An important additional consideration when using a tunneled conduit is the added length that the delivery sheath must traverse to reach the diseased segment of the thoracic aorta. Therefore, one must make sure that

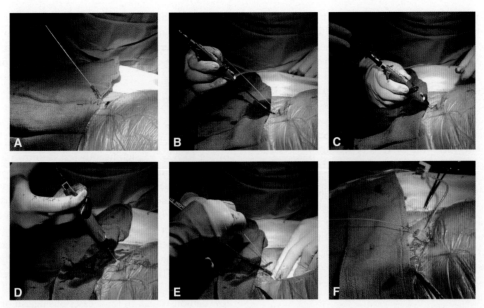

FIGURE 56.8 The preclose technique to allow for totally percutaneous placement of thoracic aortic stent graft. **A.** Percutaneous needle access of the femoral artery is obtained in standard fashion. **B.** Following dilation of the puncture tract with 8 French dilator, the Proglide is advanced over the wire into the femoral artery. **C.** Following wire removal the Proglide is advanced into the artery until there is flow through the side port. **D.** The Proglide is then rotated either medially or laterally and deployed in a numbered stepwise fashion. **E.** The device is then partially removed and the wire is readvanced through the delivery port to allow for placement of a second device rotated in the opposite direction from the first. **F.** "Preclosed groin" with replaced 8 French sheath and surgical clamps on preplaced prolene sutures.

the delivery system is of appropriate length to reach the desired deployment location before using a tunneled conduit.

COMPLICATIONS

Neurologic Complications

Neurologic complications continue to be a rare but devastating complication of TEVAR. Spinal cord ischemia, both immediate and delayed, resulting in paraplegia has been reported to occur in about 3% to 5% of patients in multiple series and is clearly a multifactorial event.[32] Multiple risk factors have been implicated, including exclusion of greater than 20 cm in aortic length, coverage of the LSCA, exclusion of the distal thoracic aorta (especially the T8-L2 region), and a history of prior

abdominal aortic repair.[33] Perioperative hypotension (mean arterial pressure [MAP] <70) has also been implicated as a risk factor for both immediate and delayed spinal cord injury.[34] Like many authors, we advocate the use of prophylactic CSF drainage in patients with these preoperative risk factors. Meticulous maintenance of blood pressure above an MAP of greater than 90 mm Hg beginning immediately after exclusion of the TAA in the postprocedural period is highly recommended. What is

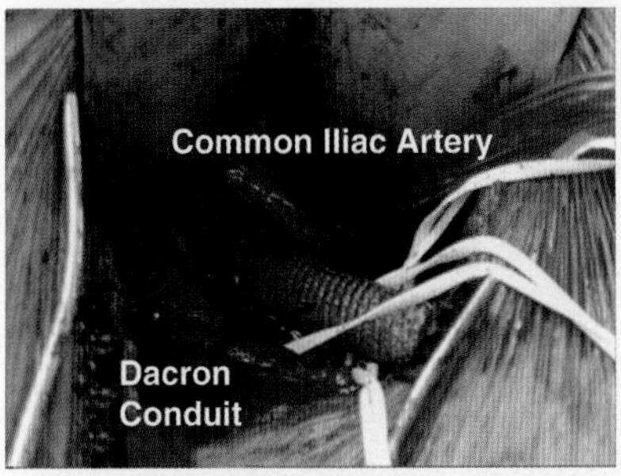

FIGURE 56.9 Surgical conduit for placement of thoracic stent graft. Intraoperative photograph demonstrating the proximal end-to-side anastomosis of 10-mm polyester conduit to the common iliac artery through a small retroperitoneal incision.

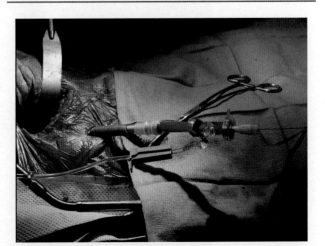

FIGURE 56.10 Surgical conduit for placement of thoracic stent graft. Intraoperative photograph illustrating the technique of side wall needle cannulation of the surgical conduit directed through a separate counter incision to lessen the degree of angulation, which the large delivery sheaths must traverse.

more disconcerting, however, are the significant numbers of reports in the literature of patients presenting with spinal cord ischemia weeks after the procedure, likely representing further loss of collateral pathways superimposed on transient episodes of hypotension.[32,33] The spontaneous resolution of some endoleaks over time further emphasizes the potentially dynamic state of the perianeurysmal circulatory bed and its significant role in the outcomes in certain patients.

Cerebrovascular accidents (CVA) have also been reported in 3% to 5% of patients following TEVAR procedures.[6,16,20,24] Patients with severe atheromatous disease in the aortic arch region or those patients requiring extensive aortic arch manipulation or extension of endografting into zones 0 through 2 may be at particular risk for a CVA.[35] Specifically, coverage of the LSCA (zone 2 deployment) has been reported to have an associated CVA rate of 8.6% as reported by Woo et al.[22] in their review of 70 patients undergoing zone 2 TEVAR and appears to pose a higher stroke risk than TEVAR performed within zones 3 and 4. Risks of embolic cerebrovascular events are likely related to the severity and composition of the aortic atherosclerotic plaques and the extent of wire, catheter, and device manipulation within the arch, including balloon molding of the endograft.

Vascular Complications

Vascular complications have been reported in 9.2% to 22% of cases in the initial pivotal trials and are almost all related to the access sites or attempting to use an "inadequate" iliofemoral artery for device delivery.[6,16,20] Decreasing vascular complications secondary to access site issues can be accomplished by using

a graft conduit as a preemptive measure rather than a bailout after a vascular injury has occurred. Indeed, in the pivotal trial with the lowest vascular complication rate, conduits were used in 15% of the cases in which TEVAR was performed.[20]

Device-Related Complications

Endoleaks

Although much has been written on the subject of endoleaks following EVAR,[36–38] significantly less is known about the natural history of endoleaks following TEVAR. Earlier studies, including single-center series and multicenter registries, have reported overall endoleak rates of 5% to 29%, a value similar to that reported for EVAR.[6,16,20,39] In our experience, however, the incidence of type II endoleaks after TEVAR appears to be less than after EVAR, likely due to the absence of the robust collaterals as seen in the retroperitoneum and absence of an artery analogous to the inferior mesenteric artery.[40] The anatomy around the aortic arch has led to more type IA endoleaks, some of which have been small or with very slow flow demonstrated. In these cases of sluggish or very diminutive type IA endoleaks, follow-up imaging has usually demonstrated resolution of most of these endoleaks, likely due to the resolution of the anticoagulation effect in the periprocedural period and the absence of an outflow collateral vessel in the TAA sac.[41]

Aneurysm Sac Enlargement

Aortic remodeling with interval decrease in aneurysm sac diameter is a good indicator that endovascular exclusion of the aneurysm has been successful (FIGURE 56.11). Even in the absence

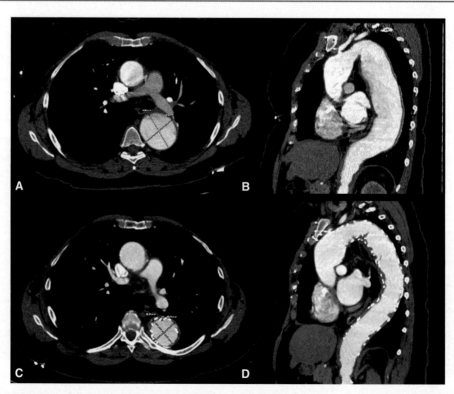

FIGURE 56.11 Five-year follow-up of patient with TAA treated with thoracic aortic stent-graft. Contrast-enhanced CTA axial and multiplanar reconstruction of a patient prior to (**A, B**) and 5 years following (**C, D**) placement of thoracic aortic device, demonstrating significant aneurysm sac shrinkage.

of a visualized endoleak on follow-up imaging, however, aneurysm sac enlargement should suggest continued pressurization of the aneurysm sac and, therefore, inadequate stand-alone therapy. The incidence of aneurysm sac enlargement of greater than 5 mm has been reported in all three pivotal trials at 1 year, ranging from 7% to 9%.[6,16,20]

Device Integrity and Migration

Stent fractures and graft material failure have been infrequently reported with the currently available FDA-approved devices. Experience with the original TAG device demonstrated that the longitudinal support bar may be susceptible to fracture with a reported 14% fracture rate at 5 years of follow-up.[15] Four fractured Talent devices have been reported, including one longitudinal bar.[19,20] The longitudinal bars have been removed from the current TAG, the cTAG, and the investigational Valiant devices. No stent fracture, barb separation, stent-to-stent separation, or component separation has been reported in the TX2 device through 1 year of follow-up.[17]

Device migration of greater than 10 mm is not common, ranging from 0.5% to 3.9% of the pivotal trial patients.[15,17,19,20] Fortunately, device migration has rarely been associated with clinically relevant adverse events and has not commonly required subsequent intervention.

▌ CONCLUSION

This chapter serves as a review of the use of endovascular stent-grafts for treatment of the descending TAAs. Currently, three devices are FDA approved for the treatment of descending thoracic aneurysms. Outcomes highly depend on good case planning and patient selection and will likely continue to improve as newer-generation devices and delivery systems are designed and made available.

▌ REFERENCES

1. DeBakey ME, Cooley DA. Successful resection of aneurysm of the thoracic aorta and replacement by graft. *JAMA* 1953;152:673–676.
2. Achneck HE, Rizzo JA, Tranquilli M, et al. Safety of thoracic aortic surgery in the present era. *Ann Thorac Surg* 2007;84:1180–1185.
3. Parodi JC, Palmaz JC, Barone HD. Transfemoral intraluminal graft implantation for abdominal aortic aneurysms. *Ann Vasc Surg* 1991;5:491–499.
4. Dake MD, Miller DC, Semba CP, et al. Transluminal placement of endovascular stent-grafts for the treatment of descending thoracic aortic aneurysms. *N Engl J Med* 1994;331:1729–1734.
5. Dake MD, Miller DC, Mitchell RS, et al. The "first generation" of endovascular stent-grafts for patients with aneurysms of the descending thoracic aorta. *J Thorac Cardiovasc Surg* 1998;116:689–703.
6. Makaroun MS, Dillavou ED, Kee ST, et al. Endovascular treatment of thoracic aortic aneurysms: results of the phase II multicenter trial of the GORE TAG thoracic endoprosthesis. *J Vasc Surg* 2005;41:1–9.
7. Greenberg R, Resch T, Nyman U, et al. Endovascular repair of descending thoracic aortic aneurysms: an early experience with intermediate-term follow-up. *J Vasc Surg* 2000;31:147–156.
8. Czerny M, Grimm M, Zimpfer D, et al. Results after endovascular stent graft placement in atherosclerotic aneurysms involving the descending aorta. *Ann Thorac Surg* 2007;83:450–455.
9. Dagenais F, Shetty R, Normand JP, et al. Extended applications of thoracic aortic stent grafts. *Ann Thorac Surg* 2006; 82:567–572.
10. Verhoye JP, de Latour B, Heautot JF, et al. Mid-term results of endovascular treatment for descending thoracic aorta diseases in high-surgical risk patients. *Ann Vasc Surg* 2006;20:714–722.
11. Ince H, Rehders TC, Petzsch M, et al. Stent-grafts in patients with marfan syndrome. *J Endovasc Ther* 2005;12:82–88.
12. Ehrlich M, Grabenwoeger M, Cartes-Zumelzu F, et al. Endovascular stent graft repair for aneurysms of the descending thoracic aorta. *Ann Thorac Surg* 1998;66:19–25.
13. Mitchell R, Dake M, Semba C, et al. Enodvascular stent-graft repair of thoracic aortic aneurysms. *J Thorac Cardiovasc Surg* 1996;111:1054–1062.
14. Coady M, Chueng T, Matsumoto AH, et al. Surgical management of thoracic aortic disease: open and endovascular approaches. *Circulation* 2010;121:2780–2804.
15. Makaroun MS, Dillavou ED, Wheatley GH, et al. Five-year results of endovascular treatment with the Gore TAG device compared with open repair of thoracic aortic aneurysms. *J Vasc Surg* 2008;47:912–918.
16. Greenberg RK, O'Neill S, Walker E, et al. Endovascular repair of thoracic aortic lesions with the Zenith TX1 and TX2 thoracic grafts: intermediate-term results. *J Vasc Surg* 2005; 41:589–596.
17. Matsumura JS, Cambria RP, Dake MD, et al. International controlled clinical trial of thoracic endovascular aneurysm repair with the Zenith TX2 endovascular graft: 1-year results. *J Vasc Surg* 2008;47:247–257.
18. Leurs LJ, Bell R, Degrieck Y, et al. Endovascular treatment of thoracic aortic diseases: combined experience from the EUROSTAR and United Kingdom Thoracic Endograft registries. *J Vasc Surg* 2004;40:670–680.
19. Fattori R, Nienaber CA, Rousseau H, et al. Results of endovascular repair of the thoracic aorta with the Talent Thoracic stent graft: the Talent Thoracic Retrospective Registry. *J Thorac Cardiovasc Surg* 2006;132:332–339.
20. Fairman RM, Criado F, Farber M, et al. Pivotal results of the Medtronic Vascular Talent Thoracic Stent Graft System: the VALOR trial. *J Vasc Surg* 2008;48:546–554.
21. Criado F, Abul-Khoudoud O, Domer G, et al. Endovascular repair of the thoracic aorta: lessons learned. *Ann Thorac Surg* 2005;80:857–863.
22. Woo EY, Carpenter JP, Jackson BM, et al. Left subclavian artery coverage during thoracic endovascular repair: a single-center experience. *J Vasc Surg* 2008;48:555–560.
23. Noor N, Sadat U, Hayes PD, et al. Management of the left subclavian artery during endovascular repair of the thoracic aorta. *J Endovasc Ther* 2008;15:168–176.
24. Buth J, Harris PL, Hovo R, et al. Neurologic complications associated with endovascular repair of thoracic aortic pathology: incidence and risk factors. A study from the European Collaborators on Stent/Graft Techniques for Aortic Aneurysm Repair (EUROSTAR) Registry. *J Vasc Surg* 2007;46:1103–1111.
25. Woo EY, Bavaria JE, Pochettino A, et al. Techniques for preserving vertebral artery perfusion during thoracic aortic stent grafting requiring aortic arch landing. *Vasc Endovascular Surg* 2006;40(5):367–373.
26. Reece TB, Gazoni LM, Cherry KJ, et al. Reevaluating the need for left subclavian artery revascularization with thoracic endovascular aortic repair. *Ann Thorac Surg* 2007;84(4):1201–1205.
27. Lee WA, Brown MP, Nelson PR, et al. Total percutaneous access for endovascular aortic aneurysm repair ("Preclose" technique). *J Vasc Surg* 2007;45:1095–1101.
28. Haas PC, Kracjer Z, Dietrich EB. Closure of large percutaneous access sites using the Prostar XL percutaneous vascular surgery device. *J Endovasc Surg* 1999;6:168–170.
29. Lee WA, Brown MP, Nelson PR, et al. Midterm outcomes of femoral arteries after percutaneous endovascular aortic repair using the Preclose technique. *J Vasc Surg* 2008;47:919–923.
30. Arslan B, Turba UC, Sabri S, et al. Current status of percutaneous endografting. *Semin Intervent Radiol* 2009;26(1): 67–73.
31. Arthurs ZM, Starnes BW, Sohn VY, et al. Ultrasound-guided access improves rate of access related complications for totally percutaneous aortic aneurysm repair. *Ann Vasc Surg* 2008; 22:736–741.
32. Gravereaux EC, Faries PL, Burks JA, et al. Risk of spinal cord ischemia after endograft repair of thoracic aortic aneurysms. *J Vasc Surg* 2001;34: 997–1003.
33. Baril DT, Carroccio A, Ellozy SH, et al. Endovascular thoracic aortic repair and previous or concomitant abdominal aortic repair: is the increased risk of spinal cord ischemia real? *Ann Vasc Surg* 2006;20:188–194.
34. Chiesa R, Melissano G, Marrocco-Trischitta MM, et al. Spinal cord ischemia after elective stent-graft repair of the thoracic aorta. *J Vasc Surg* 2005;42:11–17.
35. Feezor RJ, Martin TD, Hess PJ, et al. Risk factors for perioperative stroke during thoracic endovascular aortic repairs (TEVAR). *J Endovasc Ther* 2007;14:568–573.
36. White GH, Yu W, May J, et al. Endoleak as a complication of endoluminal grafting of abdominal aortic aneurysms: classification, incidence, diagnosis, and management. *J Endovasc Surg* 1997;4:152–168.

37. Faries PL, Cadot H, Agarwal G, et al. Management of endoleak after endovascular aneurysm repair: cuffs, coils, and conversion. *J Vasc Surg* 2003;37:1155–1161.

38. Sampaio SM, Panneton JM, Mozes GI, et al. Proximal type I endoleaks after endovascular abdominal aortic aneurysm repair: predictive factors. *Ann Vasc Surg* 2004;18:621–628.

39. Parmer SS, Carpenter JP, Stavropoulos W, et al. Endoleaks after endovascular repair of thoracic aortic aneurysms. *J Vasc Surg* 2006;44:447–452.

40. Adams JD, Angle JF, Matsumoto AH, et al. Endovascular repair of the thoracic aorta in the post-FDA approval era. *J Thorac Cardiovasc Surg* 2009;137:117–123.

41. Adams JD, Tracci MC, Sabri S, et al. Real-world experience with type I endoleaks after endovascular repair of the thoracic aorta. *Am Surg* 2010;76(6):599–605.

Abdominal Aortic Aneurysms

DAI YAMANOUCHI and JON S. MATSUMURA

INTRODUCTION

Abdominal aortic aneurysm (AAA) is a common condition of increasing prevalence, particularly among older men. In 1951, Dubost first replaced an AAA with a thoracic aortic homograft. Open repair was refined over the next four decades, and then endovascular repair of AAAs (endovascular aneurysm repair [EVAR]) in humans was introduced by Parodi and colleagues in 1991 using a graft fashioned from prosthetic grafts and expandable stents.[1] There followed a rapid progression from a tube graft design to the currently used bifurcated systems. Recent data show that 73% of AAA repairs in the United States were done via an endovascular approach from 1998 to 2004, and this proportion is increasing with newer devices.[2] Although long-term outcomes of EVAR compared to open repair is still controversial, the three published principal randomized trials comparing endovascular and open repair have shown a marked benefit of EVAR with respect to 30-day operative mortality.[3–6] Like many new techniques, the field of EVAR is still evolving. This chapter reviews the basic concepts, indication, devices, techniques, and complications of EVAR.

PATIENT SELECTION AND PREOPERATIVE PLANNING

Definition of Abdominal Aortic Aneurysm

Aneurysms are defined as a focal dilatation at least 50% or greater than normal arterial diameter.[7] Lederle and colleagues reported that advancing age, male gender, black race, and increasing height, weight, body mass index, and body surface area were associated with a larger infrarenal aortic diameter but that the effect of all these variables was small.[8] Because the average infrarenal aortic diameter was 2 cm in these patients, use of a 3-cm definition for an infrarenal AAA was recommended. In clinical practice with individual patients, it is more common to define an aneurysm as a 50% or greater enlargement over the diameter of the adjacent, nonaneurysmal artery.[7]

Most AAAs involve the infrarenal aorta, but about 5% to 15% of those undergoing surgical repair also involve the suprarenal aorta.[9,10] Although 25% of AAAs involve the iliac arteries,[10] isolated iliac artery aneurysms are rare.[11] Peripheral aneurysms of the femoral or popliteal artery are present in approximately 4% of patients with AAA.[12]

Indication for Aneurysm Repair

Although it is impossible to set a single threshold diameter for intervention that can be generalized to all patients, based on the best available current evidence, 5.5 cm is the most common threshold for repair of AAA in an "average" patient. Repair of selected smaller AAAs may be justified in subsets of good-risk patients with aneurysms at higher rupture risk; for example, intervention at 5-cm diameter may be indicated in women with AAA. Conversely, delaying repair until the diameter is larger may be best for older, higher-risk patients.[13] There is no justification at present for different indications for endovascular repair, such as earlier treatment of smaller AAAs.[3,4,14]

Anatomic Considerations for Endovascular Aneurysm Repair

Current indications for AAA repair include a diameter greater than 5.5 cm, an increase in size greater than 0.5 cm in 6 months, or a symptomatic aneurysm.[15] Because large clinical trials have shown reduced aneurysm-related deaths with EVAR compared to open repair, EVAR is a preferred treatment option when anatomy is suitable.[3]

There are certain morphologic features that are taken into consideration in determining if there is anatomic suitability for EVAR. Preoperative assessment and planning are typically performed by thin collimation, contrast-enhanced CT scan with postprocessing image analysis. Magnetic resonance angiography (MRA) or angiography sometimes serves as alternatives. Precise measurement of diameters and lengths is critical to plan and perform this procedure safely and have the appropriate devices available. Each of the commercially available devices has its own indications and contraindications including distance and angulation of the aortic neck, diameter of the proximal and distal implantation sites, and minimum diameter of the iliac arteries. Typical anatomic indications of major commercial devices are shown in Table 57.1.

Aortic Neck

Aortic neck is defined as a distance from the lowest renal artery to the beginning of the aneurysmal aorta. This is required for the proper fixation and sealing of the proximal attachment of the endografts to avoid migration and endoleak. Currently, the minimum distance required ranges from 10 to 15 mm (FIGURE 57.1 and Table 57.1).

Because angulation is commonly seen in the aneurysmal aorta, the angle of the aortic neck is also an important consideration. This is caused by the difficulties of endograft alignment within the angulated proximal neck and precise positioning of the delivery system through the angulation. Typical ranges of the maximum angulation are from 45 to 60 degrees (FIGURE 57.1 and Table 57.1).

The shape and characteristics of the neck are another factor. The "reverse taper" or "reverse funnel" neck that enlarges caudally is more challenging. Additionally, excessive intramural thrombus involving landing site also needs to be considered as a relative contraindication because it may cause embolic complications.

Table 57.1				
Characteristics of FDA-Approved Abdominal Aortic Endografts				
	Excluder/C3 (W. L. Gore)	Endurant II (Medtronic)	Zenith Flex (Cook)	AFK (Endologix)
Proximal neck length	≥15 mm	≥10 mm	≥15 mm	≥15 mm
Aortic neck diameter [a]	19–32 mm	19–32 mm	18–32 mm	18–32 mm
Iliac diameter	8–18.5 mm	8–25 mm	7.5–20 mm	10–23 mm
Angulation of the neck	≤60 degrees	≤60 degrees	≤60 degrees	≤60 degrees
Ipsilateral crossing profile: OD (the aortic neck)	20.4 French (19–32 mm)	18 French (18–25 mm) 20 French (26–32 mm)	21 French (18–22 mm) 23 French (23–28mm) 26 French (29–32 mm)	19 French (all sizes)

[a] Inner wall to inner wall for Excluder, Endurant, and AFK. Outer wall to outer wall for Zenith.

The Ilio-Femoral Artery

The anatomic characteristics of the ilio-femoral artery also need to be carefully evaluated. These arteries serve both as access vessels and distal implantation sites. Devices are placed through a large-diameter delivery system or sheath, and excessive calcification combined with tortuosity and stenosis are challenging. When severe, they may be contraindications for EVAR because of the difficulty to deliver endograft systems. The minimal sizes of these vessels depend on each device (Table 57.1). To overcome the limitations of the access vessels, additional procedures need to be considered; that is, an angioplasty without stenting, a covered stent ("endoconduit"), or an open conduit through a flank retroperitoneal incision using a prosthetic graft sewn to the common iliac artery. If aneurysmal changes extend into the iliac arteries, the common iliac artery is sometimes not appropriate to be a distal sealing zone. In these cases, the distal limb of the endograft may be extended to the external iliac artery. If this is expected in planning the stage, embolization of the hypogastric artery is considered to avoid a backfilling hypogastric endoleak. The femoral artery, including aneurysmal, stenotic change, and/or high bifurcation of the profunda femoral artery, also needs to be evaluated, especially when planning percutaneous EVAR with large hole closure devices.

Preintervention Planning and Measurement

Planning takes into account all of the above-mentioned anatomic characteristics, including detailed and accurate measurement of the diameter of the proximal and distal implantation sites, distance and angulation of the proximal aortic neck, maximum diameter of the aneurysm, minimum diameter of the aortic bifurcation, and distance from the proximal to the distal implantation site. Having the implanting physician involved is critical to selecting the sizes of the devices, sizes of the backup devices, and the procedural strategy because different strategies may require alternative sizing. For example, if the main trunk implantation is switched from one side to the other because access is troublesome on the first side, the diameter and length of

the required iliac components may be different. Careful measurement is important with some devices that are more tolerant than others to sizing discrepancy. In general, endograft diameters are oversized for aneurysm indications by 10% to 20% compared to the actual diameter of the implantation site. Note that the method of measurement, the ranges, and the indications depend on each device (Table 57.1).

▌ COMMERCIALLY AVAILABLE DEVICES

There are many commercially available devices for EVAR worldwide (FIGURE 57.2). As of March 2013, there are eight devices from six manufacturers approved by the United States Food and Drug Administration (FDA). There are many features to consider when selecting an EVAR system, including proximal positive fixation, suprarenal components, ipsilateral and contralateral crossing profile, graft material, flexibility, and ease of device deployment. This section provides a brief review of the features of each FDA-approved system.

Excluder/C3

The Excluder/C3 is a product of W. L. Gore & Associates, Inc. (Flagstaff, AZ). The device was initially approved by the FDA in 2002,[16] followed by the approval for C3, a newer delivery system, in 2010. These devices are a modular stent-graft system with nitinol stent exoskeleton and multilayer expanded polytetrafluoroethylene (ePTFE) graft material. Aortic neck diameters of 19 to 29 mm and iliac diameters of 8 to 18.5 mm are indicated. The outer diameter (OD) of the ipsilateral sheath is 20.4 to 23 French with contralateral sheath sizes between 12 and 18 French inner diameter (ID). Advantages of this platform are the longer device lengths requiring fewer components, established data on performance, positive fixation, ability to perform sheath injections for arteriographic control immediately before deployment, and the simple deployment system. The newer C3 delivery system provides the ability to reposition the device prior to final release from the delivery catheter for more accurate positioning and easier gate cannulation.

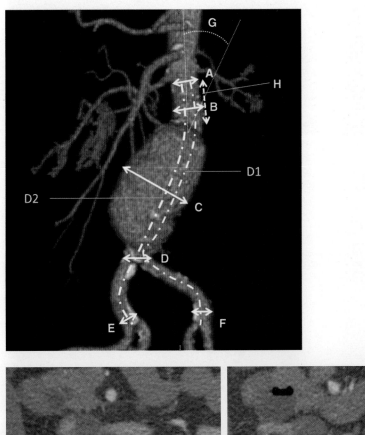

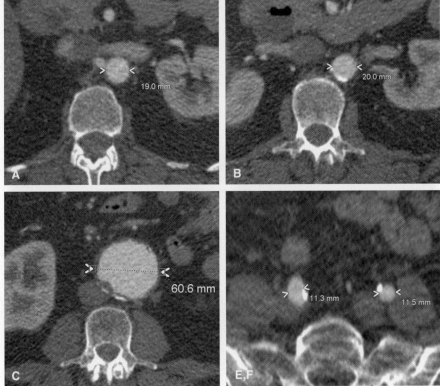

FIGURE 57.1 Preoperative measurements for EVAR. **A.** Aortic diameter at proximal implantation site. **B.** Aortic diameter at 15 mm inferior to proximal implantation site. **C.** Maximum diameter of aneurysm. **D.** Minimum diameter of the aortic bifurcation. **E, F.** Iliac diameter at distal landing site. **G.** Angle of proximal aortic neck. **H.** Distance of proximal aortic neck. *D1, D2:* Distance from proximal to distal implantation site.

Zenith Flex

The Zenith Flex endovascular graft system is a product manufactured by Cook Inc. (Bloomington, IN) and was approved by the FDA in 2003.[17] The Zenith is a bifurcated, modular system with stainless steel stents covered with woven polyester graft material. Each device has a suprarenal proximal stent with large barbs for positive fixation. Aortic neck diameters of 18 to 32 mm and iliac diameters of 7.5 to 20 mm are indicated. The ipsilateral crossing OD is available in 21, 23, and 26 French sizes with contralateral sheaths ranging from 14 to 16 French sizes (ID). This endovascular graft is preloaded in the introduction system with a staged deployment system, providing very precise

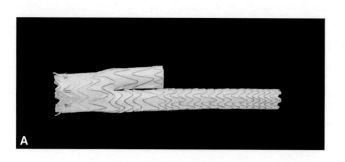
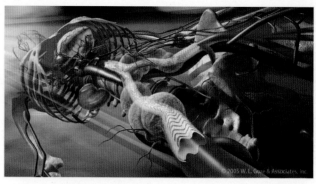
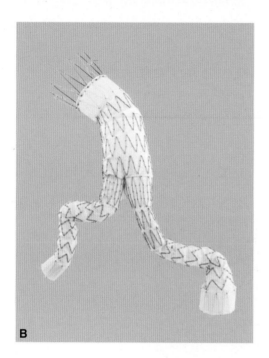
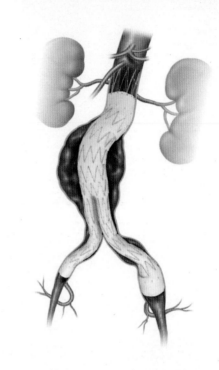
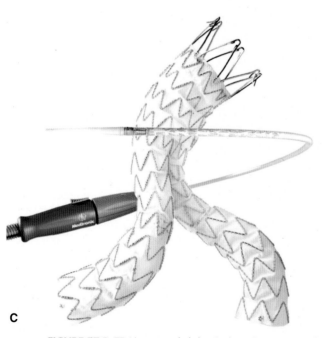
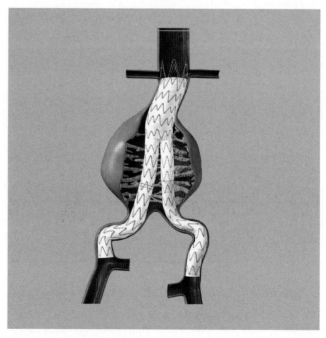

FIGURE 57.2 FDA-approved abdominal aortic commercial devices. **A:** Excluder, **B:** Zenith Flex, **C:** Endurant, **D:** AFX

(A: Courtesy of WL Gore & Associates, Inc.; C: Courtesy of Medtronic)

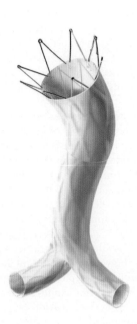

D

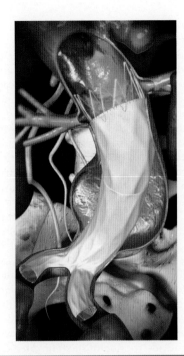

FIGURE 57.2 *(Continued)*

positioning. The advantages of this device are the ability to treat with a wide spectrum of device lengths and neck sizes, a familiar platform with long-term data, suprarenal fixation, and active fixation with anchoring barbs.[18,19] A lower-profile nitinol version is available outside the United States.

Endurant II

The Endurant stent-graft system is a product manufactured by Medtronic Inc. (Santa Rosa, CA) and was approved by the FDA in 2010.[20] This system is a modular endograft with nitinol stent and low-profile polyester graft material. Aortic neck diameters of 19 to 32 mm and iliac diameters of 8 to 25 mm are indicated. The ipsilateral OD is 18 to 20 French with contralateral sheaths available in 14 to 16 French sizes (ID). This platform has advantages including the ability to treat a very wide spectrum of AAA caused by a large range of sizes, a familiar delivery system, and suprarenal fixation with anchor pins to provide positive fixation.[21,22]

AFX

The AFX endovascular system is a product manufactured by Endologix Inc. (Irvine, CA) and was approved by the FDA in 2011 (the original device was approved in 2004).[23] AFX is a newer generation of the Powerlink endograft system that has a unibody bifurcated stent-graft system using ePTFE with self-expanding endoskeleton cobalt-chromium stents. The graft is attached to the stent with surgical suture at each end only. The device does not have barbs and is seated on the aortic bifurcation and built up from this position, and a larger-diameter aortic cuff is almost always required. Aortic neck diameters of 18 to 32 mm and iliac diameters of 10 to 23 mm are indicated. The OD of ipsilateral sheath is 19 French, and contralateral access is 9 French ID. Advantages of this device are the low profile of the ipsilateral

delivery system, the very low profile of the contralateral access, and a precannulated contralateral limb.[24,25]

■ PROCEDURAL TECHNIQUES

General, regional, and local anesthesia can be used for EVAR. Local anesthesia is beneficial when treating a frail or hemodynamically unstable patient. A large field image intensifier and digital subtraction are very useful for this procedure. Ideally, these procedures are performed with a multiaxis robotic flat detector with advanced features like fusion imaging and fluoro-CT (computed tomography) in a hybrid room with standby operating room capability for conversions and iliac conduits. A dedicated team and a well-stocked supply room are essential to manage the many challenges that may arise during an EVAR procedure.

Access

Access is typically obtained through the common femoral artery (CFA) via the cut-down or percutaneous technique using a preclosure device. When selecting the percutaneous technique, it is helpful to evaluate the character of the CFA carefully and making sure that it has an anterior puncture, using ultrasound or radiographic guidance (FIGURE 57.3A).[26] If a cut-down is performed in the groin, an oblique incision just above or below the skin crease may reduce wound complications. A short 6 French sheath is initially used to place measurement catheters and perform arteriography when necessary. Often, stiff 0.035″ guide wires are exchanged for delivery of the large sheath or EVAR delivery system. The size of the large sheath depends on each device (Table 57.1).

If there is difficulty advancing the device or large sheath to the aorta, it is necessary to carefully consider the options. These include even stiffer wires or a brachial femoral guide wire to address severe tortuosity, angioplasty of a focal stenotic lesion, usage of an expandable sheath for small arteries, or endoconduit placement with a covered stent if rupture of the iliac artery is likely. Sometimes, the best option is aborting the procedure or performing open surgical placement of a conduit sewn directly to the common iliac artery through a flank incision. When there is a difficult access problem, careful evaluation of the iliac artery with the wire still in place is useful when pulling the sheath or delivery system out at the end of the procedure to detect any injury of the access vessel. If signs of rupture of the iliac artery are noted, prompt insertion of an aortic occlusion balloon or reinsertion of the sheath to obtain the hemostasis is necessary followed by covered stent repair or conversion to open repair of the iliac artery.

Endograft Placement and Deployment

After placing the large sheath or delivery system into the aorta, an aortography is performed, centering on the renal arteries and optimizing gantry angle, to accurately place the proximal end of the graft and obtain the longest infrarenal sealing zone. It is helpful to know from the preoperative imaging which oblique craniad projection is ideal to demonstrate the renal artery origins (FIGURE 57.3B). After the proper imaging and adjustment of the device, the proximal portion of the stent-graft is deployed (FIGURE 57.3C). Some devices have a feature that permits readjustment of the positioning just before or after the initial deployment of the main body to maximize the infrarenal sealing length. Some devices with suprarenal fixation

allow staged deployment of the main body. The unibody device with a bottom-up deployment strategy requires careful attention to the second aortic cuff. Next the short docking limb of the main body is catheterized from the contralateral side. The cannulation step can be facilitated by frequently changing the image projection and positioning of the docking limb near the contralateral iliac artery and sheath prior to deployment. If selecting the limb from the contralateral side with a variety of shaped catheters is not possible, then a snaring technique may be performed. This technique involves inserting a reverse curve catheter and extra-long guide wire from the ipsilateral side through up and over the graft bifurcation into the short limb followed by snaring and pulling out from the contralateral side. To confirm the retrograde selection of the contralateral limb, it is important to routinely rotate the pigtail catheter in the main trunk seal zone (FIGURE 57.3D). By visualizing free spinning of the pigtail catheter, the catheter is confirmed to be inside the graft and not trapped between the graft and aortic neck wall. Intravascular ultrasound, multiple oblique imaging, and angiography through that catheter can further verify gate cannulation, if indicated. Some devices provide a precannulated contralateral wire that is snared during initial insertion of the bifurcated component. A stiff wire is then placed through the catheter confirmed in the contralateral gate, and an appropriate sheath or delivery system introduced into the short limb. The length of the contralateral graft limb can be measured with a marker catheter (FIGURE 57.3E) after an arteriogram demonstrates the location of the iliac bifurcation,

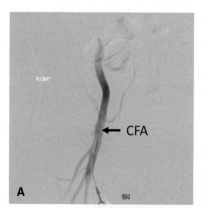
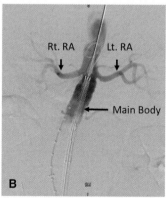
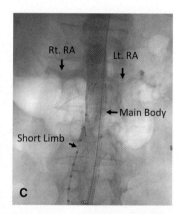
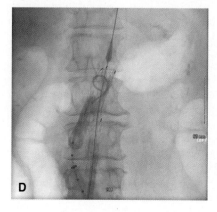
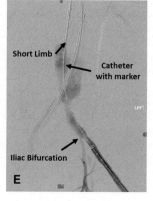
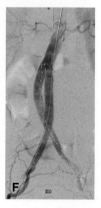

FIGURE 57.3 Intraoperative images. **A.** Common femoral artery puncture for percutaneous EVAR. **B.** Predeployment image of the renal artery. **C.** Postdeployment image of the main body. **D.** Catheterization of the short limb. **E.** Measurement of the contralateral limb. **F.** Completion.

which may be displaced by stiff wires and with manipulation. After deployment of the contralateral limb (with or without extensions) and the limb of the ipsilateral side, some devices may be gently balloon dilated at the proximal sealing site, each connection site, and the distal sealing, although this is not always indicated.

Completion and Closure

Completion angiogram is performed to look for proper placement of the endograft, endoleaks, and other complications including occlusion of essential branches, extravasation caused by rupture of the iliac artery, and kinking of unsupported segments of the iliac limbs. The latter may be performed with stiff wires replaced with soft catheters if there is high suspicion for kinking in ecstatic iliac arteries. Longer runs with slow frame rates may be helpful to evaluate endoleaks accurately. Usually, large types I and III endoleaks are treated at the initial procedure (FIGURE 57.4), whereas type II endoleaks are observed. After satisfactory completion of the arteriography, the sheath is removed and the arteriotomy closed with a preclosure device or direct suture.

▌ COMPLICATIONS

Access Site

Complications related to the access are most common for this procedure. If at any time during or after the procedure, there is a sudden drop of blood pressure or tachycardia, this should prompt suspicion and imaging to identify the arterial injury while preparing to place an occlusion balloon and repair of the damaged access artery. When a preclose technique is used, conversion to a cut-down of the femoral artery is necessary when hemostasis is inadequate or distal pulses are lost. When open cut-down is used, careful closure of the femoral artery is necessary. Often an endarterectomy or a patch closure is required to address the frequent severe atherosclerotic changes in the femoral artery. Wound closure should be meticulous to reduce the risks of lymphatic leaks, hematoma, and infection. Distal embolization to the lower extremities may occur with manipulation in the diseased aortoiliac system. Careful evaluation of the distal pulses preoperatively is necessary to precisely identify and adequately address this complication. If there are significant reductions of the distal pulses or pressures, intraoperative

angiography and therapeutic intervention should be performed immediately.

Endoleak

Endoleak is defined as a persistent flow into the aneurysm sac outside the stent-graft. There are four main types of endoleaks depending on the sources and mechanisms.

Type I

Type I endoleak is an endoleak into the aneurysm sac from around the proximal or distal end of the graft. It typically occurs when an adverse or even off-label anatomy is treated and there is incomplete sealing of the proximal implantation site and persistent flow between the graft and arterial wall causes AAA pressurization. A persistent type I endoleak needs to be treated because it may cause continuous expansion of the aneurysm. Aortic balloon angioplasty, additional aortic cuff placement, or bare metal stent placement may be performed (FIGURES 57.4 A and B). Occasionally, this complication may occur later from graft migration, particularly when older devices without positive fixation were used. Rarely, late neck dilation will lead to a late type I endoleak.

Type II

Type II endoleak is an endoleak from the smaller branches into the aneurysm. Lumbar arteries, an inferior mesenteric artery, a middle sacral artery, or an aberrant renal artery are typically the source and outflow of this endoleak. Most of these leaks seal spontaneously. If there is a sac enlargement caused by a persistent endoleak, embolization of the branches through a superselective catheterization or a translumbar approach may be performed (FIGURES 57.5 A, B).

Type III

Type III endoleak is an endoleak from the connection of the component or fabric tear of the stent-graft. These endoleaks are typically treated by the placement of an additional stent-graft.

Type IV

Type IV endoleak is an endoleak from the graft fabric without any signs of tear or erosion. This also is called as "endotension." This usually happens when the graft material is highly porous. This endoleak typically is observed without any intervention.

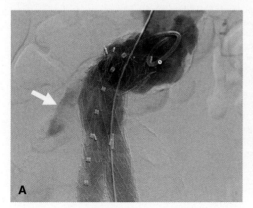
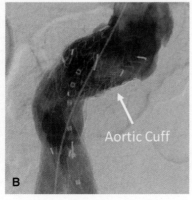

FIGURE 57.4 A. Type I endoleak. **B.** Aortic cuff placement for type I endoleak.

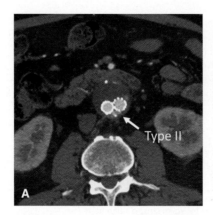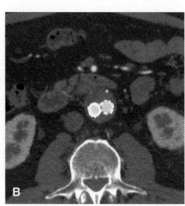

FIGURE 57.5 A. Type II endoleak at 1-month follow-up. **B.** Sealing of type II endoleak at 6-month follow-up.

Migration

Distal migration of the device is a serious complication of EVAR because it may not be detected by slow sac enlargement, and it may be missed if serial imaging is not compared to baseline after initial placement. Migration is defined as greater than or equal to 10-mm movement of the device or any endograft displacement associated with new symptoms, an endoleak, or requiring a secondary procedure,[27,28] Migration often causes acute type I or III endoleaks and is a significant contributor to late rupture after EVAR.

Others

Graft limb occlusion is typically seen as an acute complication and seems to occur in very small calcified vessels and in large ecstatic vessels with unsupported iliac limbs. Metal fatigue fracture is also a risk for stent-grafts. Because regulatory trials of each device are poorly powered to detect fracture and other late device failure modes, postmarketing surveillance is of particular importance to identify these rare complications.[29] Air embolism, proximal aortic and cardiac perforations caused by guide wires, radiation injuries, contrast allergy, and contrast nephrotoxicity are additional complications prevented and managed with standard interventional techniques.

▌ POSTPROCEDURAL MONITORING ALGORITHMS

Initially, frequent follow-up with imaging study is generally required after EVAR.[30] This included contrast-enhanced CT follow-up at 1 month, 6 months, 12 months, and yearly after EVAR. More recently, longer intervals are being used for EVAR with proven late data and long attained seal zones. Some are substituting duplex ultrasound or noncontrast volumetric analysis for some intervals.[31]

▌ CONCLUSION

Since the first human placement of the endovascular stent-graft in the1980s, EVAR has evolved with improved deployment systems and modified implants. It has now become a preferred option for aneurysm repair when anatomy is favorable. Continuation of device innovation and accumulation of clinical evidence will further define the future of endovascular repair of AAA.

▌ REFERENCES

1. Parodi JC, Palmaz JC, Barone HD. Transfemoral intraluminal graft implantation for abdominal aortic aneurysms. *Ann Vasc Surg* 1991;5:491–499.
2. Hill JS, McPhee JT, Messina LM, et al. Regionalization of abdominal aortic aneurysm repair: evidence of a shift to high-volume centers in the endovascular era. *J Vasc Surg* 2008;48:29–36.
3. Kent KC. Endovascular aneurysm repair—is it durable? *N Engl J Med* 2010;362:1930–1931.
4. Greenhalgh RM, Brown LC, Kwong GP, et al. Comparison of endovascular aneurysm repair with open repair in patients with abdominal aortic aneurysm (EVAR trial 1), 30-day operative mortality results: randomised controlled trial. *Lancet* 2004;364:843–848.
5. Prinssen M, Verhoeven EL, Buth J, et al. A randomized trial comparing conventional and endovascular repair of abdominal aortic aneurysms. *N Engl J Med* 2004;351:1607–1618.
6. Lederle FA, Freischlag JA, Kyriakides TC, et al. Outcomes following endovascular vs open repair of abdominal aortic aneurysm: a randomized trial. *JAMA* 2009;302:1535–1542.
7. Johnston KW, Rutherford RB, Tilson MD, et al. Suggested standards for reporting on arterial aneurysms. Subcommittee on Reporting Standards for Arterial Aneurysms, Ad Hoc Committee on Reporting Standards, Society for Vascular Surgery and North American Chapter, International Society for Cardiovascular Surgery. *J Vasc Surg* 1991;13:452–458.
8. Lederle FA, Johnson GR, Wilson SE, et al. Relationship of age, gender, race, and body size to infrarenal aortic diameter. The Aneurysm Detection and Management (ADAM) Veterans Affairs Cooperative Study Investigators. *J Vasc Surg* 1997;26:595–601.
9. Back MR, Bandyk M, Bradner M, et al. Critical analysis of outcome determinants affecting repair of intact aneurysms involving the visceral aorta. *Ann Vasc Surg* 2005;19:648–656.
10. Olsen PS, Schroeder T, Agerskov K, et al. Surgery for abdominal aortic aneurysms. A survey of 656 patients. *J Cardiovasc Surg (Torino)* 1991;32:636–642.
11. Brunkwall J, Hauksson H, Bengtsson H, et al. Solitary aneurysms of the iliac arterial system: An estimate of their frequency of occurrence. *J Vasc Surg* 1989;10:381–384.
12. Dent TL, Lindenauer SM, Ernst CB, et al. Multiple arteriosclerotic arterial aneurysms. *Arch Surg* 1972;105:338–344.
13. Brewster DC, Cronenwett JL, Hallett JW Jr., et al. Guidelines for the treatment of abdominal aortic aneurysms. Report of a subcommittee of the Joint Council of the American Association for Vascular Surgery and Society for Vascular Surgery. *J Vasc Surg* 2003;37:1106–1117.
14. Cao P, De Rango P, Verzini F, et al. Comparison of surveillance versus aortic endografting for small aneurysm repair (CAESAR): results from a randomised trial. *Eur J Vasc Endovasc Surg* 2011;41:13–25.
15. Lederle FA, Wilson SE, Johnson GR, et al. Immediate repair compared with surveillance of small abdominal aortic aneurysms. *N Engl J Med* 2002;346:1437–1444.
16. U.S. Food and Drug Administration. Excluder™ bifurcated endoprosthesis - P020004. Retrieved from *http://www.fda.gov/MedicalDevices/ ProductsandMedicalProcedures/DeviceApprovalsandClearances/Recently-ApprovedDevices/ucm083074.htm*

17. U.S. Food and Drug Administration. Zenith® AAA endovascular graft - P020018. Retrieved from *http://www.fda.gov/MedicalDevices/ProductsandMedicalProcedures/DeviceApprovalsandClearances/Recently-Approved-Devices/ucm082436.htm*

18. Bos WT, Tielliu IF, Zeebregts CJ, et al. Results of endovascular abdominal aortic aneurysm repair with the Zenith stent-graft. *Eur J Vasc Endovasc Surg* 2008;36:653–660.

19. Forbes TL, Harris JR, Lawlor DK, et al. Midterm results of the Zenith endograft in relation to neck length. *Ann Vasc Surg* 2010;24:859–862.

20. U.S. Food and Drug Administration. Endurant stent graft system - P100021. Retrieved from *http://www.fda.gov/MedicalDevices/ProductsandMedicalProcedures/DeviceApprovalsandClearances/Recently-ApprovedDevices/ucm240094.htm*

21. Makaroun MS, Tuchek M, Massop D, et al. One year outcomes of the United States regulatory trial of the Endurant stent graft system. *J Vasc Surg* 2011;54:601–608, e601.

22. Bockler D, Fitridge R, Wolf Y, et al. Rationale and design of the Endurant stent graft natural selection global postmarket registry (ENGAGE): interim analysis at 30 days of the first 180 patients enrolled. *J Cardiovasc Surg (Torino)* 2010;51:481–491.

23. U.S. Food and Drug Administration. Endologix Powerlink® system - P040002. Retrieved from *http://www.fda.gov/MedicalDevices/ProductsandMedicalProcedures/DeviceApprovalsandClearances/Recently-ApprovedDevices/ucm080664.htm*

24. Coppi G, Silingardi R, Tasselli S, et al. Endovascular treatment of abdominal aortic aneurysms with the Powerlink endograft system: influence of placement on the bifurcation and use of a proximal extension on early and late outcomes. *J Vasc Surg* 2008;48:795–801.

25. Qu L, Hetzel G, Raithel D. Seven years' single center experience of Powerlink unibody bifurcated endograft for endovascular aortic aneurysm repair. *J Cardiovasc Surg (Torino)* 2007;48:13–19.

26. Krajcer Z, Gregoric I. Totally percutaneous aortic aneurysm repair: methods and outcomes using the fully integrated Intuitrak endovascular system. *J Cardiovasc Surg (Torino)* 2010;51:493–501.

27. Dawson DL, Hellinger JC, Terramani TT, et al. Iliac artery kinking with endovascular therapies: technical considerations. *J Vasc Interv Radiol* 2002;13:729–733.

28. Hovsepian DM, Hein AN, Pilgram TK, et al. Endovascular abdominal aortic aneurysm repair in 144 patients: correlation of aneurysm size, proximal aortic neck length, and procedure-related complications. *J Vasc Interv Radiol* 2001;12:1373–1382.

29. Rutherford RB, Krupski WC. Current status of open versus endovascular stent-graft repair of abdominal aortic aneurysm. *J Vasc Surg* 2004;39:1129–1139.

30. Dias NV, Riva L, Ivancev K, et al. Is there a benefit of frequent CT follow-up after EVAR? *Eur J Vasc Endovasc Surg* 2009;37:425–430.

31. Bley TA, Chase PJ, Reeder SB, et al. Endovascular abdominal aortic aneurysm repair: nonenhanced volumetric CT for follow-up. *Radiology* 2009;253:253–262.

Thoracoabdominal Aneurysms

TARA M. MASTRACCI and ROY K. GREENBERG

THORACOABDOMINAL ANEURYSM: A HISTORICAL PERSPECTIVE

The investigation and treatment of thoracoabdominal aneurysms has captivated vascular and cardiothoracic surgeons for almost a century. Although recognized as a pathologic entity much earlier, the first operative interventions were performed in the 1950s using aortic homografts and, eventually, prosthetic grafts for bypass or repair.[1-3] Advances in operative techniques have included the use of left atrial bypass first and then cardiopulmonary bypass to decrease the impact of proximal cross clamping of the aorta and make repair of proximal complex aneurysms possible.[4,5] Also, cerebral spinal fluid (CSF) drainage and attention to spinal cord perfusion have decreased the incidence of neurologic injury during and after surgery, although no single technique has been effective in completely removing this risk.[6,7] Finally, a better understanding of aortic disease has seen the treatment of individual branches instead of using carrel patch technique to reduce the risk of patch aneurysm, especially in patient populations where a connective tissue disorder is suspected. The surgical community has also come to appreciate the importance of a center's operative volume in the outcome and mortality of these repairs. Many large centers have published outcomes that are unparalleled in smaller centers' experience.[8,9] Most compelling, however, have been the reports of large administrative databases[10,11] that show poorer outcomes in low-volume centers and operative volume as a variable independently associated with mortality.

Despite the known complications and drawbacks of open surgery for thoracoabdominal aneurysm, it was the mainstay of treatment for many patients from the 1950s to present day, and thus these outcomes stand as the gold standard by which other modalities of treatment must be judged. The 30-day mortalities reported by many of the larger centers of excellence are shown in Table 58.1. The most commonly reported morbidities associated with repair of thoracoabdominal aneurysms are spinal cord injury and renal dysfunction, and their incidence is also demonstrated in Table 58.1. The incidence of renal dysfunction is a critical variable because, preoperatively, it serves as a predictor of poor outcome.[8] Spinal cord injury is a catastrophic event and is linked to a markedly decreased long-term outcome.[12] Other morbidities are less consistently reported; however, it is thought that pulmonary dysfunction is the most common complication after open thoracoabdominal repair and occurs in up to 45% of patients undergoing an intervention.[9,13,14] Myocardial infarction and cardiac events are also thought to occur, in some reports as frequently as 5% of patients undergoing repair; however, these statistics are not routinely available and many authors do not routinely test.

Table 58.1

Outcomes of Thoracoabdominal Aneurysm Repair Using Conventional Open Techniques as Reported by Centers of Excellence and Large Administrative Databases

	N	Perioperative mortality %
Jacobs et al.[13]	279	9
Safi et al.[20]	1,106	15
Schepens et al.[21]	571	9
Fehrenbacher et al.[22]	110	4
Achneck et al.[17]	130	26
Chiesa et al.[14]	178	17
Coselli et al.[9]	2,286	5
Soukiasian et al.[23]	20	15
Quinones-Baldrich[24]	47	4
Conrad et al.[16]	455	9
Kieffer et al.[25]	171	12
Kawanishi et al.[26]	92	3
Greenberg et al.[19]	372	8
Rigberg et al.[10]	1,010	19
Cowan et al.[11]	1,542	22

IMAGING FOR THORACOABDOMINAL ANEURYSM

The identification and definitive diagnosis of thoracoabdominal aneurysm has evolved as rapidly as the understanding of the disease. Early surgeons relied on plain films, capitalizing on the common calcific deposition in the wall of the aorta to provide a radiopaque marker, or the mass effect that large aneurysms would have on displacement of the carina or other intrathoracic/mediastinal structures. After clinical suspicion was put forth, angiography was historically a second-line modality; however, luminal filling and the presence of thrombus may thwart true and accurate measurements of aneurysm diameter. Indications for repair in early surgery were largely symptom based. A classification system was created by Crawford that attempted to categorize the extent of the disease (FIGURE 58.1) based on plain film and angiographic imaging. In these patients, he designated the border of the 6th rib to distinguish between group II and group III aneurysms because this is the rib commonly removed in repair of both, hence providing a permanent radiographic marker for formal classification.

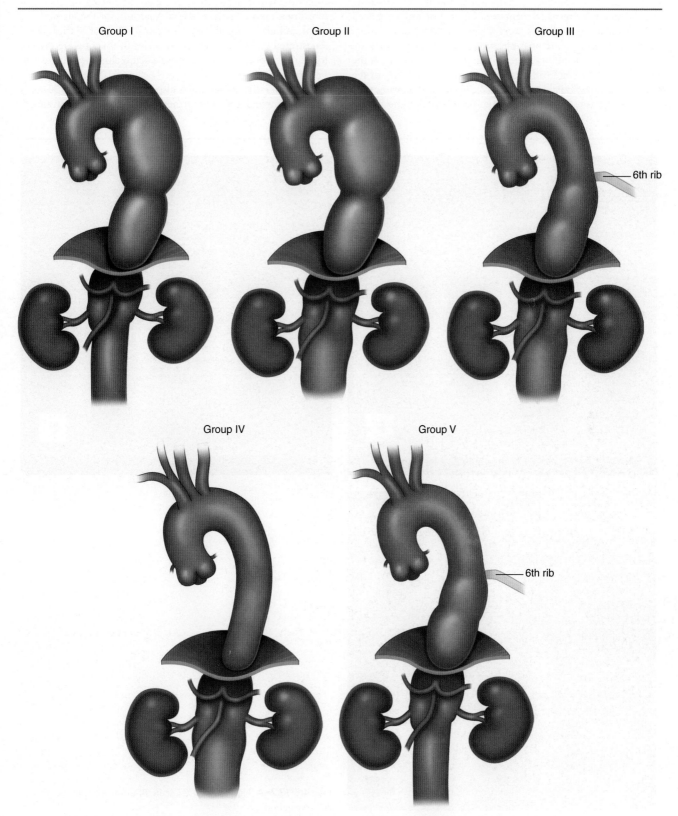

FIGURE 58.1 Crawford classification of thoracoabdominal aneurysms. This figure is "adapted from" reference 35.

With the advent of cross-sectional imaging, the anatomy of thoracoabdominal aneurysm was much more clear and accurate surveillance could be undertaken. Initially, computed tomographic (CT) imaging provided only axial views, making three-dimensional interpretation challenging, and often providing skewed diameter measurements. As CT technology advanced and isovoxel DICOM data were available, three-dimensional reconstruction became possible, and postprocessing software then provided the ability to manipulate and interact with the images so that a better understanding of the complexity of the disease was now available (FIGURE 58.2). The postprocessing software server has now become an irreplaceable tool in the thither

of vascular and cardiovascular surgeons. Multiplanar reconstructions and algorithms calculating center line of flow (CLF) is the final and important advance in preoperative thoracoabdominal aneurysm imaging. Moving from conventional open surgery to endovascular modalities, using a CLF allows for precision in estimating the relative branch anatomy for the visceral segment and allows for the planning and sizing of branched and fenestrated endografts. These advances in imaging are integral to the development of new endovascular techniques that require precise imaging (FIGURE 58.3).

Intraoperative imaging has also evolved in the last 50 years. Whereas angiography was formerly the only modality available,

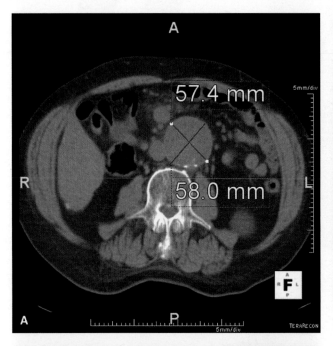

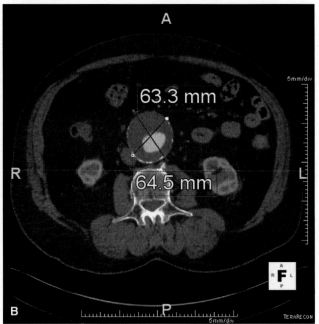

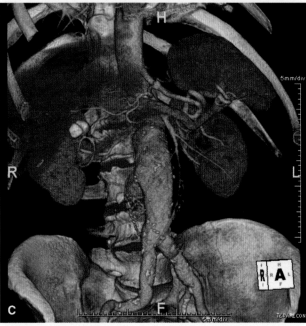

FIGURE 58.2 A. Noncontrast CT scan. **B.** Contrast scan. **C.** 3D reconstruction.

current surgeons have a much broader choice.[15] Both cone beam CT (CBCT) and intravascular ultrasound (IVUS) have expanded in the treatment of complex aneurysms.

The use of CBCT in the operating room both expands the scope of diagnostic media available to the surgeon and allows for use of fusion techniques to minimize radiation dose during complex aneurysm repair. CBCT can be fused with three-dimensional renderings of preoperative multidetector computed tomography (MDCT) scans to assist in the localization of branch vessels during repair (FIGURE 58.4).[15] This allows the surgeon to cannulate branch vessels without angiography, which results in a substantial reduction in the amount of contrast required (94 cc [95% confidence interval 72 to 131cc], vs. 136 cc [95% confidence interval 72 to 131cc],) in one series comparing 40 contemporary patients with interventions conducted in a modern hybrid endovascular suite versus recent historical controls. There was also a nonstatistically significant trend toward lower operative times and shorter fluoro times with the use of fusion imaging. As these techniques are refined, the ability to predict the behavior of branch vessels to wire or stent placement may further decrease the need for real-time fluoroscopy, increasing the safety of the procedure and making previously impossible interventions a reality.

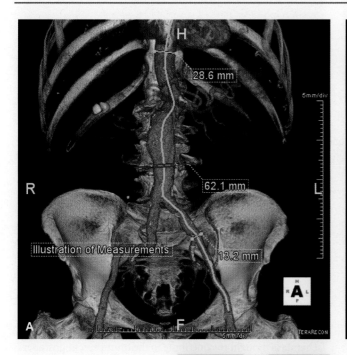

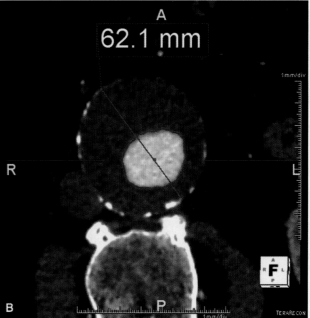

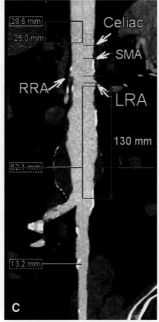

FIGURE 58.3 A. Depiction of centre line of flow (CLF) vector superimposed on 3D image; **B.** Perpendicular image generated by CLF view, showing aneurysm diameter measurement; **C.** Stretched view of aorta using the CLF projection, demonstrating the relative anatomy of branched vessels.

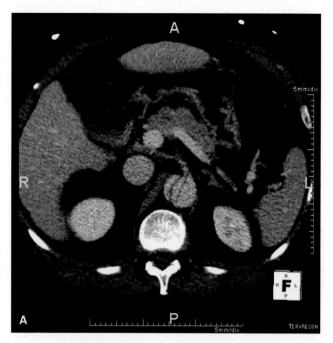
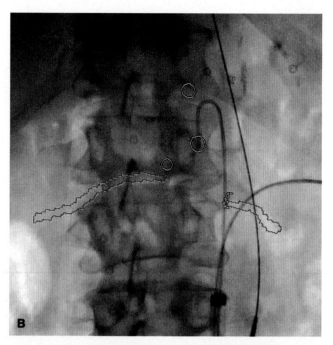

FIGURE 58.4 Fusion imaging depicting real-time fluoroscopic image with markers based on preoperative CT scans (**A**) superimposed in three dimensions. **B.** These markers aid in locating branch vessel ostia without additional contrast/angiography.

The use of IVUS has been most explored in the setting of aortic dissection. The ability to image the aortic wall, and the relative relationship of branch vessels, as well as confirm placement in the true lumen makes it another important adjunct for the aortic surgeon. Although a full description of IVUS use in aortic surgery is beyond the scope of this chapter, it is becoming clear that reduction in radiation dose for endovascular complex aneurysm repair will be a major thrust of future development of imaging modalities.

OPERATIVE MANAGEMENT: OPEN REPAIR

Conventional surgery for thoracoabdominal aneurysm was first described in the middle of the 20th century, and the techniques have only marginally improved since that time. A patient deemed fit for surgery will be brought to the operating room and placed in a left lateral position (FIGURE 58.5). A thoracoabdominal incision will be made, at the level of the sixth interspace for aneurysm with a long thoracic component, and likely in the ninth interspace for group IV thoracoabdominal aneurysms, which come to the level of the crus. Proximal and distal clamp sites are determined based on the level of aorta involved. In the modern era, atriofemoral bypass or full cardiopulmonary bypass is used to maintain perfusion to distal territories as the proximal anastomoses are performed. Commonly, when the aneurysm spans the intercostal vessels from T6 to T12, a patch will be fashioned and sewn separately to the graft to maintain blood flow to these important spinal cord feeders. Depending on the age of the patient, and the presence of connective tissue disease, visceral vessels will be reattached using a Carrel patch or with individual bypasses. In younger patients, where the prevalence

of connective tissue disease is greater and the expected life span is longer, the small amount of residual aortic tissue that remains with a Carrel patch technique may lead to the development of patch aneurysms, which would favor an alternate approach in this group. Once the distal anastomosis is completed, the process of restoring normal coagulation function is undertaken—usually with the use of supplemental blood products. The large incision leads to hypothermia and this combined with hepatic ischemia is thought to contribute to the omnipresent postoperative coagulopathy commonly seen after extensive aortic repair. Patients are recovered in an intensive care unit with a spinal drain in situ for at least 48 hours after the procedure.

OPERATIVE MANAGEMENT: ENDOVASCULAR REPAIR

Endovascular repair of thoracoabdominal aneurysms requires the custom design of a fenestrated or branched endograft prior to the repair. Using CLF measurements, the relative anatomy for branch vessels is determined, and a device is designed to appropriately fit the patient's anatomy. In the current market, there is a single manufacturer of custom endografts (Cook Zenith, Inc. Bloomington, Indiana) and the production of products globally occurs in Australia. There are two different iterations of branch devices for thoracoabdominal aneurysms available (FIGURE 58.6). This leads to a manufacturing delay for repair of aneurysms using endovascular techniques.

Once the device is constructed, the patient is brought to the operating room and, again, a spinal drain is placed. Common femoral arteries are exposed, as is the brachial or axillary artery in cases where branches require access in an antegrade

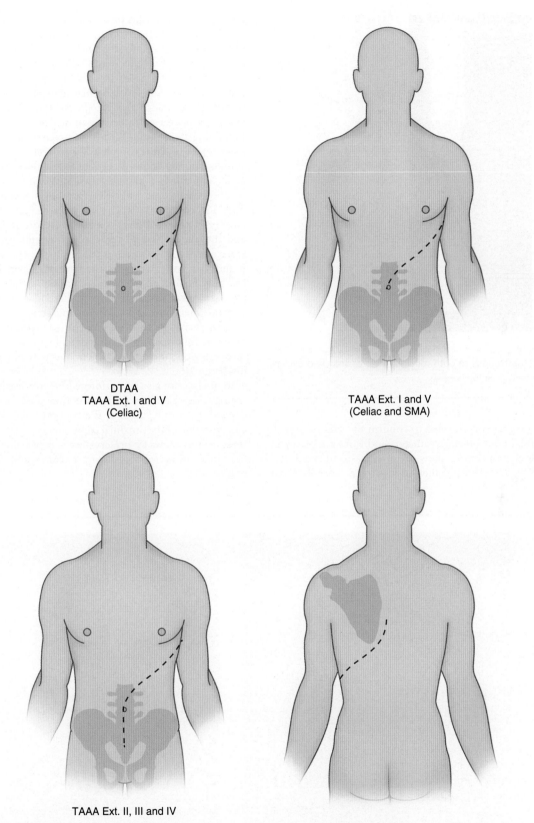

DTAA
TAAA Ext. I and V
(Celiac)

TAAA Ext. I and V
(Celiac and SMA)

TAAA Ext. II, III and IV

FIGURE 58.5 Depiction of Incisional placement for open thoracoabdominal aneurysm repair.
DTAA (Descending thoracic aortic aneurysm)

Redrawn from Townsend CM Jr, Beauchamp RD, Evers BM, et al. *Sabiston Textbook of Surgery: The Biological Basis of Modern Surgical Practice.* 18th ed. Philadelphia, PA: Saunders/Elsevier; 2007.

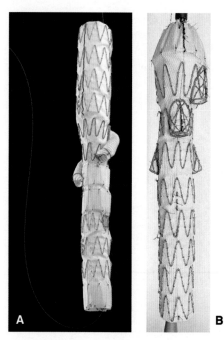

FIGURE 58.6 Thoracoabdominal branched devices. **A.** Helical device with fenestrations to both renal arteries. **B.** Branched devices with branches for all four vessels.

fashion. Imaging is performed to confirm the sites of branch vessels, and, in our practice, catheters and wires are placed in at least three branches to allow for orientation of the device (FIGURE 58.7). The device is then inserted and, once oriented

appropriately, is unsheathed to allow cannulation of fenestration/branches and then subsequent branch vessels (FIGURE 58.7). Once access is gained to all branches from within the graft, the constraining wires reducing the diameter of the graft are released, as are the trigger wires holding the graft to the delivery system (FIGURE 58.8). Small branch stent-grafts are then placed in each of the branch vessels to bridge to the main body of the device (FIGURE 58.9). In the case of helical branched graft, self-expanding stents are placed from brachial access in the arm. After this segment is completed, proximal or distal bifurcated components are added according to the anatomy of the aneurysm. Sometimes, if branch vessels have a great deal of tortuosity, they are bridged with self-expanding stents to increase the durability of repair (FIGURE 58.10). Once the catheters and wires have been removed from the aorta, arteriotomies are closed, and the patient is also returned to the intensive care unit. Once again, a spinal drain is left in situ for 48 hours. We have found that, for extensive aortic coverage, coagulopathies can also develop for endovascular repair despite the small incisions and lack of aortic cross clamping. Careful attention is paid to patients' metabolic and hemodynamic status in the first hours after surgery to be sure this is corrected expeditiously. The patients are followed with CT angiography to ensure the integrity of the devices, the first of which is usually obtained prior to discharge (FIGURE 58.11).

Branches can also be performed for hypogastic or iliac pathology. There are two different devices used for this purpose, depending on the length of the common iliac artery and the configuration of the proximal components (FIGURE 58.12). Use of these devices allows for preservation of pelvic blood flow, which has ramifications for spinal cord outcomes and patient quality of life (FIGURE 58.13).

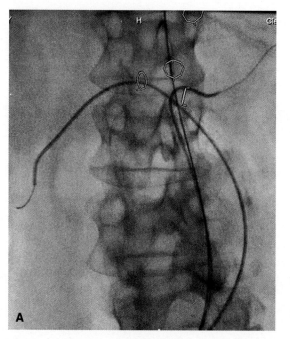
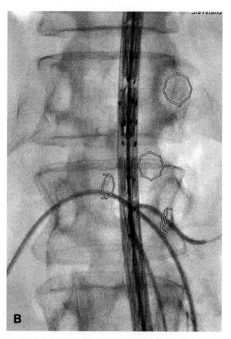

FIGURE 58.7 Succession of fenestrated repair. **A.** Cannulation of branch vessels to provide fixed markers for orientation. **B.** Placement of the undeployed device into the aorta with orientation at the level of the fixed markers. **C.** Unsheathing of the device. **D.** Access to renal arteries through fenestrations.

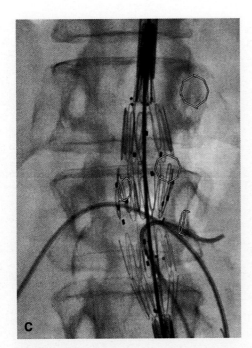
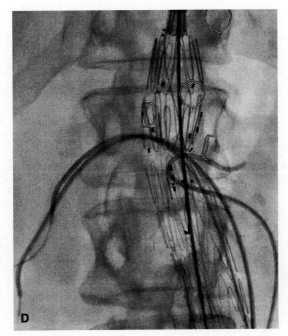

FIGURE 58.7 *(Continued)*

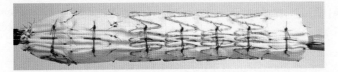

FIGURE 58.8 Posterior constraining wires on fenestrated and branched main bodies allow for manipulation of the device within the aorta after unsheathing.

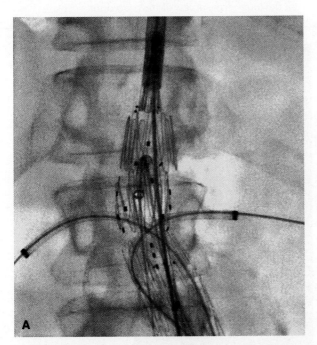
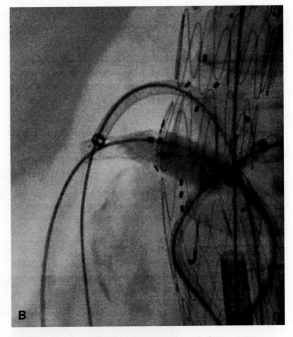

FIGURE 58.9 Branched stents. **A.** Placement of sheaths into renals/superior mesenteric artery through fenestrations. **B.** Deployment of balloon-expandable stent-grafts into branches to complete repair. **C.** Completion angiography of fenestrated stent-graft. *(continued)*

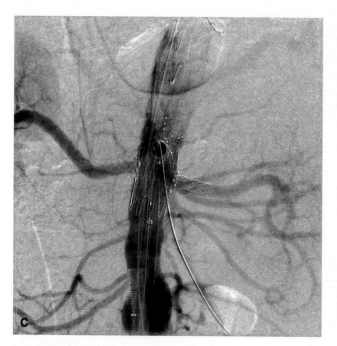

FIGURE 58.9 *(Continued)*

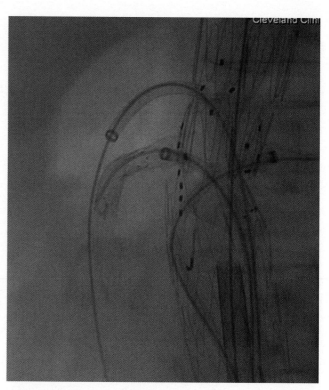

FIGURE 58.10 Kink in right renal artery, which is bridged with an uncovered self-expanding stent to prevent long-term intimal hyperplasia.

THORACOABDOMINAL ANEURYSMS: PUBLISHED OUTCOMES

Initial series of conventional open thoracoabdominal repair report 25% perioperative mortality,[1] and despite advances in perioperative care, some groups continue to report similar mortality rates (Table 58.1). Success of this procedure is likely linked to higher volume practices[10] because of the level of expertise required to manage the complexity of comorbidities that are often present. There is limited guidance in the literature to develop this expertise: most series focus on only mortality and spinal cord ischemia as outcomes. The rate of other complications, such as cardiac event rates, clinically significant coagulopathy, or renal insufficiency, are less often reported but have a bearing on the long-term success of the procedure.

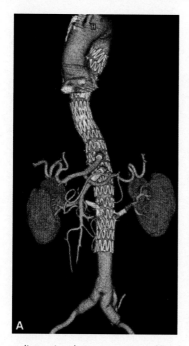
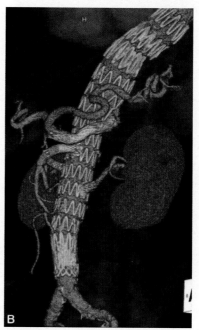

FIGURE 58.11 Three-dimensional reconstruction of implanted fenestrated (**A**) and helical (**B**) device. Note the unkinked path of the stent into the branch vessels in **B**.

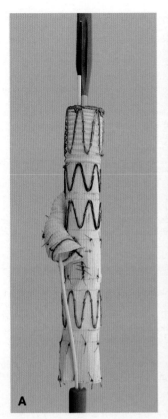
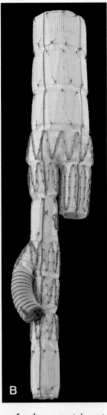

FIGURE 58.12 Helical branched devices for hypogastric arteries. **A.** The IBG device. **B.** The bifurcated-bifurcated device.

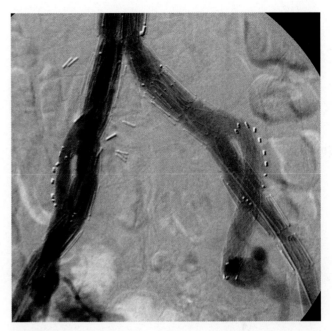

FIGURE 58.13 Completion angiogram of bilateral hypogastric branched device.

The excellence achieved by some larger centers are not likely to reflect the true efficacy of the operation: aggregate data that include outcomes from institutions with lower volume or limited expertise, such as reported by Rigberg et al.,[10] do not reflect the same perioperative success. In Rigberg's report, the elective operative mortality (30 days) was 19%, and follow-up at 1 year revealed a mortality of 31%. Other morbidity can also occur with open thoracoabdominal aortic aneurysm (TAAA) repair, including spinal cord injury (1% to 9.6%) 2 to 10, perioperative myocardial infarction (4% to 8%) 2 to 6, and clinically significant coagulopathy (2% to 14%).[9,16,17]

Complex aneurysm morphology implies that the visceral segment of the aorta is involved in the aneurysmal dilation; thus the devices needed to provide suitable exclusion from circulatory flow become more complex. Different iterations of branched devices customized to bridge aneurysmal aorta have been used.[18] Outcomes for the worldwide experience are difficult to collect because of the heterogeneity of the patient population and the variety of devices uses but are presented in Table 58.2. The Cleveland Clinic currently has the largest single center experience with treatment of TAAAs using endovascular repair worldwide. Under the specifications of an Investigational Device Exemption (IDE), these devices are only used to treat high-risk individuals who are not candidates and, thus, have been turned down for conventional open surgery. The perioperative mortality in the most recent published series is 5.7%, which compares favorably to the 8.3% perioperative mortality of a concurrent group of low-risk patients

Table 58.2

Outcomes of Branched Devices as Reported in the Literature

	30-day mortality	Median F/U (months)	Late mortality
Semmens et al.[27]	2/58 (3.4%)	16.8 (3–30)	6/58 (10.3%)
O'Neill et al.[28]	1/119 (0.8%)	19 (0–42)	15/119 (12.6%)
Muhs et al.[29]	1/30 (3.3%)	25.8 (13–39)	—
Halak et al.[30]	0/15 (0%)	20.5 (4–40)	1/15 (6.7%)
Ziegler et al.[31]	0/59 (0%)	23 (5–41)	14/63 (22%)
Scurr et al.[32]	1/45 (2.2%)	24 (1–48)	4/45 (8.8%)
Bicknell et al.[33]	0/11 (0%)	12 (9–14)	1/11 (9%)
Kristmundsson et al.[34]	2/54 (3.7%)	25 (12–32)	12/54 (22%)

treated with conventional open repair.[19] Furthermore, the rate of spinal cord ischemia was 4.3% in the endovascular group and 7.5% in the open group. No further data were available on major adverse events, either in the perioperative period or long term, because of the retrospective nature of the project. In the context of a very high-risk patient population, we are encouraged for the potential of this technology in all patients with thoracoabdominal aneurysm, but certainly more research is needed.

THE FUTURE OF THORACOABDOMINAL REPAIR

There is no question that the treatment of thoracoabdominal aneurysm disease has been revolutionized with the advent of endovascular treatment. The understanding of aortic pathology has also evolved and the current-day management is markedly different than that of only 20 years ago. As the concept of connective tissue diseases is further explored, there will soon be medical options for aneurysm treatment that may delay or even obviate intervention. Until that time, however, we will continue refining the indications for operative and endovascular repair.

REFERENCES

1. Debakey ME, Crawford ES, Garrett HE, et al. Surgical considerations in the treatment of aneurysms of the thoraco-abdominal aorta. *Ann Surg* 1965;162:650–662.
2. Creech O Jr, Debakey ME, Morris GC Jr. Aneurysm of thoracoabdominal aorta involving the celiac, superior mesenteric, and renal arteries; report of four cases treated by resection and homograft replacement. *Ann Surg* 1956;144:549–573.
3. Crawford ES, Debakey ME, Blaisdell FW. Simplified treatment of large, sacciform aortic aneurysms with patch grafts. Experiences with 5 cases. *J Thorac Cardiovasc Surg* 1961;41:479–491.
4. Weiss AJ, Lin HM, Bischoff MS, et al. A propensity score-matched comparison of deep versus mild hypothermia during thoracoabdominal aortic surgery. *J Thorac Cardiovasc Surg* 2012;143:186–193.
5. Jex RK, Schaff HV, Piehler JM, et al. Early and late results following repair of dissections of the descending thoracic aorta. *J Vasc Surg* 1986;3:226–237.
6. Safi HJ, Miller CC III, Reardon MJ, et al. Operation for acute and chronic aortic dissection: recent outcome with regard to neurologic deficit and early death. *Ann Thorac Surg* 1998;66:402–411.
7. Bischoff MS, Di LG, Griepp EB, et al. Spinal cord preservation in thoracoabdominal aneurysm repair. *Perspect Vasc Surg Endovasc Ther* 2011;23:214–222.
8. Huynh TT, van Eps RG, Miller CC III, et al. Glomerular filtration rate is superior to serum creatinine for prediction of mortality after thoracoabdominal aortic surgery. *J Vasc Surg* 2005;42:206–212.
9. Coselli JS, Bozinovski J, LeMaire SA. Open surgical repair of 2286 thoracoabdominal aortic aneurysms. *Ann Thorac Surg* 2007;83:S862–S864.
10. Rigberg DA, McGory ML, Zingmond DS, et al. Thirty-day mortality statistics underestimate the risk of repair of thoracoabdominal aortic aneurysms: a statewide experience. *J Vasc Surg* 2006;43:217–222.
11. Cowan JA Jr, Dimick JB, Henke PK, et al. Surgical treatment of intact thoracoabdominal aortic aneurysms in the United States: hospital and surgeon volume-related outcomes. *J Vasc Surg* 2003;37:1169–1174.
12. Wong DR, Coselli JS, Amerman K, et al. Delayed spinal cord deficits after thoracoabdominal aortic aneurysm repair. *Ann Thorac Surg* 2007;83:1345–1355.
13. Jacobs MJ, Mommertz G, Koeppel TA, et al. Surgical repair of thoracoabdominal aortic aneurysms. *J Cardiovasc Surg (Torino)* 2007;48:49–58.
14. Chiesa R, Marone EM, Brioschi C, et al. Open repair of pararenal aortic aneurysms: operative management, early results, and risk factor analysis. *Ann Vasc Surg* 2006;20:739–746.
15. Dijkstra ML, Eagleton MJ, Greenberg RK, et al. Intraoperative C-arm cone-beam computed tomography in fenestrated/branched aortic endografting. *J Vasc Surg* 2011;53:583–590.
16. Conrad MF, Crawford RS, Davison JK, et al. Thoracoabdominal aneurysm repair: a 20-year perspective. *Ann Thorac Surg* 2007;83:S856–S861.
17. Achneck HE, Rizzo JA, Tranquilli M, et al. Safety of thoracic aortic surgery in the present era. *Ann Thorac Surg* 2007;84:1180–1185.
18. Chuter TA, Rapp JH, Hiramoto JS, et al. Endovascular treatment of thoracoabdominal aortic aneurysms. *J Vasc Surg* 2008;47:6–16.
19. Greenberg RK, Lu Q, Roselli EE, et al. Contemporary analysis of descending thoracic and thoracoabdominal aneurysm repair: a comparison of endovascular and open techniques. *Circulation* 2008;118:808–817.
20. Safi HJ, Estrera AL, Azizzadeh A, et al. Progress and future challenges in thoracoabdominal aortic aneurysm management. *World J Surg* 2008;32:355–360.
21. Schepens MA, Kelder JC, Morshuis WJ, et al. Long-term follow-up after thoracoabdominal aortic aneurysm repair. *Ann Thorac Surg* 2007;83:S851–S855.
22. Fehrenbacher J, Siderys H, Shahriari A. Preservation of renal function utilizing hypothermic circulatory arrest in the treatment of distal thoracoabdominal aneurysms (types III and IV). *Ann Vasc Surg* 2007;21:204–207.
23. Soukiasian HJ, Raissi SS, Kleisli T, et al. Total circulatory arrest for the replacement of the descending and thoracoabdominal aorta. *Arch Surg* 2005;140:394–398.
24. Quinones-Baldrich WJ. Descending thoracic and thoracoabdominal aortic aneurysm repair: 15-year results using a uniform approach. *Ann Vasc Surg* 2004;18:335–342.
25. Kieffer E, Chiche L, Godet G, et al. Type IV thoracoabdominal aneurysm repair: predictors of postoperative mortality, spinal cord injury, and acute intestinal ischemia. *Ann Vasc Surg* 2008;22:822–828.
26. Kawanishi Y, Okada K, Matsumori M, et al. Influence of perioperative hemodynamics on spinal cord ischemia in thoracoabdominal aortic repair. *Ann Thorac Surg* 2007;84:488–492.
27. Semmens JB, Lawrence-Brown MM, Hartley DE, et al. Outcomes of fenestrated endografts in the treatment of abdominal aortic aneurysm in Western Australia (1997–2004). *J Endovasc Ther* 2006;13:320–329.
28. O'Neill S, Greenberg RK, Haddad F, et al. A prospective analysis of fenestrated endovascular grafting: intermediate-term outcomes. *Eur J Vasc Endovasc Surg* 2006;32:115–123.
29. Muhs BE, Verhoeven EL, Zeebregts CJ, et al. Mid-term results of endovascular aneurysm repair with branched and fenestrated endografts. *J Vasc Surg* 2006;44:9–15.
30. Halak M, Goodman MA, Baker SR. The fate of target visceral vessels after fenestrated endovascular aortic repair—general considerations and mid-term results. *Eur J Vasc Endovasc Surg* 2006;32:124–128.
31. Ziegler P, Avgerinos ED, Umscheid T, et al. Branched iliac bifurcation: 6 years experience with endovascular preservation of internal iliac artery flow. *J Vasc Surg* 2007;46:204–210.
32. Scurr JR, Brennan JA, Gilling-Smith GL, et al. Fenestrated endovascular repair for juxtarenal aortic aneurysm. *Br J Surg* 2008;95:326–332.
33. Bicknell CD, Cheshire NJ, Riga CV, et al. Treatment of complex aneurysmal disease with fenestrated and branched stent grafts. *Eur J Vasc Endovasc Surg* 2009;37:175–181.
34. Kristmundsson T, Sonesson B, Malina M, et al. Fenestrated endovascular repair for juxtarenal aortic pathology. *J Vasc Surg* 2009;49:568–574.
35. Crawford ES, Crawford JL, Safi HJ, et al. Thoracoabdominal aortic aneurysms: preoperative and intraoperative factors determining immediate and long-term results of operations in 605 patients. *J Vasc Surg* 1986;3(3):389–404.

Renal Aneurysms

ULKU CENK TURBA, ONUR SILDIROGLU, LEANNE DORÉ LESSLEY, MICHAEL D. DAKE, and ALAN H. MATSUMOTO

INTRODUCTION

Renal arterial aneurysms (RAA) can be divided into two major categories: true RAA and renal pseudoaneurysms (RPA). With a true RAA, all three layers of the arterial wall are intact, whereas with RPAs, there may be absence of one or more layers of arterial wall, or, in some instances, the blood is contained by the surrounding tissues. Most RAAs are degenerative in etiology due to a deficiency of the arterial media with loss of elastic fibers and smooth muscle. Atherosclerosis, fibromuscular dysplasia (FMD), segmental medial arteriopathy, and collagen disorders are other common causes of RAAs. Pseudoaneurysms most often develop secondary to trauma, but an infection, FMD, or a vasculitis can be a cause.[1,2] True RAAs may be further classified into four subgroups: saccular (70%), fusiform (22%), dissecting (7%), or mixed (<1%) (FIGURE 59.1).[3,4]

INCIDENCE AND NATURAL HISTORY

RAAs are discovered during 0.3% to 0.7% of autopsies and in as many as 1% of renal arteriographic procedures.[3] RAAs have a female predilection in many studies[2]; however, RAAs in women tend to be treated more aggressively, which may bias some of these reports because other studies have suggested no gender differences in the incidence of RAAs.[3] The right renal artery (60% to 65%) appears to be affected more often than the left.[3,5] Most RAAs have noncalcified walls and are saccular in shape and are located extraparenchymally at renal artery branch points.[2,3,6]

Most RAAs and RPAs are asymptomatic (55%); however, patients with RAAs or RPAs could present with flank pain, hypertension, hematuria, a retroperitoneal hematoma, distal renovascular emboli, thrombosis, rupture, an arteriovenous fistula (AVF), and renal ischemia and/or infarction.[7]

The natural history of an RAA is poorly understood. A 10-year experience involving 36,656 autopsies, including most of the sudden deaths from southern Sweden, showed no cases of ruptured RAAs.[3] In the same study, 83 RAAs were detected at the time of selective renal angiography in 8,525 patients (slightly less than a 1% incidence of RAA detection with renal angiography). These patients were asymptomatic and 83% (69 of 83) of them were managed conservatively without the development of symptoms at a mean follow-up of 4.3 years. Of the 14 patients who underwent surgery, 7 had hypertension and the remaining 7 patients were asymptomatic.[3] In another series from a New York City hospital involving 19,600 autopsies, there were no cases of RAA ruptures.[8] During the same time period at that hospital, there were 180,000 term pregnancies and childbirths. If the incidence of an RAA is about 0.1% to 1.0%, then by extrapolation, an occurrence of 18 to 180 patients would have been expected to have an RAA, yet none of the 180,000 women

experienced rupture of an RAA.[8] In a report by Hageman et al.,[9] 36 patients with RAAs were followed. In 25 patients, the RAAs were less than 2 cm in diameter and at a mean follow-up of 8 years, no adverse sequelae had occurred. In eight of the patients, serial angiograms were performed for at least 5 years with no change in size of the RAA seen. Hidai et al.[10] reviewed 43 cases of RAA ruptures. Of the 43 patients, 35 (81.4%) were female and 18 were pregnant at the time of RAA rupture. Three of the RAAs were less than 15 mm in diameter, whereas 70% of the ruptures were with RAAs that were greater than 3 cm in diameter. All but 1 of these 43 patients survived. In summary, the natural history of an RAA is not clearly defined. The literature would suggest that although rupture can occur in an RAA less than 2 cm in diameter, it is very rare in a nonpregnant patient. Mortality from rupture of an RAA is not common, but pregnant patients who present with a ruptured RAA may be at greatest risk for a bad outcome. Most RAAs that are less than 2 cm in diameter will remain stable in size and are unlikely to enlarge or cause problems. Females of childbearing age with an RAA should be monitored more closely, however, and perhaps treated more aggressively.

TREATMENT

The decision of when to treat an RAA is complex and involves the evaluation of the clinical history, symptoms, and laboratory and imaging findings. In most cases of symptomatic or enlarging RAAs or RPAs, intervention is strongly entertained regardless of its size. In patients with asymptomatic RAAs, when to intervene becomes less well defined, however, because of the lack of good natural history studies. If an RAA ruptures, a retroperitoneal hemorrhage and/or an arterial to venous fistula (AVF) may result or it may be contained within the renal parenchyma as a pseudoaneurysm. Autopsy series suggest, however, that death caused by rupture of an RAA is very rare.[3,7] One exception to this general understanding is in women of childbearing age. Due to the hemodynamic, blood volume, and systemic hormonal level changes that occur during pregnancy, the risk of rupture of all visceral aneurysms increases, even at smaller size diameters.[7,10]

The American College of Cardiology/American Heart Association consensus guidelines suggest that once a visceral aneurysm is greater than 2 cm in diameter, including an RAA, there should be strong consideration for its repair even in asymptomatic patients.[11,12] This recommendation is less well defined for RAAs, however, unless the patient is a woman of childbearing age. In general, stability in RAA size for several years, the absence of symptoms, and an intraparenchymal location of the RAA may obviate the need for aggressive therapy and allow for a more conservative course of observation.[3,8,10] In most instances,

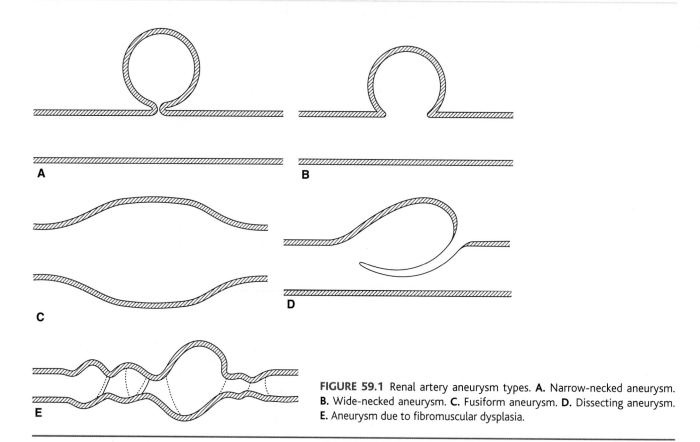

FIGURE 59.1 Renal artery aneurysm types. **A.** Narrow-necked aneurysm. **B.** Wide-necked aneurysm. **C.** Fusiform aneurysm. **D.** Dissecting aneurysm. **E.** Aneurysm due to fibromuscular dysplasia.

RPAs that are the result of traumatic or iatrogenic etiologies are typically treated regardless of their size.

RAAs can be repaired by either surgical or endovascular techniques and, on occasion, by using a combination of the two approaches. The type of aneurysm and the anatomic location of the RAA or RPA usually will dictate which endovascular or surgical technique can be employed in its treatment (FIGURE 59.2).

ENDOVASCULAR TREATMENT OPTIONS

Historically, the treatment of an RAA was surgical, including an aneurysmectomy, ex vivo repair of the RAA and kidney with reimplantation of the kidney, direct repair of the affected segmental artery, exclusion of the aneurysm with a bypass graft, or partial or complete nephrectomy.[7] Open surgery for RAA repair is associated with higher morbidity and a greater risk of parenchymal loss. The availability of a wider variety of devices has resulted in endovascular treatment being a more viable therapeutic option in a broader array of RAA cases. Therefore, when possible, endovascular techniques should be employed as the first line of therapy for RAAs or RPAs. The specific choice of endovascular treatment will depend on the type and anatomy of the RAA or RPA. In a report by Henke et al.[7] involving 185 angiographically demonstrated RAAs, the most common aneurysm location was at the renal artery bifurcation (60%), followed by the distal renal arterial branches and the main renal artery. Most of the RAAs were noncalcified (63 %) and saccular (79%).

If an RAA or RPA is saccular or fusiform in shape but involves the main renal artery without involvement of any branches, exclusion of the RAA or RPA can be best accomplished with a covered stent (FIGURE 59.3). If a saccular RAA has branches originating from its aneurysmal sac, it may be best to embolize the aneurysm sac itself with coils, including its parent artery, while preserving the main renal artery and its other branches. If the RAA is fusiform and involves only a small arterial branch that provides perfusion to a minimum amount of renal parenchyma, the RAA and its parent artery can also be completely occluded with embolization materials. A saccular RPA can be treated with off-label use of thrombin (Gentrac, Middleton, WI), which can be injected into the RPA, if the flow in the parent artery can be balloon occluded to minimize spilling of the thrombin into the parent or downstream branch arteries. Additionally, direct puncture embolization of an RPA can be performed using thrombin or cyanoacrylate glue (Trufil, Cordis Endovascular, Warrenton, NJ).

Dissecting aneurysms or pseudoaneurysms of the main renal artery are best treated with covered stents (used in an off-label application). Covered stents have the advantage of completely excluding the neck of the aneurysm, but it requires good preprocedural planning and the availability of good landing zones for the stent. On occasion, complex RAAs that involve the hilum of the kidney can be treated using a combination of stents and coils to preserve the key segmental arterial branches while excluding the RAA (FIGURE 59.4).

TECHNICAL AND DEVICE CONSIDERATIONS

The endovascular approach and type of devices used for treating an RAA will vary significantly depending on the location and type of RAA (FIGURE 59.5). Detailed anatomic mapping

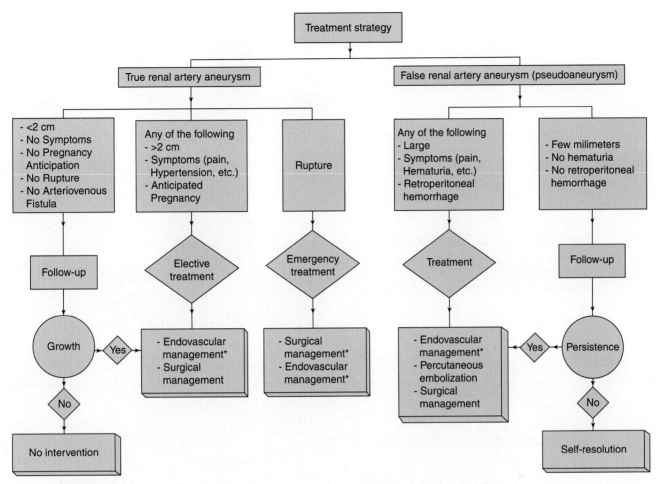

FIGURE 59.2 Current management strategies for renal artery aneurysms and pseudoaneurysms.

*Preferred Treatment

of the RAA is performed with a CT angiogram (CTA) or MR angiogram (MRA) to allow for preprocedural treatment planning. Often, subtleties that cannot be defined with cross-sectional imaging studies will have to be further delineated with catheter-based angiography. In these cases, an aortogram is obtained with a flush catheter and then selective renal arteriography is performed using a 5 French (F) cobra or RC 2 catheter (Cook Inc., Bloomington, IN) or a reverse curve catheter, such as an SOS Omni 2 (AngioDynamics, Queensbury, NY) in multiple planes using the projection that best profiles the RAA as determined from the previously reviewed CTA or MRA studies.

TREATMENT SELECTION STRATEGIES

Management decisions should be based on the indications for treatment, the anatomic characteristics of the RAA, and the patient's symptoms and age. If the patient is a female, the desire for future pregnancy will also affect the management algorithm (FIGURE 59.2). A variety of guide catheters and sheaths; microcatheters; microcoils; 0.035″, 0.014″, or 0.018″ platforms of bare metal and covered stents; and liquid embolic agents allow for the use of a wide array of technology to treat simple or complex

RAAs or RPAs. Complex cases that preclude an endovascular approach may be managed with laparoscopic nephrectomy, extracorporeal repair with autotransplantation, or complex revascularization surgery with excellent results.[13]

PLANNING THE INTERVENTIONAL PROCEDURE

Previously obtained cross-sectional imaging with CTA and MRA, especially with the review of multiplanar reformatted images, provide excellent tools to define the complexity of the lesion and plan the endovascular treatment. In addition to cross-sectional imaging, the use of three-dimensional (3D) rotational angiography or conebeam CT (DynaCT, Siemens Medical, Erlangen, Germany) in the angiographic suite are invaluable tools for helping to define the RAA anatomy and the adjacency of renal artery branches for these sometimes complex lesions.[14]

SPECIFIC INTRAPROCEDURAL TECHNIQUES

The technique used for the endovascular treatment of an RAA or RPA will be based on the anatomy of the lesion (FIGURE 59.5).

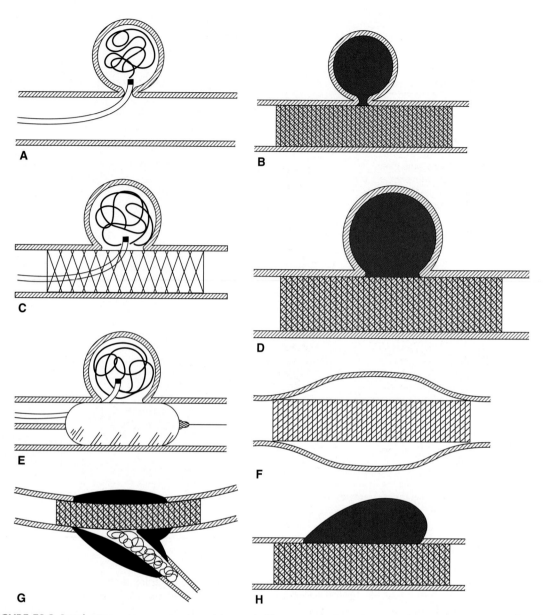

FIGURE 59.3 Renal artery aneurysm treatment types. **A.** Narrow-necked renal artery aneurysm treatment with coils. **B.** Narrow-necked renal artery aneurysm covered with renal stent. **C.** Wide-necked renal artery aneurysm treatment with coils using bare stent assistance. **D.** Wide-necked renal artery aneurysm treatment with covered stent. **E.** Wide-necked renal artery aneurysm treatment with coils using balloon assistance. **F.** Fusiform renal artery aneurysm treatment with covered stent. **G.** Fusiform renal artery aneurysm at the branching point treatment with embolization of the smaller branch and preserving the larger branch while excluding the aneurysm. **H.** Dissecting renal artery aneurysm treatment with covered stent.

Renal Arterial Aneurysm

Determination of the anatomy of the RAA is important because treatment methods will differ based on the presence, size, and number of branches entering and exiting it. Occasionally, a distal branch will need to be embolized for successful exclusion of the RAA from collateral circulation, even though most renal branches are end arteries. This type of embolization requires catheterizing the small branch via the aneurysm sac and coiling the small artery before exclusion of the RAA.

The most common type of RAA is the saccular type. It can be treated using a variety of methods depending on the location of the aneurysm and on whether the aneurysm neck is wide or narrow. Although there is no consensus regarding when the neck of a saccular RAA is considered to be wide versus narrow, a neck that is more than 4 to 5 mm is considered to be a wide-necked aneurysm.[15] The most common location of a saccular RAA is at the main renal artery bifurcation where embolization is the best method of endovascular management, especially if the aneurysm neck is narrow. Embolization of a narrow-necked saccular RAA has been consistently reported to be successful in case reports using coils and/or a combination of other embolization materials, such as thrombin, gelfoam, particles, glue,

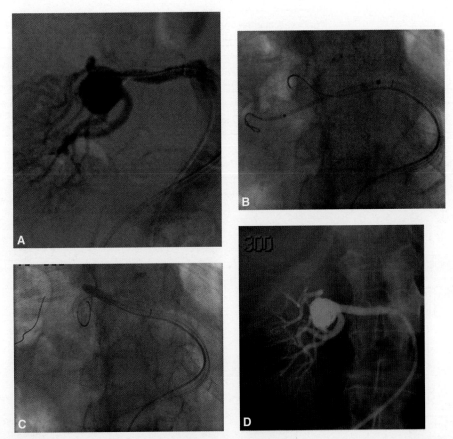

FIGURE 59.4 Complex renal artery aneurysm involving multiple renal artery branches located at the renal artery bifurcation. Coil embolization using balloon and stent assistance. **A.** Renal artery angiogram showed saccular aneurysm at the bifurcation point. Dual arterial access was gained for treatment with coils with one access, bare stent, and/or balloon assistance. **B.** Self-expanding bare stent was placed across the aneurysm neck. **C.** Following placement of a bare stent, temporary inflation of a balloon catheter was performed at the neck of the renal artery aneurysm while deploying the coils. **D.** Follow-up renal arteriogram shows complete exclusion of the saccular aneurysm while preserving the renal artery branches.

or ethanol (Table 59.1).[4,14–44] Covered stents are not advisable at bifurcations because of the potential need to exclude significant branches with the resultant sacrifice of significant renal parenchyma.

Covered stents are particularly attractive for treating saccular RAAs that involve the main renal artery in which there are adequate proximal and distal seal zones without compromising segmental branch perfusion. Covered stents are increasingly being used to treat visceral aneurysms and more and more cases are being reported (Table 59.1). In most case reports, however, follow-up is poor and long-term patency of such covered stents is unknown. Use of covered stents in distal small branches of the renal arteries is technically not feasible in most situations and embolization may be performed when the vessel occlusion will result in minimal sacrifice of renal parenchymal tissue.

Wide-necked saccular RAAs located at renal arterial bifurcations may be best treated with detachable coils. The Guglielmi Detachable Coil (GDC) (Boston Scientific Corp, Natick, MA) is an example of a detachable coil that can be used in an RAA. Several other types of detachable coils for peripheral interventions have become available. One such coil (Azur hydrocoil,

Terumo, Somerset, NJ) has hydrogel coating on the coil that undergoes limited expansion within the first 3 to 5 minutes of its deployment and fully expands to a volume four times its original volume within 20 minutes. The GDC, Azur, and a recently released 0.035″ (Boston Scientific Corp) platinum coil possess a circular memory and are available in various helical diameters and lengths. In a wide-necked RAA, detachable coils are advantageous over pushable coils because of the better control with deployment. Framing coils are specifically designed to reduce compartmentalization and provide greater coverage with a three-dimensional configuration for embolization of aneurysms. Additionally, framing coils provide stability of the system at the beginning of the embolization by conforming to the diverse morphologies of RAAs while minimizing prolapse of the coil material into the parent artery. Framing coils also provide even distribution of coil loops within the sac.

There are other maneuvers to overcome technical challenges associated with the treatment of wide-necked aneurysms. Balloon-assisted coil embolization (BACE) requires a second arterial access, which allows use of a temporary balloon catheter that can be inflated at the neck of the aneurysm and provides

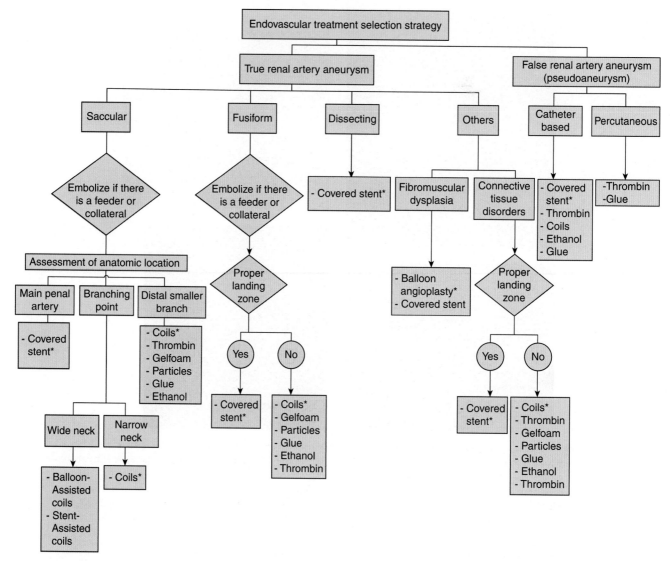

FIGURE 59.5 Endovascular strategies and techniques for treatment of renal artery aneurysms and pseudoaneurysms.

*Preferred Treatment

additional stability while embolization material is delivered into the RAA sac. BACE procedures reduce the chance of unintentional occlusion of the parent vessel by coils or other embolization materials.

Another method developed for treating wide-necked RAAs is stent-assisted coil embolization (SACE). The SACE procedure may be performed with a self-expanding bare metal stent deployed across the wide neck of the RAA so that coil embolization can be performed through the stent struts. The SACE procedure provides stability of the coil while preventing prolapse of the coil material into the parent artery, similar to the BACE procedure (FIGURE 59.4). In some cases, coils may be combined with other embolization agents, such as thrombin. For example, coils may be dipped in the thrombin to enhance thrombogenicity, or glue may be injected to fill the space in between the coils.

Management of fusiform RAAs depends on its location and the presence of branch artery involvement. Treatment choices are very similar to the decision process made with saccular aneurysms.

A dissecting RAA has different features compared to saccular or fusiform RAAs. A dissecting aneurysm is associated with intimal disruption and a weakened vessel and secondary aneurysmal dilatation. This type of aneurysm may have some compromise to the distal blood flow due to the relative stenosis created by the obstructing dissection flap. The preferred treatment for this type of lesion is a balloon expandable covered stent, which treats the aneurysm by sealing the intimal disruption while also eliminating the stenosis. If the dissecting aneurysm is chronic, calcified, and associated with a thick dissection flap and there is no landing zone for a covered stent, coil embolization may be an option just like for the saccular type of RAA.

Treatment of RAAs caused by FMD is based on the size, symptoms, and location of the RAA. The most common type of FMD is medial fibrodysplasia, and aneurysmal dilatation adjacent to areas of stenosis may be present. Treatment usually involves balloon angioplasty to disrupt the internal webs causing hemodynamic obstruction of renal blood flow. Often, the

Table 59.1

Renal Artery Aneurysm Endovascular Treatment Literature Review and Procedural Details

Study	Year	Demographics	No. of patient/lesion/treated	Rupture	AVF	Indication	Symptoms	Embolization	Location	Size (mm)	Success	Mean follow-up (months)	Complication	30-day mortality
Mali et al.[16]	1989	58/M	1/1/1	No	No	Hypertension	Headache	Stent	Right	N/A	100%	0	None	No
Routh et al.[17]	1990	79/M	1/1/1	Yes	No	Hypertension	N/A	PVA	Left	30	100%	9	None	No
Sueyoshi et al.[18]	1996	42/M	1/1/1	Yes	No	Behcet	Pain, RPH	Coils	Right	N/A	100%	0	None	Yes[a]
Bui et al.[19]	1995	50/F	1/1/1	No	No	Hypertension, FMD	N/A	Stent	Right	15	100%	12	None	No
Tateno et al.[20]	1996	76/M	1/1/1	No	No	Postoperative	Hematuria	Coils	Left	13	100%	0	None	No
Prabulos et al.[21]	1997	28/F	1/2/1	Yes	No	hypertension, pregnancy	Pain	Coils, gelfoam	Both	30	Failure	0	None	Yes[b]
Yamamoto et al.[22]	1998	51/F	1/1/1	No	No	N/A	None	Coils	Right	35	100%	2	None	No
Klein et al.[23]	1997	48/M-F	12/12/12	No	No	Hypertension	Hematuria	Coils	Both	12	100%	28	None	No
Centenera et al.[4]	1998	42/F	1/3/1	No	No	Hypertension	N/A	Coils	Left	17	100%	6	None	No
Karkos et al.[24]	2000	53/M	1/1/1	No	No	N/A	Hematuria	Coils	Left	30	100%	12	None	No
Mounayer et al.[25]	2000	69/F	1/1/1	No	No	FMD, hypertension	N/A	Coils	Right	20	100%	0	None	No
Rikimaru et al.[26]	2001	32/F	1/1/1	No	No	None	Pain	Stent	Right	32	100%	12	None	No
Tan et al.[27]	2001	51/F	1/1/1	No	No	Hypertension	N/A	Stent	Right	30	100%	3	ES	No
Schneidereit et al.[28]	2003	86/F	1/1/1	Yes	No	Hypertension, pseudogut	Pain	Stent	Right	N/A	100%	0	None	No
Dib et al.[15]	2003	31/F	1/1/1	No	No	Hypertension	N/A	Coils	Right	7	100%	12	None	No
Fiesseler et al.[29]	2004	52/M	1/1/1	Yes	Yes	None	RPH, hematuria, Pain	Coils	Right	N/A	100%	0	MI	No
Trocciola et al.[30]	2005	48/F	1/1/1	No	No	Hypertension	Pansystolic bruit	Coils	Right	13	100%	12	None	No

(continued)

Table 59.1

Renal Artery Aneurysm Endovascular Treatment Literature Review and Procedural Details (Continued)

Study	Year	Demographics	No. of patient/lesion/treated	Rupture	AVF	Indication	Symptoms	Embolization	Location	Size (mm)	Success	Mean follow-up (months)	Complication	30-day mortality
Andersen et al.[31]	2005	67/M	1/1/1	No	No	Atherosclerosis	Pain	Stent	Right	25	100%	0	None	No
Malacrida et al.[32]	2007	58/F	1/1/1	No	No	None	None	Stent	Left	20	100%	6	None	No
Degertekin et al.[33]	2006	54/F	1/1/1	No	No	Hypertension	N/A	Stent	Right	35	100%	6	None	No
Gandini et al.[34]	2006	51/M	1/2/2	No	No	CRF, Hypertension	Pain	Stent	Both	23	100%	6	None	No
Goy et al.[35]	2007	38/F	1/1/1	No	No	Marfan Hypertension	Pain	Stent, coils	Left	N/A	100%	2	None	No
Sahin et al.[36]	2007	55/F	1/1/1	No	No	Hypertension	N/A	Stent	Left	20	100%	6	None	No
Gutta et al.[37]	2008	39/M	1/1/1	No	No	None	None	Coils	Left	100	100%	18	None	No
Clark et al.[14]	2008	56/F	1/1/1	No	No	Hypertension	N/A	Stent, coils	Right	25	100%	3	None	No
Hagihara et al.[38]	2009	66/F	1/1/1	Yes	No	Sjogren,	Pain, vomiting	Coils	Left	30	100%	0	Fever	No
Altit et al.[39]	2009	60/F	1/1/1	No	Yes	SLE, FMD, Hypertension	None	Coils	Right	40	100%	9	None	No
Hobbs et al.[40]	2009	4/M	1/Mult/Mult	No	No	FMD	Nausea, vomiting	Coils, ethanol	Left	N/A	100%	3	None	No
Sciacca et al.[41]	2009	42/F	1/1/1	No	No	Hypertension, FMD	N/A	Stent	Left	25	100%	1	None	No
Xiong et al.[42]	2010	42/M	1/1/1	No	No	None	None	Stent, coils	Left	25	100%	12	IRF	No
Gumustas et al.[43]	2010	16/M	1/1/1	No	No	Hypertension	N/A	Coils	Left	25	100%	0	None	No
Meyer et al.[44]	2011	74/M	1/1/1	No	No	Hypertension	N/A	Stent	Left	26	100%	5	None	No

[a] Patient died 3 days after embolization due to pneumonia.

[b] Patient had multiple visceral aneurysms and died from splenic aneurysm rupture.

N/A, not applicable; RPH, retroperitoneal hematoma; Mult, multiple; M, male; F, female; PVA, polyvinyl alcohol; FMD, fibromuscular dysplasia; Marfan, Marfan syndrome; Sjogren, Sjogren syndrome; CRF, chronic renal failure; Behcet, Behcet disease; MI, myocardial infarction; SLE, systemic lupus erythematosus; ES, embolization syndrome; IRF, impaired renal function..

areas of adjacent aneurysmal dilatation may improve following balloon angioplasty. In selected cases, however, a covered stent may be the best treatment option when an aneurysm of the main renal artery is the dominant finding.

Renal Pseudoaneurysms

RPAs may be treated in a similar fashion as renal aneurysms (FIGURE 59.6). Just like RAAs, a variety of endovascular methods may be employed (Table 59.2).[45–82] If the RPA is large and an endovascular treatment option is technically not possible, percutaneous needle puncture under CT or ultrasound (US) guidance can be performed with direct RPA embolization using thrombin, gelfoam, or coils.[76,77]

ENDPOINT ASSESSMENT OF THE PROCEDURE

At the conclusion of the endovascular intervention, it is expected that the RAA or RPA is completely excluded and patency of the parent artery and distal branches is maintained. Depending on the complexity of the lesion, postintervention follow-up imaging may be need at 1, 3, and 12 months. In our experience, however, once successful occlusion of an RAA or RPA is clearly documented, recanalization of the lesion rarely occurs. Immediate postprocedure care should include monitoring for access site complications, blood pressure fluctuations, evidence for renal infarction, and renal function. It is well documented in the literature that with repair or elimination of an RAA in a patient with hypertension, the hypertension may actually improve.[9] Patients should be followed for at least 12 months to ensure exclusion of the aneurysm and persistent patency of the parent vessel. If a

stent has been employed in the treatment of the lesion, appropriate antiplatelet therapy and noninvasive follow-up of stent patency are recommended. Cross-sectional imaging follow-up with MR or CT is probably the best to show morphology of the lesion and treatment outcome; however, US imaging with Doppler is also acceptable and involves less cost and no radiation.

PROCEDURAL COMPLICATIONS AND HOW TO MANAGE THEM SUCCESSFULLY

The percutaneous endovascular treatment of an RAA or RPA is relatively safe and associated with a high technical and clinical success rate. Unlike the surgical approach, endovascular treatment obviates the need for general anesthesia in most cases and can be performed using conscience sedation. To minimize the risks associated with the use of contrast media and the hazards of radiation, careful patient preparation (i.e., hydration, pregnancy screening, etc.) and use of pulsed fluoroscopy should be performed. To reduce the risk for thrombotic complications, anticoagulation with heparin 70 international units/kg intravenously should be given during the procedure to maintain the activated clotting time (ACT) greater than 220 seconds.

During covered stent deployment, one of the most concerning complications is unintended coverage of a large-vessel branch, which would lead to distal renal infarction. To avoid this complication, preplanning with cross-sectional imaging is paramount to define the anatomy properly. Even when there is a good landing zone, stent migration or maldeployment is another potential complication that can occur.

Wide-necked RAA coil embolization could be challenging, and coil migration and/or prolapses into the parent artery

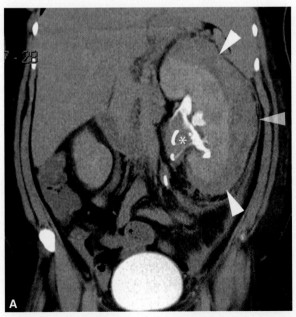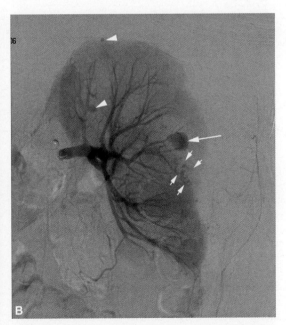

FIGURE 59.6 Treatment of a 38-year-old woman, status postneprolithototomy. **A.** CT demonstrates perirenal (*arrowheads*) and retroperitoneal hematoma. Additionally, there is some blood collection (*star*) within the renal collecting system. **B.** Selective left renal arteriogram demonstrates a large pseudoaneurysm (*long arrow*) and active hemorrhage (*small arrows*). Incidental note made of two smaller pseudoaneurysms (*arrowheads*), which were not treated. *(continued)*

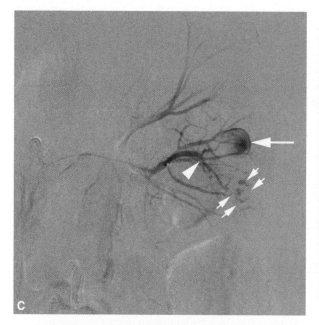

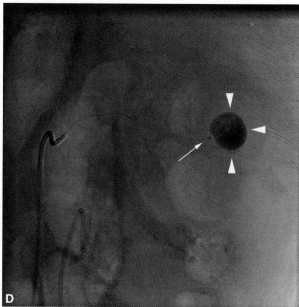

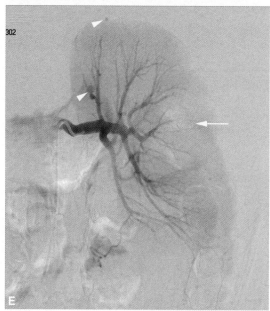

FIGURE 59.6 *(Continued)* **C.** Superselective renal arteriogram via microcatheter demonstrates pseudoaneurysm (*long arrow*) and active hemorrhage (*arrows*). Note that both pseudoaneurysm and active hemorrhage originate from the same vessel (*arrowhead*). **D.** Superselective renal arteriogram via microcatheter (arrow) at the neck of the pseudoaneurysm (*arrowheads*). **E.** Post-transcatheter coil placement; a selective left renal arteriogram demonstrates exclusion of the large pseudoaneurysm (*arrow*). Smaller pseudoaneurysms were not treated (*arrowheads*).

are possible. To avoid this complication, bare stent-assisted (through the struts) or balloon-assisted coil embolization can be performed. Additionally, detachable coils allow controlled deployment of the coil such that if a coil prolapses into the parent artery, the detachable coil may be able to be repositioned or removed easily.

One possible complication of cyanoacrylate glue (NBCA, Cordis Endovascular, Warren, NJ) use is premature polymerization of the liquid material, resulting in occlusion of the catheter lumen and/or adherence of the catheter tip to the vessel wall. To avoid this complication, timing of the catheter pull and flushing the microcatheter with dextrose 5% before the glue is delivered is important. With thrombin, the typical concentration used is approximately 500 to 2,000 units/cc. Inadvertent instillation of

thrombin into the parent artery will lead to parent vessel occlusion or distal arterial thrombosis. More recently, polyethylene vinyl alcohol (Onyx, EV3 Irvine, CA), a liquid cohesive agent, became available for use for embolization of brain arteriovenous malformations (AVMs) and has been employed in an off-label fashion for other applications, such as renal arterial lesions. In these cases, the microcatheter (i.e., Echelon, EV3) must be compatible with DMSO (dimethyl sulfoxide). DMSO is used to flush the microcatheter to prevent precipitation of the Onyx within the microcatheter.

Even though it is rare, a patient may develop a transient embolization syndrome, especially in renal infarction with ethanol, glue, or thrombin. Those patients may be managed conservatively.

Table 59.2

Renal Artery Pseudoaneurysm Literature Review and Procedural Details

Study	Year	Demographics	No. of patient/lesion/treated	Rupture	AVF	Indication	Symptoms	Embolization	Location	Size (mm)	Success	Mean follow-up (months)	Complication	30-day mortality
Chang et al.[45]	1978	45/M	1/1/1	No	No	Trauma	Hematuria	Gelfoam	Left	13	100%	8	None	No
Hall et al.[46]	1987	68/F	1/1/1	No	No	Mycotic	Hematuria	Gelfoam, coils	Right	N/A	100%	0	None	No
Steffens et al.[47]	1996	15/M	1/2/2	No	No	Trauma	Hematuria	Particles	Left	N/A	100%	36	None	No
Peh et al.[48]	1997	39/M	1/1/1	No	No	Spontaneous	RH	Coils	Right	N/A	100%	1	None	Yes[a]
Silberzweig et al.[49]	1998	41/M	1/1/1	No	No	Biopsy	Pain	PVA, coils	Left	N/A	100%	0	None	No
Miyazaki et al.[50]	1998	54/M	1/1/1	No	No	Surgery	None	Coils	A	40	100%	0	None	No
Singh et al.[51]	1998	18/F	1/1/1	No	No	PCNL	Hematuria	Ethanol	Right	N/A	100%	0	None	No
Yamakado et al.[52]	2000	54/F	1/1/1	No	No	Biopsy	RH	Coils, NBCA	N/A	N/A	100%	70	None	No
Parsons et al.[53]	2001	56/F	1/1/1	No	No	Surgery	Pain, RH	Coils	Left	N/A	100%	1	None	No
Parildar et al.[54]	2003	N/A	11/11/11	No	No	N/A	N/A	N/A	N/A	N/A	100%	N/A	N/A	No
Sharma et al.[55]	2002	61/F	1/2/2	No	No	Biopsy	Hematuria	Coils	Right	N/A	100%	0	None	No
Miller et al.[56]	2002	44/M	1/Multiple/1	No	No	Trauma	Pain, hematuria	N/A	Right	N/A	100%	3	None	No
Halachmi et al.[5]	2003	11/M	1/1/1	No	No	Trauma	Pain, hematuria	Coils	Left	10	100%	1	None	No
Nakatani et al.[58]	2003	51/F	1/1/1	No	No	Biopsy	Pain	Coils	A	20	100%	0	None	No
Cantasdemir et al.[59]	2003	32/M-F	5/5/5	No	No	Trauma	Hematuria	NBCA	Right/left/A	14	100%	12	None	No
Aston et al.[60]	2004	29/M	1/1/1	No	No	ESWL	Pain, hematuria	Coils	Left	N/A	100%	0	None	No
Giannopoulos et al.[61]	2004	25/M	1/1/1	No	No	Trauma	Pain, hematuria, RH	Coils	Left	N/A	100%	2	None	No
Singh et al.[62]	2005	59/M-F	6/6/6	No	No	Surgery	Hematuria	Coils	Right	N/A	100%	26	None	No
Saad et al.[63]	2005	11/F	1/1/1	No	No	Trauma	Pain, hematuria	Coils	Right	20	100%	0	None	No
Hidas et al.[64]	2005	63/F	1/1/1	Yes	No	Surgery	Hematuria, RH	Coils	Right	N/A	100%	0	None	No

(continued)

Table 59.2

Renal Artery Pseudoaneurysm Literature Review and Procedural Details (Continued)

Study	Year	Demographics	No. of patient/lesion/treated	Rupture	AVF	Indication	Symptoms	Embolization	Location	Size (mm)	Success	Mean follow-up (months)	Complication	30-day mortality
Lee et al.[65]	2005	52/M	1/1/1	No	No	Trauma	Pain, RH	Gelfoam	Left	N/A	100%	0	None	No
Novellas et al.[66]	2006	1/unknown	1/1/1	No	No	Biopsy	Hematuria	Coils	Right	5	100%	6	None	No
Massulo-Aguiar et al.[67]	2006	48/M	1/1/1	No	No	PCNL	Hematuria	NBCA	Right	N/A	100%	0	None	No
Cohenpour et al.[68]	2007	66/M-F	5/5/5	No	No	Surgery	Hematuria	Coils	Left	21	100%	0	None	No
Uberoi et al.[69]	2007	49/M	2/2/2	No	No	Surgery	Pain, hematuria	Coils	Left / Right	25	100%	1	None	No
Pastorin et al.[70]	2007	25/M	1/1/1	No	No	Trauma	Pain, hematuria	NBCA, coils	Left	N/A	100%	3	None	No
Gupta et al.[71]	2008	42/M	1/1/1	No	No	PCNL	Hematuria	PC-thrombin	Left	39	100%	6	None	No
Kubasiewicz et al.[72]	2008	66/F	2/2/2	No	Yes	Biopsy	Pain	Coils	Right	N/A	100%	0	None	No
Zelenak et al.[73]	2009	66/F	1/1/1	No	No	Surgery	Hematuria	Onyx	Right	N/A	100%	0	None	No
Schellhammer et al.[74]	2008	4/M-F	1/1/1	No	No	Surgery	N/A	Thrombin	Right	16	100%	0	None	No
Bozgeyik et al.[75]	2008	40/M-F	2/2/2	No	No/yes	Trauma	Pain, RH	Coil	Left / Right	20	100%	3	None	No
Lal et al.[76]	2009	43/M	1/1/0	No	No	PCNL	Hematuria	PC-NBCA	Left	9	100%	0	None	No
Sakr et al.[77]	2009	42/N/A	14/14/14	No	No	Trauma, surgery	Hematuria	PC-gelfoam	N/A	N/A	100%	8	Rebleeding	No
Mima et al.[78]	2009	37/M	1/1/1	Yes	No	Biopsy	Pain, hematuria	Coils	Left	10	100%	0	None	No
Watanabe et al.[79]	2010	19/M	1/1/1	No	No	PCNL	Hematuria	Coils	Left	42	100%	1	None	No
Schlunz-Hendann et al.[80]	2011	50/F	1/1/1	No	No	Trauma	None	Coils	Right	15	100%	0	None	No
Caughlin et al.[81]	2010	27/F	1/1/1	No	No	Spontaneous	Hematuria	NBCA	Left	25	100%	0	None	No
Shakhssalim et al.[82]	2010	26/F	1/1/1	No	Yes	Surgery	Hematuria	N/A	Left	25	100%	2	None	No

a Died of sepsis.

M, male; F, female; N/A, not applicable; A, allograft; PCNL, percutaneous nephrolithotomy; ESWL, extracorporeal shock wave lithotripsy; RH, retroperitoneal hematoma; PC, percutaneous; PVA, polyvinyl alcohol; NBCA, n-butyl cyanoacrylate; Onyx (eV3 Plymouth, MN).

OUTCOMES/PROGNOSIS

Measured postintervention outcomes include technical success, length of hospital stay, blood pressure effect, number of hypertensive medications, renal function, pain, evidence for renal infarction, and follow-up imaging studies.

If the RAA or RPA is complex, fusiform, and involves multiple branches and endovascular treatment is technically not possible, surgical options include direct surgical repair of the lesion using in vivo or ex vivo techniques or a partial or total nephrectomy.

Although most RAAs and RPAs can be treated endovascularly with immediate high-technical and clinical success rates, long-term follow-up experience remains sparse (Tables 59.1 and 59.2). Short and intermediate follow-up data, however, show excellent technical and clinical success rates.

Patients with RAAs may be at risk for developing other visceral aneurysms.[21] Therefore, they may benefit from surveillance for the development of more visceral aneurysms, especially if they have an underlying connective tissue disorder.

DISEASE SURVEILLANCE AND TREATMENT MONITORING ALGORITHMS

Regardless of which treatment is chosen, careful postprocedural surveillance is required to ensure that there is no reperfusion of the aneurysm. On follow-up, it should be documented that there is no expansion of the aneurysm. Even after successful exclusion of the aneurysm, there is possibility of regrowth or new aneurysm development. For this reason, interval noninvasive follow-up is mandatory to ensure that aneurysm expansion or recurrence is not happening. On clinical follow-up, symptomatic recurrence should be sought and clinical, laboratory, and imaging investigation should be performed. In most instances, once exclusion of the RAA is demonstrated, follow-up can be performed with ultrasound unless the patient develops recurrent symptoms or unless more detailed anatomic information is needed. If an RPA is excluded, recurrence is very unlikely in the absence of chronic anticoagulation.

EARLY FAILURES AND OPTIONS FOR MANAGEMENT

In surgery, a technical failure of the attempted renal artery reconstruction usually leads to nephrectomy or occlusion of the reconstructed artery. Most patients who experience technical failure of an attempted endovascular treatment still have an option of having surgical revascularization, aneurysmectomy, or partial or complete nephrectomy.

There is a potential risk of aneurysm rupture during an attempted endovascular treatment; however, to our knowledge, there is no report available in the literature of the occurrence of such a complication. Patients with a ruptured RAA can be treated fairly easily using catheter-directed embolization, although they may undergo surgical treatment depending on the clinical scenario.

LATE FAILURES AND OPTIONS FOR MANAGEMENT

Patients who underwent endovascular treatment should be under follow-up to ensure there is no aneurysm regrowth (very unlikely) or no new lesion development. Although there are no reports of late failures, in theory, like a cerebral aneurysm, coil contraction or aneurysm growth could lead to a recurrence. In cases in which a covered stent has been used, unless the stent migrates, recurrence would be very unlikely once the RAA has been excluded (Tables 59.1 and 59.2). In theory, however, a new lesion may develop in time depending on the underlying etiology for the RAA.

PRACTICAL ADVANTAGES AND LIMITATIONS

Surgery has been a historical treatment method for RAAs and endovascular treatment has been available recently. Therefore, the results of open repair and endovascular treatment are difficult to compare. Many endovascular reports are anecdotal case reports with excellent results. Multicenter, randomized studies are unlikely to be initiated due to the relative rarity of RAAs, and the multitude of endovascular and open repair treatment options would also make outcomes analysis very difficult.

Endovascular and open surgical treatment of an RAA or RPA requires an experienced interventionist and a vascular surgeon, respectively.

RELATIVE THERAPEUTIC EFFECTIVENESS COMPARED TO MEDICAL AND SURGICAL MANAGEMENT

Although the outcomes of surgical intervention for RAAs are good, surgery has been the most prevalent type of treatment in the past.[7] Advances in catheter-based interventions, however, have allowed for the successful treatment of even complex RAAs and RPAs. Furthermore, most of the RPAs are the result of trauma or an iatrogenic complication. Therefore, endovascular treatment has been used with great success and is now being employed more often than open repair. Hislop et al.[83] reviewed a New York State database and noted that by 2003, the number of RAA repairs performed using endovascular techniques was equal to the number of open repairs and that the trend toward endovascular repair was increasing. The length of hospital stay and rates of being discharged to home (versus a skilled nursing facility) also were statistically better with endovascular therapy as compared to open surgery.

THE FUTURE

With improvement in endovascular devices, the ability to treat most of the complex RAAs and RPAs is now feasible.

The interventional techniques and most of the devices used to treat RAAs, however, were originally designed for the treatment of intracranial aneurysms. In this respect, neurointerventional procedures are possibly making the best contribution to the technical development of RAA treatment. Therefore, close attention to neurointerventional procedure development is one of the keys for the development of future treatment methods for RAAs. Other developments involving stent technology improvements, which may allow branch vessel perfusion, will impact the treatment of RAAs.[41,80]

CONCLUSION

Renal artery pseudoaneurysm is an uncommon but potentially life-threatening complication. Presentation is often delayed. Following partial nephrectomy, open or laparoscopic, a high index of suspicion and an understanding of its typical clinical presentation will enable rapid diagnosis. Selective angiographic embolization should be the initial treatment of choice in those patients.

RAAs and RPAs are increasingly being diagnosed due to the more routine use of CTA and MRA imaging. The clinical presentation and characterization of the aneurysmal lesions help to determine the etiology and the potential need for treatment. Emergent treatment is required in the setting of a ruptured RAA or actively bleeding RPAs. Defining the specific anatomy of the RAA, including its size, stability, and the presence of branches emanating from the aneurysm, and if there are associated symptoms will drive the direction of therapy. More aggressive therapy should be pursued in women of childbearing age who have a desire to become pregnant, in the presence of an enlarging or symptomatic RAA, for an RAA with a diameter of more than 2 cm, and for an RPA secondary to trauma or an iatrogenic complication. Whenever possible, endovascular therapy should be the first line of therapy for the treatment of an RAA or RPA because surgery is associated with more morbidity.

REFERENCES

1. Hossain A, Reis ED, Dave SP, et al. Visceral artery aneurysms: experience in a tertiary-care center. *Am Surg* 2001;67(5):432–437.
2. Nosher JL, Chung J, Brevetti LS, et al. Visceral and renal artery aneurysms: a pictorial essay on endovascular therapy. *Radiographics* 2006;26(6):1687–1704; quiz.
3. Tham G, Ekelund L, Herrlin K, et al. Renal artery aneurysms. Natural history and prognosis. *Ann Surg* 1983;197(3):348–352.
4. Centenera LV, Hirsch JA, Choi IS, et al. Wide-necked saccular renal artery aneurysm: endovascular embolization with the Guglielmi detachable coil and temporary balloon occlusion of the aneurysm neck. *J Vasc Interv Radiol* 1998;9(3):513–516.
5. Panayiotopoulos YP, Assadourian R, Taylor PR. Aneurysms of the visceral and renal arteries. *Ann R Coll Surg Engl* 1996;78(5):412–419.
6. Cura M, Elmerhi F, Bugnogne A, et al. Renal aneurysms and pseudoaneurysms. *Clin Imaging* 2011;35(1):29–41.
7. Henke PK, Cardneau JD, Welling TH, 3rd, et al. Renal artery aneurysms: a 35-year clinical experience with 252 aneurysms in 168 patients. *Ann Surg* 2001;234(4):454–462; discussion 62–63.
8. McCarron JP, Jr., Marshall VF, Whitsell JC, 2nd. Indications for surgery on renal artery aneurysms. *J Urol* 1975;114(2):177–180.
9. Hageman JH, Smith RF, Szilagyi E, et al. Aneurysms of the renal artery: problems of prognosis and surgical management. *Surgery* 1978;84(4):563–572.
10. Hidai H, Kinoshita Y, Murayama T, et al. Rupture of renal artery aneurysm. *Eur Urol* 1985;11(4):249–253.
11. Hirsch AT, Haskal ZJ, Hertzer NR, et al. ACC/AHA guidelines for the management of patients with peripheral arterial disease (lower extremity, renal, mesenteric, and abdominal aortic): a collaborative report from the American Associations for Vascular Surgery/Society for Vascular Surgery, Society for Cardiovascular Angiography and Interventions, Society for Vascular Medicine and Biology, Society of Interventional Radiology, and the ACC/AHA Task Force on Practice Guidelines (writing committee to develop guidelines for the management of patients with peripheral arterial disease)—summary of recommendations. *J Vasc Interv Radiol* 2006;17(9):1383–1397; quiz 98.
12. Rundback JH, Rizvi A, Rozenblit GN, et al. Percutaneous stent-graft management of renal artery aneurysms. *J Vasc Interv Radiol* 2000;11(9):1189–1193.
13. Shirodkar SP, Bird V, Velazquez O, et al. Novel management of complicated renal artery aneurysm: laparoscopic nephrectomy and ex-vivo repair with heterotopic autotransplant. *J Endourol* 2010;24(1):35–39.
14. Clark TW, Sankin A, Becske T, et al. Stent-assisted Gugliemi detachable coil repair of wide-necked renal artery aneurysm using 3-D angiography. *Vasc Endovascular Surg* 2007–2008;41(6):528–532.
15. Dib M, Sedat J, Raffaelli C, et al. Endovascular treatment of a wide-neck renal artery bifurcation aneurysm. *J Vasc Interv Radiol* 2003;14(11):1461–1464.
16. Mali WP, Geyskes GG, Thalman R. Dissecting renal artery aneurysm: treatment with an endovascular stent. *AJR Am J Roentgenol* 1989;153(3):62–64.
17. Routh WD, Keller FS, Gross GM. Transcatheter thrombosis of a leaking saccular aneurysm of the main renal artery with preservation of renal blood flow. *AJR Am J Roentgenol* 1990;154(5):1097–1099.
18. Sueyoshi E, Sakamoto I, Hayashi N, et al. Ruptured renal artery aneurysm due to Behcet's disease. *Abdom Imaging* 1996;21(2):166–167.
19. Bui BT, Oliva VL, Leclerc G, et al. Renal artery aneurysm: treatment with percutaneous placement of a stent-graft. *Radiology* 1995;195(1):181–182.
20. Tateno T, Kubota Y, Sasagawa I, et al. Successful embolization of a renal artery aneurysm with preservation of renal blood flow. *Int Urol Nephrol* 1996;28(3):283–287.
21. Prabulos AM, Chen HH, Rodis JF, et al. Angiographic embolization of a ruptured renal artery aneurysm during pregnancy. *Obstet Gynecol* 1997;90(4 pt 2):663–665.
22. Yamamoto N, Ishihara S, Yoshimura S, et al. Endovascular embolization of a renal artery aneurysm using interlocking detachable coils. *Scand J Urol Nephrol* 1998;32(2):143–145.
23. Klein GE, Szolar DH, Breinl E, et al. Endovascular treatment of renal artery aneurysms with conventional non-detachable microcoils and Guglielmi detachable coils. *Br J Urol* 1997;79(6):852–860.
24. Karkos CD, D'Souza SP, Thomson GJ, et al. Renal artery aneurysm: endovascular treatment by coil embolisation with preservation of renal blood flow. *Eur J Vasc Endovasc Surg* 2000;19(2):214–216.
25. Mounayer C, Aymard A, Saint-Maurice JP, et al. Balloon-assisted coil embolization for large-necked renal artery aneurysms. *Cardiovasc Intervent Radiol* 2000;23(3):228–230.
26. Rikimaru H, Sato A, Hashizume E, et al. Saccular renal artery aneurysm treated with an autologous vein-covered stent. *J Vasc Surg* 2001;34(1):169–171.
27. Tan WA, Chough S, Saito J, et al. Covered stent for renal artery aneurysm. *Catheter Cardiovasc Interv* 2001;52(1):106–109.
28. Schneidereit NP, Lee S, Morris DC, et al. Endovascular repair of a ruptured renal artery aneurysm. *J Endovasc Ther* 2003;10(1):71–74.
29. Fiesseler FW, Riggs RL, Shih R. Ruptured renal artery aneurysm presenting as hematuria. *Am J Emerg Med* 2004;22(3):232–234.
30. Trocciola SM, Chaer RA, Lin SC, et al. Embolization of renal artery aneurysm and arteriovenous fistula—a case report. *Vasc Endovascular Surg* 2005;39(6):525–529.
31. Andersen PE, Rohr N. Endovascular exclusion of renal artery aneurysm. *Cardiovasc Intervent Radiol* 2005;28(5):665–667.
32. Malacrida G, Dalainas I, Medda M, et al. Endovascular treatment of a renal artery branch aneurysm. *Cardiovasc Intervent Radiol* 2007;30(1):118–120.
33. Degertekin M, Bayrak F, Mutlu B, et al. Images in cardiovascular medicine. Large renal artery aneurysm treated with stent graft. *Circulation* 2006;113(23):e848–849.
34. Gandini R, Spinelli A, Pampana E, et al. Bilateral renal artery aneurysm: percutaneous treatment with stent-graft placement. *Cardiovasc Intervent Radiol* 2006;29(5):875–878.
35. Goy JJ, Tinguely F, Poncioni L, et al. Aneurysm of the renal artery in a patient with the Marfan syndrome, treated by stenting and coils implantation. *Catheter Cardiovasc Interv* 2007;69(5):701–703.
36. Sahin S, Okbay M, Cinar B, et al. Wide-necked renal artery aneurysm: endovascular treatment with stent-graft. *Diagn Interv Radiol* 2007;13(1):42–45.
37. Gutta R, Lopes J, Flinn WR, et al. Endovascular embolization of a giant renal artery aneurysm with preservation of renal parenchyma. *Angiology* 2008;59(2):240–243.
38. Hagihara M, Kitagawa A, Izumi Y, et al. Emergent coil embolization for ruptured renal artery aneurysm. *Jpn J Radiol* 2009;27(7):275–279.
39. Altit R, Brown DB, Gardiner GA. Renal artery aneurysm and arteriovenous fistula associated with fibromuscular dysplasia: successful treatment with detachable coils. *J Vasc Interv Radiol* 2009;20(8):1083–1086.
40. Hobbs DJ, Barletta GM, Mowry JA, et al. Renovascular hypertension and intrarenal artery aneurysms in a preschool child. *Pediatr Radiol* 2009;39(9):988–990.
41. Sciacca L, Ciocca RG, Eslami MH, et al. Endovascular treatment of renal artery aneurysm secondary to fibromuscular dysplasia: a case report. *Ann Vasc Surg* 2009;23(4):536, e9–12.
42. Xiong J, Guo W, Liu X, et al. Renal artery aneurysm treatment with stent plus coil embolization. *Ann Vasc Surg* 2010;24(5):695, e1–3.
43. Gumustas S, Ciftci E, Bircan Z. Renal artery aneurysm in a hypertensive child treated by percutaneous coil embolization. *Pediatr Radiol* 2010;40(7):1285–1287.
44. Meyer C, Verrel F, Weyer G, et al. Endovascular management of complex renal artery aneurysms using the multilayer stent. *Cardiovasc Intervent Radiol* 2011;34(3):637–641.

45. Chang J, Katzen BT, Sullivan KP. Transcatheter gelfoam emboliza-tion of posttraumatic bleeding pseudoaneurysms. *AJR Am J Roentgenol* 1978;131(4):645–650.

46. Hall CL, Cumber P, Higgs CM, et al. Life threatening haemorrhage from a mycotic renal pseudoaneurysm treated by segmental renal artery embolisa-tion. *Br Med J (Clin Res Ed)* 1987;294(6586):1526.

47. Steffens MG, Bode PJ, Lycklama à Nijeholt AA, et al. Selective embolization of pseudo-aneurysms of the renal artery after blunt abdominal injury in a patient with a single kidney. *Injury* 1996;27(3):219–220.

48. Peh WC, Yip KH, Tam PC. Spontaneous renal pseudoaneurysm rup-ture presenting as acute intraabdominal haemorrhage. *Br J Radiol* 1997;70(839):1188–1190.

49. Silberzweig JE, Tey S, Winston JA, et al. Percutaneous renal biopsy complicated by renal capsular artery pseudoaneurysm. *Am J Kidney Dis* 1998;31(3):533–535.

50. Miyazaki T, Saitoh R, Doi T, et al. Embolization of a pseudoaneurysm in the transplanted kidney. *AJR Am J Roentgenol* 1998;171(6):1617–1618.

51. Singh B, Sudan D, Singh P, et al. Intraarterial ethanol for the manage-ment of iatrogenic renal artery pseudoaneurysm. *Cathet Cardiovasc Diagn* 1998;45(4):442–444.

52. Yamakado K, Nakatsuka A, Tanaka N, et al. Transcatheter arterial emboli-zation of ruptured pseudoaneurysms with coils and n-butyl cyanoacrylate. *J Vasc Interv Radiol* 2000;11(1):66–72.

53. Parsons JK, Schoenberg MP. Renal artery pseudoaneurysm occurring after partial nephrectomy. *Urology* 2001;58(1):105.

54. Parildar M, Oran I, Memis A. Embolization of visceral pseudoaneu-rysms with platinum coils and n-butyl cyanoacrylate. *Abdom Imaging* 2003;28(1):36–40.

55. Sharma AK, Sunil S, Rowlands P, et al. Pseudoaneurysm with severe hae-maturia in renal allograft after renal biopsy treated by percutaneous embo-lization. *Nephrol Dial Transplant* 2002;17(5):934–935.

56. Miller DC, Forauer A, Faerber GJ. Successful angioembolization of renal ar-tery pseudoaneurysms after blunt abdominal trauma. *Urology* 2002;59(3):444.

57. Halachmi S, Chait P, Hodapp J, et al. Renal pseudoaneurysm after blunt renal trauma in a pediatric patient: management by angiographic emboliza-tion. *Urology* 2003;61(1):224.

58. Nakatani T, Uchida J, Han YS, et al. Renal allograft arteriovenous fistula and large pseudoaneurysm. *Clin Transplant* 2003;17(1):9–12.

59. Cantasdemir M, Adaletli I, Cebi D, et al. Emergency endovascular emboli-zation of traumatic intrarenal arterial pseudoaneurysms with n-butyl cya-noacrylate. *Clin Radiol* 2003;58(7):560–565.

60. Aston W, Whiting R, Bultitude M, et al. Pseudoaneurysm formation after flexible ureterorenoscopy and electrohydraulic lithotripsy. *Int J Clin Pract* 2004;58(3):310–311.

61. Giannopoulos A, Manousakas T, Alexopoulou E, et al. Delayed life-threat-ening haematuria from a renal pseudoaneurysm caused by blunt renal trauma treated with selective embolization. *Urol Int* 2004;72(4):352–354.

62. Singh D, Gill IS. Renal artery pseudoaneurysm following laparoscopic par-tial nephrectomy. *J Urol* 2005;174(6):2256–2259.

63. Saad DF, Gow KW, Redd D, et al. Renal artery pseudoaneurysm second-ary to blunt trauma treated with microcoil embolization. *J Pediatr Surg* 2005;40(11):e65–67.

64. Hidas G, Croitoru S, Wolfson V, et al. Renal artery pseudoaneurysm af-ter partial nephrectomy complicated by rupture into the collecting sys-tem, managed by selective angiographic embolization. *Isr Med Assoc J* 2005;7(6):410–411.

65. Lee DG, Lee SJ. Delayed hemorrhage from a pseudoaneurysm after blunt renal trauma. *Int J Urol* 2005;12(10):909–911.

66. Novellas S, Chevallier P, Motamedi JP, et al. Superselective embolization of a post-biopsy renal pseudoaneurysm in a 13-month-old infant. *Pediatr Radiol* 2006;36(8):874–876.

67. Massulo-Aguiar MF, Campos CM, Rodrigues-Netto N, Jr. Intrarenal pseudoaneurysm after percutaneous nephrolithotomy. Angiotomographic assessment and endovascular management. *Int Braz J Urol* 2006;32(4):440–442; discussion 3–4.

68. Cohenpour M, Strauss S, Gottlieb P, et al. Pseudoaneurysm of the renal artery following partial nephrectomy: imaging findings and coil emboliza-tion. *Clin Radiol* 2007;62(11):1104–1109.

69. Uberoi J, Badwan KH, Wang DS. Renal-artery pseudoaneurysm after lapa-roscopic partial nephrectomy. *J Endourol* 2007;21(3):330–333.

70. Pastorin R, Rodriguez N, Polo AM, et al. Posttraumatic giant renal pseu-doaneurysm. *Emerg Radiol* 2007;14(2):117–121.

71. Gupta V, Galwa R, Khandelwal N, et al. Postpyelolithotomy renal artery pseudoaneurysm management with percutaneous thrombin injection: a case report. *Cardiovasc Intervent Radiol* 2008;31(2):422–426.

72. Kubasiewicz L, Maleux G, Oyen R, et al. Pseudoaneurysm complicat-ing protocol renal transplant biopsies: case reports. *Transplant Proc* 2008;40(5):1397–1398.

73. Zelenak K, Sopilko I, Svihra J, et al. Successful embolization of a renal artery pseudoaneurysm with arteriovenous fistula and extravasations using Onyx after partial nephrectomy for renal cell carcinoma. *Cardiovasc Intervent Ra-diol* 2009;32(1):163–165.

74. Schellhammer F, Steinhaus D, Cohnen M, et al. Minimally invasive therapy of pseudoaneurysms of the trunk: application of thrombin. *Cardiovasc In-tervent Radiol* 2008;31(3):535–541.

75. Bozgeyik Z, Ozdemir H, Orhan I, et al. Pseudoaneurysm and renal arte-riovenous fistula after nephrectomy: two cases treated by transcatheter coil embolization. *Emerg Radiol* 2008;15(2):119–122.

76. Lal A, Kumar A, Prakash M, et al. Percutaneous cyanoacrylate glue in-jection into the renal pseudoaneurysm to control intractable hematu-ria after percutaneous nephrolithotomy. *Cardiovasc Intervent Radiol* 2009;32(4):767–771.

77. Sakr MA, Desouki SE, Hegab SE. Direct percutaneous embolization of renal pseudoaneurysm. *J Endourol* 2009;23(6):875–878.

78. Mima A, Toma M, Matsubara T, et al. Angio-embolization of re-nal artery pseudoaneurysm after renal biopsy: a case report. *Ren Fail* 2009;31(8):753–755.

79. Watanabe M, Padua HM, Nguyen HT, et al. Renal pseudoaneurysm fol-lowing laser lithotripsy: endovascular treatment of a rare complication. *J Pediatr Urol* 2010;6(4):420–422.

80. Schlunz-Hendann M, Wetter A, Landwehr P, et al. Stent-assisted coil em-bolization of a traumatic wide-necked renal segmental artery pseudoaneu-rysm. *Cardiovasc Intervent Radiol* 2011;34(5);1065–1068. Epub 2011 Feb 8.

81. Caughlin CE, Simons ME, Robinette MA. Direct percutaneous emboliza-tion of a renal pseudoaneurysm with use of n-butyl cyanoacrylate. *J Vasc Interv Radiol* 2010;21(8):1317–1318.

82. Shakhssalim N, Nouralizadeh A, Soltani MH. Renal artery pseudoaneurysm following a laparoscopic partial nephrectomy: hemorrhage after a success-ful embolization. *Urol J* 2010;7(1):12–14.

83. Hislop SJ, Patel SA, Abt PL, et al. Therapy of renal artery aneurysms in New York State: outcomes of patients undergoing open and endovascular repair. *Ann Vasc Surg* 2009;23(2):194–200.

Mesenteric Aneurysms

SEBASTIAN KOS, DAVID M. LIU, and AUGUSTINUS L. JACOB

INTRODUCTION

Visceral arterial aneurysms (VAAs) are rare entities with a described incidence of less than 0.2%, thereby representing only 0.1% to 0.2% of all arterial aneurysms.[1,2] VAAs may involve different vascular territories with the splenic artery being the most commonly affected (60%). Hepatic artery (20%) and superior mesenteric artery (SMA; 5.5%) aneurysms are more common than those of the celiac artery (4%), gastric arteries (4%), ileal/jejunal/colic arteries (3%), gastroduodenal artery (1.5%), and inferior mesenteric artery (1%) (FIGURE 60.1).[2–4]

The distribution of hepatic artery aneurysms reveals a disproportionate representation of the right hepatic artery (79%) as compared to the middle (10%) and left (8%) artery.

In patients with a known aneurysm incidence of a second splanchnic aneurysm may be as high as 38%.[5]

VAAs may measure up to 20 cm in size with mean diameters measuring 2 to 5 cm.[6,7]

Splenic aneurysms represent the most common of VAAs with a female predominance (4:1) and higher incidence amongst multiparous women.[8,9]

Visceral aneurysms, especially when small (<2 cm), commonly remain asymptomatic. In a series of 217 patients with splenic artery aneurysms, 93.7% remained asymptomatic.[8] In another study on 18 patients with celiac artery aneurysms, 13 (72%) remained asymptomatic.[10] Abdominal pain and discomfort, tenderness, flank pain, gastrointestinal bleed or

hemosuccus pancreaticus, and signs of rupture including hemodynamic instability can be encountered in symptomatic patients.

The high percentages of clinically asymptomatic VAAs imply that those entities often had not been detected prior to the advent of modern cross-sectional imaging. In the last decades, however, widespread use especially of computed tomography (CT) and CT angiography has resulted in earlier, and frequently incidental, depiction of such aneurysms.[11,12] Whether the increased identification of subclinical aneurysms has changed the course of the disease as a result of earlier intervention remains controversial, especially within lesions of less than 2 cm.

On ultrasound imaging, which of course is time-consuming and operator dependent, those typical VAAs present as anechoic/hypoechoic collections when using grayscale imaging. Flow can be detected on color Doppler with classic signs being described as *ying-yang* configuration of the turbulent flow in the aneurysm and *to-and-fro* biphasic flow within the aneurysm neck.

On CT noncontrast imaging, VAAs usually present as rounded structures of fluid attenuation with or without calcification. Contrast-enhanced arterial phase images should be obtained using thin slices (1 to 3 mm) with the VAA being equal in attenuation when compared with the adjacent artery. Three-dimensional reformations may allow for better anatomic orientation and detection of very small aneurysms (1 to 2 mm).

For its availability magnetic resonance imaging (MRI) is usually not the first imaging modality and therefore may detect VAAs either incidentally or help characterize them as an adjunct

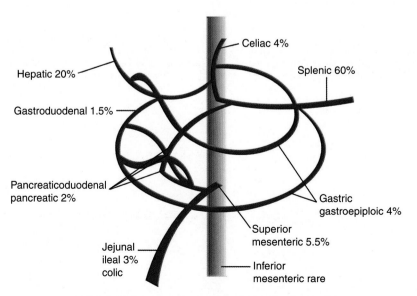

FIGURE 60.1 Schematic synopsis of VAA distribution.[2–4]

to diagnostic ultrasound or in patients with contraindications to CT (e.g., pregnancy, iodine allergy). Again contrast-enhanced sequences should be obtained and the VAA signal should be of equal intensity when compared with the adjacent artery.

For better and earlier detection of VAAs, the need for a therapeutic plan allowing for patient risk stratification and management became evident. For the purpose of stratification, all detected VAAs should be classified into two pathophysiologically separate entities and, therefore, groups. Pseudoaneurysms, also termed *false aneurysms,* are histologically areas of focal hemorrhage that occur within the vessel wall. The term *pseudoaneurysm*, according to one definition, describes partial disruption of the artery with patent flow in a defined space beyond the confines of the vessel.[13] The external wall of the pseudoaneurysm consists of perivascular tissue, outer arterial wall layers, blood clot, and reactive fibrosis. As opposed to acute extravasation, arterial pressurized blood recirculates into the feeding artery through the aneurysm neck, resulting in the turbulence and classic ying-yang sign.

The second entity, true aneurysms, comprise all three arterial wall layers. VAAs may have a broad variety of causes including hereditary, inflammatory, tumor associated, traumatic, and iatrogenic. For a synopsis of VAA etiologies FIGURE 60.2.

PATIENT SELECTION

Due to the rather sporadic nature of VAA presentation, and improved detection of subclinical VAA (especially <2 cm), little literature exists as to its true pathophysiology or natural history. Thus, the rationale in support of intervention has been based on symptomatic patient presentation and post hoc analysis of rupture characteristics as opposed to prospective observational data that would potentially reflect the true nature of the VAA.

For pseudoaneurysms in single series, spontaneous thrombosis has been described.[14] Extraorganic visceral pseudoaneurysms that are not treated may rupture, with a mortatlity rate of up to 100%.[7] Therefore, because of the high risk of rupture (up to 25%) and high mortality rates consecutively (16% to 100%) all pseudoaneurysms require treatment.[6,7,15,16]

Current literature suggests that true aneurysms have a lower risk of rupture but long-term data from surveillance studies are still lacking. In current clinical practice, a decision to treat is typically based on individual factors, which include the detection of aneurysm growth, affected vascular territory, aneurysm size, patient symptoms, and overall patient condition.[17,18] For a proposed VAA stratification algorithm, FIGURE 60.3.

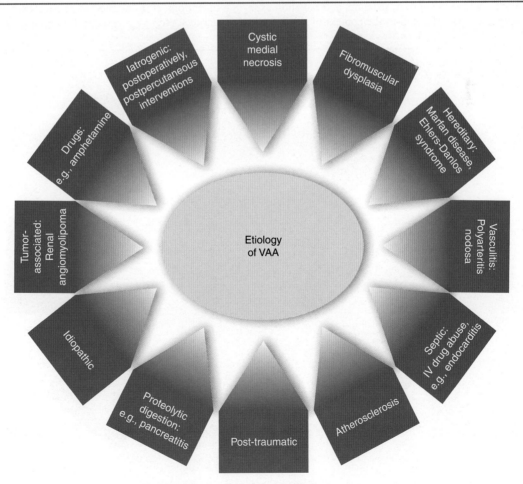

FIGURE 60.2 Synopsis of VAA etiologies.

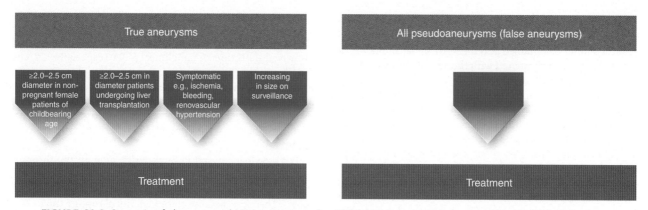

FIGURE 60.3 Synopsis of the proposed VAA treatment algorithm. Note: According to a guideline published by the American College of Cardiology and American Heart Association, a treatment threshold of 2.0 cm diameter is recommended, whereas other authorities and organizations suggest a threshold of 2.5 cm diameter.

CONTRAINDICATIONS

There are no absolute contraindications for endovascular aneurysm repair, if indicated, according to the criteria published by the American College of Cardiology and American Heart Association. Patients with known severe renal impairment, hyperthyroidism, and/or known allergy to iodinated contrast media should not undergo the procedure if other therapeutic options exist because of the possible adverse effects of the contrast media used. The use of contrast, sedation, and radiation exposure requires special attention in the context of the pregnant and pediatric populations. For a list of relative contraindications see FIGURE 60.4.

PLANNING THE INTERVENTIONAL PROCEDURE

Comprehensive prepocedural patient assessment includes evaluation of patient history (symptoms, allergies, previous operations, etc.) and focused physical examination (pulses, tenderness, etc.). A computed tomography angiogram (CTA) is

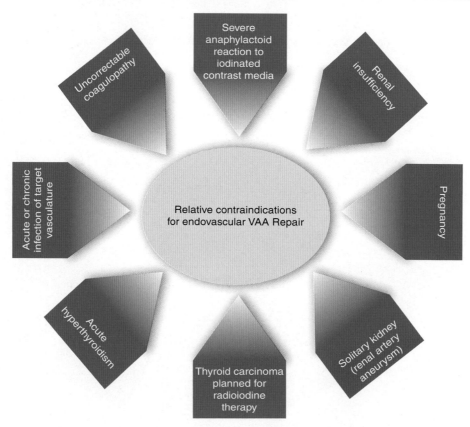

FIGURE 60.4 Synopsis of relative contraindications for endovascular VAA treatment.

recommended prior to the procedure to allow for depiction of the vascular anatomy and anatomic relationships and to exclude aberrant or unusual vasculature. Three-dimensional and maximum intensity projection (MIP) reconstructions from either a CTA or the new generation of volumetric magnetic resonance angiogram (MRA) techniques allow for more advanced planning in terms of embolic (coil, plug, or glue) as well as selective platform (sheath, guide catheter, catheter, and microcatheter), making the possibility of better assessment of the aneurysm(s) in relation to arterial branch anatomy (FIGURE 60.5). Recent blood work has to be obtained including complete blood count (CBC), International Normalized Ratio (INR), creatinine, glomerular filtration rate (GFR), platelets, partial thromboplastin time (PTT), and C-reactive protein (CRP). Written informed consent is to be obtained.

▌ PROCEDURE

Patients should be prepared in a standardized fashion. Prior to the procedure, patients should be NPO for 6 hours. Oral medications may be administered with minimal amounts of water. Intravenous (IV) access has to be established to allow for sufficient hydration of the patient and conscious sedation if needed. Monitoring of the patient's vital signs including blood pressure, heart rate, and pulse oximetry should be available and active during the procedure. The skin at the access site has to be prepared and draped in a standard sterile fashion. Conscious sedation should be administered at the operator's discretion in the individual setting.

In most cases the procedure can be performed using a transfemoral access route. A transbrachial, transradial, or transaxillary access also can be used, however, in cases where a safe transfemoral access (e.g., iliac artery occlusion) cannot be obtained or when it may provide an easier access according to anatomic considerations (e.g., massive iliac elongation and kinking or acute angulation of the SMA or celiac trunk origin).

Having obtained the transfemoral arterial access, some authors routinely position a 6 or 7 French guiding sheath within the abdominal aorta to stabilize the catheter system and potentially allow for easier visceral artery sounding.[13] At our institution a short 6 French access sheath is used in most cases and longer guide sheaths (45 cm) are inserted whenever significant kinking and arterial elongation interfere with catheter advancement and rotation.

In those cases in which a CTA was not obtained prior to the procedure, diagnostic aortography using a flush catheter is helpful to determine vascular anatomy and potentially detect other pathologies or normal variants.

Selective catheterization of the targeted visceral artery is performed next. For first- and second-degree branches, a 4 or 5 French selective catheter (cobra, vertebral, or sidewinder shape) in combination with a hydrophilic guide wire are mostly used. For third- or fourth-order branches a combination of a superselective microcatheter (2.3 to 2.9 French) and microwire is usually required. With the catheter in selective position IV administration of hyoscine butylbromide (Buscopan) can minimize bowel movement (20 to 40 mg bolus). Selective arteriograms are performed in multiple projections or in modern suites, as 3D rotational digital subtraction arteriography (DSA) (FIGURE 60.6). Vascular assessment includes the dimensions and morphology of the aneurysm and also of the afferent/efferent arterial segment. Presence of branching vessels and normal arterial variants has to be evaluated.

More recently, new cone beam CT technology has been integrated into state-of-the-art angiography suites. This technique allows for volumetric data acquisition within a single rotation of the detector and X-ray source. The intra-arterial contrast-enhanced cone beam CT (e.g., DynaCT digital angiography; Siemens Medical Systems, Erlangen, Germany) can simplify angiographic assessment, particularly in cases in which the anatomy is not clearly defined.[19,20]

For intra-arterial contrast-enhanced cone beam CT, the following parameters have been described[21]: a 48-cm field of view with the isocenter of the volume being positioned at the selectively positioned catheter tip; contrast media injection rate of 3 cc/second for 8 seconds; and a 2-second X-ray delay, 3 degrees/frame, single breath hold, 200-degree arc rotation (30 degrees/second) are favorable. Images should be reconstructed on a dedicated workstation. Three-dimensional reformations and reconstructions including MIPs should be performed.

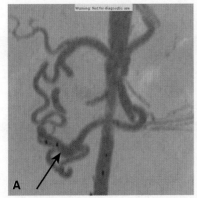 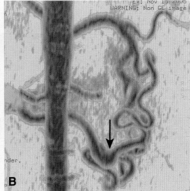 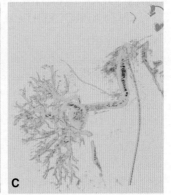

FIGURE 60.5 CTA reformations, including maximum intensity projection (*arrows*) (**A**) and volume rendering (*arrow*) technique (**B**), of an aneurysm involving the inferior pancreaticoduodenal artery. Volume rendering technique provides clear depiction of a right renal artery aneurysm (**C**).

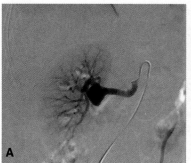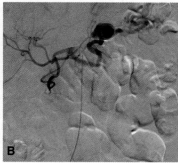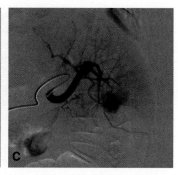

FIGURE 60.6 Digital subtraction angiograms depicting a right renal artery aneurysm (**A**), a proximal splenic artery aneurysm (**B**), and an intraparenchymal splenic artery aneurysm (**C**).

DEVICE SELECTION STRATEGIES

Meticulous knowledge of the embolic material applied is of utmost importance for procedural success. For embolization and occlusion of VAAs a vast variety of embolic agents have been applied and described in the literature. This includes covered stents, coils, combinations of coils (e.g., Hilal, Nester, Tornado; Cook, Bloomington, IN) and bare stents, glue, and Amplatzer plug (AGA Medical, Plymouth, MN).[15,16,21] As previously discussed, preprocedural planning requires careful consideration for the platform of delivery and type of embolic (e.g., plug with sheath/catheter compatibility, catheter and glue compatibility, microcathether and microcoil system compatibility).

To date, no device has been shown to be superior in outcome or complication rate and, as such, the access, experience of the operator, and availability of the system generally dictate the embolic approach.

ANATOMIC OR LESION CONSIDERATIONS

In general, to avoid stasis and arterial occlusion, the selective (micro-)catheter should not be advanced into arteries that are less than twofold the catheter's diameter in size.

This implies that for safe and distal purchase, especially in target vessels that are small and/or tortuous, a coaxial microcatheter should be considered.

ENDOVASCULAR TREATMENT OPTIONS AND SPECIFIC INTRAPROCEDURAL TECHNIQUES

Isolation Technique

The isolation technique (commonly referred to as front-and-backdoor embolization) may be applied to a VAA in the proximal mesenteric bed (e.g., proximal to the arc of Riolan, or in vascular territories that may potentially be sacrificed, such as the splenic artery). The aneurysm's arterial outflow is considered the back door and the proximal feeding arteries are referred to as the front door. After positioning of the selective catheter distal to the aneurysm, embolization is performed from a distal-to-proximal approach, completely occluding the aneurysm. Techniques utilizing coils, glue, and vascular plug have been described (FIGURE 60.7).[21,22] It is of utmost importance that the outflow (back door) is occluded first and completely. This total occlusion should be angiographically documented because reaccessing cases with incomplete distal occlusion and

sufficient proximal embolization will be technically demanding, if not impossible. Following distal embolization, occlusion of the proximal, inflow vessel should be completed.

In such cases in which the back door cannot be accessed and is occluded (e.g., vasospasm), isolated front-door occlusion may be performed but angiographic controls are mandatory and should be comprehensive to rule out retrograde filling after the embolization (FIGURE 60.8). As an important variation of the isolation technique, a scaffold can be created using a large coil being deployed as a distal anchor beyond the aneurysmal sac. This scaffold allows for tight deployment and packing of smaller (micro-) coils on top of it with another larger coil occluding the proximal inflow.

Covered Stent Placement Across the VAA Neck

In recent years technical developments have made smaller delivery platforms for covered stents available. Therefore, placement of such covered stents has become more popular.[23,24] The ultimate goal of this technique and approach is to exclude the aneurysmal sac while maintaining adequate perfusion distal to the VAA (FIGURE 60.9).

When comparing covered stents with other devices (e.g., microcoils) it becomes evident that the deployment platforms

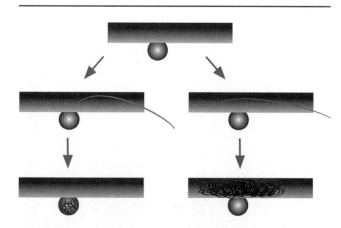

FIGURE 60.7 Illustration of the isolation technique with the right side with occlusion of the front and back doors of the VAA by deploying coils distal to the aneurysm and then occluding the proximal afferent artery. On the left side, occlusion of the aneurysm by coil packing is demonstrated. Note: This technique should only be applied in true aneurysms.

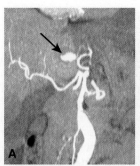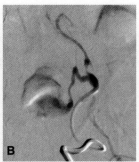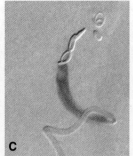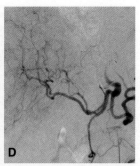

FIGURE 60.8 A. Spontaneous pseudoaneurysm of the left hepatic artery (*arrow*) branching from the left gastric artery as an anatomic variant (CT maximum intensity projection, coronal view). The left gastric artery was selectively catheterized (**B**) but due to significant vasospasm the back door was not accessible. Therefore, front-door occlusion was performed using coils (**C**). Postembolization angiography revealed no signs of retrograde aneurysm filling (**D**).

are still larger, less flexible, and more rigid. These features imply that this technique is best suited for VAAs in larger, straight vessels. Because deployment of a covered stent may not only cover and occlude the aneurysm but also the adjacent branches, these side branches close to the aneurysmal sac must be identified prior to deployment to minimize the risk of ischemic complications.

As another limitation in aneurysms resulting from systemic diseases (e.g., vasculitis) or inflammation (e.g., pancreatitis) it may be difficult or even impossible to angiographically determine the precise length of the diseased arterial wall segment. In these cases other techniques should be considered.

Coil Packing of the Aneurysm Sac

Using a selective catheter directed toward/into the aneurysmal sac, coils are sequentially deployed to complete packing and exclusion from blood flow (FIGURE 60.7).[25] This technique should only be applied in true aneurysms. As opposed to this, in false aneurysms, the already weakened arterial wall may perforate when being coiled or during the postoperative course, potentially resulting in dislodgment of the coil pack. The coil packing technique itself may well be combined with the above-mentioned front- and backdoor occlusion (isolation technique), thereby not only occluding the aneurysmal sac but also decreasing/eliminating the flow within the afferent and afferent arteries.

Uncovered Stent Placement and Coil Packing

As another modification of coil packing technique, an uncovered stent is initially deployed to cover the aneurysm's neck (FIGURE 60.10). Following this and using a coaxial microcatheter, coils are sequentially packed into the sac through the covering stent's struts.[26] As a theoretical limitation (see above) again in our opinion pseudoaneurysms should not be packed as a stand-alone measure for the increased risk of rupture and coil dislodgment.

Liquid Occlusive Agents

Embolization of vessels, endoleaks, arteriovenous (AV) malformations, and aneurysms using liquid embolic agents is widely performed. In general occlusion with cyanoacrylates (histoacryl) or ethylene vinyl alcohol (Onyx, EV3, Plymouth, MN) has been described. We highly recommend limiting its usage to the hands of experienced operators, because these liquid agents have to be

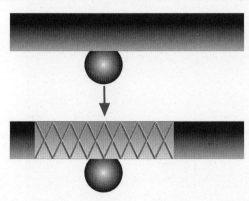

FIGURE 60.9 Illustration of aneurysm exclusion from blood flow by a covered stent. Because of the size and relative rigidity of such covered stent platforms, this technique is typically considered in large and relatively straight vessels.

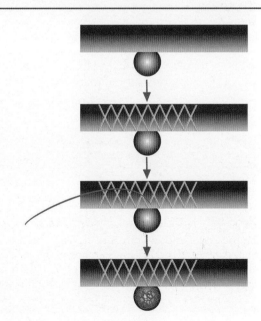

FIGURE 60.10 Illustration of aneurysm exclusion by segmental coverage using an uncovered stent and, subsequently, coil packing through the struts of the deployed stent.

precisely controlled and meticulous knowledge of the substances is mandatory to allow for safe processing and usage.[27,28] Unique to the use of glues, the rate of polymerization should be taken into consideration to avoid incomplete occlusion of the target vessel resulting from rapid polymerization, or alternatively, profound distal embolization as a result of incomplete or slow polymerization. As with any other embolic device it is furthermore of utmost importance to occlude the arterial segments both proximal and distal to the VAA. We do not recommend using glue in pseudoaneurysms without occluding the adjacent segments.

Some operators have tried to minimize collateral ischemic damage by applying transient balloon occlusion across the aneurysm neck when injecting the liquid occlusive agent.[29,30]

Thrombin Injection

Besides the transarterial techniques previously discussed, percutaneous thrombin injection has been described for the management of aneurysms.[31–33] This technique has proven its value in VAA management, particularly in cases where access is limited or impossible, such as previously coiled aneurysms or aneurysms distal to occluded arterial segments.[34,35] For this purpose percutaneous puncture of the aneurysmal sac can be performed under

fluoroscopic, ultrasound or CT guidance with a small-caliber (e.g., 22-gauge Chiba) needle. Even in cases being performed using ultrasound or CT for primary guidance, having adjunct fluoroscopy available may simplify the procedure and allow for better confirmation of intra-arterial needle positioning by contrast injection. To minimize the risk of ischemic complications, a minimal dose and volume of thrombin should be injected, just allowing for safe occlusion of the aneurysm. Normally 500 units of thrombin diluted in 1 to 2 mL of normal saline are sufficient to thrombose most aneurysmal sacs, particularly those that are (partially) reperfused after initial endovascular intervention.

▌ ORGAN-SPECIFIC COMMENTS

Splenic Artery Aneurysms[17,36,37]

Among VAAs, splenic aneurysms are the most common, accounting for 60% of all cases. Due to the tortuous nature of the vessel, adequate support catheter selection is required to allow for distal tracking of the terminal embolic device or technique (FIGURE 60.11 and 60.12). For this a selective catheter (e.g., Sos, Sim) or even providing more stable access, a 6 French renal double curve sheath (RDC-CCV; Terumo Destination,

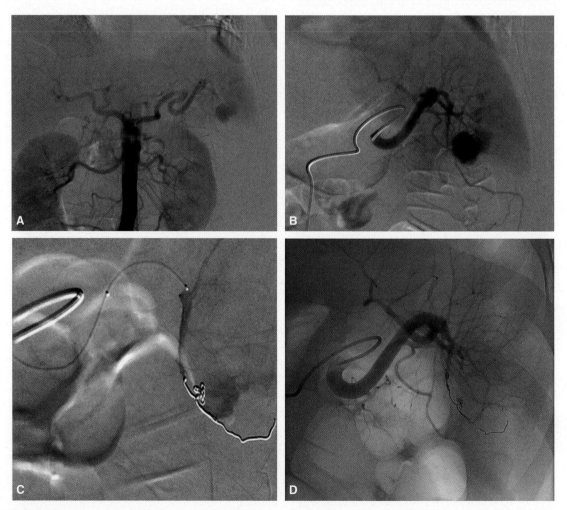

FIGURE 60.11 Aortography depicting an intraparenchymal splenic artery aneurysm (**A**). This aneurysm was then selectively treated using a combination of selective guide catheter and a coaxial microcatheter (**B**). Embolization was then performed using microcoils and isolation technique for occlusion of the front and back doors (**C,D**).

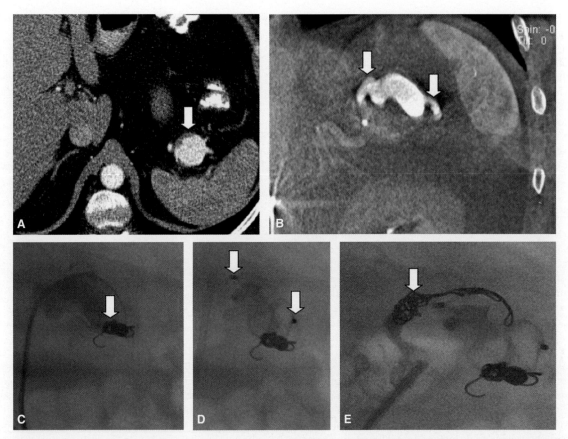

FIGURE 60.12 CT angiography (axial view) revealed the 3.6-cm measuring prehilar splenic artery aneurysm (*arrow* in **A**). Cone beam CT (coronal view) documented the extent of the aneurysmal sac and the afferent and efferent arterial segments of the splenic artery (*arrows* in **B**). Embolization was performed in a three-step approach. First, the arterial "back door" was occluded using two 6-mm diameter, 14-cm long Nester coils (Cook Medical, Inc., Bloomington, IN) (*arrow* in **C**). Second, the aneurysmal sac was occluded using a 22-mm diameter, 18-mm long Amplatzer vascular plug II (AGA Medical Inc., Plymouth, MN) (*arrows* in **D**). Third, the afferent "front door" was occluded using two 8-mm diameter, 14-cm long Nester coils (*arrow* in **E**).

Reprinted with permission from Kos et al. Endovascular management of complex splenic aneurysm with the "amplatzer" embolic platform: application of cone-beam computed tomography. *Can Assoc Radiol J* 2010;61(4):230–232.

Terumo Medical Corp., Elkton, MD) can be used. Through the latter sheath, for example a combination of a 0.035″ hydrophilic guide wire (Standard Glidewire; Terumo Medical Corp, Tokyo, Japan) and a 4 to 5 French hydrophilic catheter (e.g., vertebral catheter, Terumo Medical Corp) can be advanced into the splenic artery. In many cases of hilar aneurysms, microcatheterization is required to allow for adequate control of both the distal and proximal neck.

The embolization technique may depend on the location of the aneurysm and the size of the splenic artery and its degree of elongation. Because many aneurysms occur distally at the level of the splenic hilum, they are mainly treated using the isolation technique by embolization of the artery proximal and distal to the aneurysm neck. This implies that some degree of splenic infarction will occur. Those aneurysms presenting in the more proximal portion, thereby usually larger and straighter, of the artery can be considered for treatment using a covered stent or by total occlusion of the aneurysm sack using coils, thus decreasing the risk of partial splenic infarction.

Hepatic Artery Aneurysms[34,38,39]

Hepatic artery aneurysms are the second most common VAAs, accounting for 20% of them. Precise knowledge of vascular anatomy is essential because anatomic variants are common; for example, replaced right hepatic (up to 15%) and replaced left hepatic variants (up to 10%).[40] The dual blood supply of the liver parenchyma through either portal vein or hepatic artery allows for safe occlusion of hepatic arterial branches in patients with a patent portal venous system. Therefore, and prior to any embolization, patency of the portal vein should be confirmed by angiography to limit the risk of hepatic infarction. Proximal aneurysms may rupture into the abdominal cavity, thereby potentially resulting in rapid development of shock or exsanguination. As opposed to this, intrahepatic rupture of the aneurysm may also result in hemobilia by contained rupture into the biliary system.

For the regular anatomy selective reverse curved catheters (e.g., Sos, Simmons) are mostly used to engage the celiac trunk. The same can be applied for the SMA in cases presenting with a replaced right hepatic artery. In rare cases with a shallow, almost horizontal branching of the celiac trunk even a cobra-type catheter can be considered. In patients which do not allow for femoral access of the celiac trunk, a transbrachial approach can be applied. Nevertheless, for most cases with an intrahepatic aneurysm, a coaxial microcatheter will be needed and is recommended.

Usually single intrahepatic aneurysms can be safely excluded using coils proximal and distal to the aneurysm, thereby isolating the aneurysm from blood flow. In contrast, in cases with multiple pseudoaneurysms (mainly post-traumatic), diffuse shower embolization using gelfoam should be considered and is more effective.

Renal Artery Aneurysms[35,36,41]

As described for splenic artery aneurysms, a coaxial approach using a combination of a guide sheath with an inner diameter (ID) of 5 to 6 French (e.g., renal double curve), a 4 to 5 French diagnostic catheter (e.g., Sos Omni or cobra), and a hydrophilic guide wire can be used for most cases. Through this stable access, additional usage of microcatheters may be necessary for small- and distal branch aneurysms. Having obtained stable access, selective angiography should be performed with optimal angulation (e.g., 10- to 15-degree ipsilateral oblique) to allow for better assessment of the renal vasculature.

Embolic occlusion of renal artery branches invariably leads to a certain extent of ischemic infarction, which is almost always smaller than those that result after surgical approaches. Therefore, front- and backdoor occlusion may not be a suitable option. In such patients with already impaired renal function, sac exclusion techniques using glue or coils may be an option, but other surgical options should be considered interdisciplinarily.

In such cases where aneurysms are associated with an angiomyolipoma, the aneurysm should be excluded first; thereafter, gelfoam or particle embolization of the tumor can be considered.

Mesenteric Aneurysms[28,34,38,42]

As rare entities, mesenteric aneurysms account for only 6% of all visceral aneurysms. The gastroduodenal artery is most frequently involved, but generally all mesenteric branches can be affected. Aneurysms of the gastroduodenal artery (GDA) are mostly caused by pancreatitis or duodenal ulceration. Those of the pancreaticoduodenal artery are caused by pancreatitis or may present secondary to increased flow in cases with stenotic/occluded celiac trunks or SMA. SMA aneurysms are frequently mycotic or atherosclerotic in nature and the celiac trunk itself can be affected by cystic medial degeneration and median arcuate ligament syndrome. The collateral pathways present normally allow for sufficient collateral perfusion and even total embolic occlusion of the GDA. Pre-embolization angiograms have to precisely rule presence of celiac trunk or proximal proper hepatic stenosis, however, thereby decreasing the risk of malperfusion and ischemic complications (FIGURE 60.13).

ENDPOINT ASSESSMENT OF THE PROCEDURE

To allow for safe endpoint determination of endovascular treatment of the VAA, selective diagnostic angiographies, again from different angles or using rotational angiography (e.g., Dyna-DSA,

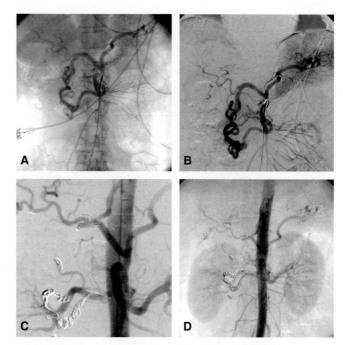

FIGURE 60.13 Tubular aneurysm of the inferior pancreaticoduodenal arcade (**A,B**). This aneurysm was then treated using a combination of selective guide catheter and a coaxial microcatheter. Embolization was performed using microcoils and isolation technique for occlusion of the front and back doors (**C,D**).

cone beam CT), should be obtained (FIGURE 60.14). These additional angiographies should confirm complete aneurysm exclusion from blood flow and successful treatment prior to removal of the endovascular devices (FIGURE 60.11 and 60.13).

If available, we recommend performing contrast-enhanced cone beam CT (e.g., injected through microcatheter or selective catheter), again allowing for further 3D reformations and precise depiction of the aneurysmal sac and relevant branch vessels.

■ POSTPROCEDURE MANAGEMENT

Most institutions monitor the patient and have a regimen for postembolization bed rest and observation. The duration of this period should be related to the course of the intervention, its degree of success, potentially encountered and/or expected complications, and the recovery from conscious sedation.

In cases with confirmed or expected postembolization syndrome, analgesic therapy (perchlorpromazine and acetaminophen) should be considered. Antiemetic therapy can be administered for symptomatic patients (ondansetron and dexamethasone).

Prior to discharge, or (depending on the technical success) after up to 4 weeks, cross-sectional imaging (CT or MRI) should be performed. This allows for noninvasive assessment of therapeutic success. It should depict and document occlusion or potentially (re-)perfusion of the aneurysmal sac and, if present, the extent of distal ischemia. The overall and individual length of the hospital stay is determined by the aneurysm's etiology, the potential occurrence of postembolization

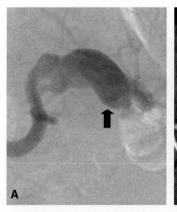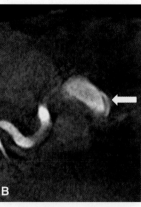

FIGURE 60.14 Two-dimensional DSA revealed the extent of the aneurysmal sac (*arrow* in **A**) and visualized the afferent and efferent arterial segments of the splenic artery aneurysm. A short gastric artery originating from the aneurysmal sac was not seen on DSA images, however, but was revealed on cone beam CT (*arrow* in **B**).

Reprinted with permission from Kos et al. Endovascular management of complex splenic aneurysm with the "amplatzer" embolic platform: application of cone-beam computed tomography. *Can Assoc Radiol J* 2010;61(4):230–232.

syndrome resulting from organ infarction, and the presence of complications.

OUTCOMES/PROGNOSIS

With the overall incidence of VAAs being low, data on endovascular VAA repair are limited. The literature mainly consists of small retrospective single-center experiences commonly summarizing data on multiple vascular territories or even different therapeutic approaches.[15,16,23,27,28,34,36–39,41–43] The data are promising, however, because overall technical success rates for VAA treatment are as high as 90% to 100%. Unfortunately, as a significant limitation, comparative data and studies between techniques or comparisons with surgical options are not available.

PRACTICAL ADVANTAGES AND LIMITATIONS

For the relatively high rupture risk, medical management and surveillance is not feasible for many VAAs, as described earlier in the stratification algorithm (FIGURE 60.3).

There are no studies available that prospectively compare the relative therapeutic effectiveness of endovascular treatments with medical and surgical management. Little data suggest that endovascular treatment may be superior when comparing technical success on an intention-to-treat basis (less than 10% of the endovascular treatments failed, compared to 18.5% in the surgical group).[44]

In many institutions and for the minimally invasive nature of the procedure, thus the usually quick remobilization of patients and its high technical success rates, endovascular therapy is primarily considered for VAAs. If, for example, anatomic variants, arterial stenoses, or occlusions should not allow for appropriate access to the aneurysm, then surgical techniques (e.g., resection, aneurysmorrhaphy) are valuable and alternative options.

MANAGEMENT (INCLUDING CLINICAL, PATHOPHYSIOLOGIC, AND ANATOMIC MEASURES)

For the proposed VAA stratification algorithm, based on clinical, anatomic, and pathophysiologic variables, FIGURE 60.3 and the above-mentioned criteria for patient selection.

COMPLICATIONS

As for any endovascular therapy, arterial puncture site complications may be encountered (e.g., hematoma, false aneurysm). Related to the embolization therapy and predominantly with embolization of renal, hepatic, and splenic hilar aneurysms, partial, segmental, or subsegmental organ infarction may develop, especially when using the above-described isolation technique.

Manifestations of postembolization syndrome are frequently seen (fever, pain, nausea). Abscess formation, mostly within infarcted organ tissue, however, is a rare complication of embolization (<1%).

All technique-related complications (e.g., aneurysm perforation, nonselective embolization with necrosis of the gastric wall/bowel, pancreatitis) can be minimized by meticulous technique, precise understanding and depiction of the vascular anatomy, and operator experience.

Management of Complications

Infectious complications after embolization including abscess formation are rare and when encountered can mainly be managed by antibiotic therapy and, if necessary, percutaneous drainage. For postembolization syndrome, symptomatic treatment with hydration and antiemetic and analgesic drugs is recommended. For technical complications like intra- or perioperative aneurysm perforation, emergent treatment is essential, mostly again by endovascular therapy. In rare cases, operative repair may become necessary.

Disease Surveillance and Treatment Monitoring Algorithms

There are no proven international guidelines on surveillance and monitoring established. All regimens have to encounter individual risk factors for disease progression including VAA etiology and initial therapeutic success.

Early and Late Failures and Options for Management

Therapeutic failures of VAA occlusion or exclusion are mostly related to (re-)perfusion of the VAA. Further therapeutic options are related to the individual anatomy as well as the length and location of the reperfused VAA and its afferent and efferent vessels. In such cases allowing for reaccess of the VAA (as documented on CTA, MRA, and/or angiography) using an endovascular route, this should be attempted. For all therapeutic failures not allowing for endovascular re-access surgery or percutaneous treatments (glue, thrombin), injection should be considered.

THE FUTURE

Newer, smaller, and more flexible generations of embolization devices allow for even better vascular access and safer endovascular treatment of VAAs. In conjunction with state-of-the art angiography suites allowing for cone beam CT and rotational angiography, endovascular management should be able to prove its high value and efficacy in treatment algorithms for VAAs. Integrating MR scanner into angio-suites may potentially allow for intra- or peri-interventional MRA, thereby enabling functional (perfusion, oxygenation, etc.) tissue assessment before, during, and after the procedure. Some groups have furthermore developed MR-safe vascular devices including an MR-safe guide wire, which in the future may even allow vascular interventions in the MR suite.[45,46]

▌ CONCLUSION

Today endovascular management is considered a safe and efficient first-line treatment for VAAs in suitable patients and as determined by interdisciplinary algorithms.

▌ REFERENCES

1. Drescher R, Koster O, von Rothenburg T. Superior mesenteric artery aneurysm stent graft. *Abdom Imaging* 2006;31:113–116.
2. Ozbulbul NI. CT angiography of the celiac trunk: anatomy, variants and pathologic findings. *Diagn Interv Radiol* 2011;17(2):150–157.
3. Stanley JC, Thompson NW, Fry WJ. Splanchnic artery aneurysms. *Arch Surg* 1970;101:689–697.
4. Horton KM, Smith C, Fishman EK. MDCT and 3D CT angiography of splanchnic artery aneurysms. *AJR Am J Roentgenol* 2007;189:641–647.
5. Knox R, Steinthorsson G, Sumpio B. Celiac artery aneurysms: a case report and review of the literature. *Int J Angiol* 2000;9:99–102.
6. Tessier DJ, Fowl RJ, Stone WM, et al. Iatrogenic hepatic artery pseudoaneurysms: an uncommon complication after hepatic, biliary, and pancreatic procedures. *Ann Vasc Surg* 2003;17:663–669.
7. Tessier DJ, Stone WM, Fowl RJ, et al. Clinical features and management of splenic artery pseudoaneurysm: case series and cumulative review of literature. *J Vasc Surg* 2003;38:969–974.
8. Abbas MA, Stone WM, Fowl RJ, et al. Splenic artery aneurysms: two decades experience at Mayo clinic. *Ann Vasc Surg* 2002;16:442–449.
9. Trastek VF, Pairolero PC, Joyce JW, et al. Splenic artery aneurysms. *Surgery* 1982;91:694–699.
10. Stone WM, Abbas MA, Gloviczki P, et al. Celiac arterial aneurysms: a critical reappraisal of a rare entity. *Arch Surg* 2002;137:670–674.
11. Adaletli I, Ozpeynirci Y, Kurugoglu S, et al. Abdominal manifestations of polyarteritis nodosa demonstrated with CT. *Pediatr Radiol* 2010;40:766–769.
12. Ozaki K, Miyayama S, Ushiogi Y, et al. Renal involvement of polyarteritis nodosa: CT and MR findings. *Abdom Imaging* 2009;34:265–270.
13. Kapoor BS, Haddad HL, Saddekni S, et al. Diagnosis and management of pseudoaneurysms: an update. *Curr Probl Diagn Radiol* 2009;38:170–188.
14. Raghavan A, Wong CK, Lam A, et al. Spontaneous occlusion of posttraumatic splenic pseudoaneurysm: report of two cases in children. *Pediatr Radiol* 2004;34:355–357.
15. Lookstein RA, Guller J. Embolization of complex vascular lesions. *Mt Sinai J Med* 2004;71:17–28.
16. Larson RA, Solomon J, Carpenter JP. Stent graft repair of visceral artery aneurysms. J Vasc Surg 2002;36:1260–1263.
17. Madoff DC, Denys A, Wallace MJ, et al. Splenic arterial interventions: anatomy, indications, technical considerations, and potential complications. *Radiographics* 2005;25 (suppl 1):S191–211.
18. Hirsch AT, Haskal ZJ, Hertzer NR, et al. ACC/AHA 2005 guidelines for the management of patients with peripheral arterial disease (lower extremity, renal, mesenteric, and abdominal aortic): executive summary a collaborative report from the American Association for Vascular Surgery/Society for Vascular Surgery, Society for Cardiovascular Angiography and Interventions, Society for Vascular Medicine and Biology, Society of Interventional Radiology, and the ACC/AHA Task Force on Practice Guidelines (writing committee to develop guidelines for the management of patients with peripheral arterial disease) endorsed by the American Association of Cardiovascular and Pulmonary Rehabilitation; National Heart, Lung,
and Blood Institute; Society for Vascular Nursing; TransAtlantic Inter-Society Consensus; and Vascular Disease Foundation. *J Am Coll Cardiol* 2006;47:1239–1312.
19. Orth RC, Wallace MJ, Kuo MD. C-arm cone-beam CT: general principles and technical considerations for use in interventional radiology. *J Vasc Interv Radiol* 2008;19:814–820.
20. Wallace MJ, Kuo MD, Glaiberman C, et al. Three-dimensional C-arm cone-beam CT: applications in the interventional suite. *J Vasc Interv Radiol* 2008;19:799–813.
21. Kos S, Burrill J, Weir G, et al. Endovascular management of complex splenic aneurysm with the "amplatzer" embolic platform: application of cone-beam computed tomography. *Can Assoc Radiol J* 2010;61(4):230–232. Epub 2009 Dec 31.
22. Lagana D, Carrafiello G, Mangini M, et al. Indications for the use of the Amplatzer vascular plug in interventional radiology. *Radiol Med* 2008;113:707–718.
23. Rossi M, Rebonato A, Greco L, et al. Endovascular exclusion of visceral artery aneurysms with stent-grafts: technique and long-term follow-up. *Cardiovasc Intervent Radiol* 2008;31:36–42.
24. Carrafiello G, Rivolta N, Fontana F, et al. Combined endovascular repair of a celiac trunk aneurysm using celiac-splenic stent graft and hepatic artery embolization. *Cardiovasc Intervent Radiol* 2010;33:352–354.
25. Ikeda O, Tamura Y, Nakasone Y, et al. Nonoperative management of unruptured visceral artery aneurysms: treatment by transcatheter coil embolization. *J Vasc Surg* 2008;47:1212–1219.
26. Assali AR, Sdringola S, Moustapha A, et al. Endovascular repair of traumatic pseudoaneurysm by uncovered self-expandable stenting with or without transstent coiling of the aneurysm cavity. *Catheter Cardiovasc Interv* 2001;53:253–258.
27. Bratby MJ, Lehmann ED, Bottomley J, et al. Endovascular embolization of visceral artery aneurysms with ethylene-vinyl alcohol (Onyx): a case series. *Cardiovasc Intervent Radiol* 2006;29:1125–1128.
28. Tulsyan N, Kashyap VS, Greenberg RK, et al. The endovascular management of visceral artery aneurysms and pseudoaneurysms. *J Vasc Surg* 2007;45:276–283; discussion 283.
29. Rautio R, Haapanen A. Transcatheter embolization of a renal artery aneurysm using ethylene vinyl alcohol copolymer. *Cardiovasc Intervent Radiol* 2007;30:300–303.
30. Gulati GS, Gulati MS, Makharia G, et al. Percutaneous glue embolization of a visceral artery pseudoaneurysm in a case of sickle cell anemia. *Cardiovasc Intervent Radiol* 2006;29:665–668.
31. Perek B, Urbanowicz T, Zabicki B, et al. CT-guided thrombin injection to control rapid expansion of ascending aortic false aneurysm 15 months after Bentall-Bono operation. *Cardiovasc Intervent Radiol* 2011;34(suppl 2):S83–85.
32. Lee GS, Brawley J, Hung R Complex subclavian artery pseudoaneurysm causing failure of endovascular stent repair with salvage by percutaneous thrombin injection. *J Vasc Surg* 2010;52:1058–1060.
33. Poloczek A, Amann-Vesti B, Thalhammer C, et al. Successful treatment of a mycotic pseudoaneurysm of the brachial artery with percutaneous ultrasound-guided thrombin injection and antibiotics. *Vasa* 2010;39:181–183.
34. Lagana D, Carrafiello G, Mangini M, et al. Multimodal approach to endovascular treatment of visceral artery aneurysms and pseudoaneurysms. *Eur J Radiol* 2006;59:104–111.
35. Corso R, Carrafiello G, Rampoldi A, et al. Pseudoaneurysm after spontaneous rupture of renal angiomyolipoma in tuberous sclerosis: successful treatment with percutaneous thrombin injection. *Cardiovasc Intervent Radiol* 2005;28:262–264.
36. Vallina-Victorero Vazquez MJ, Vaquero Lorenzo F, Salgado AA, et al. Endovascular treatment of splenic and renal aneurysms. *Ann Vasc Surg* 2009;23:258, e213–257.
37. Sadat U, Dar O, Walsh S, et al. Splenic artery aneurysms in pregnancy—a systematic review. *Int J Surg* 2008;6:261–265.
38. Ferrero E, Gaggiano A, Ferri M, et al. Visceral artery aneurysms: series of 17 cases treated in a single center. *Int J Angiol* 2010;29:30–36.
39. Berceli SA. Hepatic and splenic artery aneurysms. *Semin Vasc Surg* 2005;18:196–201.
40. Liu DM, Salem R, Bui JT, et al. Angiographic considerations in patients undergoing liver-directed therapy. *J Vasc Interv Radiol* 2005;16:911–935.
41. Nosher JL, Chung J, Brevetti LS, et al. Visceral and renal artery aneurysms: a pictorial essay on endovascular therapy. *Radiographics* 2006;26:1687–1704, quiz 1687.

42. Carr SC, Mahvi DM, Hoch JR, et al. Visceral artery aneurysm rupture. *J Vasc Surg* 2001;33:806–811.

43. Parildar M, Oran I, Memis A. Embolization of visceral pseudoaneurysms with platinum coils and n-butyl cyanoacrylate. *Abdom Imaging* 2003;28:36–40.

44. Huang YK, Hsieh HC, Tsai FC, et al. Visceral artery aneurysm: risk factor analysis and therapeutic opinion. *Eur J Vasc Endovasc Surg* 2007;33:293–301.

45. Kos S, Huegli R, Bongartz GM, et al. MR-guided endovascular interventions: a comprehensive review on techniques and applications. *Eur Radiol* 2008;18:645–657.

46. Kos S, Huegli R, Hofmann E, et al. Feasibility of real-time magnetic resonance-guided angioplasty and stenting of renal arteries in vitro and in swine, using a new polyetheretherketone-based magnetic resonance-compatible guidewire. *Invest Radiol* 2009;44:234–241.

Iliac Artery Aneurysms

ADNAN Z. RIZVI and ANDREW H. CRAGG

EPIDEMIOLOGY

Iliac artery aneurysms (IAAs) are most commonly associated with infrarenal abdominal aortic aneurysms (AAAs). This pattern is seen in 10% to 20% of all AAAs. There is variability in the reported prevalence of isolated IAAs in the population. Autopsy studies report the incidence of isolated IAAs ranging from 0.03%[1] to more recent studies showing an incidence of 1.4% to 4%.[2,3] Isolated common iliac artery aneurysms (CIAAs) occur in less than 2% of all aneurysms involving the aortoiliac distribution.[4-6] Aneurysms limited to the CIA are seen in approximately 70% of patients presenting with isolated IAAs and fewer than 20% are isolated to the internal iliac artery. Silver et al.[7] reported on 671 aortoiliac artery aneurysms and identified only 3 aneurysms isolated to the internal iliac artery. Isolated external iliac artery (EIA) aneurysms are uncommon, usually occurring in conjunction with CIAAs or common femoral artery aneurysms. Isolated IAAs have a male preponderance with a male-to-female ratio of 7:1 and tend to present later in life.

ETIOLOGY

The exact etiology of IAAs is unknown but is felt to be similar to that of AAAs. Most are related to degenerative atherosclerosis caused by proteolytic degradation, inflammation, and wall stress. Less common causes include anastomotic graft failures (pseudoaneurysms), arterial trauma, infectious or mycotic aneurysms related to bacterial infections (*Salmonella*, *Staphylococcus aureus*, and *Klebsiella*), connective tissue disorders (Marfan or Ehlers-Danlos syndrome), and various vasculitides (Behcet disease, Kawasaki disease, and Takayasu arteritis).

NATURAL HISTORY

The natural history of IAAs is not as well described as that of AAAs. Santilli et al.[8] followed a large population of patients with IIAAs and found that IAAs less than 3 cm in size tend to grow at a slower rate (0.11 ± 0.02 cm/year) compared with IAAs measuring between 3 and 5 cm (0.26 ± 0.1 cm/year). In a study from the Mayo Clinic, 104 CIAAs were followed with at least 2 imaging studies and they found the mean growth was 0.29 cm per year.[9] On multivariate analysis, only hypertension predicted faster expansion (0.32 versus 0.14 cm/year, $p = .01$). Similar to AAAs, the risk of rupture of IIAAs correlates with diameter. The range of IIAA size when they present with rupture varies by study, but the mean range is 5.8 to 7.8 cm.[5,6,10,11] Both Santilli et al.[8] and Huang et al.[9] found in their series of CIAAs that there were no ruptures in aneurysms measuring less than 3.8 cm. There are fewer data on the natural history of isolated IIAAs. Most reports in the literature describe rupture as the presenting symptom in a large percentage of patients. Dix et al.[12] recently reviewed the current literature on isolated IIAAs and 40% of patients presented with rupture. The median size of ruptured IIAAs was 7.0 cm (range 5 to 13 cm) and that of nonruptured IIAAs was 6.0 cm (range 2 to 11 cm).[12]

CLINICAL PRESENTATION

Most IAAs are discovered incidentally while undergoing an imaging modality for a separate indication. Patients presenting with rupture develop acute onset lower abdominal pain and may be hypotensive. Other symptoms if present and not related to rupture are typically caused by compression of adjacent structures, such as adjacent nerves, colon/rectum, ureter, or iliac vein. If the ureter is involved, the patient may have ureteral obstruction or repeating urinary tract infections. Colon or rectum compression can cause tenesmus or constipation. Compression of the lumbosacral nerves can cause neurogenic lower extremity pain or paresthesias. Finally, compression of the iliac vein can cause a deep venous thrombosis and erosion results in an arterial-venous fistula.

DIAGNOSIS

The diagnosis of an IAA is difficult on physical examination, especially in the obese individual. Occasionally, on plain abdominal X-ray, a calcified ring in the pelvis outlining the iliac vessels may suggest an IAA. Imaging modalities to further define an IAA include ultrasonography (US), computed tomography (CT), and magnetic resonance imaging (MRI). US is readily available and can accurately diagnose an IAA. It may be difficult to visualize an isolated IIAA by US. CT or MR angiography are the imaging modalities of choice to delineate IAAs and offer great detail in determining size and the overall iliac artery anatomy for case planning.

INDICATIONS FOR INTERVENTION

When to intervene on IAAs has typically been based on the maximum diameter. Based on studies that have not demonstrated a rupture of a CIAA less than 3.5 cm in size,[8,11] the current recommendations is to intervene once a CIAA exceeds 3.5 cm because the rupture risk increases at this point. Reported risk of mortality after repair of a ruptured IAA remains high. Past surgical series report a mortality rate ranging from 0% to 40% (Table 61.1).[6,10,13-15] Patients with symptomatic IAAs should be considered for repair regardless of the size of the aneurysm. For patients with CIAAs less than 3.5 cm in size, surveillance

Table 61.1

Results of Open Surgical Repair of Iliac Artery Aneurysms

Author	Year	Nonruptured n	Mortality %	Ruptured/ symptomatic n	Mortality %
Richardson and Greenfield[6]	1988	25	11	30	33
Weimann et al.[14]	1990	15	0	7	40
Nachbur et al.[15]	1991	7	0	51	20
Krupski et al.[13]	1998	9	0	12	0
Kasirajan et al.[10]	1998	21	6	4	0
Soury et al.[26]	2001	33	3	5	40

imaging with either US or CT should be performed. Similar to CIAAs, IIAAs have a propensity to rupture once they enlarge.

Data on a size threshold regarding when to intervene on IIAAs are limited. Based on data from small observational series, current recommendations suggest that IIAAs should be repaired once they exceed 3 cm in diameter.[4]

In addition to the aneurysm size, patient factors must be considered when deciding to intervene. These include underlying comorbidities, prior abdominal or pelvic surgery, stomas, pelvic radiation, and obesity. Traditionally, repair of IAAs has been performed surgically via a variety of techniques. More recently with the advent of endovascular AAA repair, similar minimally invasive catheter-based techniques have been adopted to address IAAs. Although long-term data are not available on the

endovascular repair of IAAs, there is a significant reduction in morbidity and mortality compared to open techniques. There are a wide variety of techniques to treat IAAs by an endovascular approach and they vary based on the location and anatomy of the aneurysm.

Endovascular Treatment and Techniques

Preoperative planning is critically important when deciding on an endovascular repair (Table 61.2). CT angiography provides detailed anatomy on the length of the proximal and distal landing or "seal zone," the tortuosity of the iliac artery, and the overall length of the vessels to be treated. The technique and method of repair depend on the location and number of aneurysms involved. Fahrni et al.[16] devised anatomic criteria for IAAs that help simplify how to manage these using an endovascular approach. The following is a modification of Fahrni et al.'s classification scheme and a description of how to manage anatomic variations of IAAs.

Type 1a: Isolated CIAA with Adequate Proximal and Distal Neck

The anatomic configuration is suitable for an endovascular repair. The minimum length of proximal and distal neck needed for a commercially available stent graft is 1 cm. These can be treated with a variety of devices, including a Viabahn graft (W. L. Gore, Flagstaff, AZ), Excluder (W. L. Gore), Zenith (Cook, Bloomington, IN), Aneurx (Medtronic, Minneapolis, MN), and Talent (Medtronic). The stent-graft is typically deployed from the ipsilateral retrograde approach and imaging is obtained from the contralateral femoral artery (FIGURE 61.1).

Type 1b: Isolated CIAAs with Inadequate Distal Neck

Similar to a type 1a CIAA, this can be treated with a single stent-graft from the proximal CIA and extending into the EIA. There may be a size discrepancy between the CIA and EIA, thus proper device sizing is critical. The IIA is typically treated with embolization using either an Amplatzer vascular plug (AGA Medical, Plymouth, MN) or coils. Our preference is to use a single Amplatzer plug because it preserves the distal IIA collateral branches. The IIA embolization is typically performed from a contralateral approach (FIGURE 61.2). If there is involvement

Table 61.2

Results of Endovascular Repair of Iliac Artery Aneurysms

Author	Year	Nonruptured n	Mortality %	Ruptured/symptomatic n	Mortality %	Patency and follow-up/ secondary interventions
Sanchez et al.[27]	1999	39	2.5	0	0	94.5% (4 y)/15.8%
Casana et al.[28]	2003	16	0	0	20	100% (18 mo)/6.2%
Caronno et al.[29]	2006	20	0	5	0	91% (32 mo)/23.8%
Tielliu et al.[30]	2006	30	0	5	0	98% (31 mo)/5.7%
Boules et al.[31]	2006	40	0	5	0	95% (2 y)/12%
Patel et al.[32]	2009	31	0	1	0	96% (5 y)/3%
Chemelli et al.[33]	2010	79	1.2	12	0	97% (45.9 mo)/13.2%
Hechelhammer et al.[34]	2010	0	0	11	18	100% (23 mo)/9%

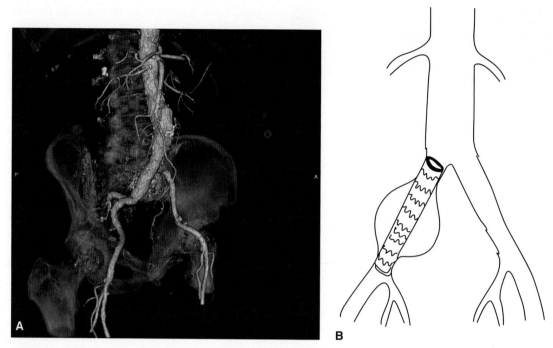

FIGURE 61.1 A. CT reconstruction of a 4.3-cm right common iliac artery aneurysm suitable for endovascular repair using a single iliac stent-graft. **B.** Drawing demonstrating use of a single stent-graft sealing in the proximal and distal common iliac artery and successfully excluding an isolated common iliac artery aneurysm.

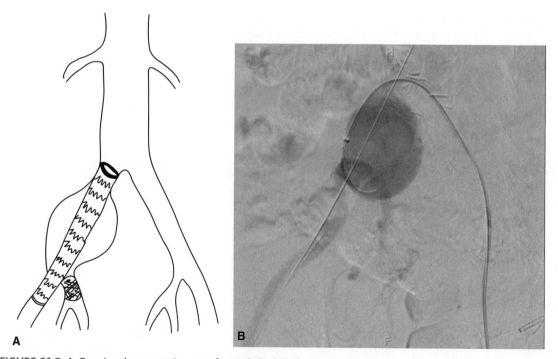

FIGURE 61.2 A. Drawing demonstrating use of a single limb and embolization of the origin of the internal iliac artery to allow for an adequate distal seal. **B.** Angiography demonstrating a large right common iliac aneurysm extending to the iliac bifurcation.

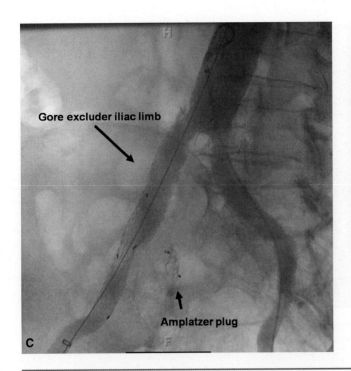

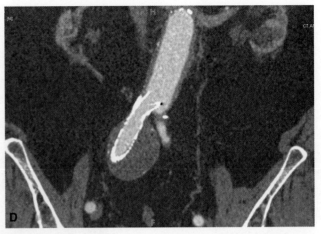

FIGURE 61.2 *(Continued)* **C.** Completion angiogram after embolizing the internal iliac artery with an Amplatzer vascular plug (*short arrow*) and placing a single Gore Excluder iliac limb (*long arrow*). **D.** 3-Month follow-up CTA demonstrating good proximal seal and no endoleak.

of the proximal IIA with aneurysmal disease and there is not adequate neck for placement of a proximal IIA plug or coil, then the more distal branches of the IIA need to be treated with either a vascular plug or coil embolization.

Type 1c: Single or Bilateral CIAA without Adequate Proximal and/or Distal Neck

This type of anatomic configuration presents a much more challenging repair and may require concurrent surgical intervention. For isolated common iliac aneurysms without adequate proximal seal zone, this can be addressed two ways. One approach entails placing an aorto-uni-iliac stent-graft (Cook Zenith) on the ipsilateral side. The IIA can be treated by techniques already described if the distal landing zone in the CIA is inadequate. The contralateral CIA should be occluded with either an Amplatzer vascular plug or a Cook Zenith iliac plug. A femoral-to-femoral artery bypass is necessary to maintain antegrade and retrograde perfusion to the contralateral femoral artery and IIA, respectively (FIGURE 61.3). If the infrarenal aortic neck is of adequate diameter, another approach is to place a commercially available bifurcated stent-graft used to treat AAAs. The contralateral limb extending into the CIA is placed in the typical standard fashion. Care must be taken as to not "jail" the contralateral gate during deployment of the main body. If the contralateral gate is "jailed" after deployment, this can typically be cannulated from the brachial approach and eventually both iliac limbs will need to be treated with "kissing" balloon angioplasty (FIGURE 61.4).

For patients with bilateral CIAa, exclusion of the aneurysms can be performed using a modular bifurcated stent-graft. In this scenario, management of the IIA is not standardized. We will discuss the incidence of buttock claudication with bilateral IIA embolization later. Our preference has been to maintain patency to at least one IIA to prevent the complications of bilateral IIA embolization. Traditionally this has been performed with a

retrograde surgical bypass (Dacron or polytetraethylfluorene graft) off the ipsilateral common femoral artery to the IIA in an end-to-end fashion and extension of the iliac limb of the

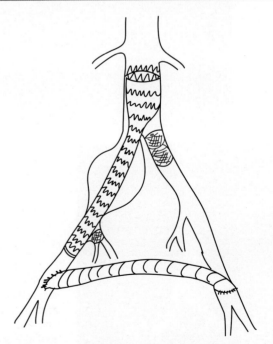

FIGURE 61.3 Drawing demonstrating use of a commercially available aorto-uniliac stent-graft to exclude a right common iliac artery aneurysm without adequate proximal or distal seal zone. The right internal iliac artery is embolized with an Amplatzer vascular plug at the origin of the contralateral common iliac artery. A right-to-left femoral-femoral bypass graft maintains perfusion to the left leg.

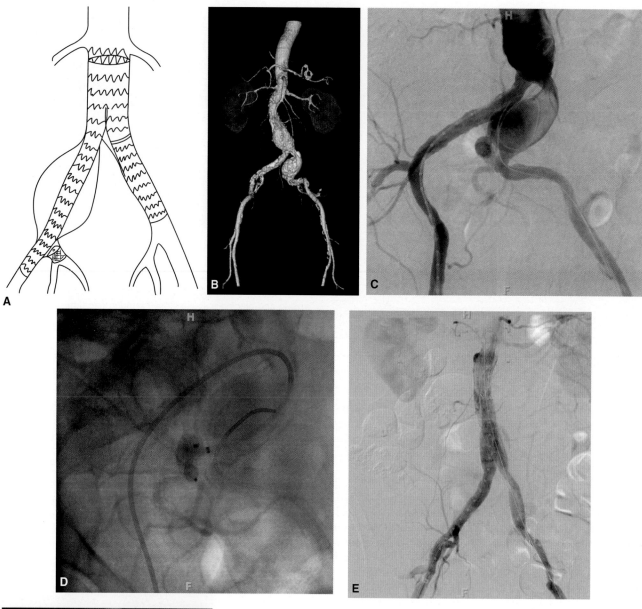

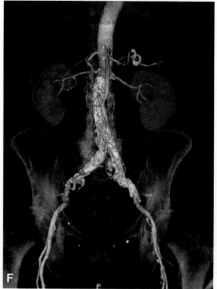

FIGURE 61.4 A. Drawing demonstrating a common iliac artery aneurysm without adequate proximal or distal common iliac seal zone and placement of a modular bifurcated stent-graft with one limb extending into the external iliac artery after coil embolization of the ipsilateral internal iliac artery. **B.** Preop reformatted CTA demonstrating a 3.5-cm infrarenal AAA and a 4.3-cm left common iliac artery aneurysm. **C.** Angiography demonstrating the AAA and left common iliac artery aneurysm. **D.** Cannulation of the internal iliac artery with placement of an Amplatzer vascular plug into the origin of the internal iliac artery. **E.** Completion angiogram after left internal iliac artery embolization and placement of a Gore Excluder graft with the left limb extending into the proximal external iliac artery. **F.** 3-Month follow-up CTA showing successful treatment of the AAA and large left common iliac aneurysm with no endoleak. The right internal iliac artery remains patent.

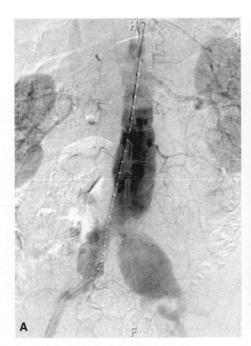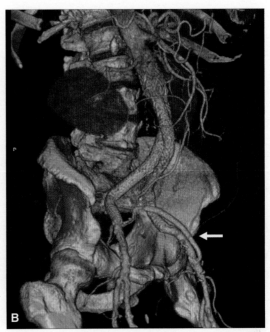

FIGURE 61.5 A. Angiography demonstrating a small infrarenal AAA with bilateral large common iliac artery aneurysms extending to the iliac bifurcation. **B.** 3-Month post-CTA demonstrating successful exclusion of the AAA and iliac aneurysms. The right internal iliac artery was treated with coil embolization to allow for a distal landing zone. Perfusion to the left internal iliac artery was maintained with a retrograde left common femoral to internal iliac artery bypass via a retroperitoneal approach (*arrow* indicates bypass graft).

stent-graft into the proximal EIA (FIGURE 61.5). Novel endovascular techniques to maintain IIA perfusion are discussed later.

Type 2a–c: Internal Iliac Artery Aneurysms with or without Adequate Proximal or Distal Necks

The endovascular management of IIAAs also depends on the proximal and distal aspects of the vessels. For IIAAs with an adequate proximal neck beyond the iliac bifurcation, these can typically be occluded using an Amplatzer plug. The management of the outflow vessels depends on their size and location. If one or two large outflow vessels are present, these can be treated either with an Amplatzer plug or with coils (FIGURE 61.6). The advantage of the Amplatzer plug is it typically will not encroach on the smaller branch/collateral vessels. Often, the IIAA gives off small collateral vessels that are difficult to cannulate to embolize. Options for this scenario include leaving the branches alone and hoping they will thrombose with time or packing the aneurysm sac with coils or wires to promote sac thrombosis.

If the anatomy of the IIAA proximal neck does not allow for placement of an Amplatzer plug, occlusion of inflow can typically be treated by bridging the distal CIA and proximal EIA with a covered stent (FIGURE 61.7).

Buttock Claudication with Bilateral Internal Iliac Artery Embolization

Certain patients with bilateral CIAAs (typically in the setting of aortoiliac aneurysmal disease) may need both IIAs treated with embolization to obtain an adequate distal landing zone

for stent grafting. There is considerable controversy in regard to the safety of bilateral IIA embolization for planned stent-graft repair. The complications associated with bilateral IIA embolization include buttock claudication, colon ischemia, erectile dysfunction, spinal cord ischemia, gluteal compartment syndrome, decubitus ulcers, and bladder dysfunction.[17–20] Lin et al.[21] recently reviewed the literature of pelvic complications following IIA embolization in conjunction with endovascular repair or aortoiliac aneurysmal disease. The incidence of buttock claudication after bilateral IIA embolization varied from 1.6% to 56%. The incidence was lower (28%) in patients undergoing unilateral IIA embolization compared to those undergoing bilateral IIA embolization (42%). A less common complication is colonic ischemia. Typically the inferior mesenteric artery is covered if an aortoiliac aneurysm is treated with a stent-graft. With bilateral IIA embolization, important pelvic collaterals are sacrificed. The overall incidence in the literature of colonic ischemia after bilateral IIA embolization is 3.4%.[21] Finally, the incidence of spinal cord ischemia after bilateral IIA embolization is rare, occurring less than 0.1% in the reported literature. Anatomic risk factors for developing complications after bilateral IIA embolization have been identified. Patients with severe contralateral IIA disease or ostial stenosis or severe profunda femoris disease may have underlying compromised pelvic circulation.[22,23] Identification of these patients and appropriate adjunctive management (i.e., maintaining patency to one IIA or repairing a diseased profunda femoris artery) at the time of intervention for the iliac aneurysmal disease may prevent pelvic ischemic complications during IIA embolization.

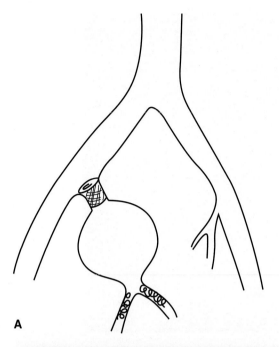

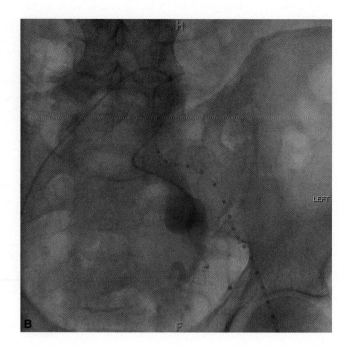

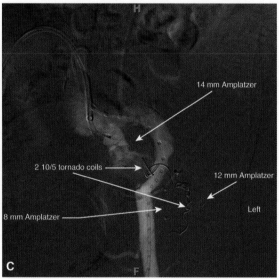

FIGURE 61.6 A. Drawing representing placement of an Amplatzer vascular plug in the origin of the internal iliac artery and placement of coils in the main branch vessels of the outflow IAA vessels. **B.** Selective angiogram of a large left internal iliac artery aneurysm. There is an adequate proximal neck, two large outflow vessels, and two smaller outflow vessels (not seen in this image). **C.** Final completion angiogram after placement of a 14-mm Amplatzer plug in the IIA origin, and an 8-mm and a 12-mm Amplatzer plug in the two main outflow vessels. Two 10-mm diameter, 5-cm long coils were placed in a medium-sized outflow branch.

Novel Techniques to Preserve the Internal Iliac Artery

In the setting of bilateral CIAA without an adequate distal landing zone, various endovascular techniques have been described to maintain perfusion to the IIA to prevent complications of pelvic ischemia after IIA embolization. Using the Zenith AAA platform, Cook has designed custom branched iliac endografts with a separate IIA limb that maintains antegrade IIA perfusion (FIGURE 61.8). The iliac branched graft is deployed from the ipsilateral side and a preloaded catheter over a 0.035″ wire is snared from the contralateral approach. This allows access into the internal iliac branch graft, which is positioned into the IIA. From here the branch graft and IIA is bridged with a commercial covered stent. Midterm results of compiled series using iliac branched grafts demonstrate occlusion of the IIA branch

graft occurring in 13% of treated vessels at greater than 30 days follow-up.[24]

Unfortunately, the branched iliac endografts are not commercially available and currently are limited to clinical trials. Interventionists have devised other techniques with commercially available devices to obviate this issue. One technique ("Trifurcated Technique")[25] entails placing a standard bifurcated stent-graft in the infrarenal aorta. In the limb of the infrarenal graft with the CIAA, an additional modular bifurcated stent-graft is placed. The longer limb is extended into the EIA, and from the brachial or axillary approach, the gate is accessed and bridged to the IIA with an appropriately sized Viabahn or similar covered self- or balloon-expanding stent (FIGURE 61.9). Another technique described as the "snorkel technique or chimney technique" has been described for treating aortic arch and paravisceral aortic pathology. A similar technique has been

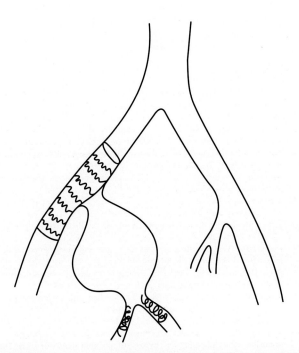

FIGURE 61.7 Drawing demonstrating an internal iliac artery aneurysm without an adequate proximal neck to place a vascular plug or coil. A covered stent has been placed across the origin to exclude inflow and the outflow vessels have been treated with coil embolization.

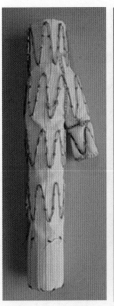
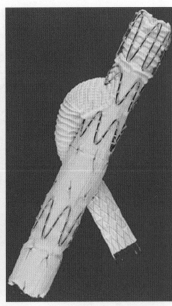

FIGURE 61.8 Left image shows a Cook Zenith bifurcated iliac side device (Cook Inc., Bloomington, IN) with the short side branch for the preservation of the internal iliac artery. Right image shows a helical Branch Endograft (Cook Inc.) with a directional side branch for preservation of the internal iliac artery.

Reprinted with permission: Minion DJ, Xenos E, Sorial E, et al. The trifurcated endograft technique for hypogastric preservation during endovascular aneurysm repair. *J Vasc Surg* 2008;47(3):658–661.

FIGURE 61.9 Steps for treating a large right common iliac artery aneurysm using the "Trifurcated Technique." In this example a Gore Excluder graft is used. Note the left internal iliac artery has been treated with coil embolization with the limb extended into the left external iliac artery. **A.** Deployment of a standard bifurcated main body graft. **B.** Deployment of a right iliac extension limb with the distal portion measuring 20mm in diameter. This will act as a landing zone for a second main body graft. **C.** Second main body graft deployed from the right femoral approach with the contralateral gate oriented towards the right hypogastric artery. **D.** The right hypogastric extension is deployed from the brachial approach. These are covered self-expanding stents. **E.** The left hypogastric artery is coil-embolized from the brachial approach. **F.** The left iliac extension limb into the left external iliac artery is deployed from the left femoral approach and final ballooning of the seal zones and graft overlap sites is performed.

Reprinted with permission: Minion DJ, Xenos E, Sorial E, et al. The trifurcated endograft technique for hypogastric preservation during endovascular aneurysm repair. *J Vasc Surg* 2008;47:658–661.

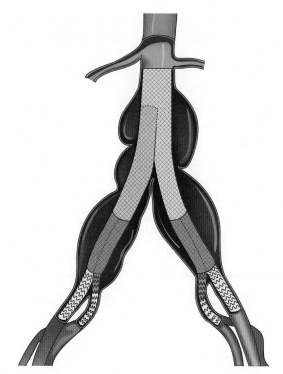

FIGURE 61.10 Drawing demonstrating use of the "snorkel/chimney technique" to treat bilateral large common iliac artery aneurysms with preservation of antegrade flow into both internal iliac arteries.

of the anatomy, a thorough understanding of the devices available to treat aortic and iliac aneurysmal disease, and careful preprocedural planning.

REFERENCES

1. Brunkwall J, Hauksson H, Bengtsson H, et al. Solitary aneurysms of the iliac arterial system: an estimate of their frequency of occurrence. *J Vasc Surg* 1989;10:381–384.
2. Lederle FA, Johnson GR, Wilson SE, et al. Prevalence and associations of abdominal aortic aneurysm detected through screening. Aneurysm Detection and Management (ADAM) Veterans Affairs Cooperative Study Group. *Ann Intern Med* 1997;126:441–449.
3. Bengtsson H, Bergqvist D, Sternby NH. Increasing prevalence of abdominal aortic aneurysms. A necropsy study. *Eur J Surg* 1992;158:19–23.
4. McCready RA, Pairolero PC, Gilmore JC, et al. Isolated iliac artery aneurysms. *Surgery* 1983;93:688–693.
5. Lowry SF, Kraft RO. Isolated aneurysms of the iliac artery. *Arch Surg* 1978;113:1289–1293.
6. Richardson JW, Greenfield LJ. Natural history and management of iliac aneurysms. *J Vasc Surg* 1988;8:165–171.
7. Silver D, Anderson EE, Porter JM. Isolated hypogastric artery aneurysm. Review and report of three cases. *Arch Surg* 1967;95:308–312.
8. Santilli SM, Wernsing SE, Lee ES. Expansion rates and outcomes for iliac artery aneurysms. *J Vasc Surg* 2000;31:114–121.
9. Huang Y, Gloviczki P, Noel AA, et al. Early complications and long-term outcome after open surgical treatment of popliteal artery aneurysms: is exclusion with saphenous vein bypass still the gold standard? *J Vasc Surg* 2007;45:706–713; discussion 13–15.
10. Kasirajan V, Hertzer NR, Beven EG, et al. Management of isolated common iliac artery aneurysms. *Cardiovasc Surg* 1998;6:171–177.
11. Huang Y, Gloviczki P, Duncan AA, et al. Common iliac artery aneurysm: expansion rate and results of open surgical and endovascular repair. *J Vasc Surg* 2008;47:1203–1210; discussion 10–11.
12. Dix FP, Titi M, Al-Khaffaf H. The isolated internal iliac artery aneurysm—a review. *Eur J Vasc Endovasc Surg* 2005;30:119–129.
13. Krupski WC, Selzman CH, Floridia R, et al. Contemporary management of isolated iliac aneurysms. *J Vasc Surg* 1998;28:1–11; discussion 11–13.
14. Weimann S, Tauscher T, Flora G. Isolated iliac artery aneurysms. *Ann Vasc Surg* 1990;4:297–301.
15. Nachbur BH, Inderbitzi RG, Bar W. Isolated iliac aneurysms. *Eur J Vasc Surg* 1991;5:375–381.
16. Fahrni M, Lachat MM, Wildermuth S, et al. Endovascular therapeutic options for isolated iliac aneurysms with a working classification. *Cardiovasc Intervent Radiol* 2003;26:443–447.
17. Mehta M, Veith FJ, Darling RC, et al. Effects of bilateral hypogastric artery interruption during endovascular and open aortoiliac aneurysm repair. *J Vasc Surg* 2004;40:698–702.
18. Bratby MJ, Munneke GM, Belli AM, et al. How safe is bilateral internal iliac artery embolization prior to EVAR? *Cardiovasc Intervent Radiol* 2008;31:246–253.
19. Lin PH, Bush RL, Chaikof EL, et al. A prospective evaluation of hypogastric artery embolization in endovascular aortoiliac aneurysm repair. *J Vasc Surg* 2002;36:500–506.
20. Karch LA, Hodgson KJ, Mattos MA, et al. Adverse consequences of internal iliac artery occlusion during endovascular repair of abdominal aortic aneurysms. *J Vasc Surg* 2000;32:676–683.
21. Lin PH, Chen AY, Vij A. Hypogastric artery preservation during endovascular aortic aneurysm repair: is it important? *Semin Vasc Surg* 2009;22:193–200.
22. Queral LA, Whitehouse WM Jr, Flinn WR, et al. Pelvic hemodynamics after aortoiliac reconstruction. *Surgery* 1979;86:799–809.
23. Yano OJ, Morrissey N, Eisen L, et al. Intentional internal iliac artery occlusion to facilitate endovascular repair of aortoiliac aneurysms. *J Vasc Surg* 2001;34:204–211.
24. Ghosh J, Murray D, Paravastu S, et al. Contemporary management of aorto-iliac aneurysms in the endovascular era. *Eur J Vasc Endovasc Surg* 2009;37:182–188.
25. Minion DJ, Xenos E, Sorial E, et al. The trifurcated endograft technique for hypogastric preservation during endovascular aneurysm repair. *J Vasc Surg* 2008;47:658–661.
26. Soury P, Brisset D, Gigou F, et al. Aneurysms of the internal iliac artery: management strategy. *Ann Vasc Surg* 2001;15:321–325.

described for maintaining IIA perfusion. In this setting the contralateral limb of a standard bifurcated AAA stent-graft is accessed from both the ipsilateral femoral approach and brachial/axillary approach. From the brachial/axillary approach, the IIA is cannulated. Simultaneously, two covered stent-grafts are positioned and deployed such that they are sandwiched in the contralateral gate. Distally one stent-graft seals in the IIA and the other in the EIA. The area where the two stent-grafts are "sandwiched" within the contralateral gate are simultaneously ballooned and sealed (FIGURE 61.10). It should be noted that both of these described techniques are "off-label" and long-term durability has not been addressed.

CONCLUSION

With the advent of endovascular technology to address AAAs, the same principles have been applied to the management of iliac artery aneurysms, and currently endovascular techniques to repair these have, in many instances, supplanted traditional open surgical repair. Midterm results show equal patency and low morbidity and mortality for elective repair and substantially lower mortality for symptomatic or ruptured presentation. Depending on the location of the aneurysm and extent of involvement of the infrarenal aorta or internal iliac artery, the interventionist can tailor the approach to each anatomic scenario. Preservation of the IIA is important to avoid pelvic ischemic complications and a variety of techniques are available to maintain perfusion to this important vessel. The key to successful endovascular repair of IAAs depends on thorough knowledge

27. Sanchez LA, Patel AV, Ohki T, et al. Midterm experience with the endovascular treatment of isolated iliac aneurysms. *J Vasc Surg* 1999;30: 907–913.
28. Casana R, Nano G, Dalainas I, et al. Midterm experience with the endovascular treatment of isolated iliac aneurysms. *Int Angiol* 2003;22:32–35.
29. Caronno R, Piffaretti G, Tozzi M, et al. Endovascular treatment of isolated iliac artery aneurysms. *Ann Vasc Surg* 2006;20:496–501.
30. Tielliu IF, Verhoeven EL, Zeebregts CJ, et al. Endovascular treatment of iliac artery aneurysms with a tubular stent-graft: mid-term results. *J Vasc Surg* 2006;43:440–445.

31. Boules TN, Selzer F, Stanziale SF, et al. Endovascular management of isolated iliac artery aneurysms. *J Vasc Surg* 2006;44:29–37.
32. Patel NV, Long GW, Cheema ZF, et al. Open vs. endovascular repair of isolated iliac artery aneurysms: a 12-year experience. *J Vasc Surg* 2009;49:1147–1153.
33. Chemelli A, Hugl B, Klocker J, et al. Endovascular repair of isolated iliac artery aneurysms. *J Endovasc Ther* 2010;17(4):492–503.
34. Hechelhammer L, Rancic Z, Pfiffner R, et al. Midterm outcome of endovascular repair of ruptured isolated iliac artery aneurysms. *J Vasc Surg* 2010;52(5):1159–1163.

Popliteal Artery Aneurysms

HEIKO UTHOFF and BARRY T. KATZEN

INTRODUCTION

Over 4,000 years ago, the Ebers Papyrus already described features of peripheral artery aneurysms. Popliteal artery aneurysm (PAA) is reported to be the most frequent type of peripheral artery aneurysm.[1,2] PAA is often diagnosed as a result of screening tests or other imaging studies in patients who do not have obvious symptoms of vascular disease. When symptoms are present, they are often acute limb threatening caused by thrombosis or acute peripheral thromboembolism. Thus, the main goal in PAA management is early diagnosis and treatment of (asymptomatic) PAAs to prevent the occurrence of potential limb-threatening complications.

PAA management has changed over time. Until the start of the 20th century, the management of PAA was to induce thrombosis within the aneurysm either by ligation or compression.[3] Today, the aim of treatment is to prevent (limb-threatening) thrombosis, although how to achieve this remains controversial.

Current treatment options, screening, and surveillance recommendation for the management of PAA are discussed in this chapter.

ANATOMIC ISSUES

Anatomy

The popliteal artery is in continuity with the superficial femoral artery. Its anatomic landmarks include the tendinous insertion of the adductor magnus muscle in the distal femur superiorly, and the bifurcation of the popliteal artery into the anterior tibial artery and tibioperoneal trunk at the level of the tibial tuberosity inferiorly. The popliteal artery lies posterior to the femur and anterior to the popliteal vein. The popliteal artery and vein are normally located between the two heads of the gastrocnemius muscle.

Normal Popliteal Artery Diameter

The diameter of the normal popliteal artery is not uniform throughout its length and is affected by a person's gender, age, height, and weight. Reports show that a normal popliteal artery diameter varies between 5 and 11 mm. In a recent duplex ultrasound study including 104 healthy men and 100 women, the mean midpopliteal external arterial diameters were 6.8 ± 0.8 mm in men and 6.0 ± 0.7 mm in women.[4] Proximal popliteal diameters were nearly identical, but the distal diameters were significantly smaller at 4.9 ± 0.6 mm and 4.4 ± 0.6 mm, respectively.

DEFINITION OF POPLITEAL ARTERY ANEURYSM, RISK FACTORS, AND EXPANSION RATES

The popliteal artery is defined as aneurysmal when a minimal focal dilation of 12 mm is identified and the diameter of the vessel is increased more than 50% relative to the proximal normal vessel segment.

Most PAAs are of atherosclerotic origin. Rare causes include infection, trauma, congenital, or those associated with Marfan or Behcet disease. PAAs are true aneurysms involving all layers of the vessel wall (intima, media, adventitia). Pseudoaneurysm formation in the popliteal artery has also been described but is rare and usually associated with trauma (i.e., blunt trauma, massage, acupuncture) or local infiltrative processes (i.e., osteochondromas). Common risk factors for true PAAs include male gender, smoking, hypertension, and advancing age. Repeated flexion and extension of the knee or upstream obstruction (i.e., popliteal entrapment) causing turbulent flow in the popliteal artery may contribute to arterial wall degeneration and aneurysm formation. Growth of ectatic popliteal arteries is typically slow (<1 mm/year) but variable and difficult to predict. Published expansion rates for small (15 to 20 mm) PAAs range from 0.7 to 1.5 mm/year, whereas rates for larger PAAs range from 1.5 to 3.7 mm/year.[5–7] PAA in patients with previously treated contralateral PAA and those with aneurysms at other locations as well as patients with hypertension were reported to have a faster than average growth rate. It is noteworthy that diabetes mellitus appears to provide "protective effect" with slower aneurysm growth rates, similar to that seen in abdominal aortic aneurysm (AAA).[5,8] Although time intervals between surveillance imaging should be based on the individual patient, they are largely defined by the expected expansion rate and threshold diameter for intervention. In contrast to AAA, however, rupture is uncommon in PAA; thus not only the diameter but also several other parameters should be borne in mind when planning surveillance and treatment. These are discussed below in detail.

Epidemiology

PAAs account for roughly 80% of all peripheral aneurysms. The real prevalence of PAA is difficult to determine and ranges from 1% in men aged 65 to 80 years to 0.001% in women of all ages.[1,9] Men are consistently more affected than women with a reported male-to-female ratio ranging from 10:1 to 30:1 and present at younger ages (mean age at presentation is 65 years).[10,11]

In approximately 50% of patients, PAA are bilateral and are also associated with aneurysms in other locations. A PAA can be found in 9% to 14% of patients with diagnosed AAA and, conversely, if a PAA is diagnosed, an AAA is simultaneously present in 30% to 50% of cases.[2] These associations have important implications. Therefore, patients with PAA should be screened for contralateral PAA and AAA and vice versa. In contrast, a community-based aneurysm screening for PAA cannot be recommended due to the low prevalence of PAA.

Presentation and Natural History

The risk of limb-threatening thrombotic complications implicates the importance to diagnose even asymptomatic PAAs as early as possible. With increasing awareness among physicians and more widespread use of imaging for other indications with coincidental PAA discovery, up to 80% of diagnosed PAAs are asymptomatic. The natural history of PAA is variable, but when left untreated there is a high incidence of thromboembolic complications (mean reported incidence 35%) with associated amputation rates of up to 67% (mean 25%).[12–14] Asymptomatic PAAs become symptomatic at a rate of approximate 14% per year.[15] Symptoms include nonspecific pain or discomfort behind the knee, intermittent claudication from thrombosis, repeated microemboli, or combined occlusive arterial disease and leg swelling, with or without deep venous thrombosis secondary to compression of the popliteal vein.[16] The clinical presentation of embolic events from PAA can be diverse, depending on the size and location of the embolism, and the collateral circulation in the leg. Large emboli usually manifest as acute leg ischemia and are diagnosed easily. By contrast, smaller emboli occluding only one of the three tibial arteries can be silent, particularly in inactive patients. Thus, a significant number of patients with asymptomatic aneurysms are likely to have had incidental distal occlusions or silent embolic events. Severe pain behind the knee because of aneurysm rupture is rare and often confined to the popliteal space.[17,18]

Diagnosis

As part of a routine vascular examination, palpation of the popliteal fossa can reveal a pulsatile popliteal mass in up to 60% of patients with PAA. A popliteal aneurysm may not be palpable if the aneurysm is less than 20 mm or thrombosed, however. All patients should also be examined for clinical signs of distal embolization and pedal pulse status. In general, ultrasound is the most commonly used and best imaging modality for diagnosing PAAs. Ultrasound can help determine the presence and patency of an aneurysm and whether the aneurysm contains thrombus. Duplex ultrasound also can help to distinguish an aneurysm from a popliteal mass, such as a Baker cyst, or demonstrate a simultaneous arteriovenous fistula. Additional computed tomography (CT) or magnetic resonance (MR) angiography is recommended depending on institutional resources and the clinical presentation. Duplex, CT, and MR angiography have major advantages over conventional arteriography due to their ability to accurately delineate the aneurysmal sac, mural thrombus, and surrounding structures. Unless emergent arteriography is needed to identify a suitable outflow vessel for lower extremity revascularization, conventional arteriography has no role in the diagnosis of PAA. FIGURES 62.1 and 62.2 demonstrate typical PAAs as seen in ultrasound, CTA, and digital subtraction angiography.

Patient Selection

Cardiovascular risk factors of all patients with PAA should be treated as discussed in current guidelines.[19,20] Table 62.1 summarizes the indications for PAA repair.

Symptomatic Patients

There is consensus that all patients with symptomatic PAA, regardless of size, should be referred for vascular evaluation and PAA repair (AHA guidelines grade 1A recommendation) because these patients have a high risk of developing acute ischemic complications that are associated with a high risk for limb loss.[19] In patients with PAA and evidence of acute thrombosis, distal embolization, or chronic limb ischemia, immediate initiation of therapeutic dose intravenous (IV) heparin is recommended while awaiting revascularization.[20–22] The treatment choices, including thrombolysis and surgical and endovascular treatment options, are discussed in detail later.

Asymptomatic Patients

Patients with large asymptomatic aneurysms (>30 mm) should undergo repair. Controversy remains regarding the management of asymptomatic smaller (<30 mm) PAAs.[16,23,24] The decision to treat a PAA requires weighing the risks and results of treatment against the risks of continued follow-up.

Elective Repair Versus Emergent Repair

PAAs treated electively seem to have superior outcomes in terms of limb loss, graft patency, and patient mortality than those presenting as an emergency. In the emergency setting, limb loss has been described as high as 20% to 59% and operative mortality rates of 5.4% to 11.8% compared to no limb loss or perioperative mortality in the elective setting.[18,25–27] Thus, historically, the management of PAA in the elective setting has been considered crucial. Comparable outcomes may be achieved for PAA in some tertiary care centers that have the capacity to provide both prompt evaluation and complex intervention.[28]

Risk Factors Favoring Early Repair

Size, distortion, presence of thrombus, and the runoff status have all been suggested as means of identifying a high-risk PAA, and their evaluation may provide some guidance in the decision process.

It is problematic to base treatment decisions on diameter alone, as opposed to the case of an AAA where there is a more defined causality linkage between diameter and aneurysm complications. In a review of 34 PAAs, small aneurysms (<20 mm) were shown to be less benign than previously suggested with a high incidence of thrombosis, clinical symptoms, and distal occlusive disease.

Nevertheless, using a cutoff value of less than 20 mm in diameter will subject an unacceptably large number of patients to unnecessary intervention and possibly related morbidity and mortality. It is generally agreed that although increased scrutiny and vigilance are required in these patients, operating on PAAs of less than 20 mm confers no clear benefit for most. In contrast, ongoing controversy surrounds management of PAAs in the 20- to 30-mm range. Facing 18% to 35% of PAA patients becoming symptomatic with conservative management, some clinicians feel that outcomes are improved with elective repair.

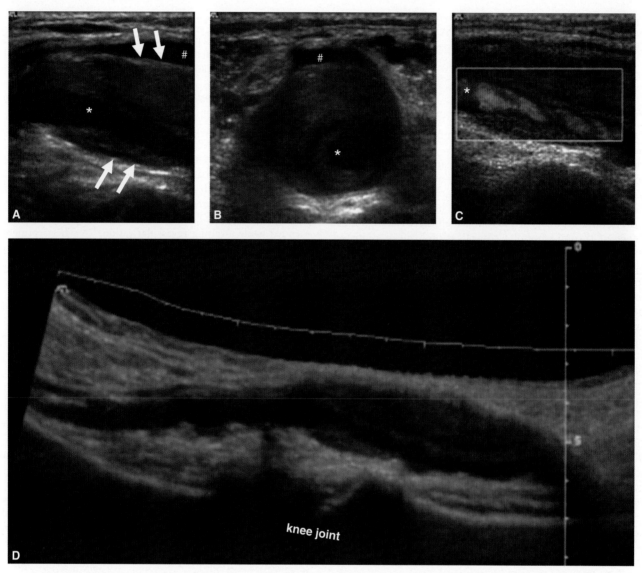

FIGURE 62.1 B-mode images in axial (**A**) and sagittal (**B**) views and sagittal F-mode color imaging (**C**) detail persistent luminal patency (*asterisk*), outer wall of popliteal artery aneurysms (*arrows*), and adjacent compressed popliteal vein (*hash*). B-mode longitudinal image centered at the knee (**D**) provides an extended view of the course and contour of the aneurysm.

Courtesy of Markus Aschwanden (University of Basel, Switzerland).

The ACC/AHA Practice Guidelines recommend treatment of any asymptomatic PAA with a diameter greater than 20 mm,[19] whereas others argue that PAAs that are less than 30 mm, in the absence of other risk factors (excessive distortion, mural thrombus, no distal pulses), could be observed safely using ultrasound and potentially antithrombotic therapy.[29] Obviously, size alone is not a reliable prognostic factor; combining risk factors may instead be more useful. The combination of size and distortion (>45 degrees) had been shown in one small study to be associated with the rate of acutely thrombosed PAAs, especially in PAAs greater than 30 mm, but these findings have not been reproduced to date.[30]

Ultrasound scanning revealed that in up to 70% of PAAs, a mural thrombus was present and that PAA thrombi are generally larger.[27] Because the popliteal artery is subject to continual flexion and extension, it has been postulated that PAA thrombus is at greater risk of disintegration and embolization compared with AAA thrombus. The presence of mural thrombus within the PAA in fact is associated with complications in several trials, and thus considered a high-risk factor by most clinicians.[6,31] Dawson et al. reported that 40% of asymptomatic PAA patients have absent pedal pulses, which appears to be a strong predictor of adverse outcome. These patients have an 86% likelihood of symptoms developing at 3 years compared with 34% in asymptomatic patients with intact pulses.[13] Absent pedal pulses may indicate repeated silent peripheral thrombosis and is likely to increase the likelihood of acute PAA thrombosis due to impaired outflow. With ongoing microembolism of the peripheral circulation, treatment options might be progressively worse over time; thus early intervention seems to be reasonable

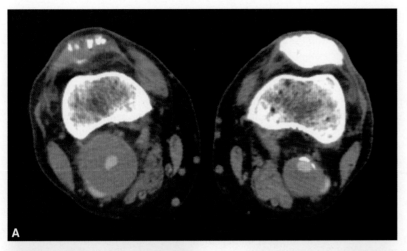

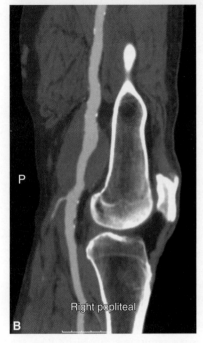

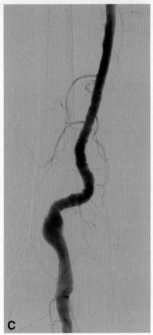

FIGURE 62.2 A. Axial contrast-enhanced CT view demonstrating bilateral PAA with mural thrombus. **B.** Sagittal MIP reconstruction of the right popliteal artery. **C.** Digital subtraction angiogram of the same PAA.

in these patients. The role of anticoagulation in the conservative management of small PAA with thrombus has not been defined but may be an alternative. Some clinicians advocate that small aneurysms in patients with low operative risk, acceptable run-off, adequate venous conduit, and mural thrombus should be considered for repair. Although surgical repair in these patients shows generally excellent results, with a long-term patency greater than 95%, perioperative deaths occur (approximately 1% to 2%) and limb swelling after surgical repair can be very troublesome for some patients. So careful decision making is

Table 62.1				
Strategies for Management of Popliteal Artery Aneurysms				
Presentation	Symptomatic		Asymptomatic	
Diameter	Regardless of diameter	<20 mm	20–30 mm	>30 mm
Treatment	(Thrombolysis &) repair	Conservative[a]	Consider repair[b]	Repair

[a]Duplex ultrasound surveillance every 6 to 12 months, antiplatelet therapy, consider anticoagulation.

[b]Factors favoring early repair: young age, high thrombus load, distorsion greater than 60 degrees, absent pedal pulse, saphenous vein available, previous contralateral PAA repair.

mandatory in every patient because the patient's limb or even life is at stake.

In summary, the retrospective character of all data and the rather small sample sizes make it difficult to give clear recommendations. The key is to identify PAAs with a high potential to cause acute limb ischemia and to discuss the pros and cons of early intervention accordingly with individual patients.

TREATMENT OPTIONS

In general, four treatment options are possible in patients with PAAs.

Conservative Treatment

In patients with a small, low-risk PAA, conservative treatment includes serial physical exam and duplex ultrasonography every 6 to 12 months. The time interval between examinations depends on the patient's risk factors for expansion. Antiplatelet therapy should be initiated, and anticoagulation may be reasonable in patients with a mural thrombus. Only one small study found a lower incidence of thrombus formation in patients with PAA who were treated with warfarin compared with antiplatelet therapy.[6] Data are largely lacking, however, and randomized trials are needed to determine the role of antithrombotic therapy in the conservative management of PAA.

Thrombolytic Therapy

In most centers thrombolysis is performed as rescue or bridging therapy in patients with acutely thrombosed PAA and limb-threatening ischemia before definitive repair. Lysis can clear the thrombosed PAA as well as runoff arteries effectively and therefore might relieve persistent ischemia. Outcome in these patients is generally poor, however, with a major amputation rate within 30 days of at least 14%.[14] Low-dose intra-arterial thrombolysis was first used in an attempt to clear a thrombosed PAA in the early 1980s.[32] According to a recent Cochrane meta-analysis of fibrinolytics in acute peripheral arterial ischemia, intra-arterial delivery of thrombolytic agents appeared to be more effective than IV administration.[33] Using streptokinase, urokinase, or recombinant tissue plasminogen activator (rt-PA), preoperative thrombolysis has been shown to improve the angiographically assessed runoff in 87% of critical limbs and to improve primary patency rates compared to thrombectomy and bypass alone (e.g., at 5 years 74% vs. 45%).[14,34,35]

There is no evidence that one fibrinolytic agent is more effective than others in this setting. However, data indicate that high-dose regimens (e.g., rt-PA bolus of 5 to 10 mg, followed by an infusion of up to 5 mg/hour) may provide more rapid initial lysis but cause more hemorrhagic complications and do not appear to improve limb salvage rates. Thrombolysis protocols are varying substantially between centers. Thrombolysis seems to be more effective when an angiographic lysis catheter is placed within the thrombus. A reasonable protocol consists of the infusion of 0.25 to 1 mg/hour of rt-PA via the lysis catheter and simultaneous infusion of 300 international units/hour of heparin via the sheath side port to prevent catheter-related thrombus. In addition to close clinical surveillance for signs of bleeding, coagulation parameters should be monitored at least every 6 hours with subsequent adjustment of the infusion rate

(e.g., fibrinogen 150 to 100 mg/dL, continue rt-PA with half the dosage; fibrinogen <100 mg/dL, pause rt-PA infusion). Lysis effects should be evaluated after 24 hours by means of an angiographic assessment. The maximum duration is not defined, but thrombolysis is rarely necessary beyond 48 hours.

In summary, intra-arterial thrombolytic therapy (catheter directed or direct intraoperative) may be indicated if no target vessel or multiple distal emboli are present. However, dissolution of the thrombus with distal showering and subsequent limb deterioration in up to 13% of cases as well as major bleeding complications including intracranial bleeding in 1% of cases remain a concern and may result in an unacceptably high risk of thrombolysis.[36,37]

Surgical Repair

The surgical management of PAAs has been in evolution for centuries and was described as early as the third century AD in Greece.

Options include simple bypass of the aneurysm, aneurysm exclusion and bypass, vein or prosthetic graft bypass, and bypass by lateral or posterior approach. The optimal open surgical approach for repair of PAA has not been standardized but overwhelming data suggest that (saphenous) vein bypass grafting should be used over prosthetic bypass grafting whenever possible. In a recent prospective study, primary patency of open surgical repair at 12, 36, and 48 months was 100%, 90.9%, and 81.8%, respectively.[38] Although reported outcomes vary widely due to inconsistent patient populations, treatment, and patency definitions, most studies report bypass graft patency of 81% to 100% at 1 year, 69% to 85% at 5 years, and limb salvage rates between 75% and 100%.[39–41] In general, clinical outcomes are negatively influenced by the presence of ischemic symptoms, poor runoff, and prosthetic bypass grafting. Periprocedural mortality rates were around 1% to 2%, and significant rates of perioperative complications, such as neurologic, infection, seroma, and hematoma, were reported.[40,42] Troublesome leg swelling has been documented in up to 50% of patients following bypass surgery and aneurysmal expansion over time is reported in up to 30% of patients despite open repair.[40,43,44]

In summary, compressive symptoms caused by PAA are likely best treated with an open repair that includes sac decompression. Furthermore, for young, active patients bypass using a saphenous vein is certainly a valid option because long-term data (>10 years) of endovascular approaches are pending.

Endovascular Repair

Several recent reports have advocated endovascular treatment of PAAs over surgical repair.[29,38,45–47] Endovascular treatment provides shorter operative time, shorter hospital stays with less perioperative morbidity, and faster recovery.[38,48] The first report of endovascular PAA repair was published in 1994, in which a vascular graft was sewn to two balloon-expandable stents and then deployed.[49] Since then, many different approaches to endovascular repair have been reported, including both ePTFE (expanded polytetrafluoroethylene), vein, or Dacron attached to balloon-expandable stents and commercial Dacron stent-grafts. Early outcomes with these devices were mixed, primarily due to high rates of thrombosis and mechanical failure.[50–52] More recent studies, predominantly using the Hemobahn/Viabahn endoprosthesis device (W.L. Gore and Associates, Inc., Flagstaff,

AZ), report mid- to long-term (5 to 10 years) clinical outcomes comparable to traditional surgical bypass.[38,53,54] The devices were primarily tested for a life cycle of 10 years; thus concerns regarding the long-term durability of the devices exist. In fact, during a median follow-up of 50 months, stent fractures were reported in up to 17% in 78 studied Hemobahn/Viabahn.[55] No significant association between stent fracture and device occlusion rate was demonstrated but the power of the study was limited. Younger age, most likely a proxy for a high-activity level, was the major risk factor for stent-graft fracture; thus life expectancy should be kept in mind during evaluation of the treatment options.

Table 62.2 shows a summary of recent endovascular PAA repair studies. Furthermore, there is not much debate that endovascular therapy of PAA is attractive to many of our patients.

In summary, the endovascular approach, with its clear advantage of reduced peri-interventional morbidity, has replaced open repair as the gold standard for PAA therapy, at least in frail patients with limited life expectancy.

PLANNING THE INTERVENTIONAL PROCEDURE

Comprehensive preprocedural patient assessment includes patient history and focused physical examination. The ankle brachial index and segmental pulse volume recordings should be obtained at baseline so that pre- and postprocedure functional status can be compared objectively. The patient should be screened for contralateral PAA and concurrent AAA. AAA is generally treated first, followed by repair of the PAA, unless limb-threatening ischemia is present. Contralateral PAAs are usually treated in a staged fashion. Duplex ultrasound of the PAA and the in- and outflow vessels should be performed for evaluation of concurrent peripheral occlusion disease (e.g., significant ipsilateral superficial femoral artery stenosis) and anatomic features as described next. CTA or MRA using thin slices (1 to 3 mm) with 3D reformations may allow for better anatomic orientation and procedure planning. Routine blood work, including assessment of renal function and coagulation parameters, should be performed together with the history of contrast allergy before the procedure.

Anatomic and Technical Considerations

Proximal arterial occlusive disease; the distortion/tortuosity of the popliteal artery; the length, diameter, and presence of thrombus of the PAA; as well as the length and diameter of the proximal and distal landing zone are important anatomic criteria to take into consideration. Table 62.3 displays the (anatomic) criteria for a suitable endovascular PAA treatment (derived from inclusion criteria for endovascular repair studies and own experiences).

Unique forces are exerted on the popliteal artery during knee flexion, including bending, torsion, and radial and longitudinal extension and compression. Therefore, stents and stent-grafts that are intended to be used in the popliteal artery must have great flexibility to conform to the artery during motion without subjecting the adjacent artery to kinking or undergoing fracture due to local stress. Two major devices have been used in the past, the Hemobahn/Viabahn and the Wallgraft endoprosthesis. The latter is composed of a braided polyester graft, which is bonded to the outside of a commercially available wallstent with a thin layer of a Corethane (Boston Scientific/Meditech, Newton,

Table 62.2					
Study Overview—Endovascular Repair of PAAs[53–56,58,61–68]					
Author	Year	Number of limbs	Latest follow-up (years)	Primary patency (%)	Study type
Mohan et al.[53]	2006	30	3.5	75	Retrospective, multicenter
Rajasinghe et al.[62]	2006	23	1	93	Retrospective, single center
Antonello et al.[54]	2007	21	6	71	Prospective, randomized/comparative, single center
Maru et al.[63]	2008	50	2	60	Retrospective, single center
Idelchik et al.[64]	2009	33	4.5	85	Prospective, single center
Thomazinho et al.[65]	2008	11	1.7	90	Retrospective, single center
Ascher et al.[61]	2010	15	2.5	80	Retrospective, single center
Etezadi et al.[58]	2010	18	1	86	Retrospective, single center
Jung et al.[66]	2010	15	6	85	Retrospective, single center
Tielliu et al.[55]	2010	78	10	58	Prospective, single center
Le et al.[67]	2010	21	0.6	95	Retrospective, single center
Kim et al.[68]	2010	24	1	91	Retrospective, comparative, single center
Midy et al.[56]	2010	57	3	82	Retrospective, multicenter

Table 62.3

Anatomic and Clinical Criteria for Endovascular Popliteal Artery Aneurysm Treatment

Anatomic Criteria

- Proximal/distal landing zone length >10 mm, best results >20 mm
- Distal landing zone 30 mm from the trifurcation
- Distal diameter >4 mm
- No excessive tortuosity
- PAA <50 mm in diameter and <10 cm in length
- At least one patent runoff vessel
- Absence of untreated stenotic iliac or SFA lesion
- Absence of noncompliant lesion

Clinical Criteria

- Absence of severe renal insufficiency and/or contrast allergy
- Absence of bacteremia and untreated infection
- No contraindications for dual antiplatelet therapy for at least 6 weeks
- No allergies against graft components
- (Limited life expectancy of <10 years)

MA). Cumulative complication rate (occlusion and endoleak) has been reported to be higher using the Wallgraft endoprosthesis,[56] but no randomized controlled comparison exists. The most frequently used device for PAA treatment in current literature, as well as in our institute, is the Viabahn endoprosthesis, a more flexible, self-expanding endoluminal prosthesis consisting of an ePTFE lining with an external nitinol support extending along its entire length. The device is approved and has been used for PAA treatment in Europe for over 10 years. In contrast to Europe, however, there is no current device approved by the U.S. Food and Drug Administration (FDA) for PAA treatment. In the United States, the Viabahn endoprosthesis is currently only indicated for improving blood flow in superficial artery lesions with reference vessel diameters ranging from 4 to 7.5 mm and iliac artery lesions from 4 to 12 mm; off-label use is common for PAA indications. The current version of the device (Viabahn 3) is available with a labeled diameter of 5 to 13 mm and length of 2.5 to 15 cm delivered over a 6 to 12 French introducer sheath. Excessive endograft oversizing (>20%) was associated with endograft occlusion[54]; thus it is preferable to limit oversizing to 10% to 15% to ensure proximal sealing. Therefore, a proximal artery measuring less than 12 mm in diameter is an important determinant for successful endovascular PAA exclusion. The supragenicular segment of the popliteal artery has been demonstrated as the flexion zone of the knee, with accordant greatest twisting of the stent-graft in this location.[57] Stent-graft fracture has been attributed to overlapping two stent-grafts in the knee flexion zone at the level of the adductor tubercle.[45,56]

Because of the tendency for endografts to shorten or plicate in larger aneurysm sacs without thrombus and distal migration, it is important to select a device length that ensures a proximal and distal landing zone of greater than 20 mm. A proper landing zone is an adjacent healthy arterial segment with no mural thrombus or evidence of aneurysmal changes in this segment. Occasionally, there is a significant mismatch between distal and proximal landing zone diameters, requiring the implantation of more than one endograft sequentially to achieve the appropriate diameters. The ultimate length of the endografts is dictated by the need of a 2- to 3-cm overlap of the endografts within each other and the avoidance of an overlap in the bending zone.

Contraindications

Relative contraindications to an endoluminal covered stent strategy for the management of PAAs include severe renal failure and contrast allergy. Absolute contraindications currently include bacteremia, an untreated infection, or an allergy to a stent-graft component. The Viabahn endoprosthesis is contraindicated for noncompliant lesions where full expansion of an angioplasty balloon catheter cannot be achieved during predilatation, or where lesions cannot be dilated sufficiently to allow passage of the delivery system. Because of its heparin bioactive surface, Viabahn devices should not be used in patients with known hypersensitivity to heparin, including those patients who have had a previous incidence of heparin-induced thrombocytopenia (HIT) type II.

Procedure

Prior to the procedure, patients should be NPO for 6 hours, although oral medications may be administered with minimal amount of clear water. A secure IV access has to be established and euvolemia established to prevent contrast-induced nephropathy. Periprocedural blood pressure, heart rate, and pulse oximetry monitoring are standard. Conscious sedation should be administered at the operator's discretion in the individual setting.

After preparing the access site in a sterile fashion, immediately before the start of the procedure, a short time-out should be performed. Reviewing and checking the patient's name, presence of the informed consent, planned procedure, history of allergies, and main lab results enhances patient safety.

Most cases can be performed using an ipsilateral antegrade transfemoral access route. However, in patients with large body habitus or heavily calcified access vessels, a contralateral approach or surgical cut down can be performed to gain safe access. A 6 French sheath for initial access is suggested. A weight-adjusted heparin bolus (approximately 5,000 international units) is administered intravenously followed by a continuous infusion of heparinized saline (500 international units/500 mL). Generally, a guide wire is used to traverse the superficial femoral artery and popliteal artery and the guide wire is passed distally to the level of the tibioperoneal trunk. Injection of contrast agent is performed and a 5 French calibrated marker catheter is used to measure length and diameters at various segments of the artery (FIGURE 62.3). Using intravascular ultrasound measurements as gold standard, it has been reported that catheter-based angiography diameter measurements are more appropriate than CT angiography diameter measurements.[58]

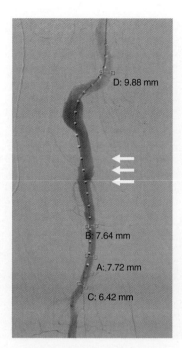

FIGURE 62.3 A calibrated marker catheter is used to measure diameters at various segments of the artery previously illustrated in FIGURE 62.2. The *arrows* indicate the knee bending zone slightly proximal to the joint space.

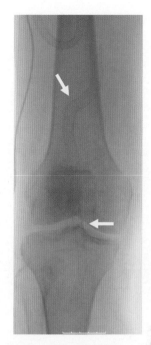

FIGURE 62.4 Radiograph of the knee shows the deployed Viabahn covered stents (W.L. Gore and Associates, Flagstaff, AZ) placed within the popliteal artery aneurysm presented in **FIGURES 62.2 and 62.3**. Because of the mismatch between the distal (6.5 mm) and proximal (9.9 mm) landing zone diameters, three Viabahn stents (8, 9, and 10 mm) were sequentially implanted. The *arrows* indicate the overlap areas, created intentionally to avoid the knee bending zone.

Both preoperative duplex ultrasound scanning and intraoperative calibrated angiography are generally used in the decision making. If necessary, the 6 French sheath can be replaced by a larger introducer sheath to accommodate the selected stent-graft size. To attempt percutaneous closure at the end of the procedure, suture-medicated closure systems (e.g., Perclose ProGlide, Abbott Vascular, Santa Clara, CA) can be placed. Some interventionists use a 30-cm-long sheath to enhance stability and precision during deployment. The guide wire provides critical support to prevent the endograft from bending into the aneurysm during deployment[58,59]; thus the recommendation is to use a stiff guide wire of the appropriate diameter. The deployment starts distally and to minimize the risk of migration, the endograft is deployed to cover at least 2 cm of the distal landing zone but placed no closer than 10 mm to the origin of the anterior tibial artery (FIGURE 62.4). After deployment of the endografts, a low-pressure balloon expansion is performed to achieve optimal wall apposition as well as apposition of the overlap zones.

Endpoint Assessment of the Procedure

Completion angiography from different angles is performed in flexed and extended knee positions to confirm the absence of a sealing endoleak or collateral endoleak and absence of distal embolization (FIGURE 62.5).

Postprocedure Management and Disease Surveillance

Patients should be prescribed and counseled to take a lifelong daily regimen of aspirin (100 to 325 mg) and daily clopidogrel (75 mg) for at least 6 weeks. Dual antiplatelet therapy has been

demonstrated to decrease early occlusion rates significantly,[45,56] but prolonged dual antiplatelet therapy is also associated with a higher incidence of bleeding complications and should be used more cautiously, especially in the elderly. Most institutions have a regimen for postinterventional observation, and time of hospitalization should be related to the course of the intervention and the patient's performance status. Routine follow-up includes clinical examination, ankle brachial and pulse-volume measurements, color duplex, and plain radiography of the knee in flexion/extension views. Further assessment using CTA or digital subtraction angiography should be restricted to patients with worsening clinical symptoms or abnormal physical/noninvasive findings. There are no proven international guidelines on surveillance; follow-up scheduling depends on initial therapeutic success and individual risk factors for disease progression. A 30-day, 3-month, 6 month, 1-year, and annually thereafter follow-up regimen is reasonable but could be adjusted to the patient's needs and preferences.

EARLY AND LATE FAILURES AND OPTIONS FOR MANAGEMENT

Occlusion

Stent-graft occlusion is reported in 7% to 27% and is mostly related to in-stent restenosis, stent fracture, or problems in the initial procedure to deploy the endograft correctly.[38,45,55] Although rare cases of asymptomatic occlusion have been

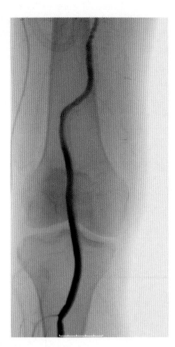

FIGURE 62.5 Angiographic result after placement of the Viabahn stents with preserved patency of the popliteal artery and runoff vessels.

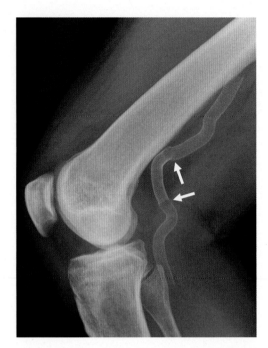

FIGURE 62.6 Lateral radiograph shows a stent-graft fracture and dislocation both at the upper and lower borders of an overlap zone (*arrows*).

Reprinted with permission from Tielliu IF, Zeebregts CJ, Vourliotakis G, et al. Stent fractures in the Hemobahn/Viabahn stent graft after endovascular popliteal aneurysm repair. *J Vasc Surg* 2010;51(6):1413–1418.

reported, most patients are acutely symptomatic. Emergent thrombolysis with subsequent endovascular reintervention in the presence of a restenosis of distal graft dislocation was reported, but the failure rate is around 33%.[45] In these cases, open thrombectomy or bypass surgery is often inevitable.

Stent Fracture

Reported stent fracture in the PAA setting rates vary widely, from 1% to 17%, maybe caused by different surveillance protocols, as well as the amount and type of stent-grafts used. FIGURE 62.6 shows a complete fracture of a stent-graft. In contrast to experiences in the femoropopliteal segment, Tielliu et al. reported a nonsignificant difference in the cumulative primary patency rate for patients with stent fracture compared to patients without stent fracture (38.5% vs. 24.6%, $p = .284$).[55,60] Due to the small sample size, however, the power to detect a difference was low and the problem of stent fractures after endovascular repair of PAA may be globally underestimated. Whether detected stent fractures should be treated when diagnosed, before occurrence of an occlusion, is unclear, but currently no data support this approach. If dislodged struts cause a significant stenosis, percutaneous transluminal angioplasty (PTA) with deployment of a stent with higher radial forces may be performed but concerns regarding refracture exist.

Stent Migration

Early graft migration with disconnection of overlapping stent-grafts and a type III endoleak, as well as late graft migration with type I endoleak caused by short sealing zones, has been described.[45] Repair with a bridging stent or extension are viable options in these cases.

Endoleak

Late expansion caused by a phenomenon similar to that of type II endoleak after endovascular aneurysm repair (EVAR) was recognized in up to one-third of PAAs that were surgically repaired (with the median approach) and monitored for a median of 7 years.[40] This expansion was symptomatic in most of the patients (88%) and resulted in reoperation in 14% of those affected. In a retrospective analysis of 38 endovascular treated PAAs, only four endoleaks were detected with aneurysm growth in two of them. Both enlarged aneurysms could be treated with an ultrasound-guided percutaneous thrombin injection (e.g., 250 to 500 international units). Obviously, collaterals originating from the aneurysm itself rarely cause type II endoleaks and sealing apposition of the stent-graft to the landing zone's vessel wall may explain the low incidence of type II endoleaks observed. Thus we do not recommend routine embolization of predeployment angiographically detected genicular branches.

▌ THE FUTURE

Length and diameter restrictions of the available stent-grafts have thus led to the use of multiple devices and eventually to a number of stent fractures related to overlap zones. In the future, tapered and longer devices will largely solve this problem, and lowering the number of cases in which two (or even more) devices are required. Further design and material improvements are likely to improve both primary patency rates and device durability. Duplex-guided endovascular repair of PAAs has been shown to be feasible and may largely reduce the need for contrast and radiation and its associated complications.[61]

CONCLUSION

PAAs are a rare but serious potentially limb-threatening condition, often requiring treatment in an asymptomatic state. Thus vigilance and knowledge about PAA is mandatory for every physician. Endovascular PAA exclusion has been proven to be a promising alternative to open repair. In patients with a limited life expectancy and high operative risk due to associated comorbidities, endovascular PAA treatment may replace the gold standard of surgical repair. In younger patients, stent-graft durability remains a concern, and bypass using a saphenous vein is certainly a valid option in these patients.

KEY REFERENCES

- Antonello M, Frigatti P, Battocchio P, et al. Open repair versus endovascular treatment for asymptomatic popliteal artery aneurysm: results of a prospective randomized study. *J Vasc Surg* 2005;42:185–193.
- Kropman RH, Schrijver AM, Kelder JC, et al. Clinical outcome of acute leg ischaemia due to thrombosed popliteal artery aneurysm: systematic review of 895 cases. *Eur J Vasc Endovasc Surg* 2010;39:452–457.
- Cross JE, Galland RB, Hingorani A, et al. Nonoperative versus surgical management of small (less than 3 cm), asymptomatic popliteal artery aneurysms. *J Vasc Surg* 2011;53:1145–1148.
- Tielliu IF, Zeebregts CJ, Vourliotakis G, et al. Stent fractures in the Hemobahn/Viabahn stent graft after endovascular popliteal aneurysm repair. *J Vasc Surg* 2010;51:1413–1418.
- Midy D, Berard X, Ferdani M, et al. A retrospective multicenter study of endovascular treatment of popliteal artery aneurysm. *J Vasc Surg* 2010;51:850–856.

ACKNOWLEDGMENT

We would like to thank Constantino Pena and Margaret Kovacs (both of Baptist Cardiac & Vascular Institute, FL) for their critical revisions of the manuscript.

REFERENCES

1. Lawrence PF, Lorenzo-Rivero S, Lyon JL. The incidence of iliac, femoral, and popliteal artery aneurysms in hospitalized patients. *J Vasc Surg* 1995;22:409–415; discussion 15–16.
2. Diwan A, Sarkar R, Stanley JC, et al. Incidence of femoral and popliteal artery aneurysms in patients with abdominal aortic aneurysms. *J Vasc Surg* 2000;31:863–869.
3. Galland RB. History of the management of popliteal artery aneurysms. *Eur J Vasc Endovasc Surg* 2008;35:466–472.
4. Wolf YG, Kobzantsev Z, Zelmanovich L. Size of normal and aneurysmal popliteal arteries: a duplex ultrasound study. *J Vasc Surg* 2006;43:488–492.
5. Magee R, Quigley F, McCann M, et al. Growth and risk factors for expansion of dilated popliteal arteries. *Eur J Vasc Endovasc Surg* 2010;39:606–611.
6. Stiegler H, Mendler G, Baumann G. Prospective study of 36 patients with 46 popliteal artery aneurysms with non-surgical treatment. *Vasa* 2002;31:43–46.
7. Pittathankal AA, Dattani R, Magee TR, et al. Expansion rates of asymptomatic popliteal artery aneurysms. *Eur J Vasc Endovasc Surg* 2004;27:382–384.
8. Golledge J, Karan M, Moran CS, et al. Reduced expansion rate of abdominal aortic aneurysms in patients with diabetes may be related to aberrant monocyte-matrix interactions. *Eur Heart J* 2008;29:665–672.
9. Trickett JP, Scott RA, Tilney HS. Screening and management of asymptomatic popliteal aneurysms. *J Med Screen* 2002;9:92–93.
10. Crawford ES, DeBakey ME. Popliteal artery arteriosclerotic aneurysm. *Circulation* 1965;32:515–516.
11. Wright LB, Matchett WJ, Cruz CP, et al. Popliteal artery disease: diagnosis and treatment. *Radiographics* 2004;24:467–479.
12. Dawson I, Sie R, van Baalen JM, et al. Asymptomatic popliteal aneurysm: elective operation versus conservative follow-up. *Br J Surg* 1994;81:1504–1507.
13. Dawson I, Sie RB, van Bockel JH. Atherosclerotic popliteal aneurysm. *Br J Surg* 1997;84:293–299.
14. Kropman RH, Schrijver AM, Kelder JC, et al. Clinical outcome of acute leg ischaemia due to thrombosed popliteal artery aneurysm: systematic review of 895 cases. *Eur J Vasc Endovasc Surg* 2010;39:452–457.
15. Michaels JA, Galland RB. Management of asymptomatic popliteal aneurysms: the use of a Markov decision tree to determine the criteria for a conservative approach. *Eur J Vasc Surg* 1993;7:136–143.
16. Cross JE, Galland RB, Hingorani A, et al. Nonoperative versus surgical management of small (less than 3 cm), asymptomatic popliteal artery aneurysms. *J Vasc Surg* 2011;53:1145–1148.
17. Illig KA, Eagleton MJ, Shortell CK, et al. Ruptured popliteal artery aneurysm. *J Vasc Surg* 1998;27:783–787.
18. Anton GE, Hertzer NR, Beven EG, et al. Surgical management of popliteal aneurysms. Trends in presentation, treatment, and results from 1952 to 1984. *J Vasc Surg* 1986;3:125–134.
19. Hirsch AT, Haskal ZJ, Hertzer NR, et al. ACC/AHA 2005 practice guidelines for the management of patients with peripheral arterial disease (lower extremity, renal, mesenteric, and abdominal aortic): a collaborative report from the American Association for Vascular Surgery/Society for Vascular Surgery, Society for Cardiovascular Angiography and Interventions, Society for Vascular Medicine and Biology, Society of Interventional Radiology, and the ACC/AHA Task Force on Practice Guidelines (Writing Committee to Develop Guidelines for the Management of Patients with Peripheral Arterial Disease): endorsed by the American Association of Cardiovascular and Pulmonary Rehabilitation; National Heart, Lung, and Blood Institute; Society for Vascular Nursing; TransAtlantic Inter-Society Consensus; and Vascular Disease Foundation. *Circulation* 2006;113:e463–e654.
20. Tendera M, Aboyans V, Bartelink ML, et al. ESC guidelines on the diagnosis and treatment of peripheral artery diseases: document covering atherosclerotic disease of extracranial carotid and vertebral, mesenteric, renal, upper and lower extremity arteries: The Task Force on the Diagnosis and Treatment of Peripheral Artery Diseases of the European Society of Cardiology (ESC). *Eur Heart J* 2011;32:2851–2906.
21. Norgren L, Hiatt WR, Dormandy JA, et al. Inter-society consensus for the management of peripheral arterial disease (TASC II). *J Vasc Surg* 2007;45(suppl S):S5–S67.
22. Sobel M, Verhaeghe R; Physicians ACoC. Antithrombotic therapy for peripheral artery occlusive disease: American College of Chest Physicians evidence-based clinical practice guidelines (8th edition). *Chest* 2008;133:815S–843S.
23. Cross JE, Galland RB. Part one: for the motion asymptomatic popliteal artery aneurysms (less than 3 cm) should be treated conservatively. *Eur J Vasc Endovasc Surg* 2011;41:445–448; discussion 9.
24. Hingorani A, Ascher E. Part two: against the motion asymptomatic popliteal artery aneurysms (less than 3 cm) should be repaired. *Eur J Vasc Endovasc Surg* 2011;41:448–449; discussion 9.
25. Bouhoutsos J, Martin P. Popliteal aneurysm: a review of 116 cases. *Br J Surg* 1974;61:469–475.
26. Mahmood A, Salaman R; Sintler M, et al. Surgery of popliteal artery aneurysms: a 12-year experience. *J Vasc Surg* 2003;37:586–593.
27. Varga ZA, Locke-Edmunds JC, Baird RN. A multicenter study of popliteal aneurysms. Joint Vascular Research Group. *J Vasc Surg* 1994;20:171–177.
28. Aulivola B, Hamdan AD, Hile CN, et al. Popliteal artery aneurysms: a comparison of outcomes in elective versus emergent repair. *J Vasc Surg* 2004;39:1171–1177.
29. Forbes TL, Ricco JB. Editors' commentary. *J Vasc Surg* 2011;53:1148–1149.
30. Galland RB, Magee TR. Popliteal aneurysms: distortion and size related to symptoms. *Eur J Vasc Endovasc Surg* 2005;30:534–538.
31. Ascher E, Markevich N, Schutzer RW, et al. Small popliteal artery aneurysms: are they clinically significant? *J Vasc Surg* 2003;37:755–760.
32. Schwarz W, Berkowitz H, Taormina V, et al. The preoperative use of intra-arterial thrombolysis for a thrombosed popliteal artery aneurysm. *J Cardiovasc Surg (Torino)* 1984;25:465–468.

33. Kessel DO, Berridge DC, Robertson I. Infusion techniques for peripheral arterial thrombolysis. *Cochrane Database Syst Rev* 2004;(1):CD000985.

34. Dorigo W, Pulli R, Turini F, et al. Acute leg ischaemia from thrombosed popliteal artery aneurysms: role of preoperative thrombolysis. *Eur J Vasc Endovasc Surg* 2002;23:251–254.

35. Ravn H, Björck M. Popliteal artery aneurysm with acute ischemia in 229 patients. Outcome after thrombolytic and surgical therapy. *Eur J Vasc Endovasc Surg* 2007;33:690–695.

36. Galland RB, Earnshaw JJ, Baird RN, et al. Acute limb deterioration during intra-arterial thrombolysis. *Br J Surg* 1993;80:1118–1120.

37. Galland RB. Popliteal aneurysms: from John Hunter to the 21st century. *Ann R Coll Surg Engl* 2007;89:466–471.

38. Antonello M, Frigatti P, Battocchio P, et al. Open repair versus endovascular treatment for asymptomatic popliteal artery aneurysm: results of a prospective randomized study. *J Vasc Surg* 2005;42:185–193.

39. Huang Y, Gloviczki P, Noel AA, et al. Early complications and long-term outcome after open surgical treatment of popliteal artery aneurysms: is exclusion with saphenous vein bypass still the gold standard? *J Vasc Surg* 2007;45:706–713; discussion 13–15.

40. Ravn H, Wanhainen A, Björck M, et al. Surgical technique and long-term results after popliteal artery aneurysm repair: results from 717 legs. *J Vasc Surg* 2007;46:236–243.

41. Davies RS, Wall M, Rai S, et al. Long-term results of surgical repair of popliteal artery aneurysm. *Eur J Vasc Endovasc Surg* 2007;34:714–718.

42. Johnson ON, Slidell MB, Macsata RA, et al. Outcomes of surgical management for popliteal artery aneurysms: an analysis of 583 cases. *J Vasc Surg* 2008;48:845–851.

43. Soong CV, Barros B'Sa AA. Lower limb oedema following distal arterial bypass grafting. *Eur J Vasc Endovasc Surg* 1998;16:465–471.

44. Ebaugh JL, Morasch MD, Matsumura JS, et al. Fate of excluded popliteal artery aneurysms. *J Vasc Surg* 2003;37:954–959.

45. Tielliu IF, Verhoeven EL, Zeebregts CJ, et al. Endovascular treatment of popliteal artery aneurysms: results of a prospective cohort study. *J Vasc Surg* 2005;41:561–567.

46. Tielliu IF, Verhoeven EL, Zeebregts CJ, et al. Endovascular treatment of popliteal artery aneurysms: is the technique a valid alternative to open surgery? *J Cardiovasc Surg (Torino)* 2007;48:275–279.

47. Moore RD, Hill AB. Open versus endovascular repair of popliteal artery aneurysms. *J Vasc Surg* 2010;51:271–276.

48. Curi MA, Geraghty PJ, Merino OA, et al. Mid-term outcomes of endovascular popliteal artery aneurysm repair. *J Vasc Surg* 2007;45:505–510.

49. Marin ML, Veith FJ, Cynamon J, et al. Transfemoral endovascular stented graft treatment of aorto-iliac and femoropopliteal occlusive disease for limb salvage. *Am J Surg* 1994;168:156–162.

50. Howell M, Krajcer Z, Diethrich EB, et al. Waligraft endoprosthesis for the percutaneous treatment of femoral and popliteal artery aneurysms. *J Endovasc Ther* 2002;9:76–81.

51. Shames ML, Rubin BG, Sanchez LA, et al. Treatment of embolizing arterial lesions with endoluminally placed stent grafts. *Ann Vasc Surg* 2002;16:608–612.

52. Barry MC, Mackle T, Joyce L, et al. Endoluminal graft stenting of peripheral aneurysms: questionable results compared with conventional surgery. *Surgeon* 2003;1:42–44.

53. Mohan IV, Bray PJ, Harris JP, et al. Endovascular popliteal aneurysm repair: are the results comparable to open surgery? *Eur J Vasc Endovasc Surg* 2006;32:149–154.

54. Antonello M, Frigatti P, Battocchio P, et al. Endovascular treatment of asymptomatic popliteal aneurysms: 8-year concurrent comparison with open repair. *J Cardiovasc Surg (Torino)* 2007;48:267–274.

55. Tielliu IF, Zeebregts CJ, Vourliotakis G, et al. Stent fractures in the Hemobahn/Viabahn stent graft after endovascular popliteal aneurysm repair. *J Vasc Surg* 2010;51:1413–1418.

56. Midy D, Berard X, Ferdani M, et al. A retrospective multicenter study of endovascular treatment of popliteal artery aneurysm. *J Vasc Surg* 2010;51:850–856.

57. Wensing PJ, Scholten FG, Buijs PC, et al. Arterial tortuosity in the femoropopliteal region during knee flexion: a magnetic resonance angiographic study. *J Anat* 1995;187(pt 1):133–139.

58. Etezadi V, Fuller J, Wong S, et al. Endovascular treatment of popliteal artery aneurysms: a single-center experience. *J Vasc Interv Radiol* 2010;21:817–823.

59. Ranson ME, Adelman MA, Cayne NS, et al. Total Viabahn endoprosthesis collapse. *J Vasc Surg* 2008;47:454–456.

60. Scheinert D, Scheinert S, Sax J, et al. Prevalence and clinical impact of stent fractures after femoropopliteal stenting. *J Am Coll Cardiol* 2005;45:312–315.

61. Ascher E, Gopal K, Marks N, et al. Duplex-guided endovascular repair of popliteal artery aneurysms (PAAs): a new approach to avert the use of contrast material and radiation exposure. *Eur J Vasc Endovasc Surg* 2010;39:769–773.

62. Rajasinghe HA, Tzilinis A, Keller T, et al. Endovascular exclusion of popliteal artery aneurysms with expanded polytetrafluoroethylene stent-grafts: early results. *Vasc Endovascular Surg* 2006;40:460–466.

63. Maru S, Anain P, Harris L, et al. Mid-term results of endovascular repair of popliteal artery aneurysms with covered stents: the significance of run-off score on primary patency. In: Society of Vascular Surgery Annual Meeting; San Diego, CA; 2008.

64. Idelchik GM, Dougherty KG, Hernandez E, et al. Endovascular exclusion of popliteal artery aneurysms with stent-grafts: a prospective single-center experience. *J Endovasc Ther* 2009;16:215–223.

65. Thomazinho F, da Silva J, Sardinha W, et al. Endovascular treatment of popliteal artery aneurysm. *Jornal Vascular Brasileiro* 2008;7:38–43.

66. Jung E, Jim J, Rubin BG, et al. Long-term outcome of endovascular popliteal artery aneurysm repair. *Ann Vasc Surg* 2010;24:871–875.

67. Le H, Reil T, Santilli S, et al. Endovascular repair of popliteal artery aneurysms with Gore Viabahn stent-graft: early results. In: Society of Interventional Radiology 35th Annual Scientific Meeting; Tampa, FL. *J Vasc Interv Radiol* 2010;21:S81–S82.

68. Kim B, Garg K, Rockman C, et al. Comparison of endovascular and open popliteal artery aneurysm repair. In: Vascular Annual Meeting; Boston, MA. *J Vasc Surg* 2010;51:60S–61S.

Other Aortic Diseases and Endovascular Management

Aortic Dissection: Classification, Imaging Evaluation, Indications for Intervention

MATTHEW D. FORRESTER and MICHAEL D. DAKE

INTRODUCTION

Aortic dissection is a disruption of the media of the aorta with intramural bleeding and resultant separation of the intima and adventitia.[1] Thus, a dissection flap separating a true and a false lumen is created along a variable length of the aorta. This pathology was originally described in the 16th century.[2] However, an accurate description and the term *aortic "dissection"* were first described in detail by Maunoir in 1802.[3] Despite remaining a challenging, controversial, and often lethal disease process, there has been considerable evolution of the identification and management of aortic dissection. Initial attempts at repair involved surgical fenestration for malperfusion[4] and prevention of aneurysmal dilatation by wrapping the aorta in cellophane.[5,6] It was not until the 1950s, with the advent of cardiopulmonary bypass, that primary surgical repair became a viable option.[7–9] Open surgical techniques initially resulted in very high operative mortality.[10–12] Despite extensive improvements in surgical outcome,[10] aortic dissection remains a difficult clinical entity with significant early and late morbidity and mortality. The development of endovascular techniques for treatment of aortic dissection has provided additional treatment options, yet there remains considerable debate regarding the treatment for various forms of dissection. Appropriate patient selection for open surgical repair, endovascular techniques, and medical management requires a thorough understanding of the disease process including classification of various lesions, imaging evaluation, and current indications for intervention.

CLASSIFICATION

Aortic dissection exists along a continuum of aortic disease with involvement ranging from a localized intimal tear to a dissection along the entire aorta and, ultimately, to rupture either through the intimal flap and back into the true lumen or through the adventitia. Various classification systems have been devised historically to describe the wide variety of dissections and to assist in categorizing lesions based on treatment. These systems are based on the location and extent of disease with further categorization related to the time from onset of initial symptoms.

Aortic dissections can be categorized temporally from the onset of symptoms into acute, subacute, and chronic. Acute dissection is defined as presentation within 2 weeks of onset of symptoms; subacute, between 2 and 6 weeks; and chronic, more than 6 weeks from onset.[1] The temporal relationship of symptoms and presentation is important in determining the best management strategy and is discussed in detail later in this chapter.

As mentioned earlier, aortic dissection is in reality an entity along a continuum of disease processes. Although, classically, aortic dissection involves an intimal tear and subsequent separation of aortic layers creating a true and a false lumen, aortic intimal lesions have a wide variety of presentation. The classic aortic dissection is present in 90% of patients.[1] Subtle differences in aortic intimal lesions, however, are the basis of a classification system describing five intimal variants of dissection proposed in 1999 by Svensson et al.[13] and later supported in 2001 by the Task Force on Aortic Dissection organized by the European Society of Cardiology[14] (FIGURE 63.1).

Type I. *Classic aortic dissection* (FIGURE 63.2) represents an intimal tear and true and false lumens separated by a septum (intimal flap). Communication is often seen between lumens and at sheared-off intercostal arteries or distal reentry sites.

Type II. *Intramural hematoma (IMH)* (FIGURE 63.3) consists of fresh thrombus within the aortic wall without imaging identification of blood flow in a false lumen or of an intimal defect. Typically, a preserved cylindrical aortic lumen is evident. Some authors believe that an IMH arises from hemorrhage of the vasa vasorum located within the medial layers of the aorta,[15,16] whereas others feel that it is a result of microscopic aortic intimal tears. Up to 15% of patients with a suspected aortic dissection have an apparent IMH without evidence of an intimal tear on noninvasive

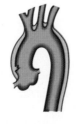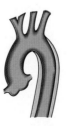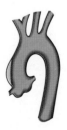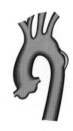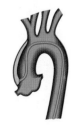

| Type I | Type II | Type III | Type IV | Type V |

FIGURE 63.1 Intimal tear classification. **Type I.** Classic aortic dissection. **Type II.** Intramural hematoma. **Type III.** Intimal tear without medial hematoma (limited dissection). **Type IV.** Penetrating atherosclerotic ulcer. **Type V.** Iatrogenic/traumatic aortic dissection.

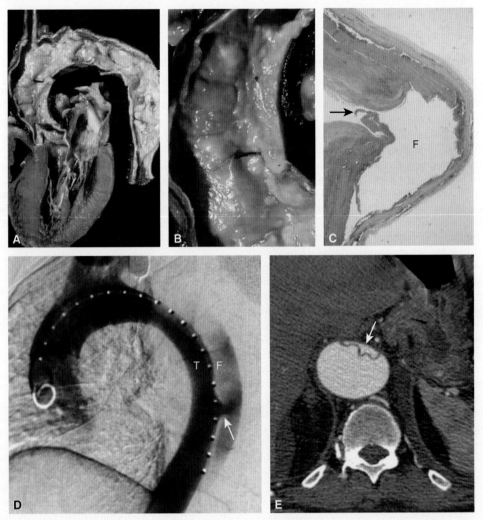

FIGURE 63.2 Views of aortic dissection. **A.** Surgical specimen with classical elements of type A aortic dissection: transverse intimal tear in the midascending aorta, false lumen along the outer curve of the thoracic aorta with extension into the innominate artery, and left ventricular hypertrophy secondary to chronic hypertension. **B.** Close-up view of the ascending aorta displays 1-cm primary intimal tear. The primary entry tear in aortic dissection is typically linear and transverse in orientation, perpendicular to the course of blood flow. **C.** Histologic display of intimal entry tear (*arrow*) with mural cleavage plan typical of aortic dissection and presence of false lumen channel (*F*). **D.** Conventional aortogram in the left anterior projection shows intimal disruption (*arrow*) and flow of contrast media between the true lumen (*T*) along the inner curve and false lumen (*F*) around the outer curve in type B aortic dissection. **E.** Axial CT scan at the level of the diaphragms with near circumferential extension of dissection septum and associated true lumen collapse (*arrow*) surrounded by large, dominant false lumen.

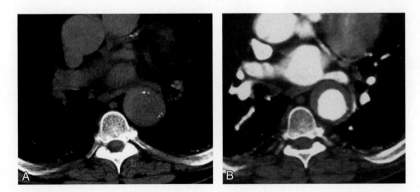

FIGURE 63.3 Intramural hematoma of the descending thoracic aorta. **A.** Axial CT scan precontrast administration at the mid/lower thoracic level shows characteristic features of intramural hematoma of the aorta with a higher attenuating circumferential rim surrounding a circular lower-density lumen. This precontrast higher attenuation mantle represents acute or subacute hematoma within the aortic wall. Also noted is displacement of calcified foci within the wall by the subjacent intramural clot as well as preservation of the normal round luminal contour. **B.** Postcontrast administration axial CT image with thickened aortic wall typical of intramural hematoma, slightly irregular luminal margin but, essentially, preservation of circular aortic channel.

imaging, whereas autopsy studies demonstrate that only 4% of patients have no intimal tear. Moreover, a tear is found in most patients at the time of open surgical intervention.[17] Both of these findings largely support the latter hypothesis. An IMH most commonly occurs in the descending aorta and in older patients and clinically can mimic classic aortic dissection.[18,19] Approximately 10% of IMHs resolve,[20] whereas others may convert into a classic dissection (16% to 36%[21]).[1] Given the propensity for IMHs to propagate to classic aortic dissection, these lesions are typically classified under the Stanford or DeBakey classification systems described next.

Type III. *Intimal tear without medial hematoma (limited dissection)*—these lesions are characterized by a localized intimal tear and exposure of the media without propagation of a dissection flap. Such intimal tears are difficult to diagnose by noninvasive methods and even catheter aortography. Patients with Marfan syndrome are prone to this type of lesion.[13] If aortic dissection is highly suspected, different imaging modalities should be considered in succession because a combination of imaging studies separated by a short interval (24 to 48 hours) will often yield a diagnosis.

Type IV. *Penetrating atherosclerotic ulcer (PAU)* (FIGURE 63.4) refers to an atherosclerotic ulceration that penetrates the internal elastic lamina to a varying degree from intimal ulceration, ulceration through the media and contained by the adventitia (contained rupture or pseudoaneurysm), and frank rupture. They may also lead to hematoma formation

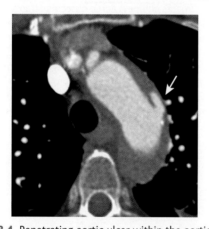

FIGURE 63.4 Penetrating aortic ulcer within the aortic arch with intramural hematoma. Contrast-enhanced axial CT image through the aortic arch ulcer-like projection (*arrow*) along the lateral aspect of the distal arch/proximal descending aorta associated with a thick rind of intramural hematoma. It is difficult to determine the evolutionary relationship between these coexisting findings with only an isolated imaging study at a single snapshot in time. A primary penetrating aortic ulcer may lead to an intramural hematoma and, conversely, a patient presenting with pain and a fundamental process of intramural hematoma may rapidly develop a luminal erosion or secondary ulceration. Thus, without a series of imaging exams commencing shortly after the onset of symptoms, it may be very difficult in some patients to ascertain the precise pathogenic etiology.

within the media of the aortic wall (IMH) and classic aortic dissection.[22] Because atherosclerotic changes are more common in the descending thoracic aorta, approximately 90% of PAUs are found in this region.[23] Similar to classic aortic dissection, an important distinction must be made between symptomatic and asymptomatic PAUs, which assists in directing treatment strategy.

Type V. *Iatrogenic/traumatic aortic dissection* may occur after coronary angiography, aortic balloon dilatation, and other catheter-based and operative interventions (i.e., aortic cross clamp injury). Traumatic aortic dissection is typically located at the level of the aortic isthmus and is usually a result of rapid deceleration.

Originally described in 1970,[24] the Stanford classification system is based on the anatomic segments of the aorta involved in the dissection. It is the simplest system and most widely used because it delineates between locations of dissection that have very different prognoses based on the natural histories of disease and the anatomic sites involved.

Type A. Involvement of the ascending aorta (proximal to the innominate artery) regardless of distal extent and location of primary intimal tear.

Type B. Dissection does not involve the ascending aorta and is thus limited to the aorta distal to the innominate artery (FIGURE 63.5).

Classically, surgical intervention is recommended for dissections involving the ascending aorta, and nonsurgical management is usually indicated if the ascending aorta is not involved. The Stanford system does not take into account the extent of the dissection or the location of the primary intimal tear. Type B dissections are further subcategorized into *complicated* and *uncomplicated* dissections. Complicated dissections are defined by rupture, impending rupture, visceral or extremity malperfusion, rapid false lumen expansion, persistent pain, or uncontrollable hypertension (FIGURE 63.6). Uncomplicated type B dissections are usually managed medically. Naturally, complicated dissections generally warrant intervention. Aortic dissections with a primary intimal tear distal to the innominate artery with retrograde extension and involvement of the ascending aorta are often termed *retro-type A* dissections.

The DeBakey classification system categorizes aortic dissections based on the location of the intimal tear and the extent of the dissection. The original classification was described in 1964 and 1965 with three basic types: type I refers to a dissection involving the ascending and descending aorta, type II refers to involvement of only the ascending aorta, and type III refers to a dissection of only the thoracic (type IIIA) or thoracoabdominal aorta (type IIIB).[12,25] In 1975, Reul further classified dissections originating in the descending thoracic aorta into four subtypes, adding DeBakey IIIC and IIID to DeBakey's original description.[26] In Reul's modification of the DeBakey system, types IIIA–C describe dissections involving varying lengths of the thoracoabdominal aorta with type IIIA limited to the upper thoracic aorta, type IIIB extending to the diaphragm, and type IIIC extending below the diaphragm. Type IIID refers to a dissection originating in the thoracic aorta and extending retrograde to involve the ascending aorta. Although the exact description of the classification system varies slightly in various historical publications, the currently favored version of

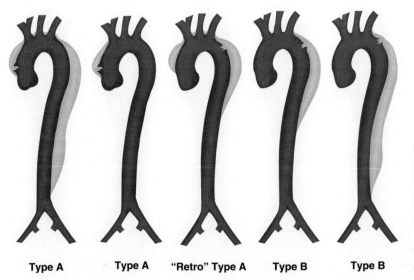

FIGURE 63.5 Stanford classification. **Type A.** Dissection involving the ascending aorta (proximal to the innominate artery) regardless of the distal extent and location of the primary intimal tear. **"Retro" Type A.** Intimal tear within the descending aorta with retrograde dissection involving the ascending aorta. **Type B.** Dissection does not involve the ascending aorta and is thus limited to the aorta distal to the innominate artery.

Type A   Type A   "Retro" Type A   Type B   Type B

the DeBakey classification was described in 1982[2] with three types (types I, II, IIIA–B). With the addition of type IIID, the DeBakey classification system used today is as follows (note that type IIIC is encompassed by types IIIA and IIIB and is thus not used):

Type I. Dissection involving the ascending aorta and extending distally for a variable distance
Type II. Dissection limited to the ascending aorta
Type IIIA. Dissection limited to the descending thoracic aorta

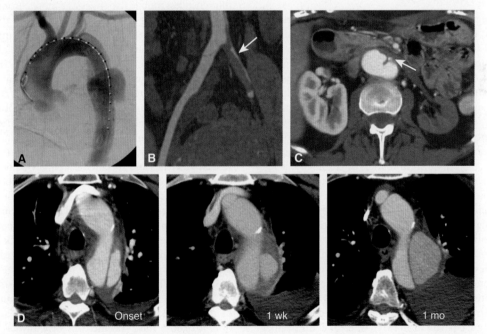

FIGURE 63.6 Medley of complications associated with acute type B aortic dissection. **A.** Oblique aortogram with type B aortic dissection associated with false lumen rupture and shock. **B.** Pelvic arteriogram shows false lumen extension into the left common iliac artery without distal reentry. Consequently, the blind pouch false lumen within the left iliac artery compresses the true lumen to near obliteration (string-like contrast column along the lateral wall of the common iliac, *arrow*). This was associated with acute ischemic symptoms, including a cold, painful leg without palpable pulses. The right iliac artery is exclusively perfused via the true lumen. **C.** Axial CT scan of aortic dissection at the level of the kidneys shows asymmetric nephrograms. The right kidney is perfused by a large aortic false lumen. whereas the aortic true lumen is collapsed to a punctuate channel (*arrow*) with associated dynamic branch vessel involvement of the left renal artery, which originates from the true lumen and an abnormal left nephrogram. **D.** Series of axial CT images through the same level of the aortic arch demonstrate progressive dilatation of the false lumen and enlarging pleural effusion in type B aortic dissection over a 1-month interval after diagnosis.

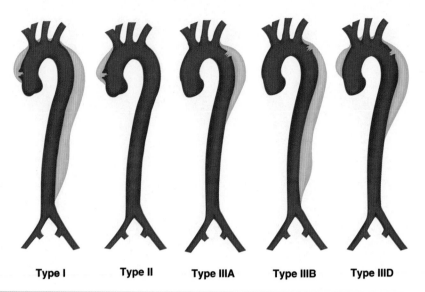

FIGURE 63.7 DeBakey classification. **Type I.** Dissection involving the ascending aorta and extending distally for a variable distance. **Type II.** Dissection limited to the ascending aorta. **Type IIIA.** Dissection limited to the descending thoracic aorta. **Type IIIB.** Dissection involving the descending aorta and extending into the abdominal aorta. **Type IIID.** Dissection within the descending thoracic aorta with retrograde extension into the ascending aorta.

Type I   Type II   Type IIIA   Type IIIB   Type IIID

Type IIIB. Dissection involving the descending aorta and extending into the abdominal aorta

Type IIID. Dissection within the descending thoracic aorta with retrograde extension into the ascending aorta (FIGURE 63.7)

▌ IMAGING EVALUATION

Appropriate imaging of the aorta is critical in diagnosing and managing aortic dissection. Available imaging modalities include computed tomography (CT), magnetic resonance imaging (MRI), transthoracic and transesophageal echocardiography (TTE/TEE), and catheter aortography. The appropriate exam varies with patient- and disease-related factors and institutional availability. Not surprisingly, it has been demonstrated that a delay in diagnostic imaging can affect mortality in patients with a high clinical suspicion of aortic dissection.[27] Ultimately, dedicated aortic imaging can assist the clinician with diagnosis, detailed definition of the anatomy, determination of chronicity, assessment of need for intervention, and planning an intervention.

Computed tomographic scanning has become the gold standard imaging modality for aortic dissection. It is widely available, provides highly detailed imaging of the entire aorta, and allows for definitive inclusion or exclusion of aortic disease. Newer-generation multidetector helical CT scanners demonstrate sensitivities of up to 100% and specificities of 98% to 99%.[28,29] Further, electrocardiogram (ECG)-gated techniques now provide motion-free images of the aortic root and coronary arteries. Noncontrast CT imaging can be useful in detecting subtle high-attenuation changes of an IMH, whereas contrast imaging can delineate the presence of a dissection flap, demonstrate contrast extravasation, identify potential malperfusion, and provide detailed vascular anatomy, furnishing sufficient information to plan surgical or endovascular treatment.[1] Two- and three-dimensional reconstructions, such as maximum intensity projections, multiplanar and curved multiplanar reformations, and volume rendering, may assist with interpretation, communication, and procedural planning (FIGURE 63.8).[30]

CT scanning can also assist the clinician in determining the chronicity of dissection. Acute Stanford type A dissections usually represent a surgical emergency, and complicated type B dissections often require urgent or emergent intervention. Those patients who fall into the subacute or chronic categories often can be addressed on a more elective basis. Thus, subtle CT findings in addition to history and physical examination are important in determining appropriate management. For example, the intimal flap can be viewed in systole and diastole. Significant movement of the flap with the cardiac cycle is indicative of an acute process, whereas a thickened less mobile flap suggests a more chronic process.

It is important to obtain imaging from the thoracic inlet through the pelvis including the iliac and femoral vessels. Not only can an accurate diagnosis be made, but also detailed procedural planning can be performed prior to intervention. Access vessels, extent of calcification, involvement of the dissection process, and its extension into branch vessels can all be assessed with high-resolution CT scanning. Thus, appropriate intervention can be planned, and accurate measurements can be made for device selection.

MRI is also very accurate in diagnosing aortic dissection[29,31,32] with sensitivities and specificities that are equivalent or may exceed CT. Similar to CT, MRI can provide detailed imaging of the entire vascular tree. MRI can also provide useful information regarding the aortic valve and left ventricular function. One obvious advantage of MRI over CT is the lack of exposure to radiation. Its biggest disadvantages, however, include longer time for acquisition of images and lack of widespread availability on an emergency basis.[1]

TTE and TEE can also provide useful information. Although TTE can often make the diagnosis, its use is limited by the quality of images, making it less sensitive than TEE. TTE has a sensitivity of 77% to 80% and a specificity of 93% to 96% for identification of proximal aortic dissection (much lower for more distal aortic dissection), whereas TEE has a sensitivity for proximal aortic dissection of 88% to 98% and a specificity of 90% to 95%.[33] TEE can provide high-quality dynamic images of the aorta. It is highly sensitive and allows for direct evaluation of the aortic valve, pericardial space, and coronary ostia. Echocardiography, however, has limited use in descending aortic dissections, although TEE can visualize relatively high descending thoracic aortic pathology.

Although catheter aortography was once considered the gold standard for diagnosis of aortic dissection, noninvasive imaging modalities, such as CT and MRI, are now more commonly used.

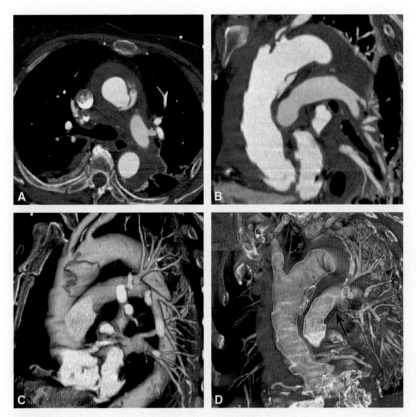

FIGURE 63.8 Series of CT renderings of the thoracic aorta from an 89-year-old patient with acute type A intramural hematoma and associated rupture into the mediastinum and communication with the lumen at a site along the lesser curve of the arch opposite the origin of the innominate artery. The image displays presented include: (**A**) axial; (**B**) oblique maximum intensity projection (MIP), which shows a diffuse aortic intramural hematoma and extensive hemorrhage throughout the mediastinum; (**C, D**) multiplanar reformation (MPR) and volume rendering (VR). The MIP presents high-quality angiographic resolution while displaying calcified foci and extravascular detail. MPR and VR projections ignore vessel calcium and, thus, may offer the most accurate CT techniques to determine the exact degree of any luminal stenosis. In this case, these complementary techniques present a complete depiction of the process, including the size and location of the intramural communication with the lumen.

Aortography is an invasive test requiring percutaneous arterial access. In diagnosing aortic dissection, it has a reported sensitivity as low as 88% and a specificity of 94%.[34] Aortography is limited by its invasive nature, contrast requirement (although arguably lower that CT angiography in some cases), difficulty in identifying IMHs and a thrombosed false lumen, and difficulty visualizing the intimal flap when the true and false lumens are simultaneously opacified.[34] This modality may be useful in identifying branch vessel and coronary involvement as well as aortic regurgitation.

INDICATIONS FOR INTERVENTION

Appropriate treatment for an aortic dissection is determined by a combination of location and extent of the dissection, time from onset of symptoms, comorbid risk factors, and dissection-related conditions, such as visceral malperfusion or impending rupture. Although most patients present with acute aortic dissections, up to one-third present with symptoms greater than 2 weeks in duration.[35] This distinction between acute and chronic dissection is of therapeutic significance because patients with acute aortic dissections are at highest risk for life-threatening complications. In the current era, treatment options can be divided into three main categories: medical management, surgical intervention, and endovascular intervention. Recommendations for management of thoracic aortic dissection have been made by the 2010 ACCF/AHA task force for the diagnosis and management of patients with thoracic aortic disease.[1] The initial management in all acute aortic dissections should include the following principles: stabilization of the degree of dissection, reduction of dynamic aortic vessel obstruction, minimization of intimal flap mobility, and reduction of the risk of aortic rupture.[36] These objectives

are accomplished by careful monitoring in an intensive care unit setting; immediate administration of antihypertensive medications to reduce heart rate, systemic blood pressure, and rate of rise blood pressure (dP/dT); and adequate pain control to reduce sympathetic stimulation.[36] It is important to initiate beta-blockade prior to a vasodilating agent to prevent reflex tachycardia and, thus, increased aortic shear stress.

Ascending aortic dissections (Stanford Type A, DeBakey I, II) comprise approximately 60% of all dissections[37] and are at high risk of acute complication including cardiac tamponade (5%), myocardial ischemia (7% to 19%), acute aortic regurgitation (45%), heart failure (5%), stroke (8%), and ultimately death.[38] The mortality rate for acute type A dissections without intervention is estimated to be approximately 1% per hour after patients arrive in the hospital with mortalities of 38%, 50%, 70%, and 90% at 24 hours, 48 hours, 1 week, and 2 weeks, respectively.[39,40] In general, type A dissections require emergent surgical repair. Presently, there are no endovascular devices for the ascending aorta that have been approved by the Food and Drug Administration (FDA).[1]

There remains some controversy over the treatment strategy of type B aortic dissections. In 1965, DeBakey et al.[25] published a large series of 179 aortic dissection patients treated surgically with an operative mortality of 21% and a 5-year mortality of 50%. In comparison to large series of patients with aortic dissections who had undergone nonoperative treatment, DeBakey and colleagues concluded that all patients with aortic dissections should undergo surgical intervention.[11,12] Later, Wheat and colleagues[41] advocated a selective approach based on the observation that surgical intervention carried a 25% early mortality, whereas patients treated pharmacologically had a 16% early mortality.[11] It was not until 1970, when Daily and colleagues[24] at Stanford introduced the Stanford dissection classification, that the importance of distinguishing ascending and descending aortic dissections became apparent. It was thus widely held that type B dissections ought to be treated medically unless life-threatening complications were present. Although operative mortality for type B dissections significantly improved over time (57% to 13% in the Stanford series),[10] several risk factors including visceral ischemia, aortic rupture, and older age portended dramatically increased risk with surgical repair.[11,42] In the current era of endovascular stent-grafts, it seems intuitive that less invasive techniques for stabilization of acute type B dissections, which carry a high risk of mortality with and without surgical intervention, could provide an opportunity to improve outcomes in this very ill patient population.

Although 20% to 50% of uncomplicated type B aortic dissections demonstrate eventual aneurysmal dilatation within 3 to 5 years of diagnosis,[43,44] there is small risk of rupture in the acute setting with a 30-day mortality of about 10% in contemporary studies. Most authors advocate medical treatment with blood pressure control and close follow-up with interval imaging.[14] Many of these patients will ultimately require intervention beyond the acute setting and, thus, some authors have suggested that asymptomatic descending aortic dissections be treated with stent-grafts to prevent late complications.[45] There is not yet sufficient long-term data comparing medical treatment and stent-grafts in uncomplicated acute type B dissections to define the appropriate treatment strategy. The INSTEAD trial attempted to answer a similar debate in subacute and chronic type B dissections (within 2 to 52 weeks of onset) by randomizing patients to either medical therapy or stent-graft placement.[46] The trial found no difference in all-cause and aorta-related mortality at 1-year follow-up, but 91% of those in the stent-graft group demonstrated evidence of aortic remodeling as compared to only 19% of those in the medical group.[46] Even though the INSTEAD trial did not include acute aortic dissections (<2 weeks from onset), the trial did reveal a potential for stent-grafts to promote aortic remodeling and potentially prevent late aneurysmal

degeneration. It is important to note that based on this trial, it appears that stent-graft treatment of patients with subacute or chronic aortic dissection offers no benefit in terms of reducing the risk of aortic rupture or enhancing life expectancy. Longer follow-up is necessary, however, to understand the true benefit or lack thereof for stent-grafts in asymptomatic type B dissections.

In contradistinction, complicated type B aortic dissections, defined by the presence of visceral or peripheral malperfusion, rupture, rapid false lumen expansion, persistent pain, or uncontrollable hypertension, often require intervention. Despite significant improvement in operative mortality for acute type B dissections, operative mortality in the presence of visceral ischemia and rupture remains as high as 70% to 80%.[11,47] The addition of endovascular interventions has provided an opportunity for a less invasive, more expeditious procedure to stabilize the dissection, prevent rupture, and restore true lumen perfusion.

Endovascular treatment options include aortic stent-graft placement (FIGURE 63.9), dissection flap fenestration (FIGURE 63.10), and branch-vessel stenting (FIGURE 63.11).[48] Each technique aims to achieve one or both of the two major goals in treatment of an acute aortic dissection: prevent aortic rupture and restore end-organ perfusion. The current indications for intervention encompass life-threatening complications of acute aortic dissection, hence the term *complicated*. As mentioned previously, complicated dissections are defined by visceral or limb malperfusion, aortic rupture or impending rupture (e.g., rapid false lumen expansion), or evidence of an unstable dissection plane (e.g., persistent pain, uncontrollable hypertension).

Malperfusion syndrome is defined by obstruction of one or more aortic branches, resulting in critical ischemia of the vascular territory.[48] Obstruction may result from either a *static* (FIGURES 63.12 and 63.13) or a *dynamic* (FIGURE 63.14) obstruction. A static obstruction occurs when the dissection directly enters a branch vessel. As the dissection process extends into a branch, it may terminate with false lumen reentry with a tear in the flap

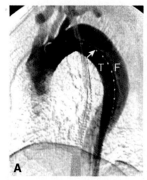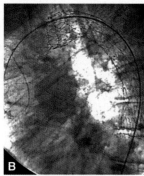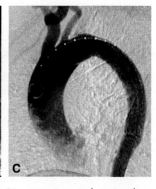

FIGURE 63.9 Aortograms of acute type B aortic dissection with large entry tear pre- and postendovascular repair. **A.** Oblique aortogram demonstrates simultaneous filling of the true (*T*) and false (*F*) aortic lumens (note the angiographic catheter within the true lumen against the dissection septum (*arrows*). The simultaneous contrast opacification of both lumens implies the presence of a large communication through a gaping entry tear without appreciable delay in false lumen flow or easy angiographic definition of the tear. Large proximal entry tears are commonly associated downstream with true lumen collapse and dynamic branch vessel ischemia. Here the aortic true lumen progressively tapers as it courses distally. **B.** Stent-graft after deployment. **C.** Aortogram postendograft placement of the entry tear shows complete coverage of the proximal communication with exclusive contrast filling of the true lumen. Note the angiographic catheter position against the outer curve of the aortic true lumen. Distally, the true lumen collapse was immediately reversed and the acute symptoms of branch vessel ischemia resolved without further intervention required.

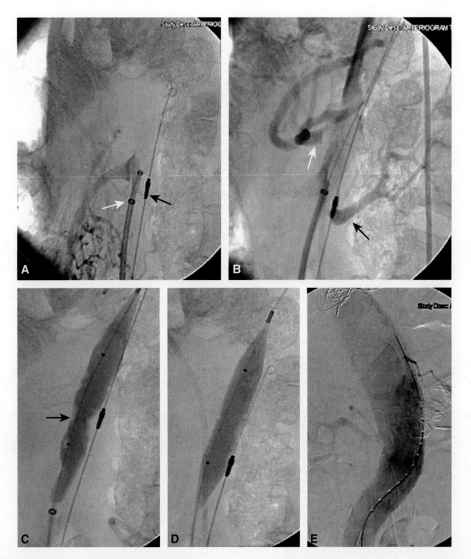

FIGURE 63.10 Percutaneous balloon fenestration of the aortic septum in acute type B dissection. **A.** Oblique image from an abdominal aortography shows the relative position of the intravascular ultrasound transducer (*black arrow*) and precurved metallic TIPS cannula (*white arrow*) prior to flap fenestration in a 67-year-old man with aortic dissection that occurred distal to a thoracic aortic endograft placed for treatment of a degenerative aneurysm. **B.** Aortography in the same position after needle puncture of the septum and guide wire placement across it from the true to false lumen. Contrast outlines a collapsed aortic true lumen anteriorly with effacement of the channel outlined by contrast and resultant dynamic branch vessel ischemia involving the celiac (*white arrow*), left renal (*black arrow*), and superior mesenteric (not shown) arteries. The dissection originated from an acute junction between the distal margin of a previously placed endograft and a severely angled segment of supraceliac aorta. **C.** After transgression of the flap from the collapsed true lumen to the large surrounding false lumen under ultrasound guidance (with the imaging catheter in the target false lumen) and fluoroscopic monitoring (with the imaging plane oriented parallel to the course of the flap), a 15-mm angioplasty balloon was inflated over a 0.035-inch guide wire. The flap location is appreciated by the waist on the balloon adjacent to the ultrasound probe (*arrow*). **D.** Upon application of further pressure the waist is obliterated with enlargement of the septal fenestration. **E.** Frontal projection during simultaneous contrast injections of both the true and false aortic lumens shows good filling of the entire abdominal aorta. Postprocedure, the patient's acute abdominal pain resolved.

at the distal extent of the false channel or it may terminate without a reentry tear in the false lumen. The former scenario with branch vessel reentry of the false lumen is more common and results in double-barrel or dual channel flow to the vascular bed supplied by the involved branch. The other form of static branch vessel involvement with no reentry of the false lumen is less common and is typically associated with tissue malperfusion. Without

a reentry tear, there is no flow via the blind sac of the false lumen, which progressively enlarges to its distal extent and may critically obstruct or markedly narrow the true lumen. Thus, the vascular territory supplied by the affected branch is frequently ischemic and tissue necrosis may occur without expeditious intervention with reperfusion. Alternatively, dynamic obstruction occurs when the aortic true lumen is collapsed and flow to its

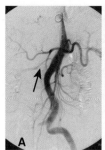 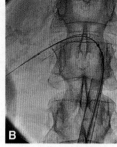 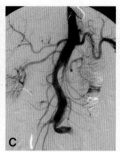 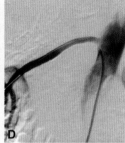

FIGURE 63.11 Static branch vessel involvement of the right renal artery postendograft management of a 64-year-old woman with acute type B dissection complicated by aortic true lumen collapse and dynamic branch vessel involvement. **A.** Postendograft true lumen aortogram shows good filling of the previously compromised aortic true lumen and abdominal branches originating exclusively from it (celiac, superior mesenteric, and left renal arteries). The right renal artery is supplied by both the true and false lumens; however, the false lumen in the right renal artery does not have a reentry tear. Consequently, it functions as blind wind sock or sausage casing that compresses and obstructs the true lumen flow within the branch (*arrow*). **B.** Despite the remote coverage of the aortic entry tear with an endograft and the resultant reversal of aortic true lumen collapse and dynamic branch vessel ischemia, coexisting static involvement of one or more branches by direct extension of the aortic dissection flap into the branch may persist as a cause of malperfusion—especially if the false lumen extension does not terminate with a distal reentry within the affected artery. Without a tear at the distal extent of the false lumen within the branch, the dead-end channel expands to compress the true lumen. This often results in acute branch vessel ischemia and potential organ necrosis regardless of the adequacy of aortic true lumen flow. Here, a self-expanding nitinol stent has been placed via the aortic true lumen into the true lumen of the right renal artery to expand the channel. **C.** Postdeployment of the branch stent, good flow is observed and intrarenal branch opacification is evident. **D.** Following reperfusion of the right kidney, the stent will continue to expand with time over the length of the thrombosed false lumen, which slowly resorbs.

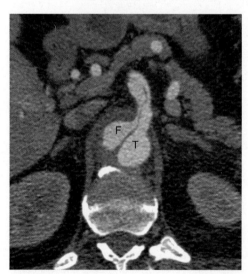

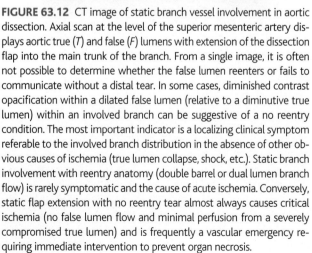

FIGURE 63.12 CT image of static branch vessel involvement in aortic dissection. Axial scan at the level of the superior mesenteric artery displays aortic true (*T*) and false (*F*) lumens with extension of the dissection flap into the main trunk of the branch. From a single image, it is often not possible to determine whether the false lumen reenters or fails to communicate without a distal tear. In some cases, diminished contrast opacification within a dilated false lumen (relative to a diminutive true lumen) within an involved branch can be suggestive of a no reentry condition. The most important indicator is a localizing clinical symptom referable to the involved branch distribution in the absence of other obvious causes of ischemia (true lumen collapse, shock, etc.). Static branch involvement with reentry anatomy (double barrel or dual lumen branch flow) is rarely symptomatic and the cause of acute ischemia. Conversely, static flap extension with no reentry tear almost always causes critical ischemia (no false lumen flow and minimal perfusion from a severely compromised true lumen) and is frequently a vascular emergency requiring immediate intervention to prevent organ necrosis.

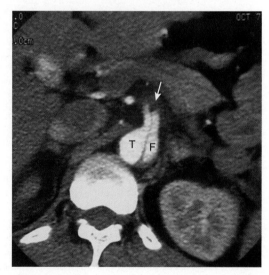

FIGURE 63.13 Axial CT scan of aortic dissection complicated by static involvement of the superior mesenteric artery with no branch reentry tear. Contrast-enhanced CT shows aortic true (*T*) and false (*F*) lumens with aortic septum coursing into the proximal aspect of the superior mesenteric artery. A rounded filling defect within the false lumen is evident at the distal extent of the imaged vessel (*arrow*). This is likely a clot within the terminal extent of the false lumen cul-de-sac that does not have a distal reentry. Typically, stagnant blood clots within the blindly occluded false lumen. It appears on CT as a low attenuating mass that causes a progressively tapered compression of the true lumen with maximum obstruction at the distal terminus of the false lumen. Distal to the false lumen, the branch is only composed of a nondissected true lumen and the diameter of the contrast-filled lumen at that point may increase. This appearance is perhaps more apparent on multiplanar or curved planar CT reconstructions of the involved branch or with conventional selective catheter arteriography.

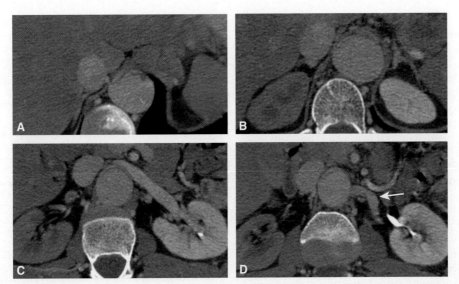

FIGURE 63.14 CT imaging of acute aortic dissection complicated by dynamic branch vessel involvement in a 36-year-old patient with Marfan syndrome. Axial images from the level of the celiac artery (**A**) to the left renal artery (**D**) show a dilated aorta (**B**) with near circumferential dissection and aortic true lumen collapse (**A–D**). The dissection flap is plastered against the anterior aortic wall with a typical appearance of dynamic branch vessel involvement. Consequently, the dissection septum covers all abdominal branches originating from the true lumen like a curtain. The combination of in-flow via a slit-like aortic true lumen and an obstructing flap prolapsed over the origins of true lumen branches results in ischemia. At the level of the left renal artery (**D**), note the asymmetric nephrograms with a normal appearing left kidney fed by a renal artery originating from the false lumen (*arrow*) and a poorly perfused right kidney supplied by an artery originating from a wafer-thin crescentic aortic true lumen.

branches is compromised by the dissection flap and a usually much larger false lumen. Dynamic branch vessel obstruction is frequently associated with a large proximal primary entry tear and a relatively circumferential intimal dissection. The extent of true lumen obliteration is commonly greatest at the levels of the distal descending and proximal abdominal segments. A slit-like aortic true lumen below the diaphragm often courses anteriorly to give origin to the celiac trunk and superior mesenteric arteries. In these cases, the true lumen may be barely perceptible as a wafer-thin crescent with the dissection septum prolapsed over the origins of true lumen branches like a curtain. The severity of dynamic obstruction may be variable owing to constant motion of the dissection flap, particularly in the acute phase, and to hemodynamic changes in blood pressure and heart rate.[49,50] In an individual patient, both static and dynamic mechanisms of branch vessel involvement with or without resultant ischemia may coexist. Branch vessel malperfusion occurs in approximately 30% to 50% of all aortic dissections[51,52] and yields an almost threefold increase in risk of in-hospital mortality with acute type B dissection.[53] Given the markedly high operative mortality rate with malperfusion, endovascular options are attractive. Malperfusion syndrome can be treated by thoracic aortic stent-grafting and coverage of the primary intimal tear, distal aortic intimal flap fenestration, branch-vessel stenting, or a combination of all three.

Surgical intervention for rupture or impending rupture in type B dissections also carries an extremely high operative mortality.[47] Acutely, coverage of the intimal tear with an appropriately sized stent-graft may effectively exclude a rupture or stabilize the dissection while improving true lumen flow. Moreover, exclusion of the primary intimal tear and precluding false lumen patency may reduce some of the late sequelae of type B

dissections (aneurysmal dilatation, rupture, and mortality) by promoting false lumen thrombosis.[54–56] The feasibility of successful stent-grafting depends on appropriate patient selection with suitable aortic anatomy, which ideally includes a sufficient proximal landing zone (usually 15 to 20 mm) in a relatively disease-free segment of nondissected aorta.

One of the earliest endovascular treatments in the setting or acute type B dissection was performed in 1935 by Gurin,[4] who fenestrated an intimal flap distally to treat lower extremity ischemia. This strategy treats a non-reentry aortic false lumen and dynamic obstruction of the aortic true lumen by decreasing resistance to false lumen outflow rather than treating the proximal tear.[57] Similar to Gurin's original attempt, flap fenestration can be applied for lower extremity ischemia. Limitations include continued false lumen flow, which may expose patients to increased late complications of aortic dissection.[58] Fenestration may provide a treatment option in patients with malperfusion who are poor surgical candidates or who have unsuitable anatomy for stent-grafting.

Finally, uncovered stent placement either within the aorta or more typically within compromised aortic branch vessels may further improve flow to an ischemic region. Indications for an uncovered stent include inadequate relief of an obstruction after surgery, stent-grafting, or fenestration, and static obstruction of a branch vessel.[56,57] Uncovered stent placement may also be used alone or as an adjunct to percutaneous balloon fenestration of the dissection septum to increase aortic true lumen diameter.

Dissection variants, such as IMHs and PAUs, add additional complexity to treatment and indications for intervention for acute aortic disease. As mentioned, 16% to 36% of IMHs progress to classic aortic dissection.[21] Moreover, because a significant percentage of patients with IMH and no apparent intimal tear on noninvasive imaging actually have a visible tear at the time of operation or autopsy, it is difficult to clearly distinguish IMH and aortic dissection. There is a general consensus that an IMH be treated similar to classic aortic dissection in the corresponding aortic segment.[1,21] Similarly, PAUs, which are often associated with IMHs[59] and pseudoaneurysm, may be amenable to surgical or endovascular intervention. Such patients, however, are often very ill and have significant atherosclerotic disease throughout the vascular tree, which may lead to difficulty with endovascular access and stent-graft deployment.[21]

It is important to note that acute aortic dissection in patients with Marfan syndrome or other connective tissue disorders should be treated uniquely. Although initial management of the acute dissection follows the same overall principles, there is a general consensus that stent-grafts and other endovascular interventions be used with extreme caution, if at all.[1,36,60] Not only are these patients often young and the long-term durability of stent-grafts is not yet known, but also there is significant concern regarding the continuous radial forces on a diseased aortic wall induced by stent-grafts. Further, stent-grafts may promote aortic dissection in some genetic aortopathies. Thus, endovascular intervention in patients with connective tissues disorders is not recommended unless there is a clear indication for intervention and the patient presents with prohibitive operative risk factors as deemed by a cardiovascular surgeon.[21]

CONCLUSION

Aortic dissection is a potentially lethal entity that demands high clinical suspicion, accurate and prompt diagnosis, a thorough understanding of anatomy and natural history, and a multidisciplinary approach to management of this highly variable disease process. As clinical experience and understanding of aortic pathology grows, various classification systems have been developed to assist in categorizing aortic lesions, which may behave quite differently and, therefore, require patient and complication-specific approaches to management. The Stanford and DeBakey classification systems are most commonly used today to describe aortic dissections and help guide treatment. Subtle variants of aortic dissection, however, are increasingly common as noninvasive imaging improves.

Although catheter aortography was once considered the gold standard for diagnosis of aortic dissection, computerized tomographic scanning has clearly become the preferred imaging modality today for both diagnosis and treatment planning because it is highly sensitive and specific. Many invasive and noninvasive imaging modalities may be useful, however.

Management of aortic dissection is complex and is directed by multiple patient- and disease-specific factors. Initial blood pressure and heart rate control and monitoring in the intensive care unit setting are critical. Ascending aortic dissections (Stanford A, DeBakey I and II) generally require emergent surgical intervention, whereas descending aortic dissections (Stanford B, DeBakey III) present a more difficult challenge in terms of management decision making. Type B dissections complicated by rupture, rapid false lumen expansion, tissue malperfusion, or intractable pain or uncontrollable hypertension are likely to require acute intervention. Conversely, uncomplicated type B dissections are typically treated medically. With the advent and evolution of endovascular techniques, more, often less invasive, treatment options are becoming available to the clinician. There

is no clear consensus yet regarding open surgical repair versus stent-graft and other adjunctive interventions, however. Further clinical investigation is clearly needed and is ongoing. Ultimately, treatment of aortic dissection will likely employ multiple techniques and more patient- and disease-specific approaches.

REFERENCES

1. Hiratzka LF, Bakris GL, Beckman JA, et al. 2010 ACCF/AHA/AATS/ACR/ASA/SCA/SCAI/SIR/STS/SVM guidelines for the diagnosis and management of patients with thoracic aortic disease: a report of the American College of Cardiology Foundation/American Heart Association Task Force on Practice Guidelines, American Association for Thoracic Surgery, American College of Radiology, American Stroke Association, Society of Cardiovascular Anesthesiologists, Society for Cardiovascular Angiography and Interventions, Society of Interventional Radiology, Society of Thoracic Surgeons, and Society for Vascular Medicine. *Circulation* 2010;121(13): e266–e369.
2. DeBakey ME, McCollum CH, Crawford ES, et al. Dissection and dissecting aneurysms of the aorta: twenty-year follow-up of five hundred twenty-seven patients treated surgically. *Surgery* 1982;92(6):1118–1134.
3. Maunoir JP. *Mâemoires Physiologiques Et Pratiques Sur l'Anâevrisme Et La Ligature Des Artâeres.* Geneva, Switzerland; 1802.
4. Gurin D. Dissecting aneurysms of the aorta: diagnosis and operative relief of acute arterial obstruction due to this cause. *NY State J Med* 1935;35:1200.
5. Abbott OA. Clinical experiences with application of polythene cellophane upon aneurysms of thoracic vessels. *J Thorac Surg* 1949;18:435.
6. Paullin JE, James DF. Dissecting aneurysm of aorta. *Postgrad Med* 1948;4:291–299.
7. De Bakey ME, Cooley DA, Creech O Jr. Surgical considerations of dissecting aneurysm of the aorta. *Ann Surg* 1955;142:586, discussion 611.
8. Cooley DA, Creech O Jr, De Bakey ME. Surgical treatment of dissecting aneurysm. *JAMA* 1956;162:1654.
9. Creech O Jr, De Bakey ME, Cooley DA. Surgical treatment of dissecting aneurysm of the aorta. *Tex State J Med* 1956;52:287.
10. Fann JI, Smith JA, Miller DC, et al. Surgical management of aortic dissection during a 30-year period. *Circulation* 1995;92:113–121.
11. Umania JP, Lai DT, Mitchell RS, et al. Is medical therapy still the optimal treatment strategy for patients with acute type B aortic dissections? *J Thorac Cardiovasc Surg* 2002;124:896–910.
12. De Bakey ME, Henly WS, Cooley DA, et al. Surgical management of dissecting aneurysm involving the ascending aorta. *J Cardiovasc Surg* 1964;5:200.
13. Svensson LG, Labib SB, Eisenhauer AC, et al. Intimal tear without hematoma. *Circulation* 1999;99:1331–1336.
14. Erbel R, Alfonso F, Boileau C, et al. Diagnosis and management of aortic dissections. *Eur Heart J* 2001;22:1642–1681.
15. Nienaber CA, Sievers HH. Intramural hematoma in acute aortic syndrome: more than one variant of dissection? *Circulation* 2002;106:284–285.
16. O'Gara PT, DeSanctis RW. Acute aortic dissection and its variants. Toward a common diagnostic and therapeutic approach. *Circulation* 1995;92:1376–1378.
17. Roberts CS, Roberts WC. Aortic dissection with the entrance tear in the descending thoracic aorta. *Ann Surg* 1991;213:356–368.
18. Vilacosta I, San Roman JA, Ferreiros J, et al. Natural history and serial morphology of aortic intramural hematoma: a novel variant of aortic dissection. *Am Heart J* 1997;134:495–507.
19. Von Kodolitsch Y, Csosz SK, Koschyk DH, et al. Intramural hematoma of the aorta: predictors of progression to dissection and rupture. *Circulation* 2003;107:1158–1163.
20. Moizumi Y, Komatsu T, Motoyoshi N, et al. Clinical features and long-term outcome of type A and type B intramural hematoma of the aorta. *J Thorac Cardiovasc Surg* 2004;127:421–427.
21. Svensson LG, Kouchoukos NT, Miller DC, et al. Expert consensus document on the treatment of descending thoracic aortic disease using endovascular stent-grafts. *Ann Thorac Surg* 2008;85:S1–S41.
22. Stanson AW, Kazmier FJ, Hollier LH, et al. Penetrating atherosclerotic ulcers or the thoracic aorta: natural history and clinicopathologic complications. *Ann Vasc Surg* 2986;1:15–23.
23. Cho KR, Stanson AW, Potter DD, et al. Penetrating atherosclerotic ulcer of the descending thoracic aorta and arch. *J Thorac Cardiovasc Surg* 2004;127:1393–1399.
24. Daily PO, Trueblood HW, Stinson EB, et al. Management of acute aortic dissections. *Ann Thorac Surg* 1970;10:237.

25. DeBakey ME, Henley WS, Cooley DA, et al. Surgical management of dissecting aneurysms of the aorta. *J Thorac Cardiovasc Surg* 1965;49:130–149.

26. Reul GJ, Hallman GL, et al. Dissecting aneurysm of the descending aorta. *Arch Surg* 1975;110:632–640.

27. Sarasin FP, Louis-Simonet M, Gaspoz JM, et al. Detecting acute thoracic aortic dissection in the emergency department: time constraints and choice of optimal diagnostic test. *Ann Emerg Med* 1996;28:278–288.

28. Yosdhida S, Akiba H, Tamakawa M, et al. Thoracic involvement of type A aortic dissection and intramural hematoma: diagnositc accuracy: comparison of emergence helical CT and surgical findings. *Radiology* 2003;228:430–435.

29. Sommer T, Fehske W, Holzknecht N, et al. Aortic dissection: a comparative study of diagnosis with spiral CT, multiplanar transesophageal echocadiography, and MR imaging. *Radiology* 1996;199:347–352.

30. Quint LE, Francis IR, Williams DM, et al. Evaluation of thoracic aortic disease with the use of helical CT and multiplanar reconstructions: comparison with surgical findings. *Radiology* 1996;201:37–41.

31. Francois CJ, Carr JC. MRI of the thoracic aorta. *Cardiol Clin* 2007;25:171–184, vii.

32. Kapustin AJ, Litt HI. Diagnostic imaging for aortic dissection. *Semin Thorac Cardiovasc Surg* 2005;17:214–223.

33. Shiga T, Wajima Z, Apfel CC, et al. Diagnostic accuracy of transesophageal echocardiography, helical computed tomography, and magnetic resonance imaging for suspected thoracic aortic dissection: systemic review and meta-analysis. *Arch Intern Med* 2006;166:1350–1356.

34. Cigarroa JE, Isselbacher EM, DeSanctis RW, et al. Diagnostic imaging in the evaluation of suspected aortic dissection. Old standards and new directions. *N Engl J Med* 1993;328:35–43.

35. Spittell PC, Spittell JA, Joyce JW, et al. Clinical features and differential diagnosis of aoric dissection: experience with 236 cases (1980 through 1990). *Mayo Clin Proc* 1993;68:642–651.

36. Lin PH, Huynh TT, Kougias P, et al. Descending thoracic aortic dissection: evaluation and management in the era of endovascular technology. *Vasc Endovasc Surg* 2009;43(1):5–24.

37. Pretre R, Alfonso E, Boileau C, et al. Aortic dissection. *Lancet* 1997;349:1461–1464.

38. Pape LA, Tsai TT, Iselbacher EM, et al. Aortic diameter greater than or equal to 5.5 cm is not a good predictor of type A aortic dissection: observations from the International Registry of Acute Aortic Dissection (IRAD). *Circulation* 2007;116:1120–1127.

39. Anagnostopoulos CE, Prabhakar MJ, Kittle CF. Aortic dissections and dissecting aneurysms. *Am J Cardiol* 1972;30:263–273.

40. Ehrlich MP, Ergin MA, McCullough JN, et al. Results of immediate surgical treatment of all acute type A dissections. *Circulation* 2000;102:III248–III252.

41. Wheat MW Jr, Harris PD, Malm JR, et al. Acute dissecting aneurysms of the aorta: treatment results in 64 patients. *J Thorac Cardiovasc Surg* 1969;58:344–351.

42. Miller DC, Mitchell RS, Oyer PE, et al. Independent determinants of operative mortality for patients with aortic dissectons. *Circulation* 1984;70(suppl 1):I153–I164.

43. Wheat MW Jr. Acute dissection of the aorta. *Cardiovasc Clin* 1987;17:241–262.

44. Doroghazi RM, Slater EE, DeSanctis RW, et al. Long-term survival of patients with treated aortic dissection. *J Am Coll Cardiol* 1984;3:1026–1034.

45. Nienaber CA, Zannetti S, Barbieri B, et al. Investigation of stent grafts in patients with type B aortic dissections: design of the INSTEAD trial—a prospective, multicenter European randomized trial. *Am Heart J* 2005;149:592–599.

46. Nienaber CA, Kische S, Akin I, et al. Strategies for subacute/chronic type B aortic dissection: the investigation of stent grafts in patients with type B aortic dissection (INSTEAD) trial 1-year outcome. *J Thorac Cardiovasc Surg* 2010;149(suppl 6):S101–S108.

47. DC Miller. The continuing dilemma concerning medical versus surgical management of patients with acute type B dissections. *Semin Thorac Cardiovasc Surg* 1993;5:33–46.

48. Swee W, Dake MD. Endovascular management of thoracic dissections. *Circulation* 2008;117:1460–1473.

49. Chung JW, Elkins C, Sakai T, et al. True-lumen collapse in aortic dissection: part I, evaluation of causative factors in phantoms with pulsatile flow. *Radiology* 2000;1(214):87–98.

50. Chung JW, Elkins C, Sakai T, et al. True-lumen collapse in aortic dissection: part II, evaluation of treatment methods in phantoms of pulsatile flow. *Radiology* 2000;1(214):99–106.

51. Fann JI, Sarris GE, Mitchell RS, et al. Treatment of patients with aortic dissection presenting with peripheral vascular complications. *Ann Surg* 1990:705–713.

52. Cambria RP, Brewster DC, Gertler JG, et al. Vascular complications associated with spontaneous aortic dissection. *J Vasc Surg* 1988;7:199–209.

53. Suzuki T, Mehta RH, Ince H, et al. Clinical profiles and outcomes of acute type B aortic dissection in the current era: lessons from the International Registry of Aortic Dissection (IRAD). *Circulation* 2003;108(suppl II):II312–II317.

54. Resch TA, Delle M, Falkenberg M, et al. Remodeling of the thoracic aorta after stent grafting of type B dissection: a Swedish multicenter study. *J Cardiovasc Surg* 2006;47:503–508.

55. Kusagawa H, Shimono T, Ishida M, et al. Changes in false lumen after transluminal stent-graft placement in aortic dissection: six years' experience. *Circulation* 2005;111:2951–2957.

56. Dake MD, Kato N, Mitchell RS, et al. Endovascular stent-graft placement for the treatment of acute aortic dissection. *N Engl J Med* 1999;340:1546–1552.

57. Williams DM, Lee DT, Hamilton BH, et al. The dissected aorta: percutaneous treatment of ischemic complications: principles and results. *J Vasc Interv Radiol* 1997;8:605–625.

58. Erbel R, Oelert H, Meyer J, et al. Effect of medical surgical therapy on aortic dissection evaluated by transesophageal echocardiography: implications for prognosis and therapy. *Circulation* 1993;87:1604–1615.

59. Cho KR, Stanson AW, Potter DD, et al. Penetrating atherosclerotic ulcer of the descending thoracic aorta and arch. *J Thorac Cardiovasc Surg* 2004;127:1393–1401.

60. Milewicz DM, Dietz HC, Miller DC. Treatment of aortic disease in patients with Marfan syndrome. *Circulation* 2005;111:e150–e157.

Aortic Dissection: Principles of Endovascular Treatment

DAVID M. WILLIAMS, HIMANSHU J. PATEL, and G. MICHAEL DEEB

INTRODUCTION

The management of aortic dissection is in a period of rapid evolution. Until recently, standard treatment of aortic dissection still relied on principles from landmark articles by DeBakey et al.[1] in 1955 and Wheat et al.[2] in 1965, which laid the groundwork for the surgical and medical treatment of acute aortic dissection. Indeed, administration of antihypertensive and chronotropic medication is still the first step in treating newly recognized acute dissection, and urgent prophylactic open repair of the ascending aorta is still standard of care for acute type A dissections. Endovascular techniques using fenestration, stents, and stent-grafts have recently begun to replace or supplement surgical repair of certain complications of dissection.

Mortality from acute aortic dissection is mostly caused by tamponade or exsanguination from false lumen rupture or by organ ischemia from the malperfusion syndromes.[1–7] These conditions comprise the targets of complication-specific endovascular approaches to treating acute dissection, which include percutaneous fenestration and endograft implantation. Proper and effective application of these new endovascular techniques requires detailed anatomic and physiologic characterization of the aorta and its branches, including the anatomic extent of dissection, identification of true and false lumens, location of entry and reentry tears, sources of critical vessel perfusion, assessment of the adequacy of perfusion of critical aortic branches, identification of the mechanisms of malperfusion, technical details of the two procedures, and relative merits of endograft versus fenestration; these topics comprise the subject of this chapter, which is greatly expanded from an earlier chapter in reference 8. Before elaborating on these details of fenestration and endografts, it is worthwhile to review briefly the pathoanatomy and pathophysiology of false lumen rupture and the malperfusion syndromes.

PATHOANATOMY OF FALSE LUMEN RUPTURE

In a model of aortic dissection with no flow and equal pressures in the true and false lumens, the true lumen contracts and the false lumen dilates, resulting in an overall increase in aortic cross section.[9] The normal aorta expands because of blood pressure until the wall tension generated by elastic recoil of wall constituents balances blood pressure. In aortic dissection, the dissection flap typically contains the intima and two-thirds of the media, and the outer wall of the false lumen contains the remaining one-third of the media and the adventitia. Because it is thinner and less elastic than the outer wall of the undissected aorta, the outer wall of the false lumen must expand to a larger diameter to generate, at a given blood pressure, the same wall tension. The dissection flap, which lies between isobaric lumens, has been relieved of transmural pressure and therefore undergoes passive elastic collapse. Thus, false lumen dilation and true lumen collapse are expected from purely structural considerations of the aortic wall and are confirmed in those cases of dissection with fortuitous computed tomography (CT) scans prior to acute dissection (FIGURE 64.1). Rapid flow through a narrow true lumen can lead to further collapse caused by the Bernoulli principle. Finally, if false lumen pressure exceeds true lumen pressure, the true lumen may also be compressed.

When an endograft is implanted so as to cover the entry tear of a dissection, in a sense, the pathoanatomy of dissection is reversed. The transmural pressure is at least partially restored to the dissection flap and is reduced on the outer wall of the false lumen. The true lumen expands, and the false lumen contracts, to a degree depending on residual transluminal communications through other intimal "reentry" tears (FIGURE 64.2). Obviously, achieving this hemodynamic reversal of the dissection process requires accurate identification of the location and

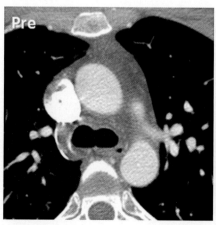
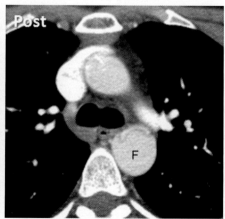

FIGURE 64.1 A 47-year-old woman with a history of hypertension and smoking. CT 1 year before (**left panel**) and immediately after (**right panel**) acute type B aortic dissection shows true lumen collapse and false lumen expansion in the mid-descending thoracic aorta. *F*, false lumen.

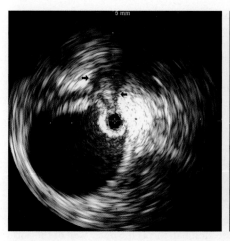
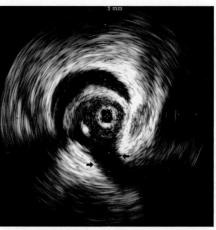

FIGURE 64.2 Intravascular ultrasound images of the abdominal aorta at the level of the superior mesenteric artery before (**left frame**) and immediately after (**right frame**) placement of an endograft across the thoracic aortic entry tear of an acute type B dissection, showing immediate reexpansion of the true lumen at the expense of the false lumen. Echogenic material within the SMA (*arrows*, **right frame**) is ultrasound artifact caused by sluggish flow, which disappears after restoration of SMA perfusion.

extent of the entry and reentry tears and accurate placement of the endograft.

Necropsy studies suggest that in acute dissection the location of false lumen rupture is near the entry tear of the dissection.[10,11] Furthermore, it appears that the endograft deployed across the entry tear of an acute dissection induces localized thrombosis of the nearby false lumen.[12] Thus, there is a sound anatomic and physiologic basis for treating the entry tear of a dissection, restoring flow and transmural pressure, even apart, to the true lumen.

PATHOANATOMY OF BRANCH ARTERY OBSTRUCTION

The Michigan classification of branch artery obstruction[13] is based on the anatomic relationship of the dissection flap to the branch artery in question (FIGURE 64.3). It is an intuitively appealing classification because this anatomic distinction forms the basis of distinct diagnostic and treatment strategies. The causes of obstruction are listed in Table 64.1. As noted, the critical challenge in characterizing an arterial obstruction is to distinguish whether it is caused by an aortic problem or a branch artery problem.

In static obstruction, the dissection flap intersects the origin of a branch and encroaches on the lumen. If the dissection flap enters a vessel origin, but the false lumen reenters the true lumen distally through a large intimal tear (ending the dissection), then the false lumen can completely compensate for a narrowed true lumen and no pressure gradient may be present. If the dissection flap enters the vessel origin but the false lumen does not reenter, the true lumen of the vessel is narrowed if not obliterated and a pressure gradient may be measured across the stenosis between the aorta and the arterial trunk. Treatment is aimed at relieving the branch artery stenosis.

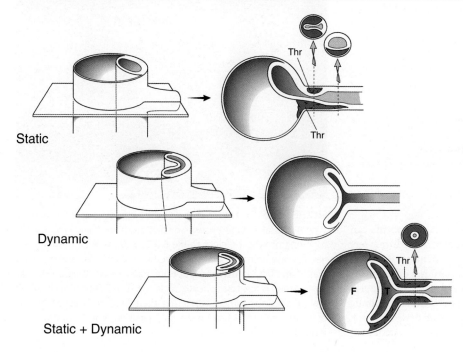

Static

Dynamic

Static + Dynamic

FIGURE 64.3 Diagram illustrating mechanisms of arterial obstruction causing malperfusion specific to acute aortic dissection. In static obstruction, the dissection enters the branch artery and narrows the true lumen. In dynamic obstruction, the dissection flap spares the branch artery trunk but lies across the origin like a curtain. Mixed static and dynamic obstruction also occurs.

Reprinted with permission from Williams DM, Lee DY, Hamilton B, et al. The dissected aorta: III, anatomy and radiologic diagnosis of branch-vessel compromise. *Radiology* 1997;203:37–44.

Table 64.1
Classification of Arterial Obstruction in Aortic Dissection
Static obstruction
Dynamic obstruction
Mixed static and dynamic obstruction
Miscellaneous
• Related to dissection: thrombosis, embolism
• Unrelated to dissection: atherosclerosis, fibromuscular dysplasia

In dynamic obstruction, the dissection flap spares the vessel origin but prolapses across it like a washcloth over a bathtub drain. Unlike static obstruction, which is a branch arterial problem, dynamic obstruction is an aortic problem. This obstruction is dynamic in two senses. It is observed only during cross-sectional imaging with the aorta pressurized and conducting flow; it disappears when the aorta is observed at aortotomy or at necropsy. Furthermore, it may disappear during medical treatment with antihypertensives and beta blockers and recur during hypertensive episodes. Treatment must be directed at the dissection flap in the aorta. Two approaches are feasible: covering the entry tear by means of an endograft, thereby restoring true lumen flow and partially collapsing the false lumen, and fenestrating the dissection flap, thereby establishing flow across the flap into the compromised true lumen.

IDENTIFICATION OF THE TRUE AND FALSE LUMENS

Identification of the true and false lumens is crucial in the endovascular treatment of aortic dissection. The true and false lumens behave differently. As noted previously, the false lumen is prone to ectasia and is at risk of rupture, and the true lumen is prone to collapse and is at risk of compromise of its branch arteries. Numerous steps in the endovascular treatment of dissection require real-time knowledge of which lumen the guide wire, the diagnostic catheter, and of course treatment devices lie within. These steps include:

Deploying an endograft across the entry tear within the true lumen
Stenting a branch artery to the aortic true lumen
Stenting the aortic true lumen after fenestration to reduce a prolapsing flap
Aligning both iliac arteries with the aortic true lumen during aortoiliac stenting

Injudicious placement of aortic or branch artery stents can complicate subsequent transfemoral catheter procedures, retrograde aortic perfusion, or endograft treatment of the aorta. Endovascular treatment of aortic dissection requires distinguishing the true and false lumens based on local features of the aorta cross section when it is not possible to consult a global anatomic study, such as a CT scan. Furthermore, in acute dissection, the baseline cross-sectional configuration of the aortic true lumen

may change because of the hemodynamic effects of endovascular interventions. In chronic dissections, the distinction between the true and false lumens is usually straightforward. For patients with chronic dissections, the interventionist will have the benefit of a chest, abdomen, and pelvis CT. With the anatomic information garnered from the CT, and with the real-time help of intravascular ultrasound (IVUS), it is easy to stay oriented with respect to true and false lumens in a chronic dissection because dramatic changes in luminal diameters are not encountered in dissections that are months old. In acute dissections, a complete CT exam may not be available. Local aortic features identifying the false lumen include aortic cobwebs and the "beak" sign.[14–16] Aortic cobwebs are remnants of media stretching (like cobwebs) between the dissection flap and the outer wall of the false lumen (FIGURE 64.4). The beak sign is the acute angle (the beak) with which the dissection flap meets the outer wall of the aorta (FIGURE 64.4). As such, it is the imaging correlate of the cleaving wedge of hematoma as it splits the medial layers to form the false lumen. These signs are highly reliable local identifiers of the false lumen. Generally reliable characteristics of the true lumen are continuity with the aortic root, which remains the source of most of the large-diameter aortic branches, and continuity with the femoral arteries. Although these global features are not themselves conveniently available during interventions, they do provide orientation in terms of identifying which branch artery arises from true and false lumens.

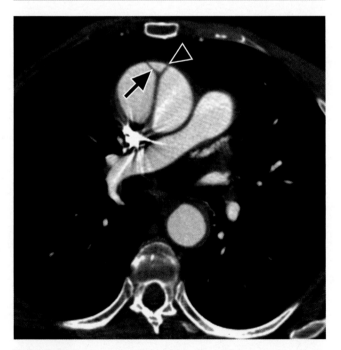

FIGURE 64.4 CT section through the ascending aorta in chronic type A (DeBakey type 2) aortic dissection shows the dissection flap running from the 1 o'clock to the 6:30 positions. A cobweb (*arrowhead*), present on one slice only, runs between the flap and the outer wall of the false lumen and is specific for the false lumen. The beak sign (*arrow*) refers to the acute angle the flap makes with the outer wall of the false lumen. Note that the beak sign is absent at the opposite end of the flap (in the 6:30 position) due to thrombus or intimal hyperplasia.

Once the lumens are identified on the CT scan, they should be traced from root to groin. A reliable anatomic rule to use while drawing a mental path within the aorta from slice to slice on a CT exam is that every time the path crosses the flap it changes the lumen. A second reliable anatomic rule is that, in acute dissections, the lumens are continuous. If two lumens are observed in the chest and two are observed in the pelvis, then two are present in the abdomen, although one of them may be difficult to identify. Sources of branch artery perfusion are identified as exclusively true lumen, exclusively false lumen, or shared true and false lumens. Branches with shared perfusion are further characterized as with or without reentry tears. This classification of branch artery perfusion is a critical part of the anatomic survey that should precede endovascular treatment. Cross-sectional imaging and knowledge of the mechanisms of branch artery obstruction largely determine which branches are susceptible to malperfusion and by what mechanism.

DIAGNOSIS OF BRANCH ARTERY OBSTRUCTION

Although the clinical indication for endovascular treatment is usually organ or limb malperfusion, it should be recognized that the premise of both fenestration/stenting and endograft implantation is that hemodynamically significant arterial obstruction is present or at least is an imminent threat at the time of angiography. Malperfusion can be transient, intermittent, or fixed. A kidney with acute tubular necrosis may have suffered ischemic injury caused by malperfusion early in the dissection process, but subsequent reentry of the dissection within the renal artery might restore normal perfusion. Transient malperfusion such as this does not benefit from endovascular treatment. Fixed malperfusion is documented by manometry showing a significant perfusion pressure deficit in a branch artery or by arteriographic evidence of thrombosis, embolism, or stenosis (FIGURE 64.5). A second premise of the angiographic evaluation is that the hemodynamic status of the patient at angiography is representative of the patient on the ward or in the emergency department (ED). Intermittent malperfusion is a state of recurring arterial obstruction caused by alterations in the configuration of the dissection flap. This phenomenon accounts for the occasional paradoxical finding of losing a femoral pulse when the patient becomes hypertensive and is one explanation (the other being development of an iliac artery reentry tear) of the missing femoral pulse when the patient presents hypertensive in the ED that reappears after initiation of beta-blocker and antihypertensive medication. Intermittent malperfusion is a cause for false negative angiographic evaluation for arterial obstruction when the physiologic circumstances of the angiogram are different from those obtained at the time of the clinical diagnosis.

It would be useful at this point to summarize the anatomic details required to direct endovascular treatment of malperfusion. These must be established by cross-sectional imaging, such as by preoperative CT or by intraoperative IVUS and arteriography, and include:

Anatomic extent (dissection type)
Location of entry tear
Location of reentry tears
Identification of true and false lumens throughout the aorta
Identification of arteries at risk of malperfusion

Identification of mechanism of obstruction
Features of prospective landing zone of endograft

Cross-sectional imaging is useful to rule out "ischemic anatomy." If the true lumen is of reasonable caliber from entry tear to termination, and if the dissection flap spares every major branch artery, then branch artery obstruction is unlikely. If the flap crosses a vessel origin, however, or the true lumen is collapsed, then malperfusion may be present. In cases of acute type B dissection, the aorta and at-risk arteries should be evaluated by angiography, where malperfusion is either ruled out or confirmed and treated. In cases of acute type A dissection, the decision to postpone open repair depends on the clinical status of the patient and the CT vascular assessment.

Angiographic evaluation begins with inspection of the flap in relation to branch artery origins. This can be done most expeditiously using IVUS. Pressure measurements are made simultaneously in the aortic root and abdominal aortic true and false lumens. If these are equal, subsequent pressures can be measured using the abdominal aortic pressure as a surrogate for root pressure. If they are unequal, the commonest explanation is collapse of the aortic true lumen with dynamic obstruction of infradiaphragmatic vessels. Less commonly, such gradients can be caused by a coarctation-like obstruction within the aorta, such as at an aortic graft anastomosis or area of aortic false lumen thrombosis.

Aortic pressures should be compared to arterial trunk pressures in the organ of interest clinically as well as in those branches suspected of being compromised on the basis of

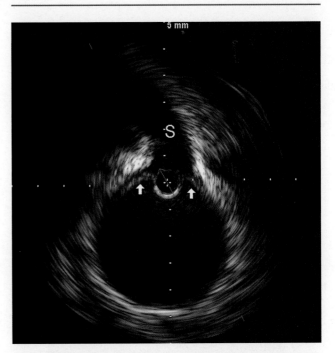

FIGURE 64.5 Intravascular ultrasound image shows complete collapse of the abdominal aortic true lumen with prolapse of the flap across the superior mesenteric artery (SMA) origin (*arrows*). Manometry (not shown) documented a 66 mm Hg pressure deficit in the SMA compared to the aortic root with an absolute SMA pressure of 29 mm Hg; the gradient was eliminated after placement of an endograft. *S*, SMA.

imaging. Equal pressures in a false lumen and a collapsed true lumen do not mean that the branch artery pressures are also equal. Pressure measurements within a branch artery should be followed by selective arteriography to make sure that the measurement is representative of the perfusion pressure at the organ level. This precaution is necessary in instances of static obstruction, wherein the reentry tear may be several centimeters deep in the trunk; unless the measurement is distal to the reentry tear, it may underestimate the branch artery deficit in perfusion pressure (FIGURE 64.6).

Dynamic obstruction that is intermittent is sometimes demonstrably pressure dependent. In cases where this is suspected, especially when the clinical history suggests that the patient is noncompliant with medications or clinical follow-up, a negative workup for malperfusion is followed by reassessment after tapering down the dose of the beta blocker. For this reason, we request patients with subacute dissection and a history suggesting sporadic episodes of malperfusion be converted to short-acting beta blockers, antihypertensives, and sedation. Patients with acute dissection are, ordinarily, already being treated with short-acting drugs.

Management

The DeBakey and Stanford classifications provide anatomic criteria for stratifying patients into immediate surgical or medical management based on involvement of the ascending aorta. Initiation of anti-impulse and antihypertensive medication in all patients is paramount before considering the logistics and

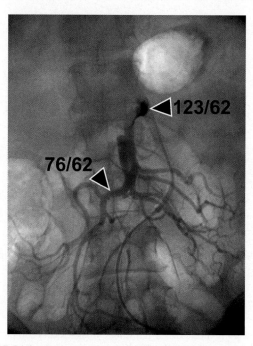

FIGURE 64.6 Manometry proximal and deep in the superior mesenteric artery (SMA) shows the importance of measuring pressures distal to the terminal point of the dissection. Reliance on proximal trunk pressures would have missed the 47 mm Hg pressure drop across the SMA dissection. Pressure in the distal SMA was normalized after placement of overlapping self-expanding stents.

details of endovascular therapy. Treatment of the leaking type A false lumen (impending rupture or tamponade), coronary artery obstruction, and severe acute aortic insufficiency takes precedence over suspected mesenteric, renal, lower extremity, or spinal cord malperfusion, and open repair should proceed immediately in patients with reasonable operative risk. Patients with prolonged malperfusion of gut or lower extremity may be unsuitable for immediate repair even with type A dissection, and in such cases the first priority is to restore flow to critical vessels. The anatomy of the dissection, location of the entry tear, and mechanism of arterial obstruction determine the appropriate treatment in a given case; therefore, the first principle of treatment is to define arterial anatomy and assess visceral perfusion. In particular, ensuring the integrity of the superior mesenteric artery (SMA), or restoring perfusion to the compromised SMA, has the highest priority of any endovascular goal in this group of patients. Even when resection of dead bowel is necessary, preoperative endovascular restoration of SMA perfusion will give the general surgeon reliable margins between viable and unsalvageable bowel.

Setting Priorities

Treatment priorities depend on patient characteristics, anatomy of the aortic dissection including complications, and resources of the institution. Is an emergent procedure indicated? And if so, does the patient require open aortic reconstruction or endovascular treatment? With current endograft technology, patients with uncomplicated type A dissection undergo immediate open reconstruction of the ascending aorta. Patients with type A complicated by wide-open aortic insufficiency, false lumen rupture, or coronary artery involvement with myocardial ischemia should also undergo immediate open repair. Patients with type A dissection complicated by prolonged organ ischemia, but who are otherwise stable, may undergo endovascular treatment of their malperfusion by fenestration, and, if they survive their reperfusion injury and do not rupture their aorta, have delayed aortic repair.[17–19] Whether this course of action (fen-sten, then operate) is feasible for type A dissections depends on the referral pattern of the institution, the philosophy of the thoracic surgeon, the current state of the art in endovascular devices, and the experience of the interventionist. Many endovascular options are available to patients with complicated type B aortic dissections.[20–30]

When open aortic reconstruction is not indicated, and a patient is being considered as a candidate for endovascular treatment, certain procedural priorities should be observed. As of 2011, there has been no evidence that patients with uncomplicated acute type B dissections will benefit from endograft treatment[31] compared to medical treatment. Because endograft placement can treat complications of the degenerating false lumen simultaneously as well as malperfusion, the first priority, if appropriate endovascular devices are available, is to establish whether the patient is anatomically suitable for an endograft. With endograft trials for aortic dissection in 2011, general anatomic criteria require 2 cm between the left common carotid origin and the proximal edge of the entry tear. In patients with an acute type B dissection and rupture of the false lumen, there is a clear indication for endograft placement in anatomically appropriate patients. In patients with an acute type B dissection and clinical malperfusion, there is presently no general consensus on how much effort should be made to confirm ongoing arterial obstruction in a patient clinically suspected of malperfusion. Our own approach is to measure pressures in the aortic root and in branch arteries to establish the presence of ongoing arterial obstruction before we conclude that endovascular treatment is indicated. Because placement of an endograft is a global treatment for the degenerating false lumen as well as malperfusion, it is a reasonable approach, having established that endograft treatment is indicated, to place the endograft first and then evaluate for end-organ malperfusion after placement. When the only endovascular option is fenestration and stenting, then the target arteries must be evaluated and treated regionally: (1) superior mesenteric and celiac arteries, (2) bilateral renal arteries, and (3) bilateral common iliac arteries. In this case, the first priority, regardless of the organ clinically suspected of malperfusion, is to establish the integrity of SMA perfusion and restore perfusion if the artery is obstructed. Succeeding priorities are the spinal cord, solitary kidney, and lower extremity.

Two other groups of patients with aortic dissections present with malperfusion. A small group of patients who have undergone open repair of the ascending aorta for acute type A dissection have persistent malperfusion after the operation. The approach in these patients is the same as in those without operation: the anatomy of the dissection and pattern of suspected malperfusion determine the treatment. Occasionally, postoperative patients must be evaluated for malperfusion after femoral artery cutdown for embolectomy or bypass. In these cases, access for diagnosis can be achieved using two tandem femoral artery accesses in the unoperated groin. If endovascular treatment needs access through the postsurgical groin, then ultrasound-assisted access may be repaired operatively.

Finally, malperfusion can be present in patients with chronic type B or repaired type A dissections. In dissections a few months old, we have encountered dynamic obstruction of the iliac arteries. In older dissections, dynamic obstruction is uncommon, and malperfusion is typically caused by branches arising from an anatomically isolated portion of the true lumen, stenoses or kinks at aortic graft anastomoses, or static obstruction from the dissection flap entering a branch artery without adequate reentry.

In summary, four treatment algorithms or decision trees can be envisioned. The first is the conventional stratification between type A versus type B dissections. If endografts are not available, the primary question is, "Is prolonged malperfusion suspected?" Here, patients are stratified between immediate angiography to correct malperfusion and treatment determined by the conventional algorithm (FIGURE 64.7A). In the era of endografts restricted to conventional indications for surgical intervention, namely, impending rupture or malperfusion, the first question is, "Is an endograft indicated?" followed by "Is an endograft anatomically feasible?" (FIGURE 64.7B). In the era of unrestricted use of endografts, the first question is, "Is an endograft anatomically feasible?" (FIGURE 64.7C).

Vascular Access

In general, bilateral femoral artery access is both desirable and possible in endovascular treatment of aortic dissection. Great effort should be made to enter the femoral artery true lumen. In cases where we anticipate performing aortic fenestration, bilateral 8 French × 30-cm sheaths are inserted. These are large enough in diameter to accommodate IVUS and long enough to extend above the aorta bifurcation, which is obviously cephalad to entry tears at the aorta bifurcation or iliac arteries. This allows catheter exchange without constantly needing to verify which lumen a newly advanced catheter lies within. Once the sheaths are placed, our practice is to advance the IVUS catheter into the femoral artery, confirming its location within the true or false lumen, and proceed to examination of the entire aorta. If the catheter enters the true lumen at the groin but crosses the dissection flap through a reentry tear into the false lumen in the common iliac or abdominal aorta, the IVUS catheter is withdrawn back into the true lumen, then a guide wire and catheter are used to systematically explore the vessel, advancing and readvancing the IVUS until the reentry tear is passed and the ultrasound catheter continues within the true lumen. At this point,

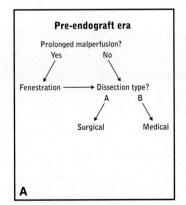

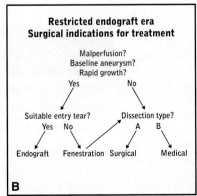

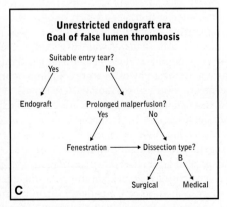

FIGURE 64.7 Decision trees for endovascular treatment of an aortic dissection, including for fenestration and stenting of an acute aortic dissection (**A**), for endovascular treatment of aortic dissections in the era of endografts available through clinical trials (**B**), and for endovascular treatment of dissections in the era of unrestricted endografts (**C**).

Reprinted with permission from Williams DM. Aortic dissection: evaluation and management—choosing the right intervention. In Lumsden A, et al. eds. *Advanced Endovascular Therapy of Aortic Disease.* Malden, MA: Blackwell Futura; 2007:117–122.

the access sheath is advanced over the IVUS, securing progress within the true lumen achieved by the IVUS catheter. This same technique is occasionally used to enter the false lumen deliberately to evaluate, for example, a renal artery inaccessible from the true lumen, or to place a balloon catheter in the false lumen for the occasional need to target the balloon during fenestration.

Three variations of femoral artery involvement by the dissection deserve additional comments. When one common femoral artery is dissected, but the other is not, then the uninvolved femoral artery is accessed first. True lumen location at the aorta bifurcation is confirmed by IVUS, and a Cobra or similar catheter is passed across the bifurcation to the contralateral groin. Again, IVUS is used to confirm true lumen location in the contralateral external iliac and common femoral arteries. When this is secured, a 6 × 4 balloon catheter or similar device is advanced into the common femoral artery true lumen and used as a target for direct fluoroscopic guided puncture. A second variation is when both common femoral arteries are dissected. In these cases we have secured access into nondissected superficial femoral artery with a 4 French sheath, through which a 0.018 or 0.014 wire and balloon are used as a fluoroscopic target for true lumen access in the common femoral artery.

A third variation is when access into the common femoral artery enters a thrombosed common femoral or external iliac artery. In these cases, even using IVUS with a 6 French catheter, it may be difficult to tell whether the access and surrounding thrombus are within true or false lumen. If the sandwiched intimal flap is not conspicuous on the IVUS image, we generally assume we are in the false lumen. Maneuvers to confirm this include extending the wire into the aorta, where the true lumen is generally more conspicuous, or advancing a catheter from the contralateral groin antegrade from the aorta bifurcation as described previously. The thrombosed and dissected iliac artery not only presents an inconvenience for vascular access, but also a challenge that is critical to evaluate and possibly treat before treating more central problems in the aorta. If the iliac thrombus is within true lumen, then restoring aortic true lumen flow by covering the entry tear with an endograft may result in showering the leg with iliac thrombus fragments. If the thrombus is within false lumen, then endograft placement or aortic fenestration can be performed first, and the iliac artery dissection treated secondarily if leg malperfusion persists following the aortic intervention.

Occasionally, bilateral femoral artery access is not desirable. For example, some patients with suspected malperfusion present for angiographic evaluation following groin exploration and Fogarty thrombectomy of an acute cold limb or after open aortic reconstruction using femoral artery bypass. A large-caliber sheath inserted into such a femoral artery would require removal in the operating suite. In circumstances where anatomic features of the dissection allow placement of an endograft to cover a dissection entry tear, the surgeon may wish to secure access from an unoperated groin. In these circumstances, tandem punctures and placement of 8 French sheaths in a single femoral artery will allow evaluation of the patient's anatomic suitability and clinical indication for endograft placement. If the patient is suitable for an endograft, then femoral artery cutdown proceeds in the unused groin. If the patient is not anatomically suitable for an endograft, and yet aortoiliac reconstruction is necessary to eliminate lower extremity malperfusion, then a third puncture can be made in the unused groin when appropriate.

TECHNIQUE OF ENDOVASCULAR TREATMENT

Implantation of endografts for aortic dissection follows the general principles of endovascular treatment of aneurysms. In procedures to treat the false lumen, the endograft is deployed so as to cover the intimal tear, allowing communication of flow and perfusion pressure between the two lumens. In procedures to treat malperfusion, endograft treatment presents the opportunity to treat all the malperfused territories simultaneously, recognizing that individual vascular territories must be assessed following endograft deployment. Fenestration and true lumen stenting, however, treats vascular territories piecemeal. For example, fenestration and stenting may relieve dynamic obstruction of the celiac artery and SMA, partially relieve dynamic obstruction of the renal arteries, and leave iliac artery malperfusion unaltered. Because significant but unsuspected mesenteric malperfusion may accompany clinically apparent leg ischemia, our practice is to assess gut perfusion as a first priority in every case where the local true lumen is collapsed. In practice, a CT scan may show an uncollapsed true lumen at the level of the SMA with no sign of distal occlusion, and this may lower the priority of SMA assessment during the angiographic workup. Tables 64.2 and 64.3 and FIGURE 64.8 describe the basic steps in the endovascular treatment of dissection.

Several techniques of fenestration have been described. All of them entail crossing the dissection flap at some chosen site, then creating the tear. Generally the puncture is made from the smaller lumen into the larger lumen; that is, usually from the true lumen into the false lumen. Wire passage can be accomplished using a TIPS or other needle or reentry device and IVUS and fluoroscopic guidance to puncture the flap, or else placing a guide wire in the false lumen (via a distal reentry tear, if available) and poising an inflated balloon or loop-snare at the desired level and puncturing the target. The IVUS method can be used with both accesses in the true lumen, or one in the true lumen and the other in the false lumen. The target methods require one access in the false lumen, which in practice is not always possible (for example, when the dissection extends into the internal iliac artery and no reentry tear is accessible).

To extend the guide wire hole into a transverse tear, we inflate a 14- or 16-mm balloon centered on the puncture site.

Table 64.2
Steps in Endograft Treatment
Define the anatomy of arch vessels and intimal tear
Establish the extent of dissection
Inspect the relation of the dissection flap to branch origins
Identify the length of the proximal landing zone
Size the endograft according to the proximal landing zone diameter
Confirm guide wire placement exclusively in the true lumen
Deploy the endograft
Assess branch artery perfusion based on clinical history, laboratory findings, and imaging

Table 64.3
Steps in Fenestration and Stenting

Define the anatomy of dissection

Establish the extent of dissection

Identify the source of branch artery perfusion from the true lumen or false lumen, or both, with or without reentry

Inspect the relation of the dissection flap to branch origins: anatomy of possible malperfusion

Identify dynamic obstruction

Identify static obstruction

Identify mixed dynamic and static obstruction

Confirm malperfusion (ongoing arterial obstruction)

Perform simultaneous pressure measurements between the aortic root and branch arteries

Perform branch arteriography

　To document manometry is distal to reentry and reflects organ perfusion

　To rule out other causes of malperfusion (emboli, fibromuscular dysplasia, atherosclerosis)

Perform fenestration

Monitor using IVUS (from either lumen)

Use a Rosch-Uchida set or other steerable needle to cross the dissection flap

Extend the hole from the crossing needle into a window in the flap, using a 14-mm balloon

If true lumen collapse persists, place the stent in the aortic true lumen (16- to 18-mm self-expending stent)

　Fenestration sites: celiac, just below the renal arteries, just above the bifurcation

　Aorta stent sites: supramesenteric, infrarenal, aortoiliac

Reassess branch artery perfusion, stenting static obstruction as necessary

A distinct waist is unusual. The balloon should not be retracted during inflation, lest the intimal cast be torn loose and intussuscept. Others have described a more dramatic, if less controlled, method of creating the tear. In one variation, the operator punctures the flap and crosses it with a guide wire then snares the wire from the opposite lumen and extracts it from the groin. Then both ends of the wire are retracted, like reins on a horse. An alternate method places a wire in the true lumen and, with a second side-by-side wire, crosses the flap distally. The sheath is then advanced forcefully over the two wires together. It has been suggested that these guide wire maneuvers result in longitudinal tearing of the dissection flap, although I am not aware of anatomic proof of that claim. It should be recalled that the acute aorta dissection flap tears easily in the circumferential or transverse direction and resists tearing longitudinally.[32] A more plausible mechanism is that both techniques convert the guide wire hole into a circumferential tear and then, rather than tear the now-cylindrical intimal flap, cause it to intussuscept: distally when the guide wire loop is retracted, proximally when the sheath is advanced over the crossing guide wire.

Intramural Hematoma With or Without Ulcerlike Intimal Tears

The acute aortic syndrome includes classical double-barrel aortic dissection, the entity discussed in detail in this chapter, as well as intramural hematoma (IMH), penetrating atherosclerotic ulcer, and leaking thoracic aortic aneurysms. These lesions are also amenable to endovascular treatment[33–35] and fall into the scope of this chapter when an IMH is present.

An IMH can occasionally present with static obstruction of a renal or mesenteric artery. When an IMH extends into a branch artery origin, the vessel is narrowed by the thrombosed false lumen; these obstructions can be directly treated with branch artery self-expanding stents. Balloon expansion should be avoided, or at least significantly undersized, because the intimal flap overlying the thrombosed false lumen is easily torn, resulting in extrusion of thrombus into the true lumen and distal embolization.

When an IMH is accompanied by an intimal tear, a treatment target is well defined and, when anatomically suitable with respect to landing zone and critical aortic branches, appropriate for treatment with an endograft. Unlike in classical dissection, when the true lumen expansion and reciprocal false lumen collapse occur after the entry tear is covered, in an IMH true lumen expansion is countered by the thrombus in the false lumen. The friable intimal flap covering the thrombus-filled false lumen is easily torn. Consequently, if medical management successfully controls pain, heart rate, and blood pressure, endograft treatment is generally delayed to allow some resolution of the hematoma and healing of the flap.

Complications

Endovascular treatment of aortic dissection entails a number of component procedures including femoral artery puncture or cutdown, branch artery cannulation, use of large sheaths, and so on, which are associated with the angiographic procedure as such, as well as complications specific to treating the aortic dissection. We will discuss the second group of complications.

The most feared complication of endovascular treatment of aortic dissection is conversion of a type B dissection to an acute type A dissection, which generally requires urgent open repair of the ascending aorta. To my knowledge, this is associated with the endograft treatment of dissection and has not been observed with fenestration. It is uncertain whether this complication is related to traumatic injury of the fragile aortic wall by the rather stiff endograft delivery catheter or to conversion of the stable false lumen to an expanding false lumen after covering the decompressing "entry" tear. Traumatic injury of the aortic wall can be minimized by adhering to the traditional angiographic technique: advancing devices over atraumatic guide wires, not forcing a device that has snagged on a plaque or vessel origin, never deploying a device unless certain of the guide wire location, and so forth. The relevance of the second mechanism,

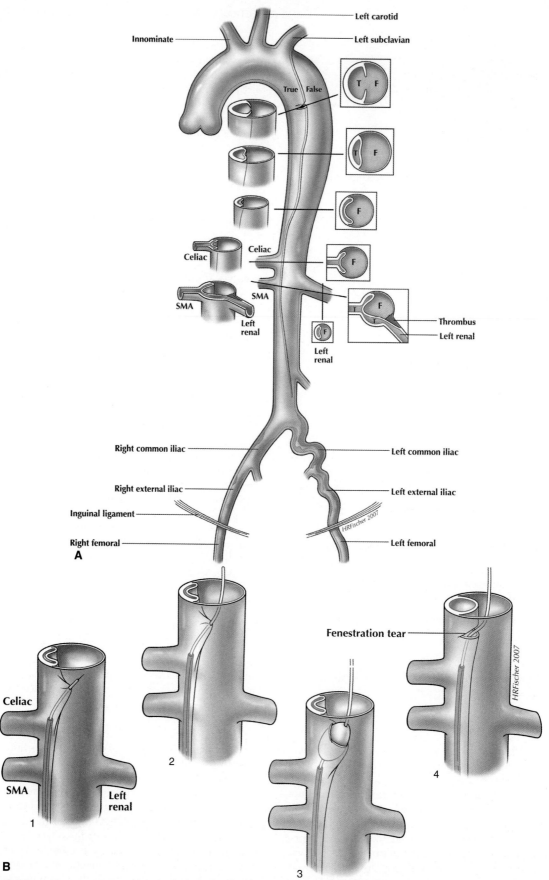

FIGURE 64.8 Drawings illustrating an acute type B aortic dissection with entry tear several centimeters distal to the left subclavian artery (**1**) as it would be treated by fenestration and stenting (**2,3**) or by endograft (**4**). (B) shows steps in the fenestration procedure. (C) and (D) show residual renal artery stenosis after fenestration and endograft treatment, respectively. If hemodynamically significant, the renal artery narrowing would be treated with a true lumen bare metal stent.

Reprinted with permission from Patel HJ, Williams DM. Endovascular therapy for malperfusion in acute type B aortic dissection. *Oper Tech Thorac Cardiovasc Surg* 2009;14(1):2–11.

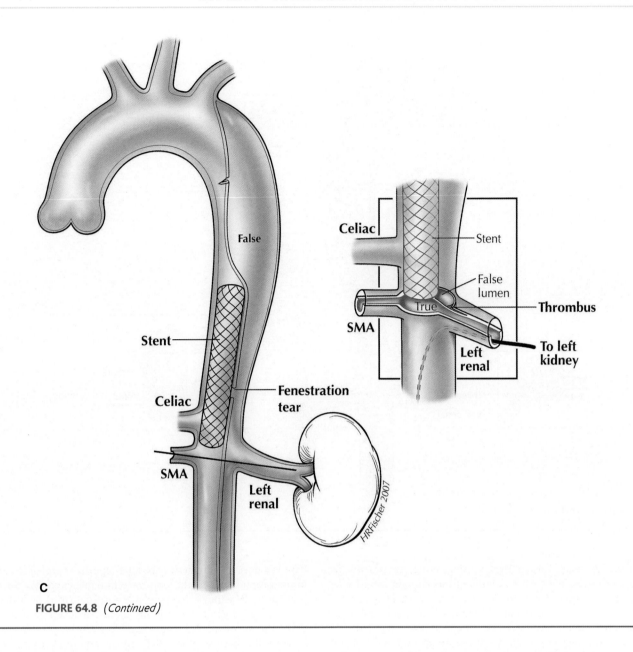

C

FIGURE 64.8 *(Continued)*

which potentially restores the expansile nature of the developing false lumen, will become evident as we accumulate further experience in endograft treatment.

Complications of the fenestration/stenting procedure are related either to the flap puncture, creating the tear in the dissection flap, and misadventures in stent placement. Partial solutions for complications are summarized in the following section on bailout procedures. Flap puncture has been remarkably safe. We have had one case of self-limited and nonfatal hemothorax after needle passage, when the crossing was made at the T10 level, but no instance of clinically evident retroperitoneal bleeding after needle passage in the abdominal aorta.

A relatively common complication is encountered when the initial malperfusion consists of static obstruction of the SMA or common iliac artery. Restoring flow to vessels that are nearly totally obstructed can result in collapse of the true lumen more proximally. Early in our experience, we treated several patients with leg malperfusion caused by a dissected common iliac

artery. Stenting the isolated iliac dissection resulted in collapse of the infrarenal aortic true lumen, necessitating infrarenal fenestration. This, in turn, caused collapse of the supramesenteric aortic true lumen, requiring a second fenestration. Presently when we are faced with isolated occlusion of an iliac artery, our first choice is to perform an iliac artery fenestration if the false lumen is patent. In the case of the SMA or when the iliac artery false lumen is thrombosed, the most straightforward treatment is to stent the vessel and to treat any aortic true lumen collapse that may ensue.

Misadventures in the placement of aortic stents can complicate the remainder of the endovascular treatment. For example, placement of the aortic stent through the fenestration tear, rather than entirely within the true lumen alongside the tear, diverts all transfemoral guide wires and devices from the true lumen caudal to the stent into the false lumen cephalic to the stent. This biluminal placement thus complicates future transfemoral access to the coronary or brachiocephalic vessels and

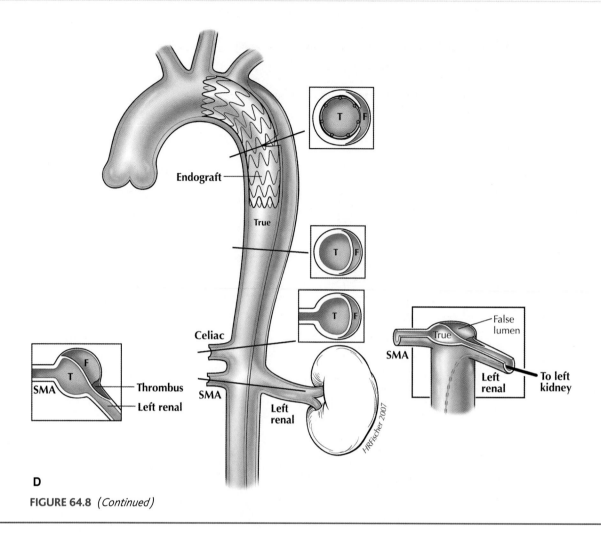

D

FIGURE 64.8 *(Continued)*

precludes future cardiac bypass using retrograde transfemoral perfusion. We have encountered this complication twice: once in a patient transferred to us with persistent malperfusion despite fenestration and biluminal stent placement at an outside hospital, and once when the guide wire inadvertently passed through an intercostal artery origin on the dissection flap and biluminal placement of the self-expanding stent after fenestration was discovered using IVUS while investigating why the stent failed to expand after release. Instead, the stent should be deployed entirely within the aortic true lumen, and confirmation of guide wire location entirely within the true lumen at the level of treatment is mandatory. A similar problem can occur when the edge of the true lumen stent abuts a fenestration or reentry tear: here the competent true lumen, held open by the stent on one side of the tear, may lose continuity with the collapsed true lumen on the other side of the tear. Although we have not encountered such an instance during endograft deployment, one would anticipate that an endograft expanding in a collapsed true lumen might tear the flap at the edge of the prosthesis with loss of continuity of the true lumen on the other side of the iatrogenic tear.

Probably the most dramatic complication of the fenestration procedure is causing the cylindrical intimal cast to intussuscept into the distal aorta. We have not encountered this complication when creating the tear by inflating the angioplasty across the flap. We have encountered anecdotal reports of probable flap intussusception during the loop-retraction maneuver described previously. Whether using proximal-to-distal (p-d) or distal-to-proximal (d-p) intussusception, these maneuvers are inherently uncontrolled. P-d intussusception can be complicated by aortoiliac occlusion, and d-p intussusception can result in unpredictable hemodynamics if the patient subsequently needs cardiopulmonary bypass from the femoral access. Both can lead to unpredictable changes in the SMA or renal arteries, especially if these vessels are dissected with thrombosed false lumens. We have encountered flap intussusception only once in over 400 angiographic procedures on patients with aortic dissection. During the diagnostic evaluation of a patient with acute type B dissection and an intimal tear in the mid-descending aorta, we inadvertently cannulated the tear with a Simmons-1 catheter. Slight traction on the catheter extended the tear to full circumferential dehiscence, and the force of blood flow folded the intimal cast and caused it to intussuscept distally, creating a large wad of balled-up intimal tissue that lay across the celiac artery and SMA origins. Fortunately, this complication responded to fenestration at the level of the celiac trunk and placement of a large self-expanding stent in the intimal cast on the diaphragmatic side of the dehiscence (FIGURE 64.9).

Although correcting life-threatening malperfusion is the goal of these procedures, the endovascular physician should bear in

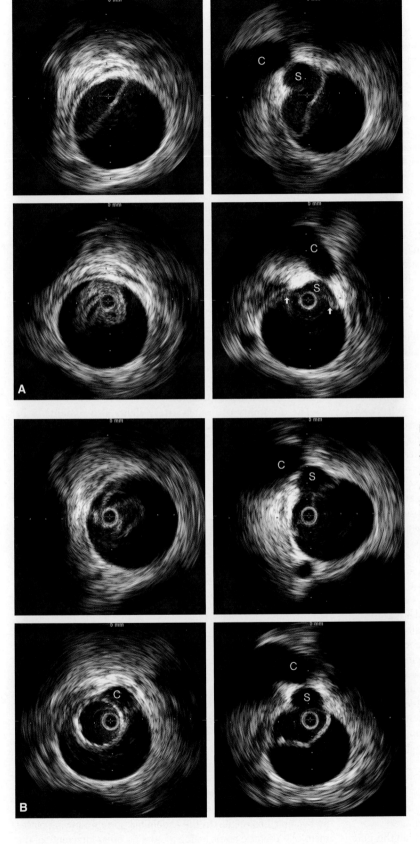

FIGURE 64.9 Intravascular ultrasound pictures from a 31-year-old man with Marfan syndrome and entry tear of acute type B dissection in the mid-descending aorta. Baseline IVUS (**A, top row**) just above the celiac origin and at the level of the SMA shows a small true lumen with a mobile flap intermittently baffling the SMA origin with a 32 mm Hg systolic pressure deficit in the SMA compared to the aortic root. IVUS at the same levels following inadvertent cannulation of the entry tear with intussusception of the cylindrical intimal flap (**A, bottom row**) showed intussuscepted mass of densely folded intimal flap and fixed collapse of the true lumen with SMA obstruction. It was not technically possible to cannulate the SMA, but cannulation of similarly affected right renal artery documented a 69 mm Hg pressure deficit. Following fenestration (**B, top row**) the tangled flap has unfolded and the true lumen at the SMA is less compromised. Finally, after true lumen stenting (**B, bottom row**), the flap has resumed its cylindrical configuration with widely patent SMA without aortomesenteric gradient. *C*, celiac artery; *S*, SMA.

Reprinted with permission from Mirick AL, Patel HJ, Deeb GM, Williams DM. Aortic intussception complicating diagnostic angiography: Recognition and management. *Ann Thorac Surg*. In press.

mind that additional endovascular procedures may be necessary in the future. This is especially important when treating patients with type A dissections complicated by malperfusion in whom aortic root reconstruction may be delayed. As noted earlier, deploying a self-expanding stent through a fenestration tear, from the false lumen above to the true lumen below, may effectively treat the malperfusion. Because the stent compresses the true lumen as it crosses the dissection flap at the tear, however, the biluminal configuration would channel flow from the transfemoral cardiac bypass from the true lumen in the groin into the false lumen at the level of the stent. A second consideration is the ideal location of the fenestration tear. Our practice has been to fenestrate close to the level of the branch arteries we are trying to rescue because, occasionally, fenestration without an aortic stent is sufficient to reduce the obstructing flap; but the proximity of the tear to the vessel origin inherently complicates a subsequent endograft procedure to devascularize a growing false lumen. Obviously, the immediate life-threatening problem must be corrected, but one should keep in mind that the dissected aorta is a degenerating organ with lifelong vascular complications.

Bailout Procedures

Conversion of type B to type A aortic dissection currently requires open aortic reconstruction to prevent rupture of the ascending component. Complications and misadventures that may allow for endovascular solutions include misplacement of stent-grafts, biluminal placement of the self-expanding stent after fenestration, collapse of the proximal aortic true lumen after restoration of perfusion to distal obstructed branch arteries, and distal intussusception of the circumferentially torn dissection flap. The principles of bailout procedures are: demonstrate the altered vascular anatomy (for which IVUS is invaluable), restore or maintain aortic true lumen continuity, and perfuse critical vessels. In the instances of endograft or stent prolapsing through an iatrogenic or reentry tear, entry into the adjoining collapsed true lumen on the cephalic end can be problematic from the femoral approach. If patient and systematic attempts to cannulate the collapsed true lumen from below are unsuccessful, transbrachial access from above can deliver a wire into the endograft or stent, and continuity from below can be reestablished then secured with a bridging endograft or self-expanding stent. When the stent is centered on the tear, cephalic half in the false lumen and caudal half in the true lumen, a guide wire is directed through the wall of the stent at the level of the tear into the true lumen above the tear; stent and tear are expanded and secured with a new self-expanding stent. This creates a "Y" stent, one arm in the false lumen, one arm in the true lumen, and the single leg in the true lumen. Management of true lumen collapse following restoration of perfusion into obstructed branches is achieved by fenestration and true lumen stenting as described previously. Our single instance of intussusception of the circumferential dissection flap was also successfully managed by fenestration and stenting.

AREAS OF UNCERTAINTY AND FUTURE DEVELOPMENT

Certain principles of treatment remain to be clarified in this new era of endovascular treatment of dissection. At the present time, although there has been a suggestion that stent-graft treatment of uncomplicated dissection in anatomically suitable patients may result in increased survival compared to medical treatment, there is no consensus that this is so. Sizing of aortic endografts remains an issue. In general, these are sized according to the diameter of the undissected landing zone, although this may be grossly oversized for a collapsed true lumen, especially if thrombus prevents it from immediately reexpanding after the entry tear is covered.

As noted, the premise of endovascular treatment of malperfusion is that the endograft or fenestration is treating ongoing arterial obstruction. In general, the medical literature regarding how to establish the presence and severity of correctible obstruction is scant. The effect of endograft placement on static obstruction of the iliac or SMA by a thrombosed false lumen is indeterminate. In one instance in our experience an aortic endograft relieved such obstruction without the need for an iliac artery stent (FIGURE 64.10). Fenestration and aortic stenting do not relieve such branch artery obstruction, which typically requires stenting of the branch artery beyond the terminal involvement by the dissection. When the thrombosed false lumen obliterates the iliac and femoral arteries down to the common femoral artery bifurcation, stenting of the true lumen down to the inguinal ligament must be followed by open false lumen thrombectomy of the common femoral artery or, if there is no alternative, by extension of stents into the femoral artery bifurcation. Whether central aortic endograft placement will typically need branch artery touch-up such as this will become evident with further experience.

The durability of branch artery stents also remains to be determined. In our experience, the dissection arteriopathy of these patients is characterized by lack of intimal hyperplasia in visceral and iliac artery stents.

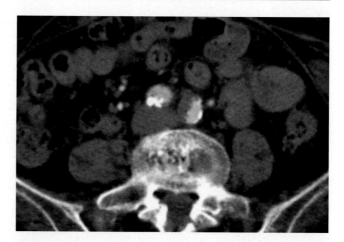

FIGURE 64.10 CT slice in a 69-year-old woman with acute type B dissection shows extension of the dissection into the left common iliac artery. The false lumen is thrombosed and acts as a fixed stenosis with a 69 mm Hg gradient between the aortic root and the left external iliac artery, of which approximately 20 mm Hg was caused by dynamic obstruction in the abdominal aorta. Following placement of a thoracic aortic endograft and no other intervention, the aortoiliac gradient was reduced to 15 mm Hg, which was considered acceptable.

There are two developments that may profoundly change our approach to managing aortic dissection. The first is the possible demonstration that covering the entry tear provides a long-term benefit to all patients, not just those presenting with malperfusion or impending rupture. In this scenario, the angiographic search for arterial obstruction in endograft candidates is superfluous in the preoperative phase but appropriate to document the adequacy of perfusion after deployment of the endograft. The second is development of a valved conduit for the ascending aorta, which can be anchored at the valve ring, sealed at the coronary ostia, and anchored in the aortic arch.

CONCLUSION

New endovascular treatments of acute aortic dissection impose new challenges and opportunities for diagnostic cross-sectional imaging to define the individual patient's vascular pathoanatomy and plan treatment strategy. The integration of clinical assessment, contemporary high-resolution imaging with computed tomography angiogram and IVUS, and new endovascular treatments are changing the management of acute and chronic aortic dissection.

REFERENCES

1. DeBakey ME, Cooley DA, Creech O. Surgical considerations of dissecting aneurysm of the aorta. *Ann Surg* 1955;142:586–610.
2. Wheat MW, Palmer RF, Bartley TD, et al. Treatment of dissecting aneurysms of the aorta without surgery. *J Thorac Cardiovasc Surg* 1965;50:364–373.
3. Gore I, Seiwert VJ. Dissecting aneurysm of the aorta: pathological aspects: an analysis of eighty-five fatal cases. *AMA Arch Pathol* 1952;53:121–141.
4. Hirst AE, Johns VJ, Kime SW. Dissecting aneurysm of the aorta: a review of 505 cases. *Medicine (Baltimore)* 1958;37:217–279.
5. Miller DC, Mitchell RS, Oyer PE, et al. Independent determinants of operative mortality for patients with aortic dissections. *Circulation* 1984;70:I153–I164.
6. Mehta RH, Suzuki T, Hagan PG, et al. Predicting death in patients with acute type A aortic dissection. *Circulation* 2002;105:200–206.
7. Suzuki T, Mehta RH, Ince H, et al. Clinical profiles and outcomes of acute type B aortic dissection in the current era: lessons from the International Registry of Aortic Dissection (IRAD). *Circulation* 2003;108(suppl 1):II312–II317.
8. Williams DM. Aortic dissection: evaluation and management—choosing the right intervention. In: Lumsden A, et al, eds. *Advanced Endovascular Therapy of Aortic Disease*. Malden, MA: Blackwell Futura; 2007:117–122.
9. Williams DM, LePage MA, Lee DY. The dissected aorta: I, early anatomic changes in an in vitro model. *Radiology* 1997;203:23–31.
10. Roberts CS, Roberts WC. Aortic dissection with the entrance tear in the descending thoracic aorta. Analysis of 40 necropsy patients. *Ann Surg* 1991;213:356–368.
11. Roberts WC. Aortic dissection: anatomy, consequences, and causes. *Am Heart J* 1981;101:195–214.
12. Nienaber CA, Fattori R, Lund G, et al. Nonsurgical reconstruction of thoracic aortic dissection by stent-graft placement. *N Engl J Med* 1999;340:1539–1545.
13. Williams DM, Lee DY, Hamilton B, et al. The dissected aorta: III, anatomy and radiologic diagnosis of branch-vessel compromise. *Radiology* 1997;203:37–44.
14. Lee DY, Williams DM, Abrams GD. The dissected aorta: II, differentiation of the true from the false lumen with intravascular US. *Radiology* 1997;203:32–36.
15. Williams DM, Joshi A, Dake MD, et al. Aortic cobwebs: an anatomic marker identifying the false lumen in aortic dissection-imaging and pathologic correlation. *Radiology* 1994;190:167–174.
16. LePage MA, Quint LE, Sonnad SS, et al. Aortic dissection: CT features that distinguish true lumen from false lumen. *Am J Roentgenol* 2001;77:207–211.
17. Deeb GM, Williams DM, Bolling SF, et al. Surgical delay for acute type A dissection with malperfusion. *Ann Thorac Surg* 1998;64:1669–1677.
18. Patel HJ, Williams DM, Dasika NL, et al. Operative delay for peripheral malperfusion syndrome in acute type A aortic dissection: a long-term analysis. *J Thorac Cardiovasc Surg* 2008;135:1288–1295.
19. Deeb GM, Patel HJ, Williams DM. Treatment for malperfusion syndrome in acute type A and B aortic dissection: a long-term analysis. *J Thorac Cardiovasc Surg* 2010;140:S98–S100.
20. Williams D, Lee D, Hamilton B, et al. The dissected aorta: percutaneous management of ischemic complications with endovascular stents and balloon fenestration. *J Vasc Interv Radiol* 1997(8):605–625.
21. Dake M, Kato N, Mitchell R, et al. Endovascular stent-graft placement for the treatment of acute aortic dissections. *N Engl J Med* 1999;340:1546–1552.
22. Nienaber CA, Fattori R, Lund G, et al. Nonsurgical reconstruction of thoracic aortic dissection by stent-graft placement. *N Engl J Med* 1999;340:1539–1545.
23. Song T, Donayre C, Walot I, et al. Endograft exclusion of acute and chronic descending thoracic aortic dissections. *J Vasc Surg* 2006;43:247–258.
24. Patel HJ, Williams DM, Meekov M, et al. Long-term results of percutaneous management of malperfusion in acute type B aortic dissection: implications for thoracic aortic endovascular repair. *J Thorac Cardiovasc Surg* 2009;138:300–308.
25. Barnes D, Williams DM, Dasika NL, et al. A single-center experience treating renal malperfusion after aortic dissection with central aortic fenestration and stenting. *J Vasc Surg* 2008;47:903–911.
26. Henke PK, Williams DM, Upchurch GR, et al. Acute limb ischemia associated with type B aortic dissection: clinical relevance and therapy. *Surgery* 2006;140(4):532–539.
27. Chavan A, Rosenthal H, Luthe L, et al. Percutaneous interventions for treating ischemic complications of aortic dissection. *Eur Radiol* 2009;19:488–494.
28. Park K, Do Y, Kim S, et al. Endovascular treatment of acute complicated aortic dissection: long-term follow-up of clinical outcomes and CT findings. *J Vasc Interv Radiol* 2009;20:334–341.
29. Szeto W, McGarvey M, Pochettino A, et al. Results of a new surgical paradigm: endovascular repair for acute complicated type B aortic dissection. *Ann Thorac Surg* 2008;86:87–94.
30. Patel HJ, Williams DM. Endovascular therapy for malperfusion in acute type B aortic dissection. *Oper Tech Thorac Cardiovasc Surg* 2009;14(1):2–11.
31. Nienaber C, Rousseau H, Eggebrect H, et al. Randomized comparison of strategies for type B aortic dissection; The INvestigation of STEnt Grafts in Aortic Dissection (INSTEAD) trial. *Circulation* 2009;120:2519–2528.
32. Williams DM, Andrews JC, Marx MV, et al. Creation of reentry tears in aortic dissection by means of percutaneous balloon fenestration: gross anatomic and histologic considerations. *J Vasc Interv Radiol* 1993;4:75–83.
33. Hiratzka L, Bakris G, Beckman J, et al. 2010 ACCF/AHA/AATS/ACR/ASA/SCA/SCAI/SIR/STS/SVM guidelines for the diagnosis and management of patients with thoracic aortic disease. *Circulation* 2010;121:e266–e369.
34. Nordon IM, Hinchliffe RJ, Loftus IM, et al. Management of acute aortic syndrome and chronic aortic dissection. *Cardiovasc Intervent Radiol* 2011;34:890–902.
35. Monnin-Bares V, Thony F, Rodiere M, et al. Endovascular stent-graft management of aortic intramural hematomas. *J Vasc Interv Radiol* 2009;20:713–721.

Acute Intramural Hematoma

CYNTHIA E. WAGNER and JOHN F. ANGLE

INTRODUCTION

Aortic intramural hematoma (IMH) is a distinct entity along the spectrum of acute aortic syndromes, a group of disorders including aortic dissection, penetrating atherosclerotic ulcer, and IMH.[1] These aortic disorders produce similar clinical symptoms. Most patients with IMH present with the acute onset of chest or back pain[2,3] but less often with the symptoms of branch occlusion seen with dissection. In a meta-analysis of 143 reported cases of IMH, 5% to 20% of patients presenting with symptoms suggestive of aortic dissection were diagnosed with IMH.[2] Classification is also similar with type A aortic IMH or dissection involving the ascending aorta and type B IMH or aortic dissection involving only the descending aorta.[4] The underlying pathology among these disease processes is different. IMH is thought to result from spontaneous rupture of the vasa vasorum into the medial layer of the aorta without disruption of the intimal layer.[5] As a result, IMHs often do not have the long abdominal extension seen in dissection.

CLINICAL FEATURES

Hypertension is the most common risk factor for the development of IMHs and is found in most patients with IMH and aortic dissection.[3] An IMH is more likely to involve the descending aorta compared to ascending aortic involvement in patients presenting with aortic dissection.[3] The median age of patients presenting with type B IMH is significantly higher than the median age of those presenting with type A IMH.[6] These findings influence treatment options, and endovascular stent-grafting of the descending aorta can be offered as an alternative to medical management to a group of older patients with comorbidities who may not be operative candidates but would benefit from intervention.

The overall in-hospital mortality of aortic IMH is 21%,[2] which is not significantly different from the 24% overall mortality reported for aortic dissection.[3] This similar mortality may be related to the fact that although an IMH can spontaneously regress and resolve completely, it can also degenerate into aortic dissection, develop into an aortic aneurysm, or lead to aortic rupture.[7] These complications have been reported in 32% of patients within 24 to 72 hours of diagnosis of an IMH.[6] In another series of 66 patients with IMH, complications occurred in 59% within 30 days.[8] Complications are more common with type A IMH,[9] and involvement of the ascending aorta is an independent predictor of early progression.[8] The in-hospital mortality has been shown to increase as the IMH becomes closer to the aortic valve, independent of treatment modality.[3] Aortic aneurysm development can occur years after complete resolution of an IMH, likely secondary to structural weakening of the aortic

wall, necessitating long-term follow-up imaging to identify potentially asymptomatic complications of the IMH.[7] Late progression will occur in 21% of patients with IMH.[8] Absence of beta-blocker therapy during follow-up is an independent risk factor for late progression. Survival at 1 year is improved from 67% without beta-blocker therapy to 95% with it.[8] Late complications are expected to occur in 50% of patients by 5 years.[9] Complications within the first 6 months are usually caused by disruption of the intima, aortic dissection, whereas complications after 1 year are more often secondary to progressive dilatation of the aorta, potentially leading to aortic rupture.[9] Such individual variation in the natural history of IMHs precludes a universal treatment algorithm.

DIAGNOSTIC EVALUATION

Computed tomography (CT) is the imaging modality of choice in the diagnosis of IMHs,[7] and most cases are initially diagnosed with CT.[2,3] With superior resolution provided by multidetector row CT angiography, the sensitivity and specificity of identifying pathology within the acute aortic syndrome approach 100%.[10] The optimal sequence to visualize an aortic IMH and to distinguish this entity from the clinically identical aortic dissection consists of an unenhanced transverse CT followed by contrast enhancement.[7] The findings of a crescentic hyperattenuated region of aortic wall thickening greater than 7 mm on noncontrast CT that does not enhance and the absence of an intimal flap are diagnostic of an aortic IMH (FIGURES 65.1 and 65.2).[6,8]

PATIENT SELECTION (DEMOGRAPHIC, FUNCTIONAL, PHYSIOLOGIC CONSIDERATIONS)

Several findings on CT have prognostic significance: location, maximal hematoma thickness, and maximal aortic diameter are all associated with increased rates of progression of aortic IMH to aortic dissection and other complications.[4,10] An initial aortic diameter greater than 55 mm and an initial hematoma thickness greater than 16 mm are independent predictors of progression of type A IMH to aortic dissection,[11] whereas an initial aortic diameter greater than 40 mm and an initial hematoma thickness greater than 10 mm are predictive of type B IMH progression.[12]

TREATMENT SELECTION STRATEGIES (DECISION-MAKING FLOWCHARTS)

Most patients with type A IMH, like type A aortic dissection, undergo surgery, whereas most of those with type B IMH or uncomplicated dissection receive medical management.[3] Patients

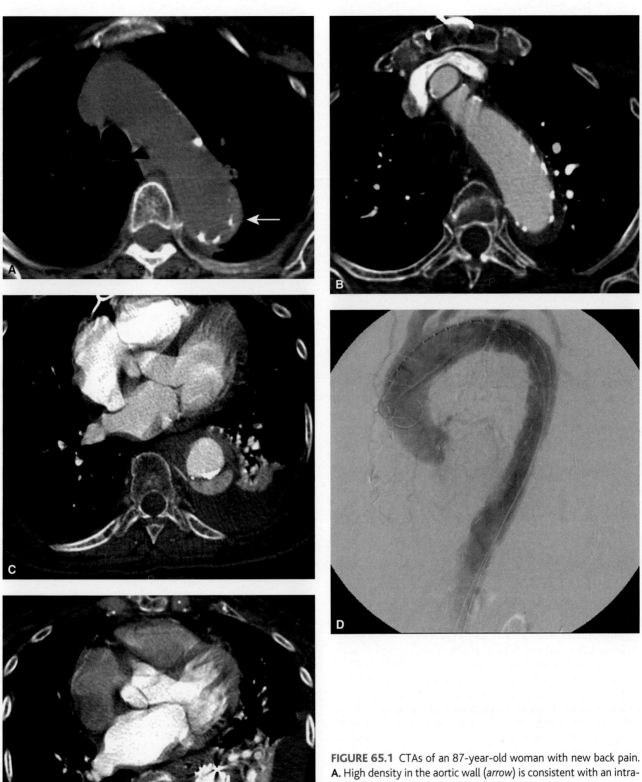

FIGURE 65.1 CTAs of an 87-year-old woman with new back pain. **A.** High density in the aortic wall (*arrow*) is consistent with an intramural hematoma. **B.** CTA does not demonstrate any contrast entry into the hematoma. **C.** Seven days later the patient had new chest pain and there is now contrast entering the hematoma, suggesting a new tear in the intima. **D.** Thoracic endograft placed from the left subclavian artery to near the celiac artery. **E.** Follow-up CTA 3 days postendograft demonstrates some persistent filling of the false lumen by retrograde intercostal artery flow (*arrow*), but the chest pain has resolved.

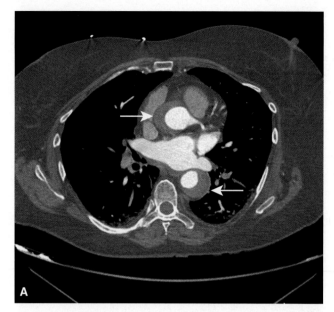
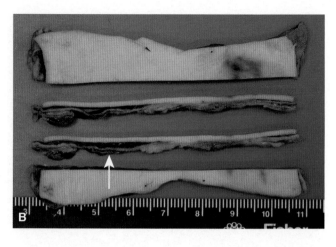

FIGURE 65.2 A. CTA of a 61-year-old woman with diaphoresis and chest pain. Upon presentation, she was bradycardic and the CTA demonstrated an acute type A IMH (*arrows*) with extension to the renal arteries. **B.** Transverse sections of a surgical specimen of the ascending aorta demonstrate a hematoma in the aortic wall (*arrow*) with no fenestrations.

Images courtesy of David A. Williams, M.D., Professor of Radiology, University of Michigan.

with type A IMH who receive surgical treatment have a significantly lower mortality compared with those with type A IMH who undergo medical therapy.[2,8] The outcome in patients with type B IMH who undergo surgical treatment versus medical therapy is similar, however.[2,6] These patients are often elderly with multiple comorbidities and surgery may not be a possibility. Treatment with an endovascular stent-graft can be offered as an alternative in many of these patients if an intervention is indicated. There is little debate that IMH with complications, as for complicated dissection, should be managed aggressively with endograft placement.[4] Examples include rupture, rapidly expanding aortic diameter, conversion to a dissection with antegrade extension leading to abdominal or lower extremity hypoperfusion, and perhaps even for retrograde extension. What remains unclear is whether or not a minimally symptomatic IMH (e.g., persistent back pain, or low-density left pleural effusion) or an IMH with minimal intimal changes on CTA (e.g., focal dissection or penetrating ulcer) should be managed with an endograft. Even less well defined is whether intervention is indicated based on aorta or hematoma size alone to prevent early and late complications, but early investigations suggest treatment in these cases that are likely to become complicated may be indicated.[13]

PLANNING THE INTERVENTIONAL PROCEDURE

It is the author's personal observation that the proximal end of the endograft should be placed in normal aorta. There have been reports of proximal erosions leading to a new dissection.[14] Obtaining a normal segment of aorta for the distal landing zone is more challenging in cases where the IMH extends to near the diaphragm. It appears that extending the endograft to near the diaphragm is an acceptable treatment plan in many patients. It is also a common belief that distal barbs or uncovered struts are more likely to lead to a distal dissection.

Specific Intraprocedural Techniques

As with all endograft placements, planning is the key to a successful procedure. The IMH may not be visible angiographically so intravascular ultrasound (IVUS) and access to preprocedure CTA images are important in the procedure room.

As with dissection, grafts are sized to the normal aorta. Infolding of grafts seen immediately after placement may need balloon dilatation. Balloon dilatation of the proximal and distal landing zones should be avoided, however, to reduce the risk of inducing a dissection.

As with treatment of a dissection, it is probably safest to build the endograft from a proximal to distal manner to avoid pressuring the false lumen by blocking an undetected distal reentry point while leaving a small proximal entry point uncovered.

Endpoint Assessment of the Procedure

Because the IMH is often not visible on angiography, the endpoint is less clear than when treating an aneurysm or dissection with an endograft. The endpoint will usually involve angiography to confirm that the proximal and distal ends are opposed to the wall, that there are no type III junctional leaks, and to exclude graft infolding if there was significant oversizing.

In most cases of IMHs, visceral reperfusion will not be necessary, but consideration should be given to a completion angiogram to evaluate the abdominal aortic branches.

Procedural Complications and How to Manage Them Successfully

Diagnosis and management of endoleaks using CTA is an important component of clinical follow-up. The postprocedure imaging must also include evaluation for the development of a new dissection at the proximal or distal end of the endograft. Graft extensions may exclude these problems, but essential aortic branches may make extension impossible. A snorkel procedure, a fenestrated graft, or a branched graft may rescue a procedure, but all these procedures remain investigational. In some circumstances, operative repair may be the only alternative.

Infolding of oversized grafts can often be remedied with balloon dilatation. Occasionally a balloon expandable stent (Palmaz XL, Cordis, NJ) may be required to reexpand a collapsed stent.[15]

■ OUTCOMES/PROGNOSIS

Outcomes of stent-graft repair and medical management for patients with type B IMH have recently been reported. In one prospective study, 33 of 56 patients with type B IMH underwent elective stent-graft repair if the IMH was associated with a penetrating atherosclerotic ulcer, if the maximum aortic diameter was greater than 45 mm, if the hematoma thickness was greater than 10 mm, or if persistent chest pain and/or back pain occurred in spite of maximal medical therapy. The remaining patients received continuation of medical therapy. In all 33 patients undergoing endovascular repair, each stent-graft was successfully placed, no complications occurred during the procedure, hematoma thickness was reduced on follow-up imaging of each patient, and the mortality was 0%. In those receiving medical therapy alone, however, IMH progression occurred in 26% of patients and mortality was 9%.[13]

Stent-graft repair was reported in another series of 15 patients with promising results. Most of these patients underwent endovascular treatment for IMH progression after a trial of medical management, although several patients received a stent-graft because of acute complications. The 30-day mortality was 0%, and the IMH partially regressed in 8 patients and resolved completely in 7 patients. These authors reported a success rate of 93% because 1 patient developed a type I endoleak. They also reported a 20% complication rate secondary to late aneurysm development and a 7% late mortality.[16] However, 4 of their patients treated with a descending endograft had an ascending component, and 11 of the 15 were treated as IMH complications developed.

Disease Surveillance and Treatment Monitoring Algorithms

Because of the potential for early and late complications, follow-up imaging is essential in all patients. In those managed medically, early reimaging should be performed to screen for degeneration to dissection or aneurysm formation. In our practice, these patients have several days of inpatient observation and serial CTA confirming stability or regression. In patients where the IMH has proven stable and are discharged without open or endovascular repair, additional short interval imaging should be performed. It has been recommended to perform routine surveillance imaging, usually a CTA, at 1, 3, 6, 9, and 12 months after discharge and then annually to detect asymptomatic complications of IMH.[3] For patients treated with endograft, we routinely perform a predischarge CTA to exclude formation of a dissection. We then perform follow-up CTAs starting at 1 month.

Early Failures and Options for Management

Dissection formation at the proximal or distal end is the most dreaded early complication. This complication may be associated with rapid increases in aortic diameter or even rupture. Endograft extension and operative repair of the aorta are the only options. Type II endoleaks can also occur, but the natural history and management of these remain unclear.

Late Failures and Options for Management

As for early failures, dissection and aneurysm formation are the most important late complications of IMHs. Depending on the source of the leak, additional stent-graft placement, embolization of feeding arteries to the aneurysm, or aneurysm sac puncture should be considered.[16]

Practical Advantages and Limitations

Endografts can be placed for IMHs with low complication rates.[13] Many patients presenting with an IMH do not have persistent symptoms but do have other indications for endograft placement, such as aortic size, hematoma size, or the development of dissection. The risk-benefit ratio of endograft placement depends not only on symptoms related to the IMH, but also on the patient's age, comorbidities, and factors that may increase the risk of the procedure, such as chronic renal insufficiency or unfavorable access.

Relative Therapeutic Effectiveness Compared to Medical and Surgical Management (Clinical, Pathophysiologic, Anatomic Measures)

Outcomes in the available literature suggest reduced morbidity and mortality with early endograft placement in patients with any complicating features to the IMH. However, a significant proportion of asymptomatic patients without aortic enlargement or a large false lumen may be managed medically.

■ THE FUTURE

Patient selection needs further refinement, particularly in the subset of minimally symptomatic IMHs, or defining what degree of aortic enlargement or false lumen size should be managed with an endograft.

Device technology needs to be refined. Perhaps more than with any other aortic disease, graft injury to the aorta can occur at the proximal or distal landing zone. Grafts that are relatively atraumatic to the aortic wall without sacrificing radial force and device fixation are needed. Iliac artery size, tortuosity, and calcification all remain potential risk factors for endograft treatment, and future grafts that are lower profile and more flexible will allow more patients to be treated more safely.

▎CONCLUSION

Aortic IMH is a unique etiology of acute aortic syndrome and has increasingly become recognized as a distinct clinical entity as well. The typical patient is hypertensive presenting with the acute onset of chest pain and/or back pain. Noncontrast CT followed by contrast-enhanced CT is the preferred diagnostic imaging series, which classically reveals a crescentic hyperattenuated region of aortic wall thickening that does not enhance and is not associated with an intimal flap. Natural history of IMH is variable, although most type A IMHs are treated surgically and most type B IMHs are treated medically. IMH in the descending aorta can degenerate into a dissection or become aneurysmal and rupture. Close imaging follow-up and intervention in complicated IMHs is indicated. The role of endovascular stent-grafts in the treatment of a type B IMH is emerging as a safe and effective option for elderly patients with multiple comorbidities at high surgical risk.

▎REFERENCES

1. Tsai TT, Nienaber CA, Eagle KA. Acute aortic syndromes. *Circulation* 2005;112(24):3802–3813.
2. Maraj R, Rerkpattanapipat P, Jacobs LE, et al. Meta-analysis of 143 reported cases of aortic intramural hematoma. *Am J Cardiol* 2000;86(6):664–668.
3. Evangelista A, Mukherjee D, Mehta RH, et al. Acute intramural hematoma of the aorta: a mystery in evolution. *Circulation* 2005;111(8):1063–1070.
4. Nordon IM, Hinchliffe RJ, Loftus IM, et al. Management of acute aortic syndrome and chronic aortic dissection. *Cardiovasc Intervent Radiol* 2011;34(5):890–902. Epub 2010 Nov 12.
5. Baikoussis NG, Apostolakis EE, Papakonstantinou NA, et al. The implication of vasa vasorum in surgical diseases of the aorta. *Eur J Cardiothorac Surg* 2011;40(2):412–417.
6. Nienaber CA, von Kodolitsch Y, Petersen B, et al. Intramural hemorrhage of the thoracic aorta. Diagnostic and therapeutic implications. *Circulation* 1995;92(6):1465–1472.
7. Chao CP, Walker TG, Kalva SP. Natural history and CT appearances of aortic intramural hematoma. *Radiographics* 2009;29(3):791–804.
8. von Kodolitsch Y, Csösz SK, Koschyk DH, et al. Intramural hematoma of the aorta: predictors of progression to dissection and rupture. *Circulation* 2003;107(8):1158–1163.
9. Moizumi Y, Komatsu T, Motoyoshi N, et al. Clinical features and long-term outcome of type A and type B intramural hematoma of the aorta. *J Thorac Cardiovasc Surg* 2004;127(2):421–427.
10. Buckley O, Rybicki FJ, Gerson DS, et al. Imaging features of intramural hematoma of the aorta. *Int J Cardiovasc Imaging* 2010;26(1):65–76.
11. Song JK, Yim JH, Ahn JM, et al. Outcomes of patients with acute type A aortic intramural hematoma. *Circulation* 2009;120(21):2046–2052.
12. Sueyoshi E, Imada T, Sakamoto I, et al. Analysis of predictive factors for progression of type B aortic intramural hematoma with computed tomography. *J Vasc Surg* 2002;35(6):1179–1183.
13. Li DL, Zhang HK, Cai YY, et al. Acute type B aortic intramural hematoma: treatment strategy and the role of endovascular repair. *J Endovasc Ther* 2010;17(5):622–623.
14. Zipfel B, Buz S, Laube H, et al. Type A dissection after implantation of a stent-graft triggered by an intramural hematoma. *J Endovasc Ther* 2009;16(2):243–250.
15. Tadros RO, Lipsitz EZ, Chaer RA, et al. A multicenter experience of the management of collapsed thoracic endografts. *J Vasc Surg* 2011;53(5):1217–1222.
16. Monnin-Bares V, Thony F, Rodiere M, et al. Endovascular stent-graft management of aortic intramural hematomas. *J Vasc Interv Radiol* 2009;20(6):713–721.

CHAPTER 66

Penetrating Atheromatous Aortic Ulcer: Diagnosis and Management

ROBERT A. LOOKSTEIN, KEVIN HERMAN, and JOHN H. RUNDBACK

INTRODUCTION

Penetrating atheromatous ulcer or penetrating aortic ulcer (PAU) of the thoracic aorta is a distinct clinical entity with characteristic clinical, radiographic, and histopathology features. In 1934, Shennan[1] recognized a separate entity from classic aortic dissection that involved atheroma directly related to the site of primary rupture or dissection. It was not until 1986 when Stanson et al.[2] demonstrated the natural history of this pathology that an initial recommendation of early surgical intervention in patients diagnosed with a PAU was made. Advances in imaging technologies have led to increased recognition of aortic pathologies including PAU. Since the initial report of PAU, advances in endovascular therapy for the treatment of thoracic aortic disease has been made as well. The optimal management of this entity remains controversial, however.

Definition/Epidemiology

Penetrating Atherosclerotic Ulcer (PAU) is an ulcerating atherosclerotic lesion that penetrates the internal elastic lamina into the media.[2,3] PAU is generally associated with hematoma formation in the media of the aortic wall.[2,3] The true incidence of PAU is unknown and is most likely higher than previously reported.[2] Most patients with diagnostic findings of a PAU are asymptomatic; however, 2.3% to 6.7% of patients evaluated for suspected acute aortic syndromes were found to have a PAU[2,4] in previous studies. Most aortic ulcers are small and limited to the intima.[5] Most PAUs involve the mid- to distal descending thoracic aorta (86.7%) and are uncommon in the aortic arch and ascending aorta (13.3%).[4]

CLASSIFICATIONS OF DISEASE

The task force on the diagnosis and management of aortic dissection of the European Society of Cardiology adopted a novel classification of aortic disease that considers PAUs as a class 4 aortic dissection.[6–8] This classification scheme differentiates aortic disease by the form of dissection in the aortic wall. Class 1 is the classical aortic dissection with intimal flap between the true and false lumens. Class 4 aortic disease is considered when plaque ruptures and leads to aortic ulceration and a penetrating aortic atherosclerotic ulcer with surrounding hematoma.[8] Additionally, some authors utilize the Stanford classification to categorize PAUs according to the location of ulcerative disease, with type A in the ascending aorta and type B in the descending aorta.[7]

PATHOPHYSIOLOGY AND DISEASE PROGRESSION

The process and formation of PAUs is distinct from aneurysm formation and aortic dissection. Initially, an atheromatous ulcer develops in patients with atherosclerosis. When the ulcer is confined to the intimal layer the patient is generally asymptomatic. With disease progression the ulcer may then penetrate through the elastic intima into the media generally accompanied with hematoma formation.[2] The exact mechanism of hematoma propagation is unclear and based on pathology studies. Intramural hematoma (IMH) formation may extend proximally or distally for varying lengths of the aorta.[2] It is believed that in many cases the propagation of IMH is limited by coexisting aortic wall fibrosis from longstanding atherosclerosis.[9]

The natural history of PAU is one of progressive aortic enlargement commonly resulting in saccular and fusiform aortic aneurysms. Six penetrating aortic ulcers with a mean follow-up of 4.6 years progressed to aneurysms at an annual growth rate of 0.31 cm/year.[9] Additionally, up to 40% of patients with PAU may have concomitant but separate aortic aneurysms in the thoracic or abdominal aorta.[4,9] The PAU itself may also heal spontaneously. The disease course of PAU can be complicated by aortic dissection, aortic rupture, and/or embolization.[2,3,9]

CLINICAL FEATURES (INCLUDING PRESENTING SYMPTOMS AND SIGNS)

The typical clinical presentation of a symptomatic PAU occurs in an elderly patient with multiple risk factors for atherosclerotic cardiovascular disease.[2–4,10–12] The differentiation of PAU from classic aortic dissection at initial presentation is of paramount importance for optimal treatment of these patients. In comparison to patients with type A or B aortic dissections, patients with a symptomatic PAU have a mean age of at least 72 years.[2–4,10–12] The initial clinical presentation of PAU is abrupt chest, epigastric, or back pain. PAU may also present with symptoms of distal ischemia caused by emboli arising from the ulcerated atheroma. Many authors have reported a high prevalence of hypertension and other cardiovascular risk factors, such as hyperlipidemia and tobacco abuse.[2–4,10–12]

The initial clinical impression in these patients is that of aortic dissection. In distinction to aortic dissection, however, the patient suffering from PAU does not have pulse deficits, compromise of flow to the visceral vessels, cerebrovascular insufficiency, and/or aortic valve insufficiency.[4] Patients with symptomatic PAU are generally stabilized with antihypertensive medications and afterload-reducing agents in an intensive care unit (ICU) setting until pain relief and hemodynamic stability is preserved.[13]

The initial clinical course despite aggressive medical intervention in patients with PAU may be complicated with persistent or recurrent pain and hemodynamic instability. The worsening clinical situation is often related to a contained or transmural rupture of the PAU and hematoma. In one study, 40% of patients diagnosed with PAU presented with acute aortic rupture, highlighting the malignant nature of this disease and need for urgent intervention.[14] The high percentage of patients presenting with acute rupture can be attributed to the location of the PAU. In that study 46% of the patients had a type A PAU. PAU in the ascending thoracic aorta is known to have a more virulent clinical course.[4]

RELATIONSHIP BETWEEN PENETRATING AORTIC ULCER AND AORTIC DISSECTION

Although the signs and symptoms of patients with classic aortic dissection and PAU are similar, there are several differentiating characteristics that can be used to separate the two entities. The typical patient, diagnostic features, extent of the lesion, and treatment options differentiate PAU from aortic dissection. Classic aortic dissection usually occurs at sites in the aorta not complicated by significant atherosclerosis (Table 66.1).

Table 66.1

Relationship Between Penetrating Aortic Ulcer (PAU) and Aortic Dissection

Characteristic	PAU	Aortic dissection
Typical patient	Elderly with hypertension	Often young with hypertension Occasionally with bicuspid aortic valve Marfan syndrome
Symptoms or signs	Chest or back pain	Chest or back pain Aortic insufficiency (type A) Pulse inequality Neurologic deficits Compromise of blood flow to visceral vessels
Diagnostic features	No intimal flap Localized ulceration penetrating internal elastic lamina Intramural hematoma	Intimal flap with contrast filling false lumen
Extent of lesion	Focal	Usually extensive
Degree of atherosclerosis	Always severe	Variable (often minimal)

DIAGNOSTIC EVALUATION STRATEGIES AND RECOMMENDATIONS

The use of diagnostic imaging to identify or exclude a PAU is crucial in the workup of patients with suspected acute aortic syndrome. The spectrum of imaging modalities includes the use of plain chest radiography, computed tomography angiography (CTA), magnetic resonance angiography (MRA), conventional digital subtraction angiography (DSA), and transesophageal echocardiography (TEE).

The key imaging differential diagnostic considerations are acute aortic dissection, IMH without PAU, and aortic aneurysm with irregular mural thrombus. The first two conditions should be readily distinguishable via cross-sectional imaging by identifying an ulcerated atheromatous plaque underlying the aortic wall hematoma in patients with PAU.

Chest Radiography

Many patients with acute aortic syndrome including PAU have abnormal chest X-ray findings. Findings may include focal or diffuse enlargement of the descending aorta, unilateral or bilateral pleural effusions, and/or mediastinal widening.[11] Patients with suspected acute aortic syndrome must undergo cross-sectional imaging, such as a dynamic enhanced CT for further evaluation.

Computed Tomography

Multidetector CT (MDCT) is generally the first-line imaging test in the assessment of acute aortic syndromes. CT and CTA findings include focal aortic ulceration, IMH, and a calcified displaced intima.[2,3,11,15,16] It is important to initially evaluate the extent of an IMH in both its longitudinal and its radial course to assess for disease progression when evaluating the follow-up imaging studies.[15] If an IMH is identified, a search for a culprit PAU is necessary because patients with an IMH associated with PAU have a more progressive disease course than patients with an IMH not associated with PAU.[15] Thorough evaluation for other sites of aortic ulceration and other aortic pathologies, such as concomitant thoracic or abdominal aortic aneurysms, should be sought.[13] Additional relevant imaging findings include pleural effusions, mediastinal fluid collections, and contained perforations.

Once a PAU is identified, the clinician should also evaluate the maximum diameter and maximum depth of the ulcer crater. If the maximum diameter of the ulcer was measured at 20 mm or greater, the positive and negative predictive values for disease progression were 100% and 71%, respectively.[15] If the maximum depth of the ulcer was measured at 10 mm or greater, the positive and negative predictive values for disease progression were 80% and 88%, respectively.[15] In another study there were no differences found in CT findings between the groups of patients treated surgically versus those treated conservatively.[11] In one study the only CT feature predictive of clinical outcome was the lack of pleural effusion seen correlating with clinical stability.[16] Disease progression should be considered in patients with persistent or recurrent pain despite aggressive treatment and/or interval increase in pleural effusions.[15]

Magnetic Resonance Imaging

Magnetic resonance imaging (MRI) has been proven to be accurate in the diagnosis of aortic dissection.[17] MR findings in patients with PAU are similar to those of CT findings including aortic ulcers and IMHs. MR may be superior to CT in its ability to differentiate acute IMH from atherosclerotic plaque and chronic intraluminal thrombus.[17] Magnetic resonance may be limited in its ability to depict displaced intimal calcification, however. Additional MRI finding includes a localized area of high signal intensity that was seen on the aortic wall on both T1- and T2-weighted images. This finding is indicative of subacute hematoma in the wall of the aorta.[17] MRA is also a valuable tool in the evaluation of patients with PAU; findings would be similar to those seen on CTA.[18]

Transesophageal Echocardiography

TEE is a proven imaging tool for the evaluation of patients with aortic disease and can be used reliably to detect patients with PAU.[19-22] TEE is readily available, relatively noninvasive, and does not utilize contrast agents. The expected findings on TEE include an atherosclerotic aorta, a craterlike ulcer with jagged edges, and an echolucent center and possibly aortic wall thickening. On pulsed wave Doppler there is color flow within the PAU. This finding indicates that the lesion is likely a PAU and not simply an IMH. One author suggests that the disappearance of flow and a change in the "craterlike" shape of the ulcer may be a sign of plaque stabilization.[22]

Angiography

Angiography was once considered the gold standard for diagnosing PAUs; however, it is limited by its two-dimensional projectional nature. Imaging characteristics include localized ulceration predominantly in the mid- to distal thoracic aorta, the appearance of which is similar to an ulcer found on barium examination.[2] Of the number of cases, 70% to 90% may show associated aortic wall thickening and IMH; however, the extent of IMH evaluation is limited.[2,9] No false lumen is identified on angiography.[2,3,9] However, a localized intimal flap may be detected when PAU is complicated by aortic dissection.[2]

Summary

In general, the characteristic imaging findings in patients with PAU are not able to reliably predict disease progression and separate out those patients in need of early surgical intervention. Rather, the clinical scenario along with imaging findings and other factors will generate the treatment plan. Close interval follow-up is crucial to evaluate these patients for radiographic evidence of deterioration, such as worsening pleural effusions, increased hematoma formation, propagation to aortic dissection, and/or aortic rupture. Once the acute episode of PAU has resolved, imaging at 1, 3, 6, and 12 months is recommended.

▌ CLASSIFICATIONS OF THERAPY

The treatment strategies in the acute setting for patients diagnosed with PAU include nonoperative medical management alone, endovascular treatment, and surgical intervention. The controversy surrounding how best to treat PAUs hinges on the argument and scientific findings related to the natural progression of the disease.[23] On one hand, PAU is believed to behave in an aggressive and malignant fashion with a high rate of mortality caused by aortic rupture if not treated surgically.[2-4,9] On the other hand, several authors suggest that PAU behaves in a less aggressive manner and can be managed nonoperatively in many situations.[10-12]

In 1986, Stanson et al.[2] initially described the natural history of PAUs of the thoracic aorta in 16 patients and concluded that PAUs behaved in an aggressive and malignant fashion with high mortality, thereby warranting an aggressive surgical approach. In 1989, based on their series of five patients, Hussain et al.[10] concluded that nonoperative management of these patients was initially appropriate because the natural course of the disease was not as aggressive as believed. Based on a series of 15 patients in 1998 Coady et al.[4] concluded that, in fact, surgical management is advocated for patients with PAU who exhibit early clinical or radiologic signs of deterioration. In 2002, 26 patients with PAU were studied and the authors confirmed earlier suspicions that due to a high early rupture rate surgical replacement of the aorta was warranted as long as the patient's comorbidities did not preclude them from surgical intervention.[14] More recently, a retrospective study based on 25 years of experience at the Mayo clinic concluded that many PAUs of the thoracic aorta can be managed nonoperatively in the acute setting; however, careful follow-up is necessary.[12]

Medical Management

Nonoperative management of PAUs includes aggressive medical therapy aimed at controlling blood pressure, close observation, and serial follow-up of the aorta with imaging tests to detect complications. Because of the potential for serious complications these patients are monitored very closely and may require early or late surgical intervention despite aggressive medical therapy.

Surgical Management

The indications for surgical intervention in patients with PAU are controversial but include hemorrhage, recurrent chest or back pain, embolization, enlarging pseudoaneurysm, and progressive aneurysmal dilatation.[9] The operative technique for PAU is much different than for surgical management of classic aortic dissection. The operative technique for patients with classic aortic dissection is local graft interposition at the site of intimal tear.[2] If the cause of an extensive IMH is a penetrating ulcer of the lower thoracic aorta, however, proximal grafting of the thoracic aorta would be ineffective. Rather, graft replacement of the aorta, including the site of penetration, is mandatory for patients with PAU.[2] The mortality rates for the surgical repair of patients with symptomatic PAU range from 15% to 40%.[24]

PAU that involves the ascending arch (type A) is believed to behave in a particularly aggressive manner and, therefore, according to most authors should be treated early with a surgical and/or endovascular approach.[4,23,25]

Endovascular Management

As our diagnostic capabilities increase, individualization of therapy is necessary in managing patients with symptomatic PAU. With the advent of endovascular stent grafting, the debate on optimal treatment and timing of treatment for symptomatic PAU persists. The therapeutic goal for treatment of PAU is to reduce wall stress and provide stabilization of the diseased aortic segment to prevent complications, such as aneurysm formation, aortic dissection, and/or ruptured or distal embolus.[7] The PAU is generally a focal lesion that is limited to a short aortic segment. Treatment goals and physical characteristics of the PAU make it very suitable for the treatment with endovascular stent-grafts. Additionally, the patients presenting with PAU are typically at a high surgical risk and, therefore, a less invasive option would be beneficial.

Thoracic endovascular aortic repair (TEVAR) was initially reported in 1994 for the treatment of thoracic aortic aneurysms.[26,27] Given the high morbidity and mortality associated with surgical repair of PAU an endovascular approach if feasible would be very appealing. Initial case reports describing the use of stent-grafts for repair of PAUs were favorable and technically successful.[28,29]

The current experience with endovascular repair in PAU is summarized in Table 66.2. The procedural success rate was 96% out of a total of 134 patients.[24,26,28–40] Complete sealing of the ulcer was achieved in 95% of the patients. Incomplete seal was usually caused by a type I endoleak that was either treated with stent-graft extension or balloon fixation or followed closely.[24,28,38] In-hospital mortality was 6.7% and neurologic complications occurred in 3.7%. Neurologic complications included paresthesia, transient paraplegia, and minor stroke. Neurologic complication rates with stent grafting are lower than those associated with open repair of the descending aorta.

PLANNING THE INTERVENTIONAL PROCEDURE

All patients should undergo CTA scanning with three-dimensional reconstruction prior to stent-graft placement to determine the location, length, and diameter of the diseased aortic

Table 66.2

Published Results of Endovascular Treatment of Patients with PAU

Study	N	Technical success	Complete sealing of PAU	Neurologic complications	In-hospital mortality	Additional endovascular procedures required	Aorta-related mortality during follow-up	Mean duration of follow-up, months
Dake et al.[26]	5	5/5 (100%)	Not spec	0	0	0	0	11.6
Murgo et al.[28]	4	4/4 (100%)	3/4 (75%)	1/4 (25%)	1/4 (25%)	1/4 (25%)	1/4 (25%)	7.7
Brittenden et al.[29]	2	2/2 (100%)	2/2 (100%)	0	0	0	0	12
Maruyama et al.[41]	1	1/1 (100%)	1/1 (100%)	0	1/1 (100%)	0	—	—
Sailer et al.[34]	4	4/4 (100%)	4/4 (100%)	0	0	0	0	8.5
Haulon et al.[35]	2	2/2 (100%)	Not spec	0	0	NS	0	7.3
Pitton et al.[36]	1	1/1 (100%)	1/1 (100%)	0	0	0	0	12
Schoder et al.[37]	8	8/8 (100%)	8/8 (100%)	1/8 (13%)	0	0	1/8 (12.5%)	14.1
Kos et al.[38]	10	10/10 (100%)	9/10 (90%)	1/10 (10%)	0	1/10 (10%)	0	9
Faries et al.[39]	1	1/1 (100%)	1/1 (100%)	0	0	0	0	18
Ganaha et al.[30]	6	6/6 (100%)	6/6 (100%)	0	1/6 (17%)	NA	NA	NA
Eggebrecht et al.[32]	10	10/10 (100%)	9/10 (90%)	0	0	1/10 (10%)	0	24.4
Crane et al.[42]	1	1/1 (100%)	1/1 (100%)	0	0	0	0	12
Demers et al.[31]	26	23/26 (92%)	NA	0	3/26 (12%)	1/26 (4%)	1/26 (4%)	51
Brinster et al.[40]	21	21/21 (100%)	21/21 (100%)	0	0	1/21 (5%)	0	14
Girn et al.[24]	11	10/11 (90.9%)	10/11 (91%)	1/11	3/11 (27%)	0	0	32.5
Eggebrecht et al.[33]	22	21/22 (96%)	NA	1/22 (5%)	0	1/27 (4%)	0	27
Total	134	129/134 (96%)	76/80 (95%)	5/134 (3.7%)	9/134 (6.7%)	6/126 (4.8%)	3/128 (2.3%)	17.4

N/A. Not available.

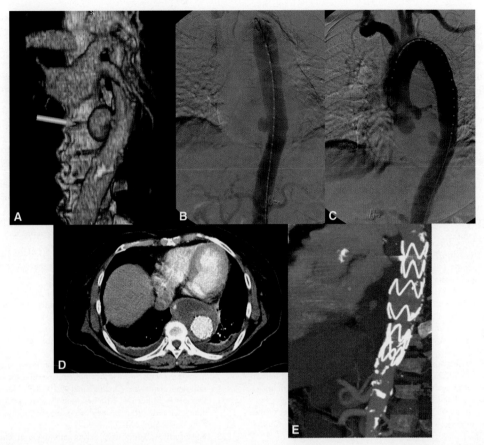

FIGURE 66.1 Fifty eight year old female with crushing back pain undergoes computed tomographic angiogram (CTA) demonstrating a descending thoracic penetrating atherosclerotic ulcer (PAU) [**A**]. Subsequent calibrated aortagram confirms the localization of the ulcer to the descending thoracic aorta [**B**]. Following Thoracic Endovascular Aneurysm Repair (TEVAR), there is no perfusion seen in the PAU [**C**]. CTA at follow up demonstrates no perfusion to the ulcer [**D-E**].

segment. Stent-graft dimensions are calculated from the CTA image. The endoprosthesis should be oversized 10% to 15% compared to the landing zone diameter and be 30 to 40 mm longer than the target lesion to ensure an adequate seal.[7] Additionally, location and size of intercostal arteries should be assessed during the planning phase to minimize the number of intercostal arteries covered, especially in the lower third of the descending thoracic aorta. One should evaluate the femoral arteries and iliac vessels for size and atherosclerotic disease because the currently available devices employ relatively large delivery systems (FIGURE 66.1).

SPECIFIC INTRAPROCEDURAL TECHNIQUES

Bilateral femoral access is necessary with either percutaneous techniques or surgical femoral arteriotomies. Initially a flush aortogram in multiple projections usually including anteroposterior and left anterior oblique views is obtained from the aortic valve to the celiac artery to delineate the treatment zone of the aorta. The projection that most clearly delineates the proximal seal zone should be chosen to deliver the stent-graft device. The contralateral access is used to deliver the device under direct fluoroscopic vision. The proximal seal zone can be visualized using angiography through the flush catheter positioned at the proximal seal zone. Once the device has been delivered and positioned at the proximal seal zone, it is imperative to visualize the distal

seal zone to ensure that an aortic branch is not inadvertently covered. Once the device is deployed, the flush catheter is removed. The introducer system for the stent-graft is then exchanged for a dilatation balloon catheter to affix the device to the aortic wall in a uniform manner. Once the device has been postdilated along its entire course, a completion angiogram must be performed. The dilatation catheter is exchanged for a flush catheter that is usually placed in the ascending aorta to perform a completion arch aortogram. The completion study must pay particular attention to the proximal and distal seal zones and to the treatment area to diagnose any endoleaks. The most common type of endoleak following endovascular repair of PAUs is an attachment site or type 1 leak. This is usually managed intraprocedurally with more dilatation of the device to optimize wall apposition. Rarely the device needs to be extended proximally or distally with another piece to optimize the seal zone. In the rare case a type 2 endoleak is seen at the end of the procedure, the procedure is completed. A type 2 endoleak is routinely observed in the follow-up period.

CONCLUSION

Penetrating aortic ulcer is a common form of acute aortic syndrome that can result in devastating complications including aortic dissection and aortic rupture. This entity is frequently diagnosed with the more widespread use of cross-sectional imaging in the evaluation of the patient with an acute chest pain. The patient with PAU must be closely observed for stability of his or her aortic lesion. Those patients who fail medical management tailored to control hypertension and stabilize the ulcerated lesion warrant urgent repair with endovascular stent grafting. This technique has rapidly emerged as the standard of care for the treatment of this devastating cardiovascular diagnosis. The endovascular procedure is characterized by excellent technical success and low morbidity. Further research will focus on early identification of risk factors for this entity and predicting those patients who will fail medical management and undergo aortic repair.

▌ REFERENCES

1. Shennan T. *Dissecting Aneurysm* (Medical Research Council, Special Report Series, No. 193). London, England: HMSO; 1934.
2. Stanson AW, Kazmier FJ, Hollier LH, et al. Penetrating atherosclerotic ulcers of the thoracic aorta: natural history and clinicopathologic correlations. *Ann Vasc Surg* 1986;1:15–23.
3. Cooke JP, Kazmier FJ, Orszulak TA. The penetrating aortic ulcer: pathologic manifestations, diagnosis, and management. *Mayo Clin Proc* 1988;63:718–725.
4. Coady MA, Rizzo JA, Hammond GL, et al. Penetrating ulcer of the thoracic aorta: what is it? How do we recognize it? How do we manage it? *J Vasc Surg* 1998;27:1006–1016.
5. Kazmier FJ. Penetrating aortic ulcer. *Cardiovasc Clin* 1992;22:201–217.
6. Svensson LG, Labib SB, Eisenhauer AC, et al. Intimal tear without hematoma: an important variant of aortic dissection that can elude current imaging techniques. *Circulation* 1999;99:1331–1336.
7. Eggebrecht H, Baumgart D, Schermund A, et al. Penetrating ulcer of the aorta: treatment by endovascular stent-graft placement. *Curr Opin Cardiol* 2003;18:431–435.
8. Erbel R, Alfonso F, Boileau C, et al. Diagnosis and management of aortic dissection. *Eur Heart J* 2001;22:1642–1681.
9. Harris JA, Bis KG, Glover JL, et al. Penetrating atherosclerotic ulcers of the aorta. *J Vasc Surg* 1994;19:90–99.
10. Hussain S, Glover JL, Bree R, et al. Penetrating atherosclerotic ulcers of the thoracic aorta. *J Vasc Surg* 1989;9:710–717.
11. Kazerooni EA, Bree RL, Williams DM. Penetrating atherosclerotic ulcers of the descending thoracic aorta: evaluation with CT and distinction from aortic dissection. *Radiology* 1992;183:759–765.
12. Cho KR, Stanson AW, Potter DD, et al. Penetrating atherosclerotic ulcer of the descending thoracic aorta and arch. *J Thorac Cardiovasc Surg* 2004;127:1393–1401.
13. Braverman AC. Penetrating atherosclerotic ulcers of the aorta. *Curr Opin Cardiol* 1994;9:591–597.
14. Tittle SL, Lynch RJ, Cole PE, et al. Midterm follow-up of penetrating ulcer and intramural hematoma of the aorta. *J Thorac Cardiovasc Surg* 2002;123:1051–1059.
15. Levy JR, Heiken JP, Gutierrez FR. Imaging of penetrating atherosclerotic ulcers of the aorta. *AJR Am J Roentgenol* 1999;173:151–154.
16. Quint LE, Williams DM, Francis IR, et al. Ulcerlike lesions of the aorta: imaging features and natural history. *Radiology* 2001;218:719–723.
17. Yucel EK, Stainberg FL, Egglin TK, et al. Penetrating aortic ulcers: diagnosis with MRI imaging. *Radiology* 1990;177:779–781.
18. Mohiaddin RH, McCrohon J, Francis JM, et al. Contrast-enhanced magnetic resonance angiogram of penetrating aortic ulcer. *Circulation* 2001;103:e18–e19.
19. Mohr-Kahaly S, Erbel R, Kearney P, et al. Aortic intramural hemorrhage visualized by transesophageal echocardiography: findings and prognostic implications. *J Am Coll Cardiol* 1994;23:658–664.
20. Movsowitz HD, David M, Movsowitz C, et al. Penetrating atherosclerotic aortic ulcers: the role of transesophageal echocardiography in diagnosis and clinical management. *Am Heart J* 1993;126:745–747.
21. Movsowitz HD, Lampert C, Jacobs LE, et al. Penetrating atherosclerotic aortic ulcers. *Am Heart J* 1994;128:1210–1217.
22. Atar S, Nagai T, Birnbaum Y, et al. Transesophageal echocardiographic Doppler findings in patients with penetrating aortic ulcers. *Am J Cardiol* 1999;83:133–135.
23. Sundt TM III. Intramural hematoma and penetrating ulcer. In: *VIII International Symposium on Advances in Understanding Aortic Diseases*. 2007; 143–151.
24. Girn HRS, McPherson S, Nicholson T, et al. Short series of emergency stent-graft repair of symptomatic penetrating thoracic aortic ulcers. *Vasc Med* 2009;14:123–128.
25. Nienaber CA, von Kodolitsch Y, Petersen B, et al. Intramural hemorrhage of the thoracic aorta: diagnosis and therapeutic implications. *Circulation* 1995;92:1465–1472.
26. Dake MD, Miller C, Semba CP, et al. Transluminal placement of endovascular stent grafts for the treatment of descending thoracic aortic aneurysms. *N Engl J Med* 1994;331:1729–1734.
27. Fanelli F, Dake MD. Standards of practice for the endovascular treatment of thoracic aortic aneurysm and type B dissections. *Cardiovasc Intervent Radiol* 2009;32:849–860.
28. Murgo S, Dussaussois L, Golzarian J, et al. Penetrating atherosclerotic ulcer of the descending thoracic aorta: treatment by endovascular stent-graft. *Cardiovasc Intervent Radiol* 1998;21:454–458.
29. Brittenden J, McBride K, McInnes G, et al. The use of endovascular stents in the treatment of penetrating ulcers of the thoracic aorta. *J Vasc Surg* 1999;30:1946–1949.
30. Ganaha F, Miller DC, Sugimoto K, et al. Prognosis of aortic intramural hematoma with and without penetrating atherosclerotic ulcer: a clinical radiological analysis. *Circulation* 2002;106:342–348.
31. Demers P, Miller DC, Mitchell S, et al. Stent-graft repair of penetrating atherosclerotic ulcers in the descending thoracic aorta: mid-term results. *Ann Thorac Surg* 2004;77:81–86.
32. Eggebrecht H, Baumgart D, Schmermund A, et al. Endovascular stent-graft repair for penetrating atherosclerotic ulcer of the descending aorta. *Am J Cardiol* 2003;91:1150–1153.
33. Eggebrecht H, Herold U, Schmermund A, et al. Endovascular stent-graft treatment of penetrating aortic ulcer: results over a median follow-up of 27 months. *Am Heart J* 2005;151:530–536.
34. Sailer J, Peloschek P, Rand T, et al. Endovascular treatment of aortic type B dissection and penetrating ulcer using commercially available stent-grafts. *AJR Am J Roentgenol* 2001;177:1365–1369.
35. Haulon S, Koussa M, Beregi JP, et al. Stent-graft repair of the thoracic aorta: short-term results. *Ann Vasc Surg* 2002;16:700–707.
36. Pitton MB, Duber C, Neufang A, et al. Endovascular repair of a non-contained aortic rupture caused by a penetrating aortic ulcer. *Cardiovasc Intervent Radiol* 2002;25:64–67.
37. Schoder M, Grabenwoger M, Holzenbein T, et al. Endovascular stent-graft repair of complicated penetrating atherosclerotic ulcers of the descending thoracic aorta. *J Vasc Surg* 2002;36:720–726.
38. Kos X, Bouchard L, Otal P, et al. Stent-graft treatment of penetrating thoracic aortic ulcers. *J Endovasc Ther* 2002;9:II25–II31.
39. Faries PL, Lang E, Ramdev P, et al. Endovascular stent-graft treatment of a ruptured thoracic aortic ulcer. *J Endovasc Ther* 2002;9:II20–II24.
40. Brinster DR, Wheatley GH III, Williams J, et al. Are penetrating aortic ulcers best treated using an endovascular approach? *Ann Thorac Surg* 2006;82:1688–1691.
41. Maruyama K, Ishiguchi T, Kato K, Naganawa S, Itoh S, Sakurai T, Ishigaki T. Stent-graft placement for pseudoaneurysm of the aorta. *Radiat Med*. 2000.
42. Crane JS, Cowling M, Cheshire NJ. Endovascular stent grafting of a penetrating ulcer in the descending thoracic aorta. *Eur J Vasc Endovasc Surg*. 2003 Feb;25(2):178–9. May–Jun;18(3):177–85.

Aortic Connective Tissue Disorders

CHASE R. BROWN and ROY K. GREENBERG

INTRODUCTION

The endovascular management of connective tissue disorders (CTDs) involving the aorta is in its infancy. Historically, the use of endovascular procedures in these patients have been viewed critically and, perhaps, rightly so. The arguments against endovascular management are based on concern for the stability of the interface between the implant and the artery in the absence of extensive follow-up data. Over the last several years, however, endovascular treatments have been used successfully in many patients with CTDs, and treatment paradigms are beginning to evolve. One of the most important aspects of treating these patients successfully is to have a solid understanding of interventional techniques, surgical techniques, and the pathophysiology of the disease.

OVERVIEW OF CONNECTIVE TISSUE DISEASES CAUSING ANEURYSMS AND DISSECTIONS

CTDs occur as a result of mutations in specific genes that are responsible for maintaining tissue integrity and/or regulating the cell's extracellular matrix. The clinical manifestations of these mutations can vary and often overlap between differing clinical diagnoses. Controversy exists with respect to whether the clinical characteristics of the patient define the disease (frequently in the absence of a known genetic mutation) or whether the detected gene abnormality determines the diagnosis (independent of the clinical characteristics of the patient). This dichotomy occurs as a result of variable penetrance of the mutations, even in patients with identical genetic mutations. We tend to refer to the specific genetic mutation, rather than the clinical syndrome that may be caused by that mutation, in an effort to provide some clarity to what is now becoming a very confusing field. Thus, the patients, in this chapter, are all classified by a gene abnormality that has, in some manner, guided our clinical decision making.

MARFAN SYNDROME

Marfan syndrome (MFS) is an autosomal dominant disorder with pleotropic manifestations of the connective tissue defects caused by mutation in the FBN-1 gene. Typically, this systemic disease affects the ocular, skeletal, and cardiovascular systems with an incidence of 2 to 3 per 10,000 individuals.[1] The most common cause of death in patients afflicted with MFS relates to the progressive dilatation of the aortic root and ascending aorta with subsequent dissection and/or rupture resulting in cardiac collapse.[2]

Genetics and Pathogenesis of Marfan Syndrome

The FBN-1 gene is found on chromosome 15 and encodes for a large glycoprotein, fibrillin-1, which is a component within microfibrils located in the extracellular matrix of connective tissue. Microfibrils are found in elastic fibers that constitute the medial layer of the ascending aorta as well as in other connective tissues.[3] The pathogenesis of aortic disease in MFS is more complex than the inherent weakening of the extracellular matrix scaffolding due to abnormal fibrillin-1. The latent TGF-β binding protein interacts with FBN-1, causing sequestration of TGF-β. FBN-1 mutations lead to the loss of this ability, resulting in an overabundance of TGF-β. TGF-β is a peptide growth factor that is important in the regulation of angiogenesis, cell proliferation, cell differentiation, and apoptosis and is a modifier of the structure and function of the extracellular matrix.[4] The dysregulation in the TGF-β pathway creates abnormalities within the extracellular matrix of the vessel walls, which leads to aortic and vascular disease.[5]

Diagnosis of Marfan Syndrome

It is important to understand that MFS remains a syndrome today, despite the broad availability of FBN-1 testing. The newly revised Ghent nosology, which outlines the diagnostic criteria for MFS, relies most heavily on aortic root dilatation and ectopia lentis—dislocation of the lens of the eyes—for diagnosis.[6] Over 90% of patients meeting the Ghent nosology will have an FBN-1 mutation, so, importantly, some patients without FBN-1 mutations can be considered to have MFS. Other genetic mutations have been found in FBN-1-negative MFS patients. The most prominent example results from mutations in transforming growth factor-beta type II receptor (TGFBR2, discussed later), but this accounts for less than 10% of MFS patients. The distinction is clinically relevant, however, when considering the treatment of the proximal aorta. In patients with an FBN-1 mutation, the risk for aneurysm rupture or dissection in the ascending aorta is low when the aneurysm is less than 5 cm, which represents the threshold for intervention.[7] In contrast, patients with TGFBR2 mutations appear to be at a greater risk for aneurysm rupture and/or dissection and the surgical threshold for intervention is now considered to be an aortic diameter greater than 4.2 cm.[8] Thus, even in patients who clearly meet the Ghent nosology for the diagnosis of MFS, knowledge of the genetic defect remains important.

Cardiovascular Complications of Marfan Syndrome

Aortic root dilatation and sequelae of aortic dissections were the cause of over 90% of all deaths in MFS patients.[9] The disease typically begins with dilatation of the aortic root, which occurs in an estimated 60% to 80% of patients with MFS, potentially resulting in aortic regurgitation and proximal dissection.[10] Ventricular dysrhythmias are also common in Marfan patients (20%) and are associated with early mortality and sudden death.[11] When aortic dissection occurred in Marfan patients, 37% were limited to the ascending aorta, 43% were involved in the entire aorta, and 20% were limited to the descending aorta.[12] Marfan patients can also present with abdominal aortic aneurysms (AAA) and aneurysms of the subclavian arteries; however, such manifestations are less frequently observed. The preponderance of aortic pathology compared with aneurysmal disease in other vessels relates to the pathophysiology of the disease, specifically caused by an increased density of microfibrils in the aorta. The risk for aneurysmal rupture or dissection in the ascending aorta appears to be low when the aneurysm is less than 5 cm, which is now considered to be the threshold for surgical intervention.[7]

TGFBR1 AND TGFBR2 MUTATIONS (LOEYS-DIETZ SYNDROME)

Mutations in the transforming growth factor beta receptors (TGFBR1 and TGFBR2) cause both syndromic and nonsyndromic forms of aneurysmal disease. The most severe manifestation of TGFBR1/2 mutations is sometimes referred to as Loeys-Dietz syndrome (LDS), an autosomal dominant disorder affecting the connective tissue with multisystemic involvement. TGFBR1/2 mutations are characterized by hypertelorism (widely space eyes), cleft palate, bifid uvula, or generalized arterial tortuosity with affected patients having a high incidence of aortic aneurysms or dissections. On the other end of the spectrum, patients can have a TGFBR1/2 mutation in the setting of an aortic aneurysm and/or dissection but without any evidence of other connective tissue problems. Thus, the phenotype and expressivity of TGFBR1/2 mutations vary widely among patients. The median survival for patients with TGFBR1/2 mutations is only 37 years, compared with a median survival of 48 years in Elhers-Danlos type IV syndrome or 70 years in treated MFS patients.[13]

Genetics of TGFBR1 and TGFBR2 Mutations

Mutations in TGFBR1 (chromosome 9) or TGFBR2 (chromosome 3) are inherited in an autosomal dominant pattern. Approximately 75% of patients develop a *de novo* mutation, whereas the remaining 25% inherit the mutation directly from a parent. The most commonly mutated gene is TGFBR2, affected in about 75% of patients. To date, there have not been any well-described genotype-phenotype associations with these gene mutations because the same genetic variant can result in vastly different phenotypes among individuals. How the same mutation can cause a severe phenotype in one patient and only an uncomplicated aortic aneurysm in another patient continues to remain elusive to investigators.

Mutations in TGFBR1/2 lead to aneurysms and dissections through the dysregulation of TGF-β signaling. TGF-β transduces its signal to the cell's nucleus through two transmembrane receptors (TGFBR1 and TGFBR2). When TGF-β growth factor binds to TGFBR2, they form a complex with TGFBR1 and together activate a downstream signaling pathway, which is ultimately responsible for the regulation of the extracellular matrix. Mutations in either the TGFBR1 or TGFBR2 gene interrupt this normal signaling pathway. This leads to an enhancement in the TGF-β signaling pathway and an overabundance of TGF-β, resulting in disorganization of the elastic fibers, medial degeneration, and increased collagen deposition in the aortic media.[14,15] TGF-β overabundance and signal dysregulation is also present in MFS but occurs by a different mechanism and pathway, allowing one to better understand why LDS patients have altered extracellular matrix throughout the arterial system whereas patients in MFS have primarily aortic pathology.

Diagnosis of TGFBR1 and TGFBR2 Mutations

Due to the wide spectrum of features in patients with TGFBR1/2 mutations, many have questioned what clinical characteristics are necessary to make a diagnosis. It has recently been demonstrated that TGFBR1 and TGFBR2 mutations can cause familial thoracic aortic aneurysms and dissections in the absence of any connective tissue disease manifestations.[16] For this reason, no minimal diagnostic criteria have been developed as there are in MFS and Ehlers-Danlos type IV syndrome (EDS-IV). It is important to understand that the genetics dictates the diagnosis rather than the clinical manifestations at the time of presentation. Due to the aggressive natural history of this disease, surgical intervention is recommended at diameter thresholds of 4.2 cm for the ascending aorta.[8] These guidelines are even applied to patients with TGFBR1/2 mutations that may be otherwise phenotypically silent.

Vascular Complications of TGFBR1 and TGFBR2 Mutations

The most common cardiovascular complication is aortic root dilatation, occurring in 98% of patients classified as having a TGFBR1/2 mutation.[13] Aortic root dilatation often leads to aortic dissection, which is the primary cause of death in these individuals. In the study by Loeys et al., 84% of patients with TGFBR1/2 mutations had an ascending aortic aneurysm, 31% had aneurysms of the thoracic arterial branches, 10% had aneurysms in the head or neck arterial branches, 10% had a descending thoracic aneurysm, and 10% had an AAA.[13] In addition to aneurysms of the aorta, 52% had aneurysms in other arteries, most commonly in the subclavian. Additionally, arterial tortuosity was prevalent throughout the arterial tree in 84% of patients, often in the cerebral circulation. Although there are no genotype-phenotype associations, one correlation that prevails is that the severity of craniofacial abnormalities predicts the age of the first cardiovascular event.[13]

EHLERS-DANLOS TYPE IV SYNDROME (VASCULAR TYPE)

There exist several types of Ehlers-Danlos syndrome (EDS), of which type IV (vascular type) is the most clinically relevant to cardiovascular pathology. EDS-IV has an estimated incidence of 1 in 5,000 to 20,000 live births.[17] Patients with EDS-IV have major complications of arterial and bowel rupture and clinical features, such as thin and translucent skin, characteristic facial features, and easy bruising.[18] Mean life expectancy is less than 50 years. Over 70% of the patients with EDS-IV die as a result of arterial complications.[18]

Genetics of Ehlers-Danlos Type IV Syndrome

EDS-IV arises from the production of abnormal type III collagen caused by a mutation in the COL3A1 gene, located on chromosome 2.[19] The COL3A1 gene encodes for type III procollagen, a major component of the vascular extracellular matrix.[20] Specifically, collagen type III is found in the elastin lamella of the media and the collagenous network of the adventitia of the vessel wall. Type III procollagen is a molecule formed by three alpha-1 (III) chains that contain the repeating amino acid sequence glycine-X-Y. Proper assembly of these alpha-1 (III) chains is crucial to ensuring its correct function.[18] If mutations interrupt the normal glycine-X-Y repeats or change the length of one of the three monomers, a nonfunctional type III collagen will result. This results in the accumulation of the defective type III collagen molecules in the rough endoplasmic reticulum of cells, which impedes normal trafficking and processing of other proteins and molecules.[21] The most common mutation in EDS-IV is the substitution of another amino acid for glycine, whereas deletion/duplication mutations occur in only 2% of cases. To date, there has not been any association between the type of missense mutation and frequency of major complications. Additionally, if the defective type III collagen gets secreted into the extracellular matrix, its abnormal arrangement is unable to form proper collagen fibrils, thus affecting the structure and function of the tissue. Given that type III collagen is a major component of the vasculature, vascular abnormalities are frequently seen in these patients.

In addition to substitution and splice site mutations, COL3A1 null mutations have recently been reported.[22] The COL3A1 null mutation results in a premature termination codon. Instead of abnormal type III collagen being produced as in substitution or splice site mutations, a null mutation causes the production of only half the amount of normal type III collagen. Such patients have a milder phenotype than those with missense or splice site mutations. Such patients have an extended life span and a delayed age of first complication as compared to those with EDS-IV. The major complications appear to be limited to vascular events and no bowel or organ rupture is present.

Diagnosis of Ehlers-Danlos Type IV Syndrome

A clinical diagnosis of EDS-IV is based on having at least two of the four diagnostic criteria—arterial, intestinal, and/or uterine rupture, or a family history of EDS-IV.[17] These patients may also have easy bruising, thin skin with visible veins, and characteristic facial features. In patients who meet the diagnostic criteria, genetic testing for COL3A1 mutations is highly recommended. Over 95% of patients who meet the diagnostic criteria will have an identified COL3A1 mutation through gene sequencing. If the mutation is not identified by sequencing, biochemical testing using patient fibroblasts can confirm diagnosis.[23] This is a genetically based disorder and abnormalities (mutations, deletions,

duplications) in the COL3A1 gene will always be present in a patient with EDS-IV.

Vascular Complications of Ehlers-Danlos Type IV Syndrome

Pepin et al. studied 419 patients with EDS-IV, and 46% of had an arterial complication as their initial presenting symptom at the mean age of 23. Over half of the abnormalities involved the trunk vessels, whereas disease in the remaining arteries (cerebral vasculature or extremities) was less commonly seen.[18] In a study by Oderich et al.,[23] 30 patients with EDS-IV were analyzed and 77% had vascular complications, which comprised arterial dissections and dissecting aneurysms (48%), arterial ruptures (38%), true fusiform aneurysms (14%), and cerebral aneurysms (10%). Patients are usually unaware of their diagnosis until they develop complications, making early detection and treatment difficult.

PATIENT SELECTION FOR ENDOVASCULAR MANAGEMENT

Very little evidence exists in the literature to help guide decision making regarding the surgical or interventional management of CTD patients. The most important concept is based on the perceived risk-to-benefit ratio of treating versus not treating the disease. Even in the setting of exceptionally high risks of rupture or dissection, the decision regarding an optimal treatment strategy is difficult. Guidelines are essentially nonexistent, further stressing the need for an understanding of the disease and clinical judgment. Considerations include an understanding of the quality of the vascular tissues, comorbid conditions, knowledge regarding the specifics of planned procedure, and an understanding of the patient's CTD because arterial tissue fragility frequently seen with EDS-IV is not generally encountered with MFS or TGFBR1/2 mutations. The physiologic status of the patient must also be carefully evaluated. CTDs are systemic diseases, which can cause cardiopulmonary abnormalities that must be considered. Importantly, one must consider the interface of the proposed endovascular device to the arterial wall in the CTD patient. Surgically implanted grafts make excellent proximal and distal landing zones—essentially bypassing any concern for the endovascular device to arterial wall interface, whereas caution is warranted when landing such devices in the native diseased arteries.[24–26] Any type of intervention planned in patients with a CTD must be viewed as a segway to the next because most of these individuals will undergo several operations during their lifetime.[27–29] Thus, endovascular procedures are usually considered in the context of specific anatomic defects following or in anticipation of subsequent procedures.

ANATOMIC OR LESION CONSIDERATIONS FOR ENDOVASCULAR MANAGEMENT

Each patient with CTD disease is unique. Consequently, there is no single endovascular strategy to treating this population. The endovascular approaches must be based on the location and extent of the anatomic lesion and in conjunction with the type of CTD present. We have categorized our endovascular approaches based on the arterial location of the aneurysm and/or dissection as follows: supra-aortic trunk vessels, aortic, and other arteries.

Endovascular Management of Aneurysms in the Supra-Aortic Trunk Vessels

The size criteria for treatment of aneurysms in the carotid, subclavian, axillary, and vertebral arteries are poorly defined. Generally, aneurysms that are greater than or equal to 2 to 2.5 cm for subclavian and extracranial carotid warrant consideration for treatment, whereas smaller vertebral aneurysms may be considered significant. Two endovascular approaches exist to treat subclavian artery aneurysms. One approach is to occlude the aneurysm both proximally and distally in conjunction with an extra-anatomic bypass. An alternative method involves the use of a stent-graft to maintain inline flow, excluding the aneurysm akin to endovascular aortic aneurysm repair. The specific morphology of the aneurysm will often dictate the optimal approach. Given the potential for future arterial complications, we usually attempt to preserve antegrade flow into the subclavian and vertebral arteries when possible. The specifics of the endovascular strategy relate to the detailed analysis of the anatomy. FIGURES 67.1 and 67.2 depict two patients with MFS and right subclavian artery aneurysms with differing proximal morphology. The patient depicted in FIGURE 67.1A precludes the use of a stent-graft repair, given the absence of a distal landing zone proximal to the brachial artery, whereas the patient depicted in FIGURE 67.2A has no proximal landing zone. If possible, vertebral artery integrity should be maintained, given the potential for degeneration in the contralateral vessels or late cerebral vascular complications. Subclavian side branches can be readily managed with supraselective catheterization and embolization techniques, whereas the larger arteries requiring occlusion are often treated with occluding plugs (FIGURES 67.1B and 67.2B) or other devices. In the setting of a long landing zone, this is a straightforward procedure (FIGURE 67.1B); yet when the morphology is complex,

as in FIGURE 67.2A, this can be quite challenging, resulting in incomplete aneurysm exclusion, plug migration, endoleak, and the potential for aneurysm rupture, as seen in FIGURE 67.2B. Ultimately, such failed endovascular techniques may require surgical resolution, resulting in a true hybrid approach. The patient illustrated in FIGURE 67.3 was initially treated endovascularly; however, failure of the proximal plug to exclude the aneurysm (FIGURE 67.2B) resulted in explantation and surgical ligation.

When sufficient proximal and distal landing zones are present, a stent-graft can be used to exclude the aneurysm. FIGURE 67.4 depicts a patient with a TGFBR2 mutation with a left subclavian artery aneurysm. Unlike the right subclavian artery, the left subclavian artery has no relationship to the common carotid artery. This allows the stent-graft to be deployed along the entire length of the left subclavian artery aneurysm.

The management of vertebral pathology will depend on the extent of the disease, status of the contralateral vertebral artery, and potential for late complications of any cerebrovascular vessel. Distal vertebral artery aneurysms are relatively uncommon (FIGURE 67.5A) and require management with extra-anatomic bypass grafting from the ipsilateral common carotid artery to C1/C2 (FIGURE 67.5B). Proximally these vertebral arteries are simply ligated. If the aneurysm is isolated to the proximal vertebral artery, the proximal artery can be ligated, and the midvertebral artery can be mobilized and anastomosed to the common carotid artery in an end-to-side fashion (FIGURE 67.5C).

Endovascular Management of Aneurysms and Dissections in the Aorta

Aortic aneurysms and dissections are the most common type of vascular pathology in patients with CTDs. The endovascular management of these patients has greatly evolved over the last

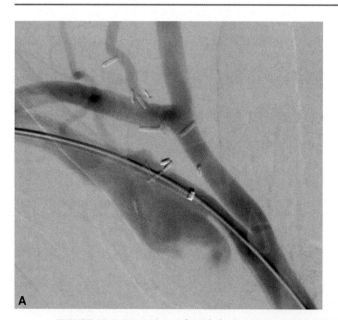
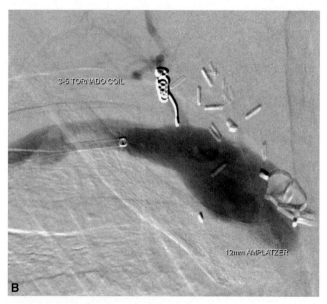

FIGURE 67.1 Extensive right subclavian artery aneurysm in patient with MFS. The status of the proximal subclavian in conjunction with the relationship to the common carotid artery (i.e., right vs. left subclavian artery) will dictate treatment options. The image in **(A)** demonstrates a right subclavian artery aneurysm with a sufficient proximal landing zone to allow for an occluder to be placed **(B)** following an extra-anatomic bypass procedure. Note coils placed in the subclavian artery branch to prevent retrograde leak into aneurysms.

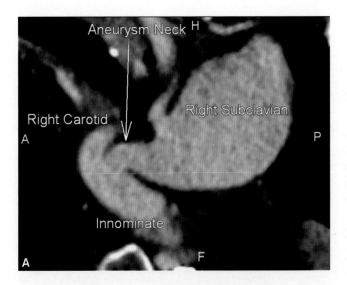

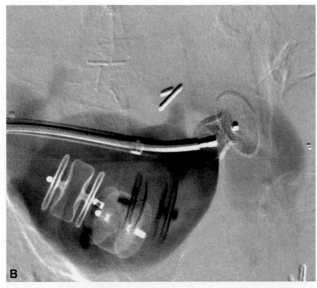

FIGURE 67.2 **Large right subclavian artery aneurysm in MFS patient. A.** CT image shows a right subclavian artery aneurysm in a patient with MFS that has an insufficient proximal landing zone for a stent-graft. Endovascular plugging was attempted **(B)** in an attempt to avoid any future chest incisions but failed (FIGURE 67.3).

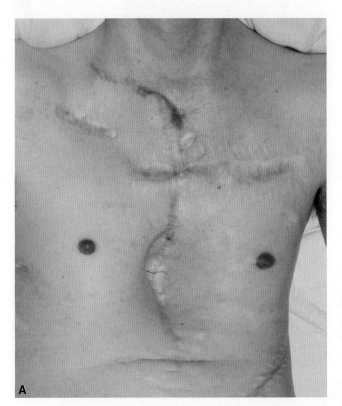

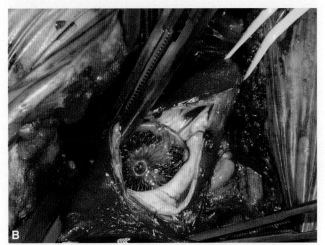

FIGURE 67.3 **Complications of subclavian artery aneurysm occlusion.** In an effort to avoid a chest incision caused by severe deformity (pectus), multiple prior surgeries **(A)**, and respiratory compromise, a septal occluder device was placed into the small proximal neck of the right subclavian artery aneurysm in this MFS patient (FIGURE 67.2). Note the persistent leak that was present following proximal occlusion (FIGURE 67.2B). This required an explantation of the occluder from the right subclavian artery and surgical ligation of the aneurysm **(B)**.

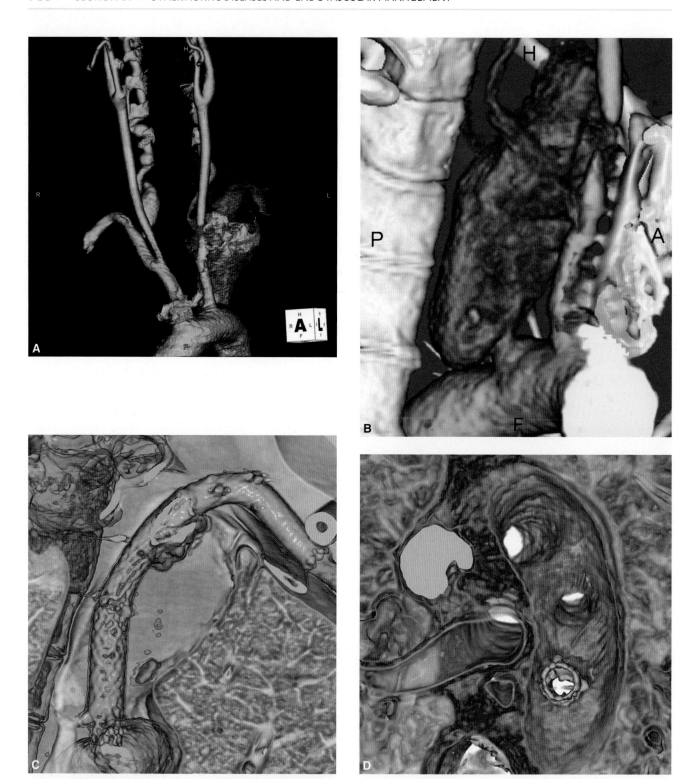

FIGURE 67.4 Patient with a TGFBR2 mutation and a left subclavian artery aneurysm. CT images demonstrate a short and narrow, yet sufficient, proximal landing zone **(A, B)**. This allowed for stent-graft placement **(C)**. An inferior view of the aortic arch **(D)** with the stent-graft seen in the left subclavian extending several millimeters into the lumen of the arch.

decade. The most important concept for treating aortic aneurysms endovascularly in patients with a CTD is selecting good proximal and distal fixation sites. When planning the procedure, there are several options to consider. The first option includes mating the endovascular stent-graft onto an existing graft from a previous aortic repair. Patients who have had previous aortic surgery, such as an elephant trunk graft (FIGURE 67.6A), thoracoabdominal aortic aneurysm (TAAA), or a visceral patch aneurysm (FIGURE 67.6B) repair can be treated using this approach. When placing the proximal seal and fixation in the

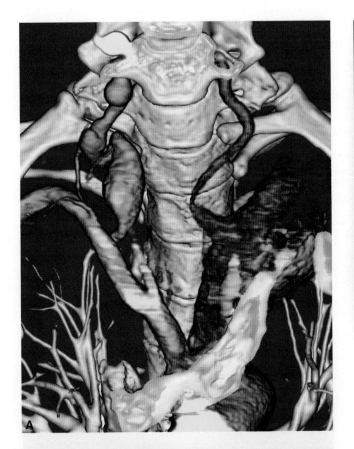

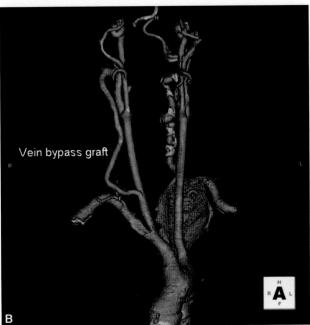

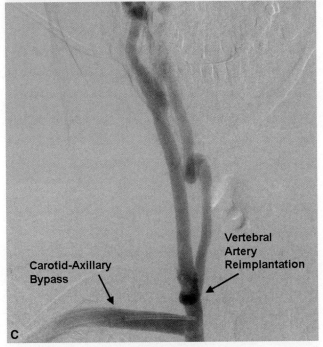

FIGURE 67.5 Managing vertebral artery aneurysms. When possible, vertebral artery preservation is desirable. The status of the distal vertebral artery dictates the strategy for preservation. With extensive distal vertebral artery aneurysms, as in the patient with a TGFBR2 mutation **(A)**, a bypass can be constructed using a saphenous vein from the common carotid artery to the C1/C2 vertebral artery segment **(B)**. Alternatively, if only the subclavian artery or proximal vertebral artery disease is present, the vertebral artery can be transected and reimplanted in an end-to-side fashion to the proximal common carotid artery **(C)**. Other branches arising from the aneurysmal subclavian artery can be coiled as seen previously in FIGURE 67.1B.

native aortic tissue of a patient with a CTD, however, there is concern with regard to the long-term integrity of the device-artery relationship. Yet it is apparent that not all patients can or should undergo a preliminary surgical procedure to ensure the secure placement of an endovascular device. In such situations, one strategy that we utilize is to deploy a short thoracic graft and use this as the fixation site for the branched/fenestrated stent-graft (FIGURES 67.6C and 67.6D). The thoracic grafts utilized are completely covered and have no bare springs, and the only regions of active fixation (barbs) arise distal to the proximal sealing region. This approach avoids placing active fixation mechanisms required for branched devices on the native aorta

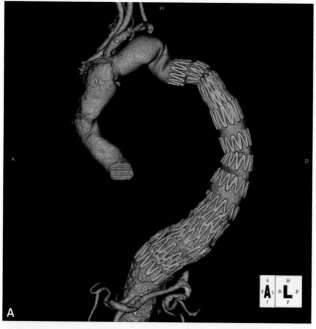

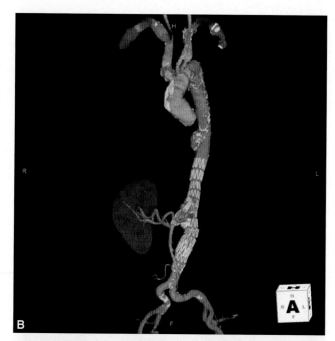

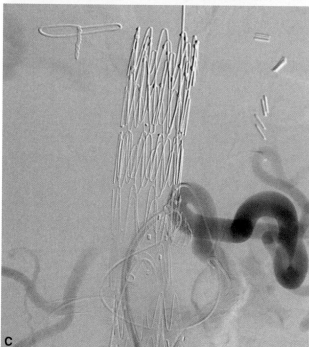

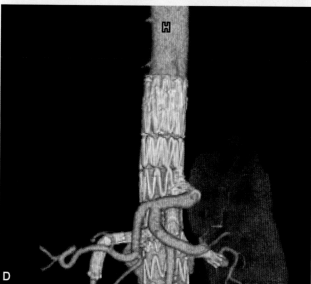

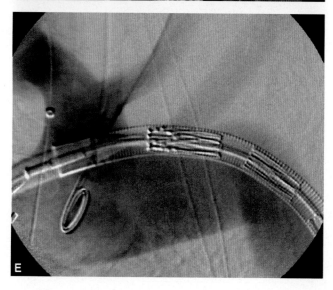

FIGURE 67.6 Aortic stent-graft to arterial interface. Fundamentally, the point of proximal sealing and fixation is paramount to the long-term success of an endovascular aortic repair in a patient with a CTD. Options include landing an endovascular graft into a previously placed surgical graft, such as an elephant trunk graft (**A**), or graft from a previous repair of a visceral patch aneurysm or thoracoabdominal aortic aneurysm (**B**—note the patent intercostal patch that was not covered in an attempt to decrease the risk for paraplegia). In the absence of a surgical graft, the native aorta may be protected from radial force and fixation systems by placing a short thoracic graft (**C**), into which the branched/fenestrated device may be placed (**D**). Additionally, attention should be directed at aligning the stent-graft with straight portions of the aorta to provide good apposition in the setting of tortuosity, as in this MFS patient (**E**).

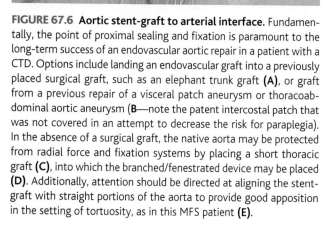

and also provides a double layer of fabric at any region of interface. A second important concept to consider when planning the proximal fixation site of the device is how to align the stent-graft with the walls of the aorta such that no sections of the device sit proud along a curved arterial segment (FIGURE 67.6). This ensures that a circumferential seal is established and is of critical importance when dealing with the aortic arch (FIGURE 67.6E). In such circumstances, the aortic morphology should dictate the location of the proximal sealing zone, rather than the location of the supra-aortic trunk vessels. If the aortic morphology mandates placement of a thoracic device proximal to the supra-aortic trunk vessels, then those vessels should be incorporated into the endovascular repair or treated with an extra-anatomic bypass procedure.

Endovascular Management of Aneurysms in Other Arteries

Although less common than aortic manifestations, individuals with a CTD may also present with aneurysms or dissections in arteries, such as the common iliac arteries or the visceral branches off the aorta. In patients with iliac and internal artery aneurysms, one must first assess the patient's risk for buttock claudication and paraplegia. This will help determine whether the internal iliac arteries should be preserved or simply occluded. This decision is in part limited by the morphology of the aneurysm, recognizing that many of the new therapies allow for extremely distal placement of stent-grafts, such that patients with deep internal iliac artery aneurysms can have preservation of antegrade perfusion if desired. This becomes particularly relevant when the disease is coupled with aortic aneurysms because the risk for paraplegia is linked to the status of antegrade internal iliac perfusion (FIGURE 67.7). As seen in FIGURE 67.7, the patient's left internal iliac artery aneurysm extended distally through the sciatic notch. Even though the aneurysm was very distal, a stent-graft can be used in such cases to exclude the aneurysm and preserve blood flow. This was especially important because the patient's right internal iliac artery was occluded during the previous endovascular aortic repair.

In addition to iliac artery aneurysms, visceral artery aneurysms may also be present in CTD patients. FIGURES 67.7C and 67.7D show a patient with EDS-IV with a pseudoaneurysm of the posterior branch of the left renal artery. One month prior, the patient had a mirror image aneurysm (in the right renal artery) rupture following a spontaneous dissection. Patients with EDS-IV constitute the most concerning group of patients, given that severity of their tissue fragility is unpredictable and the fear of intervening must be balanced against an unknown risk of rupture. The patient in FIGURE 67.7 was treated electively, as we opt to do with most EDS-IV patients with concerning lesions. Yet the interface between the endovascular device and artery is always a concern. In this case, the posterior branch of the left renal artery was occluded proximally and distally to the aneurysm using coil embolization techniques (FIGURE 67.7E).

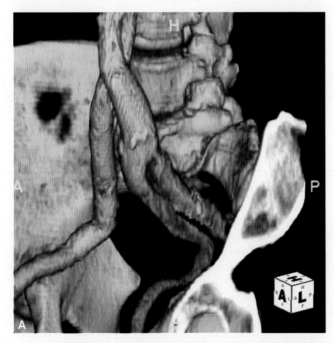
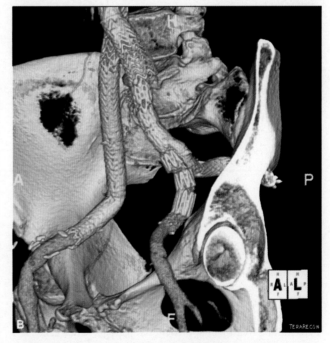

FIGURE 67.7 Other aneurysms. Smaller arteries that have aneurysmal involvement must be assessed for the potential need for preservation versus ability for simple exclusion. Distal internal iliac aneurysms may still be suitable for preservation with an endovascular stent-graft, as in this patient with a dissection and an aneurysm of the abdominal aorta, where antegrade flow was desired through the remaining left internal iliac artery to minimize paraplegia risk **(A)**. Note that the left internal iliac artery stent-graft is long and exits the greater sciatic notch **(B)**. Alternatively, sequential renal artery aneurysms as in the EDS type IV patient can be coil embolized electively, particularly following a prior mirror image rupture in the right renal artery **(C, D, E)**. *(continued)*

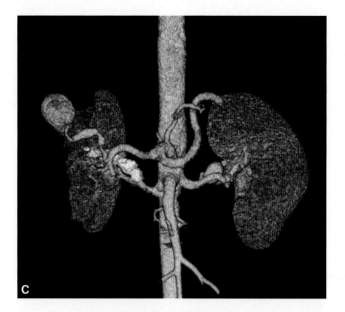

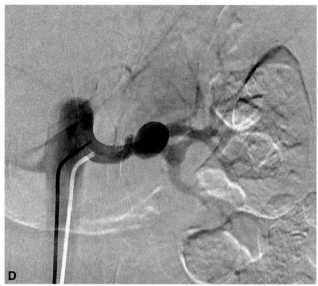

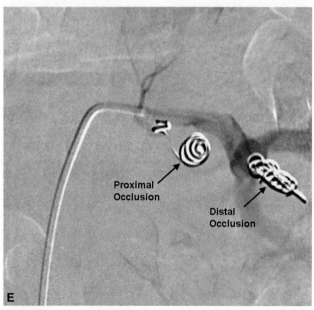

FIGURE 67.7 *(Continued)*

CONCLUSION

Endovascular approaches to patients with a CTD have an important role in the management of arterial aneurysms. Endovascular techniques will continue to evolve, understanding that open surgery still represents the mainstay of the management of most arterial aneurysms. Basic principles of endovascular repair in CTD patients must be underscored. First, when determining treatment approaches in patients with a CTD, it is critical to have a strong understanding of the pathophysiology of the patient's disease and to appreciate the importance of clinical intervention based on the gene mutation and not only on the phenotype. Second, these patients should be assessed for aneurysm and dissections throughout their entire vascular bed, scanning from the intracranial viscerals to the lower extremities. Third, if endovascular treatment is an option, one must critically evaluate the proximal and distal landing zones. This must be stressed because most endovascular failures will be caused by interface problems between devices and arteries that may result in endoleaks or device migration. Fourth, reoperations appear to be the rule in CTD patients. Endovascular repair and open surgical repair represent treatments, not cures for these diseases. Thus, when planning any procedures in such patients one must always strategize for future reoperations.

REFERENCES

1. Judge DP, Dietz HC. Marfan's syndrome. *Lancet* 2005;366(9501):1965–1976.
2. van Karnebeek CD, Naeff MS, Mulder BJ, et al. Natural history of cardiovascular manifestations in Marfan syndrome. *Arch Dis Child* 2001;84(2):129–137.

3. Dietz HC, Pyeritz RE. Mutations in the human gene for fibrillin-1 (FBN1) in the Marfan syndrome and related disorders. *Hum Mol Genet* 1995;4(spec no):1799–1809.

4. Brown KA, Pietenpol JA, Moses HL. A tale of two proteins: differential roles and regulation of Smad2 and Smad3 in TGF-beta signaling. *J Cell Biochem* 2007;101(1):9–33.

5. Byers PH. Determination of the molecular basis of Marfan syndrome: a growth industry. *J Clin Invest* 2004;114(2):161–163.

6. Loeys BL, Dietz HC, Braverman AC, et al. The revised Ghent nosology for the Marfan syndrome. *J Med Genet* 2010;47(7):476–485.

7. Milewicz DM, Dietz HC, Miller DC. Treatment of aortic disease in patients with Marfan syndrome. *Circulation* 2005;111(11):e150–e157.

8. LeMaire SA, Pannu H, Tran-Fadulu V, et al. Severe aortic and arterial aneurysms associated with a TGFBR2 mutation. *Nat Clin Pract Cardiovasc Med* 2007;4(3):167–171.

9. Murdoch JL, Walker BA, Halpern BL, et al. Life expectancy and causes of death in the Marfan syndrome. *N Engl J Med* 1972;286(15):804–808.

10. Roman MJ, Devereux RB, Kramer-Fox R, et al. Comparison of cardiovascular and skeletal features of primary mitral valve prolapse and Marfan syndrome. *Am J Cardiol* 1989;63(5):317–321.

11. Yetman AT, Bornemeier RA, McCrindle BW. Long-term outcome in patients with Marfan syndrome: is aortic dissection the only cause of sudden death? *J Am Coll Cardiol* 2003;41(2):329–332.

12. Mimoun L, Detaint D, Hamroun D, et al. Dissection in Marfan syndrome: the importance of the descending aorta. *Eur Heart J* 2011;32(4):443–449.

13. Loeys BL, Schwarze U, Holm T, et al. Aneurysm syndromes caused by mutations in the TGF-beta receptor. *N Engl J Med* 2006;355(8):788–798.

14. Loeys BL, Chen J, Neptune ER, et al. A syndrome of altered cardiovascular, craniofacial, neurocognitive and skeletal development caused by mutations in TGFBR1 or TGFBR2. *Nat Genet* 2005;37(3):275–281.

15. Maleszewski JJ, Miller DV, Lu J, et al. Histopathologic findings in ascending aortas from individuals with Loeys-Dietz syndrome (LDS). *Am J Surg Pathol* 2009;33(2):194–201.

16. Tran-Fadulu V, Pannu H, Kim DH, et al. Analysis of multigenerational families with thoracic aortic aneurysms and dissections due to TGFBR1 or TGFBR2 mutations. *J Med Genet* 2009;46(9):607–613.

17. Beighton P, De Paepe A, Steinmann B, et al. Ehlers-Danlos syndromes: revised nosology, Villefranche, 1997. Ehlers-Danlos National Foundation (USA) and Ehlers-Danlos Support Group (UK). *Am J Med Genet* 1998;77(1):31–37.

18. Pepin M, Schwarze U, Superti-Furga A, et al. Clinical and genetic features of Ehlers-Danlos syndrome type IV, the vascular type. *N Engl J Med* 2000;342(10):673–680.

19. Smith LT, Schwarze U, Goldstein J, et al. Mutations in the COL3A1 gene result in the Ehlers-Danlos syndrome type IV and alterations in the size and distribution of the major collagen fibrils of the dermis. *J Invest Dermatol* 1997;108(3):241–247.

20. Arteaga-Solis E, Gayraud B, Ramirez F. Elastic and collagenous networks in vascular diseases. *Cell Struct Funct* 2000;25(2):69–72.

21. Byers PH. Ehlers-Danlos syndrome: recent advances and current understanding of the clinical and genetic heterogeneity. *J Invest Dermatol* 1994;103(5 suppl):47S–52S.

22. Leistritz DF, Pepin MG, Schwarze U, et al. COL3A1 haploinsufficiency results in a variety of Ehlers-Danlos syndrome type IV with delayed onset of complications and longer life expectancy. *Genet Med* 2011;13(8):717–722.

23. Oderich GS, Panneton JM, Bower TC, et al. The spectrum, management and clinical outcome of Ehlers-Danlos syndrome type IV: a 30-year experience. *J Vasc Surg* 2005;42(1):98–106.

24. Ince H, Rehders TC, Petzsch M, et al. Stent-grafts in patients with Marfan syndrome. *J Endovasc Ther* 2005;12(1):82–88.

25. Baril DT, Carroccio A, Palchik E, et al. Endovascular treatment of complicated aortic aneurysms in patients with underlying arteriopathies. *Ann Vasc Surg* 2006;20(4):464–471.

26. Geisbüsch P, Kotelis D, von Tengg-Kobligk H, et al. Thoracic aortic endografting in patients with connective tissue diseases. *J Endovasc Ther* 2008;15(2):144–149.

27. de Oliveira NC, David TE, Ivanov J, et al. Results of surgery for aortic root aneurysm in patients with Marfan syndrome. *J Thorac Cardiovasc Surg* 2003;125(4):789–796.

28. Alexiou C, Langley SM, Charlesworth P, et al. Aortic root replacement in patients with Marfan's syndrome: the Southampton experience. *Ann Thorac Surg* 2001;72(5):1502–1507; discussion 1508.

29. Gott VL, Cameron DE, Alejo DE, et al. Aortic root replacement in 271 Marfan patients: a 24-year experience. *Ann Thorac Surg* 2002;73(2):438–443.

Aortic Inflammatory Disease (Mycotic Lesions, Fistulas, Anastomotic Disruptions)

SAHER S. SABRI and MARGARET CLARKE TRACCI

▌ INTRODUCTION

Mycotic Aneurysm

The term *mycotic aneurysm* is used to describe any infected aneurysm, regardless of its pathogenesis. In fact most infected aneurysms are of bacterial etiology. The aneurysms can develop secondary to weakening of the arterial wall, which can result from superinfection of diseased and atherosclerotic surfaces from bacteremia and embolization of infectious material, or, less commonly, colonization of normal wall through the vasa vasorum.[1-4] One other mechanism for formation of infected aneurysms involves direct penetration of the vascular wall from an extravascular source, such as a perivertebral abscess. Alternatively, an extravascular infectious focus, such as vertebral osteomyelitis, may penetrate directly or through the lymphatic tissue into an adjacent vascular structure, leading to necrosis, bleeding, and formation of a pseudoaneurysm.[3,4]

Anastomotic Pseudoaneurysm

Degeneration of the anastomotic suture line following surgical repair of the aorta typically results in pseudoaneurysm formation. Anastomotic pseudoaneurysms may represent sterile degeneration of the arterial wall at the anastomosis, a technical defect in the anastomosis, or be the result of either frank or occult infection.[5] They should, however, be distinguished from progressive growth of true aneurysms of the aorta above or the iliac arteries below an aortic graft, a disease process that is well described but is beyond the scope of this chapter. It has been observed that pseudoaneurysms may occur after surgery for either occlusive or aneurysmal disease, but that true aneurysms tend to occur more frequently following surgery for aortic aneurysms.[6] Predisposing factors appear to include hypertension, chronic obstructive pulmonary disease (COPD), tobacco use, hyperlipidemia, suture type, technical failures, and a history of groin wound complications.[5,7,8]

Aortoenteric Fistula

Aortoenteric fistulas may rarely arise as a primary process, generally manifesting as erosion of an aneurysmal abdominal aorta into the adjacent duodenum. A minority of primary fistulas are associated with mycotic aneurysm, aortitis, neoplastic invasion, or adjacent gastrointestinal (GI) disease. Most of these lesions occur as postprocedural complications, however, and may be considered to represent one end of a clinical spectrum of complications that ranges from uninfected anastomotic pseudoaneurysms to frank graft infection to aorto- or graft-enteric fistulae.

Secondary aortoenteric fistulae may either involve the classic "herald bleed" presentation associated with erosion of a graft anastomosis into the GI tract, most commonly at the duodenum, or sepsis associated with the development of a fistulous communication between a portion of the graft and the gut.[9]

▌ INCIDENCE AND NATURAL HISTORY

Mycotic Aneurysm

The infected aneurysms are estimated to comprise 1% to 2% of all thoracic and abdominal aneurysms.[4,10,11] This condition is associated with high morbidity and mortality and is more common in immunocompromised patients, such as those with known malignancies and those receiving corticosteroids or cytotoxic drugs. The thoracic aorta is involved in 42% to 66% of cases, whereas the abdominal aorta is involved in 17% to 39% of cases.[4,11] Less likely involved arteries include the iliac, infrainguinal, and visceral.[10] The source of infection is found in only 50% of cases and may be related to (1) previous arterial intervention, such as catheterization, endovascular, or open vascular interventions; (2) an existing infection, such as endocarditis, spondylodiskitis, pneumonia, or intra-abdominal infections; or (3) arterial-enteric fistula, the presence of which is usually associated with worse outcome.[4,10] Additionally, blood cultures may be negative in 25% to 40% of cases. It is worth mentioning that in a third of the patients, the source of infection may not be identified but the blood cultures may be positive.[4] Salmonella species is the most common organism and can be cultured in up to 60% of cases, followed by *Staphylococcus aureus* in a third of patients. Other less common infectious etiologies include gram-negative bacilli and *Mycobacterium* and streptococcus species.[10-12] Secondary to the increased prevalence of methicillin-resistant *S. aureus* (MRSA), however, this organism has been increasingly implicated as the source of infection in mycotic aneurysms.[13-16]

Anastomotic Pseudoaneurysm

Pseudoaneurysm formation at graft-native artery anastomoses represents one of the most frequently reported graft-related complications of aortic surgery. In the Mayo Clinic series of 307 patients treated surgically for infrarenal aortic aneurysm, the authors detected anastomotic pseudoaneurysms in 3% of patients.[17] Following aortic surgery, these occur in decreasing order of frequency at the femoral, iliac, and aortic anastomoses.[17-19]

It is worth noting that anastomotic complications in the aortic and iliac positions are almost certainly underreported because they are less clinically evident than those presenting in the groin. Indeed, most of the reported series either predate the routine use of computed tomography (CT) imaging for surveillance or relied either on symptomatic presentation or incidental discovery of anastomotic disruptions. Prospective studies utilizing routine imaging of arterial grafts in all positions have suggested much higher rates that appear to increase over time. Limited data with regard to pseudoaneurysms occurring at the proximal or distal anastomoses of infrarenal aortic grafts seem to support similar trends.[18] Routine surveillance with ultrasound, for instance, demonstrated para-anastomotic pseudoaneurysms in 6.3% of aortic anastomoses following abdominal aortic graft placement at a mean interval of 12 years from operation.[6]

Aortoenteric Fistula

Primary abdominal aortoenteric fistula (AEF) is exceedingly uncommon with incidence ranging from 0.02% to 0.07% in autopsy studies,[20] whereas secondary fistula is relatively so, affecting 1% to 2% of aortic grafts in large series.[17] Primary fistula seems to occur with greater frequency in the thoracic than the abdominal aorta.[20] Secondary AEF is typically a relatively late complication, presenting, in one series, a mean of 36 months postoperatively.[21]

CLINICAL PRESENTATION AND PATIENT SELECTION

Mycotic Aneurysm

Compared to noninfected aneurysms, the patients with mycotic aneurysms are more commonly to be symptomatic, presenting with symptoms, such as back and abdominal pain (76%), fever (28% to 48%), or septic shock (7%). Elevated C-reactive protein (CRP) or white count is noted in 47% to 79% of patients. Additionally, 15% to 37% of patients present with ruptured aneurysm requiring emergency intervention. Primary AEF can be demonstrated in approximately 12% of patients at the time of presentation.[4,10–12]

When a mycotic aneurysm is suspected, cross-sectional imaging is usually performed with CT (FIGURE 68.1). Findings may include stranding in fat tissue, irregular-shaped aneurysm, multiple focal aneurysms in different locations in the aorta, fluid collection, or periaortic gas. A new developing aneurysm with rapid increase in size over a short period should raise suspicion for mycotic aneurysm. Magnetic resonance (MR) may similarly demonstrate periaortic fluid or surrounding inflammation, although its ability to detect gas is limited.

Diagnostic angiography provides excellent visualization of vascular anatomy and focal aneurysms and may be useful for

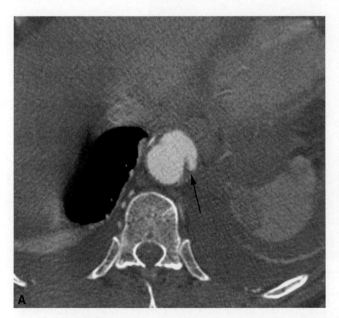

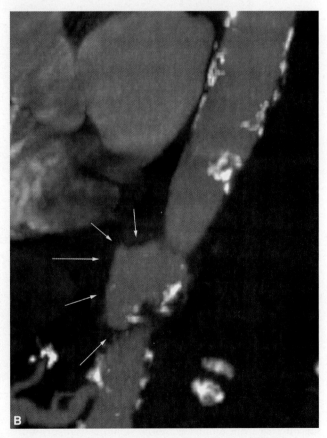

FIGURE 68.1 A 56-year-old man with new-onset abdominal and chest pain 3 weeks postcolonic resection for diverticulitis. Axial and sagittal CT angiograms of the descending aorta (**A, B**) show an irregular outpouching consistent with a mycotic pseudoaneurysm (*arrows*). The patient was afebrile and the blood cultures were negative. Angiogram (**C**) shows the pseudoaneurysm (*arrows*) prior to stent-graft deployment. Axial and sagittal CT angiograms (**D, E**) 4 weeks poststent-graft deployment show exclusion of the pseudoaneurysm. *(continued)*

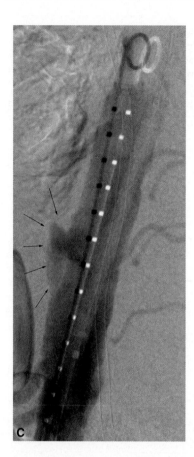

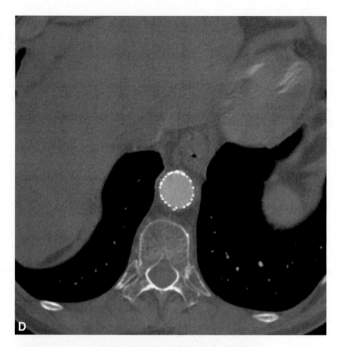

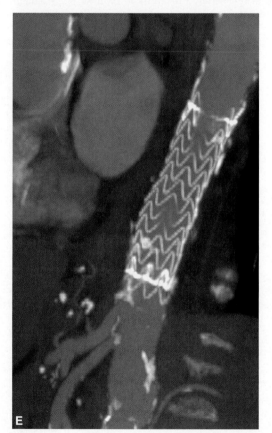

FIGURE 68.1 *(Continued)*

procedural planning, but its utility is limited in distinguishing infected from uninfected aorta. Gallium scans or, more recently, indium-111 (^{111}In) or ^{99}Tc tagged WBC scans have become a mainstay of diagnosis where CT findings are not definitive and may be quite useful in defining the extent of the infection.

Predictors for posttreatment aneurysm-related morbidity and mortality in one study included advanced age, salmonella species infection, AEF, fever, leukocytosis, and shock at the time of intervention.[12] Other studies concluded that nonsalmonella species infection is associated with worse mortality and morbidity[22–25] compared to salmonella species infection. Protective factors included adjunctive procedures to control or drain the infection and preprocedural use of intravenous antibiotics for more than 1 week.[10,11]

Anastomotic Pseudoaneurysm

The key distinction, once the diagnosis of anastomotic disruption has been made, is between sterile and infected pseudoaneurysm. An infected pseudoaneurysm following surgical placement of an aortic graft is, for clinical purposes, a graft infection.

A careful history may elicit evidence of fever, chills, weight loss, or other signs of infection. Physical examination may demonstrate erythema, induration, a fluid collection, or purulent drainage in the groin or a tender mass in the abdomen or pelvis. The laboratory evaluation is also useful in distinguishing an infected from a noninfected pseudoaneurysm and may, in this regard, include a complete blood count with differential, blood cultures, fluid cultures, and markers of inflammation, such as CRP or erythrocyte sedimentation rate.

Ultrasound may detect a pseudoaneurysm and may even be able to visualize perigraft fluid beyond the immediate postoperative period that is suggestive of graft infection. Typically, ultrasound examination is utilized to evaluate groin masses or as a routine screening examination for the intra-abdominal portion of the repair. Once a pseudoaneurysm is detected by ultrasound, CT or MR is utilized to evaluate for further evidence of infection followed by a WBC scan as described for mycotic aneurysms. Detection of perigraft fluid or gas on cross-sectional imaging confirmed with increased uptake on the WBC scan are key findings in establishing the diagnosis of an infected pseudoaneurysm.

Identification of bacteria or yeast on Gram stain or speciation on culture may guide therapy, but the pathogens typical of graft infections, such as *S. epidermidis*, frequently yield multiple negative cultures in the setting of a clinical infection. Because operative drainage and debridement are generally considered obligatory when graft infection is suspected, cultures may be obtained of fluid, debrided tissue, and graft at operation with a potentially higher diagnostic yield.

Whereas some series describe a relatively benign course in anastomotic pseudoaneurysms managed expectantly, others have described a high (44%) mortality rate associated with rupture of untreated anastomotic pseudoaneurysms.[17,26] This far exceeds the observed mortality rate for either elective or emergent open operative repair or for endovascular therapy.[7] In any case, a large, enlarging, or symptomatic pseudoaneurysm should be treated expeditiously.[8]

Aortoenteric Fistula

Aortoenteric fistula remains a diagnostic challenge because the clinical presentation may vary widely depending on the anatomic characteristics of the fistula. In a secondary AEF, frank aortoenteric communication typically occurs at the anastomoses and is more likely to present with gastroenteric hemorrhage than a simple fistulous communication between the GI tract and graft. At least one large series has found that a minority of patients (22%) in the former group actually offer the classic presentation of a "herald" upper GI bleed followed by hematemesis and hypotension. In fact, recurrent self-limiting GI hemorrhage, most typically melena, was the most common presenting symptom.[21] The same group found that patients, on average, experienced 25 days of bleeding prior to establishment of the diagnosis of an AEF.

Contrast-enhanced CT may demonstrate perigraft fluid or gas in conjunction with thickened intestinal wall or even frank extravasation of contrast into the GI tract (FIGURE 68.2). Esophagogastroduodenoscopy (EGD) may demonstrate lesions in the typical position in the third or fourth portion of the duodenum or, in the case of an enteric-graft communication, permit visualization of exposed graft through a defect in the intestinal wall. A negative examination does not, however, exclude the diagnosis of an AEF.

The utility of magnetic resonance imaging and nuclear medicine studies is somewhat limited by the duration of these examinations. The sensitivity of catheter angiography in this setting is poor because it is unable to detect perigraft fluid or sinus or bowel thickening or proximity and, consistent with CT findings, is rarely able to demonstrate contrast filling of the actual fistula.

It is clear that the clinician must maintain a high index of suspicion where GI bleeding develops in a patient with a prior aortic graft. Because failure to make the correct diagnosis in the event of an AEF is almost invariably fatal, immediate surgical or endovascular intervention without further investigation is appropriate if an AEF is suspected and the patient is unstable.[9]

▌ TREATMENT SELECTION STRATEGIES

Traditionally, the mainstay of treatment of mycotic aneurysm, infected pseudoaneurysm, and AEF has been surgical debridement of infected material and tissue with in situ or extra-anatomic arterial reconstruction. Although sterile pseudoaneurysms have been surgically repaired in a similar fashion, more recent data support the use of endovascular therapy for noninfected lesions.[27] Based on these data, endovascular treatment is the appropriate first-line therapy for pseudoaneurysms presenting without any evidence of infection, including fever, leukocytosis, or perigraft fluid or gas. Endovascular therapy may yield durable results in uncomplicated mycotic aneurysms and may be used as a first-line option. The endovascular approach also can be utilized as a temporizing measure reserved for poor surgical candidates in the setting of a complicated mycotic aneurysm, an infected pseudoaneurysm, or an AEF. A proposed management flow chart is presented in FIGURE 68.3.

Surgical Management

Several surgical techniques are typically utilized for the management of anastomotic pseudoaneurysms. In an uninfected setting, the most frequently utilized is simple debridement and interposition grafting. Where infection is apparently limited to a single limb of the graft, resection limited to the limb or its involved portion has been described, followed by in situ or extra-anatomic reconstruction. This may be followed by ongoing antibiotic irrigation of the retroperitoneal field through operatively placed drains.[28]

Anastomotic pseudoaneurysm with evidence of extensive graft infection and secondary aortoduodenal fistula are

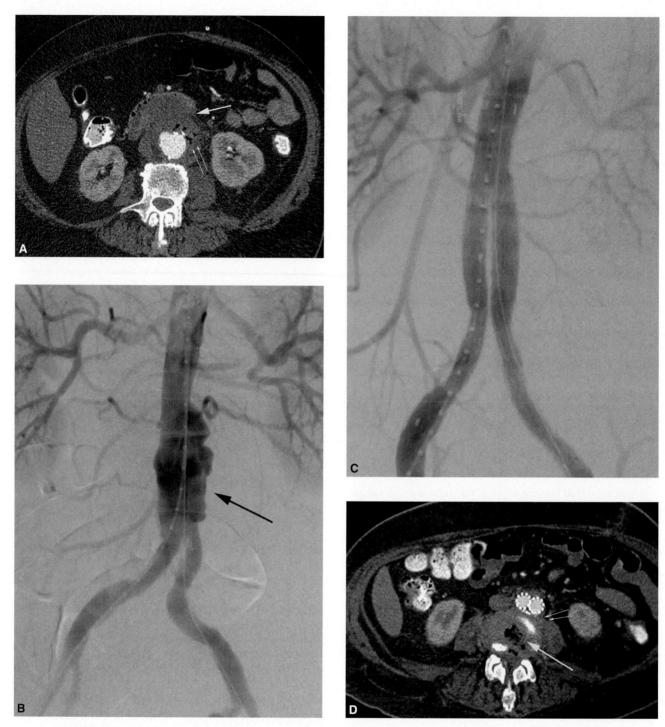

FIGURE 68.2 A 74-year-old man presented with gastrointestinal bleeding. Axial CT angiogram (**A**) shows an irregular abdominal aortic aneurysm (*arrow*) that contains air (*small arrows*). There is fat stranding and loss of fat plain between the aorta and third portion of the duodenum consistent with an aortoenteric fistula. Abdominal aortogram (**B**) shows the irregular aneurysm (*arrow*). Angiogram postbifurcated aortic stent-graft (**C**) shows exclusion of the aneurysm. Follow-up CT angiogram 6 weeks postprocedure (**D**) shows fluid accumulation and loss of fat plains posterior to the aorta with gas present within the vertebral body (*arrow*), indicating osteomyelitis. The patient underwent surgical resection with extra-anatomic bypass and lifelong antibiotics.

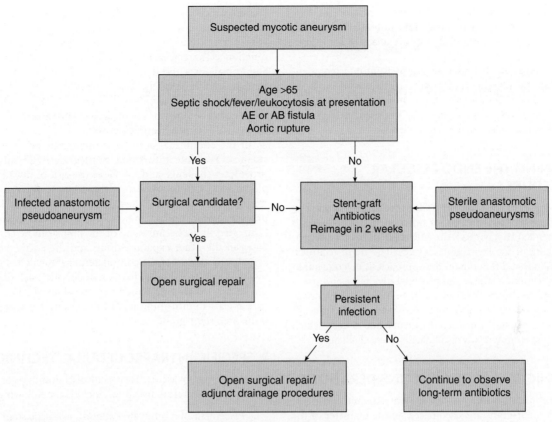

FIGURE 68.3 Management flow chart for suspected mycotic aneurysm.

managed by removal of the entire graft with generous irrigation and debridement of involved tissue. Traditionally, axillobifemoral bypass grafting accompanied by graft excision and closure of the aortic stump has been considered the gold standard of therapy. Staging of this approach by performing the extra-anatomic reconstruction first, followed either the same day or after an interval of up to several days by graft excision resulted in significantly improved survival compared with the earlier approach of excision prior to reconstruction.[29] Recurrent graft infection, graft thrombosis, and the nearly invariably fatal complication of aortic stump infection or disruption continue to contribute to significant morbidity, mortality, and limb loss following this operation, however. Thorough debridement, layered closure, and vascularized pedicle flap coverage of the aortic stump are considered of paramount importance in avoiding the latter complication.

Infected aortic graft or mycotic aneurysms may also be replaced in situ using antibiotic-impregnated synthetic graft, cryopreserved arterial allograft, or saphenofemoral vein autograft.[30–32] The neoaortoiliac system (NAIS) venous autograft reconstruction described by Clagett represents a longer, more demanding procedure often undertaken using a full second surgical team so that vein harvest may be conducted simultaneously with the generally difficult dissection required for graft explant. The other principal distinction among these approaches has been the rate of reinfection with synthetic graft generally demonstrating the highest rate of reinfection, cryopreserved arterial allograft an intermediate rate, and autogenous vein consistently

the lowest. Those utilizing synthetic graft typically utilize adjunctive measures, such as antibiotic impregnation of the graft, wrapping of the graft and new anastomoses with well-vascularized pedicle flaps, retroperitoneal antibiotic irrigation, or retroperitoneal tunneling through a clean tissue plane.

In an aortoduodenal fistula, the duodenum should then be primarily repaired with consideration given to local drainage, proximal decompression via nasogastric or gastrostomy tube, and provisions for eventual resumption of distal enteral nutrition.

ENDOVASCULAR MANAGEMENT

Stent-graft repair of infected aneurysms was first proposed by Semba et al.[24] as an alternate approach to open surgical repair. This was followed by several subsequent reports providing evidence that endovascular management is a viable, less invasive treatment approach with promising results.[12,25,33–35]

Similar to any other aortic intervention, endovascular management provides the potential benefit of shorter operation time, less blood loss, avoidance of cross-clamping of the aorta and the ischemic risks associated with it, as well as avoidance of other postoperative complications, such as adhesions and abdominal wall hernias. Unique to the infectious aneurysms, endovascular repair provides the additional benefit of avoiding a major open surgery and associated comorbidities in critically ill patients, provides a temporizing measure to treat or prevent a catastrophic aortic rupture, and potentially delays a definitive surgery, if needed, once the patient's condition stabilizes. One other potential benefit is avoidance of the potential risk of aortic stump leak and anastomotic dehiscence in an infected surgical bed.

Disadvantages of endovascular treatment in infected aneurysms include the placement of the stent-graft as a foreign body in an infected bed. Additionally, the stent-graft will potentially prevent or treat aortic rupture but does not manage the infection, which surgical debridement provides.

PLANNING THE ENDOVASCULAR PROCEDURE

The planning steps for the stent-graft procedure are similar to planning stent-graft placement for other aortic pathologies. It is recommended to have a CT or MR angiograms for preprocedural sizing of the stent-graft devices. The main technical consideration that differentiates the approach to mycotic aneurysms, aortoenteric fistulas, and postoperative leaks and pseudoaneurysms to degenerative aortic aneurysms is the adequacy of landing zones. The landing zone (proximal and distal neck) sizes are usually smaller than that for aneurysmal disease, which makes placing commercially available devices a challenge.

TECHNICAL AND DEVICE CONSIDERATIONS

In the thoracic aorta, similar to aortic aneurysms and aortic dissection, the stent-grafts are sized based on the diameter of the proximal and distal landing zone in the aorta. In the absence of aneurysmal disease, the aortic diameter may be as small as

20 mm, which may be too small to accommodate some thoracic stent-graft devices. This has led to the off-label use of iliac limb stent-graft extensions or aortic stent-graft cuff extensions to function as thoracic stent-grafts. Such devices, designed for the abdominal aorta and iliac arteries, respectively, would accommodate smaller-sized thoracic aortas (FIGURE 68.4).[36] Recently, several thoracic stent-grafts with sizes as small as 22 mm in diameter have become commercially available and may prove useful in small-diameter thoracic aortas.

In the abdominal aorta, a similar issue arises where the smallest available bifurcated stent-graft is 22 mm, which provides a challenge and increases the risk of infolding when placed in an abdominal aorta with a diameter less than 18 mm. Additionally, the size of the distal aorta at its bifurcation can provide another limitation for the ability to accommodate two bifurcated limbs because one of the limbs can be compressed between the other expanded limb and the aortic wall or the actual cannulation of the contralateral gate may be prohibited by the inability of the gait to open due to the small diameter of the aorta. It is recommended that the abdominal aortal measure at least 15 mm at the aortic bifurcation to accommodate a bifurcated stent-graft.

SPECIFIC INTRAPROCEDURAL TECHNIQUES

Methods of endovascular treatment of abdominal aortic infections and postsurgical disruption include the following:

1. Placement of a bifurcated abdominal aortic stent-graft for proximal neck diameters greater than 18 mm and aortic bifurcation greater than 15 mm.

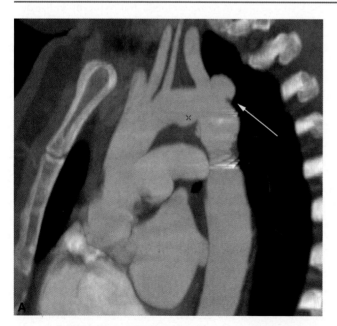
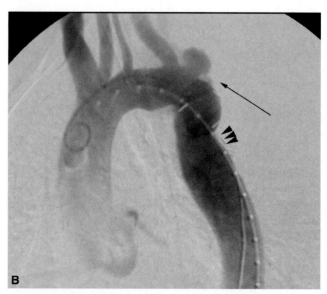

FIGURE 68.4 A 32-year-old man postaortic coarctation repair. Sagittal CT angiogram (**A**) shows a pseudoaneurysm arising at the proximal surgical graft anastomosis (*arrow*). This was thought to be a sterile pseudoaneurysm. Thoracic aortogram (**B**) shows the pseudoaneurysm (*arrow*) as well as the constriction at the site of the surgically corrected coarctation (*arrowheads*). Iliac stent-graft components were utilized as thoracic stent-graft (**C**) with exclusion of the pseudoaneurysm and intentional coverage of the adjacent left subclavian artery. The constricion at the site of the surgically corrected coarctation is still noted (*arrow*). Follow-up sagittal CT angiogram 6 months postprocedure (**D**) shows no filling of the pseudoaneurysm.

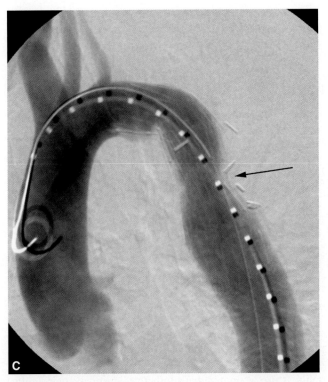

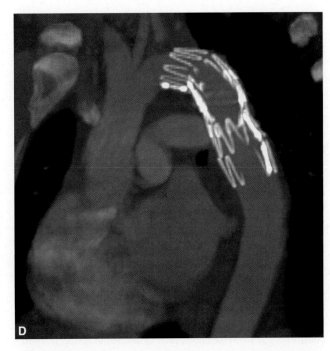

FIGURE 68.4 *(Continued)*

2. Placement of an aortic cuff extension or iliac limb extension used as a " tube" stent-graft in the infrarenal aorta provided there is an adequate proximal landing zone (>15-mm distance from the lowest renal artery) and adequate distal landing zone (>15-mm distance from the aortic bifurcation) where the diameter of the aorta at these zones accommodates the intended stent-grafts.

3. Placement of an aorto-uni-iliac stent-graft, embolization of the contralateral common iliac artery, and performing a surgical femoral-femoral bypass. This method is used if the distal aortic size is small (<15 mm) and there is concern that the distal aorta will not accommodate a bifurcated stent-graft.

It is encouraged to extend the stent-graft coverage of the aortic wall for long segments beyond the area of apparent infection more so than usually applied in noninfected aneurysms. Many authors advocate such modification of the stent-graft implantation technique because of the likelihood of inflammatory changes affecting the aortic wall beyond the area of apparent infection on imaging, which makes such areas prone to formation of pseudoaneurysms, endoleaks, or rupture at the points of contact of the stent-graft with the involved and weakened aortic wall.[35,36]

PROCEDURAL COMPLICATIONS AND HOW TO MANAGE THEM SUCCESSFULLY

The most significant procedure-related complication specific to the endovascular therapy of mycotic aneurysm, para-anastomotic pseudoaneurysm, and aortoduodenal fistula is persistent or recurrent infection. This may present as a local infection with the potential to invade adjacent retroperitoneal structures, such as the psoas muscle or spine, as generalized sepsis, or even as septic embolization.

OUTCOMES/PROGNOSIS

Mycotic Aneurysm

The results from multiple series on endovascular management of infected aneurysms have shown initial clinical success and sustained long-term outcomes. Recent studies compare favorably with the surgical series where the 1-year survival rate for patients with no persistent infection is as high as 94% compared with the 70% 1-year survival rate for traditional surgical management of infected aortic aneurysms. Patients with persistent infection after endovascular aneurysm repair (EVAR) have a much lower 1-year survival at 39%. These results suggest that a successful stent-graft procedure with appropriate control of pre- and postprocedure infection can result in preferable outcome compared to a traditional surgical approach. Several factors have been proposed to explain such preferable outcomes, the most important of which is the proper identification of the causative organism and aggressive antibiotic treatment preprocedure. Kan et al.[12] have shown in their series as well as their review of published data that at least a week-long antibiotic treatment was proven to be a protective measure against early mortality and persistent infection. In fact, obtaining a negative blood culture in hemodynamically stable patients, if possible, is considered a prerequisite to performing the stent-graft procedure by some authors.[25,33] As mentioned earlier, up to 40% of patients will have negative blood cultures at the time of presentation and the risk of infection recurrence is believed to be low in this group. Postoperative antibiotics are a mainstay of treatment and are recommended to be administered parenterally for up to 8 weeks. Many authors recommend a total duration of antibiotic therapy of 3 months but others advocate a lifelong antibiotic therapy.[12,25,33–35,37,38] Antibiotic-coated stent-grafts have also been proposed by some authors, who describe favorable outcomes with such technique.[33] This has not been widely adopted, however.

One other major factor in controlling the infectious process is to perform adjunct procedures, such as percutaneous drainage of infected fluid collections or subsequent surgical debridement of the infected bed. Such measures, although not always required, have been shown to be associated with lower mortality and lower frequency of recurrent persistent infections.

The factors that have been associated with worse mortality rates and higher rates of postprocedure infections included age above 65 years, fever at the time of the procedure, aortic rupture, and the presence of aortoenteric or aortobronchial fistulas (Table 68.1).

Delaying the stent-graft procedure to obtain negative blood cultures is not always feasible, such as in cases of acute GI bleeding from an AEF or presence of aortic rupture. In these cases, stent-graft placement can be considered as a temporizing measure because open surgical repair has been associated with high periprocedure mortality. As mentioned earlier, the presence of such condition where there is frank violation of the aortic wall increases the risk of infections to persist postprocedure. Once the patient's condition is stabilized, definitive surgical repair with in situ graft can be performed.

Anastomotic Pseudoaneurysm

Intervention for anastomotic pseudoaneurysm, whether sterile or infected, is mandatory because mortality rates of 44% secondary to rupture have been reported in patients with untreated anastomotic pseudoaneurysms.[39] It has been established that the incidence of both intra-abdominal (aortic or iliac) and extracavitary (femoral) anastomotic aneurysms increases with time.

Operative mortality rates that have been reported for the repair of pseudoaneurysms in the aortic position are 17% for elective cases and 24% or higher for emergent cases.[27]

Endovascular repair of intra-abdominal or intrathoracic para-anastomotic aneurysms has been reported with 3.8%

perioperative mortality and 49% overall mortality over a mean follow-up of 18 months.[27] Technical success was reported in 52 of 53 patients (98%); endoleaks are thought to occur more commonly following emergent repair.

Aortoenteric Fistula

The standard of practice for open repair of an AEF was initially resection of the infected aorta or graft with ligation of the aortic stump, intestinal repair, and revascularization via an extra-anatomic axillofemoral bypass graft. Operative mortality rates exceeding 50% were common and typically were higher in those for whom this operation was performed for AEF than for graft infection alone. Amputation rates of 25% to 43% were also reported.[9,29] The evolution of sequential (axillofemoral bypass graft immediately followed by debridement) or staged (axillofemoral bypass graft followed 1 to 5 days later or more by debridement) approaches to this procedure yielded lower mortality and amputation rates.

In a recent meta-analysis of reported cases of endovascular treatment of aortoenteric fistulas, decreased 30-day mortality was noted (8.5%) compared to the most reported results of open repair (Table 68.2). A significant number of patients developed recurrent bleeding (19%) or persistent/recurrent sepsis (32%), both of which are associated with increased mortality. It also was noted that adjunctive intestinal repair significantly reduced the combined rate of recurrent bleeding and sepsis (0% vs. 48%). Factors associated with poor outcomes included perioperative sepsis, colon fistula, tube graft placement, no intestinal repair, and recurrent AEF.[40]

■ THE FUTURE

With continued improvement in endovascular devices, the ability to treat most of the inflammatory aortic conditions and anastomotic leaks is now feasible. The stent-graft devices currently used for this application were originally designed to treat noninfectious abdominal aortic aneurysms (AAAs) or thoracic aortic aneurysms (TAAs). Introduction of a wider size range for stent-graft components will allow for more endovascular treatment options. Additionally, the availability of antibiotic-impregnated devices may prove beneficial in limiting recurrent infections. Aortic anastomotic disruptions and infectious pseudoaneurysms located adjacent to branch vessels remain a challenge to treat by endovascular means. The availability and continued development of fenestrated and branched stent-graft components may allow for treatment of such entities.

■ CONCLUSION

Endovascular management of inflammatory aortic conditions including mycotic aneurysms, anastomotic disruptions, and aortoenteric fistulas is increasingly utilized as the primary treatment in patients with uninfected anastomotic disruptions or uncomplicated mycotic aneurysms. Surgical management remains the primary treatment for patients with infected surgical grafts, aortoenteric fistulas, or complicated mycotic aneurysms. Endovascular management can serve as a temporizing measure for this population and function as a bridge to more definitive surgical management.

Table 68.1
Predictors for Postprocedural Mortality and Morbidity
Age >65
Septic shock
Presence of aortoenteric or aortobronchial fistula
Aortic rupture
Fever and leukocytosis at the time of presentation

Table 68.2

Outcomes of Different Management Strategies for Aortoenteric Fistula

Approach	Number of patients	Operative/ 30-day mortality (%)	Limb loss	1-Year survival (%)	Recurrent infection (%)	Recurrent bleeding (%)	Follow-up (months)
Historic axillofemoral bypass[29]	7	43	43	—	43	—	36.8
Staged axillofemoral bypass[29]	57	24–26	11–16	—	16–18	—	36.8
Cryopreserved aortic allograft[31]	56	13	5	75% at average of 5.3 mo	9	9	5.3
NAIS (saphenofemoral vein)[41]	187	10	7.4	52% at 5 y	5	5	32
Rifampin-soaked graft[42]	54	9	0	59% at 5 y	4	—	51
Endovascular (meta-analysis)[40]	59	8.5	—	68	32	19	

REFERENCES

1. Anderson CB, Butcher HR, Ballinger WF. Mycotic aneurysms. *Arch Surg* 1974;109:712–717.
2. Reddy DJ, Ernst CB. Infected aneurysms. In: Rutherford RB, ed. *Vascular Surgery*. 4th ed. Philadelphia, PA: W. B. Saunders; 1995:1139–1153.
3. Parrellada JA, Monill JM, Zidan A, et al. Mycotic aneurysm of the abdominal aorta: CT findings in three patients. *Abdom Imaging* 1997;22:321–324.
4. Muller BT, Wegener OR, Grabitz K, et al. Mycotic aneurysms of the thoracic and abdominal aorta and iliac arteries: experience with anatomic and extraanatomic repair in 33 cases. *J Vasc Surg* 2001;33:106–113.
5. Youkey JR, Clagett PG, Rich NM, et al. Femoral anastomotic false aneurysms. An 11-year experience analyzed with a case-control study. *Ann Surg* 1984;199(6):703–708.
6. Edwards JM, Teefey SA, Zierler RE, et al. Intraabdominal paraanastomotic aneurysms after aortic bypass grafting. *J Vasc Surg* 1992;15(2):344–350.
7. Ylonen K, Biancari F, Leo E, et al. Predictors of development of anastomotic femoral pseudoaneurysms after aortobifemoral reconstruction for abdominal aortic aneurysm. *Am J Surg* 2004;187:83–87.
8. Chaikof EL, Brewster DC, Dalman RL, et al. The care of patients with an abdominal aortic aneurysm: the Society for Vascular Surgery practice guidelines. *J Vasc Surg* 2009;50(suppl 8S):2S–49S.
9. Kashyap VS, O'Hara PJ. Local complications: aortoenteric fistulae. In: Cronenwett J, Johnston JL, eds. *Rutherford's Vascular Surgery*. 7th ed. Philadelphia, PA: W. B. Saunders; 2010.
10. Razavi MK, Razavi MD. Stent-graft treatment of mycotic aneurysms: a review of the current literature. *J Vasc Interv Radiol* 2008;19:S51–S56.
11. Kan CD, Lee HL, Yang YJ. Outcome after endovascular stent graft treatment for mycotic aortic aneurysm: a systematic review. *J Vasc Surg* 2007;46:906–912.
12. Kan CD, Lee HL, Luo CY, et al. The efficacy of aortic stent grafts in the management of mycotic abdominal aortic aneurysm—institute case management with systemic literature comparison. *Ann Vasc Surg* 2010;24:433–440.
13. Corso JE, Kasirajan K, Milner R. Endovascular management of ruptured, mycotic abdominal aortic aneurysm. *Am Surg* 2005;71:515–517.
14. Gonzalez-Fajardo JA, Gutierrez V, Martin-Pedrosa M, et al. Endovascular repair in the presence of aortic infection. *Ann Vasc Surg* 2005;19:94–98.
15. Froeschl M, Wolfsohn A, Beauchesne LM. Ruptured mycotic pseudoaneurysm of the thoracic aorta. *Cardiovasc Pathol* 2006;15:116–118.
16. Nishimoto M, Hasegawa S, Asada K, et al. Stent-graft placement for mycotic aneurysm of the thoracic aorta: report of a case. *Circ J* 2004;68:88–90.
17. Hallett JW Jr, Marshall DM, Petterson TM, et al. Graft-related complications after abdominal aortic aneurysm repair: reassurance from a 36 year population-based experience. *J Vasc Surg* 1997;25(2):277–286.
18. Bianchi P, Nano G, Cusmai F, et al. Uninfected para-anastomotic aneurysms after infrarenal aortic grafting. *Yonsei Med J* 2009;50(2):227–238.

19. Szilagyi DE, Elliot JP Jr, Smith RF, et al. A thirty-year survey of the reconstructive surgical treatment of aortoiliac occlusive disease. *J Vasc Surg* 1986;3(3):421–436.
20. Antoniou GA, Koutsias S, Antoniou SA, et al. Outcome after endovascular stent graft repair of aortoenteric fistula: a systematic review. *J Vasc Surg* 2009;49:782–789.
21. Champion MC, Sullivan SN, Coles JC, et al. Aortoenteric fistula: incidence, presentation, recognition, and management. *Ann Surg* 1982;195(3):314–317.
22. Hsu RB, Chen RJ, Wang SS, et al. Infected aortic aneurysms: clinical outcome and risk factor analysis. *J Vasc Surg* 2004;40:30–35.
23. Oderich GS, Panneton JM, Bower TC, et al. Infected aortic aneurysms: aggressive presentation, complicated early outcome, but durable results. *J Vasc Surg* 2001;34:900–908.
24. Semba CP, Sakai T, Slonim SM, et al. Mycotic aneurysms of the thoracic aorta: repair with use of endovascular stent-grafts. *J Vasc Interv Radiol* 1998;9:33–40.
25. Jones KG, Bell RE, Sabharwal T, et al. Treatment of mycotic aortic aneurysms with endoluminal grafts. *Eur J Vasc Endovasc Surg* 2005;29:139–144.
26. Mulder EJ, van Bockel JH, Maas J, et al. Morbidity and mortality of reconstructive surgery of noninfected false aneurysms detected long after aortic prosthetic reconstruction. *Arch Surg* 1998;133:45–49.
27. Sachdev U, Baril DT, Morrissey NJ, et al. Endovascular repair of paraanastomotic aortic aneurysms. *J Vasc Surg* 2007;46:636–641.
28. Calligaro KD, Veith FJ, Yuan JG, et al. Intra-abdominal aortic graft infection: complete or partial graft preservation in patients at very high risk. *J Vasc Surg* 2003;38(6):1199–1205.
29. Reilly LM, Stoney RJ, Goldstone J, et al. Improved management of aortic graft infection: the influence of operation sequence staging. *J Vasc Surg* 1987;5:421–431.
30. Oderich GS, Bower TC, Cherry KJ Jr, et al. Evolution from axillofemoral to in situ prosthetic reconstruction for the treatment of aortic graft infections at a single center. *J Vasc Surg* 2006;43(6):1166–1174.
31. Noel AA, Gloviczki P, Cherry KJ Jr, et al. Abdominal aortic reconstruction in infected fields: early results of the United States Cryopreserved Aortic Allograft Registry. *J Vasc Surg* 2002;35(5):847–852.
32. Clagett GP, Valentine RJ, Hagino RT. Autogenous aortoiliac/femoral reconstruction from superficial femoral-popliteal veins: feasibility and durability. *J Vasc Surg* 1997;25:255–266.
33. Ting AC, Cheng SW, Ho P, et al. Endovascular stent graft repair for infected thoracic aortic pseudoaneurysms—a durable option? *J Vasc Surg* 2006;44:701–705.
34. Lee KH, Won JY, Lee do Y, et al. Stent-graft treatment of infected aortic and arterial aneurysms. *J Endovasc Ther* 2006;13:338–345.
35. Ishida M, Kato N, Hirano T, et al. Limitations of endovascular treatment with stent-grafts for active mycotic thoracic aortic aneurysm. *Cardiovasc Intervent Radiol* 2002;25:216–218.

36. Kaufman JA, Song HK, Ham BB, et al. Traumatic thoracic aortic transection in small-diameter aortas: percutaneous endograft repair. *J Vasc Interv Radiol* 2007;18(11):1429–1433.

37. Luo CY, Ko WC, Kan CD, et al. In situ reconstruction of septic aortic pseudoaneurysm due to *Salmonella* or *Streptococcus* microbial aortitis: long-term follow-up. *J Vasc Surg* 2003;38:975–982.

38. Sayed S, Choke E, Helme S, et al. Endovascular stent graft repair of mycotic aneurysms of the thoracic aorta. *J Cardiovasc Surg* 2005;46:155–161.

39. Mulder EJ, van Bockel H, Maas J, et al. Morbidity and mortality of reconstructive surgery of noninfected false aneurysms detected long after aortic prosthetic reconstruction. *Arch Surg* 1998;133:45–59.

40. Kakkos SK, Papadoulas S, Tsolakis IA. Endovascular management of arterioenteric fistulas: a systemic review and meta-analysis of the literature. *J Endovasc Ther* 2011;18(1):66–77.

41. Ali AT, Modrall JG, Hocking J, et al. Long-term results of the treatment of aortic graft infection by in situ replacement with femoral popliteal vein grafts. *J Vasc Surg* 2009;50(1):30–39.

42. Oderich GS, Bower TC, Hofer J, et al. In situ rifampin-soaked grafts with omental coverage and antibiotic suppression are durable with low reinfection rates in patients with aortic graft enteric erosion or fistula. *J Vasc Surg* 2011;53(1):99–106.

Traumatic Arterial Injuries

Aortic Injuries

NAVEED U. SAQIB, RABIH A. CHAER, and MICHEL S. MAKAROUN

INTRODUCTION

Aortic trauma can result from penetrating, blunt, or iatrogenic injuries. Each is associated with a different mechanism of injury and with a variable degree of surrounding organ and tissue damage as well as a different extent of aortic wall damage. In this chapter, aortic injuries and their treatment are broadly classified and discussed based on the injured segment and mechanism of injury.

TRAUMATIC THORACIC AORTIC INJURY

Traumatic thoracic aortic injury (TAI) is a highly lethal condition.[1] Its most common form, traumatic transection, has been implicated as the second most common cause of death in trauma patients. It is estimated that approximately one-fifth of all deaths from motor vehicle collisions result from TAI and is surpassed only by 60% of deaths caused by intracranial hemorrhage. More than 80% of patients with this condition usually die at the accident scene, and of those who survive to reach a hospital, one-third die of their aortic injury early in their hospital course.[2] Prompt diagnosis and treatment are therefore critical.

The sudden deceleration associated with blunt trauma creates a shear force between a relatively mobile part of the aorta and the adjacent fixed segment of the descending thoracic aorta.[3] This shear force causes a transverse tear in the aortic wall, ranging from partial tear in the intima to complete transection.[3] The most common location for thoracic aortic transection is the descending aorta just distal to the left subclavian artery at the aortic isthmus. Parmley et al.[1] reported that 50% to 71% of lesions occur at the isthmus, 18% in the ascending aorta, and 14% in the distal aorta. The most common mechanisms of injury include motor vehicle collisions (68%), followed by motorcycle accidents (13%), falls from height (7.3%), auto versus pedestrian (6.3%), and other blunt mechanisms (5.7%).[6]

TAI typically affects young (mean age 40) males (75%)[4,5] and is highly associated with multisystem trauma including head, facial, thoracic, abdominal, pelvic, and extremity injuries.[6] The most common presenting symptom is interscapular or retrosternal pain, but it is seen in only one-fourth of patients because many of them have associated closed head injury or other factors that make a clinical diagnosis difficult. Routine helical computed tomographic angiogram (CTA) of the mediastinum in blunt trauma patients with severe deceleration injury has resulted in early and frequent diagnosis of TAI.[7,8] Despite high suspicion and advances in imaging technology, however, TAI remains undiagnosed in 1% to 2% of the cases at the time of injury because some patients present months later with *chronic traumatic pseudoaneurysms*.[1] Chronic traumatic aortic pseudoaneurysms are usually localized, calcified, saccular in appearance, and located distal to the left subclavian artery. Approximately

half of these patients will develop symptoms within 5 years, including one-third who will die of rupture or other complications, if untreated.[10]

Acute rupture or expansion of the hematoma associated with TAI usually presents with worsening midscapular back pain, unexplained hypotension, upper extremity hypertension, bilateral femoral pulse deficits, or initial chest tube output in excess of 750 mL.[11] A high index of suspicion is required because the patients usually have other injuries that may mask the acute nature of the problem.

Penetrating injuries to the ascending thoracic aorta are commonly caused by stab wounds. Gunshot wounds, on the other hand, can cause injury to any portion of the aorta but more commonly involve the descending portion of the thoracic aorta. Most patients with penetrating injuries present with hemodynamic instability and require emergent repair of the aortic tear and other associated injuries.

Diagnostic Modalities

The management of TAI has undergone major changes in the last decade and has resulted in early diagnosis and treatment.

Chest roentgenographic (CXR) signs (FIGURE 69.1) suggestive of TAI include widened paratracheal stripe, deviation of the nasogastric tube or central venous pressure line, blurring of the aortic knob, abnormal paraspinous stripe, apical capping, and rightward tracheal deviation. Mediastinal widening of greater than 8 cm has 92% sensitivity but a low specificity of 10% in diagnosing TAI.[11] In the past, these radiologic signs were indications for angiographic evaluation in hemodynamically stable patients. TAI may be present even in the absence of mediastinal abnormality on chest radiography. In a review of 52 articles with 656 patients with aortic or brachiocephalic artery injuries, the mediastinum was normal in 7.3% of the patients.[12] In another multicenter study of 274 patients with traumatic aortic rupture, Fabian et al.[2] reported similar findings.

Aortography (FIGURE 69.2) was considered as the gold standard for diagnosis for many years in patients with blunt trauma and a high suspicion of TAI. It has several drawbacks, however, which include the invasive, time-consuming nature and associated expense and resource utilization, along with a rather low yield. Routine use of angiography may overwhelm busy trauma centers, interfere with the care of other patients, and present a potential risk for a severe multitrauma patient away from the optimal environment of the resuscitation room, the intensive care unit (ICU), or the operating room. Because of these concerns, most centers practiced a policy of selective angiographic evaluation based on the mechanism of injury and chest radiographic findings, which has a significant risk of missing aortic injuries.

Aortography has largely been replaced by helical computed tomographic (CT) scan for the evaluation of the thoracic aorta in

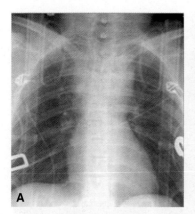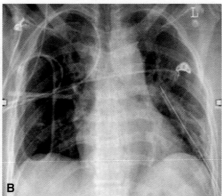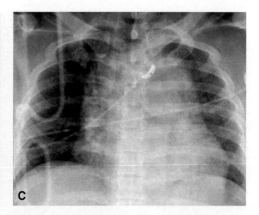

FIGURE 69.1 Chest radiographs revealing radiologic signs of traumatic thoracic aortic transection: widening of paratracheal stripe (**A**), blurring of aortic knob (**B**), and widened mediastinum (**C**).

settings of blunt trauma.[8] The development of helical CT scans in the early 1990s has revolutionized imaging for trauma with its speed and superior definition. Its ubiquitous presence in most emergency departments and trauma centers also provides rapid and complete diagnostic evaluation of the polytrauma-injured patient. The ability to perform three-dimensional reconstructions has further enhanced the diagnostic value of the helical CT scans for aortic assessment. Fabian et al.[13] conducted a comparative prospective study, which concluded the sensitivity, specificity, accuracy, positive predictive value, and negative predictive value of helical CT scan to be 100%, 83%, 86%, 50%, and 100%,

respectively, higher than reported with angiography. Currently, it is recommended that all patients with severe deceleration injury undergo helical CT scan to screen for TAI. Absence of CT findings indicative of TAI is sufficient to exclude the diagnosis with no further testing required. A repeat CT scan for indeterminate findings can be performed after the patient is stable from other injuries.[14] CT scans are also particularly helpful in preoperative planning of thoracic endovascular aneurysm repair (TEVAR), allowing accurate measurements of important anatomic details at the landing zones as well as the access vessels (FIGURE 69.3).

Transesophageal echocardiography (TEE) provides high-quality imaging of different cardiac and vascular structures with speed, low risk of complications, and ability to perform at the patient's bedside and even in the emergency department. Because of these advantages TEE has also emerged as a potential additional valuable diagnostic tool. Some authors have proposed TEE as a routine frontline examination for screening for TAI during the initial evaluation of severe trauma patients involved in severe deceleration blunt injuries to rule out TAI. Because of limited access and operator dependability, however, TEE has not been widely used.[15] A systematic review conducted by Cinnella et al.[16] of seven studies with 758 patients revealed a maximum joint sensitivity and specificity of TEE of 97%, which corresponds to a false-positive and false-negative rate of 3%. TEE can also be used intraoperatively to guide endovascular stent-graft placement.

Intravascular ultrasound (IVUS) has also been described and used as an intraoperative adjunct to localize the extent of the injury and for precise stent-graft placement during TEVAR and for further evaluation of injury in indeterminate TAI.

SPECTRUM AND CLASSIFICATION OF THORACIC AORTIC INJURY

The severity of TAI ranges from intimal flap, hematoma, dissection, transaction, and pseudoaneurysm to free rupture. Based on imaging, Azzizadeh et al.[17] proposed a classification scheme for TAI based on the severity of injury. TAI is classified in four categories, grades I through IV, in severity. Grade I represents an *intimal tear*; grade II, *intramural hematoma*; grade III, *aortic pseudoaneurysm*; and grade IV, *free rupture*.

FIGURE 69.2 Traumatic aortic injury just distal to the left subclavian artery identified on an arch aortogram.

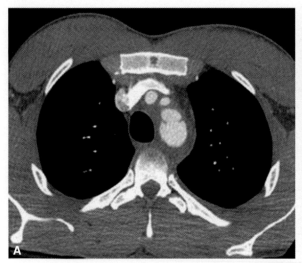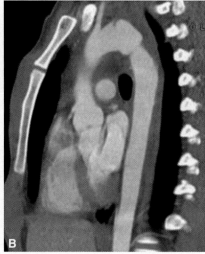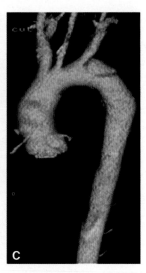

FIGURE 69.3 Helical contrast-enhanced CT angiogram facilitates the diagnosis and preoperative planning of TAI repair by presenting anatomic information in multiple planes. In addition to the standard axial image (**A**), coronal, sagittal (**B**), and 3D reconstructive views are now routinely created (**C**).

TREATMENT

Open Surgical Repair

Traditional open surgical repair (OR) of TAI involves a high left posterolateral thoracotomy, single lung ventilation, systemic anticoagulation with heparin, and aortic cross clamping. Depending on the degree and extent of the injury, the injured segment of the descending thoracic aorta is either replaced with an interposition graft or repaired primarily. The clamp and sew technique and surgical adjuncts (Gott shunt, partial left heart bypass and cardiopulmonary bypass) have been utilized but they are associated with significant postoperative mortality and morbidity including a significant risk of paraplegia.

Surgical repair has also been historically offered to patients with chronic traumatic thoracic pseudoaneurysm presenting with symptoms or aortic expansion on follow-up.[10] This repair is reported to be associated with 4% to 17% operative mortality and a 1% to 5% risk of paraplegia.[23]

Medical Management

Medical management with blood pressure control and interval imaging has been used to prioritize and address treatment of other visceral injuries and, in some cases of minimal injury, as the only method of management. Nonoperative options have a significant incidence of rupture, estimated to occur in 30% of patients with others remaining stable over time. These patients as well as those with unrecognized transections may present with late pseudoaneurysms at the isthmus, providing support for medical management in certain clinical situations with severe associated trauma and low-grade aortic injuries.

Endovascular Repair

TEVAR is a rapidly evolving therapy for the treatment of a variety of thoracic aortic pathology. Although TEVAR has only been approved and developed for the treatment of degenerative aneurysmal disease, applications for other pathologies including dissections and transections are emerging. TEVAR involves placement of an endovascular stent-graft under imaging guidance into the thoracic aorta by accessing the femoral or iliac arteries (FIGURE 69.4).

TEVAR allows definitive repair without the morbidity of a thoracotomy, aortic cross clamping, and cardiopulmonary bypass. It can be performed rapidly and even percutaneously under local anesthesia and often without systemic anticoagulation. It simplifies the management of the multisystem-trauma and critically ill patients who previously might not have tolerated open repair.

Comparative Analysis of Outcomes in Different Treatment Modalities for Thoracic Aortic Injury

Historically, open repair of traumatic aortic injuries has been associated with a 28% mortality rate and a 16% paraplegia rate.[18] A study conducted by the American Association for the Surgery of Trauma (AAST$_1$) in 1997 reflecting outcomes in 50 major trauma centers in the United States reported a mortality rate of 15% with open repair. Paraplegia rates of approximately 16% with the clamp and sew technique were only reduced to 8.2% with the variety of adjunct temporary bypass procedures.[2]

The clinical experience of large-volume trauma centers and the addition of technical adjuncts have played a pivotal role in diminishing paraplegia rates but not operative mortality.[19,20] The presence of associated nonaortic injuries also causes difficulties with conventional open repair. About one-fifth of patients have associated thoracic and cervical spine fractures that make proper positioning difficult. The use of systemic heparin may aggravate intracranial hemorrhage, solid organ bleeding, and blood loss from extremities and associated fractures. Delaying aortic repair in those patients who otherwise would not tolerate immediate surgery used to be the only alternative[22] option, and when applied judiciously actually did improve the survival in selected

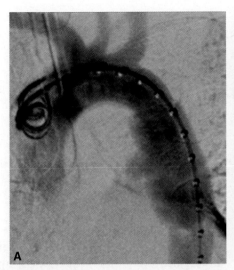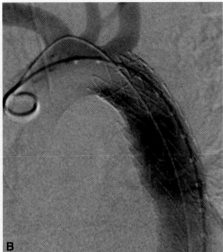

FIGURE 69.4 Thoracic endovascular repair of traumatic thoracic aortic transection (**A**) by deployment of a TAG thoracic aortic stent-graft (**B**).

cases.[21,22] This delay, however, comes at a cost; some patients with untreated transection do progress to exsanguination before undergoing repair. Delay of definitive repair is associated with a high 6.7% risk of rupture and mortality in this subset of patients.[2]

Kato et al.[9] and Semba et al.[24] reported their initial experience with homemade aortic endografts in the treatment of acute TAI. The early reports of success highlighted that treatment strategy of TEVAR can be performed with a low mortality rate and decreased paraplegia rate. This was followed by multiple more recent series[68–71] documenting the high technical success and low mortality and morbidity rates associated with TEVAR.

The American Association for the Surgery of Trauma sponsored a prospective multicenter trial conducted over a period of 26 months between 2005 and 2007 (AAST$_2$)[6] and demonstrated changing therapeutic practices and outcomes in TAI in the United States. AAST$_2$ was conducted in 18 centers and included 193 patients as compared to 274 patients in AAST$_1$.

A review by the American Association for the Surgery of Trauma comparing AAST$_1$ and AAST$_2$ summarized the status of TEVAR use for traumatic aortic transections in late 2007. The review found a relentless trend to replace open aortic repair with TEVAR; it cited a 1997 study showing that two-thirds of all patients with transection in 2007 in the United States were then being managed with TEVAR with significantly decreased mortality and paraplegia rates. The mortality rate, after exclusion of patients presenting in extremis or treated nonoperatively, was 22% (53 of 241) AAST$_1$ and 13% (25 of 193) in AAST$_2$ ($p = .02$). Murad et al.[25] conducted a systematic review commissioned by the Society for Vascular Surgery (SVS) to compare the effectiveness of different modalities for the treatment of patients with TAI. This systematic review of 7,768 patients included 139 previously published studies. The outcomes and effectiveness of nonoperative, open aortic repair (OR), or endovascular repair (TEVAR) were compared. Nonoperative management was associated with the highest mortality rate (46%) and TEVAR with the lowest (9%), whereas open repair had a mortality of 19%. No difference in stroke rates was noted between groups. Compared with the open approach, TEVAR was also associated with lower rates of spinal cord ischemia (SCI), end-stage renal disease, and systemic and graft infections. The endovascular options, however, were associated with a trend for more secondary procedures.

Based on that review[25] and utilization of Grading of Recommendations Assessment, Development, and Evaluation (GRADE) methods, the SVS recommends endovascular repair for TAI.[26] In developing the specific recommendation as a practice guideline that endovascular repair should be performed preferentially over open surgical repair or nonoperative management, the committee placed a significantly higher value on preventing catastrophic complications of thoracic aortic repair (death, stroke, and SCI) and a lower value on potential adverse events, such as endoleaks, need for reintervention, and device failures. The committee also placed less value on possible late-term outcomes that remain unknown at this time. Furthermore, the committee acknowledged the off-label use of a medical device in the context of endovascular repair of TAI, which was tolerated, given the mortality advantage associated with TEVAR.

Limitations of Endovascular Repair

The lack of endografts designed specifically for TAI presents some concerns because the application of a technology to clinical entities not part of preclinical testing and stress analysis raises durability and performance issues. Younger patients experiencing TAI have smaller and more elastic aortas when compared to patients with degenerative aneurysmal disease. A tight arch distal to the left subclavian artery presents challenges in proper stent-graft positioning to achieve exclusion of the injury. The lack of inner curve apposition in these aortas may be associated with serious complications, such as graft collapse.[38] Smaller iliac arteries may also prevent the introduction of the larger sheaths necessary for large endografts. The most challenging question, however, remains the issue of ongoing follow-up after TEVAR with radiographic imaging that might prove to be burdensome in this young population, exposing them to the risks of radiation for a prolonged period along with possible late device failures.

Despite all the potential drawbacks of TEVAR in transection, its application has been spreading because of its perceived benefits. Early reports clearly suggested that this approach to the treatment of transection is a safer alternative to open repair.

THE UPMC EXPERIENCE IN THE TREATMENT OF THORACIC AORTIC INJURY

We performed the first TEVAR in our institution for a patient with a chronic traumatic thoracic aortic pseudoaneurysm in 1999 and our first acute TAI case in 2004. The last open procedure for traumatic transection was in January 2007 after which all TAI cases were treated with TEVAR.

We have treated 90 patients (69 males, mean age 39.2 years, range 16 to 84) with TAI between January 1999 and January 2011. The most common cause of injury was motor vehicle accident (86.5%). Of these patients, 41 underwent open repair (OR) and 49 underwent TEVAR. There was no significant difference between the two groups in baseline characteristics (age, gender) and injury severity score (ISS). Mortality rate was significantly higher in the OR group (8/42, 19.5%) when compared to the TEVAR group (3/46, 6.1%). Pulmonary complications were similar (28/41, 68.3% vs. 27/49, 55.1%). A trend toward a shorter stay in the ICU and shorter periods of ventilator dependence was observed among patients who underwent TEVAR. Two patients (4.7%) developed paraplegia after OR compared with none after TEVAR.

In 49 patients treated with TEVAR, 37 were treated with commercially available thoracic stent-grafts (TSGs) and 12 patients were treated with a series of stacked proximal aortic extension cuffs (AECs). Two patients developed a puncture site pseudoaneurysm, one with a retroperitoneal hematoma. Ten stent-graft–related complications occurred in eight patients (16.3%). All of these occurred before 2008 and were associated with the use of a TSG related to poor apposition to the lesser curve of the aortic arch. Two occurred within 30 days of the procedure and the rest (six) occurred later. Four patients required secondary

TEVAR for TSG collapse. Conversion to OR was performed in a total of four patients. Three had already undergone secondary TEVAR. The indications for open conversion in this subgroup of patients included an aortoesophageal fistula, recurrent collapse, and physiologic aortic coarctation. In two patients open conversion was done without a secondary TEVAR. The indication for conversion in these patients was graft impingement on the left common carotid artery based on duplex ultrasound and neurologic symptoms. There were no deaths in the patients who underwent open conversion.

Since 2008, we modified our endovascular approach and have preferentially used AEC instead of TSG (FIGURE 69.5). There have been no instances of graft collapse or need for open conversion in this subset of patients.

SPECIFIC CONSIDERATIONS FOR THORACIC ENDOVASCULAR ANEURYSM REPAIR IN THORACIC AORTIC INJURY

Management of Different TAI Categories

Expectant management with serial imaging for type I injuries in TAI is recommended. This is based on early evidence that most type I injuries heal spontaneously. The decision to intervene and its timing should be guided by progression of the initial radiographic abnormality and/or symptoms.[17] Types II to IV injuries should all be repaired. Patients with type IV TAI usually succumb to the injury and may not survive to the emergency department.

Timing of TEVAR in TAI

Hemodynamically unstable patients who have no other source of obvious bleeding should undergo emergent repair. These patients should undergo urgent (<24 hours) repair barring other serious concomitant nonaortic injuries, or immediate repair after other injuries have been treated or stabilized, but at the latest prior to hospital discharge. This is consistent with the available

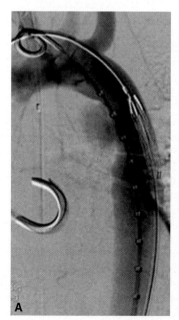
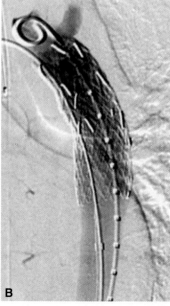

FIGURE 69.5 TEVAR for traumatic thoracic aortic transection (**A**) using proximal Excluder aortic extension cuffs (AECs) (**B**).

evidence in which mortality was 46% in those managed nonoperatively. As mentioned previously, expectant management with follow-up imaging is appropriate.

Murad et al.[25] reported that the lag time between aortic injury and performing the endovascular or open procedure correlated with improved survival, suggesting both ecologic and survival biases.

Choice of Endograft

There are three commercially available thoracic endografts: TX2 (Cook, Bloomington, IN), TAG (W. L. Gore, Flagstaff, AZ), and Talent (Medtronic, Santa Rosa, CA). These endografts have been tested and approved for safety and efficacy in clinical trials for thoracic aneurysmal disease. Although none of the current devices was designed for the treatment of TAI, off-label use is common despite previously mentioned limitations. There are other ongoing clinical trials investigating the safety and efficacy of TEVAR using modified devices designed to overcome the shortcomings of current endografts when used for TAI.[17]

Most modifications used pertain to device conformability and diameter. The currently available thoracic endograft sizes mostly reflect the larger aortic diameters that would be typically encountered in an older cohort with degenerative aneurysms. The aortic diameters are relatively smaller in the younger subset of trauma patients. Excessive oversizing has been implicated with endoleak, device infolding, endograft collapse, and even death from acute aortic occlusion.[31] There is no consensus regarding the optimal oversizing for TAI cases, and opinions were equally divided among minimal to no oversizing, 5% to 10% oversizing, and standard oversizing per manufacturer's recommendations.

Aortic Extension Cuffs

We have switched to the preferential use of abdominal AECs in the treatment of TAI because we reported better adaptation of the anatomy by short segments and better apposition to both aortic curvatures near the subclavian artery.[29]

Inability of thoracic endografts to conform to the thoracic aortic curvature can result in device malaposition, which can lead to endoleak and endograft collapse.[27] AECs have been used as an alternative to overcome such anatomic limitations. Although use of AECs helps in obtaining better conformation to the contour of the thoracic aortic arch, it has potential drawbacks. These devices may not reach the site of injury from a femoral access due to the short delivery system, necessitating either use of a longer makeshift delivery system or access through a more proximal site, typically the distal external iliac artery that can be exposed under the inguinal ligament. Additionally, AECs are typically short, therefore necessitating the use of multiple overlapping pieces. Such an intercalating construction allows slightly improved conformation to the arch but at the same time introduces multiple junctions with a potential for a type 3 endoleak.

Next-Generation Thoracic Devices

A number of next-generation devices are presently undergoing clinical trials that may address some of the unmet needs of TEVAR for TAI. Cook (Bloomington, IN) recently introduced the TX2 Proform delivery system, which is intended to improve arch conformability, and is introducing TX2 LP (low profile) in the near future, which will decrease the profile of the delivery catheter and broaden the range of available diameters. Medtronic

(Santa Rosa, CA) will introduce Valiant thoracic endograft with the Captivia delivery system, which should enhance the stability and reliability of the deployment mechanism. W. L. Gore (Flagstaff, AZ) recently finished enrollment in a clinical trial for TAI, testing its conformable C-TAG device with which preliminary experience outside the United States appears to show improved arch conformability and greater tolerance to device oversizing.

Anatomic Considerations

There are several fundamental differences in the anatomic morphology between patients with atherosclerotic thoracic aortic aneurysm and traumatic aortic injuries that may have an impact on the choice of endograft devices and deployment techniques.[31]

The main anatomic challenges for TEVAR in the treatment of TAI are the small aortic diameter and small access vessels in younger victims. The mean aortic diameters adjacent to an aortic injury are reported to be 19.3 mm.[35] This normally requires smaller endografts that are typically used for aneurysmal applications. Small access vessels may theoretically require a retroperitoneal access with creation of iliac artery conduits for passage of 20 to 21 French introducer sheaths for TSG. This is important to avoid additional iliac injuries. We have not yet encountered any patients who required such proximal access because of vessel size, however. The soft distensible nature of these arteries with a very short indwelling time for the sheaths has allowed rather uniform femoral access in the cases we have treated.

The proximal landing zone is critical and is generally near the left subclavian artery because of the location of TAI. A rapid decision must be made whether to cover the subclavian artery or not and whether a prophylactic carotid-subclavian bypass is required. Those decisions follow established criteria with aneurysmal disease, namely, the need to maintain forward vertebrobasilar flow through at least one vertebral artery. Although it is reported that 30% of TAI cases require left subclavian artery coverage, we have not found that to be the case.[32] A complicating factor in these patients is the difficulty of evaluating the exact landing zone length distal to the left subclavian artery because of the surrounding hematoma on CT scan. The standard 2 cm landing zone also may not be necessary in all these cases with relatively healthy aortas that are not usually completely severed circumferentially. As such, we currently do not believe that subclavian coverage is needed in most patients and have only used it in five of ours and mostly earlier in our experience. We currently attempt to reach only the distal ostium of the left subclavian artery, which facilitates the procedure and decreases the problem of poor apposition to the lesser curve of the arch. The distal landing zone, on the other hand, is usually not a critical factor because the long segment of the normal descending thoracic aorta is more than sufficient to permit proper device fixation.

Choice of Repair in a Young Patient

The anatomic suitability is important for TEVAR but age should not be a factor in deciding the modality of repair. It has been demonstrated that the risks of death and SCI are significantly lower in all age groups after TEVAR compared with open surgery, and that these early benefits outweigh the concerns of potential late complications. We currently preferentially perform TEVAR in TAI in our institution for all patients. Our experience so far indicates that open surgical conversion for endograft complications at a later date has lower complications in an elective situation and is well tolerated. TEVAR may therefore serve in these cases as a bridge to a later elective open repair, and this should not be considered a failure of the technique.

Systemic Anticoagulation

The decision to administer systemic anticoagulation must be individualized based on the balance of the perceived risks of bleeding in a particular organ system versus the thromboembolic complications. The safety of systemic anticoagulation using heparin during endovascular repair in a multitrauma patient with a closed head injury or abdominal solid organ injury is a controversial issue.

Most of the SVS review committee[17] indicated that they routinely use systemic heparin but at a lower dose than in elective TEVAR. A minority opinion was expressed that heparin may not be necessary because most of these cases can be performed relatively rapidly and the risk of a thrombotic event is likely small if performed via a percutaneous approach.[33] Should that approach be chosen, care must be taken to flush the sheaths regularly and perform the procedure expeditiously, which can usually be done in less than 15 minutes of indwelling sheath time.

Spinal Drainage

Spinal drainage has been the mainstay of management of SCI after endovascular or open repair of thoracic or thoracoabdominal aneurysms. The issue of prophylactic spinal drainage with TEVAR is controversial even for treatment of degenerative thoracic aneurysms. We have not used it at all in our TAI patients because the incidence of SCI in these cases is very low (3%).[25] Additionally, the proximal location of the injury, the limited coverage of the thoracic aorta, and the risk of epidural hematoma in a coagulopathic patient present serious drawbacks to this prophylactic maneuver. The SVS recommendation is that spinal drainage not routinely used in TAI was unanimous, suggesting that its use be restricted to symptoms of SCI.[26]

Choice of Anesthesia (General Versus Regional Versus Local)

It is possible to perform TEVAR under local anesthesia, especially if using a percutaneous approach. Unreliable cooperation of an agitated trauma patient and the presence of concomitant injuries, however, may make local anesthesia less favorable. We use local anesthesia in these cases very selectively and only in patients where airway management is not a major problem. Regional anesthesia may not be practical in the trauma setting, therefore favoring the use of general anesthesia.

Considerations for Gaining Access

Percutaneous TEVAR using suture-mediated closure devices can be performed safely with very low rates of early and late limb or life-threatening events.[34] We preferentially use femoral access and favor a percutaneous approach with the use of closure devices (Prostar XL, Abbott Vascular, Santa Clara, CA) given the fact that most trauma patients have noncalcified access vessels.

In emergent settings, percutaneous access can also facilitate the expeditious insertion of the endograft by obviating the need for surgical exposure of the femoral artery. We believe that this technique may allow a more rapid endograft delivery and repair in a hemodynamically unstable patient.[33,34] In this case we differ from the SVS committee recommendations to favor open femoral exposure to minimize potentially avoidable complications related to percutaneous closure of large-bore access sites.[26]

Adjunctive Maneuvers to Facilitate Endograft Placement in Complex Cases

Several adjunctive endovascular techniques have been described that may facilitate the deployment of a TSG in difficult cases and can be used for TAI as well as for aneurysmal disease. These include concomitant brachial artery access, femoral artery guide wire placement, controlled hypotension, and transient asystole induced pharmacologically or by rapid ventricular pacing. We typically have not found the need to use any of these techniques in most TAI cases.[36,37,65,66]

Follow-Up Strategy

Yearly follow-up imaging leads to the concerns of cumulative radiation, iodinated contrast exposure, and the late endograft-related complications; hence the optimal strategy for long-term follow-up of these patients post-TEVAR is still in evolution. The opinions on frequency and types of imaging to be utilized remain varied.[26] In the absence of any abnormalities on imaging (i.e., stable endograft position, no endoleak) in the first 12 to 36 months, some have suggested decreasing the frequency to 2 to 5 years, whereas others have expressed that, lacking any evidence to the contrary, follow-up for TAI should be no different than for those treated with TEVAR for other pathologies. The combination of multiview chest X-ray and a magnetic resonance angiography (MRA) may be preferred over conventional contrast CTA for long-term imaging with due consideration of the metallic composition of the endograft.[26]

Early and Late Complications

Death, paraplegia (SCI), stroke, end-stage renal disease, graft infection, and access site complications are known early complications. Device-related late complications include endoleak, stent-graft collapse, physiologic coarctation of the aorta, stent-graft migration, dynamic obstruction of the left subclavian artery or left common carotid artery, erosion through the aortic wall, and aortoenteric fistula.

In the recent meta-analysis by Murad et al.,[25] secondary interventions were required in 83 patients (5.4%). The most common indications for secondary interventions were *endoleak* (50, 60%), *stent-graft collapse* (9, 11%), intraoperative rupture (2, 2%), iliac artery injury (1, 1%), and penetration of metal stent (1, 1%); the remaining 20 (25%) were described as device-related failures that required secondary intervention. Of the 50 endoleaks reported in literature, only 15 were specifically described as type 1 endoleak, and the rest were nonspecified. The outcomes of the 50 endoleaks were only described in 13 patients. One was treated with coil embolization, two resolved spontaneously, five required open conversion, and five required placement of additional cuffs.

In our series, device-related complications, such as graft collapse, physiologic aortic coarctation, stent migration, and subclavian coverage requiring reintervention, were found in eight

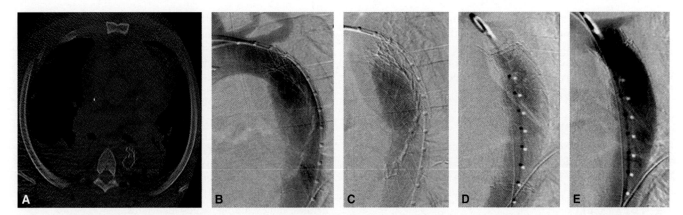

FIGURE 69.6 Thoracic stent-graft collapse. Diagnosis is made by CT of the chest (**A**), confirmed by aortography (**B, C**), followed by successful treatment with secondary TEVAR (**D, E**).

patients. We observed five incidences of graft collapse (8.6%), which is similar to previous reports ranging from 0.03% to 10%. Collapse was detected at 1, 4, 20, 36 weeks, and 3 years[28] postoperatively from the initial graft placement and were treated with a secondary TEVAR (FIGURE 69.6) placement of an additional TSG or by open conversion.[38]

Physiologic aortic coarctation, as previously described by our group, is caused by protrusion of the TSG into the aortic arch without stent infolding.[29] This is an infrequent phenomenon but can be life threatening.[30] Patients present with symptoms of proximal hypertension, left upper extremity ischemia, or left carotid or vertebral insufficiency. Obstruction of the left subclavian artery and left common carotid artery has been shown to occur when the ostium is partially obstructed. These can be treated by additional stent placement in the left subclavian artery or the left common carotid artery or by carotid-subclavian or right carotid-carotid bypass surgery. In a younger fit patient, conversion to open repair with stent-graft explanation may be a more durable option.

Erosion of the aortic wall and aortoesophageal fistula can occur as well, and this necessitates open conversion and TSG explantation. Secondary infection in TSGs in patients treated for TAI has not been reported. Heyer et al.[64] reported a 4.77% (5/105 TEVAR) incidence of secondary stent-graft infections. One of the five patients underwent endograft removal and reconstruction using a rifampin-impregnated Dacron graft. The remaining four patients were treated medically; one patient survived and was placed in hospice care, two died of rupture of the mycotic aneurysm, and one died of multiorgan system failure.

The above-mentioned findings underscore the importance of lifelong follow-up for the early diagnosis and treatment of such potentially fatal complications.

▌ TRAUMATIC ABDOMINAL AORTIC INJURY

The abdominal aorta is the second most common injured vessel in the setting of abdominal vascular injury. In a review of 302 abdominal vascular injuries, the aorta was involved in 63 cases (21%) followed by inferior vena caval injuries (25%).[44] The most common cause of abdominal aortic injury (AAI) is penetrating trauma. AAI was reported in 33 patients from a series of 1,218 injuries (2.7%) with abdominal gunshot wounds.[42] The incidence

of AAI in stab wounds is lower and is reported to be at 1.5% (8 out of 529 patients).[42]

Blunt injury to the abdominal aorta is extremely rare. The incidence of blunt AAI is reported to be 0.04% of all blunt trauma admission or 0.07% of patients with an ISS greater than 15.[39] Motor vehicle collisions account for 50% of these cases. Direct blows to the abdomen, falls from height, and explosions are responsible for the rest of the cases. Thoracolumbar spine fractures and seat-belt injuries are associated with high risk for blunt aortic injuries of the abdominal aorta.[41]

Clinical Presentation

Most patients with major abdominal vascular injuries die at the scene. The clinical presentation depends on the mechanism of the injury, the specific type of injury, the presence of free intraperitoneal hemorrhage or retroperitoneal hematoma, the time lag since the injury, and the presence of other associated injuries.

The presentation of penetrating AAIs is usually dramatic. Of the patients presenting to a trauma room, about 28% have non-recordable blood pressure and 21% undergo emergency resuscitative thoracotomy.[45] In approximately one-fifth of the cases there is temporary tamponade by the retroperitoneum.[46] These patients may present with hemodynamic stability on admission only to decompensate a few minutes later.

Similar to TAIs, on rare occasions, initially missed AAIs can manifest as future pseudo-aneurysms or aortocaval fistulas. Blunt injuries may often be missed on initial examination or even during the initial hospitalization, unless they are associated with significant bleeding or early ischemic changes. Mesenteric, renal, or extremity ischemia can occur depending on the location of the injury. It is reported that in 33% of patients with blunt aortic trauma, the diagnosis may be made months to years from the initial injury.[47]

Diagnostic Modalities

Because of the critical condition and need for immediate laparotomy most of the patients with AAIs from penetrating injuries do not need investigative studies. In hemodynamically stable patients with gunshot wounds, radiographic evaluation of the chest and abdomen might assist in the operative planning or in diagnosing associated extra-abdominal injuries.

There is minimal or no role of CT scans in suspected AAIs secondary to penetrating injury; however, the findings of dissection, pseudoaneurysm, occlusion, or large hematoma in blunt trauma help in the diagnosis. An elective CT scan with intravenous contrast may also help in the diagnosis of an aortocaval fistula or pseudoaneurysm.[43]

Spectrum of Injuries

AAIs can range from free rupture, contained hematoma, pseudoaneurysm, focal dissection, aortocaval fistula, or focal mural hematoma.

▌TREATMENT

Open Surgical Repair

Surgical repair of infrarenal aortic injuries requires laparotomy with suprarenal or infrarenal aortic clamping, depending on the extent of the injury. For injuries of the visceral aorta, a left thoracotomy and cross clamping of the aorta is sometimes necessary. After control of the hemorrhage the associated intra-abdominal injuries are addressed.

Lateral aortorrhaphy is possible in some cases due to the relative healthy aorta and limited injury in the trauma population. In patients with high-velocity missiles the extent of the injury may not be fully appreciated by visual inspection and care must be taken not to leave behind devitalized tissue. In these and other extensive aortic wall injuries a prosthetic graft repair may be needed. In cases where enteric spillage is encountered it is recommended that the spillage be controlled and the peritoneum be washed out prior to the use of a prosthetic graft. Although suboptimal, several reports do not consider the presence of enteric spillage a contraindication for the use of a prosthetic graft for aortic repair in trauma.

Acute renal failure, intraoperative blood loss, morbidity of associated injuries, pulmonary failure, pulmonary infections, graft infections, aortoenteric fistulas, and incisional hernia have all been reported complications with open surgical repair of aortic injuries.

Endovascular Treatment

Endovascular aortic repair has a limited role in most AAIs. In select cases with a CT diagnosis of a blunt trauma away from visceral branches, it offers definitive management without the associated morbidity and mortality of open repair. Endovascular treatment of selected traumatic vascular injuries is particularly promising for restoring luminal continuity, closing aortocaval fistulas, and excluding pseudoaneurysms.

We have treated patients with limited infrarenal traumatic aortic dissection, focal traumatic pseudoaneurysm (FIGURE 69.7), or traumatic aortocaval fistula (FIGURE 69.8) at our institution with placement of abdominal endografts or covered stent-grafts. Others have similarly reported on the efficacy of endovascular repair in the setting of blunt trauma to infrarenal abdominal aorta.[40,48–50]

▌OUTCOMES

The reported mortality after blunt AAIs (27%)[51] is lower than after penetrating AAIs (67%).[42,52] Suprarenal aortic injuries have significantly worse outcomes,[53] and the reported mortality of emergent resuscitative thoracotomy was 100%.[42]

▌IATROGENIC AORTIC INJURY

Iatrogenic injury to the aorta is a rare but well-recognized complication of a variety of interventions and procedures, including intra-aortic balloon pump (IABP) placement, spine

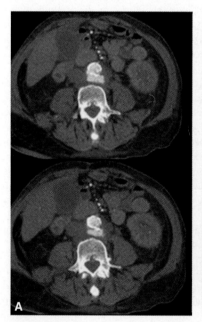
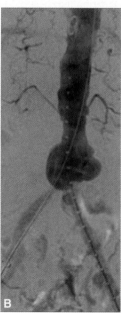
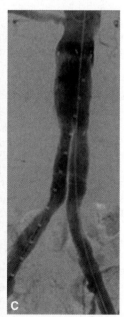

FIGURE 69.7 Blunt abdominal aortic injury. Contrast-enhanced axial CT scan of the abdomen and pelvis reveals a pseudoaneurysm above the aortic bifurcation (**A, B**). Pre- and postaortography (**C**) document successful exclusion of the pseudoaneurysm after endovascular aortic repair with a bifurcated stent-graft.

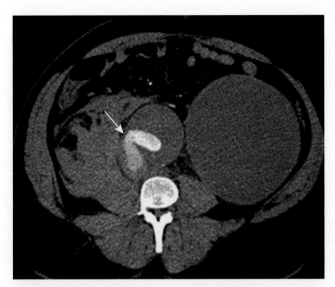

FIGURE 69.8 Blunt abdominal aortic injury resulting in traumatic aortocaval fistula (*arrow*).

surgery, and trocar injuries during laparoscopic and gynecologic procedures. Acute aortic perforation results in hemorrhage, leading to either hemodynamic instability in case of free rupture or rapid hematoma formation, or both. Iatrogenic aortoiliac trauma can also lead to pseudoaneurysm or aortocaval fistula formation.

Iatrogenic Aortic Injuries During Laparoscopic Procedures

Retroperitoneal vascular injuries resulting from trocar placement during gynecologic and general surgery operations have an incidence of approximately 0.1%.[62] Several studies suggest that almost all of the major vascular injuries occurred during the primary trocar placement.[63]

The comparison of different techniques for placing the initial trocar has not revealed superiority of a particular approach. Open Hasson technique, Blind Veress Needle technique, and Optical trocars have all been associated with a small incidence of major vascular injury.[62] Most of the injuries involve iliac vessels, the distal aorta, or the distal inferior vena cava because most of the initial trocars are placed at the umbilicus.

These injuries are typically identified by a retroperitoneal hematoma or an active hemorrhage requiring open conversion. The aortic injuries can be managed by primary repair, patch, or interposition graft. The pseudoaneurysms identified later can be managed by endovascular aneurysm repair (EVAR).[63]

Injury from Aortic Perforation by Intra-Aortic Balloon Pump

Aortic perforation or acute aortoiliac dissections are extremely rare but known vascular complications related to the placement and prolonged use of IABP. Arafa et al.[61] reported 41 (8%) major vascular complications in their series of 509 consecutive patients undergoing open heart bypass with concomitant IABP, including 2 iatrogenic aortic injuries.

We successfully treated one patient at our institution with acute aortic perforation secondary to IABP with EVAR. Given the focal nature of the injury, and the associated comorbidities often present in this patient population, endovascular repair, when feasible, should be considered the first-line treatment in most IABP or catheter-related iatrogenic aortic injuries.

Injury from Perforation or Impingement by Spinal Pedicle Screws

Several CT scanning studies have demonstrated a significant (4% to 25%) incidence of screw malposition after posterior spinal instrumentation.[56–58] Because the aorta and the iliac arteries are in close proximity to the spine, the malpositioned pedicle screws can perforate or impinge on the aorta. The reported incidence of aortic injury after such spinal instrumentations is less than 0.0005%.[54] Mortality after these iatrogenic aortic injuries is as high as 61%.[55]

Mechanism of Injury

Penetration of a malpositioned pedicle screw can cause penetrating injury to the aorta at the time of operation. Studies have shown that actual pedicle screw penetration of the aorta is not necessary to cause delayed iatrogenic aortic injury. Mere impingement on the aorta by the fixation screw can lead to aortic wall weakening and the potential for eventual erosion as the aorta continues to pulsate and cause repeated trauma with every heartbeat. Proximity of the screw tip to the aortic wall has been reported in 2% to 12% of iatrogenic aortic injuries.[59] The time frame and the natural course of impingement of the aorta by the tip of a screw from the development to the pathologic aortic change is not well known.

Clinical Presentation

Iatrogenic aortic injuries can present as immediate intraoperative or perioperative hemorrhage requiring emergent vascular intervention. More commonly, these injuries present as a symptomatic (back pain) pseudoaneurysm or an incidentally detected pseudoaneurysm on CT scan performed for follow-up.

Treatment

Intraoperative and perioperative hemodynamic instability necessitate emergent repair. All iatrogenic aortic pseudoaneurysms should be repaired urgently to prevent rupture. The management of identification of spinal screw tip impingement without pseudoaneurysm is not clearly defined and, currently, these injuries are either empirically treated to avoid rupture on removal of the screw or patients are closely followed with serial imaging.[55,60]

Traditionally, repair of iatrogenic aortic injuries involved a thoracotomy or laparotomy depending on the location of the injury. Types of repair include primary repair, patch angioplasty, or interposition grafting depending on the extent of the injury.[59] Open repair can carry a morbidity rate of up to 50%, including SCI, renal ischemia, mesenteric ischemia, pulmonary failure, and intraoperative hemorrhage.[60] In select cases where previous spinal instrumentation was performed in the setting of osteomyelitis (methicillin-resistant *Staphylococcus aureus* [MRSA] or Pott disease) and there is suspicion of an infected pseudoaneurysm, open repair is favored. Extra-anatomic reconstruction may be favored in these situations.

Successful endovascular repair of iatrogenic aortic injury from spinal instrumentation with a covered stent-graft has been reported in several isolated reports. EVAR can provide repair with low associated morbidity and mortality in selected cases.[59,60]

In case of screw tip penetration, tip removal is necessary to avoid the risk of tearing the stent-graft material and recurrent injury. Simple burring of the screw tip usually suffices. Full hardware removal is reserved for infected cases, followed by a secondary fixation if spinal instability occurs.

■ THE FUTURE

In the future, the development of stent-grafts specific for transection injuries might help in decreasing device-related complications. The development and use of branched or fenestrated stent-grafts will increase the utility of endovascular repair in paravisceral aortic injuries. The continuing surveillance will also provide more information regarding the long-term outcomes and issues encountered.

■ CONCLUSION

Thoracic endovascular aortic repair has replaced open surgical repair for traumatic TAI/transection to a great extent. This paradigm shift has resulted in a major reduction of mortality and procedure-related paraplegia but also an increase in graft-related complications. Even with endografts not specifically designed and approved for traumatic thoracic aortic transection, the results of thoracic endovascular aortic repair in the acute setting are superior to open thoracotomy and surgical procedures. The open conversion can always be done safely later in more elective stable situation if needed. In the trauma patients who typically are in their third or fourth decade of life, long-term follow-up is essential, and device improvement will need to occur before TEVAR can become a standalone procedure for the treatment of aortic transection. Most abdominal aortic injuries are repaired primarily. Endovascular repair is emerging and offers the potential for definitive repair in hemodynamically stable and select injuries. The future development and universal availability of fenestrated or branched grafts might expand the applicability of endovascular repair to a variety of injuries in the paravisceral abdominal aorta.

■ REFERENCES

1. Parmley LF, Mattingly TW, Manion WC, et al. Nonpenetrating traumatic injury of the aorta. *Circulation* 1958;17:1086–1101.
2. Fabian TC, Richardson JD, Croce MA, et al. Prospective study of blunt aortic injury: multicenter trial of the American Association for the Surgery of Trauma. *J Trauma* 1997;42:374–380.
3. Richens D, Field M, Neale M, et al. The mechanism of injury in blunt traumatic rupture of the aorta. *Eur J Cardiothorac Surg* 2002;21:288–293.
4. Hunt JP, Baker CC, Lentz CW, et al. Thoracic aorta injuries: management and outcomes off 144 patients. *J Trauma* 1996;40:547–555.
5. Greendyke RM. Traumatic rupture of aorta: special reference to automobile accidents. *JAMA* 1966;195:527–530.
6. Demetriades D, Velmahos GC, Scalea TM, et al. Operative repair or endovascular stent graft in blunt traumatic thoracic aortic injuries: result of an American Association for the Surgery of trauma multicenter study. *J Trauma* 2008;64:561–571.
7. Garant ML, Flick P, Menke P, et al. CT angiography of thoracic aortic rupture. *Am J Roentgenol* 1996;166:955–961.
8. Demetriades D, Gomez H, Velmahos G, et al. Routine helical computed tomographic evaluation of the mediastinum in high risk blunt trauma patients. *Arch Surg* 1998;133:1084–1088.
9. Kato N, Dake MD, Miller DC, et al. Traumatic thoracic aortic aneurysm: treatment with endovascular stent grafts. *Radiology* 1997;205:657–662.
10. Finkelmeier BA, Mentzer RM Jr, Kaiser DL, et al. Chronic traumatic thoracic aneurysm. Influence of operative treatment on natural history: an analysis of reported cases, 1950–1980. *J Thorac Cardiovasc Surg* 1982;84:257–266.
11. Kram HB, Wohlmulth DA, Appel PL, et al. Diagnosis of traumatic aortic rupture: a 10 year retrospective analysis. *Ann Thorac Surg* 1989;47:282–286.
12. Woodring JH. The normal mediastinum in blunt traumatic rupture of the thoracic aorta and brachiocephalic arteries. *J Emerg Med* 1990;8:467–476.
13. Fabian TC, Davis KA, Gavant ML, et al. Prospective study of blunt aortic injury: helical CT is diagnostic and antihypertensive therapy reduces rupture. *Ann Surg* 1998;227:666–677.
14. Nagy K, Fabian T, Rodman G, et al. Guidelines for the diagnosis and management of blunt aortic injury. An EAST practice management guidelines work group. *J Trauma* 2000;48:1128–1143.
15. Vignon P, Boncoeur MP, François B, et al. Comparison of multiplane transesophageal echocardiography and contrast-enhanced helical CT in the diagnosis of blunt traumatic cardiovascular injuries. *Anesthesiology* 2001;94:615–622.
16. Cinnella G, Dambrosio M, Brenza N, et al. Transesophageal echocardiography for diagnosis of traumatic aortic injury: an appraisal of the evidence. *J Trauma* 2004;57:1246–1255.
17. Azzizadeh A, Keyhani K, Estrera AL, et al. Blunt traumatic aortic injury: initial experience with endovascular repair. *J Vasc Surg* 2009;49:1403–1408.
18. Cowley RA, Turney SZ, Hankins JR, et al. Rupture of thoracic aorta caused by blunt trauma. A fifteen year experience. *J Thorac Cardiovasc Surg* 1990;100:652–660.
19. Jahromi AS, Kazemi K, Safar HA, et al. Traumatic rupture of the thoracic aorta: cohort study and systemic review. *J Vasc Surg* 2001;34:1029–1034.
20. Attar S, Cadarelli MG, Downing SW, et al. Traumatic aortic rupture: recent outcome with regard to neurologic deficit. *Ann Thorac Surg* 1999;67(4):959–964.
21. Tehrani HY, Peterson BG, Katariya K, et al. Endovascular repair of thoracic aortic tears. *Ann Thorac Surg* 2006;82:873–877.
22. Hoornweg LL, Dinkelman MK, Goslings JC, et al. Endovascular management of traumatic ruptures of the thoracic aorta: a retrospective multicenter analysis of 28 cases in The Netherlands. *J Vasc Surg* 2006;43:1096–1102.
23. Bennett DE, Cherry JK. The natural history of traumatic aneurysms of the aorta. *Surgery* 1967;61:516–523.
24. Semba CP, Kato N, Kee ST, et al. Acute rupture of the descending thoracic aorta: repair with use of endovascular stent-grafts. *J Vasc Interv Radiol* 1997;8:337–342.
25. Murad MH, Rizvi AZ, Malgor R, et al. Comparative effectiveness of the treatments for thoracic aortic transection. *J Vasc Surg* 2011;53(1):193–199.e1–21.
26. Lee WA, Matsumura JS, Mitchell RS, et al. Endovascular repair of traumatic thoracic aortic injury: clinical practice guidelines of the Society for Vascular Surgery. *J Vasc Surg* 2011;53(1):187–192.
27. Raupach J, Ferko A, Lojik M, et al. Endovascular treatment of acute and chronic thoracic aortic injury. *Cardiovasc Intervent Radiol* 2007;30:1117–1123.
28. Shukla AJ, Jeyabalan G, Cho JS. Late collapse of thoracic endoprosthesis. *J Vasc Surg* 2011;53(3):798–801.
29. Go MR, Makaroun MS, Cho JS, et al. Thoracic endovascular aortic repair for traumatic aortic transection. *J Vasc Surg* 2007;46:928–933.
30. Go MR, Siegenthaler MP, Rhee RY, et al. Physiologic coarctation of the aorta resulting from protrusion of thoracic aorta stent grafts into the arch. *J Vasc Surg* 2008;48:1007–1011.
31. Lin PH, Bush RL, Zhou W, et al. Endovascular treatment of traumatic thoracic aortic injury – should this be the new standard of treatment? *J Vasc Surg* 2006;43:22A–29A.
32. Matsumura JS, Lee WA, Mitchell RS, et al. The Society for Vascular Surgery Practice Guideline: management of the left subclavain artery with thoracic endovascular aortic repair. *J Vasc Surg* 2009;50:1155–1158.
33. Peterson BG, Matsamura JS, Morasch MD, et al. Percutaneous endovascular repair of blunt thoracic aortic transection. *J Trauma* 2005;59:1062–1065.
34. Lee WA, Brown MP, Nelson PR, et al. Midterm outcomes of femoral arteries after percutaneous endovascular aortic repair using the Preclose technique. *J Vasc Surg* 2008;47:919–923.

35. Bosra JJ, Hoffer EK, Karmy-Jones R, et al. Angiographic description of blunt traumatic injuries to the thoracic aorta with specific relevance to endovascular repair. *J Endovasc Ther* 2002;9:1184–1191.

36. Kahn RA, Marin ML, Hollier L, et al. Induction of ventricular fibrillation to facilitate endovascular stent graft repair in thoracic aortic aneurysms. *Anesthesiology* 1998;88:534–536.

37. Dorros G, Cohn JM. Adenosine-induced transient cardiac asystole enhances precise deployment of stent-grafts in the thoracic and abdominal aorta. *J Endovasc Surg* 1996;3:270–272.

38. Tadros RO, Faries P, Cho JS, et al. A multicenter experience of the management of collapsed thoracic endograft. *J Vasc Surg* 2011;53(5):1217–1222.

39. Asensio JA, Forno W, Roldan G, et al. Abdominal vascular injuries: injuries to the aorta. *Surg Clin North Am* 2001;81:1395–1416.

40. Naude GP, Back M, Perry MO, et al. Blunt disruption of the abdominal aorta: a case report and review of literature. *J Vasc Surg* 1997;25:931–935.

41. Coimbra R, Yang J, Hoyt DB. Injuries to the abdominal aorta and inferior vena cava in association with thoracolumbar fractures: a lethal combination. *J Trauma* 1996;41:533–535.

42. Demetriades D, Theodorou D, Murray J, et al. Mortality and prognostic factors in penetrating injuries of the aorta. *J Trauma* 1996;40:761–763.

43. Coimbra R, Hyot D, Winchell R, et al. The ongoing challenge of retroperitoneal vascular injuries. *Am J Surg* 1996;172:541–545.

44. Asensio TA, Chahwan S, Hanpeter D, et al. Operative management and outcomes of 302 abdominal vascular injuries. *Am J Surg* 2000;180:524–534.

45. Frykberg ER, Vines FS, Alexandar RH. The natural history of clinically occult arterial injuries: a prospective evaluation. *J Trauma* 1989;29:577–583.

46. Frykberg ER, Crump JM, Dennis JW, et al. Non-operative observation of clinically occult arterial injuries: a prospective evaluation. *Surgery* 1991;109:85–96.

47. Nanobashvili J, Kopadze T, Tavaldze M, et al. War injuries of major extremity arteries. *World J Surg* 2003;27:134–139.

48. White R, Donayre C, Walot I, et al. Endograft repair of an aortic pseudoaneurysm following gunshot wound injury: impact of imaging on diagnosis and planning of intervention. *J Endovasc Ther* 1997;4:344–351.

49. Waldrop JL Jr, Dart BW IV, Barker DE, et al. Endovascular stent graft treatment of a traumatic aorto-caval fistula. *Ann Vasc Surg* 2005;19:562–565.

50. Tucker S Jr, Row VL, Rao R, et al. Treatment options for traumatic pseudoaneurysms of paravisceral abdominal aorta. *Ann Vasc Surg* 2005;19:613–618.

51. Inaba K, Kirkpatrick W, Finkelstein AJ, et al. Blunt abdominal aortic trauma with association with thoracolumbar spine fractures. *Injury* 2001;35:385–389.

52. Accola KD, Feliciano DV, Mattox KL, et al. Management of injuries to the suprarenal aorta. *Am J Surg* 1987;154:613–618.

53. Degiannis E, Levy RD, Florizone MG, et al. Gunshot injuries of the abdominal aorta: a continuing challenge. *Injury* 1997;28:195–197.

54. Szolar DH, Preidler KW, Steiner H, et al. Vascular complications in disk surgery: report of four cases. *Neuroradiology* 1996;38:521–525.

55. Bingol H, Cingoz F, Yilmaz AT, et al. Vascular complications related to lumbar disc surgery. *J Neurosurg* 2004;100:249–253.

56. Wiesner L, Kothe R, Schulitz, et al. Clinical evaluation and computed tomography scan analysis of screw tracts after percutaneous insertion of pedicle screws in the lumbar spine. *Spine* 2000;25:615–621.

57. Suk SI, Kim WJ, Lee SM, et al. Thoracic pedicle screw fixation in spinal deformities: are they really safe? *Spine* 2001;26:2049–2057.

58. Kuklo TR, Lenke LG, O'Brien MF, et al. Accuracy and efficacy of thoracic pedicle screws in curves more than 90 degrees. *Spine* 2005;30:222–226.

59. Kakkos SK, Shepard AD. Delayed presentation of aortic injury by pedicle screws: report of two cases and review of the literature. *J Vasc Surg* 2008;47:1074–1082.

60. Loh SA, Maldonaldo TS, Rockman CB, et al. Endovascular solutions to arterial injury due to posterior spine surgery. *J Vasc Surg* 2012;55(5):1477–1481.

61. Arafa OE, Pedersen TH, Svennevig JL, et al. Vascular complications of the intra-aortic balloon pump in patients undergoing open heart operations: a 15 year experience. *Ann Thorac Surg* 1999;67:645–651.

62. Fuller J, Scott W, Ashar B, et al. *Laparoscopic Trocar Injuries: A Report from a U.S. Food and Drug Administration (FDA) Center for Devices and Radiological Health (CDRH) Systematic Technology Assessment of Medical Products (STAMP) Committee.* Silver Spring, MD: U.S. Food and Drug Administration; 2003.

63. Bhoyrul S, Vierra MA, Nezhart CR, et al. Trocar injuries in laparoscopic surgery. *J Am Coll Surg* 2001;192(6):677–683.

64. Heyer KS, Modi P, Matsumura JS, et al. Secondary infections of thoracic and abdominal aortic endografts. *J Vasc Interv Radiol* 2009;20:173–179.

65. Nienaber CA, Kische S, Rehders TC, et al. Rapid pacing for better placing: comparison of techniques for precise deployment of endografts in the thoracic aorta. *J Endovasc Ther* 2007;14:506–512.

66. Murphy JJ. Current practice: complications of temporary transvenous cardiac pacing. *BMJ* 1996:312–314.

67. Demetriades D, Velmahos GC, Scalae TM, et al. Diagnosis and treatment of blunt thoracic aortic injuries: changing perspectives. *J Trauma* 2008;64(6):1415–1419.

68. Yamane BH, Tefera G, Acher CW, et al. Blunt thoracic aortic injury: open or stent graft repair? *Surgery* 2008;144(4):575–580.

69. Bent CL, Matson MB, Sobeh M, et al. Endovascular management of acute blunt traumatic thoracic aortic injury; a single center experience. *J Vasc Surg* 2007;46(5):920–927.

70. Xenos ES, Abedi NN, Endean ED, et al. Meta-analysis of endovascular open repair for traumatic descending thoracic aortic rupture. *J Vasc Surg* 2008;48(5):1343–1351.

71. Tang GL, Tehrani HY, Usman A, et al. Reduced mortality, paraplegia, and stroke with stent graft repair of blunt aortic transections: a modern meta-analysis. *J Vasc Surg* 2008;47(3):671–675.

Traumatic Arterial Injuries: Arch Vessels

JOHN R. GAUGHEN, JR. and MARY E. JENSEN

▌ INTRODUCTION

Trauma involving the cervical region can result in either blunt or penetrating injury to the brachiocephalic vessels with attendant hemorrhagic and/or neurologic sequelae. Recently, the use of liberal screening protocols have determined a higher prevalence of blunt cervical vascular injury (BCVI) than previously thought with a reported incidence of 1.2% to 1.6% of carotid or vertebral artery injury in all trauma patients[1–3] and an associated risk of acute cerebral ischemia in 12% to 15% of affected patients.[1,4] This chapter is intended to promote a heightened awareness of cervical vascular injury (CVI) in trauma patients through a discussion of the risk factors, pathologic processes, anatomic considerations, clinical screening, and radiographic imaging associated with traumatic lesions.

▌ RISK FACTORS

Blunt Cervical Vascular Injury

The risk of CVI is increased in the setting of cervical spine, basilar skull, or severe facial fractures; spinal cord and traumatic brain injury; and major thoracic injuries.[1,5,6] Screening for BCVI is proposed in the presence of these risk factors. Vertebral artery injuries are more common than carotid artery injuries (0.53% vs. 0.32%) in all patients with BCVI, most likely caused by impaction on bony structures as it courses through the intervertebral foramina.[7,8] Injury of the carotid or vertebral artery has been reported in 2.7% of patients with severe, multisystem trauma.[9]

Mechanism of injury is another risk factor for BCVI, and it is associated with severe cervical hyperextension/rotation or hyperflexion injury, near-hanging with cerebral anoxia, and seat belt abrasion or other soft-tissue injury of the anterior neck resulting in significant cervical swelling or altered mental status.[6] However, it is important to recognize that about 20% of patients with BCVI demonstrate none of these "classic" risk factors.[1,6]

Vascular injury, usually in the form of a dissection, can occur after trivial trauma, or in otherwise healthy individuals with no clinically evident risk factors. The average annual incidence of these "spontaneous" occurrences is between 2.6 and 2.9 per 100,000 people[10] and accounts for 13% to 22% of ischemic strokes in patients younger than 45 years of age.[11] Collagen-vascular disorders, such as Ehlers-Danlos syndrome (type IV), fibromuscular dysplasia, Marfan syndrome, osteogenesis imperfecta, pseudoxanthoma elasticum, and cystic medial necrosis, are associated with the development of spontaneous dissection.[6,12] Even in the absence of an identified collagen-vascular disease, however, most skin biopsies in patients with spontaneous dissection demonstrate structural abnormalities of the connective tissue, indicative of an underlying genetic predisposition.[12] These affected individuals with a generalized weakness of their vessel walls may be more prone to injury from insignificant trauma associated with exercise, coughing, or vomiting.[6]

Penetrating Cervical Vascular Injury

Damage from penetrating cervical vascular injury (PCVI) trauma is less common than blunt trauma with carotid and vertebral artery injuries accounting for only 3% and 0.5%, respectively, of arterial injuries treated in civilian trauma centers in the latter part of the last century.[13] In the same population, greater than 15% of venous injuries were penetrating injuries to the jugular vein.[13] Severe injuries in patients with gunshot and stab wounds have been reported as 50% and 10% to 20%, respectively, although other investigators have found the incidence of serious injury in this setting to be much lower.[14] In military combatants, neck injuries caused by explosive fragments account for 8.7% of all battle injuries, and 41% of neck injuries from explosive fragments are fatal. The most common cause of death in explosive fragment injury to the neck is from vascular trauma (85%),[15] and when the cause of death is from airway compromise it is usually due to hemorrhage into the airway from an adjacent structure.[16]

▌ ANATOMIC CONSIDERATIONS

Historically, the approach to diagnosis and treatment of PCVI started by determining the location of the injury within a well-defined anatomic region. The most widely used classification is by Monson et al.[17] and divides the neck into three anatomic zones anterior to the sternocleidomastoid muscles. Zone I is the area between the inferior margin of the clavicles and the cricoid cartilage and contains the origins of the brachiocephalic vessels and the subclavian and innominate veins. Zone II is the area between the cricoid cartilage and the angle of the mandible and includes the distal common carotid arteries, the proximal internal and external carotid arteries, the vertebral arteries, and the internal jugular veins. Zone III is the area between the angle of the mandible and the base of the skull and holds the distal cervical internal carotid arteries, the external carotid artery (ECA) branches, the distal vertebral arteries, and the proximal internal jugular veins. Corresponding vertebral levels in this scheme are the body of T1 to the body of C6 in zone I, the body of C6 to the upper border of C3 in zone II, and the upper border of C3 to the skull base in zone III.[18]

The vertebral artery remains narrow and the furthest from the skin surface, and is protected by 4 to 6 mm of bone throughout its course except in zone I.[18] The diameter of all three vascular structures (vertebral artery, carotid artery, and internal jugular vein) is greater, and their location more superficial as the anatomic plane moves caudally. Thus the zone I vascular structures are most vulnerable to small fragments and shallow wounds, and penetrating injuries in this location carry the highest morbidity and mortality. Zone III posteriorly is the least common area of the neck to be injured by penetrating trauma.[18] Additionally, the carotid artery and internal jugular vein are less vulnerable in zone III due to protection from the mandible and smaller size of the vessels.[18]

Specific anatomic features are also important in the evaluation of blunt trauma. The internal carotid artery (ICA) ascends ventral to the transverse processes of the C1–C3 vertebral bodies before it enters the petrous canal at the skull base. Stretch injury to the ICA from hyperextension and contralateral rotation occurs when the vessel impinges on the lateral articular processes and pedicles of the upper cervical spine.[6,19] The ICA is also vulnerable to dissection at the skull base from deceleration injury or petrous canal fractures. Less common causes of blunt carotid trauma include a direct blow to the neck (e.g., hanging), intraoral trauma from a foreign object, or a posteriorly displaced mandibular fracture.[6,19]

The vertebral artery ascends through the transverse foramina from C2 to C6. Stretching from rotation or subluxation, or transverse process fractures can result in dissection or occlusion at these levels. The distal cervical segment of the vertebral artery may be crushed against the C1 vertebral or the dural edge in cases of craniocervical junction distraction or dislocation.[19]

In conclusion, the decision to perform surgical exploration versus radiographic evaluation depends on the type of injury and the clinical condition of the patient. Penetrating injuries in zone II usually present with overt signs, such as external or oral bleeding, expanding or stable hematoma, difficulty breathing, bruit or thrill, and loss of carotid pulsation with or without neurologic deficits. Immediate surgical exploration is appropriate in life-threatening hemorrhage, hemoptysis, hematemesis, expanding hematoma, airway compromise, or loss of the carotid pulse with a neurologic deficit.[13,14] Injuries that penetrate the platysma carry the potential for vascular damage; however, surgical exploration carries a significant morbidity and patients with stable vital signs are usually evaluated first by noninvasive imaging, such as ultrasound or computed tomographic angiography (CTA).[14] All three zones can be rapidly assessed using CTA, which has led to the markedly decreased use of more invasive studies, such as catheter angiography. Furthermore, multiplanar reconstruction of the study using bone windows also detects vertebral, skull base, and/or facial fractures associated with vascular injury, either in blunt or penetrating trauma.

PATHOPHYSIOLOGY

The final common pathway for vascular injury, regardless of the mechanism of action, is intimal damage. Although seemingly innocuous, even minimal intimal disruption may promote platelet aggregation, leading to clot formation with distal embolization or vascular thrombosis. At its most insignificant, focal spasm may be all that is noted. More substantial injury includes subintimal dissection with intramural thrombus (FIGURE 70.1A), raised intimal flap (FIGURE 70.1B), pseudoaneurysm formation (FIGURE 70.1C), transection with active extravasation (FIGURE 70.1D), occlusion (FIGURE 70.1E), and arteriovenous fistula (AVF) development (FIGURE 70.1D).[6,19] Progression of subintimal thrombus in a false lumen (FIGURE 70.1A) or a subendothelial tear with pseudoaneurysm enlargement (FIGURE 70.1C) may lead to luminal stenosis with subsequent hemodynamic compromise and cerebral ischemia. Multivessel injury has been reported in

18% to 38% of cases[20–23]; combinations of injuries may occur in the same vessel, along with rapid change in the appearance of the vascular injury.[19]

In 1999, Biffl et al.[24] devised a grading scale for blunt carotid injury based on angiographic features of the lesion in an effort to predict the risk of stroke. The scale was revised in 2002[22] to include AVFs and to endorse the same scale for classifying blunt vertebral artery injury (Table 70.1). The most severe injury identified in a vessel is used to determine its Biffl score, although all the injuries in a particular vessel, and not just the one used for grading purposes, should be reported.[19] In general, the higher the Biffl grade for the carotid artery, the higher the risk of stroke. In the vertebral artery, grade II lesions were associated with the highest risk of stroke.

In 2012, Seth et al.[25] proposed a modification to the scale in which grades II and III carotid abnormalities were subclassified into (a) less than 70% stenosis (non–flow-limiting) and (b) greater than 70% stenosis (flow-limiting). Patients with high-grade stenoses, progressive pseudoaneurysm enlargement, or marked intimal irregularity associated with grade IIa injuries were considered for endovascular stenting provided antiplatelet therapy could be utilized.

PATIENT SCREENING

The creation of the Biffl scale was a major advancement in the care of patients with BCVI in that it created a "shorthand" method of describing vascular injury used and understood across multiple disciplines and identified patients who were at high risk for stroke. Another key development that affected patient care was the implementation of standardized screening protocols for detecting "at-risk" patients for BCVI prior to the onset of neurologic dysfunction.[26] Patients with BCVI are often asymptomatic at presentation and only develop neurologic deficits after a latent period, which can span from 1 hour to several weeks.[22,27,28] Morbidity and mortality for blunt carotid artery injury (BCI) are high, ranging from 32% to 67% and 17% to 38%, respectively.[19] Morbidity and mortality is lower in blunt vertebral artery injury (BVI) but still significant, ranging from 14% to 24% and 8% to 18%, respectively.[19]

Prior to the mid-1990s, the diagnosis of BCVI was usually made only when a stroke became clinically apparent.[29] In 2001, Miller et al.[30] reported a 0.9% incidence of BCVI after initiation of an aggressive screening program. Improved stroke and survival rates were also noted after the institution of anticoagulation therapy. In this retrospective series, the stroke rate for carotid artery injury (CAI) decreased from 64% to 6.8% and for vertebral artery injury (VAI) from 54% to 2.6% when systemic heparinization was used in appropriate candidates. Earlier studies had also supported improved outcomes in patients with BCI-related stroke treated with anticoagulants.[27,28,30,31] Given this success, investigators were keen to identify BCVI in asymptomatic patients so treatment could be initiated before a neurologic deficit occurred.

Aggressive screening protocols designed to identify patients at high risk for BCVI have developed over time with the initial protocol devised at the Denver Health Medical Center by Biffl and colleagues[31] in 1998. The list of screening criteria has expanded over time as new studies have identified more conditions associated with an increased incidence of BCVI. Factors associated with injury are listed in Table 70.2[29] and include mechanism of injury, presence of facial, skull base, and cervical

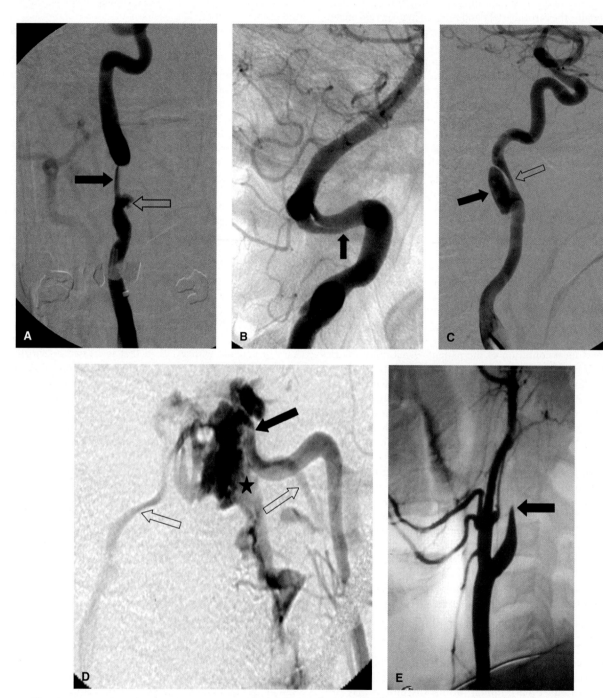

FIGURE 70.1 Selected images from cerebral angiograms performed on patients with blunt cervical trauma demonstrate the various injuries that may be seen. **A.** AP oblique DSA image of a focal dissection flap (*open arrow*) of the internal carotid artery (ICA) shows thrombus in the false lumen compressing the true lumen (*solid arrow*). **B.** Lateral DSA image of the vertebral artery shows a free-floating flap arising from the vessel wall (*solid arrow*) with contrast seen on both sides of the flap. **C.** Lateral view of the ICA demonstrating a large pseudoaneurysm (*open arrow*) compressing the true lumen (*solid arrow*). **D.** AP DSA image of the left ICA in a patient with a gunshot wound through the mouth. The ICA is transected within the cavernous sinus (*solid arrow*) with extravasation into the mouth (*star*) and fistulous flow through both cavernous sinuses into the inferior petrosal sinuses bilaterally (*open arrows*). **E.** Lateral DSA image of an acute ICA occlusion showing the classic flame-shaped tapering (*black arrow*).

Table 70.1

Biffl Grading Scale for Carotid and Vertebral Artery Injury

Grade	Description
I	Luminal irregularity (i.e., intimal injury) or dissection with <25% luminal narrowing
II	Dissection or intraluminal hematoma with ≥25% luminal narrowing, intraluminal thrombus, raised intimal flap, or hemodynamically insignificant AVF
III	Pseudoaneurysm
IV	Occlusion
V	Transection or hemodynamically significant AVF

Biffl WL, Moore EE, Offner PJ, et al. Blunt carotid arterial injuries: implications of a new grading scale. *J Trauma* 1999;47:845–853.

fractures, and the patient's Glasgow Coma Scale (GCS) score and injury severity score (ISS) as criteria for consideration. In the Denver experience, patients with GCS less than or equal to 6, evidence of diffuse axonal injury, and Lefort 2 or 3 fractures had a 93% probability of CAI. Cervical spine fractures were associated with VAI in 33% of patients.[8,24] Other series have shown that the BCVI is present in 60% of cervical spine fractures and 18% of skull base fractures.[4,19,29]

Table 70.2

Modified Denver Health Medical Center Screening Criteria

Signs/symptoms

Arterial hemorrhage

Expanding hematoma

Cervical bruit in patients <50 y of age

Focal neurologic deficit

Neurologic examination inconsistent with head CT findings

Stroke on secondary head CT

Risk factors

LeForte II or III fracture pattern

Cervical spine fracture patterns

Subluxation

Fractures extending into the transverse process

Fractures of the C1–C3 vertebrae

Basilar skull fracture with involvement of the carotid canal

Diffuse axonal injury with GCS <6

Near-hanging with anoxic brain injury

Anaya C, Munera F, Bloomer CW, et al. Screening multidetector computed tomography angiography in the evaluation on blunt neck injuries: an evidence-based approach. *Semin Ulrasound CT MRI* 2009;30:205–214.

As the use of aggressive screening protocols took hold, debate over the liberal use of cervicocerebral angiography arose, centered around the added risk of morbidity and mortality and the cost to the health care system. This argument was countered by the fact that systematic heparinization in selected asymptomatic patients with "positive" findings resulted in improved neurologic outcome and survival.[21,22,30–33] The issue became less contentious as further studies confirmed the increased detection rate of injury, the improved outcomes with treatment, and the replacement of catheter angiography with noninvasive imaging, such as CTA, as part of routine trauma protocols. In fact, some investigators believe that routine screening should be performed in all patients with significant trauma regardless of the results of the screening protocol.[9,19]

▌ IMAGING MODALITIES

As noted earlier, blunt and penetrating CVIs represent two distinct disease entities that carry significantly different mechanisms of injury, diagnostic algorithms, and treatment paradigms. Both diseases, however, rely heavily on medical imaging as a central component of the diagnostic evaluation, and both possess a common endpoint of vascular injury that results in a well-defined group of potential imaging findings.

Digital Subtraction Angiography

Traditionally heralded as the gold standard, catheter angiography (also known as digital subtraction angiography [DSA]) has historically represented the workhorse in the diagnostic evaluation of PCVI and BCVI. Over the past 20 years, however, continued improvements in noninvasive vascular imaging have caused a shift away from this invasive technology for the bulk of the diagnostic evaluation of CVI.

Two major limitations in catheter angiography contribute to this shifting diagnostic paradigm. First, catheter angiography allows for intricate endovascular evaluation but an extremely limited assessment of the extravascular structures and mural integrity. Second, although "relatively" safe, diagnostic cervicocerebral DSA carries definite risks to the patient, including exposure to ionizing radiation and a number of potential neurologic and non-neurologic complications. Current literature reports an estimated rate of neurologic complication associated with diagnostic cerebral catheter angiography of 0.9% to 4% and associated permanent morbidity of 0.2% to 1.3%.[34–43] In a retrospective review of 19,826 consecutive diagnostic cerebral angiograms performed at the Mayo Clinic, Kaufmann et al.[34] found a 0.06% mortality rate.

Although no longer central in the diagnostic triage of CVI, DSA remains an important component in the workup and treatment in a subset of these patients. It allows for very high spatial resolution and two- and three-dimensional endovascular imaging, as well as for temporal information relating to the rate and amount of blood flow through the cerebrovascular tree. Indeed, DSA remains the test of choice for detecting flow-related complications of cervical and cerebral vascular injury, such as AVF (FIGURE 70.1D), and for the evaluation of collateral circulation to compromised vascular territories. DSA is often used as a problem-solving modality when noninvasive imaging is inconclusive and routinely employed for preoperative planning. Finally, catheter angiography offers a minimally invasive and increasingly utilized treatment alternative to open surgical approaches for vascular injury repair.

Duplex Sonography

Duplex sonography, commonly used in the screening evaluation of nontraumatic cervical vascular disease, represents a powerful noninvasive instrument for cervical vascular imaging. Duplex sonography employs a combination of gray scale, color flow, and spectral imaging to interrogate the integrity of the vascular system. Its portable nature and lack of need of intravenous contrast media make it ideal for use in the emergency department. Doppler imaging allows for detailed evaluation of endoluminal flow characteristics, whereas gray scale imaging allows for detailed imaging of the vessel wall and extraluminal structures. Vessel injury, manifested as occlusion, dissection, intramural hematoma, pseudoaneurysm, laceration, transection, or AVF, has been well described and reliably identified in several studies[44–48] with a reported sensitivity as high as 92% to 100%[49,50] in penetrating neck trauma. Indeed, Montalvo et al.[51] found no significant difference in accuracy between Doppler sonography alone and catheter angiography in screening of certain subsets of patients with penetrating injuries of the neck.

Despite the above-described list of positive attributes, several limitations of sonography inhibit widespread usage of vascular ultrasound for diagnostic triage of CVIs. First, the technology is highly operator dependent and can be time consuming. Additionally, metallic foreign bodies, subcutaneous gas, and osseous structures can limit visibility of the vascular structures. Detailed evaluation is particularly difficult for the upper cervical ICA, residing above the angle of the mandible (zone III), and the vertebral arteries,[52] which are housed in the osseous transverse processes through much of their cervical course. Finally, ultrasound is limited in its role as a triage tool in cervical and thoracic trauma due to its inability to adequately evaluate the osseous and air-filled structures.

Magnetic Resonance Imaging

Magnetic resonance imaging (MRI) employs the application of a radiofrequency pulse to tissue within a strong magnetic field to produce dynamic changes in the tissue that manifest as characteristic imaging appearances. MRI technology offers a high degree of tissue contrast and spatial resolution that allow for reliable disease detection. In the setting of blunt and penetrating cervical trauma, MRI is the test of choice to evaluate the spinal cord, peripheral nervous system (brachial plexus), and musculotendinous and ligamentous elements, although its utility is limited in the detailed evaluation of the osseous structures as well as the air-filled structures of the aerodigestive tract and thoracic cavity. MRI also provides the most effective evaluation of the intracranial compartment for ischemic (FIGURE 70.2D) and hemorrhagic complications of CVI.

A variety of imaging sequences are available for vascular imaging, including two- and three-dimensional time-of-flight and contrast-enhanced MR angiography (MRA), as well as fat-saturated T1- and T2-weighted sequences, which are effective at evaluating arterial wall integrity and are often included in the workup of suspected arterial dissection (FIGURE 70.2A–C).

Although literature pertaining specifically to the MR evaluation of the cervical vasculature in blunt and penetrating cervical trauma is limited, researchers have evaluated the utility of the modality in the setting of suspected arterial dissection (FIGURE 70.2). In the largest of these studies, Levy et al.[53] reported an overall sensitivity and specificity of 83% and 99%, respectively, using three-dimensional time-of-flight angiography, although sensitivity was much lower for the vertebral arteries (20%). Several studies have indeed shown similarities between CTA and MRA in the detection of cervical arterial dissection,[22,33] and a meta-analysis of CTA and MRA[54] discovered sensitivities in detection of cervical arterial dissection ranging between 50% and 100% and specificities ranging from 29% and 100%.

In everyday practice, there are several obstacles that limit the utility of MR imaging in the diagnostic evaluation of BCVI and PCVI. Metallic fragments can contraindicate the use of MRI, particularly in penetrating cervical trauma, and MRI can be cumbersome in acutely ill patients. MR imaging also is often more time consuming than CT, particularly in patients with multisystem trauma, and detailed evaluation of the osseous structures is limited. For these reasons, emergency department imaging of penetrating and blunt cervical trauma in the United States has evolved to largely revolve around computed tomography (CT).

Computed Tomography

CT utilizes ionizing radiation to produce cross-sectional imaging based on differences in density between different tissues. Over the past two decades, continued advancements in CT technology have allowed for significant expansion in its application as a triage tool in trauma patients. The advent of multidetector CT (MDCT) technology allows for noninvasive imaging of a large volume in a very short time with a high spatial resolution. Isometric voxelation allows for seamless multiplanar reconstructions and volume-rendered three-dimensional imaging.

As it pertains to cervical trauma, MDCT offers the ability to image the entire cervicocerebral vascular system within a few seconds with a spatial resolution that rivals catheter angiography. A recent evaluation of CTA with 16-slice MDCT scanners demonstrated 97.7% sensitivity and 100% specificity compared with the criteria standard of conventional angiography.[55] MDCT also simultaneously allows assessment of the adjacent nonvascular structures, including detailed evaluation of the osseous cervical spine. Unlike MRI, CT imaging carries no absolute contraindications and very few relative contraindications (including contrast allergy and renal insufficiency/failure), which allows for reliably safe and rapid performance of the procedure. Because of these attributes, MDCTA has usurped catheter angiography as the predominant imaging modality in the diagnosis of PCVI and BCVI.

Pertinent disadvantages of utilizing CT technology in the diagnosis of CVI include the use of ionizing radiation and potentially nephrotoxic contrast agents as well as the low sensitivity that CT possesses for the detection of acute ischemic stroke.

▌ PATTERNS OF DISEASE

As discussed previously, both penetrating and blunt cervical trauma can result in vascular injuries that manifest in a relatively limited number of imaging patterns, including vasospasm, intimal injury, dissection, pseudoaneurysm, AVF, and vessel occlusion.

Occlusion

Vascular occlusion represents a clinically dangerous manifestation of vascular injury, which unfortunately also appears to be one of the most common. It has been reported to be the most

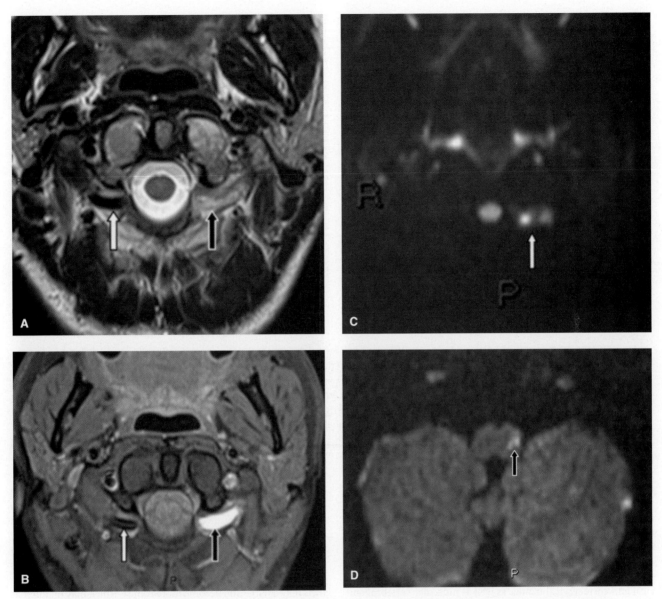

FIGURE 70.2 MRI in a 37-year-old male in motor vehicle accident with sudden onset of dizziness and vomiting. Axial T2-weighted (**A**) and fat-saturated T1-weighted (**B**) images show normal flow-related signal void in the right vertebral artery (*white arrow*) and abnormal hyperintensity in the left vertebral artery (*black arrow*) consistent with intramural thrombus, which is also noted by the *white arrow* on the diffusion-weighted image (DWI) (**C**). Axial DWI image *black arrow* (**D**) also shows restricted diffusion in the left lateral medulla.

common imaging appearance of cervical carotid arterial injury in both blunt and penetrating cervical trauma with a prevalence as high as 33%[27] and 36%,[56] respectively.

The imaging appearance of occlusion varies relative to the acuity and etiology of the event. In situ thrombosis or embolic disease often manifests as an abrupt, blunt occlusion (FIGURE 70.3A), sometimes accompanied by a "meniscus" sign or "tram-tracking" related to the intraluminal thrombus. Conversely, occlusive dissection often manifests as a tapered, flame-shaped occlusion (FIGURE 70.1E).

In CTA, arterial occlusion is usually readily apparent as an abrupt termination of the contrast column in the affected vessel. Depending on the timing of imaging and location of the

obstruction, contrast opacity within the affected vessel may vary. For example, occlusion of the ICA or vertebral artery in the early arterial phase may show no contrast enhancement within its lumen, simulating a proximal vascular occlusion; whereas more delayed imaging would show contrast opacification in the vessel to the level of the occlusion due to the percolation of contrast material into the stagnant column.

In the acute phase of cervical arterial occlusion, there is no antegrade flow through the obstruction, although collateral channels may allow for vessel reconstitution distal to the occlusion. Patterns of collateralization vary depending on the vessel and location injured. In common carotid artery occlusion, retrograde filling of the ECA from the contralateral ECA collaterals

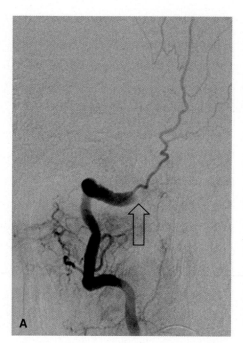 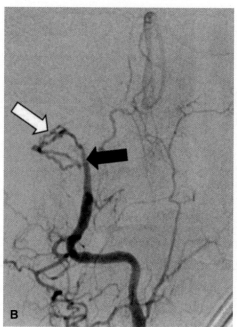

FIGURE 70.3 Vertebral artery occlusion. **A.** DSA imaging of the right vertebral artery immediately following a motor vehicle accident demonstrates abrupt occlusion of the right vertebral artery (*open arrow*) at the craniocervical junction just distal to the origin of the posterior meningeal artery. **B.** DSA imaging performed 6 months later demonstrates diminution of the right vertebral and a chronic, tapered occlusion (*black arrow*) that terminates in the posterior meningeal artery. Note the irregular multichannel appearance of the distal cervical right vertebral artery (*white arrow*), a common finding in the chronic stage of vessel occlusion, possibly representing recanalized channels within the vertebral artery or vaso vasorum.

or from muscular branch vertebral artery collaterals can result in antegrade cervical ICA opacification. In cervical ICA occlusion, antegrade filling of the intracranial ICA can occur through ECA collaterals, with the petrous and cavernous segments of the ICA, and ophthalmic arteries. In cervical vertebral artery occlusion, multiple potential collateral pathways exist for reconstituting the cervical vertebral artery, including collaterals from the thyrocervical and costocervical trunks, as well as muscular vertebral and occipital artery collaterals. In fact, the robustness of these collateral pathways and the intactness of the Circle of Willis influence the brain's ability to tolerate an acute cervical arterial occlusion.

In the setting of acute CVI, differentiating between occlusion and severe stenosis is of paramount importance because of the implications related to future thromboembolic risks and treatment option. As a noninvasive study, CTA shows a high degree of accuracy for differentiating these two entities but, occasionally, the results are inconclusive. In these instances, catheter angiography remains the gold standard for evaluation and can be performed to delineate between the two with a high degree of certainty.

Contrast-enhanced MRA, which entails intravenous administration of a gadolinium-based contrast agent, results in similar imaging characteristics to those described earlier for CTA. With currently commercially available MRI equipment and software, however, contrast-enhanced MRA of the neck offers a lower spatial resolution than CTA and, as such, can have more difficulty differentiating between occlusion and severe stenosis. Time-of-flight (2D and 3D) MR angiographic techniques have shown historically lower sensitivity and specificity than contrast-enhanced MRA.

In the chronic stage of cervical occlusion (FIGURE 70.3B), the affected vessel typically thromboses from the site of occlusion down to the level of the most distal arterial branch arising from the patent vessel with the patent vessel becoming more diminutive in caliber to reflect the decreased demand. If there is no branch arising proximal to the occlusion, the thrombosis usually extends proximally to the origin of the vessel. Over time, collateral channels may enlarge and become more robust, which may manifest as increased opacification of the affected vessel at follow-up imaging.

Vasospasm

Vasospasm represents the mildest form of vascular injury following blunt or penetrating cervical trauma. In fact, vasospasm is not a form of injury as much as it is a physiologic response of the arterial wall to mechanical or chemical irritation, resulting in contraction of the smooth muscle within the arterial wall and segmental areas of associated vascular narrowing. Vasospasm in the cervical vasculature is a uniformly reversible and self-limited event and usually responds favorably to vasodilators, such as nitroglycerin, papavarine, and calcium channel blockers.

The diagnosis of vasospasm can be difficult in the setting of cervical trauma. Vasospasm can be indistinguishable from subtle intimal injury, which can manifest as segmental narrowing, but vasospasm should never be associated with an intimal flap or a pseudoaneurysm. It can also be indistinguishable from mild forms of connective tissue disorders, particularly fibromuscular dysplasia, and can be subtle enough to be overlooked or be undetectable on CTA and MRA.

Intimal Flap

An intimal flap represents arterial injury that results in the separation of a short segment of the intimal layer from the medial layer of the arterial wall. This entity, which represents the *forme fruste* of arterial dissection, presents on imaging as a linear intraluminal filling defect that is in continuity with arterial wall without an associated wall hematoma or discreet false lumen (FIGURE 70.1B). Intimal flaps have similar imaging characteristics on CTA and MRI, but they are more reliably detected with CTA. Because they are focal and often subtle imaging findings, the ability to detect them is impaired by adjacent metallic foreign bodies or other sources of beam-hardening artifact (such as venous contrast reflux into the internal jugular vein), and they can present as diagnostic dilemmas in the lower cervical region due to quantum mottle at the level of the shoulders.

There is considerable debate over the incidence, significance, and appropriate treatment of intimal flaps. Theoretically, they can be a nidus for thromboembolic material (and indeed, an intimal flap and nonocclusive intraluminal thrombus can mimic each other identically), and they possess the potential of progressing to frank dissection. In practice, most minor intimal injuries heal spontaneously without sequelae.

Dissection and Pseudoaneurysm

Etiologically, cervical arterial dissections are the most common vascular injury following blunt cervical trauma, representing as many as 76% of these injuries,[32] but they can also occur after mild trauma (e.g., chiropractic manipulation, roller coaster riding) or spontaneously without an identifiable inciting traumatic event. There is clearly an association between spontaneous dissections and hereditary connective tissue disorders, as described previously, although the estimates of the prevalence in the spontaneous dissection population vary dramatically, ranging from 0% to 18%.[57] Cervical arterial dissections can also arise as an extension in aortic aneurysms involving the aortic arch.

Pathophysiologically, arterial dissection represents a separation or tearing of the intimal layer of the arterial wall away from the medial layer. Blood then flows into the damaged medial layer, creating a false channel. The evolution of this false channel ultimately dictates the imaging appearance of the dissection. Radiographically, the cervical arterial dissections demonstrate a variety of appearances ranging from an uncomplicated intimal flap to complete occlusion. As described previously, an intimal flap appears on vascular imaging as a linear intraluminal filling defect and without demonstrable medial disruption is not truly considered a dissection.

Early imaging of a dissection may demonstrate this as a blind-ended pouch with varying degrees of contrast opacification. If blood in the false channel creates a "re-entrance" intimal tear, or fenestration, the vessel takes on the "double barrel" appearance of two parallel vascular channels. In fact, this can often represent a stable state in which the vessel heals, giving the vessel a permanent double barrel appearance (FIGURE 70.4). If the hemorrhage does not create a fenestration, the false lumen can progress to cause stenosis, occlusion, or pseudoaneurysm. The evolution of this false channel depends on the location within the medial layer in which the dissection occurs. If the dissection involves the subintimal media, it will evolve into stenosis or occlusion (FIGURE 70.3B), whereas if the dissection involves the

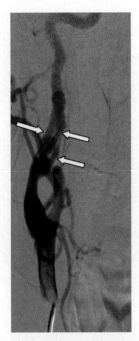

FIGURE 70.4 A 50-year-old male was involved in a snowboarding accident resulting in multiple vascular injuries. Follow-up DSA study several months later shows the chronic dissection of the right ICA with three separate parallel channels (*white arrows*) involving the midportion of the carotid lumen. All three channels reconstitute the true lumen distally without flow limitation or turbulent flow.

subadventitial media, it will evolve into pseudoaneurysm formation (FIGURES 70.1C and 70.7).

If hemorrhage in the subintimal false channel thromboses due to stagnant flow, the patient is left with an intramural hematoma that invariably results in some degree of stenosis or even occlusion (FIGURE 70.1A). Stenosis usually appears as a smooth, tapered narrowing that varies in severity and length depending on the extent of the dissection. DSA imaging can elucidate the luminal narrowing associated with dissection, but cross-sectional imaging optimizes visibility of the vessel wall to demonstrate the offending intramural hematoma. On CTA, this manifests as vessel luminal narrowing with paradoxical enlargement of the total diameter of the vessel (FIGURES 70.5 and 70.6). Intramural hematoma may appear iso- or mildly hyperdense to adjacent muscle. On MR, the intramural hematoma becomes even more conspicuous, demonstrating the hyperintense "crescent" sign on fat-saturated T1-weighted images (FIGURE 70.6). Intramural hematoma also restricts diffusion on diffusion-weighted imaging (FIGURE 70.2C), which can occasionally be seen in patients with craniocervical dissection undergoing brain MRI. These findings are more reliably conspicuous in the carotid artery than the vertebral artery because normal sluggish flow in the closely approximated vertebral venous channel can mimic the "crescent" sign of vertebral dissection.

Occlusive dissection possesses a characteristic flame-shaped, tapered luminal narrowing (FIGURE 70.1E). The wall hematoma will possess the same imaging characteristics as described earlier, but differentiating intramural hematoma from intraluminal thrombus can be difficult, if not impossible, in the setting of occlusion.

Pseudoaneurysms resulting from subadventitial dissection, represent saccular outpouching projecting beyond the expected

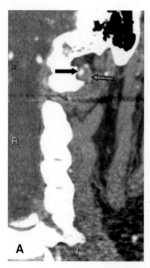
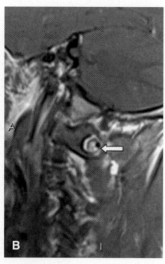

FIGURE 70.5 Vertebral artery dissection. **A.** Sagittal CTA image shows irregularity of the vertebral artery at the level of the C1 posterior arch, manifest as an eccentric, narrowed lumen (*black arrow*) with a surrounding crescent of soft tissue (*open arrow*) representing an intramural hematoma that dilates the overall size of the vertebral artery. These findings are consistent with acute dissection. **B.** Sagittal T2-weighted MR at the same level again shows enlargement of the vessel size with a large crescent of hyperintense material (hematoma) surrounding the eccentric, narrow flow void of patent lumen (*white arrow*).

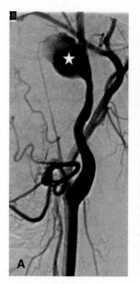
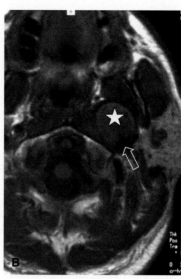

FIGURE 70.7 Following a high-speed motor vehicle accident. **A.** DSA imaging performed immediately following the accident demonstrates the development of a large left ICA pseudoaneurysm (*star*) seen on DSA imaging. **B.** Follow-up T1-weighted image shows the large, partially thrombosed pseudoaneurysmal sac (*star*) compressing the true lumen (*open arrow*).

confines of the vessel wall. The term *pseudoaneurysm* is applied due to the fact that the aneurysmal outpouching fails to possess all three vascular wall layers. On DSA and cross-sectional vascular imaging, pseudoaneurysms appear as contrast-filled outpouchings adjacent to and in continuity with the vessel lumen (FIGURE 70.7). On cross-sectional imaging, adjacent hematoma may be evident. Characteristic findings on color Doppler include the "yin-yang" appearance of swirling flow within the pseudoaneurysm sac.

In blunt trauma, dissection is the most common cause for pseudoaneurysm, but penetrating trauma can result in a laceration of the vessel wall that can also cause a pseudoaneurysm. Pseudoaneurysms caused by penetrating trauma much more commonly involve the carotid arterial system than the vertebral arteries. Unlike dissecting pseudoaneurysms, those caused by laceration contain no vessel wall with the sac instead being comprised of perivascular connective tissue and/or surrounding hematoma. This results in an instability that invariably leads to pseudoaneurysm growth and could lead to a vascular "blowout." For these reasons, pseudoaneurysms related to vessel laceration are usually treated surgically or endovascularly.

Follow-up imaging in cervical arterial dissections is imperative because dissections show a variable evolution. Many dissections heal without evident abnormality, rendering follow-up imaging normal; however, some dissections heal with chronic stenosis or pseudoaneurysm (FIGURE 70.8B). Occlusive dissections may recanalize, and dissecting pseudoaneurysms may enlarge. Understanding these changes aids in treatment decisions both in the acute and chronic stages of the disease.

Arteriovenous Fistulas

AVFs represent abnormal communication between arteries and veins that result in arterialization of the venous systems. Traumatic cervical AVFs almost always arise from penetrating

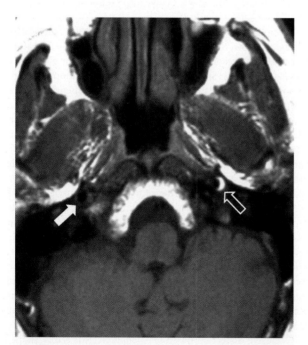

FIGURE 70.6 Axial T1-weighted image in a woman in a high-speed motor vehicle accident shows the classic "crescent" sign of an acute dissection with thrombus in the false lumen represented as eccentric hyperintensity in the left ICA (*open arrow*) and narrowing of the true lumen. The overall diameter of the left ICA is wider than the normal right ICA (*white arrow*).

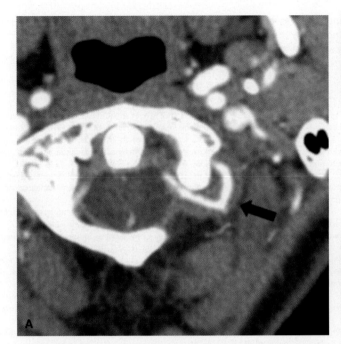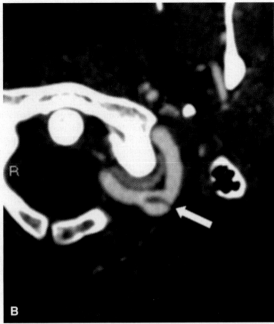

FIGURE 70.8 Left vertebral artery dissection and subsequent pseudoaneurysm formation. **A.** Axial CTA image performed immediately following a motor vehicle accident demonstrates luminal narrowing and eccentric wall thickening of the left vertebral artery (*black arrow*), indicative of acute dissection. **B.** Follow-up axial CTA image performed 1 month later demonstrates improvement in the overall luminal caliber of the left vertebral artery and resolution of the wall thickening. However, there has been the development of a small pseudoaneurysm (*white arrow*) that results in moderate focal stenosis of the left vertebral artery. No associated thrombus is evident.

traumas (FIGURE 70.1D), although rarely, blunt trauma can result in carotid-cavernous and vertebrovenous fistulas. Although not always the case, AVFs usually do not manifest at the time of initial injury, but rather mature and enlarge over time to present symptoms in a delayed fashion. Symptoms may be as innocuous as an audible bruit or neck pain but could present with more sinister signs and symptoms, such as those related to cerebral ischemia or venous hypertension.

Noninvasive vascular imaging may be able to detect evident AVFs, but catheter angiography remains the gold standard for evaluating these lesions. Cross-sectional imaging may show the fistulous connection as well as a caliber change of the affected artery and enlargement of the affected vein. Time-resolved CT and MR technologies offer some degree of temporal information, but sensitivity for detection and characterization of these lesions noninvasively remains suboptimal. With AVFs, color flow and spectral Doppler demonstrate the fistulous communication as well as showing low-resistance arterial and arterialized venous waveforms. On DSA, these lesions become apparent with rapid arteriovenous transit time and early filling of the affected veins. Depending on the size of the fistula, there may be a caliber change of the affected artery at the level of the lesion, and the artery may show no antegrade flow beyond the fistula.

Transection

Transection represents the most severe form of cervical arterial injury and occurs much more commonly in penetrating trauma (FIGURE 70.1D). Severe blunt trauma can occasionally cause vessel transection, as exemplified by VAI following severe cervical spinal fractures[58] and intracranial ICA injury following extensive skull base fractures. Indeed, many of the blunt traumas that cause this degree of injury are lethal.

Radiographically, arterial transections can present with any of three imaging appearances: vessel occlusion, active extravasation, or AVF (all described previously). Cervical arterial transections carry high morbidity and mortality.

▌ TREATMENT

A detailed discussion of treatment options for traumatic CVI resides well beyond the scope of this chapter, but it should be noted that image-guided therapy has evolved into the first line of treatment for traumatic CVI. Appropriate diagnosis using the imaging modalities listed earlier allows for appropriate treatment, whether in the form of surveillance, conservative medical management, or endovascular or open surgical intervention. Of the previously described imaging techniques, DSA can play a role not only in triage and diagnosis but also in the treatment of CVI. Flow-limiting or symptomatic dissections can be treated with balloon angioplasty and/or endovascular stenting[25]; pseudoaneurysms can be treated with coil embolization with or without stent assistance[25]; transections and active extravasation can be treated with vessel sacrifice; and AVFs can be treated with transarterial or transvenous embolization.

▌ CONCLUSION

Over the past 25 years, our understanding of both PCVI and BCVI has evolved dramatically, and minimally invasive and noninvasive imaging continues to play a significant role in the triage and treatment of these patients. A strong understanding of the imaging spectrum in traumatic CVI and of the imaging tools available to diagnose these diseases allows for the optimization of treatment and improvement in patient outcomes.

❚ REFERENCES

1. Stein DM, Boswell S, Sliker CW, et al. Blunt cerebrovascular injuries: does treatment always matter? *J Trauma* 2009;66:132–143; discussion 143–144.
2. Langner S, Fleck S, Krisch M, et al. Whole-body CT trauma imaging with adapted and optimized CT angiography of the craniocervical vessels: do we need an extra screening examination? *AJNR Am J Neuroradiol* 2008;29:1902–1907.
3. Berne JD, Reuland KS, Villarreal DH, et al. Sixteen-slice multi-detector computed tomographic angiography improves the accuracy of screening for blunt cerebrovascular injury. *J Trauma* 2006;60:1204–1209.
4. Eastman AL, Muraliraj V, Sperry JL, et al. CTA-based screening recudes time to diagnosis and stroke rate in blunt cervical vascular injury. *J Trauma* 2009;67:551–556.
5. Berne JD, Cook A, Rowe SA, et al. A multivariate logistic regression analysis of risk factors for blunt cerebrovascular injury. *J Vasc Surg* 2010;51:57–64.
6. Biffl WL, Moore EE, Offner PJ, et al. Blunt carotid and vertebral arterial injuries. *World J Surg* 2001;25:1036–1043.
7. Prall JA. Incidence of unsuspected blunt carotid artery injury. *Neurosurgery* 1998;42:495–498; discussion 498–499.
8. Biffl WL. The devastating potential of blunt vertebral arterial injuries. *Ann Surg* 2000;231:672–681.
9. Mutze S, Rademacher G, Mathes G, et al. Blunt cerebrovascular injury in patient with blunt multiple trauma: diagnostic accuracy of duplex Doppler US and early CT angiography. *Radiology* 2005;237:884–892.
10. Schievink WI, Mokri B, Whisnant JP. Internal carotid artery dissection in a community: Rochester, Minnesota, 1987–1992. *Stroke* 1993;24:1678–1680.
11. Schievink WI, Mokri B, O'Fallon WM. Recurrent spontaneous cervical artery dissection. *N Engl J Med* 1994;330:393–397.
12. Gdynia HJ, Kuhnlein P, Ludoph AC, et al. Connective tissue disorders in dissections of the carotid or vertebral arteries. *J Clin Neurosci* 2008;15:489–494.
13. Feliciano DV. Management of penetrating injuries to carotid artery. *World J Surg* 2001;25:1028–1035.
14. Munera F, Danton G, Rivas LA, et al. Multidetector row computed tomography in the management of penetrating neck injuries. *Semin Ultrasound CT MRI* 2009;30:195–204.
15. Breeze J, Allanson-Bailey LS, Hunt NC, et al. Mortality and morbidity from combat neck injury. *J Trauma* 2012;72:969–974.
16. Mabry RL, Edens JW, Pearse L, et al. Fatal airway injuries during Operation Enduring Freedom and Operation Iraqi Freedom. *Prehosp Emerg Care* 2010;14:272–277.
17. Monson DO, Saletta JD, Freeark RJ. Carotid vertebral trauma. *J Trauma* 1969;9:987.
18. Breeze J, West A, Clasper J. Anthropometric assessment of cervical neurovascular structures using CTA to determine zone-specific vulnerability to penetrating fragmentation injuries. *Clin Radiol* 2013;68:34–38.
19. Sliker CW, Mirvis SE. Imaging of blunt cerebrovascular injuries. *Eur J Radiol* 2007;64:3–14.
20. Kerwin AJ, Bynoe RP, Murray J, et al. Liberalized screening for blunt carotid and vertebral injuries is justified. *J Trauma* 2001;51:308–314.
21. Cothren CC, Moore EE, Biffl WL, et al. Anticoagulation is the gold standard therapy for blunt carotid injuries to reduce stroke rate. *Arch Surg* 2004;139:540–545.
22. Biffl WL, Ray CE, Moore EE, et al. Treatment-related outcomes from blunt cerebrovascular injuries: importance of routine follow-up arteriography. *Ann Surg* 2002;235:699–706.
23. Berne JD, Norwood SH, McAuley CE, et al. Helical computed tomographic angiography: an excellent screening test for blunt cerebrovascular injury. *J Trauma* 2004;57:11–17.
24. Biffl WL, Moore EE, Offner PJ, et al. Blunt carotid arterial injuries: implications of a new grading scale. *J Trauma* 1999;47:845–853.
25. Seth R, Obuchowski AM, Zoarski GH. Endovascular repair of traumatic cervical internal carotid artery injuries: a safe and effective treatment option. *AJNR Am J Neuroradiol* 2012 Dec 6. [Epub ahead of print]
26. Arthurs AM, Starnes BW. Blunt carotid and vertebral artery injuries. *Injury* 2008;39:1232–1241.
27. Cogbill TH, Moore EE, Meissner M, et al. The spectrum of blunt injury to the carotid artery: a multicenter perspective. *J Trauma* 1994;37:473–479.
28. Davis JW, Holbrook TL, Hoyt DB, et al. Blunt carotid artery dissection: incidence, associated injuries, screening, and treatment. *J Trauma* 1990;30:1514–1517.
29. Anaya C, Munera F, Bloomer CW, et al. Screening multidetector computed tomography angiography in the evaluation on blunt neck injuries: an evidence-based approach. *Semin Ulrasound CT MRI* 2009;30:205–214.
30. Miller PR, Fabian TC, Bee TK, et al. Blunt cerebrovascular injuries: diagnosis and treatment. *J Trauma* 2001;51:279–285.
31. Biffl WL, Moore EE, Ryu RK, et al. The unrecognized epidemic of blunt carotid arterial injuries: early diagnosis improves neurologic outcome. *Ann Surg* 1998;228:462–470.
32. Fabian TC, Patton JH Jr, Croce MA, et al. Blunt carotid injury: importance of early diagnosis and anticoagulant therapy. *Ann Surg* 1996;223:513–525.
33. Miller PR, Fabian TC, Croce MA, et al. Prospective screening for blunt cerebrovascular injuries: analysis of diagnostic modalities and outcomes. *Ann Surg* 2002;236:389–393.
34. Kaufmann TJ, Huston J III, Mandrekar JN, et al. Complications of diagnostic cerebral angiography: evaluation of 19,826 consecutive patients. *Radiology* 2007;243(3):812–819.
35. Heiserman JE, Dean BL, Hodak JA, et al. Neurologic complications of cerebral angiography. *AJNR Am J Neuroradiol* 1994;15:1401–1407.
36. Dion JE, Gates PC, Fox AJ, et al. Clinical events following neuroangiography: a prospective study. *Stroke* 1987;18:997–1004.
37. Earnest F IV, Forbes G, Sandok BA, et al. Complications of cerebral angiography: prospective assessment of risk. *AJR Am J Roentgenol* 1984;142: 247–253.
38. Willinsky RA, Taylor SM, TerBrugge K, et al. Neurologic complications of cerebral angiography: prospective analysis of 2,899 procedures and review of the literature. *Radiology* 2003;227:522–528.
39. Waugh JR, Sacharias N. Arteriographic complications in the DSA era. *Radiology* 1992;182:243–246.
40. Hankey GJ, Warlow CP, Sellar RJ. Cerebral angiographic risk in mild cerebrovascular disease. *Stroke* 1990;21:209–222.
41. Hankey GJ, Warlow CP, Molyneux AJ. Complications of cerebral angiography for patients with mild carotid territory ischaemia being considered for carotid endarterectomy. *J Neurol Neurosurg Psychiatry* 1990;53:542–548.
42. Leffers AM, Wagner A. Neurologic complications of cerebral angiography: a retrospective study of complication rate and patient risk factors. *Acta Radiol* 2000;41:204–210.
43. Johnston DC, Chapman KM, Goldstein LB. Low rate of complications of cerebral angiography in routine clinical practice. *Neurology* 2001;57:2012–2014.
44. Bluth EI, Shyn PB, Sullivan MA, et al. Doppler color flow imaging of carotid artery dissection. *J Ultrasound Med* 1989;8:149–153.
45. Gardner DJ, Gosink BB, Kallman CE. Internal carotid artery dissections: duplex ultrasound imaging. *J Ultrasound Med* 1991;10:607–614.
46. Steinke W, Schwartz A, Hennerici M. Doppler color flow imaging of common carotid artery dissection. *Neuroradiology* 1990;32:502–505.
47. Sturzenegger M. Ultrasound findings in spontaneous carotid artery dissection: the value of duplex sonography. *Arch Neurol* 1991;48:1057–1063.
48. Panetta TF, Hunt JP, Buechter KJ, et al. Duplex ultrasonography versus arteriography in the diagnosis of arterial injury: an experimental study. *J Trauma* 1992;33:627–636.
49. Ginzberg E, Montalvo B, LeBlang S, et al. The use of duplex ultrasonography in penetrating neck trauma. *Arch Surg* 1996;131:691–693.
50. Fry WR, Dort JA, Smith S, et al. Duplex scanning replaces arteriography and operative exploration in the diagnosis of potential cervical vascular injury. *Am J Surg* 1994;168:693–696.
51. Montalvo BM, LeBlanq SD, Nuñez DB Jr, et al. Color Doppler sonography in penetrating injuries of the neck. *AJNR Am J Neuroradiol* 1996;17:943–951.
52. Trattnig S, Schwaighofer B, Hübsch P, et al. Color-coded Doppler sonography of vertebral arteries. *J Ultrasound Med* 1991;10:221–226.
53. Levy C, Laissy JP, Raveau V, et al. Carotid and vertebral artery dissections: three-dimensional time-of-flight MR angiography and MR imaging versus conventional angiography. *Radiology* 1994;190:97–103.
54. Provenzale JM, Sarikaya B. Comparison of test performance characteristics of MRI, MR angiography, and CT angiography in the diagnosis of carotid and vertebral artery dissection: a review of the medical literature. *AJR Am J Roentgenol* 2009;193(4):1167–1174.
55. Eastman AL, Chason DP, Perez CL, et al. Computed tomographic angiography for the diagnosis of blunt cervical vascular injury: is it ready for primetime? *J Trauma* 2006;60:925–929.
56. Kuehne JP, Weaver FA, Papanicolau G, et al. Penetrating trauma of the internal carotid artery. *Arch Surg* 1996;131:942–948.
57. De Bray JM, Baumgartner RW. History of spontaneous dissection of the cervical carotid artery. *Arch Neurol* 2005;62(7):1168–1170.
58. Baerlocher MO, Zakrison TL, Tien H, et al. Traumatic cervical vertebral artery transection associated with a dural tear leading to subarachnoid extravasation. *Eur J Trauma Emerg Surg* 2009;35(1):67–70.

Abdominal Trauma

KEI YAMADA, SHAUN LOH, and DAVID M. HOVSEPIAN

INTRODUCTION

According to the U.S. Center for Disease Control and Prevention (CDC), unintentional injuries and accidents are the leading cause of death in the age group of 1 to 44 years with 51,587 reported deaths in 2007. Of these injuries, nearly half, or 24,829, are caused by motor vehicle collisions and resultant abdominal trauma.

In hemodynamically stable patients, the nonoperative management of hepatic, splenic, and renal injuries has steadily improved over the past 25 years and consistently results in lower transfusion requirements, fewer postoperative infections, and reduced lengths of hospital stay when compared to surgery.[1] Currently over 80% of hepatic injures are managed nonoperatively,[2] and the success of splenic conservation reaches rates of 90% or above.[3] In all instances of severe trauma, rapid and successful control of arterial hemorrhage plays a key role in improved survival.

This chapter explores the evolution of the management of abdominal trauma as it parallels the advances in catheter-based minimally invasive interventions. Specifically, we will review the current state-of-the-art diagnosis and treatment of hepatic, splenic, and renal trauma.

HEPATIC TRAUMA

The liver is a common site of traumatic injury due to its anatomic location and points of attachment. Injuries include subcapsular hematoma, laceration, intrahepatic hematoma, and contusion. The right lobe is injured more frequently than the left, and injuries often occur in association with right-sided rib fractures, pulmonary contusion, and pneumothorax and injuries to the right kidney and/or adrenal gland. Anatomically, the liver is attached to the diaphragm superiorly; to the coronary, triangular, and falciform ligaments anteriorly; and to the lesser curve of the stomach medially.[4]

Characteristic patterns of injury are observed based on the forces involved. For instance, crush injuries that result in focused blunt trauma to the right upper quadrant typically push the ribs into the liver, causing a stellate laceration involving the dome and anterior surface of the right lobe that has been termed a *bear-claw injury*.[5] On the other hand, deceleration injuries typically cause tears at sites of fixation. Forces directed in an anterior to posterior direction commonly split the liver along the plane existing between the anterior and posterior segments of the right hepatic lobe. If the forces are concentrated on the median fissure—the line of Cantlie—from the inferior vena cava to the gallbladder fossa, the liver can be divided into right and left halves.

Diagnosis of Hepatic Injuries

Unstable patients following abdominal trauma are generally taken immediately to the operating room for surgical exploration. In hemodynamically stable patients, suspicion of liver injury may be confirmed by diagnostic peritoneal lavage (DPL), aspirate (DPA), or ultrasound, often referred to as FAST (Focused Assessment for Sonography in Trauma). However, computed tomography (CT) scanning, if it is readily available, should be considered. Sensitivity for CT in suspected liver injury ranges from 92% to 97% with a very high specificity of almost 99%.[6] CT also allows one to characterize and grade liver injuries, assess the volume of hemoperitoneum, and detect active hemorrhage as extravasation of contrast (FIGURE 71.1).

The American Association for the Surgery of Trauma (AAST) has developed a grading system of hepatic injuries that is based on CT scanning. Injuries range from grades I to VI, from least to most severe, based on the estimated size of the hematoma and depth of laceration (Table 71.1). Although the AAST grading system reflects the relative extent of parenchymal damage, by itself it does not help predict the outcome of conservative treatment. For instance, even grade IV hepatic injuries can be safely observed without intervention in some patients. The decision to perform angiography and embolization in hemodynamically stable patients should not be based solely on CT findings, but rather on clinical circumstance and associated injuries.[7]

Management Considerations

The accepted criteria for hemodynamic stability are systolic blood pressure (SBP) greater than 90 mm Hg and heart rate less than 100 beats per minute initially or after resuscitation with 2 L of crystalloid. As is to be expected, the need for surgical intervention increases with the severity of the injury because hemodynamic instability becomes more likely as fracture severity increases.

Of patients with grade I injury, only 18% will require operative intervention, as compared to 68% for those presenting with a grade V laceration, in which case the liver is shattered. As the grade of liver injury increases, so does operative mortality, because of the increased likelihood of injuries to other organs. The operative mortality for grade I hepatic laceration is only 6.5%, whereas it may be as high as 92% for grade V injury.[8]

The overall mortality from hepatic trauma has declined over the past 25 years, which is caused by multiple factors. Not only has surgical technique improved, but CT scanning has also had a significant impact by reducing the number of unnecessary exploratory surgeries for what were non–life-threatening venous injuries and by triaging to emergent angiography and embolization when

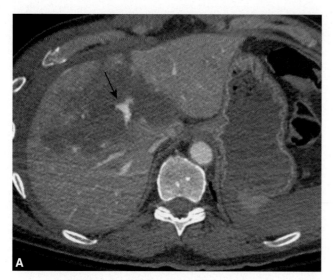
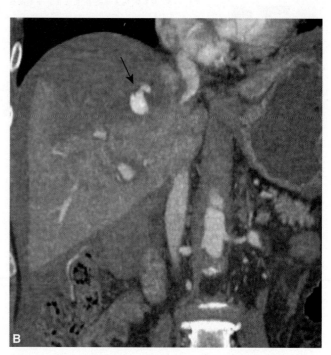

FIGURE 71.1 Contrast-enhanced abdominal CT of hepatic injury following motor vehicle collision. **A.** An arterial phase axial image of the liver shows a grade IV liver laceration—as seen by a large low-attenuation area that transects the right and left hepatic lobes. There is extravasation of contrast (*arrow*) in the area of injury. **B.** Coronal reformatted image again demonstrating significant injury. A gap is visible along the contour of the dome of the liver with contrast extravasation (*arrow*), indicating arterial injury.

arterial extravasation is identified.[2] The technical success rate for endovascular intervention for arterial injury is greater than 90% with overall success rate of nonoperative management of hepatic trauma ranging from 80% to 100%.[5]

In addition to potentially life-threatening hemorrhage, traumatic injuries of the liver frequently involve bile duct laceration and biloma formation. In fact, delayed arterial hemorrhage in trauma has been suggested to occur because of the inflammation that results from bile in contact with arteries that leads to erosion, pseudoaneurysm formation, and rupture.[9] Drainage of any sizable fluid collections is therefore advisable because bilomas may not be readily distinguishable from other post-traumatic fluid collections, such as hematomas and seromas, and the consequences of leaving a biloma undrained can be severe. Biliary diversion, whether by percutaneous catheter placement or endoscopic stenting, is often a necessary adjunct for uncomplicated and full recovery.

As mentioned earlier, transcatheter embolization has become an essential part of the treatment of hepatic arterial injuries. Indications for angiography in hemodynamically stable patients include active extravasation of contrast on a contrast-enhanced computed tomography (CECT) scan, high-grade liver injury by AAST criteria, and continued postoperative hemorrhage after laparotomy.

A CT scan depicting active extravasation portends a 20-fold increase in the likelihood of an arterial injury over a scan that does not. Approximately 60% of patients whose CECT scans show active extravasation will have angiographic evidence of arterial injury that requires embolization.[10,11]

CT evidence of major hepatic venous involvement, in addition to serving as a marker for severity of injury, is also predictive of concurrent arterial hemorrhage. Injuries involving one or more of the major hepatic veins were shown to be 3.5 times more frequently associated with arterial injury than those without hepatic venous injury.[10]

Hepatic angiography is generally not recommended for patients with grades II and III injuries in the absence of active extravasation on CT, but no consensus exists about whether angiography is necessary for patients with grade IV or V in the absence of signs of active bleeding. Some contend that angiography in this setting, even without evidence of vascular injury on CT, will reveal sites of hemorrhage.[10] Others go even further and advise that hepatic angiography should be mandatory in all patients with hepatic injuries of CT grade III or higher (FIGURE 71.2).[12]

Current surgical consensus supports the use of hepatic angiography and embolization as an adjunct to staged surgical techniques or emergent ("damage control") laparotomy, including perihepatic packing and temporary closure.[13] In one study, 52% of hemodynamically unstable patients who had undergone staged laparotomy showed continued postoperative intrahepatic bleeding on angiogram requiring embolization.[11] This suggests that hepatic arterial hemorrhage can continue despite successful operative packing, especially in the setting of deep liver parenchymal injury, which is potentially difficult and dangerous to approach surgically.[14]

Hepatic Arteriography and Intervention

Once a patient is deemed a candidate for angiography and possible transarterial embolization (TAE), an abdominal aortogram is obtained first to evaluate the anatomy, including anatomic

Table 71.1

AAST Liver Injury Scale

Grade[a]	Type	Description of injury[b]
I	Hematoma	Subcapsular, nonexpanding, <10% surface area
	Laceration	Capsular tear, nonbleeding, <10 cm parenchymal depth
II	Hematoma	Subcapsular, nonexpanding, 10%–50% surface area; intraparenchymal, nonexpanding, <2 cm in diameter
	Laceration	Capsular tear, active bleeding, 1–3 cm parenchymal depth, <10 cm in length
III	Hematoma	Subcapsular, >50% surface area or expanding: ruptured subcapsular hematoma with active bleeding; intraparenchmal hematoma >2 cm or expanding
	Laceration	>3 cm parenchymal depth
IV	Hematoma	Ruptured intraparenchymal hematoma with active bleeding
	Laceration	Parenchymal disruption involving >50% of hepatic lobe
V	Hematoma	Parenchymal disruption involing >50% of hepatic lobe
	Vascular	Juxthepatic venous injuries, that is, retrohepatic vena cava/major veins
VI	Vascular	Hepatic avulsion

[a]Advance one grade for multiple injuries to the same organ.
[b]Base on most accurate assessment at autopsy, laparotomy, or radiologic study.

Reprinted with permission from Moore EG, Cogbill TH, Jurkovich GJ, et al. Organ injury scaling: spleen and liver. *J Trauma* 1995;38:323–324.

variants, and identify apparent sites of bleeding to direct further therapy. Following the aortogram, selective catheterization of the hepatic artery is typically performed using a preshaped 4 or 5 French catheter. Anatomic variations are common in the liver, and selective catheterization of the celiac and superior mesenteric arteries is necessary for complete assessment of the hepatic arterial supply. If a CECT scan is available, it may depict normal or variant arterial anatomy and sites of arterial injury in advance.

If a source of bleeding is identified, superselective catheterization is typically performed using a microcatheter. Digital subtraction angiography (DSA), with two or more projections (or cone beam CT), should be performed and filming should be sufficient (3 to 4 frames per second) for temporal resolution of the site of origin. Embolization can then be performed (FIGURE 71.3).

Active extravasation, pseudoaneurysm, and arteriovenous fistulae are all amenable to TAE. The more selective the embolization, the less likely the risk of infarction of healthy tissue. The embolic strategy for focal arterial injuries is to use coils because they allow precise delivery and minimize nontarget embolization. When injuries are multiple or the injuries on CT appear greater than they do on the angiogram, a wider target is chosen and a nonfocal agent, such as gelfoam slurry, is used. The agent(s) used and technical details may vary with operator preference with no significant impact on outcomes.[15]

Outcomes and Complications

Approximately 30% of patients who undergo hepatic embolization experience delayed complications.[11] These commonly include hepatic necrosis, abscess formation, and bile leak, as well as gallbladder ischemia, which all may be managed percutaneously or require operation.[16]

Patients with CT findings of major hepatic venous involvement are more prone to persistent and/or recurrent hepatic bleeding and delayed complications are more frequently encountered in this group.[10] Complicated fluid collections, particularly biloma, are at risk for erosive vascular complications, and as mentioned earlier, intervention is warranted.

■ SPLENIC TRAUMA

The spleen is the most commonly injured organ following blunt abdominal trauma. It is a highly vascular organ that holds 40 to 50 mL of red cells and as much as 25% of the circulating platelets in reserve. It filters 10% to 15% of the total blood volume every minute and serves an immunologic function as well. Because of these important roles, interventions that potentially conserve the spleen are advisable to avoid impaired immune function and a predisposition to sepsis.[17]

The splenic artery supplies the spleen, stomach, and portions of the pancreas via the dorsal and greater pancreatic arteries. Distally, the splenic artery typically divides into superior and inferior branches, which further subdivide into four to six segmental branches (FIGURE 71.4).

Diagnosis of Splenic Injuries

Noninvasive investigation of splenic injury is the same as for all abdominal trauma, either in the emergency department by FAST or DPL/DPA if access to CT is limited. As with hepatic injuries, CT scanning rapidly provides specific diagnosis and grading of

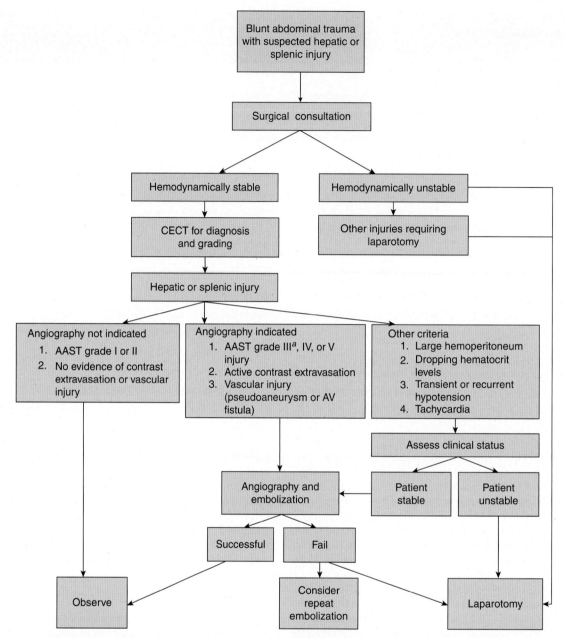

FIGURE 71.2 Treatment algorithm for blunt abdominal and splenic trauma.

[a]It is controversial as to whether angiography is indicated for grade III liver injury in the absence of active contrast extravasation or vascular injury.

Reprinted with permission from Raikhlin A, Baerlocher MO, Asch MR, et al. Imaging and transcatheter arterial embolization for traumatic splenic injuries: review for literature. *Can J Surg* 2008;51(6):464–472.

splenic injuries and helps triage patients to appropriate management, be it TAE or surgery (FIGURE 71.5).

Splenic injuries are also graded according to AAST guidelines, which are based on the degree of anatomic disruption and resultant hematoma found at CT or during laparotomy (Table 71.2). According to the AAST, splenic injuries are graded from I to V from least to most severe. Despite the high sensitivity of CT for detection of vascular injury, in more severe injuries a negative study does not preclude the need for angiography. In fact, one retrospective study showed that 23% of those patients who underwent angiography for AAST grades III to V splenic

injury were found to have a vascular injury requiring embolization, despite no extravasation seen on CT.[18]

Using two criteria for contrast-enhanced spiral CT, specifically contrast extravasation and splenic pseudoaneurysm, there is an overall sensitivity of 81% and a specificity of 84% in predicting the need for splenic arteriography and subsequent TAE or surgery.[19] In fact, the presence of arteriovenous fistulae on arteriogram predicts a failure rate for nonsurgical management at around 40%, even including angiography and embolization.[20]

The multi-institutional study of the Eastern Association for the Surgery of Trauma (EAST) reported an overall failure rate

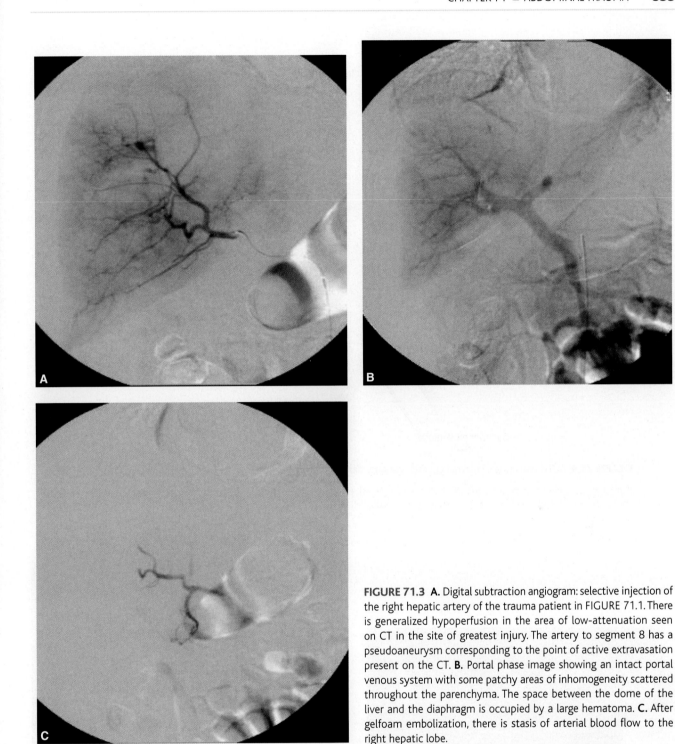

FIGURE 71.3 A. Digital subtraction angiogram: selective injection of the right hepatic artery of the trauma patient in FIGURE 71.1. There is generalized hypoperfusion in the area of low-attenuation seen on CT in the site of greatest injury. The artery to segment 8 has a pseudoaneurysm corresponding to the point of active extravasation present on the CT. **B.** Portal phase image showing an intact portal venous system with some patchy areas of inhomogeneity scattered throughout the parenchyma. The space between the dome of the liver and the diaphragm is occupied by a large hematoma. **C.** After gelfoam embolization, there is stasis of arterial blood flow to the right hepatic lobe.

of nonoperative management of 11%. Failure rates increased significantly for each AAST grade of splenic injury, 4.8% failure for grade I, 9.5% for grade II, 19.6% for grade III, 33.3% for grade IV, and 75% for grade V.[21] The numbers obtained in this retrospective review are based on conservative use of angiography and embolization, however, and the rates of successful nonoperative management of splenic trauma have been shown to improve when angiography and embolization are more aggressively used.[22]

Management Considerations

Standard nonoperative observational management for hemodynamically stable patients includes bed rest, serial hemoglobin/hematocrit checks, and monitoring of hemodynamic parameters. The success of this strategy increases with higher blood pressure, higher hematocrit, higher Glasgow Coma Scale, less severe injury based on the injury severity score (ISS), and lower grade of splenic injury.

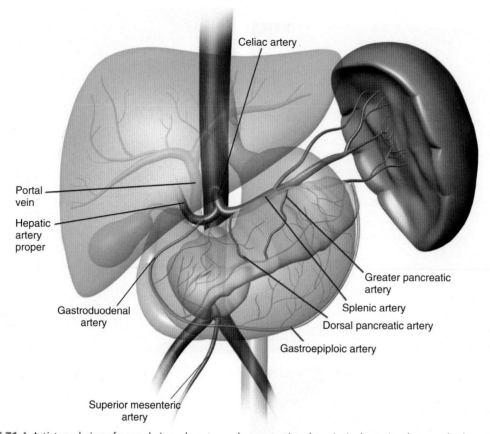

FIGURE 71.4 Artist rendering of normal visceral anatomy demonstrating the principal arteries that supply the pancreas.

Reprinted with permission from Madoff DC, Denys A, Wallace MJ, et al. Splenic arterial interventions: anatomy, indications, technical considerations, and potential complications. *Radiographics* 2005;25:S191–S211.

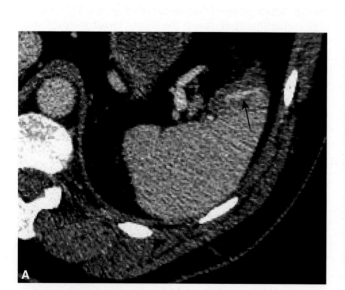

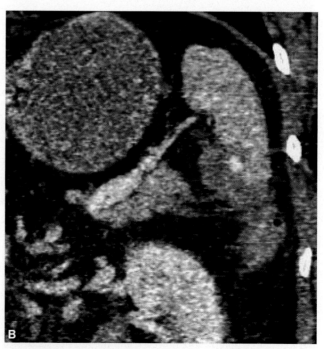

FIGURE 71.5 Contrast-enhanced abdominal CT after splenic injury from blunt trauma. **A.** This arterial phase axial image demonstrates a splenic laceration at the inferior pole with contrast extravasation (*arrow*) at the site of injury. **B.** Coronal reformatted image provides another view of the lower pole with no obvious injury elsewhere in the spleen.

Table 71.2		
AAST Spleen Injury Scale		
Grade[a]	Type	Description of injury[b]
I	Hematoma	Subcapsular, nonexpanding, <10% surface area
	Laceration	Capsular tear, nonbleeding, <1 cm parenchymal depth
II	Hematoma	Subcapsular, nonexpanding, 10%–50% surface area; intraparenchymal, nonexpanding, <5 cm in diameter
	Laceration	Capsular tear, active bleeding, 1–3 cm parenchymal depth which does not involve a trabecular vessel
III	Hematoma	Subcapsular, >50% surface area or expanding: ruptured subcapsular hematoma with active bleeding; intraparenchmal hematoma <5 cm or expanding
	Laceration	>3 cm parenchymal depth or involving trabecular vessels
IV	Hematoma	Ruptured intraparenchymal hematoma with active bleeding
	Laceration	Laceration involving segmental or hilar vessels producing major devascularization (>25% of spleen)
V	Hematoma	Completely shattered spleen
	Vascular	Hilar vascular injury which devascularizes the spleen

[a]Advance one grade for multiple injuries to the same organ.
[b]Base on most accurate assessment at autopsy, laparotomy, or radiologic study.

Reprinted with permission from Moore EG, Cogbill TH, Jurkovich GJ, et al. Organ injury scaling: spleen and liver. *J Trauma* 1995;38:323–324.

Follow-up CT scans are frequently performed 24 to 72 hours after the initial injury. There is little evidence to support repeating a CT in clinically stable patients with low-grade (I to III) injuries.[23]

Angiography and TAE have improved the success rates of nonoperative management, even among those with high-grade injuries.[22] Indications for angiography and possible embolization include active contrast extravasation on CT, splenic vascular injuries, AAST grades III to V injury and large (>1,500 mL) hemoperitoneum. The overall splenic salvage rate for embolization is over 90%, which drops to 80% to 90% for grades IV and V injuries.[20] In 1995, Sclafani et al. reported the results of a study of 172 patients who suffered blunt splenic trauma, 60 of whom underwent splenic arterial embolization. Rescue splenectomy was required in only 7%.[24]

Splenic Arteriography and Embolization

Angiography frequently demonstrates areas of focal blush that correspond to intraparenchymal hematomas, often without evidence of gross extravasation (FIGURE 71.6). The tissue phase of the arteriogram may show disruption of the normal contours, hypovascular regions that correspond to clefts in the spleen, or areas of hypoperfusion caused by vascular injury (FIGURE 71.7).

Transarterial treatment options fall into two broad categories: proximal and distal splenic artery embolization, each with its potential risks and benefits, and each with accepted indications but no clear, evidence-based consensus or treatment algorithm.

In proximal splenic artery embolization, as the name suggests, a proximal region in the splenic artery is occluded, preferably beyond the origin of any pancreatic artery branches.

The agents used are generally large coils or vascular occluders, such as the Amplatzer. Patients who are considered at high risk for delayed rupture of the spleen are candidates for main splenic artery embolization because this strategy is thought to reduce the perfusion pressure to the splenic parenchyma and promote hemostasis while preserving collateral blood flow via the short gastric and gastroepiploic arteries, which may help avoid infarction. Patients with diffuse parenchymal injury or large parenchymal hematoma on CT would fall into this category.

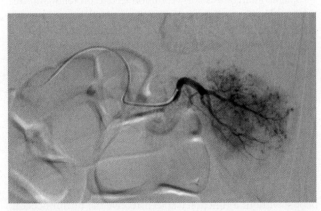

FIGURE 71.6 A selective injection of the distal splenic artery of the patient in FIGURE 71.5 shows myriad punctate hemorrhages or contusions. Because of the diffuse nature of the injury, gelfoam embolization was performed (not shown).

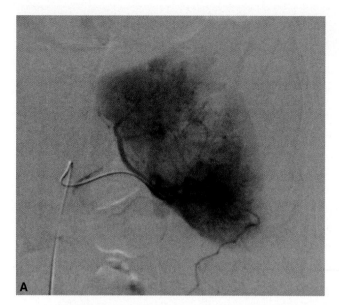
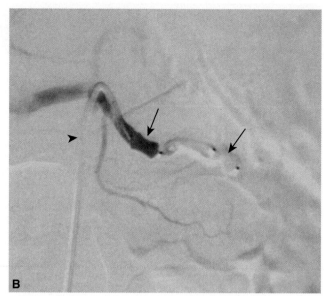

FIGURE 71.7 A different patient with a blunt splenic injury. **A.** Digital subtraction angiogram shows a diagonal band of hypoperfused tissue corresponding to a grade IV laceration. **B.** After deposition of two Amplatzer II occluders (*arrows*) beyond the dorsal pancreatic artery (*arrowhead*), there is no direct flow to the spleen. Gastroepiploic and other natural collateral pathways provide continued perfusion.

When the injury is focal, and arterial laceration(s) and extravasation are seen, then more distal occlusion may be sufficient for treatment (FIGURE 71.8). Agents that can be delivered through a microcatheter are typically used due to the size of the vessels involved. These include microcoils, glue, Onyx, and gelfoam. Parenchymal perfusion is largely preserved, as is immune function, but occult injuries may go untreated and result in delayed hemorrhage.

Outcomes and Complications

Overall, complications following splenic artery embolization occur in about 30% of patients.[20,25] Both techniques—proximal and distal embolization—fail to control bleeding in approximately 10% of patients, although re-embolization is only necessary in about 2%.[18]

Splenic infarction is fairly common to find on follow-up imaging, although most patients are asymptomatic or nearly so. A large multicenter review of splenic embolization found that distal embolization alone was associated with infarction in close to 30% of patients, as compared to only 20% who underwent proximal embolization.[20] If splenic artery embolization is performed both proximally and distally, infarction is even more likely to occur.

Abscess formation following embolization is rare and accounts for only 3% of complications. Proximal embolization is less likely to result in abscess formation than is superselective (distal) embolization.[18]

Pneumococcal sepsis is a recognized complication in unvaccinated patients following splenectomy with a lifetime risk of 1% to 2%.[26] In the surgical literature, it is recommended that people without a functional spleen receive the pneumococcal, *Haemophilus influenzae* B, and meningococcal vaccines at least 14 days before a scheduled splenectomy or within 14 days following emergent removal of the spleen. Annual influenza vaccination is recommended as well.

The issue of long-term antibiotics is more controversial, but some would advise that a prophylactic dose be given to all patients after splenectomy, especially in the first two postoperative years, those under 16 years of age, and those who are immunocompromised. Despite these recommendations, there are little published data on the need for vaccines or prophylactic antibiotics following splenic artery embolization as well as inconsistent compliance with published guidelines for immunization and antibiotic prophylaxis in many surgical practices.[27] Overall, it is generally recommended to offer vaccinations for patients who have undergone splenic embolization.

■ RENAL TRAUMA

The kidneys are retroperitoneal organs that are generally protected from blunt injury by the ribs, a thick fascial layer, and a cushion of perirenal fat. As with the liver and spleen, common mechanisms of injury to the kidneys include lacerations caused by rapid deceleration and/or puncture by the overlying ribs. Some preexisting conditions increase the vulnerability of the kidneys to blunt trauma.[28] These include hydronephrosis, cysts, tumors, and anatomic variations of location or orientation.

Renal injuries occur in approximately 8% to 10% of blunt or penetrating abdominal trauma.[29] Like the AAST grading system for hepatic and splenic injuries, a similar scale exists for renal traumatic injuries.

Diagnosis of Renal Injuries

As with other suspected solid-organ injuries in trauma, CECT scanning is the imaging modality of choice to evaluate the kidneys. CECT can provide accurate and detailed information

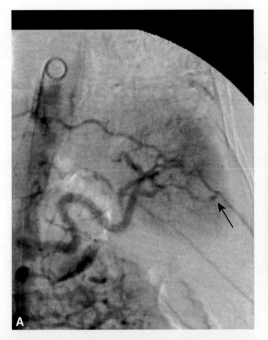

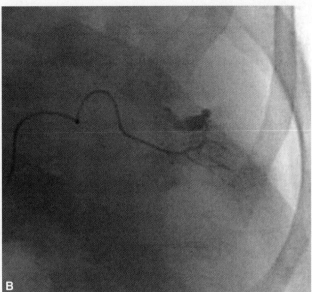

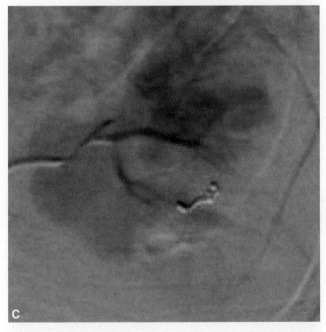

FIGURE 71.8 Patient with a focal laceration after splenic trauma. **A.** An aortogram of the upper abdomen shows a small focus of contrast extravasation in the lower pole (*arrow*), which was also seen on CT. **B.** Superselective injection of the injured lower pole branch defines the extravasation. The catheter was advanced right to the point of leak and two microcoils were deposited, which can be seen as misregistration artifact in (**C**), which also shows patchy enhancement in the remainder of the spleen indicative of multiple contusions.

regarding the presence and location of renal laceration, hematoma, or whether there is active arterial or urinary extravasation.

Overall, hematuria is common in patients with renal injury and is present in 80% to 94% of cases, but there is no correlation between the presence, absence, or degree of hematuria with the severity of renal injury.[30] In the absence of renal insufficiency, CECT of the urinary tract in adults is indicated for any penetrating injury that is associated with hematuria.

In the setting of blunt trauma and suspected renal injury, CECT is indicated when there is gross hematuria. When the hematuria is microscopic, the indication for CECT scanning is hypotension (SBP <90 mm Hg) or any significant associated injury.[31] The grade of renal injury, the overall ISS, and need for blood transfusion(s) are the primary criteria used

to determine the need for nephrectomy and prediction of overall outcome.[32]

Renal injuries are classified into five categories (Table 71.3). Grade I includes minor trauma, such as contusion and subcapsular hematoma. This category of injury is the most common, representing approximately 80% of all renal injuries, and is managed conservatively.[33] Grade II injuries include minor renal laceration or nonexpanding perirenal hematoma. Grade III injuries are deeper lacerations that extend deeper than 1 cm into the renal cortex. Grade IV lacerations extend into the medulla or have a contained hemorrhage resulting from injury to the main renal artery or vein. Grade V injuries are the most severe and are characterized by devascularization of the kidney from avulsion of the renal hilum or the kidney is shattered.

Table 71.3		
AAST Kidney Injury Scale		
Grade[a]	Type	Description of injury[b]
I	Contusion	Hematuria, imaging studies normal
	Hematoma	Subcapsular hematoma (nonexpanding)
II	Hematoma	Perirenal hematoma (contained, nonexpanding)
	Laceration	Cortical lacerations (<1 cm) without urinary extravasation, nonexpanding perirenal hematoma
III	Hematoma	Perirenal hematoma (contained, nonexpanding)
	Laceration	Corticomedulllary laceraton deeper than 1 cm without extravasation
IV	Laceration	Corticomedullary laceration deeper than 1 cm with collecting system injury
	Vascular	Injury to main renal artery or vein with contained hemorrhage
V	Vascular	Avulsion of renal hilum, devascularizing kidney

[a]Advance one grade for bilateral injuries up to grade III.
[b]Base on most accurate assessment at autopsy, laparotomy, or radiologic study.

Reprinted with permission from Moore EG, Shackford SR, Pachter HL, et al. Organ injury scaling: spleen, liver, and kidney. *J Trauma* 1989;29(12):1664.

Most minor renal contusions and lacerations can be managed with observation alone.[34] There are few absolute indications for surgical treatment of renal injury—renal pedicle avulsion, pulsatile or expanding hematoma, and persistent life-threatening hemorrhage are among them.[35]

Urinary extravasation, with the exception of obvious ureteral or renal pelvic injury, alone is not an absolute indication for surgery because it resolves spontaneously in about 80% of cases.[36] Percutaneous or endoscopic intervention is only required when there is a persistent leak, urinoma formation, or in the setting of sepsis.[37]

Typical CT evaluation of the kidneys includes both early and delayed scans. The early phase is timed for optimal vascular enhancement, which will help to determine the presence of active bleeding. The delayed or excretory phase is important for evaluating injuries to the collecting system (FIGURE 71.9).

Renal angiography is used to evaluate suspected renal vascular injuries in hemodynamically stable patients who either have ongoing hemorrhage or who have complications of injury, such as arteriovenous fistula or pseudoaneurysm (FIGURE 71.10). Grades I and II injuries are typically managed conservatively.

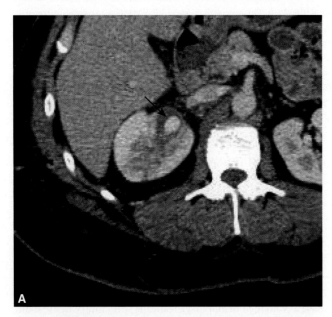
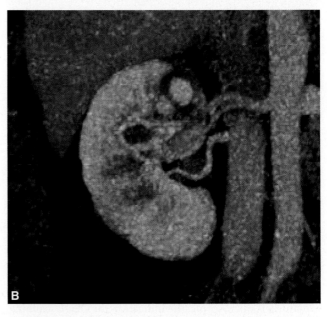

FIGURE 71.9 Contrast-enhanced abdominal CT following blunt renal trauma. **A.** This arterial phase axial image demonstrates a severe injury to the right kidney. The laceration is a large low-attenuation area that bisects the kidney with frank extravasation of contrast (*arrow*) near the hilum. **B.** Coronal reformatted image again shows the upper pole injury with a rounded focus of arterial extravasation and hypoperfusion of most of the medulla.

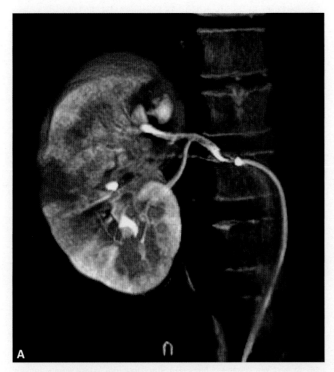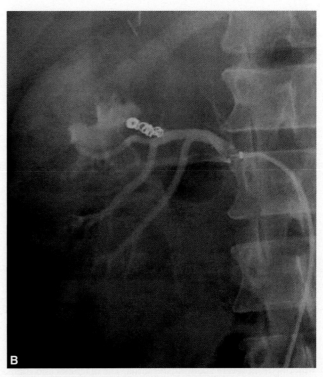

FIGURE 71.10 Treatment of the patient in FIGURE 71.9. **A.** A 3D reconstruction during catheter angiography helps to localize the injury for selective catheterization. **B.** The completion angiogram after placement of stainless steel coils confirms successful hemostasis. Excreted contrast opacifies the renal collecting system, which appears intact.

Grades III and IV injuries that do not have extravasation evident on CT are also treated conservatively. Occasionally they may require surgical management because of the hemodynamic status of the patient or the presence of a coexisting abdominal or pelvic injury requiring surgical exploration. Grade IV injuries with vascular involvement and grade V injuries are typically catastrophic and generally require surgical management, often nephrectomy.

The most significant vascular injury to the kidney following trauma is thrombosis of the main renal artery, which occurs in the setting of deceleration injuries that result in stretching and tearing of the intima and exposure of luminal substrates to tissue factor. The success of revascularization of a post-traumatic occlusion of the renal artery is poor with the literature showing that only 14% who undergo attempted revascularization have return of normal renal function, and only if the duration of ischemia was less than 12 hours.[38]

One subset of patients who may benefit from angiography and intervention are those who have discontinuity of Gerota fascia and expanding hematoma. When the fascia has been disrupted, potential tamponade of the arterial injury can no longer be performed. In one small study, 79% of patients with discontinuity of Gerota fascia and concurrent pararenal hematoma on CT required angiography and embolization. In that same study, 92% of patients who had an intact fascia did not have evidence of active bleeding at angiography.[39]

Superselective renal artery embolization for management of arterial hemorrhage in stable patients following blunt or penetrating renal trauma is often successful. Given that functioning renal parenchyma may be lost whether surgical or conservative treatment has been chosen, TAE has been shown to have lower

morbidity than surgery,[40] even after taking into account the possibility of contrast nephrotoxicity.

Most commonly, selective renal DSA is performed transfemorally using a preshaped 4 or 5 French catheter. Once the site of arterial injury is identified, a microcatheter is advanced coaxially to the target artery. Branches as small as third and fourth order divisions may be successfully catheterized and embolized.

Active extravasation, pseudoaneurysm, and arteriovenous fistula are all amenable to transcatheter embolization. The embolic strategy for focal arterial injury is again to use coils, whether trapping a pseudoaneurysm or blockading an end artery. Success rates for embolization of isolated renal branch injuries are 70% to 80%.[41] When injuries are multiple or distal, gelfoam or a particulate agent may be used. Occasionally, a small amount of ethanol may also be necessary to treat the affected subsegment because of the risk of residual hypoperfusion of downstream territory resulting in the development of hypertension via the renin-angiotensin system.

Complications

Technical complications associated with endovascular treatment of renal trauma include nontargeted embolization, iatrogenic vascular damage, and bleeding at the arterial access site. Renal artery dissection, which historically has been described to occur in up to 7% of patients,[42] is probably a much rarer occurrence these days, given the increasingly widespread use of microcatheters and microcoils for this purpose.

Immediate or short-term clinical complications related to embolization include postembolic syndrome, worsened renal function, and arterial hypertension. Postembolization syndrome results in fever, pain, nausea, and leukocytosis. These symptoms have been reported in up to 10% of cases and can be severe.[30] Symptoms are likely the result of an inflammatory response to necrotic tissue after embolization. Although it is more commonly seen following total renal devascularization, it can be seen with even selective embolization. Management of postembolization syndrome is supportive.

Post-traumatic renovascular hypertension has been described in the setting of renal artery stenosis and occlusion, renal artery compression, arteriovenous fistula, pseudoaneurysm formation, and subcapsular hematoma.[43] After renal artery embolization, especially proximal renal artery branch occlusion,[44] renin-mediated hypertension may be triggered. The true incidence of renal hypertension after trauma embolization is unknown, but the likelihood may be reduced with as superselective an embolization as possible. Subcapsular hematomas resulting in arterial hypertension, often referred to as "Page" kidney, can be managed via surgical or percutaneous evacuation. Evacuation of the hematoma may restore renal function, but results depend on the timing of intervention.[45]

▌ SUMMARY

Interventional radiologists play a vital role among the team of medical professionals who are entrusted with the care of patients suffering from severe abdominal trauma. The diagnosis and management of hepatic, splenic, and renal injuries encompass a broad set of complex skills. Overall better outcomes for trauma patients are the result of many who have devoted years and careers to this goal. It is the authors' hope that this chapter serves as a foundation for interventional radiologists who wish to engage in this important service, knowing that these few pages have only touched the surface.

▌ REFERENCES

1. Malhotra AK, Latifi R, Fabian TC, et al. Multiplicity of solid organ injury: influence on management and outcomes after blunt abdominal trauma. *J Trauma* 2003;54:925–929.
2. Richardson DJ, Franklin GA, Lukan JK, et al. Evolution in the management of hepatic trauma: a 25-year perspective. *Ann Surg* 2000;232:324–330.
3. Pachter HL, Guth AA, Hofstetter SR, et al. Changing patterns in the management of splenic trauma: the impact of nonoperative management. *Ann Surg* 1998;227:708–717; discussion 17–19.
4. Skandalakis JE, Skandalakis LJ, Skandalakis PN, et al. Hepatic surgical anatomy. *Surg Clin North Am* 2004;84:413–435, viii.
5. Piper GL, Peitzman AB. Current management of hepatic trauma. *Surg Clin North Am* 2010;90:775–785.
6. Hoff WS, Holevar M, Nagy KK, et al. Practice management guidelines for the evaluation of blunt abdominal trauma: the East practice management guidelines work group. *J Trauma* 2002;53:602–615.
7. Becker CD, Gal I, Baer HU, et al. Blunt hepatic trauma in adults: correlation of CT injury grading with outcome. *Radiology* 1996;201:215–220.
8. Christmas AB, Wilson AK, Manning B, et al. Selective management of blunt hepatic injuries including nonoperative management is a safe and effective strategy. *Surgery* 2005;138:606–610; discussion 10–11.
9. Hagiwara A, Yukioka T, Shimazaki S, et al. Delayed hemorrhage following transcatheter arterial embolization for blunt hepatic injury. *Cardiovasc Intervent Radiol* 1993;16:380–383.
10. Poletti PA, Mirvis SE, Shanmuganathan K, et al. CT criteria for management of blunt liver trauma: correlation with angiographic and surgical findings. *Radiology* 2000;216:418–427.
11. Misselbeck TS, Teicher EJ, Cipolle MD, et al. Hepatic angioembolization in trauma patients: indications and complications. *J Trauma* 2009;67:769–773.
12. Hagiwara A, Yukioka T, Ohta S, et al. Nonsurgical management of patients with blunt hepatic injury: efficacy of transcatheter arterial embolization. *AJR Am J Roentgenol* 1997;169:1151–1156.
13. Johnson JW, Gracias VH, Gupta R, et al. Hepatic angiography in patients undergoing damage control laparotomy. *J Trauma* 2002;52:1102–1106.
14. Buckman RF Jr, Miraliakbari R, Badellino MM. Juxtahepatic venous injuries: a critical review of reported management strategies. *J Trauma* 2000;48:978–984.
15. Sclafani SJ, Shaftan GW, McAuley J, et al. Interventional radiology in the management of hepatic trauma. *J Trauma* 1984;24:256–262.
16. Mohr AM, Lavery RF, Barone A, et al. Angiographic embolization for liver injuries: low mortality, high morbidity. *J Trauma* 2003;55:1077–1081; discussion 81–82.
17. Holden A. Abdomen—interventions for solid organ injury. *Injury* 2008;39:1275–1289.
18. Haan JM, Bochicchio GV, Kramer N, et al. Nonoperative management of blunt splenic injury: a 5-year experience. *J Trauma* 2005;58:492–498.
19. Shanmuganathan K, Mirvis SE, Boyd-Kranis R, et al. Nonsurgical management of blunt splenic injury: use of CT criteria to select patients for splenic arteriography and potential endovascular therapy. *Radiology* 2000;217:75–82.
20. Haan JM, Biffl W, Knudson MM, et al. Splenic embolization revisited: a multicenter review. *J Trauma* 2004;56:542–547.
21. Peitzman AB, Heil B, Rivera L, et al. Blunt splenic injury in adults: multi-institutional study of the Eastern Association for the Surgery of Trauma. *J Trauma* 2000;49:177–187; discussion 87–89.
22. Rajani RR, Claridge JA, Yowler CJ, et al. Improved outcome of adult blunt splenic injury: a cohort analysis. *Surgery* 2006;140:625–631; discussion 31–32.
23. Lawson DE, Jacobson JA, Spizarny DL, et al. Splenic trauma: value of follow-up CT. *Radiology* 1995;194:97–100.
24. Sclafani SJ, Shaftan GW, Scalea TM, et al. Nonoperative salvage of computed tomography-diagnosed splenic injuries: utilization of angiography for triage and embolization for hemostasis. *J Trauma* 1995;39:818–825; discussion 26–27.
25. Ekeh AP, McCarthy MC, Woods RJ, et al. Complications arising from splenic embolization after blunt splenic trauma. *Am J Surg* 2005;189:335–339.
26. Webb CW, Crowell K, Cravens D. Clinical inquiries. Which vaccinations are indicated after splenectomy? *J Fam Pract* 2006;55:711–712.
27. Ramachandra J, Bond A, Ranaboldo C, et al. An audit of post-splenectomy prophylaxis—are we following the guidelines? *Ann R Coll Surg Engl* 2003;85:252–255.
28. Brower P, Paul J, Brosman SA. Urinary tract abnormalities presenting as a result of blunt abdominal trauma. *J Trauma* 1978;18:719–722.
29. Gillenwater JY. *Adult and Pediatric Urology*. 4th ed. Philadelphia, PA: Lippincott Williams & Wilkins; 2002:3 v. (xii 2760, 68 p.) ill. 29 cm. + 1 CD-ROM (4 3/4 in.).
30. Santucci RA, Wessells H, Bartsch G, et al. Evaluation and management of renal injuries: consensus statement of the renal trauma subcommittee. *BJU Int* 2004;93:937–954.
31. McAndrew JD, Corriere JN Jr. Radiographic evaluation of renal trauma: evaluation of 1103 consecutive patients. *Br J Urol* 1994;73:352–354.
32. Kuo RL, Eachempati SR, Makhuli MJ, et al. Factors affecting management and outcome in blunt renal injury. *World J Surg* 2002;26:416–419.
33. Dunnick NR. *Textbook of Uroradiology*. 4th ed. Philadelphia, PA: Lippincott Williams & Wilkins; 2008.
34. Cass AS, Luxenberg M. Conservative or immediate surgical management of blunt renal injuries. *J Urol* 1983;130:11–16.
35. McAninch JW, Carroll PR. Renal exploration after trauma. Indications and reconstructive techniques. *Urol Clin North Am* 1989;16:203–212.
36. Matthews LA, Smith EM, Spirnak JP. Nonoperative treatment of major blunt renal lacerations with urinary extravasation. *J Urol* 1997;157:2056–2058.
37. Meng MV, Brandes SB, McAninch JW. Renal trauma: indications and techniques for surgical exploration. *World J Urol* 1999;17:71–77.
38. Spirnak JP, Resnick MI. Revascularization of traumatic thrombosis of the renal artery. *Surg Gynecol Obstet* 1987;164:22–26.
39. Fu CY, Wu SC, Chen RJ, et al. Evaluation of need for angioembolization in blunt renal injury: discontinuity of Gerota's fascia has an increased probability of requiring angioembolization. *Am J Surg* 2010;199:154–159.
40. Dinkel HP, Danuser H, Triller J. Blunt renal trauma: minimally invasive management with microcatheter embolization experience in nine patients. *Radiology* 2002;223:723–730.
41. Kantor A, Sclafani SJ, Scalea T, et al. The role of interventional radiology in the management of genitourinary trauma. *Urol Clin North Am* 1989;16:255–265.
42. Corr P, Hacking G. Embolization in traumatic intrarenal vascular injuries. *Clin Radiol* 1991;43:262–264.
43. Kawashima A, Sandler CM, Corl FM, et al. Imaging of renal trauma: a comprehensive review. *Radiographics* 2001;21:557–574.
44. Bertini JE Jr, Flechner SM, Miller P, et al. The natural history of traumatic branch renal artery injury. *J Urol* 1986;135:228–230.
45. Babel N, Sakpal SV, Chamberlain RS. The Page kidney phenomenon secondary to a traumatic fall. *Eur J Emerg Med* 2010;17:24–26.

Angiographic Management of Hemorrhage in Pelvic Fractures

KHASHAYAR FARSAD, JOHN A. KAUFMAN, and ARTHUR C. WALTMAN

Retroperitoneal arterial bleeding from pelvic trauma is ideally suited for management with angiographic embolization techniques. Uncontrolled pelvic hemorrhage is associated with a high mortality rate, despite aggressive transfusion.[1,2] Open surgical procedures are extremely difficult because of the confined space of the pelvis and difficulty of localizing bleeding vessels in the presence of an extensive retroperitoneal hematoma.[3–5] Proximal ligation of the hypogastric arteries is frequently unsuccessful because of the rich collateral arterial supply within the pelvis.[1,6,7] Furthermore, incision of the retroperitoneum with evacuation of the hematoma can be counterproductive because release of the tamponading effect of the thrombus permits more bleeding and may predispose to infection.[8]

Angiographic localization and embolization of pelvic arterial bleeding in blunt trauma were first described by Margolies et al. in 1972.[9] Angiography permits rapid, precise identification of arterial injury without disruption of the retroperitoneum. Transcatheter embolization effectively controls bleeding with success rates that approach 90%.[10–13] This technique is now generally accepted as the treatment of choice in patients with pelvic trauma and uncontrolled retroperitoneal bleeding.[14–28]

HEMORRHAGE IN PELVIC FRACTURE

Exsanguination into the retroperitoneum has long been recognized as a major problem in patients with pelvic fractures.[1,2] Historically, 60% of early deaths in patients with crush injuries of the pelvis were attributed to bleeding.[2,19] Most patients with severe pelvic fractures can be managed successfully with pelvic fixation devices or binders, resulting in mortality rates that approach 10% to 20%.[29–33] However, 5% to 15% of all patients with pelvic fractures continue to require angiographic intervention to control pelvic hemorrhage.[14,15,34,35]

The etiology of retroperitoneal hemorrhage in patients with pelvic fracture is multifactorial. Bleeding may be from fractured cancellous bone, severed arterial and venous structures, or crushed soft tissues.[14,36–38] Coagulopathic states induced by massive transfusion or iatrogenic lesions created during resuscitation of the patient can also contribute to bleeding.[14,36–38]

Injury to arteries can occur from shearing against a fixed ligamentous structure, avulsion of a vessel attached to a displaced pelvic segment, or penetrating injury from a shard of bone.[14] In a postmortem study of 27 individuals who had died from pelvic fractures, Huittinen et al.[36] found retroperitoneal extravasation of contrast material from internal iliac artery injections in 23 cases. Leakage was unilateral in 6, bilateral in 17, and from multiple vessels in 14.[36] Discrete sources of arterial extravasation could be identified at dissection in only 14 cases, however, and the remaining 9 hematomas were attributed to bleeding from fractured cancellous bone.[36]

Internal iliac artery ligation was suggested in the early 1960s in response to the dismal outcomes noted with supportive management of patients with obvious hemodynamic instability resulting from retroperitoneal hemorrhage.[39] This technique was extrapolated from experience in elective pelvic surgery during which bilateral internal iliac artery ligation was performed with a low incidence of ischemic injury to the pelvic viscera or soft tissues.[39–41] Successful outcomes were described in several small trauma series, but the technique did not achieve lasting popularity.[15,39–41] Not only was the ligation difficult to perform in the setting of a massive retroperitoneal hematoma and active bleeding, but serious concerns were expressed regarding the utility of the technique and the morbidity of disturbing the retroperitoneal hematoma.[4,42,43] In particular, critics of proximal ligation of both internal iliac arteries argued that it would not stop hemorrhage from vessels that had uninterrupted collateral supply from lumbar, femoral, and inferior mesenteric arteries, and that the risk of infection of the pelvic hematoma was increased.[6]

The potential value of angiography in the evaluation and management of hemodynamically unstable patients with pelvic trauma was suggested in 1971 and described in a small series in 1972.[9,44] In the first reported case, autologous blood clot was used to embolize the right obturator artery after a pitressin infusion failed to control bleeding in an elderly patient.[9] Although two of the three patients in this series died of multiorgan system failure, there was dramatic hemodynamic stabilization immediately after embolization.[9] The clinical utility of the technique was confirmed in a larger series from the same institution, which showed that early embolization markedly reduced transfusion requirements in patients with pelvic fractures.[22] Embolization was successfully applied by several other authors with similarly encouraging results.[8,10,23–27] In some centers, angiographic evaluation assumed an early and primary role in the management of patients with pelvic fractures.[20] However, it was recognized that angiographic techniques had limitations in that the bleeding sites could not be identified in as many as 29% of patients, and embolizations could not be performed in 10% of patients in whom bleeding was visualized because of technical difficulties.[10,20]

Early stabilization of pelvic fractures to control pelvic bleeding and facilitate recuperation was proposed because of evidence suggesting that a large amount of the bleeding was a result of fractured cancellous bone.[36] This technique has since become a basic component of the management of pelvic fractures. Initial studies employed the pneumatic antishock garment (the "MAST-suit" or "G-suit").[17] This apparatus was supplanted in the 1980s by externally or internally applied fixation devices.[29–32] More recently, pelvic binders and C-clamps have been utilized to provide simple and rapid means for stabilization. Early stabilization is believed to reduce the bleeding associated with pelvic fractures by reapproximating bone fragments and reducing the volume of the bony pelvis.[14,15] A 3-cm diastasis of the symphysis pubis is estimated to double the potential volume of the pelvis to 8 L.[14] In addition to reducing transfusion requirements, pelvic fixation has other benefits, such as early and simpler mobilization of the patient, which decreases overall morbidity.[31,32] Rapid stabilization of the pelvis has dramatically improved the mortality and morbidity rates associated with pelvic fracture when compared with the conservative management techniques of the 1960s.

Despite the application of early pelvic stabilization, some patients continue to exsanguinate from their fractures. Between 5% and 20% of all patients with pelvic fractures will still have uncontrolled retroperitoneal bleeding after pelvic fixation.[14,15,18,34,35] Several studies have suggested that the patients at risk for continued bleeding can be identified by the mechanism of pelvic fracture.[15,34,35,45] Pelvic fractures are caused by (a) lateral compression, (b) anteroposterior compression, (c) vertical shear, and (d) combined mechanisms.[15,35,44] In civilian trauma, the mechanism of injury in 65% of patients is lateral compression.[14,44] Lateral compression fractures are graded on a scale of 1 to 3 with higher grades indicative of increased severity of injury.[35] With the application of lateral force, the side of the pelvis folds inward, preserving the pelvic ligaments.[44] In general, this is a stable injury with a reduced pelvic volume and intact ligaments that contain the retroperitoneal hematoma.[34] Transfusion requirements are usually low with angiographic intervention needed in only 1% of patients, most of whom have grade 2 or 3 fractures.[35] An uncommon but severe form of lateral compression injury in which the contralateral side of the pelvis rotates externally, the so-called wind-swept pelvis, typically results in greater blood loss with embolization necessary in 7% of instances.[35] Anteroposterior compression, vertical shear, and combined force injuries to the pelvis are less common than lateral compression fractures but typically result in more unstable injuries.[15,34,35,44]

Anteroposterior injuries may involve disruption of the sacrotuberous, sacrospinous, and sacroiliac ligaments and widening of the symphysis pubis and/or pubic rami fractures.[35] These are also graded on a scale of 1 to 3 with grade 2 and 3 injuries most likely to require transfusion.[46,47] Vertical shear injuries involve symphysial diastasis or fracture of the pubic rami, rupture of the sacroiliac ligaments and/or a vertical fracture through the sacrum or ilium, and vertical displacement of the affected hemipelvis.[44] Combined injuries involve multiple force vectors, but usually one predominates.[35] Vertical shear and combined injuries require angiographic intervention more often than do lateral or anterior compression injuries.[12,47]

Patients with these mechanisms of injury are more likely to be hemodynamically unstable than patients with lateral compression fractures.[34] The potential volume of the pelvis is increased because of the disrupted ligaments, allowing unchecked retroperitoneal bleeding.[14] As a group, these patients have a higher transfusion requirement than patients with lateral compression fractures.[34] Percutaneous embolization is required as well as early pelvic fixation in 18% to 28% of patients with anteroposterior compression, vertical shear, and combined force injuries.[12,15,34,35]

The current management of hemodynamically unstable patients with pelvic fractures involves vigorous fluid resuscitation, rapid assessment to determine the sources of bleeding, and rapid intervention.[4,14] Survival of patients with severe pelvic fractures can be predicted by transfusion requirements with risk of death increasing 62% for each 1 unit per hour increase in blood

transfusion during the initial resuscitation.[48] This process is complicated by the fact that patients with severe pelvic fractures frequently have multiple injuries because of the high energy of the trauma.[4,5,15,18,20,49] Because associated intra-abdominal injury is found in as many as 31% of these patients, peritoneal lavage, or, more often, abdominal computed tomography (CT) or ultrasound, is performed early in the evaluation of patients with pelvic fractures.[1,50]

Conventional contrast-enhanced CT had an 80% sensitivity and 98% specificity for identification of bleeding from pelvic fractures based on visualization of a large hematoma or extravasation of contrast.[51] The sensitivity improves to over 90% with multichannel CT and may allow distinction between arterial and venous bleeding.[52] If bleeding is suspected from a primarily intra-abdominal source, such as a liver laceration, the patient proceeds to emergent laparotomy.[4,10,14] Patients with massive pelvic bleeding should undergo angiographic evaluation and embolization prior to laparotomy because opening the abdomen results in decompression of the peritoneal cavity and increased retroperitoneal bleeding. Patients who are more stable undergo pelvic stabilization as soon as possible.[31,32] If the patient has a persistent transfusion requirement that exceeds 4 to 6 units in 24 hours, angiography is performed emergently as both a diagnostic and therapeutic procedure.[10,14,15,22] In all unstable patients, an important reason for early angiography is that the embolization can be performed before the patient develops a coagulopathic diathesis secondary to massive transfusion.[15,22] When angiography is delayed, mortality can exceed 18% despite successful embolization.

■ ANGIOGRAPHY

Angiography in hemodynamically unstable patients with pelvic fractures has two goals: (a) rapid but thorough diagnostic evaluation of potential sources of arterial bleeding, and (b) expeditious embolization of bleeding vessels. Whenever possible, plain films and CT scans of the pelvis should be reviewed to identify the location of fractures and potential ligamentous injuries. The sites of arterial trauma may be suggested by the pattern of pelvic fracture and the location of hematomas (FIGURE 72.1).[18,34,35,53] Extravastion or a pseudoaneurysm may be seen on the CT scan (FIGURE 72.2). Abdominal and chest studies, if available, should also be reviewed to determine whether angiographic evaluation of the abdomen or thorax is also indicated. Angiography is indicated in the absence of a fracture in patients with blunt pelvic trauma if there is CT and/or clinical evidence of uncontrolled retroperitoneal bleeding. Arterial injury in the pelvis without bony injury has been reported.[54–56]

The internal iliac branches that are most commonly injured are (in descending order of frequency) the superior gluteal; the internal pudendal; the obturator; the inferior gluteal; the lateral sacral; and the iliolumbar arteries.[15,20,22] Complete transection of the internal iliac artery trunk occurs less frequently than injury to a branch vessel.[20] Less common bleeding sites include lumbar arteries (particularly in patients with vertical shear injuries); branches of the inferior epigastric artery, such as accessory or replaced obturator and external pudendal arteries; and the iliac circumflex arteries[22] (FIGURE 72.3). Spasm is commonly observed in the external iliac artery as a result of either vasoconstriction or trauma, but the predominant injury to this vessel is intimal tear rather than transection.[20,57]

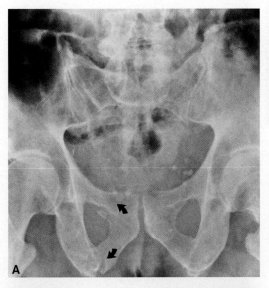

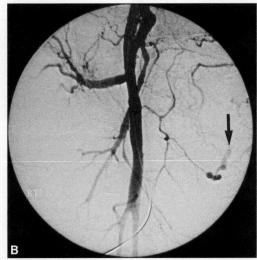

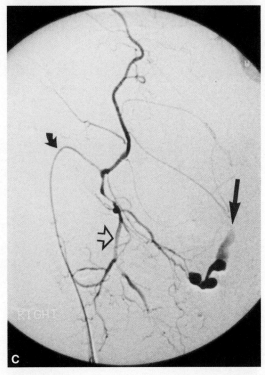

FIGURE 72.1 Examination of the plain films may predict the site of bleeding. Elderly man with a stable pelvic fracture but a massive pelvic hematoma. **A.** Plain film of the pelvis shows fractures of the right pubic rami (*arrows*). **B.** Digital subtraction angiogram of the right common iliac artery (left posterior oblique) shows extravasation in the region of the fractures (*arrow*). **C.** Selective right inferior epigastric artery injection shows extravasation from the external pudendal artery (*straight arrow*). In this patient, the obturator artery is replaced to the inferior epigastric artery (*open arrow*). The injection was performed through a 5 French Cobra-2 catheter from the ipsilateral approach (*curved arrow*).

The full range of arterial injuries occurs in patients with pelvic trauma, including complete transection, partial transection, intimal disruption, intramural hematoma, acute arteriovenous communication, and spasm. These injuries manifest angiographically as free extravasation, contained extravasation or pseudoaneurysm, abrupt vessel occlusion, intimal flap, arteriovenous fistula, and focal arterial spasm (FIGURE 72.3).

Angiography should be performed from the femoral approach if possible.[15–28] The short distance from the femoral access site to the internal iliac arteries facilitates selective catheterization. In some patients, a femoral pulse may not be palpable because of overlying soft-tissue swelling, vasospasm, or hypotension. In

these instances, ultrasonographically guided puncture is usually successful. If the femoral vein is inadvertently punctured, an angiographic guide wire should be inserted. This guide wire can then be used as an indirect guide to fluoroscopically localize the femoral artery for a more lateral puncture. The axillary approach may be necessary in patients with extensive soft-tissue trauma to the groins.[15,21,28] In this instance, the left axillary approach is preferred to minimize the risk to the great vessels and to provide the most direct access to the descending thoracic aorta. Regardless of the approach, insertion of an angiographic sheath is recommended early in the procedure to protect the arterial access during catheter exchanges and the embolization procedure.[15]

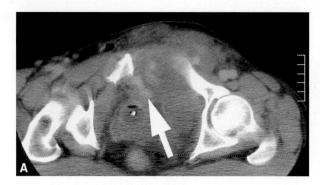

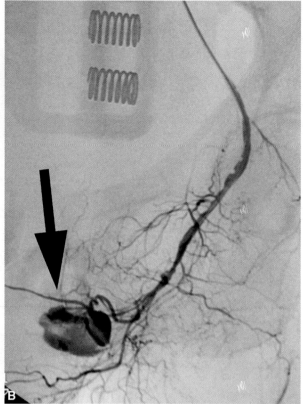

FIGURE 72.2 Patient with hypotension following motorcycle accident. **A.** Contrast-enhanced CT image showing diastasis of the pubic symphysis and extravasation of contrast (*arrow*) in the pelvis. **B.** Selective left internal pudendal angiogram showing extravasation (*arrow*).

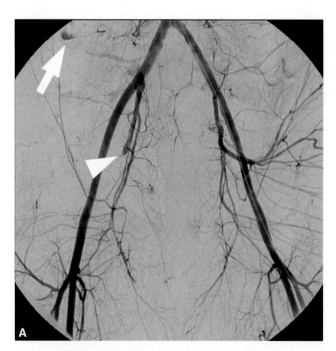

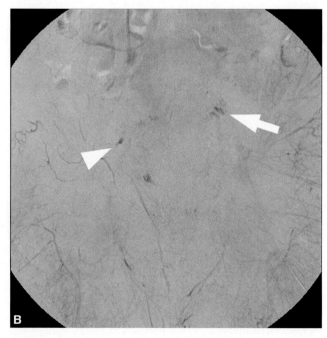

FIGURE 72.3 Patient with pelvic crush injury. **A.** Pelvic angiogram shows multiple areas of extravasation and arterial occlusion. The *white arrow* shows extravasation from a lumbar artery branch. The *arrowhead* shows occlusion of the right superior gluteal artery. **B.** Later image from the same injection. Note the persistent contrast at the site of the right superior gluteal artery occlusion (*arrowhead*) and the contrast stain (*arrow*) in the region of the left superior gluteal artery. **C.** Selective left superior gluteal artery angiogram using a Waltman loop shows massive extravasation (*arrow*). **D.** Prior to the embolization blood was noted at the urethral meatus and a Foley catheter could not be advanced into the bladder. During embolization the bladder distended, suggesting urethral avulsion (*arrow*), which was subsequently confirmed with an on-table retrograde urethrogram when the embolization was completed. A percutaneous suprapubic cystostomy tube was placed. **E.** Digital spot film showing coils in the right superior gluteal stump, the right internal pudendal artery, and the left superior gluteal artery. The right L5 lumbar artery was also embolized with coils. The suprapubic catheter is in place.

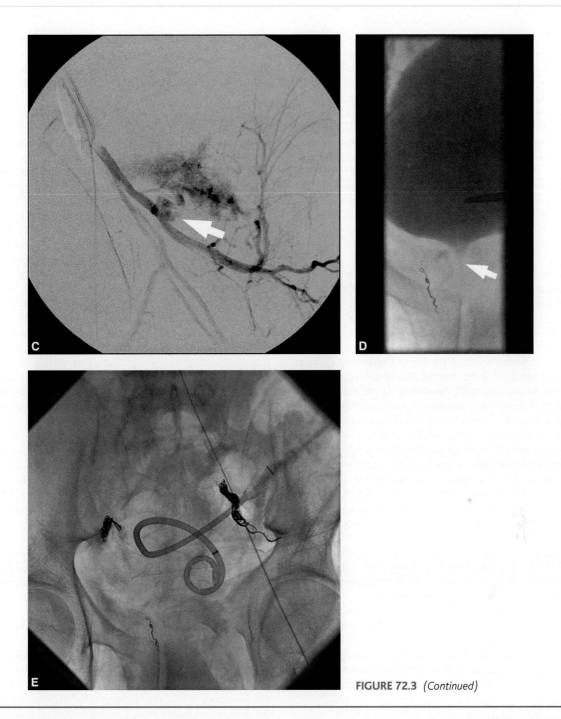

FIGURE 72.3 (Continued)

Drainage of the bladder by a Foley catheter or a cystostomy tube is helpful to prevent a contrast-filled bladder from obscuring the pelvic vessels during the angiogram (FIGURE 72.3). However, this may not be feasible before angiography in hemodynamically unstable patients with suspected urethral injury. The potentially lifesaving angiographic procedure should not be delayed to drain the patient's bladder.[15,21,22] An initial pelvic arteriogram should be performed with a 5 or 6 French pigtail catheter positioned above the aortic bifurcation to fill the lower lumbar and pelvic arteries. Contrast material should be injected at a rate of 8 to 12 mL/second for 3 to 4 seconds. The purpose of the pelvic arteriogram is to determine the arterial anatomy and to detect extravasation. Therefore, adequate volumes of contrast

and extended filming are essential. Important arterial variants, such as obturator arteries replaced to the inferior epigastric artery and occlusive disease in older patients, may be detected on the pelvic arteriogram. Brisk arterial bleeding from an internal iliac artery branch can frequently be visualized from injection in the distal aorta, but an absence of this finding on the pelvic angiogram does not exclude its presence.

Selective bilateral internal and external iliac artery angiograms should then be routinely performed in patients with pelvic trauma.[15] A selective catheter should be positioned in the proximal internal iliac artery most closely associated with the fracture or hematoma. Angiograms in both the posterior and anterior oblique projections should be obtained with injection of contrast material at a rate of 5 to 8 mL/second for 3 seconds. In some cases, selective anterior and posterior division branch injections may be required to evaluate questionable areas of extravasation. Multiple views are commonly necessary to completely evaluate patients with metallic external pelvic fixation because of the bulky metal components of the device.

The importance of selective angiography in patients with pelvic trauma cannot be overstated. Selective arteriography is necessary before embolization when extravasation is present on the initial pelvic angiogram to precisely localize the bleeding. When extravasation is not demonstrated on the initial pelvic angiogram, selective arteriography is essential to conclusively exclude arterial injury (FIGURE 72.4). Finally, selective injections are required to evaluate extravasation that occurs in a site supplied by multiple vessels, such as the sacrum and the iliac wing (FIGURE 72.5).

Several techniques can be used for performing selective internal iliac artery angiography.[10,15,21,28] From the femoral approach, the authors favor a 5 French braided Cobra-2 catheter and an angled hydrophilic guide wire for both the ipsilateral and contralateral arteries.[10] A loop is formed for catheterization of the ipsilateral iliac arteries (FIGURE 72.3). The precise torque control and cephalad angle of the tip of the looped catheter permit rapid selection of the internal iliac artery trunk and the branches of the anterior and posterior divisions. Alternatively, an angled or recurved selective catheter can be used to select the ipsilateral internal iliac artery directly. In elderly patients with a steep aortic bifurcation or tortuous iliac arteries, a long, curved sheath placed over the aortic bifurcation improves the stability and control of the selective catheter for the contralateral arteries. Bilateral femoral artery punctures with bilateral selection of the contralateral internal iliac artery may be required in patients with tortuous or diseased iliac arteries. The catheterization from the axillary approach requires a long, angled catheter, such as a Headhunter 1.[28]

Extended filming may be necessary to visualize pelvic arterial extravasation.[21,28] Digital subtraction angiography (DSA) allows for rapid examination of hemodynamically unstable patients.[18] An important pitfall of DSA is pseudoextravasation caused by misregistration artifacts from bowel gas, ureteral peristalsis, and patient movement. Careful selection of the mask, pixel shifting, or review of the unsubtracted digital angiogram may reveal the true nature of the suspected extravasation. Neither the normal uterine blush in menstruating women nor the stain at the base of the penis in males should be confused with extravasation.[58]

▌ EMBOLIZATION

Once bleeding has been identified, a selective catheter should be securely positioned to allow embolization of the target vessel. The primary goal of embolization in patients with pelvic fractures is to expeditiously decrease or arrest the flow of arterial blood to the injured vessel to allow hemostasis to occur.[15] Superselective catheterization should be used judiciously in patients who are unstable because the time spent manipulating a microcatheter into a small vessel may unnecessarily prolong the procedure and limit the operator to small embolic materials. Rapid embolization of the entire anterior or posterior division is preferable to an elegant but long superselective embolization. Complete occlusion of the internal iliac artery is an acceptable alternative to exsanguination.

The embolic material should be easy to use, widely available, and able to rapidly occlude medium-size arteries. Temporary occlusion on the order of several weeks is ideal because this allows recanalization of the vessel after healing of the injury.[15] Materials that are difficult to use, such as tissue adhesives, are inappropriate because of the emergent nature of the procedure. Materials that embolize the terminal arterial branches, such as gelfoam powder or other fine particles, should not be used because of the risk of ischemia to the pelvic viscera, soft tissues, and nerves.[59,60] Absolute alcohol is contraindicated because of tissue necrosis and poor control of the liquid embolic agent within the richly anastomotic pelvic circulation. The original pelvic embolizations for trauma employed autologous blood clot formed in a sterile bowl during the procedure.[9] Formation of clot can take a long time in coagulopathic patients, requiring the use of topical thrombin.[25] This is no longer a first-line agent because it is difficult to control the size of the emboli and because recanalization can occur within days.

The agent of choice in pelvic trauma is gelfoam cut into pieces to match the vessel to be embolized.[10,15,20,21,28] Gelfoam is readily available, easy to use, quickly tailored to the individual patient, flow directed to the injured vessel when there is rapid extravasation, and a temporary agent that permits later recanalization. The dimensions of the pledget should be sized to the diameter of the vessel at the bleeding site. Proximal embolization of the vessel may allow continued bleeding via collateral supply. Typical pledget dimensions range from 1-mm cubes to 1 mm × 2 mm × 5 mm rectangles. Long gelfoam strips up to 5 cm long may be necessary for large vessels.[12] The gelfoam pledget is first soaked in contrast and then loaded into a 1-mL Luer-Lok syringe. Embolization is accomplished by injection of the pledget through the selective catheter. Use of tuberculin syringes should be avoided because they lack Luer-Loks and dislodge from the catheter during injection of the embolus. Large strips of gelfoam are injected using 5- to 10-mL Luer-Lok syringes and must be injected through 5 French or larger catheters.[15] Multiple pledgets of varying sizes may be required, depending on the progress of the embolization. Embolization continues until extravasation is no longer visualized.

When numerous bleeding sites are present or selection beyond the internal iliac trunk cannot be accomplished, the scatter technique described by Ben-Menachem et al.[15] may be used (FIGURE 72.4). Numerous 2-mm gelfoam cubes suspended in contrast material are injected in a pulsatile fashion into the internal iliac artery, resulting in occlusion of multiple vessels.[21] The low resistance within the bleeding vessels favors distribution of the gelfoam emboli to these branches. Bilateral embolization is well tolerated and has been advocated as an empiric therapy in the absence of demonstrable extravasation for unstable patients with severe fractures.[61]

Coils are useful adjuncts in pelvic embolization procedures. When large vessels are transected, the gelfoam may be swept into the retroperitoneum. Coils can provide an intravascular substrate on which gelfoam pledgets can be packed (FIGURE 72.3). In patients with pseudoaneurysms or arteriovenous fistulas, where a precise embolization may be desirable, coils are the embolic material of choice. In contrast to gelfoam pledgets, which are injected in a relatively uncontrolled manner, coils can be pushed through the catheter with a floppy wire and deposited in a more deliberate fashion. In patients with pelvic hemorrhage, some authors have used proximal coil blockade

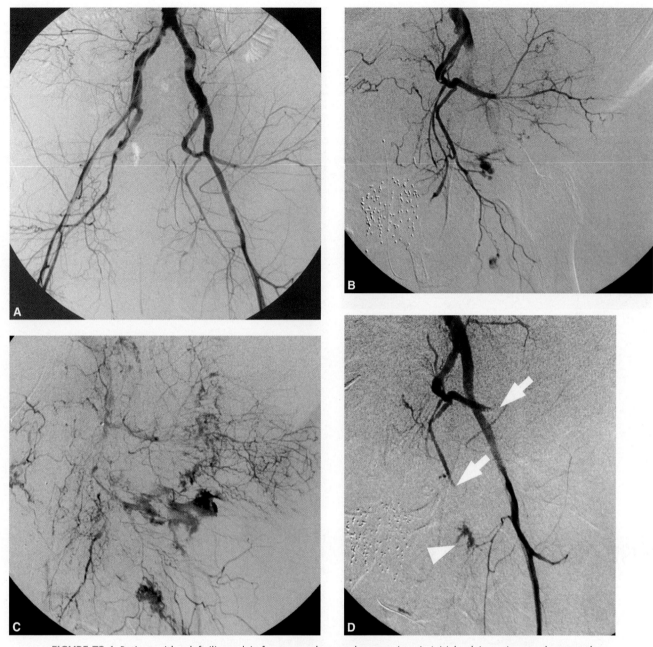

FIGURE 72.4 Patient with a left iliac pelvic fracture and severe hypotension. **A.** Initial pelvic angiogram does not show extravasation. The patient had a blood pressure of 60/30 mm Hg at the time of this injection. **B.** While the patient was resuscitated, a selective superior gluteal artery angiogram was performed showing extravasation from multiple sites. **C.** Later image from the same injection showing the massive nature of the extravasation. **D.** Embolization was performed with a slurry of gelatin sponge cubes of the entire left internal iliac to gain rapid control. There is occlusion of the anterior and posterior divisions (*arrows*). Bleeding from a profunda femoris branch (*arrowhead*). This was also embolized with gelatin cubes after selective catheterization.

to protect normal vessels during injection of small pieces of gelfoam.[10] This practice is suitable only in stable patients in whom the pace of the embolization can be slower and is of unproven benefit. A variety of coil sizes and shapes are available for both standard selective and superselective microcatheters. In most cases, however, coils are not the primary embolization material in hemodynamically unstable patients because of the time needed for careful placement and occasional incomplete vascular occlusion.[15]

Balloon occlusion catheters positioned in the internal iliac artery can temporarily control hemorrhage in exsanguinating patients.[9,15,21,28,62] Embolization can then be performed through

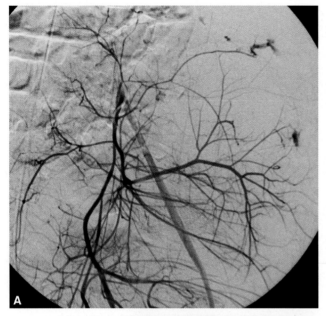

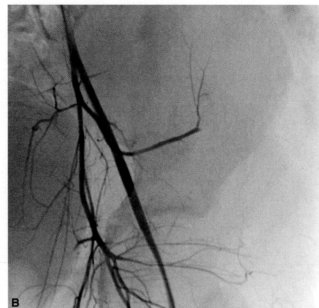

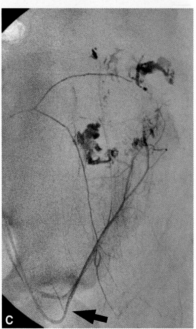

FIGURE 72.5 Collateral supply to a bleeding site in a patient with a fracture of the left hemipelvis. **A.** Left internal iliac artery angiogram shows multiple sites of extravasation. **B.** After gelatin sponge embolization of the posterior division, bleeding is no longer visualized. The patient remained hypotensive. **C.** Injection of the left deep iliac circumflex artery (*arrow*) shows massive extravasation distal to the embolized posterior division branches. This was successfully embolized with gelatin cubes.

the lumen of the occlusion catheter using 3 French microcatheters. Balloon occlusion techniques may also be useful when hemorrhage is discovered from a vessel that cannot be safely embolized, such as the common or external iliac arteries. The balloon remains inflated while a stent-graft is deployed or the patient is transferred to the operating room for open repair.[63]

The role of embolization in the presence of traumatic occlusions of internal iliac artery branches is not well defined. These occlusions may represent thrombosed arterial transections or areas of spasm. Differentiation is impossible from the diagnostic angiograms because both lesions appear as abrupt arterial cutoffs. Probing of the occlusion with a guide wire is ill advised because of the risk of converting an intact but spastic artery into a perforated vessel. Some authors recommend prophylactic embolization of the occluded vessels to prevent possible future hemorrhage, particularly in patients who are hemodynamically unstable[15,21] (FIGURE 72.3). This may be technically difficult if only a short stump of the vessel remains patent. In this instance, placement of a coil is preferred to the less-controlled injection of gelfoam pledgets. An alternative management strategy in hemodynamically stable patients is to follow transfusion requirements without embolization with prompt return to the angiographic suite for evidence of resumed bleeding (transfusion of more than 4 to 6 units of packed red cells in fewer than 24 hours). Patients who are not embolized should be monitored carefully because the rate of clot lysis is unpredictable.

Successful embolization is frequently clinically evident with sudden improvement in the patient's hemodynamic status during the procedure. Angiographically, extravasation ceases, and vasospasm improves. Completion angiography is necessary to document cessation of bleeding and to screen for previously unsuspected sites of extravasation or collateral supply (FIGURE 72.4). A pelvic angiogram is mandatory. If extravasation was visualized with only selective injections, these should be repeated. Bilateral internal iliac angiograms should be performed if extravasation was from a midline vessel. When embolization in the pelvis is complete but the patient remains hemodynamically unstable, angiographic evaluation of the abdomen or thorax for another source of bleeding may be warranted.[15]

The complications of percutaneous embolization of bleeding in pelvic trauma should be compared with the morbidity associated with attempted operative repair or conservative management with massive transfusion.[27] Patients should never be considered "too unstable" to undergo this procedure if the suspected etiology of hemodynamic collapse is uncontrolled pelvic hemorrhage. Concerns regarding contrast material, such as renal failure, are legitimate but should never prevent the procedure. Patients who undergo angiography for diagnosis and treatment of pelvic bleeding are dying. Most complications are acceptable alternatives to exsanguinations.

Nontarget embolization is an important procedure-specific complication of pelvic embolization. Fortunately, the most common site of nontarget embolization is another branch of the internal iliac artery. This is usually of little clinical consequence because the bladder, rectum, and pelvic soft tissues have multiple sources of blood supply, including the opposite internal iliac artery and sources originating outside the anatomic boundaries of the pelvis. As long as the embolic material is of appropriate size and composition, ischemic complications are rare.[59,60] Reflux of embolic material into the ipsilateral lower extremity can occur if the catheter is not well seated in the internal iliac artery or the pledget is injected with excessive force. Emboli that lodge in the profunda femoris artery or other muscular branches are usually clinically silent unless these are sources of collateral supply to the lower limb. Occlusion of a runoff vessel, such as the superficial femoral or popliteal artery, may result in a severely ischemic limb that requires urgent revascularization (FIGURE 72.6).[21] These complications can usually be quickly managed with suction embolectomy of Gelfoam or snare retrieval of coils.

Impotence in men and inability to achieve pregnancy in women may be perceived as potential complications of embolization by referring physicians. Before the widespread application of percutaneous embolization in pelvic trauma, impotence was closely linked to urethral injury with an incidence of 30% to 50%.[64,65] The etiologies of impotence following pelvic fracture

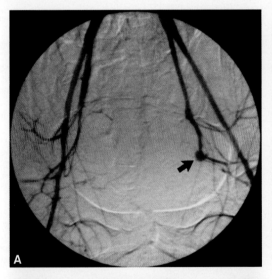
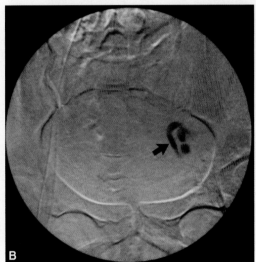
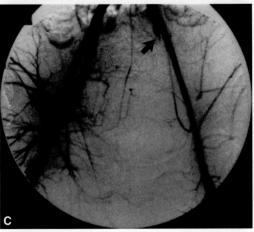

FIGURE 72.6 Distal embolization resulting from reflux of gelfoam pledgets, complicating pelvic embolization for post-traumatic bleeding. **A, B.** Early and late images from the digital subtraction angiogram of the pelvis show extravasation from the anterior division of the left internal iliac artery (*arrow*). **C.** The postembolization digital subtraction angiogram shows complete occlusion of the left internal iliac artery (*arrow*). **D.** After the embolization, the patient was noted to have new onset of left foot ischemia. Cut-film angiogram of the left lower leg shows embolic occlusion of the proximal anterior tibial artery and the tibioperoneal trunk (*arrows*). Gelfoam strips and thrombus were recovered at surgery. *(continued)*

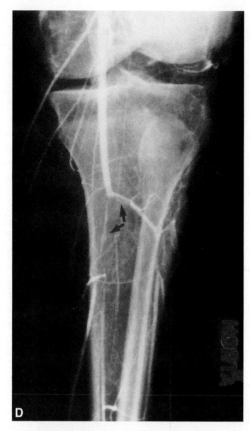

FIGURE 72.6 *(Continued)*

are predominantly vascular and neurologic insults that occur at the time of the original trauma.[66,67] In women, conception with successful pregnancies has been documented after surgical devascularization of the uterus and ovaries.[68] The use of a temporary embolic agent, such as gelfoam, may permit future recanalization of pudendal, uterine, and ovarian arteries. No studies prove that pelvic embolization in trauma does not cause impotence in men or infertility in women, however. These concerns should be weighed against the immediate needs of an exsanguinating patient.

SUMMARY

Percutaneous embolization of uncontrolled retroperitoneal pelvic hemorrhage is a lifesaving technique for which no adequate alternative procedure exists. Early intervention in hemodynamically unstable patients with pelvic fractures is essential to reduce the morbidity of the injury. Embolization can be quickly and safely performed using widely available embolic materials. Angiography is likely to continue to have an important role in the management of pelvic trauma.

REFERENCES

1. Patterson FP, Morton KS. The cause of death in fractures of the pelvis: with a note on treatment by ligation of the hypogastric (internal iliac) artery. *J Trauma* 1973;13:849–856.
2. Rothenberger DA, Fischer RP, Strate RG, et al. The mortality associated with pelvic fractures. *Surgery* 1978;84:356–361.
3. Ravitch MM. Hypogastric artery ligation in acute pelvic trauma. *Surgery* 1964;56:601–602.
4. Mucha P, Farnell MN. Analysis of pelvic fracture management. *J Trauma* 1984;24:379–386.
5. Reed RA, Teitelbaum GP, Katz MD, et al. Early management of the trauma patient with pelvic fracture: a medical perspective. *Semin Intervent Radiol* 1992;9:1–3.
6. Brotman S, Soderstrom CA, Oster-Granite M, et al. Management of severe bleeding in fractures of the pelvis. *Surg Gynecol Obstet* 1981;153:823–826.
7. Yellin AE, Lundell CJ, Finck EJ. Diagnosis and control of posttraumatic pelvic hemorrhage: transcatheter angiographic embolization techniques. *Arch Surg* 1983;118:1378–1383.
8. Ayella RJ, DuPriest RW Jr, Khaneja SC, et al. Transcatheter embolization of autologous clot in the management of bleeding associated with fractures of the pelvis. *Surg Gynecol Obstet* 1978;147:849–852.
9. Margolies MN, Ring EJ, Waltman AC, et al. Arteriography in the management of hemorrhage from pelvic fractures. *N Engl J Med* 1972;287:317–321.
10. Panetta T, Sclafani SJ, Goldstein AS, et al. Percutaneous transcatheter embolization for massive bleeding from pelvic fractures. *J Trauma* 1985;25:1021–1029.
11. Flint L, Cryer HG. Pelvic fracture: the last 50 years. *J Trauma* 2010;69:483–488.
12. Jeske HC, Larndorfer R, Krappinger D, et al. Management of hemorrhage in severe pelvic injuries. *J Trauma* 2010;68:415–420.
13. Velmahos GC, Toutouzas KG, Vassiliu P, et al. A prospective study on the safety and efficacy of angiographic embolization for pelvic and visceral injuries. *J Trauma* 2002;53:303–308.
14. Papakostidis C, Kanakaris N, Dimitriou R, et al. The role of arterial embolization in controlling pelvic fracture haemorrhage: a systematic review of the literature. *Eur J Radiol* 2012;81:897–904.
15. Ben-Menachem Y, Coldwell DM, Young JWR, et al. Hemorrhage associated with pelvic fractures: causes, diagnosis, and emergent management. *AJR Am J Roentgenol* 1991;157:1005–1014.
16. Brown JJ, Greene FL, McMillan RD. Vascular injuries associated with pelvic fractures. *Am Surg* 1984;50:150–154.
17. Evers BM, Cryer HM, Miller FB. Pelvic fracture hemorrhage: priorities in management. *Arch Surg* 1989;124:422–424.
18. Flint LW, Brown A, Richardson JD, et al. Definitive control of bleeding from severe pelvic fractures. *Ann Surg* 1979;189:709–714.
19. Gilliland MD, Ward RE, Barton RM, et al. Factors affecting mortality in pelvic fractures. *J Trauma* 1982;22:691–693.
20. Kam J, Jackson H, Ben-Menachem Y. Vascular injuries in blunt pelvic trauma. *Radiol Clin North Am* 1981;19:171–186.
21. Katz MD, Teitelbaum GP, Pentecost MJ. Diagnostic arteriography and therapeutic transcatheter embolization for post-traumatic pelvic hemorrhage. *Semin Intervent Radiol* 1992;9:4–12.
22. Matalon TS, Athanasoulis CA, Margolies MN, et al. Hemorrhage with pelvic fractures: efficacy of transcatheter embolization. *AJR Am J Roentgenol* 1979;133:859–864.
23. Maull KI, Sachatello CR. Current management of pelvic fractures: a combined surgical-angiographic approach to hemorrhage. *South Med J* 1976;69:1285–1289.
24. Poole GV, Ward EF, Muakkassa FF, et al. Pelvic fracture from major blunt trauma: outcome is determined by associated injuries. *Ann Surg* 1991;213:532–538.
25. Ring EJ, Athanasoulis CA, Waltman AC, et al. Arteriographic management of hemorrhage following pelvic fracture. *Radiology* 1973;109:65–70.
26. Ring EJ, Waltman AS, Athanasoulis CA, et al. Angiography in pelvic trauma. *Surg Gynecol Obstet* 1974;139:375–380.
27. Smith K, Ben-Menachem Y, Duke JH Jr, et al. The superior gluteal: an artery at risk in blunt pelvic trauma. *J Trauma* 1976;16:273–279.
28. Stock JR, Harris WH, Athanasoulis CA. The role of diagnostic and therapeutic angiography in trauma to the pelvis. *Clin Orthop Relat Res* 1980;151:31–40.
29. Davidson BS, Simmons GT, Williamson PR, et al. Pelvic fractures associated with open perineal wounds: a survivable injury. *J Trauma* 1993;35:36–39.
30. Riemer BL, Butterfield SL, Diamond DL, et al. Acute mortality associated with injuries to the pelvic ring: the role of early patient mobilization and external fixation. *J Trauma* 1993;35:671–677.
31. Latenser BA, Gentilello LM, Tarver AA, et al. Improved outcomes with early fixation of skeletally unstable pelvic fractures. *J Trauma* 1991;31:28–31.
32. Goldstein A, Phillips T, Sclafani SJ, et al. Early open reduction and internal fixation of the disrupted pelvic ring. *J Trauma* 1986;26:325–333.

33. Biffl WL, Smith WR, Morre EE, et al. Evolution of a multidisciplinary clinical pathway for the management of unstable patients with pelvic fractures. *Ann Surg* 2001;233:843–850.

34. Cryer HM, Miller FB, Evers BM, et al. Pelvic fracture classification: correlation with hemorrhage. *J Trauma* 1988;28:973–979.

35. Burgess AR, Eastridge BJ, Young JWR, et al. Pelvic ring disruptions: effective classification system and treatment protocols. *J Trauma* 1990;30:848–856.

36. Huittinen V-M, Slätis P. Postmortem angiography and dissection of the hypogastric artery in pelvic fractures. *Surgery* 1973;73:454–462.

37. Motsay GJ, Manlove C, Perry JF. Major venous injury with pelvic fracture. *J Trauma* 1969;9:343–346.

38. Ben-Menachem Y. Delayed, exsanguinating pelvic hemorrhage after blunt trauma without bony fracture: case report. *J Trauma* 1991;31:1018.

39. Seavers R, Lynch J, Ballard R, et al. Hypogastric artery ligation for uncontrollable hemorrhage in acute pelvic trauma. *Surgery* 1964;55:516–519.

40. Horton RE, Hamilton GI. Ligature of the internal iliac artery for massive haemorrhage complicating fracture of the pelvis. *J Bone Joint Surg Br* 1968;50:376–379.

41. Fleming WH, Bowen JC. Control of hemorrhage in pelvic crush injuries. *J Trauma* 1973;13:567–570.

42. Ger R, Condrea H, Steichen FM. Traumatic intrapelvic retroperitoneal hemorrhage: an experimental study. *J Surg Res* 1969;9:31–34.

43. Ravitch MM. Hypogastric artery ligation in acute pelvic trauma. *Surgery* 1964;56:601–602.

44. Athanasoulis CA, Duffield R, Shapiro JH. Angiography to assess pelvic vascular injury. *N Engl J Med* 1971;285:1539.

45. Young JW, Resnik CS. Fracture of the pelvis: current concepts and classification. *AJR Am J Roentgenol* 1990;155:1169–1175.

46. Eastridge B, Starr A, Minei JP, et al. The importance of fracture pattern in guiding therapeutic decision-making in patients with hemorrhagic shock and pelvic ring disruptions. *J Trauma* 2002;53:446–450.

47. Bassam D, Cephas GA, Ferguson KA, et al. A protocol for the initial management of unstable pelvic fractures. *Am Surg* 1998;64:862–867.

48. Wong YC, Wang LJ, Ng CJ, et al. Mortality after successful transcatheter arterial embolization in patients with unstable pelvic fractures: rate of blood transfusion as a predictive factor. *J Trauma* 2000;49:71–75.

49. Ochsner MG, Hoffman AP, DiPasquale D, et al. Associated aortic rupture-pelvic fracture: an alert for orthopedic and general surgeons. *J Trauma* 1992;33:429–434.

50. Demetriades D, Karaiskakis M, Toutouzas K, et al. Pelvic fractures: epidemiology and predictors of associated abdominal injuries and outcomes. *J Am Coll Surg* 2002;195:1–10.

51. Stephen DJ, Kreder HJ, Day AC, et al. Early detection of arterial bleeding in acute pelvic trauma. *J Trauma* 1999;47:638–642.

52. Kertesz JL, Anderson SW, Murakami AM, et al. Detection of vascular injuries in patients with blunt pelvic trauma by using 64-channel multidetector CT. *Radiographics* 2009;29:151–164.

53. Blackmore CC, Jurkovich GJ, Linnau KF, et al. Assessment of volume of hemorrhage and outcome from pelvic fracture. *Arch Surg* 2003;138:504–508.

54. Brumback RJ. Traumatic rupture of the superior gluteal artery, without fracture of the pelvis, causing compartment syndrome of the buttock. A case report. *J Bone Joint Surg* 1990;72:134–137.

55. Baumgartner F, White GH, White RA, et al. Delayed, exsanguinating pelvic hemorrhage after blunt trauma without bony fracture: case report. *J Trauma* 1990;30:1603–1605.

56. Belley G, Gallix BP, Derossis AM, et al. Profound hypotension in blunt trauma associated with superior gluteal artery rupture without pelvic fracture. *J Trauma* 1997;43:703–705.

57. Birchard JD, Pichora DR, Brown PM. External iliac artery and lumbosacral plexus injury secondary to open book fracture of the pelvis: report of a case. *J Trauma* 1990;30:906–908.

58. Schrumpf JD, Sommer G, Jacobs RP. Bleeding simulated by the distal internal pudendal artery stain. *AJR Am J Roentgenol* 1978;131:657–659.

59. Braf ZF, Koontz WW Jr. Gangrene of the bladder: complication of hypogastric artery embolization. *Urology* 1977;9:670–671.

60. Hare WS, Holland CJ. Paresis following internal iliac artery embolization. *Radiology* 1983;143:47–51.

61. Velmahos GC, Chahwan S, Hanks SE, et al. Angiographic embolization of bilateral internal iliac arteries to control life-threatening hemorrhage after blunt trauma to the pelvis. *Am Surg* 2000;66:858–862.

62. Paster SB, Van Houten FX, Adams DF. Percutaneous balloon catheterization: a technique for the control of arterial hemorrhage caused by pelvic trauma. *JAMA* 1974;230:573–575.

63. Balogh Z, Voros E, Suveges G, et al. Stent graft treatment of an external iliac artery injury associated with pelvic fracture. A case report. *J Bone Joint Surg Am* 2003;85:919–922.

64. Gibson GR. Impotence following fractured pelvis and ruptured urethra. *Br J Urol* 1970;42:86–88.

65. King J. Impotence following fractures of the pelvis. *J Bone Joint Surg* 1975;57:1107–1109.

66. Ellison M, Timberlake GA, Kerstein MD. Impotence following pelvic fracture. *J Trauma* 1988;28:695–696.

67. Sharlip ID. Penile arteriography in impotence after pelvic trauma. *J Urol* 1981;126:477–481.

68. Mengert WF, Burchell RC, Blumstein RW, et al. Pregnancy after bilateral ligation of the internal iliac and ovarian arteries. *Obstet Gynecol* 1969;34:664–666.

Peripheral Trauma

REHAN HUSSAIN, SHAWN SARIN, and ANTHONY C. VENBRUX

Adverse consequences of arterial injury in extremity trauma include pseudoaneurysm, arteriovenous fistulas (AVFs), ischemia, gangrene, limb loss, high-flow cardiac output, and differential limb growth in children. Prompt and accurate diagnosis is vital to minimize these adverse effects when traumatic injuries to vascular structures are suspected.[1] Limb salvage rates are generally greater than 90% when rapid treatment is provided.[2] For many years, arteriography has been an important part of the management of patients with suspected vascular injury, both for diagnosis and for treatment. Recent literature has also supported the use of computed tomography angiography (CTA) as a sensitive and specific test for diagnosing vascular injury within the extremities, and some studies have suggested that CTA should supplant conventional angiography as the diagnostic modality of choice in evaluating for acute peripheral vascular injuries.[3]

PATIENT EVALUATION AND INDICATIONS FOR ARTERIOGRAPHY

The clinical situation, physical findings, and mechanism of injury play a major role in directing trauma management. In all forms of trauma—penetrating, iatrogenic, and blunt—physical examination is key to patient selection. Not all patients require arteriography for extremity trauma. For example, a patient with a through-and-through gunshot wound in the distal thigh, an expanding hematoma, and no distal pulses clearly has a superficial femoral artery injury, precisely localized by the wound. This injury requires prompt surgical repair rather than arteriography. Arteriography is indicated when an injury is suspected but not certain, or when endovascular therapy is to be attempted.[1] In the presence of a normal vascular exam, routine arteriography for proximity of injury is unnecessary. Arteriography should be reserved to identify those few patients with an abnormal vascular examination and an unclear injury who may require vascular repair.[4]

Significant clinical findings in extremity trauma that increase suspicion for arterial injury "hard signs" include pulse deficit, active bleeding, bruit, thrill, and an expanding hematoma. Pulse deficit, the most important finding, indicates arterial injury in 56% to 87% of cases.[5,6] Although uncommon, the presence of a bruit or thrill, suggestive of an AVF, yields a positive arteriogram rate of almost 100%.[5,6] An expanding hematoma is associated with arterial injury in 38% of cases.[6] Patients who present with these findings typically undergo immediate operative wound exploration and arterial repair. Emergency arteriography may be performed in these patients when they have multiple potential vascular injury sites, when the exact location of injury is not clear (e.g., when it involves a long path through the limb), when

surgical access is difficult (e.g., at the thoracic outlet), when significant atherosclerosis limits the pulse exam, or when an injury might be amenable to transcatheter therapy.[7]

"Soft signs" for extremity arterial trauma include injury to the anatomically related nerve, a small, stable hematoma, or a history of either hypotension or significant bleeding. A neurologic deficit has been found to be associated with a high percentage of vascular injuries in some studies, but this finding has not been confirmed by others.[5,8] Other physical signs, such as long bone fracture or large areas of soft-tissue injury, are of lesser yield.[5,6] These patients may be observed for the interval development of more concrete signs, or urgent arteriography may be requested.

The greatest controversy exists as to the need for arteriography for wounds near major neurovascular bundles.[9–13] A proximity wound is usually defined as being within 1 cm of the expected location of the vessels concerned. As many as 95% of arteriograms performed for proximity alone are negative.[2] Efforts have been directed toward identifying subgroups of proximity wounds that are at higher risk for vascular injury. The Doppler-derived ankle brachial index (ABI) or wrist brachial index (WBI) has been adopted at several centers as an extension of the physical examination for this purpose.[8,14,15] An ABI or WBI of less than 0.9 has been associated with a positive arteriography rate of 30%.[8] Such arteriograms need not be performed on an emergent basis but can be delayed up to 24 hours unless surgical intervention is planned earlier for another indication.[11] Doppler examinations miss lesions that do not decrease distal flow: branch arterial injuries, small AVFs, and nonobstructing arterial defects.

Other approaches have been reported for stable patients with suspicion of vascular injury. Alternate imaging modalities have been suggested to replace arteriography. Duplex ultrasound has been recommended as a screening tool to identify traumatic arterial injury. The sensitivity of ultrasound for detection of arterial injury has been reported from a poor 50% to an excellent 99%.[16–18] It is useful for flow analysis and for follow-up after treatment. Because of limitations inherent to sonography (such as bones, air, casts, and skin burns), however, magnetic resonance imaging (MRI), CTA, and catheter angiography may be necessary for further evaluation in selected cases.[19] Atherosclerotic disease, anatomic variants, and vasoconstriction resulting from hypotension may make interpretation difficult. The role of ultrasonography is somewhat limited for several additional reasons. It is an operator-dependent examination that is tedious when more than a single anatomic region needs evaluation. Open wounds and orthopedic hardware limit access for scanning.

A few authors have advocated CTA for the evaluation of extremity trauma because CT scanning is the cornerstone of trauma diagnosis elsewhere in the body.[20,21] CTA provides accurate peripheral vascular imaging while being noninvasive and immediately available. Studies have shown the sensitivity of CTA to be 90% to 95.1% and its specificity 98.7% to 100% for detecting arterial injury to the extremities after trauma.[22] The increasingly widespread use of 64-row multidetector CT technology offers considerable benefits in the trauma setting. These include the ability to generate isotropic data sets of long vascular territories with the acquisition performed in a short time. Isotropic voxels make CT a fully multiplanar modality, a capability that is particularly useful for evaluating tortuous vessels. Sixty-four-row multidetector CTA of the extremities has the ability to demonstrate a variety of vascular injuries, such as occlusion, pseudoaneurysm, active extravasation, and intimal dissection. Radiologists should be aware of the various potential pitfalls and limitations of extremity CTA in evaluation of trauma patients suspected to have extremity vascular injuries, including inadequate arterial enhancement, motion artifact, inadequate positioning, and streak artifact. By demonstrating the extent, location, and type of injury, CTA aids in the decision-making process to determine the appropriate management for each injury in the trauma patient.[23]

Rarely, limited arteriography performed in the emergency department has been described. A single, plain film is obtained following contrast injection, by hand, via a small needle.[24] The advantage here is primarily the speed of diagnosis. Such an exam is limited to only one vascular territory, and injection timing errors could miss injuries.

The mechanism of injury is also an important factor in the decision to perform arteriography. All high-velocity wounds, such as those from assault weapons and rifles, should undergo exploration or arteriography because of the greater force and possibility of remote concussive damage. High-speed missiles are preceded by a shock wave and followed by an area of decreased pressure called the temporary cavity, which can produce extensive damage. Such high-velocity wounds have the highest incidence of arterial injury, followed in decreasing order by gunshot wounds and stab wounds, which must penetrate the vessel directly.[10] Shotgun wounds have a high rate of arterial injury (46% to 62%) because of the multiplicity of projectiles and the larger area of trauma from pellet scatter.[10]

Although in urban centers, most extremity arterial injuries are a result of penetrating trauma, blunt trauma can also cause significant vascular injuries, accounting for 17% of arterial injuries.[25] Manifestations of blunt vascular injury can develop in a delayed manner and present with more subtle findings, such as a pulse deficit or diminished ankle brachial pressure index.[26] Early limb loss is more common with blunt distal vascular injury, especially to the popliteal and tibial arteries.[27] Knee dislocations carry a 23% to 43% rate of popliteal artery injury. Dislocations produce stretch injuries, which may cause isolated intimal damage. As with other forms of trauma, it remains controversial whether arteriography is indicated in all patients with knee dislocation or only in those with physical or Doppler signs of injury.[28,29] Open elbow dislocations and supracondylar humeral fractures also have a high incidence of vascular injury. Long bone fracture, however, is a poor indicator of arterial injury. Among patients with fractures requiring admission, the arterial injury rate is only 0.3%.[25] Blunt injury to the distal extremities is more likely to produce significant arterial injury than more proximal injuries because of the

smaller quantity of surrounding soft tissues. Complex fractures of the tibia and fibula are frequently associated with vascular injury. Blunt trauma may produce internal penetrating injury from fracture fragments. Identification of these injuries is important because isolated tibial arterial injuries, when associated with extensive soft-tissue damage, should be repaired to avoid limb loss, nonunion of fractures, and poor wound healing.[30]

Historically, all patients with abnormal arteriograms underwent surgical exploration without regard for the type of angiographic abnormality. Even small injuries were explored because of fear of subsequent thrombosis and possible distal embolization. Advances in endovascular therapy have brought into question such practices. Large and even multisegmental injuries heal after angioplasty, and small AVFs often close. Accordingly, doubt exists regarding the necessity to explore or treat small arterial injuries. Many of these asymptomatic injuries may not require surgical or radiologic intervention but rather can heal spontaneously.[10,11,31,32] Minor arterial injuries are followed conservatively at many centers, and clinical deterioration has rarely occurred.[31,33] The benign nature of these injuries remains unpredictable, however. Tufaro et al.[34] have reported multiple significant delayed complications, which included major vessel thrombosis, following such observational management, and they advise caution.

When observation is the chosen management, clinical follow-up is essential because of the unpredictability of injury healing. Areas of segmental narrowing and small intimal flaps are best suited to such follow-up. Small pseudoaneurysms (<2 to 5 mm) and small AVFs can also be managed conservatively. CTA or catheter angiography can be performed one to several weeks after the initial injury. Observation needs to be maintained until the injury completely heals or until definitive therapy is provided. Therefore, improving but incompletely healed or stable injuries require serial follow-up examinations.[6,31,32] Platelet inhibitors may be used in these patients because of concern for thrombosis.[32] An alternative method for follow-up in selected patients is color Doppler ultrasound.[16,35] If an injury is to be treated expectantly and it can be identified well by ultrasound, this modality can be used to monitor wound healing.

Alternatively, some trauma specialists believe that because major vascular injuries can result in limb loss and functional disability in characteristically young victims, diagnosis and repair of all injuries is critical. The cost and legal ramifications of a missed diagnosis motivate some surgeons to request arteriography on all penetrating trauma patients.[9,36,37] Arteriography has been shown to be cost effective when the incidence of injury is greater than 1% to 2%.[38]

Although arteriography is both sensitive (98%) and specific (98%), occult injuries do occur and may have a delayed presentation.[6] Even surgical exploration does not identify all injuries[39,40] (FIGURE 73.1). Missed injuries requiring delayed intervention may not be as difficult to repair, nor complications as frequent, as previously thought.[10,31] Although long-term delays in treatment may result in large AVFs or pseudoaneurysms, which would complicate treatment, most delays are of short duration, and definitive therapy is not usually more difficult.[31,33]

▌ TECHNIQUE OF ARTERIOGRAPHY

The site of arterial access depends on clinical evaluation of the patient. For isolated extremity trauma, the preferred access is femoral. With lower-extremity injuries, the contralateral

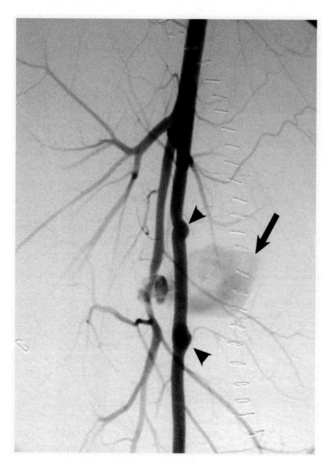

FIGURE 73.1 Patient following gunshot wound to thigh presents with a pulse deficit. Injury of the proximal superficial femoral artery was treated with surgical vein graft (*arrowheads*). A large pseudoaneurysm arising from the deep portion of the profunda femoris artery was missed (*arrow*). This injury was successfully treated by transcatheter embolization.

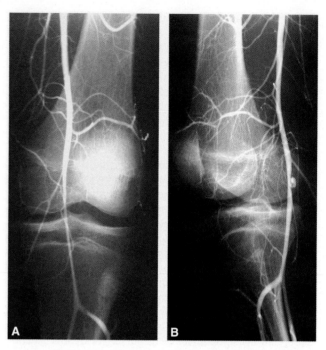

FIGURE 73.2 **A.** Frontal arteriogram after through-and-through gunshot wound to the knee reveals smooth tapering of the popliteal artery initially thought to be caused by spasm. **B.** The lateral view reveals a popliteal artery pseudoaneurysm and demonstrates the importance of orthogonal views.

common femoral artery access is preferred for endovascular therapy. Occasionally, radial, brachial, or an axillary approach may be required. Both subtraction and nonsubtraction images should be reviewed.

The arteriogram should include all potential sites of injury. Sequential images are essential with early rapid images required to identify the site of a high-flow AVF, whereas delayed images are needed to identify sites of extravasation. At least two views, preferably orthogonal, should be obtained to exclude injury (FIGURE 73.2). When large foreign bodies are present, fluoroscopy and test injections can allow positioning of the vessel of interest away from obscuring metallic material. Vessels proximal and distal to the potential injury site should be evaluated as well.

Careful positioning of the catheter is important so that all arteries in the potential injury path are evaluated. Knowledge of both the entrance and exit wounds, if present, is therefore required. The catheter should be positioned proximal enough to the injury site to allow for common anatomic variants (e.g., high takeoff of the radial artery).

Significant findings on extremity arteriography for trauma include arterial occlusion, extravasation, pseudoaneurysms, and AVFs. Occlusions may be caused by extrinsic vessel compression

or by thrombosis associated with arterial laceration or intimal flap. Luminal narrowing may be secondary to arterial spasm, intramural hematoma, extrinsic compression, or atherosclerosis. Intraluminal filling defects indicate nonocclusive thrombi or intimal injuries. Intimal flaps appear as a thin strip or globule attached to the arterial wall in at least one view[41] (FIGURE 73.3). The vessel course may be altered because of hematoma or associated long bone fracture displacement. Slow flow is an important finding and may be the sole arteriographic indication of a compartment syndrome.[41]

Of the many findings seen arteriographically, luminal narrowing is the most difficult to evaluate because vasospasm and intimal injury may be impossible to differentiate. Luminal narrowing may be a result of arterial spasm, which appears as a focal area of smooth concentric narrowing and is particularly prevalent in pediatric patients.[42] Some authors recommend the use of vasodilators when such lesions are encountered to exclude more significant lesions. Calcium channel blockers, nitroglycerin, as well as papaverine have been used as vasodilators, although their effectiveness is unreliable.[32,42] Areas of narrowing that are not concentric should raise concern for intimal injury.

ENDOVASCULAR MANAGEMENT OF ARTERIAL INJURIES

Although surgery remains the gold standard in the management of vascular extremity injuries, it has significant morbidity rates. Endovascular techniques are increasingly being used for the treatment of vascular traumatic injuries. Various techniques including balloon occlusion, embolization, and stent/stent-graft

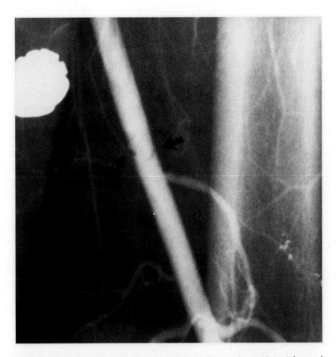

FIGURE 73.3 Two appearances of intimal flaps: a linear band (*arrow*) or a globule attached to the vessel wall (*curved arrow*).

Reprinted with permission from Hanks SE, Pentecost MJ. Angiography and transcatheter treatment of extremity trauma. *Semin Intervent Radiol* 1992;9:20–25.

placement have been described.[43] A review of the National Trauma Data Bank, found an increase from 2.1% in 1994 to 8.1% in 2003 in the use of endovascular interventions for vascular trauma.[44]

Before undertaking transcatheter therapy for arterial lesions, it is important to understand the surgical alternatives for treatment, along with their risks and benefits. Arteries may be ligated, primarily repaired, patched by vein, bypassed by vein, or, rarely, bypassed by prosthetic graft. Percutaneous treatment includes embolization as well as transcatheter placement of bare or covered stents.

The ideal candidate for endovascular intervention is a patient with a low-velocity injury (stab wound or handgun blast) in an anatomic region where surgical exposure may prolong ischemia or bleeding complications, or in a region with an increased risk of iatrogenic nerve injury during exposure of the vessel, such as the subclavian or internal carotid artery (ICA). Injuries that require surgical intervention, such as debridement for high-velocity gunshot wounds or contamination, embolectomy, or compartment syndrome, may not benefit as much from definitive endovascular repair. These injuries may benefit from angiography and proximal balloon occlusion to limit blood loss. In addition to balloon occlusion, hemorrhage control interventions include embolization and deployment of a covered stent. Pseudoaneurysms and AVFs are excluded with either covered stents or coil embolization with or without a stent. Dissections have been managed with balloons, bare metal stents, or covered stents.[44]

Previously, radiologic management was primarily limited to embolotherapy, the intentional occlusion of a vessel. Vessels

to be treated by this percutaneous means need to be expendable. These are vessels that are likely to be ligated surgically as an alternative treatment. Transcatheter embolization is usually used for nonaxial arteries (e.g., profunda femoris artery, geniculate artery, etc.) or distal axial arteries that are multiple (e.g., tibial arteries).

Each patient and each injury need to be considered individually with respect to treatment choice. Transcatheter embolization of significant injuries is preferable to surgical intervention in sites where surgical exposure and/or vascular control are difficult to achieve (e.g., in distal profunda femoris arteries).[45] In such cases, surgical dissection may require division of important collateral vessels supplying the distal extremity. In older individuals, caution should be exercised to avoid obliterating such collaterals.

The technique of embolization depends on the type and location of the vascular lesions. In general, the extremities have an extensive collateral network. It is important, therefore, to embolize both proximal and distal to the injury to prevent retrograde arterial filling or recruitment of collaterals (FIGURE 73.4). Occlusion of the proximal segment is satisfactory if the distal artery is thrombosed (FIGURE 73.5). For extremely peripheral branch arteries, embolization of the proximal portion of the injured artery may be sufficient (FIGURE 73.6).

A variety of materials are available for embolization. Choice of an agent is often based on personal preference and experience. In trauma, a temporary occluding agent, such as gelatin sponge,

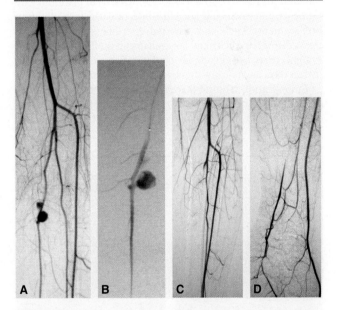

FIGURE 73.4 A. Leg arteriogram following stab wound reveals a pseudoaneurysm of the posterior tibial artery with normal peroneal and anterior tibial arteries. **B.** Selective catheterization of the PTA with a microcatheter demonstrates that coils must be placed distal to the pseudoaneurysm to prevent retrograde filling of the pseudoaneurysm. **C.** Leg arteriogram after transcatheter embolization of the PTA with microcoils both proximally and distally to the injury site. The proximal PTA, including the pseudoaneurysm, no longer fills. **D.** Lateral foot arteriogram demonstrates that the distal portion of the PTA fills via the plantar arch.

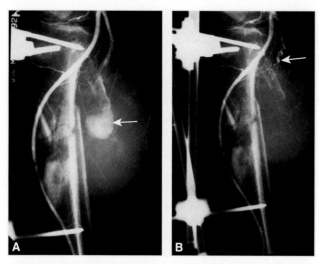

FIGURE 73.5 A. Lower-extremity arteriogram following gunshot injury demonstrates a large pseudoaneurysm of the tibioperoneal trunk (*arrow*) with occlusion of the distal arterial segment. **B.** Successful embolization of the tibioperoneal trunk with steel coils only in the proximal arterial segment (*arrow*).

is theoretically advantageous because many of these lesions will heal. Alternatively, fibered coils, although permanent, offer the advantage of precise positioning. In the extremities, exact placement is usually of foremost concern, and, therefore, coils are favored. Standard coils are 0.038-inch or 0.035-inch steel or platinum wire segments, and microcoils are 0.018-inch or 0.010-inch platinum wire segments. These coils have polyester fibers attached to increase thrombogenicity and are available in multiple sizes and in straight, curved, and complex configurations. Liquid embolics, such as onyx and *N*-butyl cyanoacrylate, are possible alternatives.

Embolization requires placement of a catheter at the injury site. After identification of an arterial injury suitable for transcatheter embolization, a diagnostic catheter must be manipulated

to the target vessel. Achieving adequate catheter position can be the limiting factor for embolization success. If the catheter is stable, coils of an appropriate size may be used.

It may be unsafe to embolize in too close proximity to essential arteries. If the target vessel is small or tortuous, or if the diagnostic catheter is unstable, a microcatheter can be used coaxially. Microcatheters allow for rapid catheterization of branches that are unreachable by diagnostic catheters. They minimize vasospasm and the risk of nontarget embolization by providing added stability. Superselective coaxial systems maximize the amount of preserved blood supply.[46,47] The recent advent of partially detachable and detachable coils facilitates complex embolization procedures.

For AVFs or pseudoaneurysms, coils should be placed so that there are no arterial branches between the coils and the injury site. It is not necessary to occlude the pseudoaneurysm or AVF itself, but rather the artery proximal and distal to the injury (FIGURES 73.7 and 73.8). Coils may be placed directly across the injury, beginning distally and progressing more proximally (FIGURE 73.9). Initial placement of a large coil can provide a network for retaining smaller coils.[48] If the artery distal to the injury is patent and access to this distal segment cannot be achieved from the proximal vessel, alternative strategies should be employed to prevent distal retrograde filling. For pseudoaneurysms, small gelfoam pledgets can be used to occlude the distal arterial segment. If pseudoaneurysms are superficial, ultrasound-guided thrombin injection has been used.[49] For AVFs,

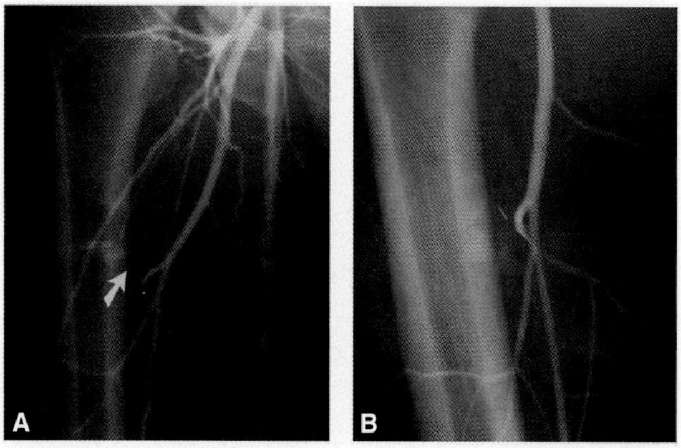

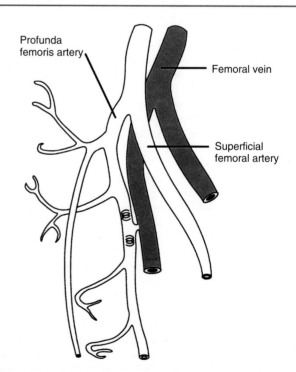

FIGURE 73.7 Diagrammatic representation of ideal coil placement for occlusion of an arteriovenous fistula (AVF). The coils are placed both distal and proximal to the AVF with no intervening arterial branches.

Reprinted with permission from Hanks SE, Pentecost MJ. Angiography and transcatheter treatment of extremity trauma. *Semin Intervent Radiol* 1992;9:20–25.

FIGURE 73.6 A. Lower-extremity arteriogram following thigh stab wound demonstrates extravasation from a distal branch of the profunda femoris artery (*arrow*). **B.** Successful superselective embolization of the bleeding muscular branch with two straight platinum microcoils.

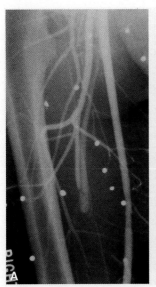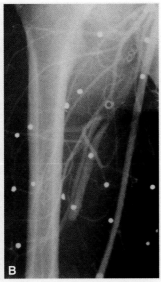

FIGURE 73.8 A. Lower-extremity arteriogram following shotgun injury demonstrates arteriovenous fistula (AVF) from the distal profunda femoris artery. **B.** Arteriogram following poor placement of occlusion coils. Isolated proximal placement of the coils has allowed for distal reconstitution of the distal profunda femoris artery and persistence of the AVF. Distal occlusion could have been accomplished with a microcatheter.

Reprinted with permission from Hanks SE, Pentecost MJ. Angiography and transcatheter treatment of extremity trauma. *Semin Intervent Radiol* 1992;9:20–25.

a transvenous approach or direct percutaneous puncture of the distal artery can be performed (FIGURE 73.10).

The success rate for transcatheter embolization has been reported to be between 85% and 100%.[45–47,50,51] These high rates can be achieved safely with modern catheters and coaxial systems. Complications from transcatheter embolization are identical to those of diagnostic arteriography but also include nontarget embolization. With careful technique and, when necessary, the use of microcatheters and microcoils, nontarget embolization is infrequent.[47,50] If coil maldeployment occurs, multiple retrieval devices have been developed to enable coil removal. Infection following embolization rarely occurs. Significant limb ischemia should not occur with appropriate lesion selection. Local infarction of tissue can be avoided by using gelatin sponge or coils rather than agents that permeate to the arteriolar or capillary level, such as gelfoam powder or alcohol. Transcatheter embolization is effective and safe and can be definitive therapy for suitable arterial injuries in both the upper and lower extremities.[52,53]

For injuries to arteries that cannot be safely sacrificed by embolic occlusion, operative intervention remains the usual therapy. Occasionally, massive hemorrhage may be identified on an arteriogram from an essential artery (e.g., superficial femoral artery). If the clinical situation is appropriate, an occlusion balloon can be used for short-term occlusion to decrease blood loss during transit to the operating room.[54]

Surgery can be avoided in some cases of injured axial vessels. Advances in stents and covered stent-grafts have increased

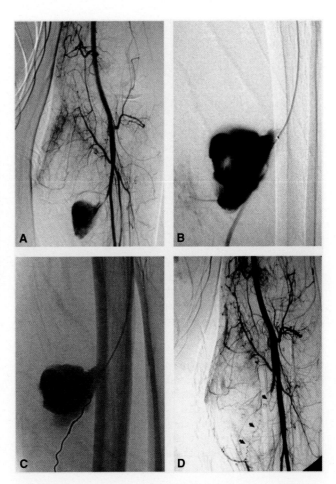

FIGURE 73.9 A. Patient with an enlarging forearm mass following gunshot wound. Upper-extremity arteriogram demonstrates a laceration of the radial artery with a large pseudoaneurysm (PA). The radial artery is not seen distal to the PA. **B.** Because surgical treatment would likely be radial artery ligation, transcatheter embolization of the radial artery was requested. Selective microcatheter placement at the site of the injury reveals there is communication of the distal radial artery with the PA. The radial artery distal to the PA must be occluded to prevent retrograde filling. **C.** Occlusion of the distal segment has been achieved with the placement of platinum microcoils. **D.** Additional microcoils have been placed as the microcatheter was withdrawn across the injury (*arrows*). The proximal radial artery is now completely occluded. Flow to the hand is via the ulnar artery. There is no filling of the PA.

transcatheter therapy to include the management of arterial injuries in vessels that are essential conduits. A percutaneous approach may reduce blood loss, decrease length of stay, involve fewer iatrogenic nerve injuries, and facilitate shorter recovery time, as compared with open approaches.[55] Recent case reports suggest that bare or, more frequently, covered stents can successfully treat injuries in axial vessels in which embolization would be inappropriate.[55–62] Bare stents have been used to treat pseudoaneurysms and traumatic flow-limiting dissection. Stent-grafts have been used to manage selected arterial injuries with excellent results, including AVFs and pseudoaneurysms in the subclavian, axillary, brachial, iliac, common, and superficial femoral arteries

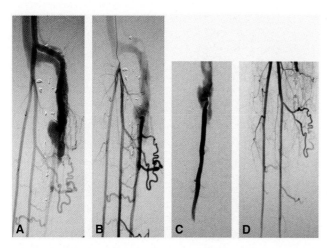

FIGURE 73.10 A. Two years following gunshot wound to the leg, patient returns with pain and swelling. Lower-extremity arteriogram demonstrates a large arteriovenous fistula (AVF) from a hypertrophied anterior tibial artery. No antegrade flow is demonstrated in the distal ATA. **B.** Selective injection of the tibioperoneal trunk reveals filling of the distal ATA via collateral vessels. The distal ATA has retrograde filling into the AVF. Treatment of this injury will require ligation or occlusion of both ends of the transected artery. **C.** The distal ATA could not be accessed from the proximal route. Ultrasound guidance was utilized to perform a retrograde puncture of the distal ATA at the ankle. Injection of the distal ATA demonstrates retrograde flow and filling of the AVF. **D.** Coils were placed near the AVF site from both the antegrade and retrograde catheters. Arteriogram following embolization documents complete occlusion of the AVF.

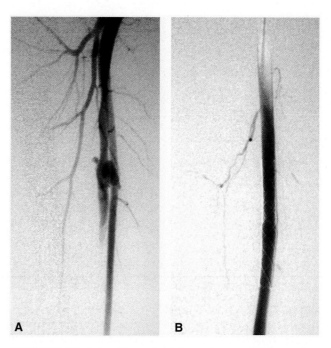

FIGURE 73.12 A. A midsuperficial femoral artery (SFA) pseudoaneurysm with associated AVF is present following gunshot to the thigh. **B.** A covered stent preserves SFA patency and prevents filling of the pseudoaneurysm and AVF.

(FIGURES 73.11 and 73.12). Additionally, Stampfl et al.[63] have shown balloon-expandable stent-grafts to be a safe and effective option in treating patients with acute hemorrhage from pseudoaneurysms, vessel erosion, or iatrogenic vessel injury. Given the young patient population in whom these traumatic vascular injuries most often occur, the long-term patency of a stent-graft is essential. Large studies addressing long-term patency and overall limb salvage rates are lacking at this time.[55]

Percutaneous treatment may be preferred in polytrauma patients because of associated major injuries or for patients

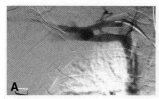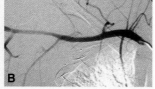

FIGURE 73.11 A. Polytrauma patient with gunshots to the face, neck, chest, abdomen, and pelvis. Right subclavian arteriogram demonstrates a large arteriovenous fistula. It was advantageous to avoid thoracic surgery because this patient had already undergone multiple abdominal surgeries. **B.** Following placement of a covered stent from an axillary approach, arteriography confirms exclusion of the fistula from the circulation.

in which vessels are difficult to access surgically, such as the subclavian arteries, which require thoracotomy. Treatment of these patients by placement of a bare or covered stent may be indicated because 40% to 50% of penetrating axillosubclavian trauma is amenable to endovascular management.[64] In addition to femoral access, axillosubclavian injuries are accessible through retrograde brachial or radial access, which allows for a direct approach to the injury while other injuries are being treated by the trauma team. Endovascular management, where feasible, has shown a significant reduction in operating room time and estimated blood loss when compared with similar surgical cohorts.[65]

There are several cases where blunt trauma to the brachial artery was treated with balloon angioplasty (percutaneous transluminal angioplasty [PTA]) to fixate the dissected intima to the vessel wall. The "tacking" of the intimal flap was effective in giving a long lasting patency.[66]

Both blunt and penetrating trauma to the popliteal artery have been associated with significant morbidity and high amputation rates.[67] Penetrating and blunt injuries to the popliteal artery have mortalities of 10.5% and 27.5%, respectively, and injuries to the tibial arteries have an amputation rate of 38%.[68,69] Endovascular techniques have been used with caution in the popliteal artery because of the instability of a rigid stent across the motion of the knee joint.[70] Injuries to tibial arteries with foot ischemia must involve repair of one of the tibial vessels with a tibial artery bypass to avoid amputation. Endovascular techniques have been employed safely with 2-year patency in a patient with foot ischemia and thrombosis of the anterior tibial, peroneal, and posterior tibial arteries treated with self-expanding coronary stents to maintain patency of the posterior tibial artery. Endovascular intervention in this case avoided surgical dissection posterior to the tibia in a surgical field with an open tibia fracture, hematoma, and orthopedic hardware to reduce the fracture.[68]

▌SUMMARY

The management of extremity trauma continues to evolve as the natural history of nonsurgically explored arterial injuries is reported. Clinical findings form the basis for extremity trauma management. Although arteriography is both sensitive and specific for the diagnosis of arterial injury, the indications for arteriography in extremity trauma remain in flux. Review of the recent literature indicates that, for most trauma specialists, proximity is no longer an indication for arteriography. Recent studies have supported the expanding role of CTA in diagnosing peripheral arterial injury. CTA is less invasive than arteriography and has similar high sensitivity and specificity. The increasing endorsement of expectant management of minor vascular injuries has caused surgeons and radiologists to question whether diagnosis of small injuries is necessary. By decreasing surgical and angiographic exploration, it is clear that additional arterial injuries will be missed regardless of the screening method. These injuries can be treated at the time of clinical manifestation. It remains unclear whether this triage is clinically sound, primarily because the natural history of such arterial lesions, particularly small injuries, is unknown. Resolution of this controversy depends on the difficult task of obtaining adequate follow-up in a largely noncompliant, unreliable patient population. The utility of arteriography, however, goes beyond diagnostic purposes and can be reserved for a situation where endovascular therapy is planned.

▌REFERENCES

1. Katz MD, Hanks SE. Arteriography and transcatheter management of extremity trauma. In: Baum S, Pentecost MJ, eds. *Abram's Angiography: Interventional Radiology*. 2nd ed. Philadelphia, PA: Lippincott Williams & Wilkins; 2006.
2. Frykberg ER. Advances in the diagnosis and treatment of extremity vascular trauma. *Surg Clin North Am* 1995;75:207–223.
3. Wallin D, Yaghoubian A, Rosing D, et al. Computed tomographic angiography as the primary diagnostic modality in penetrating lower extremity vascular injuries: a level I trauma experience. *Ann Vasc Surg*. 2011;25(5):620.
4. Gahtan V, Bramson RT, Norman J. The role of emergent arteriography in penetrating limb trauma. *Am Surg* 1994;60(2):123–127.
5. Weaver FA, Yellin AE, Bauer M, et al. Is arterial proximity a valid indication for arteriography in penetrating extremity trauma? A prospective analysis. *Arch Surg* 1990;125:1256–1260.
6. Trooskin SZ, Sclafani S, Winfield J, et al. The management of vascular injuries of the extremity associated with civilian firearms. *Surg Gynecol Obstet* 1993;176:350–354.
7. Lipchik EO, Kaebnick HW, Beres JJ, et al. The role of arteriography in acute penetrating trauma to the extremities. *Cardiovasc Intervent Radiol* 1987;10:202–204.
8. Schwartz MR, Weaver FA, Bauer M, et al. Refining the indications for arteriography in penetrating extremity trauma: a prospective analysis. *J Vasc Surg* 1993;17:116–124.
9. King TA, Perse JA, Marmen C. Utility of arteriography in penetrating extremity injuries. *Am J Surg* 1991;162:163–165.
10. Dennis JW, Frykberg ER, Crump JM. New perspectives on the management of penetrating trauma in proximity to major limb arteries. *J Vasc Surg* 1990;11:84–93.
11. Frykberg ER, Crump JM, Vines FS, et al. A reassessment of the role of arteriography in penetrating proximity extremity trauma: a prospective study. *J Trauma* 1989;29:1041–1052.
12. Modrall JG, Weaver FA, Yellin AE. Vascular considerations in extremity trauma. *Orthop Clin North Am* 1993;24:557–563.
13. Gonzalez RP, Falimirski ME. The utility of physical examination in proximity penetrating extremity trauma. *Am Surg* 1999;65:784–789.
14. Johansen K, Lynch K, Paun M, et al. Non-invasive vascular tests reliably exclude occult arterial trauma in injured extremities. *J Trauma* 1991;31:515–522.
15. Nassoura ZE, Ivatury RR, Simon RJ, et al. A reassessment of Doppler pressure indices in the detection of arterial lesions in proximity penetrating injuries of extremities: a prospective study. *Am J Emerg Med* 1996;14:151–156.
16. Schwartz M, Weaver F, Yellin A, et al. The utility of color flow Doppler examination in penetrating extremity arterial trauma. *Am Surg* 1993;59:375–378.
17. Kuzniec S, Kauffman P, Molnar LJ, et al. Diagnosis of limbs and neck arterial trauma using duplex ultrasonography. *Cardiovasc Surg* 1998;6:358–366.
18. Bynoe RP, Miles WS, Bell RM, et al. Noninvasive diagnosis of vascular trauma by duplex ultrasonography. *J Vasc Surg* 1991;14:346–352.
19. Gaitini D, Razi NB, Ghersin E, et al. Sonographic evaluation of vascular injuries. *J Ultrasound Med* 2008;27(1):95–107.
20. Busquets AR, Acosta JA, Colon E, et al. Helical computed tomographic angiography for the diagnosis of traumatic arterial injuries of the extremities. *J Trauma* 2004;56:625–628.
21. Soto JA, Munera F, Morales C, et al. Focal arterial injuries of the proximal extremities: helical CT arteriography as the initial method of diagnosis. *Radiology* 2001;218:188–194.
22. Miller-Thomas MM, West OC, Cohen AM. Diagnosing traumatic arterial injury in the extremities with CT angiography: pearls and pitfalls. *Radiographics* 2005;25(suppl 1):S133–S142.
23. Pieroni S, Foster BR, Anderson SW, et al. Use of 64-row multidetector CT angiography in blunt and penetrating trauma of the upper and lower extremities. *Radiographics* 2009;29(3):863–876.
24. Itani KMF, Rotheberg SS, Brandt ML, et al. Emergency center arteriography in the evaluation of suspected peripheral vascular injuries in children. *J Pediatr Surg* 1993;28:677–680.
25. Sturm JT, Bodily KC, Rothenberger DA, et al. Arterial injuries of the extremities following blunt trauma. *J Trauma* 1980;20:933–936.
26. Peck MA, Rasmussen TE. Management of blunt peripheral arterial injury. *Perspect Vasc Surg Endovasc Ther* 2006;18(2):159–173.
27. Kauvar DS, Sarfati MR, Kraiss LW. National trauma databank analysis of mortality and limb loss in isolated lower extremity vascular trauma. *J Vasc Surg* 2011;53(6):1598–1603. Epub 2011 Apr 22.
28. Kaufman SL, Martin LG. Arterial injuries associated with complete dislocation of the knee. *Radiology* 1992;184:153–155.
29. Applebaum R, Yellin AE, Weaver FA, et al. Role of routine arteriography in blunt lower-extremity trauma. *Am J Surg* 1990;160:221–225.
30. Shah DM, Corson JD, Karmody AM, et al. Optimal management of tibial arterial trauma. *J Trauma* 1988;28:228–234.
31. Stain SC, Yellin AE, Weaver FA, et al. Selective management of nonocclusive arterial injuries. *Arch Surg* 1989;124:1136–1141.
32. Hoffer EK, Sclafani SJ, Herskowitz MM, et al. Natural history of arterial injuries diagnosed with arteriography. *J Vasc Interv Radiol* 1997;8:43–53.
33. Frykberg ER, Crump JM, Dennis JW, et al. Nonoperative observation of clinically occult arterial injuries: a prospective evaluation. *Surgery* 1991;109:85–96.
34. Tufaro A, Arnaold T, Rummel M, et al. Adverse outcome of nonoperative management of intimal injuries caused by penetrating trauma. *J Vasc Surg* 1994;20:656–659.
35. Knudson MM, Lewis FR, Atkinson K, et al. The role of duplex ultrasound arterial imaging in patients with penetrating extremity trauma. *Arch Surg* 1993;128:1033–1038.
36. Cikrit DF, Dalsing MC, Bryant BJ, et al. An experience with upper-extremity vascular trauma. *Am J Surg* 1990;160:229–233.
37. Perry MO. Complications of missed arterial injuries. *J Vasc Surg* 1993;17:399–407.
38. Keen JD, Dunne PM, Keen RR, et al. Proximity arteriography: cost-effectiveness in asymptomatic penetrating extremity trauma. *J Vasc Interv Radiol* 2001;12:813–821.
39. Richardson JD, Vitale GC, Flint LM. Penetrating arterial trauma. *Arch Surg* 1987;122:678–683.
40. Feliciano DV, Cruse PA, Burch JM, et al. Delayed diagnosis of arterial injuries. *Am J Surg* 1987;154:579–584.
41. Rose SC, Moore EE. Angiography in patients with arterial trauma: correlation between angiographic abnormalities, operative findings, and clinical outcome. *AJR Am J Roentgenol* 1987;149:613–619.

42. Sclafani SJA, Cooper R, Shaftan GW, et al. Arterial trauma: diagnostic and therapeutic angiography. *Radiology* 1986;161:165–172.

43. Doody O, Given MF, Lyon SM. Injury. Extremities—indications and techniques for treatment of extremity vascular injuries. *Injury* 2008;39(11):1295–1303. Epub 2008 Oct 8.

44. Johnson CA. Endovascular management of peripheral vascular trauma. *Semin Intervent Radiol* 2010;27(1):38–43.

45. Sclafani SJA, Shaftan GW. Transcatheter treatment of injuries to the profunda femoris artery. *AJR Am J Roentgenol* 1982;138:463–466.

46. Kaufman SL, Martin LG, Zuckerman AM. Peripheral transcatheter embolization with platinum microcoils. *Radiology* 1992;184:369–372.

47. Teitelbaum GP, Reed RA, Larsen D, et al. Microcatheter embolization of non-neurologic traumatic vascular lesions. *J Vasc Interv Radiol* 1993;4:149–154.

48. Butto F, Hunter DW, Castaneda-Zuniga W, et al. Coil-in-coil technique for vascular embolization. *Radiology* 1986;161:554–555.

49. Arthurs ZM, Sohn VY, Starnes BW. Vascular trauma: endovascular management and techniques. *Surg Clin North Am* 2007;87(5):1179–1192, x–xi.

50. Levey DS, Teitelbaum GP, Finck EJ, et al. Safety and efficacy of transcatheter embolization of axillary and shoulder arterial injuries. *J Vasc Interv Radiol* 1991;2:99–104.

51. Clark RA, Gallant TE, Alexander ES. Angiographic management of traumatic arteriovenous fistulas: clinical results. *Radiology* 1983;147:9–13.

52. Aksoy M, Taviloglu K, Yanar H, et al. Percutaneous transcatheter embolization in arterial injuries of the lower limbs. *Acta Radiol* 2005;46(5):471–475.

53. Levey DS, Teitelbaum GP, Finck EJ, et al. Safety and efficacy of transcatheter embolization of axillary and shoulder arterial injuries. *J Vasc Interv Radiol* 1991;2(1):99–104.

54. Ben-Menachem Y. Embolotherapy in extremity trauma. In: Neal MP, Tisnado J, Cho SR, eds. *Emergency Interventional Radiology.* Boston, MA: Little, Brown; 1989:79–90.

55. Stewart DK, Brown PM, Tinsley EA Jr, et al. Use of stent grafts in lower extremity trauma. *Ann Vasc Surg* 2011;25(2):264.e9–264.e13.

56. Marin ML, Veith FJ, Panetta TF, et al. Transluminally placed endovascular stented graft repair for arterial trauma. *J Vasc Surg* 1994;20:466–471.

57. Schmitter SP, Marx M, Bernstein R, et al. Angioplasty-induced subclavian artery dissection in a patient with internal mammary artery graft: treatment with endovascular stent and stent-graft. *AJR Am J Roentgenol* 1995;165:449–451.

58. Pfammatter T, Kunzli A, Hilfiker P, et al. Relief of subclavian venous and brachial plexus compression syndrome caused by traumatic subclavian artery aneurysm by means of transluminal stent-grafting. *J Trauma* 1998;45:972–974.

59. Althaus SJ, Keskey TS, Harker CP, et al. Percutaneous placement of self-expanding stent for acute traumatic arterial injury. *J Trauma* 1996;41:145–148.

60. Dinkel HP, Eckstein FS, Triller J, et al. Emergent axillary artery stent-graft placement for massive hemorrhage from an avulsed subscapular artery. *J Endovasc Ther* 2002;9:129–133.

61. Uflacker R, Elliott BM. Percutaneous endoluminal stent-graft repair of an old traumatic femoral arteriovenous fistula. *Cardiovasc Intervent Radiol* 1996;19:120–122.

62. Maynar M, Baro M, Qian Z, et al. Endovascular repair of brachial artery transection associated with trauma. *J Trauma* 2004;56:1336–1341.

63. Stampfl U, Somner CM, Bellemann N, et al. The use of balloon-expandable stent grafts for the management of acute arterial bleeding. *J Vasc Interv Radiol* 2012;23(3):331–337.

64. Danetz JS, Cassano AD, Stoner MC, et al. Feasibility of endovascular repair in penetrating axillosubclavian injuries: a retrospective review. *J Vasc Surg* 2005;41(2):246–254.

65. Xenos ES, Freeman M, Stevens S, et al. Covered stents for injuries of subclavian and axillary arteries. *J Vasc Surg* 2003;38(3):451–454.

66. Lönn L, Delle M, Karlström L, et al. Should blunt arterial trauma to the extremities be treated with endovascular techniques? *J Trauma* 2005;59(5):1224–1227.

67. Frykberg ER. Popliteal vascular injuries. *Surg Clin North Am* 2002;82(1):67–89.

68. Alvarez-Tostado J, Tulsyan N, Butler B, et al. Endovascular management of acute critical ischemia secondary to blunt tibial artery injury. *J Vasc Surg* 2006;44(5):1101–1103.

69. Hutto JD, Reed AB. Endovascular repair of an acute blunt popliteal artery injury. *J Vasc Surg* 2007;45(1):188–190.

70. Arthurs ZM, Sohn VY, Starnes BW. Vascular trauma: endovascular management and techniques. *Surg Clin North Am* 2007;87(5):1179–1192, x–xi.

Gastrointestinal Hemorrhage

FREDERICK S. KELLER and JOSEF RÖSCH

▌ INTRODUCTION

Selective angiographic diagnosis and interventional treatment of gastrointestinal (GI) bleeding are among the earliest procedures performed by vascular and interventional radiologists. Interventional treatment for GI bleeding has continued to be an active area of interest and investigation.

It was in 1960 that Margulis et al.[1] first reported that operative angiography was effective in demonstrating the site of GI bleeding that had not been detected by conventional barium studies. Within a few years, selective angiography became established as a safe, accurate technique for preoperative localization of bleeding GI lesions.[2,3] It did not take long, however, for adventurous angiographic pioneers to expand the role of the angiographic catheter from a diagnostic tool designed solely for the presurgical localization of GI bleeding into a therapeutic instrument intended to arrest the hemorrhage and obviate the need for major surgery.

Initially, interventional therapy for GI bleeding consisted of infusing vasoconstrictor drugs, such as vasopressin or a combination of epinephrine and propranolol, into the artery supplying the bleeding lesion.[4,5] Then, in 1972, Rösch et al.[6] first used selective arterial embolization to control an acutely bleeding gastric ulcer. During the intervening years, introduction and refinement of digital angiography, microcatheters, micro guide wires, microcoils, and other embolic materials led to the rapid improvement in interventional treatment of GI bleeding, transforming it from a last-ditch procedure reserved for only desperate circumstances to a front-line therapy.

▌ ACUTE GASTROINTESTINAL BLEEDING

Clinical Considerations

The needs of a patient undergoing angiography and interventional treatment for GI bleeding are best met by a hospital equipped with a well-trained interventional team consisting of interventional radiologists, interventional radiology technologists and nurses, and a modern interventional suite. The interventional team must be available and ready to respond within a short time at any hour of the day or night. Not every patient with acute GI bleeding requires interventional treatment or, for that matter, even diagnostic angiography. With aggressive medical treatment consisting of blood replacement, intravenous fluids, correction of coagulation defects, sedation, and bed rest, GI hemorrhage will cease in approximately 75% to 80% of patients.[7]

Today, endoscopy is both the primary diagnostic and therapeutic method for investigation of acute *upper* GI tract hemorrhage. Arterial bleeding can be treated through the endoscope with epinephrine injection, heater probe application, and electrocoagulation. Bleeding varices can be differentiated from arterial bleeding; and, when discovered, the patient can be either referred for transjugular intrahepatic portosystemic shunt (TIPS) or treated with endoscopic sclerosis or banding. Angiography is reserved for those patients who continue to bleed from lesions in the upper GI tract that fail attempts at endoscopic control. In these patients, the endoscopist can place clips adjacent to the bleeding lesion to provide guidance for the interventional radiologist. Because the nature of the bleeding lesion and its location in the upper GI tract has already been established by endoscopy in this group of patients, the interventional radiologist's role is directed toward stopping the hemorrhage with transcatheter therapy.

Endoscopy is less useful for acute *lower* GI bleeding. Because blood travels both proximally and distally to a bleeding colonic or small-bowel lesion, often the site of bleeding will be obscured. Additionally, because endoscopy during acute lower GI bleeding is performed on an emergency basis the colon is unprepared, leading to a less than satisfactory examination. Similarly, bleeding sites in the small bowel are difficult to detect. At present, capsule endoscopy and multidetector computed tomography (MDCT) enterography may be useful in determining the location of these lesions.[8] Neither of these examinations is capable of giving a rapid answer in an actively bleeding patient, however, and is more suited for those with occult chronic small-bowel bleeding.

The pathognomonic angiographic sign of acute arterial hemorrhage is extravasation of contrast material into the GI lumen (FIGURE 74.1). Because acute GI bleeding is frequently intermittent, often stopping and starting, several conditions must be present for the extravasation to be demonstrated on the angiogram. First, the patient must be bleeding actively at a rate equal to or greater than 0.5 mL/minute when the angiographic contrast material is injected. Second, the contrast material must be injected into the specific artery that supplies the bleeding lesion; and third, the site of hemorrhage must be included within the area imaged (FIGURE 74.2). Therefore, the timing of the angiographic study is crucial. If the patient has stopped bleeding actively, extravasation will not be present. Lesions, such as tumors and angiodysplasias, can usually be identified on the angiogram by their morphologic changes on the arteries even when the patient is not bleeding acutely and extravasation is absent. For many of the more common lesions causing GI bleeding, such as ulcers and diverticulae, structural changes in the arteries supplying the lesion are not present and, therefore, without the presence of extravasation the angiogram will be negative. Occasionally, the location of an ulcer found on endoscopy that had stopped bleeding is indicated angiographically by a subtle

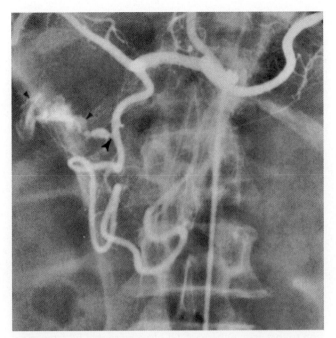

FIGURE 74.1 Extravasation. Contrast material extravasates into the duodenal lumen (*small arrowheads*) from a hole in the gastroduodenal artery (*large arrowhead*) caused by a duodenal ulcer.

pseudoaneurysm, occluded arterial branch, or sharply angulated artery. Superselective catheterization of these branches and injection of contrast material will often reactivate acute bleeding and result in extravasation, allowing the interventionists to definitively know which artery to treat.

Gastric lavage is useful in timing the angiogram for upper GI bleeding. If the lavage return continues to be bloody after evacuation of clots, bleeding is active and the angiogram will likely be positive. However, it is more difficult to determine the activity of lower GI bleeding. Passage of bloody stools may occur hours after the patient has stopped bleeding. In patients with lower GI bleeding, clinical signs and symptoms of ongoing activity include continuous hematochezia, tachycardia, and a falling hematocrit.

NONINVASIVE IMAGING FOR ACUTE GASTROINTESTINAL BLEEDING

Radionuclide Scanning

Because of the difficulty in determining activity of lower GI bleeding, several strategies have been developed to improve the timing of angiography to coincide with an episode of active bleeding, thus increasing the chances for a positive angiogram and some form of interventional therapy. Intravenous administration of radionuclide prior to angiography has been useful to demonstrate active bleeding. Scanning with ^{99m}Tc sulfur colloid can show extravasation of radionuclide in the bowel at rates as low as 0.1 mL/second. Extravasation may be evident within 2 to 3 minutes after isotope injection. Because Tc sulfur colloid accumulates in the liver and spleen, bleeding lesions in the hepatic and splenic flexures of the colon may be obscured. Scanning with ^{99m}Tc sulfur colloid has been used as a screening procedure, allowing selection of patients to progress on to catheter angiography.[9,10]

An alternative nuclear medicine technique is the use of ^{99m}Tc tagged red blood cells as the scanning agent. After administration, the patient is scanned every 5 minutes. This agent stays in the bloodstream for a long time. Therefore, the

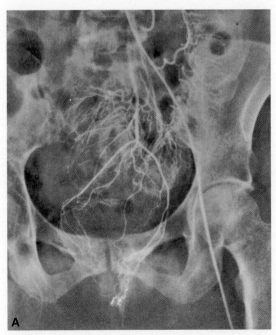
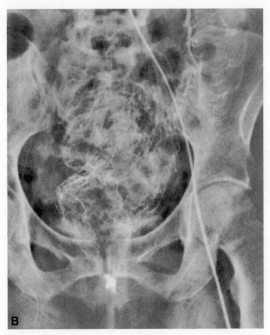

FIGURE 74.2 Acute lower GI bleeding from the anus (early phase **[A]** and late phase **[B]**) that was missed on the first arteriogram because this area was not included in the field of imaging.

patient can be brought back to the nuclear medicine department for up to 6 hours following its administration if the early scans were negative and clinically the patient started to bleed again. Because blood travels proximally and distally in the bowel, however, scanning with tagged red cells indicates that the patient had active bleeding since the last scan but it is considerably less precise in determining the location of the responsible lesion.[11,12]

Multidetector Computed Tomography Angiography

The most significant new development in demonstrating the presence and location of extravasation in patients with obscure lower GI bleeding prior to angiography is MDCT angiography.[13–18] Unlike radionuclide scanning, MDCT angiography is readily available at all hours of the day, is rapid, and is easy to perform. Sensitivity in detecting the presence of acute hemorrhage requires a bleeding rate between that of angiography (0.5 mL/minute) and nuclear medicine scanning (0.1 mL/minute).[19,20] For MDCT angiography, contrast is administered intravenously and, therefore, the entire arterial supply to the GI tract is simultaneously opacified with contrast during the few seconds it takes to scan the entire alimentary tract, from the esophagus to the anus.

Initially when MDCT angiography was introduced a single scan was performed during the arterial phase. However, it rapidly became evident that any preexisting high-attenuating material within the GI tract could easily be confused with extravasation. This potential source of false positive diagnosis can be eliminated by performing an unenhanced scan immediately prior to contrast administration. Today, in most institutions, an unenhanced scan is performed followed by scans in the arterial and portal vein phases. The latter shows continuing accumulation of extravasated contrast material that occurs in the time interval between the arterial and portal vein phases.

Use of MDCT angiography to detect the presence and location of active lower GI hemorrhage has been rapidly adopted as extremely useful in reducing the number of patients who have negative catheter angiography (FIGURE 74.3). Overall sensitivity and specificity has been reported between 79% and 89% and 85% and 95%, respectively.[14,15] In one study of 74 patients the positive predictive value was 86% and MDCT angiography's negative predictive value was an impressive 92%. There were no cases in which the results of MDCT angiography were negative and subsequent catheter angiography within the next 24 hours was positive.[14] In addition to detecting the presence of acute GI bleeding, MDCT is able to demonstrate other abdominal pathology outside the alimentary tract and vascular pathology that can influence the performance of the angiogram, such as stenoses or occlusions of visceral arteries or the presence of an abdominal aortic aneurysm.

The quality of MDCT angiography has reached the level where the individual branch supplying a bleeding lesion can be identified and used as a guide for embolization even when extravasation is not present on the diagnostic catheter angiogram.[21] Presently, in most institutions, MDCT angiography has replaced radionuclide scanning as the noninvasive method of choice to determine whether active bleeding is present and the location of the bleeding lesion.

PREANGIOGRAPHIC WORKUP

Before angiography and possible intervention is undertaken the patient should be visited by the interventional radiologist for an explanation of the procedure, its risks, and potential complications. Informed consent is obtained at this time. A limited physical examination with notation of the femoral and peripheral pulses should be done. The patient's chart and all pertinent laboratory results, imaging exams, and endoscopic reports need to be reviewed. Factors that may increase the procedural risk, such as renal insufficiency, hypertension, and severe atherosclerotic disease of the peripheral arteries or coagulopathy, should be recorded along with the rationale for proceeding with the examination in the presence of increased risk. Because visceral arteriography and interventional treatment of acute GI bleeding are expensive, invasive procedures with a low but definite risk, the procedure must be geared toward maximizing patient benefit.

PERFORMANCE OF THE ANGIOGRAM

If the bleeding lesion has been localized by endoscopy or noninvasive imaging, the interventional radiologist can focus attention to that area. Otherwise, GI bleeding should be categorized as "upper" or "lower." If the patient has hematemesis, upper GI bleeding is present. Bloody return from a nasogastric lavage indicates upper GI bleeding; however, non-bloody return does not exclude it. Patients with a bleeding duodenal ulcer and a competent pylorus may present with rectal bleeding and clear gastric aspirates. Therefore, angiographic examination of the stomach and duodenum should be performed if negative superior and inferior mesenteric angiograms are obtained in a patient presenting with lower GI bleeding.

It is important that imaging cover the entire GI tract. In patients with upper GI bleeding, this extends from the distal esophagus to the ligament of Treitz. For lower GI bleeding, the entire small bowel and colon to the level of the anus should be imaged.

It is equally important to take into account the anatomy of the vascular arcades that are present in the visceral circulation. The left gastric artery (a branch of the celiac artery) forms an arcade along the lesser curvature of the stomach with the right gastric artery (a branch of the hepatic artery). Another arcade is formed along the greater gastric curvature by the right gastroepiploic artery (branch of the gastroduodenal artery) and the left gastroepiploic artery (branch of the splenic artery). The superior pancreaticoduodenal artery (branch of the gastroduodenal artery) forms an arcade along the medial aspect of the duodenum with the inferior pancreaticoduodenal artery (branch of the superior mesenteric artery). An arcade also extends along the transverse and descending colon formed by the middle colic artery (branch of the superior mesenteric artery) joining the left colic artery (branch of the inferior mesenteric artery). Finally, there are anastomoses between the superior hemorrhoidal arteries (branches of the inferior mesenteric artery) and the middle hemorrhoidal arteries (branches of the internal iliac arteries).

Provocative Angiography

Because of its intermittent, minute-to-minute nature acute lower GI bleeding often stops between a positive MDCT angiogram or nuclear medicine scan and the angiogram. If clinically active

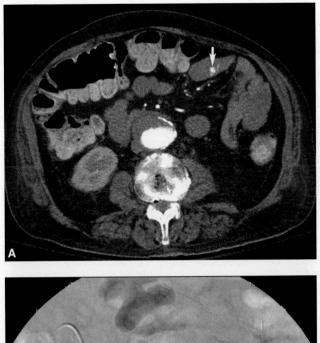

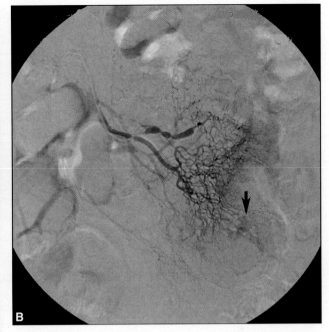

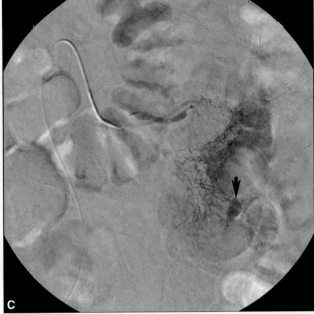

FIGURE 74.3 Acute jejunal bleeding (*arrows*). Multidetector CT angiography (**A**) localizes the active bleeding for arteriography (early phase [**B**] and late phase [**C**]).

lower GI bleeding is present just before a negative angiographic examination, provocative measures, such as vasodilators, anticoagulants, or fibrinolytics, can be used to reactivate the bleeding.[22–28] These aggressive measures should be reserved for patients who are diagnostic problems and for whom the risk of prolonging or reactivating bleeding is outweighed by the potential benefit. Interventions to prolong or reactivate bleeding should be performed only on hemodynamically stable patients for whom replacement blood is available. In one report, the use of provocative measures increased the percentage of positive angiograms for lower GI hemorrhage with extravasation from 32% to 69%.[29]

Intraoperative Localization of Small-Bowel Bleeding

Pathologic lesions in the stomach or colon that are responsible for bleeding are easy to locate during surgery because these structures are relatively fixed. However, peristalsis in the small bowel causes loops of intestine to shift in the abdomen. A small-bowel lesion demonstrated at angiography to be in one location may shift dramatically by the time of surgery. Frequently, it is difficult to know angiographically in which loop of small bowel the lesion is located exactly. Precise preoperative localization of lesions, such as angiodysplasias, is required because they usually cannot be seen or palpated at surgery. In addition, jejunal and ileal angiodysplasias are difficult to find at surgery because once the bowel is eviscerated for inspection the spatial relationship between individual bowel loops change. Placing a microcatheter in the small-bowel branch supplying the pathologic lesion just before surgery is one method to ensure that the correct loop of bowel is resected. Once the abdomen is opened and the small bowel exposed, methylene blue is injected through the microcatheter, staining the abnormal area and making it readily distinguished from adjacent normal bowel (FIGURE 74.4).[30,31] An alternative technique is to deploy a metallic embolization coil that is easy for the surgeon to palpate in the branch supplying the pathologic lesion.[32]

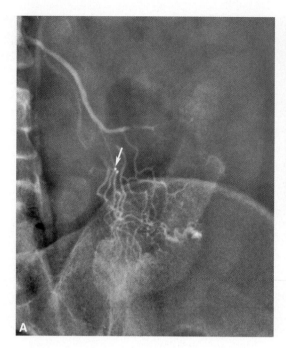

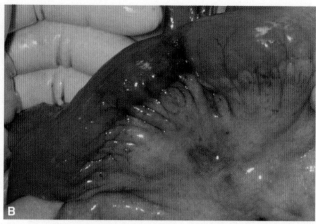

FIGURE 74.4 Intraoperative localization of small-bowel bleeding. A microcatheter (*arrow*) has been placed in the jejunal arterial branch supplying an angiodysplasia (**A**). At surgery, methylene blue has been injected through the microcatheter (**B**).

INTERVENTIONAL TREATMENT OF ACUTE GASTROINTESTINAL BLEEDING

Precise localization of the bleeding artery is the first step in catheter therapy of acute GI hemorrhage. In patients with gastric bleeding it has been reported that arterial supply to the bleeding lesion is from the left gastric artery in 85% of cases.[33] The right and short gastric arteries each supplied the bleeding gastric lesion in 5% of cases. The remaining 5% of cases had supply from the gastroepiploic arteries (3%), phrenic artery (1%), and gastroduodenal artery (1%). Duodenal bleeding can be supplied by the gastroduodenal artery or the inferior pancreaticoduodenal artery or often a combination of both. Small-bowel and colonic hemorrhage originate from various branches of the superior or inferior mesenteric arteries. A bleeding colonic lesion in the "watershed" area of the splenic flexure can be supplied by branches of both the superior and inferior mesenteric arteries. Distal rectal or anal bleeding may also have a dual supply: superior hemorrhoidal branches from the inferior mesenteric artery and/or middle hemorrhoidal branches from the internal iliac artery.

Once the exact bleeding site has been established, the interventional radiologist has two available methods of transcatheter control of arterial GI hemorrhage: vasopressin infusion and embolization.

Vasopressin Infusion

Vasopressin infusion is used occasionally today and is the method of choice when an angiographic catheter cannot be advanced to a position that is satisfactory for safe embolization or when bleeding is from a diffuse area. Vasopressin is an octapeptide produced in the neurohypophysis. It has a variety of pharmacologic actions. One of these, smooth muscle contraction, is most useful in controlling GI bleeding. Vasopressin causes smooth muscle contraction in the walls of arterioles, resulting in vasoconstriction. Additionally, it induces smooth muscle contraction in the bowel wall, compressing the penetrating blood vessels.

Vasopressin is infused selectively into the bleeding artery at a dose of 0.1 to 0.4 unit/minute, depending on the rate of bleeding and arterial size. An angiogram can be repeated after a trial infusion of 20 minutes. If the bleeding has stopped, the infusion can be continued at its present rate. If bleeding persists on this trial, however, the dose can be increased but should not exceed 0.4 unit/minute. Once bleeding is controlled in the interventional suite, the patient is sent to the intensive care unit (ICU) for long-term infusion. Infusion continues for 24 to 36 hours as the dose is tapered. If bleeding does not recur after that time, the catheter may be kept open with saline or 5% dextrose for another 12 hours before its removal.

Vasopressin infusion is frequently successful in controlling bleeding from superficial gastric lesions, such as erosive gastritis, Mallory Weiss tears, and stress ulcers.[34–37] Colonic diverticulae and angiodysplasias, the lesions most responsible for acute lower GI bleeding, are also responsive to vasopressin infusion.[34,36,37] For bleeding lesions near the splenic flexure, vasopressin infusions in both the superior and inferior mesenteric arteries may be required to control hemorrhage.

Vasopressin infusion is substantially less effective in controlling bleeding from duodenal ulcers.[38] Several reasons account for this difference. First, there is a dual blood supply to the duodenum from both the celiac and superior mesenteric arteries. Infusion of only one side of the arcade is usually not effective because the lesion can continue to bleed from the opposite side. Secondly, vasopressin has its maximum effect on small vessels. However, duodenal hemorrhage is predominately caused by ulcers with erosion into larger arteries that are less responsive to vasopressin. Also, chronic inflammation associated with peptic disease limits both the ability of small arteries in proximity to the ulcer to constrict as well as contractability of the adjacent duodenal wall. Finally, if endoscopic control of a bleeding duodenal ulcer has been attempted with electrocoagulation or heater probe, vascular contractability will be impaired.[39]

Interventionists involved in the management of GI bleeding must be familiar with the potential side effects of vasopressin therapy. These may be categorized as systemic, cardiovascular, peripheral vascular, and GI. Because vasopressin is the same substance as antidiuretic hormone (ADH) systemic side effects include water retention, hyponatremia, and hypertension. Cardiovascular complications of vasopressin are myocardial ischemia, decreased cardiac output, and arrhythmias. Acrocyanosis leading to gangrene of the digits and of the penis has been reported to occur during vasopressin infusion.[38] Because vasopressin causes smooth muscle contraction of the bowel wall, GI cramping is very common. Both bowel infarction and thrombosis of the superior mesenteric and portal veins have been reported with vasopressin infusion when the dose exceeds 0.4 unit/minute.

Embolotherapy

Since the early 1970s when embolization was introduced to control acute GI hemorrhage, its indications have expanded.[6,40,41] Initially embolization was reserved for patients with life-threatening hemorrhage who failed a trial vasopressin infusion. Today, however, most interventional radiologists prefer to use embolotherapy as initial therapy and limit vasopressin infusion to those few instances where the angiographic catheter cannot be placed close enough to the bleeding lesion to avoid unwanted and potentially dangerous nontarget embolization. The goal of embolization is to reduce the blood pressure at the bleeding site and allow a stable clot to form without causing tissue ischemia or necrosis. Compared to vasopressin infusion, embolotherapy has the advantages of rapid control of bleeding without the problems of maintaining long-term arterial catheterization and the undesirable pharmacologic side effects of vasopressin. Embolization is not without its risks, however. Unlike vasopressin, which can be decreased or discontinued at the first sign of untoward side effects, embolic particles and most embolic devices cannot be retrieved once they are released.

Particle Embolization

Autologous blood clot was the first material used to control active GI bleeding.[6] Today, the choice of embolic material varies with the preference of the interventional radiologist and the anatomy and size of the vessels to be embolized. Many lesions causing acute GI bleeding are benign and self-limiting and will heal with medical treatment. Use of temporary agents like gelfoam sponge is preferred. Recanalization of arteries occluded with gelfoam usually occurs within 1 to 3 weeks. The gelfoam sponge is cut into small pledgets, mixed with contrast material, and carefully injected into the bleeding artery to avoid reflux. If deeper penetration of gelfoam is desired, the pledgets can be mixed with contrast material and passed between two syringes with a three-way stopcock interposed. This will result in a fine mixture of gelfoam that can be injected through microcatheters. Gelfoam powder, on the other hand, penetrates too far distally, occluding arteries as small as 50 to 60 μm in diameter, making it unacceptable as an embolic material for interventional management of GI bleeding. Both acute and chronic superficial and perforating gastric ulcers occurred in swine whose left gastric arteries were embolized with gelfoam powder.[42]

Polyvinyl alcohol foam or calibrated acrylic particles are preferred by some interventionists. The diameters of these particles range in size from 100 to 1,000 μm. Interventionists can choose the appropriate diameter particle depending on the desired depth of penetration. These agents cause permanent occlusion and are especially indicated when GI hemorrhage is caused by invasion of the GI tract by primary or secondary malignancies. The particles are suspended in a syringe containing dilute contrast material and carefully delivered under fluoroscopic monitoring. Because they are soft and conformable, they can easily pass through microcatheters.

Coil Embolization

Occlusion coils are mechanical devices that are also very effective in controlling GI hemorrhage. They may be used for bleeding from large vessels for which gelfoam or other particles may be ineffective. Unlike particles that embolize distally from the catheter, coils remain where they are deployed at the site of the lesion. Occlusion coils are indicated when peptic erosion has caused a large arterial defect, frequently seen in the gastroduodenal artery in a patient with an acutely bleeding duodenal ulcer. With this situation, particulate embolics will likely pass directly through the hole in the artery into the lumen of the duodenum. To function as intended, occlusion coils require an intact coagulation system. In patients with a focal bleeding site originating from a large artery, the interventional strategy is to "bracket" the lesion by placing coils just proximal and distal to it (FIGURE 74.5). To accomplish this with bleeding duodenal ulcers, both sides of the pancreaticoduodenal arcade may require catheterization and occlusion.[43] Refinement in occlusion coil technology resulted in the development of detachable coils, microcoils capable of being delivered through a microcatheter, and metallic coils that do not degrade magnetic resonance (MR) or CT images (FIGURE 74.6).

Liquid Embolic Agents

Liquid embolic agents also have a role in interventional therapy of GI bleeding. N-butyl cyanoacrylate (Trufill) is a type of glue that is mixed with Ethiodol and polymerizes upon contact with ions in the blood. The rapidity of polymerization depends on the ratio of the mixture. This material is useful when a permanent occlusion is desired and the angiographic catheter cannot be advanced close enough to the pathologic lesion for placement of a coil and for which vasopressin infusion or particulate embolization has decreased chances of success.[44] Use of N-butyl cyanoacrylate is not intuitive. Because proper usage requires a moderate amount of training in either an animal lab or on a model, it is not an embolic material that can be pulled off the shelf and used for the first time to embolize an acutely bleeding patient. Absolute ethanol is another liquid embolic agent that has been used in interventional radiology for specifically limited indications. However, because absolute ethanol denatures protein and infarcts tissue, it has absolutely no role in the interventional therapy of acute GI bleeding.

Empiric Embolization

In most instances embolization for acute GI bleeding occurs following the demonstration of extravasation of contrast material from the offending lesion on the initial angiogram. Empiric embolization is the practice of performing embolization based

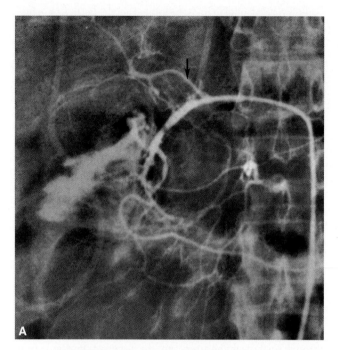
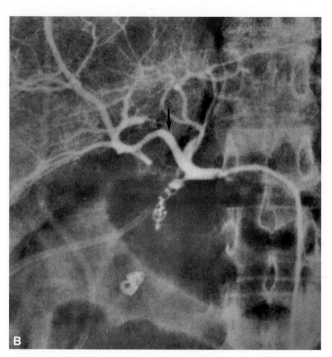

FIGURE 74.5 Massive bleeding from a duodenal ulcer. Contrast material extravasates from the gastroduodenal artery. The patient is in shock with profound vasoconstriction of the common hepatic artery (*arrow*) (**A**). After placing occlusion coils in the gastroduodenal artery, both proximal and distal to the bleeding site, hemorrhage is controlled. Return to normal size of the common hepatic artery (*arrow*) corresponded with return to normal blood pressure (**B**).

on either the endoscopic or MDCT angiography findings in the absence of extravasation. The endoscopist may place a clip next to the bleeding site to help guide the interventional radiologist. Used almost exclusively in patients with upper GI bleeding, empiric embolization has essentially the same overall good results as embolization performed in the presence of extravasation.[45–47] One large study concluded that stopping upper GI hemorrhage with embolization had a significantly positive effect on

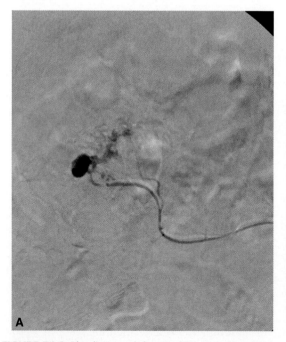
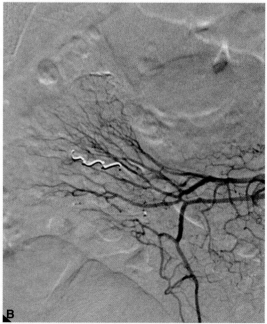

FIGURE 74.6 Bleeding cecal diverticulum. Extravasation into a bleeding cecal diverticulum in a coagulopathic patient. **A.** Following embolization of the vasa recta supplying the bleeding site with microcoils and *N*-butyl cyanoacrylate, the bleeding has ceased. **B.** Superficial ulceration of the cecum at the mouth of the previously bleeding diverticulum is present on endoscopy 2 days after embolization. **C.** The ulceration is caused by the use of *N*-butyl cyanoacrylate.

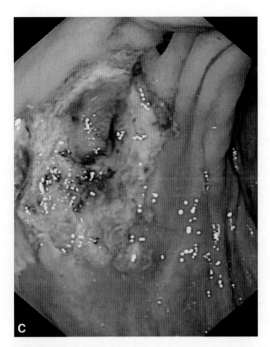

FIGURE 74.6 *(Continued)*

survival independent of demonstrable extravasation at the time of embolization.[45]

For patients with endoscopically identified gastric bleeding who do not have active extravasation at angiography, the left gastric artery is embolized empirically.[45,46] If the endoscopic exam reveals duodenal bleeding and no angiographic extravasation is present, the gastroduodenal artery is empirically embolized in its entirety. Furthermore, depending on the endoscopic findings, the anterior or posterior superior pancreaticoduodenal arteries and sometimes the inferior pancreaticoduodenal artery are also empirically embolized.[45,48]

CHRONIC GASTROINTESTINAL BLEEDING

Unlike acute GI hemorrhage with its dramatic presentations of hematemesis, hematochezia, or melena, patients with chronic GI bleeding present with occult fecal blood and iron deficiency anemia. Occasionally, there are recurrent brief episodes of acute and sometimes massive hemorrhage. Usually some type of tumor will be diagnosed in these patients by endoscopy or noninvasive imaging. Angiography is reserved for patients with chronic GI bleeding who continue to bleed despite endoscopies including capsule endoscopy, CTs, and barium studies. For patients with chronic GI bleeding, a positive angiogram reveals some type of hypervascular lesion rather than extravasation into the lumen of the GI tract. The diagnosis in a significant percentage of patients with chronic or recurrent lower GI hemorrhage remains unknown even after well-performed angiography.[49]

Angiodysplasia

Known variously as telangiectasias, angiomas, vascular ectasias, angiodysplasias, and vascular malformations, these lesions are commonly responsible for lower GI bleeding, especially in the elderly.[50,51] They are often associated with mitral and aortic

valvular disease and hereditary hemorrhagic telangiectasia. Morphologically, angiodysplasias are foci of ectatic submucosal vascular spaces. As such, the angiographic appearance is that of a tangle of vessels, sometimes quite subtle, in the bowel wall that fills earlier than the rest of the bowel. An early filling and densely draining vein is also present (FIGURE 74.7). Angiodysplasias are usually removed surgically; however, embolization has been used successfully to treat these lesions.[52] As already stated, precise presurgical localization of small-bowel angiodysplasias is important.[31,32]

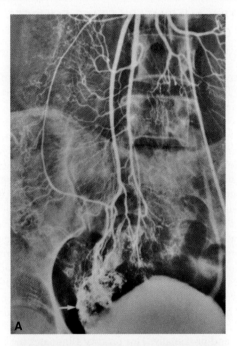
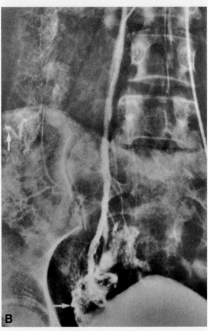

FIGURE 74.7 Angiodysplasias. Early (**A**) and late (**B**) phases of a superior mesenteric arteriogram in a patient with a large cecal angiodysplasia and a small ascending colon angiodysplasia (*arrows*).

Meckel Diverticulum

Meckel diverticulum is a common cause of both chronic and acute GI bleeding in young patients. Arteriography performed during an episode of acute bleeding from a Meckel diverticulum reveals extravasation. If the angiogram is done in the absence of active bleeding, a long, nonbranching, embryonic ileal artery leading to the diverticulum is often seen (FIGURE 74.8). Other angiographic findings may include irregular arteries in the wall of the diverticulum that are the remnants of vitelline arteries and an increased parenchymal blush arising from the gastric mucosa within the wall of the Meckel diverticulum.[53]

EXTRA-ALIMENTARY TRACT SOURCES OF GASTROINTESTINAL BLEEDING

Hemobilia

Once considered an extremely rare source of GI hemorrhage, hemobilia, bleeding into the biliary tract, has been encountered more frequently in recent years.[54] Trauma, including iatrogenic trauma occurring either in the recent or remote past, is the most common cause. Although blunt trauma with liver lacerations and penetrating trauma from stab wounds are well-known causes of hemobilia, invasive diagnostic and therapeutic procedures, such as percutaneous liver biopsies and transhepatic biliary drainages, are the greatest causes of hemobilia today.[55]

Traditional therapy for hemobilia was either surgical resection of the hepatic lobe or segment containing the involved lesion or hepatic artery ligation.[53] Today, however, both surgeons and interventional radiologists agree that superselective transcatheter occlusion of the intrahepatic artery (or portal vein branch) that supplies the pathologic lesion responsible for hemobilia is the current therapy of choice.[56–58] If a pseudoaneurysm in a large central hepatic artery exists, the interventional radiologist should try to isolate it by bracketing it with occlusion coils placed just distally and proximally. This practice eliminates the chance of

rebleeding from perfusion of the pseudoaneurysm in a retrograde fashion from intrahepatic collaterals. For peripheral hepatic lesions causing hemobilia, simple placement of occlusion coils as close as possible to the lesion is the best approach (FIGURE 74.9).

Gastrointestinal Hemorrhage of Pancreatic Origin

Digestion of the arterial walls by enzymes released during an episode of acute pancreatitis can cause formations of pseudoaneurysms that may communicate with the lumen of various segments of the alimentary tract, the pancreatic duct (hemosuccus pancreaticus), or pseudocysts. Patients may present with massive GI hemorrhage.

In these patients, CT often demonstrates a pseudoaneurysm filled with blood and may show extravasation of contrast material into the GI tract if the patient is bleeding acutely at the time of the CT. The CT serves as a guide for the interventional treatment of these lesions. Surgical intervention is often required to manage the complications of pancreatitis. Preoperative embolization in patients needing surgery reduces the chances of serious hemorrhage during the operation and frequently obviates the need for surgery altogether. Interventional treatment of pseudoaneurysms from pancreatitis that cause acute GI bleeding consists of isolating the pseudoaneurysm by placing occlusion coils both distally and proximally to it. *N*-butyl cyanoacrylate is also a useful embolic agent for management of hemorrhagic complications of pancreatitis.[59–62]

Aortoenteric and Arterioenteric Fistulas

Vascular graft anastomoses, aneurysms, and pseudoaneurysms that lie near and eventually erode into a portion of the alimentary tract as a result of continuous pulsations against it are rare causes of acute GI bleeding. Often these problems are diagnosed by CT and the patient goes directly to surgery. If the patient is bleeding actively at the time of angiography, extravasation of

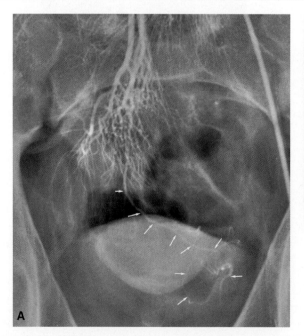

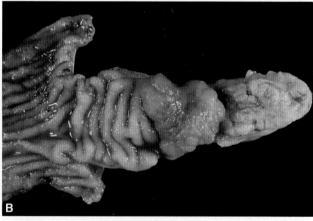

FIGURE 74.8 Meckel diverticulum. Long, nonbranching, embryonic ileal artery leading to a rounded mass (*arrows*) in the pelvis (**A**). Resected specimen (**B**).

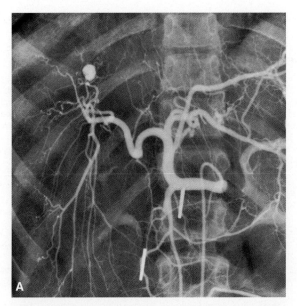 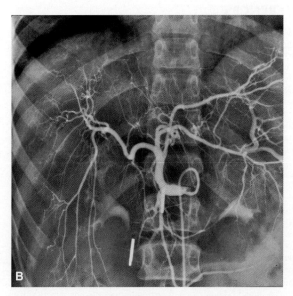

FIGURE 74.9 Hemobilia. Peripheral intrahepatic arterial pseudoaneurysm in a 9-year-old girl who had six episodes of upper GI bleeding after a traumatic liver injury and surgery (**A**). Follow-up angiogram 2 months after embolization (**B**).

contrast material is present on an aortogram (FIGURE 74.10). The interventional radiologist, however, must have a high index of suspicion for an aortoenteric or iliac artery enteric fistula based on a history of aneurysms of these vessels or aortic or iliac artery surgery. In these cases, the first contrast injection should be an aortogram. Typical findings of arterial (aortic) enteric fistulas when active bleeding is not present are either a pseudoaneurysm or a defect in the wall of the artery at the site of the fistula.[63]

Traditional therapy for these lesions is vascular surgery. If the patient is bleeding actively, an occlusion balloon can be placed in the aorta or iliac artery at the site of the fistula and inflated to tamponade the hemorrhage prior to operation. If, however, the patient is a poor operative candidate, either embolization or interventional placement of an aortic or iliac artery endograft has successfully managed hemorrhage from these lesions.[64,65]

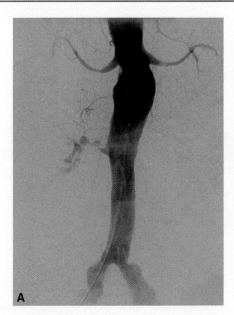 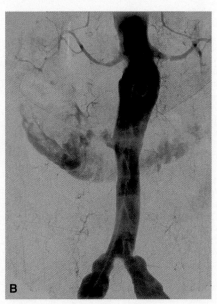

FIGURE 74.10 Aortoduodenal fistula. Early (**A**) and late (**B**) phases of an aortogram show massive extravasation of contrast material from the aorta into the duodenum.

‖ REFERENCES

1. Margulis AR, Heinbecker P, Bernard HR. Operative mesenteric arteriography in the search for the site of bleeding in unexplained gastrointestinal hemorrhage. *Surgery* 1960;48:534.
2. Baum S, Stein GN, Nussbaum M, et al. Selective arteriography in the diagnosis of hemorrhage in the gastrointestinal tract. *Radiol Clin North Am* 1969;7:131.
3. Baum S, Nusbaum M, Clearfield HR, et al. Angiography in the diagnosis of gastrointestinal bleeding. *Arch Intern Med* 1967;119:16.
4. Rösch J, Dotter CT, Antonovic R. Selective vasoconstrictor infusion in the management of arteriocapillary gastrointestinal hemorrhage. *AJR Am J Roentgenol* 1972;116:279.
5. Rösch J, Gray RK, Grollman JH, et al. Selective arterial drug infusions in the treatment of acute gastrointestinal bleeding. *Gastroenterology* 1970;59:341.
6. Rösch J, Dotter CT, Brown M. Selective arterial embolization. A new method for control of gastrointestinal bleeding. *Radiology* 1972;102:303.
7. Rösch J, Antonovic R, Dotter CT. Current angiographic approach to diagnosis and therapy of gastrointestinal bleeding. *Fortschr Röntgenstr* 1976;125:310.
8. Lee SS, Oh TS, Kim HJ, et al. Obscure gastrointestinal bleeding: diagnostic performance of multidetector CT enterography. *Radiology* 2011;259:739.
9. Alavi A, Dann RW, Baum S, et al. Scintigraphic detection of acute gastrointestinal bleeding. *Radiology* 1977;124:753.
10. Alavi A, Ring EJ. Localization of gastrointestinal bleeding: superiority of ^{99m}Tc sulfur colloid compared with angiography. *AJR Am J Roentgenol* 1981;137:741.
11. Orrechia PM, Hensley EK, McDonald PT, et al. Localization of lower gastrointestinal hemorrhage: experience with red blood cells labeled in vitro with Tc^{99m}. *Arch Surg* 1985;120:621.
12. Dolezal J, Vizd'a J, Rures J. Detection of acute gastrointestinal bleeding by means of technetium-99m in vivo labeled red blood cells. *Nucl Med Rev Cent East Eur* 2002;5:151.
13. Tew K, Davies RP, Jadun CK, et al. MDCT of acute lower gastrointestinal bleeding. *AJR Am J Roentgenol* 2004;182:427.
14. Kennedy DW, Laing CJ, Tseng LH, et al. Detection of active gastrointestinal hemorrhage with CT angiography: a 4½ year retrospective review. *J Vasc Interv Radiol* 2010;21:848.
15. Wu LM, Xu JR, Yin Y, et al. Usefulness of CT angiography in diagnosing acute gastrointestinal bleeding: a meta-analysis. *World J Gastroenterol* 2010;16:3957.
16. Heiss P, Zorger N, Hamer O, et al. Optimized multidetector computed tomographic protocol for the diagnosis of active gastrointestinal bleeding: a feasibility study. *J Comput Assist Tomogr* 2009;33:698.
17. Geffroy Y, Rodallec MH, Boulay-Coletta I, et al. Multidetector CT angiography in gastrointestinal bleeding: why, when and how. *Radiographics* 2011;31:831.
18. Yoon W, Jeong YY, Shin SS, et al. Acute massive gastrointestinal bleeding: detection and localization with arterial phase multi-detector row helical CT. *Radiology* 2006;239:160.
19. Zink SI, Ohki SK, Stein B, et al. Noninvasive evaluation of active lower gastrointestinal bleeding: comparison between contrast enhanced MDCT and ^{99m}Tc RBC scintigraphy. *AJR Am J Roentgenol* 2008;191:1107.
20. Kuhle WG, Scheiman RG. Detection of active colonic hemorrhage with use of helical CT: findings in a swine model. *Radiology* 2003;228:743.
21. Feld RS, Zink S, Rosteraro A. Empiric embolization of a diverticular bleed with CT angiographic mapping: enlarging the therapeutic window for transcatheter arterial interventions. *J Vasc Interv Radiol* 2010;21:593.
22. Rösch J, Keller FS, Wawrukiewicz A, et al. Pharmacoangiography in the diagnosis of recurrent massive gastrointestinal bleeding. *Radiology* 1982;145:615.
23. Ryan JM, Key SM, Dumbleton SA, et al. Nonlocalized lower gastrointestinal bleeding: provocative bleeding studies with intraarterial tPA, heparin and tolazoline. *J Vasc Interv Radiol* 2001;12:1273.
24. Johnston C, Tuite D, Pritchard R, et al. Use of provocative angiography to localize site in recurrent gastrointestinal bleeding. *Cardiovasc Intervent Radiol* 2007;30:1042.
25. Malden ES, Hicks ME, Royal HD, et al. Recurrent gastrointestinal bleeding: use of thrombolysis with anticoagulation in diagnosis. *Radiology* 1998;201:147.
26. Bloomfield RS, Smith TP, Schneider AM, et al. Provocative angiography in patients with gastrointestinal hemorrhage of obscure origin. *Am J Gastroenterol* 2000;95:2807.
27. Kim CY, Suhocki PV, Miller MJ, et al. Provocative mesenteric angiography for lower gastrointestinal hemorrhage: results from a single-institution study. *J Vasc Interv Radiol* 2010;21:477.
28. Glickerman DJ, Knowdley, Rösch J. Urokinase in gastrointestinal tract bleeding. *Radiology* 1988;168:375.
29. Rösch J, Kozak BE, Keller FS. Interventional diagnostic angiography in acute lower gastrointestinal bleeding. *Semin Intervent Radiol* 1988;5:10.
30. Remzi FH, Dietz DW, Unal E, et al. Combined use of preoperative provocative angiography and highly selective methylene blue injection to localize an occult small-bowel bleeding site in a patient with Crohn's disease: report of a case. *Dis Colon Rectum* 2003;46:260.
31. Athanasoulis CA. Therapeutic applications of angiography. *N Engl J Med* 1980;302:1117.
32. Schmidt SP, Boskind JF, Smith DC, et al. Angiographic localization of small bowel angiodysplasias with use of platinum coils. *J Vasc Interv Radiol* 1993;4:737.
33. Kelemouridis V, Athanasoulis CA, Waltman AC. Gastric bleeding sites: an angiographic study. *Radiology* 1983;149:643.
34. Athanasoulis CA, Waltman AC, Novelline RA, et al. Angiography: its contribution to the emergency management of gastrointestinal hemorrhage. *Radiol Clin North Am* 1976;14:265.
35. Eckstein MR, Kelemouridis V, Athanasoulis CA, et al. Gastric bleeding: therapy with intraarterial vasopressin and transcatheter embolization. *Radiology* 1984;152:643.
36. Kadir S, Athanasoulis CA. Angiographic management of gastrointestinal bleeding with vasopressin. *Fortschr Röntgenstr* 1977;127:111.
37. Keller FS, Rösch J. Angiography in the diagnosis and therapy of acute upper gastrointestinal bleeding. *Schweiz Med Wochenschr* 1979;109:586.
38. Twiford TW, Granmayeh M, Tucker MJ. Gangrene of the feet associated with mesenteric intraarterial vasopressin. *AJR Am J Roentgenol* 1978;130:558.
39. Waltman AC, Greenfield AJ, Novelline RA, et al. Pyloroduodenal bleeding and intraarterial vasopressin: clinical results. *AJR Am J Roentgenol* 1979;133:643.
40. Gomes AS, Lois JF, McCoy RD. Angiographic treatment of gastrointestinal hemorrhage: comparison of vasopressin infusion and embolization. *AJR Am J Roentgenol* 1986;146:1031.
41. Lieberman DA, Keller FS, Katon RM, et al. Arterial embolization for massive upper gastrointestinal tract bleeding in poor surgical candidates. *Gastroenterology* 1984;86:876.
42. Rösch J, Keller FS, Kozak BE, et al. Gelfoam powder embolization of the left gastric artery in treatment of massive small vessel gastric bleeding. *Radiology* 1984;151:365.
43. Ring EJ, Oleaga JA, Freeman D, et al. Pitfalls in angiographic management of hemorrhage: hemodynamic considerations. *AJR Am J Roentgenol* 1977;129:1007.
44. Jae HJ, Chung JW, Jung AY, et al. Transcatheter arterial embolization of nonvariceal upper gastrointestinal bleeding with N-butyl cyanoacrylate. *Korean J Radiol* 2007;8:48.
45. Schenker MP, Duszak R, Soulen MC, et al. Upper gastrointestinal hemorrhage and transcatheter embolotherapy: clinical and technical factors impacting success and survival. *J Vasc Interv Radiol* 2001;12:1263.
46. Lang EV, Picus D, Marx MV, et al. Massive upper gastrointestinal hemorrhage with normal findings on arteriography: value of prophylactic embolization of the left gastric artery. *AJR Am J Roentgenol* 1992;158:547.
47. Padia SA, Geisinger MA, Newman JS, et al. Effectiveness of coil embolization in angiographically detectable versus non-detectable sources of upper gastrointestinal hemorrhage. *J Vasc Interv Radiol* 2009;20:461.
48. Ichiro I, Shushi H, Akihiko I, et al. Empiric transcatheter arterial embolization for massive bleeding from duodenal ulcers: efficacy and complications. *J Vasc Interv Radiol* 2011;22:911.
49. Sheedy PF, Fulton RE, Atwell DT. Angiographic evaluation in a patient with chronic gastrointestinal bleeding. *AJR Am J Roentgenol* 1975;123:338.
50. Sprayregen S, Boley SJ. Vascular ectasias of the right colon. *JAMA* 1977;239:962.
51. Baum S, Athanasoulis CA, Waltman AC. Angiodysplasia of the right colon: a cause of gastrointestinal hemorrhage. *AJR Am J Roentgenol* 1977;129:789.
52. Sebrechts C, Bookstein JJ. Embolization in the management of lower gastrointestinal hemorrhage. *Semin Intervent Radiol* 1988;5:39.
53. Routh WD, Lawdahl RB, Lund E, et al. Meckel's diverticula: angiographic diagnosis in a patient with non-acute hemorrhage and negative scintigraphy. *Pediatr Radiol* 1990;20:152.
54. Sandblom P. *Hemobilia (Biliary Tract Hemorrhage): History, Pathology, Diagnosis, Treatment.* Springfield, IL: Charles C. Thomas; 1972.

55. Hovells J, Nelsson U. Intrahepatic vascular lesions following non-surgical percutaneous transhepatic bile duct intubation. *Gastrointest Radiol* 1980:5:127.

56. Mitchell SE, Shuman LS, Kaufman SL, et al. Biliary catheter drainage complicated by hemobilia: treatment by balloon embolotherapy. *Radiology* 1985;157:5645.

57. Vaughan R, Rösch J, Keller FS, et al. Treatment of hemobilia by transcatheter vascular occlusion. *Eur J Radiol* 1984;4:1983.

58. Sclafani SJA, Shaftan GW, McAuley I. Interventional radiology in the management of hepatic trauma. *J Trauma* 1984;4:183.

59. Izaki K, Yamaguchi M, Kawasaki R, et al. N-butyl cyanoacrylate embolization for pseudoaneurysms complicating pancreatitis or pancreatectomy. *J Vasc Interv Radiol* 2011;22:302.

60. Hyare H, Desigan S, Brookes JA, et al. Endovascular management of major arterial hemorrhage as a complication of inflammatory pancreatic disease. *J Vasc Interv Radiol* 2007;18:591.

61. Nicholson AA, Patel J, McPherson S, et al. Endovascular treatment of visceral aneurysm associated with pancreatitis and a suggested classification with therapeutic implications. *J Vasc Interv Radiol* 2006;17:1297.

62. Yamakado K, Nakatsuka A, Tanaka N, et al. Transcatheter arterial embolization of ruptured pseudoaneurysms with coils and N-butyl cyanoacrylate. *J Vasc Interv Radiol* 2000;11:66.

63. Thompson WM, Jackson DC, Johnsrude IS. Aortoenteric and para prosthetic-enteric fistulas: radiologic findings. *AJR Am J Roentgenol* 1976;127:235.

64. Verhey P, Best A, Lakin P, et al. Successful endovascular treatment of aortoenteric fistula secondary to eroding duodenal stent. *J Vasc Interv Radiol* 2006;17:1345.

65. Finch L, Heathcock B, Quigley T, et al. Emergent treatment of a primary aortoenteric fistula with N-butyl 2-cyanoacrylate and endovascular stent. *J Vasc Interv Radiol* 2002;13:841.

Renal Hemorrhage

SIDDHARTH A. PADIA and KARIM VALJI

INTRODUCTION

Urinary tract injuries occur in up to 10% of patients with abdominal trauma, and the kidneys are the most commonly injured urologic organ. The overall incidence of renal injury in patients with abdominal trauma is 1.2% to 3.25%.[1,2] The most frequent presenting clinical sign is hematuria, but the degree of bleeding is usually a poor indicator of the degree of renal injury. In renal pedicle injuries, hematuria may be absent in over one-third of cases. Conversely, the presence of microscopic hematuria is a poor indicator of significant renal injury. Imaging is essential for further evaluation to stage the degree of injury and plan appropriate therapy. For evaluation of renal trauma, the use of computed tomography (CT) has largely replaced conventional radiography and ultrasound. Management of renal trauma often is taken into consideration with injuries to other abdominal organs, which may dictate therapy. Fortunately, 75% to 80% of renal injuries are minor and represent contusions or superficial lacerations that can be managed conservatively. Major renal injuries are rare (grade V lesions, see later) and are usually surgical emergencies. The remaining are serious injuries, and it is here where catheter-based intervention has played the most significant role. Furthermore, the current trend toward more conservative (nonsurgical) management of renal trauma,[3] the routine use of microcatheters, and advances in embolic agents may increase the use of interventional techniques.

PATIENT SELECTION

Mechanisms of Injury: Blunt Renal Trauma

Most injuries to the kidney are a result of blunt renal trauma, most commonly caused by motor vehicle collisions. Other common causes included assault, trauma secondary to sporting activities, and falls. Injuries by street trauma, firearms, or surgery can potentially damage a broad volume or "wide tract" in the kidney or even involve its entire volume. Superficial or deep lacerations with intrarenal or perinephric hematomas or even renal rupture can occur. Intrarenal bleeding often results in direct bleeding into the collecting system, resulting in hematuria. Wide tract blunt trauma, as in deceleration in the setting of motor vehicle collision, can result in intimal disruption of the main renal arteries or avulsion. Because the kidneys are relatively mobile, the more securely anchored vessels are stretched to the point of injury. In a study of the National Trauma Data Bank,[4] renal artery injury occurred in 0.05% of blunt trauma cases. Of renal traumas, 2.5% to 4% involve the renal artery—more common in instances of penetrating trauma.[1,5,6] Hematuria is often absent in renal artery injury, and therefore diagnosis can be delayed. In the 517 cases in the National Trauma Data Bank, mortality was high at 21% with the majority of the deaths resulting from associated injuries.[4] In the few cases of surgical renal artery revascularization, mortality was only slightly lower at 15%. In renal artery thrombosis, trauma to the artery likely results in an intimal tear or dissection, followed by platelet aggregation. Via the thrombotic cascade, there is resulting occlusion of the renal artery. On CT, a complete absence of renal enhancement is suggestive. After several hours, a cortical rim sign may be identified due to collateral perfusion via capsular branches. In the rare cases of complete renal artery tears, a hematoma may be identified in the periaortic region.

Mechanisms of Injury: Penetrating Renal Trauma

Injuries from street assaults (gunshot or stab injuries), biopsies, and nephrostomies leave a narrower, sharply defined residual tract. The potential for arterial injury is very high, especially with street assaults, and there is a propensity for pseudoaneurysm formation with or without an associated arteriovenous fistula (AVF). Typically patients have persistent gross hematuria, severe enough in some to cause shock. However, most renal bleeding is iatrogenic secondary to such procedures as renal biopsy, nephrostomy, and nephrolithotripsy. Although these procedures are relatively safe with low rates of hemorrhage, their prevalent use results in a high incidence of renal hemorrhage. Additionally, biopsies of renal transplants are frequently performed to determine the cause of declining renal function. Vascular complications following biopsy in renal transplants has been reported as high at 15%.[7] The surgical evaluation of a narrow wound tract has its limitations because it does not allow proper assessment of the depth of injury. Penetrating renal trauma can be associated with a nonsterile condition, however, necessitating the need for surgical debridement or even nephrectomy.

Evaluation: Imaging

Traditionally, imaging assessment consisted of retrograde or conventional intravenous urography. These have largely been replaced because they are time-consuming and nonspecific.[8] Additionally, they have limited evaluation of the renal parenchyma. Ultrasound is advantageous because of its portability and widespread availability. Frequently, a focused assessment with sonography for trauma (FAST) is performed in emergency departments. Its use lies in the assessment of intra-abdominal hemorrhage, which often necessitates immediate surgical intervention. Its role in evaluating specific organ injury is limited, and its sensitivity for retroperitoneal hemorrhage is also limited. Because of its low sensitivity for renal pathology, a negative ultrasound does not exclude a renal injury.[9,10] Contrast-material-enhanced CT has become the imaging technique of choice in cases of suspected renal trauma.[11,12] CT is widely available in emergency departments, can be performed quickly, and its images and interpretation are more reproducible due to decreased operator dependence. With contrast medium enhancement, CT has a high sensitivity and specificity in assessing the presence and degree of renal parenchymal damage. Additionally, delayed imaging allows for assessment of the urinary collecting system. Finally, because most renal traumas also have concurrent injury to another abdominal organ, CT is useful in providing a more global assessment.

Although CT is performed for a wide variety of indications in the setting of trauma, certain situations in trauma exist where CT is mandatory[13,14]: gross hematuria, hematuria with hypotension, and blunt trauma secondary to a mechanism known to be associated with renal injury (e.g., high-speed motor vehicle accident).

Angiography traditionally was used to primarily diagnose renal injury. This is now rare, and angiography is only used as a primary diagnostic tool when it is already being performed to diagnose and/or treat another injury, such as pelvic trauma. However, angiography is becoming more common in renal trauma to perform endovascular treatment.

Renal Injury Classification

Table 75.1 provides the classification of acute renal injuries developed by the Organ Injury Scaling Committee of the American Association for Surgery of Trauma.[15] This grading system has been validated by several studies, including a study of 2,467 patients, which demonstrated high correlation between lesion classification and the need for surgical repair or nephrectomy (Santucci, Validation of the American Association). Another study[16] showed worse outcomes with increasing levels of lesion severity. Appropriate categorization of renal injuries will allow for appropriate therapy.[17] Renal injury severity based on this scale has been the strongest predictor of nephrectomy.[18]

Grade I lesions represent the most common renal injury, comprising 75% of all renal injuries.[17] Grade I injuries represent a renal contusion or nonexpanding subcapsular hematoma. Grade II lesions are nonexpanding perirenal hematomas or cortical lacerations less than 1 cm deep. Grade III lesions represent cortical lacerations greater than 1 cm deep without urinary extravasation. These are often associated with larger perinephric hematomas. Grade IV injuries represent lacerations that extend into the renal collecting system (FIGURE 75.1). Additionally, renal artery or vein injury with contained hemorrhage is classified as grade IV lesions. Grade V lesions, the most severe injuries, are shattered kidneys or avulsion of the renal pedicle. Of note, segmental renal artery injuries are not classified in this system.

▌ TREATMENT OPTIONS

Minimizing hemorrhage and preserving renal function are the main goals in the treatment of renal trauma. Therefore, conservative management is used for most cases. Many patients already undergo exploratory laparotomy for a concurrent solid organ injury, which has been reported to be present in 61% of renal stab wounds.[19] In patients who undergo exploratory laparotomy for repair, nephrectomy is more common compared to observation. Additionally, renal function is often compromised after surgical repair. The increasing use of conservative management is largely due to increased use of CT, improved care in the intensive care unit, and the availability of catheter-directed therapy.

The management of renal trauma has evolved over the last two decades. Where surgical exploration was typically performed in most cases, a conservative nonoperative approach is now taken for most cases.[20] Because grades I and II renal lesions are often self-limited, observation is recommended. In a prospective observational series of 200 patients presenting with renal stab wounds, 96% of grade I and 73% of grade II lesions were successfully managed nonoperatively.[19] The

Table 75.1

Classification of Acute Renal Injuries Developed by the Organ Injury Scaling Committee of the American Association for Surgery of Trauma

Grade	Type	Description
I	Contusion	Microscopic or gross hematuria, urologic studies are normal
	Hematoma	Nonexpanding subcapsular hematoma with no laceration
II	Hematoma	Nonexpanding perirenal hematoma confined to the retroperitoneum
	Laceration	<1-cm parenchymal depth of the renal cortex with no urinary extravasation
III	Laceration	>1-cm parenchymal depth of the renal cortex with no urinary extravasation
IV	Laceration	Parenchymal laceration extending through the renal cortex, medulla, and collecting system
	Vascular	Main renal artery or vein injury with contained hemorrhage
V	Laceration	Completely shattered kidney
	Vascular	Avulsion or thrombosis of the renal artery or vein that devascularizes the kidney

Reprinted with permission from Moore EE, Shackford SR, Pachter HL, et al. Organ injury scaling: spleen, liver, and kidney. *J Trauma* 1989;29(12):1664–1666.

xt:

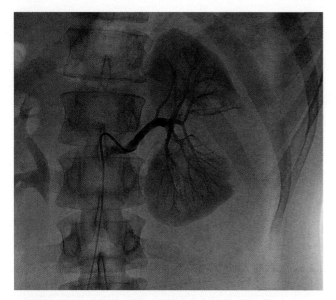

FIGURE 75.1 A 22-year-old man who sustained a blunt injury while playing football and presented with gross hematuria, hypotension, and decreasing hematocrit. CT (not shown) showed a grade IV laceration through the renal parenchyma. Selective left renal arteriogram demonstrates a single laceration through the entire parenchymal width of the kidney, extending centrally to the collecting system. By the time he underwent angiography, he became hemodynamically stable and no contrast extravasation was identified. Therefore, embolization was not performed.

remainder required either immediate or delayed surgical intervention. Treatment of grades III and IV lesions is controversial and often institution dependent. Many grade III lesions heal without intervention, whereas others require surgical correction. Many physicians opt for a conservative approach when the patient is hemodynamically stable.[21] Although most grades III and IV lesions can be treated conservatively, delayed renal bleeding can occur.[1] Grades III and IV lesions are likely the most appropriate situations where angiographic evaluation with embolization can make a significant impact to avoid surgical intervention and decrease the incidence of delayed rebleeding (FIGURE 75.2). Within these categories, the presence of large perirenal hematomas or active contrast extravasation has been associated with the need for angiographic embolization.[22] In cases of severe hemodynamic instability, severe injury to other abdominal organs, the presence of urine leaks, or when there is greater than 50% involvement of the kidney, surgical intervention is often warranted. Overall mortality for grades I through IV lesions is low, approximately 5%.[23] Moreover, there is no significant difference in mortality between grades I and IV lesions.[23] Proposals have been made to stratify grade IV lesions into high risk and low risk, based on three CT features: increased perirenal hematoma size, contrast extravasation, and a medial site of renal laceration.[24] Grade V renal injuries are relatively uncommon[23] and usually require surgical intervention. Additionally, these are often associated with significant injury to other abdominal organs, and surgical intervention is

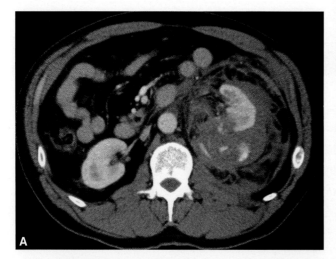
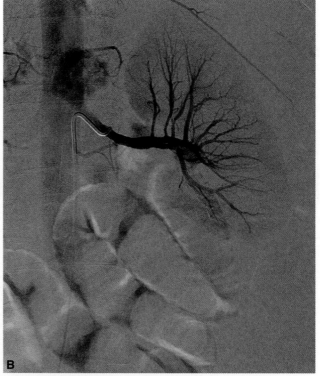

FIGURE 75.2 A 37-year-old man involved in a motorcycle accident. CT (A) demonstrates multiple grade IV lesions involving the left kidney with a perirenal hematoma. The patient had a decreasing hematocrit, so angiography was performed. Selective catheterization and angiography (B) of the left renal artery demonstrates a pseudoaneurysm arising off a central branch (C, arrow). After the feeding artery was coil embolized, repeat angiography (D) showed active contrast extravasation off a separate branch (arrow). This branch was subsequently coil embolized (E). As a result, approximately 50% of the renal parenchyma was infarcted.

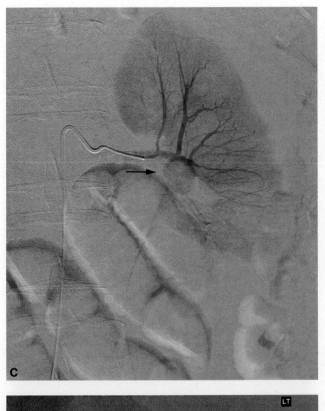

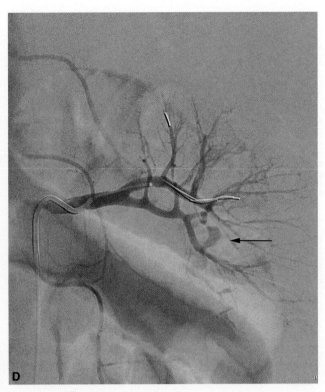

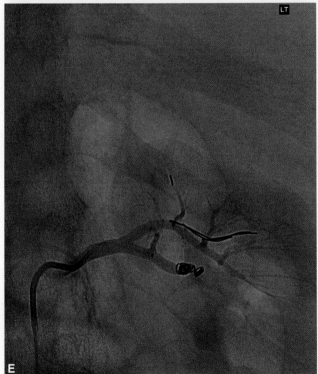

FIGURE 75.2 *(Continued)*

warranted to treat the concomitant injuries. However, renal injuries may also be overlooked during emergency laparotomy for other solid visceral intraperitoneal injuries unless they are suspected clinically and/or demonstrated radiographically before surgery. In grade V lesions, mortality reaches 29%[23] and is often caused by associated abdominal organ injuries.

However, catheter-directed therapy has been performed with success.[25,26]

Various therapeutic options for the treatment of renal artery injury (grades IV and V injuries) exist. Options include nephrectomy, surgical repair, catheter-directed therapy, and observation. Warm ischemia can result in irreversible renal damage, even after 2 hours.[27,28] Because the warm ischemic time of the kidney should not exceed a few hours, repair of the artery (either surgical or endovascular) often cannot be performed. In the cases of bilateral renal artery injury or solitary kidney, however, arterial repair may be warranted even if the ischemic time exceeds several hours. If a unilateral injury is incomplete or is recognized early, revascularization is warranted (either surgical or endovascular). Surgical revascularization of the renal artery has traditionally had poor outcomes[29,30] with limited restoration of parenchymal flow. In a series of 36 patients presenting with renal artery injury, 6 underwent immediate nephrectomy. Nine patients underwent attempted repair of the artery with only two of the nine patients with achieved complete renal preservation.[5]

Renal vascular injuries from a biopsy or nephrostomy may be destabilizing; therefore, immediate angiographic diagnosis and prompt treatment are required. However, most heal spontaneously. If there is hemodynamic instability or if hematuria should persist for 2 to 3 days, angiographic investigation and possible embolization are warranted. On the other hand, a few injuries may remain clinically silent and present with hematuria and/or hypertension months to years later as the result of an undiagnosed AVF (FIGURE 75.3). Additionally, hematuria is not seen in up to 36% of renal pedicle injuries and in 24% of renal artery occlusions.[6,31]

Embolotherapy is more likely to be used in the treatment of narrow tract vascular injuries. Patient stability and the absence of suspected concomitant bowel injury are essential considerations in selecting patients for interventional management. However, emergency angiography and embolization could potentially stabilize a patient with poorly controlled shock and decrease the risk of subsequent exploratory surgery. Interventional procedures should be encouraged as a viable alternative to surgery in selected patients, particularly in those with narrow tract penetrating trauma because most reported cases of successful embolization of these specific injuries have been in patients in which surgery had failed to achieve permanent hemostasis. Alternatively, most injuries resulting from biopsy or nephrostomy have been treated primarily with embolization, thus avoiding surgery (FIGURE 75.3). These injuries tend to be less urgent and typically involve only the kidney. Furthermore, hemorrhage from renal biopsies is often pursued after 2 to 3 days of persistent or recurrent hematuria because many stop bleeding spontaneously.

One must also be aware of secondary hemorrhage. This is observed more commonly in cases of deep laceration, grade V trauma or conservatively managed trauma. It can happen at any time after the primary incident and most often occurs 2 to 3 weeks after trauma. This is usually caused by a post-traumatic

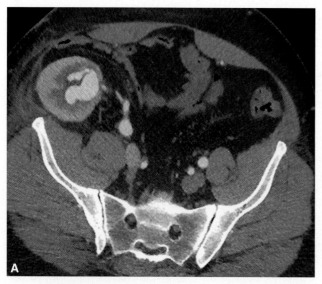

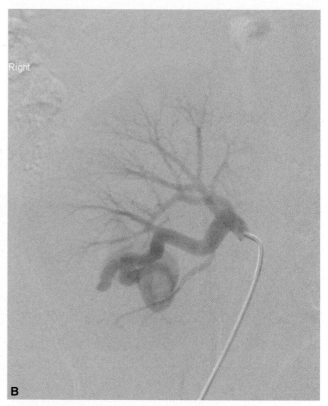

FIGURE 75.3 A 56-year-old man who underwent a percutaneous biopsy of his renal transplant and developed persistent gross hematuria. Axial (**A**) CT demonstrates a large pseudoaneurysm in the lower pole of the transplant kidney. Selective catheterization of the renal artery was performed, and an arteriogram (**B**) confirms the diagnosis. After catheterization of the lower pole branch with a microcatheter (**C**), coil embolization of the feeding artery was performed. Final angiogram (**D**) demonstrates resolution of the pseudoaneurysm with minimal nonperfusion of the associated parenchyma.

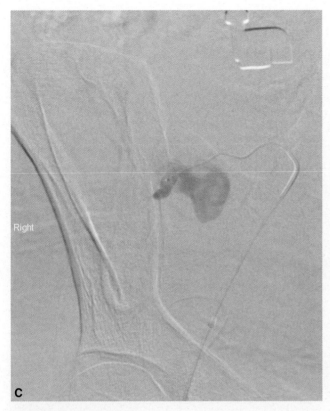

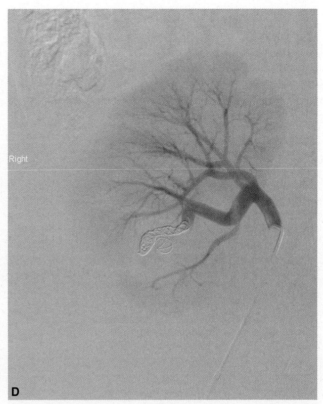

FIGURE 75.3 *(Continued)*

pseudoaneurysm or AVF. Because these entities are the most common causes, penetrating trauma has a higher incidence of secondary trauma compared to blunt trauma.

The criteria for embolization begin with clinical findings of post-traumatic hematuria and/or a dropping hematocrit or the demonstrated presence of a large intrarenal or perinephric hematoma by CT. Ideally, patients should be sufficiently stable to permit an angiographic investigation. The presence of hemodynamic instability should not significantly delay angiography, however, because angiography may control hemorrhage and result in stabilization. Extravasation, pseudoaneurysms, AVFs, and arterial calyceal fistulas, occurring individually or in combination, are potentially controllable with embolization (FIGURES 75.2 and 75.3). On occasion, one also may consider empirically embolizing a large transected renal artery branch to avoid a future unexpected hemorrhage that may require management in less controlled circumstances (FIGURE 75.4).

▌ TECHNICAL CONSIDERATIONS

Various arterial injuries can result from trauma, including main renal artery intimal disruption or avulsion, renal artery branch transection without or with extravasation, pseudoaneurysm formation, and AVF. Multiple injuries are also possible. Through a sheath in the femoral artery, evaluation of the abdominal aorta should be performed with a pigtail catheter to assess the location and number of renal arteries. Depending on their configuration, renal arteries can be selected with standard 4 or 5 French catheters (e.g., Cobra, Sos, Renal Double Curve). Digital subtraction

angiography should be performed in multiple projections to pinpoint the exact source of bleeding and to plan a route and projection for vessel selection.

When treating segmental or subsegmental renal arterial branches, a coaxial microcatheter system provides a safe and user-friendly platform for embolization.[32] This is typically performed with a 2 to 3 French microcatheter, which can allow for embolization with microcoils, particles, gelfoam, or glue. The size of coils and particles that can be used is dictated by the inner diameter of the microcatheter. Specific selection of the injured renal artery branch is ideal before embolization because some degree of renal infarction usually occurs. The choice of embolic is based on several factors. These include the nature of the vascular injury, the size of the injured artery, and the flow dynamics of the vessel. Gelatin sponge has been used most commonly for embolization because of its utility, absorbability, ease of use, and familiarity to operators.[33] Recently, *N*-butyl cyanoacrylate glue has been used successfully in treating distal arterial hemorrhage. This allows for embolization of the selected branch of the renal artery as well as its small distal tributaries with minimal associated nontarget embolization. The presence of larger vessel injuries or AVF often requires a more aggressive approach, necessitating the use of coils for occlusion. If high-flow AVFs are present, there is a risk of downstream dislodgment of coils, which could then flow into the venous system. In these cases, the use of detachable coils (e.g., Trufill, Guglielmi) allows for safer delivery of embolic. Alternatively, the venous outflow tract can be temporarily stopped with a balloon occlusion catheter.

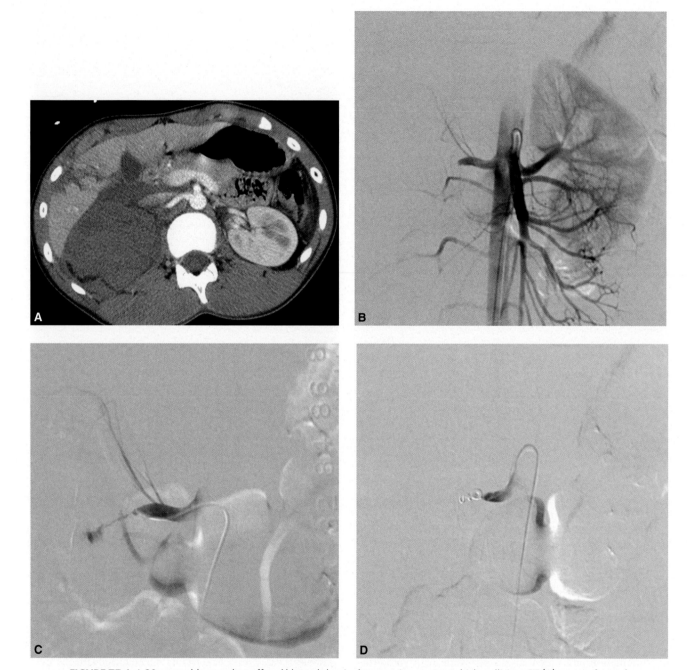

FIGURE 75.4 A 30-year-old man who suffered blunt abdominal trauma in a motor vehicle collision. CT (**A**) was performed immediately upon arrival to the emergency department, demonstrating nonperfusion of the right kidney with a perirenal hematoma. There is an abrupt occlusion of the right main renal artery with surrounding hematoma. The patient also had a hepatic laceration (not shown). Abdominal aortogram (**B**) demonstrates abrupt cutoff of the main renal artery with non-perfusion of the right kidney. After the occlusion was carefully traversed with a guide wire, advancement of the catheter into the renal artery (**C**) revealed avulsion of the artery with free extravasation of contrast material and no filling of the distal renal artery. Therefore, the renal artery was coil embolized (**D**).

Alternatively, direct injection of thrombogenic material can be performed via an ultrasound-guided percutaneous approach. This could be performed if the bleeding vessel cannot be accessed with a microcatheter. In a series of 14 patients, direct

percutaneous embolization of traumatic pseudoaneurysms with gelatin sponge was successful in 13 patients.[34]

In the cases of traumatic injury to the main renal artery, various approaches can be used (FIGURE 75.5). Again, abdominal

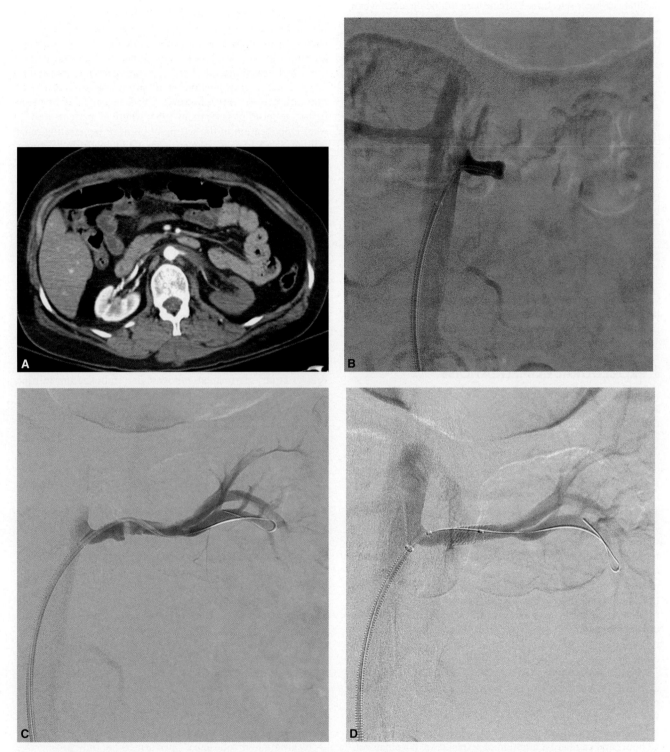

FIGURE 75.5 A 48-year-old woman who jumped in front of a moving automobile. She sustained multiple pelvic fractures. CT (**A**) was performed immediately upon arrival to the emergency department, demonstrating nonperfusion of the left renal artery and kidney. Angiography was performed 90 minutes after the trauma, showing complete occlusion of the left main renal artery with selective catheterization (**B**). After the renal artery was successfully traversed with a 0.014-inch wire (**C**), a balloon-expandable stent was deployed across the site of injury (**D**) with adequate flow to the renal parenchyma.

Courtesy of Marouane Bouchareb, MD, Austin Radiological Association.

aortography allows for assessment of renal artery location to facilitate catheter selection. Extreme care should be taken when selecting the renal artery with a diagnostic catheter so as not to cause further injury or vasospasm. In the case of a renal artery dissection, attempts should be made to cross the dissection with a wire. Low-profile systems with 0.014-inch wires (often with a 3 French microcatheter) are often used because they are less traumatic. Once the artery is traversed, a 6 French sheath (e.g., Ansel curved sheath) can be advanced to the ostia of the renal artery using a 4 or 5 French catheter as inner support. Once the diagnostic catheter is removed, angiography through the sheath can be performed to plan for potential stent placement. Balloon-expandable stents (e.g., Palmaz Blue, Formula) are a viable option in this setting because of their high radial force and precise deployment.[35] Polytetrafluoroethylene (PTFE)-covered balloon-expandable stents (e.g., Atrium iCast) can be considered for focal main renal artery lacerations as well.

Contraindications

There are no absolute contraindications to renal embolization. Caution is advised in patients with renal dysfunction or infection. In patients with single kidneys, attempts should be made to perform selective embolization to avoid complete renal failure.

▌ PROCEDURAL COMPLICATIONS

Potential complications of renal embolotherapy include those at the puncture site, such as hemorrhage or arterial damage. Contrast reaction or contrast-induced nephropathy may occur. Nephropathy secondary to contrast use may be challenging to diagnose because concurrent renal injury is also present. Perhaps of greatest concern is nontarget embolization with material inadvertently distributing to alternate areas of the kidney or to other locations downstream in the aorta. Furthermore, the actual placement of coils may displace the catheter and result in a more central occlusion, producing a larger area of infarction. Coils placed in an undesired location can often be snared with retrieval devices. Additionally, detachable coils (e.g., Guglielmi detachable coil, Trufill, Interlock) can be used if precise placement is a concern. Postembolic hypertension is a rare complication that has been observed after surgical treatment. However, there have been no reported cases in the literature following catheter-directed therapy. Postembolic infection has not been a factor, but application of good sterile technique continues to be essential in any embolization procedure.

After large volume embolization, moderate-severe pain can be expected. This requires aggressive hydration and pain control with narcotics via patient-controlled analgesia if not contraindicated. Postembolization infarction syndrome manifests as pain, leukocytosis, and transient low-grade fever. This often begins within 48 hours and can have a duration of several days. If a small volume of tissue is infarcted, the syndrome is uncommon. Treatment is supportive, consisting of hydration, antipyretics, antiemetics, and narcotics. In the case of complete renal embolization, surgical nephrectomy can be performed when the patient stabilizes.

A delay in diagnosis can also complicate angiography and embolization. Deformity of the kidney by a large intrarenal hematoma can occur with stretching of vessels, which in turn may prevent subselection and necessitate a more proximal embolization with more tissue loss caused by infarction.

▌ OUTCOMES

The first reported series was in 1973 by Bookstein and Goldstein, where three cases of post-biopsy AVF were successfully embolized.[36] In most reported larger series, embolization was successful in most cases. Since then, numerous series have been published describing the success of transarterial embolization (Table 75.2). Authors' definition of "clinical success" varied significantly between series, however. Uflacker et al.[37] described the first large series of patients in 1984, where 17 patients underwent embolization in the setting of blunt or penetrating renal trauma. Size 5 French catheters were used to perform gelatin or steel coil embolization of AVFs, pseudoaneurysms, and arteries with active contrast extravasation. They achieved an 82% clinical success rate.

In 1991, Corr and Hacking[38] reported the largest series of embolization in 40 patients with traumatic AVF or pseudoaneurysms. Size 5 or 7 French catheters were used for vessel selection. Gelatin sponge pledgets were used for the smaller lesions, whereas steel coils were used for the larger ones. Technical success was obtained in 88%. However, 90% demonstrated some degree of parenchymal infarction, including 33% of cases with greater than 50% parenchymal infarction. At that time, microcatheters were not in routine use, which could have allowed for superselective catheterization, reducing the degree of parenchymal infarction.

Although most grade V lesions are treated surgically, Brewer et al.[25] performed endovascular embolization in nine hemodynamically unstable patients with grade V renal trauma. All patients had injuries in addition to renal trauma. Four of the nine patients had injury to the main renal artery, whereas the remainder had injury to the renal parenchyma. Of the nine patients, seven underwent complete embolization of the main renal artery and two patients underwent selective embolization. Gelatin or coils were used for embolization. The operators obtained both clinical and technical success in all cases with no patients requiring further intervention, including surgery. At the time of long-term follow-up (mean 32 months) there were no cases of renal failure.[26] Only one patient had hypertension, and the degree was mild and could not be definitively attributed to the patient's renal trauma. In contrast, Breyer et al.[39] had no success in treating five patients with a grade V injury.

Embolization of vascular injuries in renal transplants has also been reported.[40,41] In a retrospective series of 21 patients with vascular complications after renal transplant biopsy, technical success was achieved in 95% of the patients and clinical success in 88%.[41] One patient eventually required a transplant nephrectomy due to persistent labile hypertension and progressively declining renal function. In another retrospective series of 13 patients,[42] both technical and clinical successes were achieved in 100% of the patients. Microcoils were used in all cases with the addition of glue in a single case.

Hagiwara and colleagues[43] performed the only prospective study evaluating angiography with embolization in this setting. The authors instituted a protocol where all hemodynamically stable patients with grades III to V lesions underwent angiography within 3 hours of their diagnostic CT. Embolization was performed if contrast extravasation or an AVF was identified. Endovascular treatment was not performed for main renal artery or vein injury. In 21 patients, angiography was performed. Of those, eight demonstrated contrast extravasation or AVF and these were all successfully embolized. One of the 21 patients

Table 75.2

Published Series on Catheter-Directed Treatment for Traumatic Renal Injury

Lead author, year	N	Type of injury	Angiographic findings	Embolic material	Clinical success (%)
Uflacker, 1984[37]	17	Blunt and penetrating trauma	AVF, PSA, contrast extravasation	Gelatin, coils	82
Fisher, 1989[33]	15	Stab wound (8), biopsy (4), nephrolithotomy (2), nephrostomy (1)	AVF, PSA, contrast extravasation	Gelatin, coils	100
Corr, 1991[38]	40	Stab wound (23), blunt trauma (9), biopsy (7), other (1)	AVF, PSA	Gelatin, coils, glue, alcohol, occluding balloon	87.5
Eastham, 1992[47]	16	Stab wound	AVF, PSA	Gelatin, coils	81
Heyns, 1992[48]	11	Stab wound	AVF, PSA	Gelatin, coils	82
Beaujeux, 1995[32]	6	Biopsy (1), nephrolithotomy (1), ruptured AVM (1), nephrostomy (2), AML (1)	AVF, PSA, arteriocalyceal fistula	Coils, glue	100
Dorffner, 1998[40]	7	Renal transplant biopsy	AVF, PSA, arteriocalyceal fistula	Coils, glue, gelatin, PVA	71
Perini, 1998[41]	21	Renal transplant biopsy	AVF, PSA	Coils, gelatin	88
Hagiwara, 2001[43]	21	Blunt trauma: grade III (4), grade IV (10), grade V (7)	AVF, contrast extravasation	NA	100
Dinkel, 2002[49]	9	Blunt trauma: grade III (5), grade IV (1), grade V (3)	AVF, PSA, contrast extravasation	Coils, PVA	100
Maleux, 2003[42]	13	Renal transplant biopsy	AVF, PSA, contrast extravasation	Coils, glue	100
Chatziioannou, 2004[50]	6	Blunt trauma (2), nephrolithotomy (2), partial nephrectomy (1), AML (1)	AVF, PSA, contrast extravasation	Coils	100
Vignali, 2004[51]	15	Nephrolithotomy (8), nephrostomy (4), endopyelotomy (2), biopsy (1)	AVF, PSA hematoma	Coils, gelatin, homologous blood clot	100
Sofocleous, 2005[52]	22	Blunt trauma (12) and penetrating trauma (10)	AVF, PSA, arteriocalyceal fistula, contrast extravasation, pedicle rupture	Coils, gelatin, PVA	82
Breyer, 2008[39]	26	Blunt trauma (10), penetrating trauma (6), iatrogenic (6), renal mass (4)	NA	Coils, gelfoam, PVA, stent	65; success in 0/5 in grade V lesions
Brewer, 2009[25]	9	Grade V renal injury caused by blunt trauma	Renal artery occlusion, shattered kidney	Coils, gelatin slurry	100
Sakr, 2009[34]	14	Penetrating trauma (5), renal biopsy (2), nephrolithotripsy (7)	PSA	Direct percutaneous gelatin injection	93

AVF, arteriovenous fistula; PSA, pseudoaneurysm; AVM, arteriovenous malformation; AML, angiomyolipoma; PVA, polyvinyl alcohol; NA, not available.

required laparotomy with nephrectomy after angiography due to avulsion of the renal vein. Two of the 21 patients died secondary to multitrauma and multiorgan failure. Overall, the authors were able to avoid exploratory laparotomy in greater than 90% of the patients.

Renal artery stent placement in the setting of renal artery injury in trauma was initially described in 1995 by Whigham.[35] The authors used a Palmaz balloon-expandable stent to treat an intimal tear in the renal artery. Other reports have had similar success with Palmaz balloon-expandable stents.[44,45] In both cases, distal flow was maintained after stent placement, and perfusion defects in the renal parenchyma were not present. Self-expanding wallstents have also been used with success.[46]

■ THE FUTURE

Because the trend over the last decade has been to take a more conservative approach toward patients with renal trauma, angiography with embolization may play a larger role to avoid surgical intervention. Additionally, endovascular restoration of the renal artery in renovascular trauma may be considered more. With the arrival of more precise embolics and interventional radiologists' increasing use and comfort level, embolization may prove to be more effective with even greater sparing of normal renal parenchyma.

■ CONCLUSION

Most renal traumas are managed conservatively without any interventions. In severe cases (grade V), most patients are intervened surgically, often with nephrectomy. In the remainder of cases, catheter-based therapy can play a significant role in treating hemorrhage and stabilizing patients. Its increasing use, increasing amount of evidence, and the more conservative approach taken toward kidney trauma will result in a greater role for the interventional radiologist in this setting. In the rare cases of renal artery injury, catheter-directed therapy can play a significant role if intervention can be performed in a timely manner.

■ REFERENCES

1. Wessells H, Suh D, Porter JR, et al. Renal injury and operative management in the United States: results of a population-based study. *J Trauma* 2003;54(3):423–430.
2. Herschorn S, Radomski SB, Shoskes DA, et al. Evaluation and treatment of blunt renal trauma. *J Urol* 1991;146(2):274–276; discussion 6–7.
3. Wessells H, McAninch JW, Meyer A, et al. Criteria for nonoperative treatment of significant penetrating renal lacerations. *J Urol* 1997;157(1):24–27.
4. Sangthong B, Demetriades D, Martin M, et al. Management and hospital outcomes of blunt renal artery injuries: analysis of 517 patients from the National Trauma Data Bank. *J Am Coll Surg* 2006;203(5):612–617.
5. Carroll PR, McAninch JW, Klosterman P, et al. Renovascular trauma: risk assessment, surgical management, and outcome. *J Trauma* 1990;30(5):547–552; discussion 53–54.
6. Cass AS, Bubrick M, Luxenberg M, et al. Renal pedicle injury in patients with multiple injuries. *J Trauma* 1985;25(9):892–896.
7. Plainfosse MC, Calonge VM, Beyloune-Mainardi C, et al. Vascular complications in the adult kidney transplant recipient. *J Clin Ultrasound* 1992;20(8):517–527.
8. Cass AS, Vieira J. Comparison of IVP and CT findings in patients with suspected severe renal injury. *Urology* 1987;29(5):484–487.
9. McGahan JP, Richards JR, Jones CD, et al. Use of ultrasonography in the patient with acute renal trauma. *J Ultrasound Med* 1999;18(3):207–213; quiz 15–16.
10. Perry MJ, Porte ME, Urwin GH. Limitations of ultrasound evaluation in acute closed renal trauma. *J R Coll Surg Edinb* 1997;42(6):420–422.
11. Bretan PN, McAninch JW, Federle MP, et al. Computerized tomographic staging of renal trauma: 85 consecutive cases. *J Urol* 1986;136(3):561–565.
12. McAninch JW, Federle MP. Evaluation of renal injuries with computerized tomography. *J Urol* 1982;128(3):456–460.
13. Goldman SM, Sandler CM. Urogenital trauma: imaging upper GU trauma. *Eur J Radiol* 2004;50(1):84–95.
14. Alonso RC, Nacenta SB, Martinez PD, et al. Kidney in danger: CT findings of blunt and penetrating renal trauma. *Radiographics* 2009;29(7):2033–2053.
15. Moore EE, Shackford SR, Pachter HL, et al. Organ injury scaling: spleen, liver, and kidney. *J Trauma* 1989;29(12):1664–1666.
16. Kuo RL, Eachempati SR, Makhuli MJ, et al. Factors affecting management and outcome in blunt renal injury. *World J Surg* 2002;26(4):416–419.
17. Carpio F, Morey AF. Radiographic staging of renal injuries. *World J Urol* 1999;17(2):66–70.
18. Wright JL, Nathens AB, Rivara FP, et al. Renal and extrarenal predictors of nephrectomy from the national trauma data bank. *J Urol* 2006;175(3, pt 1):970–975; discussion 5.
19. Armenakas NA, Duckett CP, McAninch JW. Indications for nonoperative management of renal stab wounds. *J Urol* 1999;161(3):768–771.
20. Broghammer JA, Fisher MB, Santucci RA. Conservative management of renal trauma: a review. *Urology* 2007;70(4):623–629.
21. Matthews LA, Smith EM, Spirnak JP. Nonoperative treatment of major blunt renal lacerations with urinary extravasation. *J Urol* 1997;157(6):2056–2058.
22. Nuss GR, Morey AF, Jenkins AC, et al. Radiographic predictors of need for angiographic embolization after traumatic renal injury. *J Trauma* 2009;67(3):578–582; discussion 82.
23. Santucci RA, McAninch JW, Safir M, et al. Validation of the American Association for the Surgery of Trauma organ injury severity scale for the kidney. *J Trauma* 2001;50(2):195–200.
24. Dugi DD, Morey AF, Gupta A, et al. American Association for the Surgery of Trauma grade 4 renal injury substratification into grades 4a (low risk) and 4b (high risk). *J Urol* 2010;183(2):592–597.
25. Brewer ME, Strnad BT, Daley BJ, et al. Percutaneous embolization for the management of grade 5 renal trauma in hemodynamically unstable patients: initial experience. *J Urol* 2009;181(4):1737–1741.
26. Stewart AF, Brewer ME, Daley BJ, et al. Intermediate-term follow-up of patients treated with percutaneous embolization for grade 5 blunt renal trauma. *J Trauma* 2010;69(2):468–470.
27. Bruce LM, Croce MA, Santaniello JM, et al. Blunt renal artery injury: incidence, diagnosis, and management. *Am Surg* 2001;67(6):550–554; discussion 5–6.
28. Culp DA. Renal arterial block. *Surg Gynecol Obstet* 1969;129(1):114–115.
29. Knudson MM, Harrison PB, Hoyt DB, et al. Outcome after major renovascular injuries: a Western trauma association multicenter report. *J Trauma* 2000;49(6):1116–1122.
30. Brown MF, Graham JM, Mattox KL, et al. Renovascular trauma. *Am J Surg* 1980;140(6):802–805.
31. Wilson RF, Ziegler DW. Diagnostic and treatment problems in renal injuries. *Am Surg* 1987;53(7):399–402.
32. Beaujeux R, Saussine C, al-Fakir A, et al. Superselective endo-vascular treatment of renal vascular lesions. *J Urol* 1995;153(1):14–17.
33. Fisher RG, Ben-Menachem Y, Whigham C. Stab wounds of the renal artery branches: angiographic diagnosis and treatment by embolization. *AJR Am J Roentgenol* 1989;152(6):1231–1235.
34. Sakr MA, Desouki SE, Hegab SE. Direct percutaneous embolization of renal pseudoaneurysm. *J Endourol* 2009;23(6):875–878.
35. Whigham CJ, Bodenhamer JR, Miller JK. Use of the Palmaz stent in primary treatment of renal artery intimal injury secondary to blunt trauma. *J Vasc Interv Radiol* 1995;6(2):175–178.
36. Bookstein JJ, Goldstein HM. Successful management of postbiopsy arteriovenous fistula with selective arterial embolization. *Radiology* 1973;109(3):535–536.
37. Uflacker R, Paolini RM, Lima S. Management of traumatic hematuria by selective renal artery embolization. *J Urol* 1984;132(4):662–667.
38. Corr P, Hacking G. Embolization in traumatic intrarenal vascular injuries. *Clin Radiol* 1991;43(4):262–264.
39. Breyer BN, McAninch JW, Elliott SP, et al. Minimally invasive endovascular techniques to treat acute renal hemorrhage. *J Urol* 2008;179(6):2248–2252; discussion 53.
40. Dorffner R, Thurnher S, Prokesch R, et al. Embolization of iatrogenic vascular injuries of renal transplants: immediate and follow-up results. *Cardiovasc Intervent Radiol* 1998;21(2):129–134.

41. Perini S, Gordon RL, LaBerge JM, et al. Transcatheter embolization of biopsy-related vascular injury in the transplant kidney: immediate and long-term outcome. *J Vasc Interv Radiol* 1998;9(6):1011–1019.
42. Maleux G, Messiaen T, Stockx L, et al. Transcatheter embolization of biopsy-related vascular injuries in renal allografts. Long-term technical, clinical and biochemical results. *Acta Radiol* 2003;44(1):13–17.
43. Hagiwara A, Sakaki S, Goto H, et al. The role of interventional radiology in the management of blunt renal injury: a practical protocol. *J Trauma* 2001; 51(3):526–531.
44. Goodman DN, Saibil EA, Kodama RT. Traumatic intimal tear of the renal artery treated by insertion of a Palmaz stent. *Cardiovasc Intervent Radiol* 1998;21(1):69–72.
45. Paul JL, Otal P, Perreault P, et al. Treatment of posttraumatic dissection of the renal artery with endoprosthesis in a 15-year-old girl. *J Trauma* 1999; 47(1):169–172.
46. Villas PA, Cohen G, Putnam SG, et al. Wallstent placement in a renal artery after blunt abdominal trauma. *J Trauma* 1999;46(6):1137–1139.
47. Eastham JA, Wilson TG, Larsen DW, et al. Angiographic embolization of renal stab wounds. *J Urol* 1992;148(2, pt 1):268–270.
48. Heyns CF, van Vollenhoven P. Increasing role of angiography and segmental artery embolization in the management of renal stab wounds. *J Urol* 1992;147(5):1231–1234.
49. Dinkel HP, Danuser H, Triller J. Blunt renal trauma: minimally invasive management with microcatheter embolization experience in nine patients. *Radiology* 2002;223(3):723–730.
50. Chatziioannou A, Brountzos E, Primetis E, et al. Effects of superselective embolization for renal vascular injuries on renal parenchyma and function. *Eur J Vasc Endovasc Surg* 2004;28(2):201–206.
51. Vignali C, Lonzi S, Bargellini I, et al. Vascular injuries after percutaneous renal procedures: treatment by transcatheter embolization. *Eur Radiol* 2004;14(4):723–729.
52. Sofocleous CT, Hinrichs C, Hubbi B, et al. Angiographic findings and embolotherapy in renal arterial trauma. *Cardiovasc Intervent Radiol* 2005; 28(1):39–47.

Nasopharyngeal Hemorrhage

RICARDO D. GARCIA-MONACO

INTRODUCTION

The most common clinical presentation of nasopharyngeal hemorrhage is epistaxis. This type of bleeding is rather common, benign, and self-limiting in most cases. Up to 60% of the population experiences at least one episode of nasal bleeding, but only 6% require medical care.[1]

Epistaxis has been classified as anterior or posterior depending on the bleeding site. Anterior epistaxis is the most common type and is located at the conjunction of the anterior septum vessels, an area known as Kiesselbach plexus. This location is readily accessible and treatable with simple measures, such as manual compression, anterior nasal packing, or cautery. The prognosis is excellent and usually does not require any further treatment.

Posterior epistaxis occurs in 5% of patients with nasopharyngeal bleeding and usually originates in the posterior branches of the sphenopalatine artery (SPA), although some other vessels may also be involved. Because it is located in a relatively inaccessible region, treatment is not so simple and usually requires posterior nasal packing and hospitalization.[2] Failure to stop the bleeding despite correct medical treatment or early recurrence after nasal packing removal is rather common, and this condition is defined as intractable epistaxis. In such a situation, occlusion of the arteries supplying the posterior nasal fossa is necessary to stop the bleeding; therapy could be performed either by surgery or by endovascular embolization.[3–5]

Embolization for intractable posterior epistaxis was first described by Sokoloff et al.[6] in 1974 and was later refined by Lasjaunias et al.[7] in 1979, whose therapeutic protocol has remained so far almost unchanged. Although still controversial in some institutions, embolization has gained increased acceptance and large series with excellent results have been reported.[8–10]

PATIENT SELECTION

Epistaxis affects males and females in similar frequency. Although it may occur at any age, there is a mild peak of onset before 20 years of age and a more remarkable age-related increase after 40 years of age.[11] The latter increase may reflect the prominence of vascular disease, hypertension, iatrogenic and pathologic bleeding, and falls as a cause of trauma.[12]

Regarding the etiology of posterior epistaxis, multiple causes have been reported in different pathologic entities. In many cases, the cause of bleeding cannot be determined—so-called idiopathic epistaxis—but hypertension, heavy smoking, alcohol consumption, and hypercholesteremia have been described as associated factors.[3] Most patients with idiopathic posterior epistaxis are relatively healthy individuals with a sudden onset of posterior nasal bleeding in which imaging modalities, including angiography, are usually regarded as normal.

In other circumstances, there is a well-recognized etiology of nasopharyngeal bleeding that may be diagnosed by proper anamnesis, clinical examination, or imaging modalities: vascular malformations, trauma, hypervascular tumors, and systemic coagulopathy are among the most common.

Indeed, severe and recurrent epistaxis is a common symptom in patients with hemorrhagic hereditary telangiectasia (HHT) where multiple telangiectasias in the nasal mucosa are the source of bleeding.[13] Diagnosis is easy in patients with a family history of bleeding (epistaxis, gastrointestinal, etc.) and presence of mucocutaneous telangiectasias in the tongue, ears, fingers, or toes. Other vascular malformations causing epistaxis are less common but aneurysms, arteriovenous, or venous malformations should be considered.[3,4,14]

Blunt or penetrating trauma is another cause of posterior epistaxis, usually secondary to facial or skull base injuries or otherwise to iatrogenic procedures, such as maxillofacial or transsphenoidal surgery.[4,15,16]

Hypervascular nasopharyngeal tumors, such as juvenile angiofibroma, angiomatous polyp, or hypervascular primary or metastatic cancer may also induce severe posterior epistaxis.[3,4,7]

Whatever the etiology, posterior epistaxis should be initially treated with posterior nasal packing and hospitalization to achieve hemodynamic and medical stabilization while enabling medical workup. It should be noted that packing is painful and stressful for the patient and its prolonged use may be complicated by infection, alar necrosis, aspiration, and respiratory disorders.[17] Indeed, complication rates up to 20% to 60% have been reported in the literature and, therefore, early removal (48 hours) is recommended to prevent complications.[3,18] Additionally, failure of posterior nasal packing to control posterior epistaxis was reported as high as 50%.[12,18]

Persistent epistaxis despite nasal packing or recurrence of bleeding after packing removal—as a consequence of complications or due time—needs an alternative treatment and is the main indication for arterial occlusion of the nasopharyngeal vascular supply.

VASCULAR ANATOMY OF THE NASOPHARYNGEAL REGION

Knowledge of the functional vascular anatomy of the nasopharyngeal region and understanding of its variations improve the reliability and safety of embolization. Indeed, the main danger in head and neck embolization lies in lack of familiarity with the anatomic vascular arrangement in a given patient. The transosseous arteries at the base of the skull that communicate the extra-intracranial circulation are of utmost concern and therefore should be clearly recognized by the interventional radiologist.

The blood supply to the nasopharyngeal region is complex (FIGURE 76.1) and it derives from both the external (ECA) and the internal carotid arteries (ICA).[7,19] The SPA is the dominant vessel and is responsible for posterior epistaxis in most clinical situations. It originates from the pterygopalatine segment of the internal maxillary artery (IMA) and exits the pterygopalatine fossa via the sphenopalatine foramen to enter the nasal cavity behind and above the middle concha (FIGURE 76.2). It ramifies into two major groups, the medial branches that supply the nasal septum and the lateral branches that supply the turbinates and the paranasal sinuses.

The anterior (AEA) and posterior ethmoidal (PEA) arteries, which branch off the intraorbital segment of the ophthalmic artery (OphA), supply the roof of the nasal cavity and anastomoses with the SPA (FIGURE 76.3). The ethmoidal arteries may be the primary source of epistaxis or otherwise bleeding recurrence because of anastomotic reconstitution of the SPA caused by proximal arterial therapeutic occlusion.

The ascending palatine artery (APA) and descending palatine artery (DPA), usually branches of the facial artery (FA) and IMA, supply the floor of the nasal cavity and are more commonly involved in epistaxis secondary to hypervascular nasopharyngeal tumors.

The superior labial artery (SLA), a distal branch of the FA, gives off the alar branch and the anterior septum branch. These arteries are not commonly a main source of severe epistaxis but may be involved in some type of vascular malformations or act as collateral pathways to reconstitute the SPA after surgical or endovascular proximal occlusion.

The anterior branches of the ascending pharyngeal artery (APhA) supply the nasopharynx but are usually not involved in the origin of epistaxis except in the case of hypervascular nasopharyngeal tumors or traumatic lesions.

The ICA does not supply the nasal cavity directly but gives off a transcranial branch—the mandibular artery—which supplies the lymphatic tissue in the vicinity of the Rosenmuller foramen and may be involved in the vascular supply of nasopharyngeal hypervascular tumors.[19,20] In some uncommon but life-threatening clinical situations the cavernous, petrous, or cervical segments of the ICA could be the direct source of nasopharyngeal hemorrhage, especially in patients with skull base trauma.[4,16]

Additional possible vascular supply to the nasopharyngeal region is by collateral circulation through transmedian anastomoses of the SPA, accessory meningeal arteries, and transcranial vessels, especially after proximal arterial ligations reconstituting blood supply to the mucoperiosteum.[3,19]

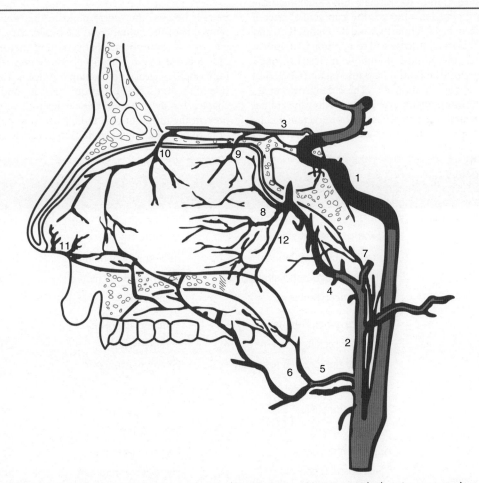

FIGURE 76.1 Schematic drawing of arterial nasal supply (modified from Willems et al (12) with permission).

1, internal carotid artery; 2, external carotid artery; 3, ophthalmic artery; 4, internal maxillary artery; 5, facial artery; 6, ascending palatine artery; 7, ascending pharyngeal artery; 8, sphenopalatine artery; 9, posterior ethmoidal artery; 10, anterior ethmoidal artery; 11, superior labial artery; 12, descending palatine artery.

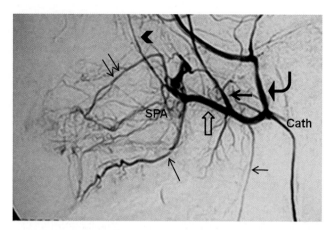

FIGURE 76.2 Angiography of the internal maxillary artery (*open arrow*) and its branches: middle meningeal artery (*curve arrow*), accessory meningeal artery (*large arrow*), descending palatine artery (*arrow*), infraorbital artery (*double arrow*), inferior alveolar artery (*short arrow*), anterior deep temporal artery (*arrowhead*).

SPA, sphenopalatine artery; *Cath*, 4 French catheter.

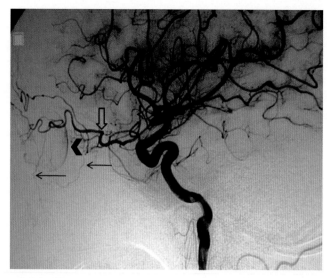

FIGURE 76.3 Angiography of the internal carotid artery (lateral view) shows the ophthalmic artery (*open arrow*) as well as the anterior and posterior ethmoidal arteries (*arrows*). Notice the choroidal blush (*arrowhead*).

A special consideration to the vascular functional anatomy of the nasopharyngeal region addresses the transcranial arterial anastomoses between the ECA branches and the OphA, ICA, and vertebral artery (VA). Its knowledge and recognition is of utmost importance because the passage of embolic material through these vessels may reach the central nervous system (CNS) and lead to catastrophic complications.[12,21] These dangerous anastomoses are usually low flow tiny arteries that follow the cranial nerves along the neural foramen. These extra-intracranial connections, although not always seen at angiography, are always present because they correspond to the vascular embryologic remnants of the neural crest.[19] As such, they may occasionally give rise to anatomic arterial variations that the interventional radiologist needs to recognize because they represent a hazard for nasopharyngeal embolization.[19] A detailed anatomic description of the transcranial anastomoses is beyond the scope of this chapter, but awareness of these dangerous vessels is essential to prevent the interventional radiologist from potential complications of nasopharyngeal embolization (Table 76.1).

Table 76.1			
Dangerous Transcranial Anastomosis			
ECA trunk	**Specific dangerous branch**	**Specific course**	**Intracraneal anastomosis**
	Infraorbital (orbital branch)	Inferior orbital fissure	
	MMA (meningo-ophthalmic)	Superior orbital fissure	Ophtalmic artery
	Anterior deep temporal	Transmalar	
Internal maxillary	MMA (cavernous ramus)	Foramen spinosum	
	Accessory meningeal	Foramen ovale	Cavernous ICA
	Artery of the foramen rotundum	Foramen rotundum	
	MMA (petrosal branch)	Petrosal canal	
	Anterior tympanic	Anterior tympanic canal	Intrapetrous ICA
	Vidian artery	Vidian canal	
Ascending pharyngeal	Superior pharyngeal	Foramen lacerum	Cavernous ICA
	Hypoglossal (odontoid arterial arch)	Hypoglossal foramen	Vertebral artery
		III cervical space	
	Musculospinal artery	III, IV cervical spaces	

ECA, external carotid artery; MMA, middle meningeal artery; ICA, internal carotid artery.

The IMA has dangerous anastomoses with the OphA as well as the ICA in both its cavernous and petrous segments. The meningo-OphA that courses the superior orbital fissure, the infraorbital artery that courses the inferior orbital fissure, and the anterior deep temporal artery that has a transmalar course connect the IMA with the OphA and, therefore, may potentially supply the retinal artery. In few occasions, these vessels may represent an anatomic variation, giving the main vascular supply to the OphA through the ECA instead of the ICA.

The artery of the foramen rotundum that runs the homonymous foramen connects the cavernous ICA through the infero-lateral trunk or clival arteries (FIGURE 76.4). The cavernous ramus of both the middle meningeal artery (MMA) and the accessory meningeal artery, branches arising from the IMA, connect the ICA siphon through the foramen spinosum and the foramen ovale, respectively. Other IMA transcranial anastomoses with the ICA, but in the petrous segment, are the petrosal branch of the MMA, the vidian artery (anastomoses the mandibular artery), and the anterior tympanic that run through the petrosal canal, the vidian canal, and the anterior tympanic canal.

The APhA has dangerous anastomoses with both the ICA and VA (FIGURE 76.5). The superior pharyngeal branch, usually supplying hypervascular nasopharyngeal tumors, is an anterior branch of the APhA that connects to the ICA through the cavernous artery that runs in the foramen lacerum. The anastomoses with the VA arise from the posterior or neuromeningeal trunk of the APhA, through the hypoglossal and cervical nerves arteries, but the posterior trunk is usually not approached in nasopharyngeal bleeding embolization.

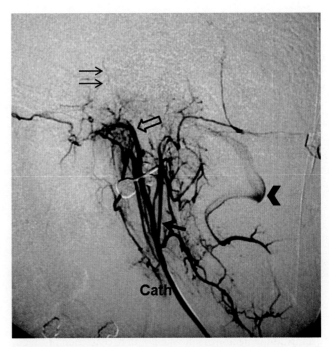

FIGURE 76.5 Angiography of the ascending pharyngeal artery with an enlarged superior pharyngeal artery (*open arrow*) showing the cavernous ramus (*double arrows*) that anastomoses to the internal carotid artery and the neuromeningeal trunk (*arrow*) with its anastomoses to the vertebral artery (*arrowhead*).

Cath, 4 French catheter.

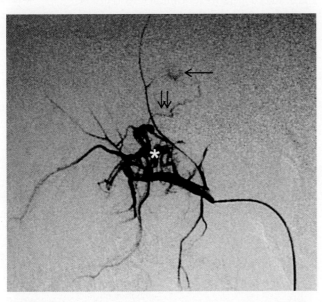

FIGURE 76.4 Angiography of the internal maxillary artery before embolization of a juvenile nasopharyngeal angiofibroma (*asterisk*), shows the artery of the foramen rotundum (*double arrows*) anastomosing the infero-lateral trunk and the internal carotid artery (*arrow*).

TECHNICAL/DEVICE CONSIDERATIONS

The angiography and embolization are performed in the angiographic suite under standard endovascular technique. An ordinary 5 French sheath is needed to gain femoral access as well as a cerebral catheter to approach the ICA and ECA. In young individuals or patients with hypervascular nasopharyngeal lesions, a single diagnostic 4 French catheter could be used for both diagnostic angiography and embolization. Otherwise, a 4 or 5 French catheter with a 0.038-inch lumen may be used for the pretherapeutic angiography and combined with a 3 French microcatheter (00.21- or 00.25-inch lumen) for superselective catheterization of ECA arteries and embolization.

In older patients with a tortuous and elongated brachiocephalic trunk or carotid artery, a Simmons IV-type catheter is sometimes better to gain rapid carotid access.

In cases where the epistaxis is suspected to be secondary to laceration or rupture of the ICA, a 6 or 7 French catheter with a larger lumen is preferred to allow the coaxial insertion of latex detachable balloons or stent-grafts.

The guide wires that are commonly used depend on the catheter scheduled, usually a 0.032-inch hydrophilic for 4 or 5 French catheters and a 0.018 inch for microcatheters.

The embolic material varies depending on the etiology of the epistaxis and the angioarchitecture of a given lesion. The most widely used embolic materials are particulate agents, such as trisacryl microspheres or polyvinyl alcohol (PVA) particles ranging from 150 to 500 μm.[12] Pledgets of gelatin sponge are occasionally used supplementary to particulate embolization or less commonly as a sole agent when there are large and visible transcranial anastomoses at angiography.[22,23]

Platinum coils and gelfoam powder or particles less than 150 μm are not recommended at all.[3,22] The former produce proximal arterial occlusion; therefore, collateral circulation leading to early rebleeding is likely. The latter may embolize too distally with an increased risk of necrosis, cranial palsy, and undesired passage to transcranial anastomoses.

In epistaxis secondary to ICA rupture, detachable latex balloons are usually used to achieve vessel occlusion by a trapping technique, frequently the endovascular treatment of choice.[4,22] In some cases an endoluminal stent-graft may be used to repair the arterial wall while maintaining lumen patency, although it is technically troublesome to approach the intracranial ICA.[12]

TREATMENT SELECTION STRATEGIES

Patients with severe posterior epistaxis usually consult in emergency and are managed by multidisciplinary approach, usually led by the ear, nose, and throat (ENT) department. Clinical care (transfusions, hemodynamic stabilization, correction of coagulation disorders, etc.) and posterior nasal packing with hospitalization are the standard of care in most severe cases. If bleeding stops, the nasal packing is removed 48 hours after placement, and if there is no recurrence the patient is discharged with further medical control as an outpatient.[2,5]

In the case of complication of nasal packing that needs early removal, symptomatic recurrence after packing removal, or continuous bleeding despite the packing, further treatment with arterial occlusion of the bleeding vessels is necessary. In such a case either endoscopic surgery or transarterial embolization is currently the best way to achieve this goal.[5,8–10,12,14] On occasion, and depending on the clinical history or etiology suspicion, a craniofacial computed tomography (CT) or magnetic resonance

imaging (MRI) is performed. The treatment algorithm followed at our institution is summarized in FIGURE 76.6.

Treatment strategy selection depends on many factors, such as type of bleeding, hemodynamic situation of the patient, arterial source, clinical history, as well as medical expertise and/or local preferences. In institutions where skull base endovascular therapy is commonly performed, embolization is usually the preferred treatment because of its multiple advantages.[4,9,10]

A thorough clinical history and a correct physical and/or eventually an imaging evaluation (CT, MR) are recommended to determine the type of nasopharyngeal bleeding—either idiopathic (70% of cases[9,10]) or due to an organic disease—because planning of the interventional procedure may be different.

PLANNING THE INTERVENTIONAL PROCEDURE

As in any other endovascular procedure a complete blood test laboratory, including creatinine serum levels and coagulation tests, should be obtained for proper care and to avoid predictable complications.

The procedure, including angiography and embolization, is performed in the angiographic suite with the nasal packing in place. The patient should be well hydrated by intravenous (IV) infusion and, preferably, general anesthesia is utilized. Although a conscious sedation or local anesthesia may be alternative possibilities, it should be remembered that the nasal packing is uncomfortable and could lead to respiratory insufficiency or aspiration in these anxious patients. General anesthesia ensures a quiet patient, controlled respiration, and decreased vascular spasm (common in ECA catheter manipulation) and also provides a more comfortable task for the interventional radiologist.[3,12,22]

Conscious sedation or local anesthesia is reserved for patients in whom general anesthesia entails high risk or in patients where an ICA occlusion is foreseen. In the latter, patients need to be awake and cooperative for clinical test occlusion.[20,22]

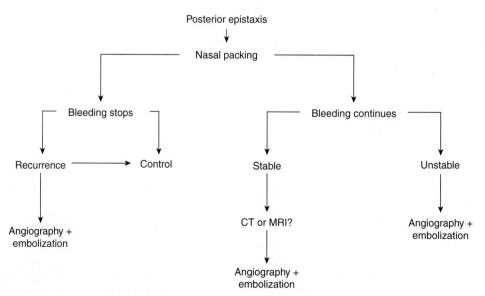

FIGURE 76.6 Algorithm of nasopharyngeal hemorrhage management and indications for angiography and embolization.

Table 76.2	
Angiographic and Embolization Protocol	
Angiography of the ipsilateral ICA	• Verify supply to the OphA and choroidal blush • Rule out ICA source of bleeding • Check for prominent EA • Check for anatomic variants
Angiography and embolization of the ipsilateral IMA	• Rule out ICA visualization or choroidal blush • Check for anatomic variants • Free-flow embolization
Angiogram and embolization of the ipsilateral FA	• Check for nasal mucosa supply • Alar artery • Septum artery • Inferior palatine artery • Free-flow embolization
Repeat same sequence on the contralateral side	
Angiogram and embolization of APhA	• To be considered in special clinical situations (JNA, trauma?)

ICA, internal carotid artery; OphA, ophthalmic artery; EA, ethmoidal artery; IMA, internal maxillary artery; FA, facial artery; APhA, ascending pharyngeal artery; JNA, juvenile nasopharyngeal angiofibroma.
Modified from Lasjaunias P, Marsot-Dupuch J, Doyon D. The radio-anatomical basis of arterial embolization of epistaxis. *J Neuroradiol* 1979;6:45–52.

Diagnostic pretherapeutic angiography and therapeutic embolization are performed not in a random fashion but following a standardized protocol that may vary depending on the clinical suspicion of bleeding site and type of epistaxis. The standardized angiographic and embolization protocol that is employed at our institution for idiopathic epistaxis is widely used and has been previously described.[4,7,12] The angiographic protocol is important to follow, not only to prevent skipping any artery involved with the epistaxis but also to check for visible anastomoses and/or anatomic variants that could jeopardize the safety of the procedure. The angiographic and embolization protocol and its key points are summarized in Table 76.2.

The ipsilateral ICA is catheterized and injected first, not only to rule out a bleeding source but also to check for both the OphA and choroidal blush, for the possibility of a huge AEA or PEA vascular supply to the nasal fossa, as well as for the presence or absence of anatomic variations (FIGURE 76.3).

Then the ipsilateral IMA is catheterized and injected to check the expected anatomy, including the visualization of the SPA as well as the DPA, and to rule out visualization of the ICA or choroidal blush through patent transcranial anastomoses (FIGURE 76.2). Angiography is then followed by free-flow embolization of the SPA, usually the prominent vascular supply to the bleeding mucosa.

The next step is catheterization and injection of the ipsilateral FA to check or rule out important nasal vascular supply (FIGURE 76.7). This may happen occasionally due to reconstitution of distal branches of the SPA through its anastomoses from the alar and anterior septal branches of the SLA. If important nasal vascular supply is present, embolization is immediately performed; if not, some authors do not embolize but others prefer embolization anyway to decrease the risk of early recurrence of epistaxis.[7,8]

The same sequence is then performed on the contralateral side; thus bilateral embolization is planned every time (even if the epistaxis has been proved to be unilateral) to decrease the risk of revascularization and recurrence through the transmedian anastomoses.[4,7,12]

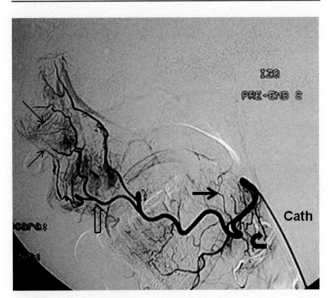

FIGURE 76.7 Angiography of the facial artery and its branches: submandibular artery (*curve arrow*), ascending palatine artery (*large arrow*), superior labial artery (*open arrow*), anterior septum artery (*short thin arrow*), alar artery (*long thin arrow*).

Cath, 4 French catheter.

The nasal packing should be left in place during the whole procedure, and it is usually removed after the embolization or a few hours later by the ENT specialist.[3,4,23]

Although the aforementioned protocol of angiography and embolization is used in most cases of intractable epistaxis, the suspicion or finding of a particular cause or source of bleeding may alter the treatment protocol. Indeed, when the ICA or even other arteries, such as the AphA, APA, and/or DPA, are suspected to be involved, they may need to be catheterized and embolized.[16,20,22] In the next paragraphs we discuss different etiologies of epistaxis, commenting on the angiographic findings and their implications for the planning of the endovascular strategy.

Idiopathic Epistaxis

This is the most common type of intractable epistaxis and usually the angiographic findings are normal. It is not expected, as is the case in other severe hemorrhages (gastrointestinal, splenic, etc.), to see extravasation or active bleeding at angiography. Occasionally, congestion or hyperemia in the nasal mucosa may be identified due to local inflammatory changes and the presence of the nasal packing. The aforementioned protocol of angiography and embolization is recommended to achieve a successful result to stop this type of bleeding.

Hereditary Hemorrhagic Telangiectasia

This entity, also known as Rendu-Osler-Weber disease, is a systemic autosomal dominant hereditary disorder involving vascular abnormalities in various organs.[4,13,24] Epistaxis from telangiectasias of the nasal mucosa is a common manifestation of this disease and can be an extremely difficult management issue for the ENT specialist. This is reflected by the multitude of treatment options available including local or systemic hormonal therapy, local cauterization, topical medications, brachytherapy, bleomycin injection, septal dermoplasty, nasal obturators, and others.[3,12] None of these provide a definitive cure, so the aim of treatment is to reduce the frequency and severity of bleedings as much as possible. Embolization may be indicated in intractable epistaxis, in the need for blood transfusions, or when the bleeding episodes are so frequent that they alter the patient's quality of life considerably.[4,23] It should be noted, however, that recurrence is rather high and repetitive procedures are needed.[25]

Angiography typically shows multiple mucosal telangiectasias, identified as vascular spots in the late arterial and parenchymatous phases (FIGURE 76.8). An extensive embolization with preservation of the proximal vessels for future procedures is recommended because of the high incidence of symptomatic recurrence. For the same reasons, surgical proximal arterial ligations need to be avoided. Early recurrence after embolization may be caused by prominent vascular supply through the ethmoidal arteries, which is rather common in HHT.[25]

Trauma

Massive intractable epistaxis may be a consequence of maxillofacial or skull base trauma. Etiologic diagnosis is easy after blunt or penetrating trauma as well as iatrogenic injuries because of the apparent causal relationship.

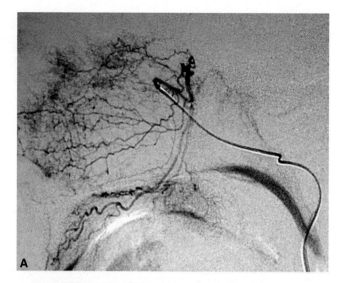

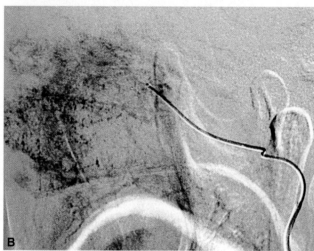

FIGURE 76.8 Pre-embolization angiography of the distal internal maxillary artery in arterial (**A**) and parenchymal phase (**B**) shows multiple telangiectasias in the nasal mucosa and soft palate, typical of Rendu-Osler-Weber disease. The patient was embolized with microspheres and the intractable epistaxis immediately stopped.

The ECA branches may be lacerated in cases of severe blunt maxillofacial trauma with bone fractures. Thus, in trauma, unlike idiopathic epistaxis, angiography may occasionally show a bleeding vessel that can be easily identified because of contrast extravasation (FIGURE 76.9). Arterial dissection, pseudoaneurysms, and arteriovenous fistulas are also possible angiographic findings in severe vascular trauma.[22]

The mechanism of trauma may lead to the suspicion of the injured artery causing the intractable epistaxis: an ICA laceration in the case of skull base trauma or recent transsphenoidal surgery or an AphA injury after complex maxillofacial surgery.[15,16,22] In these cases the endovascular treatment strategy will depend not only on the injured vessel but also on the angioarchitecture of the traumatic lesion.

An ICA source of epistaxis after trauma is uncommon but life threatening; therefore, it should not remain unsuspected in cases of severe skull base blunt trauma. The cavernous segment

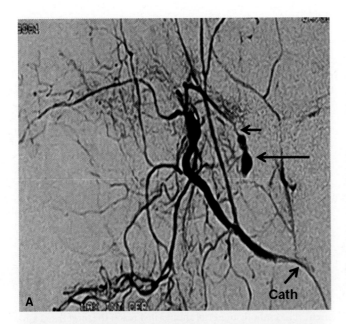

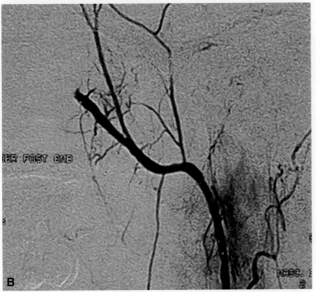

FIGURE 76.9 **A.** Angiography of the internal maxillary artery (IMA) shows nasopharyngeal hemorrhage (*long arrow*) and arterial dissection (*short arrow*) in a patient with blunt maxillofacial trauma. **B.** Control angiography after embolization shows a stump in the distal IMA with no longer signs of bleeding with clinical correlation.

Cath, 3 French microcatheter.

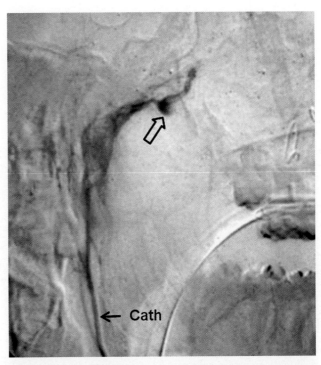

FIGURE 76.10 Angiography of the ascending pharyngeal artery in a young patient with intractable epistaxis after plastic surgery (anterior maxillofacial traction) shows the site of bleeding and a pseudoaneurysm (*open arrow*). Embolization with a gelfoam strip resulted in complete and permanent hemostasis.

Cath, 4 French catheter.

rupture may also occur like in any traumatic event. Although the SPA or ethmoidal artery could be involved in cases of septorhinoplasty, the APhA may be the cause of epistaxis after complex maxillofacial surgery (FIGURE 76.10) or the ICA after transsphenoidal surgery (FIGURE 76.11). The diagnostic and treatment strategy of the ICA source of bleeding is somewhat different from the endovascular treatment of other types of intractable epistaxis and is addressed later in the chapter.

Vascular Malformations

Except in patients with HHT, nasopharyngeal hemorrhage caused by vascular malformations is uncommon. Angiographic findings are related to the type of vascular malformation. If the nidus or the venous drainage of an arteriovenous malformation (AVM) involves the nasopharyngeal region, epistaxis may occur and treatment to the malformation itself needs to be addressed as in any other type of AVM.[4,12,14] Venous malformations may involve the nasopharyngeal region but intractable epistaxis is uncommon, therefore not requiring treatment as a consequence of bleeding.

Aneurysms are rare in the ECA branches but those located at the intracavernous or petrous segment of the ICA may manifest as intractable epistaxis.[12] Progressive sphenous bone weakening and further aneurysmal rupture may lead to severe epistaxis in the former; epistaxis in the latter may be caused by direct communication with the nasopharynx through the eustachian tube.[4,12] Anyway, in most clinical situations there is a history

is more prone to be injured because of the cutting edge of the dura at that location and pseudoaneurysm formation is likely.[4] Epistaxis usually presents in a delayed fashion due to pseudoaneurysm rupture into the sphenous sinus, typically 2 to 3 weeks after trauma.[4,12] ICA injury needs to be suspected in patients recovering from skull base trauma that presents with recurrent episodes of epistaxis, even if it is mild.[4,12,22]

Surgical trauma can also lead to severe epistaxis. The diagnosis is straightforward when the hemorrhage develops shortly after surgery, but delayed epistaxis caused by pseudoaneurysmal

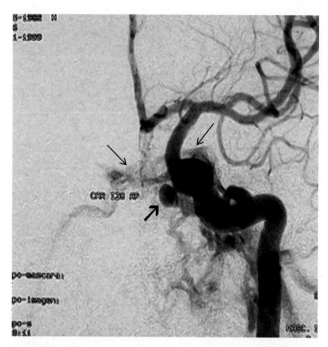

FIGURE 76.11 Angiography of the ICA in Towne position in a patient with intractable epistaxis after transsphenoidal surgery. ICA rupture identified by a pseudoaneurysm (*thick arrow*) and a carotid-cavernous fistula with ipsilateral and contralateral venous drainage (*thin arrows*). Endovascular ICA occlusion with trapping balloon technique was immediately performed and bleeding stopped.

of head injury and diagnosis of a chronic pseudoaneurysm is more likely. Idiopathic aneurysms of the ICA causing nasopharyngeal epistaxis do exist, however, and, although uncommon, are life threatening. The diagnostic and treatment strategy of ICA aneurysms are different from conventional epistaxis of the ECA branches and are addressed later in the chapter.

Nasopharyngeal Tumors

The most common tumor that presents with epistaxis is juvenile nasopharyngeal angiofibroma (JNA). This is a benign tumor but with potential aggressive behavior that occurs almost exclusively in young males around puberty. It is a highly vascular tumor that originates in the sphenopalatine foramen and spreads through the foramina and fissures into the skull base. Angiography typically shows an intense but inhomogeneous tumor blush that appears during the arterial phase and remains until the late venous phase.[4,20] There are no arteriovenous shunts, the draining veins appearing at the venous phase. The feeding vessels depend on the tumor size and extension but usually recruit nasopharyngeal branches of the IMA (SPA, accessory meningeal, DPA), the AphA (pharyngeal anterior trunk), the FA (APA), and even from the ICA if there is intracranial or orbital extension (mandibular, infero-lateral trunk, OphA, etc.). Embolization of the ECA feeding vessels in JNA can be performed to control intractable epistaxis and/or prevent excessive hemorrhage during surgical resection. ICA vessels feeding the JNA are considered too risky to be accessed and embolized for presurgical devascularization procedures and may be controlled during surgery.[2]

A deep description of the endovascular treatment of this tumor is beyond the scope of the chapter, but embolization needs to occlude the intratumoral vessels and not just the supplying feeders (FIGURE 76.12). Indeed, proximal embolization should be avoided to preclude recruitment of intracranial vessels that may reconstitute the vascular tumor supply at the skull base that will make the surgical resection difficult.[20] The angiographic and embolization protocol previously described is relevant but adding the exploration and embolization of the involved APhA branches bilaterally.[4,19]

Other nasopharyngeal tumors that may cause intractable epistaxis or may need presurgical devascularization are hypervascular metastasis or hemangiomas, but these are uncommon in clinical practice.

▌ SPECIFIC INTRAPROCEDURAL TECHNIQUES

Caution when performing catheterization and embolization of the ECA branches is crucial for successful bleeding control and to avoid predictable complications of the endovascular treatment. The embolic material should just reach the target area and not dangerous vessels, such as those that connect with the OphA or ICA. Therefore, special intraprocedural techniques should be kept in mind, especially to maintain normal antegrade arterial flow and to avoid undesired passage of the embolic material to nontarget areas. The particles should be suspended in diluted contrast medium and injected under fluoroscopic control until significant flow reduction is noted in the distal arterial branches. Prior to injection of the embolic material, various hand test injections are recommended with contrast alone to determine the tolerance and/or pressure needed not to fill the anastomoses.[22]

Because free-flow embolization is mandatory when using particles, arterial spasm needs to be avoided. Careful and gentle endovascular navigation with catheters and wires is a must because ECA vessels are very prone to spasm. For this reason some authors recommend the use of microcatheters for superselective catheterization of ECA branches. However, just a 4 French catheter may be used in experienced hands regarded that flow should be overweighed to catheter selectivity.[22,23]

To achieve free-flow embolization, the particles just need to be gently expelled from the distal tip of the catheter during systole and blood flow should carry them to the target arterial branches. A wedge catheter position should therefore be avoided. Indeed, embolization is forbidden in the absence of free flow because the injection pressure may lead the particles to undesired vessels, such as transcranial anastomoses.[26] It is also important when using particles to rotate continuously or to change the syringe position to prevent sedimentation or aggregation of the particles to any part of the syringe, which may result in catheter occlusion or the need for powerful injection of the embolic material.[22]

Another key issue besides free-flow embolization for safe occlusion is avoidance of overembolization. It should be noted that ongoing embolization increases the resistance of the embolized territory and that after significant flow reduction the particles may divert to undesired vessels or dangerous anastomoses.[4,12,22]

Although the SPA gives the main vascular supply to the nasal fossa in idiopathic epistaxis, there is no need to access this artery selectively for embolization. Catheterization of the IMA

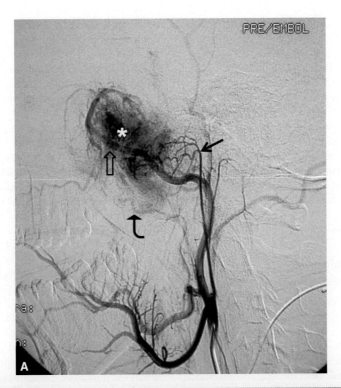

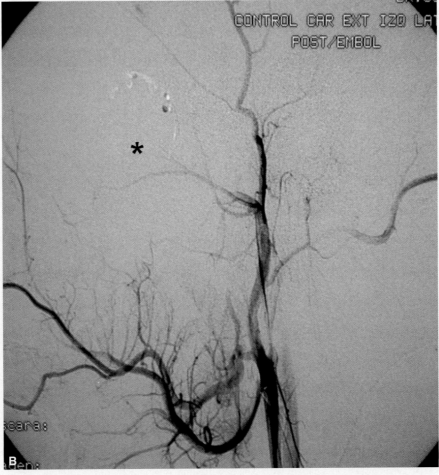

FIGURE 76.12 Angiography of the external carotid artery before (**A**) and after (**B**) embolization from branches of the internal maxillary artery (*open arrow*), ascending pharyngeal artery (*arrow*), and ascending palatine artery (*curve arrow*) supplying a juvenile nasopharyngeal angiofibroma (*asterisk*) shows excellent presurgical tumor devascularization. The patient was operated the following day with complete tumor removal and very little intraoperative blood loss.

followed by free-flow particle embolization is usually enough. The FA is embolized subsequently from its proximal origin with few particles or otherwise with a gelfoam strip because the goal is to avoid collateral circulation through the SLA.[23,26] Then the same procedure is performed on the contralateral side.[4,7]

The visualization of transcranial dangerous anastomoses at pre-embolization angiography precludes the use of small particles.[4,26] In such a case larger particles or gelfoam strips not amenable to pass through the anastomoses should be considered. After embolization, the lumen of the catheter needs to be washed to clear out any remaining embolic agent inside the catheter or otherwise backflushed and rinsed to ensure that it is free of material.[4,22,26] This is of outmost importance when a postembolization angiographic control is performed through the same catheter used for embolization.

Specific Technique Considerations for Internal Carotid Artery Occlusion

Epistaxis from an ICA origin is uncommon but potentially fatal. It must be suspected in cases of repeated epistaxis that become more severe in time, in hemodynamic unstable patients with massive epistaxis, or in the presence of persistent bleeding despite bilateral SPA surgical ligation. ICA source of epistaxis may occur after skull base trauma, complications of transsphenoidal surgery, previous ENT infections all of which have formation of a pseudoaneurysm, or otherwise in healthy individuals as a consequence of a giant intracranial aneurysm.[4,12,16,26]

A selective embolization of the pseudoaneurysm with detachable microcoils keeping the patency of the ICA should not be attempted. It is highly risky because of the fragile nature of the pseudoaneurysmal wall and will probably induce its rupture with recurrent massive bleeding.[4,27] The proper way to stop the bleeding is not to treat the pseudoaneurysm but the ICA itself. The best and faster procedure is to occlude the parent vessel, including the pseudoaneurysm, using a trapping technique with detachable balloons.[4,20] In this way, two balloons are positioned proximal and distal to the pseudoaneurysm or injured ICA wall (FIGURE 76.13). The procedure is preferably performed with the patient awake, so that neurologic condition can be continuously assessed. Before detaching the balloons, a tolerance test, while the ICA is transiently occluded, should be performed both clinically and angiographically. In the case of an angiographically demonstrated adequate brain hemispheric ipsilateral collateral supply, including symmetric venous drainage, and in the absence of any neurologic deficit during the test period, the balloons are detached.[4,22,26] Following the procedure the patient should be closely monitored for at least 12 hours in the intensive care unit. During this time special care is taken to avoid a fall in blood pressure below the systolic level of 100 mm Hg because this may cause ischemia in the occluded cerebral hemisphere.[20]

Endovascular stent-grafts are an alternative treatment to repair the injured ICA while keeping its patency and preventing pseudoaneurysm rupture and early rebleeding.

However, this is technically difficult and troublesome to deploy intracranially, so it is preferably reserved for extracranial ICA cases of epistaxis (FIGURE 76.14).

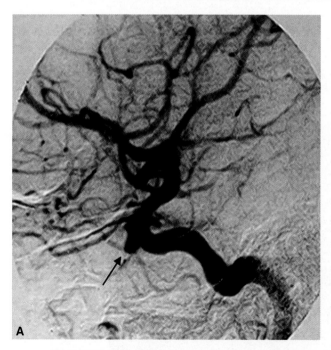
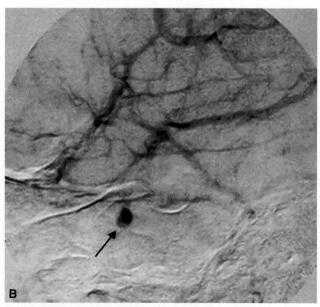

FIGURE 76.13 Delayed epistaxis in a patient with skull base trauma. Angiography of the internal carotid artery (ICA) in arterial (**A**) and venous (**B**) phase shows the pseudoaneurysm (*arrow*). Angiography of the ipsilateral common carotid artery (**C**) and vertebral artery (**D**) postendovascular occlusion of the ICA shows collateral circulation to the brain hemisphere. **E**. Plain skull X-ray shows the occlusion balloons. Epistaxis stopped completely with uneventful follow-up.

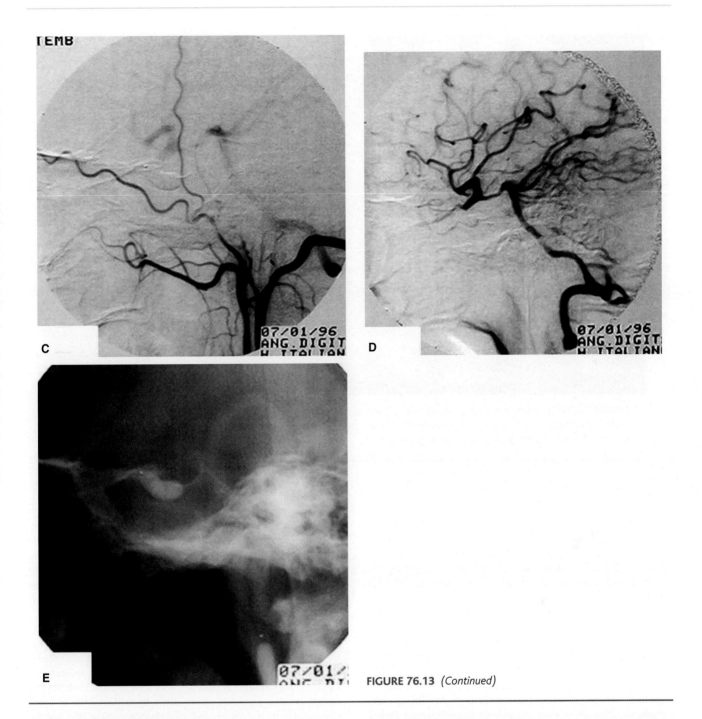

FIGURE 76.13 *(Continued)*

ENDPOINT ASSESSMENT OF THE PROCEDURE

The endpoint of embolization is crucial to achieve a good result while avoiding predictable complications. In the case of idiopathic epistaxis, the endpoint is considered when bilateral significant flow reduction of the nasal branches of the IMA is noticed as well as no visible reconstitution of the nasal arteries through the FA.[3,4,12] It should be noted that in idiopathic cases, differently than in organic epistaxis, there is not a target lesion to check for disappearance after postembolization control angiography. Therefore, an angiographic control of both the ECA and ICA by common carotid artery (CCA) injection is not necessary in idiopathic epistaxis.[4,26]

Prominent AEA and/or PEA at angiography may predict further bleeding. This is more frequent in cases of vascular malformations or in HHT.[25] Although selective catheterization could sometimes be achieved,[28] embolization of these arteries is risky and not recommended. On the contrary, surgical clipping is very easy and considered the treatment of choice to stop bleeding from this source.[29]

PROCEDURAL COMPLICATIONS

The complications of angiography and embolization of nasopharyngeal hemorrhage may be secondary to the arterial access, the use of contrast media, the carotid catheterization, and/or embolization.

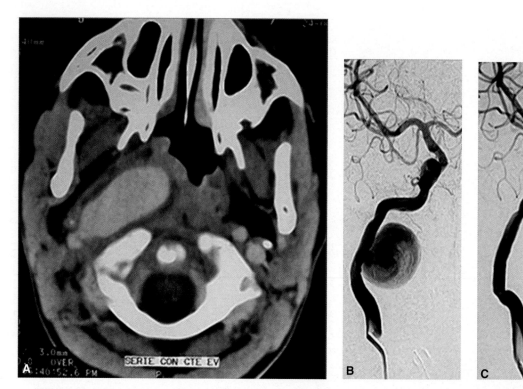

FIGURE 76.14 Epistaxis in a young patient with a cervical internal carotid artery (ICA) pseudoaneurysm secondary to a subacute throat infection that was successfully treated by endovascular stent graft. **A**. CT scan. **B**. ICA angiography. **C**. Control ICA angiography after stent-graft placement.

Groin hematoma and/or other complications at the femoral puncture site are uncommon, but usual precautions are necessary, especially in elderly patients. Contrast media complications may be decreased by proper patient selection, IV hydration, and a correct anamnesis and/or premedication in patients with a history of allergy.

Catheterization of the carotid arteries and their branches needs to be performed by skilled interventionists, and cautious endovascular navigation is a must to avoid arterial dissection, plaque disruption, or any other complication that may lead to brain injury.

In high-risk patients for endovascular navigation, such as elderly patients with severe atheromatosis of the supra-aortic vessels, the hazards of endovascular treatment should be balanced with other alternative therapies, such as nasal endoscopy.

Embolization of the ECA arteries is the main step of endovascular treatment and carries the risks of minor and self-limited complications or otherwise severe major complications, both of which can be prevented with knowledge of the vascular functional anatomy and a proper procedure technique.[19,26]

Minor complications secondary to embolization are possible if the embolic particles reach nontarget areas. Headache, facial pain, jaw pain, or trismus may occur as a consequence of muscular ischemia when the particles reach the distal branches of the middle deep temporal or deep masseteric arteries, both arising from the proximal IMA. Sialadenitis of the submandibular gland after FA embolization with particles has also been reported due to gland ischemia, although this may also happen

as a reaction to contrast media.[12] These symptoms are usually mild, self-limiting, and well controlled with nonsteroidal anti-inflammatory drugs (NSAIDs). However, pre-embolization placement of the microcatheter in the IMA beyond the origin of the aforementioned muscular arteries and in the FA beyond the submandibular branch, respectively, may avoid these minor complications.

Major complications, such as stroke or monocular blindness, are the most frightful but are uncommon in skilled operators (<1%).[4,9,22,26] Indeed, the main hazard of nasopharyngeal embolization is the undesired passage of embolic material to intracranial nontarget vessels that may lead to those catastrophic complications. This may occur either by reflux of the embolic material to the ICA or because of its passage to the ICA and/or OphA through transcranial anastomoses.[4,19,22,26]

Proper catheter position in the ECA branches, correct choice of the embolic material, and cautious embolization technique are deemed necessary to avoid the complications of ICA reflux, which is exceptionally uncommon nowadays.

Thus, the main cause of major complications (blindness and/or stroke) are a result of retinal or CNS embolization as a consequence of intracranial passage of the embolic material through transcranial arterial anastomoses as well as embolization of non-recognized dangerous anatomic variations.[7,19] Blindness may occur as a major complication in cases where the OphA is supplied by branches of the ECA instead of the ICA (FIGURE 76.15). In such an anatomic variation, the choroidal blush is visualized only in the ECA angiography and absent in that of the ICA.

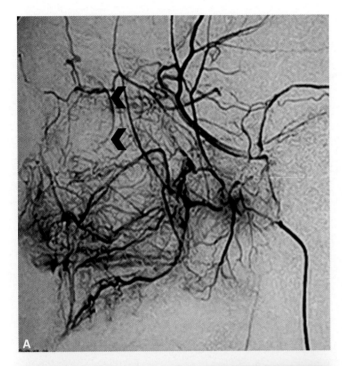

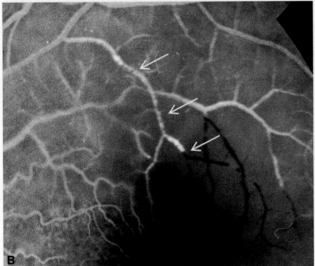

FIGURE 76.15 A. Pre-embolization angiography of the internal maxillary artery in a patient with intractable epistaxis. In the late arterial phase the choroidal blush is clearly seen (*arrowheads*) because of a meningo-ophthalmic anatomic variation. However, this anatomic condition was not recognized by the operator and embolization with particles was performed. **B.** Fluorescein angiography performed the following day because of monocular blindness show a retinal arterial occlusion and microspheres inside the vascular lumen (*arrows*).

This is one of the reasons that ICA and ECA angiography is performed before injecting the embolic particles into the IMA toward the SPA, as discussed previously in procedure planning.[7]

Another possibility of monocular blindness is the inadvertent passage of particles through the transorbital anastomoses that arise from the IMA when performing embolization.[21] The

visualization of transcranial dangerous anastomoses at angiography does not represent a strict contraindication to embolization but precludes the use of small particles.[4,22,26] In such a case, larger particles or gelfoam strips should be considered.[22]

It should be remembered that these anastomoses are embryologic remnants and therefore are always present, even if not visible at angiography.[4] These dangerous anastomoses may open in case of increased pressure during embolization. To avoid this complication, free-flow embolization is mandatory. Embolization should not be performed if there is no antegrade blood flow or if the catheter is in wedge position. It should also be noted that during ongoing embolization, the sump effect of the distal capillary bed is decreased; therefore, overembolization may divert the particles to nontarget vessels, including the transcranial anastomoses.[3,12,22]

Stroke may also occur as a major complication in the case of inadvertent embolization of the ICA through the transcranial anastomoses (FIGURES 76.4 and 76.5). Keeping the rule of free-flow embolization described earlier and avoiding overembolization will prevent this complication in most cases. Because some ECA-ICA anastomoses arise from the MMA and the accessory MMA, an additional safety measure is placement of a microcatheter in the IMA beyond the origin of these arteries.[12] However, in patients with previous carotid stenosis or in some anatomic variants, a prominent artery of the foramen rotundum may supply the ICA.[19] In such a case embolization may be performed from the IMA with large gelfoam strips to avoid ICA passage of the embolic material through the aforementioned anastomoses. Ipsilateral ICA supply should be ensured from other arteries different from the ECA, such as the intracranial collaterals of the circle of Willis.[19,26]

In some unfavorable vascular anatomic arrangements or in high-risk patients not deemed for endovascular procedures, an alternative treatment, such as endoscopic electrocoagulation, may be considered.[12,30] Although this situation is unlikely in operators familiarized with endovascular skull base procedures, it should be kept in mind for less experienced interventional radiologists.

Major complications of nasopharyngeal embolization do not have good functional prognoses despite any available treatment. Therefore, all efforts should not be addressed to manage the major complications but rather to avoid them. A detailed knowledge of the functional vascular anatomy of the ECA—especially the dangerous anastomoses—as well as the use of specific technical tips of embolization previously discussed is essential to avoid predictable major complications (Table 76.3).

■ OUTCOMES/PROGNOSIS

The aim of embolization is to stop the bleeding in cases of intractable epistaxis, and the outcomes are generally excellent. The clinical success immediately following the procedure has been reported as high as 93% to 100%.[8–10,12,31] Permanent and/or severe complications that may worsen the outcome are uncommon and have been reported less than 1%.[9,10,12,22,31]

The prognosis is different in cases of idiopathic epistaxis than in cases with a well-recognized underlying disease. In the former, the prognosis is excellent with a low rate of recurrence provided there is adequate control of associated factors, such as hypertension.

In a trauma setting, embolization of the bleeding artery, either the ECA branches or ICA pseudoaneurysms, usually

Table 76.3

Dangerous Anastomoses: How to Deal with Them and Stay Out of Trouble

- Beware of dangerous anastomoses
- Follow the protocol
- Embolize with particles >250 μm
- Look for them, both at angiography and fluoroscopy
- If seen, consider bigger particles or gelfoam strips
- Although not seen they are always there
- Invisible anastomoses carry invisible risks
- Always free flow embolization
- Do not perform forceful embolization
- Avoid vasospasm
- Do not embolize if there is vasospasm
- Do not ever overembolize

allows immediate hemorrhagic control without recurrence, and healing of the injured vessel is the rule.[4,15,16] Patient overall outcome depends also on the evolution of associated traumatic lesions.

In the case of AVM-related epistaxis, nasal bleeding is usually controlled with proper embolization, but recurrence cannot be completed spared in the presence of residual compartments of the malformation.[14,26] Otherwise, when complete anatomic AVM occlusion is granted, the long-term outcome is excellent.

In the case of JNA, where the goal is just to prevent surgical blood loss during surgical resection, the outcome is not only measured by the absence of complications but also by the important reduction of surgical hemorrhage. If proper capillary tumor vessels are embolized, the surgical conditions improve so much that the ENT surgeon will indicate it any time possible.[20]

Outcome in patients with HHT is generally good in the acute setting, allowing epistaxis control and nasal packing removal. However, the long-term outcome is not so good in terms of epistaxis recurrence, and, frequently, patients will require further re-embolization and/or surgery because nasal telangiectasias cannot be completed cured by any treatment so far.[25]

EARLY AND LATE FAILURES

Early failure of embolization to halt nasopharyngeal embolization is unlikely but if it does happen, in most cases, it is caused by incomplete endovascular treatment. It has been suggested that the success rate and early failure depend on the embolization protocol used.[4,8] Unilateral and/or single IMA embolization has theoretically more risk of rebleeding than bilateral embolization of both the IMA and FA.[8] Indeed, in the former the SPA is more prone to be reconstituted by transmedian or distal FA anastomoses, especially if proximal IMA embolization has been performed instead.

In the case of early failure of embolization, the patient is sent back to the angiographic room to check the nasopharyngeal arteries and a new embolization is performed. In this second look procedure a thorough study of all potential bleeding arteries, including the APhA, is mandatory.

Another reason that early failure may occur even when the suggested protocol of embolization has been followed is the prominent supply to the nasal cavity from the AEA or PEA. This is more prone to occur in patients with HHT, although it may also happen in idiopathic epistaxis.[3,25] Visualization of prominent ethmoidal arteries at pre-embolization angiography may predict further bleeding and/or failure of the embolization procedure.[3] In such a case these arteries should not be embolized but instead referred to the ENT for open surgical clipping, which is a very easy and straightforward procedure.[4,29]

Late failures of embolization are rather common in patients with HHT, where epistaxis recurrence is likely.[3,4,25] This does not preclude embolization in these patients because the goal is not to achieve a definitive cure but rather to stop an intractable bleeding or otherwise reduce the frequency of bleeding episodes in these patients. This issue should be discussed with the patient as well as with the referring physician at preprocedure consultation.

THERAPEUTIC EFFECTIVENESS COMPARED TO SURGICAL MANAGEMENT

Embolization is indicated when no medical or supportive therapies are sufficient to halt nasopharyngeal bleeding. The alternative treatment is surgical management either by transmalar arterial ligation or by the most recently developed endoscopic approach. The complication rate of transmalar approach is as high as 40% with a failure rate of 15% for bleeding control.[18] With the advent of endoscopy procedures, complication rates of surgery have decreased but the failure rate is still as high as 12% to 33%.[30,32] The main underlying causes of surgical failure rates are inadequate arterial ligation, incorrect vessel selection, anatomic variations, alternate dominance of blood supply, and reconstitution of nasal mucosa flow through collateral circulation.[3]

Endovascular procedures have many advantages compared to surgery because they may explore and occlude all potentially involved vessels in nasopharyngeal hemorrhage, including those not accessible to surgery, such as the APhA and ICA. There are no randomized control trials comparing embolization with surgery; however, large series have shown good results for both treatments but the outcome is better with embolization in terms of clinical success.[8–10,12,31]

Nevertheless the outcome of both endovascular and surgical procedures is strongly related to operator skill and experience. The selection of the treatment in a given institute is influenced by local logistics and preferences but embolization is usually preferred if available. Indeed the effectiveness, simplicity, and safety of the embolization procedure, in trained hands, make it the preferred primary modality of treatment in intractable epistaxis.

CONCLUSION

Angiography and embolization have been definitely incorporated into the multidisciplinary treatment strategy of nasopharyngeal hemorrhages. The advantages compared to surgery are noteworthy, which mainly are the possibility of diagnosing a bleeding site different from the SPA and to treat all possible sources of hemorrhage in the same session, independently of its intracranial or extracranial location. It is, however, associated with a small risk of serious morbidity if embolic material inadvertently enters the ICA or OphA. Therefore, clinical and functional vascular anatomic knowledge of this complex region, as well as experience with embolization techniques, is the basis for therapeutic success. Clinical knowledge will lead to adequate patient selection and treatment strategy. Thorough anatomic knowledge and mastery of endovascular techniques will avoid predictable complications. Provided these conditions are met, embolization of nasopharyngeal hemorrhage yields rewarding therapeutic and clinical results.

▌REFERENCES

1. Small M, Murray JA, Maran AG. A study of patients with epistaxis requiring admission to hospital. *Health Bull (Edinb)* 1982;40:20–29.
2. Viducich RA, Blanda MP, Gerson LW. Posterior epistaxis: clinical features and acute complications. *Ann Emerg Med* 1995;25:592–596.
3. Valavanis A, Setton A. Embolization of epistaxis. In: Valavanis A, ed. *Interventional Neuroradiology*. Berlin, Germany: Springer-Verlag; 1993.
4. Lasjaunias P, Berenstein A. *Surgical Neuroangiography: Endovascular Treatment of Craniofacial Lesions*. Vol 2. Berlin, Germany: Springer-Verlag; 1987.
5. Cullen M, Tami T. Comparison of internal maxillary artery ligation versus embolization for refractory posterior epistaxis. *Otolaryngol Head Neck Surg* 1998;118:636–642.
6. Sokoloff J, Wickbom I, McDonald D, et al. Therapeutic percutaneous embolization in intractable epistaxis. *Radiology* 1974;111:285–287.
7. Lasjaunias P, Marsot-Dupuch J, Doyon D. The radio-anatomical basis of arterial embolization of epistaxis. *J Neuroradiol* 1979;6:45–52.
8. Vitek J. Idiopathic intractable epistaxis: endovascular therapy. *Radiology* 1991;181:113–116.
9. Elden L, Montanera W, Terburgge K, et al. Angiographic embolization for the treatment of epistaxis: a review of 108 cases. *Otolaryngol Head Neck Surg* 1994;111:44–50.
10. Tseng E, Narducci C, Willing S, et al. Angiographic embolization for epistaxis: a review of 114 cases. *Laryngoscope* 1998;108:615–619.
11. Pallin D, Chng Y, McKay M, et al. Epidemiology of epistaxis in US emergency departments, 1992 to 2001. *Ann Emerg Med* 2005;46:77.
12. Willems P, Farb R, Agid R. Endovascular treatment of epistaxis. *Am J Neuroradiol* 2009;30:1637–1645.
13. Faughnan M, Palda V, García-Tsao G, et al. International guidelines for the diagnosis and management of hereditary haemorrhagic telangiectasia. *J Med Genet* 2011;48:73–87. Epub 2009 Jun 23.
14. De Tilly L, Willinsky R, TerBrugge K, et al. Cerebral arteriovenous malformation causing epistaxis. *Am J Neuroradiol* 1992;13:333–334.
15. Bynoe R, Kerwin A, Parker H, et al. Maxillofacial injuries and life-threatening hemorrhage: treatment with transcatheter arterial embolization. *J Trauma* 2003;55:74–79.
16. Raymond J, Hardy J, Czepko R. Arterial injuries in transsphenoidal surgery for pituitary adenoma; the role of angiography and endovascular treatment. *Am J Neuroradiol* 1997;18:655–665.
17. Monte E, Belmont M, Wax M. Management paradigms for posterior epistaxis: a comparison of costs and complications. *Otolaryngol Head Neck Surg* 1999;121:103–106.
18. Schaitkin B, Strauss M, Houck J, et al. Epistaxis: medical surgical therapy—a comparison of efficacy, complications and economic considerations. *Laryngoscope* 1987;97:1392–1397.
19. Lasjaunias P, Berenstein A. *Surgical Neuroangiography: Functional Anatomy of Craniofacial Arteries*. Vol 1. Berlin, Germany: Springer-Verlag; 1987.
20. Valavanis A. Embolization of intracranial and skull base tumors. In: Valavanis A, ed. *Interventional Neuroradiology*. Berlin, Germany: Springer-Verlag; 1993.
21. Ashwin PT, Mirza S, Ajithkumar N, et al. Iatrogenic central retinal artery occlusion during treatment for epistaxis. *Br J Ophthalmol* 2007;91:122–123.
22. García-Mónaco R, Lasjaunias P, Alvarez H, et al. Embolization of vascular lesions of the head and neck. In: Valavanis A, ed. *Interventional Neuroradiology*. Berlin, Germany: Springer-Verlag; 1993.
23. Alvarez H, Théobald M, Rodesch G, et al. Endovascular treatment of epistaxis. *J Neuroradiol* 1998;25(1):15–18.
24. García-Mónaco R, Taylor W, Rodesch G, et al. Pial arteriovenous fistula in children as presenting manifestation of Rendu-Osler-Weber disease. *Neuroradiology* 1995;37:60–64.
25. Layton KF, Kallmes DF, Gray LA, et al. Endovascular treatment of epistaxis in patients with hereditary hemorrhagic telangiectasia. *AJNR Am J Neuroradiol* 2007;28:885–888.
26. Berenstein A, Lasjaunias P, Terbrugge K. *Surgical Neuroangiography: Clinical and Endovascular Treatment Aspects in Adults*. Berlin, Germany: Springer-Verlag; 2004.
27. Garcia-Monaco R, Rodesch G, Alvarez H, et al. Pseudoaneurysms within ruptured intracranial arteriovenous malformations: diagnosis and early endovascular management. *AJNR Am J Neuroradiol* 1993;14:315–321.
28. Alvarez H, Rodesch G, García-Mónaco R, et al. Embolization of the ophthalmic artery branches distal to its visual supply. *Surg Radiol Anat* 1990;12:293–297.
29. Melia L, McGarry G. Epistaxis: update on management. *Curr Opin Otolaryngol Head Neck Surg* 2011;19:30–35.
30. Nouraei S, Maani T, Hajioff D, et al. Outcome of endoscopic sphenopalatine artery occlusion for intractable epistaxis: a 10-year experience. *Laryngoscope* 2007;117:1452–1456.
31. Fukutsuji K, Nishiike S, Aihara T, et al. Superselective angiographic embolization for intractable epistaxis. *Acta Otolaryngol* 2008;128:556–560.
32. Rockey JG, Anand R. A critical audit of the surgical management of intractable epistaxis using sphenopalatine artery ligation/diathermy. *Rhinology* 2002;40:147–149.

SECTION XII

Embologenic Arterial Lesions

Aortic Sources of Emboli

ANDREW D. MCBRIDE, RIPAL GANDHI, HEIKO UTHOFF, and JAMES F. BENENATI

▌ EMBOLIC SOURCES

Aortic atherosclerotic plaques are a source of embolic phenomena that can present with cerebral, visceral, or peripheral manifestations. Cerebral manifestations include transient ischemic attacks and stroke, whereas visceral/peripheral manifestations may include renal ischemia, bowel necrosis, splenic/hepatic infarction, and acute limb ischemia. In 1966 Edwards et al.[1] detailed 82 patients with peripheral embolization, and although the source was cardiac in 94% of the patients, 3 patients had emboli associated with atherosclerotic ulceration of the aorta. Atherosclerotic plaques develop in a specific evolutionary sequence from foam cells into atheromas, followed by the formation of overlying fibrous plaques. The fibrous cap is then destabilized in an inflammatory environment with potential for rupture and exposure of the thrombotic core. This can lead to acute thrombosis and possible embolization. Some of the early investigation into the thoracic aorta as a source of embolization was performed by Karalis et al. in 1991.[2] Their study identified intra-aortic complex atherosclerotic plaque protruding into the vessel lumen in 7% of patients undergoing transesophageal echocardiography. Embolic events were identified in 31% of these patients in the study and 27% of patients undergoing an invasive aortic procedure (FIGURE 77.1).

Ulcerative changes, in addition to being associated with advancing age, are thought to have a particularly high correlation to embolic disease. These lesions typically form in regions of low wall shear stress and in the setting of increased capillary permeability. The shape and thickness of the plaque, in part, contribute to the likelihood of embolization. In a small retrospective study by Karalis et al.,[2] pedunculated and mobile plaque was more likely to embolize than layered and immobile plaque. Thicker plaque embolizes more readily than thinner plaque, particularly plaque greater than 4 mm in thickness. These findings were later supported in subsequent studies including the French Study of Aortic Plaques in Stroke Group.[3] Their conclusion was that in the aortic arch, the presence of plaques greater than 4-mm thickness was a strong independent predictor of vascular events of all types. A potential explanation for this finding is that thicker plaque tends to be more lipid-laden with overlying thrombi, both of which increase the chance of embolization.

▌ MACROEMBOLIC SOURCES

Atherosclerotic plaque comprises two embolic forms. Thromboembolism is the more common form, and it arises from thrombus that overlies an atheromatous plaque in the aorta or a large artery. These embolic fragments tend to be fewer but larger and

can lead to mesenteric or peripheral ischemia. Clinical manifestations depend on the arterial segment affected by embolic disease. Emboli originating from the ascending aorta or arch are likely to lead to cerebral or upper extremity emboli. Therefore, such patients will present with transient ischemic attacks or stroke symptoms and upper extremity ischemia, respectively. A review of 44 years of arterial embolic disease by Abbott et al.[4] demonstrated the following frequencies: femoral (28%), arm (20%), aortoiliac (18%), popliteal (17%), visceral/other (9%). Descending thoracic aortic emboli may lead to visceral, renal, or distal extremity emboli. Embolic locations most commonly include areas of stenosis as well as the femoral, iliac, and popliteal bifurcations (FIGURE 77.2).

Shaggy Aorta Syndrome and Additional Entities Associated with Thromboembolism

Diffuse aortic atherosclerotic disease with multiple, ulcerated, atherosclerotic plaques have been called a shaggy aorta and can act as a source of spontaneous atheromatous embolization (FIGURE 77.3). Many patients demonstrate diffuse aortic thombus without embolic episodes; shaggy aorta syndrome diagnosis therefore requires the combination of both clinically evident embolic episodes as well as ulcerated lesions on imaging studies. Thromboembolic disease from a shaggy aorta can cause peripheral ischemia, renal failure, bowel infarction, and pancreatitis, among many additional clinical manifestations. Shaggy aorta syndrome has no proven medical treatment; however, Illuminati et al.[5] described a case of shaggy aorta syndrome that was treated with a stent-graft in the thoracic aorta in combination with aortofemoral bypass. Hollier et al.[6] described 88 patients who demonstrated spontaneous embolization in the setting of a shaggy aorta. In these patients, 40.9% demonstrated visceral embolization. In their experience, management options with the lowest morbidities and mortalities involved surgical repair including extra-anatomic bypass with ligation of the distal external iliac arteries. Although anticoagulation has been investigated in the past as a treatment option, it is thought to enhance the instability of aortic plaques, which can increase the risk of embolization.[7]

Aortic aneurysms are a known but uncommon source of emboli. The formation of thrombus and atheroma within aortic aneurysms are a potential source of both visceral/mesenteric as well as peripheral emboli. Early descriptions in the literature include an article by Darling et al.,[8] who reported that of 260 patients with arterial emboli, in 1.5% of patients the source was determined to be mural thrombus in either an abdominal aortic or iliac aneurysm. Subsequently in 1973, Lord et al.[9] reported on their experience with an abdominal aortic aneurysm

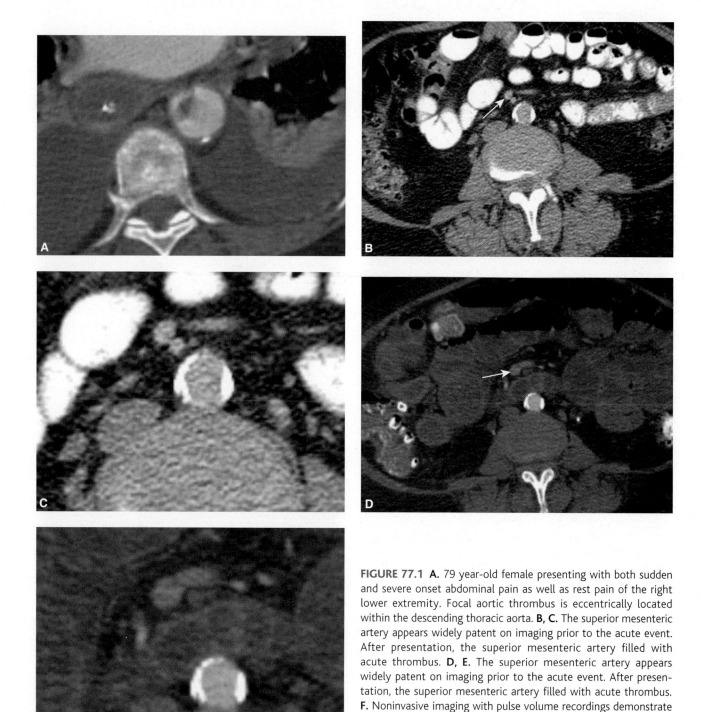

FIGURE 77.1 A. 79 year-old female presenting with both sudden and severe onset abdominal pain as well as rest pain of the right lower extremity. Focal aortic thrombus is eccentrically located within the descending thoracic aorta. **B, C.** The superior mesenteric artery appears widely patent on imaging prior to the acute event. After presentation, the superior mesenteric artery filled with acute thrombus. **D, E.** The superior mesenteric artery appears widely patent on imaging prior to the acute event. After presentation, the superior mesenteric artery filled with acute thrombus. **F.** Noninvasive imaging with pulse volume recordings demonstrate dampening of the left above- and below-knee waveforms consistent with femoral-popliteal disease. **G.** Angiogram demonstrates an abrupt cutoff of the profunda in addition to a distal superficial femoral artery occlusion.

(AAA) with mural thrombus as an unsuspected source of embolism. Ascending thoracic aortic aneurysms (TAA) are possible sources of cerebral emboli as described by Toyoda et al.[10] No strong evidence exists as to whether saccular, fusiform, or mycotic aneurysms carry any greater likelihood of emboli. However, case reports suggest that rapid enlargement, which can occur with inflammatory and mycotic aneurysms, can dislodge thrombus.

■ MICROEMBOLIC SOURCES

Cholesterol embolization, or atheroembolism, is the less common form of embolism from atherosclerotic plaque, and its prevalence is often underappreciated. In patients with severe atherosclerosis of the ascending aorta, atheroemboli were discovered in 22% of postcardiac surgery autopsy cases.[11] Meanwhile,

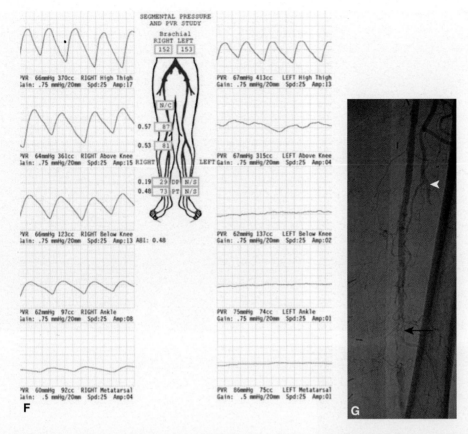

FIGURE 77.1 *(Continued)*

Thurlbeck and Castleman[12] found postmortem evidence for atheroembolism in 77% of their patients following AAA resection.

Atheroemboli, most commonly from the abdominal aorta, include atheromatous plaque fragments containing cholesterol crystals as well as platelet and fibrin thrombi, which lead to a shower of microemboli. The microembolic fragments cause an inflammatory reaction in addition to mechanical occlusion, which in combination can lead to ischemia, necrosis, and/or infarction. Cholesterol emboli can also be liberated in aortic inflammatory conditions, including cases of Behcet syndrome, retroperitoneal fibrosis, aortitis syndrome, and bacterial infections.[13] Cholesterol emboli can also complicate catheter-directed procedures or anticoagulant therapy. It has been reported after placement of an intra-aortic balloon pump, percutaneous coronary intervention, percutaneous transluminal angioplasty, and thoracic/abdominal aortic stent placement.

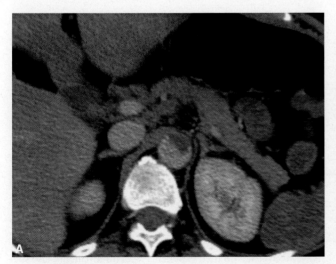
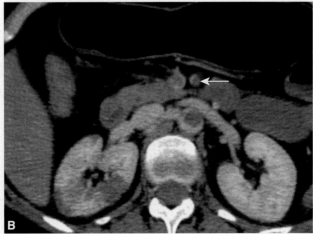

FIGURE 77.2 A, B. 44 year-old female presenting with diffuse abdominal pain and acute renal failure. There is eccentric aortic thrombus proximal to thrombus within the superior mesenteric artery (see *arrowhead*) Focal thrombus is also present at the level of the renal arteries with multiple right-sided renal infarctions.

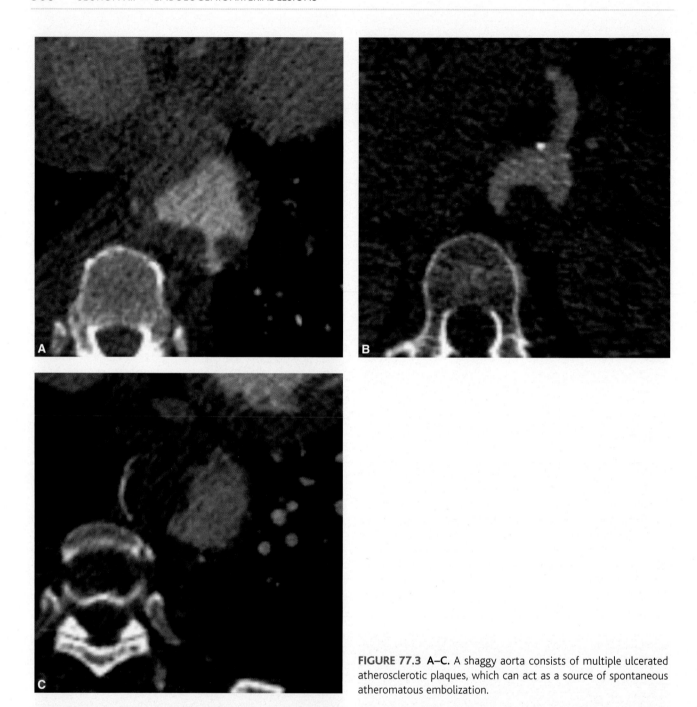

FIGURE 77.3 A–C. A shaggy aorta consists of multiple ulcerated atherosclerotic plaques, which can act as a source of spontaneous atheromatous embolization.

Jones and Iannaccone[14] even described a 1% incidence of atheromatous emboli in the setting of a renal biopsy. The criteria for "Definitive" and "Possible" cholesterol embolization syndrome (CES) have been defined by Fukumoto et al. in 2003.[15] "Definite CES" is defined as development of cutaneous signs including livedo reticularis, blue toe syndrome, and digital gangrene with or without renal impairment. "Possible CES" is defined as the presence of only renal impairment, that is, a postcatheterization serum creatinine greater than 1.3 mg/dL, 2 weeks after the procedure in the presence of normal preprocedural renal function without skin lesions.[15,16] As previously discussed, the abdominal aorta is the most common area for atherosclerotic plaques; however, Fukumoto et al. found that there

were no significant differences in the prevalence of cholesterol embolization between the brachial and the femoral approach for invasive aortic procedures. The diagnosis is predominantly clinical, but a definitive diagnosis can be made by muscle, skin, or renal biopsy. Biopsy specimens reveal "ghost" crystals lodged within vascular spaces.[17] Laboratory findings are nonspecific, but the strongest correlation has been made with eosinophilia.

The association between anticoagulation and atheroembolic disease was first described by Feder and Auerbach in 1961.[18] Nevelsteen et al.,[19] in their experience with three patients, also suggested a causal relationship between blue toe syndrome and the initiation of oral anticoagulation. The suspected pathophysiology is that anticoagulation prevents the formation of thrombus over atherosclerotic plaques, increasing the possibility of embolization.[20] Some controversy persists regarding the effect of anticoagulation on atheroembolism. The cessation of low-molecular-weight heparin has been associated with the improvement in clinical manifestations of atheroembolism.[21] The French Study of Aortic Plaques in Stroke Group found no significant difference in cerebral infarction in patients on warfarin or aspirin as long as the plaque thickness was less than 4 mm.[3] Fukumoto et al.[15] evaluated 25 patients out of 1,786 with cholesterol emboli complicating cardiac catheterization, an overall incidence of 1.4%. Of the 25 patients, 48% presented with cutaneous signs, whereas 64% had renal insufficiency. The study concluded that there was no association between anticoagulation and CES. This further complicates the decision point of stopping or continuing anticoagulation in the setting of clinical manifestations of atheroembolism with evidence available to support both courses of action. Liew and Bartholomew[20] concluded that based on the limited data, clinicians should continue anticoagulation in the setting of "compelling indications."

CES has a variety of clinical presentations, commonly with multiorgan involvement. Cholesterol emboli originating in both the thoracic and abdominal aorta may lead to renal failure, bowel ischemia, myocardial infarction, stroke, limb ischemia and emboli to the skeletal muscles and skin. The most commonly affected organs are the skin and the kidneys, and the association of renal and cutaneous disease should prompt further investigation for atheroembolic disease. Although gastrointestinal manifestations are thought to be common, they rarely present clinically. Fine et al.[22] evaluated 221 cases and concluded that the kidney is the most frequently affected organ with the skin, spleen, pancreas, bowel, adrenal glands, and liver also commonly affected. Purpuric rash, livedo reticularis, and myalgias are common presentations. Gutiérrez Solís et al.[23] reviewed 45 cases of cholesterol embolism and found that most patients were male (93.3%), elderly smokers with a history of hypertension. They concluded that both renal and individual outcomes are poor with 55.6% requiring long-term dialysis and 64.4% of patients not surviving a follow-up time of 12 ± 16.3 months. Given the mechanism of embolic phenomena, it is likely that any risk factor that increases the likelihood of atherosclerotic plaque also increases the risk of cholesterol embolization.

Microembolic Sources: Renal

Atheroembolic renal disease (AERD) is the result of cholesterol crystal embolization and is felt to be related to the degree of aortic atherosclerosis. The cholesterol crystal is thought to obstruct the arteriole lumen and incite a local granulomatous reaction with subsequent inflammation, endothelial damage, and intimal proliferation. The resulting fibrosis obstructs the vascular lumen. Cholesterol crystal embolization may be secondary to aortic manipulation, anticoagulation, or spontaneous embolization from an atherosclerotic plaque.[24] AERD has been reported to be the primary etiology for 5% to 10% of all cases of acute renal failure in the hospital setting as well as 4% of all nephrology consultations. Even more alarming, of the cases thought to be "probable" for atheroembolism, the mortality rate was over 50%.[25] There is a spectrum of clinical presentations for AERD including end-stage disease, varying degrees of renal insufficiency, uncontrolled hypertension, hematuria, infarction, and proteinuria.[20] The timeline for presentation is usually distinct from that seen with contrast-induced nephropathy (CIN). AERD has been

found to present several weeks to months after the inciting event, peaking in the third to the eighth week.[26] It is believed to result in dialysis in up to 30% of patients.[27] Lye et al.[28] reported that only 20% of patients were able to discontinue dialysis once initiated.

Overall the prognosis is poor both for the restoration of renal function as well as overall patient mortality. The clinical presentation includes acute renal failure usually in combination with eosinophilia. Fukumoto et al.[15] reported that patients with CES had significantly elevated eosinophil counts compared to post-cardiac catheterization patients without symptoms. Furthermore, those patients with renal dysfunction demonstrated even higher eosinophil counts than patients with CES and no renal dysfunction. Lastly, this prospective study also demonstrated an in-hospital mortality of 16% and found that renal dysfunction was present in all of the fatal outcomes. In a separate small study of 15 patients with atheroembolism, Scolari et al.[27] reported peripheral eosinophilia in 76% of patients, all of whom also had a negative antineutrophil cytoplasmic antibodies (ANCA) test.

The clinical manifestations of AERD significantly overlap with that of numerous vasculitides, complicating the treatment plan for both diagnoses.[29] Cutaneous manifestations of livedo reticularis and purpura can be seen in both entities. Unfortunately, there is also overlap in the laboratory testing of both vasculitides and AERD. Peat and Mathieson[30] describes a case of AERD that was associated with a laboratory finding of ANCA, a common diagnostic test for systemic vasculitis, and one that has already been described in the setting of cholesterol crystal embolization.[31] Although peripheral eosinophilia is strongly associated with AERD, Churg-Strauss also typically presents with eosinophilia. It has been suggested that hypocomplementaemia may provide some assistance in distinguishing between these entities because this condition can be seen in the setting of cholesterol embolism but is rare in systemic vasculitis.[32] However, Scolari et al.[27] reported that none of the patients they evaluated for AERD had hypocomplementaemia. Overall, despite the overlap of both clinical manifestations and laboratory data, distinguishing between these two entities is essential given the preferred treatment of steroids for systemic vasculitis and the controversial results of steroid administration in the setting of AERD.

Microembolic Sources: Dermatologic Manifestations

Dermatologic manifestations most commonly include livedo reticularis, blue toe syndrome, cyanosis, and gangrene. The frequency of cutaneous findings ranges from 35% to 96%.[33] Livedo reticularis is a blue-red mottled discoloration in a net-like pattern that is usually confined to the lower extremities but can extend superiorly to involve the chest or abdomen. The pathophysiology is a delay in superficial venous drainage caused by the obstruction of capillaries and venules by cholesterol emboli.[34] Livedo reticularis is not specific for atheroembolism and the differential diagnosis includes multiple types of vasculitides. Microvascular ischemia of the distal extremities from cholesterol emboli has been called blue toe syndrome (FIGURE 77.4). Patients present with cyanotic, cool, and painful toes with palpable distal pulses. The cyanosis is more prominent in dependent leg areas, typically with asymmetrical presentation if both extremities are involved. The degree of severity depends on the degree of microvascular obstruction with tissue necrosis, ulceration, and gangrenous changes present in the most severe cases.

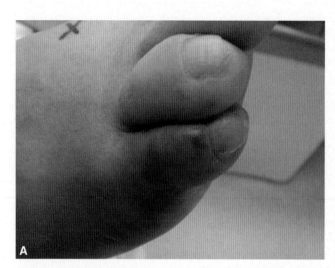
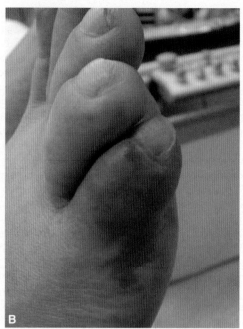

FIGURE 77.4 A, B. Patient presenting with clinical manifestations of atheroembolism. These pictures demonstrate microvascular ischemia, blue toe syndrome, in a patient with palpable distal pulses.

Large arteries are unaffected by the microemboli and remain palpable; however, given the association with atherosclerotic disease it is not uncommon for the dorsalis pedis and posterior tibial arteries to be nonpalpable from coexisting disease.

Microembolic Sources: Additional Sequelae of Atheroembolism

Atheroembolism can also present with gastrointestinal, central nervous system, and pulmonary manifestations, although these are less common than the cutaneous and renal presentations. Gastrointestinal atheroembolic disease can present with bleeding, pain, or diarrhea, most commonly involving the colon.[35] Hepatic involvement can present with elevated transaminase levels. Although rare, Moolenaar and Lamers[36] also described acute inflammatory disease of both the pancreas and gallbladder from cholesterol embolization. Atheroemboli to the central nervous system can present with cerebral infarction, retinal artery occlusion, or transient ischemic attack. Spinal cord infarction has been described and is commonly associated with iatrogenic causes. Retinal atheroembolism is defined by the presence of a Hollenhorst plaque, and, therefore, fundoscopy should be included in the workup for CES.[37] Pulmonary hemorrhage is a rarely reported presentation of cholesterol embolization; however, Vacher-Coponat et al.[38] presented a case of pulmonary hemorrhage in the setting of renal failure thought to be secondary to cholesterol emboli. Supportive treatment options are limited with steroids, statins, antiplatelet agents, and low-density lipoprotein (LDL) apheresis all described in the literature. The use of steroids remains highly controversial with some of the literature describing the beneficial effects of steroids in the setting of AERD and others describing their potentially devastating effects. Gutiérrez Solís et al.[23] reported that steroids actually reduced the mean time

to dialysis and increased the likelihood of both dialysis and death. In 1987 Fine et al.,[22] concluded that the administration of steroids in the setting of AERD increased the risk of death with 100% mortality in all patients who received steroids. In general, Liew and Bartholomew[20] do not recommend the use of steroids in the treatment of atheroembolism. Statins, despite having an association with plaque stabilization,[39] were described to have no benefit on patient outcome.[23] A large prospective review by Scolari et al.[40] demonstrated a benefit of statin therapy with decreased risk of end-stage renal disease. Dipyridamole and aspirin have been used in the setting of lower extremity ischemia but no strong evidence supports their use with atheroembolic disease. Finally, LDL apheresis has been reported by Tamura et al.[41] to improve dermatologic manifestations and pain from peripheral ischemia.

Primary treatment options include decreasing the risk factors for atheromatous embolization including blood pressure control, the avoidance of hypercholesterolemia, and smoking cessation. Protection devices during endovascular intervention, stent placement in the setting of ulcerative atherosclerotic plaques, and open surgical repair are all potential treatment options for patients with significant atherosclerotic disease at risk for atheroembolism. The patient's history should involve interrogation regarding potential vasculitides, trauma, hypercoagulable states, and recent catheter-directed therapy, including recent endograft repair, cardiac catheterization, or peripheral vascular disease intervention.

▌ IATROGENIC

Aortic atherosclerosis is a source of systemic embolism in patients undergoing percutaneous interventions. Endovascular procedures can be a source of both thromboembolism and atheroembolism. Common procedures include percutaneous coronary intervention, abdominal or thoracic stent placement, intra-aortic balloon pump placement, and percutaneous transluminal angioplasty with or without intervention. Aortoembolic phenomena caused by dislodging of debris from the aortic wall may occur when a catheter or wire traverse an aorta containing atherosclerotic plaque. A prospective evaluation by Keeley and Grines[42] designed to quantify the aortic debris that exited the guide catheter during its advancement around the aortic arch concluded that more than 50% of percutaneous revascularization procedures are associated with scraping debris during guide catheter placement. Despite such a common occurrence, Noto et al.[43] reported an incidence of clinically apparent embolism and stroke of less than 1% after cardiac catheterization. Endovascular procedures outside of cardiac intervention also have significant risk of atheromatous embolization. There have been numerous studies evaluating ischemic complications after open infrarenal aortic reconstruction. The complication rate has been estimated to be between 1% and 3% but with an associated mortality of up to 40%.[44,45] Endovascular repair of AAAs is also associated with ischemic complications. Vascular complications can be related either to the endograft complex itself or to the vascular access. In a retrospective review of 48 patients treated with an endograft for AAAs, Aljabri et al.[46] found that 9.6% of patients had a thromboembolic complication. This included only one patient with an embolic complication, whereas the rest of the patients presented with graft thrombosis. Görich et al.[47] describes a complication rate of infarctions alone of 9.2% including renal, splenic, and mesenteric. In 2004 Maldonado et al.[48] concluded that ischemic complications after endovascular aneurysm repair (EVAR) may exceed the incidence with open surgical repair, most often resulting from limb occlusion. A total of 311 patients were included in this study, which demonstrated peripheral atheroembolic complications in just 1% of the patients. Although ischemic complications from inferior mesenteric artery or hypogastric artery occlusion have been associated with EVAR, Maldonado et al. also described a case of paraparesis from conus medullaris atheroembolism. Overall, early studies between 2001 and 2004 have estimated the rate of complication to be 3% to 10%. Recently, the use of lower-profile endografts and sheaths may be associated with lower embolization rates. Given the embolic risks during endograft repair and any angiographic intervention, preoperative examination before and after the procedure should at least include a distal vascular exam that includes evaluation of the lower extremity pulses.

Spinal cord ischemia and infarction are additional complications of aortic aneurysm repair. Szilagyi et al.[49] have estimated the incidence of spinal cord infarction to be approximately 1 case in 400 after open AAA repair and 1 case in 5,000 after arterial reconstruction for aortoiliac occlusive disease. A few years later Dormal et al.[50] described cord infarction as a complication of aneurysm repair or rupture with an estimated incidence to be 1% to 2% in all infrarenal surgery. More recently, spinal cord ischemia has been described as a complication after EVAR, and EUROSTAR database analysis including 2,862 patients who had undergone EVAR found an incidence of 0.21% for spinal cord ischemia.[51] Although the exact etiology is not well understood, Kouvelos et al.[52] suggested that potential etiologies for cord ischemia after open AAA repair include prolonged aortic occlusion, intraoperative hypotension, atheromatous embolization, and interruption of the great radicular artery or collateral circulation. Atheromatous embolization as a cause of spinal

cord ischemia is likely related to catheter manipulation in areas of atherosclerotic plaque. In the EUROSTAR registry, factors associated with intraoperative microembolization included procedure time greater than 150 minutes, extensive intravascular handling, and preoperative or perioperative embolizations of the hypogastric and lumbar arteries.[51] Management strategies have developed from experience with TAA repairs where cerebral spinal fluid (CSF) drainage has been shown to offer neurologic protection. Partially limiting this strategy is the risk of complication, however, because Wynn et al.[53] reported a rate of neurologic deficit of 1% and a mortality rate of 0.6% with CSF drainage. Additional strategies include hypothermia, steroids, and arterial pressure augmentation.[52]

❚ NEOPLASM

Thrombotic events are not infrequent in patients with malignancy and may be multifactorial in nature, including etiologies such as immobilization, surgery, invasive procedures, chemotherapy, hormonal therapy, dehydration, and a neoplasia-induced hypercoagulable state. Although venous thrombosis is common in cancer patients, arterial thromboembolic disease and particularly aortic thromboembolic disease are rare. Aortic thrombus has been documented in patients with lymphoma, leukemia, and pancreatic adenocarcinoma. In a report by Poirée et al.,[54] the malignant lesions were in immediate proximity of the aorta when aortic thrombus occurred without any other precipitating factors. Nonocclusive aortic thrombus in the setting of neoplastic disease often resolves with anticoagulation alone; however, surgical thomboembolectomy or stent-graft placement may be necessary in selected patients.

Chemotherapy has been implicated as an independent risk factor for thrombosis; patients with malignancy undergoing chemotherapy are at increased risk of venous and arterial thromboembolic events compared to patients not receiving chemotherapy. Although there are several chemotherapy agents that increase the risk of thromboembolism, cisplatin is the agent most commonly implicated in cancer patients who develop arterial thrombosis.[55] There are several reports of isolated aortic thrombosis occurring in patents as a result of cisplatin chemotherapy. Hahn et al.[56] published a rare case of ascending aortic thrombosis and renal infarction occurring in a 74-year-old man treated with cisplatin and etoposide for non–small-cell lung cancer. Cisplatin often causes spontaneous aortic thrombosis in patients without cardiac disease or underlying aortic atherosclerotic or aneurysmal disease. The precise mechanism by which cisplatin administration triggers vascular toxicity is not clear, but potential etiologies include hypomagnesemia, direct endothelial damage injury, reduction of left ventricular function, vasospasm, and increases in von Willebrand factor concentrations.[57]

Primary neoplasms of the aorta are exceedingly rare and usually are malignant. Aortic involvement by retroperitoneal tumors, abdominal tumors, or thoracic tumors is more common than primary involvement. Patients most commonly present with vascular occlusion or arterial tumor embolization. Because aortic tumors may mimic other pathologies, such as aortic thrombus, ulcerated plaque, vasculitis, dissection, and other extra-aortic malignancies, they are usually diagnosed at surgery or autopsy.[58,59] Malignant histologic types of primary aortic tumors reported in the literature include malignant fibrous histiocytoma, fibrosarcoma, angiosarcoma, myxosarcoma, fibromyxosarcoma, fusiform cell sarcoma, leiomyosarcoma, epithelioid sarcoma, and unclassified sarcoma. Benign histologies comprise myxoma and fibromyxoma. If there is clinical suspicion for aortic malignancy, magnetic resonance imaging with and without gadolinium is the most sensitive diagnostic imaging modality and may optimize evaluation of tumor enhancement.[60] Additionally, the multiplanar imaging and superior contrast resolution may help exclude other aortic diseases.

Patients with epithelioid angiosarcoma may present with constitutional symptoms, weight loss, and high sedimentation rate, which may result in a presumptive diagnosis of vasculitis.[61] Vascular malignancy should be considered in patients presenting with signs and symptoms of vasculitis that do not improve with steroids. The prognosis of patients with malignant primary aortic tumors is poor and metastatic disease usually results in the patient's demise. According to one report, metastatic disease was identified postmortem in 71.2% of patients. In patients in whom a diagnosis could be established, mean survival was 14 months.[62]

Although sarcomas of the aorta are rare and often difficult to prospectively identify, an association has been described between primary aortic tumors and Dacron graft material. Most aortic sarcomas are diagnosed during microscopic evaluation of thromboemboli, but Fehrenbacher et al. described a patient with an angiosarcoma originating near a Dacron graft and then went on to review three additional previously described patients with similar findings.[63]

▌ HYPERCOAGULABLE STATE

Hypercoagulable states, such as those seen in malignancy, sepsis, disseminated intravascular coagulation, pregnancy, polycythemia, antiphospholipid syndrome (APS), heparin-induced thrombocytopenia (HIT), and protein C or S deficiency, may precipitate thromboembolic disease of the aorta.[64,65] Hypercoaguable disorders are rare causes of aortic thrombus with protein C and S deficiencies, APS, and hyperhomocysteinemia all linked to the formation of mural thrombus within the aorta. Although most cases of aortic thromboembolic disease occur in the setting of underlying disease of the aorta, such as atherosclerosis, dissection, aneurysm, or cardiac thrombus, there are reports in the literature in which aortic thrombus occurs in the absence of aortic pathology. One should suspect a hypercoaguable state when thrombosis occurs in patients of young age, few vascular risk factors, and female gender.

APS is an autoimmune, hypercoagulable state resulting from antibodies against cell-membrane phospholipids that causes recurrent venous and arterial thrombosis and may manifest clinically with fetal demise.[64,66] APS may be primary when it occurs in the absence of other disease or secondary when it develops in the setting of other autoimmune disorders, such as systemic lupus erythematosus. Although venous thrombosis predominates in patients with this disease, APS has a greater prevalence of arterial thrombosis than other hypercoagulable states. Even though arterial occlusion predominates in the cerebral circulation, there are reports of aortic thromboembolic disease. It is important to consider this diagnosis in young women who present with aortic thrombus; however, it is unusual for patients with APS to present in this manner. Anticoagulation is the recommended therapy in patients who present with arterial thrombosis, although more aggressive interventions may be warranted with extensive disease and resulting ischemic complications.

HIT is an immune-mediated disorder that usually occurs secondary to heparin exposure and results in venous and arterial thromboembolism.[67] A few cases of aortic occlusion secondary to HIT have been described in the literature.[68,69] In patients with aortic thrombus without underlying pathology, HIT should be suspected when thrombocytopenia occurs 5 to 14 days after exposure to heparin. Diagnosis is made by detecting antibodies against heparin-PF4 complexes. Heparin should be immediately discontinued in patients with HIT, and treatment with direct thrombin inhibitors is indicated. Aortic occlusion caused by HIT is associated with a high mortality and cases have traditionally been treated with open surgery. Karkos et al.[70] describe a case of acute infrarenal aortic thrombus secondary to HIT that was treated with endovascular treatment with stents.

▌ SUMMARY

Embolic sources of the aorta include aneurysms, atherosclerotic plaques, trauma, aortic neoplasm, and coagulopathies. However, less commonly reported is primary mural aortic thrombus, which can act as a source for embolic disease involving both cerebral ischemia and peripheral/visceral arterial embolization. The most commonly reported sources of aortic emboli are from atherosclerotic plaque with superimposed thrombus and subsequent embolization. Embolization can be in the form of atheroembolic disease or thromboembolism. Finally, atherosclerosis of the thoracic aorta is a strong predictor of peripheral atherosclerosis. Vascular risk factors including smoking, hypercholesterolemia, plasma fibrinogen, and homocysteinaemia relate to the severity of atherosclerotic lesions. Homocysteine may either directly induce endothelial dysfunction and atheroma progression, or it may be a risk marker of atherosclerosis. Diagnostic evaluation includes a combination of computed tomography (CT) angiogram, magnetic resonance (MR) angiogram, or transesophageal echocardiogram. During evaluation of the lower extremity ischemia, distal emboli should be suspected when a noninvasive evaluation reveals an asymmetrical distribution of disease severity.

▌ REFERENCES

1. Edwards EA, Tilney N, Lindquist RR. Causes of peripheral embolism and their significance. *JAMA* 1966;196:133–138.
2. Karalis DG, Chandrasekaran K, Victor MF, et al. Recognition and embolic potential of intraaortic atherosclerotic debris. *J Am Coll Cardiol* 1991;17:73–78.
3. Atherosclerotic disease of the aortic arch as a risk factor for recurrent ischemic stroke. The French Study of Aortic Plaques in Stroke Group. *N Engl J Med* 1996;334:1216–1221.
4. Abbott WM, Maloney RD, McCabe CC, et al. Arterial embolism: a 44 year perspective. *Am J Surg* 1982;143:460–464.
5. Illuminati G, Bresadola L, D'Urso A, et al. Simultaneous stent grafting of the descending thoracic aorta and aortofemoral bypass for "shaggy aorta" syndrome. *Can J Surg* 2007;50:E1–E2.
6. Hollier LH, Kazmier FJ, Ochsner J, et al. "Shaggy" aorta syndrome with atheromatous embolization to visceral vessels. *Ann Vasc Surg* 1991;5:439–444.
7. Hyman BT, Landas SK, Ashman RF, et al. Warfarin-related purple toes syndrome and cholesterol microembolization. *Am J Med* 1987;82:1233–1237.
8. Darling RC, Austen WG, Linton RR. Arterial embolism. *Surg Gynecol Obstet* 1967;124:106–114.
9. Lord JW, Rossi G, Daliana M, et al. Unsuspected abdominal aortic aneurysms as the cause of peripheral arterial occlusive disease. *Ann Surg* 1973;177:767–771.
10. Toyoda K, Yasaka M, Nagata S, et al. Aortogenic embolic stroke: a transesophageal echocardiographic approach. *Stroke* 1992;23:1056–1061.

11. Blauth CI, Cosgrove DM, Webb BW, et al. Atheroembolism from the ascending aorta. An emerging problem in cardiac surgery. *J Thorac Cardiovasc Surg* 1992;103:1104–1111; discussion 11–12.
12. Thurlbeck WM, Castleman B. Atheromatous emboli to the kidneys after aortic surgery. *N Engl J Med* 1957;257:442–447.
13. Nakamura S, Misumi I, Koide S. Cholesterol embolism as a complication of aortic dissection. *Circulation* 1999;100:e48–e50.
14. Jones DB, Iannaccone PM. Atheromatous emboli in renal biopsies. An ultrastructural study. *Am J Pathol* 1975;78:261–276.
15. Fukumoto Y, Tsutsui H, Tsuchihashi M, et al. The incidence and risk factors of cholesterol embolization syndrome, a complication of cardiac catheterization: a prospective study. *J Am Coll Cardiol* 2003;42:211–216.
16. Shaikh AH, Hanif B, Hasan K, et al. Cholesterol emboli syndrome— a rare complication of cardiac catheterization. *J Pak Med Assoc* 2010;60: 492–494.
17. Vidt DG. Cholesterol emboli: a common cause of renal failure. *Annu Rev Med* 1997;48:375–385.
18. Feder W, Auerbach R. "Purple toes": an uncommon sequela of oral coumarin drug therapy. *Ann Intern Med* 1961;55:911–917.
19. Nevelsteen A, Kutten M, Lacroix H, et al. Oral anticoagulant therapy: a precipitating factor in the pathogenesis of cholesterol embolization? *Acta Chir Belg* 1992;92:33–36.
20. Liew YP, Bartholomew JR. Atheromatous embolization. *Vasc Med* 2005; 10:309–326.
21. Belenfant X, d'Auzac C, Bariéty J, et al. Cholesterol crystal embolism during treatment with low-molecular-weight heparin [in French]. *Presse Med* 1997;26:1236–1237.
22. Fine MJ, Kapoor W, Falanga V. Cholesterol crystal embolization: a review of 221 cases in the English literature. *Angiology* 1987;38:769–784.
23. Gutiérrez Solís E, Morales E, Rodríguez Jornet A, et al. Atheroembolic renal disease: analysis of clinical and therapeutic factors that influence its progression [in Spanish]. *Nefrologia* 2010;30:317–323.
24. Scolari F, Tardanico R, Zani R, et al. Cholesterol crystal embolism: a recognizable cause of renal disease. *Am J Kidney Dis* 2000;36:1089–1109.
25. Mayo RR, Swartz RD. Redefining the incidence of clinically detectable atheroembolism. *Am J Med* 1996;100:524–529.
26. Thadhani RI, Camargo CA, Xavier RJ, et al. Atheroembolic renal failure after invasive procedures. Natural history based on 52 histologically proven cases. *Medicine (Baltimore)* 1995;74:350–358.
27. Scolari F, Bracchi M, Valzorio B, et al. Cholesterol atheromatous embolism: an increasingly recognized cause of acute renal failure. *Nephrol Dial Transplant* 1996;11:1607–1612.
28. Lye WC, Cheah JS, Sinniah R. Renal cholesterol embolic disease. Case report and review of the literature. *Am J Nephrol* 1993;13:489–493.
29. Young DK, Burton MF, Herman JH. Multiple cholesterol emboli syndrome simulating systemic necrotizing vasculitis. *J Rheumatol* 1986;13:423–426.
30. Peat DS, Mathieson PW. Cholesterol emboli may mimic systemic vasculitis. *BMJ* 1996;313:546–547.
31. Baslund B, Segelmark M, Wiik A, et al. Screening for anti-neutrophil cytoplasmic antibodies (ANCA): is indirect immunofluorescence the method of choice? *Clin Exp Immunol* 1995;99:486–492.
32. Systemic vasculitis. *Lancet* 1985;1:1252–1254.
33. Kronzon I, Saric M. Cholesterol embolization syndrome. *Circulation* 2010;122:631–641.
34. Colt HG, Begg RJ, Saporito JJ, et al. Cholesterol emboli after cardiac catheterization. Eight cases and a review of the literature. *Medicine (Baltimore)* 1988;67:389–400.
35. Moolenaar W, Lamers CB. Cholesterol crystal embolisation to the alimentary tract. *Gut* 1996;38:196–200.
36. Moolenaar W, Lamers CB. Cholesterol crystal embolization to liver, gallbladder, and pancreas. *Dig Dis Sci* 1996;41:1819–1822.
37. Slavin RE, Gonzalez-Vitale JC, Marin OS. Atheromatous emboli to the lumbosacral spinal cord. *Stroke* 1975;6:411–415.
38. Vacher-Coponat H, Pache X, Dussol B, et al. Pulmonary-renal syndrome responding to corticosteroids: consider cholesterol embolization. *Nephrol Dial Transplant* 1997;12:1977–1979.
39. Libby P, Aikawa M. Mechanisms of plaque stabilization with statins. *Am J Cardiol* 2003;91:4B–8B.
40. Scolari F, Ravani P, Pola A, et al. Predictors of renal and patient outcomes in atheroembolic renal disease: a prospective study. *J Am Soc Nephrol* 2003;14:1584–1590.
41. Tamura K, Umemura M, Yano H, et al. Acute renal failure due to cholesterol crystal embolism treated with LDL apheresis followed by corticosteroid and candesartan. *Clin Exp Nephrol* 2003;7:67–71.

42. Keeley EC, Grines CL. Scraping of aortic debris by coronary guiding catheters: a prospective evaluation of 1,000 cases. *J Am Coll Cardiol* 1998;32:1861–1865.
43. Noto TJ, Johnson LW, Krone R, et al. Cardiac catheterization 1990: a report of the Registry of the Society for Cardiac Angiography and Interventions (SCA&I). *Cathet Cardiovasc Diagn* 1991;24:75–83.
44. Brewster DC, Franklin DP, Cambria RP, et al. Intestinal ischemia complicating abdominal aortic surgery. *Surgery* 1991;109:447–454.
45. Diehl JT, Cali RF, Hertzer NR, et al. Complications of abdominal aortic reconstruction. An analysis of perioperative risk factors in 557 patients. *Ann Surg* 1983;197:49–56.
46. Aljabri B, Obrand DI, Montreuil B, et al. Early vascular complications after endovascular repair of aortoiliac aneurysms. *Ann Vasc Surg* 2001;15:608–614.
47. Görich J, Krämer S, Tomczak R, et al. Thromboembolic complications after endovascular aortic aneurysm repair. *J Endovasc Ther* 2002;9:180–184.
48. Maldonado TS, Rockman CB, Riles E, et al. Ischemic complications after endovascular abdominal aortic aneurysm repair. *J Vasc Surg* 2004;40: 703–709; discussion 9–10.
49. Szilagyi DE. A second look at the etiology of spinal cord damage in surgery of the abdominal aorta. *J Vasc Surg* 1993;17:1111–1113.
50. Dormal PA, Delberghe X, Roeland A. Infrarenal aortic aneurysm and spinal cord ischaemia. A new case and review of the literature. *Acta Chir Belg* 1995;95:136–138.
51. Berg P, Kaufmann D, van Marrewijk CJ, et al. Spinal cord ischaemia after stent-graft treatment for infra-renal abdominal aortic aneurysms. Analysis of the Eurostar database. *Eur J Vasc Endovasc Surg* 2001;22:342–347.
52. Kouvelos GN, Papa N, Nassis C, et al. Spinal cord ischemia after endovascular repair of infrarenal abdominal aortic aneurysm: a rare complication. *Case Report Med* 2011;2011:954572.
53. Wynn MM, Mell MW, Tefera G, et al. Complications of spinal fluid drainage in thoracoabdominal aortic aneurysm repair: a report of 486 patients treated from 1987 to 2008. *J Vasc Surg* 2009;49:29–34; discussion 34–35.
54. Poirée S, Monnier-Cholley L, Tubiana JM, et al. Acute abdominal aortic thrombosis in cancer patients. *Abdom Imaging* 2004;29:511–513.
55. Fernandes DD, Louzada ML, Souza CA, et al. Acute aortic thrombosis in patients receiving cisplatin-based chemotherapy. *Curr Oncol* 2011;18:e97–e100.
56. Hahn SJ, Oh JY, Kim JS, et al. A case of acute aortic thrombosis after cisplatin-based chemotherapy. *Int J Clin Oncol* 2011;16:732–736.
57. Doll DC, Ringenberg QS, Yarbro JW. Vascular toxicity associated with antineoplastic agents. *J Clin Oncol* 1986;4:1405–1417.
58. Das AK, Reddy KS, Suwanjindar P, et al. Primary tumors of the aorta. *Ann Thorac Surg* 1996;62:1526–1528.
59. Mason MS, Wheeler JR, Gregory RT, et al. Primary tumors of the aorta: report of a case and review of the literature. *Oncology* 1982;39:167–172.
60. Higgins R, Posner MC, Moosa HH, et al. Mesenteric infarction secondary to tumor emboli from primary aortic sarcoma. Guidelines for diagnosis and management. *Cancer* 1991;68:1622–1627.
61. Böhner H, Luther B, Braunstein S, et al. Primary malignant tumors of the aorta: clinical presentation, treatment, and course of different entities. *J Vasc Surg* 2003;38:1430–1433.
62. Seelig MH, Klingler PJ, Oldenburg WA, et al. Angiosarcoma of the aorta: report of a case and review of the literature. *J Vasc Surg* 1998;28:732–737.
63. John W. Fehrenbacher, William Bowers, Randall Strate, et al. Angiosarcoma of the Aorta Associated with a Dacon Draft. *Ann Thorac Surg.* 1981 Sep;32(3):297–301.
64. Insko EK, Haskal ZJ. Antiphospholipid syndrome: patterns of life-threatening and severe recurrent vascular complications. *Radiology* 1997;202:319–326.
65. Hazirolan T, Perler BA, Bluemke DA. Floating thoracic aortic thrombus in "protein S" deficient patient. *J Vasc Surg* 2004;40:381.
66. Soubrier M, Carrie D, Urosevic Z, et al. Aortic occlusion in a patient with antiphospholipid antibody syndrome in systemic lupus erythematosus. *Int Angiol* 1995;14:233–235.
67. Warkentin TE, Levine MN, Hirsh J, et al. Heparin-induced thrombocytopenia in patients treated with low-molecular-weight heparin or unfractionated heparin. *N Engl J Med* 1995;332:1330–1335.
68. Chevalier J, Ducasse E, Dasnoy D, et al. Heparin-induced thrombocytopenia with acute aortic and renal thrombosis in a patient treated with low-molecular-weight heparin. *Eur J Vasc Endovasc Surg* 2005;29:209–212.
69. Klemp U, Bisler H. Case report: acute infrarenal aortic occlusion and leg vein thrombosis in heparin-induced thrombocytopenia [in German]. *Vasa Suppl* 1991;33:289–290.
70. Karkos CD, Mandala E, Gerogiannis I, et al. Endovascular management of acute infrarenal aortic thrombosis caused by heparin-induced thrombocytopenia in a patient treated with low molecular weight heparin. *J Vasc Interv Radiol* 2011;22:581–582.

Peripheral Sources of Distal Embolic Disease

FRANCISCO J. CONTRERAS and ALEX POWELL

INTRODUCTION

It is estimated that in the general population, the incidence of acute arterial insufficiency secondary to arterial thromboembolism ranges from 13 to 17 per 100,000.[1] With proper care, acute limb ischemia is a highly treatable condition, but despite significant advances in both surgical and endovascular techniques, the mortality associated with tissue ischemia from arterial occlusion remains high, typically averaging 10% to 25%.[2,3] The term *embolus* was first introduced in the 19th century by Virchow, who used the term to describe a sudden obstruction of arterial blood flow by any material arising from a distal site. It has been discovered that these occlusive plugs can consist of platelet-fibrin thrombus, cholesterol debris, laminated aneurysmal thrombus, or even a foreign body attaining access to a person's circulation.[2]

Early in the evolution of medical management of arterial embolic disease, treatment was strikingly conservative. It commonly involved observation that would lead to limb loss or patient death. It was not until the early 20th century that early surgical techniques were developed, allowing for physical removal of emboli.[4] Therapy was revolutionized after the introduction and accepted use of intravenous heparin infusion before, during, and, eventually, after surgical interventions.[5] It was at this point that the medical and surgical communities learned that prompt treatment with heparin decreased the propagation of thrombus, stabilized existing clot burden, and established the necessary environment for the recruitment of collateral vessels to bypass areas of arterial occlusion. Despite significant advances in surgical techniques and operator ability to completely excise thromboembolic plugs, the removal of large propagated thrombus remained significantly problematic. Early methods of treatment employed the use of suction catheters, vigorous arterial flushing with distal control, and external compression of affected limbs.[6-8] Surgical and endovascular techniques have continued to evolve through the years, currently allowing thromboembolic material to be removed quickly with relatively little trauma to vessels.

In the current era of management, it has been well established that the risks of mortality from arterial occlusive disease remains proportionally related to the degree of limb ischemia suffered by the patient. The deleterious effects of this sudden arterial insufficiency arise from the consequences of both tissue ischemia and associated reperfusion injury. These two factors are strongly influenced by the altered balance between blood supply and the tissue demands of the affected limbs.[1] Only in the setting of prompt diagnosis, rapid initiation of pharmacologic therapy, and hasty intervention does one achieve improvement in a 37% amputation rate and mortality associated with this vascular emergency.[9]

CLASSIFICATION OF PERIPHERAL ARTERIAL EMBOLI

Arterial emboli are traditionally classified by size, content, and site of its origin. An understanding of this classification is paramount because it strongly influences a patient's clinical presentation and natural history of the disease as well as determines a patient's management. In general, embolic phenomenon in arterial vasculature is broadly considered either microembolic or macroembolic. The latter of these categories can be further subclassified into those arising from a cardiac source, a noncardiac source, and those of unknown origin.

Microemboli

Microemboli arise from a variety of lesions ranging in locations but most commonly from the infrarenal aorta to the popliteal artery. It has long been established that popliteal artery aneurysms (PAAs) have a favored predisposition for the release of microemboli. Iliac and common femoral aneurysms are uncommon in isolation and rarely produce distal embolization. These vessels are more commonly associated with acute thrombotic occlusive disease as is often seen in peripheral vascular disease (PVD). In significant contrast, though, atherosclerotic plaques of the iliac, common femoral, and superficial femoral vessels do provide fertile ground for microembolic material. Lesions in these arteries that predispose to microemboli typically include stenotic, irregularly luminal contoured, and ulcerated plaques.[10]

Microemboli arise from fragmentation of atheromatous plaques and the subsequent dislodgement of the fragmented debris then traveling to distal sites.[11] Atherosclerotic plaques are composed of a fibrous cap containing a dynamic mixture of macrophages, necrotic debris, and cholesterol crystals. Plaques at highest risk of rupture are those with a thin fibrous cap containing a lipid-rich core. Because of their relatively low-density and hydrophobic characteristics, cholesterol crystals rapidly pass through the circulation until they encounter arterial bifurcations or reach the end of an arterial bed.[12] Atheromatous cholesterol-containing emboli (also sometimes composed of fibrinoplatelet or thrombotic material) are the ones often found in digital arteries as well as those smaller arteries of calf muscles.[13] In general, distal embolization of atheromatous debris, fibrinoplatelet fragments, or other thrombotic material tend to lodge in muscular arteries as well as digital arteries averaging 100 to 200 μm in size.[14] In contrast, material embolized from aneurysmal sources are composed of laminated thrombus that are ejected downstream as they are exposed to the turbulent laminar flow within aneurysmal vessels.

Adding to the clinical problem is that autopsy examinations have consistently shown that atherothrombotic microembolization is generally under-recognized as the etiology of distal arterial occlusions.[15] Cholesterol emboli terminating in arterioles cause an immediate inflammatory response that is characterized by the recruitment of both polymorphonuclear and eosinophilic elements. Within a month, a chronic inflammatory infiltrate develops as cholesterol crystals become embedded within the intimal smooth muscles of vessels.[16] The inevitable endothelial proliferation caused by this chronic inflammation leads to the formation of a fibrous cap.

The most important risk factor for the development of atheroembolism is to have pre-established atherosclerosis. Significant risk factors therefore include hypertension, older age, coronary artery disease (CAD), and PVD.[17] There are also multiple precipitating factors to consider when dealing with atheroembolic disease and specifically with plaque instability that has been documented to occur after trauma, vascular surgery, endovascular interventions, anticoagulation, as well as thrombolysis.

Macroemboli—Cardiac Origin

By definition, macroemboli arise from the dislodgment of a large plaque or mural thrombus, resulting in an acute large, single-vessel occlusion. In approximately 80% to 90% of cases, the heart serves as the source of arterial macroemboli with a shift in the underlying etiology of heart disease from rheumatic heart disease previously to atherosclerotic coronary vascular disease presently. Atherosclerotic heart disease is now implicated in approximately 60% to 70% of all cases of emboli with rheumatic mitral valve disease and more commonly atrial fibrillation (AF) deemed the causative factor in the remaining 30% to 40% of cases.[18]

As a direct result of stasis, especially in the left atrial appendage, AF is currently associated with the highest risk of peripheral embolization. After AF, myocardial infarction is the next leading cause of potential peripheral emboli because ventricular wall akinesis or hypokenesis leads to the development thrombus formation. Although much less frequent, cardiac valvular prostheses can act as a source of emboli, requiring lifelong anticoagulation. Embolic complications in this subset of patients is common when anticoagulation is either inadequate or discontinued. Of note, it has been reported that biosynthetic valves are not as thrombogenic as prosthetic valves, sometimes not requiring any anticoagulation on the part of the patient.[19] Intracardiac tumors, such as atrial myxomas are a rare but possible source of peripheral emboli. This etiology can be suspected in younger patients and those without a significant history of atherosclerosis. Although transesophageal echocardiography (TEE) offers the most accurate evaluation of the heart, its sensitivity is still less than ideal. As a result, in the absence of detectable thrombus by TEE, one cannot entirely exclude a cardiac source of arterial emboli.

Macroemboli—Noncardiac Origin

Peripheral arterial emboli from noncardiac sources only account for approximately 5% to 10% of cases of arterial occlusive disease.[18] Large embolic fragments commonly originate from mural erosions/irregular ulcerations of atherosclerotic disease in more proximal vessels. Noncardiac sources include aortic and peripheral aneurysms; vascular anatomic variants, such as persistent sciatic arteries (PSAs); arterial dissection; foreign bodies; tumor cells; aortoiliac stents; primary aortic mural thrombus; hematologic conditions; and thoracic outlet syndrome.[1]

Hematologic conditions predisposing to peripheral arterial emboli should always be screened for with a thorough patient history. Causes include deficiencies of cellular anticoagulants, disorders of the fibrinolytic cascade, the presence of antiphospholipid antibodies, and disorders of platelet aggregation. Surgical intervention in these patients can have catastrophic results if the underlying disorder proceeds either unrecognized or untreated.

Another consideration for a noncardiac source of peripheral embolization is that associated with paradoxical emboli. Venous thrombosis can be ejected into the arterial circulation via a right-to-left shunt, which commonly occurs as a result of a patent foramen ovale—a condition found in 35% of the general population.[20] Especially in cases of unexplained arterial occlusion, a high degree of clinical suspicion is needed to include this category of emboli.

Macroemboli—Unknown Origin

Cryptogenic emboli comprise an additional 5% to 10% of cases of peripheral embolic disease that originate from a source that remains undetermined despite exhaustive interrogation.[21] The incidence of this entity is significantly decreasing as the resolution of current clinical imaging tools continues to improve. Also contributing to the decreasing incidence of this subcategory of macroemboli is the increased recognition of noncardiac sources of emboli that are now more commonly considered in differential diagnoses. As mentioned earlier, particularly in younger patients without evidence of previous PVD and in those with known malignancies, hypercoagulable states should always be entertained as the etiologic agent of peripheral emboli.

▌ PATHOPHYSIOLOGY

Clinically, approximately 20% of emboli affect the cerebrovascular circulation and 10% involve visceral organ vessels.[21] The upper and lower extremities therefore account for more than 70% of vascular beds affected by arterial occlusive disease. It should also be noted that emboli terminate in the lower extremities five more times than in the upper extremities. Overall, the abrupt change in vessel diameter that occurs at bifurcations makes these areas the most common site of occlusions with the femoral bifurcation being the most frequent site of embolization.

The outcome of patients with arterial occlusive disease depends on several important factors including the size of the vessel involved, the degree of obstruction achieved, and, most importantly, the preexisting collateral pathways present. The effects of a sudden cessation of blood flow in a previously normal vessel are more likely to produce profound ischemia because there is no significant collateral network in place. In contrast, the sudden occlusion of a severely stenotic vessel may likely only produce mild clinical symptoms, owing to the presence of collateral pathway recruitment.

The physiologic state of an ischemic limb is the best predictor of limb salvage potential. This is largely determined by the metabolic supply and demand of the affect limb, rather than on the time from onset of symptoms. Regardless, the presence of preexisting collaterals is the most influential factor. After an acute arterial occlusion, limb ischemia can be significantly worsened by three main issues. The first, and arguably the most detrimental, is clot propagation. As the site of embolic occlusion extends, there is a greater chance of irreversible tissue damage because established collateral pathways may become compromised. Early and aggressive treatment is aimed at the prevention of thrombus propagation and protection of collateral flow. A second event that can occur in embolic phenomena is that of clot fragmentation causing distal emboli from a distal embolic source, leading to a larger affected vascular territory. In some instances, though, partial disintegration of embolic material can be the mechanism by which spontaneous clinical resolution occurs in a patient. Lastly, the development of a concomitant venous thrombosis can cause further reduction of arterial blood flow. It is suggested that the sluggish flow in the thrombosed vein in addition to the ischemia in the intima of the affected vein results in worsening tissue damage as well as significant edema after revascularization.

Besides the morbidity and mortality associated with limb loss, patients with severe limb ischemia from embolism are at increased risk for severe systemic metabolic complications that typically occur after reperfusion. Elevated levels of potassium, lactic acid, myoglobin, and cellular debris pooling in devitalized vascular territories can have profound consequences. The sudden release of these elements back into the systemic circulation often leads to reperfusion syndrome characterized by peripheral muscle infarction, myoglobinemia, and renal failure. Patients with this syndrome suffer from severe hyperkalemia, metabolic acidosis, and myoglobinuria.

Even with successful embolectomy, local inflammatory effects after ischemic reperfusion can lead to limb loss and mortality. The largest contributor to local inflammation is the edema that often follows revascularization. The disintegration of capillary walls following vessel ischemia is directly responsible for the large degree of edema. As large quantities of free radicals are released, the bodies' intracellular oxidation scavenger systems become overwhelmed, leading to extensive damage of cellular membranes and resulting in the transudation of cellular fluid into the interstitial spaces. The presence of hydrostatic pressure increases from edema leads to further reduction in perfusion and worsening tissue injury. A local compartment syndrome can develop that worsens vascular obstruction. Although fasciotomy can correct some of the effects of compartment syndrome, it does little to alleviate small-vessel obstruction.

▌ CLINICAL PRESENTATION

There is a large variability in clinical presentations owing to several factors including the location of the embolic source, the extent of vascular compromise, the size of the embolization, the degree of arterial occlusion, and the existence or lack of collateral circulatory pathways in the region affected. Acute occlusive arterial macroembolization is typified by a sudden onset of pain associated with loss of a previously palpable pulse.[22] Presenting symptoms can often be both subtle and nonspecific to include fever, myalgias, headache, and weight loss. Commonly though, the vascular bed compromised by an embolic event can be accurately identified on physical examination.

When macroemboli are present the physical examination typically demonstrates loss of pulses below the level of the embolic occlusion. When only microembolic disease is present, however, the examination frequently reveals palpable pulses. Clinical cases 1 and 3 both had easily palpable pedal (case 1) and wrist (case 3) pulses in spite of obvious embolic disease. Delayed capillary refill can help to distinguish microemboli from other

potential sources of a painful, discolored limb when palpable pulses are present.

The pain associated with an acute arterial occlusion is characteristically severe and persistent. The muscle groups below the level of occlusion are the first to become symptomatic followed by progression to involve locations increasingly distal to the site of obstruction. Muscular tenderness is usually a worrying sign, indicating advancing muscle ischemia and possible infarction. The overlying skin distal to the area of obstruction will often demonstrate pallor that can progress to mottled area of cyanosis. When left untreated, necrosis and desquamation can ensue. Temperature changes associated with arterial occlusion are normally noted one joint distal to the point of obstruction.

In certain patients, a sensory disturbance may predominate, masking the complaints of pain. In these instances, the complaint of paresthesia occurs because of ischemic sensory nerve tissues and may present without any significant pain component. When ischemia affects motor nerve tissue, paralysis can develop. This is usually a late manifestation of symptomatology. The extent of motor deficit can be seen as a good index of the degree of tissue anoxia. Complete motor loss is a late development that often heralds impending gangrene because it marks a severe combination of end-stage muscle and neuronal ischemia. When paralysis progresses to rigor (i.e., involuntary muscle contracture), irreversible limb ischemia has developed. It is at this point that, although the affected limb may be salvaged with significant functional compromise, the risk of fatal systemic metabolic consequences from revascularization is highest.

A careful history and meticulous physical examination is paramount in stratifying ischemic limbs for the purposes of therapeutic management. In combination with clinical findings, Doppler signals from both arterial and venous sources allow peripheral embolic disease to be categorized into three relevant groups as recommended by the Society for Vascular Surgery/International Society for Cardiovascular Surgery (SVS/ISCVS) committee.[23]

Viable: Not immediately threatened. There is no ischemic pain, no neurologic deficit present; there is adequate skin capillary circulation; and clearly audible Doppler pulsatile flow signal is present in pedal arteries (ankle pressure >33 mm Hg).

Threatened Viability: Indicates a state of reversible ischemia provided arterial obstruction is promptly relieved. Ischemic pain or mild and incomplete neurologic deficit is present. Doppler pulsatile flow in pedal arteries is not audible, but venous signals are demonstrable.

Irreversible Ischemic Change: Profound sensory loss and muscle paralysis is present; there is absent capillary skin flow; muscle rigor has developed; and skin marbling is present. Neither arterial nor venous Doppler flow is audible. A major amputation is required regardless of therapy.

▌ DIAGNOSTIC IMAGING

Noninvasive Imaging

The combination of a bedside, hand-held Doppler with physical examination findings can produce a quick and sensitive way to determine the severity of peripheral ischemia. The quick availability to interrogate arterial blood flow helps greatly in formulating an initial treatment plan. Insonation allows for immediate assessment for the presence of blood flow, the spectral waveform characteristics (i.e. monphasic, biphasic, or triphasic), and calculation of ankle brachial indices (ABIs). The SVS/ISCVS has recommended standards of stratifying limb ischemia as follows [23]:

Class I: Audible Doppler signals; no motor or sensory deficits
Class IIa: No audible Doppler signal; paresthesias and/or limited digit sensory loss
Class IIb: Persistent pain; greater sensory loss; any level of motor deficit
Class III Early: Complete anesthesia and paralysis
Class III Late: Muscle rigor; skin marbling; no detectable venous flow, even with compressive maneuvers

Class I and IIa patients have viable limbs or areas that are only marginally threatened. Further diagnostic studies can be pursued to help shape continued management. Class IIb and early class III limbs are immediately threatened and require immediate revascularization. Late class III limbs are unsalvageable.

Duplex Ultrasound and Pulse Volume Recordings

In patients with viable limbs in which further imaging may help influence management and therapy, the use of duplex ultrasound can be valuable. Modern-day ultrasonography can easily demonstrate the distribution and extent of thrombosis in the peripheral vasculature. It can detect aneurysms or plaques proximal to affected vascular beds, which can determine the source of emboli when caused by artery-to-artery mechanisms. Patients with both arterial and venous obstructions may also be accurately diagnosed.

In the absence of significant atherosclerosis, an acute thrombus can easily be distinguished from the arterial wall by duplex ultrasound. In this instance, the outer layer of the thrombus appears echogenic because of its high concentration of fibrin as compared to the underlying smooth muscle arterial wall. Areas proximal to a complete thrombosis can show sharp, short duration spikes depicting a water-hammer effect as forward flowing blood flow comes to an abrupt cessation at the edge of thrombus.

In addition to duplex ultrasound, pulse volume recordings (PVRs) can help to determine the location and severity of the occlusion. Macroemboli will dampen PVRs below the level of obstruction (case 2). It should be kept in mind, however, that microemboli can present with normal PVRs (cases 1 and 3). In these cases additional studies including digital waveforms (case 3) are helpful to confirm the diagnosis.

Computed Tomographic and Magnetic Resonance Arteriography

Whereas the diagnosis of peripheral emboli is usually made based on physical examination and duplex imaging, computed tomography (CT) and magnetic resonance imaging (MRI) can serve to diagnose the cause and severity of an underlying source lesion. As illustrated in case 2, CT imaging (FIGURES 78.1B, C) was the means of diagnosing a persistent sciatic artery. The aneurysm of this aberrant artery that was the source of the emboli was easily detected as was the extent of the distal macroembolization. In case 1, CT angiography (FIGURE 78.2B) confirmed

the diagnosis of a PAA but also provided critical information regarding the extent of the aneurysm as well as vessel sizing prior to aneurysm repair.

Invasive Imaging

Diagnostic arteriography (FIGURE 78.1D) has multiple advantages in the evaluation of peripheral embolic disease. It can often determine the cause of thrombosis as well as provide detailed information regarding the state of circulation proximal to areas of occlusion. It can accurately map the extent of collateral pathways and provide information as to the extent of blood flow distal to areas of embolic occlusions.

▎LOWER EXTREMITIES

Blue Toe Syndrome

Blue toe syndrome (BTS) is used to describe a spectrum of findings seen in patients suffering from distal arterial occlusions in small arteries of the lower extremities.[24] The syndrome is characterized by focal, painful, cyanotic areas in the distal extremities that are sharply demarcated from adjacent normally perfused tissue.[25] This is associated with preserved patency of the larger arteries supplying the affected vascular bed as well as demonstrating preservation of distal pulses. As emboli break off and shower distal vascular territories, end arterioles in the feet occlude, leading to toe ischemia and then clinical manifestation of BTS are unmasked. FIGURE 78.3 demonstrates the multiple punctuate areas of discoloration in the toe and plantar aspect of the foot often seen in patients with BTS. It is important to distinguish BTS from other nonembolic entities that may present similarly, such as Raynaud's disease, thermal injury from hypothermic exposure, and idiopathic digital artery thrombosis. The importance of establishing the presence of embolic disease in BTS is that episodes are often recurrent and could result in limb loss and death if the extent of embolic disease becomes large enough.

Traditionally, the treatment of patients with BTS and an upstream arterial lesion is surgical endarterectomy or bypass. Because of the poor outcomes of patients with BTS, there continues to be much debate and concern as to how best to treat these lesions. Many patients still present with an identifiable stenotic atherosclerotic lesion that can promote fibrinoplatelet aggregation and fragmentation. The resolution of pressure gradients across significantly stenotic lesions should greatly aid in the prevention of future thrombus fragmentation and subsequent embolization. For this reason, the focus of recent trials has been in the treatment of these structurally obstructing lesions. Placement of endovascular stents has proven quite successful in treating these arterial stenoses and obstructions. Intra-arterial stents also provide a scaffold for preventing future plaque embolization and also promote plaque remodeling.[26–28] Although there is concern for producing more distal emboli during the placement of stents and angioplasty, clinical evidence has shown that in most patients treated with endovascular revascularization, there is no significant clinical evidence that new emboli are deposited distally in the immediate period following stent placement.[25,26] To this end, a growing accepted practice is thrombus stabilization with anticoagulation and/or antiplatelet therapy prior to performing PTA with or without stent placement (PTA).[24–26]

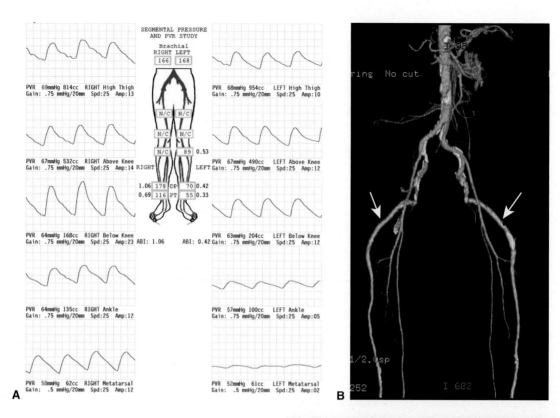

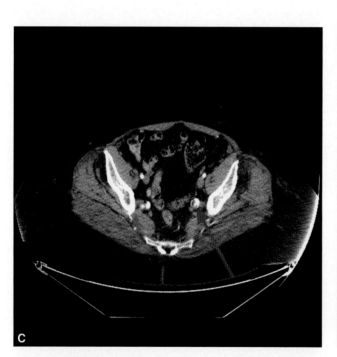

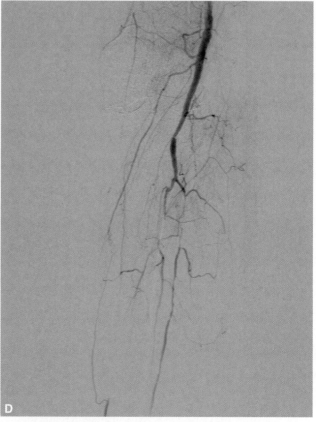

FIGURE 78.1 **A.** Noninvasive pulse volume recording demonstrates inadequate augmentation in the left lower extremity from the high thigh to below the knee as well as dampening of waveforms in the ankle and metatarsals consistent with mild femoral popliteal and moderate tibial occlusive disease. **B.** Three-dimensional volume-rendered images from a contrast-enhanced CT demonstrating bilateral persistent sciatic arteries (*arrows*). **C.** Contrast-enhanced CT reveals an embolic source from an aneurysm of the persistent left sciatic artery (*arrow*). **D.** Tibial occlusions secondary to emboli are evident on the subsequent digital subtraction angiogram.

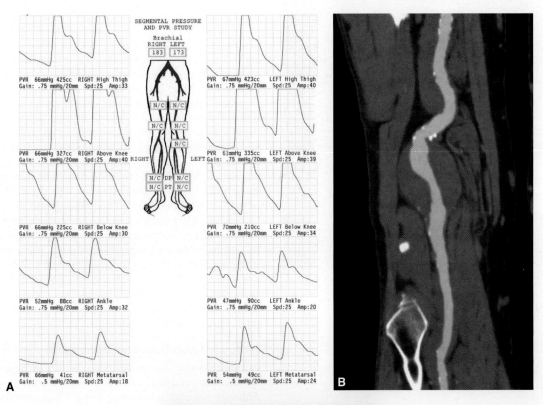

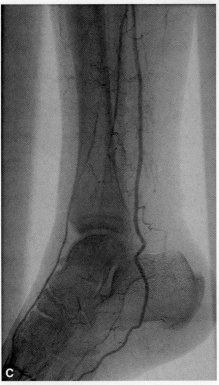

FIGURE 78.2 **A.** Noninvasive pulse volume recordings demonstrating no significant abnormality in a patient with clinically evident distal embolic disease/BTS. **B.** Center-line reformatted imaging from a contrast-enhanced CT angiogram demonstrated a large popliteal artery aneurysm. **C.** Digital subtraction angiogram taken immediately before endovascular aneurysm repair demonstrates collateral filling of the anterior tibial artery but otherwise preserved tibial vessels, indicating a massive microembolic load.

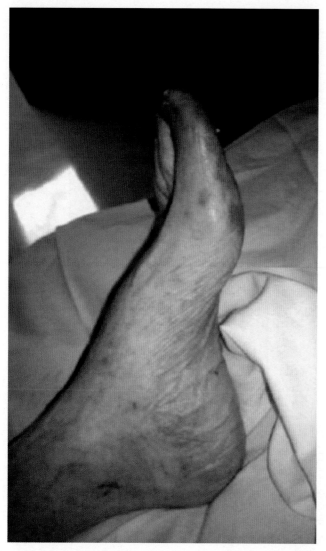

FIGURE 78.3 Image demonstrates the classical findings of multiple punctuate areas of discoloration on the toe and plantar aspect of the foot in a patient with great toe pain.

Peripheral Artery Aneurysms of the Lower Extremities

Femoral Arteries

True aneurysms of the common femoral arteries are uncommon. They are the second most common site of peripheral lower extremity aneurysms after those of the popliteal artery. In the initial evaluation, care must be taken to make sure that aneurysms are not pseudoaneurysms arising after trauma or previous endovascular catheterization because pseudoaneurysms have a completely different treatment algorithm and are not common sources of distal embolic disease. True femoral artery aneurysms have a higher prevalence in elderly men (>55 years of age) with a smoking history.[29] In approximately half of these patients, aneurysms are bilateral and also often associated with abdominal aortic aneurysms (AAAs).[30] The pathogenesis of aneurysms in this location is still not well established but is often ascribed to the degeneration of the arterial wall caused by atherosclerosis.

On occasion, femoral artery aneurysms are a manifestation of a more global arteriomegaly, in which there is diffuse enlargement of several arterial segments with extensive aneurysmal dilatation of vessels below the level of the renal arteries. In the setting of diffuse aneurysms of the lower extremities, an exhaustive search for etiologies, such as inflammatory arteritis, Behcet syndrome, arterial dysplasia, and idiopathic primary aneurysms should be conducted. In general, most femoral artery aneurysms are clinically silent unless they produce distal embolic disease. When large enough, though, aneurysms in the femoral arteries can cause neurovascular compression leading to symptomatology, such as edema, pain, or paresthesias caused by compression of adjacent femoral veins and nerve, respectively. More concerning is the potential of these aneurysms to produce acute or chronic thrombosis leading to distal embolization and, on rare occasions, rupture.

Femoral artery aneurysms can be detected by physical examination, most of which present with asymptomatic swelling in the groin. When the diagnosis of femoral artery aneurysms is made, evaluation of the aorta and popliteal vessels needs to be undertaken. Both CT and MR angiography can be helpful in the evaluation of lower extremity vessels for other sites of involvement. Significant limb-threatening complications are seen in only approximately 3% of patients.[30]

Profunda Femoris Artery Aneurysms

Aneurysms isolated to the profunda femoris are rare, accounting for only about 0.5% of cases of peripheral artery aneurysms.[31] Although rare, when present, there is a high complication rate at presentation of approximately 58% demonstrating distal embolisms and rupture.[32] Because there is little known about the natural history of aneurysms in this location and that they are not usually detected until quite large (owing to their deep location), surgical intervention is usually indicated even if an aneurysm is asymptomatic.

Superficial Femoral Artery Aneurysms

Isolated degenerative aneurysms of the superficial femoral artery (SFA) are also rare and make up only approximately 1% of all femoral aneurysms.[29] Again, there are a limited number of reported cases in the literature. As with all peripheral aneurysms of the lower extremities, SFA aneurysms may be complicated by thrombosis, distal embolization, and rupture.

Popliteal Artery Aneurysms

Aneurysms of the popliteal artery are uncommon but constitute the most common peripheral artery aneurysm. They make up approximately more than 70% of all peripheral aneurysms.[29] Although the exact prevalence and incidence of PAAs is not well established, they are strongly associated with the concomitant presence of AAA. The popliteal artery is a direct extension of the SFA as it exits through the adductor hiatus. Its location directly behind the knee in the popliteal fossa places it in a unique anatomic space in which it is subject to repetitive external compression from the adjacent adductor and gastrocnemius muscles as well as the femur. Its position in this tight anatomic space can produce popliteal artery entrapment syndrome (PAES). As in other locations, aneurysms of the popliteal artery are most commonly degenerative from chronic repetitive trauma.

Patients present with a variety of symptoms. It is estimated that asymptomatic PAAs can range as high as 37%.[33] Even in asymptomatic patients, the absence of distal pedal pulses often indicate silent distal embolic disease and usually results in a much less favorable evolution of PVD. In the remaining patients with PAA, limb ischemia is the leading presenting symptom in about 55% of cases with local compression accounting for 6.5% of cases, and ruptures only 1.4%.[33] The popliteal artery is considered to be aneurysmal when it exceeds a diameter of 7 mm. Clinical symptoms have a higher occurrence in aneurysms larger than 2 cm.

Duplex ultrasound is a very powerful tool in accurately diagnosing PAAs. Ultrasound can easily detect thrombus within popliteal aneurysms, which, depending on their chronicity, appear as varying echogenic material adhered to the vessel wall. Because of its accuracy, ultrasound is a more cost-effective imaging modality when compared to comparably accurate cross-sectional imaging, such as MR and CT angiography. Ultrasound also offers advantages over diagnostic angiography in that the true extent of a thrombosed aneurysmal sac can be visualized. In most cases, angiography will only image the residual flow lumen in a partially thrombosed PAA.[34]

Traditionally, surgical techniques for treatment for PAA have been proximal ligation with bypass reconstruction with either harvested vein or synthetic grafts. Important factors in employing this treatment algorithm are evaluating the conditions of inflow and outflow channels that determine the long-term durability of any bypass. More recently, endovascular techniques with the placement of covered stent-grafts has gained favor, especially in patients with a risk of operative morbidity. Regardless of the technique used, operators must be cognizant of the possibility of dislodging existing thrombus in partially occluded PAA, which can worsen distal limb ischemia and lead to devastating tissue loss. When this occurs, catheter-directed thrombolysis is indicated and can more easily and speedily be deployed in the setting of endovascular repair of PAA.

Clinical Case Correlation

Case 1: PAA as a source of microemboli:

This is a 74-year-old man who presented with extreme calf pain and a cyanotic right. Although ABIs could not be obtained secondary to noncompressible vessels, the PVRs to the level of the ankle were normal (FIGURE 78.2A). Subsequent CTA (FIGURE 78.2B) demonstrated a large PAA. An angiogram (FIGURE 78.2C) taken immediately before endovascular aneurysm repair demonstrates the relatively preserved runoff.

Tibial Artery Aneurysms

Aneurysms of the tibial vessels are exceedingly rare and typically caused by traumatic pseudoaneurysms. Traumatic etiologies that should be considered are fractures, iatrogenic injury from external fixation of fractures, and gunshot wounds. Bone tumors can also be included in the differential diagnosis. Symptoms are usually absent, especially because these aneurysms can be small. As with other peripheral aneurysms, duplex ultrasound is usually the first deployed imaging tool with digital subtraction angiography performed to confirm the diagnosis. Management of these aneurysms is surgical ligation with occasional reconstruction.

Anatomic Vascular Variants

Persistent Sciatic Arteries

An uncommon, but important, diagnostic consideration in the evaluation of peripheral embolic disease is the presence of vascular anomalies, such as PSAs. The existence of this anomaly

was first described in 1831 with an overall incidence of 0.01% to 0.06%.[35,36] Embryologically, circulation to the developing lower extremities starts from the dorsal root of the umbilical artery, running along the dorsal surface of the limb bud as the thigh, knee, and leg form.[37] As the native femoral artery continues to develop, it becomes the dominant ventral vascular channel. The growing femoral artery stimulates capillary plexi that connect it to the external iliac artery. This developing connection signals the sciatic artery to being its involution.[38] Portions of the sciatic artery due persist as the inferior gluteal, popliteal, and peroneal arteries. If the femoral artery does not develop appropriately, the sciatic artery remains running through the posterior compartment of the lower extremity, eventually giving rise to the popliteal artery.

There are two main types of PSAs. A complete type occurs when the sciatic artery is the primary arterial circulation to the lower extremity and exists in direct continuity with the popliteal artery. In this instance, there is an absent femoral pulse with a strong popliteal pulse. The incomplete type has no connection with the popliteal artery. Distal circulation is achieved through collateral pathways.[39]

Aneurysms of PSA is common with an incidence of approximately 15%.[37] Aneurysms are commonly located under the gluteal muscle at the level of the greater trochanter where it is prone to repetitive trauma and aneurysm formation. As in all cases of peripheral embolic disease from aneurysm emboli, treatment is strongly influenced by the type of PSA and the severity of limb ischemia. The incomplete type of PSA usually does not require revascularization if the extent of collateral circulation is sufficiently preserved. In the complete type, revascularization either by surgical or endovascular techniques is needed, especially as primary prevention of further embolic phenomenon.

Clinical Case Correlation

Case 2: Persistent sciatic artery presenting with macro- and microembolic emboli.

This is a 65-year-old woman who presented with left foot discoloration. The patient reported 4 days of progressively increasing pain and burning in her foot, which now has become severe. Noninvasive imaging (FIGURE 78.1A) demonstrates mild femoral popliteal and moderate tibial occlusive disease. CT images (FIGURES 78.1B, C) reveal an embolic source from a persistent sciatic artery aneurysm. Tibial occlusions secondary to emboli are evident on the subsequent angiogram (3d).

▌ UPPER EXTREMITIES

Peripheral Artery Aneurysms of the Upper Extremities

Subclavian Arteries

Aneurysms of the upper extremity are much less common compared to the incidence in the lower extremities. Their diagnosis and treatment is important because embolisms in the upper extremities can cause major disability, limb and digit loss, and can result in death if rupture occurs. Aneurysms of the subclavian artery arise from three main etiologies that include degenerative disease, thoracic outlet obstruction, and trauma. Approximately 30% to 50% of patients presenting with subclavian artery aneurysms also have aortoiliac or other peripheral aneurysms.[40]

Patients can present with a variety of symptoms including chest, neck, and/or shoulder pain from acute expansion of the arterial wall or from rupture. Patients can also experience acute and chronic ischemic symptoms from multiple episodes of distal embolization. Distal retrograde embolic disease can be seen in the carotid and vertebral arteries, leading to transient ischemic attacks and stroke. Compressive symptoms are also seen leading to upper extremity pain, neurologic dysfunction if the brachial plexus is affected, and hoarseness when the recurrent laryngeal nerve is impinged. Patients can experience respiratory insufficiency from tracheal compression. When aneurysms are large enough, they can erode into the adjacent lung apex to cause hemoptysis.[41]

Physical exam findings include the presence of a supraclavicular bruit, absent or diminished upper extremity pulses, normal pulses with signs of microemboli similar to that seen in BTS, and sensory and motor dysfunction from compression of the brachial plexus. Diagnosis should be confirmed with imaging. Ultrasound and CT are valuable in establishing an accurate diagnosis. It is important to always also include an evaluation of the aortic arch in upper extremity imaging to completely delineate the extent of the aneurysm. Because of the potential for significant disability associated when there is loss of function in the upper extremity, prompt surgical treatment is usually necessary with proximal ligation used in combination with bypass reconstruction.

Subclavian-Axillary Arteries—Thoracic Arterial Outlet Compression

Complications for thoracic outlet syndrome are uncommon but usually seen in younger women. Arterial injury is generally the result of osseous anomalies or exaggerated development of shoulder girdle muscles that cause compression and repetitive trauma on the underlying arterial vasculature.[42] Diagnosis and prompt intervention are needed to prevent potential severe debilitating limb loss. Aneurysms that can lead to distal embolic disease related to this group of disorders are usually located at the junction between the subclavian and axillary arteries.

The most common cause of arterial aneurysms associated with thoracic arterial outlet compression (TAOC) is the presence of cervical ribs followed by compression caused by hypertrophied anterior scalene muscle. Arterial compression from the pectoralis minor tendon and even the humeral head can also lead to degenerative aneurysms of the subclavian-axillary arteries. Other sources of compression include the clavicle and fibrocartilaginous bands. Besides the symptoms of digit ischemia from distal embolisms, symptoms caused by compression of the adjacent neurologic and venous structures are also common.

The diagnosis and treatment in patients with TAOC starts with ultrasound and CT or MR angiographic evaluation to determine the arteries involved and the extent of injury. It is important to realize that in neutral positions, the offending compression is often not identified. For this reason, diagnostic imaging in suspected cases of outlet obstruction requires that patients be scanned in varying positional views (abduction-external rotation or hyperabduction) to demonstrate the actual source of compression.[42]

A special subset of patients in whom disorders of thoracic outlet obstruction should be routinely excluded is in high-performance athletes. Athletes who perform rigorous repetitive shoulder motion can develop TAOC. In these patients, bony anomalies are less commonly the cause of injury. Instead, hypertrophy of the pectoralis minor and anterior scalene muscles is more often the cause.[43] Athletes also suffer compression

secondary to the humeral head, especially in the throwing motion of pitchers. Other athletes to be considered are those engaged in golf, handball, Frisbee, kayaking, and weight lifting. An early and important sign of injury to the arterial system to look out for is early fatigue of the upper extremity in a conditioned athlete.[43] When diagnosis is accomplished early, retraining with respect to changes in the mechanics of their repetitive motions is highly effective. Surgical intervention is usually reserved for those with more advanced stages of upper extremity and hand ischemia.

Treatment needs to be geared at effectively relieving the source of arterial compression, which can include complete resection of bony, cartilaginous, and fibrous portions of a cervical rib where it attaches to the first thoracic rib as well as complete resection of the anterior scalene muscle. Endovascular and surgical techniques also focus on revascularization of affected arteries to promptly restore distal circulation to maintain limb viability.

Ulnar Arteries—Hypothenar Hammer Syndrome

Aneurysms of the ulnar artery are mostly commonly found in men younger than 50 years of age.[41] Although rare, ulnar artery aneurysms are a common cause of peripheral limb ischemia limited to the digits of the hand. Prompt diagnosis and early intervention are important to prevent digit necrosis and severe disability. This syndrome develops in patients who use their palms for pushing, pounding, or excessive twisting. This disorder can also be seen in athletes who undergo repetitive trauma to the hand, such as in volleyball, skiing, cycling, and martial arts.

The pathophysiology is based on the vascular anatomy of the hand in which the ulnar artery and nerve enter the hand through Guyon canal, defined by a medial border of the pisiform bone, dorsally by the transverse carpal ligament, and superficially by the volar carpal ligament. In this anatomic space, portions of the ulnar artery lie anterior to the hook of the hamate and is covered only by the palmaris brevis muscle and overlying skin and subcutaneous tissue.[44–46] With little protection from adjacent structures as well as that the artery is fixed by the course of its deep branches, chronic compression leads to arterial degeneration, which can form thrombus and fragment embolic material distally into the digits.[41] It has been shown that damage to the intima alone results in vessel thrombosis, but that injury to the arterial media results in aneurysm formation.

Although the syndrome typically involves chronic repetitive trauma, cases have been reported in which a single acute event has led to digit embolism. At the time of injury, patients often complain of pain and tenderness over the hypothenar eminence. Ischemic changes will typically follow after weeks or months from the initial injury. Ischemic signs include pain, cold sensation, paresthesias, cyanosis, and mottling of the digits. Anatomically the fourth and fifth digits are most commonly affected, but any digit can be involved with the exception of the thumb.

Diagnostic imaging evaluation should include digital plethysmography, Doppler digital pressures, and duplex ultrasound. This is a unique syndrome in which conventional angiography is often mandated to most accurately map out the vascular beds affected. Angiography will show luminal irregularity, aneurysmal dilatation, or occlusion of the ulnar artery, which is pathognomonic for the disorder. Treatment is surgical revascularization with or without ligation of the ulnar artery to preserve flow to the digits. Microsurgical reconstruction can be accomplished but is usually reserved for patients with poor collateral pathways.

Clinical Case Correlation

Case 3: Microemboli to the hand as a result of hypothenar hammer syndrome

This is a 46-year-old man who presented with painful, discolored third and fourth digits of the left hand following a long bike ride (riding style was outstretched hands on the handlebars). Upper extremity PVRs (FIGURE 78.4A) demonstrate the typical, normal appearance with microembolic disease. Left-sided depressed finger waveforms (FIGURE 78.4B) correspond to the asymmetrically affected digits on physical exam. MRA imaging (FIGURE 78.4C) demonstrates a small aneurysm of the ulnar artery and the occlusion of the digital arteries to the third and fourth digits. The ulnar artery aneurysm was subsequently resected.

Fibromuscular Dysplasia

Fibromuscular dysplasia (FMD) is a well-established non-inflammatory, fibrotic tissue proliferation occurring within arterial walls. It is an uncommon disorder predominantly affecting younger women and most often involving the renal and carotid arteries. It can uncommonly present with hand ischemia secondary to distal emboli typically when it affects the brachial arteries.[47]

The affected arterial walls are segmentally thickened with areas of multifocal aneurysmal dilatation. It is associated with marked medial smooth muscle hypertrophy and elastic tissue deposition in the adventitia of affected vascular beds. Angiography is typified by multiple constricting lesions interspersed with areas of aneurysms. Thrombus formation within these aneurysms is the source of distal embolic material.

The definitive treatment of FMD involving long segments of vessels is surgical excision with bypass reconstruction to allow

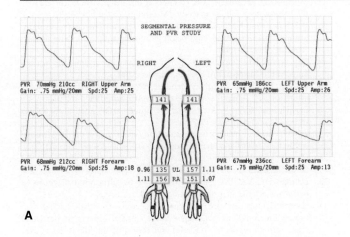

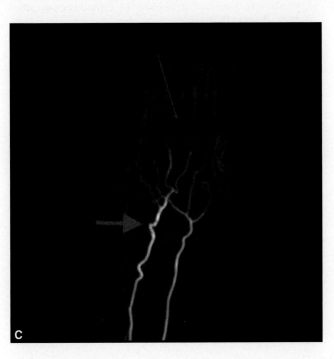

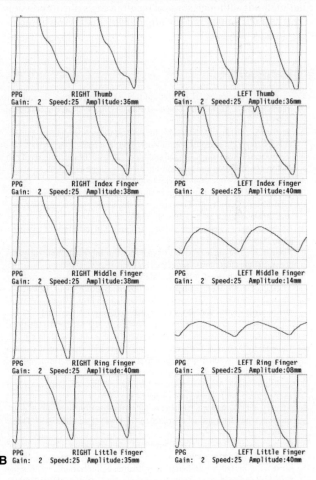

FIGURE 78.4 **A.** Noninvasive pulse volume recordings demonstrating no significant abnormality in the upper extremities. **B.** Noninvasive digital plethysmography reveals depressed finger waveforms in the third and fourth digits, which correspond to the affected digits on physical exam. **C.** Time-resolved contrast-enhanced MR angiogram demonstrates a small aneurysm of the ulnar artery (*large arrow*) and occlusion of the digital arteries to the third and fourth digits (*small arrow*).

restoration of normal circulation while eliminating the bed of embolic source. Short-segment disease can be amenable to percutaneous transluminal angioplasty (PTA), which is the treatment of choice in the renal arteries as well to disrupt the areas of fibrotic stricturing.

▌CONCLUSION

As can be seen with all types of embolic sources leading to peripheral artery occlusions, the initial presentation is hardly a diagnostic dilemma if macroembolization has occurred. one must remain aware, however, that microembolization can have maintained distal pulses. Digital noninvasive imaging can frequently help to confirm the diagnosis in these cases. Once diagnosed, a search for the underlying source lesion must be undertaken. CT and MRI can often be helpful to achieve this goal.

Once the source of embolic lesion and the extent of vascular occlusion have been determined, treatment can be initiated. Frequently, lesions can be successfully treated through endovascular methods, although surgical repair in cases of compression at the thoracic outlet and for ulnar artery aneurysms remains the standard.

▌REFERENCES

1. Leon LR Jr, Rodriguez HE, Labropoulos N. Arterial occlusion: thrombotic versus embolic. In: *Vascular Diagnosis*. Philadelphia, PA: Elsevier Saunders; 2005.
2. Fecteau SR, Darling RC III, Roddy SP. Arterial thromboembolism. In: *Vascular Surgery*. Philadelphia, PA: Elsevier Saunders; 2005.
3. Becquemin J, Kovarsky S. Arterial emboli of the lower limbs: analysis of risk factors for mortality and amputation. *Ann Vasc Surg* 1995;9:S32.
4. Moynihan B. An operation for embolus. *BMJ* 1907;2:823.
5. Murray D. The use of heparin in thrombosis. *Ann Surg* 1938;108:163.
6. Crawford E, DeBakey M. The retrograde flush procedure in embolectomy and thrombectomy. *Surgery* 1956;40:737.
7. Keely J, Rooney J. Retrograde milking: an adjunct in technique of embolectomy. *Ann Surg* 1951;134:1022.
8. Dale W. Endovascular suction catheters: for thrombectomy and embolectomy. *J Thorac Cardiovasc Surg* 1962;44:557.
9. Blaisdell FW, Steele M, Allen RE. Management of acute lower extremity arterial ischemia due to embolism and thrombosis. *Surgery* 1978;84:822.
10. Shah D, Leather RP. Arterioarterial atherothrombotic microemboli of the lower limb. In: Veith FJ, Hobson RW, William RA, et al, eds. *Vascular Surgery: Principles and Practice*. New York, NY: McGraw-Hill;1994: 397–408.
11. Carvajal JA, Anderson WR, Weiss L, et al. Atheroembolisms: an etiological factor in renal insufficiency, gastrointestinal hemorrhages, and peripheral vascular disease. *Arch Intern Med* 1977;119:593.
12. Hollenhorst RW. Vascular status of patients who have cholesterol emboli in the retina. *Am J Ophthalmol* 1966;61:1159.
13. Maurizi CP, Barker AE, Trueheart RE. Atheromatous emboli: a postmortem study with special reference to the lower extremities. *Arch Pathol* 1968;86:528.
14. Kempczinski R. Lower-extremity emboli from ulcerating atherosclerotic plaques. *JAMA* 1979;241:807.
15. Gore I, Collins DP. Spontaneous atheromatous embolization: review of the literature and a report of 16 additional cases. *Am J Clin Pathol* 1960;33:416.
16. Jose DB, Iannaccone PM. Atheromatous emboli in renal biopsies: an ultrastructural study. *Am J Pathol* 1975;78:261.
17. Blauth CI, Cosgrove DM, Webb BW, et al. Atheroembolism from the ascending aorta: an emerging problem in cardiac surgery. *J Thorac Cardiovasc Surg* 1992;103:1104.
18. Abbott W, Maloney R, McCabe C, et al. Arterial embolism: a 44-year perspective. *Am J Surg* 1982;143:460.
19. Pipkin R, Buch W, Fogarty T. Evaluation of aortic valve replacement with porcine xenograft without long-term anticoagulation. *J Thorac Cardiovasc Surg* 1976;71:179.
20. Ward R, Jones D, Haponik EF. Paradoxical embolism: an under-recognized problem. *Chest* 1995;108:549.
21. Darling R, Austen W, Linton R. Arterial embolism. *Surg Gynecol Obstet* 1967;124:106.
22. Rutherford R. Acute limb ischemia: clinical assessment and standards of reporting. *Semin Vasc Surg* 1992;5:4.
23. Rutherford R, Flanigan D, Gupta S, et al. Suggested standards for reports dealing with lower extremity ischemia. *J Vasc Surg* 1986;64:80.
24. Brewer ML, Malonnie LK, Perler BA, et al. Blue toe syndrome: treatment with anticoagulants and delayed percutaneous transluminal angioplasty. *Radiology* 1988;166:31.
25. Kumpe DA, Zwerdlinger S, Griffin DJ. Blue digit syndrome: treatment with percutaneous transluminal angioplasty. *Radiology* 1988;166:37.
26. Matchett WJ, McFarland DR, Eidt JF, et al. Blue toe syndrome: treatment with intra-arterial stents and review of therapies. *J Vasc Interv Radiol* 2000;11:585.
27. Murphy KD, Encarnacion CE, Le VA, et al. Iliac artery stent placement with the Palmaz stent: follow-up study. *J Vasc Interv Radiol* 1995;6:321.
28. Bosch JL, Hunink MG. Meta-analysis of the results of percutaneous transluminal angioplasty and stent placement for aortoiliac occlusive disease. *Radiology* 1997;204:87.
29. Van Bockel JH, Hamming JF. Lower extremity aneurysms. In: *Vascular Surgery*. Philadelphia, PA: Elsevier Saunders; 2005.
30. Graham LM, Zelenock GB, Whitehouse WM, et al. Clinical significance of arteriosclerotic femoral artery aneurysms. *Arch Surg* 1980;115:502.
31. Levi N, Schroeder TV. Arteriosclerotic femoral artery aneurysms: a short review. *J Cardiovasc Surg* 1997;38:335.
32. Yahel J, Witz M. Isolated true atherosclerotic aneurysms of the deep femoral artery. Case report and literature review. *J Cardiovasc Surg* 1996;37:17.
33. Dawson I, Sie RB, van Bockel JH. Atherosclerotic popliteal aneurysm. *Br J Surg* 1997;84:293.
34. Nelman HL, Yao JST, Silver TM. Gray-scale ultrasound diagnosis of peripheral arterial aneurysms. *Radiology* 1979;130:413.
35. Green PH. On a new variety of the femoral artery. *Lancet* 1831;1:730.
36. Bower EB, Smullens SN, Parke WW. Clinical aspects of persistent sciatic artery: report of two cases and review of the literature. *Surgery* 1977;81:558.
37. Thomas ML, Blakeney CG, Browse NL. Arteriomegaly of persistent sciatic arteries. *Radiology* 1978;128:55.
38. Nicholson FL, Pastershank SP, Bharadwaj BB. Persistent primitive sciatic artery. *Radiology* 1977;122:687.
39. Binkert CA, Barton RE, Keller FS. SCVIR annual meeting film panel session: diagnosis and discussion of case 7. *J Vasc Interv Radiol* 2001;12:662.
40. Pairolero PC, Walls JT, Payne WS, et al. Subclavian-axillary artery aneurysms. *Surgery* 1981;90:757.
41. Clagett GP. Upper extremity aneurysms. In: *Vascular Surgery*. Philadelphia, PA: Elsevier Saunders; 2005.
42. Durham JR, Yao JST, Pearce WH, et al. Arterial injuries in the thoracic outlet syndromes. *J Vasc Surg* 1995;21:57.
43. McCarthy WJ, Yao JST, Schafer MF, et al. Upper extremity arterial injury in athletes. *J Vasc Surg* 1989;9:317.
44. Loring LA, Hallisey MJ. Arteriography and interventional therapy for diseases of the hand. *Radiographics* 1995;15:1299.
45. Modari B, McIrvine A. The hypothenar hammer syndrome. *J Vasc Surg* 2008;47:1350.
46. Smith JW. True aneurysms of traumatic origin in the palm. *Am J Surg* 1962;104:7.
47. Cheu HW, Mills JL. Digital artery embolization as a result of fibromuscular dysplasia of the brachial artery. *J Vasc Surg* 1991;14:225.

Vascular Complications in Solid Organ Transplantation Part 1: Liver Transplantation

SECTION XIII

Transplant-Related Vascular Diseases

Vascular Complications after Solid Organ Transplantation: Part 1: Liver Transplantation

WAEL E. SAAD

INTRODUCTION

Solid organ transplants include liver, renal, and pancreatic transplantation. Recipients of these transplanted organs represent a growing population worldwide. Vascular complications are not uncommon after solid organ transplantation and may lead to graft dysfunction and, ultimately, graft loss. Understanding the relative surgical anatomy, the causes and types of vascular complications, their presentation, and the options for therapy is important for managing solid organ transplant recipients. Endovascular management of these vascular complications also has had a growing role in managing these postoperative complications owing to the minimal invasiveness of the endovascular management and that these techniques usually do not preclude subsequent surgical bailout.

Liver transplantation, in particular, is a large and complex surgery with two inflows (arterial and portal) and the hepatic venous outflow and invariable surgical anatomy. The regulatory mechanism of the hepatic inflow (hepatic artery buffer response), if intact, adds to the complexity of the transplant's hemodynamics.

This chapter discusses the surgical anatomy, the postoperative vascular complications of liver transplantation, and the endovascular management options of these vascular complications. It is followed by another chapter discussing the vascular complications of renal and pancreatic transplants.

LIVER TRANSPLANTATION

Surgical Anatomy

Most complications after liver transplantation are related to the surgery and are not primary anatomic or pathologic issues related to the recipient or the donor graft.[1] Moreover, posttransplant vascular surgical anatomy is crucial to reporting of endovascular and surgical management of vascular complications. There are numerous variables in the vascular surgical anatomy.[1] This is caused by the varying surgical techniques, types of hepatic grafts, types of transplant surgeries and their complexities, and different requirements and sizes of donors (children vs. small adults vs. larger adults). A detailed anatomy discussion is beyond the scope of this chapter; however, basic surgical anatomy is described to introduce the principles of liver transplant surgical anatomy.

Arterial Surgical Anatomy

The posttransplant arterial supply to the hepatic graft is divided into two main categories: (1) conduits or jump-grafts and (2) end-to-end visceral anastomoses (FIGURE 79.1). The conduits can be subclassified according to the type (material) of the jump-graft/conduit and where the takeoff of the conduits are. Conduit materials usually include preserved arterial autologous grafts (iliac arteries usually) or venous conduits from cadaveric donors. Many other arteries and veins (even from the recipients) can be used, such as saphenous veins and radial arteries.[1] Classification of conduits based on anastomoses can be classified into infrarenal aortohepatic conduits (most common) or supraceliac aortohepatic conduits. Infrarenal aortohepatic conduits can be further classified into retroperitoneal anterior to the pancreas and posterior to the pancreas.[1] End-to-end visceral anastomoses are classified based on the source recipient artery, which can be the hepatic artery (most common), splenic artery, gastroduodenal artery (GDA), and replaced right hepatic artery off the recipient superior mesenteric artery (SMA) (FIGURE 79.2).[1]

Focal anatomic defects (hepatic artery stenoses, kinks, and/or dissections, for example) are subclassified according to the site relative to the anastomosis. This is especially practiced in the setting of hepatic artery stenosis (HAS) (see HAS and hepatic artery thrombosis (HAT) below) (FIGURE 79.3). The GDA can be ligated or can be left intact depending on the transplant surgeon's preferences.[1]

Portal Inflow Venous Surgical Anatomy

Portal venous surgical anatomy is usually not as complex and variable as is the arterial surgical anatomy. Commonly, it is an end-to-end recipient portal vein to donor portal vein anastomosis. The donor portal vein can be the main portal vein of a whole cadaveric graft or the right main portal vein or left portal vein of split grafts (whether living or deceased donor grafts). Another variable is the length of the donor stump in a whole graft. The stump may be long and intact from harvesting and this makes an easier end-to-end portal anastomosis that is somewhat a distance from the porta hepatis and the portal bifurcation. If the graft/donor portal vein stump is short or damaged during harvesting, however, the anastomosis can be very close or even involve the portal bifurcation. In that instance, portal vein stenoses can be complex and involve the portal bifurcation. Another variable on the recipient side of the portal circulation is the presence of preexisting (pretransplant) left-sided (mesenterico-renal, mesenterico-caval, gastrorenal, gastro-caval) portosystemic collaterals. These collaterals may persist despite a successful well-sized hepatic transplant. They are in existence because of the prior (pretransplant) portal hypertension. Obviously, the latter variable (existence of left-sided portosystemic collaterals) is part of the recipient's portal anatomy and not a "surgical" anatomic variable.

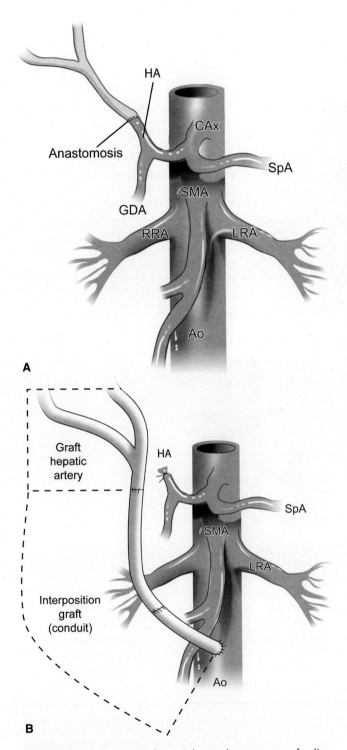

FIGURE 79.1 Basic surgical arterial vascular anatomy of a liver transplant comparing between an end-to-end hepatic artery anastomosis (**A**) and an infrarenal aortohepatic conduit (**B**).

Ao, abdominal aorta; CAx, celiac axis/trunk; SMA, superior mesenteric artery; LRA, left renal artery; RRA, right renal artery; SpA, splenic artery; HA, hepatic artery (recipient hepatic artery); GDA, gastroduodenal artery.

Hepatic Venous Outflow Surgical Anatomy

The hepatic graft venous outflow includes the hepatic veins proper and the donor and/or recipient vena cava. FIGURE 79.4 illustrates the varying hepatic venous outflow surgical anatomy.

Steno-Occlusive Complications of the Hepatic Artery

Occlusive or *steno-occlusive disease of hepatic artery* is a collective term referring to HAS, hepatic artery kinks (HAK), and HAT.[1,2] Additionally, a poorly described and rare entity is short-segment (<2 cm in length) hepatic artery occlusion without thrombosis. This hepatic artery occlusion is more like a long-segment 99% to 100% stenosis and not HAT. Steno-occlusive hepatic artery complications represent over 95% of arterial complications of the hepatic artery after liver transplantation.[1–5] In general, the incidence of posttransplant steno-occlusive hepatic artery complications probably depends on the degree and frequency of noninvasive imaging.[2] The more thorough the posttransplant imaging, the more likely the incidence of arterial complications will be documented, particularly HAS, and thus the incidence will probably rise within a particular institution. HAT is the most common at 58% of arterial complications, followed by HAS (31%), HAK (6%), and the rarely described short-segment hepatic artery occlusion.[1,2,5,6] HAS and HAK can progress to HAT,[2–4,6] implicating at least in part, that HAS and HAT are two contiguous components of the broader allograft ischemic spectrum.[2–4,7]

Hepatic Artery Stenosis

HAS occurs in 5% to 13% of liver transplants.[4,7–11] The incidence probably depends on the degree and frequency of noninvasive imaging.[1,2] The more thorough the posttransplant imaging, the more likely the incidence of HAS is going to rise within a particular institution. Hepatic artery stenoses are classified according to their location and multiplicity.[1–4,10,12] Location based classification is relative to the surgical anastomosis.[1–4,10,12] As a result, HAS is classified into (1) anastomotic HAS (A-HAS), occurring at the surgical anastomosis; (2) proximal HAS (P-HAS), occurring proximal to the surgical anastomosis in the recipient arteries; and (3) distal HAS (D-HAS), which occurs distal to the anastomosis in the graft or donor vessels (FIGURE 79.3C).[1–3] D-HAS can be subclassified into distal extrahepatic (main graft hepatic artery) and distal intrahepatic (branch graft hepatic artery) artery stenosis (FIGURE 79.3C).[1–3] The major etiologies of HAS based on location are demonstrated in FIGURE 79.5.

HAS usually is asymptomatic and is either detected and diagnosed incidentally by noninvasive imaging (Doppler ultrasound [DUS] or computed tomographic angiography [CTA] usually) or suspected by abnormal laboratory values representing liver function tests (LFTs). However, LFTs or even symptomatic graft dysfunction are not specific for HAS. In fact, hepatic graft dysfunction can represent a myriad of posttransplant hepatic graft complications, such as all vascular complications, biliary abnormalities, graft rejections, graft ischemia not related to anatomic vascular defects, and significant infections/sepsis. HAS less commonly presents as biliary strictures, biliary necrosis, or intrahepatic parenchymal breakdown and abscess formation.

In the setting of HAS, DUS demonstrates a tardus pravus ("blunted") waveform signified by a high acceleration time (>0.08 second) and a reduced or decreasing (decreasing trend over time) arterial resistive index (RI).[13,14] When using an arterial RI of less than 0.50 the sensitivity and specificity for detecting steno-occlusive hepatic arterial disease is 53% and 86%, respectively.[13,14] If the acceleration time (>0.08 second) is considered in combination to an RI less than 0.50, the sensitivity and specificity in detecting steno-occlusive disease become 53% and 86%, respectively.[14] However, in the current author's experience

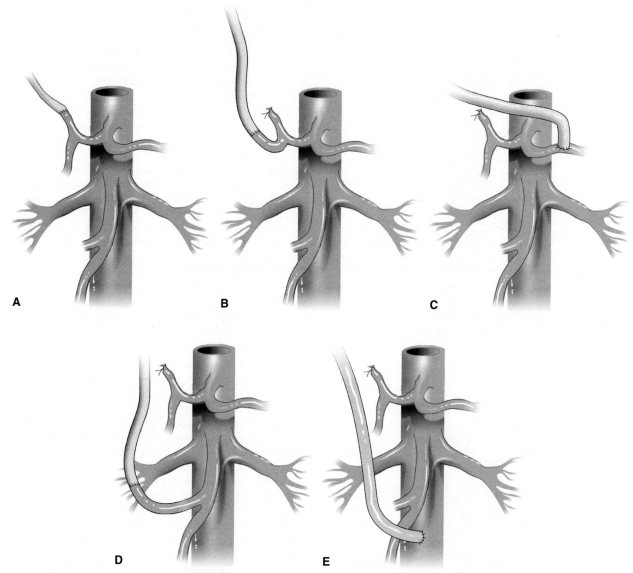

FIGURE 79.2 Varying surgical arterial vascular anatomy of a liver transplant. For labeling comparison please see FIGURE 79.1. **A.** Demonstrates straightforward end-to-end recipient hepatic artery to graft hepatic artery anastomosis. **B.** Demonstrates an end-to-end recipient gastroduodenal artery to graft hepatic artery anastomosis. **C.** Demonstrates an end-to-side recipient splenic artery to graft hepatic artery anastomosis. **D.** Demonstrates an end-to-end recipient replaced hepatic artery, which is off the recipient superior mesenteric artery to graft hepatic artery anastomosis. **E.** Demonstrates an infrarenal aortohepatic interposition graft/bypass. These can be anterior or posterior to the pancreas. Moreover, aorto-hepatic conduits can be supraceliac (not drawn).

accurately measuring the acceleration time is poor (poor intra- and interobserver agreement)[15]; and thus the arterial RI is used solely as a screening method for detecting hepatic arterial abnormality requiring further imaging, such as conventional angiography or CTA.[1,2,13] With multidetector technology, CTA (in patients with no renal dysfunction) has had an increasing role in evaluating for HAS after suspected DUS. Its advantages over angiography are that it is noninvasive and it evaluates beyond the artery, such as intrahepatic collections, possibly gross biliary abnormalities, as well as portal vein abnormalities, among others. However, unlike conventional angiography, it is not a dynamic study and, thus, it cannot detect flow/dynamic

abnormalities, such as splenic steal syndrome (nonocclusive hepatic artery hypoperfusion [NOHAH] syndrome) (*see below*).

There are no randomized studies to prove that management of HAS, whether surgically or by endovascular means, has an improved outcome on patient morbidity and/or graft survival. Such a study would be difficult to design, hard to implement, and require large subject numbers involving multiple centers enrolling study subjects over years. This is because of the relative rarity of the complication and the numerous surgical, anatomic, medical, and transplant-related variables that need to be considered for a comprehensive outcome analysis. Orons and coworkers[4] showed that poor liver function was a poor prognostic sign regardless of

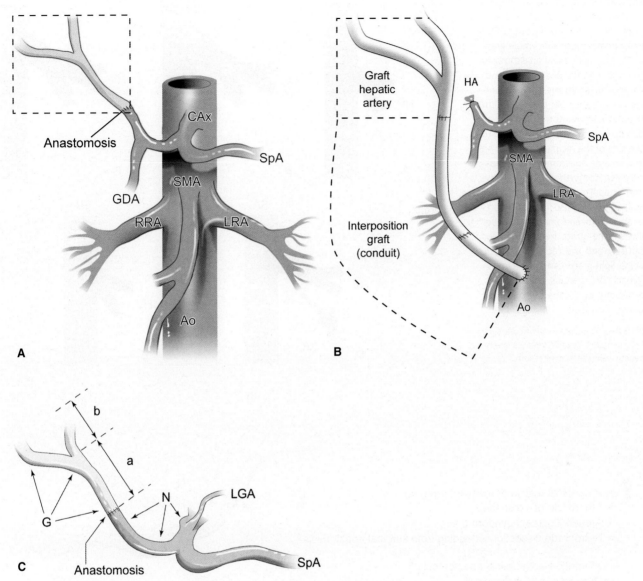

FIGURE 79.3 Basic surgical arterial vascular anatomy of a liver transplant comparing between an end-to-end hepatic artery anastomosis (**A**) and an infrarenal aortohepatic conduit (**B**). In addition, detailed surgical anatomic terminology for the hepatic artery is provided (**C**). **C.** Demonstrates an end-to-end anastomosis. Proximal to the surgical anastomosis (*anastomosis*) is the native (*N*) or recipient vasculature. Distal to the surgical anastomosis (*anastomosis*) is the donor or graft (*G*) vasculature. The graft (*G*) hepatic artery is subdivided into the extrahepatic hepatic artery (*a*) and the intrahepatic/branch hepatic arteries (*b*).

Ao, abdominal aorta; CAx, celiac axis/trunk; SMA, superior mesenteric artery; LRA, left renal artery; RRA, right renal artery; SpA, splenic artery; HA, hepatic artery (recipient hepatic artery); GDA, gastroduodenal artery; LGA, left gastric artery.

the success or failure of percutaneous transluminal angioplasty (PTA). This is contrary to the findings of an anecdotal case report prior to the work of Orons et al.[4] that showed resolution of initial hepatic dysfunction or intrahepatic parenchymal collections.[2,16–19] Another opinion, however, is to treat HAS regardless if symptoms are present in an attempt to reduce the risk of developing HAT, which may have a greater morbidity and a higher graft mortality.[1,2] Saad and coworkers[3] showed that HAT developed in 65% of patients with untreated HAS at 6 months, and that this was a greater than threefold thrombosis rate compared to treated (by PTA) HAS, which had a HAT rate of 19% at 6 months.

Traditionally, the treatment of HAS includes anticoagulation, surgical revascularization, and even retransplantation.[2,10,20–22] With the advent of low-profile endovascular therapy, angioplasty and/or stent placement has taken the larger share of managing HAS in the last 25 years.[2–4,6,8,10,16,17,19,23–28] FIGURE 79.6 demonstrates a straightforward hepatic artery angioplasty. Overall, the technical success rate of angioplasty is 80% to 81%.[2–4] Intraprocedural complications occur in 7% to 10% of cases and include arterial spasm (most common complications), arterial dissection (4% to 5% of cases), arterial perforation/rupture (2% to 5% of cases), and HAT (0% to 2% of cases).[2–4] When stratifying

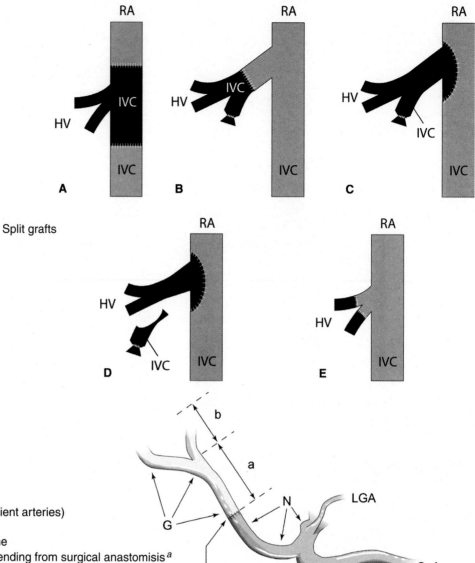

FIGURE 79.4 Variable venous vascular anatomy of a liver transplantation. **A.** An interposition caval anastomosis in a whole graft. **B, C.** Piggyback caval anastomoses for whole grafts: **B** is with an end-to-end anastomosis with the recipient hepatic vein after recipient hepatic vein venotomy, and **C** is an end-to-side with a graft patch to the side of the recipient cava. **D.** An end-to-side anastomosis with possible venotomy/triangulation of the graft hepatic venous outflow for split grafts. **E.** Also for split grafts is an end-to-end anastomosis between the graft hepatic venous outflow and the recipient hepatic veins. Split grafts can also have piggyback IVC venous anastomoses, especially right-lobe living related donor transplants.

Black IVC, donor inferior vena cava; Gray IVC, recipient inferior vena cava; HV, hepatic vein(s); RA, right atrium.

Proximal-HAS (native or recipient arteries)
- Atherosclerotic disease
- Arcuate ligament syndorme
- Retrograde dissection extending from surgical anastomisis [a]

Anastomotic-Has (surgical anastomosis) [a]
- Over-sewing/faulty sewing [a]
- Angulations between afferent (native) and efferent (graft) arteries [a]
- Focal intimal flap (focal dissection) [a]
- Proximal clamp injury [a]

Distal-Has (graft or donor arteries)
- Extrahepatic D-Has:
    Distal clamp injury [a]
    Retrograde dissection extending from surgical anastomosis [a]
- Intrahepatic/branch D-HAS
    Ischemia (compromise of the vasa vasorum)
    Graft rejection
    Graft infection

FIGURE 79.5 Demonstrates the celiac axis/trunk with an end-to-end anastomosis and the etiologies of hepatic artery stenosis (HAS) depending on lesion location. HAS that occurs at the surgical anastomosis are called anastomotic-HAS (A-HAS). Proximal to the surgical anastomosis (*anastomosis*) is the native (*N*) or recipient vasculature and HAS in these vessels are called proximal-HAS (P-HAS). Distal to the surgical anastomosis (*anastomosis*) is the donor or graft (*G*) vasculature and HAS in these vessels are called distal-HAS (D-HAS). The graft (*G*) hepatic artery is subdivided into the extrahepatic hepatic artery (*a*) and the intra-hepatic/branch hepatic arteries (*b*).

SpA, Splenic artery; LGA, Left gastric artery.
[a]Signifies surgical/technical etiologies.

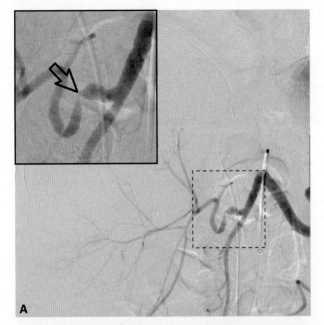

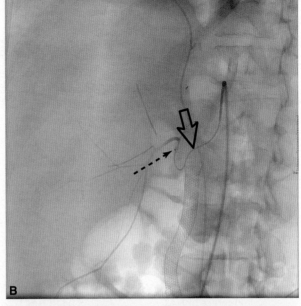

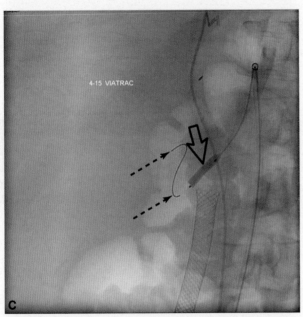

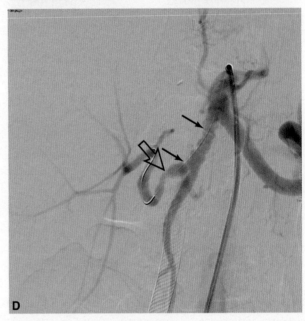

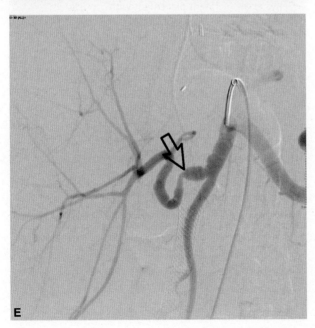

FIGURE 79.6 Balloon angioplasty of an anastomotic transplant hepatic artery stenosis (A-HAS). A. Initial celiac axis angiogram with magnified inset (*top left corner*) demonstrating a hepatic artery stenosis (HAS) at the surgical anastomosis (*hollow arrow*). A decision was made to perform a hepatic artery angioplasty. **B.** Fluoroscopic image showing a 2.7 French microcatheter (*dashed arrow*) has been advanced coaxially through the diagnostic angiographic catheter, which is also placed coaxially through a reinforced 5 French sheath. The hollow arrow points to the site of arterial narrowing (hepatic artery stenosis). **C.** Fluoroscopic image during balloon angioplasty of the anastomotic hepatic artery stenosis (*hollow arrow*). The 4-mm semicompliant balloon (*hollow arrow*) was inflated to 4.3 mm over a 0.014-inch stiff wire (*dashed arrows*). **D.** Postangioplasty digital subtraction angiogram of the celiac axis (trunk) via the reinforced sheath demonstrating a corrugated appearance to the recipient common hepatic artery due to spasm (*between solid arrows*). There is less than 30% residual stenosis (*hollow arrow*) at the anastomosis. The operator gave the patient 300 μg of intra-arterial nitroglycerin via the sheath, followed by 20 cc of warm 0.9% saline to help resolve the spasm. **E.** Completion digital subtraction angiogram of the celiac axis (trunk) via the reinforced sheath after removal of the wire and intra-arterial nitroglycerin injection demonstrating less spasm and the less than 30% residual stenosis at the anastomosis (*hollow arrow*).

Table 79.1

Technical Results from Angioplasty of Hepatic Artery Stenosis (HAS) Based on Multiplicity, HAS Locations, and Presence or Absence of Hepatic Arterial Kinks (HAK)

Lesion description and associations with HAK		Technical success rate	Complication rate
Presence of HAK	**HAS descriptions**		
No HAK	Solitary A-HAS	100%	0%
	Solitary D-HAS	80%	0%
No HAK	A-HAS (solitary or tandem)	100%	8%
	D-HAS (solitary or tandem)	85%	23%
No HAK	Solitary HAS (all locations)	95%	0%
	Tandem HAS (all locations)	90%	30%
No HAK	All HAS (without HAK)	94%	10%
Presence of HAK	All HAS (with HAK)	14%	29%
Overall results of all lesions (all comers)		**81%**	**7%**

Data from Saad WE. Management of hepatic artery steno occlusive complications after liver transplantation. *Tech Vasc Interv Radiol* 2007;10:207–220. Saad WE, Davies MG, Sahler LG, et al. Hepatic artery stenosis in liver transplant recipients: primary treatment with percutaneous transluminal angioplasty. *J Vasc Interv Radiol* 2005;16:795–805.

lesions according to multiplicity, location relative to the surgical anastomosis, and the presence of concomitant HAK, Saad et al.,[2,3] demonstrated that anastomotic lesions (solitary or in tandem) without HAK had a 95% to 100% technical success rate with a 0% to 8% complication rate (Table 79.1). This demonstrates that lesion selection or favorable surgical anatomy and HAS pathology in a particular institution is very important for improved technical results. Additionally, it is probably the reason for improved technical results is particular studies where the technical success rate ranges 93% to 100% and the complication rate ranges 0% to 6.7%.[8,27,28] In fact these three studies in particular did not mention the presence of HAK or the presence of tandem lesions.[8,27,28] The restenosis rate and HAT rate after angioplasty and/or stent placement range between 31% and 41% and 8% and 19%, respectively.[2,3,8,10,27,28] The 1-year primary unassisted patency and assisted patency range from 44% to 65% and 60% to 83%, respectively.[2,3,8,27,28] Saad et al. demonstrated that with selective lesions (no HAK and HAS predominantly anastomotic), the 1-year primary unassisted patency can be improved from 44% (all comers) versus 65% (selected cases).[2,3] Similarly, the primary assisted patency (repeat angioplasty) also improved with lesion selection from 60% (all comers) to 83% (selected cases).[2,3] The graft survival of patients with HAS and subsequent endovascular management exceeds 70% at 1 year.[2,3,8,27,28] Saad et al. demonstrated that the assisted patency of angioplasty with surgery as a bailout for complicated and/or failed angioplasty attempts was 74%.[2,3] Table 79.2 demonstrates the 6- to 12-month HAT rate after the treatment of HAS by angiography, stent placement, or surgical revascularization.

Hepatic Artery Kinks

HAK are arterial anatomic defects related to sharp bends in the hepatic arterial course.[2,3] HAK occur in 0.4% of liver transplants, 6% of abnormal hepatic angiograms, and represent up

Table 79.2

Hepatic Artery Thrombosis (HAT) Rate Following Different Treatment Methods (If Any) of Hepatic Artery Stenosis

Study	Treatment method (if any)	6- to 12-month HAT rate
Saad[2]	No treatment (no anticoagulation)	65%–74%[a]
Saad[2]	Primary angioplasty (no anticoagulation)	19%
Denys et al.[8]	Stent placement with anticoagulation	8%
Ueno et al.[28]	Stent placement with anticoagulation	14%
Saad[2]	Surgical revascularization	26%
Abassoglu[10]	Surgical revascularization	27%

[a]Seventy-four percent is when hepatic arterial kinks are included.

Data from Saad WE. Management of hepatic artery steno-occlusive complications after liver transplantation. *Tech Vasc Interv Radiol* 2007;10:207–220. Saad WE, Davies MG, Sahler LG, et al. Hepatic artery stenosis in liver transplant recipients: primary treatment with percutaneous transluminal angioplasty. *J Vasc Interv Radiol* 2005;16:795–805. Denys AL, Qonadli SD, Durand F, et al. Feasibility and effectiveness of using coronary stents in the treatment of hepatic artery stenosis after liver transplantation: preliminary report. *AJR Am J Roentgenol* 2002;178:1175–1179. Abassoglu O, Levy MF, Vodapally MS, et al. Hepatic artery stenosis after liver transplantation: incidence, presentation, treatment and long-term outcome. *Transplantation* 1997;63:250–255. Ueno T, Jones G, Martin A, et al. Clinical outcome from hepatic artery stenting in liver transplantation. *Liver Transpl* 2006;12:422–427.

to 13% to 19% of hepatic arterial defects.[2,3,5] HAK are less likely a result of outer compression caused by drains and are more commonly related to arterial redundancy.[2,3,22] Arterial redundancy is most commonly a technical problem (long/redundant donor and/or recipient arterial stumps) and are less commonly caused by hepatic graft growth and rotation. Significant HAK (significantly reducing arterial diameter >50%), if left alone without treatment, may progress to HAT as do HAS.[2,3] Saad[2] demonstrated that the 6-month HAT rate following untreated HAS only versus untreated HAS and/or HAK was 65% and 74%, respectively. As discussed previously, the presence of HAK can wreak havoc on the endovascular management procedure of HAS if HAS and HAK are associated (Table 79.1).[2,3] Saad et al.[3] also demonstrated that there is a learning curve for the endovascular management of HAS in transplant recipients and that institutions with less than 28 endovascular cases of HAS have a higher rate of complications (18% compared to 0%) and lower technical success rate (75% compared to 93%) compared to experiences that exceed 28 endovascular cases. They speculated that this learning curve was a result of lesion selection and possibly the avoidance of performing hepatic artery angioplasty on HAS that were associated with HAK (Table 79.1).[2,3]

If the cause of HAK is an adjacent drain that has contorted the hepatic artery (not common), then the removal or repositioning of the drain most likely will resolve the HAK.[2,3,22] If the HAK is not associated with an adjacent surgical or percutaneous drain, however, then anticoagulation or surgical revision are usually the best options.[2,3] The current authors do not advise the endovascular management of HAK without recognizing that it is a higher-risk procedure. The risks include recoil to simple angioplasty (high technical failure), arterial dissection, spasm and/or thrombosis.[2,3] If endovascular management is sought, the current author recommends a relatively long self-expanding coronary stent placement with or without a short balloon-expandable stent placed in the middle of the self-expanding stent. The two greater concerns when attempting to manage the HAK is arterial dissection when attempting to cross the HAK and propagation of the arterial kink to the ends of the deployed self-expanding stents.

Short-Segment Hepatic Artery Occlusion

This is rare and is the most underdescribed arterial complication after liver transplantation. Most are amalgamated with either HAS series or HAT series, and there is a good reason for that. It acts like a significant (>98% to 99% diameter reduction) and relatively long-segment (under 2 cm in length) HAS; however, it appears as a relatively short-segment (under 2 cm in length) occlusion that may be caused by HAT. Its etiology is unknown and we can only speculate the causes. Anecdotally, intrahepatic or branch hepatic artery lesions (most common locations) are more likely severe distal-HAS (FIGURE 79.5: D-HAS) due to vessel wall ischemia (vaso vasorum injury) or infections. Extrahepatic lesions (less common) would probably be short-segment thrombus or a focal ischemic injury. One may argue that this entity is a matter of semantics; however, in the author's opinion it should be identified and reported separately (at least disclosed) when reporting results of endovascular management of HAS and/or HAT. This is because these lesions are recalcitrant to balloon angioplasty and recoil immediately, requiring stent bailout. In other words, they are difficult lesions to treat with a high failure rate when reporting

the results of angioplasty alone. Conversely, they usually do not need catheter-directed pharmaco-fibrinolysis and resolve simply by stent placement. That is, they are easy "HAT" cases to treat because the "thrombosis," or better yet hepatic artery occlusion, may not be a true thrombus or may be an old localized clot that is easily treated with stent placement. This may very well be one of the more important reasons for why there are widely variable results for the endovascular management of HAT (see below).

Hepatic Artery Thrombosis

HAT is blood clot occlusion of the main hepatic artery and usually extends into or significantly reduces flow in the intrahepatic arterial branches. As mentioned earlier, short, less than 2-cm, occlusions may not necessarily be thrombus, but nonfocal (long segment) severe (occlusive or near-occlusive) HAS. HAT is the most common and usually most devastating of hepatic arterial complications. It represents 58% of arterial complications and is twice as likely to occur in pediatric recipients compared to adult whole graft recipients: 4% to 11% versus 11% to 26%, respectively.[2–5,12,29]

Most HAT cases present within the first 3 months after a transplant and can be classified into early HAT (within 30 days from transplant) or late HAT (after 30 days).[5–7,30,31] HAT can be asymptomatic and is either detected and diagnosed incidentally by noninvasive imaging (DUS or CTA usually) or suspected by abnormal laboratory values representing LFTs. However, LFTs or even symptomatic graft dysfunction are not specific (see above). If not clinically silent, there are three equally common ways HAT can clinically present. They include: (1) intermittant relapsing bacteremia, (2) biliary ischemia (biliary strictures, biliary cast syndrome, biliary necrosis), and (3) fulminant hepatic failure (rapidly deteriorating graft function).[7,23,32,33] Eventually, the most prevalent finding is biliary ischemic complications. HAT is associated with a high mortality rate of approximately 33% (ranging between 27% and 75%).[7,20,30–39] Despite having a higher incidence of HAT, pediatric transplants appear to do better than adult transplants in the setting of HAT[7,12,32,33,40] with an estimated mortality within the same institution of adults with HAT of 83% compared to 38% in children with HAT.[32,33] This most likely is due to better arterial collateralization in pediatric recipients. For years this theory hinged on the age-related ability of the pediatric recipient population to create arterial collaterals.[7,12] However, in recent years with the advent of living donor right lobe liver transplants, it appears that HAT is also tolerated by adult recipients. This brings further speculation as to the cause of increased arterial collaterals beyond the mere age of the recipients. The common denominator of pediatric transplants and adult living donor right lobe transplants is that they are split grafts. As a result, the speculative theories of increased collateral formation may hinge on split grafts and not only pediatric recipients. These theories include: (1) The cut surface of split graft has numerous severed arterioles and venules that may release angiogenesis mediators, which promote arterial neogenesis and collateral formation; (2) The cut surface of the liver heals by fibrosis, which may adhere to surrounding tissue and/or acts as a medium for entry of newly formed collaterals (no capsule) from adjacent structures (roux-en-Y loops and mesentery, omentum, upper gastrointestinal vessels); (3) The neohilum of the split graft is closer to the recipient's native vasculature (visceral arteries) and adjacent to the vascular omentum of the recipient.

HAT can be detected by CTA, which has a sensitivity, specificity, and accuracy for detecting HAS that exceeds 90%, 89%, and 95%, respectively.[13,30,34,35] The main diagnostic screening modality for evaluating for HAT is DUS, however.[13] HAT by DUS typically shows no intrahepatic arterial flow and has a sensitivity and negative predictive value of greater than 80% and greater than 90%, respectively.[12,13,41-45] However, due to arterial collateral formation, arterial flow can be detected and may even have a relatively "normal" arterial RI of 0.45 to 0.50.[12,41] Because of this, the radiologist and transplant service should be vigilant to accompanying ischemic findings, such as ischemic biliary complications, parenchymal perfusion defects by contrast-enhanced CT or magnetic resonance (MR), and/or intrahepatic fluid collections. These secondary radiographic findings may increase the sensitivity and specificity of imaging, as a whole, in diagnosing HAT. The mere presence of parenchymal abnormalities (including intrahepatic fluid collections) has a sensitivity for detecting HAT of greater than 80%.[46]

Despite the high morbidity associated with HAT, in recent years, prompt revascularization of the thrombosed graft has been described and this may salvage up to 70% of hepatic grafts with early HAT without hepatic parenchymal necrosis.[12] This, in conjunction with percutaneous biliary drainage and percutaneous fluid-collection drainage, may prolong allograft survival and temporize both recipient and graft to allow retransplantation in more favorable settings.[11,46-49] Transcatheter endovascular management of HAT may be an alternative or a prelude to prompt surgical revascularization.[6,19,25,30,31,40,50-62] Revascularization of the thrombosed hepatic artery by any means (endovascular or surgically) is mostly uncharted. The role of endovascular therapy is further unclear in the literature because the experience is scant, inconsistent, and thus largely anecdotal. Techniques, vascular anatomy, the status of the graft at time of therapy, and the time lapse between transplant and endovascular therapy (age of the thrombus) are some of the variables that are inconsistently reported. Furthermore, there is a definite mix of two separate vascular entities within the literature: (1) short-segment hepatic artery occlusion (not necessarily thrombosis, but may be coined HAT by reporting authors) treated simply by angioplasty/stent placement only (*please see above under: Short-Segment Hepatic Artery Occlusion*) and (2) true HAT with thrombus requiring thrombolysis with or without angioplasty/stent placement. Moreover, another variable that is not discussed in the literature that may have considerable impact on the outcome of thrombolysis of HAT is the varying anatomy between recipients with end-to-end hepatic artery anastomosis and aortohepatic conduits. Thrombolysis of aortohepatic conduits, all variables being the same, may (in theory) be easier to thrombolyse because the conduit in line with the hepatic artery vascular bed is an end artery and pharmacolytics have nowhere to go but into the liver. However, in the setting of end-to-end hepatic artery anastomoses off a branch of the celiac axis, administered phamacolytic agents may preferentially go to patent visceral arteries, such as the splenic artery, GDA, and/or left gastric artery.

The preceding is the current author's explanation for the significant disparity in the results of transcatheter endovascular therapy of "HAT or hepatic artery occlusion" in the literature (Table 79.3).[6,19,25,30,40,50-62] Table 79.3 summarizes the literature of endovascular management of HAT.[6,19,25,30,40,50-62] Overall, 75 "HAT cases" (an undisclosed number are short-segment focal

occlusions) have been reported with a definitive endovascular technical success rate of 62% (n = 47/76).[6,19,25,30,40,50-62] Three additional patients had successful surgical revascularization with excellent long-term results (artery patency and graft survival) (Table 79.3).[50,62] By the Kaplan-Meier method the intent-to-treat primary assisted patency of the hepatic arteries utilizing endovascular means only at 1, 3, 6, and 12 months was 54% ±4, 54% ±7, 48% ±8, and 48% ±10, respectively (Table 79.3).[6,19,25,30,40,50-62] Not all of these 76 cases are HAT proper and if focal/short-segment hepatic artery occlusion cases are excluded, such as in cases reported in the two studies of Cotroneo et al.[25] and Boyvat et al.,[59] the technical success rate for HAT proper will probably decrease. Moreover, operators who have technical successes are more likely to report their cases compared to operators who had failures. Furthermore, in the current author's opinion, the disparity of the results (Table 79.3, 0% to 100% success rates), the numerous variables, and the nonstandardization of reporting make it impossible to conclude the exact success rate as well as the anatomic and clinical applications of this practice. Saad et al.[50] anecdotally suggested that thrombolysis may be best applied for the management of HAT diagnosed 1 to 3 weeks to 1 to 3 months after the transplantation. Before 1 week (early postoperative period), there is an increased risk for bleeding and after 3 months from the transplant, the graft has a better chance tolerating HAT possibly due to collateralization.[50] In the 76 cases in the literature, 46 were performed within 21 days of the transplant with a hemorrhagic complication rate of 33% (n = 15/46), and all hemorrhagic complications reported (n = 15) occurring in HAT-thrombolysis cases were performed within 21 days of the transplant.[6,19,25,30,40,50-62] In addition (and just like other vascular surgical connections/conduits/grafts), finding an underlying anatomic defect (HAS and/or HAK) after resolving the thrombus and reestablishing hepatic arterial inline flow is cautiously a good sign (identifying an anatomic reason for thrombosis) rather than finding no reason (hemodynamic problem and/or hypercoagulable problem). Moreover, once an anatomic defect is unmasked after pharmacolysis, it must be resolved (either by endovascular means or surgical revascularization) to obtain definitive therapy.[50] Indeed, 30 of the 47 (64%) technically successful cases required balloon angioplasty (n = 4) or stent placement (n = 26) (Table 79.3).[6,19,25,30,40,50-62] Even in the face of failing to resolve underlying anatomic defects, reestablishing inline arterial flow to the graft allows time for the surgical team to mobilize and to plan for the most adequate revascularization (identifying anatomic defects and plan to how to resolve them surgically).[50]

Nonocclusive Hepatic Artery Hypoperfusion Syndrome (Splenic Steal Syndrome)

Splenic steal syndrome is a controversial diagnosis of hepatic artery hypoperfusion and is an under-recognized cause of graft ischemia.[63,64] Splenic steal syndrome presents nonspecifically as graft dysfunction (including ascites months after the liver transplant) that may progress to graft failure.[65,66] Its incidence ranges widely from 0.6% to 10.1% of liver transplant recipients[64,65,67-74] and has been treated in up to 26% of them.[73,74] The wide range in the incidence is possibly because of the lack of objective diagnostic imaging criteria. The author speculates that the condition is probably under-recognized in certain institutions and is probably overcalled in others. The gold standard diagnostic

Table 79.3

Technical and Anatomic Outcomes of Endovascular Therapy as a Definitive Treatment for Hepatic Artery Thrombosis

Study and year	Patients	Technical success	PTA or stent placement in successful cases	Patency
Zajko et al.,[40] 1985	$n = 1$	$n = 0/1$	NA	Failed ($n = 1$)
Hidalgo et al.,[51] 1989	$n = 2$	$n = 2/2$	PTA ($n = 2$), stents ($n = 0$)	<1 mo HAT ($n = 1$) >1 mo F/U ($n = 1$)
Raby et al.,[19] 1991	$n = 1$	$n = 0/1$	NA	Failed ($n = 1$)
Figueras et al.,[52] 1995	$n = 1$	$n = 1/1$	None ($n = 1$)	<1 mo F/U ($n = 1$)
Bjerkvik et al.,[53] 1995	$n = 1$	$n = 1/1$	PTA ($n = 1$)	Restenosed at 4 mo ($n = 1$)
Cotroneo et al.,[25] 2002	$n = 2$	$n = 2/2$	Stents ($n = 2$)	Re-HAT at 4 mo ($n = 1$) 18 mo F/U ($n = 1$)
Zhou et al.,[54] 2005	$n = 8$	$n = 8/8$	None ($n = 8$)	0–27mo F/U ($n = 8$)
Wang et al.,[55] 2006	$n = 9$	$n = 7/9$	Stents ($n = 6$), none ($n = 1$)	Failed ($n = 2$) Re-HAT <1 mo ($n = 1$) >1 mo F/U ($n = 6$)
Kim et al.,[56] 2006	$n = 2$	$n = 2/2$	None ($n = 2$)	>7 mo F/U ($n = 2$)
Li et al.,[57] 2007	$n = 9$	$n = 6/9$	Stents ($n = 5$), none ($n = 1$)	Failed ($n = 3$) >12 mo F/U ($n = 6$)
Saad et al.,[50] 2007	$n = 5$	$n = 0/5^a$	NA	Failed ($n = 5$)
Reyes-Corona et al.,[58] 2007	$n = 3$	$n = 3/3$	Stents ($n = 3$)	Re-HAT at 4 mo ($n = 1$) Restenosed at 12 mo ($n = 1$) Restenosed at 26 mo ($n = 1$)
Boyvat et al.,[59] 2008	$n = 9$	$n = 9/9$	Stents ($n = 9$)	<1 mo F/U ($n = 9$)
Yang et al.,[60] 2008	$n = 3$	$n = 2/3$	None ($n = 2$)	Failed ($n = 1$) Re-HAT <1 mo ($n = 1$) <1 mo F/U ($n = 1$)
Lopez et al.,[61] 2008	$n = 1$	$n = 1/1$	PTA ($n = 1$)	>8 mo F/U ($n = 1$)
Jeon et al.,[62] 2008	$n = 4$	$n = 1/4$	None ($n = 1$)	>1 mo F/U ($n = 1$)
Duffy et al.,[30] 2009	$n = 9$	$n = 1/9$	None ($n = 1$)	<1 mo F/U ($n = 1$)
Sabri et al.,[6] 2011	$n = 6$	$n = 1/6$	Stents ($n = 1$)	Restenosed at >3 mo then >17 mo F/U ($n = 1$)

HAT, hepatic artery thrombosis; PTA, percutaneous transluminal angioplasty; NA, not applicable. No technical successes from a definitive endovascular therapy standpoint; Re-HAT, rethrombosis of the hepatic artery after and initially successful procedure.

^{a}Saad et al. had four patients revascularized surgically after reestablishing inline arterial flow. These patients did well with a patency rate in all four patients exceeding 1 year following revascularization.

modality is angiography.[63–65,67–73] It is defined by sluggish flow in the hepatic artery (subjective slow flow in the hepatic artery relative to the flow in the splenic artery) in the absence of significant (>50% arterial diameter reduction) arterial anatomic defects, such as HAS and/or HAK.[63–65,67–73]

The most objective angiographic finding was described by Uflacker et al.,[68] who diagnosed splenic steal syndrome when there was visualization of the hepatic artery during the portal-venous phase of the angiogram. This finding represents very slow hepatic arterial flow and, in this case, the threshold may be set high, to the extent that the sensitivity of this angiographic finding is low.

Certain studies have evaluated the incidence of splenomegaly (>830 mL has a 75% accuracy), nominal splenic artery diameters (>4 mm is considered significant), and/or the ratio of the splenic artery to the hepatic artery (>1.5 is considered significant).[70,73] However, most transplant patients have had chronic cirrhosis prior to their transplantation and all these splenomegaly and splenomegaly-related findings are not uncommon.

DUS findings are not specific and are not consistently described in reported splenic steal syndrome cases.[66,72,75,76] The most common Doppler finding described is an abnormally high arterial RI (>0.80).[66,68,72,74–77] Not uncommonly, when Doppler parameters are mentioned, the RI of the hepatic artery is 1.00

due to reversed end-diastolic volume.[74,75,78] Self-limiting abnormally high RI in the immediate postoperative period, when many splenic steal syndrome cases are diagnosed, is not uncommon. Furthermore, the pathogenesis is not fully understood. However, it is theorized that there is increased resistance in the peripheral hepatic arterial bed in the early postoperative period.[72,75] Splenic steal syndrome is commonly (up to 82% of cases) described within 60 days of transplantation,[65,67,69,72,76,79] and some of these cases may have a splenic steal component to them.

Portal vein velocities are sporadically reported splenic steal syndrome cases. When reported, portal vein velocities have been valued at greater than 50 (up to 150) cm/second[66,74,76] (*see significance of this below*). However, portal vein velocities have also been reported between 13 and 37 cm/second.[72,78,80]

It is important to understand the hemodynamics of the splanchnic vasculature and the various hypotheses behind the cause of splenic steal syndrome. Unfortunately, the splanchnic hemodynamics are partly understood, and this adds to the difficulty in making this diagnosis. There is a controversy regarding the exact cause of the hepatic artery hypoperfusion in splenic steal syndrome. Initially when it was first described (1990–1993), it was considered a true arterial flow phenomenon with flow preferentially going to the splenic artery and being diverted from the hepatic artery (a true steal phenomenon); hence the original name of the syndrome.[81–84] Recently (in 2008) it has been proposed that the hepatic arterial hypoperfusion is in response to portal venous hyperperfusion, mediated by the hepatic arterial buffer response (HABR).[74,85] The authors who proposed this were rather dogmatic,[74] and for the past 3 years (2009–2011) their hypothesis for the etiology of "splenic steal syndrome" has gone undisputed.[71–73] However, the important finding of high portal venous velocity/flow could be a secondary effect or contributing effect and not necessarily the cause. The current author agrees with Quintini et al. that adequate response by occluding the splenic artery does not necessarily support the steal theory over the portal hyperperfusion theory because occluding the splenic artery leads to reduction of the portal venous flow.[72,74]

When considering hepatic artery hypoperfusion, there are two issues that were overlooked with the theory suggested by Quintini et al.[74] First is the gastroduodenal arterys (GDA) steal cases. GDA steal is a recognized steal phenomenon similar to splenic steal that represents up to 18% of steal cases in liver transplant recipients.[65,69,72,81,86] The current authors doubt that embolizing the GDA has a significant effect on the portal venous flow. As a result, one cannot explain that splenic steal syndrome is just a portal venous hyperperfusion phenomenon. Furthermore, Nishida et al.[77] described a GDA steal case with pre- and post-GDA ligation disclosing arterial DUS parameters. From pre- to post-GDA ligation: the peak systolic velocity (PSV) increased from 13 to 79 cm/second, the end diastolic velocity (EDV) increased from 0 to 23 cm/second, the mean arterial velocity (MAV) increased from 4 to 49 cm/second, and the RI decreased from 1.0 to 0.71.[77] These findings mimic those Doppler findings that are typical of post splenic artery embolization for splenic steal syndrome.[66,74,76] The second aspect that does not fit the Quintini hyperperfusion theory is that arterial steal phenomena (GDA and/or splenic) do not occur in liver transplant recipients with direct aortohepatic conduits/jump-grafts.[63,72] In fact, aortohepatic conduits/jump-grafts are a treatment of posttransplant arterial steal.[67,68,75,82] If the arterial hypoperfusion is in response to the portal hyperperfusion, then the arterial flow in the conduit should also respond to

splenic embolization. Unfortunately, there are so many variables affecting the splanchnic circulation that it is impossible to make any assertion as to the cause(s) of splenic steal syndrome.

The complexity of the hemodynamics of the splanchnic circulation can be simplified in the following manner (FIGURE 79.7). Simply, it is a partly reciprocal relationship between: (**A**) two arterial components in balance and (**B**) two venous components that are relative to one another. The arterial (**A**) and venous (**B**) components are intertwined/mediated by the partly reciprocal HABR. The details and hypotheses of the HABR are beyond the scope of this chapter.[87–91]

From the arterial standpoint, there is a hypothetical balance between the resistance of the splenic arterial bed and the resistance of the hepatic arterial bed (FIGURE 79.7). A low-resistant splenic bed relative to a higher-resistant hepatic bed would favor flow toward the spleen (splenic steal). This has been partly discussed by prior authors, where they proposed that causes of increased hepatic arterial resistance may aggravate the splenic steal condition.[63–65,68,69,75,77] Posttransplant conditions include: (1) poorly compliant graft, (2) large subcapsular hematoma, (3) postoperative edema, (4) preservation

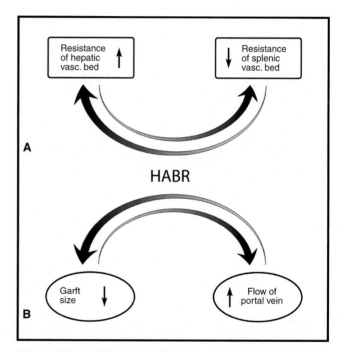

FIGURE 79.7 Influencing factors of the hepatic arterial inline flow (components of the nonocclusive hepatic artery hypoperfusion [NOHAH] syndrome). There is a partly reciprocal relationship between the arterial half (**A**, top half of illustration) and the porto-venous half (**B**, lower half of illustration) of the illustration. The reciprocal relationship is mediated by the hepatic artery buffer response (*HABR*). The arterial half of the system (**A**, top half of illustration) is a balance between the peripheral arterial resistance of the splenic vascular bed (*resistance of splenic vasc. bed*) and the hepatic vascular bed (*resistance of hepatic vasc. bed*). The porto-venous half of the system (**B**, lower half of illustration) is a balance between the size and quality of the hepatic graft and the degree of portal venous flow. The *arrows* in the eclipses and curved-corner boxes denote what would promote hepatic arterial hypoperfusion; in other words, promote NOHAH syndrome.

injury, (5) graft rejection, and (6) abdominal compartment syndrome.[63–65,68,69,75,77] Rarely have authors included HAS as a superadded condition causing increased hepatic arterial resistance and thus accentuating splenic steal syndrome.[65] The current authors, as do most prior authors, consider splenic steal syndrome and hemodynamically significant HAS (>50% diameter reduction) as mutually exclusive.[63,75,77]

From the portal venous standpoint, there is a relative balance between the portal venous inflow to the hepatic graft and the size of the graft. The problem can be an undersized graft or portal venous hyperperfusion, or both (it is relative). The relative portal venous hyperperfusion (hyperdynamic portal circulation), irrespective of the cause, would induce a reduction in the hepatic arterial inflow mediated by the HABR. Again, this has been partly proposed by prior authors.[72,74,92–95] Mogl et al. proposed that a known problem in split grafts, called undersized grafts (small-for-size-syndrome), where there is relative portal venous hyperperfusion, may induce arterial hypoperfusion mediated by the HABR.[9] They speculated that this phenomenon may exist in whole grafts where the portal inflow is relatively higher than the whole graft size.[72]

As can be deduced from the above and delineated by the illustration in FIGURE 79.7, all these variables are relative and the hemodynamic descriptions and associations in the literature are fragmented. No one study has proof of cause. However, this problem, with all its relative variables, has not been discussed globally as it is discussed here. We can only speculate that "splenic steal syndrome" may have several causes and, if certain causes predominate, there may be several types. Furthermore in the speculation, there may be predisposing factors, such as splenomegaly relative to hepatic graft size/quality with a dual hypoperfusion effect on the hepatic artery: (1) HABR-mediated response precipitated or accentuated by increased peripheral arterial resistance and (2) true arterial steal. Furthermore, there may be degrees of severity of this or these hypoperfusion phenomena. The current author does agree, however, with Quintini et al., in that "splenic artery steal syndrome" may be a misleading name because we are not sure whether it is actually a steal phenomenon in all cases or in none at all. The current author proposes a new name based on what we do know: Posttransplant "NOHAH syndrome" allowing all the potential and relative hypothetical causes to be included without a commitment to a particular concomitant finding, cause, predisposing/precipitating factors, and/or type.

Management of NOHAH syndrome is to attempt to identify the problem(s) and treat it. Careful evaluation of the celiac angiogram to look for underlying anatomic defects (HAS and/or HAK) is the first step.[63] Allograft rejection should be diagnosed by biopsy, immune-suppressant serum values, and clinical suspicion, and it should be managed medically. Large subcapsular hematomas should be evacuated or percutaneously decompressed. Abdominal compartment syndrome should be relieved by celiotomy. Unfortunately, other causes of increased hepatic arterial peripheral resistance are not easy to diagnose and manage.[63]

In cases of GDA steal syndrome, a lateral aortogram looking at significant SMA stenosis is required with resolution of the SMA stenosis with angioplasty/stenting or arcuate ligament release with or without GDA embolization.[63] Direct aortohepatic conduits/jump-grafts can also be utilized for any of the NOHAH syndrome cases.[67,68,75,82]

If there is preferential flow to the splenic artery, then methods at reducing flow to the splenic artery are utilized.[63–65,67–74] These include splenic artery banding, ligation, embolization, and, rarely, hour-glass stents.[63–65,67–74] Splenic artery ligation or banding are usually resorted to as prophylactic measures although they can be utilized if the diagnosis is made posttransplant.[73,74] Splenic artery embolization is the predominant method for reducing the preferential flow to the splenic artery and redirecting flow to the hepatic artery after transplantation.[63–65,67–74,81–83,86,96] The technical results are excellent and the risk of splenic infarction is minimized by embolizing the splenic artery proximally.[63–65,67–74,81–83,86,96] If the hepatic artery hypoperfusion is suspected along with hypersplenism (large spleen in the presence of pancytopenia, especially thrombocytopenia), graduated particular distal splenic artery embolization can be performed to reduce the size of the spleen, which also helps with the NOHAH syndrome. This particular embolization would utilize standard microcatheter techniques and available bland particulate embolic products. Usually two to three sessions are required to help reduce the splenic volume with decreased risk of splenic infarction with superadded abscess formation. Thirty percent to 40% of the spleen is embolized every session.[63]

Intrahepatic Arterial Injuries: Fistulae and Pseudoaneurysms

The causal relationship between intrahepatic arterial injuries and percutaneous procedures (such as liver biopsies and percutaneous transhepatic cholangiograms) is well described.[97–102] Of the 280 reported arterioportal fistulas (APF) in livers, 60% are directly associated with prior percutaneous procedures.[63,97,100,101] Arterial injuries resulting from percutaneous transhepatic procedures include: (1) parenchymal contusions, (2) active arterial bleeding, (3) intrahepatic pseudoaneurysms (PsA), and (4) arteriovenous fistulas.[63,97–101] The most prevalent (because it is the most enduring and insidious) injury is the APF. APFs represent 37%, 86%, and 100% of all arterial injuries immediately after a biopsy, 1 week after the biopsy, and 4 weeks after the biopsy, respectively.[97–99] Extrahepatic PsA are not included in this section with the intrahepatic PsA because their predisposing factors, etiology, prognosis, and management are completely different (*see next section below*). Intrahepatic PsA have similar etiology, prognoses, and management as other intrahepatic arterial injuries.[12,63]

Arterioportal Fistulas

This is the most prevalent intrahepatic arterial injury on the long-run (*see above*) and represents an iatrogenic communication between hepatic artery branch(es) and adjacent portal venous branch(es). They vary significantly from simple APFs (one arterial branch to one portal branch) to complex APFs with multiple arterial branches involved. They also vary considerably depending on through-put from the miniscule that is barely and accidentally noticed by imaging (angiograms and contrast-enhanced CT) to large hemodynamically significant APFs that alter the hemodynamics of the main branches of the portal vein and may alter the function of the hepatic graft.[102,103] In fact, most APFs are small, irrelevant, and asymptomatic and, as a result, they are most likely the least documented arterial complication.[63,103] APFs (significant or not) are found in 0% to 5.4% of abnormal angiograms in liver transplant recipients.[7,23,40,63,102] Up to 17%

of APFs detected by imaging are actually significant.[63,102] In a recent article, Saad et al.[103] demonstrated an incidence rate of significant APFs (hemodynamically significant with or without symptoms) in the general transplant population of 0.2%.[103] Additionally, there is speculation that APFs may be more prevalent in native livers compared to transplanted livers.[63,102,103]

Some APFs may heal and others may progress to large fistulas.[63,97,98,100,102] The reason why some progress and others heal is unknown, but the discrepancy in the APF incidence between transplants and native (nontransplanted) livers may shed light on this.[63,97,98,102] Figueras et al.[104] suggested that increased arterial flow might raise the risk of developing significant APFs. It has been speculated that the relative compromise of the arterial circulation in liver transplants relative to native livers may reduce the risk of APFs.[102] Furthermore, the relative "stiffness" or poor compliance of transplanted grafts may not allow tract formation, development, and growth.[102] It remains unclear how and why some arterial injuries develop into significant shunts and whether high tissue (parenchymal) compliance or low tissue compliance may be the higher risk. Furthermore, some native livers may be poorly compliant due to cirrhosis, chemoembolization, and liver fibrosis.

By angiography, an APF is defined as visualizing a portal venous radical adjacent to a hepatic arterial branch early in the arterial phase of the angiogram. A fistulous tract is usually not seen.[102,103] Hemodynamically significant APF by angiography are defined as visualizing (contrast enhancement) of the main portal vein or its first-order branch during a hepatic arteriogram.[102,103] By contrast-enhanced CT (CE-CT) the findings are similar. There also can be paucity of enhancing arteries in the vicinity (hepatic segment-s-) of the affected portal vein in the early arterial phase of the CE-CT. This represents the sump effect of the APF on the hepatic artery.[63] In the late arterial phase of the CE-CT, there is early portal venous enhancement of the parenchyma in the vicinity of the affected portal vein.[63] The affected liver segment is "ahead and out of synch" compared to the rest of the liver.[63] After successful embolization of the APF, all hepatic segments become in synch when it comes to arterial and porto-venous enhancement.[63]

DUS is a useful screening tool for vascular complications of liver transplants.[102] It only detects 50% of APFs; however, it does detect all hemodynamically significant APFs.[102] DUS findings of hemodynamically significant APFs include: reduced RIs of the hepatic artery, reversed flow in particular portal vein radicals (considered a rare finding,) and an arterialized portal vein waveform.[102] Occasionally a small focus of turbidity and Doppler aliasing is noticed at the exact site of the fistulous tract of the APF.[102] Features of hemodynamic significance of an APF by Doppler include reversal and/or arterialization of the portal flow in the main portal vein or its first-order branch.[63,102,103] After successful embolization of the APF, the DUS findings are reversed.[63] The endpoint of a successful APF embolization does not have to be complete obliteration of the APF by angiography and DUS, but to reduce the reversed arterialized portal venous flow (reversal of hemodynamically significant findings).[63,103]

Most APFs are asymptomatic.[63,97,98,100,102] APFs in transplanted and nontransplanted livers have been known to cause a variety of symptoms and clinical findings, such as portal hypertension, hemobilia, biliary obstruction, sepsis, pain, and even pulmonary hypertension.[63,100,102,104–111] In contrast to systemic arteriovenous fistulas, APFs have not been described as causing congestive heart failure[100] probably because the outflow is actually not systemic

but portal and the portal vascular bed acts as an impeding barrier that prevents "a short circuit" that leads to the hyperdynamic circulation leading to eventual congestive heart failure. Due to the rarity of the complication in transplants, we can only glean from the literature what these significant APFs present with. From 11 of the 13 cases of significant APFs in liver transplants with clinical detail, abnormal LFTs are the most common (64%, $n = 7/11$) presentation with or without other symptoms or findings, followed by bleeding (45%, $n = 5/11$) and pain (36%, $n = 4/11$).[100,103–111] The most likely source/presentation of bleeding is hemobilia (27%, $n = 3/11$). However, broadly, the most prevalent clinical character of APFs in transplants is graft dysfunction (73%, $n = 8/11$), which rises either in the LFTs only (45%, $n = 5/11$) or in LFTs accompanied by ascites (27%, $n = 3/11$).[100,103–111]

The indications for treatment of APFs remain unclear. However, the discovery of a high flow APF in a graft with signs of ischemia or other dysfunction should be considered for therapy. The options include open surgery or endovascular management. Traditionally, the management of APF was open surgery including segmentectomy, ligation, and retransplantation.[112,113] There appears to be a paradigm shift toward endovascular management in the last 10 to 15 years, however.[100,104–111] This is because the APF are located deep within the parenchyma, are most likely difficult to identify surgically, and require tedious surgical dissection with significant blood loss.[105,112,113] One of the 13 cases in this review underwent a failed surgery after a failed embolization attempt. The patient was subsequently retransplanted.[111] On evaluating the 13 cases in the literature, there were 16 attempts at embolization: 3 patients underwent 2 attempts, 2 cases were a success after the second attempt, and 1 case had a failed second attempt.[100,106] The cumulative technical success rate is 63% to 77% ($n = 10/13$ patients and $n = 10/16$ attempts) with a complication rate (intraprocedural HAT and dissection) of 12% to 15% ($n = 2/13$ cases and $n = 2/16$ attempts).[100,103–111] The 6-month graft loss in the 11 cases with follow-up is 36% ($n = 4/11$).[100,103–111]

The endovascular management of APF is more difficult compared to the APF in native (nontransplanted) livers. The hepatic graft is more susceptible to ischemia, and embolization should be used in the most selective catheterization as possible. The problem is that the fistulous tract is usually not seen (is very short) and, usually, embolization of the entire feeding artery is unavoidable. Endovascular case selection can be divided into high ischemic risk APF embolization compared to low ischemic risk APF embolization procedures. Smaller and more peripheral APFs are lower risk because if the small feeding artery is sacrificed (completely embolized) the ischemia will be confined to that particular region and intrahepatic arterial collaterals most likely will cover the ischemic segment or subsegment. If the APF is large and central, however, then sacrificing the involved artery (which is usually a major artery) would probably lead to a larger ischemic parenchymal volume of the graft. Furthermore, large through-put fistulas may make it difficult to embolize the fistula, specifically due to concerns for the embolic agent passing through the fistula, which may lead to portal vein branch thrombosis. Incidentally, portal vein branch thrombosis after APF has been described but without clinical consequences.[109] Due to the higher risk of embolizing large APFs (by requiring to block a larger arterial territory) and in addition to the ischemic steal phenomenon associated with large APFs, some authors advocate treating only those that are symptomatic or those that are progressing rapidly from a hemodynamic standpoint.[63,102] In fact, out of the 13 significant APFs in this review, 2 (15%) were not treated initially and were observed by DUS on a monthly basis showing progression of hemodynamic findings over 2.5 and 9 months.[103,110]

Intrahepatic Pseudoaneurysms

PsA in liver transplant recipients are classified into intrahepatic and extrahepatic.[63,114–118] Extrahepatic PsA are more common than intrahepatic PsA: 69% to 100% and 0% to 31% of all post-liver transplant PsA, respectively[114–118] (Table 79.4). By convention, intrahepatic PsA are iatrogenic (percutaneous transhepatic procedures, such as percutaneous transhepatic cholangiography and biopsies), and extrahepatic PsA are "spontaneous" and thus are not considered to be due to iatrogenic causes related to minimally invasive procedures, such as biopsies, percutaneous transhepatic cholangiograms, endoscopically placed biliary stents, and hepatic artery balloon angioplasty.[63,115] "Spontaneous" extrahepatic PsA are considered secondary to infection thought to be caused by postoperative infectious arteritis.[12,63] Intrahepatic PsA have the same etiology and management as APFs and have a better prognosis compared to extrahepatic PsA.[12,63,115] As a result of this, the intrahepatic PsA are placed in the intrahepatic arterial injury section and the extrahepatic PsA are discussed separately. Moreover, certain intrahepatic PsA can rupture into adjacent portal vein radicals, forming a complex injury with a PsA component and an APF component.[12,63] Conversely, an undisclosed percentage of intrahepatic PsA may be associated with intrahepatic infections.[12,63,115]

Management of intrahepatic PsA is similar to that of APFs. An ideal approach would be selective microcatheter embolization of

---

Table 79.4

Incidence of Intra- and Extrahepatic Pseudoaneurysms as a Percentage of All Posttransplant Hepatic Artery Pseudoaneurysms

Study	Intrahepatic pseudoaneurysm	Extrahepatic pseudoaneurysm
Kim et al.[114]	n = 0/13 (0%)	n = 13/13 (100%)
Marshall et al.[115]	n = 4/13 (31%)	n = 9/13 (69%)
Fistouris et al.[116]	n = 1/12 (13%)	n = 11/12 (87%)
Leelaudomlipi[117]	n = 0/8 (0%)	n = 8/8 (100%)
Harman[118]	n = 2/9 (22%)	n = 7/9 (78%)
Saad et al.[194]	n = 3/23 (13%)	n = 20/23 (87%)
Total of six studies	n = 10/78 (13%)	n = 68/78 (87%)

Data from Kim HJ, Kim KW, Kim AY, et al. Hepatic artery pseudoaneurysms in adult living-donor liver transplantation: efficacy of CT and Doppler sonography. *AJR Am J Roentgenol* 2005;184:1549–1555. Marshall MA, Muiesan P, Srinivasan P, et al. hepatic artery pseudoaneurysms following liver transplantation: incidence, presenting features and management. *Clin Radiol* 2001;56:579–587. Fistouris J, Herlenius L, Backman L, et al. Pseudoaneurysm of the hepatic artery following liver transplantation. *Transplant Proc* 2006;38:2679–2682. Leelaudomlipi SL, Bramhall SR, Gunson BK, et al. Hepatic-artery aneurysm in adult liver transplantation. *Transpl Int* 2003;16:257–261. Harman A, Boyvat F, Hasdogan B, et al. Endovascular treatment of active bleeding after liver transplant. *Exp Clin Transplant* 2007;5:1–4. Saad WE, Dasgupta N, Lippert AJ, Turba UC, et al. Extrahepatic pseudoaneurysms and ruptures of the hepatic artery in liver transplant recipients: endovascular management and a new iatrogenic etiology. *Cardiovasc Intervent Radiol.* 2013 Feb;36(1):118–27. doi: 10.1007/s00270-012-0408-y. Epub 2012 May 31.

---

the PsA sac itself with sparing of the injured/affected artery.[63] This is particularly important if the injured artery is large and central, and sparing of the arterial vasculature of the graft is paramount. However, if the injured artery is small, peripheral, and thus dispensable and the operator is unable to selectively catheterize the PsA itself, then embolization of the actual injured artery is performed both distally and proximally to prevent backfilling of the PsA sac by collaterals reconstituting the distal hepatic artery.[63] If the injured artery cannot be selectively catheterized or is only embolized proximally with backfilling for the distal artery, direct transhepatic needle puncture of the PsA sac under ultrasound (or, less likely, CT) guidance can be performed with obliteration of the sac utilizing, thrombin, coils, glue, or any combination of these embolic agents.[63] As always, the primary intention (best endpoint) is to treat the lesion with minimal collateral damage to the arterial vasculature of the graft.

Extrahepatic Arterial Rupture and/or Pseudoaneurysms

Extrahepatic disruption has been described as two entities reflecting the same posttransplant complication: either as a contained rupture (PsA) or an uncontained rupture (true rupture).[63] The two terms are used interchangeably in the transplant literature, with "PsA" being the more common term used.[5,22,114–139] Disruption of the extrahepatic graft artery after liver transplantation, whether termed PsA or rupture, is rare.[5,114–117,120–124] In 10 studies in the last 12 years evaluating a total of 7,328 consecutive liver transplants, 57 (0.8%) were observed (Table 79.5).[5,114–117,120–124] The range for each individual study is 0.4% to 2.5%.[5,114–117,120–124]

The etiology of extrahepatic PsA include infection (mycotic aneurysms or postoperative infectious arteritis) caused by bacterial contamination (predisposed by biliary leaks, biliary-enteric anastomoses, and repeat surgeries) or defective surgical techniques, leading to delayed rupture (dissecting PsA).[63,115,120,125,126,133] This classification is despite rare reports of iatrogenic extrahepatic PsA/ruptures being the result of minimal invasive procedures.[3,4,26,27,50,115,118,123,124,133,138–140] Several reports have described immediate (hepatic arterial rupture) or delayed (dissecting PsA) during or after hepatic artery angioplasty for the treatment of HAS or HAT.[3,4,26,27,50,115,118,138–140] In fact, hepatic artery angioplasty studies consistently place a rupture risk of approximately 5% (Table 79.6).[3,4,27] In addition, iatrogenic extrahepatic PsA have been described as a result of percutaneous biopsy[123,124] and endoscopically placed prostheses.[133] Unfortunately, most studies describing the management of iatrogenic extrahepatic PsA do not place their incidence within the broader hepatic artery PsA/rupture incidence by including the entire institutional transplant experience/population as a denominator nor by including "spontaneous" (not related to minimally invasive procedural iatrogenic injury) posttransplant PsA.[3,4,26,27,50,118,138–140] Harman et al.[118] studied eight extrahepatic posttransplant PsA. One (13%) of them was spontaneous and seven (87%) were iatrogenic from hepatic artery angioplasty.[118] Obviously, the ratio of iatrogenic versus spontaneous PsA would vary from one institution to the next depending on the extent of the transplant services utilization of the interventional radiologic and endoscopic services within the institution.

Extrahepatic PsA/rupture (historically spontaneous) have been associated with other pathologies in the hepatic artery and

Table 79.5

Incidence of Intra- and Extrahepatic Pseudoaneurysms as a Percentage of All Posttransplant Hepatic Artery Pseudoaneurysms

Study and year	Number of extrahepatic pseudoaneurysm (spontaneous)	Percentage (spontaneous)
Lowell et al.,[123] 1999	$n = 2/263$ ($n = 1/263$)	0.7% (0.4%)
Stange et al.,[124] 2000	$n = 6/964$ ($n = 5/964$)	0.6% (0.5%)
Marshall et al.,[115] 2001	$n = 9/1327$	0.7%
Leelaudomlipi et al.,[117] 2003	$n = 8/1575$	0.5%
Kim et al.,[114] 2005[a]	$n = 13/530$	2.5%[a]
Finley et al.,[121] 2005	$n = 2/200$	1.0%
Alamo et al.,[120] 2005	$n = 2/450$	0.4%
Jain et al.,[5] 2006	$n = 4/1000$	0.4%
Fistouris et al.,[116] 2006	$n = 11/825$	1.3%
Jones et al.,[122] 2008	$n = 2/194$	1.0%
Total of 10 studies	$n = 57/7,328$	0.8%

[a]This study involved 530 living related liver transplant recipients, both left and right lobe hepatic grafts.[114] Most of the grafts of the remaining studies are cadaveric whole grafts.[5, 114–117,120–124]

in the biliary tract.[114,115,117] Posttransplant hepatic artery PsA have been found to be associated with other vascular complications such as partial-HAT (15% to 22%), complete HAT (0% to 22%), and HAS (0% to 23%).[114,115] We can only speculate as to the etiology of associated HAT. There may be multiple factors, such as (1) external compression on the artery and secondary thrombosis, (2) partial thrombosis of the PsA with distal thromboembolization of the intrahepatic arterial branches, (3) flow phenomenon and turbulence due to the PsA predisposing to thrombus formation, and (4) HAT associated with sepsis, which is not uncommon with spontaneous PsA. In the

Table 79.6

Hepatic Artery Rupture Risk During Angioplasty for Managing of Hepatic Artery Stenosis

Study and year	Rupture per patient/artery	Rupture per angioplasty procedure
Orons et al.,[4] 1995	$n = 1/19$ (5.3%)	$n = 1/21$ (4.8%)
Saad et al.,[3] 2005	$n = 2/37$ (5.4%)	$n = 2/42$ (4.8%)
Kodama et al.,[27] 2006	$n = 1/18$ (5.6%)	$n = 1/24$ (4.2%)
Total 1995–2006	$n = 4/74$ (5.4%)	$n = 4/87$ (4.6%)

Data from Orons PD, Zajko AB, Bron KM, et al. Hepatic artery angioplasty after liver transplantation: experience in 21 allografts. *J Vasc Interv Radiol* 1995;6:523–529. Saad WE, Davies MG, Sahler LG, et al. Hepatic artery stenosis in liver transplant recipients: primary treatment with percutaneous transluminal angioplasty. *J Vasc Interv Radiol* 2005;16:795–805. Kodama Y, Sakuhara T, Abo D, et al. Percutaneous transluminal angioplasty for hepatic artery stenosis after liver donor liver transplantation. *Liver Transpl* 2006;12:465–469.

biliary tract, historically spontaneous extrahepatic PsA have had a higher association with biliary-enteric anastomoses, particularly constructed with a Roux-en-Y limb, with an incidence of 63% to 78%.[115,117] In fact, biliary-enteric anastomoses are considered to be predisposing factors for posttransplant spontaneous extrahepatic PsA.[115,117]

Posttransplant extrahepatic PsA present in various ways. The most common presentation is hypotension or hemodynamic instability, which occurs in 50% to 67% of cases, followed by gastrointestinal bleeding including hemobilia, which occur in 22% to 25% of cases, and no-specific symptoms/findings, if any (varying from sepsis, increased LFTs, and drop in hematocrit), which occur in 11% to 25% of cases.[115,117] Nonspecific graft dysfunction (increased LFTs) may be caused by (1) associated HAT, (2) biliary obstruction (external compression by PsA),[123] (3) response to sepsis secondary to PsA, or (4) coincidental.

Regardless of the clinical presentation, conventionally, posttransplant extrahepatic PsA present within 30 to 60 days of the transplant[20,21,23,115–117,120,123,126,133] and more frequently within the first 20 to 30 days posttransplant.[20,21,23,115,123,126] However, with iatrogenic PsA, which are not directly related to the transplant surgery itself, the presentation can occur at any time following transplantation. They typically occur during or soon after the minimally invasive procedure.

Due to the high risk of rupture and potential life-threatening bleeding, intervention, whether surgical or by endovascular means, is mandatory.[120] Unfortunately, in the presence of active bleeding, sacrifice of the hepatic artery may be unavoidable,[115,120] which sometimes equates with graft loss. Surgical techniques are the traditional methods of managing spontaneous extrahepatic PsA.[115,120–131] These include: (1) hepatic artery ligation only, (2) hepatic artery ligation or excision with extra-anatomic autologous bypass, and (3) retransplantation.[115,120–131]

A rarely mentioned surgical option when describing hepatic artery PsA is simply primary repair of the artery in the case of uncontaminated postangioplasty rupture.[3,4,123] An interposition graft in this setting would probably not be due to concerns of field contamination but for arterial stump length adequacy after the injured ends of the donor and recipient arteries are excised. One controversy is whether to perform an immediate revascularization or just ligate the artery without reestablishing inline arterial flow to the graft.[20,63,115,117,119,121,123–128,130,141] Supporters of revascularization stress the importance of arterial flow to the hepatic graft, particularly in the early posttransplant period (given the graft's biliary dependence on arterial flow) when most PsA present.[20,63,117,123–126,141] The lack of arterial flow may cause graft ischemia, leading to biliary necrosis, parenchymal ischemia and tissue breakdown, and/or graft ischemia with fulminant hepatic failure and death.[117,123,133] With or without revascularization there is a high mortality, ranging between 33% and 78%[115–117,119,120,122,124,125] and there is no clear outcome to conclude whether revascularization or arterial ligation is superior particularly, when considering the numerous variables involved with liver transplantation and the small sample size of studies.[117]

In recent years (2001 to present) transcatheter embolization has been described as an alternative to arterial ligation[115,122,132] (FIGURE 79.8) and seems to be a valid and lower morbidity minimally invasive alternative.[63] The five transcatheter occlusive (ligation alternative) embolization cases described were successful.[115,122,132] To the best of our knowledge, there are no reports of successful selective transcatheter embolization of a PsA with the intention of preserving arterial inline flow to the graft. A failed selective embolization has been described where the PsA was finally treated successfully utilizing a stent-graft.[137]

Recently (2005 to present), additional minimal invasive techniques have been used successfully for the definitive management of extrahepatic PsA by obliterating the PsA while preserving the graft arterial inflow.[118,133–139] These include two cases of direct percutaneous coil or thrombin injection[133,134] and 11 endovascular stent-graft placement attempts.[116,118,135–139] Nine of the 11 (82%) stent-graft placement attempts in the literature were successful.[116,118,135–139] One declared failure was

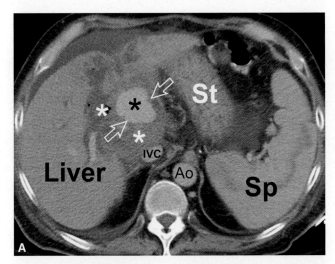
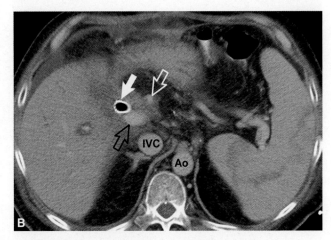

FIGURE 79.8 Hepatic artery pseudoaneurysm with coil embolization of the hepatic artery. A, B. Axial images of a contrast-enhanced CT demonstrating a large pseudoaneurysm (*black asterisk*, and in-between *hollow white arrows*) in the vicinity of the hepatic hilum. There is hematoma (*white asterisks*) around the pseudoaneurysm. The patient is status-post liver transplantation and has gastrointestinal bleeding, hypovolemic shock, and pain. A more caudad axial image (**B**) shows a self-expanding metal stent (*solid white arrow*) adjacent to the intact proximal hepatic artery (*hollow white arrow*) and the main portal vein (*hollow black arrow*). **C.** Coronal reformat of a contrast-enhanced CT demonstrating the large pseudoaneurysm (*black asterisk*) in the vicinity of the hepatic hilum. There is an outer layering hematoma (*white asterisk*) around the pseudoaneurysm. The proximal hepatic artery (*hollow white arrow*) is seen but not the distal hepatic artery. **D.** Initial digitally subtracted angiogram of the celiac trunk demonstrating the large pseudoaneurysm (*black asterisk*) in the vicinity of the hepatic hilum and involving the hepatic anastomosis (*hollow arrow points*) to the site of the arterial surgical anastomosis where the hepatic artery truncates. The distal hepatic artery is thrombosed (not visualized). **E.** Fluoroscopic spot image (unsubtracted angiogram) of the proximal hepatic artery through a 5 French catheter (*dashed arrow*) in the hepatic artery, again demonstrating the large pseudoaneurysm (*black asterisk*) in the vicinity of the hepatic hilum and the truncated proximal hepatic artery at the surgical anastomosis (*hollow arrow*). **F.** Fluoroscopic spot image (unsubtracted angiogram) of the proximal hepatic artery through a 5 French catheter in the hepatic artery after coil embolization and occlusion (*dashed white arrows*) of the proximal hepatic artery. Two initial coils (*hollow arrow*) were undersized and actually ended up in the pseudoaneurysm (*asterisk*). Complete (occlusive) coil embolization of the proximal hepatic artery is the surgical equivalent to surgical ligation and is not unreasonable in the emergent setting of hypovolemia and shock, particularly when the hepatic artery is thrombosed.

IVC, inferior vena cava; Ao, aorta; St, stomach; Sp, spleen. *(continued)*

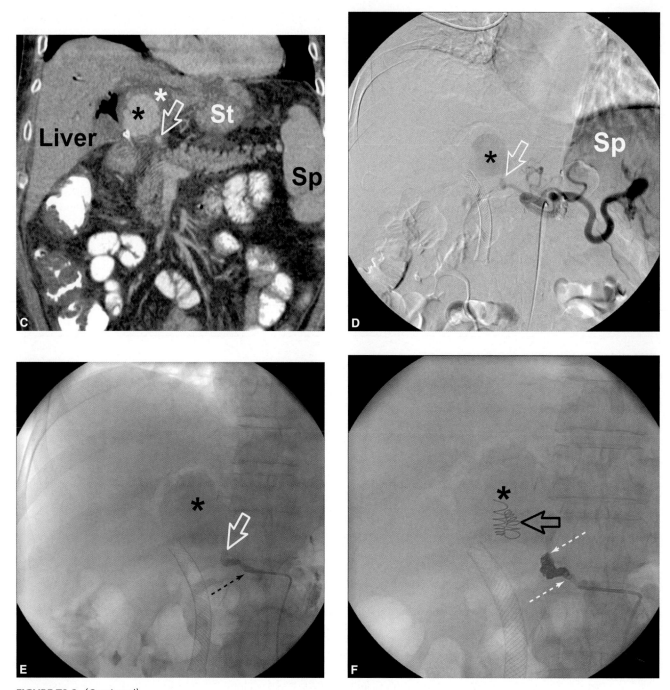

FIGURE 79.8 *(Continued)*

actually not attempted because of vessel tortuosity and the other failure was a successful deployment; however, the stent-graft did not seal the arterial leak.[116,118] Eight of the 11 stent-graft cases (73%) in the literature had PsA/arterial ruptures as a result of balloon angioplasty during the treatment of HAS and/or HAT.

One must be cautious, however, regarding the above stent-graft analysis and the anecdotal case reports in the literature.[116,118,135–139] Additionally, one must also be cautious about the utilization of stent-grafts in post-liver transplant PsA in general. Stent-grafts require a stiffer platform (delivery system and larger/stiffer guiding sheaths) and they do not track easily

through tortuous vessels, which is not uncommon to encounter in liver transplant visceral arteries. Not all transplant hepatic arteries are amenable to stent-graft placement. Furthermore, the long-term patency of stent-grafts in small visceral arteries (<3 to 4 mm) is unknown and probably reduced.[116,133] Also, a large percentage of these PsA are mycotic and a stent-graft may act as an infectious nidus. As a result, the current authors view stent-grafts in the setting of mycotic/spontaneous post-transplant PsA as a temporizing measure, preventing further bleeding and, in the short-term, maintaining arterial flow to the allograft. This allows the transplant team to evaluate the graft and whether it is salvageable. Furthermore, this allows planning for elective revascularization of the graft or retransplantation of a new hepatic graft. Stent-grafts in the setting of iatrogenic postangioplasty hepatic artery rupture is most likely to be more technically feasible (the catheter and guiding wire system is already across the defect, albeit may need to be upsized) and more of a definitive long-term therapy (if successful) than spontaneous PsA.

More readily we need to address minimal invasive procedures versus primary surgical management and discuss temporizing measures and definitive management. As Leelaudomlipi et al.[117] concluded in their analysis of their experience as well as their review of the literature on arterial ligation versus immediate revascularization, no clear method is superior due to the rarity of the complication and the numerous variables in the literature. However, we disagree with the assertion by Alamo et al.[120] that endovascular management should be reserved for stable patients, which is contrary to that of Marshall et al. Their findings suggested that occlusive embolization stabilized previously hemodynamically compromised patients and once stable, those patients may have had a better outcome.[115] Interventional radiology, particularly in liver transplant institutions, can mobilize quickly, and endovascular measures (embolization or stent-graft placement) can be used to temporize and stabilize patients. The dilemma arises when discussing definitive long-term management. Anecdotally, the current author believes that definitive management in the setting of mycotic/spontaneous PsA is surgical (either revascularization for salvageable grafts or retransplantation for unsalvageable grafts). Endovascular measures in this potentially infected setting are temporizing or terminal measures. Regardless of the initial management, retransplantation is commonly required albeit with a high mortality.[115,126,130] The retransplant rate ranges between 33% and 45% and the overall mortality of post-liver transplant PsA (retransplanted or not) is 33% to 78%.[115–117,119,120,122,124,125]

Portal Venous Inflow Disease

Portal Venous Stenosis

Portal venous stenosis (PVS) is the most common portal vein complication, but, overall, it is an uncommon complication, occurring in 1% to 2% of transplants.[7,20,142,143] PVS almost always occurs at the anastomosis. Its distance from the portal bifurcation depends on the proximity of the surgical anastomosis to the graft portal bifurcation. Early PVS (occurring within 6 months of the transplantation) is probably technical. Most PVS occur late (after 6 months) and present with symptoms of portal hypertension, such as ascites and variceal bleeding.[144–147] Many of the PVS cases in the literature have been reported in pediatric liver transplant recipients[19,144,145,148–151] with a PVS reported in up to 8% of pediatric recipients.[150,151] In this age group, the recipient portal vein usually has a relatively small diameter, which usually requires plication of the relatively larger donor portal vein, which possibly predisposes to anastomotic stenosis.[142,148] Furthermore, in living donor split hepatic grafts, the portal vein anastomosis is technically challenging because the donor portal vein segment(s) is relatively short and not infrequently requires interposition grafts or multiple/complex anastomotic reconstructions.[152] These interposition grafts are usually venous (maternal gonadal vein, paternal mesenteric vein, or a cryo-preserved iliac vein).[150]

Significant PVS is difficult to ascertain by nondynamic cross-sectional studies, such as CT and MR. It is particularly difficult to accurately assess the portal anastomosis when there is a size mismatch between the diameter of the recipient and graft portal vein with or without angulation.[12] DUS may be the most accurate noninvasive modality and suggests significant stenosis where peak portal velocities are three- to fourfold higher at the anastomosis.[12,13] A focal increase of portal velocity greater than threefold and/or a peak velocity greater than 125 cm/second has a 73% sensitivity and a 95% to 100% specificity to PVS.[13,153] Unlike posttransplant arterial complications, however, angiography (in this case portography) remains, by far, the most accurate and gold standard exam along with portal pressure gradient measurement across the anastomosis.[12,13,154] However, the gradient that signifies a significant anastomotic stenosis is exactly unknown and controversial.[150] Most operators use a gradient of greater than 4 to 5 mm Hg as significant and others use an 8 mm Hg gradient or a 3 mm Hg gradient.[150,155] The author can only speculate why this controversy exists. **First**, the case numbers are small and there are numerous variables with liver transplantation. This is compounded by the fact that graft dysfunction normalization after treatment may not occur quickly and may be coincidental if it occurs. **Second**, it is difficult to make a nominal gradient cutoff of a relative measurement, particularly when there can be considerable variation in the portal pressure that affect the nominal gradient. For example, a 20% to 25% gradient across the anastomosis in a patient with a portal pressure of 20 mm Hg (4 to 5 mm Hg) is equally as significant as a 20% to 25% gradient across the anastomosis in a patient with a portal pressure of 12 mm Hg (≤3 mm Hg). **Third**, there may be portosystemic collaterals (porto-azygous left gastric to esophageal varices, meso-caval or splenorenal or gastrorenal shunts to name the most common significant ones) that decompress the portal circulation of the recipient distal to the anastomosis and thus reduce the portal pressure gradient across the portal anastomosis.

The percutaneous transhepatic approach is preferred over the "TIPS approach" for portal vein access[12] (FIGURE 79.9). The TIPS approach is longer and more cumbersome and does not give enough "running room" to the anastomoses because the TIPS portal access site is usually close to the anastomosis. If it is not, and the portal access from the transjugular approach is more intrahepatic, then there is probably a curved hepatic parenchymal tract that is not aligned with the anastomosis. Most portal veins also are easily accessed under ultrasound and/or fluoroscopy. The right intercostal approach is more common than a left-sided sub-xyphoid approach in whole grafts. The short direct tract through the liver provides the best mechanical advantage for negotiating severe stenoses.[12,144] However, the right intercostal approach most likely has a higher risk of bleeding and pleural injury compared to the left portal approach. Intravenous heparin is given to help reduce the risk of thrombosis during the angioplasty. Postangioplasty anticoagulation is occasionally used for 24 to 72 hours after the procedure but is not usually used in the long-term.[144] Self-expanding bare stents are usually used, such as wallstents,[144] although personally the current author has, on rare occasions, used balloon-expandable bare- and covered-stents.

Funaki and coworkers found in 30 patients that one-third recoiled immediately after angioplasty and required immediate stent placement. Of the remaining two-thirds of patients who responded well to balloon angioplasty, half (one-third of the overall population) restenosed 1 to 31 months (mean 6 months)

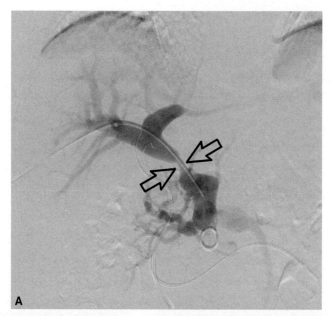

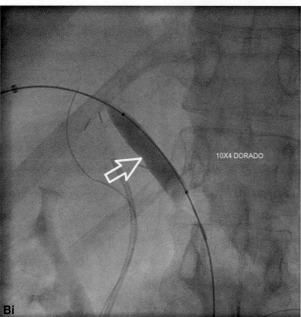

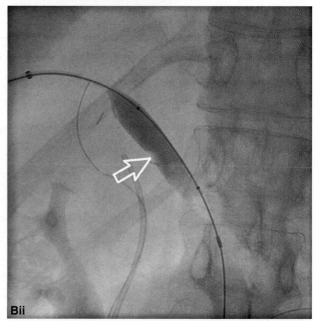

FIGURE 79.9 Portal vein stenosis at the surgical anastomosis treated with balloon angioplasty. A. Digitally subtracted portogram of a liver transplant recipient obtained from a percutaneous transhepatic approach. There is a portal stenosis at the surgical anastomosis (between *hollow arrows*). The patient complained of persistent graft dysfunction and mild ascites. The portal venous gradient across the stenosis was 9 mm Hg. **B**. Fluoroscopic spot images during balloon dilation of the portal anastomosis utilizing a 10-mm balloon (**Bi**) and a 12-mm balloon (**Bii**). The *hollow arrows* point to waists on the balloons. These waists were eventually effaced (lost with further balloon dilation). **C**. Completion digitally subtracted portogram demonstrating resolution of the anastomotic stenosis with less than 30% residual stenosis (the residual stenosis extends between the two *hollow arrows*). The portal venous gradient across this residual stenosis was 3 mm Hg. **D**. Digitally subtracted portograms before (**Di**) and after (**Dii**) balloon angioplasty demonstrating resolution of the anastomotic stenosis with less than 30% residual stenosis (**Dii**). The gradient across the stenosis has been reduced from 9 to 3 mm Hg. This, by definition, is a technically successful angioplasty.

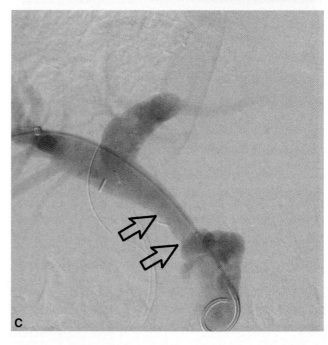

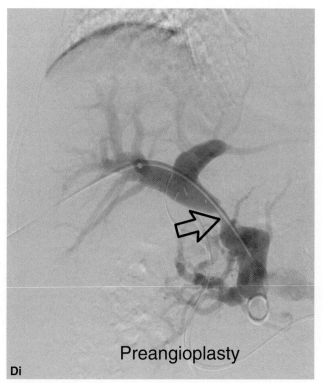
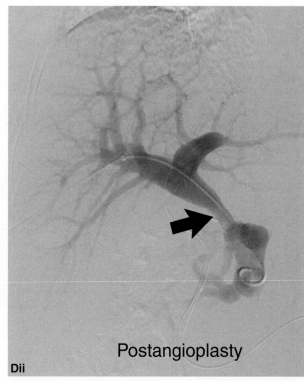

FIGURE 79.9 *(Continued)*

after the initial angioplasty[144] (FIGURE 79.9). Failures of angioplasty (intraprocedural or delayed restenoses) were treated with stent placement with good long-term results.[144] Two complications (7%) occurred in their experience and both were portal vein thromboses.[12,144] Both complications responded favorably to transcatheter thrombolysis.[12,144] When considering the long-term success of a single balloon dilation without stent placement, the results are variable with a long-term patency/success of 36% to 71% at 2 to 3 years.[144,151] Stents are reserved usually for intraprocedural recoil and early restenosis (probably within 6 months) after a technically successful angioplasty. This is because stents may impede future surgeries (retransplantation) and, in the pediatric recipient population, may cause focal narrowing at the stent edge due to graft and recipient growth (stents do not grow with the patient and graft and thus form a relative narrowing).[150,156] The patency results of stents in portal veins is even more scant. Most stents are self-expanding and the patency appears to be as high as 100% over 3 to 5 years.[144,157]

Portal Venous Thrombosis

Portal venous thrombosis (PVT) is an uncommon complication, occurring in 1% to 4% of transplants.[144,151,158] PVT usually occurs within a month from the transplant[12,144,158,159]; however, it has been described as iatrogenic from intraprocedural angioplasty[144] or on top of previously placed stents for PVS.[149] Similar to severe PVS, PVT presents with signs of portal hypertension (*see above*) if symptomatic. If asymptomatic, nonspecific LFT abnormalities maybe encountered.[12,146,158] DUS demonstrates lack of flow or echogenic thrombus may be seen.[12,41] Acute thrombus may cause increase in caliber of the portal vein, which can be seen on DUS, CT, or MR. Some authors feel the urgency

that immediate treatment should be performed because graft loss is imminent.[158] Anecdotally, this may be a function of time. For example, early PVT (within 30 days from the transplant) may cause rapid graft decline and not necessarily delayed PVT after years from the transplant.

Unlike PVS, the portal venous approach varies from one operator/institution and from one circumstance to the other. The TIPS approach has advantages because it may cause less risk of intraperitoneal bleeding once it is established. Additionally, creating a TIPS shunt can provide outflow to the portal vein, especially if the intrahepatic portal radicals are occluded with thrombus that is recalcitrant to fibrinolysis. Furthermore, a percutaneous thrombectomy can be performed through the TIPS from a transjugular approach by dragging a Fogarty from the portal vein and into the inferior vena cava (IVC). The disadvantages are that a TIPS is a more involved procedure and that there is no "running room" to the anastomosis in case a stent needs to be placed. The advantages of a percutaneous transhepatic approach are discussed above. The disadvantage is that it may have an increased bleeding risk. Various combinations of mechanical and pharmaceutical thrombolytic devices, drugs, and techniques have been described. Adjunct stent deployment has been utilized to avoid, if not reduce, pharmaceutical thrombolysis and thus reduce the length of the procedure and the bleeding risk.[160] The additional advantage of stent placement in the setting of PVT is that it addresses underlying PVS, if any is to be found.[144,160]

Portal vein thrombolysis experience in the literature is very scant,[144,146,151,158–163] and little conclusions can be drawn regarding complications, technical successes, and longevity of successful procedures. The technical success is probably around

55% to 70% and long-term patency is 50% to 60%.[151,159] Iatrogenic PVT from PVS balloon angioplasty is very successful because the clot is fresh and the underlying anatomic defect/PVS is already identified and is being treated.

Hepatic Venous Outflow Disease

Hepatic venous outflow disease following liver transplantation is classified into (1) hepatic vein disease occlusive disease proper (more common in split grafts) and (2) IVC occlusive disease.[1,12,164,165]

Hepatic Venous Occlusive Disease Proper

Stenosis of the hepatic veins (HVS) after transplantation is a rare complication in whole grafts; however, it occurs in 4% to 7% of split grafts.[156,164–167] The rarity of HVS in whole grafts is obviously caused by lack of hepatic venous anastomoses in whole grafts, especially in interposition (non-piggyback anastomoses) IVC anastomoses.[41] However, HVS proper can occur without anastomoses due to graft edema, graft rotation (torsion), and/or impingement.[12,41,166] This may partly explain why HVS is more common in undersized grafts, which typically rotate as they hypertrophy to fulfill recipient requirements; the rotation and segmental hypertrophy may torse or impinge on the hepatic veins.[156,166] Hepatic vein thrombosis (HVT) is caused by HVS/IVC stenosis, sepsis, and hypercoagulable states (including dehydration), especially in children.[12,41]

Hepatic venous occlusive disease (HVS or HVT) presents with iatrogenic Budd-Chiari syndrome (ascites, hepatic hydrothorax, coagulopathy, and/or hepatic graft dysfunction/abnormal LFTs).[12] DUS demonstrates decrease hepatic vein velocities and reduced respiratory phasicity of the waveform.[13,164] The respiratory phasicity of the hepatic veins in native (nontransplanted) livers is normally triphasic and normally (postsurgical norm) become biphasic posttransplant.[13] Significant hepatic vein occlusive disease degrades the posttransplant biphasic waveform to a dampened biphasic or monophasic waveform.[13,164,166,168] Other Doppler findings include increased velocity with turbulance/aliasing, reversed hepatic venous flow, and direct visualization of the stenosis on gray scale ultrasound.[13] Portal vein velocities may also be reduced secondarily to the iatrogenic Budd-Chiari syndrome.[13] By CT or MR direct visualization of the stenosis can be seen, although, anecdotally, this can be overcalled.[13,164] Furthermore, nonspecific perfusion anomalies can also be seen.[13] The definitive diagnosis is by venography and, specifically, transcatheter manometry. Only 77% of cases are positive by venography and manometry after noninvasive imaging suspicion of HVS.[169] However, as in the portal vein, the degree of pressure gradient for the diagnosis is not agreed upon and varies widely from greater than 3 to 20 mm Hg.[19,166,170,171] A common threshold is 10 mm Hg, although in the setting of high clinical suspicion the current author utilizes 4 mm Hg as did Weeks et al.,[171] who utilized pressure gradient thresholds as low as 3 mm Hg for the diagnosis.

Endovascular management is the treatment of choice.[12,164–166] Primary treatment is by balloon angioplasty with stent placement reserved for recalcitrant lesions.[12,165] The transjugular approach is usually the more common approach. However, when this fails a transhepatic/combined transjugular-transhepatic approach can be used.[12,166,170] A femoral approach may be needed if the angulation of a piggyback anastomosis is downward and not upward.[172] Balloons are typically oversized and may be kept inflated for 1 or 2 minutes.[166] Cutting balloons may be used especially to lesions that are recalcitrant to conventional balloon dilation.[166,173] Alternatively, bare-stents are placed for lesions with immediate recoil or, with certain operators, early recurrence.[12,165]

Technical success of endovascular therapy is high (including stent placement), ranging from 94% to 100%; however, recurrences (restenoses) are common and can occur as early as 1 week.[165,166,174] These require multiple sessions of balloon angioplasty with an assisted primary patency approaching 100%.[12,165,166] Major complications are extremely rare (0%).[149,166,175] Minor complications can occur in up to 10% of cases and are mostly related to arrhythmias and transient hypotension.[149,166] Anastomotic disruption with catastrophic bleeding, in theory, is a potential complication, although it has not been reported.[166] Clinical response after technically successful treatment is usually quick (as early as days postdilation) and is approximately 73%.[12,165,166] Clinical failure despite technical success may be caused by chronic untreated hepatic venous stenosis, which leads to irreversible damage to the liver (posthepatic cirrhosis, fibrosis, necrosis) with the development of portal hypertension.[166,176]

Inferior Vena Cava Stenosis

Overall, IVC stenoses posttransplantation occur in 0.8% to 2.6% of transplants.[11,12,142,166,167,170,171,177–182] Again, pediatric and split grafts are more likely to have a higher incidence rate of IVC stenoses.[142,178–180] IVC (hepatic graft outflow) stenosis includes (1) recipient IVC stenosis in interposition anastomoses and (2) hepatic graft venous outflow in piggyback IVC anastomoses (FIGURES 79.4B, C and 79.10). Piggyback anastomoses are designed to reduce the hepatic venous outflow obstruction in whole grafts, although the rate of piggyback anastomotic stenoses has been reported in up to 3.4% of piggyback transplants.[156,166,183] Anatomically, and clinically, piggyback anastomoses look, are oriented (obliqued horizontally), and present like HVS proper (usually do not obstruct infrahepatic recipient venous outflow) and are technically treated in similar ways (see above).[1] Interposition IVC stenoses are oriented vertically and are subclassified into suprahepatic (at the suprahepatic IVC) and subhepatic (below the liver, between the hepatic veins/outflow veins and the renal veins).

Posttransplant IVC occlusive disease does not affect the hepatic graft only. In fact, true IVC occlusive disease affects the subdiaphragmatic venous return with (suprahepatic stenosis/occlusion) or without (subhepatic stenosis/occlusion) hepatic graft dysfunction. Subdiaphragmatic venous return occlusion can cause renal dysfunction and lower extremity swelling.[12,178,184,185] When the suprahepatic IVC is involved, the hepatic graft outflow is affected and patients present, additionally, with hepatic graft dysfunction, which ranges from abnormal LFTs to ascites/pleural effusion to posthepatic cirrhosis and graft failure.[12,178,184,185] Suprahepatic IVC stenosis is more common than infrahepatic IVC, although this may be a function of the unforgiving/susceptible nature of the hepatic graft, which brings suprahepatic IVC stenoses to the attention of the transplant team.[12,182,185]

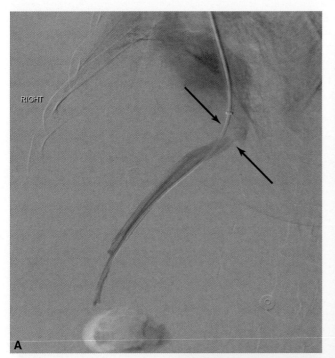

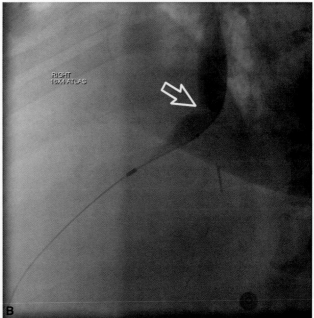

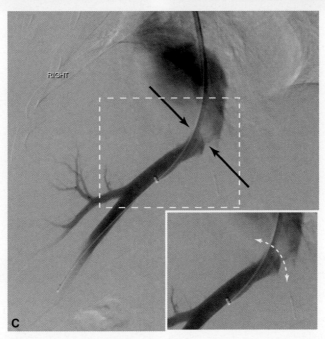

FIGURE 79.10 **Hepatic venous outflow stenosis at the surgical anastomosis with a piggyback IVC anastomosis. This was refractory to conventional balloon angioplasty and was treated with stent placement. A**. Digitally subtracted hepatic venogram of a liver transplant recipient obtained from a transjugular approach. There is a hepatic venous stenosis at the surgical anastomosis, which is a piggyback inferior vena cava anastomosis (see FIGURE 79.4B, C). The patient complained of persistent graft dysfunction. The venous gradient across the stenosis was 10 mm Hg. **B**. Fluoroscopic spot images during balloon dilation of the hepatic venous outflow anastomosis utilizing a 16-mm balloon. This was after a serial dilation sequentially with a 10-, 12-, and 14-mm balloon. All balloon waists were effaced. The hollow arrows point to waists on the balloon. This waist was eventually effaced (lost with further balloon dilation). **C**. Digitally subtracted venogram with inset (*bottom right corner*) demonstrating persistence of the anastomotic stenosis (between *black arrow* in the main image and *curved bidirectional arrow* in inset) with a venous gradient across this residual stenosis of 7 mm Hg. **D**. Fluoroscopic images during a balloon-expandable stent (Palmaz stent) placement (between *solid white arrows*). The stent is advanced through a deeply placed reinforced sheath (**Di**. *dashed arrow* at needle tip). The sheath is pulled back to "unsheath" the balloon-mounted stent (**Dii**. *dashed arrow* at needle tip). The stent (between solid white arrows) is then balloon opened (**Dii**). **E**. Digitally subtracted venogram (**Ei**) and a fluoroscopic spot image (**Eii**) after the balloon-expandable stent (Palmaz stent) has been placed (**Eii**. between *solid white arrows*). The outflow venous stenosis (**Ei**. between *solid black arrows*) has resolved and the gradient across the narrowing is 2 mm Hg. *(continued)*

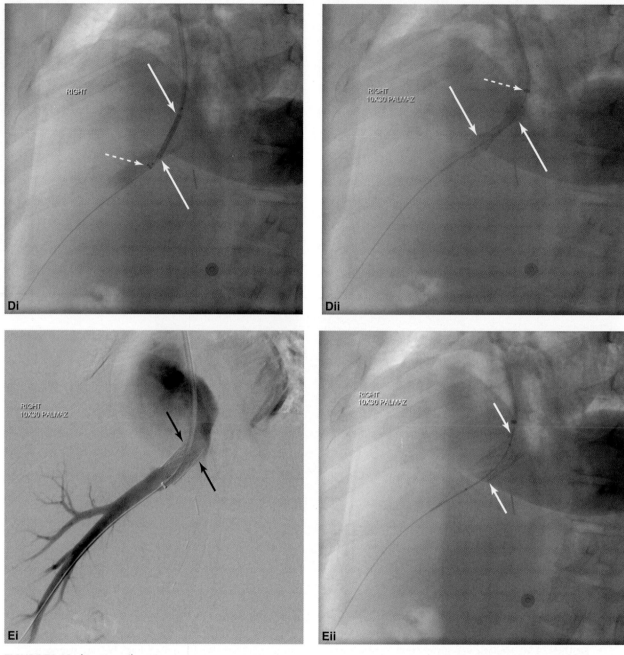

FIGURE 79.10 *(Continued)*

IVC stenoses can present in the early (within a month) post-transplant period or later (after a month from transplantation). Both early and late are equally as prevalent (56% vs. 44%, respectively).[12,185] Early IVC stenosis/narrowing are commonly caused by (1) technical reasons (tight anastomotic suture line and caval redundancy), (2) IVC external compression (posttransplant edema and/or oversized grafts), and (3) IVC torsion due to graft rotation.[12,149,179–182,185–190] IVC torsion is caused by posttransplant graft edema, oversized grafts, initially undersized grafts with subsequent hypertrophy, remodeling and graft rotation as the graft regenerates (not necessarily uniformly with some hepatic segments growing relatively faster than others) and rotates to accommodate the space within the abdominal cavity.[12,185] Late IVC stenosis (>1 month from transplant) results from (1) fibrosis/scarring, (2) intimal hyperplasia, or (3) chronic thrombus.[12,149,181,182,187–190] IVC thrombosis occurs secondary to IVC narrowing (stenosis proper, compression, or torsion), particularly in the setting of hypercoagulable states.[12,179,180]

DUS findings are not specific and are similar to the findings with HVS (*see above*).[12,185] In critical suprahepatic IVC stenosis, reversal of flow can be seen in the hepatic veins with slowing of the flow in the portal vein.[41] MRA and CTA are valuable tools and may suggest the presence or absence of IVC stenoses and at what level (supra- or infrahepatic); however, they are nondynamic studies. The gold standard for the diagnosis is cavography (IVC venography) with pressure gradient measurements.[41,185]

Cavography should be performed in the frontal and lateral projections to accurately identify any IVC stenoses. The exact value of a pressure gradient that signifies a hemodynamically significant IVC stenosis is not known. Certain authors consider a pressure gradient of 8 to 10 mm Hg as significant[19,184]; however, others consider a pressure gradient of less than 8 mm Hg.[184,185] The current authors utilize a pressure gradient of greater than 4 mm Hg as significant. Torsion appears like a "ribbon-like" twisted narrowing of the IVC, which may require multiple projections to verify the diagnosis. Unfortunately, the diagnosis of torsion is usually made after stent placement where the narrowing is found to propagate inferior to the newly placed stent (FIGURE 79.11).[12,185,191]

As in almost all posttransplant vascular complications, endovascular therapy has become the primary management of posttransplant IVC complications.[19,108,149,178,181–190,192,193] Traditionally, surgical therapy was performed, which included cavotomy, thrombectomy, patch-venoplasty, and liver retransplantation.[39,142,178–180] Pharmaceutical and mechanical catheter-directed thrombectomy/thrombolysis is utilized to remove thrombus.[178,179,184] Once the thrombus is cleared balloon angioplasty or stent placement is utilized to resolve underlying anatomic defects (IVC stenosis and narrowing).[12] The initial intraprocedural technical success of angioplasty alone for the resolution of IVC stenoses is 29% with a high restenosis rate of 40% to 50%.[19,149,178,181,184,186] Many of the lesions that were

refractory to IVC angioplasty are probably IVC torsion and external compression and not IVC stenoses proper.[12] Borsa and coworkers[184] suggested that early IVC narrowing, because it was probably due to torsion, compression, postoperative edema, and kinking (*see above*), was ideally treated with stent placement. They reserved angioplasty for delayed IVC stenoses because they probably were caused by scarring/intimal hyperplasia.[184]

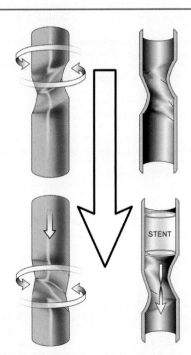

FIGURE 79.11 Illustration depicting the problem with endovascular management (stent placement) of inferior vena cava (IVC) torsion. The two drawings on the right are drawings of the outer IVC and the two drawings on the left are longitudinal sectional cuts along the IVC. The above two drawings are before stent placement and the bottom two drawings are after stent placement (stent placement depicted by central directional *arrow*). There is a twist depicted in the IVC and this level of torsion (twist) propagates downward (or upward) when a stent is placed.

■ REFERENCES

1. Saad WE, Orloff MC, Davies MG, et al. Postliver transplantation vascular and biliary surgical anatomy. *Tech Vasc Interv Radiol* 2007;10:172–190.
2. Saad WE. Management of hepatic artery steno-occlusive complications after liver transplantation. *Tech Vasc Interv Radiol* 2007;10:207–220.
3. Saad WE, Davies MG, Sahler LG, et al. Hepatic artery stenosis in liver transplant recipients: primary treatment with percutaneous transluminal angioplasty. *J Vasc Interv Radiol* 2005;16:795–805.
4. Orons PD, Zajko AB, Bron KM, et al. Hepatic artery angioplasty after liver transplantation: experience in 21 allografts. *J Vasc Interv Radiol* 1995;6:523–529.
5. Jain A, Costa G, Marsh W, et al. Thrombotic and nonthrombotic hepatic artery complications in adults and children following primary liver transplantation with long-term follow-up in 1000 consecutive patients. *Transpl Int* 2006;19:27–37.
6. Sabri SS, Saad WE, Schmitt TM, et al. Endovascular therapy for hepatic artery stenosis and thrombosis following liver transplantation. *J Vasc Endovasc Surg* 2011;45(5):447–452.
7. Wozney P, Zajko AB, Bron KM, et al. Vascular complications after liver transplantation: a 5 year experience. *AJR Am J Roentgenol* 1986;147:657–663.
8. Denys AL, Qonadli SD, Durand F, et al. Feasibility and effectiveness of using coronary stents in the treatment of hepatic artery stenosis after liver transplantation: preliminary report. *AJR Am J Roentgenol* 2002;178:1175–1179.
9. Zajko AB, Campbell WL, Logsdon GA, et al. Cholangiographic findings in hepatic artery occlusion after liver transplantation. *AJR Am J Roentgenol* 1987;149:485–489.
10. Abassoglu O, Levy MF, Vodapally MS, et al. Hepatic artery stenosis after liver transplantation: incidence, presentation, treatment, and long-term outcome. *Transplantation* 1997;63:250–255.
11. Orons PD, Zajko AB, Bron KM, et al. Angiography and interventional procedures in liver transplantation. *Radiol Clin North Am* 1995;33:541–558.
12. Saad WE, Waldman DL. Endovascular repair of vascular lesions in solid organ transplantation. In: Oriel K, Katzen BT, Rosenfield K, eds. *Complications in Endovascular Therapy*. New York, NY: Taylor & Francis Informa; 2006:223–252.
13. Saad WE, Lin E, Ormanoski M, et al. Noninvasive imaging of liver transplant complications. *Tech Vasc Interv Radiol* 2007;10:191–206.
14. Dodd GD III, Memel DS, Zajko AB, et al. Hepatic artery stenosis and thrombosis in transplant recipients: Doppler diagnosis with resistive index and systolic acceleration time. *Radiology* 1994;192:657–661.
15. Gottlieb RH, Snitzer EL, Hartley DF, et al. Interobserver and intraobserver variation in determining intrarenal parameters by Doppler sonography. *AJR Am J Roentgenol* 1997;168:627–631.
16. Abad J, Hidalgo EG, Cantarero JM, et al. Hepatic artery anastomotic stenosis after transplantation: treatment with percutaneous transluminal angioplasty. *Radiology* 1989;171:661–662.
17. Castaneda F, Samuel KS, Hunter DW, et al. Reversible hepatic transplant ischemia: case report and review of the literature. *Cardiovasc Interv Radiol* 1990;13:88–90.
18. Mondragon JB, Karani JB, Haetn ND, et al. The use of percutaneous transluminal angioplasty in hepatic artery stenosis after transplantation. *Transplantation* 1994;57:228–231.
19. Raby N, Karoni J, Thomas S, et al. Stenoses of vascular anastomoses after hepatic transplantation: treatment with balloon angioplasty. *AJR Am J Roentgenol* 1991;157:167–171.
20. Langras AN, Marujo W, Stratta RJ, et al. Vascular complications after orthotopic liver transplantation. *Am J Surg* 1991;161:76–83.
21. Merion RM, Burtch GD, Ham JM, et al. The hepatic artery in liver transplantation. *Transplantation* 1989;48:438–443.
22. Hesselink EJ, Sloof MJH, Schuur KH, et al. Consequences of hepatic artery pathology after orthotopic liver transplantation. *Transplant Proc* 1987;19:2476–2477.

23. Karatzas T, Lykaki-Karatzas M, Webb JN, et al. Vascular complications, treatment and outcome following orthotopic liver transplantation. *Transplant Proc* 1997;29:2853–2855.

24. Stein M, Radich SM, Riegler JL, et al. Dissection of an iliac artery conduit to liver allograft: treatment with an endovascular stent. *Liver Transpl Surg* 1999;5:252–254.

25. Cotroneo AR, DiStasi C, Cina A, et al. Stent placement in four patients with hepatic artery stenosis or thrombosis after liver transplantation. *J Vasc Interv Radiol* 2002;13:619–623.

26. Narumi S, Osorio RW, Freise CE, et al. Hepatic artery pseudoaneurysm with hemobilia following angioplasty after liver transplantation. *Clin Transplant* 1998;12:508–510.

27. Kodama Y, Sakuhara T, Abo D, et al. Percutaneous transluminal angioplasty for hepatic artery stenosis after liver donor liver transplantation. *Liver Transpl* 2006;12:465–469.

28. Ueno T, Jones G, Martin A, et al. Clinical outcome from hepatic artery stenting in liver transplantation. *Liver Transpl* 2006;12:422–427.

29. Cheng TF, Chen YS, Huang TL, et al. Interventional radiographic procedures in liver transplantation. *Transpl Int* 2001;14:223–229.

30. Duffy JP, Hong JC, Farmer DG, et al. Vascular complications of orthotopic liver transplantation: experience in more than 4,200 patients. *J Am Coll Surg* 2009;208:896.

31. Singhal A, Stokes K, Sebastian A, et al. Endovascular treatment of hepatic artery thrombosis following liver transplantation. *Transpl Int* 2010;23:245–256.

32. Tzakis AG, Gordon RD, Shaw BW, et al. Clinical preservation of hepatic artery thrombosis after liver transplantation in the cyclosporin era. *Transplantation* 1985;40:667–671.

33. Tzakis AG. The dearterialized liver graft. *Semin Liver Dis* 1985;5:375–376.

34. Bekker JS, Ploem S, de Jong KP. Early hepatic artery thrombosis after liver transplantation: a systematic review of the incidence, outcomes, and risk factors. *Am J Transpl* 2009;23:245–256.

35. Singhal A, Stokes K, Sebastian A, et al. Endovascular treatment of hepatic artery thrombosis following liver transplantation. *Transpl Int* 2009;23:245–256.

36. Blumgardt G, Ringe B, Lauchart W, et al. Vascular problems in liver transplantation. *Transplant Proc* 1987;19:2412.

37. Tisone G, Gunson BK, Buckels JAC, et al. Raised hematocrit: a contributing factor to hepatic artery thrombosis following liver transplantation. *Transplantation* 1988;46:162–163.

38. Shaw BW Jr, Gordon RD, Iwatsuki S, et al. Hepatic transplantation. *Transplant Proc* 1985;17:264–271.

39. Lerut J, Gordon RD, Iwatsuki S, et al. Surgical complications in human orthotopic liver transplantation. *Acta Chir Belg* 1987;87:193–204.

40. Zajko AB, Bron KM, Starzl TE, et al. Angiography of liver transplantation patients. *Radiology* 1985;157:305–311.

41. Glokner JF, Forauer AR. Vascular or ischemic complications after liver transplantation: pictorial essay. *AJR Am J Roentgenol* 1999;173:1055–1059.

42. Dravid VS, Shapiro MJ, Needleman L, et al. Arterial abnormalities following orthotopic liver transplantation: arteriographic findings and correlation with Doppler sonographic findings. *AJR Am J Roentgenol* 1994;163:585–589.

43. Flint EW, Sumkin JH, Zajko AB, et al. Duplex sonography of hepatic artery thrombosis after liver transplantation. *AJR Am J Roentgenol* 1988;151:481–483.

44. Defranc J, Trotteur G, Dundelinger RF. Duplex ultrasonographic evaluation of liver transplants. *Acta Radiol* 1993;34:478–481.

45. Segel MC, Zajko AB, Bowen A, et al. Hepatic artery thrombosis after liver transplantation: radiological evaluation. *AJR Am J Roentgenol* 1986;146:137–141.

46. Ozaki CF, Katz SM, Monsour HPJ, et al. Surgical complications of liver transplantation. *Surg Clin North Am* 1994;74:1155–1167.

47. Bhattacharja S, Gurson BK, Mirza DF, et al. Delayed hepatic artery thrombosis in adult orthotopic liver transplantation: 12-year experience. *Transplantation* 2001;71:1592–1596.

48. Kaplan SB, Zajko AB, Koneru B. Hepatic bilomas due to hepatic artery thrombosis in liver transplant recipients: percutaneous drainage and clinical outcomes. *Radiology* 1990;174:1031–1035.

49. Robkin JM, Orlott SL, Corless CL, et al. Hepatic allograft abscess with hepatic arterial thrombosis. *Am J Surg* 1998;175:354–359.

50. Saad WE, Davies MG, Saad NE, et al. Trans-catheter thrombolysis of thrombosed hepatic arteries in liver transplant recipients: predictors of definitive endoluminal success and the role of pre-operative thrombolysis. *Vasc Endovasc Surg* 2007;41:19–26.

51. Hidalgo EG, Abad J, Canterero JM, et al. High-dose intra-arterial urokinase for the treatment of hepatic artery thrombosis in liver transplantation. *Hepatologastroenterology* 1989;36:529.

52. Figueras J, Busquets J, Diminguez J, et al. Intraarterial thrombosis in the treatment of acute hepatic artery thrombosis after liver transplantation. *Transplantation* 1995;59:1356.

53. Bjerkvik PS, Vante K, Mathisen O, et al. Percutaneous revascularization of postoperative hepatic artery thrombosis in a liver transplant. *Transplantation* 1995;59:1746.

54. Zhou J, Fan J, Wang JH, et al. Continuous transcatheter arterial thrombolysis for early hepatic artery thrombosis after liver transplantation. *Transplant Proc* 2005;37:4426.

55. Wang XH, Yan LN, Zhang F, et al. Early experiences on living donor liver transplantation in China: multicenter report. *Chin Med J* 2006;119:1003.

56. Kim BW, Won JH, Lee BM, et al. Intraarterial thrombolytic treatment for hepatic artery thrombosis immediately after living donor liver transplantation. *Transplant Proc* 2006;28:3128.

57. Li ZW, Wang WQ, Zhou NX, et al. Interventional treatment of acute hepatic artery occlusion after liver transplantation. *Hepatobiliary Pancreat Dis Int* 2007;6:474.

58. Reyes-Corona J, Gonzalez-Huezo MS, Zea-Medina MV, et al. Paclitaxel coated-stent for early onset thrombosis after liver transplantation. *Ann Hepatol* 2007;6:272.

59. Boyvat F, Aytekin C, Harman S, et al. Endovascular stent placement in patients with hepatic artery stenosis or thrombosis after liver transplantation. *Transplant Proc* 2008;12:606.

60. Yang Y, Hua LI, Sheng FU, et al. Hepatic artery complication after orthotopic liver transplantation: interventional treatment or retransplantation? *Clin Med J* 2008;12:1997.

61. Lopez BR, Schlieter M, Hallscheidt PJ, et al. Successful arterial thrombolysis and percutaneous transluminal angioplasty for early hepatic artery thrombosis after split transplantation in a 4-month-old baby. *Pediatr Transpl* 2008;12:606.

62. Jeon GS, Won JH, Wanh HJ, et al. Endovascular treatment of acute arterial complications after living donor liver transplantation. *Clin Radiol* 2008;63:1099.

63. Saad WE. Management of nonocclusive hepatic artery complications after liver transplantation. *Tech Vasc Interv Radiol* 2007;10:221–232.

64. Rassmussen A, Hjortrup A, Kirkegaard P. Intraoperative measurement of graft blood flow: a necessity in liver transplantation. *Transpl Int* 1997;10:74–77.

65. Nussler NC, Settmacher U, Haase R, et al. Diagnosis and treatment of arterial steal syndrome in liver transplant recipients. *Liver Transpl* 2003;9:596–602.

66. Lima CX, Mandil A, Ulhoa AC, et al. Splenic artery steal syndrome after liver transplantation: an alternative technique of embolization. *Transplant Proc* 2009;41:1990–1993.

67. Geissler I, Lamesch P, Witzigmann H, et al. Splenohepatic arterial steal syndrome in liver transplantation: clinical features and management. *Transpl Int* 2002;15:139–141.

68. Uflacker R, Selby JB, Chavin K, et al. Transcatheter splenic artery occlusion for treatment of splenic artery steal syndrome after orthotopic liver transplantation. *Cardiovasc Intervent Radiol* 2002;25:300–306.

69. Sevmis S, Boyvat F, Aytekin C, et al. Arterial steal syndrome after orthotopic liver transplantation. *Transplant Proc* 2006;38:3651–3655.

70. Kirbas I, Ulu EMK, Ozturk A, et al. Multidetector computed tomographic angiography findings of splenic artery steal syndrome in liver transplantation. *Transplant Proc* 2007;39:1178–1180.

71. Granov AM, Tarazov PG, Granov DA, et al. Role of interventional radiology in pre- and post-operative periods of liver transplantation. *Khirurgiia (Mosk)* 2010;3:31–36.

72. Mogl MT, Nussler NC, Presser SJ, et al. Evolving experience with prevention and treatment of splenic artery syndrome after orthotopic liver transplantation. *Transpl Int* 2010;23:831–841.

73. Grieser C, Denecke T, Steffen IG, et al. Multidetector computed tomography for preoperative assessment of hepatic vasculature and prediction of splenic artery steal syndrome in patients with liver cirrhosis before transplantation. *Eur Radiol* 2010;20:108–117.

74. Quintini C, Hirose K, Hashimoto K, et al. "Splenic artery steal syndrome" is a misnomer: the cause is portal hyperperfusion, not arterial siphon. *Liver Transpl* 2008;14:374–379.

75. Sanyal R, Shah SN. Role of imaging in the management of splenic artery steal syndrome. *J Ultrasound Med* 2009;28:471–477.

76. Shimizu K, Tashiro H, Fudaba T, et al. Splenic artery steal syndrome in living donor liver transplantation: a case report. *Transplant Proc* 2007;39:3519–3522.

77. Nishida S, Kadono J, Werviston D, et al. Gastroduodenal artery steal syndrome during liver transplantation: intraoperative diagnosis with Doppler ultrasound and management. *Transpl Int* 2005;18:350–353.

78. Umeda Y, Yagi T, Sadamori H, et al. Preoperative splenic artery embolization: a safe and efficacious portal decompression technique that improves the outcome of liver donor liver transplantation. *Transpl Int* 2007;20:947–955.

79. Choa CP, Nguyen JH, Paz-Fumagalli R, et al. Splenic embolization in liver transplant recipients: early outcomes. *Transplant Proc* 2007;39:3194–3198.

80. Barcena R, Moreno A, Foruny JR, et al. Improved graft function in liver-transplanted patients after partial splenic embolization: reversal of splenic artery steal syndrome. *Clin Transplant* 2006;20:517–523.

81. Langer R, Langer M, Scholz A, et al. The splenic steal syndrome and the gastroduodenal steal syndrome in patients before and after liver transplantation. *Aktuelle Radiol* 1992;2:55–58.

82. De Carlis L, Sansalone CV, Rondinara GF, et al. Splenic artery steal syndrome after orthotopic liver transplantation: diagnosis and treatment. *Transplant Proc* 1993;25:2594–2596.

83. Manner M, Otto G, Senninger N, et al. Arterial steal: an unusual cause for hepatic hypoperfusion after liver transplantation. *Transpl Int* 1991;4:122–124.

84. Langer R, Langer M, Neuhaus P, et al. Angiographic diagnosis in liver transplantation-II: angiography after transplantation. *Digitale Bilddiagn* 1990;10:92–96.

85. Lautt WW. Regulatory process interacting to maintain hepatic blood flow constancy: vascular compliance, hepatic arterial buffer response, hepatorenal reflex, liver regeneration, escape from vasoconstriction. *Hepatol Res* 2007;37:891–903.

86. Vogl TJ, Pegios W, Balzer JO, et al. Arterial steal syndrome in patients after liver transplantation: transarterial embolization of the splenic and gastroduodenal arteries. *Rofo* 2001;173:908–913.

87. Lautt WW. Mechanism and role of intrinsic regulation of hepatic arterial blood flow: hepatic arterial buffer response. *Am J Physiol* 1985;249:G549–G556.

88. Jakab F, Sugar I, Rath Z, et al. The relationship between portal venous and hepatic arterial blood flow: I, experimental liver transplantation. *HPB Surg* 1996;10:21–26.

89. Jakab F, Rath Z, Schmal F, et al. The interaction between hepatic and portal venous blood flows: simultaneous measurement by transit time ultrasonic volume flowmetry. *Hepatogastroenterology* 1995;42:18–21.

90. Kito Y, Nagino M, Nimura Y. Doppler sonography of hepatic arterial blood flow velocity after percutaneous transhepatic portal vein embolization. *AJR Am J Roentgenol* 2001;176:909–912.

91. Richter S, Vollmar B, Mucke I, et al. Hepatic arteriolo-portal venular shunting guarantees maintenance of nutritional microvascular supply in hepatic arterial buffer response. *J Physiol* 2001;1:193–201.

92. Lo CM, Liu CL, Fan ST. Portal hyperperfusion injury as the cause of primary nonfunction in a small-for-size liver graft: successful treatment with splenic artery ligation. *Liver Transpl* 2003;9:626–630.

93. Troisi R, Cammu G, Militerno G, et al. Modulation of portal graft inflow: a necessity in adult living-donor liver transplantation? *Ann Surg* 2003;237:429–436.

94. Tucker ON, Heaton N. The "small for size" liver syndrome. *Curr Opin Crit Care* 2005;11:150–155.

95. Umeda Y, Yagi T, Sadamori H, et al. Effects of prophylactic splenic artery modulation on portal overperfusion and liver regeneration in small-for-size graft. *Transplantation* 2008;86:673–680.

96. Farges O, Belghitti J. Editorial on "diagnosis and treatment of arterial steal syndromes in liver transplantation recipients." *Liver Transpl* 2003;9:603–604.

97. Saad WE, Davies MG, Ryan CK, et al. Incidence of arterial injuries detected by angiography following percutaneous right-lobe ultrasound-guided core liver biopsies in human subjects. *Am J Gastroenterol* 2006;101:2641–2645.

98. Hellenkant C. Vascular complications following needle puncture of the liver. *Acta Radiol Diagn* 1976;17:209–222.

99. Okuda K, Moyha H, Makajima Y, et al. Frequency of intrahepatic arteriovenous fistulas as a sequela to percutaneous puncture of the liver. *Gastroenterology* 1978;74:1204.

100. Jabour N, Reyes J, Zajko AB, et al. Arterioportal fistula following liver biopsy: three cases occurring in liver transplant recipients. *Dig Dis Sci* 1995;40:1041–1044.

101. Hellenkant C, Olint T. Vascular complications following needle puncture of the liver: an angiographic investigation in the rapid. *Acta Radiol Diagn* 1973;14:577.

102. Saad WE, Davies MG, Rubens DJ, et al. Endoluminal management of arterioportal fistulae in liver transplant recipients: a single center experience. *Vasc Endovasc* 2006;40:451–459.

103. Saad WE, Lippert AJ, Davies MG, et al. Prevalence, presentation, and endovascular management of hemodynamically or clinically significant arterioportal fistulae in living- and cadaveric-donor liver transplant recipients. *Clin Transplant* 2012;26(4):532–538.

104. Figueras J, Soubrane O, Pariente D, et al. Fatal hemobilia after liver graft biopsy in a transplanted child. *Gastroenterol Clin Biol* 1994;18:786–788.

105. Chavan A, Harms J, Picjlmayr R, et al. Transcatheter coil occlusion of an intrahepatic arterioportal fistula in a transplanted liver. *Bildgebung* 1993;60:215–218.

106. Vivas S, Palacio MA, Lomo J, et al. Arterioportal fistula and hemobilia in a patient with hepatic transplant. *Gastroenterol Hepatol* 1998;21:88–89.

107. Charco R, Margarit C, Lopez-Talavera JC, et al. Outcome and hepatic hemodynamics in liver transplant patients with portal vein arterialization. *Am J Transplant* 2001;1:146–151.

108. Karatzas T, Lykaki-Karatzas M, Webb JN, et al. Vascular complications, treatment and outcome following orthotopic liver transplantation. *Transplant Proc* 1997;29:2853–2855.

109. Botelberge T, Van Vlierberghe H, Voet D, et al. Detachable balloon embolization of an arterioportal fistula following liver biopsy in a liver transplant recipient: a case report and review of the literature. *Cardiovasc Intervent Radiol* 2005;28:832–835.

110. Detry O, De Roover A, Delwaide J, et al. Selective coil occlusion of a large arterioportal fistula in a liver graft. *Liver Transpl* 2006;12:888–889.

111. Otobe Y, Hashimoto T, Shimizu Y, et al. Formation of a fatal arterioportal fistula following needle biopsy in a child with a living-related liver transplant: a report of a case. *Surg Today* 1995;25:916–919.

112. Strodel E, Eckhauser FE, Lemmer JH, et al. Presentation and perioperative management of arterioportal fistulas. *Arch Surg* 1987;122:563–571.

113. Agha FP, Raji MR. Successful transcatheter embolic control of significant arterioportal fistula: a serious complication of liver biopsy. *Radiology* 1983;56:277–280.

114. Kim HJ, Kim KW, Kim AY, et al. Hepatic artery pseudoaneurysms in adult living-donor liver transplantation: efficacy of CT and Doppler sonography. *AJR Am J Roentgenol* 2005;184:1549–1555.

115. Marshall MA, Muiesan P, Srinivasan P, et al. hepatic artery pseudoaneurysms following liver transplantation: incidence, presenting features and management. *Clin Radiol* 2001;56:579–587.

116. Fistouris J, Herlenius L, Backman L, et al. Pseudoaneurysm of the hepatic artery following liver transplantation. *Transplant Proc* 2006;38:2679–2682.

117. Leelaudomlipi SL, Bramhall SR, Gunson BK, et al. Hepatic-artery aneurysm in adult liver transplantation. *Transpl Int* 2003;16:257–261.

118. Harman A, Boyvat F, Hasdogan B, et al. Endovascular treatment of active bleeding after liver transplant. *Exp Clin Transplant* 2007;5:1–4.

119. Houssin D, Ortega D, Richardson A, et al. Mycotic aneurysm of the hepatic artery complicating human liver transplantation. *Transplantation* 1988;46:469–471.

120. Alamo JM, Gomez MA, Tamayo MJ, et al. Mycotic pseudoaneurysm after liver transplantation. *Transplant Proc* 2005;37:1512–1514.

121. Finley DS, Hinojosa MW, Paya M, et al. Hepatic artery pseudoaneurysm: a report of seven cases and a review of the literature. *Surg Today* 2005;35:543–547.

122. Jones VS, Chennapragada MS, Lord DJE, et al. Post-liver transplant mycotic aneurysm of the hepatic artery. *J Ped Surg* 2008;43:555–558.

123. Lowell JA, Coopersmith CM, Shenoy S, et al. Unusual presentations of nonmycotic hepatic artery pseudoaneurysms after liver transplantation. *Liver Transpl Surg* 1999;5:200–203.

124. Stange B, Settmacher U, Glanemann M, et al. Aneurysm of the hepatic artery after liver transplantation. *Transplant Proc* 2000;32:533–534.

125. Fischelle JM, Colacchio G, Castaing D, et al. Infected false hepatic aneurysm after orthotopic liver transplantation treated by resection and reno-hepatic vein graft. *Ann Vasc Surg* 1997;11:300–303.

126. Bonham CA, Kapur S, Geller D, et al. Excision and immediate revascularization for hepatic artery pseudoaneurysm following liver transplantation. *Transplant Proc* 1999;31:443.

127. Bussenius-Kammerer M, Ott R, Wutke R, et al. Pseudoaneurysm of the hepatic artery: a rare complication after orthotopic liver transplantation. *Chirurg* 2001;72:78–81.

128. Madariaga J, Tzakis A, Zajko AB, et al. Hepatic artery pseudoaneurysm ligation after orthotopic liver transplantation: a report of 7 cases. *Transplantation* 1992;54:824–828.

129. Goss JA, Shackleton CR, McDiarmid SV, et al. Long-term results of pediatric liver transplantation: an analysis of 569 transplants. *Ann Surg* 1998;228:411–420.

130. Settmacher U, Stange B, Haase R, et al. Arterial complications after liver transplantation. *Transpl Int* 2000;13:372–378.

131. Marujo WC, Langnas AN, Wood RP, et al. Vascular complications following orthotopic liver transplantation: outcome and the role of urgent revascularization. *Tranplant Proc* 1991;23:1484–1486.

132. Almogy G, Bloom A, Verstandig A, et al. Hepatic artery pseudoaneurysm after liver transplantation: a result of transhepatic biliary drainage for primary sclerosing cholangitis. *Transpl Int* 2002;15:53–55.

133. Patel JV, Weston MJ, Kessel DO, et al. Hepatic artery pseudoaneurysm after liver transplantation: treatment with percutaneous thrombin injection. *Transplantation* 2003;75:1755–1757.

134. Millonig G, Graziadi IW, Waldenberger P, et al. Percutaneous management of a hepatic artery aneurysm: bleeding after liver transplantation. *Cardiovasc Intervent Radiol* 2003;75;1755–1757.

135. Elias G, Rastellini C, Nsier H, et al. Successful long-term repair of hepatic artery pseudoaneurysm following liver transplantation with primary stent-grafting. *Liver Transpl* 2007;13:1346–1348.

136. Muraoka N, Uematsu H, Kinoshita K, et al. Covered coronary stent graft in the treatment of hepatic artery pseudoaneurysm after liver transplantation. *J Vasc Intervent Radiol* 2005;16:300–302.

137. Maleux G, Pirenne J, Aerts R, et al. Hepatic artery pseudoaneurysm after liver transplantation: definitive treatment with a stent-graft after failed coil embolization. *Br J Radiol* 2005;78:453–456.

138. Ginat DT, Saad WEA, Waldman DL, et al. Stent-graft placement for the management of iatrogenic hepatic artery branch pseudoaneurysm after liver transplantation. *Vasc Endovasc Surg* 2009;43:513–517.

139. Yamakado K, Nakatsuka A, Takaki H, et al. Stent-graft for the management of hepatic arterial rupture subsequent to transcatheter thrombolysis and angioplasty in a liver transplant recipient. *Cardiovasc Intervent Radiol* 2008;31:S104–S107.

140. Sheng R, Orons PD, Ramos HC, et al. Dissecting pseudoaneurysm of the hepatic artery: a delayed complication of angioplasty in a liver transplant. *Cardiovasc Intervent Radiol* 1995;18:112–114.

141. Jarzembowski TM, Sankary HN, Bogetti D, et al. Living donor liver graft salvage after rupture of hepatic artery pseudoaneurysm. *Int Surg* 2008;93:300–303.

142. Lerut J, Tzakis AG, Bron K, et al. Complications of venous reconstruction in human orthotopic liver transplantation. *Ann Surg* 1987;205:404–414.

143. Settmacher U, Nussler NC, Glanemann M, et al. Venous complications after othotopic liver transplantation. *Clin Transplant* 2000;14:235–241.

144. Funaki B, Rosenblum JD, Leef JA, et al. Percutaneous treatment of portal venous stenosis in children and adolescents with segmental hepatic transplants: long-term results. *Radiology* 2000;215:147–151.

145. Funaki B, Rosenblum JD, Leef JA, et al. Angioplasty treatment of portal vein stenosis in children with segmental liver transplants: mid-term results. *AJR Am J Roentgenol* 1997;169:551–554.

146. Cherukuri R, Haskal ZJ, Naji A, et al. Percutaneous thrombolysis and stent placement for the treatment of portal vein thrombosis after liver transplantation: long-term follow-up. *Transplantation* 1998;65:1124–1126.

147. Mathias K, Bolder U, Lohlein D, et al. Percutaneous transhepatic angioplasty and stent implantation for prehepatic portal vein obstruction. *Cardiovasc Intervent Radiol* 1993;16:313–315.

148. Rollins NK, Sheffield EG, Andrews WS. Portal vein stenosis complicating liver transplantation in children: percutaneous transhepatic angioplasty. *Radiology* 1992;182:731–734.

149. Zajko AB, Sheng R, Bron K, et al. Percutaneous transluminal angioplasty of venous anastomotic stenoses complicating liver transplantation: intermediate-term results. *J Vasc Interv Radiol* 1994;5:121–126.

150. Woo DH, LaBerge JM, Gordon RL, et al. Management of portal venous complications after liver transplantation. *Tech Vasc Interv Radiol* 2007;10:233–239.

151. Ueda M, Egawa H, Uryuhara K, et al. Portal vein complications in long-term course after pediatric living donor liver transplantation. *Transplant Proc* 2007;37:1138–1140.

152. Millis JM, Seaman DS, Piper JB, et al. Portal vein thrombosis and stenosis in pediatric liver transplantation. *Transplantation* 1996;62:748–754.

153. Chong WK, Beland JC, Weeks SM. Sonographic evaluation of venous obstruction in liver transplants. *AJR Am J Roentgenol* 2007;188:515–521.

154. Quiroga S, Sebastia MC, Margarit C, et al. Complications of orthotopic liver transplantation: spectrum of findings with helical CT. *Radiographics* 2001;21:1085–1102.

155. Shibata T, Itoh K, Kubo T, et al. Percutaneous transhepatic balloon dilation of portal venous stenosis in patients with living donor liver transplantation. *Radiology* 2005;235:1078–1083.

156. Buell JF, Funaki B, Cronin DC, et al. Long-term venous complications after full-size and segmental pediatric transplantation. *Ann Surg* 2002;236:658–666.

157. Ko GY, Sung KB, Yoon HK, et al. Early posttransplantation portal vein stenosis following living donor liver transplantation: percutaneous transhepatic primary stent placement. *Liver Transpl* 2007;13:530–536.

158. Baccarani U, Gasparini D, Risaliti A, et al. Percutaneous mechanical fragmentation and stent placement for the treatment of early post-transplatation portal vein thrombosis. *Transplantation* 2001;15:1572–1582.

159. Durham JD, LaBerge JM, Altman S, et al. Portal vein thrombolysis and closure of competitive shunts following liver transplantation. *J Vasc Interv Radiol* 1994;5:611–615.

160. Gibson M, Dick R, Burroughs A, et al. Incidence, risk factors, management and outcome of portal vein abnormalities at orthotopic liver transplantation. *Transplantation* 1994;57:1174.

161. Ciccarelli O, Goffette P, Laterre PF, et al. Transjugular intrahepatic portosystemic shunt approach and local thrombolysis for treatment of early post-transplant portal vein thrombosis. *Transplantation* 2001;72:159–161.

162. Haskal ZJ, Naji A. Treatment of portal vein thrombosis after liver transplantation with percutaneous thrombolysis and stent placement. *J Vasc Interv Radiol* 1993;4:789–792.

163. Olcott EW, Ring EJ, Roberts JP, et al. Percutaneous transhepatic portal vein angioplasty and stent placement after liver transplantation: early experience. *J Vasc Interv Radiol* 1990;1:17–20.

164. Egawa H, Tanaka K, Uemoto S, et al. Relief of hepatic vein stenosis by balloon angioplasty after living-related donor liver transplantation. *Clin Transplant* 1993;7:306–311.

165. Ko GY, Sung KB, Yoon HK, et al. Endovascular treatment of hepatic venous outflow obstruction after living-donor liver transplantation. *J Vasc Interv Radiol* 2002;13:591–599.

166. Darcy MD. Management of venous outflow complications after liver transplantation. *Tech Vasc Interv Radiol* 2007;10:240–245.

167. Kraus TW, Rohren T, Manner M, et al. Successful treatment of complete inferior vena cava thrombosis after transplantation by thrombolytic therapy. *Br J Surg* 1992;79:568–569.

168. Fujimoto M, Moriyassu F, Someda H, et al. Recovery of graft circulation following percutaneous transluminal angioplasty for stenotic venous complications in pediatric liver transplantation: assessment with Doppler ultrasound. *Transpl Int* 1995;8:119–125.

169. Kubo T, Shibata T, Itoh K, et al. Outcome of percutaneous transhepatic venoplasty for hepatic venous outflow obstruction after living donor liver transplantation. *Radiology* 2006;239:285–290.

170. Borsa JJ, Daly CP, Fontaine AB, et al. Treatment of inferior vena cava anastomotic stenoses with the Wallstent endoprosthesis after orthotopic liver transplantation. *J Vasc Interv Radiol* 1999;10:17–22.

171. Weeks SM, Gerber DA, Jaques PF, et al. Primary Gianturco stent placement for inferior vena cava abnormalities following liver transplantation. *J Vasc Interv Radiol* 2000;11:177–187.

172. Saad WE, Darwish WM, Davies MG, et al. Transjugular intrahepatic portosystemic shunt in liver transplant recipients: technical analysis and clinical outcome. *AJR Am J Roentgenol* 2013;200(1):210–218.

173. Narumi S, Hakamada K, Totsuka E, et al. Efficacy of cutting balloon for anastomotic stricture of the hepatic vein. *Transplant Proc* 2004;36:3093–3095.

174. Totsuka E, Hakamada K, Narumi S, et al. Hepatic vein anastomotic stricture after living donor liver transplantation. *Transplant Proc* 2004;36:2252–2254.

175. Cheng TF, Chen YS, Huang TL, et al. Angioplasty treatment of hepatic vein stenosis in pediatric liver transplants. *Transpl Int* 2005;18:556–561.

176. Narumi S, Hakamada K, Toyoki Y, et al. Hepatic clearance improves after angioplasty of the hepatic vein. *Transplant Proc* 2004;36:3091–3092.

177. Nghiem H. Imaging of hepatic transplantation. *Radiol Clin North Am* 1998;36:429–442.

178. Pfammatter T, Williams DM, Lane KL, et al. Suprahepatic caval anastomotic stenosis complicating orthotopic liver transplantation: treatment with percutaneous transluminal angioplasty, Wallstent placement, or both. *AJR Am J Roentgenol* 1997;168:477–480.

179. Brouwers MAN, de Jong KP, Peeters PMJG, et al. Inferior vena cava obstruction after orthotopic liver transplantation. *Clin Transplant* 1994;8:19–22.

180. Boillot O, Sarfati PO, Bringier J, et al. Orthotopic liver transplantation and pathology of the inferior vena cava. *Transplant Proc* 1990;22:1567–1568.
181. Berger H, Hilbertz T, Zuhlke F, et al. Balloon dilation and stent placement of supra hepatic caval anastomotic stenosis following liver transplantation. *Cardiovasc Intervent Radiol* 1993;16:384–387.
182. Zajko AB, Calus D, Clapuyt P, et al. Obstruction of hepatic venous drainage after liver transplantation: treatment with balloon angioplasty. Radiology 1989;170:763–765.
183. Sze DY, Semba CP, Razavi MK, et al. Endovascular treatment of hepatic venous outflow obstruction after piggyback technique liver transplantation. *Transplantation* 1999;68:446–449.
184. Borsa JJ, Daly CP, Fontaine AB, et al. Treatment of inferior vena cava anastomotic atenoses with the Wallstent Endoprosthesis after orthotopic liver transplantation. *J Vasc Interv Radiol* 1999;10:17–22.
185. Weeks SM, Gerber DA, Jaques PF, et al. Primary Gianturco stent placement for inferior vana cava abnormalities following liver transplantation. *J Vasc Interv Radiol* 2000;11:177–187.
186. Cardella JF, Casraneda-Zuniga WR, Hunter D, et al. Amplatzer K. Angiographic and interventional radiologic considerations in liver transplantation. *AJR Am J Roentgenol* 1986;146:143–153.
187. Cardella JF, Amplatzer K. Postoperative angiographic and interventional radiologic evaluation of liver recipients. *Radiol Clin North Am* 1987;25:309–321.
188. Simo G, Echenagusia A, Camunez F, et al. Stenosis of the inferior vena cava after liver transplantation: treatment with Gianturco expandable metalic stents. *Cardiovasc Intervent Radiol* 1995;18:212–216.
189. Rose BS, VanAman ME, Simon DC, et al. Transluminal balloon angioplasty of intrahepatic caval anastomotic stenosis following liver transplantation: case report. *Cardiovasc Intervent Radiol* 1998;11:79–81.
190. Althaus SJ, Perkins JD, Soltes G, et al. Use of a Wallstent in successful treatment of IVC obstruction following liver transplantation. *Transplantation* 1996;61:669–672.
191. Venbrux AC, Mitchell SE, Savader SJ, et al. Long-term results with the use of metallic stents in the inferior vena cava for treatment of Budd-Chiari syndrome. *J Vasc Interv Radiol* 1994;5:411–416.
192. Orons PD, Zajko AB. Angiography and interventional procedures in liver transplantation. *Radiol Clin North Am* 1995;33:541–558.
193. Orons PD, Hari AK, Zajko AB, et al. Thrombolysis and endovascular stent placement for inferior vena caval thrombosis in a liver transplant recipient. *Transplantation* 1997;64:1357–1361.
194. Saad WE, Dasgupta N, Lippert AJ, Turba UC, et al. Extrahepatic pseudoaneurysms and ruptures of the hepatic artery in liver transplant recipients: endovascular management and a new iatrogenic etiology. *Cardiovasc Intervent Radiol.* 2013 Feb;36(1):118-27. doi: 10.1007/s00270-012-0408-y. Epub 2012 May 31.

Vascular Complications after Solid Organ Transplantation: Part 2: Renal and Pancreatic Transplantation

WAEL E. SAAD

INTRODUCTION

Currently performed solid organ transplants below the diaphragm include liver, renal, and pancreatic grafts. Recipients of these transplanted organs represent a growing population worldwide. Vascular complications are not uncommon after solid organ transplantation and may lead to graft dysfunction and, ultimately, graft loss. Understanding the relative surgical anatomy, the causes and types of vascular complications, their presentation, and the options for therapy is important for managing solid organ transplant recipients. Additionally, endovascular management of these vascular complications has assumed a growing role in managing these postoperative complications owing to the minimal invasiveness of the endovascular management and that these techniques usually do not preclude subsequent surgical bailout. This chapter discusses the surgical anatomy, the vascular complications, and the endovascular management options of these vascular complications in solid organ transplant recipients.

Liver transplantation, in particular, is a large and complex surgery with two inflows (arterial and portal) and the hepatic venous outflow and invariable surgical anatomy. The regulatory mechanism of the hepatic inflow (hepatic artery buffer response), if intact, adds to the complexity of the transplant's hemodynamics.

This chapter discusses the surgical anatomy, the postoperative vascular complications of renal and pancreatics transplantation, and the endovascular management options of these vascular complications. It is preceded by Chapter 79 which discusses the vascular complications of liver transplantation.

RENAL TRANSPLANTATION

Surgical Anatomy

The many of complications after kidney transplantation are related to the surgery and are not primary anatomic or pathologic issues related to the recipient or the donor graft.[1,2] Furthermore, post-transplant vascular surgical anatomy is crucial to reporting of endovascular and surgical management of vascular complications. There are several variables in the vascular surgical anatomy.[1,2] This is due to the varying surgical techniques and types of hepatic grafts. A detailed anatomy discussion is beyond the scope of this chapter; however, basic surgical anatomy is described to introduce the principles of liver transplant surgical anatomy.

Arterial Surgical Anatomy

In most cases, the arterial communications of the recipient to the graft in renal transplants is from the recipient iliac arteries to the graft renal artery(s). The recipient iliac to graft renal anastomosis most commonly is either (1) end-to-end internal iliac artery to graft renal artery or (2) end-to-side external iliac artery to graft renal artery (FIGURE 80.1). The latter is more common than the former. A maximum of two to three graft renal arteries can be connected to the recipient iliac system depending on the number of accessory renal arteries in the renal graft. Transplant renal arterial stenoses (TRAS) are classified according to their site relative to the surgical anastomosis.[2] Extremes of arterial communications can be demonstrated in an example where the aorta (with its anatomic renal artery branches to both kidneys in a diseased infant donor) is connected end-to-side to either the recipient infrarenal abdominal aorta or one of the common iliac arteries.

Venous Surgical Anatomy

The venous surgical anatomy commonly follows the arterial surgical anatomy (*see above*) (FIGURE 80.1).

Iliac Inflow Arterial Stenosis

This is not a complication of the renal transplant procedure but is almost always underlying (preexisting or progressing) atherosclerotic disease of the recipient.[1-9] It is occasionally referred to as proximal transplant renal artery stenosis (prox-TRAS) or pseudo-TRAS.[2,3] It occurs in 0% to 2.4% of renal transplants[1,2,9] and represents 0% to 30% of vascular stenoses in renal transplants.[7-9] Early prox-TRAS (occurring within 30 days from the renal transplants) can represent up to 25% of prox-TRAS[5] and is most likely caused by poor pretransplant workup and proactive management of iliac atherosclerotic disease. Indeed, the incidence of prox-TRAS after renal transplantation can decrease with careful surveillance and management of native/recipient atherosclerotic iliac arterial disease prior to renal transplantation. Early prox-TRAS most likely presents with poor graft function from the offset and continuing hypertension (*see below*).

Delayed prox-TRAS (occurring after 30 days and up to years after the transplant) represents at least 75% of all prox-TRAS cases.[5] This is not uncommon because many renal transplants are performed with diabetes mellitus and hypertension as

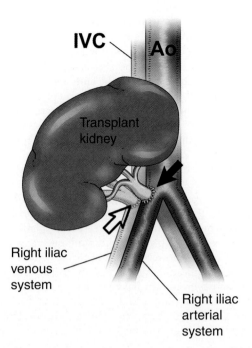

FIGURE 80.1 Basic surgical vascular anatomy of a right lower quadrant kidney transplant. Both the transplant renal artery and vein are surgically connected (anastomosed) end to side to the right iliac arterial (*solid arrow*) and venous systems (*hollow arrow*), respectively. The iliac vessels of the recipient are usually the right external iliac artery and vein and not the common iliac artery and vein.

Ao, abdominal aorta; IVC, inferior vena cava.

underlying causes of the failure of the native kidneys of their recipients. Both these diseases are known to contribute and accelerate the development and progression of aortoiliac atherosclerotic disease. Indeed, the incidence of prox-TRAS after renal transplantation increases with increased recipient age.[3–5] Moreover, the longer the renal transplant and its recipient survive, the more likely atherosclerotic iliac inflow disease is to develop/progress to form significant aortoiliac stenoses.

Prox-TRAS presents similarly to renal artery stenosis (RAS) of the renal graft (TRAS-proper), hence the name pseudo-TRAS (*see below*).[1–9] In addition to symptoms of TRAS-proper there are lower extremity symptoms, such as claudication or rest pain. The management of prox-TRAS is best by endovascular means, which include balloon angioplasty with or without stent placement.[1–9]

Steno-Occlusive Complications of the Transplant Renal Artery

Occlusive or steno-occlusive disease of the renal artery is a collective term referring to transplant renal artery stenosis proper (TRAS-proper), transplant renal artery kinks, and transplant renal artery thrombosis (RAT).[10] TRAS-proper is the most common complication, representing at least 30% of these.[10] Renal artery kinks and thrombosis are rare and represent, at most, 10% to 15% of vascular complications following renal transplantation.[10]

Transplant Renal Artery Stenosis Proper

TRAS-proper occurs in 3% to 12.5% of renal transplants but has been reported in up to 23% of renal transplant recipients.[2,4,11–14] The incidence probably depends on the degree and frequency of noninvasive imaging.[1,2,15] The more thorough the post-transplant imaging, the more likely the incidence of TRAS is going to rise within a particular institution. Wong and coworkers[15] demonstrated that the incidence of "documented" TRAS within the same institution increased by more than fivefold from 2.4% in the era prior to Doppler ultrasound (DUS) surveillance to 12.4%.

TRAS are classified according to their location and multiplicity.[2] Location-based classification is relative to the surgical anastomosis into preanastomotic, anastomotic, and postanastomotic.[1,2,4,14–17] The latter can also be classified into extrarenal and segmental/lobar renal artery stenoses.[1,2] Early TRAS (probably occurring within the first 1 to 2 months after the transplant) most likely occurs due to surgical technical problems and complications, including suturing (oversewing/faulty suturing), clamp injury, trauma during harvesting (including clamp injury and focal dissection), focal dissection with super-added neointimal hyperplasia, cyclosporine toxicity, increased cold ischemia time, cytomegalovirus (CMV) infection, overlooked fibromuscular dysplasia (FMD) in the renal allograft, and acute rejection.[2,4,7,9,11,15,18–21] Delayed (probably occurring 1 to 2 months after the transplant) TRAS usually is caused by vascular ischemia (vaso-vasorum ischemia) and, more commonly, progression of atherosclerotic disease.[9,18,22,23] In an evaluation by Voiculescu and coworkers,[7] 27% of TRAS was due to progression of atherosclerotic disease, 41% was due to neointimal hyperplasia, 8% was due to focal dissection, and less than 3% was due to FMD. Predisposing factors that increase the risk of TRAS is end-to-end anastomoses, diseased graft donors, aging recipients, and acute rejection.[2,9,10,18,22,24,25]

Most TRAS occur within 2 to 24 months of the renal transplant with 25% and 60% of TRAS diagnosed at 2 months and 4 to 5 months after the transplantation, respectively.[9,15] The clinical presentation of TRAS depends on the timing of its development/diagnosis after transplantation.[2,14,18,19,26] In the immediate post-transplant period (within 1 to 2 weeks of the transplant), TRAS presents with anuria and continued dialysis dependence.[2,24] After the first 1 to 2 weeks post-transplantation, however, TRAS can present in two ways, which are both mediated by the renin-angiotensin system secondary to renal parenchymal ischemia due to TRAS.[19] The primary presentation is accelerated renovascular hypertension, which occurs, solely or in combination with renal insufficiency, in over 80% of cases.[2,4,24] Renovascular hypertension may vary in acuity form of sudden-onset malignant hypertension to a more insidious refractory hypertension that usually requires more antihypertensive medications than prior to transplantation.[19] Rarely, paradoxical hypotension can occur due to TRAS.[16] The less common presentation (associated with the salt-avid conditions mediated by the renin-angiotensin system) is fluid retention. However, its eventual prevalence probably equals that of renovascular hypertension where fluid-retention symptoms occurs, solely or in combination with renal-vascular hypertension, in over 80% of cases.[2,4,24] Fluid retention can present as diuretic-resistant edema, flash pulmonary edema, and congestive heart failure.[16,19,27] Unfortunately, systemic hypertension with or without graft dysfunction has a wide clinical differential diagnosis, which includes chronic rejection, steroid use, cyclosporine toxicity, recurrent glomerulonephritis, and disease of the native kidneys.[4,24] Because of this, noninvasive imaging is important to the diagnosis of TRAS.[1,2]

Noninvasive imaging includes DUS, magnetic resonance (MR), and radioisotope renal scans.[2,9,10,19,25,27–36] Contrast-enhanced computed tomography (CT) has a negligible role due to the high intravenous contrast dose and the ionizing radiation dose, particularly when there is suspicion of TRAS, which has a high association with renal insufficiency. Radioisotope renal scans have a moderate sensitivity (75%) and specificity (67%).[9,10,27] The utilization of radioisotope renal scans for evaluating TRAS is probably on the decline as improvement in technology in DUS and MR occur (*see below*). As a result, DUS and MR are the primary noninvasive imaging modality for evaluating TRAS.[2,19]

DUS is often the initial modality utilized in the evaluation of potential TRAS because of its availability and cost-effectiveness.[2] The relatively large and superficial nature of the transplanted renal artery makes DUS an ideal screening modality.[2] DUS findings suggestive of TRAS are a peak systolic velocity of greater than 2.0 to 2.5 m/second, a low pulsatility index of 0.9 ± 0.1, and a parvus tardus waveform with a systolic acceleration time greater or equal to 0.1 second.[2,29,30] In addition, color Doppler aliasing at the stenotic segment with a velocity gradient of more than 2:1 between the stenotic segment and prestenotic segment.[2] Utilizing these criteria, DUS has a sensitivity and specificity range of 87% to 94% and 86% to 100%, respectively.[9,31] However, DUS examination is not consistent (operator dependent) and the examination may not be complete by not visualizing the entire transplant renal artery.[2,19] Magnetic resonance imaging (MRI) is a more consistent examination and with improved technology (high-resolution contrast-enhanced MR angiography) its sensitivity and specificity can be increased significantly.[19,32–34] The overall sensitivity and specificity ranges for MR are 67% to 100% and 75% to 100%, respectively.[9,35,36] The advantages of MR is that it can characterize TRAS, define anatomic details, and evaluate the transplant renal parenchyma, inflow aortoiliac disease, and other vascular and nonvascular complications.[2,19,25] Despite the technologic advances of noninvasive imaging, the gold standard radiologic examination for TRAS continues to be conventional transcatheter angiography.[2,9,19,37]

The primary method of choice for the management of TRAS is transcatheter angioplasty with or without stent placement[4,7–9,15,16,20,38–48] (FIGURE 80.2). Even the studies that suggested that surgical repair had better clinical success and less morbidity still recommend percutaneous angioplasty as the first-line therapy.[38] Historically (when end-to-end internal iliac to transplant renal artery anastomoses were more popular), end-to-side anastomoses (91% technical success) were found to be more technically amenable than end-to-end anastomoses (75% technical success) to percutaneous angioplasty.[39] Also historically (prior to the popular use of stents), TRAS refractory to percutaneous transluminal angioplasty (PTA) was observed in 10% of cases.[38] However, in recent years primary stent placement has been reported in up to 32% to 38% of TRAS cases.[7,40] Unfortunately, given the retrospective nature of studies, it is not clear whether operator preference or strict recalcitrant (refractory to angioplasty alone) lesions went on to stent placement.[7,40] Certain studies have shown a higher rate of stent-placement increases

in restenotic lesions (44% stent rate) compared to primary stent placement for first-time lesions (7% stent rate).[41] Moreover, other authors have clearly defined a policy toward stent placement where stents are placed for first-time TRAS recalcitrant to PTA and restenotic lesions.[16] In the author's institution most (>70% of cases) TRAS cases end up with stent placement despite having balloon angioplasty as the primary treatment (unpublished data).

The overall technical success has probably increased over the past 30 years. Prior to the year 2000, the technical success ranged from 69% to 99% (overall, 79% [$n = 249/316$]),[15,39,42–47] compared to post-2000, where the technical success ranges from 88% to 100% (overall, 92% [$n = 216/234$]).[4,8,9,16,20,40,48] We can only speculate that the reason may be due to improved technology with more flexible and lower-profile platforms. The overall "anatomic vascular complication" rate ranges for 0% to 10.3%.[16,20,38–40,48] However, when nephrotoxicity is included, the overall complication rate exceeds 10%. The rate of clinically evident nephrotoxicity has been reported in up to 5.9%.[48] Anatomic vascular complications include RAT (occurs: 0% to 6.9%), flow-limiting renal artery dissection (occurs: 0% to 9.8%), and renal artery rupture/pseudoaneurysm (occurs: 0% to 2.3%).[16,20,38–40,48]

The restenosis rate of TRAS following successful angioplasty and/or stenting ranges between 20% and 36%.[15,20,39,41] Voiculescu and coworkers[7] placed the restenosis rate after angioplasty only, primary stent placement, and surgical repair for the management of TRAS at 62%, 30%, and 14%, respectively. Most restenoses occur within 8 to 9 months following the endovascular procedure.[10,13,23,26,38,39,46,47] The Kaplan-Meier primary unassisted and primary assisted patency at 12 months following angioplasty and/or stenting is 72% to 85% and 85% to 95%, respectively.[16,40]

Renal graft loss from endovascular complications has been described in up to 10% of cases[20] and the long-term graft survival following treated TRAS is 56% to 76%.[15,40,43] The overall clinical success rate is 60% to 75%.[8,20,38,39,48] Furthermore, the early (within 1 month of the endovascular procedure) and long-term (3 months and later) clinical success rates are 58% to 82% and 41% to 75%, respectively,[1,4,7,8,38,39,46,47] with the peak of clinical success occurring 3 months after the endovascular procedure.[8] When considering response to hypertension only, the clinical success rate is 63% to 83%.[39,42,43,45–48] When considering renal dysfunction (serum creatinine level reduction >15%),[1,4] however, the clinical success is 45% to 67%.[40,45,48]

Transplant Renal Artery Kinks

Transplant renal artery kinks are arterial anatomic defects related to sharp turns in the transplant arterial course. Transplant renal kinks occur in up to 0.4% of renal transplants and represent up to 15% of renal transplant arterial defects.[10] Arterial redundancy is the most common cause and is a technical problem (long/redundant donor and/or recipient arterial stumps).[10] A less common cause is post-transplant graft shifting or shifting of adjacent pelvic contents.[10] The consequences of transplant renal artery kinks are similar to those of TRAS. These include renovascular hypertension, salt-and-water retention, graft dysfunction, and even graft loss. Similar to the transplant hepatic artery, transplant renal artery kinks are notoriously recalcitrant to endovascular therapy. Furthermore, the

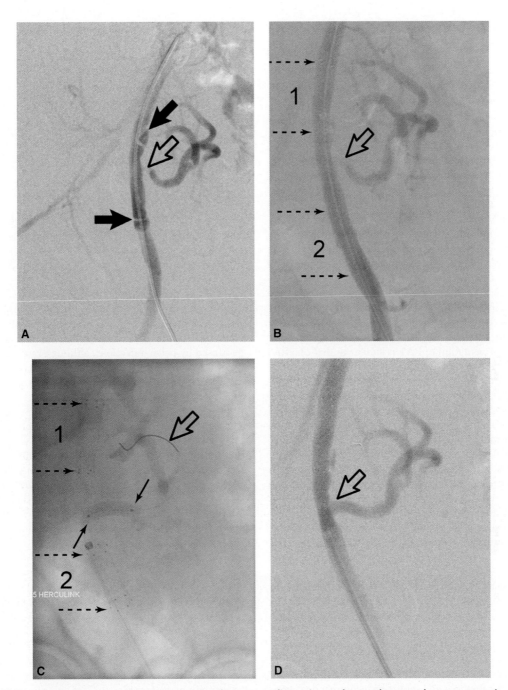

FIGURE 80.2 Stent placement for postoperative iliac artery dissection and transplant renal artery stenosis.
A. Initial oblique right iliac artery angiogram demonstrating external iliac artery dissection (*solid arrows*) above and below the transplant renal artery. There is also an anastomotic stenosis of the transplant renal artery (*hollow arrow*). The angiogram is performed from an ipsilateral right femoral approach utilizing a straight-flush multi-sidehole diagnostic angiographic catheter. The dissection is not from the endovascular access. **B**. Right iliac artery angiogram after self-expanding stent placement to resolve the external iliac artery dissection noted proximal (*1* between upper paired *dashed arrows*) and distal (*2* between lower pair of *dashed arrows*) to the transplant renal artery. Again noted is the anastomotic stenosis of the transplant renal artery (*hollow arrow*). **C**. Fluoroscopic image during after self-expanding stent placement to resolve the external iliac artery dissection noted above (*1* between *dashed arrows*) and below (*2* between second and lower pair of *dashed arrows*) and during the balloon-expandable stent placement for the anastomotic stenosis of the transplant renal artery (between *solid arrow*). The balloon-expandable stent (between *solid arrow*) is passed over a 0.014-inch wire (*hollow arrow*). **D**. Completion right iliac artery angiogram after stent placement to resolve the external iliac artery dissection noted above and the anastomotic transplant renal artery stenosis. Both iliac dissections and the anastomotic transplant renal artery stenosis (*hollow arrow*) are resolved.

endovascular procedure is considered high-risk (high-risk for dissection) in the presence of arterial kinks.[10] The ideal treatment, if feasible, is open surgical repair and ridding the renal artery of its redundancy.

Transplant Renal Artery Thrombosis

Transplant RAT is part of an entity referred to as renal graft thrombosis, which includes RAT and/or renal vein thrombosis (RVT).[1,10] Transplant RAT occurs in 0.3% to 1.9% of renal transplants and represents up to 10% of renal transplant arterial defects and 31% to 43% of renal graft thrombosis.[10,49,50] Moreover, RAT coexists with RVT in 11% to 15% of cases.[1,49,51] RAT occurs mostly within 2 weeks of the transplant with 80% occurring within a month of the renal transplant.[1,52] RAT occurring after 1 month of renal transplantation is usually associated with graft rejection or high-grade TRAS.[1,10,53] In addition, recipients receiving cyclosporine have a higher risk of RAT (1.8% to 7.0% in recipients with cyclosporine versus 0% to 1.0% in recipients without cyclosporine).[54,55] This is because cyclosporine contributes to vascular thrombosis by reducing blood flow, enhancing platelet aggregation, and causing endothelial damage.[56,57]

The clinical presentation of RAT is similar to that of TRAS from a hypertension/renal dysfunction standpoint. However, the usual time proximity to the transplant, the usually occlusive nature of RAT, and the possibility of evolving into global renal graft thrombosis (combined RAT and RVT) makes RAT's presentation more of an urgent nature.[58–60] The maximum duration of normothermic ischemia compatible with complete recovery of renal function in native kidneys is estimated to be 30 to 45 minutes.[58,59] Severe renal damage followed by irrecoverable renal damage can be expected as early as 1 to 2 hours and 3 hours, respectively.[60] Conversely, anecdotal case reports have reported successful renal graft salvage (recovery of renal function) within 48 hours (all but one within 24 hours).[53,61–68] Some of the cases that recover may have been due to the fact that RAT was actually partial and not complete as well as the formation of collaterals.[53,63,66,67]

Once a renal artery complication is suspected, a DUS evaluation of the transplant renal artery should be performed. By DUS, RAT shows lack of or diminished arterial flow with possible thrombus filling defects in the renal artery.[1,69,70] Once RAT is confirmed by imaging, an urgent revascularization should be performed as soon as possible to optimize the chances of graft recovery (*see above*). Surgical thrombectomy is certainly quicker than endovascular methods and should be recommended, especially in the immediate post-transplant period where there is the additional risk of bleeding from thrombolytics.[1] Certainly, transcatheter thrombolysis has the advantage of reestablishing flow while the surgical team mobilizes. In addition, transcatheter thrombolysis can uncover underlying anatomic defects (kinks or TRAS) that may have caused or contributed to the RAT.[1,53] Rouviere and coworkers[53] had the largest case series (*n* = 4) of transplant renal artery transcatheter thrombolysis where three of four (75%) were technically successful with reestablishment of inline arterial flow to the graft within 10 to 22 hours (mean of 16 hours) of urokinase transcatheter infusion. Two of the three had established renal graft recovery (50% clinical success rate).[53] The technically failed case was caused by a heavy clot burden where the arterial thrombus had propagated to the

iliac arteries.[53] Certainly, cases of minimal clot burden, such as segmental RAT, have also been described.[50,71] Once inline arterial flow has been established, careful interrogation of the renal artery is warranted to evaluate for underlying anatomic defects (renal artery kinks and TRAS).[1,53] These underlying anatomic defects should be resolved either surgically or by endovascular means.[1,53] In two of the three technically successful transcatheter thrombolysis cases by Rouviere, two (67%) had underlying anatomic defects: one was a kink and the other was a significant TRAS, which was resolved by angioplasty alone.[53]

Renal Arterial Injuries

Renal artery injuries include: (1) flow-limiting arterial dissections, (2) renal artery pseudoaneurysms (PsA), (3) renal artery to renal vein arteriovenous fistulas (AVFs), and (4) renal artery to urinary arteriocalyceal fistulas.[1] Dissections can be iatrogenic from the transplant surgery or from endovascular procedures, AVFs and arteriocaliceal fistulas are probably all from percutaneous biopsies whether pre-, intra-, or post-transplantation.[1,72,73] PsA can be iatrogenic from endovascular procedures (uninfected contained ruptures) but may not be due to injuries: They may be caused by pelvic infections, although rarely reported. These injuries may coexist, particularly AVFs, PsA, and arteriocaliceal fistulas, in up to 30% of arterial injury cases.[1,72]

Renal Artery Dissection

This entity, in the absence of endovascular procedures, is rarely reported after renal transplantation.[69,74] It is either spontaneous, but is most likely, or iatrogenic. "Spontaneous" renal artery dissection is most likely actually iatrogenic from the surgery itself, starting as a small intimal flap that enlarges when inline arterial flow is established and then propagates distally to become an arterial blood flow limiting anomaly.[1,9,11,18,69] Superadded RAT may ensue.[1,69] Significant renal artery dissection with or without superadded RAT presents within the first 2 to 7 days following transplantation and usually presents with anuria and dialysis dependence. Small intimal flaps/arterial dissections that do not grow and propagate may be the cause and location of neointimal hyperplasia, which may evolve into significant TRAS at a later date (probably weeks to months after the renal transplantation).[1,9] Certainly, many transplant renal artery dissections may be from endovascular procedures (primarily TRAS-renal artery angioplasty and/or stent placement) where the dissection rate has been described in up to 10% of cases of transplant renal artery angioplasty (*see above*).[16,20,38–40,48] The presence of arterial kinks in a transplant artery adds to the risk of creating dissection during angioplasty and stent placement.[1,2,10,75,76]

It is difficult for operators utilizing DUS to detect dissections; however, they can identify renal artery flow compromise or thrombosis and they should suggest an angiogram to further define the arterial flow anomaly.[1,69] Non-flow-limiting dissection should be left alone: they do not need treatment because they do not compromise flow and are high risk for propagating and becoming significant. The endovascular management of transplant renal dissection is to cross the dissection flap starting from the true lumen and returning distally into the true lumen and attempting to stabilize the dissection flap up against the renal artery wall by either "tacking" it with a balloon or placing a stent (usually a self-expanding stent).[1,69]

Renal Artery Pseudoaneurysms

This entity, in the absence of endovascular procedures, is rarely reported after renal transplantation.[72,73] PsA may be related to biopsies, postoperative infections, or as contained ruptures after endovascular procedures.[1,16,39,72,73] They may coexist with AVF in up to 30% of cases.[1,73] Intrarenal PsA may be small and asymptomatic and may even resolve spontaneously.[1,73] However, they may present (like AVF, *see below*) with hematuria.[1,73] Extrarenal PsA, like most extravisceral PsA, carry the potential of rupture with catastrophic consequences.[77]

DUS may have difficulty identifying small PsA, especially in the setting of small (or largely thrombosed) extrarenal PsA associated with arterial tortuosity. Intrarenal, particularly cortical or medullary lesions, can be spotted by DUS. Small asymptomatic PsA can be left alone, untreated, however, with careful imaging follow-up.[1] Large and/or symptomatic PsA require endovascular management: either coil embolization (intrarenal PsA) or stent exclusion (usually extrarenal or segmental lesions.[1]

Renal Artery to Vein Fistulas

Renal AVFs occur in 0.2 to 2.0% of renal transplants.[72,73] It is well reported that AVFs are related to or caused by percutaneous biopsies of the renal parenchyma whether pre-, intra-, or post-transplantation.[1,10,72,73,78] They occur after 1% to 18% of percutaneous biopsies of renal transplants[1,10,73,78–80] and usually become evident within 2 to 3 months after a biopsy.[1,73] They may coexist with PsA in up to 30% of cases.[1,73] They occur, almost always, intra renal.[2] Small AVFs are usually asymptomatic and many, up to 70%, resolve within 1 to 2 years from the diagnosis.[1,10,72] However, they may present with gross hematuria (up to 90% of cases), renal insufficiency (graft dysfunction), hypertension, and high cardiac output failure.[1,2,10,72,81–83]

DUS would probably show what is seen in many other transplant fistulas. This includes: decreased arterial resistive indices, arterialization (increased velocity and arterial waveform) of the renal vein and its involved tributaries, turbulence and aliasing at the site of the AVF in the renal parenchyma, and (if the AVF is hemodynamically significant) lack of arterial Doppler flow in the involved renal parenchyma distal to the AVF.[84,85] Contrast-enhanced MR will probably detect only large AVFs showing a perfusion defect in the renal parenchyma, may visualize the fistula itself, and show a large renal vein that fills early in the arterial phase of the enhancement. Conventional transcatheter angiography is still the gold standard. It is a dynamic study that can evaluate the hemodynamic significance of the AVF. Conventional angiography can also detect the most minuscule of AVFs, especially when using carbon dioxide as a contrast agent because it is volatile and passes through the region of the vascular bed with the least resistance (the AVF).[2] Typically, the fistula site is visualized with a dilated, high-velocity, early draining vein(s).[2]

Endovascular management is the first-choice management option[1,2] and is indicated in symptomatic AVF only.[1,2,10,72,81–83] Endovascular management is in the form of superselective embolization (commonly microcoils) with a technical success rate of 71% to 100% of cases and alleviation of symptoms in 57% to 88%.[1,2,72,81–83] Major renal allograft infarcts involving up to 30% to 50% of the renal parenchyma with subsequent graft loss have been reported in up to 29% of cases during the embolization management of large AVFs.[83] As a result, some authors do not consider aggressive embolization of the AVF with complete obliteration,

which, although necessary at times, is a necessary endpoint.[2] The appropriate endpoint is embolization enough to alleviate symptoms and not necessarily complete angiographic results.[2]

Transplant Renal Vein Thrombosis

Transplant RVT is part of an entity referred to as renal graft thrombosis, which includes RVT and/or RAT.[1,10] Transplant RVT occurs in 0.1% to 6% of renal transplants and represents over 60% of renal graft thromboses.[10,49–50] Moreover, RVT coexists with RAT in 11% to 15% of cases.[1,49,51] RVT occurs mostly within 2 weeks of the transplant with 80% occurring within a month of it.[1,52] Recipients receiving cyclosporine have a higher risk of RVT. In addition, RVT is associated with deep venous thrombosis (DVT) extending to the iliac veins.[1,70,86,87] RVT usually represents oliguria, hematuria, graft dysfunction (rising creatinine), and, occasionally, graft pain and tenderness.[51,53,69,70,86–89] RVT with iliac DVT is associated with lower extremity edema.[1,70,86,87] In extreme cases, the graft may rupture, leading to hypovolemia and shock.[86] If RVT is associated with RAT (global graft thrombosis), urgent symptoms of RAT are evident including graft failure/anuria and hypertension (*see above*).[58–60] Global renal graft thrombosis is a serious complication. In one study renal graft thrombosis represented 45% and 37% of renal graft loss within 3 and 12 months, respectively.[49] DUS findings of RVT in the absence of RAT shows graft edema, swelling, and no venous flow.[1,69,70] Thrombus in the transplant renal vein can be visualized. In the absence of RAT, the arterial resistive index is increased with reversal of diastolic flow. If RAT is present, diminished arterial flow with possible thrombus filling defects in the renal artery is seen.[1,69,70]

Traditionally, renal graft thrombosis is managed by emergent laparotomy to evaluate for graft viability, and if the graft is viable, an emergent surgical thrombectomy is performed.[1] However, isolated partial RVT (no RAT) has been successfully treated with anticoagulation alone.[90] In isolated complete RVT (no RAT) thrombolysis can be performed in an attempt to reduce periprocedural morbidity as well as manage underlying femoroiliac venous DVT.[1,51,70,86] Successful venous transcatheter thrombolysis has been reported.[91–100] The thrombolysis catheter(s) can be placed in the veins only or the arterial side only, or both.[91–100] Hypothetically, the strategy behind placing the thrombolytic catheter on the arterial side when managing RVT is administering pharmacolytics proximal to the thrombus (including small venules, which are tributaries to the thrombosed renal vein) as well as indwelling within the main renal vein thrombus. It is important to manage the underlying/associated iliofemoral DVT because it may be the cause of the RVT and/or it may propagate, if not resolved, back into the renal vein, causing early recurrence.[1] Management of iliofemoral DVT is conventional including mechanical and pharmacolytics, iliac stents, and inferior vena cava filter placement.[1]

▍ PANCREATIC TRANSPLANTATION
Surgical Anatomy

It is not uncommon to have concomitant pancreatic and renal transplants. These transplants can by synchronous (performed simultaneously within the same operative setting) or metachronous (subsequent to one another). Many of the complications after pancreatic transplants with and without kidney transplantation are related to the surgery and are not primary anatomic or pathologic issues related to the recipient or the donor graft. Furthermore, post-transplant vascular surgical anatomy is crucial to the reporting of endovascular and surgical management of vascular complications. There are several variables in the vascular surgical anatomy.[101] This is due to the varying surgical techniques and types of hepatic grafts. A detailed anatomy discussion is beyond the scope of this chapter; however, basic surgical anatomy is described to introduce the principles of renal and pancreatic transplant surgical anatomy.

Arterial Surgical Anatomy

There are several variations in pancreatic transplant artery surgical anatomy.[101–114] However, a common surgical anatomy using a "Y-graft" is described.[101,110] In most cases, the arterial communications of the recipient to the pancreatic allograft is created using a homograft iliac Y-graft (FIGURE 80.3). The base of the Y-graft is sutured end-to-side to the recipient common or external iliac artery (less commonly aorta) (FIGURE 80.3). One limb of the bifurcated Y-graft is sutured to the allograft superior mesenteric artery (SMA). The other bifurcated Y-graft limb is sutured to the splenic artery (SpA). The gastroduodenal artery (GDA) coming off the common hepatic artery communicates with the inferior pancreatico-duodenal artery (IPDA), which anatomically arises from the SMA (FIGURE 80.3). The IPDA and GDA form the pancreatico-duodenal arcade supplying the pancreatic head. The SpA supplies most of the pancreatic body and tail.[101,110]

Venous Surgical Anatomy

Pancreatic allograft venous drainage is natural into the splenic and mesenteric vein(s), which then drain anatomically into the allograft portal vein.[101,110] The allograft portal vein is sutured systemically to the recipient inferior vena cava or iliac vein. These are not shown on the schematic (FIGURE 80.3).

VASCULAR COMPLICATIONS

Due to the scarcity of detailed reporting on different pancreatic transplant and that most pancreatic transplant vascular complications present and are worked up (clinically and by imaging) similarly, vascular complications of pancreatic transplants are discussed altogether and not separately into detailed entities as was discussed in the liver and renal transplant sections.

Vascular complications represent more than 50% of early (within 6 months of pancreatic transplantation) and less than 10% of late (after 6 months of pancreatic transplantation) pancreatic graft failure.[105] The most common and detrimental of these vascular complication is "graft thrombosis."[105,115–118] It is unclear in reviewing most of the reports in the literature whether

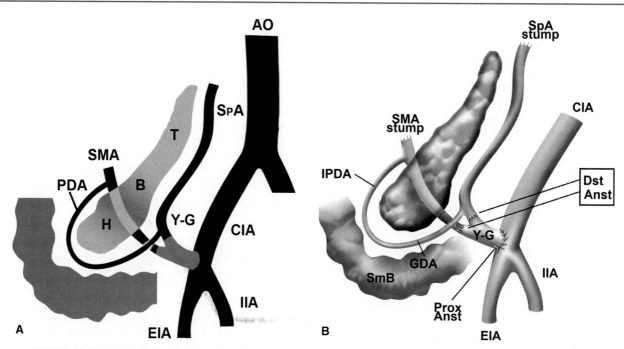

FIGURE 80.3 Basic surgical arterial anatomy of a right lower quadrant pancreatic transplant. The transplant pancreas has two primary arteries, which are the splenic artery (*SpA*) and the superior mesenteric artery (*SMA*) and their branches. The main branch off the proximal splenic (celiac axis) artery is the gastroduodenal artery (**B**, *GDA*), which contributes to the pancreatico-duodenal arcade (**A**, *PDA*), which connects to the SMA primarily by the inferior pancreatico-duodenal artery (**B**, *IPDA*). The PDA (*GDA* and *IPDA* included) supply the pancreatic head (*H*). The remainder of the splenic artery (*SpA*) runs along the pancreatic body (*B*) and tail (*T*) supplying it via the pancreatic magna. To connect the two primary arteries supplying the pancreatic transplant (*SpA* and *SMA*) to the right iliac arterial system of the recipient end-to-side via one anastomosis, a Y-graft (*Y-G*) is used as a conduit. The proximal arterial anastomosis (*Prox Anst*) of the pancreatic transplant is the end-to-side anastomosis of the Y-graft (the "base" of the Y-graft) with the recipient iliac arteries. The distal anastomoses (*Dst Anst*) are two: the mesenteric artery limb of the Y-graft with the graft SMA and the splenic artery artery limb of the Y-graft with the graft SpA.

Ao, abdominal aorta; CIA, common iliac artery; EIA, external iliac artery; IIA, internal iliac artery; SmB, small bowel.

this term refers to thrombosis that is arterial or venous, or both; or whether it represents complete/total or partial arterial or venous thrombosis.[105,115–118] In some instances it is defined clearly as arterial and/or venous thrombosis;[119] however, in many instances they are amalgamated and not clear.[105,115–118] Nevertheless, the pancreatic artery thrombosis component of the greater "graft thrombosis" complication is the most common and most serious. Because of that the definition of "graft thrombosis" in the literature is not clear[105,115–118] and may refer to slightly different severities or extents of vascular thrombosis; the incidence of pancreatic graft thrombosis in the literature ranges widely from 2% to 19%.[105,115–124]

Vascular complications present with pancreatic graft dysfunction in the form of insulin dependence.[105,115–124] This is either primary (*author's term*: never achieved insulin dependence after pancreatic transplantation), which is immediately posttransplantation, or secondary (*author's term*: after achieving insulin dependence after pancreatic transplantation), which occurs later in the post-transplantation period. Pancreatitis may also be present either as a cause and/or effect of the vascular complications (particularly pancreatic artery PsA). In addition, PsA of the pancreatic artery or adjacent recipient iliac artery and branches may present with gastrointestinal bleeding, pelvic bleeding, and hypovolemia.[101–124]

Noninvasive imaging (modalities and techniques and sequences) of vascular complications are similar to those of renal transplants (*see above*) with the exception of renal radioisotope scans, which have no role in pancreatic transplants.

However, radioisotope scans for lower gastrointestinal bleeding can be used to evaluate for (localize the bleeding: pancreatic transplant source or extrapancreatic source) potential occult insidious bleeding, which may occur from within the pancreatic transplant. Again, contrast-enhanced CT has a lesser role due to the high intravenous contrast dose and the ionizing radiation dose, particularly when considering that many pancreatic transplant recipients have a history of renal insufficiency and, not uncommonly, have concomitant renal transplants. When compared to renal transplantation, DUS has a lesser role, in the current author's opinion, because of obscurity from adjacent bowel, the not uncommon presence of pancreatitis, and (possibly) the more complex nature of the vascular surgical anatomy. This places contrast-enhanced high-resolution magnetic resonance angiography (MRA) in the forefront of noninvasive imaging evaluation of vascular complications after pancreatic transplantation.[103] The advantages of MRA is that it can characterize the vascular complication, define anatomic details, evaluate the pancreatic transplant parenchyma, evaluate concomitant renal transplants (vascular and parenchymal), and evaluate inflow aortoiliac disease.[103]

The role of endovascular interventions for the management of vascular complications of pancreatic transplants is not well established due to the rarity of the procedures and the limited literature on the subject, mainly consisting of anecdotal case reports describing technically successful procedures.[106–114] These reports include stent placement for iliac artery inflow disease,[101,106,107] percutaneous angioplasty of pancreatic artery

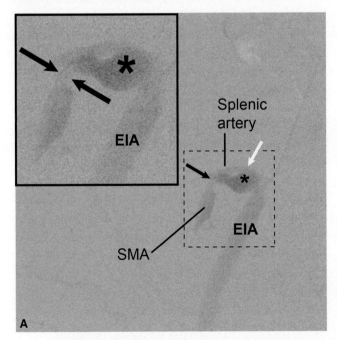
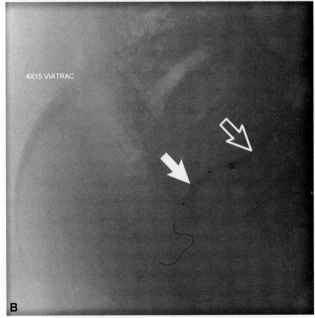

FIGURE 80.4 Balloon angioplasty of the distal anastomosis of the superior mesenteric artery and the Y-graft. **A**. Right iliac artery angiogram demonstrating a distal anastomotic stenosis (*black arrows*) of the transplant pancreas involving the Y-graft (*asterisk*) and the superior mesenteric artery (*SMA*). The distal anastomosis with the splenic artery (*white arrow*) is patent. The angiogram is performed from a contralateral left femoral approach. EIA, right external iliac artery. **B**. Fluoroscopic image during balloon angioplasty of the stenosis utilizing a 4-mm semicompliant balloon (*solid white arrow*) placed through a 6 French reinforced sheath (*hollow white arrow* at sheath tip). **C**. Completion right iliac artery angiogram after balloon angioplasty with resolution of the distal anastomotic SMA stenosis (*solid black arrow*). The difference in vessel diameter is a size mismatch (relatively undersized graft limb with a relatively oversized transplant SMA). The *asterisk* denotes the body or "base" of the Y-graft. *(continued)*

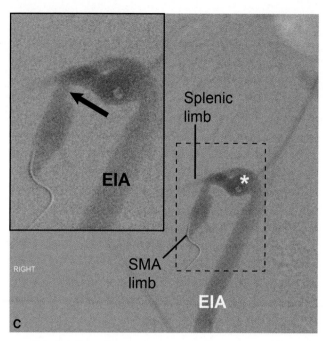

FIGURE 80.4 *(Continued)*

stenoses,[101] transcatheter thrombolysis of thrombosed pancreatic arteries,[101] and embolization for AVF,[101,108,109] PsA, or active bleeding.[101,111–114] Perhaps the most technically and clinically effective procedure is embolization for AVF.[101,108,109] PTA for pancreatic artery stenosis appears to be technically effective; however, it is difficult to evaluate PTA clinically due to the limited experience[101] (FIGURE 80.4). Transcatheter thrombolysis for pancreatic artery thrombosis/pancreatic graft thrombosis appears to be technically and clinically futile.[101] Overall, because of the limited experience in the literature, the retrospective nature of the studies, and the heterogeneous management approaches, it is difficult to determine with certainty whether endovascular interventions are clinically effective.

▪ REFERENCES

1. Saad WE, Waldman DL. Endovascular repair of vascular lesions in solid organ transplantation. In: Oriel K, Katzen BT, Rosenfield K, eds. *Complications in Endovascular Therapy.* New York, NY: Taylor & Francis Informa; 2006:223–252.
2. Hedegard W, Saad WE, Davies MG. Management of vascular and nonvascular complications after renal transplantation. *Tech Vasc Interv Radiol* 2009;12:240–262.
3. Krol R, Ziaja J, Chudek J, et al. Iliac artery stenosis as a cause of posttransplant renovascular hypertension: report of two cases. *Ann Transplant* 2005;10:66–69.
4. Patel NH, Jindal RM, Wilkin T, et al. Renal artery stenosis in renal allografts. Retrospective study of predisposing factors and outcomes after percutanoeus transluminal angioplasty. *Radiology* 2001;219:663–667.
5. Voiculescu A, Hollerbeck M, Plum J, et al. Iliac artery stenosis proximal to a kidney transplant: clinical findings, duplex sonographic criteria, treatment and outcome. *Transplantation* 2003;76:332–339.
6. Weigele JB. Iliac artery stenosis causing renal allogtaft-mediated hypertension: angiographic diagnosis and treatment. *AJR Am J Roentgenol* 1991;157:513–515.
7. Voiculescu A, Schmitz M, Hollenbeck M, et al. Management of arterial stenosis affecting kidney graft perfusion: a single-centre study in 53 patients. *Am J Transplant* 2005;5:1731–1738.
8. Hagen G, Wadstrom J, Magnusson M, et al. Outcome after percutaneous transluminal angioplasty of arterial stenosis in renal transplant patients. *Acta Radiol* 2009;50:270–275.
9. Pappas P, Zavos G, Kaza P, et al. Angioplasty and stenting of arterial stenosis affecting renal transplant function. *Transplant Proc* 2008;40:1391–1396.
10. Aktas S, Boyvat F, Sevmis S, et al. Analysis of vascular complications after renal transplantation. *Transplant Proc* 2011;43:557–561.
11. Fervenza FC, Lafayette RA, Alfey EJ, et al. Renal artery stenosis in kidney transplantation. *Am J Kidney Dis* 1998;31:142–148.
12. Mammen NI, Chacko N, Garesh G, et al. Aspects of hypertension in renal allograft recipients: a study of 1000 live renal transplants. *Br J Urol* 1993;71:256–258.
13. Roberts JP, Ascher NL, Fryd DS, et al. Transplant renal artery stenosis. *Transplantation* 1989;48:580–583.
14. Lacombe M. Arterial stenosis complicating renal allo-transplantation in man: a study of 38 cases. *Ann Surg* 1997;181:183.
15. Wong W, Fynn SP, Higgins RM, et al. Transplant renal artery stenosis in 77 patients: does it have an immunological course? *Transplantation* 1996;61:215–219.
16. Marini M, Fernandez-Rivera C, Cao I, et al. Treatment of transplant renal artery stenosis by percutaneous transluminal angioplasty and/or stenting: study in 63 patients in a single institution. *Transplant Proc* 2011;43:2205–2207.
17. Bruno S, Remuzzi G, Ruggenemti P. Transplant renal stenosis. *J Am Soc Nephrol* 2004;15:134.
18. Smellie WA, Vinik M, Hume DM. Angiographic investigation of hypertension complicating human renal transplantation. *Surg Gynecol Obstet* 1969;128:963.
19. Spinosa DJ, Isaacs RB, Matsumoto AH, et al. Angiographic evaluation and treatment of transplant renal artery stenosis. *Curr Opin Urol* 2001;11:197.
20. Audard V, Matignon M, Hemery F, et al. Risk factors and long-term outcomes of transplant renal artery stenosis in adult recipients after treatment by percutaneous transluminal angioplasty. *Am J Transplant* 2006;6(1):95–99.
21. Humar A, Ukins M, Papaluis V, et al. Is there an association between cytomegalovirus and renal artery stenosis in kidney transplant recipients? *Transplantation* 2000;69:S386.
22. Becker BN, Odorico JS, Becker YT, et al. Peripheral vascular disease and renal transplant artery stenosis: a reappraisal of transplant renovascular disease. *Clin Transplant* 1999;13:349.
23. Rengel M, Gomes-Da-Silva G, Inchaustegui L, et al. Renal artery stenosis after kidney transplantation: diagnostic and therapeutic approach. *Kidney Int Suppl* 1998;68:S99.
24. Osman Y, Shokeir A, Ali-el-Dein B, et al. Vascular complications after live donor renal transplantation: study of risk factors and effects on graft and patient survival. *J Urol* 2003;169:859–862.
25. Libicher M, Radeleff B, Grenechar L, et al. Interventional therapy of vascular complications following renal transplantation. *Clin Transplant* 2006;20:55–59.
26. Gray D. Renal artery stenosis in the transplanted kidney. *Transplantation* 1994;58:15–21.
27. Lye W, Leong S, Lee E. Transplant renal artery stenosis presenting with recurrent acute pulmonary edema. *Nephron* 1996;72:302–304.
28. Erley CM, Duda SH, Wakat J-P, et al. Noninvasive procedures for diagnosis of renovascular hypertension in renal transplant recipients: a prospective analysis. *Transplantation* 1992;54:863.
29. Cloudon M, Lefevre F, Hestin D, et al. Power Doppler imaging: evaluation of vascular complications after renal transplantation. *Am J Roentgenol* 1999;76:332–339.
30. Gottlieb RH, Lieberman JL, Pabico RC, et al. Diagnosis of renal artery stenosis in transplant kidneys: value of Doppler waveform analysis of the intrarenal arteries. *Am J Roentgenol* 1995;165:1441–1446.
31. Loubeyre P, Abidi H, Cahen R, et al. Transplant kidney renal artery: detection of stenosis with color Doppler US. *Radiology* 1997;203:661.
32. Johnson DB, Lerner CA, Prince MR, et al. Gadolinium-enhanced magnetic resonance angiography pf renal transplants. *Magn Reson Imaging* 1997;15:13–20.
33. Kelekis NL, Semelka RC, Worawattanakul S, et al. Magnetic resonance imaging of the abdominal aorta and iliac vessels using combined 3-D gadolinium-enhanced MRA and gadolinium-enhanced fat-suppressed spoiled gradient echo sequences. *Magn Reson Imaging* 1999;17:641–651.
34. Neimatallah MA, Dong Q, Schoenberg SO, et al. Magnetic resonance imaging in renal transplantation. *J Magn Reson Imaging* 1999;10:357–368.

35. Vasbinder GBC, Nelemans PJ, Kessels AGH, et al. Diagnostic tests for renal artery stenosis in patients suspected of having renovascular hypertension: a meta-analysis. *Ann Intern Med* 2001;135:401.

36. Thomsen HS. How to avoid CIN: guidelines from the European Society of Urogenital Radiology. *Nephrol Dial Transplant* 2005;20(suppl 1):18.

37. Gedroyc WM, Reidy JF, Saxton HM. Arteriography of renal transplantation. *Clin Radiol* 1987;38:239.

38. Benoit G, Moukarzel M, Hiesse C, et al. Transplant renal artery stenosis: experience and comparative results between surgery and angioplasty. *Transpl Int* 1990;3:137–140.

39. Raynaud A, Bedrossian J, Remy P, et al. Percutaneous transluminal angioplasty of renal transplant arterial stenoses. *AJR Am J Roentgenol* 1985;146:853–857.

40. Beecroft JR, Rajan DK, Clark TWI, et al. Transplant renal artery stenosis: outcome after percutaneous intervention. *J Vasc Interv Radiol* 2004;15:1407–1413.

41. Geddes CC, McManus SK, Koteswaran S, et al. Long-term outcome of transplant renal artery stenosis managed conservatively or by radiological intervention. *Clin Transplant* 2008;22:572–578.

42. Sankari BR, Geisner M, Zelch M, et al. Post-transplant renal artery stenosis: impact of therapy on long-term kidney function and blood pressure control. *J Urol* 1996;155:1860–1864.

43. Grossman RA, Dafoe DC, Shoenfield RB, et al. Percutaneous transluminal angioplasty treatment of renal transplant artery stenosis. *Transplantation* 1982;34:339–343.

44. Halimi JM, Al-Najjar A, Buchler M, et al. Transplant renal artery stenosis: potential role of ischemia/reperfusion injury and long-term outcome following angioplasty. *J Urol* 1999;161:28–32.

45. Fauchland P, Vatne K, Paulsen D, et al. Long-term clinical results of percutaneous transluminal angioplasty in transplant renal artery stenosis. *Nephrol Dial Transplant* 1992;7:256–259.

46. Greenstein SM, Verstandig A, McLean GK, et al. Percutaneous transluminal angioplasty: the procedure of choice in the hypertensive renal allograft recipient with renal artery stenosis. *Transplantation* 1987;43:29–32.

47. Matalon TA, Thompson MJ, Patel SK, et al. Percutaneous transluminal angioplasty for transplant renal artery stenosis. *J Vasc Interv Radiol* 1992;3:55–58.

48. Peregrin JH, Stribrna J, Lacha J, et al. Long-term follow-up of renal transplant patients with renal artery stenosis treated by percutaneous angioplasty. *Eur J Radiol* 2008;66:512–518.

49. Nakir N, Sluites WJ, Ploeg RJ, et al. Primary renal graft thrombosis. *Nephrol Dial Transplant* 1996;11:140–147.

50. Jsmail H, Kalicinski P, Drewniak T, et al. Primary vascular thrombosis after renal transplantation in children. *Pediatr Transplant* 1997;1:43–47.

51. Robertson AJ, Nargund V, Gray DWR, et al. Low dose aspirin as prophylaxis against renal-vein thrombosis in renal transplant recipients. *Nephrol Dial Transplant* 2002;15:1865–1868.

52. Groggel CG. Acute thrombosis of the renal transplant artery: a case report and review of the literature. *Clin Nephrol* 1991;36:42–45.

53. Rouviere O, Berger P, Beziat C, et al. Acute thrombosis of renal transplant artery: graft salvage by means of intra-arterial fibrinolysis. *Transplantation* 2002;73:403–409.

54. Rigotti P, Fleschner SM, VanBuren CT, et al. Increased incidence of renal allograft thrombosis under cyclosporine immunosuppression. *Int Surg* 1986;71:38.

55. The Canadian Multicenter Transplant Study Group: a randomized clinical trial of cyclosporine in cadaveric renal transplantation. *N Engl J Med* 1983;309:809.

56. McKenzie N, Deviveni R, Vezina W, et al. The effect of cyclosporine on organ blood flow. *Transplant Proc* 1985;17:1873–1975.

57. Brown Z, Neild GH. Cyclosporine inhibits prostacyclin production by cultured human endothelial cells. *Transplant Proc* 1987;19:1178–1180.

58. Shabanah FH, Connolly JE, Martin DC. Acute renal artery occlusion. *Surg Gynecol Obstet* 1970;131:689.

59. Collins GM, Taft P, Greer RD, et al. Aderine nucleotide levels in preserved and ischemically injured canine kidneys. *World J Surg* 1977;1:237.

60. Madden JL. Renal artery and suprarenal aortic occlusion. *Arch Surg* 1968;97:853.

61. Zajko AB, McLean GK, Grossman RA, et al. Percutaneous transluminal angioplasty and fibrinolytic therapy for renal allograft arterial stenosis and thrombosis. *Transplantation* 1982;33:447.

62. Gerard DF, Devin JB, Halsz NA, et al. Transplant renal artery thrombosis. *Arch Surg* 1982;117:361.

63. Lee HM, Mendez-Picon G, Pierce JC, et al. Renal artery occlusion in transplant recipients. *Am Surg* 1977;43:186.

64. Melzer JS, Gregorio AS, Etheredge EE, et al. Successful re-vascularization of early posttransplant renal artery occlusion. *Surgery* 1982;91:168.

65. Okiye SE, Zincke H. Renal allograft salvage after prolonged early post-transplant renal artery occlusion. *J Urol* 1983;129:1216.

66. Nicholson JD, Burleson RL, Bredenberg CE. Survival of a renal allograft after correction of an early total acute renal artery occlusion. *Transplantation* 1978;26:131.

67. Swanson DA, Sullivan MJ. Thrombo-endarterectomy for anuria 4 1/2 years post-renal transplant: a case report. *J Urol* 1976;116:799.

68. Renders L, Georig M, Schrieber M, et al. Successful surgical revascularization of a kidney transplant after PTA-induced arterial dissection of the allograft renal artery. *Nephrol Dial Transplant* 1997;12:1264.

69. Takadashi M, Humke U, Girndt M, et al. Early post-transplantation renal allograft perfusion failure due to dissection: diagnosis and interventional treatment. *AJR Am J Roentgenol* 2003;180:759–763.

70. Giustacchini O, Pisanti F, Citterio F, et al. Renal vein thrombosis after renal transplantation: an important cause of graft loss. *Transplant Proc* 2002;34:2126–2127.

71. Samara ENS, Voss BL, Pederson JA. Renal artery thrombosis associated with elevated cyclosporine levels: a case report and review of the literature. *Transplant Proc* 1988;20:119.

72. Maleux G, Messiaen T, Stockx L, et al. Transcatheter embolization of biopsy-related vascular injuries in renal allografts: long-term technical, clinical and biochemical results. *Acta Radiol* 2003;44:13–17.

73. Phadke RN, Sawlani V, Rastogi H, et al. Iatrogenic renal vascular injuries and their radiological management. *Clin Radiol* 1997;52:119.

74. Peregrin JH, Lacha J, Adamec M. Successful handling by stent implantation of postoperative renal graft artery stenosis and dissection. *Nephrol Dial Transplant* 1999;14:1004–1006.

75. Saad WEA. Management of hepatic artery steno-occlusive complications after liver transplantation. *Tech Vasc Interv Radiol* 2007;10(3):207–220.

76. Saad WEA, Davies MG, Sahler LG, et al. Hepatic artery stenosis in liver transplant recipients: primary treatment with percutaneous transluminal angioplasty. *J Vasc Interv Radiol* 2005;16(6):795–805.

77. Saad NEA, Saad WEA, Davies MG, et al. Pseudoaneurysms and the role of minimally invasive techniques in their management. *Radiographics* 2005;25:173–189.

78. Grenier N, Claudon M, Trillaud H, et al. Non-invasive radiology of vascular complications in renal transplantation. *Eur Radiol* 1997;52:119.

79. Orons PD, Zajko AB. Angiography and interventional aspects of renal transplantation. *Radiol Clin North Am* 1995;33:461.

80. Martinez T, Palomaces M, Bravo JA, et al. Biopsy-induced arteriovenous fistula and venous aneurysm in a renal transplant. *Nephrol Dial Transplant* 1998;13:2937.

81. Perini S, Gordon RL, LaBerge JM, et al. Transcatheter embolization of biopsy-related vascular injury in the transplant kidney: immediate and long-term outcome. *J Vasc Interv Radiol* 1998;9:1011–1019.

82. deSouza NM, Reidy JF, Koffman CG. Arteriovenous fistulas complicating biopsy of renal allografts: treatment of bleeding with superselective embolization. *AJR Am J Roentgenol* 1991;156:507–510.

83. Dorffner R, Thurnher S, Prokesch R, et al. Embolization of iatrogenic vascular injuries of renal transplants: immediate and follow-up results. *Cardiovasc Intervent Radiol* 1998;21:129–134.

84. Saad WEA. Management of non-occlusive hepatic artery complications after liver transplantation. *Tech Vasc Interv Radiol* 2007;10:221–232.

85. Saad WEA, Davies MG, Rubens DJ, et al. Endoluminal management of arterio-portal fistulae in liver transplant recipients: a single center experience. *Vasc Endovasc Surg* 2006;40:451–459.

86. Bedani PL, Galeotti R, Mugnani G, et al. Successful local arterial urokinase infusion to reverse late postoperative venous thrombosis of renal graft. *Nephrol Dial Transplant* 1999;14:2225–2227.

87. Karaesa FB, Audikouk K, Pappas P, et al. Late renal transplant arterial thrombosis in a patient with systemic lupus erythematosus and antiphospholipid syndrome. *Nephrol Dial Transplant* 1999;14:472–474.

88. Ramirez PJ, Gohh RY, Kestin A, et al. Renal allograft loss due to proximal extension of iliofemoral deep venous thrombosis. *Clin Transplant* 2002;16:310–313.

89. Merion RM, Calne RY. Allograft renal vein thrombosis. *Transplant Proc* 1985;17:1746–1750.

90. Herrera RO, Benitez AM, Abad MJH. Renal vein partial thrombosis in three recipients of kidney transplantation. *Arch Esp Urol* 2000;53:45–48.

91. duBuf-Vereijken PWG, Hillbrands LB, Wetzels JFM. Partial renal vein thrombosis in a kidney transplant: management by streptokinase and heparin. *Nephrol Dial Transplant* 1998;13:499–502.

92. Chiu AS, Landsberg DN. Successful treatment of acute transplant renal vein thrombosis with selective streptokinase infusion. *Transplant Proc* 1991;23:2297–2300.

93. Robinson JM, Cockrell CH, Tisnado J, et al. Selective low-dose streptokinase infusion in the treatment of acute transplant renal vein thrombosis. *Cardiovasc Intervent Radiol* 1986;9:86–89.

94. Schwiger J, Reiss R, Cohen JL, et al. Acute renal allograft dysfunction in the setting of deep venous thrombosis: a case of successful urokinase thrombolysis and a review of the literature. *Am J Kidney Dis* 1993;22:345–350.

95. Killewich LA, Pais SO, Sandager G, et al. Salvage of renal allograft function and lower extremity venous patency with thrombolytic therapy: case report and review of the literature. *J Vasc Surg* 1995;21:691–696.

96. Modrall JG, Teitelbaum GP, DiazLunn H, et al. Local thrombolysis in a renal allograft treated by renal vein thrombosis. *Transplantation* 1993;65:1101–1013.

97. Tamin W, Arous E. Thrombolytic therapy: the treatment of choice for iliac vein thrombosis in the presence of kidney transplant. *Ann Vasc Surg* 1999;13:436–438.

98. Mark MJ, Pais SO, Bartlett ST. Successful restoration of renal allograft function of urokinase thrombolysis in the setting of phlegmasia cesurae dolens. *J Vasc Interv Radiol* 1995;6:279–282.

99. Fava M, Loyola S, Flores P, et al. External iliac vein thrombosis after renal transplantation: treatment by thrombolysis and stent placement: a case report. *Transplantation* 1997;64:928–930.

100. Stella N, Rolli A, Catalano A, et al. Simultaneous urokinase perfusion in renal artery and vein in a case of renal vein thrombosis. *Minerva Cardioangiol* 2001;49:273–278.

101. Saad WEA, Darwish WM, Turba UC, et al. Endovascular management of vascular complications in pancreatic transplants. *Vasc Endovascular Surg* 2012;46:262–268.

102. Neri E, Cappelli C, Boggi U, et al. Multirow CT in the follow-up of pancreas transplantation. *Transplant Proc* 2004;36:597–600.

103. Hagspiel KD, Nandalur K, Pruett TL, et al. Evaluation of vascular complications of pancreas transplantation with high special-resolution contrast-enhanced MR angiography. *Radiology* 2007;242:590–599.

104. Eubank WB, Schmiedl UP, Levy AE, et al. Venous thrombosis and occlusion after pancreas transplantation: evaluation with breath-hold gadolinium-enhanced three-dimensional MR imaging. *AJR Am J Roentgenol* 2000;175:381–385.

105. Gruessner AC, Sutherland DER. Pancreas transplant outcomes for United States (US) and non-US cases as reported to the United Network for Organ Sharing (UNOS) and the International Pancreas Transplant Registry (IPTR) as of June 2004. *Clin Transplant* 2005;19:433–455.

106. Woo EY, Milner R, Brayman KL, et al. Successful PTA and stenting for acute iliac arterial injury following pancreas transplantation. *Am J Transplant* 2003;3:85–87.

107. Kimura T, Saito T, Tsuchiya A, et al. Treatment of external iliac artery dissection with endovascular stent placement in a patient with simultaneous pancreas and kidney transplantation. *Transplant Proc* 2005;37:3572–3573.

108. Phillips BJ, Fabrega AJ. Embolization of a mesenteric arteriovenous fistula following pancreatic allograft: the steal effect. *Transplantation* 2000;70:1529–1539.

109. Angle JF, Matsumoto AH, McGraw JK, et al. Percutaneous embolization of a high-flow pancreatic transplant arteriovenous fistula. *Cardiovasc Intervent Radiol* 1999;22:147–149.

110. Barth MM, Khwaja K, Faintuch S, et al. Transarterial and transvenous embolotherapy of arteriovenous fistulas in the transplanted pancreas. *J Vasc Interv Radiol* 2008;19:1231–1235.

111. Tan M, Di Carlo A, Stein LA, et al. Pseudoaneurysm of the superior mesenteric artery after pancreas transplantation treated by endovascular stenting. *Transplantation* 2001;72:336–338.

112. Orsenigo E, De Cobelli F, Salvioni M, et al. Successful endovascular treatment for gastroduodenal artery pseudoaneurysm with an arteriovenous fistula after pancreas transplantation. *Transpl Int* 2003;16:694–696.

113. McBeth BD, Stern SA. Lower gastrointestinal hemorrhage from an arterioenteric fistula in a pancreatorenal transplant patient. *Ann Emerg Med* 2003;42:587–591.

114. Semiz-Oysu A, Cwikiel W. Endovascular management of acute enteric bleeding from pancreas transplant. *Cardiovasc Intervent Radiol* 2007;30:313–316.

115. Decker E, Coimbra C, Weekers L, et al. A retrospective monocenter review of simultaneous pancreas-kidney transplantation. *Transplant Proc* 2009;41:3389–3392.

116. Martins L, Pedroso S, Henriques AC, et al. Simultaneous pancreas-kidney transplantation: five-year results from a single center. *Transplant Proc* 2006;38:1929–1932.

117. Michalak G, Kwiatkowski A, Czerwinski J, et al. Surgical complications of simultaneous pancreas-kidney transplantation: a 16-year experience at one center. *Transplant Proc* 2005;37:3555–3557.

118. Sansalone CV, Maione G, Aseni P, et al. Surgical complications are the main cause of pancreatic allograft loss in pancreas-kidney transplant recipients. *Transplant Proc* 2005;37:2651–2653.

119. Reddy KS, Stratta RJ, Shokouh-Amici MH, et al. Surgical complications after pancreas transplantation with portal-enteric drainage. *J Am Coll Surg* 1999;189(3):305–313.

120. Fernandez MP, Bernardino ME, Neylan JF, et al. Diagnosis of pancreatic transplant dysfunction: value of gadopentetate dimeglumine-enhanced MR imaging. *AJR Am J Roentgenol* 1991;156:1171–1176.

121. Ozak CF, Stratta RJ, Taylor RJ, et al. Surgical complications in solitary pancreas and combined pancreas-kidney transplantation. *Am J Surg* 1992;164:546–551.

122. Douzdjian V, Abecassis MM, Cooper JL, et al. Incidence, management and significance of surgical complications after pancreatic transplantation. *Surg Gynecol Obstet* 1993;177:451–456.

123. Gruessner AC, Sutherland DER, Troppman C, et al. The risk of pancreas transplantation in the cyclosporine era: an overview. *J Am Coll Surg* 1997;185:128–144.

124. Bruce DS, Newell KA, Woodle ED, et al. Synchronous pancreas-kidney transplantation with portal venous and enteric exocrine drainage: outcome in 70 consecutive cases. *Transplant Proc* 1998;30:270–271.

SECTION **XIV**
Arterial Access Closure

Device-Mediated Access Closure: Indications, Techniques, and Complications

DAVID LEE

INTRODUCTION

The Seldinger technique was first described in 1953 and marked the departure from surgical cut-down and the beginning of percutaneous femoral arterial catheter-based interventions.[1] Over the next several decades, there has been an emergence of a multitude of endovascular procedures via the percutaneous transfemoral approach. Advances in vascular interventions have led to the use of larger sheaths along with administration of potent antithrombotic and antiplatelet agents, both of which increase the risk of access site–related bleeding complications. Mechanical compression, either via manual or the use of commercially available femoral compression devices, was established as the standard for achieving hemostasis. However, concerns regarding access site complications, patient discomfort, and prolonged recumbency duration led to the development of novel approaches for facilitating hemostasis. Several arteriotomy closure devices were introduced in the 1990s as an alternative to manual or mechanical compression. These vascular closure devices (VCDs) can be categorized according to their mechanism of action: extravascular sealant-based closure, suture-based approximation, staple/clip-mediated closure, or passive vessel approximation. Each has distinct advantages and limitations. Factors that define the optimal closure device are efficacy of achieving hemostasis, complexity of deployment, cost, and risk of complications. Over the last 15 years, several novel devices have been developed and come into clinical practical with millions of devices sold each year. They have been shown to reduce time to hemostasis following sheath removal, shorten time to ambulation, and improve patient satisfaction. Controversy remains regarding their effect on the risk of vascular complications compared with manual compression.

SEALANT-BASED CLOSURE

VasoSeal

The VasoSeal (Datascope Corporation, Mahwah, NJ) was introduced in 1995 as the first sealant device to market. It utilizes an entirely extravascular collagen plug that forms a hemostatic seal over the arteriotomy in the puncture tract. The collagen plug stimulates thrombus formation and platelet aggregation, resulting in "passive" rather than "active" approximation of the vessel. The original VasoSeal VHD (Vascular Hemostatic Device) consisted of a needle measuring kit, an 11 French dilator, 11.5 French sheaths of different lengths, and two collagen delivery cartridges. Measurement of the skin-to-vessel distance was required to select the appropriate-sized sheath. Two operators, as well as a large tissue tract, were required to deploy the device. Manual compression was recommended following deployment. The next-generation VasoSeal Elite device eliminated the need for premeasurement with incorporation of a removable J-tipped wire anchor. The size of the collagen plug was reduced by 40% and manual compression was no longer a requirement.

Efficacy and safety of the VasoSeal in patients undergoing coronary angiography and angioplasty were demonstrated in a randomized, multicenter trial. In diagnostic cases, hemostasis time and time to ambulation were shorter compared to manual compression. There were no major vascular complications after diagnostic catheterization but a trend toward higher complications in patients who underwent angioplasty.[2] Subsequent comparisons against other VCDs (Perclose, Angio-Seal) have shown slightly higher complication rates.[3,4] The emergence of active arteriotomy approximation devices led to the decline in use and the eventual termination of active marketing of the VasoSeal.

Duett

The Duett Pro (Vascular Solutions, Minneapolis, MN) is composed of a low-profile, 3 French balloon catheter over a movable core wire along with an injectable procoagulant mixture of collagen and thrombin. The device is inserted into the procedural sheath and the balloon is inflated. The core wire is retracted and the balloon assumes an elliptical shape with a maximal diameter of 6 to 7 mm. Upon retraction, the balloon opposes the puncture site, serving as an intra-arterial anchor. The procoagulant mixture is then injected through the side arm of the sheath into the tissue tract to achieve hemostasis.

Upon deflation, the movable core wire is advanced to elongate the deflated balloon to allow easy removal of the catheter. The initial feasibility showed rapid hemostasis (4 minutes for diagnostic cases and 6.9 minutes for coronary interventions) with 97.7% success.[5] In the pivotal randomized SEAL trial, time to hemostasis and ambulation were significantly reduced. Major and minor complications trended higher compared to manual compression, at 2.4% and 4.1%, respectively. However, the one major complication of this device is the potential for inadvertant intra-arterial injection of the mixture, which results in acute limb ischemia. This was reported in 0.5% of cases.[6] Due to the risk of this rare but catastrophic complication, the Duett Pro has seen low market shares.

Angio-Seal

The Angio-Seal device (St. Jude Medical, St. Paul, MN), approved in 1996, incorporates an intravascular footplate and an extravascular collagen plug that are mechanically approximated over a suture to create a "sandwich-like" seal at the arteriotomy puncture site (FIGURE 81.1). Two size options are available: 6 and 8 French. The device is made up of three components: a high-molecular weight polymer anchor, a collagen plug, and a self-tightening traction suture, all of which are bioabsorbed in 60 to 90 days. Deployment is uncomplicated with a short learning curve. Over a 0.035" wire, the procedural sheath is replaced with the Angio-Seal insertion sheath. An "arteriotomy locator," with a distal blood inlet and a proximal drip hole, allows for proper positioning of the sheath tip within the intraluminal space. The arteriotomy locator and wire are then removed and the Angio-Seal device is advanced into the insertion sheath until the device cap snaps in place. The footplate is deployed upon retraction of the device cap. Upon pullback of the apparatus, the footplate is anchored against the inner vessel wall and the collagen plug is exposed. Over the suture, downward pressure is applied, with the tamper tube, onto the collagen plug to seal the arteriotomy site. Hemostasis is obtained in 2 to 4 minutes.[7,8] Time to ambulation is 1 hour, although 20 minutes is considered safe following diagnostic procedures. The rate of successful closure is high, up to 97% on glycoprotein IIb/IIIa inhibitor therapy.[9] The simple design and ease of deployment have lent to its popularity; it makes up more than half of the VCD market in the United States. The device has undergone several improvements that facilitate delivery and deployment. The latest Angio-Seal Evolution incorporates an automated collagen compaction system, which ensures consistent compaction of the collagen against the exterior wall of the vessel. Reaccess of the arteriotomy site following initial Angio-Seal deployment is not recommended within 90 days of closure, although some data suggest that it can be done safely.[10]

The Angio-Seal has been extensively studied. In a meta-analysis of prospective randomized trials involving the Angio-Seal, the device was associated with a statistically significant reduction in risk of complications following diagnostic procedures with an odds ratio of 0.51.[11] Another meta-analysis showed a nonsignificant trend toward less complications in a percutaneous coronary intervention (PCI) setting with an odds ratio of 0.46.[4] In a direct comparison with the Perclose Proglide, the Angio-Seal had higher rates of deployment success with no significant difference in major vascular complications between groups.[12]

Mynx

The Mynx device (AccessClosure, Mountain View, CA), approved by the Food and Drug Administration (FDA) in 2007, utilizes a water-soluble, nonthrombogenic, polyethylene glycol (PEG) sealant delivered onto the extraluminal surface of the artery (FIGURE 81.2). Upon contact with blood, the porous polymer material rapidly expands to fill the tissue tract. The bioinert PEG completely dissolves through hydrolysis within 30 days. The device is delivered through a standard 5, 6, or 7 French

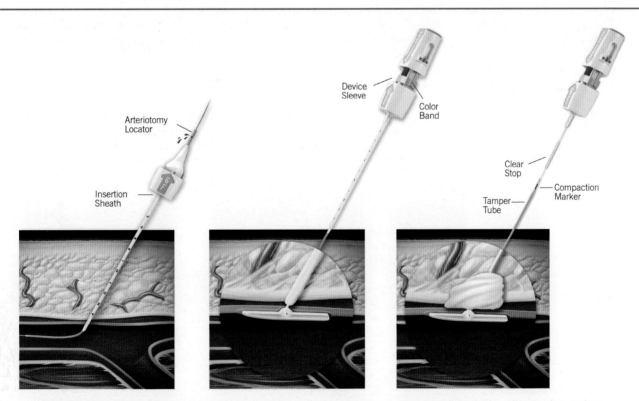

FIGURE 81.1 **Angio-Seal device**. The arteriotomy is "sandwiched" between a biodegradable collagen plug and an intravascular footplate.

Image courtesy of St. Jude Medical.

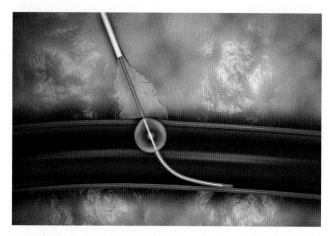

FIGURE 81.2 Mynx device. The PEG sealant is deployed in the extravascular space utilizing the removable balloon as an intravascular anchor.

Image courtesy of Access Closure.

sheath. Like the Duett, the Mynx incorporates a 6-mm balloon located at the distal tip, which, when inflated, serves as an intra-arterial anchor. The shuttle housing the sealant is advanced to the inflated balloon. The sheath hub is then retracted to expose the PEG polymer. An advancer tube is then used to tamp the sealant over the arteriotomy site. The balloon is deflated and removed, leaving no intravascular component. The Mynx is indicated for diagnostic and interventional procedures utilizing 6 or 7 French sheaths. The smaller Mynx M5 is designed for 5 French closure. The initial study showed average time to hemostasis and ambulation of 1.3 minutes and 2.6 hours, respectively.[13] In a retrospective comparison study with the Angio-Seal, vascular complication rates were identical at 2.1%, but failure rates were 2.5 times higher with the Mynx.[14] There are currently no published data regarding arteriotomy reaccess after Mynx.

SUTURE-BASED CLOSURE

The Perclose Prostar and Techstar (Abbott Vascular, Santa Clara, CA), introduced in 1994, were the first FDA-approved suture-mediated closure devices. The Prostar, indicated for 8 to 10 French closure, consists of four needles that are deployed in an outward fashion from the intra-arterial lumen. The needles are then manually extracted using a hemostat from the proximal device hub to expose four attached suture ends. Multiple intricate steps, including manual knot tying, were required for successful closure. A randomized trial comparing the Prostar to manual compression showed 97.6% successful hemostasis with a median time to hemostasis of 19 minutes and time to ambulation of 3.9 hours. The major complication rate was 2.4% (versus 1.1% in the compression arm).[15] Due to the need for a large tissue tract and the complexity of deployment, the Prostar has not captured a large market share. The Techstar, approved for 6 to 8 French closure, offered a more simplified, two-needle system that also required a manual knot tie. The initial registry study for the Techstar showed 99% efficacy with a median hemostasis of 13 minutes.[15]

The next iteration, the Closer and Closer-S, introduced a modification whereby the needles were deployed extraluminally into the vessel wall. This was further improved upon with the Perclose A-T, which incorporated a pretied polyester suture knot, allowing for rapid and more efficient deployment. The newest offering, the ProGlide, added a suture-trimming mechanism and replaced the polyester suture material with a high-tensile strength polypropylene monofilament (FIGURE 81.3). It is indicated for closure of 5 to 8 French sheaths. The device is inserted into the arteriotomy over a guide wire until blood return confirms positioning within the lumen. Lifting the lever deploys two footplates within the vessel lumen and the device is retracted until the footplates are anchored against the inner arterial wall. The plunger is depressed, deploying two nitinol needles through the vessel wall into the footplates, creating a suture loop. Two sutures tails are exposed upon removal of the needles. The footplates are retracted and the device is removed. An accompanying knot-pusher device is used to advance the pretied slipknot

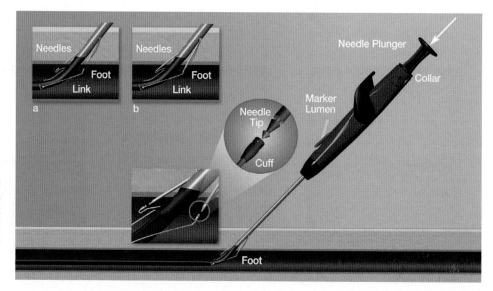

FIGURE 81.3 Perclose Proglide device. A. The needle plunger drives the two needles through the vessel wall. **B**. The suture loop is completed when the needle tips are driven into the cuffs on the footplates.

Image courtesy of Abbott Vascular.

toward the arteriotomy to achieve hemostasis. The Perclose has a steeper learning curve than the Angio-Seal device but remains popular among those who prefer the well-established surgical approach of active suture arteriotomy approximation.

An off-label, "preclosure technique" has been described for closure of large arteriotomy punctures up to 26 French in diameter. Two Proglide devices are deployed at orthogonal angles (30° medially then 30° laterally) and the two sets of suture strands are left extracorporeally. Guide wire position is maintained and the arteriotomy site is then serially dilated up to the necessary procedural sheath size. Following the completion of the procedure, the large-caliber sheath is removed and arteriotomy closure is obtained by sequentially securing the knots on the two sets of sutures.[16] The preclosure technique was studied in patients undergoing percutaneous endovascular aortic repairs. For closure of 12 to 16 French sheaths, there was 99% successful hemostasis and for 18 to 24 French closures, 91% success.[17]

With respect to postclosure reaccess, there do not appear to be any problems with immediate reaccess. In addition, off-label closure of venous access sites has been performed without any major known complications.[18]

STAPLE/CLIP-MEDIATED CLOSURE

The StarClose (Abbott Vascular, Redwood City, CA) is a clip-mediated closure device that was FDA approved in 2005. The device is a small nitinol circumferential clip that is delivered onto the extraluminal arterial surface to approximate the arteriotomy puncture site (FIGURE 81.4). Deployment involves four steps: replacement of the procedural sheath with the StarClose clip, deployment of the vessel locator, delivery of the clip to the arterial surface, and engagement of the clip. No intraluminal component remains after deployment. In the prospective, randomized CLIP study comparing the StarClose to manual compression, average time to hemostasis and to ambulation were significantly reduced (1.46 vs. 15.47 minutes, and 163 vs. 269 minutes, respectively) for patients undergoing diagnostic

coronary angiography.[19] Patients who underwent coronary interventional procedures also had significantly reduced time to hemostasis and ambulation. Rates of vascular complications were equivalent at 1.1% for both Starclose and controls. A randomized study comparing StarClose to Angio-Seal and manual compression found more frequent tract oozing and higher rates of unsuccessful hemostasis with the StarClose.[20] Immediate reaccess is both possible and safe with the StarClose device.

PASSIVE APPROXIMATION

The Catalyst II, formerly known as the Boomerang Catalyst, (Cardiva Medical, Sunnyvale, CA) has a unique mechanism of vascular closure that creates passive approximation of the tissue tract. The device is composed of a retractable biconcave 6.5-mm nitinol disc on a wire catheter. A proprietary hemostatic coating on the wire facilitates closure by stimulating coagulation and platelet adhesion. The Catalyst II wire is inserted through the procedural sheath and the distal tip is deployed, which opens the biconvex disc within the lumen of the femoral artery distal to the sheath tip. After removing the introducer sheath over the Catalyst II wire, gentle upward tension is applied on the wire to conform the disc to the inner vessel wall, thereby occluding the arteriotomy. Tension is maintained by applying an external clip to the wire at the puncture site to generate site-directed compression. The wire remains in the tissue tract to allow time for the coating to stimulate coagulation and hemostasis. The device recommended dwell time is a minimum of 15 minutes for diagnostic cases and a minimum of 2 hours for interventional cases. Following appropriate dwell time, the disc is collapsed and the device is completely removed from the artery with no material left behind, minimizing the risk of ischemic or infection complications. Final hemostasis of the puncture site occurs after a short period of manual compression. The latest version, the Catalyst III, incorporates a protamine coating for neutralization of heparin. Limited published data are available regarding the efficacy of the Catalyst device.

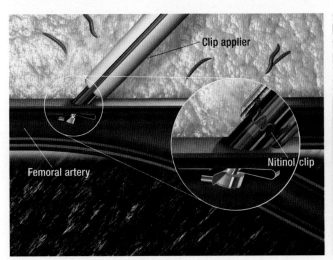 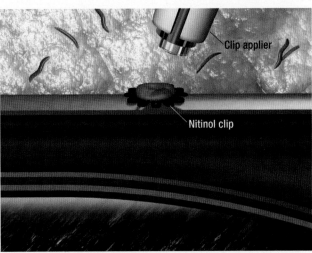

FIGURE 81.4 Starclose device. The nitinol clip is delivered into the vessel wall and remains entirely extraluminal following deployment.

Image courtesy of Abbott Vascular.

VASCULAR CLOSURE DEVICE–ASSOCIATED COMPLICATIONS

Vascular complications following device-mediate closure vary widely from small hematomas to the rare, but serious, life-threatening complications. These include retroperitoneal hemorrhage, access site infections, pseudoaneurysm formation, and device embolization leading to acute limb ischemia. Device failure may be secondary to a multitude of reasons, including operator inexperience, patient characteristics (obesity, presence of peripheral vascular disease), and procedural factors (large sheath size, antithrombotic regimen). The early experience with the first-generation VCDs raised concerns about higher complication rates. Dangas et al. evaluated vascular complications in over 5,000 individuals who underwent PCIs from 1996 to 1999. Rates of hematoma formation, surgical repair, and significant hematocrit drops were higher in the closure group.[21] A single center study involving over 2,900 patients undergoing PCIs showed higher rates of retroperitoneal hemorrhage and access site infection with VCD use.[22] Koreny et al., in their meta-analysis involving 30 studies, reported increased risk for local bleeding (odds ratio [OR] 1.48), hematoma (OR 1.14), and pseudoaneurysm (OR 1.19) with VCD use, although none were statistically significant.[23] A meta-analysis examining the use of VCDs in noncoronary, interventional radiology procedures showed equivalent complication rates compared with manual compression.[24] Overall, meta-analysis data demonstrate that complications are not significantly different between compression and VCDs. With the evolution in device technology and increased operator experience, more recent studies have suggested a trend toward improved complication rates. Applegate and colleagues[9] showed statistically significant reductions in total complications for post-PCI patients receiving either Perclose or Angio-Seal versus manual compression (1.5% vs. 2.5%, respectively, $p < .05$). In a prospective registry of nearly 13,000 patients from 2002 to 2005, the risk of vascular complications was significantly lower with closure device compared with manual compression for both diagnostic angiography (0.5% vs. 1.1%, $p = .01$) and PCI (2.4% vs. 4.9%, $p < .001$).[25]

CONCLUSION

Vascular hemostasis is of critical importance for the successful completion of percutaneous endovascular procedures. The emergence of VCDs has revolutionized postprocedure care. There is strong evidence that time to hemostasis and ambulation have been significantly reduced by device-mediated closure. VCDs are widely used following catheter-based procedures worldwide and are the mainstay of postprocedure vascular access management in many high-volume catheterization laboratories.[23] they have not become standard of care across all endovascular practitioners, however. Reasons why there has not been more widespread adoption include cost considerations, potential for device-related complications (i.e., embolization, infection), and lack of convincing evidence demonstrating reductions in access site complications when compared to manual compression. Meta-analysis data of the existing trials have not proven superiority of these devices over manual compression.[4,23,24,26,27] Currently, the decision regarding use of VCDs is not based on established guidelines and remains at the discretion of the operator. Patient characteristics as well as operator familiarity with a particular closure device are key factors in achieving successful hemostasis and avoiding access site complications. A femoral angiography should be performed prior to consideration of VCD placement and avoidance of their usage in the presence of high-risk features (i.e., high or low femoral punctures, presence of femoral artery atherosclerosis or calcifications) will likely lead to further reductions in risk of vascular complications. Continued advances in closure technologies are emerging with the hope of improving on the current armamentarium.

REFERENCES

1. Seldinger SI. Catheter replacement of the needle in percutaneous arteriography; a new technique. *Acta Radiol* 1953;39(5):368–376.
2. Sanborn TA, et al. A multicenter randomized trial comparing a percutaneous collagen hemostasis device with conventional manual compression after diagnostic angiography and angioplasty. *J Am Coll Cardiol* 1993;22(5):1273–1279.
3. Tavris DR, et al. Risk of local adverse events following cardiac catheterization by hemostasis device use—phase II. *J Invasive Cardiol* 2005;17(12):644–650.
4. Nikolsky E, et al. Vascular complications associated with arteriotomy closure devices in patients undergoing percutaneous coronary procedures: a meta-analysis. *J Am Coll Cardiol* 2004;44(6):1200–1209.
5. Mooney MR, et al. Immediate sealing of arterial puncture sites after cardiac catheterization and coronary interventions: initial U.S. feasibility trial using the Duett vascular closure device. *Catheter Cardiovasc Interv* 2000;50(1):96–102.
6. Investigators S. Assessment of the safety and efficacy of the DUETT vascular hemostasis device: final results of the safe and effective vascular hemostasis (SEAL) trial. *Am Heart J* 2002;143(4):612–619.
7. Silber S. Rapid hemostasis of arterial puncture sites with collagen in patients undergoing diagnostic and interventional cardiac catheterization. *Clin Cardiol* 1997;20(12):981–992.
8. Silber S. Hemostasis success rates and local complications with collagen after femoral access for cardiac catheterization: analysis of 6007 published patients. *Am Heart J* 1998;135(1):152–156.
9. Applegate RJ, et al. Vascular closure devices in patients treated with anticoagulation and IIb/IIIa receptor inhibitors during percutaneous revascularization. *J Am Coll Cardiol* 2002;40(1):78–83.
10. Applegate RJ, et al. Restick following initial Angioseal use. *Catheter Cardiovasc Interv* 2003;58(2):181–184.
11. Vaitkus PT. A meta-analysis of percutaneous vascular closure devices after diagnostic catheterization and percutaneous coronary intervention. *J Invasive Cardiol* 2004;16(5):243–246.
12. Martin JL, et al. A randomized trial comparing compression, Perclose Proglide and Angio-Seal VIP for arterial closure following percutaneous coronary intervention: the CAP trial. *Catheter Cardiovasc Interv* 2008;71(1):1–5.
13. Scheinert D, et al. The safety and efficacy of an extravascular, water-soluble sealant for vascular closure: initial clinical results for Mynx. *Catheter Cardiovasc Interv* 2007;70(5):627–633.
14. Azmoon S, et al. Vascular complications after percutaneous coronary intervention following hemostasis with the Mynx vascular closure device versus the AngioSeal vascular closure device. *J Invasive Cardiol* 2010;22(4):175–178.
15. Baim DS, et al. Suture-mediated closure of the femoral access site after cardiac catheterization: results of the suture to ambulate aNd discharge (STAND I and STAND II) trials. *Am J Cardiol* 2000;85(7):864–869.
16. Bhatt DL, et al. Successful "pre-closure" of 7Fr and 8Fr femoral arteriotomies with a 6Fr suture-based device (the Multicenter Interventional Closer Registry). *Am J Cardiol* 2002;89(6):777–779.
17. Lee WA, et al. Total percutaneous access for endovascular aortic aneurysm repair ("Preclose" technique). *J Vasc Surg* 2007;45(6):1095–1101.
18. Mylonas I, et al. The use of percutaneous suture-mediated closure for the management of 14 French femoral venous access. *J Invasive Cardiol* 2006;18(7):299–302.
19. Hermiller J, et al. Clinical experience with a circumferential clip-based vascular closure device in diagnostic catheterization. *J Invasive Cardiol* 2005;17(10):504–510.

20. Deuling JH, et al. Closure of the femoral artery after cardiac catheterization: a comparison of Angio-Seal, StarClose, and manual compression. *Catheter Cardiovasc Interv* 2008;71(4):518–523.

21. Dangas G, et al. Vascular complications after percutaneous coronary interventions following hemostasis with manual compression versus arteriotomy closure devices. *J Am Coll Cardiol* 2001;38(3):638–641.

22. Cura FA, et al. Safety of femoral closure devices after percutaneous coronary interventions in the era of glycoprotein IIb/IIIa platelet blockade. *Am J Cardiol* 2000;86(7):780–782, A9.

23. Koreny M, et al. Arterial puncture closing devices compared with standard manual compression after cardiac catheterization: systematic review and meta-analysis. *JAMA* 2004;291(3):350–357.

24. Das R, et al. Arterial closure devices versus manual compression for femoral haemostasis in interventional radiological procedures: a systematic review and meta-analysis. *Cardiovasc Intervent Radiol* 2011;34(4): 723–738.

25. Arora N, et al. A propensity analysis of the risk of vascular complications after cardiac catheterization procedures with the use of vascular closure devices. *Am Heart J* 2007;153(4):606–611.

26. Biancari F, et al. Meta-analysis of randomized trials on the efficacy of vascular closure devices after diagnostic angiography and angioplasty. *Am Heart J* 2010;159(4):518–531.

27. Dauerman HL, Applegate RJ, Cohen DJ. Vascular closure devices: the second decade. *J Am Coll Cardiol* 2007;50(17):1617–1626.

SECTION **XV**

Venous Disease and Endovascular Management

CHAPTER
82
Acute Lower Extremity Deep Vein Thrombosis: Classification, Imaging Evaluation, Indications for Intervention

HARALDUR BJARNASON, PHILLIP M. YOUNG, and JAMES C. MCEACHEN

Deep venous thrombosis (DVT) represents a significant worldwide health problem that has led to a *"Call to Action"* by the U.S. Surgeon General.[1] It is part of a spectrum of diseases termed *venous thromboembolism* (VTE), which includes both asymptomatic and symptomatic DVT as well as pulmonary embolus (PE). By estimates of the U.S. Department of Health and Human Services, at least 350,000, and as many as 600,000, Americans are projected to contract DVT/PE each year.[1] At least 100,000, and perhaps as many as 180,000, individuals will die directly or indirectly as a result of VTE each year.[1] The economic impact of treating DVT alone within the United States is in the billions of dollars per year.[2] Information from Europe shows a similar impact on the population. A study of six European countries has estimated the incidence of first lifetime and recurrent DVT at 148 per 100,000 person-years and PE at 95 per 100,000 person-years.[3] VTE is the third most common cardiovascular pathology in Western populations after coronary artery disease and stroke.[1,4] The incidence of total cases of VTE exceeds the total number of myocardial infarctions and strokes in the United States yearly.[5] Furthermore, the number of VTE-related deaths exceeds that of myocardial infarction- or stroke-related deaths.[5]

Imbalanced activation of the coagulation system appears to be the most important factor underlying the occurrence of an acute DVT.[5] Within the lower extremity, thrombi originate in areas where imbalanced coagulation is localized by stasis, such as in the venous sinuses and behind valve pockets.[5] Acute venous thrombosis causes an inflammatory response both in the vein wall and thrombus itself. This process involves pro- and anti-inflammatory mediators, which include leukocytes, cytokines, chemokines, and other inflammatory factors. The overall inflammatory response leads to amplification of thrombus formation, organization, and recanalization, which ultimately causes damage to the vein wall and valvular elements.

Virchow's triad of stasis, endothelial injury, and hypercoagulability encompass most, if not all, of the factors that are felt to put one at increased risk of developing acute DVT.[6–8] The most important risk factors for acute VTE are listed in Table 82.1[5]: The proportion of patients who develop an acute DVT where none of these risk factors can be identified (idiopathic DVT) has been estimated between 26% and 49%.[9–11] In many cases there is more than one risk factor identifiable, and three or more risk factors are present in up to 80% of inpatients with VTE and 30% of outpatients with DVT.[5,12,13]

The reported incidence of lower extremity DVT highly depends on the population studied, underlying risk factors, and diagnostic methods used in the evaluation.[5] Adjusting for age

Table 82.1	
Major Risk Factors for Acute Venous Thromboembolism	
• Age	• Immobilization
• Major surgery	• Central venous catheters
• Trauma	• Pregnancy
• Hypercoagulable states	• Estrogen replacement
• Malignancy	• Oral contraceptives
• In-patient care	• Hormonal treatment
• Personal or family history of VTE	• Long-distance travel

and sex, the incidence of first-time symptomatic VTE in the United States is between 71 and 117 cases per 100,000 population.[5,10] Clinically recognized first episodes of DVT occur with an age-adjusted incidence of 50 per 100,000 person-years.[14] In children, the incidence of an acute DVT is low.[15]

Older individuals are disproportionately affected by the disease. As a matter of fact, the incidence of DVT has been reported to increase by a factor of 200 between the ages of 20 and 80.[9] For persons greater than 45 years of age, the incidence is 192 per 100,000.[5] In individuals between 85 and 89 years old, the incidence increases to 310 per 100,000 population.[16] There is a strong likelihood that the incidence of DVT will increase in the future because of an aging population and increasing exposure to DVT risk factors, such as obesity, hospital admissions, oral contraceptives, and long-distance travel.[4]

CLASSIFICATION

Lower extremity DVT is classified based on anatomic location, extent of disease, and acuity because each of these factors has a bearing on the treatment approach and long-term clinical outcome. A classification based on the underlying causes for the episode of DVT has also been proposed by some authors.[17] The goal of DVT classification is to mitigate potential long-term complications by helping focus clinical decision making on an optimal, evidence-based treatment approach. The long-term clinical course of lower extremity DVT may be complicated by PE, post-thrombotic syndrome, phlegmasia alba dolens, or phlegmasia cerulea dolens.

With regard to anatomic location, lower extremity DVT has historically been divided into two broad categories based on whether or not thrombus is confined to the infrapopliteal veins (Table 82.2).

This form of classification is drawn from autopsy and imaging studies, suggesting that more than 90% of acute PE originate from the proximal lower extremity veins.[18,19] It is further supported by more recent clinical research that compared symptomatic proximal DVT to that of distal DVT. This study found that the mortality rate from proximal DVT is nearly twice that of distal DVT.[8] Additionally, proximal DVT was more frequently associated with chronic disease (i.e., active cancer, congestive heart failure, respiratory insufficiency, age >75) as compared to isolated distal DVT, which was more often associated with transient risk factors (i.e., recent surgery, immobilization, travel).[7,8]

Lower extremity DVT is also classified based on extent of the disease. Although no specific lexicon exists, broad terms (i.e., *focal, extensive, massive*) are often used to help convey the amount of thrombus burden for purposes of guiding clinical decision making. This is of particular importance in proximal DVT where the extent of thrombus may dictate whether additional imaging is necessary as well as influence which treatment approach is selected. For example, if on ultrasound evaluation an extensive proximal DVT that extends to the iliac veins is identified, additional evaluation might be considered to assess for proximal extent of the thrombosis as well as to identify possible proximal obstruction. This includes evaluation for a possible May-Thurner, tumor, inferior vena cava (IVC) abnormality, and so on. Because ultrasound visualization within the upper pelvis can be limited, the use of additional diagnostic imaging modalities, such as computed tomography (CT), magnetic resonance imaging (MRI), or contrast venography should be considered. The American Venous Forum recommends that in patients with symptomatic DVT and a large thrombus burden, particularly when the ileofemoral veins are involved, a treatment strategy involving thrombus removal should be considered.[5]

With regard to acuity, lower extremity DVT has historically been classified as acute, subacute, or chronic. Multiple factors come into play when assessing DVT acuity, including duration of symptoms, image findings (discussed in the next section), and specific laboratory values. Determination of thrombus acuity is a critical component in orchestrating the direction of DVT therapy. Although there are no absolute cutoff values to distinguish the duration of symptoms seen in acute DVT from subacute/chronic DVT, moderate quality evidence exists suggesting that thrombolysis be undertaken in patients with ileofemoral DVT with symptoms of less than 14 days.[5] Several clinical markers have been studied in an effort to help assess the age of thrombosis in patients with findings of DVT. D-dimer, endothelium- and platelet-derived microparticles, and soluble P-selectin are markers of thrombosis that are increased in patients with acute VTE.[20-23]

White and Murin proposed classification based on the underlying risk factors for the DVT. Rather than using the term *idiopathic*, which is ill-defined, they proposed a two-component descriptive system. They suggested a term, such as *temporary* or *provoking factor*, combined with a second term, such as *chronic risk factors*. The first group would then involve conditions, such as trauma or pregnancy, where a chronic risk factor would include prior VTE and severe obesity, for example.[17]

IMAGING EVALUATION

Accurate diagnostic strategies are necessary to identify an acute lower extremity DVT when it is present and safely rule it out when absent. This has borne out from the significant risks associated with not treating a patient with a proximal DVT that subsequently develops into a PE or placing a patient on anticoagulation when no DVT is present. Approximately one-third of patients with clinically suspected lower extremity DVT actually have the disease.[24,25] Patients with suspected DVT often have nonspecific signs and symptoms.[26] As such, imaging studies are commonly required to establish the diagnosis of DVT.

Table 82.2	
Classifying Lower Extremity DVT by Anatomic Location	
Proximal	**Distal**
- Described when venous thrombus has either propagated into or exists independently within the popliteal vein, femoral veins, iliac veins, or IVC	- Described when the venous thrombus is confined to the infrapopliteal veins

Table 82.3	
Contrast Venography Findings Useful in Discriminating Acute and Chronic DVT	
Acute DVT	**Chronic DVT**
Concentric, smooth intraluminal filling defect	Eccentric, irregular intraluminal filling defect
Expanded vessel size	Narrowed, irregular lumen
Venous filling defect outlined by contrast	String-like appearance and/or transverse webs
Occluded deep vein with few adjacent collaterals	Prominent collaterals in absence of deep veins
	Calcified thrombus (rare)

Several studies have shown that the diagnostic accuracy for DVT improves when the clinical probability is estimated prior to performing a diagnostic imaging test.[26–29] Several pretest probability scoring systems are available for assessing patient risk for DVT based on clinical findings. Among these are the Wells criteria with associated modifications and the Hamilton score.[28–32] Patients with a low clinical probability for DVT have less than a 5% likelihood of having DVT.[27] In patients with a high clinical probability for DVT, based on pretest probability scoring, a diagnostic imaging test should be obtained.[27]

Blood tests are often obtained to add to the clinical armamentarium for predicting DVT. The D-dimer level has been found to be the most useful. In patients who are classified as low probability for DVT based on the Wells criteria (or unlikely probability based on the Hamilton score) and have a negative D-dimer result, the diagnosis of DVT can be excluded without the need for imaging.[27–29]

Multiple minimally invasive and noninvasive diagnostic imaging techniques are available. These tests have varying degrees of sensitivity and specificity with regard to the diagnosis of lower extremity DVT. These include contrast venography (the gold standard), ultrasound, impedance plethysmography, CT, and MRI. Each of these is reviewed in terms of their specific appearance in the presence of DVT, accuracy, and limitations. As typical of most diagnostic imaging tests, the results are most useful clinically when combined with an assessment of pretest probability.

Contrast Venography

Contrast venography is the reference standard by which other imaging tests are measured in diagnosing DVT. Because the primary treatment for acute DVT is anticoagulation, the utility of this minimally invasive procedure is further enhanced by the fact that catheter-directed thrombolysis can immediately be undertaken to provide treatment in addition to diagnosis.

Acute thrombus typically forms first in a valve cusp. This is followed by central propagation of the thrombus and, ultimately, occlusion of the vessel. A nonvisualized vein during contrast venography typically implies the presence of thrombosis. Without actually identifying an intraluminal filling defect, however, the diagnosis of DVT cannot be made with certainty. In such situations, the presence of collateral vessels arising just proximal to the occlusion helps corroborate the finding of a DVT.

Contrast venography is of particular value in helping to discriminate between acute (<14 days) and chronic DVT.

The findings most often seen with both acute and chronic DVT are summarized in Table 82.3.[15]

Accuracy

Contrast venography is the most sensitive and specific examination for assessing the presence of acute DVT.[15] The most reliable finding is an intraluminal filling defect outlined by contrast on two or more views (FIGURE 82.1). If no DVT is seen on a technically adequate contrast venogram, treatment can be safely withheld.[33,34] Hull et al.[33] evaluated the clinical course of 160 patients suspected clinically of having DVT who subsequently underwent contrast venography where the results were found to be negative. Only 1.3% of these individuals developed DVT over the 6 months that followed performance of the procedure.

Limitations

Despite its status as the gold standard, contrast venography is rarely used as the initial modality for diagnosing acute DVT.

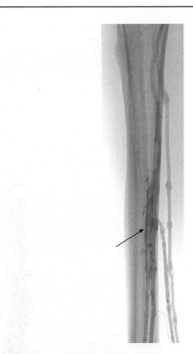

FIGURE 82.1 Intraluminal filling defect outlined by contrast (*arrow*) diagnostic for acute DVT on a lower extremity venogram.

This is due, in large part, to the near comparable accuracy of other noninvasive imaging modalities, such as compression ultrasound (CUS). Additionally, the expense, radiation exposure, and invasive nature of the procedure limit its routine use for diagnosis of DVT. Indications for use of contrast venography include the following[15,35]:

- High clinical pretest probability with negative, indeterminate, or inadequate ultrasound findings
- Conflicting results on serial ultrasound exams
- Acute symptoms in the setting of chronic venous disease

NONINVASIVE DIAGNOSTIC IMAGING TECHNIQUES

The noninvasive imaging tests proven most useful in diagnosing DVT are ultrasonography (in particular, compression ultrasonography), impedance plethysmography, CT, and MRI.

Ultrasound

The low-cost, low-risk, and widespread availability of ultrasound have made it the preferred initial choice in the workup for DVT. CUS, color Doppler ultrasound, and spectral Doppler sonographic techniques have proven to be of the greatest benefit in identifying thrombus in the lower extremity deep veins. Attempts at direct thrombus visualization are not very useful because thrombus visibility depends on the age of the clot and may potentially lead to underdiagnosis.[36] Although not validated by prospective clinical trials, gray scale ultrasound evaluation has been used to help differentiate acute from subacute/chronic thrombus based on the echogenicity of the clot whereby the subacute/chronic clot tends to appear more echogenic.[37]

Approximately 2% of patients with an initial negative ultrasound DVT study will go on to have a follow-up positive study 7 days later.[38] As such, ongoing symptoms despite a negative initial ultrasound examination may still warrant follow-up sonographic evaluation. Patients who receive a repeat negative ultrasound study within 5 to 7 days of an initial negative study have a 0.6% probability of being diagnosed with DVT within the 3 months following the initial study.[24]

The diagnosis of DVT using ultrasound is best made by a combination of compression, color Doppler, and spectral Doppler techniques. The various sonographic techniques used in assessing for thrombus are discussed next.

Compression ultrasonography

This is the most commonly used technique in evaluating for an initial lower extremity venous thrombus. It involves direct visualization and subsequent transducer compression in the transverse plane of the distal external iliac, common femoral, femoral, and popliteal veins. Evaluation of the entire extent of the vessel is performed, although stored images are only obtained along representative segmental portions of each vein. This is commonly referred to as the two-point CUS examination. The obtained images show both the noncompressed vein in the transverse plane along with its subsequent complete compression indicating a lack of thrombus (FIGURE 82.2). If a thrombus is present, the vein will not compress even with significant pressure. Incompressibility is diagnostic of DVT (FIGURE 82.3).

Accuracy

In a meta-analysis of patients with clinically suspected DVT, the finding of incompressibility in the femoral or popliteal veins is diagnostic for an acute proximal DVT with a sensitivity of 94% and specificity of 98%.[39,40] Outpatient DVT evaluation using compression ultrasonography demonstrated a sensitivity and

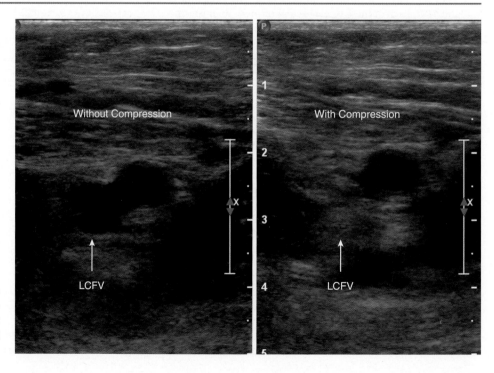

FIGURE 82.2 Compression ultrasounds of the left common femoral vein (LCFV) with and without compression demonstrating normal compressibility and no thrombus.

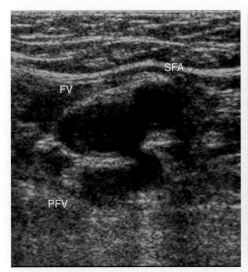
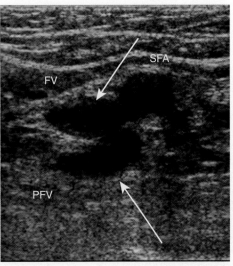

FIGURE 82.3 Femoral vein (FV), profunda femoral vein (PFV), and superficial femoral artery (SFA) without compression and with compression on the **right**. Note that the veins do not collapse upon compression (*arrows*), a positive sign for thrombus.

specificity of 100% and 99%, respectively.[41] Multiple studies have demonstrated strong interobserver agreement of findings of acute lower extremity DVT using compressive ultrasound techniques.[41,42] Compressive ultrasound is a simple and accurate diagnostic tool that has become a first-choice imaging modality in the diagnostic workup of DVT.[40,41,43]

Limitations

The utility of CUS may be limited in patients with obesity, extensive lower extremity edema, or limited access due to bandages, splints, and/or orthopedic surgical hardware. Additionally, the use of ultrasound to detect thrombus in the iliac veins and IVC is often limited by overlying bowel gas, patient body habitus,

and limited sonographic windows. Ideally, a linear transducer is used to provide more even compressibility of the vein in question. If a curved array transducer is used, extra scrutiny should be applied in the evaluation of veins showing incompressibility to ensure adequate compression in the proper direction was applied, thereby helping minimize false positive results.

Color Doppler

This ultrasound tool is used as a complement to CUS in evaluating for lower extremity DVT by providing information with regard to blood flow velocity and direction. The absence (or near complete absence) of blood flow is the criterion used to diagnose lower extremity DVT (FIGURE 82.4).

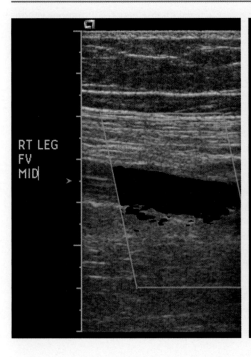
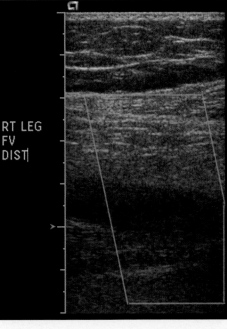

FIGURE 82.4 Color Doppler ultrasound demonstrates color flow in the mid-femoral vein but no flow in the distal femoral vein, which indicates that the vessel is thrombosed at that level.

Accuracy

The use of color Doppler in diagnosing acute proximal lower extremity DVT has a sensitivity of 95% and a specificity of 92%.[39,40]

Limitations

Slow flow, obesity, and a poor transducer angle of incidence can limit the results achieved during color Doppler sonographic analysis and may generate false positive results.

Spectral Doppler

The use of spectral Doppler allows an analysis of the frequency of the returning echo to yield important information regarding the velocity spectrum of blood flow within a vessel. In the evaluation of lower extremity DVT, spectral Doppler is most often added as a complement to performing color Doppler analysis. Spectral Doppler analysis provides both a quantitative and qualitative graphical representation of the blood flow velocity. Evaluation of the external iliac vein is often performed with spectral Doppler analysis during a Valsalva maneuver whereby the absence of variability is concerning for more central outflow occlusion. Similarly, calf compression with apparent spectral variability during the evaluation of the popliteal vein is worrisome for possible deep calf vein DVT and may warrant further evaluation. The limitations are the same as those seen with compressive and color Doppler sonographic techniques.

Additional Ultrasound Topics

In comparison to proximal lower extremity DVT, ultrasound accuracy in assessing for distal lower extremity DVT is substantially less with a reported sensitivity of approximately 70% in one study and inconclusive in other studies.[35,44,45]

Complete compression ultrasonography whereby sonographic evaluation is performed on both the proximal and distal lower extremity veins has been suggested as a means to avoid the need for repeat ultrasound in patients with an initial negative study. This approach has been evaluated in multiple studies where complete lower extremity ultrasound was used as the sole diagnostic test in patients with suspected DVT.[46–48] The results showed an incidence of DVT or symptomatic PE of less than 2% among the over 3,000 patients evaluated during the first 3 months of follow-up. The overall sensitivity and specificity of this technique are unknown because no comparison with contrast venography has been performed. Additionally, the technique is time consuming, necessitating up to 30 additional minutes per study to complete and results highly depend on the skill level of the operator.[44,45,49]

With regard to recurrent DVT, compression ultrasonography appears less useful than impedance plethysmography. Several studies have noted that less than 70% of sonographic exams return to normal at 1 year compared with over 90% with impedance plethysmography.[50–52] Research is ongoing with regard to diagnostic evaluation of recurrent DVT.

Impedance Plethysmography

Impedance plethysmography is a noninvasive method to evaluate for proximal DVT that measures blood volume changes in the leg as a function of impedance (electrical resistance).[53] There are several types of plethysmography available but the basic principle is the same: Measurement of volume changes in the

limb as a function of time as the leg is either elevated (emptied of blood) or placed in a dependent position (filled with blood). Blood pressure cuffs can also be used proximally to imitate the pooling of blood. With the patient lying still, a thigh cuff is inflated and the change in blood volume at the calf is measured from the impedance of the calf via electrodes wrapped around it.[54,55] After rapid deflation of the cuff, the change in impedance over 3 seconds is used to measure venous outflow obstruction.

This technique has been around for many years and several studies have demonstrated its utility in diagnosing DVT.[25,54] However, for the initial diagnosis of an acute DVT, the use of impedance plethysmography has largely been replaced by ultrasound as the noninvasive technique of choice.

Impedance plethysmography is used primarily in evaluating for recurrent DVT because it normalizes at a rapid and predictable rate after an initial DVT. In this regard, it has become the test of choice in evaluation of recurrent DVT. A repeat impedance plethysmography test normalizes in over 90% of patients at 9 months.[52] As compared to ultrasound, the normalization rate is less than 70% at 1 year.[50]

Accuracy

In diagnosing proximal DVT, impedance plethysmography has an overall sensitivity and specificity of 93% and 95%, respectively.[56] Two prospective studies evaluating the use of impedance plethysmography in patients suspected of having DVT showed no serious adverse events at 6 and 12 months following serial negative examinations.[25,57]

Limitations

Although relatively simple and inexpensive, impedance plethysmography has many limitations. This includes the need for the patient to lie completely still for at least 3 minutes. Positioning requirements would preclude use of patients with muscular spasm or are otherwise paralyzed.[55] Because impedance plethysmography only detects venous obstruction, false positives may result if the obstruction is caused by something other than venous thrombosis. For example, the existence of venous outflow disease or severe arterial disease may result in poor venous filling that can confound findings and lead to false positive results.

Magnetic Resonance Imaging

Multiple venography techniques have been developed that have made MRI an excellent complement to ultrasound and potential first-line diagnostic in certain clinical situations. MR venography can be performed with or without intravenously administered gadolinium chelates, and both contrast-enhanced and noncontrast techniques have been evaluated for their accuracy. Direct thrombus imaging has shown greater accuracy than compression ultrasonography for the diagnosis of recurrent DVT as noted in a recent study where all MR studies normalized over a period of 6 months, whereas ultrasound remained abnormal in nearly one-third of the patients.[58]

Accuracy

Several recent studies have shown the accuracy of MR in diagnosing DVT as comparable to contrast venography including one study where the sensitivity and specificity were determined

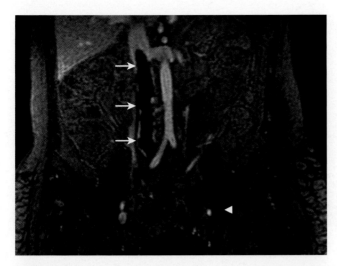

FIGURE 82.5 Contrast-enhanced MR venogram demonstrates nearly occlusive thrombus extending inferiorly from an infrarenal IVC filter (*arrows*). Thrombus extends into the left external iliac vein (*arrowhead*) but not the right external iliac vein.

to be 100% and 96%, respectively.[59–61] A meta-analysis published in 2007 estimated the sensitivity and specificity of MR to be 92% and 95% respectively.[62] Newer blood-pool contrast agents may further improve the accuracy of contrast-enhanced techniques (FIGURE 82.5). Additionally, noncontrast techniques can be performed with nearly equivalent accuracy; a study using gradient echo "bright blood" noncontrast imaging demonstrated a sensitivity of 100% and specificity of 92.9% in 66 patients[63] (FIGURE 82.6). This provides a useful alternative for imaging iliac vessels and the IVC in patients with renal insufficiency. However, outcome data are still pending.

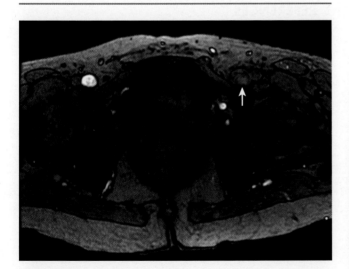

FIGURE 82.6 Noncontrast gradient recalled acquisition in the steady state (GRASS) MR sequence demonstrates lack of flow-related enhancement in the left common femoral vein (*arrow*). Saturation bands were used to suppress signal in the arteries.

Limitations

The high cost and limitations in the use of contrast agents with patients in renal failure limit the utility of MR venography. MR is also contraindicated in patients with many implanted devices, such as pacemakers, as well as most pregnant patients.

Computed Tomography

CT venography techniques show ongoing development. Most studies are performed in patients with suspected PE where the scan was subsequently extended to the legs,[53] resulting in "indirect" venography (FIGURE 82.7). "Direct" injection of diluted contrast into the affected extremity is another alternative (FIGURE 82.8). Initial results have been comparable to ultrasound evaluation in detecting femoropopliteal DVT.[62] Experience is increasing with regard to the use of CT in establishing the diagnosis of DVT and many protocols are under active investigation with the goal of evaluating for PE and DVT with no additional contrast medium and minimal added expense.[62–66]

Accuracy

In a recent meta-analysis, the pooled sensitivity and specificity for CT venography was 96% and 95%, respectively.[67]

Limitations

In a manner similar to MRI, the relative high cost and limitations in the use with patients in renal failure limit the utility of CT venography. Additionally, when performed as "indirect" venograms relying on recirculation of contrast through the leg veins after injecting through an arm vein, a high rate of nondiagnostic exams—11% in a recent study—can occur.[68] This results from dilution of the contrast bolus by essentially the entire blood pool. This has a greater deleterious effect on CT than on MR because CT is less sensitive for small amounts of iodine contrast than MR is for small amounts of gadolinium contrast.

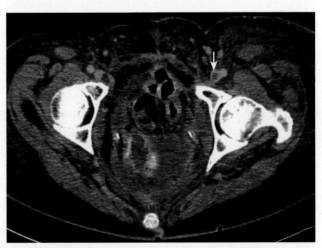

FIGURE 82.7 Indirect CT venogram demonstrates a central nonocclusive thrombus in the left common femoral vein (*arrow*).

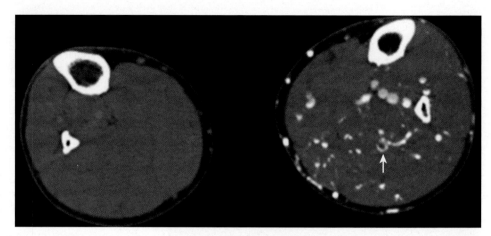

FIGURE 82.8 Direct injection CT venogram of the left leg demonstrates a small filling defect in a peroneal vein (*arrow*).

INDICATIONS FOR INTERVENTION

Most patients with acute lower extremity DVT are appropriately treated with anticoagulation alone. In the early 1990s catheter-directed thrombolysis for ileofemoral DVT was used as an adjunctive therapy to anticoagulation at many centers and a few papers were written on that topic demonstrating feasibility and reasonable safety.[68,69] This supported findings from smaller and earlier studies, which had looked at systemic delivery of thrombolytic agents for DVT.[70] These studies had indicated better resolution of thrombus with systemic delivery of thrombolytic agents than with anticoagulation alone, even long-term,[71] but with unacceptable bleeding risk with systemic delivery.[72]

Several societies have weighed in on this and given their opinion on the indications for catheter-directed thrombolysis for proximal DVT. The American College of Chest Physicians had not come out firmly in its previous guidelines, but in 2008 it says in its guidelines: "In selected patients with extensive acute proximal DVT (eg, iliofemoral DVT, symptoms for <14 days, good functional status, life expectancy >1 year) who have a low risk of bleeding, we suggest that CDT may be used to reduce acute symptoms and postthrombotic morbidity if appropriate expertise and resources are available" giving a grade 2B.[73] The Society of Interventional Radiology published in 2006 its "Guidelines for the Treatment of Lower Extremity Deep Vein Thrombosis."[74]

It appears as if a certain subset of patients may benefit from a strategy of early thrombus removal.[5] This subset comprises individuals at both ends of the clinical spectrum as described next.[5]

1. Healthy, active patients with good longevity presenting with an ileofemoral clot where early removal of thrombus helps mitigate long-term post-thrombotic complications.
2. Patients with markedly severe symptoms (i.e., massive swelling, phlegmasia) caused by extensive venous obstruction where early intervention helps to reduce morbidity and prevent progression to venous gangrene.

Patients with distal DVT (calf veins) should be treated with anticoagulation alone. Similarly, older patients with serious comorbidities who are unlikely to be active and have diminished longevity should be treated with anticoagulation alone.[5]

As the thrombus ages it becomes more difficult to treat. In general, the earlier thrombolytic treatment is applied, the more likely is the treatment to be successful. The CaVenT study, where patients were randomized to either catheter-directed thrombolysis plush anticoagulation or anticoagulation alone used 10 days of symptoms as the upper limits of symptom length for inclusion in the study. The ATTRACT trial accepts patients with up to 14 days of symptoms for inclusion in the trial.[75] No arbitrary limits can be set. At around 4 to 6 weeks, the success rate and ability to prevent venous insufficiency and establish venous patients definitely decrease significantly.

When early thrombus removal appears indicated, the American Venous Forum recommends an approach of using either catheter-directed thrombolysis (with or without percutaneous mechanical thrombolysis) over systemic thrombosis. An added benefit of catheter-directed thrombolysis is that the underlying iliac vein stenosis can be treated with balloon angioplasty or stenting, or both. Surgical thrombectomy is rarely applied and typically is reserved for patients who are unable to undergo less invasive treatment modalities, and the success depends very much on the surgeon's experience.

REFERENCES

1. U.S. Department of Health and Human Services, ed. *The Surgeon General's Call to Action to Prevent Deep Vein Thrombosis and Pulmonary Embolism.* Washington, DC: Author; 2008.
2. Hull RD, Pineo GF, Raskob GE. The economic impact of treating deep vein thrombosis with low-molecular-weight heparin: outcome of therapy and health economy aspects. *Haemostasis* 1998;28(suppl 3):8–16.
3. Cohen AT, et al. Venous thromboembolism (VTE) in Europe. The number of VTE events and associated morbidity and mortality. *Thromb Haemost* 2007;98(4):756–764.
4. Patterson BO, et al. Indications for catheter-directed thrombolysis in the management of acute proximal deep venous thrombosis. *Arterioscler Thromb Vasc Biol* 2010;30(4):669–674.
5. Gloviczki P. *Handbook of Venous Disorders Guidelines of the American Venous Forum.* 3rd ed. London, England: Edward Arnold Publishers; 2009.
6. Hirsh J, Lee AY. How we diagnose and treat deep vein thrombosis. *Blood* 2002;99(9):3102–3110.
7. Galanaud JP, et al. Comparison of the clinical history of symptomatic isolated distal deep-vein thrombosis vs. proximal deep vein thrombosis in 11 086 patients. *J Thromb Haemost* 2009;7(12):2028–2034.
8. Galanaud JP, et al. Comparative study on risk factors and early outcome of symptomatic distal versus proximal deep vein thrombosis: results from the OPTIMEV study. *Thromb Haemost* 2009;102(3):493–500.
9. Naess IA, et al. Incidence and mortality of venous thrombosis: a population-based study. *J Thromb Haemost* 2007;5(4):692–699.
10. White RH. The epidemiology of venous thromboembolism. *Circulation* 2003;107(23 suppl 1):I4–I8.

11. Agnelli G, et al. The MASTER registry on venous thromboembolism: description of the study cohort. *Thromb Res* 2008;121(5):605–610.

12. Anderson FA Jr, et al. A population-based perspective of the hospital incidence and case-fatality rates of deep vein thrombosis and pulmonary embolism. The Worcester DVT Study. *Arch Intern Med* 1991; 151(5):933–938.

13. Oger E, et al. The value of a risk factor analysis in clinically suspected deep venous thrombosis. *Respiration* 1997;64(5):326–330.

14. Fowkes FJ, Price JF, Fowkes FG. Incidence of diagnosed deep vein thrombosis in the general population: systematic review. *Eur J Vasc Endovasc Surg* 2003;25(1):1–5.

15. Kaufman JL, Lee MJ. *Vascular and Interventional Radiology: the Requisites.* Philadephia, PA: Mosby; 2004.

16. Heit JA, et al. The epidemiology of venous thromboembolism in the community. *Thromb Haemost* 2001;86(1):452–463.

17. White H, Murin S. Is the current classification of venous thromboembolism acceptable? No. *J Thromb Haemost* 2004;2(12):2262–2263.

18. Havig O. Deep vein thrombosis and pulmonary embolism. An autopsy study with multiple regression analysis of possible risk factors. *Acta Chir Scand Suppl* 1977;478:1–120.

19. Moser KM, LeMoine JR. Is embolic risk conditioned by location of deep venous thrombosis? *Ann Intern Med* 1981;94(4, pt 1):439–444.

20. Papalambros E, et al. P-selectin and antibodies against heparin-platelet factor 4 in patients with venous or arterial diseases after a 7-day heparin treatment. *J Am Coll Surg* 2004;199(1):69–77.

21. Bucek RA, et al. The role of soluble cell adhesion molecules in patients with suspected deep vein thrombosis. *Blood Coagul Fibrinolysis* 2003;14(7):653–657.

22. Blann AD, Noteboom WM, Rosendaal FR. Increased soluble P-selectin levels following deep venous thrombosis: cause or effect? *Br J Haematol* 2000;108(1):191–193.

23. Motykie GD, et al. A guide to venous thromboembolism risk factor assessment. *J Thromb Thrombolysis* 2000;9(3):253–262.

24. Birdwell BG, et al. The clinical validity of normal compression ultrasonography in outpatients suspected of having deep venous thrombosis. *Ann Intern Med* 1998;128(1):1–7.

25. Huisman MV, et al. Serial impedance plethysmography for suspected deep venous thrombosis in outpatients. The Amsterdam General Practitioner Study. *N Engl J Med* 1986;314(13):823–828.

26. Scarvelis D, Wells PS. Diagnosis and treatment of deep-vein thrombosis. *CMAJ* 2006;175(9):1087–1092.

27. Wells PS, et al. Does this patient have deep vein thrombosis? *JAMA* 2006;295(2):199–207.

28. Subramaniam RM, et al. Diagnosis of lower limb deep venous thrombosis in emergency department patients: performance of Hamilton and modified Wells scores. *Ann Emerg Med* 2006;48(6):678–685.

29. Subramaniam RM, et al. Importance of pretest probability score and D-dimer assay before sonography for lower limb deep venous thrombosis. *AJR Am J Roentgenol* 2006;186(1):206–212.

30. Wells PS, et al. Derivation of a simple clinical model to categorize patients probability of pulmonary embolism: increasing the models utility with the SimpliRED D-dimer. *Thromb Haemost* 2000;83(3):416–420.

31. Wells PS, et al. Evaluation of D-dimer in the diagnosis of suspected deep-vein thrombosis. *N Engl J Med* 2003;349(13):1227–1235.

32. Wells PS, et al. Value of assessment of pretest probability of deep-vein thrombosis in clinical management. *Lancet* 1997;350(9094):1795–1798.

33. Hull R, et al. Clinical validity of a negative venogram in patients with clinically suspected venous thrombosis. *Circulation* 1981;64(3):622–625.

34. Lensing AW, et al. Contrast venography, the gold standard for the diagnosis of deep-vein thrombosis: improvement in observer agreement. *Thromb Haemost* 1992;67(1):8–12.

35. Kearon C, et al. Noninvasive diagnosis of deep venous thrombosis. McMaster Diagnostic Imaging Practice Guidelines Initiative. *Ann Intern Med* 1998;128(8):663–677.

36. Cronan JJ, Dorfman GS. Advances in ultrasound imaging of venous thrombosis. *Semin Nucl Med* 1991;21(4):297–312.

37. Peter DJ, Flanagan LD, Cranley JJ. Analysis of blood clot echogenicity. *J Clin Ultrasound* 1986;14(2):111–116.

38. Kearon C, Ginsberg JS, Hirsh J. The role of venous ultrasonography in the diagnosis of suspected deep venous thrombosis and pulmonary embolism. *Ann Intern Med* 1998;129(12):1044–1049.

39. Goodacre S, et al. Systematic review and meta-analysis of the diagnostic accuracy of ultrasonography for deep vein thrombosis. *BMC Med Imaging* 2005;5:6.

40. Goodacre S, et al. Measurement of the clinical and cost-effectiveness of non-invasive diagnostic testing strategies for deep vein thrombosis. *Health Technol Assess* 2006;10(15):1–168, iii–iv.

41. Lensing AW, et al. Detection of deep-vein thrombosis by real-time B-mode ultrasonography. *N Engl J Med* 1989;320(6):342–345.

42. Schwarz T, et al. Interobserver agreement of complete compression ultrasound for clinically suspected deep vein thrombosis. *Clin Appl Thromb Hemost* 2002;8(1):45–49.

43. Cogo A, et al. Compression ultrasonography for diagnostic management of patients with clinically suspected deep vein thrombosis: prospective cohort study. *BMJ* 1998;316(7124):17–20.

44. Gottlieb RH, et al. Clinically important pulmonary emboli: does calf vein US alter outcomes? *Radiology* 1999;211(1):25–29.

45. Forbes K, Stevenson AJ. The use of power Doppler ultrasound in the diagnosis of isolated deep venous thrombosis of the calf. *Clin Radiol* 1998;53(10):752–754.

46. Sevestre MA, et al. Outcomes for inpatients with normal findings on whole-leg ultrasonography: a prospective study. *Am J Med* 2010;123(2):158–165.

47. Stevens SM, et al. Withholding anticoagulation after a negative result on duplex ultrasonography for suspected symptomatic deep venous thrombosis. *Ann Intern Med* 2004;140(12):985–991.

48. Subramaniam RM, et al. Deep venous thrombosis: withholding anticoagulation therapy after negative complete lower limb US findings. *Radiology* 2005;237(1):348–352.

49. Schellong SM. Distal DVT: worth diagnosing? Yes. *J Thromb Haemost* 2007;5(suppl 1):51–54.

50. Prandoni P, et al. A simple ultrasound approach for detection of recurrent proximal-vein thrombosis. *Circulation* 1993;88(4, pt 1):1730–1735.

51. Piovella F, et al. Normalization rates of compression ultrasonography in patients with a first episode of deep vein thrombosis of the lower limbs: association with recurrence and new thrombosis. *Haematologica* 2002;87(5):515–522.

52. Huisman MV, Buller HR, ten Cate JW. Utility of impedance plethysmography in the diagnosis of recurrent deep-vein thrombosis. *Arch Intern Med* 1988;148(3):681–683.

53. Tan M, et al. Diagnostic management of clinically suspected acute deep vein thrombosis. *Br J Haematol* 2009;146(4):347–360.

54. Hull R, et al. Impedance plethysmography: the relationship between venous filling and sensitivity and specificity for proximal vein thrombosis. *Circulation* 1978;58(5):898–902.

55. Grant BJ. *Diagnosis of Suspected Deep Venous Thrombosis of the Lower Extremity.* Waltham, MA: UpToDate; 2010.

56. Wheeler HB, et al., Suspected deep vein thrombosis. Management by impedance plethysmography. *Arch Surg* 1982;117(9):1206–1209.

57. Hull RD, et al. Diagnostic efficacy of impedance plethysmography for clinically suspected deep-vein thrombosis. A randomized trial. *Ann Intern Med* 1985;102(1):21–28.

58. Westerbeek RE, et al. Magnetic resonance direct thrombus imaging of the evolution of acute deep vein thrombosis of the leg. *J Thromb Haemost* 2008;6(7):1087–1092.

59. Moody AR, et al. Lower-limb deep venous thrombosis: direct MR imaging of the thrombus. *Radiology* 1998;209(2):349–355.

60. Fraser DG, et al. Diagnosis of lower-limb deep venous thrombosis: a prospective blinded study of magnetic resonance direct thrombus imaging. *Ann Intern Med* 2002;136(2):89–98.

61. Fraser DG, et al. Deep venous thrombosis: diagnosis by using venous enhanced subtracted peak arterial MR venography versus conventional venography. *Radiology* 2003;226(3):812–820.

62. Garg K, et al. Thromboembolic disease: comparison of combined CT pulmonary angiography and venography with bilateral leg sonography in 70 patients. *AJR Am J Roentgenol* 2000;175(4):997–1001.

63. Yankelevitz DF, et al. Optimization of combined CT pulmonary angiography with lower extremity CT venography. *AJR Am J Roentgenol* 2000;174(1):67–69.

64. Garg K, Mao J. Deep venous thrombosis: spectrum of findings and pitfalls in interpretation on CT venography. *AJR Am J Roentgenol* 2001;177(2):319–323.

65. Loud PA, et al. Combined CT venography and pulmonary angiography in suspected thromboembolic disease: diagnostic accuracy for deep venous evaluation. *AJR Am J Roentgenol* 2000;174(1):61–65.

66. Duwe KM, et al. Evaluation of the lower extremity veins in patients with suspected pulmonary embolism: a retrospective comparison of helical CT venography and sonography. 2000 ARRS Executive Council Award I. American Roentgen Ray Society. *AJR Am J Roentgenol* 2000;175(6):1525–1531.

67. Thomas SM, et al. Diagnostic value of CT for deep vein thrombosis: results of a systematic review and meta-analysis. *Clin Radiol* 2008;63(3):299–304.

68. Mewissen MW, et al. Catheter-directed thrombolysis for lower extremity deep venous thrombosis: report of a national multicenter registry. [Erratum appears in *Radiology* 1999;213(3):930.] *Radiology* 1999;211(1):39–49.

69. Bjarnason H, et al. Iliofemoral deep venous thrombosis: safety and efficacy outcome during 5 years of catheter-directed thrombolytic therapy. *J Vasc Interv Radiol* 1997;8(3):405–418.

70. Comerota AJ, Aldridge SC. Thrombolytic therapy for deep venous thrombosis: a clinical review. *Can J Surg* 1993;36(4):359–364.

71. Arnesen H, et al. *A prospective study of streptokinase and heparin in the treatment of deep vein thrombosis. Acta Medica Scandinavica* 1978; 203(6):457–463.

72. Goldhaber SZ, et al. Pooled analyses of randomized trials of streptokinase and heparin in phlebographically documented acute deep venous thrombosis. *Am J Med* 1984;76(3):393–397.

73. Hirsh J, et al. Antithrombotic and thrombolytic therapy: American College of Chest Physicians evidence-based clinical practice guidelines (8th ed.). [Erratum appears in *Chest* 2008;134(2):473.] *Chest* 2008;133(6 suppl):110S–112S.

74. Vedantham S, et al. Quality improvement guidelines for the treatment of lower extremity deep vein thrombosis with use of endovascular thrombus removal. [Reprint in *J Vasc Interv Radiol* 2009;20(7 suppl):S227–S239; PMID: 19560003.] *J Vasc Interv Radiol* 2006;17(3):435–447; quiz 448.

75. Vedantham S. Catheter-directed thrombolysis for deep vein thrombosis. *Curr Opin Hematol* 2010;17(5):464–468.

Acute Lower Extremity Deep Venous Thrombosis: Technical Strategies and the Roles of Regional Thrombolytic Infusions, Mechanical Thrombectomy, and Other Catheter-Based Therapies

SURESH VEDANTHAM

INTRODUCTION

Venous thromboembolism (VTE) is estimated to occur in 350,000 to 600,000 persons per year in the United States alone, of which 200,000 to 250,000 cases represent first episodes of deep venous thrombosis (DVT) that involve the lower extremity.[1] Treatment recommendations for DVT have historically been rooted in a concept of this disease as an acute condition involving a period of high risk of pulmonary embolism (PE), followed by progressively reduced risk of patient harm over time. As a result, standard treatment for DVT continues to be focused on preventing PE and reducing recurrent VTE events with use of anticoagulant drugs. For most patient groups, initial therapy consists of administration of a parenteral anticoagulant drug (unfractionated heparin, a low-molecular-weight heparin [LMWH], or fonadaparinux) with subsequent transition to long-term oral vitamin K antagonist therapy for at least 3 months with the duration of therapy depending on the presence or absence of ongoing risk factors for recurrence.[2] The preferred initial approach to most DVT patients with active cancer is LMWH monotherapy for at least 3 to 6 months.[2-4] It is worth noting that anticoagulant therapy practice is likely to evolve in the coming years with the introduction of oral direct thrombin inhibitors that can prevent recurrent VTE without the need for blood monitoring or bridging heparin therapy.[5,6] The availability of LMWHs, fonadaparinux, and direct thrombin inhibitors for outpatient therapy is viewed as a favorable trend in DVT care and has influenced endovascular DVT practice toward enabling outpatient DVT therapy, as discussed next.

THE POST-THROMBOTIC SYNDROME

Contemporary prospective studies suggest that the above concept of DVT-related health impairment needs to be modernized substantially to provide optimal late clinical outcomes for patients. Despite the use of anticoagulant therapy, prospective contemporary studies indicate that the post-thrombotic syndrome (PTS) develops in 25% to 50% of patients who suffer a first episode of proximal DVT.[7-9] PTS most commonly causes chronic, daily limb pain/aching, fatigue, heaviness, and/or swelling. In severely affected patients, limiting venous claudication, stasis dermatitis, subcutaneous fibrosis, and/or skin ulceration may develop (FIGURE 83.1). Studies have consistently shown that PTS clearly impairs DVT patients' quality of life (QOL),[10-13] and in fact the recent Venous Thrombosis Outcomes (VETO) cohort study found the presence and severity of PTS to be the leading predictors of patients' health-related QOL 2 years after a DVT episode.[14,15] PTS has also been shown to lead to venous leg ulcers that are difficult to treat and that often recur. The direct medical costs of treating PTS and the indirect costs of the related work disability have been shown to result in substantial economic burden to the health care systems of several North American and European countries.[16-19]

The pathogenesis of PTS is complex and poorly understood at a microscopic level. Studies have demonstrated that an initial inflammatory response to thrombosis strongly influences thrombus resolution, organization, and subsequent vein wall injury.[20-23] The ultimate result of this process on the composition of the adjacent vein wall appears to be an increase in thickness and reduced compliance, impaired valvular function, and other abnormalities. At a macroscopic level, the continued presence of thrombus within the deep venous system during the initial weeks after an acute DVT leads to PTS by at least two pathways. First, even with anticoagulant therapy, incomplete clearance of thrombus is common so residual thrombus that is present over the long run physically blocks venous blood flow (obstruction). Second, the inflammatory response to acute thrombosis directly damages the venous valves and alters the adjacent vein wall, leading to valvular reflux.[24,25] Uninvolved distal deep veins and superficial collaterals may dilate and become incompetent as well. When reflux and/or obstruction is present, ambulatory venous hypertension develops and ultimately leads to edema, tissue hypoxia and injury, progressive calf pump dysfunction, subcutaneous fibrosis, and skin ulceration.[26-33] Recurrent ipsilateral DVT, large initial thrombus

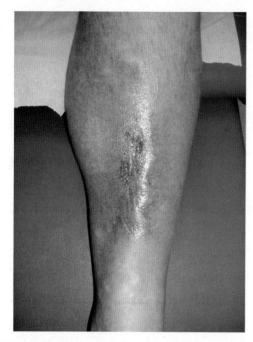

FIGURE 83.1 Post-thrombotic leg ulcer. This photograph from a 50-year-old man with a history of DVT 2 years before demonstrates brownish hyperpigmentation of a large region of skin along the left calf. There is a small round ulcer within a central area of erythema and inflammation. The ankle region, and especially its medial aspect, is the most common site of venous leg ulcers but they can also occur in the middle and lower calf, as depicted in the image.

extent (specifically, "iliofemoral DVT," which is defined as DVT involving the iliac vein and/or common femoral vein), and advancing age increase the risk of PTS, but other factors that predispose DVT patients to develop PTS are largely unknown.[7,14,15] Available studies suggest that the daily use of graduated elastic compression stockings and/or an exercise program after a DVT episode can significantly reduce the frequency of PTS, and large multicenter trials are ongoing to substantiate this.[8,9,34,35]

THROMBOREDUCTIVE THERAPIES— RATIONALE AND GOALS

It has been hypothesized for many years that rapid thrombus elimination and restoration of unobstructed deep venous flow may prevent valvular reflux, venous obstruction, and PTS. Proof-of-concept support for this "open vein hypothesis" can be found in studies of DVT patients who were treated with anticoagulation alone. In a series of ultrasound studies, Meissner et al. found that venous segments that developed valvular reflux had much longer endogenous clot clearance times than segments that did not, and that reflux developed much less frequently in veins that remained free from DVT propagation or rethrombosis.[29,33] In a secondary analysis of data from a randomized trial evaluating the use of compression therapy, Prandoni et al. found that 2-year PTS developed more frequently in proximal DVT patients who had residual venous thrombus or popliteal

valvular reflux at 6-month follow-up.[28] In 2005, Hull et al.[36] performed a meta-analysis of 11 randomized DVT treatment trials and found a strong correlation between the amount of residual thrombus after a course of anticoagulant therapy and the subsequent incidence of recurrent VTE. Finally, a small randomized trial found the use of contemporary surgical venous thrombectomy with anticoagulation to result in better venous patency and reduced PTS than anticoagulation alone.[37,38] Although this procedure is not likely to be widely adopted due to its invasiveness and dependence on specialized surgical expertise, this study certainly adds to the evidence favoring aggressive clot removal for DVT.

SYSTEMIC THROMBOLYTIC THERAPY

Systemic DVT thrombolysis, which refers to venous thrombus dissolution using a fibrinolytic drug given via an intravenous line distant from the affected limb, has been evaluated in a number of randomized trials. In studies that evaluated streptokinase, a first-generation fibrinolytic drug, greater than 50% clot lysis was observed more frequently in patients treated with streptokinase than in patients treated with heparin alone (62% versus 17%, $p < .0001$).[39] Two small follow-up studies subsequently observed that PTS developed less frequently in patients treated with streptokinase compared with heparin alone at long-term follow-up, but these studies were small and did not employ validated outcome measures of PTS.[40,41] Also, bleeding complications were frequent (14% versus 4% in a pooled analysis) in the patients treated with streptokinase.[39] For this reason, systemic streptokinase infusions are not used for DVT treatment in current practice.

Systemic infusion of recombinant tissue plasminogen activator (rt-PA), a drug with greater fibrin affinity than previous fibrinolytic agents, has also been studied for the treatment of DVT. In two early studies comprising 123 patients total, rt-PA infusions achieved greater than or equal to 50% clot lysis more often than heparin alone with a nonsignificant statistical trend toward reduced PTS in patients who had greater than 50% clot lysis.[42,43] An important observation from one of these studies was the finding that greater than 50% clot lysis occurred much more frequently in patients with nonocclusive thrombi rather than occlusive thrombi (59% versus 14%, $p < .005$), raising the possibility that the modest clot removal efficacy observed may have been related to the systemic administration route that afforded inadequate access of rt-PA to its target sites within the thrombus.[44]

The use of intermittent rt-PA injections into nearby veins in the affected leg, with or without a tourniquet system to direct the drug into the deep veins (known as "flow-directed" thrombolysis), has also been studied but were not found to be superior to systemic thrombolytic therapy either in safety or in efficacy in a randomized trial and in a large multicenter registry.[45,46]

PATIENT SELECTION—ANATOMIC AND CLINICAL CONSIDERATIONS

Given the clinical importance of PTS to the long-term health of the patient, and the invasiveness, risks, and costs of aggressive therapy, it is important for clinical decision making to be guided by rigorously performed randomized trials. However, because no adequately designed trial has been completed as yet, clinical judgment must be applied to utilize these procedures in patients who are most likely to benefit and least likely to be harmed after assessing the following factors:

1. *Projected risk of bleeding.* All patients in whom thrombolytic therapy is being considered must undergo careful evaluation for factors that may increase the risk of major bleeding complications, including (but not limited to) ongoing or recent active bleeding; recent major surgery, trauma, pregnancy, cardiopulmonary resuscitation, or other invasive procedure; thrombocytopenia or other bleeding diathesis; and the presence of bleeding-prone lesions in critical areas like the central nervous system.[47] Decisions as to whether to exclude patients from receiving thrombolytic therapy based on these risk factors should be individualized according to the clinical severity of DVT and the other factors noted next.

2. *Clinical severity of DVT.* Patients should undergo careful clinical assessment to determine what the primary intent of aggressive therapy would be and should be divided into three general categories: (a) Patients for whom *urgent endovascular thrombolysis* is indicated to prevent life-, limb-, or organ-threatening complications of acute DVT. This would include situations where limb perfusion is acutely compromised (e.g., phlegmasia cerula dolens) or when extensive/progressive inferior vena cava (IVC) thrombosis despite anticoagulation is felt to increase the risk of fatal PE or acute renal failure to unacceptably high levels. (b) Patients for whom *nonurgent second-line endovascular thrombolysis* is felt to be reasonable due to a failure of initial anticoagulation to achieve early therapeutic objectives. Such patients are those who have major anatomic DVT progression, a significant increase in clinical severity, and/or inability to tolerate ongoing major DVT symptoms (i.e., pain and swelling that are not relieved or that preclude physical activity) despite the use of initial anticoagulant therapy. In these situations, a low threshold should be applied to exclude patients if there are risk factors for bleeding. (c) Patients with symptomatic DVT for whom *nonurgent first-line endovascular thrombolysis* is being pursued as an adjunct to anticoagulant therapy with the primary purpose being to prevent late PTS. Overall, aggressive therapy for group (a) should clearly be pursued even when the patient is clinically ill due to the absence of other good treatment options, whereas a low threshold for exclusion should be applied to groups (b) and (c) when risk factors for complications exist because proof of a favorable risk-benefit ratio is lacking.

3. *Anatomic extent of DVT.* Patients with acute iliofemoral DVT, defined as DVT involving the iliac vein and/or common femoral vein, are at significantly increased risk of both PTS and recurrent VTE[13–15,48] (Table 83.1). Therefore, patients with acute iliofemoral DVT who are at low projected risk of bleeding should be provided with a balanced discussion of the risks and possible benefits of elective first-line endovascular thrombolysis for the purpose of PTS prevention. On the contrary, patients with asymptomatic DVT or isolated calf DVT should not undergo thrombolysis because the risks of developing severe PTS are low.[49] For patients with femoropopliteal DVT that does not extend to the common femoral vein level, there is little published literature to support the added efficacy of thrombolytic therapy and it therefore should be limited only to the very symptomatic with very low projected risk for bleeding. Most patients with chronic femoropopliteal DVT should not receive thrombolytic therapy because the available literature suggests that it is likely to be ineffective.[46]

4. *Life-expectancy, baseline ambulatory capacity, and comorbidities.* Patients who are chronically unable to walk or who have very short life expectancy are less likely to benefit meaningfully from aggressive therapy to prevent PTS. Additionally, some patients are likely to have difficulty in tolerating aggressive intervention—for example, patients with significant respiratory compromise who cannot lie prone and safely receive sedation for the procedure.

5. *Patients' personal values and preferences.* For aggressive therapies like DVT thrombolysis for which the benefits have not been conclusively established, it is important for the patient to receive a balanced discussion regarding the rationale, the intended benefits (and possible lack of benefits), the attendant risks and inconveniences, and treatment alternatives. Patients may arrive at different conclusions regarding their own amenability to aggressive therapy.

ENDOVASCULAR TREATMENT OPTIONS

Catheter-Directed Intrathrombus Thrombolytic Infusions

In current practice, thrombolytic drugs are delivered into peripheral thrombi using catheter-based techniques to achieve a higher local intrathrombus drug concentration (enhancing efficacy) and thereby enable successful clot lysis with a reduced drug dose (enhancing safety). Catheter-directed intrathrombus thrombolysis (CDT), which refers to the infusion of a fibrinolytic drug directly into the venous thrombus via a multi–side-hole catheter that is embedded in the thrombus using imaging guidance, was the first endovascular thrombolytic method that was applied to DVT patients.[50,51] With this technique, ultrasound guidance is used to obtain access into the deep venous system of the affected limb—whenever possible, it is ideal to access an open flowing vein below the thrombosed venous segment. A venogram is performed to define the extent of thrombus. A multi–side-hole catheter is embedded within the thrombus and attached to an infusion of a dilute solution of a thrombolytic drug. Although no drug is currently approved by the Food and Drug Administration (FDA) for the indication of DVT treatment, drugs used in clinical practice include rt-PA (0.01 mg/kg/hour up to a maximum of 1 mg/hour), reteplase (0.25 to 0.050 unit/hour), and tenecteplase (0.25 mg/hour). The infusion is typically continued for 6 to 24 hours, during which time the patient is carefully monitored for bleeding using clinical observation and laboratory testing (hematocrit, partial thromboplastin time, and fibrinogen values in some centers).

Table 83.1

Acute Iliofemoral DVT—A Distinct, High-Risk Condition

In determining initial therapy for patients with acute lower extremity DVT, physicians should group patients into three categories: (a) *distal DVT*, which is limited to the calf veins and has a low risk of PE; (b) *proximal DVT,* which does not extend above the femoral vein—this condition is associated with a significant risk of PE and a moderate risk of recurrent VTE and PTS; and (c) proximal DVT, which involves the iliac vein and/or common femoral vein (i.e., *iliofemoral DVT*), which is associated with a significant risk of PE and a high risk of recurrent VTE and PTS. Key evidence that supports a separate categorization for iliofemoral DVT is presented in this figure:

Study	Key findings
Iliofemoral DVT (IFDVT) is a high-risk condition	
Kahn et al.[14] Prospective multicenter cohort *Ann Intern Med 2008*	Patients with IFDVT have PTS scores that are two to three times higher (worse) than patients with less extensive DVT
Douketis et al.[48] Subgroup analysis of RCT *Am J Med 2001*	Patients with IFDVT have a twofold higher risk of recurrent VTE events than patients with less extensive DVT
Delis et al.[13] Prospective cohort *Ann Surg 2004*	Patients with IFDVT experience high rates of long-term exercise limitation, venous claudication, and impaired QOL
Aggressive therapy for IFDVT may offer better long-term outcome	
Plate et al.[38] Randomized controlled trial *Eur J Vasc Surg 1990*	The use of adjunctive surgical venous thrombectomy in patients with acute iliofemoral DVT was associated with reduced PTS, better venous patency, better QOL, and reduced valvular reflux at 5-y follow-up
Comerota et al.[62] Retrospective case control *J Vasc Surg 2000*	Patients with IFDVT who underwent successful CDT had fewer post-thrombotic symptoms and better QOL compared with matched patients who were treated with anticoagulant therapy alone at 16-mo follow-up
AbuRahma et al.[63] Nonrandomized trial *Ann Surg 2001*	Patients with acute IFDVT who received adjunctive CDT experienced reduced venous disease severity, better venous patency, and reduced valvular reflux at 5-y follow-up
Elsharawy and Elzayat[64] Randomized controlled trial *Eur J Vasc Endovasc Surg 2002*	Patients with acute IFDVT who received adjunctive CDT had better venous function and less valve reflux at 6-mo follow-up than patients treated with anticoagulation alone

Repeat venography is performed, the catheter is repositioned to span the remaining thrombus, and the infusion is continued. Clot maceration with an angioplasty balloon is sometimes used to facilitate thrombolysis as well.

After the acute thrombus has been eliminated, the underlying veins are evaluated by venography and any venous obstructive lesion identified is treated with balloon angioplasty and/or stent placement.[50] Typically, stents are reserved for the iliac vein if possible, although extension into the common femoral vein is sometimes necessary. Although no stent has FDA approval for this specific indication, longitudinally flexible, self-expandable bare stents are generally favored.

Limitations of the original CDT technique include the long infusion times required to obtain complete lysis of extensive DVT (typically 1 to 3 days) and the health care resources used. In an early multicenter registry, major bleeds occurred in 11% of

DVT patients treated with urokinase CDT infusions.[46] In this registry, which included a fairly unselected patient population, intracranial bleeding was observed in 0.4% of patients. Symptomatic PE and fatal PE occurred in 1.3% and 0.2% of patients, respectively. In more recent experiences using infusions of rt-PA at low doses (0.5 to 1 mg/hour), major bleeding has occurred in 2% to 4% of patients.[52–54] Reasons for this apparent difference may be improved patient selection, use of "subtherapeutic" unfractionated heparin dosing during thrombolysis, and the incorporation of routine ultrasound-guided venipuncture, which has largely eliminated the problem of local access site bleeding.

The subsequent evolution of CDT methods has been aimed at addressing the above limitations. One approach is the use of low-power ultrasound energy to disperse the thrombolytic drug within the thrombus using an ultrasound-emitting thrombolytic infusion catheter (EKOS Corporation, Bothell, WA).[55] Promising theoretical advantages of this approach are (a) the potential for relatively fast intrathrombus drug dispersion (and therefore faster thrombolysis using a lower drug dose), (b) the potential for better valvular preservation due to the ability of the ultrasound energy to access perivalvular thrombus, and (c) the potential for reduced trauma to the venous wall and valves and greater clinical practice efficiencies compared to clot removal methods that depend on use of mechanical thrombectomy devices during procedures that take several hours to perform. These potential advantages should be considered unproven until clinical studies of DVT patients verify the existence of beneficial clinical outcomes for patients.

Percutaneous Mechanical Thrombectomy

Percutaneous mechanical thrombectomy (PMT) devices are capable of macerating thrombus, and some devices ("aspirating" devices, such as the AngioJet Rheolytic Catheter System [MEDRAD Interventional, Minneapolis, MN]) can remove the macerated thrombus fragments from the venous lumen. The use of PMT increases the surface area of residual thrombus and can create a central flow channel within an occluded vein, which together may improve the efficiency of thrombolysis. However, potential disadvantages of PMT methods include the increased on-table procedure time that is required for use, the potential for displacing thrombus with mechanical manipulation, and the theoretical potential for causing venous valve injury. Published experience with stand-alone PMT (i.e., without concomitant infusion of a fibrinolytic drug) for DVT has been disappointing. In general, stand-alone PMT does not remove sufficient thrombus volumes to be clinically useful and now tends to be restricted to patients with clinically severe DVT in whom fibrinolytic drugs are contraindicated.

Pharmacomechanical Catheter-Directed Thrombolysis

The development of "pharmacomechanical" catheter-directed thrombolysis (PCDT, the combined use of CDT and PMT) has enhanced physicians' ability to efficiently remove large thrombus volumes in patients with DVT. This combination therapy is predicated on the idea that (1) PMT can increase the surface area of thrombus, accelerate pharmacologic thrombolysis, reduce the required drug dose and infusion duration, and thereby reduce bleeding complications; and that (2) CDT can dissolve PMT-created thrombus fragments that might otherwise cause PE.

Physicians have used many different combinations of drugs and devices for DVT treatment. Although each technique has its proponents and opponents, it is important to recognize that there are no rigorous studies that establish the superiority of any one technique for DVT treatment. Although many physicians have a preferred technique, most physicians appear to individualize their decisions substantially, utilizing a "toolbox" concept of tailoring their decisions on PCDT method to the specific patient. Notwithstanding the fact that there are substantial differences between the different devices and that treatment results may ultimately prove to be related to the specific drug

dosing, choice of device, and method of use, at present it may be simplest to conceive of two general categories of PCDT techniques: (1) "First-generation" PCDT methods involve the use of mechanical thrombectomy devices along with traditional infusion CDT—although these methods similarly rely on gradual thrombus dissolution, the intent is to speed this process and reduce the needed drug dose; and (2) "Single-session" PCDT methods enable rapid intrathrombus dispersion of a thrombolytic drug bolus to enable complete on-table removal of thrombus in a single 1- to 3-hour procedure, obviating the need for further drug infusion.

First-Generation Pharmacomechanical Catheter-Directed Thrombolysis

Two forms of first-generation PCDT have been used. "Infusion-first PCDT" refers to the use of an initial CDT infusion with subsequent use of PMT (with either an aspirating or nonaspirating device) at follow-up sessions to macerate and/or remove residual thrombus. The other method, termed by some *buzz-lyse*, involves use of an aspirating device to first debulk the thrombus, followed by CDT infusion. In limited studies, first-generation PCDT has resulted in (a) initial treatment safety and clot removal efficacy at least comparable to traditional stand-alone CDT; (b) 40% to 50% reductions in drug dose and treatment time compared with traditional stand-alone CDT; and (c) reduced hospital stays, intensive care unit (ICU) utilization, and hospital costs.[56]

Single-Session Pharmacomechanical Catheter-Directed Thrombolysis

An interesting development over the last few years has been the introduction of three new techniques that appear to enable single-session endovascular DVT therapy to be completed without the need for further drug infusions or ICU monitoring. Two of these techniques are performed with use of the AngioJet. With the "powerpulse" technique (FIGURE 83.2), the AngioJet is first used to forcefully pulse-spray a bolus dose of the thrombolytic drug directly into the thrombus.[57] The drug is allowed to dwell within the thrombus for 15 to 30 minutes, and then the AngioJet is used to aspirate the residual thrombus. With the "rapid lysis" technique, the thrombolytic drug is used as an infusate during simultaneous activation of the AngioJet to remove thrombus.[58] The third technique, "isolated thrombolysis," is performed using the Trellis Peripheral Infusion System (Bacchus Vascular, Santa Clara, CA).[59,60] This device features catheter-mounted balloons that are inflated to isolate a segment of vein for treatment with PCDT. With the balloons inflated, a bolus dose of a thrombolytic drug is injected directly into the thrombus. Activation of an oscillating wire for 5 to 10 minutes is then used to mechanically disperse the drug within the thrombus, then the drug may be aspirated through an aspiration port on the device. Initial reported experiences with these techniques suggest that effective DVT therapy can be accomplished in 80% to 90% of patients, of whom 50% to 80% may be treated in a single procedure session. It should be noted that the impact of these techniques on the development of PTS has not been established in multicenter randomized trials. If PTS prevention is achieved with reasonable safety, the efficiency with which these treatments can be delivered is likely to hasten their widespread adoption for DVT patients.

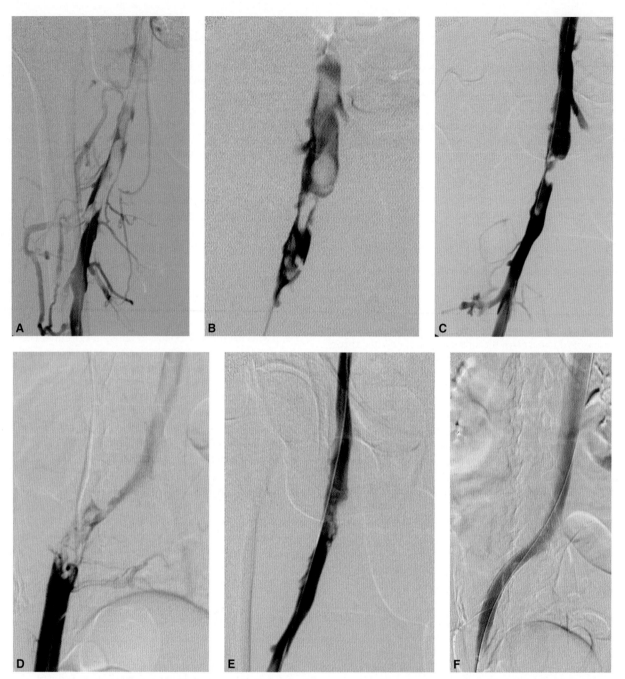

FIGURE 83.2 Powerpulse PCDT for acute iliofemoral DVT. This 30-year-old woman developed left lower extremity pain and swelling of abrupt onset 5 days before. A Duplex ultrasound exam demonstrated noncompressibility of the common femoral vein (CFV) and femoral vein (FV). Venogram performed from a left popliteal vein approach demonstrated globular filling defects consistent with acute thrombus in the **(A)** left FV and CFV and **(B)** left iliac vein. The AngioJet catheter was used to pulse-spray 10 mg of recombinant tissue plasminogen activator (rt-PA), dissolved in 50-mL normal saline, into the thrombus, and this was allowed to dwell for 30 minutes. Two passes were then made with an AngioJet DVX Catheter to aspirate residual thrombus. Follow-up venogram demonstrated clearance of most of the thrombus except for a small amount of residual thrombus in the **(C)** left FV and **(D)** left common iliac vein (CIV) in association with a tight stenosis (May-Thurner syndrome). Balloon maceration was used to facilitate additional femoral vein thrombolysis, and two 14-mm self-expandable metallic stents were placed in the left CIV. Final venogram of the **(E)** femoral and **(F)** iliac veins shows wide patency. This result was achieved in a single 2-hour procedure session with 10 mg of rt-PA.

ENDPOINT ASSESSMENT FOR ENDOVASCULAR THROMBOLYTIC PROCEDURES

The long-term clinical objective of endovascular thrombolysis is to prevent PTS via: (a) prevention of recurrent DVT, (b) maintenance of long-term venous patency, and (c) venous valvular preservation of venous valvular function. The "open vein hypothesis" holds that early thrombus elimination and restoration of venous patency will contribute to achieving these goals. However, the precise anatomic criteria that must be met to expect short- and long-term success with endovascular thrombolytic interventions are unclear. For CDT infusions, data from a large registry suggest that 1-year venous patency is approximately 80% in patients who achieve complete (>99%) clot removal, 60% in patients who achieve partial (≥50%) clot removal, and 30% in patients who achieve minimal (<50%) clot removal.[46] Additionally, a small study of patients treated with PCDT found that those in whom greater than or equal to 50% clot removal was achieved were less likely to develop PTS.[61] However, 50% clot removal in the presence of spontaneous venous flow likely has a different implication than 50% thrombus debulking without associated flow restoration. Furthermore, postprocedural recurrent thrombosis is likely to depend on a number of factors including the amount of residual thrombus, quality of venous flow, and the amount of trauma incurred by the venous system during catheter manipulations. Therefore, it may be hypothesized that PCDT methods that involve more mechanical trauma will require a better initial anatomic result to prevent PTS because recurrent thrombosis and venous valvular injury may be more likely.

RELATIVE THERAPEUTIC EFFECTIVENESS OF ENDOVASCULAR DEEP VENOUS THROMBOSIS THROMBOLYSIS

At present, there remains no published, adequately designed multicenter randomized controlled trial (RCT) that has evaluated the ability of CDT or PCDT to improve important clinical outcomes like PTS in patients with proximal DVT. The ability of CDT/PCDT to rapidly remove venous thrombus and prevent PTS in proximal DVT patients is supported by a number of comparative studies, each with significant methodologic limitations. In 2000, Comerota et al.[62] analyzed data from 68 CDT-treated acute iliofemoral DVT patients from a multicenter prospective CDT registry and found that they had fewer PTS symptoms ($p = .006$), better physical functioning ($p = .046$), less stigma of chronic venous insufficiency ($p = .033$), and less health distress ($p = .022$) at a mean follow-up of 16 months than 30 retrospectively "matched" patients who were treated with anticoagulation alone. This comparison was limited by marked age differences in the two cohorts, however. In 2001, AbuRahma et al. described a prospective study in which 51 acute iliofemoral DVT patients were permitted to choose to receive adjunctive CDT (with urokinase or rt-PA) plus anticoagulation or anticoagulation alone. The patients treated with CDT had more frequent venous patency at 6 months (83% versus 24%, $p < .0001$) and absence of symptoms at 5 years (78% versus 30%, $p = .0015$).[63] However, this study was limited by nonrandomized design, performance in a single center, and small sample size. In 2002, Elsharawy et al. described a single-center Egyptian randomized trial comparing adjunctive CDT (with streptokinase)

versus anticoagulation alone in 35 patients with acute iliofemoral DVT. At 6 months, patients treated with CDT had a higher rate of normal venous function (72% versus 12%, $p < .001$) and less valvular reflux (11% versus 41%, $p = .04$).[64] This study was limited by small sample size and performance in a single center, however, and did not evaluate clinically meaningful outcomes, such as PTS and QOL. In 2009, Enden et al.[65] described the 6-month follow-up results from the first 100 patients randomized to either CDT plus anticoagulation or anticoagulation alone in the Norwegian multicenter CaVenT Trial. Venous patency was significantly superior in the CDT-treated patients (64% versus 36%, $p < .05$), but valvular reflux was no different (60% versus 66%, $p = NS$). In 2010, Sharifi et al.[66] described the results of a 183-patient single-center RCT (the TORPEDO Trial) in which CDT plus anticoagulation proved superior to anticoagulation alone at 6 months follow-up in preventing PTS (3.4% versus 27.2%, $p < .001$) and recurrent VTE (2.3% versus 14.8%, $p < .003$). However, a validated measure of PTS was not used and follow-up period was short.

Of note, the CaVenT Trial noted previously will be assessing patients for PTS over a 2-year follow-up period. Additionally, the Acute Venous Thrombosis: Thrombus Removal with Adjunctive Catheter-Directed Thrombolysis (ATTRACT) Trial, a multicenter randomized trial sponsored by the National Heart Lung and Blood Institute (NHLBI) (www.clinicaltrials.gov, NCT00790335), is also ongoing in the United States. For this study, patients with symptomatic proximal DVT are being randomized in 50 to 60 clinical centers to receive either PCDT plus standard DVT therapy (anticoagulant therapy plus elastic compression stockings) or standard DVT therapy alone. PTS is assessed at follow-up visits every 6 months during the 2-year follow-up period using the Villalta PTS Scale, a validated measure of PTS that is endorsed by the International Society of Thrombosis and Haemostasis (ISTH).[67,68,69] Secondary outcomes being assessed include venous disease-specific and generic QOL; resolution of acute DVT symptoms (pain and swelling); rates of major bleeding, symptomatic PE, recurrent VTE, and death; and cost-effectiveness.

CONCLUSION

Acute DVT should be viewed as a chronic disease by treating physicians because the associated long-term patient disability is quite substantial. Catheter-based thromboreductive therapies offer the potential to preserve life and limb in patients with clinically severe DVT and to prevent PTS and improve QOL in patients with anatomically extensive but less clinically severe DVT. Multicenter randomized clinical trials are ongoing to determine which patients should be treated in this manner. In the meantime, patients with extensive DVT, and especially those with DVT involving the common femoral and/or iliac vein, should be considered for aggressive therapy in the context of a careful individualized assessment of risk and benefit.

REFERENCES

1. U.S. Department of Health and Human Services. *The Surgeon General's Call to Action to Prevent Deep Vein Thrombosis and Pulmonary Embolism.* Washington, DC: Author; 2008.
2. Kearon C, Kahn SR, Agnelli G, et al. Antithrombotic therapy for venous thromboembolic disease. American College of Chest Physicians Evidence-Based Clinical Practice Guidelines (8th ed.). *Chest* 2008;133:454S–545S.

3. Lee AY, Levine MN, Baker RI, et al. Low-molecular-weight heparin versus a coumarin for the prevention of recurrent venous thromboembolism in patients with cancer. *N Engl J Med* 2003;349:146–153.

4. Meyer G, Marjanovic Z, Valcke J, et al. Comparison of low-molecular-weight heparin and warfarin for the secondary prevention of venous thromboembolism in patients with cancer: a randomized controlled study. *Arch Intern Med* 2002;162:1729–1735.

5. Schulman S, Kearon C, Kakkar AK, et al. Dabigatran versus warfarin in the treatment of acute venous thromboembolism. *N Engl J Med* 2009;361(24):2342–2352.

6. EINSTEIN Investigators, Bauersachs R, Berkowitz SD, et al. Oral rivaroxaban for symptomatic venous thromboembolism. *N Engl J Med* 2010;363(26):2499–2510.

7. Prandoni P, Lensing A, Cogo A, et al. The long term clinical course of acute deep venous thrombosis. *Ann Intern Med* 1996;125:1–7.

8. Prandoni P, Lensing AW, Prins MH, et al. Below-knee elastic compression stockings to prevent the post-thrombotic syndrome. *Ann Intern Med* 2004;141:249–256.

9. Brandjes DP, Buller HR, Heijboer H, et al. Randomized trial of effect of compression stockings in patients with symptomatic proximal-vein thrombosis. *Lancet* 1997;349:759–762.

10. Beyth RJ, Cohen AM, Landefeld CS. Long-term outcomes of deep vein thrombosis. *Arch Intern Med* 1995;155:1031–1037.

11. Kahn SR, Ducruet T, Lamping DL, et al. Prospective evaluation of health-related quality of life in patients with deep venous thrombosis. *Arch Intern Med* 2005;165:1173–1178.

12. Kahn SR, Hirsch A, Shrier I. Effect of postthrombotic syndrome on health-related quality of life after deep venous thrombosis. *Arch Intern Med* 2002;162:1144–1148.

13. Delis KT, Bountouroglou D, Mansfield AO. Venous claudication in iliofemoral thrombosis: long-term effects on venous hemodynamics, clinical status, and quality of life. *Ann Surg* 2004;239:118–126.

14. Kahn SR, Shrier I, Julian JA, et al. Determinants and time course of the postthrombotic syndrome after acute deep venous thrombosis. *Ann Intern Med* 2008;149:698–707.

15. Kahn SR, Shbaklo H, Lamping DL, et al. Determinants of health-related quality of life during the 2 years following deep vein thrombosis. *J Thromb Haemost* 2008;6:1105–1112.

16. Caprini JA, Botteman MF, Stephens JM, et al. Economic burden of long-term complications of deep vein thrombosis after total hip replacement surgery in the United States. *Value Health* 2003;6:59–74.

17. Phillips T, Stanton B, Provan A, et al. A study of the impact of leg ulcers on quality of life: financial, social, and psychologic implications. *J Am Acad Dermatol* 1994;31:49–53.

18. Bergqvist D, Jendteg S, Johansen L, et al. Cost of long-term complications of deep venous thrombosis of the lower extremities: an analysis of a defined patient population in Sweden. *Ann Intern Med* 1997;126:454–457.

19. Olin JW, Beusterien KM, Childs MB, et al. Medical costs of treating venous stasis ulcers: evidence from a retrospective cohort study. *Vasc Med* 1999;4:1–7.

20. Roumen-Klappe EM, Janssen MC, Van Rossum J, et al. Inflammation in deep vein thrombosis and the development of post-thrombotic syndrome: a prospective study. *J Thromb Haemost* 2009;7:582–587.

21. Shbaklo H, Holcroft CA, Kahn SR. Levels of inflammatory markers and the development of the post-thrombotic syndrome. *Thromb Haemost* 2009;101:505–512.

22. Wakefield TW, Myers DD, Henke PK. Role of selectins and fibrinolysis in VTE. *Thromb Res* 2009;123(suppl 4):S35–S40.

23. DeRoo S, Deatrick KB, Henke PK. The vessel wall: a forgotten player in post-thrombotic syndrome. *Thromb Haemost* 2010;104:681–692.

24. Markel A, Manzo RA, Bergelin RO, et al. Valvular reflux after deep vein thrombosis: incidence and time of occurrence. *J Vasc Surg* 1992;15:377–384.

25. Caps MT, Manzo RA, Bergelin RO, et al. Venous valvular reflux in veins not involved at the time of acute deep vein thrombosis. *J Vasc Surg* 1995;22:524–531.

26. Shull KC, Nicolaides AN, Fernandes J, et al. Significance of popliteal reflux in relation to ambulatory venous pressure and ulceration. *Arch Surg* 1979;114:1304–1306.

27. Nicolaides AN, Hussein MK, Szendro G, et al. The relation of venous ulceration with ambulatory venous pressure measurements. *J Vasc Surg* 1993;17:414–419.

28. Prandoni P, Frulla M, Sartor D, et al. Venous abnormalities and the post-thrombotic syndrome. *J Thromb Haemost* 2005;3:401–402.

29. Meissner MH, Manzo RA, Bergelin RO, et al. Deep venous insufficiency: the relationship between lysis and subsequent reflux. *J Vasc Surg* 1993;18:596–608.

30. Welkie JF, Comerota AJ, Katz ML, et al. Hemodynamic deterioration in chronic venous disease. *J Vasc Surg* 1992;16:733–740.

31. Araki CT, Back TL, Padberg FT, et al. The significance of calf muscle pump function in venous ulceration. *J Vasc Surg* 1994;20:872–877.

32. Johnson BF, Manzo RA, Bergelin RO, et al. Relationship between changes in the deep venous system and the development of the postthrombotic syndrome after an acute episode of lower limb deep vein thrombosis: a one-to-six year follow-up. *J Vasc Surg* 1995;21:307–313.

33. Meissner MH, Caps MT, Bergelin RO, et al. Propagation, rethrombosis and new thrombus formation after acute deep venous thrombosis. *J Vasc Surg* 1995;22:558–567.

34. Kahn SR, Shbaklo H, Shapiro S, et al. Effectiveness of compression stockings to prevent the post-thrombotic syndrome (the SOX Trial and Bio-SOX biomarker substudy): a randomized controlled trial. *BMC Cardiovasc Disord* 2007;7:21.

35. Kahn SR, Shrier I, Shapiro S, et al. Six-month exercise training program to treat post-thrombotic syndrome: a randomized controlled two-centre trial. *CMAJ* 2011;183(1):37–44.

36. Hull RD, Marder VJ, Mah AF, et al. Quantitative assessment of thrombus burden predicts the outcome of treatment for venous thrombosis: a systematic review. *Am J Med* 2005;118:456–464.

37. Plate G, Einarsson E, Ohlin P, et al. Thrombectomy with temporary arteriovenous fistula: the treatment of choice in acute iliofemoral venous thrombosis. *J Vasc Surg* 1984;1:867–876.

38. Plate G, Akesson H, Einarsson E, et al. Long-term results of venous thrombectomy combined with a temporary arterio-venous fistula. *Eur J Vasc Surg* 1990;4:483–489.

39. Goldhaber SZ, Buring JE, Lipnick RJ, et al. Pooled analyses of randomized trials of streptokinase and heparin in phlebographically documented acute deep venous thrombosis. *Am J Med* 1984;76:393–397.

40. Elliot MS, Immelman EJ, Jeffery P, et al. A comparative randomized trial of heparin versus streptokinase in the treatment of acute proximal venous thrombosis: an interim report of a prospective trial. *Br J Surg* 1979;66:838–843.

41. Arnesen H, Hoiseth A, Ly B. Streptokinase or heparin in the treatment of deep vein thrombosis. *Acta Med Scand* 1982;211:65–68.

42. Turpie AGG, Levine MN, Hirsh J, et al. Tissue plasminogen activator (rt-PA) vs heparin in deep vein thrombosis: results of a randomized trial. *Chest Suppl* 1990;97:172S–175S.

43. Goldhaber SZ, Meyerovitz MF, Green D, et al. Randomized controlled trial of tissue plasminogen activator in proximal deep venous thrombosis. *Am J Med* 1990;88:235–240.

44. Meyerovitz MF, Polak JF, Goldhaber SZ. Short-term response to thrombolytic therapy in deep venous thrombosis: predictive value of venographic appearance. *Radiology* 1992;184:345–348.

45. Schwieder G, Grimm W, Siemens HJ, et al. Intermittent regional therapy with rt-PA is not superior to systemic thrombolysis in deep vein thrombosis (DVT)—a German multicenter trial. *Thromb Haemost* 1995;74:1240–1243.

46. Mewissen MW, Seabrook GR, Meissner MH, et al. Catheter-directed thrombolysis for lower extremity deep venous thrombosis: report of a national multicenter registry. *Radiology* 1999;211:39–49.

47. Vedantham S, Thorpe PE, Cardella JF, et al. Quality improvement guidelines for the treatment of lower extremity deep vein thrombosis with use of endovascular thrombus removal. *J Vasc Interv Radiol* 2006;17:435–447.

48. Douketis JD, Crowther MA, Foster GA, et al. Does the location of thrombosis determine the risk of disease recurrence in patients with proximal deep vein thrombosis? *Am J Med* 2001;110:515–519.

49. Ginsberg JS, Hirsh J, Julian J, et al. Prevention and treatment of postphlebitic syndrome: results of a 3-part study. *Arch Intern Med* 2001;16:2105–2109.

50. Semba CP, Dake MD. Iliofemoral deep venous thrombosis: aggressive therapy with catheter-directed thrombolysis. *Radiology* 1994;191:487–494.

51. Vedantham S, Grassi CJ, Ferral H, et al. Reporting standards for endovascular treatment of lower extremity deep vein thrombosis. *J Vasc Interv Radiol* 2006;17:417–434.

52. Shortell CK, Queiroz R, Johansson M, et al. Safety and efficacy of limited-dose tissue plasminogen activator in acute vascular occlusion. *J Vasc Surg* 2001;34:854–859.

53. Sugimoto K, Hofmann LV, Razavi MK, et al. The safety, efficacy, and pharmaco-economics of low-dose alteplase compared with urokinase for catheter-directed thrombolysis of arterial and venous occlusions. *J Vasc Surg* 2003;37:512–517.

54. Grunwald MR, Hofmann LV. Comparison of urokinase, alteplase, and reteplase for catheter-directed thrombolysis of deep venous thrombosis. *J Vasc Interv Radiol* 2004;15:347–352.

55. Parikh SR, Motarjeme A, McNamara TO, et al. Ultrasound-accelerated thrombolysis for the treatment of deep vein thrombosis: initial clinical experience. *J Vasc Interv Radiol* 2008;19(4):521–528.

56. Kim HS, Patra A, Paxton BE, et al. Adjunctive percutaneous mechanical thrombectomy for lower-extremity deep vein thrombosis: clinical and economic outcomes. *J Vasc Interv Radiol* 2006;17:1099–1104.

57. Cynamon J, Stein EG, Dym J, et al. A new method for aggressive management of deep vein thrombosis: retrospective study of the power pulse technique. *J Vasc Interv Radiol* 2006;17:1043–1049.

58. Lin PH, Zhou W, Dardik A, et al. Catheter-direct thrombolysis versus pharmacomechanical thrombectomy for treatment of symptomatic lower extremity deep vein thrombosis. *Am J Surg* 2006;192:782–788.

59. O'Sullivan GJ, Lohan DG, Gough N, et al. Pharmacomechanical thrombectomy of acute deep vein thrombosis with the Trellis-8 isolated thrombolysis catheter. *J Vasc Interv Radiol* 2007;18:715–724.

60. Hilleman DE, Razavi MK. Clinical and economic evaluation of the Trellis-8 infusion catheter for deep vein thrombosis. *J Vasc Interv Radiol* 2008;19:377–383.

61. Grewal NK, Martinez JT, Andrews L, et al. Quantity of clot lysed after catheter-directed thrombolysis for iliofemoral deep venous thrombosis correlates with postthrombotic morbidity. *J Vasc Surg* 2010;51(5):1209–1214.

62. Comerota AJ, Throm RC, Mathias SD, et al. Catheter-directed thrombolysis for iliofemoral deep venous thrombosis improves health-related quality of life. *J Vasc Surg* 2000;32:130–137.

63. AbuRahma AF, Perkins SE, Wulua JT, et al. Iliofemoral deep vein thrombosis: conventional therapy versus lysis and percutaneous transluminal angioplasty and stenting. *Ann Surg* 2001;233:752–760.

64. Elsharawy M, Elzayat E. Early results of thrombolysis vs anticoagulation in iliofemoral venous thrombosis. *Eur J Vasc Endovasc Surg* 2002;24:209–214.

65. Enden T, Klow NE, Sandvik L, et al. Catheter-directed thrombolysis versus anticoagulation alone in deep vein thrombosis: results of an open, randomized trial reporting on short-term patency. *J Thromb Haemost* 2009;7:1268–1275.

66. Sharifi M, Mehdipour M, Bay C, et al. Endovenous therapy for deep venous thrombosis: the TORPEDO Trial. *Catheter Cardiovasc Interv* 2010;76:316–325.

67. Vedantham S, Goldhaber SZ, Kahn SR, et al. Rationale and design of the ATTRACT Study: a multicenter randomized trial to evaluate pharmacomechanical catheter-directed thrombolysis for the prevention of postthrombotic syndrome in patients with proximal deep vein thrombosis. *Am Heart J* 2013; 165(4):523–553.

68. Kahn SR, Partsch H, Vedantham S, et al. Definition of post-thrombotic syndrome in the leg for use in clinical investigations: a recommendation for standardization. *J Thromb Haemost* 2009;7:879–883.

69. Kahn SR. Measurement properties of the Villalta scale to define and classify the severity of the post-thrombotic syndrome. *J Thromb Haemost* 2009;7(5):884–888.

Pulmonary Embolism: IVC Filters—Indications and Technical Considerations

MATTHEW S. JOHNSON, FRANCIS E. MARSHALLECK, and CHRISTIAN N. JOHNSON

INTRODUCTION

The exact incidence of venous thromboembolism (VTE), comprising pulmonary embolus (PE) and deep venous thrombosis (DVT), is not known. Due to difficulty in establishing its diagnosis, requiring imaging studies that are not always performed, and frequent comorbidities in patients with VTE, such as cardiac disease and malignancy, estimates of its incidence and significance vary widely. For example, it has been reported to affect 7.1 per 10,000 community residents, thus about 213,000 of 300 million U.S. citizens,[1] and it also has been reported to affect over 2 million[2] U.S. citizens each year. Further, as algorithms for the treatment of VTE have become established, the natural course of untreated VTE has become difficult to study. Older studies, including Dalen's seminal study demonstrating the value of heparin in the treatment of PE, suggest a 20% to 50% recurrence rate of untreated PE with a mortality rate of around 25%.[3,4] Regardless of the uncertainty described previously, VTE is clearly a major cause of morbidity and mortality: The U.S. Surgeon General estimates that there are 350,000 to 600,000 new cases of VTE in the United States, contributing to at least 100,000 deaths each year.[5]

PATIENT SELECTION

The American College of Chest Physicians (ACCP) provides guidelines for the treatment of people with DVT and/or PE. There is widespread agreement that the standard of care of VTE, as outlined in those guidelines, is systemic anticoagulation, which can be administered orally, subcutaneously, or intravenously.[6] There is, however, no such general agreement on the appropriate use of an inferior vena cava filter (IVCF) in the treatment of VTE. Although the ACCP guidelines state that IVCFs are appropriately placed in patients with DVT and/or PE in whom the risk of bleeding precludes anticoagulation (guidelines 1.13.2 and 4.6.2), they specifically recommend against the use of prophylactic IVCFs in trauma patients without VTE (guideline 5.1.5), and make no recommendation regarding prophylactic filters in other applications, such as in patients at risk for PE during or after bariatric or other operations. Conversely, other guidelines, such as those provided by the Society of Interventional Radiology (SIR) and the Eastern Association for the Study of Trauma (EAST), state that prophylactic filter placement is appropriate for trauma patients without VTE who are at high risk for it due to severe closed head injury, spinal cord injury with para or quadraplegia, complex pelvic and long bone fractures, and/or multiple long bone fractures, and who cannot

be anticoagulated.[7–9] The SIR guidelines state that prophylactic IVCF placement might also be appropriate in other high-risk patients, such as those at risk for VTE who are about to undergo a surgical procedure.[7]

Although the debate continues whether prophylactic IVCF placement is appropriate, there is agreement, at least in the United States, that patients with PE and/or above-knee DVT who cannot be anticoagulated, either because of contraindication to or failure or complication of that therapy, would benefit from IVCF placement. Multiple IVC filters have been cleared by the Food and Drug Administration (FDA) for use in that indication.

TREATMENT OPTIONS

Prior to the 1960s, the standard practice for IVC interruption included surgical ligation or plication of the infrarenal IVC and constriction of the IVC lumen by surgical placement of an external clip. That surgical technique was, however, associated with high morbidity and mortality rates. The first IVCF, the Mobin-Uddin Umbrella, was introduced in 1967. It was a perforated plastic cone with six supporting metal ribs that was implanted apex down via a venotomy. Although an improvement over surgical ligation, it was also associated with relatively high rates of IVC thrombosis and was eventually supplanted by the stainless steel Greenfield IVCF. In 1968, following the death of one of his patients after open pulmonary embolectomy, Lazar Greenfield approached Garman Kimmell, a prolific inventor in the oil industry, with an idea for a new IVCF. They adapted the principle of filtering sludge in oil pipelines and created the Greenfield filter (FIGURE 84.1), which obtained premarket approval (PMA) from the FDA in 1969.

Several other IVCFs have been cleared for use in the United States since 1969, all through the 510K process,[10] that is, as substantially equivalent to the predicate device, the stainless steel Greenfield filter. Despite their approval through that process, the currently available IVCFs vary considerably in their design, construction, and composition. For example, through 2001, all filters were cleared only for permanent placement. In 2002, Cook and Cordis were granted approval to market the Gunther Tulip and OptEase filters, respectively. Both were cleared for permanent placement and for removal. Thus, they were the first "retrievable" IVC filters. All filters cleared since 2002 are retrievable, approved for both permanent indication and removal if clinically desired. IVCFs (permanent and retrievable) that were previously and are currently available for use in

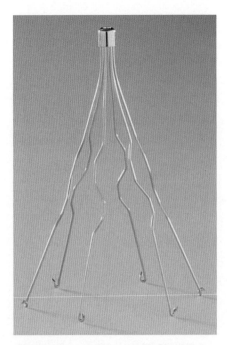

FIGURE 84.1 Stainless steel Greenfield filter.

© Boston Scientific. Used with permission.

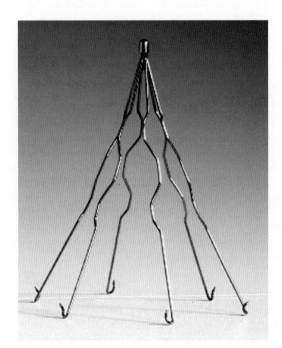

FIGURE 84.2 Titanium Greenfield filter.

© Boston Scientific. Used with permission.

the United States are listed next in order of the introduction of each company's first filter.

Boston Scientific Filters

The original 24 French (delivery sheath inner diameter [ID]) stainless steel Greenfield filter (Boston Scientific, Natick, MA) was replaced in 1989 with a titanium filter, which also had an apex-up single cone design (FIGURE 84.2). It was delivered through a 12 French ID/15 French outer diameter (OD) sheath. In 1995, the currently available stainless steel Over-the-Wire Greenfield filter, also delivered through a 12 French ID/14 French OD sheath, was introduced. All Greenfield filters are approved for permanent use only, in venae cavae up to 28 mm in diameter (FIGURE 84.2).

Cook Filters

The Gianturco-Roehm Bird's Nest Filter (Cook Medical, Bloomington, IN), introduced in 1982, comprises six wires attached to proximal and distal V-shaped barbed struts. It is delivered through a 12 French ID/14 French OD sheath. It remains the only filter cleared by the FDA for placement in venae cavae over 30 mm (up to 40 mm) in diameter. It was cleared by the FDA for permanent use only. The Günther Tulip filter, made of Elgiloy (an alloy primarily composed of cobalt, chromium, nickel, iron, and molybdenum), was introduced in 2000 as a permanent filter and later cleared as one of the first retrievable filters in 2003; it is the first of two currently available Cook filters with an apex-up single cone design. Looped wires between its four main legs are stated to facilitate capture of thrombus (FIGURE 84.3). It is packaged in a 7.5 French ID/9.5 French OD delivery system. It is approved as a permanent and retrievable filter in venae cavae up to 30 mm

in diameter. In 2007, Cook launched the Celect filter, made of Conichrome (another trademark name for the alloy described previously). The jugular and femoral deliveries for the Celect filter are packaged with a 7.0 French ID/9.5 French OD delivery sheath. It is based on the Tulip design with the Tulip's looped wires replaced by eight internal struts between Celect's four legs.

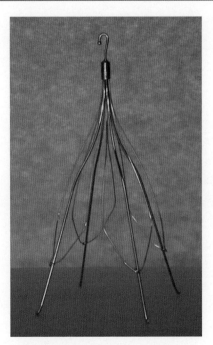

FIGURE 84.3 Günther Tulip filter.

Like its predecessor, the Celect filter's apical hook allows snare retrieval. Also like the Tulip, the Celect is approved as a permanent and retrievable filter in venae cavae up to 30 mm in diameter.

B Braun Filters

The Vena Tech LGM filter (B Braun Medical Inc., Bethlehem, PA) was introduced in 1989. Like its predecessors, it has an apex-up single cone design and is delivered through a 12 French ID/14 French OD delivery system. Made of Phynox (yet another trademark name for the Co, Cr, Ni, Fe, Mo alloy noted earlier),[11] it consists of a central cone with six side legs each containing a hook for fixation (FIGURE 84.4). In 2001, B Braun introduced the Vena Tech LP filter, also made of Phynox, but delivered through a 7 French ID/9 French OD delivery system (FIGURE 84.5). Both B Braun filters are approved for permanent use only in venae cavae up to 28 mm in diameter.

Bard Filters

The Simon Nitinol filter (Bard Peripheral Vascular, Tempe, AZ), introduced in 1990, has an apex-up design consisting of a cephalad petal component and caudal feet, providing two areas for trapping thrombus and caval contact (FIGURE 84.6). Like the Vena Tech LP filter, it is delivered through a 7 French ID/9 French OD sheath and it is approved for permanent use only in venae cavae up to 28 mm in diameter. In 2003, the Bard Recovery filter, also made of nitinol, a nickel titanium alloy, was approved as a permanent and retrievable filter in venae cavae up to 28 mm in diameter. Delivered through the same size sheath as the Simon Nitinol filter, it consisted of an apex-up conical trapping zone with six upper struts for centering and six anchoring legs with flexible hooks to facilitate removal (FIGURE 84.7).

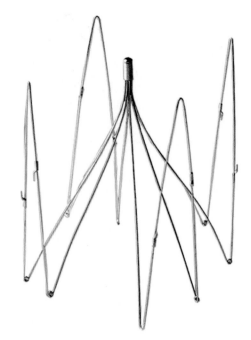

FIGURE 84.5 VenaTech LP filter.

Removal was accomplished with a 15-mm grasping cone device. The Recovery filter is no longer available, having been replaced by newer filters developed on the same background design. The G2 filter (FIGURE 84.8) which, among other modifications, has a larger resting base diameter than the Recovery filter, replaced that filter in 2007. The G2x filter, introduced in 2010, is the latest in that line of filters. Among its modifications is the addition of a hook to its apex to facilitate retrieval.

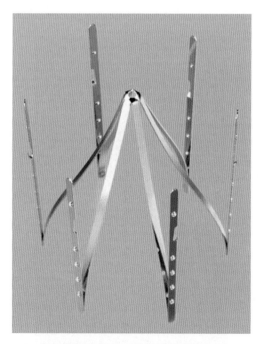

FIGURE 84.4 VenaTech LGM filter.

Courtesy of B Braun Medical, Bethlehem, PA.

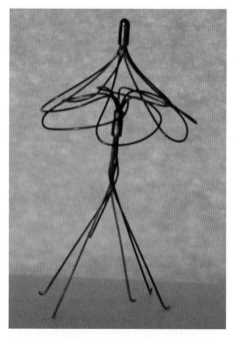

FIGURE 84.6 Simon Nitinol filter.

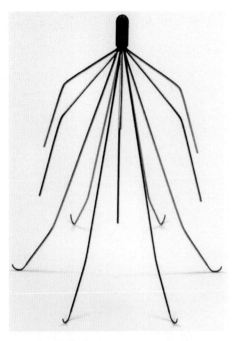

FIGURE 84.7 Bard Recovery filter.

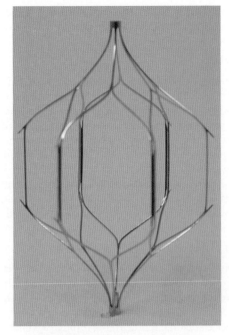

FIGURE 84.9 Cordis TrapEase filter.

Cordis Filters

The TrapEase filter (Cordis Endovascular, Miami Lakes, FL) was approved in 2000 for permanent use only in venae cavae up to 30 mm in diameter. It comprises a dual cone design, with the caudal cone apex down and the cephalad cone apex up

(FIGURE 84.9). Barbs on its side struts assist in preventing caudal or cephalad migration. It is delivered through a 6 French ID/8 French OD sheath. The OptEase filter, introduced in 2003, is similar in appearance to the TrapEase filter, also made of nitinol and delivered through the same size sheath; but whereas it has barbs to prevent cephalad migration, it does not have barbs to prevent caudal migration (FIGURE 84.10). Thus, it is retrievable from a caudal approach, unlike other retrievable filters, which are intended for removal via a cephalad approach. The OptEase

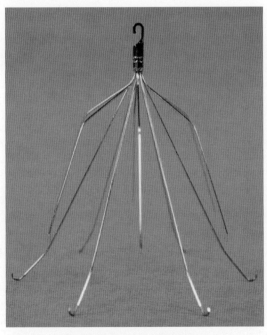

FIGURE 84.8 Bard G2 filter.

Courtesy of David Trost, MD.

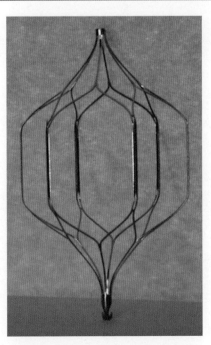

FIGURE 84.10 Cordis OptEase filter.

filter is approved for permanent and retrievable indications in venae cavae up to 30 mm in diameter.

ALN Filter

The ALN filter (Chirurgicaux, Ghisonaccia, France) is a stainless steel filter with an apex-up single cone design and nine legs (three long and six short) each of varying lengths. The six shorter legs terminate in hooks for caval fixation. It is delivered through a 7 French ID sheath. It was approved by the FDA in 2008 for permanent and retrievable indications in venae cavae up to 30 mm in diameter (FIGURE 84.11). The ALN filter is unique among the currently available retrievable filters in that its apex—the caudal apex in the case of the OptEase filter—has no hook. It is removed with a grasping device also manufactured by ALN.

Option Filter

The nitinol Option filter (Argon Medical Devices, Plano, TX) was approved in 2008 for permanent and retrievable indications in venae cavae up to 30 mm in diameter. It consists of an apex-up cone design with six legs and has a proximal hook for retrieval (FIGURE 84.12). It is delivered through a 5 French ID/6.5 French OD sheath.

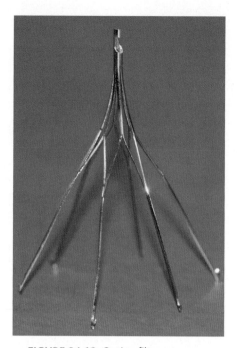

FIGURE 84.12 Option filter.

Courtesy of Rex Medical, Conshohocken, PA.

INDICATIONS AND GUIDELINES FOR INFRARENAL INFERIOR VENA CAVA FILTER INSERTION

As noted earlier, there is a lack of agreement among societal guidelines in some commonly stated indications for filter placement. Nonetheless, there is agreement on the "classic" indications for the placement of an IVCF: IVCFs are appropriate in patients with an existing PE or IVC, iliac, or femoral-popliteal DVT, and at least one of the following: contraindication to anticoagulation, complication of anticoagulation, or failure of anticoagulation, that is, recurrent PE despite adequate therapy or an inability to achieve adequate anticoagulation. Contraindications to anticoagulation include recent trauma or surgery; increased fall risk; central nervous system disorders, such as neoplasm, aneurysm, recent stroke or vascular malformation; prior bleeding complication with anticoagulation; and recent gastrointestinal hemorrhage.

In contradistinction to the ACCP, SIR and EAST guidelines[7,9] state that IVCF is appropriate in some patients in addition to those noted earlier. "Extended" indications for IVC filter insertion include patients with large, free floating iliac or caval DVT (regardless of whether anticoagulation is possible); patients with massive PE treated with embololysis and/or embolectomy, or patients with severe cardiopulmonary disease in whom another episode of PE could be fatal; patients who are poorly compliant with anticoagulation; and for protection during iliofemoral thrombolysis.

Finally, as noted previously, the guidelines conflict regarding whether to place an IVCF in a patient without proven VTE. Further research is necessary to determine whether some patients might benefit from prophylactic IVCF placement.

INDICATIONS FOR SUPRARENAL INFERIOR VENA CAVA FILTER INSERTION

Suprarenal filter insertion may be indicated when placement of an infrarenal filter is impossible or unlikely to prevent PE. Possible indications include renal vein thrombosis, IVC thrombus extending to the level of the renal veins or above, gonadal vein thrombosis, IVC duplication, low insertion of the renal veins, and thrombus extended above an existing infrarenal filter.

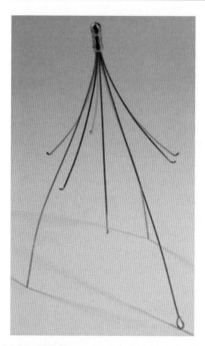

FIGURE 84.11 ALN filter.

Courtesy of ALN Implants Chirurgicaux, Bormes les Mimosas, France.

CONTRAINDICATIONS TO INFERIOR VENA CAVA FILTER INSERTION

Absolute contraindications are rare and include complete thrombosis of the IVC, which would also preclude access into the IVC. Relative contraindications include severe coagulopathy and sepsis.

TECHNIQUE OF INFERIOR VENA CAVA FILTER INSERTION

Percutaneous IVCF placement requires access into a peripheral vein. Whereas the smaller delivery sheaths of most of the currently available filters might allow filter placement through more peripheral veins, such as the basilic vein, most filters are placed through a femoral or jugular vein. Such access provides a straighter, shorter course to the infrarenal IVC. Once venous access is established, an inferior vena cavogram should be obtained to assess IVC caliber, patency, and anatomic variation; to demonstrate the level of the renal veins; and to determine whether caval thrombus is present. A flush catheter is placed within the caudal IVC near the iliac vein confluence and contrast is injected while digital subtraction images are obtained. The origins of the renal veins are usually indicated by inflow filling defects or less commonly by reflux of contrast into the main renal veins. If not properly visualized, the individual renal veins can be selected with subsequent venographic evaluation.

Classically, the IVCF is deployed with fluoroscopic guidance immediately inferior to the origin of the lowest renal vein. The tip of the filter should be positioned at the level of the renal veins for its tip to be subjected to constant flow of blood. Theoretically, such positioning decreases the incidence of thrombus formation, but there is no clinical data to support that theory. If duplication of the IVC is suspected, catheter selection is possible. The duplicated cava most commonly drains into the left renal vein. A filter may be deployed within each of the duplicated IVC or, alternatively, a suprarenal filter may be placed. Carbon dioxide can be used in patients with severe contrast allergy or renal impairment. Although filter insertion using fluoroscopic guidance remains the gold standard, IVCF insertion at the bedside with ultrasound guidance or with the use of intravascular ultrasound (IVUS) has been performed successfully.[12–15] As noted, most available filters are FDA approved for caval diameters up to 28 or 30 mm. In the uncommon patient with a larger IVC, such as up to 40 mm in diameter, a Bird's Nest filter may be placed. Alternatively, a filter may be deployed within each of the common iliac veins.

OUTCOMES

It is widely held that IVCFs prevent pulmonary embolism; however, especially outside the United States, many question their benefit: There is thus substantial international variation in IVCF placement. Most of the more than 200,000 IVCFs implanted around the world in 2010 were placed in the United States with relatively very few in Europe. Further, there is regional variation in IVCF use within the United States.[16]

The lack of agreement regarding appropriate utilization of IVCFs is in large part due to the complications related to their use, the paucity of evidence supporting that use, the quality of that evidence, and the fact that "IVCF" refers to a very heterogeneous group of devices.

That complications, such as IVC thrombosis, filter migration, filter fracture, and IVC penetration, occur is well known. However, because so few prospective studies have been performed, the true incidence of those complications is not known. Several reviews of IVCFs published prior to the introduction of most retrievable filters demonstrated not inconsequential but highly variable complication rates.[17–24]

For example, the incidence of IVC thrombosis has been reported to range from 6% to 30%, and that of filter migration from 3% to 69%. The potential of retrieval of IVCFs once they are no longer needed to reduce filter-related complications led to the enthusiasm for their placement. However, as noted by Millward in 2005,[25] modification of filters to allow their retrieval might increase the rates of some complications, such as migration; the degree to which filter retrieval lessens the rates of complications is (then and now) unknown; and the filter retrieval procedure introduces new risks, including radiation and contrast exposure during retrieval, potential retrieval procedural complications, such as damage to the IVC or filter, and recurrent PE following filter removal.

That so much about IVCFs remains unknown speaks to the paucity of high-quality studies evaluating their use. Most of the literature related to IVCFs comprise retrospective studies. Indeed, most of the filters introduced after the original Greenfield filter were cleared through the 510K process for sale in the United States despite the lack of prospective studies evaluating them. Although certainly of value, retrospective studies are limited in the data that they provide, and in the evaluation of IVCFs, the methodologies employed in those retrospective series has varied greatly, further limiting the quality of the data.

A few prospective studies evaluating single filters, and one large randomized controlled trial, in which multiple different types of filters were used, have been performed. In an effort to determine whether IVCFs were of clinical value in the treatment of patients with VTE, a prospective randomized clinical trial was performed, and its results published, initially, in the *New England Journal of Medicine* in 1998.[26] The authors of that study concluded that the initial benefit of IVCFs in preventing PE was counterbalanced by an excess of recurrent DVT, and that there was no difference in mortality between those who received an IVCF and those who did not. That study demonstrates the difficulty of performing a randomized controlled trial of IVCF use: Every one of the 400 subjects in the trial was anticoagulated prior to randomization to IVCF or no filter. Although that methodology could be defended based on the classic standard-of-care versus standard-of-care plus intervention design, it did not take appropriate clinical practice into consideration: The standard of care *is* anticoagulation; it is only those patients who cannot be anticoagulated who should be considered for IVCF placement. Placement of an IVCF in an adequately treated patient would not be expected to provide added benefit. Surprisingly, despite that negative bias, a subsequent evaluation of the subjects in the study, published in *Circulation* in 2005,[27] demonstrated a statistically significant decrease in symptomatic PE in the IVCF group (9 subjects, cumulative rate 6%) versus the control group (24 subjects, 15%, $p = .008$). DVT occurred more frequently in the IVCF group (57 patients, 36%) versus the control group (41 patients, 28%, $p = .042$), supporting the increased incidence of DVT shown in multiple prior retrospective studies. Because the authors found no significant difference on survival between groups, they recommended against routine use in patients with VTE. It is important to emphasize, however, that patients in both groups were anticoagulated; the decreased incidence of PE even in that scenario would seem to support strongly the use of IVCF in patients who cannot be anticoagulated. However, not all are in agreement with the preceding statement: In 2010, Young et al., noting that "although [IVCF] deployment seems of theoretical benefit, their clinical efficacy and adverse event profile is unclear," performed a structured review of the literature, identifying "controlled clinical trials and randomised controlled trials that examined the efficacy of filters in preventing PE." With those criteria, they identified only two studies that qualified: the previously noted PREPIC study and a smaller trial (of 129 patients with hip fractures). They concluded that no recommendations could be drawn from the two studies, and that further trials were needed to assess vena caval filter safety and effectiveness.[28] Although not available for their review because two were published at around the same time, and a third soon after, three single-arm prospective studies of retrievable filters[29–31]—the ALN, G2, and Option filters, respectively—have been published.

With the closer follow-up mandated by prospective trials, a better idea of the true incidence of recurrent PE, and of complications, is available for each of the studied devices than had been available for those for which only retrospective data were available. That notwithstanding, given the differences in study methodology—only the Johnson et al. study was performed according to published research standards[8,31] (those standards not having been published when the previous two studies were published)—uncertainty regarding the safety and efficacy of currently available filters remains. Further, the tendency to refer to all available devices as if they were all similar in safety and efficacy has interfered with their evaluation. Each device should be evaluated on its own merits.

As noted previously, societal recommendations differ in indications for IVCFs. The ACCP guidelines are arguably the most highly regarded. In addition to reserving recommendation for IVCF placement only in patients with known VTE, those guidelines recommend anticoagulation in all patients with filters once contraindication to anticoagulation no longer exists. Despite the paucity of evidence, those guidelines also recommend placement of retrievable filters in children, and their removal once the contraindication to anticoagulation no longer exists.

Currently, given the lack of data regarding their use, there are no unique indications for retrievable IVCFs that are distinct from permanent IVCFs. Additionally, retrievable filters are usually more expensive than permanent filters; therefore, the indication for placement should be justified. In 2008, Kim et al. conducted a retrospective cohort study of patients who received either retrievable or permanent filters from January 2002 through December 2006. The study concluded that both filter types provided similar protection and that the choice between permanent or retrievable filter insertion is determined by the projected duration of filtration needed.[32] However, that all retrievable IVCFs might not be retrieved, and that they become "permanent," should be considered and discussed with patients. Once a filter is placed, patients should be managed with pharmacologic methods according to their VTE status and risk of anticoagulation. Currently, there are no indications for discontinuation of filtration unless the filter itself is a source of major morbidity. Filter retrieval should only occur when the risk of clinically significant pulmonary embolism is reduced to

an acceptable level and is estimated to be less than the risk of leaving the filter in. Again, however, the quality of the literature on retrievable filters is not sufficient to support evidence-based recommendations at this time.

CONCLUSION

It is agreed that the indications for filter (permanent or retrievable) insertion include the inability to pharmacologically treat DVT and/or PE with anticoagulation. Although the preponderance of retrospective data and the relatively scarce data from prospective trials suggest that IVCFs are effective in preventing PE in appropriately selected patients, the long-term risk benefit ratio of IVCFs requires further investigation. Theoretically, the ideal filter would be one that is low profile to minimize access injury, is stable in position once placed, and is easily removed when indicated. The indications for placement of retrievable filters are still evolving. As preliminary studies indicate, there may be a role for retrievable filters in selected high-risk patients without VTE (e.g., those suffering trauma, or who are scheduled to undergo spinal or bariatric surgery) as clinically indicated. However, before the patient population who might be served is expanded to include such patients, the safety and efficacy of each available filter in its accepted indication, that is, in the treatment of patients who have known VTE and who cannot be anticoagulated, must be demonstrated.

REFERENCES

1. Snow V, Qaseem A, Barry P, et al. Management of venous thromboembolism: a clinical practice guideline from the American College of Physicians and the American Academy of Family Physicians. *Ann Fam Med* 2007;5(1):74–80.
2. Houman Fekrazad M, Lopes RD, Stashenko GJ, et al. Treatment of venous thromboembolism: guidelines translated for the clinician. *J Thromb Thrombolysis* 2009;28(3):270–275.
3. Dalen JE, Alpert JS. Natural history of pulmonary embolism. *Prog Cardiovasc Dis* 1975;17(4):259–270.
4. Silver D, Sabiston DC Jr. The role of vena cava interruption in the management of pulmonary embolism. *Surgery* 1975;77:1.
5. *The Surgeon General's Call to Action to Prevent Deep Vein Thrombosis and Pulmonary Embolism.* Office of the Surgeon General (OSG). Available at: http://www.surgeongeneral.gov/topics/deepvein/. Accessed September 28, 2011.
6. Kearon C, Kahn SR, Agnelli G, et al. Antithrombotic therapy for venous thromboembolic disease: American College of Chest Physicians Evidence-Based Clinical Practice Guidelines (8th ed.). *Chest* 2008;133(6 suppl):454S–545S.
7. Grassi C, Swan T, Cardella J, et al. Quality improvement guidelines for percutaneous permanent inferior vena cava filter placement for the prevention of pulmonary embolism. *J Vasc Interv Radiol* 2001;12(2):137–141.
8. Kaufman JA, Rundback JH, Kee ST, et al. Development of a research agenda for inferior vena cava filters: proceedings from a multidisciplinary research consensus panel. *J Vasc Interv Radiol* 2009;20(6):697–707.
9. Rogers FB, Cipolle MD, Velmahos G, et al. Practice management guidelines for the prevention of venous thromboembolism in trauma patients: the EAST practice management guidelines work group. *J Trauma* 2002;53(1):142–164.
10. *Device Advice: Comprehensive Regulatory Assistance.* U.S. Food and Drug Administration Home Page. Available at: http://www.fda.gov/medicaldevices/deviceregulationandguidance/. Accessed September 28, 2011.
11. *Specifications: Conichrome.* Fort Wayne, IN: Fort Wayne Metals. Available at: http://www.fwmetals.com Accessed September 28, 2011.
12. Benjamin M, Sandager G, Cohn E, et al. Duplex ultrasound insertion of inferior vena cava filters in multitrauma patients. *Am J Surg* 1999;178:92–97.
13. Ebaugh J, Choiu A, Morasch M, et al. Bedside vena cava filter placement guided with intravascular ultrasound. *J Vasc Surg* 2001;43:21–26.

14. Matsumura J, Morasch M. Filter placement by ultrasound technique at the bedside. *Semin Vasc Surg* 2000;13:199–203.

15. Bonn J, Liu J, Eschelman D, et al. Intravascular ultrasound as an alternative to positive contrast vena cavography prior to filter placement. *J Vasc Interv Radiol* 1999;10:843–849.

16. Dossett LA, Adams RC, Cotton BA. Unwarranted national variation in the use of prophylactic inferior vena cava filters after trauma: an analysis of the National Trauma Databank. *J Trauma* 2011;70(5):1066–1070.

17. Ray CE Jr, Kaufman JA. Complications of inferior vena cava filters. *Abdom Imaging* 1996;21(4):368–374.

18. Ballew KA, Philbrick JT, Becker DM. Vena cava filter devices. *Clin Chest Med* 1995;16:295–305.

19. Fox M, Kahn S. Postthrombotic syndrome in relation to vena cava filter placement: a systematic review. *J Vasc Interv Radiol* 2008;19(7): 981–985.e3.

20. Streiff MB. Vena caval filters: a comprehensive review. *Blood* 2000;95(12): 3669–3677.

21. Greenfield LJ, Proctor MC. The percutaneous greenfield filter: outcomes and practice patterns. *J Vasc Surg* 2000;32(5):888–893.

22. Rousseau H, Perreault P, Otal P, et al. The 6-F nitinol TrapEase inferior vena cava filter: results of a prospective multicenter trial. *J Vasc Interv Radiol* 2001;12(3):299–304.

23. Neuerberg JM, Günther RW, Vorwerk D, et al. Results of a multicenter study of the retrievable Tulip Vena Cava Filter: early clinical experience. *Cardiovasc Intervent Radiol* 1997;20(1):10–16.

24. Kinney TB. Update on inferior vena cava filters. *J Vasc Interv Radiol* 2003;14(4):425–440.

25. Millward S. Vena cava filters: continuing the search for an ideal device. *J Vasc Interv Radiol* 2005;16(11):1423–1425.

26. Decousus H, Leizorovicz A, Parent F, et al. A clinical trial of vena caval filters in the prevention of pulmonary embolism in patients with proximal deep-vein thrombosis. *N Engl J Med* 1998;338(7):409–416.

27. PREPIC Study Group. Eight-year follow-up of patients with permanent vena cava filters in the prevention of pulmonary embolism: the PREPIC (Prevention Du Risque D'Embolie Pulmonaire Par Interruption Cave) randomized study. *Circulation* 2005;112(3):416–422.

28. Young T, Tang H, Hughes R. Vena caval filters for the prevention of pulmonary embolism. *Cochrane Database Syst Rev* 2010; Feb. 17 (2):CD006212.

29. Mismetti P, Rivron-Guillot K, Quenet S, et al. A prospective long-term study of 220 patients with a retrievable vena cava filter for secondary prevention of venous thromboembolism. *Chest* 2007;131(1):223–229.

30. Binkert CA, Drooz AT, Caridi JG, et al. Technical success and safety of retrieval of the G2 filter in a prospective, multicenter study. *J Vasc Interv Radiol* 2009;20(11):1449–1453.

31. Johnson MS, Nemcek AA Jr, Benenati JF, et al. The safety and effectiveness of the retrievable option inferior vena cava filter: a United States prospective multicenter clinical study. *J Vasc Interv Radiol* 2010;21(8):1173–1184.

32. Kim H, Young M, Narayan A, et al. A comparison of clinical outcomes with retrievable and permanent inferior vena cava filters. *J Vasc Interv Radiol* 2008;19(3):393–399.

Endovascular Therapy for Acute Pulmonary Embolism

WILLIAM T. KUO

INTRODUCTION

Acute pulmonary embolism (PE) is the third most common cause of death among hospitalized patients. Treatment escalation beyond anticoagulation therapy is necessary in patients with massive PE (hemodynamic shock) as well as in many patients with submassive PE (right ventricular strain). The best current evidence suggests that modern catheter-directed therapy (CDT) to achieve rapid central clot debulking should be considered as an early or first-line treatment option for patients with acute massive PE, and emerging evidence suggests that a catheter-directed thrombolytic infusion should be considered as adjunctive therapy for many patients with acute submassive PE. This chapter reviews the current approach to endovascular therapy for acute PE in the context of appropriate diagnosis, risk stratification, and management of both acute massive and acute submassive PE.

PULMONARY EMBOLISM

Acute massive pulmonary embolism (PE), defined as hemodynamic shock from acute PE, is a common life-threatening condition and represents the most serious manifestation along the spectrum of venous thromboembolic disease. In the United States, an estimated 530,000 cases of symptomatic PE occur annually,[1] and approximately 300,000 people die every year from acute PE.[2] The mortality rate can exceed 58% in acute PE patients presenting with hemodynamic shock,[3] and most of these deaths occur within 1 hour of presentation.[4] Indeed, acute PE is believed to be the third most common cause of death among hospitalized patients,[5] and with an aging population, the number of people suffering from PE is expected to increase. For these reasons, the United States Surgeon General issued a Call to Action in 2008 recognizing venous thromboembolism as a major public health problem.[6] This chapter reviews clinical PE assessment and the rationale for performing CDT as lifesaving treatment for patients with massive PE and as adjunctive thromboreductive treatment for patients with critical right heart strain from submassive PE.

PATHOPHYSIOLOGY OF ACUTE PULMONARY EMBOLISM

To identify appropriate candidates for endovascular treatment, the interventionalist must be familiar with the clinical diagnosis of acute PE and understand its underlying pathophysiology. Life-threatening acute PE results whenever the combination of embolism size and underlying cardiopulmonary status interact to produce hemodynamic instability.[4] The pathophysiology of PE consists of direct physical obstruction of the pulmonary arteries, hypoxemic vasoconstriction, and release of potent pulmonary arterial vasoconstrictors, which further increase pulmonary vascular resistance and right ventricular (RV) afterload. Acute RV pressure overload may result in RV hypokinesis and dilation, tricuspid regurgitation, and, ultimately, RV failure. RV pressure overload may also result in increased wall stress and ischemia by increasing myocardial oxygen demand while simultaneously limiting its supply. Ultimately, cardiac failure from acute PE results from a combination of the increased wall stress and cardiac ischemia that comprise RV function and impair left ventricular (LV) output, resulting in life-threatening hemodynamic shock[4] (FIGURE 85.1). Depending on underlying cardiopulmonary reserve, patients with acute PE may deteriorate over the course of several hours to days and develop systemic arterial hypotension, cardiogenic shock, and cardiac arrest. Due to the risk of sudden death, these critically ill patients should be quickly identified as candidates for rapid endovascular treatment as a lifesaving procedure.

CLINICAL PRESENTATION OF ACUTE PULMONARY EMBOLISM

Patients with acute PE often present with dyspnea or chest pain that may be sudden in onset or evolve over a period of days to weeks. If pulmonary infarction occurs, patients may also experience pleuritic chest pain with hemoptysis. Additionally, there are many nonspecific signs and symptoms including tachypnea, tachycardia, palpitations, light-headedness, fever, cough, wheezing, and rales. These findings may or may not be associated with symptoms of acute deep venous thrombosis (DVT), and the amount of peripheral clot burden may evolve silently and then present as symptomatic or even fatal PE. The possibility of massive PE should be considered in patients who have a sudden onset of near syncope or syncope, hypotension, extreme hypoxemia, electromechanical dissociation, or cardiac arrest.[2]

Some biomarkers may offer useful clinical information. Cardiac troponin levels may be elevated, particularly in patients with acute massive or submassive PE in whom clot burden is significant enough to overwhelm the patient's underlying cardiopulmonary reserve. The enzyme becomes detectable within the bloodstream when there is enough RV strain causing leakage of enzyme from RV myocytes. An elevated troponin level is most commonly used in risk stratification in patients with established PE to help determine the presence of submassive PE, but it is not sensitive as a diagnostic tool when used alone.[2] Elevations in troponin can help clinicians suspect significant heart strain and obtain necessary confirmatory imaging, such as echocardiography, to specifically evaluate the degree of right heart

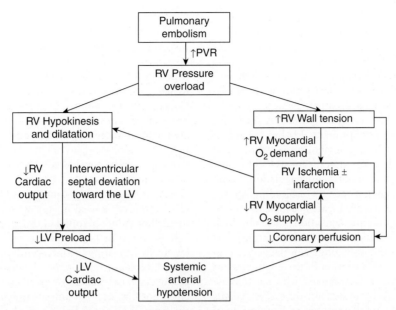

FIGURE 85.1 The pathophysiology of acute PE. *PVR* indicates pulmonary vascular resistance.

Reprinted with permission from Piazza G, Goldhaber SZ. Management of submassive pulmonary embolism. *Circulation* 2010;122:1124–1129.

dysfunction. Elevations in plasma B-type natriuretic peptide (BNP) have been also been described in patients suffering from RV dysfunction from acute PE; however, although plasma levels of brain natriuretic peptide increase with ventricular stretching and may suggest acute PE, these levels may also be elevated in patients with congestive heart failure or various other conditions that cause pulmonary hypertension.[7] The D-dimer test measures plasma levels of a specific derivative of cross-linked fibrin to indicate possible presence of DVT and/or PE. Although the enzyme-linked immunosorbent assay (ELISA)–based D-dimer tests have superior sensitivity (96% to 98%), they must be interpreted together with clinical presentation because the test alone is nonspecific and may be positive in patients with cancer, infection, injury, and underlying inflammatory conditions. When an ELISA-based D-dimer test is negative in patients with a low or moderate pretest probability, the likelihood of DVT and PE is low and precludes the need for specific imaging studies. However, in patients with a high pretest probability for acute PE, imaging should be performed instead of a screening D-dimer test.[2]

DIAGNOSTIC IMAGING OF ACUTE PULMONARY EMBOLISM

Pulmonary angiography was once considered the gold standard for diagnosing PE, but it has largely been replaced by the wide availability of cross-sectional imaging. Historically, many types of imaging studies have been used in diagnosing acute PE including ventilation–perfusion (VQ) scanning, magnetic resonance angiography (MRA), and computed tomographic angiography (CTA). CTA is the preferred modality and has proven to be advantageous due to its wide availability, superior speed, characterization of nonvascular structures, and

detection of venous thrombosis. CTA has the greatest sensitivity and specificity for detecting emboli in the main, lobar, or segmental pulmonary arteries. Systematic reviews and prospective randomized trials suggest that outpatients with suspected PE and negative CT angiographic studies have excellent outcomes without therapy.[8]

If a patient has either acute or chronic renal insufficiency and contrast administration is undesirable, echocardiography may be used to evaluate for right heart dysfunction as an indication for underlying acute PE. The echocardiogram can be performed at bedside, and the study may reveal findings that strongly support hemodynamically significant PE,[9] offering the potential to guide treatment escalation to thrombolytic or endovascular therapy. Large emboli moving from the heart to the lungs are occasionally confirmed with this technique. In addition, intravascular ultrasonography has also been used at the bedside to visualize central pulmonary emboli.[10]

MEDICAL TREATMENT OF ACUTE MASSIVE PULMONARY EMBOLISM

Acute PE causing hemodynamic shock and instability is termed *massive* and requires prompt treatment. Among acute PE patients, the diagnosis of massive PE hinges on the presence of systemic arterial hypotension (systolic blood pressure [SBP] <90 mm Hg); therefore, anatomically large PE visualized on CTA in a hemodynamically stable patient is not considered massive PE and does not carry the same mortality risk. Because the physiologic effect of massive PE is RV failure that may compromise LV preload and lead to sudden death, saline infusion for hypotension should be done with caution, and resuscitation with vasopressor therapy (e.g., dopamine) should be initiated if hypotension persists. Oxygen supplementation, intubation, and mechanical ventilation are instituted as necessary for respiratory failure. Parenteral anticoagulation with low-molecular-weight heparin, the pentasaccharide fondaparinux, or standard unfractionated heparin should be initiated unless contraindicated. Although they are not thrombolytic, these drugs can allow the patient's natural thrombolytic system to function unopposed, ultimately decreasing the thromboembolic burden.[2] Anticoagulation clearly improves survival among patients with symptomatic PE, but the risk of recurrent, nonfatal venous thromboembolism is estimated to be 5% to 10% during the first year after diagnosis.[11] If the suspicion of massive PE is high, parenteral anticoagulation should be considered prior to imaging if the risk of bleeding is low.[2] Because patients with acute massive PE are in shock, treatment escalation beyond therapeutic anticoagulation is also required. From the interventionist's standpoint, the ability to initially anticoagulate a PE patient not only influences the decision to offer inferior vena cava (IVC) filtration in these patients but it also helps to identify possible candidates who can tolerate escalation to systemic thrombolysis (full-dose tPA) versus catheter-directed thrombolytic therapy (no or low-dose local tPA). Current approved medical therapy for acute massive PE consists of systemic thrombolysis with 100 mg of alteplase (tPA; Genentech, South San Francisco, CA) infused intravenously over 2 hours,[2] and the most widely accepted indication for thrombolytic therapy in these patients is cardiogenic shock from acute PE.

RATIONALE FOR ENDOVASCULAR TREATMENT OF MASSIVE PULMONARY EMBOLISM

Although intravenous (IV) tPA is indicated for treatment of acute massive PE, many patients cannot receive systemic thrombolysis due to contraindications; and even when patients with acute PE are prescreened for absolute contraindications, the rate of major hemorrhage from systemic thrombolytic administration is approximately 20%, including a 3% to 5% risk of hemorrhagic stroke.[3,12] Furthermore, there may be insufficient time in the acute setting to infuse full-dose IV thrombolytic. For these patients, CDT with no or low-dose local tPA should be considered if available,[11,13] and the decision should be made as part of a multidisciplinary discussion involving the interventionalist and the patient's medical team. Specific indications for using CDT for acute PE have been published (Table 85.1),[14] and these should be used as guidelines to select candidates for endovascular therapy. The American College of Chest Physicians currently recommends that CDT be considered in selected highly compromised PE patients who are unable to receive thrombolytic therapy because of bleeding risk,[11] but global meta-analytic data have also demonstrated that CDT can be considered as a first-line treatment option in lieu of intravenous tPA.[13]

In patients who are candidates for all treatment options, CDT can also be used in step-wise fashion to escalate treatment after failure of initial or ongoing systemic tPA.[15] In some instances, it may be desirable to initiate IV tPA while simultaneously activating the interventional team to perform CDT. For example, in select patients who are in extremis from PE and deemed candidates for any thrombolytic treatment, some clinicians may desire to initiate urgent "medical" treatment in the form of IV thrombolytic as a bridge to escalation "surgical" treatment with CDT. When used in this fashion, IV tPA could also be less risky. For instance, the amount of IV thrombolytic could be reduced by at least 50% (from the standard 100-mg tPA dose infused over 2 hours) if catheter intervention is initiated promptly, allowing discontinuation of IV tPA within 30 to 60 minutes in patients who are candidates for systemic tPA.[16]

In a meta-analysis of 594 patients with acute massive PE treated with modern CDT, clinical success was achieved in 86.5% (FIGURE 85.2) where success was defined as the stabilization of hemodynamics, resolution of hypoxia, and survival to hospital discharge.[13] In the same study, 96% of patients received CDT as the first adjunct to heparin with no prior systemic tPA infusion, and 33% of cases were initiated with mechanical treatment alone without local thrombolytic infusion.[13] When injected locally, the required dose of tPA is likely to be lower compared to a full-dose systemic tPA infusion,[15] and there is less risk for bleeding. Indeed, the rate of major complications from modern CDT has proven to be only 2.4%.[13]

Table 85.1
The Indications for Aggressive Intervention to Treat Massive Pulmonary Embolism (at Least One of the Following Criteria Must Be Present) are as Follows

1. Arterial hypotension (<90 mm Hg systolic or drop of >40 mm Hg)
2. Cardiogenic shock with peripheral hypoperfusion and hypoxia
3. Circulatory collapse with need for cardiopulmonary resuscitation (syncope)
4. Echocardiographic findings indicating right ventricular afterload stress and/or pulmonary hypertension
5. Diagnosis of precapillary pulmonary hypertension (mean partial arterial pressure >20 mm Hg in presence of normal partial arterial pressure occlusion pressures)
6. Widened arterial-alveolar O_2 gradient (>50 mm Hg)
7. Clinically severe PE with a contraindication to anticoagulation or thrombolytic therapy

Reprinted with permission from Uflacker R. Interventional therapy for pulmonary embolism. *J Vasc Interv Radiol* 2001;12:147–164.

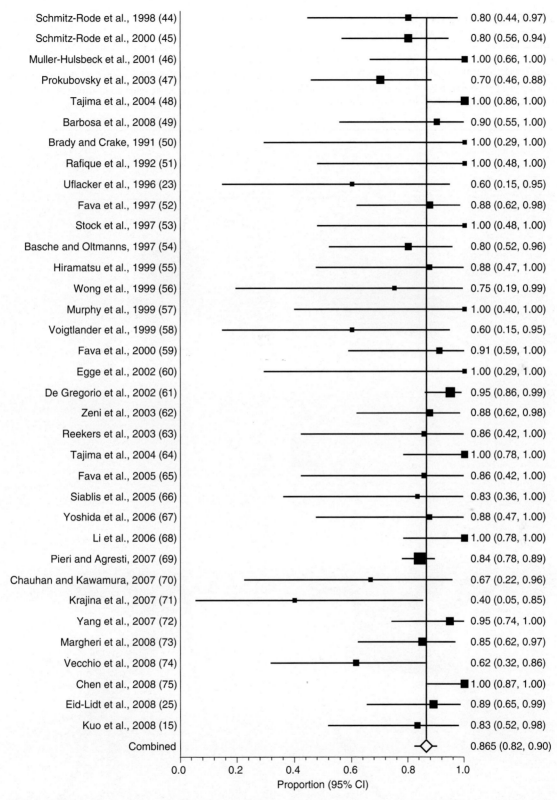

FIGURE 85.2 Forest plot shows clinical success rates from CDT and confidence intervals (CIs) from reported studies encompassing 594 patients with acute massive PE. The percentage clinical success is denoted along the x axis. Extended lines represent 95% CIs. Squares are proportional to study weight. The width of the diamonds corresponds to the 95% CI for the pooled clinical success rate of 86.5%.

Reprinted with permission from Kuo WT, Gould MK, Louie JD, et al. Catheter-directed therapy for the treatment of massive pulmonary embolism: systematic review and meta-analysis of modern techniques. *J Vasc Interv Radiol* 2009;20:1431–1440.

ENDOVASCULAR TECHNIQUES FOR MASSIVE PULMONARY EMBOLISM

Modern CDT for massive PE has been defined according to the following criteria: use of low-profile catheters and devices (≤10 French), catheter-directed mechanical fragmentation and/or aspiration of emboli using existing low-profile catheters, and intraclot thrombolytic injection if a local drug is infused.[13] Therefore, a variety of devices can be used to treat PE successfully as long as they meet these criteria for modern CDT. Depending on anticipated bleeding risk, CDT may be performed with either no or low-dose local tPA injection. The goal of all these techniques is rapid central clot debulking to relieve life-threatening heart strain and immediately improve pulmonary perfusion (FIGURES 85.3 and 85.4).

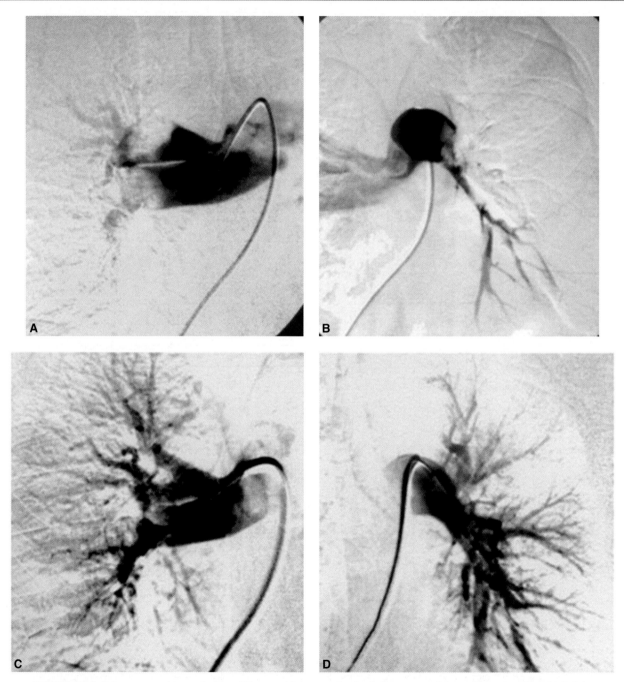

FIGURE 85.3 Pulmonary angiography in a 57-year-old woman in shock from acute bilateral massive PE. Initial right **(A)** and left **(B)** pulmonary angiograms show near-complete obstruction. Pulmonary artery pressure was 73/18 mm Hg. Final right **(C)** and left **(D)** images after suction thrombectomy and catheter-directed thrombolytic injection into each main descending pulmonary artery. Pulmonary artery pressure was reduced to 36/16 mm Hg.

From Sze DY, Carey MB, Razavi MK. Treatment of massive pulmonary embolus with catheter-directed tenecteplase. *J Vasc Interv Radiol* 2001;12:1456–1457.

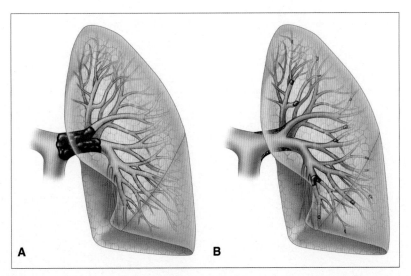

FIGURE 85.4 Large left main PE before and after catheter intervention. **A.** Prior to CDT, there is no perfusion to the lung. **B.** Following CDT, although there is some showering of distal emboli, the central obstructing embolus has been debulked and the net overall effect is increased lung perfusion.

Catheter intervention is important not only for creating an immediate flow channel through the obstruction, but also for exposing a greater surface area of thrombus to the effects of locally infused thrombolytic drug. If local thrombolysis is performed without intraclot drug injection, and if the thrombolytic is instead infused proximal to the target embolus, as performed in older studies, there is little added benefit compared to systemic IV infusion.[17] Schmitz-Rode et al.[18] demonstrated with in vitro and in vivo flow studies that an obstructing embolus causes proximal vortex formation that prevents a drug infused upstream from making rapid contact with the downstream embolus, and the eddy currents instead cause washout of thrombolytic into the nonobstructed pulmonary arteries (FIGURE 85.5). These flow studies emphasize the importance of direct intrathrombus injection as an adjunct to embolus fragmentation to achieve rapid and effective catheter-directed thrombolysis.[18]

Several devices meeting criteria for modern CDT have been used effectively (Table 85.2), but the most common technique currently employed is rotating pigtail fragmentation (FIGURE 85.6), which has been used either alone or in combination with other methods in 70% of patients worldwide receiving CDT.[13] Although pigtail clot fragmentation appears to effectively debulk proximal emboli, in some instances it has resulted in distal embolization with pulmonary artery pressure elevation requiring adjunctive aspiration thrombectomy to complete treatment.[19] Aspiration can be performed with virtually any end-hole catheter such as an 8 French JR4 catheter (Cook, Bloomington, IN). Additional clot fragmentation may also be achieved with insertion and inflation of an angioplasty balloon sized below the target arterial diameter. Thus, it is important to have adjunctive methods available to use in conjunction with pigtail rotation. The main advantage of the rotating pigtail is its

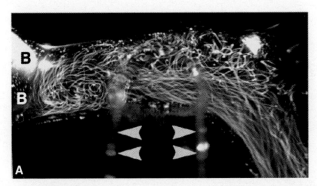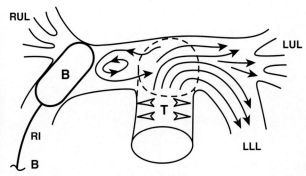

FIGURE 85.5 In vitro flow model of obstruction in the right main pulmonary artery. High-speed photo of systemically injected glass beads (**A**) and corresponding diagram (**B**) demonstrating how a vortex forms proximal to the obstruction and alters systemic drug delivery away from the target embolus. This model emphasizes the importance of intra-clot thrombolytic injection.

From Schmitz-Rode T, Kilbinger M, Günther RW. Simulated flow pattern in massive pulmonary embolism: significance for selective intra-pulmonary thrombolysis. *Cardiovasc Intervent Radiol* 1998;21:199–204.

Table 85.2

Catheter-Directed Therapy for Massive Pulmonary Embolism in 594 Patients

Author, year (reference)	Country	Patients, n	Sex-n	Age: mean, range	Technique-n	Local intra-clot lytic, during CDT-n	Local intra-clot lytic, extended infusion-n	Minor Cxs	Major Cxs	Clinical success (%)
Prospective studies										
Schmitz-Rode et al., 1998 (44)	Germany	10	M-6, F-4	54 (36–70)	PF-10	8	1	0	0	8/10 (80)
Schmitz-Rode et al., 2000 (45)	Germany	20	M-10, F-10	59 (48–60)	PF-20	0	0	1	0	16/20 (80)
Muller-Hulsbeck et al., 2001 (46)	Germany	9	M-4, F-5	55 (27–85)	ATD-9	0	5	0	0	9/9 (100)
Prokubovsky et al., 2003 (47)	Russia	20	na	51 (32–75)	PF-20	0	16	0	0	14/20 (70)
Tajima et al., 2004 (48)	Japan	25	M-8, F-17	61 (35–77)	PF&AT-25	25	21	0	0	25/25 (100)
Barbosa et al., 2008 (49)	Brazil	10	M-7, F-3	57 (39–75)	PF-10 (ATD-na)	0	0	0	0	9/10 (90)
Retrospective studies										
Brady and Crake, 1991 (50)	England	3	M-0, F-3	36 (18–71)	PF-1, MC-2	2	2	0	0	3/3 (100)
Rafique et al., 1992 (51)	South Africa	5	M-1, F-4	35 (21–47)	MC-5	5	5	1	0	5/5 (100)
Uflacker et al., 1996 (23)	U.S.A.	5	M-4, F-1	45 (25–64)	ATD-5	1	1	0	1	3/5 (60)
Fava et al., 1997 (52)	Chile	16	M-8, F-8	49 (20–68)	PF-16 (BA-na)	16	16	3	0	14/16 (88)
Stock et al., 1997 (53)	Switzerland	5	M-3, F-2	50 (21–80)	PF&BA-5	5	5	0	2	5/5 (100)
Basche and Oltmanns, 1997 (54)	Germany	15	na	na (21–73)	PF&BA-2, BA-13	na	na	0	0	12/15 (80)
Hiramatsu et al., 1999 (55)	Japan	8	M-4, F-4	58 (42–87)	AT&WD-8	0	8	0	0	7/8 (88)
Wong et al., 1999 (56)	England	4	M-2, F-2	33 (18–46)	PF-1, PF&G-1, G-2	0	4	0	1	3/4 (75)
Murphy et al., 1999 (57)	Ireland	4	M-2, F-2	60 (46–66)	MC&WD-4	4	4	0	0	4/4 (100)
Voigtlander et al., 1999 (58)	Germany	5	M-4, F-1	57 (25–72)	RT-5	0	0	4	0	3/5 (60)
Fava et al., 2000 (59)	Chile	11	M-3, F-8	61 (37–79)	Hy-11	0	4	0	0	10/11 (91)
Egge et al., 2002 (60)	Norway	3	M-2, F-1	49 (40–54)	PF-3	3	3	0	0	3/3 (100)
De Gregorio et al., 2002 (61)	Spain	59	M-25, F-34	56 (22–85)	PF-52, PF&BA-4, PF&DB-3	59	57	8	0	56/59 (95)
Zeni et al., 2003 (62)	U.S.A.	16	M-9, F-8	52 (30–86)	RT-16	0	10	2	1	14/16 (88)

Study	Country	n	Sex	Age (range)	Device					Success
Reekers et al., 2003 (63)	The Netherlands	7	M-2, F-6	46 (28–76)	Hy-6, Oa-1	7	0	0	0	6/7 (86)
Tajima et al., 2004 (64)	Japan	15	M-4, F-11	60 (27–79)	AT-15	9	0	0	0	15/15 (100)
Fava et al., 2005 (65)	Chile	7	M-3, F-4	56 (30–79)	Hy-4, Oa-3	3	3	1	1	6/7 (86)
Siablis et al., 2005 (66)	Greece	6	M-4, F-2	59 (42–76)	RT-6	4	0	2	0	5/6 (83)
Yoshida et al., 2006 (67)	Japan	8	M-4, F-4	61 (47–75)	PF&AT-8	na	na	0	1	7/8 (88)
Li et al., 2006 (68)	China	15	M-11, F-4	56 (19–73)	PF&ATD-13, PF&Hy-1, PF&Oa-1	6	0	0	0	15/15 (100)
Pieri and Agresti, 2007 (69)	Italy	164	na	68 (35–78)	PF-164	164	164	0	0	138/164 (84)
Chauhan and Kawamura, 2007 (70)	U.S.A.	6	M-2 F-4	64 (49–78)	RT-6	2	0	5	2	4/6 (67)
Krajina et al., 2007 (71)	Czech Republic	5	M-1, F-4	67 (52–80)	PF-3, PF&AT-2	3	0	0	0	2/5 (40)
Yang et al., 2007 (72)	China	19	M-13, F-6	62 (22–87)	PF-10, PF&AT-5, PF+SR-4	19	na	0	0	18/19 (95)
Margheri et al., 2008 (73)	Italy	20	M-12, F-8	66 (32–85)	RT-20	na	0	8	8	17/20 (85)
Vecchio et al., 2008 (74)	Italy	13	na	68 (54–80)	RT-13	na	0	6	8	8/13 (62)
Chen et al., 2008 (75)	China	26	M-15, F-11	53 (36–71)	ATD-17, SR-9	21	0	1	0	26/26 (100)
Eid-Lidt et al., 2008 (25)	Mexico	18	M-6, F-12	51 (47–55)	PF-5, PF&SR-13	2	0	0	0	16/18 (90)
Kuo et al., 2008 (15)	U.S.A.	12	M-7, F-5	56 (21–80)	PF&AT-6, PF&AT&BA-2, RT&AT-2, AT&IC-2	8	na	1	0	10/12 (83)
Total = 35		594		53 (18–87)		356/535	329/552	(7.9%)[a]	(2.4%)[a]	(86.5%)[a]
						67%	60%	[5.0%–11.3%]	[1.9%–4.3%]	[82.2%–90.2%]

[a]Pooled estimates from random effects model. [%] = 95% confidence intervals.

Cxs, complications; PF, pigtail fragmentation; ATD, Amplatz thrombectomy device (Microvena, White Bear Lake, MN); AT, aspiration thrombectomy; MC, multipurpose catheter; BA, balloon fragmentation; WD, wire disruption; G, Gensini (Cordis, Miami, FL); Hy, Hydrolyzer (Cordis, Miami, FL); DB, Dormia basket (Cook Europe, Bjaeverskov, Denmark); Oa, Oasis (Boston Scientific, Galway, Ireland); RT, rheolytic Angiojet thrombectomy (Possis Medical, Minneapolis, MN); SR, Straub Rotarex (Straub Medical, Wangs, Switzerland); IC, infusion catheter; na, data not available.

Reprinted with permission from Kuo WT, Gould MK, Louie JD, et al. Catheter-directed therapy for the treatment of massive pulmonary embolism: systematic review and meta-analysis of modern techniques. *J Vasc Interv Radiol* 2009;20:1431–1440.

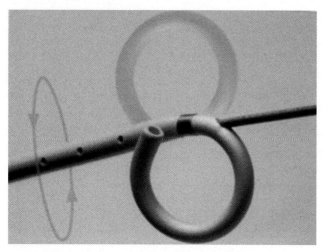

FIGURE 85.6 Photo diagram of the rotating pigtail method most commonly used to treat acute massive PE.

From Schmitz-Rode T, Janssens U, Duda SH, et al. Massive pulmonary embolism: percutaneous emergency treatment by pigtail rotation catheter. *J Am Coll Cardiol* 2000;36:375–380.

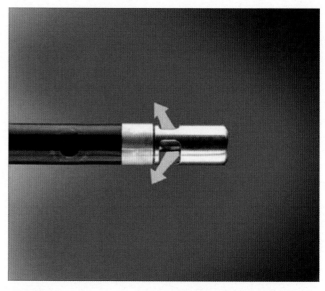

FIGURE 85.7 Photo of the Helix Thrombectomy Device. A recessed impeller is driven by a drive shaft at high speed (140,000 rpm), allowing thrombus to be aspirated through the tip, fragmented to less than 10 μm, and then expelled through the side ports (*arrows*).

Reprinted with permission from eV3 Corporation.

wide availability and low cost relative to the mechanically driven thrombectomy devices.

The use of at least one mechanical device—AngioJet Rheolytic Thrombectomy (ART) (Possis Medical, Minneapolis, MN)—has been associated with relatively higher procedure-related complications including bradyarrhythmia, heart block, hemoglobinuria, renal insufficiency, major hemoptysis, and procedure-related death. From an extensive meta-analysis,[13] the highest complication rates occurred in the 68 patients who underwent CDT with ART including 27 minor complications (40%) and 19 major complications (28%) with 5 procedure-related deaths.[13] Interestingly, 76% (19/25) of all major complications recorded in the study were directly attributed to ART despite the fact that it was used in only a small percentage (11%) of the 594 patients evaluated.[13] Conversely, the data indicate that most modern CDT (89%) has been performed worldwide with a high degree of safety and efficacy without using ART. Furthermore, AngioJet was the only device associated with bradyarrhythmia, heart block, hemoglobinuria, renal insufficiency, major hemoptysis, and procedure-related death. Several deaths related to the Angio-Jet have been recorded in the Food and Drug Administration's (FDA) MAUDE (Manufacturer and User Facility Device Experience) database.[20] As a result, the FDA has issued a block-box warning on the device label.[21] For all these reasons, unless the device can be improved, the AngioJet should probably be avoided as the initial mechanical option in future CDT protocols for acute massive PE.[16,22]

The Helix Clot Buster (eV3, Plymouth, MN), formerly known as the Amplatz Thrombectomy Device (ATD), is approved for use in both dialysis grafts and native vessel dialysis fistulas, but it has been used off-label to treat acute PE. The device is a 75- or 120-cm-long, 7 French reinforced polyurethane catheter with a distal metal tip containing an impeller that is connected to a drive shaft. The catheter is connected to an air source turbine that generates up to 140,000 rpm at

pressures between 30 and 35 psi during operation (FIGURE 85.7). Although little data are available on the new version of this device for treatment of PE, data from off-label use of the older 8 French version has been published with use in conjunction with a 10 French guide catheter.[23] The possibility of hemolytic complications exists but so far, the degree of such has not been shown to be clinically significant.[23] Despite promising results for rapid thrombectomy, production of the Helix device is currently on hold by the manufacturer (at the time of writing) with possible plans for a product re-release.

The search for an optimal thrombectomy catheter continues. A relatively new device, the Aspirex (Straub Medical, Wangs, Switzerland), has shown promising results for acute PE thrombectomy.[24,25] The catheter works on the principle of an Archimedes screw that rotates within a catheter lumen. The metallic spiral is connected to an electric motor drive and control unit. Electronic activation of the spiral coil produces aspiration from the open catheter tip, transporting material down the catheter shaft and into a collecting system (FIGURE 85.8). At the time of writing, the Aspirex is currently unavailable in the United States, but it is undergoing the evaluation process for FDA approval as a peripheral thrombectomy device. Once approved for use in the periphery, it will become available for off-label use to treat PE in the United States.

Regardless of the catheter-based technique initiated to treat acute PE, some believe that hemodynamic improvement with resolution of shock should be used as guidance to conclude initial mechanical debulking regardless of angiographic results when treating massive PE.[26] If the patient can tolerate additional thrombolysis, however, consideration can be made to treating the residual clot with a prolonged or overnight catheter-directed thrombolytic infusion, especially if there is persistent elevation of

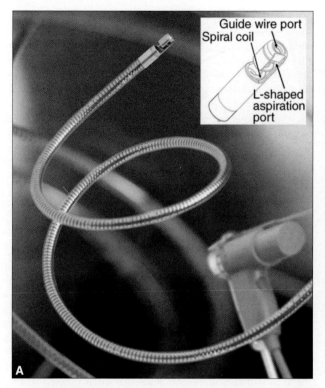
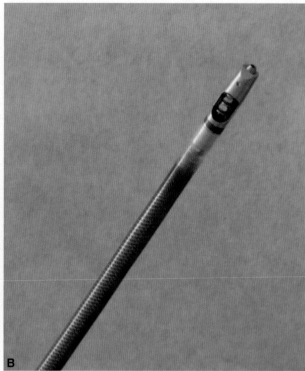

FIGURE 85.8 A. Photo and diagram of the Aspirex catheter. **B.** Close-up photo of the Aspirex device tip.

A. From Kucher N, Windecker S, Banz Y, et al. Percutaneous catheter thrombectomy device for acute pulmonary embolism: in vitro and in vivo testing. *Radiology* 2005;236:852–858.
B. Reprinted with permission from Straub Medical.

PA pressures with right heart strain and the PE has been "downstaged" from massive to submassive PE (see below). From a global meta-analysis,[13] an extended thrombolytic infusion was performed via catheter in approximately 60% of patients worldwide for treatment of residual submassive PE after initial CDT was used to resolve hemodynamic shock from acute massive PE. A possible advantage to performing a thorough thrombolytic infusion with further clot reduction and good angiographic result is the potential for reducing the risk of chronic PE formation and chronic pulmonary hypertension because data on thrombolytic therapy have suggested it may reduce the likelihood of developing chronic thromboembolic pulmonary hypertension (discussed below).

DIAGNOSIS OF SUBMASSIVE PULMONARY EMBOLISM AND RATIONALE FOR TREATMENT ESCALATION

To identify potential candidates for endovascular treatment of less severe PE, the interventionalist must be familiar with the clinical diagnosis of submassive PE (acute PE causing right heart strain without systemic hypotension) and the rationale for offering endovascular therapy. Although the diagnosis of submassive PE follows a similar workup to evaluating massive PE, these patients do not present with systemic arterial hypotension, and particular attention must be made to detecting the presence of

right heart strain, which clinches the diagnosis of submassive PE. The identification of right heart strain allows risk stratification for possible treatment escalation beyond anticoagulation in normotensive PE patients. Echocardiography is the best imaging study to detect RV dysfunction in the setting of acute PE. Characteristic echocardiographic findings in patients with submassive PE include RV hypokinesis and dilatation, interventricular septal flattening and paradoxical motion toward the LV, abnormal transmitral Doppler flow profile, tricuspid regurgitation, pulmonary hypertension as identified by a peak tricuspid regurgitant jet velocity greater than 2.6 m/s, and loss of inspiratory collapse of the IVC.[27] An RV-to-LV end-diastolic diameter ratio of 0.9 or greater, assessed in the left parasternal long-axis view or the subcostal view, is an independent predictor of hospital mortality.[28] A score based on clinical parameters, echocardiographic findings, and cardiac biomarkers can be used to stratify patients with acute PE according to risk of adverse outcomes (Table 85.3).[29] Detection of RV enlargement by chest CTA is especially convenient for diagnosis of submassive PE because it uses data acquired during the initial diagnostic scan. Submassive PE can be diagnosed when RV enlargement on chest computed tomography, defined by an RV-to-LV diameter ratio greater than 0.9, is observed[30]; and RV enlargement on chest CTA also predicts increased 30-day mortality in patients with acute PE.[30,31] Furthermore, even if shock and death do not ensue, survivors of acute submassive PE remain at increased risk for developing chronic PE and thromboembolic pulmonary hypertension.[32]

Table 85.3		
Risk Score for 30-Day Adverse Events in Acute Pulmonary Embolism Patients		
Prognostic factor	**Categories**	**Points**
Altered mental state[a]	No	0
	Yes	10
Cardiogenic shock on admission	No	0
	Yes	6
Cancer	No	0
	Yes	6
BNP (ng/L)	<100	0
	100–249	1
	250–499	2
	500–999	4
	≥1,000	8
RV/LV ratio on echocardiography	0.2–0.49	0
	0.5–0.74	3
	0.75–1.00	5
	1.00–1.25	8
	≥1.25	11

[a]Altered mental state was defined as disorientation, stupor, or coma. The calculated prognostic score can be used as a bedside tool. Range of total score, 0–41. The points assigned correspond to the following risk classes: ≤6 = class I, low risk; 7–17 = class II, intermediate risk; and ≥18 = class III, high risk. The classification correlates with the following 30-day risk of adverse events (death, secondary cardiogenic shock, recurrent venous thromboembolism): class I, low risk (predicted risk <5% or score <7); class II, intermediate risk (predicted risk 5%–30% or score 7–17); and class III, high risk (predicted risk ≥30% or score ≥18).

Reprinted with permission from Sanchez O, Trinquart L, Caille V, et al. Prognostic factors for pulmonary embolism: the PREP study, a prospective multicenter cohort study. *Am J Respir Crit Care Med* 2010;181:168–173.

Prior to obtaining cardiac imaging, patients with submassive PE can be potentially identified by the presence of RV dysfunction detected on physical examination, electrocardiogram (ECG), and cardiac biomarkers. Physical exam findings of tachycardia, elevated jugular venous pressure, right parasternal heave, accentuated sound of pulmonic valve closure (P2), and hepatomegaly suggest RV dysfunction. The ECG can provide a rapid and inexpensive indicator of RV strain and adds incremental prognostic value to echocardiographic findings of RV dysfunction, in patients with submassive PE.[33] Incomplete or complete right bundle-branch block, T-wave inversions in leads V1 through V4, and the combination of an S wave in lead I, Q wave in lead III, and T-wave inversion in lead III (S1Q3T3) signify RV strain. Elevations in cardiac biomarkers, including troponin, brain-type natriuretic peptide, and heart-type fatty acid binding protein, are associated with RV dysfunction and can help noninvasively identify patients with potential submassive PE.[34] Furthermore, these help clinicians determine the need for confirmatory imaging, such as echocardiography, to better evaluate the degree of right heart dysfunction. The identification of submassive PE for treatment escalation is important because these normotensive PE patients still demonstrate increased short-term mortality and risk of adverse outcomes when the degree of heart strain results in elevations in levels of cardiac troponins and brain-type natriuretic peptide.[35,36] Furthermore, patients with acute PE and normal heart-type fatty acid-binding protein levels have an excellent prognosis, whereas those with increased levels (≥6 ng/mL) have a higher rate of adverse events including hemodynamic collapse, respiratory failure, cardiac arrest, and death.[37,38]

TREATMENT OF SUBMASSIVE PULMONARY EMBOLISM

The use of systemic thrombolysis in submassive PE—that is, PE causing RV strain and hypokinesis without systemic hypotension—is still debated.[39–41] The optimal protocol for treatment of acute submassive PE is still in evolution, but a proposed algorithm for managing submassive PE has been published describing treatment escalation beyond anticoagulation (FIGURE 85.9). Although IV tPA infusion (100 mg administered over a 2-hour period) is FDA-approved for acute massive PE, it is still considered off-label use when infused to treat submassive PE.[34] Nevertheless, there is growing evidence that aggressive treatment of submassive PE is beneficial. The Management Strategies and Prognosis of Pulmonary Embolism Trial-3 (MAPPET-3) randomized 256 patients with submassive PE to receive 100 mg of IV tPA over a 2-hour period followed by unfractionated heparin infusion versus placebo plus heparin anticoagulation.[41] Compared with heparin anticoagulation alone, thrombolysis resulted in a significant reduction in the primary study endpoint of in-hospital death or clinical deterioration that required escalation of therapy (defined as catecholamine infusion, rescue thrombolysis, mechanical ventilation, cardiopulmonary resuscitation, or emergency surgical embolectomy).[41] The difference was largely attributable to a higher frequency of open-label thrombolysis (breaking randomized trial protocol to offer medically necessary thrombolysis) due to clinical deterioration as determined by the treating clinician.[41]

In a prospective study of 200 patients with submassive PE,[32] echocardiography was performed at the time of diagnosis and after 6 months to determine the frequency of pulmonary hypertension between two groups—one group treated with heparin and another group treated with IV tPA and heparin. The median decrease in pulmonary artery systolic pressure was only 2 mm Hg in patients treated with heparin alone compared with 22 mm Hg in those treated with tPA plus heparin.[32] At 6 months, the pulmonary artery systolic pressure increased in 27% of patients who had received heparin alone, and nearly half of these patients were moderately symptomatic.[32] These data suggest that thrombolytic therapy may reduce the likelihood of developing chronic thromboembolic pulmonary hypertension.[32]

However, the perpetual problem with systemic tPA infusion is the risk of bleeding, and it is estimated that half of all patients with acute PE have contraindications to systemic thrombolysis.[34] Furthermore, even when patients with acute

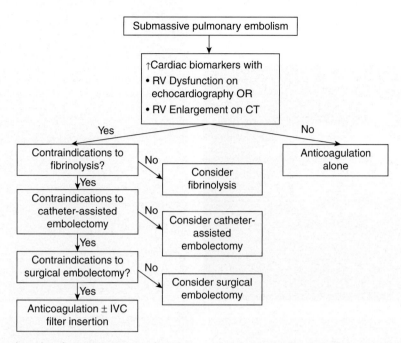

FIGURE 85.9 An algorithm for management of patients with submassive PE. CT indicates computed tomography. According to the algorithm, catheter-directed therapy should be considered in particular when there are contraindications to systemic thrombolysis.

Reprinted with permission from Piazza G, Goldhaber SZ. Management of submassive pulmonary embolism. *Circulation* 2010;122:1124–1129.

PE are carefully prescreened for absolute contraindications prior to IV tPA administration, the rate of major hemorrhage from systemic thrombolytic administration is still 20%, including a 3% to 5% risk of hemorrhagic stroke.[3,12] For patients who are not good candidates for systemic tPA, the next logical step to consider is catheter-directed intervention. That is why the incorporation of a CDT protocol (with targeted drug delivery and a lower overall thrombolytic dose) could further improve outcomes while reducing hemorrhagic risk in this submassive PE group. Indeed, when low-dose (≤30 mg) local tPA was administered to acute massive PE patients—a group at higher risk for bleeding than submassive PE patients[12]—there were no major hemorrhagic complications.[11,13]

Because submassive PE patients are hemodynamically stable, rapid mechanical clot debulking may not be necessary. For these patients, an endovascular treatment regimen should involve image-guided catheter placement into thrombosed lobar arteries for prolonged or overnight thrombolytic infusion. This can be accomplished with a multi–side-hole catheter system, such as the Unifuse (Angiodynamics, Queensbury, NY), and tPA can be infused either uni- or bilaterally at a total dose rate of 1 to 2 mg/hour (i.e., 0.5 to 1 mg/hour through each catheter) (FIGURE 85.10) depending on clot burden. Fibrinogen levels can be monitored particularly in those patients at greater risk of bleeding or if the infusion will be continued beyond 24 hours. When fibrinogen levels drop below 150 to 200 mg/dL, the infusion should be reduced, discontinued, or alternatively continued with transfusions of fresh frozen plasma if further thrombolysis is desired. Furthermore, newer modalities, such

as ultrasound-assisted catheter-directed thrombolysis, have the potential to shorten the duration of infusion and lower the total dose of thrombolytic drug in submassive PE patients.[42] The EKOS infusion catheter (EKOS Corporation, Bothell, WA) (FIGURE 85.11) uses microsonic energy designed to help loosen and separate fibrin to enhance clot permeability while increasing the availability of more plasminogen activation receptor sites for tPA. The microsonic energy is also intended to drive the thrombolytic agent deep into the blood clot to accelerate thrombolysis.[42]

FUTURE DIRECTIONS

Further research on CDT for acute PE is needed to refine existing protocols and to evaluate long-term outcomes, particularly in patients with submassive PE. In 2010, the Society of Interventional Radiology endorsed reporting standards for the endovascular treatment of PE,[43] and ongoing studies, such as the multicenter PERFECT (Pulmonary Embolism Response to Fragmentation, Embolectomy, and Catheter Thrombolysis) registry (clinicaltrials.gov identifier: NCT01097928[3]), will strive to achieve these goals.

CONCLUSION

Rapid risk stratification by identifying acute massive and acute submassive PE patients is essential in determining appropriate treatment escalation beyond anticoagulation. In the urgent clinical setting, the decision to escalate therapy should be made as part of a multidisciplinary discussion involving the

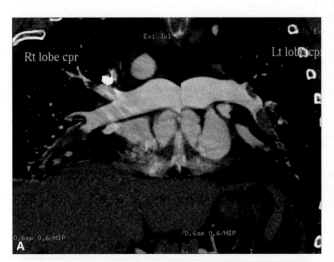

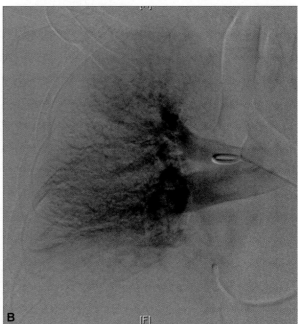

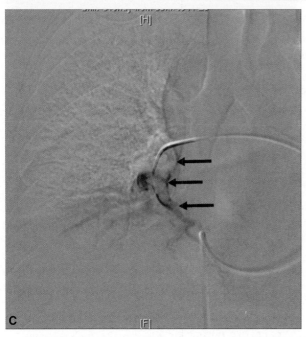

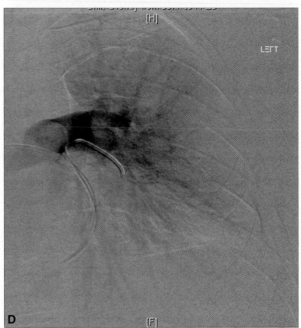

FIGURE 85.10 A 29-year-old man with an episode of DVT 12 months prior presented with a 1-day history of right flank pain made worse with inspiration. He denied fever, chills, or dysuria, but he complained of "heaviness" in his chest that made breathing difficult. His vital signs were as follows: BP 136/84 | Temp 98.2 °F | Resp 18 | SpO₂ 96%. An ELISA D-dimer test was elevated at 3244 (normal range: 68 to 494) and the patient was started on intravenous heparin. On the following day, he experienced worsening shortness of breath and could not lie flat. Echocardiography was performed showing moderate to severe right heart strain. Treatment escalation beyond heparin anticoagulation was desired, and the Interventional Radiology service was consulted for possible catheter-directed intervention. **A.** Curved planar reformats from a chest CTA showed bilateral acute PE. **B through E.** Right and left pulmonary angiograms were performed to localize large thrombosed segments (*arrows*) for infusion catheter placement. **F.** A central 8 French sheath was positioned with tip in the main pulmonary artery (*top arrows*), and the mean pulmonary pressure transduced here was 51 mm Hg. Bilateral 5 French Unifuse catheters were placed (*peripheral arrows*) and tPA infusion was initiated at 0.5 mg/hour through each catheter. **G, H.** After 24 hours and 24 mg of tPA, a follow-up chest CTA showed interval reduction of thrombus burden, and the mean pulmonary pressure transduced through the 8 French sheath was 22 mm Hg. Because the patient was still experiencing dyspnea and mild chest discomfort, the tPA infusions were continued. After 36 hours and 36 mg of tPA, the mean pulmonary pressure was reduced to 15 mm Hg, and the patient's symptoms of chest pain and shortness of breath had now resolved. The bilateral infusion catheters were removed, and a follow-up echocardiogram was performed showing normal RV function. A subsequent hematologic workup revealed the patient to be heterozygous for both Factor V Leiden and Prothrombin 20210A mutation. The patient was prescribed lifelong therapeutic anticoagulation for prevention of further venous thromboembolism.

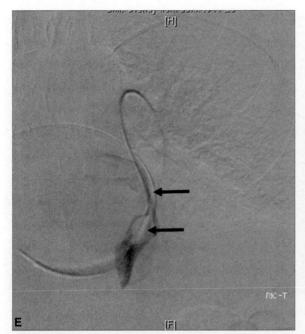

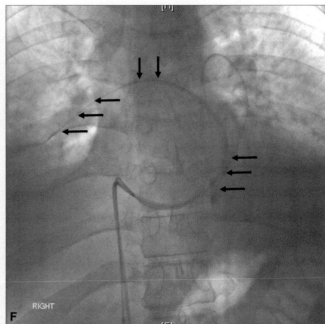

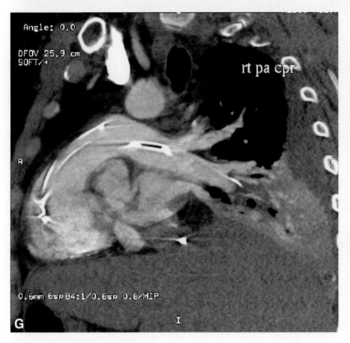

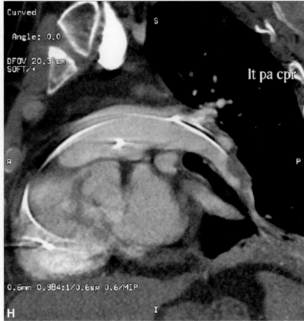

FIGURE 85.10 *(Continued)*

interventionalist and the primary medical team. For patients with less severe or submassive PE, the use of endovascular treatment in the form of local thrombolytic infusion appears to be a promising option for reducing both acute and chronic complications from PE while avoiding the bleeding risks from full-dose systemic thrombolysis. For patients in extremis from massive PE, emergent treatment escalation is necessary in the form of systemic thrombolysis, CDT, or combination therapy depending on the circumstance. If IV tPA is contraindicated or there is insufficient time for full-dose tPA, CDT may be the

only viable treatment option. Indeed, at experienced centers, the use of modern CDT has proven to be a lifesaving treatment in patients dying from acute massive PE. It is therefore recommended that all interventionalists understand the rationale for CDT and become familiar with initiating it as a lifesaving endovascular procedure.

The text in this chapter was reprinted with permission from: Kuo WT. Endovascular therapy for acute pulmonary embolism. J Vasc Interv Radiol 2012; 23:167–179.

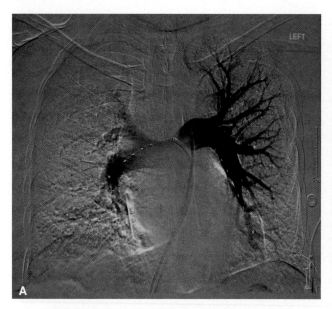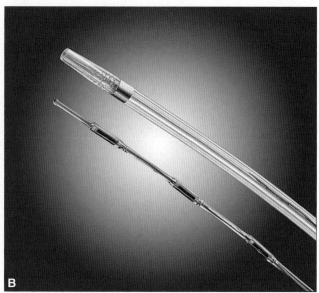

FIGURE 85.11 A. A pulmonary angiogram in a patient with submassive PE shows obstructive emboli, right greater than left. Bilateral EKOS infusion catheters have been inserted for ultrasound-assisted catheter-directed thrombolytic therapy. **B.** Close-up view of the EKOS infusion catheter and corresponding inner wire containing microtransducers.

Reprinted with permission from EKOS Corporation.

REFERENCES

1. Heit JA, Cohen AT, Anderson FA. Estimated annual number of incident and recurrent, non-fatal and fatal venous thromboembolism (VTE) events in the U.S. *Blood* 2005;106:267a.
2. Tapson VF. Acute pulmonary embolism. *N Engl J Med* 2008;358:1037–1052.
3. Goldhaber SZ, Visani L, De Rosa M. Acute pulmonary embolism: clinical outcomes in the International Cooperative Pulmonary Embolism Registry (ICOPER). *Lancet* 1999;353:1386–1389.
4. Wood KE. Major pulmonary embolism: review of a pathophysiologic approach to the golden hour of hemodynamically significant pulmonary embolism. *Chest* 2002;121:877–905.
5. Pulido T, Aranda A, Zevallos MA, et al. Pulmonary embolism as a cause of death in patients with heart disease: an autopsy study. *Chest* 2006;129:1282–1287.
6. *The Surgeon General's Call to Action to Prevent Deep Vein Thrombosis and Pulmonary Embolism.* Available at: http://www.surgeongeneral.gov/topics/deepvein/; 2008. Accessed September 2011.
7. Melanson SE, Laposata M, Camargo CA Jr, et al. Combination of d-dimer and amino-terminal pro-B-type natriuretic peptide testing for the evaluation of dyspneic patients with and without acute pulmonary embolism. *Arch Pathol Lab Med* 2006;130:1326–1329.
8. Moores LK, Jackson WL Jr, Shorr AF, et al. Meta-analysis: outcomes in patients with suspected pulmonary embolism managed with computed tomographic pulmonary angiography. *Ann Intern Med* 2004;141:866–874.
9. Goldhaber SZ, Haire WD, Feldstein ML, et al. Alteplase versus heparin in acute pulmonary embolism: randomised trial assessing right-ventricular function and pulmonary perfusion. *Lancet* 1993;341:507–511.
10. Tapson VF, Davidson CJ, Kisslo KB, et al. Rapid visualization of massive pulmonary emboli utilizing intravascular ultrasound. *Chest* 1994;105:888–890.
11. Kearon C, Kahn KR, Agnelli G, et al. Antithrombotic therapy for venous thromboembolic disease: American College of Chest Physicians Evidence-Based Clinical Practice Guidelines (8th ed.). *Chest* 2008;133:454S–545S.
12. Fiumara K, Kucher N, Fanikos J, et al. Predictors of major hemorrhage following thrombolysis for acute pulmonary embolism. *Am J Cardiol* 2006;97:127–129.
13. Kuo WT, Gould MK, Louie JD, et al. Catheter-directed therapy for the treatment of massive pulmonary embolism: systematic review and meta-analysis of modern techniques. *J Vasc Interv Radiol* 2009;20:1431–1440.
14. Uflacker R. Interventional therapy for pulmonary embolism. *J Vasc Interv Radiol* 2001;12:147–164.
15. Kuo WT, Van den Bosch MA, Hofmann LV, et al. Catheter-directed embolectomy, fragmentation, and thrombolysis for the treatment of massive pulmonary embolism after failure of systemic thrombolysis. *Chest* 2008;134:250–254.
16. Kuo WT, Hofmann LV. Optimizing endovascular therapy for acute PE: primum non nocere. *J Vasc Interv Radiol* 2010;21:1776–1777.
17. Verstraete M, Miller GAH, Bounameaux H, et al. Intravenous and intrapulmonary recombinant tissue-type plasminogen activator in the treatment of acute massive pulmonary embolism. *Circulation* 1988;77:353–360.
18. Schmitz-Rode T, Kilbinger M, Günther RW. Simulated flow pattern in massive pulmonary embolism: significance for selective intrapulmonary thrombolysis. *Cardiovasc Intervent Radiol* 1998;21:199–204.
19. Nakazawa K, Tajima H, Murata S, et al. Catheter fragmentation of acute massive pulmonary thromboembolism: distal embolisation and pulmonary arterial pressure elevation. *Br J Radiol* 2008;81:848–854.
20. FDA MAUDE database. http://www.accessdata.fda.gov/scripts/cdrh/cfdocs/cfMAUDE/search.CFM. Accessed September 2011.
21. Angiojet Xpeedior [product insert]. Minneapolis, MN: Possis Medical; 2008.
22. Kuo WT, Sze DY, Hofmann LV, et al. Catheter-directed intervention for acute pulmonary embolism: a shining saber. *Chest* 2007;133:317–318.
23. Uflacker R, Strange C, Vujic I. Massive pulmonary embolism: preliminary results of treatment with the Amplatz thrombectomy device. *J Vasc Interv Radiol* 1996;7:519–528.
24. Kucher N, Windecker S, Banz Y, et al. Percutaneous catheter thrombectomy device for acute pulmonary embolism: in vitro and in vivo testing. *Radiology* 2005;236:852–858.
25. Eid-Lidt G, Gaspar J, Sandoval J, et al. Combined clot fragmentation and aspiration in patients with acute pulmonary embolism. *Chest* 2008;134:54–60.
26. Kucher N, Goldhaber SZ. Management of massive pulmonary embolism. *Circulation* 2005;112:e28–e32.
27. Goldhaber SZ. Echocardiography in the management of pulmonary embolism. *Ann Intern Med* 2002;136:691–700.
28. Fremont B, Pacouret G, Jacobi D, et al. Prognostic value of echocardiographic right/left ventricular end-diastolic diameter ratio in patients with acute pulmonary embolism: results from a monocenter registry of 1,416 patients. *Chest* 2008;133:358–362.

29. Sanchez O, Trinquart L, Caille V, et al. Prognostic factors for pulmonary embolism: the PREP study, a prospective multicenter cohort study. *Am J Respir Crit Care Med* 2010;181:168–173.
30. Schoepf UJ, Kucher N, Kipfmueller F, et al. Right ventricular enlargement on chest computed tomography: a predictor of early death in acute pulmonary embolism. *Circulation* 2004;110:3276–3280.
31. van der Meer RW, Pattynama PM, van Strijen MJ, et al. Right ventricular dysfunction and pulmonary obstruction index at helical CT: prediction of clinical outcome during 3-month follow-up in patients with acute pulmonary embolism. *Radiology* 2005;235:798–803.
32. Kline JA, Steuerwald MT, Marchick MR, et al. Prospective evaluation of right ventricular function and functional status 6 months after acute submassive pulmonary embolism: frequency of persistent or subsequent elevation in estimated pulmonary artery pressure. *Chest* 2009;136:1202–1210.
33. Vanni S, Polidori G, Vergara R, et al. Prognostic value of ECG among patients with acute pulmonary embolism and normal blood pressure. *Am J Med* 2009;122:257–264.
34. Piazza G, Goldhaber SZ. Management of submassive pulmonary embolism. *Circulation* 2010;122:1124–1129.
35. Klok FA, Mos IC, Huisman MV, et al. Brain-type natriuretic peptide levels in the prediction of adverse outcome in patients with pulmonary embolism: a systematic review and meta-analysis. *Am J Respir Crit Care Med* 2008;178:425–430.
36. Jimenez D, Uresandi F, Otero R, et al. Troponin-based risk stratification of patients with acute nonmassive pulmonary embolism: systematic review and metaanalysis. *Chest* 2009;136:974–982.
37. Puls M, Dellas C, Lankeit M, et al. Heart-type fatty acid-binding protein permits early risk stratification of pulmonary embolism. *Eur Heart J* 2007;28:224–229.
38. Dellas C, Puls M, Lankeit M, et al. Elevated heart-type fatty acid binding protein levels on admission predict an adverse outcome in normotensive patients with acute pulmonary embolism. *J Am Coll Cardiol* 2010;55:2150–2157.
39. Witty LA, Krichman A, Tapson VF. Thrombolytic therapy for venous thromboembolism: utilization by practicing pulmonologists. *Arch Intern Med* 1994;154:1601–1604.
40. Goldhaber SZ. Thrombolytic therapy for patients with pulmonary embolism who are hemodynamically stable but have right ventricular dysfunction: pro. *Arch Intern Med* 2005;165:2197–2199.
41. Konstantinides S, Geibel A, Heusel G, et al. Heparin plus alteplase compared with heparin alone in patients with submassive pulmonary embolism. *N Engl J Med* 2002;347:1143–1150.
42. Chamsuddin A, Nazzal L, Kang B, et al. Catheter-directed thrombolysis with the Endowave System in the treatment of acute massive pulmonary embolism: a retrospective multicenter case series. *J Vasc Interv Radiol* 2008;19:372–376.
43. Banovac F, Buckley D, Kuo WT, et al. Standards of practice: reporting standards for endovascular treatment of pulmonary embolism. *J Vasc Interv Radiol* 2010;21:44–53.
44. Schmitz-Rode T, Janssens U, Schild HH, et al. Fragmentation of massive pulmonary embolism using a pigtail rotation catheter. *Chest* 1998;114:1427–1436.
45. Schmitz-Rode T, Janssens U, Duda SH, et al. Massive pulmonary embolism: percutaneous emergency treatment by pigtail rotation catheter. *J Am Coll Cardiol* 2000;36:375–380.
46. Muller-Hulsbeck S, Brossmann J, Jahnke T, et al. Mechanical thrombectomy of major and massive pulmonary embolism with use of the Amplatz thrombectomy device. *Invest Radiol* 2001;36:317–322.
47. Prokubovsky VI, Kapranov SA, Bobrov BY. Endovascular rotary fragmentation in the treatment of massive pulmonary thromboembolism. *Angiol Sosud Khir* 2003;9:31–39.
48. Tajima H, Murata S, Kumazaki T, et al. Hybrid treatment of acute massive pulmonary thromboembolism: mechanical fragmentation with a modified rotating pigtail catheter, local fibrinolytic therapy, and clot aspiration followed by systemic fibrinolytic therapy. *AJR Am J Roentgenol* 2004;183:589–595.
49. Barbosa MA, Oliveira DC, Barbosa AT, et al. Treatment of massive pulmonary embolism by percutaneous fragmentation of the thrombus. *Arq Bras Cardiol* 2008;88:279–284.
50. Brady AJB, Crake T. Percutaneous catheter fragmentation and distal dispersion of proximal pulmonary embolus. *Lancet* 1991;338:1186–1189.
51. Rafique M, Middlemost S, Skoularigis J, et al. Simultaneous mechanical clot fragmentation and pharmacologic thrombolysis in acute massive pulmonary embolism. *Am J Cardiol* 1992;69:427–430.
52. Fava M, Loyola S, Huete I. Mechanical fragmentation and pharmacologic thrombolysis in massive pulmonary embolism. *J Vasc Interv Radiol* 1997;8:261–266.
53. Stock KW, Jacob AL, Schnabel KJ, et al. Massive pulmonary embolism: treatment with thrombus fragmentation and local thrombolysis with recombinant human-tissue plasminogen activator. *Cardiovasc Intervent Radiol* 1997;20:364–368.
54. Basche S, Oltmanns G. Thrombus fragmentation in massive pulmonary embolism. *Die Medizinische Welt* 1997;48:325–327.
55. Hiramatsu S, Ogihara A, Kitano Y, et al. Clinical outcome of catheter fragmentation and aspiration therapy in patients with acute pulmonary embolism. *J Cardiol* 1999;34:71–78.
56. Wong PS, Singh SP, Watson RD, et al. Management of pulmonary thrombo-embolism using catheter manipulation: a report of four cases and review of the literature. *Postgrad Med J* 1999;75:737–741.
57. Murphy JM, Mulvihill N, Mulcahy D, et al. Percutaneous catheter and guidewire fragmentation with local administration of recombinant tissue plasminogen activator as a treatment for massive pulmonary embolism. *Eur Radiol* 1999;9:959–964.
58. Voigtlander T, Rupprecht HJ, Nowak B, et al. Clinical application of a new rheolytic thrombectomy catheter system for massive pulmonary embolism. *Catheter Cardiovasc Interv* 1999;47:91–96.
59. Fava M, Loyola S, Huete I. Massive pulmonary embolism: treatment with the hydrolyser thrombectomy catheter. *J Vasc Interv Radiol* 2000;11:1159–1164.
60. Egge J, Berentsen S, Storesund B, et al. Treatment of massive pulmonary embolism with local thrombolysis. *Tidsskr Nor Laegeforen* 2002;122:2263–2266.
61. De Gregorio MA, Gimeno MJ, Mainar A, et al. Mechanical and enzymatic thrombolyis for massive pulmonary embolism. *J Vasc Interv Radiol* 2002;13:163–169.
62. Zeni PT, Blank BG, Peeler DW. Use of rheolytic thrombectomy in treatment of acute massive pulmonary embolism. *J Vasc Interv Radiol* 2003;14:1511–1515.
63. Reekers JA, Baarslag HJ, Koolen MGJ, et al. Mechanical thrombectomy for early treatment of massive pulmonary embolism. *Cardiovasc Intervent Radiol* 2003;26:246–250.
64. Tajima H, Murata S, Kumazaki T, et al. Hybrid treatment of acute massive pulmonary thromboembolism: mechanical fragmentation with a modified rotating pigtail catheter, local fibrinolytic therapy, and clot aspiration followed by systemic fibrinolytic therapy. *Radiat Med* 2004;22:168–172.
65. Fava M, Loyola S, Bertoni H, et al. Massive pulmonary embolism: percutaneous mechanical thrombectomy during cardiopulmonary resuscitation. *J Vasc Interv Radiol* 2005;16:119–123.
66. Siablis D, Karnabatidis D, Katsanos K, et al. AngioJet rheolytic thrombectomy versus local intrapulmonary thrombolysis in massive pulmonary embolism: a retrospective data analysis. *J Endovasc Ther* 2005;12:206–214.
67. Yoshida M, Inoue I, Kawagoe T, et al. Novel percutaneous catheter thrombectomy in acute massive pulmonary embolism: rotational bidirectional thrombectomy (ROBOT). *Catheter Cardiovasc Interv* 2006;68:112–117.
68. Li J, Zhai R, Dai D, et al. Interventional mechanical thrombectomy procedure in treating acute massive pulmonary infarction. *J Intervent Radiol* 2006;15:336–338.
69. Pieri S, Agresti P. Hybrid treatment with angiographic catheter in massive pulmonary embolism: mechanical fragmentation and thrombolysis. *Radiol Med* 2007;112:837–849.
70. Chauhan MS, Kawamura A. Percutaneous rheolytic thrombectomy for large pulmonary embolism: a promising treatment option. *Catheter Cardiovasc Interv* 2007;70:121–128.
71. Krajina A, Lojik M, Chovanec V, et al. Percutaneous mechanical fragmentation of emboli in the pulmonary artery. *Ces Radiol* 2007;61:162–166.
72. Yang Z, Shi H, Li L, et al. System thrombolysis combined with percutaneous catheter fragmentation and thrombectomy in acute massive pulmonary embolism. *Chin J Radiol* 2007;41:1241–1244.
73. Margheri M, Vittori G, Vecchio S, et al. Early and long-term clinical results of Angiojet rheolytic thrombectomy in patients with acute pulmonary embolism. *Am J Cardiol* 2008;101:252–258.
74. Vecchio S, Vittori G, Chechi T, et al. Percutaneous rheolytic thrombectomy with AngioJet for pulmonary embolism: methods and results in the experience of a high-volume center. *It J Pract Cardiol* 2008;9:355–363.
75. Chen L, Gu J, Lou W, et al. Interventional mechanical thrombectomy for acute pulmonary embolism. *J Interv Radiol* 2008;17:468–471.

Chronic Lower Extremity Veno-Occlusive Disease: Medical Management and Interventional Strategies

GLORIA L. HWANG

▌INTRODUCTION

Chronic lower extremity veno-occlusive disease (VOD) most commonly arises from two etiologies: (1) post-thrombotic, in which an acute deep venous thrombosis (DVT) has failed to completely recanalize, resulting in residual stenoses and occlusions of the affected veins, and (2) nonthrombotic nonmalignant primary obstruction, typified by May-Thurner syndrome, in which compression of the left common iliac vein between the right common iliac artery and lumbar spine results in the development of endoluminal webs and spurs.[1] Many patients present with a mixed picture because the primary obstruction predisposes to development of acute DVT and its sequelae. In a series of 89 patients with chronic disabling iliocaval obstructive lesions, 34% were post-thrombotic, 58% had May-Thurner syndrome, 6% had obstruction secondary to retroperitoneal fibrosis, and 2% had congenital abnormalities of the lower extremity venous system.[2]

The prevalence of chronic lower extremity VOD in the overall population is difficult to determine. Individuals with lower extremity VOD typically present for medical attention when they develop symptoms of chronic venous insufficiency. Chronic venous insufficiency is a common medical issue; its reported prevalence is variable due to study population and definitional differences[3,4] with estimates of 2% to 7%.[5] However, not all patients with chronic venous insufficiency have VOD because the symptoms could result from reflux or obstruction, or a combination of the two.

Looking at populations at risk of developing VOD, it has been reported that 20% to 100% of patients with acute DVT develop post-thrombotic syndrome—a constellation of leg pain, swelling, skin discoloration, venous dilatation, and, in severe cases, leg ulceration—within 5 to 14 years of the acute event.[6] Patients with acute iliac vein thrombosis are particularly at risk of developing chronic obstruction: When patients diagnosed with acute iliac vein thrombus are treated with anticoagulation alone, only 20% to 30% of the iliac veins completely recanalize, whereas the remaining 70% to 80% become chronically obstructed.[7,8] Endovascular stenting represents an effective and potentially underutilized treatment for patients with VOD.

The workup of patients with chronic venous insufficiency typically includes physical exam, quality-of-life assessment, and use of noninvasive tests, such as duplex sonography and plethysmography, which can directly demonstrate occlusion of, or reflux into, the leg veins and which may indirectly

suggest occlusion of the iliac veins or inferior vena cava (IVC). Unfortunately, those studies are not entirely sensitive at diagnosing iliocaval obstruction. Although venography is considered the gold standard, noninvasive cross-sectional imaging with computed tomography (CT) and magnetic resonance imaging (MRI) are useful in preprocedure planning to better assess the status of the iliac veins, IVC, and pelvic venous collaterals. CT and MRI are excellent at assessing for venous occlusion but are limited in that they do not demonstrate the intraluminal webs often seen on venography. Even direct venography detects only 66% of lesions, when compared with intravascular ultrasound.[9] When Raju and Neglen[9] performed intravascular ultrasound in patients with severely symptomatic chronic venous disease without post-thrombotic syndrome, they found a very high incidence of obstructing or stenosing iliac vein lesions, such as webs and spurs, which they treated with stenting. Unfortunately, the expense and invasive nature of intravascular ultrasound make it prohibitive to perform on all patients with symptomatic chronic venous disease. Because noninvasive diagnostics tests are not entirely reliable at detecting potentially treatable iliac vein and IVC occlusions, the absence of noninvasive evidence of venous occlusion should not discourage the pursuit of more invasive imaging, and possibly intervention, if patients have severe symptoms of chronic venous insufficiency.

The first-line treatment for chronic venous insufficiency is compression therapy, which has been shown to be effective in clinical trials[10] and is required for 3 to 6 months by many insurers before they will consider funding other treatments.[11] However, compliance with compression therapy is poor: In a retrospective study of 3,144 referrals to a specialty clinic for chronic venous disease, only 21% of patients reported daily use of compression stockings, whereas 63% of patients reported no use at all.[11]

No oral medications are as effective as compression therapy for managing the symptoms of chronic venous insufficiency. Pentoxifylline, when used in conjunction with compression therapy, provides modest improvement in ulcer healing compared with compression alone and may provide some benefit even when used without compression therapy.[12] Micronized purified flavonoid fraction, which is not yet available in the United States, has also been shown to accelerate healing of venous ulcers and may relieve some of the symptoms of pain, heaviness, and cramps.[13]

Since the mid-1990s, metallic stents have provided a means of maintaining in-line flow in occluded iliac veins and the IVC following endovascular recanalization.[14] The first sizeable series described the use of Gianturco stents, wallstents, and Palmaz stents.[14] Whereas surgical reconstruction for large vein occlusion is technically challenging and available only at select centers, venous recanalization and stenting can be performed using common endovascular techniques and standard equipment. Multiple series with long-term follow-up have lent strong support to the important role venous stenting can play in ameliorating the symptoms of chronic lower extremity venous insufficiency.

PATIENT SELECTION

Patients with symptomatic chronic lower extremity venous occlusion present with leg pain, swelling, venous claudication, lower extremity skin changes, and/or skin ulceration. Various scoring systems have been developed and validated to grade the severity of venous disease; these rely on physician assessments or patient-reported quality-of-life assessments, or both. The CEAP classification system is a widely used scoring system that relies on the clinician's assessment of the patient (Table 86.1).[15] The Venous Clinical Severity Score[16] similarly depends on physician assessment and was designed by the American Venous Forum to supplement the CEAP classification; it allows better quantification of serial changes in the patient's condition (Table 86.2). Validated questionnaires based on patient-reported symptoms include the 20-item CIVIQ quality-of-life questionnaire (Table 86.3)[17] and the 26-item VEINES-QOL/Sym questionnaire (Table 86.4).[18] The Villalta scale, which combines five patient-rated venous symptoms and six clinician-rated physical signs, can also be used but was designed specifically for patients with history of DVT to assess the severity of post-thrombotic syndrome.[19] Patients who present as candidates for endovascular management of chronic venous insufficiency symptoms

Table 86.1

CEAP Classification for Chronic Venous Disorders (2004 Revision)

Clinical classification

C0: no visible or palpable sign of venous disease
C1: telangiectasias or reticular veins
C2: varicose veins
C3: edema
C4a: pigmentation or eczema
C4b: lipodermatosclerosis or atrophie blanche
C5: healed venous ulcer
C6: active venous ulcer
S: symptomatic, including ache, pain, tightness, skin irritation, heaviness, and muscle cramps, and other complaints attributable to venous dysfunction
A: asymptomatic

Etiologic classification

Ec: congenital
Ep: primary
Es: secondary (postthrombotic)
En: no venous cause identified

Anatomic classification

As: superficial veins
Ap: perforator veins
Ad: deep veins
An: no venous location identified

Pathophysiologic classifications

Basic CEAP
Pr: reflux
Po: obstruction
Pr,o: reflux and obstruction
Pn: no venous pathophysiology identifiable
Advanced CEAP: Same as basic CEAP, with addition that any 18 named venous segments can be used as locations for venous pathology

(continued)

Table 86.1
CEAP Classification for Chronic Venous Disorders (2004 Revision) *(Continued)*

Superficial veins
  (1) Telangiectasias or reticular veins
  (2) Great saphenous vein above knee
  (3) Great saphenous vein below knee
  (4) Small saphenous vein
  (5) Nonsaphenous veins

Deep veins
  (6) Inferior vena cava
  (7) Common iliac vein
  (8) Internal iliac vein
  (9) External iliac vein
  (10) Pelvic: gonadal, broad ligament veins, other
  (11) Common femoral vein
  (12) Deep femoral vein
  (13) Femoral vein
  (14) Popliteal vein
  (15) Crural: anterior tibial, posterior tibial, peroneal veins
  (16) Muscular: gastrocnemial, soleal veins, other

Perforating veins
  (17) Thigh
  (18) Calf

Adapted from Eklof B, Rutherford RB, Bergan JJ, et al. Revision of the CEAP classification for chronic venous disorders: consensus statement. *J Vasc Surg* 2004;40:1248–1252.

tend to have CEAP clinical scores of 3 to 6, although patients with lower clinical scores may be candidates if they have severe diffuse venous pain.[9] The severity of venous disease as assessed by physicians using the CEAP classification correlates with poor disease-specific quality of life as assessed by the VEINES-QOL/Sym questionnaire.[20]

Because no noninvasive tests can fully exclude the presence of venous obstruction, the decision to undergo intervention should be based on a patient's clinical severity. The presence of deep vein reflux is not a contraindication to stent placement. It has been shown that patients who underwent iliocaval vein recanalization and stenting showed substantial symptomatic improvement despite the fact that the degree of deep vein reflux was unchanged or worsened after treatment.[21,22]

Because of the use of fluoroscopy over the pelvic region, pregnancy is a contraindication to the procedure. Because most patients presenting with symptomatic VOD are female (female/male ratio of 2.6:1 in a series of 982 patients, with even higher ratios seen in the subset of patients with nonthrombotic nonmalignant primary obstruction),[9,23] it is important to elicit a reproductive history. The long-term safety and patency of iliac vein and IVC stents in pregnant patients is unknown; because the procedure would expose the reproductive organs to ionizing radiation, those factors should weigh in the decision to stent a female patient of childbearing years. Balloon-expandable stents in particular run the risk of compression by the gravid uterus, which could result in symptomatic venous occlusion.

Other contraindications include the typical contraindications to angiography, including allergy to iodinated contrast and renal insufficiency. Because much of the procedure may be performed with carbon dioxide as the contrast agent, with the additional use of gadolinium contrast agents for patients with allergy to iodinated contrast, those contraindications are relative. Additionally, intravascular ultrasound can be performed to assess the vessels in those patients and, according to some authors, is the procedure of choice for detecting hemodynamically significant venous stenoses; however, the cost may be prohibitive.[1]

Patients should not have contraindications to anticoagulation, which may need to be resumed or started after stent placement. Additionally, because stenting of lower extremity venous obstruction is likely to acutely increase venous return to the heart, patients with right heart failure should be approached cautiously with careful periprocedural monitoring of hemodynamic status.

ENDOVASCULAR TREATMENT OPTIONS

If occlusion of the IVC and/or iliac veins is diagnosed, recanalization and stent placement is the endovascular treatment of choice. Venoplasty alone is ineffective at maintaining long-term patency due to rapid reocclusion. The efficacy of venoplasty or stenting of occluded superficial femoral veins in the thigh remains to be seen.

Table 86.2

Revised Venous Clinical Severity Score (VCSS)

	None: 0	Mild: 1	Moderate: 2	Severe: 3
Pain				
Or other discomfort (i.e., aching, heaviness, fatigue, soreness, burning) Presumes venous origin		Occasional pain or other discomfort (i.e., not restricting regular daily activities)	Daily pain or other discomfort (i.e., interfering with but not preventing regular daily activities)	Daily pain or discomfort (i.e., limits most regular daily activities)
Varicose veins				
"Varicose" veins must be ≥3 mm in diameter to qualify in the standing position		Few: scattered (i.e., isolated branch varicosities or clusters) Also includes corona phlebectatica (ankle flare)	Confined to calf or thigh	Involves calf and thigh
Venous edema				
Presumes venous origin		Limited to foot and ankle area	Extends above ankle but below knee	Extends to knee and above
Skin pigmentation				
Presumes venous origin Does not include focal pigmentation over varicose veins or pigmentation due to other chronic diseases	None or focal	Limited to perimalleolar area	Diffuse over lower third of calf	Wider distribution above lower third of calf
Inflammation				
More than just recent pigmentation (i.e., erythema, cellulitis, venous eczema, dermatitis)		Limited to perimalleolar area	Diffuse over lower third of calf	Wider distribution above lower third of calf
Induration				
More than just recent pigmentation (i.e., erythema, cellulitis, venous eczema, dermatitis)		Limited to perimalleolar area	Diffuse over lower third of calf	Wider distribution above lower third of calf
Active ulcer number	0	1	2	≥3
Active ulcer duration				
Longest active	N/A	<3 mo	<3 mo but <1 y	Not healed for <1 y
Active ulcer size				
Diameter of largest active	N/A	<2 cm	2–6 cm	<6 cm
Use of compression therapy	Not used	Intermittent use of stockings	Wears stockings most days	Full compliance: stockings

Adapted from Vasquez MA, Rabe E, McLafferty RB, et al. Revision of the venous clinical severity score: venous outcomes consensus statement: special communication of the American Venous Forum Ad Hoc Outcomes Working Group. *J Vasc Surg* 2010;52:1387–1396.

Table 86.3
Chronic Lower Limb Venous Insufficiency Questionnaire (CIVIQ)

1. In the past four weeks, if you have felt **pain** in the **ankles** or **legs**, what was the *intensity* of this pain?

No pain	Light pain	Moderate pain	Strong pain	Intense pain
1	2	3	4	5

2. During the past four weeks, to what extend did you feel bothered/limited in your **work** or your other **daily activities because of your leg problem**?

Not bothered/ limited	A little bothered/ limited	Moderately bothered/ limited	Very bothered/ limited	Extremely bothered/ limited
1	2	3	4	5

3. During the past four weeks, did you **sleep badly** because of your leg problems, and how often?

Never	Seldom	Fairly often	Very often	Every night
1	2	3	4	5

During the past four weeks, to what extend did your **leg problems** bother/limit you **while doing the movements or activities** listed below?

Not bothered/ limited at all	A little bothered/ limited	Moderately bothered/ limited	Very bothered/ limited	Impossible to do

4. Standing for a long time

1	2	3	4	5

5. Climbing stairs

1	2	3	4	5

6. Crouching, kneeling

1	2	3	4	5

7. Walking briskly

1	2	3	4	5

8. Housework such as working in the kitchen, carrying a child, ironing, cleaning floors or furniture, doing handy work

1	2	3	4	5

9. Travel by car, bus, plane

1	2	3	4	5

10. Going to discos, weddings, parties, cocktails

1	2	3	4	5

11. Sporting activities, making physically strenuous efforts

1	2	3	4	5

Leg problems can also have an effect on one's morale. To what extent do the following sentences correspond to the way you have felt during the past four weeks?

Not at all	A little	Moderately	A lot	Absolutely

12. I feel on edge

1	2	3	4	5

13. I become tired quickly

1	2	3	4	5

14. I feel I am a burden to people

1	2	3	4	5

15. I must always take precautions (such as to stretch my legs, to avoid standing for a long time...)

1	2	3	4	5

Table 86.3

Chronic Lower Limb Venous Insufficiency Questionnaire (CIVIQ) *(Continued)*

16. I am embarrassed to show my legs

1	2	3	4	5

17. I get irritated easily

1	2	3	4	5

18. I feel handicapped

1	2	3	4	5

19. I have difficulty getting going in the morning

1	2	3	4	5

20. I do not feel like going out

1	2	3	4	5

Questions 1–4: Pain repercussions

Questions 5–8: Physical repercussions

Questions 9–11: Social repercussions

Questions 12–20: Psychological repercussions

Adapted from Launois R, Reboul-Marty J, Henry B. Construction and validation of a quality of life questionnaire in chronic lower limb venous insufficiency (CIVIQ). *Qual Life Res* 1996;5:539–554.

Table 86.4

VEINES-QOL/Sym Questionnaire

1. During the past 4 weeks, how often have you had any of the following leg problems? *(check one box on each line)*

	Every day	Several times a week	About once a week	Less than once a week	Never
1. Heavy legs	1	2	3	4	5
2. Aching legs	1	2	3	4	5
3. Swelling	1	2	3	4	5
4. Night cramps	1	2	3	4	5
5. Heat or burning sensation	1	2	3	4	5
6. Restless legs	1	2	3	4	5
7. Throbbing	1	2	3	4	5
8. Itching	1	2	3	4	5
9. Tingling sensation (e.g., pins and needles)	1	2	3	4	5

2. At what time of day is your **leg problem** most intense? *(check one)*

   1. On waking
   2. At mid-day
   3. At the end of the day
   4. During the night
   5. At any time of day
   6. Never

3. Compared to one year ago, how would you rate your **leg problem** in general now? *(check one)*

   1. Much better now than one year ago
   2. Somewhat better now than one year ago
   3. About the same now as one year ago
   4. Somewhat worse now than one year ago
   5. Much worse now than one year ago
   6. I did not have any leg problem last year

(continued)

Table 86.4

VEINES-QOL/Sym Questionnaire *(Continued)*

4. The following items are about activities that you might do on a typical day. Does your **leg problem** now limit you in these activities? If so, how much? *(check one box on each line)*

	I do not work	YES Limited a lot	YES Limited a little	NO, not limited at all
a. Daily activities at work	0	1	2	3
b. Daily activities at home (e.g., housework, ironing, doing odd jobs/repairs around the house, gardening, etc.)		1	2	3
c. Social or leisure activities in which you are standing for long periods (e.g., parties, weddings, taking public transportation, shopping, etc.)		1	2	3
d. Social or leisure activities in which you are sitting for long period (e.g., going to the cinema or the theater, travelling, etc.)		1	2	3

5. During the past 4 weeks, have you had any of the following problems with your work or other regular daily activities as a result of your **leg problem**? *(check one box on each line)*

	YES	NO
a. Cut down the **amount of time** you spent on work or other activities	1	2
b. **Accomplished less** than you would like	1	2
c. Were limited in the **kind** of work or other activities	1	2
d. Had **difficulty** performing the work or other activities (e.g., it took extra effort)	1	2

6. During the past 4 weeks, to what extent has your leg problem interfered with your normal social activities with family, friends, neighbors or groups? *(check one)*

1. Not at all
2. Slightly
3. Moderately
4. Quite a bit
5. Extremely

7. How much leg pain have you had during the past 4 weeks? *(check one)*

1. None
2. Very mild
3. Mild
4. Moderate
5. Severe
6. Very severe

8. These questions are about how you feel and how things have been with you during the past 4 weeks as a result of your **leg problem**. For each question, please give the one answer that comes closest to the way you have been feeling. How much of the time during the past 4 weeks – *(check one box on each line)*

	All of the time	Most of the time	A good bit of the time	Some of the time	A little bit of the time	None of the time
a. Have you felt concerned about the appearance of your leg(s)?	1	2	3	4	5	6
b. Have you felt irritable?	1	2	3	4	5	6
c. Have you felt a burden to your family or friends?	1	2	3	4	5	6
d. Have you been worried about bumping into things?	1	2	3	4	5	6
e. Has the appearance of your leg(s) influenced your choice of clothing?	1	2	3	4	5	6

Questions 2, 3, 6, and 7 are reverse-scored so that high scores indicate better outcomes.

Adapted from Lamping DL, Schroter S, Kurz X, et al. Evaluation of outcomes in chronic venous disorders of the leg: development of a scientifically rigorous, patient-reported measure of symptoms and quality of life. *J Vasc Surg* 2003;37:410–419.

If the patient presents initially with acute DVT, the acute thrombus should be treated with thrombolysis prior to stent placement. Depending on the clot burden and technique for thrombolysis or thrombectomy, stent placement may occur on the same day or the day following initiation of thrombolysis.

ANATOMIC OR LESION CONSIDERATIONS

One of the challenges of the endovascular management of chronic VOD is planning the approach to recanalization. In patients with May-Thurner syndrome, with isolated obstruction of the left common iliac vein just before the iliocaval confluence, the most facile approach is ipsilateral common femoral vein access and deployment of the stent across the obstructing lesion such that the stent projects into the IVC. If stenting is performed in conjunction with thrombolysis of acute DVT extending to the leg, the popliteal vein is the likely access site, and stenting can easily be performed from that approach. Although it is preferable to avoid complete coverage of the outflow of the contralateral common iliac vein with a stent, there is usually little consequence if it does occur. Unlike with common iliac artery stenting, the use of kissing stent technique is not necessary to protect the contralateral common iliac vein; the use of kissing stents can be reserved for treatment of bilateral common iliac vein lesions.[24]

Similarly, stenting across the orifice of the internal iliac vein is acceptable. If obstructing lesions are seen proximal and distal to the internal iliac vein orifice, it is preferable to stent across the vein because skip areas are likely to occlude.[21]

If stenosis or occlusion of the external iliac vein or common femoral vein is suspected, as is often the case in post-thrombotic patients, then a more upstream puncture site is required. Whereas some groups favor puncturing the superficial femoral vein in the midthigh,[25] our group prefers a popliteal approach with the patient prone.

In many cases of post-thrombotic VOD, the occluded vein segments are above inguinal ligament. At our institution, we will stent down to, but not below, the level of the lesser trochanter. Stenting across flexion points, particularly in younger patients, is discouraged because of the mechanical stresses placed on the stent. One study of 177 limbs with stenting across the inguinal ligament demonstrated fracture of a nitinol stent but no wallstent fractures, leading to the recommendation that wallstents be used in that location.[26] Unfortunately, abnormality of the veins down to the level of the lesser trochanter is often accompanied by venous abnormality more distally, such as in the superficial femoral vein. If there is poor inflow into the stented levels—as can be seen in post-thrombotic patients with poorly developed leg collaterals—there is a greater likelihood of inadequate symptom relief and development of stent thrombosis. The role of venoplasty or stenting of the superficial femoral vein remains to be determined.

When extensive occlusion of the lower IVC is present, requiring placement of a separate stent in the IVC in addition to stenting of the iliac veins, it is helpful to obtain access via the internal jugular vein because the IVC stent can then be deployed from a caudal-to-cranial direction, allowing accurate positioning of the caudal aspect of the stent. This strategy is particularly helpful when braided stents, such as wallstents, are used because the degree of stent foreshortening, which varies with the degree of stent expansion, can be difficult to predict. Additionally, jugular access places the wire across the right atrium from the superior vena cava (SVC) to the IVC; if the stent should migrate centrally during deployment, the wire can prevent its migration to the right ventricle or pulmonary arteries. If the upper IVC requires stenting, then deployment from an inferior access point (such as the common femoral vein) is preferable to allow accurate positioning of the cranial aspect of the stent relative to the right atrium. In that circumstance the wire tip should be positioned at or above the SVC, again to prevent migration into the right ventricle.

For patients with combined caval and bilateral iliac vein occlusion, Neglen et al. evaluated three different techniques of stenting and found the double barrel technique—in which a stent from each iliac vein protrudes in parallel into the IVC—to be superior (FIGURE 86.1A). The second best option is placement of stents that overlap in the IVC in a Y configuration, such that one stent is placed through the interstices of the other stent (FIGURE 86.1B). One advantage of the double barrel technique is that the total IVC diameter at the level of the double barrel stents can be larger; with Y stenting, the diameter of the IVC at the confluence of the iliac veins is limited to the diameter of a single stent. However, double barrel stenting cannot always be performed. Because it requires deployment of both stents simultaneously, the double barrel technique is not an option if contralateral vein occlusion is discovered subsequent to initial iliocaval stent placement. The least effective stent configuration is placement of a stent bridging one iliac vein and the IVC, followed by placement of a contralateral stent apposed to the wall of the first stent, leaving a gap between the two stents (FIGURE 86.1C).[24]

TECHNICAL/DEVICE CONSIDERATIONS

Self-expanding stents were used in most patients described in the literature; the wallstent was the most commonly used stent in published series. Wallstents have the advantage of being available

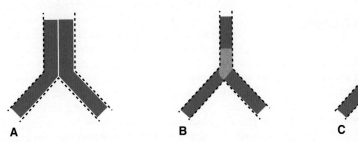

A   **B**   **C**

FIGURE 86.1 Stenting of occlusion at iliocaval junction. **A.** The double barrel technique is preferable. **B.** Placing overlapping stents in a Y configuration is an acceptable alternative. **C.** Apposing stent placement is least preferred because of the likelihood of occlusion at the iliacuein gap. Subjacent to the overriding contralateral stent.

in larger diameters, which accommodate the caliber of the IVC. Nitinol stents, which experience minimal shortening on deployment, allow more accurate stent placement in the iliac veins and are favored at our institution for stenting in those locations. The common iliac veins typically accommodate 14- to 18-mm diameter stents, the external iliac veins 12- to 16-mm stents, and the common femoral veins 10- to 14-mm stents. An occluded IVC ideally should be dilated up to accommodate a 20-mm stent. This may require predilation with high-pressure balloons with prolonged inflation. Neglen et al. suggest that wallstents are preferable to nitinol stents for stenting across the inguinal ligament because their single experience of stent fracture in that location occurred with a nitinol stent.[26] Balloon-expandable stents may be beneficial to prevent recoil in severely diseased segments but should not be used in areas where they may be compressed. Stents should be oversized to the vessel by approximately 2 to 4 mm.

Covered stents require larger sheath sizes and are significantly more expensive than bare stents. Because covered stents have the potential to disrupt communication between the stented vein and the internal iliac vein or collateral veins, there is a theoretical risk of worsening the patient's clinical status by excluding alternative drainage routes. This would be problematic, particularly if the primary drainage route should reocclude. Potential indications for covered stent use include repeat thrombosis of uncovered stents, coverage of a point of extravasation, or treatment of venous occlusion secondary to malignancy in which the extension of thrombogenic tumor into the vessel lumen is suspected.

TREATMENT SELECTION STRATEGIES

In patients with symptoms of chronic venous insufficiency, the decision to go to venography should be based on severity of symptoms because no noninvasive test is entirely sensitive in detecting hemodynamically significant venous stenoses or occlusions. Even venography in a single plane may not detect a significant lesion in 34% of cases.[9] If a hemodynamically significant lesion is suspected but not seen on venography, intravascular ultrasound can be considered, although it will add considerable cost to the procedure. Pressure measurements can be obtained. Although it is difficult to define a "significant" gradient in the venous system, absence of a gradient may be reassuring that a stenosis does not exist. If a hemodynamically significant stenosis or occlusion is detected, then stenting should be performed because angioplasty alone does not provide durable results. If balloon angioplasty is performed prior to stenting, care should be taken to limit angioplasty to the portion of vein that one expects to stent because angioplasty of a normal vein may cause injury that leads to stenosis or occlusion in the future.

PLANNING THE INTERVENTIONAL PROCEDURE

Noninvasive studies—including plethysmography and duplex sonography—are typically part of the workup of patients with symptoms of chronic venous insufficiency. Duplex sonography can assess for the presence of acute thrombus and can grade the severity of reflux. Abnormal plethysmography results can point toward a diagnosis of venous obstruction, but normal results do not exclude the possibility of obstruction.[27] CT or MR venograms are useful for assessing vascular caliber and can help gauge the extent of obstruction and hence the likelihood of successful recanalization. In our practice, we typically request that a patient obtain a CT or MR venogram extending from below the knees through the length of the IVC prior to the clinic visit. One important role of noninvasive imaging is to demonstrate the inferior and superior extent of abnormality, which will determine whether femoral, popliteal, or jugular access is needed; the choice of access site(s) determines whether the patient should lie prone or supine on the table.

If patients are being anticoagulated with warfarin, they may be transitioned to a shorter-acting agent, such as low-molecular-weight heparin, which can be held the day of the procedure. This enables the operator to titrate the patient's anticoagulation on the day of the procedure, which is useful when hemostasis needs to be achieved or if a thrombolytic infusion is required. Intraprocedurally, anticoagulation can be achieved with heparin or, if the patient has heparin-induced thrombocytopenia, an alternative anticoagulant, such as argatroban or bivalirudin. The patient should undergo a hypercoagulable workup to determine how long and how aggressively he or she should be anticoagulated after the procedure.

Although most of these procedures can be performed with moderate sedation, if the patient has significant pain medication requirements, or if it is anticipated that sharp recanalization will be necessary, then arrangements should be made for anesthesia.

SPECIFIC INTRAPROCEDURAL TECHNIQUES

At our institution, a micropuncture set is used to gain access under ultrasound guidance, and initial venography is performed through its 5 French transition dilator, prior to advancement of a 0.035" wire. The sheath should be sized appropriately for stent deployment. We often start with a standard 6 French sheath and switch to a longer sheath if further support of the catheter and wire is needed during recanalization. A short sheath is convenient if thrombolysis of acute clot is necessary because heparin can be instilled through the side arm at a low rate (400 units/hour) while the thrombolytic is administered via the multiple side holes of the infusion catheter.

A hydrophilic 0.035" angled-tip wire and 5 French angled catheter are used to recanalize the occluded vein. If necessary, as progress is made with the catheter and wire, a long sheath can be advanced to help stabilize the system and allow more directed force with the wire. When recanalizing, frequent contrast injections can be used to ensure that the wire and catheter have not taken an extraluminal course. Frequent changes of tube angulation are also helpful to ascertain that the appropriate vascular course is taken. Once a catheter has gone extraluminal, it is much more difficult to find the correct course because the catheter will often preferentially take the extraluminal course. Ascertaining the appropriate course in multiple projections will also ensure that the catheter is not taking the course of an enlarged collateral, such as a perivertebral vein.

Occasionally it is necessary to recanalize from both a jugular approach and a femoral or popliteal vein approach. An exchange-length wire can be snared from one end to gain through-and-through access, which provides mechanical advantage during angioplasty or stenting. If a very short occluded segment remains between the catheter from above and below, sharp recanalization with the back end of a wire or a long needle (such as a Hawkins needle or trans-septal needle) can be considered (FIGURE 86.2). Given the proximity of the vein to the artery,

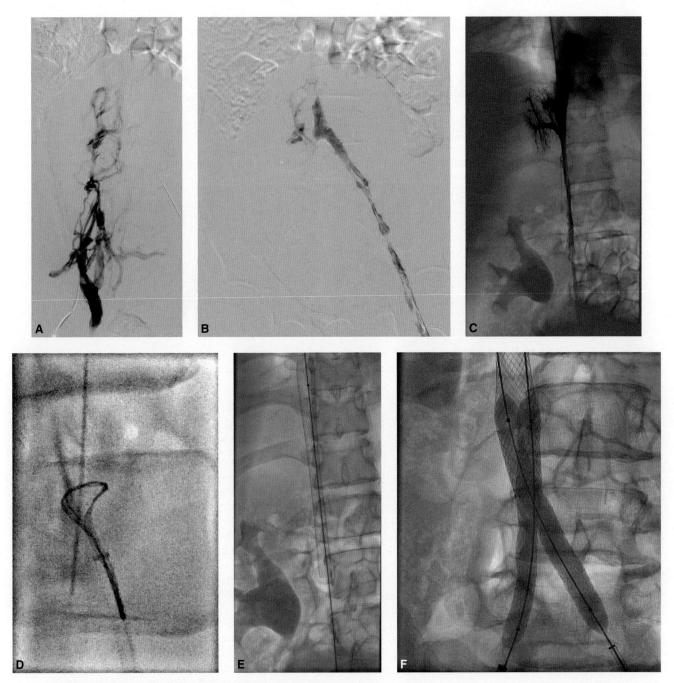

FIGURE 86.2 Complex recanalization of chronic occlusion of the inferior vena cava and iliac veins with left leg swelling. Access was obtained in the left popliteal vein, right common femoral vein, and right internal jugular vein. Venography in the prone (**A, B**) and supine (**C**) positions demonstrates (**A**) occlusion of the left external and common iliac veins, (**B**) high-grade stenosis of the right external and common iliac veins, and (**C**) occlusion of the inferior vena cava. **D.** After recanalization of bilateral iliac veins using Glidewires (Boston Scientific, Inc., Newton, MA) and catheters, sharp recanalization of the IVC was performed with the back end of a Glidewire to connect the upper and lower IVC. **E.** After balloon venoplasty of the IVC, two 20 × 80 mm wallstents (Boston Scientific, Inc.) were deployed. **F.** Given the degree of elastic recoil, kissing Palmaz Genesis (Cordis Medical, Johnson and Johnson, Inc., Warren, NJ) 10 mm diameter × 79 mm long balloon-expandable stents were simultaneously deployed in the iliocaval junction bilaterally. **G.** After self-expanding SMART stents (Cordis Medical, Johnson and Johnson, Inc.) were placed in bilateral iliac veins (12 mm diameter, 80 mm long) and the left common femoral vein (10 mm diameter, 80 mm long), completion bilateral iliofemoral venogram was performed. **H.** Completion inferior vena cavagram demonstrates in-line patency. *(continued)*

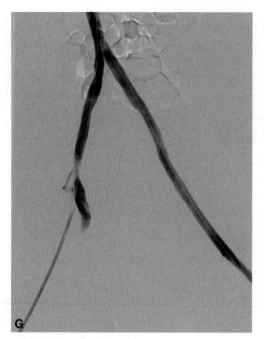
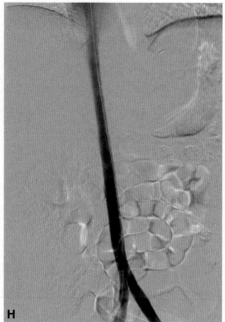

FIGURE 86.2 (*Continued*)

careful planning of the direction of needle throw is imperative. A contrast-filled balloon or snare can be used as a target for the needle. If it is available, C-arm CT imaging is useful to determine the appropriate trajectory.

Anticoagulation during the procedure is important to prevent immediate in-stent thrombosis. This is usually achieved with a heparin (5,000 units) or bivalirudin (50 mg) bolus and additional doses to maintain a target activated clotting time (ACT) of 240. The sheath can be removed and hemostasis achieved with manual compression when the ACT falls to below 200. For midthigh punctures, use of a sealing device, such as VasoSeal, has been advocated.[25]

Once the procedure is completed and hemostasis is achieved, the patient is advised to keep his legs elevated on four pillows. Compression stockings should be worn as frequently as tolerated. The patient should be administered a dose of low-molecular-weight heparin or fondaparinux prior to departure from the recovery room to maintain therapeutic levels of anticoagulation.

ENDPOINT ASSESSMENT OF THE PROCEDURE

Technical success is defined as successful recanalization of occluded segments with improved antegrade flow and decreased filling of collateral vessels. Adequate flow should be seen in both inflow and outflow vessels, although in the setting of damaged inflow vessels, the sheath itself may occlude the vessel and give the appearance of poor inflow. Compromised flow increases the likelihood of stent thrombosis. If an elevated venous pressure gradient was observed on initial venography, repeat pressure measurements should be obtained to assess for improvement.

PROCEDURAL COMPLICATIONS AND HOW TO MANAGE THEM SUCCESSFULLY

During recanalization of an occluded vein, it is not uncommon for the wire or catheter to inadvertently puncture the thin vessel wall and go extraluminal. Whenever there is a suspicion that the catheter is not within the vessel lumen, a small injection of contrast should be performed and, if necessary, the catheter retracted until the vessel lumen is again seen. Because of the low pressure of the venous system, these false passages usually do not result in significant bleeding. If persistent bleeding is seen, placement of a bare metal stent is usually adequate to seal the venotomy. If that fails, a stent-graft can be placed.

If stent migration should occur, the stent can be snared and retrieved. Ideally the wire is placed across the right atrium to bridge the SVC and IVC, so that the migrated stent is trapped by the wire and cannot travel into the right ventricle—where it is likely to cause arrhythmia—or the pulmonary arteries.

OUTCOMES/PROGNOSIS

There have been few publications with long-term follow-up of patients who have undergone iliocaval stenting for VOD. Raju and Neglen have published extensively from their prospective database of iliac vein stent placements dating back to 1997. In one study of 982 limbs in 870 patients stented for chronic, nonmalignant obstruction, they found primary, assisted primary, and secondary patency rates of 79%, 100%, and 100%, respectively, at 6 years for patients with nonthrombotic primary vein obstruction and 57%, 80%, and 86%, respectively, for patients with post-thrombotic obstruction. Early thrombosis (<30 days) occurred at a rate of 1.5%, most commonly in the stented iliac vein. Late thrombosis occurred at a rate of 3%. Factors associated with early or late stent occlusion included thrombotic etiology of lesions, long lesions requiring multiple stents, extension into the common femoral vein, and high degree of stenosis or total vein occlusion prior to stenting. The percentage of limbs free of pain improved from 24% before treatment to 62% 5 years after treatment; the percentage of limbs free from swelling improved from 18% before treatment to 32% 5 years after treatment. The cumulative rate of ulcer healing at 5 years was 58%.[23]

When they looked specifically at 528 limbs in 504 patients with deep reflux who underwent stent placement, they found a cumulative secondary patency rate of 88% for all limbs at 5 years; those with primary vein obstruction had 100% cumulative secondary patency at 5 years versus 82% for those with post-thrombotic obstruction. They also found that early DVT developed in 11/528 (2%) limbs. Improvement in pain was seen in 78% and complete pain relief was seen in 71% of patients at 5 years; for swelling, 55% of patients saw improvement and 36% had complete relief in 5 years. The cumulative rate of healing of active ulcers at 5 years was 54%.[21] In another study focusing on 319 patients stented for nonthrombotic iliac vein lesions, such as patients with May-Thurner syndrome, they found that at 2.5 years of follow-up many patients with and without reflux experienced complete relief of swelling (82% and 77%, respectively) and complete relief from pain (47% and 53%, respectively). There was an approximately 70% cumulative rate of completely healed ulcers at 2.5 years.[9]

Hartung et al. also published long-term results on 89 patients stented for chronic disabling nonmalignant obstructive iliocaval venous lesions; 13 of those patients underwent concomitant procedures, such as ovarian vein embolization and saphenous vein stripping. They experienced five complications: two stent migrations, one superficial femoral artery tear treated percutaneously, and two cases of contrast extravasation during recanalization. The technical success rate was 98%. In the subset of patients followed greater than 4 years, the primary patency rate at 4 years was 78%, the assisted-primary patency rate was 88%, and the secondary patency rate was 90%. They attributed restenoses to underestimation of the length of vein to be stented or, in one case, inadequate overlap between stents.[2]

DISEASE SURVEILLANCE AND TREATMENT MONITORING ALGORITHMS

After the procedure, patients are managed on a symptomatic basis. If new leg swelling develops, an ultrasound can quickly determine whether there is DVT. CT or MRI can assess the iliac veins and IVC if occlusion of those vessels is suspected. Venography can be performed in cases in which noninvasive imaging is inconclusive or when further intervention is warranted.

Patients should be aggressively anticoagulated and maintained at therapeutic levels from the immediate perioperative period through the first 3 to 6 months after stent placement. Continuation of anticoagulation after that period depends on the patient's history of venous thrombosis and hypercoagulable state.

On follow-up visits, compliance with compression stockings should be assessed. Objective measurements, such as calf and thigh circumference at reproducible locations, should be documented both before and after therapy. Response to therapy can be quantified using severity scores based on physician assessment and patient quality-of-life surveys.

EARLY FAILURES AND OPTIONS FOR MANAGEMENT

In certain patients with severe longstanding, long-segment venous occlusion, it may not be possible to recanalize the veins with the standard hydrophilic wires, angled catheter, and long guiding sheath. Aggressive attempts to recanalize may result in the wire creating false passages outside the vessel, making it even more difficult to recanalize the true vessel lumen. In one series of 167 limbs in 159 patients, the authors had a technical success rate of 83%.[25] Surgery may be a consideration in those patients.

Occasionally, on completion venography after stent deployment, there is poor flow within the stents. This can be caused by inadequate coverage of diseased vein by the stents; further extension of the stents may be necessary. At times, in-stent thrombosis is seen shortly after deployment. This may be caused by inadequate anticoagulation of the patient during the procedure. The ACT should be checked and additional heparin administered if appropriate. The thrombus can be treated with balloon angioplasty and/or rheolytic thrombectomy.

LATE FAILURES AND OPTIONS FOR MANAGEMENT

Patients who present with symptomatic rethrombosis of the stent or lower extremity deep veins can be managed with pharmacologic and mechanical thrombolysis. The cause of in-stent thrombosis should be determined. Potential causes include inadequate anticoagulation in the immediate postprocedural period, failure to stent the full extent of diseased vein, or mechanical stresses on the stent (such as when it is placed across the inguinal ligament). Extending the stent or placing an overlapping stent to increase radial force may be necessary. Relining the stented segment with a stent-graft is an additional consideration.

In cases refractory to endovascular management, consideration can be given to open surgical venovenous bypass grafting.

PRACTICAL ADVANTAGES AND LIMITATIONS

Given the limited surgical and medical options for patients with symptomatic chronic lower extremity VOD, endovascular management with stent placement provides an excellent minimally invasive way to treat the patient's symptoms of chronic venous insufficiency. The techniques and materials used to perform these procedures are commonly found in the interventional radiology armamentarium, making this a procedure that can easily be widely adopted.

Limitations of this procedure include difficulties in maintaining patency and adequate symptomatic relief in patients whose lesions extend below the inguinal ligament. Additionally, some patients with long-segment chronic occlusion cannot be successfully recanalized.

RELATIVE THERAPEUTIC EFFECTIVENESS COMPARED TO MEDICAL AND SURGICAL MANAGEMENT (INCLUDING CLINICAL, PATHOPHYSIOLOGIC AND ANATOMIC MEASURES)

Patients who present for iliocaval stenting typically have failed medical management, making it difficult to compare with that patient population. No randomized controlled trials have been performed to compare outcomes after venography with and without intervention.

Comparison with surgical management is also difficult because the advent of endovascular therapy has diminished the role of surgical venous bypasses, which are technically challenging and not universally available. Bypass surgeries now tend to be reserved for patients who have failed endovascular management or who are undergoing concurrent surgery for resection of malignancy.[10]

The Palma procedure is a surgical femorofemoral venous bypass technique for patients with unilateral iliac vein obstruction. The contralateral saphenous vein serves as the bypass conduit, connecting the common femoral veins through a suprapubic subcutaneous tunnel. If saphenous vein is not available, expanded polytetrafluoroethylene graft can be used, although the patency rates are much lower. A temporary arteriovenous fistula is occasionally placed to maintain graft patency. An analysis of 412 operations in nine series demonstrated a crude patency rate of 70% to 85%, although duration of follow-up and use of objective measures of graft patency varied between the studies.[10] For patients who are not candidates for the Palma procedure or who have extensive bilateral disease, in-line iliac vein or iliocaval bypass with graft can be performed, usually in conjunction with construction of an arteriovenous fistula to maintain patency. One group found the 2-year primary and secondary patency rates of 13 bypass grafts (5 iliocaval and 8 femorocaval) to be 38% and 54%, respectively.[28]

THE FUTURE

Ideally, as the medical community develops a better understanding of post-thrombotic syndrome and early interventions to prevent its development, there will be a decreased need for recanalization and stenting in patients with history of thrombosis. Whereas endovascular management of iliocaval occlusion is effective in many of those patients, the outcomes are less favorable than those for patients with primary vein obstruction.

Potential innovations that could improve the technical and long-term success of these procedures include the development of better devices to assist in recanalization of venous occlusions and the development of stents of appropriate size and radial strength for accurate placement in both the iliocaval system and, possibly, the superficial femoral vein. Stent surface treatments to prevent in-stent thrombosis could assist in maintaining primary patency.

CONCLUSION

Iliocaval recanalization and stent placement can improve pain, swelling, and clinical scores in a substantial subset of patients with chronic lower extremity venous insufficiency. Given the high prevalence of stenotic or occlusive venous lesions in the IVC and iliac veins, patients with chronic venous insufficiency refractory to conservative management should be aggressively evaluated for potential candidacy for therapies that can significantly improve their quality of life.

REFERENCES

1. Neglen P. Importance, etiology, and diagnosis of chronic proximal venous outflow obstruction. In: Bergan JJ, ed. *The Vein Book.* San Diego, CA: Elsevier Academic Press; 2007:541–548.
2. Hartung O, Loundou AD, Barthelemy P, et al. Endovascular management of chronic disabling ilio-caval obstructive lesions: long-term results. *Eur J Vasc Endovasc Surg* 2009;38:118–124.
3. Bergan JJ, Schmid-Schonbein GW, Smith PD, et al. Chronic venous disease. *N Engl J Med* 2006;355:488–498.
4. Staffa R. Chronic venous insufficiency—epidemiology. *Bratisl Lek Listy* 2002;103:166–168.
5. Van den Oever R, Hepp B, Debbaut B, et al. Socio-economic impact of chronic venous insufficiency. An underestimated public health problem. *Int Angiol* 1998;17:161–167.
6. Bernardi E, Bagatella P, Frulla M, et al. Postthrombotic syndrome: incidence, prevention, and management. *Semin Vasc Med* 2001;1: 71–80.
7. Akesson H, Brudin L, Dahlstrom JA, et al. Venous function assessed during a 5 year period after acute ilio-femoral venous thrombosis treated with anticoagulation. *Eur J Vasc Surg* 1990;4:43–48.
8. Johnson BF, Manzo RA, Bergelin RO, et al. Relationship between changes in the deep venous system and the development of the postthrombotic syndrome after an acute episode of lower limb deep vein thrombosis: a one- to six-year follow-up. *J Vasc Surg* 1995;21:307–312; discussion 313.
9. Raju S, Neglen P. High prevalence of nonthrombotic iliac vein lesions in chronic venous disease: a permissive role in pathogenicity. *J Vasc Surg* 2006;44:136–143; discussion 144.
10. Meissner MH, Eklof B, Smith PC, et al. Secondary chronic venous disorders. *J Vasc Surg* 2007;46(suppl S):68S–83S.
11. Raju S, Hollis K, Neglen P. Use of compression stockings in chronic venous disease: patient compliance and efficacy. *Ann Vasc Surg* 2007;21: 790–795.
12. Jull A, Arroll B, Parag V, et al. Pentoxifylline for treating venous leg ulcers. *Cochrane Database Syst Rev* 2007;(3):CD001733.
13. Coleridge-Smith P, Lok C, Ramelet AA. Venous leg ulcer: a meta-analysis of adjunctive therapy with micronized purified flavonoid fraction. *Eur J Vasc Endovasc Surg* 2005;30:198–208.
14. Nazarian GK, Austin WR, Wegryn SA, et al. Venous recanalization by metallic stents after failure of balloon angioplasty or surgery: four-year experience. *Cardiovasc Intervent Radiol* 1996;19:227–233.
15. Eklof B, Rutherford RB, Bergan JJ, et al. Revision of the CEAP classification for chronic venous disorders: consensus statement. *J Vasc Surg* 2004;40:1248–1252.
16. Vasquez MA, Rabe E, McLafferty RB, et al. Revision of the venous clinical severity score: venous outcomes consensus statement: special communication of the American Venous Forum Ad Hoc Outcomes Working Group. *J Vasc Surg* 2010;52:1387–1396.
17. Launois R, Reboul-Marty J, Henry B. Construction and validation of a quality of life questionnaire in chronic lower limb venous insufficiency (CIVIQ). *Qual Life Res* 1996;5:539–554.
18. Lamping DL, Schroter S, Kurz X, et al. Evaluation of outcomes in chronic venous disorders of the leg: development of a scientifically rigorous,

patient-reported measure of symptoms and quality of life. *J Vasc Surg* 2003;37:410–419.

19. Kahn SR. Measurement properties of the Villalta scale to define and classify the severity of the post-thrombotic syndrome. *J Thromb Haemost* 2009;7:884–888.

20. Kahn SR, M'Lan CE, Lamping DL, et al. Relationship between clinical classification of chronic venous disease and patient-reported quality of life: results from an international cohort study. *J Vasc Surg* 2004;39:823–828.

21. Raju S, Darcey R, Neglen P. Unexpected major role for venous stenting in deep reflux disease. *J Vasc Surg* 2010;51:401–408; discussion 408.

22. Delis KT, Bjarnason H, Wennberg PW, et al. Successful iliac vein and inferior vena cava stenting ameliorates venous claudication and improves venous outflow, calf muscle pump function, and clinical status in post-thrombotic syndrome. *Ann Surg* 2007;245:130–139.

23. Neglen P, Hollis KC, Olivier J, et al. Stenting of the venous outflow in chronic venous disease: long-term stent-related outcome, clinical, and hemodynamic result. *J Vasc Surg* 2007;46:979–990.

24. Neglen P, Darcey R, Olivier J, et al. Bilateral stenting at the iliocaval confluence. *J Vasc Surg* 2010;51:1457–1466.

25. Raju S, Neglen P. Percutaneous recanalization of total occlusions of the iliac vein. *J Vasc Surg* 2009;50:360–368.

26. Neglen P, Tackett TP Jr, Raju S. Venous stenting across the inguinal ligament. *J Vasc Surg* 2008;48:1255–1261.

27. Neglen P, Raju S. Detection of outflow obstruction in chronic venous insufficiency. *J Vasc Surg* 1993;17:583–589.

28. Jost CJ, Gloviczki P, Cherry KJ Jr, et al. Surgical reconstruction of iliofemoral veins and the inferior vena cava for nonmalignant occlusive disease. *J Vasc Surg* 2001;33:320–327; discussion 327–328.

Mesenteric Venous Thrombosis: Diagnosis, Natural History, and Interventional Strategies

RAMONA GUPTA and ROBERT K. RYU

INTRODUCTION

Mesenteric venous thrombosis is a rare cause of mesenteric ischemia. Initially described as a cause of intestinal infarction by Elliot in 1895,[1] mesenteric venous thrombosis is responsible for 5% to 15% of all mesenteric ischemic events.[2] Mesenteric venous thrombosis usually involves the superior mesenteric vein (SMV) but can extend to the splenic and portal veins and, rarely, the inferior mesenteric vein (IMV). Nonspecific symptomatology delays diagnosis and contributes to the poor outcomes associated with the condition, although improved imaging techniques have enabled more rapid recognition and detection. Additionally, improved understanding of underlying disease mechanisms has improved both treatment and outcomes. Despite a vague clinical presentation, the prompt recognition and aggressive treatment of this condition is necessitated by high morbidity and mortality rates related to intestinal infarction, bowel perforation, and high recurrence rates.[3]

ETIOLOGY

Mesenteric venous thrombosis can be classified as either primary or secondary. Primary mesenteric venous thrombosis is defined as spontaneous, idiopathic thrombosis of the mesenteric veins and accounts for approximately 25% of cases. In three-fourths of patients, an etiologic factor can be identified. As with Virchow's classic triad, the most common causes of secondary mesenteric venous thrombosis can be separated into three categories: hypercoagulable state, direct/epithelial injury, and local venous stasis (Table 87.1).[4] The number of patients with primary mesenteric venous thrombosis continues to decline as the ability to diagnose thrombotic disorders and hypercoagulable states improves.

Hypercoagulable States

Prothrombotic states are the most common cause of mesenteric venous thrombosis. There are numerous heritable coagulation disorders linked to mesenteric venous thrombosis including factor V Leiden mutation, protein C deficiency, protein S deficiency, and antithrombin III deficiency.[5] Identifying the presence of one of these is imperative because it affects long-term patient management. These patients must be managed with lifelong anticoagulation to prevent recurrence. Additional hematologic hypercoagulable states associated with mesenteric venous thrombosis include polycythemia vera, thrombocytosis, hyperfibrinogenemia, paroxysmal nocturnal hemoglobinuria, and myeloproliferative states.

Awareness of acquired hypercoagulable states is also important in the diagnosis and treatment of mesenteric venous thrombosis. Oral contraceptive use is responsible for 4% to 5% of total mesenteric venous thrombotic events, a higher percentage of cases occurring in young women.[3,6] The presence of malignancy, especially abdominal cancers and hepatic metastases, is a well-accepted risk factor for development of mesenteric venous thrombosis.[7,8] In these patients, outcomes are determined by the nature of the cancer.

Direct Injury

Direct injury is recognized as a predisposing condition for mesenteric venous thrombosis. These injuries include pancreatitis, inflammatory bowel disease, abdominal trauma, and postsurgical trauma.[4] Splenectomy, especially laparoscopic splenectomy, has a high incidence of splanchnic vein thrombosis, occurring in up to 55% of patients.[9,10] Multiple mechanisms have been suggested including venous stasis during abdominal insufflation, ligation of splenic vessels with a stapler or coagulation device as opposed to suture ligation in open procedures, and the absence of valves in the portal venous system, allowing thrombus propagation.[11]

Local Venous Stasis

Conditions causing venous stasis in the mesenteric system include cirrhosis, portal hypertension, severe congestive heart failure, and morbid obesity.[4] Cirrhotic patients often have severe impairments in coagulation caused by impaired hepatic synthesis of clotting factors; however, they are prone to thrombosis of the mesenteric venous structures due to venous stasis and portal hypertension.[12] Budd-Chiari syndrome is recognized as an important cause of mesenteric venous thrombosis associated with portal hypertension.[13]

PATHOPHYSIOLOGY

The severity of intestinal injury is determined by the location, extent, and rate of thrombus formation. The location of acute thrombus formation can be an important predictor of the underlying cause of mesenteric venous thrombosis. Intra-abdominal causes, such as splenectomy and pancreatitis, initiate thrombus formation in the large veins and spread peripherally. Hypercoagulable states often lead to thrombus formation in the vasa recta, arcuate veins, and venous arcades and progress to involve the larger veins. This is an important

---

Table 87.1

Secondary Causes of Mesenteric Venous Thrombosis

Hypercoagulable states

Factor V Leiden deficiency

Protein C deficiency

Protein S deficiency

Antithrombin III deficiency

Polycythemia vera

Hyperfibrinogenemia

Paroxysmal nocturnal hemoglobinuria

Myeloproliferative states

Sickle cell anemia

Malignancy, especially abdominal cancers and hepatic
metastases

Oral contraceptive use

Direct injury

Pancreatitis

Inflammatory bowel disease

Abdominal trauma

Postsurgical trauma

Local venous stasis

Cirrhosis

Portal hypertension

Severe congestive heart failure

Morbid obesity

Budd-Chiari syndrome

---

distinction because those patients whose disease begins in the small veins may be at greatest risk of intestinal infarction as peripheral venous drainage is immediately compromised, leading to hemorrhagic bowel infarction.[14] On the other hand, thrombus that begins in the large veins and spreads peripherally is often associated with a longer duration of symptoms and the absence of intestinal infarction until later in the disease process. Patients with subacute or chronic mesenteric venous occlusion frequently have thrombosis of the portal and/or splenic veins, sparing the vasa recta and venous arcades. These patients present less acutely because venous collaterals provide sufficient venous drainage.

Whatever the mechanism, occlusion of the mesenteric veins causes inadequate venous drainage of the bowel. The affected bowel wall becomes engorged with blood and cyanotic. Mucosal ischemia progresses to transmural infarction. Ischemic bowel becomes edematous and thickened with intramural hemorrhage, leading to rapid loss of fluid into the bowel lumen, mesentery, and peritoneal cavity. The increased venous pressure results in hemorrhage, perforation, and peritonitis.[15] Secondary arterial vasospasm may further intensify intestinal ischemia.[16] Arterial

vasospasm can occur in the presence of venous occlusion. Even after the venous obstruction has been relieved, arterial vasoconstriction can persist, adequate to cause intestinal infarction and arterial thrombosis.

▌ CLINICAL PRESENTATION

There is no sign or symptom specific for mesenteric venous thrombosis; therefore, a high index of suspicion is essential for timely diagnosis. Mesenteric ischemia usually presents with generalized midabdominal pain not explained by physical findings and is often accompanied by vomiting, abdominal distention, and constipation.[17] Presentation of mesenteric venous thrombosis can be acute, subacute, or chronic.

Acute mesenteric venous thrombosis is defined as presence of symptoms for 4 weeks' duration or less. In these cases, onset of symptoms is sudden with colicky and severe pain, out of proportion to abdominal findings on physical exam. Patients report disproportionate pain with slow progression. More than half of patients report other nonspecific symptoms, such as nausea/vomiting, anorexia, and constipation with or without bloody diarrhea.[16,18] Over 75% of patients report at least 2 days of symptoms prior to seeking medical attention. In those patients with subacute mesenteric venous thrombosis, abdominal pain is the major finding without bowel infarction or variceal hemorrhage. These patients may report constipation, diarrhea, and/or fever.

Patients with chronic mesenteric venous thrombosis have extensive venous collateral circulation and therefore less abdominal pain. The diagnosis is usually one of exclusion, after more common causes of abdominal pain, such as cholecystitis, pancreatitis, gastroesophageal reflux, and gastric disorders, have been explored.[19] These patients are asymptomatic until late complications of portal hypertension occur, such as variceal hemorrhage. These cases may demonstrate weight loss, food avoidance, and vague postprandial abdominal pain.

The differential diagnosis for acute mesenteric venous thrombosis is lengthy and includes both intravascular and extravascular causes. Arterial causes include embolic disease, occlusive/nononcclusive atherosclerotic disease, dissecting aortic aneurysm, hypoperfusion, and disseminated intravascular coagulation. Extravasular causes include incarcerated hernias, small bowel obstruction, volvulus, intussusception, and adhesive bands/scars.

▌ DIAGNOSIS

Routine blood tests are not helpful in diagnosing mesenteric venous thrombosis. A mild leukocytosis is an equivocal finding. Metabolic acidosis or elevated lactate levels are late findings associated with bowel infarction.[20] Radiographic findings are nonspecific. Findings on abdominal X-rays include dilated loops of small bowel with air-fluid levels indicative of small bowel obstruction or ileus, thickened loops of bowel or "thumbprinting" indicative of bowel wall edema, and pneumatosis intestinalis. Free intraperitoneal air is an ominous finding of bowel wall perforation.

Color Doppler ultrasonography (US) with duplex scanning can be a valuable, noninvasive tool for evaluation of portal vein patency. Generally used in the workup of other abdominal

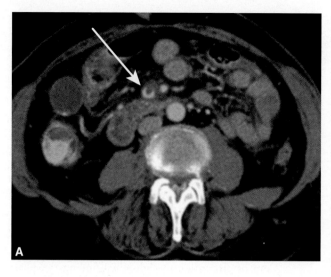

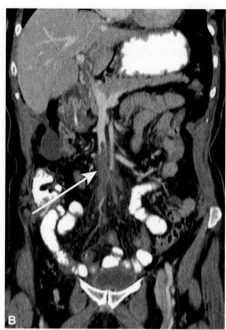

FIGURE 87.1 Axial (**A**) and coronal (**B**) images from a contrast-enhanced CT demonstrating occlusive thrombus in the SMV (*arrow*) with mesenteric edema and bowel wall thickening.

conditions including portal hypertension and gallbladder disease, portomesenteric thrombosis may be an incidental finding. This modality has several limitations: its operator-dependent nature, limited visualization due to overlying bowel gas or large patient body habitus, and sensitivity to detect slow flow.

Both contrast-enhanced computed tomography (CT) angiography and contrast-enhanced magnetic resonance (MR) angiography are highly specific and sensitive for the diagnosis of mesenteric vein thrombosis and identification of associated secondary findings.[21] In acute cases, well-defined intraluminal thrombus is visible distending the SMV (FIGURE 87.1). The mesenteric veins may have thick, enhancing walls and multivein occlusion is common. The most common finding in bowel ischemia is bowel wall thickening.[22] The bowel wall may demonstrate alternating areas of low attenuation related to edema and high attenuation from hemorrhage and hyperemia, referred to as the target or halo sign. Bowel wall dilatation is a common manifestation reflecting absence of peristalsis secondary to both arterial and venous perfusion abnormalities. Associated findings include stranding in the mesentery, collateral circulation, and ascites. Pneumatosis intestinalis, portomesenteric gas, and free intraperitoneal air are late findings of transmural infarction and perforation.[23,24] If acute clot extends into the portal vein, perfusion abnormalities in the liver can be seen (FIGURE 87.2). In patients with chronic mesenteric venous occlusion, cavernous transformation of the portal vein, abundant venous collaterals, gastroesophageal varices, and ascites can be identified in the absence of intestinal ischemia. Additionally, "ectopic" varices in the small intestine, colon, and rectum can be diagnosed. Both CT and MR techniques permit excellent detection of the portomesenteric thrombus extension and ancillary signs of mesenteric ischemia.

Because of the advances in noninvasive imaging, conventional angiography is not routinely used for the diagnosis of mesenteric venous thrombosis. Instead, it is used for equivocal cases and in conjunction with transcatheter therapies. Findings on selective mesenteric angiography with delayed venous phase imaging include thrombus in the large veins, delayed visualization of the superior mesenteric and portal veins, superior mesenteric arterial spasm, and prolonged opacification of the arterial arcades (FIGURE 87.3).[20] Both direct and indirect portography are valuable means for evaluating and treating mesenteric venous thrombosis and are discussed under endovascular intervention.

TREATMENT OPTIONS

Because of the low incidence of mesenteric venous thrombosis, management strategies are based on clinical judgment and experience. The primary aim of treatment is to avoid bowel infarction, peritonitis, and ischemia. This depends on rapid detection.

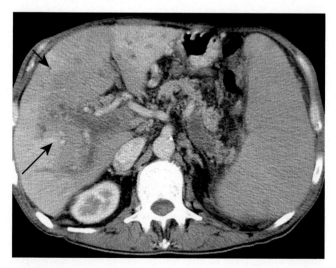

FIGURE 87.2 Axial image from a contrast-enhanced CT demonstrating thrombosis of the splenic and portal veins with perfusional changes in the liver (*black arrows*).

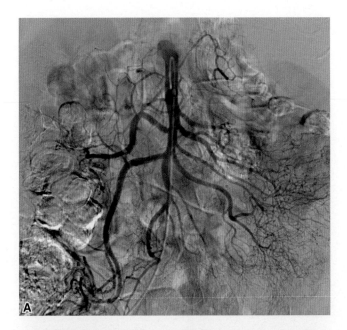

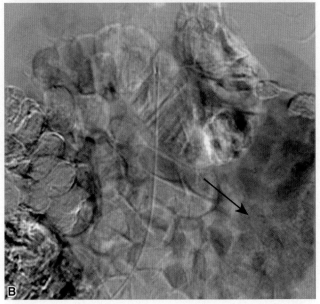

FIGURE 87.3 Initiation of SMA thrombolysis (**A**) in a patient with massive mesenteric thrombosis demonstrating prolonged opacification of the arterial arcade (**B**) on delayed phase arterial imaging (*black arrow*). Delayed filling of the SMV and portal vein was not seen.

Once the diagnosis is established, treatment should be initiated immediately.

Medical Management

Upon diagnosis of mesenteric venous ischemia, immediate heparinization is the standard of therapy, even for those patients who present with ischemia-related gastrointestinal bleeding. Heparin has been demonstrated to prevent recurrence of thrombosis after intestinal resection and lower mortality when recurrence occurs.[25] In those patients with acute thrombosis treated with anticoagulation, complete or partial vascular recanalization can

be seen in up to 90% of patients.[26] Heparin therapy is initiated with a bolus of 5,000 units followed by a continuous infusion with the dose adjusted for a goal activated partial thromboplastin time twice normal. In the absence of ongoing ischemia, oral anticoagulation with warfarin should be started and continued for 3 to 6 months or lifetime, depending on the underlying cause.[20] Supportive measures include bowel rest, nasogastric suction, and intravenous fluids. The use of anticoagulants in patients with chronic mesenteric venous ischemia is controversial; although beneficial in preventing new thromboses, it carries the risk of exacerbating variceal hemorrhage.

Surgical Management

Acute mesenteric ischemia with evidence of bowel infarction or peritonitis is an indication for emergent surgery. On CT or magnetic resonance imaging (MRI), the triad of low attenuation in the SMV, small bowel wall thickening, and peritoneal fluid indicate bowel ischemia and warrant a laparotomy. Intraoperatively, mesenteric edema and cyanotic discoloration of the bowel indicate mesenteric venous thrombosis. Once the diagnosis is established, anticoagulation should be initiated immediately and broad-spectrum antibiotics administered. Although perioperative heparin increases the risk of bleeding complications, it decreases the risk of rethrombosis and ultimately improves outcomes.[25]

Surgery involves resecting the involved segments of nonviable ischemic intestine, surgical thrombectomy, and/or delivery of transcatheter thrombolytics. In those patients who require resection, a second-look procedure should be considered 12 to 48 hours postoperatively because almost half of patients have further evidence of gangrene, requiring additional resection.[18] Surgical thrombectomy is limited in those patients who have extensive venous thrombosis extending into the venous arcades. Additionally, administration of vasodilators, such as papaverine, has been shown to improve mesenteric arterial vasoconstriction.[27] Surgical techniques are complicated by sepsis, wound infections, and short bowel syndrome in those patients who require extensive bowel resection.

In patients with chronic mesenteric venous thrombosis, therapy is directed toward the symptoms and underlying disease. Anticoagulation is initiated for those with underlying hypercoagulable disorders. Endoscopic ligation of varices and portal decompression are performed if variceal hemorrhage occurs. Patients with chronic mesenteric venous ischemia have improved survival rates as compared to those with acute thrombosis because bowel infarction is usually not present. Patients with chronic disease usually die from underlying or unrelated causes.[3]

Endovascular Intervention

As mortality rates from acute mesenteric venous thrombosis have failed to improve over the last several decades, percutaneous management strategies have evolved. The goal is rapid venous recanalization with durable venous patency, obviating the need for prolonged thrombolytic therapy. Techniques include transhepatic thrombectomy and thrombolysis, transjugular thrombectomy and thrombolysis with placement of a transjugular intrahepatic portosystemic shunt (TIPS), and transarterial thrombolysis. Patient selection is of paramount importance. CT or MRI should be used to confirm the clinical diagnosis of acute mesenteric venous thrombosis and exclude other abdominal pathology. Patients with evidence of bowel ischemia or infarction are managed surgically. The use of preoperative catheter-directed therapies is not advised given the risk of reperfusion syndrome. However, these patients may benefit from the adjunctive administration of thrombolytics postoperatively via operatively placed mesenteric vein catheters or percutaneously placed arterial catheters.[15] Written informed consent must be obtained from each patient prior to the initiation of catheter-directed therapy, including a discussion of the risks of bleeding complications and the benefits of avoiding surgical intervention and general anesthesia. Major contraindications for thrombolytic therapy should be evaluated including recent stroke, primary or metastatic central nervous system malignancies, and active bleeding diathesis. Symptomatic patients with acute mesenteric venous thrombosis confirmed on CT or MRI, without evidence of bowel ischemia, are candidates for percutaneous endovascular thrombolytic therapy.

Transhepatic Thrombectomy and Thrombolysis

Percutaneous transhepatic access into the portomesenteric veins enables direct infusion of thrombolytics into clot, mechanical thrombectomy, and venoplasty or stent placement. The transhepatic route is preferred in patients who have a larger clot burden involving the portal vein in whom transjugular access may be difficult. Transhepatic access affords a favorable angle for accessing both the portal and SMVs. This allows localized delivery of thrombolytics directly into thrombus, which enhances effectiveness. The thrombolytics can be administered at a higher dose without the complications associated with systemic exposure, thrombolysis rates are improved, and duration of treatment is reduced.[28]

Similar to percutaneous transhepatic cholangiography, transhepatic access into the portal vein is achieved using ultrasound and fluoroscopic guidance. Access into a right portal vein branch is preferred via the right midaxillary line, subcostal if possible. After accessing the portal vein, mesenteric and portal venography is performed to determine the extent of the clot (FIGURE 87.4).

Mechanical thrombectomy can be performed with a variety of techniques and devices. Suction or aspiration thrombectomy is a low-cost and easy technique. It may be performed repeatedly by advancing an angled guide catheter with a wide inner lumen and atraumatic tip through the sheath into direct contact with the clot and applying suction with a 60-mL Luer-lock syringe. The vacuum is maintained as the guiding catheter is rapidly moved back and forth across the area of clot and then removed.[29] Balloon thrombectomy can be performed using a compliant balloon, such as the Fogarty embolectomy catheter (Edwards Lifesciences, Irvine, CA). Numerous devices are available that combine both mechanical and pharmacologic thrombolysis including the AngioJet Thrombectomy Set (Possis Medical, Minneapolis, MN), the Trellis Peripheral Infusion System (Bacchus Vascular, Santa Clara, CA), the Arrow-Trerotola device (Arrow International, Reading, PA), and the Helix Clot Buster thrombectomy device (ev3, Plymouth, MN). These devices assist in more rapid dissolution of thrombus and thereby decrease duration of thrombolytic agent administration.[30] Operators should be aware that these devices can cause hemolysis, and their activation times should be limited to avoid toxicity.

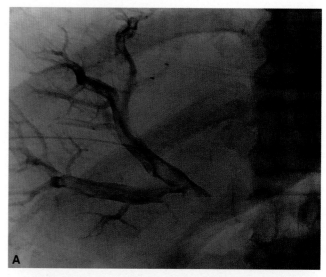

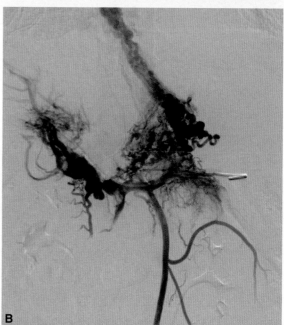

FIGURE 87.4 A. Percutaneous transhepatic access into the right portal vein demonstrating clot within the branches. **B.** Percutaneous transhepatic mesenteric venography demonstrating non-filling of the SMV, splenic vein, and portal vein. Instead, the IMV and gastroesophageal varices are noted.

Residual thromboses can be addressed with catheter-directed thrombolysis. A multi–side-hole catheter should be positioned within a thrombosed portion of the SMV. Pulse-spray thrombolysis can be performed with recombinant human tissue plasminogen activator (alteplase, Genentech, South San Francisco, CA), for example. Then a slow continuous drip of thrombolytics is initiated via the multi–side-hole catheter. Patients are monitored in the intensive care unit (ICU) for bleeding complications and restudied in the angiography suite in 24 hours. Labs, including hemoglobin, prothrombin time, partial thromboplastin time, and fibrinogen, are checked every 6 hours. If the patient experiences a bleeding complication or if the fibrinogen drops below a predefined setpoint (usually 150 mg/dL), the thrombolytic is stopped. Continuous catheter-directed thrombolysis can be continued for 48 to 72 hours; complications increase significantly if infusions last more than 72 hours.[28,31]

Following thrombolysis, any residual stenoses may be treated with venoplasty or stent placement. The goal at completion portomesenteric venography is venous patency with restoration of brisk antegrade flow. At the conclusion of the procedure, transhepatic portal vein access is removed and the tract through the liver is embolized with coils or gelfoam plugs (Gelfoam absorbable gelatin sponge; USP, Pharmacia & Upjohn Co; Kalamazoo, MI) to reduce the risk of bleeding and subcapsular hemorrhage.[32] Patients should be immediately heparinized, with a goal-activated partial thromboplastin time twice normal, and then transitioned to oral warfarin.

Transjugular Thrombectomy and Thrombolysis with Transjugular Intrahepatic Portosystemic Shunt

In the setting of ascites and coagulopathy, the transjugular approach to the portomesenteric venous system is preferred over the transhepatic approach. Avoiding the puncture of the hepatic capsule greatly decreases the risk of bleeding complication in these patients. The transjugular approach with placement of a TIPS provides direct access to the thrombus and a low-pressure conduit for the portal system. Because underlying portal hypertension is frequently a cause of mesenteric venous thrombosis, reduction of the portosystemic gradient improves venous congestion and stasis, and promotes improved mesenteric venous drainage. The procedure can be technically challenging if the clot extends into the intrahepatic portal veins but remains feasible. Transjugular portography via a wedged carbon dioxide portogram can be essential for identifying patent portal branches and a target for the intrahepatic shunt.[33,34] In difficult cases, a percutaneous transhepatic or transsplenic puncture can provide visualization and access to the portal circulation. This access can be used as a target during TIPS puncture and to facilitate venous recanalization (FIGURE 87.5). If an additional percutaneous puncture is used, embolization of the tract is necessary when the transhepatic or transsplenic sheath is removed.

Once the portal vein is accessed, the intrahepatic tract can be balloon dilated to accommodate passage of the devices required for thrombolysis and thrombectomy (FIGURE 87.6). Direct portomesenteric venography demonstrates the extent of the clot. Similar to the transhepatic technique, mechanical thrombectomy can be performed with aspiration thrombectomy (FIGURE 87.7), balloon embolectomy, or a variety of thrombectomy devices. Pharmacologic thrombolysis can be performed over several days via a multi–side-hole infusion catheter across the thrombosed veins. Placement of the TIPS stent is patient and operator dependent. In patients with sluggish flow after mesenteric venous recanalization or clotted intrahepatic portal veins, the TIPS stent may help maintain adequate blood flow by providing patent surrogate outflow.[35] For patients who rethrombose, the TIPS stent provides fast access to the mesenteric venous system for repeat intervention.

This technique has the advantage of efficiency: fast removal of thrombus, rapid reestablishment of antegrade flow, and decreased duration of thrombolytic infusion. On the other hand, the procedure can be technically complex with a high risk of periprocedural

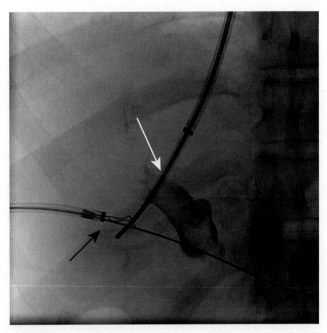

FIGURE 87.5 Percutaneous transhepatic access into the portal vein was achieved first (*black arrow*) and then used as a target for the TIPS puncture from the hepatic vein (*white arrow*). A guide wire was advanced through the TIPS needle, snared via the transhepatic access, then advanced retrograde into the portal vein.

complications, including hepatic encephalopathy, stent dysfunction, hemobilia, or infection.[36] Also, the operator must be aware if the patient is a transplant candidate because a TIPS stent can create technical issues during the transplant. The stent should extend the shortest possible distance into the main portal vein to create a portal-portal anastamosis during surgery. Similarly, the stent should not extend into the inferior vena cava or right atrium because a cuff of hepatic vein is required for anastamosis.[37]

Transarterial Thrombolysis

For patients with thrombi in the smaller veins and venules of the mesenteric system, indirect thrombolysis via the superior mesenteric artery (SMA) is a potential treatment. Via a common femoral artery approach, thrombolytics are infused into the SMA, enabling thrombolysis of multiple smaller splanchnic veins. Theoretically, the intra-arterial infusion has access to the capillaries and small venules; as these are cleared of clot, the thrombolytic agent contacts the thrombus in the larger veins.[38] Similar to the procedure described previously, thrombolytics are slowly infused via a multi–side-hole catheter placed in the SMA. Patients are monitored in the ICU with special attention toward lab parameters and bleeding complications. Every 12 to 24 hours, the patient is restudied angiographically and the clot burden is assessed on the delayed venous phase imaging. Thrombolysis can be continued for 48 to 72 hours. Angiographic endpoints include improved venous patency, lack of prolonged opacification in the arterial arcades, or symptom resolution. In many of these cases, the angiographic appearance does not significantly change but procedural success is based on clinical improvement with resolution or reduction of abdominal pain.

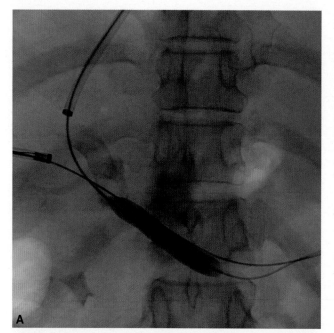

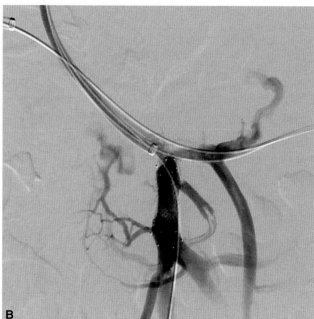

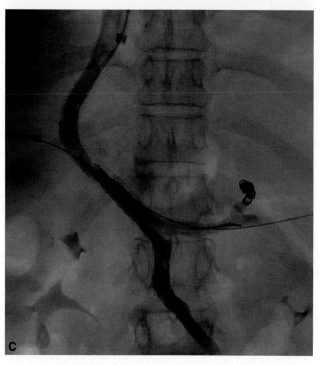

FIGURE 87.6 Following balloon dilation (**A**) of the intrahepatic shunt and main portal vein, stents were deployed within the SMV (**B**) and splenic vein. A large varix was coil embolized and the TIPS shunt was placed (**C**).

Although technically less difficult than the other approaches, this therapy has limitations. Thrombolytics are not directly infused into thrombus, which may increase duration of lytic infusion and patient bedrest. The lytic agents may be diverted into patent branches or collaterals, bypassing the clotted branches. Additionally, there are multiple risks associated with prolonged femoral arterial catheterization including infection, hematoma formation, and pseudoaneurysm.[39] This technique has been used in conjunction with direct mesenteric venous infusion of thrombolytics (either transhepatic or transjugular) to provide rapid, aggressive thrombus debulking in patients with extensive mesenteric venous thrombosis.[40,41]

COMPLICATIONS AND OUTCOMES

The most feared complication associated with endovascular techniques is hemorrhage. Overall, the focused delivery of thrombolytics is associated with fewer bleeding complications than systemic delivery. Potential complications include gastrointestinal hemorrhage, hematuria, perihepatic hematoma, intraperitoneal hemorrhage, bleeding at groin or neck puncture sites, and catheter dislodgment. These patients often respond to termination of thrombolysis and transfusion. Intracranial hemorrhage evidenced by changes in mental status or headache can be a fatal complication, occurring in approximately 1% of

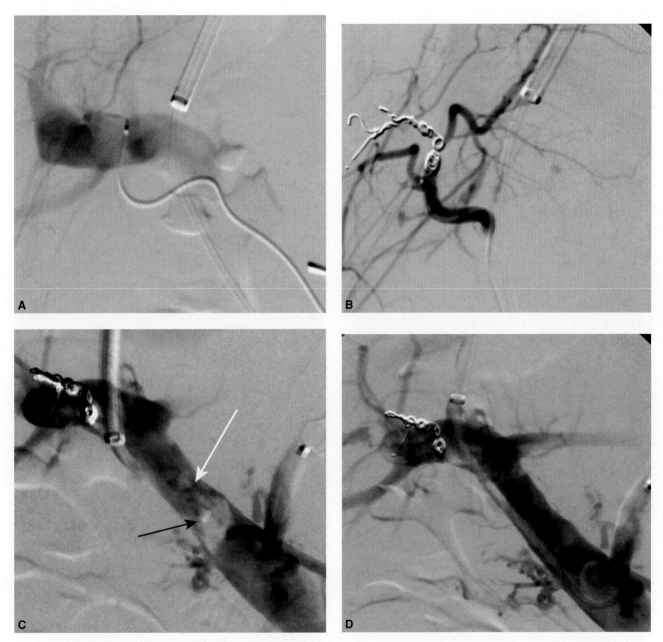

FIGURE 87.7 A. An incidental fistula between a right hepatic artery branch and a portal vein branch from a previous biopsy opacified the main portal vein and assisted in the TIPS puncture. **B.** The fistula was later coil embolized. **C.** A large filling defect is noted in the main portal vein compatible with thrombus (*black arrow*). A guiding catheter was advanced into the thrombus (*white arrow*) and used for suction thrombectomy. **D.** Post-thrombectomy venography demonstrates removal of the previously seen clot.

patients.[42] While receiving thrombolytics, all stools must be guiac tested to monitor for gastrointestinal bleeding, and IV and skin access sites should be assessed frequently. Those patients who develop gastrointestinal bleeding while on thrombolytics should be reassessed for bowel ischemia because bleeding may be the cardinal sign of worsening condition. These patients can progress rapidly to septic shock unless a laparotomy is performed. Pneumothorax or hemothorax is a reported complication if the pleural reflection is crossed during percutaneous transhepatic access.[30]

Endovascular procedures are associated with a low complication rate and a high rate of technical success. Most patients experience lysis of thrombus, whether partial or complete, with clinical improvement evidenced by decrease in abdominal pain, nausea, and distention. With careful management of long-term anticoagulation and treatment directed toward the underlying etiology, most patients fare well. Mesenteric venous thrombosis carries a better prognosis than other forms of acute mesenteric ischemia; mortality rates are primarily determined by presence of intestinal ischemia. For patients who are treated with anticoagulation, surgery, and/or endovascular techniques, mortality rates range from 20% to 50% and survival depends on multiple factors including age, coexisting conditions, timing of diagnosis, and whether surgical intervention is required. Recurrences occur most frequently in the first 30 days after presentation.[43]

Patients with chronic portomesenteric thrombosis without malignancy fare better than those with acute mesenteric venous thrombosis. Determinants of poor outcomes in chronic cases include increased bilirubin levels or presence of ascites. Variceal hemorrhage is the primary morbidity and mortality. These patients should be managed with long-term anticoagulation and beta blockade.[44]

▌CONCLUSION

Despite advances in diagnosis with contrast-enhanced CT angiography and contrast-enhanced MR angiography, mesenteric venous thrombosis remains a rare clinical entity with a high morbidity and mortality. A high index of clinical suspicion combined with early imaging is essential to improved outcomes. The treatment goals are simple: patient survival and avoidance of bowel surgery. In patients with signs of bowel infarction, immediate laparotomy is imperative with resection of necrotic bowel. In patients without imaging evidence of bowel ischemia, systemic anticoagulation and supportive care are initial treatments, although of limited value in patients with extensive thrombosis. Given the safety, efficacy, and durability of endovascular therapies, these techniques are rapidly emerging as effective alternatives.

▌REFERENCES

1. Elliot JW. II. The operative relief of gangrene of intestine due to occlusion of the mesenteric vessels. *Ann Surg* 1895;21:9–23.
2. Grendell JH, Ockner RK. Mesenteric venous thrombosis. *Gastroenterology* 1982;82:358–372.
3. Rhee RY, Gloviczki P, Mendonca CT, et al. Mesenteric venous thrombosis: still a lethal disease in the 1990s. *J Vasc Surg* 1994;20:688–697.
4. Acosta S, Alhadad A, Svensson P, et al. Epidemiology, risk and prognostic factors in mesenteric venous thrombosis. *Br J Surg* 2008;95:1245–1251.
5. Amitrano L, Brancaccio V, Guardascione MA, et al. High prevalence of thrombophilic genotypes in patients with acute mesenteric vein thrombosis. *Am J Gastroenterol* 2001;96:146–149.
6. Hassan HA. Oral contraceptive-induced mesenteric venous thrombosis with resultant intestinal ischemia. *J Clin Gastroenterol* 1999;29:90–95.
7. Douma RA, Kok MG, Verberne LM, et al. Incidental venous thromboembolism in cancer patients: prevalence and consequence. *Thromb Res* 2010;125:e306–e309.
8. Thatipelli MR, McBane RD, Hodge DO, et al. Survival and recurrence in patients with splanchnic vein thromboses. *Clin Gastroenterol Hepatol* 2010;8:200–205.
9. Stamou KM, Toutouzas KG, Kekis PB, et al. Prospective study of the incidence and risk factors of postsplenectomy thrombosis of the portal, mesenteric, and splenic veins. *Arch Surg* 2006;141:663–669.
10. Ikeda M, Sekimoto M, Takiguchi S, et al. High incidence of thrombosis of the portal venous system after laparoscopic splenectomy: a prospective study with contrast-enhanced CT scan. *Ann Surg* 2005;241:208–216.
11. Liang MK, Marks JL. Postsplenectomy portal, mesenteric, and splenic vein thrombosis. *Arch Surg* 2007;142:575.
12. Amitrano L, Guardascione MA, Brancaccio V, et al. Portal and mesenteric venous thrombosis in cirrhotic patients. *Gastroenterology* 2002;123:1409–1410.
13. Harnik IG, Brandt LJ. Mesenteric venous thrombosis. *Vasc Med* 2010;15:407–418.
14. Mc Cune WS, Keshishian JM, Blades BB. Mesenteric thrombosis following blunt abdominal trauma. *Ann Surg* 1952;135:606–614.
15. McManimon S, Ryu R, Durham JD. Mesenteric venous thrombosis. *Tech Vasc Intervent Radiol* 1998;1:209–215.
16. Harnik IG, Brandt LJ. Mesenteric venous thrombosis. *Vasc Med* 2010;15:407–418.
17. Abu-Daff S, Abu-Daff N, Al-Shahed M. Mesenteric venous thrombosis and factors associated with mortality: a statistical analysis with five-year follow-up. *J Gastrointest Surg* 2009;13:1245–1250.
18. Rhee RY, Gloviczki P. Mesenteric venous thrombosis. *Surg Clin North Am* 1997;77:327–338.
19. Moawad J, Gewertz BL. Chronic mesenteric ischemia. Clinical presentation and diagnosis. *Surg Clin North Am* 1997;77:357–369.
20. Kumar S, Sarr MG, Kamath PS. Mesenteric venous thrombosis. *N Engl J Med* 2001;345:1683–1688.
21. Shih MCP, Hagspiel KD. CTA and MRA in mesenteric ischemia: part 1, role in diagnosis and differential diagnosis. *AJR Am J Roentgenol* 2007;188:452–461.
22. Bartnicke BJ, Balfe DM. CT appearance of intestinal ischemia and intramural hemorrhage. *Radiol Clin North Am* 1994;32:845–860.
23. Horton KM, Fishman EK. CT angiography of the mesenteric circulation. *Radiol Clin North Am* 2010;48:331–345.
24. Bradbury MS, Kavanagh PV, Bechtold RE, et al. Mesenteric venous thrombosis: diagnosis and noninvasive imaging. *Radiographics* 2002;22:527–541.
25. Abdu RA, Zakhour BJ, Dallis DJ. Mesenteric venous thrombosis—1911 to 1984. *Surgery* 1987;101:383–388.
26. Condat B, Pessione F, Helene Denninger M, et al. Recent portal or mesenteric venous thrombosis: increased recognition and frequent recanalization on anticoagulant therapy. *Hepatology* 2000;32:466–470.
27. Boley SJ, Kaleya RN, Brandt LJ. Mesenteric venous thrombosis. *Surg Clin North Am* 1992;72:183–201.
28. Mewissen MW, Seabrook GR, Meissner MH, et al. Catheter-directed thrombolysis for lower extremity deep venous thrombosis: report of a national multicenter registry. *Radiology* 1999;211:39–49.
29. Ferro C, Rossi UG, Bovio G, et al. Transjugular intrahepatic portosystemic shunt, mechanical aspiration thrombectomy, and direct thrombolysis in the treatment of acute portal and superior mesenteric vein thrombosis. *Cardiovasc Intervent Radiol* 2007;30:1070–1074.
30. Kim HS, Patra A, Khan J, et al. Transhepatic catheter-directed thrombectomy and thrombolysis of acute superior mesenteric venous thrombosis. *J Vasc Interv Radiol* 2005;16:1685–1691.
31. Takahashi N, Kuroki K, Yanaga K. Percutaneous transhepatic mechanical thrombectomy for acute mesenteric venous thrombosis. *J Endovasc Ther* 2005;12:508–511.
32. Winick AB, Waybill PN, Venbrux AC. Complications of percutaneous transhepatic biliary interventions. *Tech Vasc Interv Radiol* 2001;4:200–206.
33. Sze DY, O'Sullivan GJ, Johnson DL, et al. Mesenteric and portal venous thrombosis treated by transjugular mechanical thrombolysis. *AJR Am J Roentgenol* 2000;175:732–734.
34. Ryu R, Lin TC, Kumpe D, et al. Percutaneous mesenteric venous thrombectomy and thrombolysis: successful treatment followed by liver transplantation. *Liver Transpl Surg* 1998;4:222–225.
35. Semiz-Oysu A, Keussen I, Cwikiel W. Interventional radiological management of prehepatic obstruction of [corrected] the splanchnic venous system. *Cardiovasc Intervent Radiol* 2007;30:688–695.
36. Boyer TD, Haskal ZJ. American Association for the Study of Liver Diseases Practice Guidelines: the role of transjugular intrahepatic portosystemic shunt creation in the management of portal hypertension. *J Vasc Interv Radiol* 2005;16:615–629.
37. Rosado B, Kamath PS. Transjugular intrahepatic portosystemic shunts: an update. *Liver Transpl* 2003;9:207–217.
38. Train JS, Ross H, Weiss JD, et al. Mesenteric venous thrombosis: successful treatment by intraarterial lytic therapy. *J Vasc Interv Radiol* 1998;9:461–464.
39. Babu SC, Piccorelli GO, Shah PM, et al. Incidence and results of arterial complications among 16,350 patients undergoing cardiac catheterization. *J Vasc Surg* 1989;10:113–116.
40. Rosen MP, Sheiman R. Transhepatic mechanical thrombectomy followed by infusion of TPA into the superior mesenteric artery to treat acute mesenteric vein thrombosis. *J Vasc Interv Radiol* 2000;11:195–198.
41. Sehgal M, Haskal ZJ. Use of transjugular intrahepatic portosystemic shunts during lytic therapy of extensive portal splenic and mesenteric venous thrombosis: long-term follow-up. *J Vasc Interv Radiol* 2000;11:61–65.
42. Wang MQ, Liu FY, Duan F, et al. Acute symptomatic mesenteric venous thrombosis: treatment by catheter-directed thrombolysis with transjugular intrahepatic route. *Abdom Imaging* 2011;36(4):390–398.
43. Jona J, Cummins GM Jr, Head HB, et al. Recurrent primary mesenteric venous thrombosis. *JAMA* 1974;227:1033–1035.
44. Orr D, Harrison P, Devlin J, et al. Chronic mesenteric venous thrombosis: evaluation and determinants of survival during long-term follow-up. *Clin Gastroenterol Hepatol* 2007;5:80–86.

CHAPTER

88

End-Stage Renal Disease and Dialysis Access: Epidemiology, Natural History, and Diagnostic Monitoring

BART L. DOLMATCH, MIGUEL A. VAZQUEZ, and INGEMAR J. DAVIDSON

INTRODUCTION TO END-STAGE RENAL DISEASE: A GLOBAL PERSPECTIVE

The number of individuals treated for end-stage renal disease (ESRD) throughout the world continues growing each year. Although there is no international registry of ESRD, the data from the largest international provider of dialysis services, Fresenius Medical Center (FMC), are very informative. FMC reviewed data collected from 120 countries representing 92% of the world's population and 99% of all treated ESRD patients. By their estimate, the treated global ESRD population in 2005 was 1.9 million patients.[1] Using a projected annual growth rate of 6% to 7% (the rate observed for many years), an estimated 2 million people are treated for ESRD today. Some of these patients will get a kidney transplant but most of them require dialysis therapy (peritoneal dialysis or hemodialysis). In 2005, 89% of the world's dialysis population was treated with hemodialysis. Of course, these numbers do not recognize the vast global problem of ESRD, where many people receive no treatment at all.

END-STAGE RENAL DISEASE IN THE UNITED STATES

There are excellent data regarding treatment of ESRD in the United States. The reader is encouraged to visit the U.S. Renal Data System (USRDS) website, http://www.usrds.org,[2] to review the annual comprehensive report, which is available free to all interested. Each annual report is 2 years in arrears, so the 2010 USRDS reflects data from 2008. Data from the 2010 USRDS report are cited repeatedly throughout this chapter.

Beyond a succession of individual annual reports, the USRDS provides a longitudinal perspective of trends in renal disease, including data regarding morbidity, mortality, and cost of ESRD care. But data alone does not provide the reader a comprehensive understanding of where ESRD and renal replacement have been, nor where they are going. Furthermore, the USRDS does not include important clinical trial data that can help us understand the role of different therapies. Therefore, beyond

a distillation of the 2010 USRDS data, this chapter includes a review of recent clinical trial data and prevailing opinion regarding renal replacement therapies with a predominant focus on ESRD in the United States.

The 2010 Annual USRDS report[2] demonstrates unabated growth in the number of people with ESRD in the United States between 1980 and 2008. In 1980 there were approximately 60,000 ESRD patients receiving renal replacement therapy, whereas in 2008 this population had increased to 547,982—nearly a 10-fold growth. Given a global estimate of 2 million people treated for ESRD, about one-quarter of all treated ESRD patients reside in the United States. There were 382,343 people receiving dialysis in 2008 (hemodialysis and peritoneal dialysis), up 34.7% from 2000. Hemodialysis was far more common than peritoneal dialysis with 354,600 patients undergoing hemodialysis but only 26,517 patients on peritoneal dialysis (FIGURE 88.1). Initiation of renal replacement in 2008 comprised 102,876 ESRD patients starting hemodialysis, 6,577 starting peritoneal dialysis, and 2,644 receiving a preemptive kidney transplant. On the bright side, 161,022 ESRD patients had a functioning kidney transplant by the end of 2008, accounting for nearly 30% of all ESRD patients.

ESRD is associated with high morbidity, mortality, and cost. Untreated, the survival of patients with ESRD is grim. Renal replacement consists of either dialysis or kidney transplantation. Compared to patients who receive a kidney transplant, dialysis patients have worse survival, are hospitalized more, and incur higher costs to the health care system. The 2010 USRDS annual report notes that only one in three patients who started dialysis between 1999 and 2003 survived 5 years. Overall unadjusted survival for hemodialysis is roughly the same as for peritoneal dialysis, and both cardiovascular disease and infection account for much of this mortality, although cardiovascular mortality now exceeds infection-related death. It is estimated that the annual adjusted all-cause mortality for dialysis patients was 6.4 to 7.8 times higher than for the general population, and that mortality for transplant patients was increased by a factor of 1.2 to 1.5. Higher mortality rates are seen in certain ESRD subpopulations, including both elderly patients and patients with

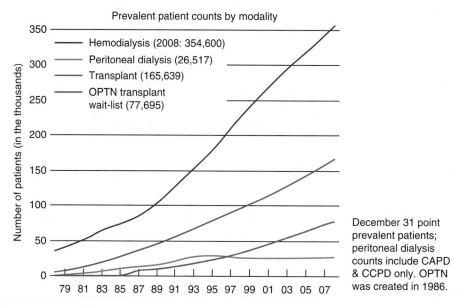

FIGURE 88.1 Prevalence of ESRD patients by modality. Hemodialysis is by far the most prevalent form of renal replacement, followed by transplant and peritoneal dialysis.

From U.S. Renal Data System. *USRDS 2010 Annual Data Report: Atlas of Chronic Kidney Disease and End-Stage Renal Disease in the United States.* Bethesda, MD: National Institutes of Health, National Institute of Diabetes and Digestive and Kidney Diseases; 2010. Available at: http://www.usrds.org.

coexistent diabetes, likely due to a higher incidence of cardiovascular disease in these subgroups.

According to the 2010 USRDS annual report the total cost for the ESRD program in the United States in 2008 was $34.96 billion with Medicare paying about three-quarters of the cost, or $26.8 billion. Most Medicare payments were for dialysis patients, of which $19.4 billion was attributable to care for

those on hemodialysis (FIGURE 88.2). Medicare-related ESRD costs increased 13.2% in 2008 from the prior year and accounted for 5.9% of the Medicare budget. Per-person per-year Medicare costs ranged from $26,668 for transplant patients to $77,506 for hemodialysis patients in 2008. Another way to look at the magnitude cost due to kidney disease in the United States is that 31% of all Medicare expenditures in 2008 were incurred by patients

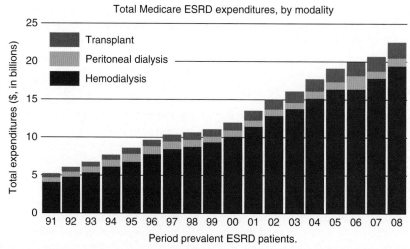

FIGURE 88.2 Medicare expenditures for ESRD, by modality, from 1991 to 2008. Modalities determined using Model 1 methodology. Includes Medicare paid claims for ESRD patients, starting at first ESRD service date & continuing until death or the end of the study period. Patients with Medicare as secondary payor are included.

From U.S. Renal Data System. *USRDS 2010 Annual Data Report: Atlas of Chronic Kidney Disease and End-Stage Renal Disease in the United States* . Bethesda, MD: National Institutes of Health, National Institute of Diabetes and Digestive and Kidney Diseases; 2010. Available at: http://www.usrds.org.

with a diagnosis of kidney disease, including patients with renal impairment not yet requiring renal replacement as well as other renal problems not requiring treatment with dialysis.

RENAL REPLACEMENT: TRANSPLANTATION

Kidney transplantation is the optimal form of renal replacement therapy. However, there are many more potential recipients than available kidneys. Furthermore, some patients are too sick or have comorbidities that preclude transplantation. In 2008 the number of patients waiting to receive a kidney reached 77,695 but there were only 17,413 transplants performed that year. The median wait time to receive a kidney transplant in 2008 was 732 days[2] during which time survival for most patients depended on dialysis. The United Network for Organ Sharing (UNOS) controls allocation of cadaveric kidneys within the United States. It has recently proposed modification to the kidney allocation program. One proposal is allocating the highest-quality kidneys to candidates with the highest estimated post-transplant survival (younger patients). Another consideration is to allocate kidneys preferentially to recipients who are within 15 years (older or younger) of the donor's age. There are ethical and practical issues in every change regarding kidney allocation. If adopted, these changes may reduce waiting times for some, whereas other people may wait much longer for a cadaveric kidney transplant. Still, the need for kidneys far exceeds the supply, and this need increases every year.

RENAL REPLACEMENT: PERITONEAL DIALYSIS

Despite the many advantages of peritoneal dialysis over hemodialysis, such as ease of implementation at home, lower cost, certain health-related benefits, and lower modality-related complication rates, peritoneal dialysis represents renal replacement therapy for only 6% of the ESRD population in the United States.[2] Furthermore, peritoneal dialysis has become less prevalent over time, down from its peak of nearly 15% of ESRD patients in 1982 to 1984. This decline is related to a number of factors including lack of financial incentives for physicians (compared to hemodialysis) as well as greater emphasis on hemodialysis during the training of nephrologists. Furthermore, many patients are not adequately informed about peritoneal dialysis, decline this therapy, or are not suitable for it. There is speculation that peritoneal dialysis may become more prevalent if ESRD reimbursement goes from a system of per-incident payment to one that provides annual capitated coverage.[2] Under a capitated system, peritoneal dialysis may become more prevalent because it is far less expensive than hemodialysis. Increased use of peritoneal dialysis, however, remains to be seen.

RENAL REPLACEMENT: HEMODIALYSIS

Human hemodialysis was first performed by Dr. Georg Haas in Giessen, Germany, in 1924 and lasted only 15 minutes.[3] Since then, many investigators and advances have contributed to the acceptance of hemodialysis as a clinically acceptable form of renal replacement. A clear and concise historical overview of hemodialysis has recently been published by Konner.[4]

Without reliable methods for accessing and cycling a patient's blood through the dialyzer, repeated hemodialysis as an effective form of renal replacement would not have developed. Today there are three types of hemodialysis access: central

venous catheters, arteriovenous fistulas (AVFs), and arteriovenous grafts (AVGs).

Catheter Access

Dual lumen catheters are the simplest and most pain-free form of hemodialysis access. But compared to AVFs, catheters are far more morbid and pose greater long-term risk to the patient. Infection is eightfold more common for ESRD patients using a nontunneled catheter and fivefold higher for cuffed catheter patients when compared to infections encountered in those using an AVF.[5] Hospitalization rates are also significantly higher in catheter patients.[6] Finally, patients who use a catheter for hemodialysis have higher mortality rates than those using an AVF or an AVG.[7,8] When catheter patients are switched to permanent access (AVF or AVG), mortality is reduced by about 50%.[9]

Cost related to catheter use is also significant. The per-person per-year total expenditure, by access type, is greatest for catheter patients, followed by patients with AVGs and AVFs ($90,110, $79,337, and $64,701, respectively) (FIGURE 88.3). Increase in cost for care from 2007 to 2008, by access type, was greatest for patients with catheters (12.8%), whereas total expenditures for patients with AVFs and AVGs increased from 8.2% to 8.6%.[2]

The high per-person per-year expenditure for catheter patients is related not only to catheter-related infections and hospitalizations, but to catheter dysfunction as well. Dysfunction occurs in a variety of ways. Complete catheter occlusion or dislodgment is easily recognized and requires correction before dialysis can be performed. For many ESRD patients, however, their catheter cannot sustain adequate flow rates for effective dialysis. In one study, inadequate dialysis, defined as poor urea clearance of less than 1.2 Kt/V, was seen in 25.2% of patients using a catheter, whereas this was seen in only 9.7% of patients with permanent access.[10] Inadequate catheter flow rates may occur when the catheter tip is enveloped by a tissue sheath, when the catheter lumen is only partially obstructed by thrombus, or when the catheter tip is malpositioned against the venous or atrial wall. To restore adequate flow, additional procedures are often performed, including catheter exchange, tissue sheath disruption, thrombolytic instillation or infusion, catheter stripping, or new catheter placement. Beyond the cost of these procedures, there is the underappreciated cost of inadequate dialysis including fluid, electrolyte, and uremic complications.

Given significant morbidity and cost for catheter-delivered hemodialysis, it is startling that 80% of patients who initiated hemodialysis in an outpatient setting in 2008 used a catheter for vascular access, and most of these patients had not yet undergone surgery for permanent AV access (FIGURE 88.4). Perhaps of even greater concern is that catheter rates in the United States and most of Western Europe have actually increased during the past decade. In the United States, between 1996 and 2007, the catheter prevalence rate had risen from 14% to 23%.[11] The reason(s) for this increase are controversial. Some attribute it to prolonged catheter dwell times related to increased AVF incidence (along with the additive effect of new ESRD patients receiving a catheter to initiate dialysis). However, Fistula First advocates counter this with data showing that increased catheter prevalence is not directly related to the success of their program creating more AVFs.[12]

The most plausible explanation for increased catheter prevalence during the past decade is lack of early AV access planning.

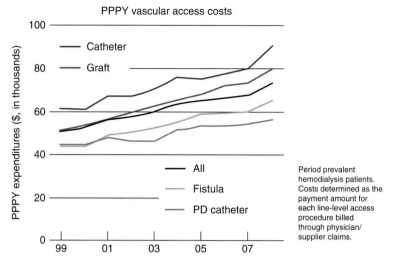

FIGURE 88.3 Per-person per-year (PPPY) vascular access costs showing that hemodialysis patients who use a catheter have the greatest cost of all dialysis patient groups by access type. The lowest cost by hemodialysis access type is for patients with an AVF. However, when considering all forms of dialysis, peritoneal dialysis has the lowest per-person per-year cost.

From U.S. Renal Data System. *USRDS 2010 Annual Data Report: Atlas of Chronic Kidney Disease and End-Stage Renal Disease in the United States*. Bethesda, MD: National Institutes of Health, National Institute of Diabetes and Digestive and Kidney Diseases; 2010. Available at: http://www.usrds.org.

The 2010 USRDS report shows that when patients had no pre-ESRD care, 83% initiated outpatient dialysis with a catheter, and only 2.8% used an AVF.[2] However, patients who were appropriately triaged for renal care in advance of their need for dialysis had much lower catheter prevalence. Only 44% of patients who had been under the care of a nephrologist for at least 12 months prior to initiation of hemodialysis used a catheter for their first outpatient dialysis treatment, whereas 30% initiated with an AVF (FIGURE 88.5). This indicates that preemptive AV access planning can effectively reduce catheter prevalence. Therefore, efforts must be directed toward the broad medical community, encouraging early referral for nephrology care long before dialysis is required. With forethought and planning it is hoped that catheter prevalence rates in the United States can be reduced.

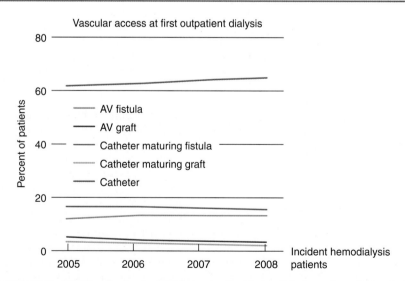

FIGURE 88.4 In 2008, 65% of ESRD patients who initiated outpatient hemodialysis used a catheter. Catheter prevalence has increased in the United States for the past decade and is also noted in this graph between 2005 and 2008.

From U.S. Renal Data System. *USRDS 2010 Annual Data Report: Atlas of Chronic Kidney Disease and End-Stage Renal Disease in the United States*. Bethesda, MD: National Institutes of Health, National Institute of Diabetes and Digestive and Kidney Diseases; 2010. Available at: http://www.usrds.org.

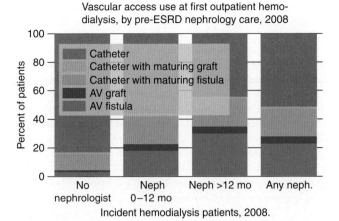

Vascular access use at first outpatient hemo-dialysis, by pre-ESRD nephrology care, 2008

FIGURE 88.5 Vascular access use at first outpatient hemodialysis is influenced by pre-ESRD nephrology care. The lowest prevalence of catheter use is seen when ESRD patients have seen a nephrologist for longer than 12 months, whereas the highest catheter prevalence is seen in the absence of nephrologist care.

From U.S. Renal Data System. *USRDS 2010 Annual Data Report: Atlas of Chronic Kidney Disease and End-Stage Renal Disease in the United States.* Bethesda, MD: National Institutes of Health, National Institute of Diabetes and Digestive and Kidney Diseases; 2010. Available at: http://www.usrds.org.

Arteriovenous Fistula Access

This form of vascular access was first described in 1966 by Brescia, Cimino, and colleagues, and led the way for broad use of hemodialysis. In their landmark publication, the authors reported creation of 14 radiocephalic AVFs for hemodialysis access.[13] In fact, the radiocephalic fistula is commonly called a Brescia-Cimino fistula, although it was third author of that paper, Kenneth Appel, who performed the surgeries. Regardless, this type of AVF has been used successfully for hemodialysis access for over 40 years. Since this initial report of the radiocephalic fistula, the brachiocephalic fistula and brachiobasilic fistula have also been popularized for vascular access. Beyond these three dominant types of endogenous AV access circuits, a number of modifications have been described using perforating arm veins and lower extremity veins to create AVFs.

There is consensus that an AVF that is usable for hemodialysis represents the best form of vascular access from cost, safety, and durability perspectives. The per-person per-year cost for patients with an AVF is roughly 60% of that for patients who used either a catheter or an AVG (FIGURE 88.3). A usable AVF also has a lower rate of infection when compared to either a catheter or an AVG.[14]

Although the advantages of a usable AVF have been appreciated for many years, AVFs were not prevalent in the United States until the past few years. Data from the Dialysis Outcomes Practice Patterns Study (DOPPS) showed the discrepancy between AVF prevalence in the United States and Western Europe.[15] During the late 1990s, AVF prevalence in the United States was only 24%, whereas it was 67% in the United Kingdom, 77% in France, 82% in Spain, 84% in Germany, and 90% in Italy. Prevalence of AVGs during that time was 58% in the United States but only 4% to 15% in Western Europe. These data, along with mounting evidence that a usable AVF was

superior to an AVG, led to the push for change in the United States. In 1997, the National Kidney Foundation (NKF) published the first Dialysis Outcomes Quality Initiative, or NKF-K/DOQI, guidelines and recommended target goals of 50% AVF incidence and 40% AVF prevalence.[16] Progress was modest until 2003, when collaboration between the ESRD networks and the Centers for Medicare and Medicaid Services (CMS) embarked on a National Vascular Access Improvement Initiative. This initiative, now called the Fistula First Breakthrough Initiative (FFBI), brought the payor (CMS) into a strategy to increase the incidence and prevalence of AVFs in the United States. The FFI website[17] now reports that the proposed 50% target prevalence for AVFs has been surpassed (57.4% AVF prevalence in the United States, November 2010) and believes that an AVF prevalence of 66% in the United States is realistic. Although the reported prevalence of AVFs now exceeds the original FFI target, the actual prevalence of usable AVFs is not known. Regardless, it is clear that the FFI has had an important impact on tilting the prevalence of permanent AV access in the United States toward the AVF and away from the AVG.

We have repeatedly stressed that a usable AVF is superior to an AVG or catheter, and it represents the best form of AV access for hemodialysis. However, not all AVFs will be usable for hemodialysis. The problem of unusable AVFs has been recognized for many years and was even described in 2 of the 14 radiocephalic AVFs in Brescia and Cimino's first report.[13] Therefore, the superiority of an AVF over an AVG (or even a catheter) is not so clear when one looks at all AVFs created, including those that cannot be used for hemodialysis.

Failure of an AVF to become usable for hemodialysis, noted during the first few months after surgery, usually leads to alternate hemodialysis access. For patients who must start dialysis, it may lead to catheter initiation of hemodialysis. For patients who have already initiated dialysis with a catheter, it may lead to extended catheter use. Some AVFs will "mature" over time without treatment, whereas others require additional intervention to allow their successful use for hemodialysis. A subset of AVFs will never be useful and must be abandoned.

There are many causes of early AVF failure, including inadequate arterial inflow, veins that do not dilate sufficiently after surgery, technical issues during surgery, anatomic factors (including small veins, deep veins, or multiple "accessory" veins), development of early postoperative venous stenosis in the precannulation zone (juxta-anastomotic stenosis), poor cardiac output, and variation in cannulation skill at the dialysis center. At least, that is the beginning of the list. At this time, a multicenter prospective study, funded by the National Institutes of Health (NIH), is underway to characterize early AVF failure in the United States. It is hoped that we will have a much clearer picture of this problem when results from that study are available.

From 1995 to 2002, most reports described early AVF failure in about 20% to 50% of all newly created fistulas, as clearly summarized in a review by Allon and Robbin.[18] However, a recent prospective, multicenter U.S. clinical trial suggests that early failure may be an even greater problem today. Using the precise definition for early failure as the inability to use the AVF for dialysis with two needles while maintaining a dialysis machine blood flow rate adequate for optimal dialysis (≥300 mL/min) during 8 of 12 dialysis sessions occurring during a 30-day suitability ascertainment period (typically 120 to 150 days after fistula surgery), Dember and colleagues found that the AVF early failure rate was about 60%.[19] Furthermore, about half of these AVFs were abandoned.

When one considers all AVFs on an "intent-to-use" basis, their patency may be not be superior to that of AVGs. In fact, Maya and colleagues reported exactly this sort of analysis regarding a series of upper arm AVFs compared with upper arm AVGs.[14] Their prospective database included 322 brachiocephalic AVFs and 289 upper arm AVGs. Retrospective review of that database found a 38% rate of early brachiocephalic fistula failure, whereas early AVG failure was only 15%. Patency analysis was performed using two methods: one excluding early failures and the other including them. When early failure was not included, the brachiocephalic AVF median cumulative survival was 3.4 years, which was statistically superior to a reported AVG survival of 1.6 years ($p = .01$). However, when all early failures were included in the analysis (looking at patency on an intent-to-use basis) the median cumulative survival for both the brachiocephalic AVF group and the AVG group was approximately 1 year, and primary patency of the AV access of each group was 40% at 2 years with overlapping rates of attrition (late AV access failure) for both groups to 900 days. So although a usable AVF (with no early failure) is superior to an AVG, the reality is that early failure is a very real problem. When successful use of an access is considered from the time of surgery rather than the time of first successful use for dialysis, cumulative patency of an AVF may be no better than an AVG.

Many more usable AVFs are needed, and various strategies have been developed to avoid early AVF failure. One approach has been preoperative vascular mapping with the hope that identification of suitable arteries and veins for AVF creation can reduce early problems. Using venography and ultrasound, preoperative vascular mapping can effectively increase the incidence of AVF creation in a surgical practice, but, unfortunately, early AVF failure rates have not been reduced.[20,21]

There are no simple explanations for the limited impact of vascular mapping on early AVF failures. Perhaps the parameters for vascular measurement have not optimized for predicting usable AVFs. Maybe there is an "information gap" where vascular mapping results obtained in the noninvasive vascular setting are not fully incorporated into the operative approach at the time of surgery. There is also the possibility that early failure will always be part of AVF creation, and that when AVF incidence increases then AVF early failures will also rise.

Data, however, suggest that early AVF failure is not a "constant," and that it indeed can be reduced. Surgical "experience" seems to be an important determinant. Ernandez et al.[22] showed that early AVF failure rates were significantly lower for surgeons who did more AVF surgery. Huijbregts et al.,[23] in a study that controlled for patient demographics, demonstrated far less early AVF failure at some of their surgical centers compared to others. The findings from these two studies, and other investigations,[24-26] show that surgical judgment and ability *do* matter and that outcomes at surgical centers where talented surgeons practice will likely be superior. Now, the challenge is to identify specific variables that, when optimized and disseminated among surgeons and centers, will lead to improved success in creating usable AVFs around the world.

In summary, a usable AVF is the best form of permanent hemodialysis access when one considers cost, safety, and durability. However, many newly created AVFs—up to 60% of them—will not be usable for hemodialysis during the first 4 to 5 months after surgery and many of them will be abandoned. Efforts to reduce early failure will be based on a greater understanding of the factors that cause it. Outcomes from an ongoing NIH study on early AVF failure are eagerly anticipated. The problem of early AVF failure, however, is not only attributable to unfavorable anatomy and physiology. More usable AVFs can be created by surgeons with greater experience, reflecting the combined value of good preoperative planning and technical skill. Therefore, achieving more usable AVFs will not likely happen because of a single recommendation, but rather a combination of changes. Toward this end, the FFBI has outlined 13 "change concepts" that they believe can increase AVF prevalence and hopefully reduce early failure.[17]

Arteriovenous Graft Access

Ten years after Brescia and colleagues described the AVF, Baker et al.[27] reported a new type of hemodialysis access, the AVG. The AVG is created by diverting flow from an artery to a vein using an interpositioned vascular conduit. Expanded polytetrafluoroethylene (ePTFE) conduit was used for their AVGs, although other conduits, such as bovine carotid heterograft, have since been reported by others. Over the ensuing 20 years, ePTFE AVGs became far more prevalent than AVFs in the United States, whereas AVFs were more prevalent than AVGs in Europe.[15] During the past decade, however, the prevalence of AVGs in the United States has been diminishing due to success of the FFBI. Still, if one assumes an AVG prevalence today of approximately 20% and there are 350,000 hemodialysis patients in the United States, then about 70,000 people depend on their AVG for dialysis access in the United States.

Unlike AVFs, where early failure is a considerable problem, most AVGs will be usable for hemodialysis within a month or two after surgery with an approximate 10% to 15% rate of early failure or abandonment.[14,18]

Although loss of AVG patency is not typical during the early months, it is a significant problem thereafter. In their recent multicenter prospective study of AVGs, Dixon et al.[28] demonstrated that only 25% of AVGs remained primarily patent 1 year after surgery (23% in the placebo group and 28% in the group taking dipyridamole-aspirin). This finding was remarkably similar to that reported 10 years earlier by Miller et al.,[29] where primary patency was 23% at 1 year in their single center review of 256 AVGs. Furthermore, primary patency at 2 years in their series was only 4%.

Loss of patency is usually caused by stenosis. Typically, patency can be restored by treating the stenosis surgically or with percutaneous transluminal angioplasty (PTA). Today, PTA is the more common type of treatment. Past literature, largely single center and retrospective, describes 6-month post-PTA primary patency of around 40% to 50% for AVGs.[30-34] Based on these, and other similar reports, the NKF-K/DOQI guidelines suggest a target 6-month primary patency rate of at least 50% after AVG angioplasty for practitioners who perform this procedure.[35]

There have been some encouraging results from trials to test interventions to prolong AVG patency after PTA. The Cutting Edge Trial[34] could not demonstrate better durability after treatment of AVGs using the peripheral cutting balloon when compared to PTA alone. Recently, though, a prospective multicenter

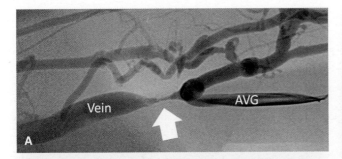

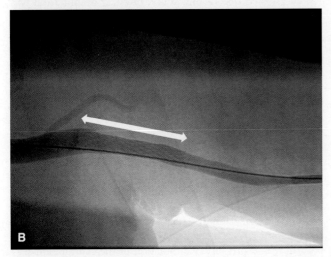

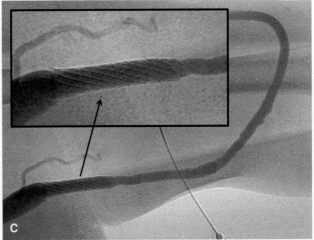

FIGURE 88.6 A. Stenosis at the venous anastomosis of an AVG (*arrow*) before treatment. AVG, arteriovenous graft; Vein, outflow vein central to the graft-to-vein anastomosis. **B.** A covered stent has been placed at the PTA site (*double-headed arrow*). **C.** Five-month angiographic follow-up (done for evaluation of a central venous stenosis that had caused arm swelling). The covered stent is patent with no appreciable restenosis (*arrow* pointing to covered stent in the **inset**).

randomized comparative trial between PTA or PTA with immediate placement of a covered stent at the PTA site demonstrated significant benefit for the covered stent group (FIGURE 88.6A–C). AVG circuit 6-month postprocedure primary patency was doubled for patients who were treated with the covered stent, and there was superior freedom from further intervention.[36] Although use of a covered stent immediately after a technically successful PTA may seem to deviate from traditional practice, it is believed that the expense of doing this will be offset by a reduction in the number of costly future interventions required to maintain AVG patency.

Another cause of patency loss is thrombosis, typically secondary to underlying stenosis. Various techniques for declotting AVGs have been described, but once clot has been successfully removed or disrupted, PTA is typically used to treat an underlying stenosis. Although declotting followed by PTA affords an 80% to a 95% success rate in returning patients for their first postprocedure dialysis session, patency thereafter is poor.[37–41] Most series describe a 3-month postprocedure clinical patency in the range of 30% to 50%. Largely based on these reports, the NKF-K/DOQI guidelines for vascular access recommend a 3-month 40% patency rate after successful treatment of a clotted graft by catheter-based technique.[35] This is probably one of the least durable vascular procedures performed anywhere in the circulatory system, although it persists because there are few alternatives beyond surgical revision or new AV access placement.

AVG patency may also be lost because of infection, with or without thrombosis. AVGs are more prone to infection compared to AVFs,[42] and although it may be possible to salvage some infected prosthetic AVGs with antibiotics alone,[43] most will need to be partially or completely resected. Most patients with an infected AVG require hospitalization. In their review of 90 infected AVGs, Minga and colleagues reported hospitalization for a mean of 7.5 days.[44] Beyond the loss of AV access, an AVG infection is expensive owing to the need for surgery and hospitalization.

Largely because of recurrent treatments for stenosis, thrombosis, and infection, the per-person per-year event costs are greatest for AVGs, followed by catheters, then AVFs (FIGURE 88.7). Frequent procedures are needed to maintain stenotic and thrombosed AVGs. Miller et al.[29] found a mean of 1.22 interventions per graft-year to maintain AVG function.

Despite disadvantages of an AVG compared to a usable AVF, some patients may not have suitable vascular anatomy for an AVF. For these patients, an AVG may be the only option for permanent hemodialysis. Beyond anatomic factors that may lead to AVG placement, there is growing awareness that certain clinical factors favor an AVG even when an AVF could be made. Lok et al.[45] determined that age of 65 or greater, presence of peripheral vascular disease or coronary artery disease, or non-Caucasian ethnicity were factors that made it less likely that an AVF would be usable for hemodialysis. Combinations of these factors further increased the risk of early AVF failure. From their initial study Lok et al. developed a risk equation, assigning scores for the presence or absence of each of these factors. Finally, they conducted a validation clinical trial in 445 patients and successfully used their equation to predict the likelihood of AVF failure in different risk groups. So although an AVF in an elderly, non-Caucasian patient with peripheral and coronary

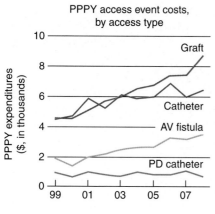

FIGURE 88.7 The per-person per-year (PPPY) cost associated with access events is greatest for an AVG.

From U.S. Renal Data System. *USRDS 2010 Annual Data Report: Atlas of Chronic Kidney Disease and End-Stage Renal Disease in the United States.* Bethesda, MD: National Institutes of Health, National Institute of Diabetes and Digestive and Kidney Diseases; 2010. Available at: http://www.usrds.org.

artery disease may successfully mature for cannulation within the first few postoperative months, many similar patients will not be so fortunate; therefore, all access options should be carefully considered.

Through success of the Fistula First program, the prevalence of AVGs has contracted over the past decade although it is not likely that they will disappear entirely. The ultimate goal is to create successful dialysis access, selecting the best option from all possibilities. For some patients, an AVG may be the most successful form of vascular access, whereas for others a tunneled hemodialysis catheter or a peritoneal dialysis may be better options. When considering renal replacement therapy, a patient-centered algorithm rather than a modality-centered approach should be used.[46]

MONITORING AND SURVEILLANCE OF PERMANENT ARTERIOVENOUS ACCESS

Monitoring is defined as using techniques or tests that are readily and routinely available in the dialysis unit to evaluate AV access, particularly physical examination. Surveillance invokes periodic use of specialized equipment or specially trained staff, or both, for AV access evaluation. Whether one uses monitoring or surveillance, the goal is to detect early signs of AV access stenosis before dialysis becomes inadequate or the AV access clots. A comprehensive review of both monitoring and surveillance of permanent AV access can be found in the 2006 NKF-K/DOQI vascular access clinical practice guidelines and recommendations with specific reference to guideline 4: Detection of Access Dysfunction: Monitoring, Surveillance, and Diagnostic Testing.[35]

Although the value of monitoring and surveillance of permanent AV access remains controversial, as discussed later in this section, current policy from CMS is unequivocal. CMS mandates routine monitoring and surveillance of both AVFs and AVGs, requiring it as a condition for Medicare coverage of ESRD facilities.[47,48] Its policy states that the facility ". . . must have an ongoing program for vascular access monitoring and surveillance for

early detection of failure and to allow timely referral of patients for intervention when indications of significant stenosis are present." For its purposes, CMS considers monitoring strategies to include physical examination, observance of changes in dialysis adequacy, as well as difficult cannulation, or difficulty in achieving hemostasis after cannulation. Surveillance includes device-based methods, such as access flow measurement, direct or derived static pressure ratios, and duplex ultrasound.

There is little argument that routine physical examination of AV access is important. It is also sensitive for detection of AV access stenosis. In one study, physical examination was as good as ultrasound for stenosis detection.[49] Other studies have validated physical examination for detection of stenosis in both AVFs and AVGs, using fistulography as the reference standard.[50,51] Examination of AV access may be done in various ways and examiner skills differ, yielding a wide range of sensitivity and specificity for detection of stenosis by different examiners. To address these issues, both Beathard[52] and Gelbfish[53] have described standardized approaches for AV access examination. The reader is directed to these two references for a review of examination techniques and discussion of significant findings.

Regardless of the precise method used for examination of permanent AV access, the exam should always include assessment of arterial inflow, the cannulation segment, and venous outflow. Early failure of an AVF may be caused by arterial stenosis or juxta-anastomotic stenosis, in which case the physical examination reveals a collapsible cannulation segment due to poor flow and pressure. Examination of the cannulation segment should include signs of impending skin breakdown or pseudoaneurysm formation where the cannulation was performed. Loss of the arteriovenous "thrill" or vibration is indicative of outflow venous stenosis and is often seen with increased pulsation of the cannulation segment. Signs and symptoms of arterial hypoperfusion, or "steal" syndrome, include diminished peripheral pulses, loss of muscle mass, and, in advanced cases, ischemic skin changes and neuropathy. Finally, central venous obstruction, often related to prior central venous dialysis catheters, is manifest as swelling of the extremity with engorged subcutaneous venous collaterals.

Overall, a physical examination has a high positive predictive value (69% to 93%) for detecting angiographically proven stenosis.[54] It costs nothing, it can be done anywhere, and it should be an integral part of care in the hemodialysis unit. It may also be useful for predicting outcome following treatment of AV access stenosis. Trerotola and colleagues[55] found that physical examination of the AV access following PTA predicts outcome as reliably as immediate post-PTA pressure measurements.

Although useful and required, the physical examination is subjective and qualitative, the skill of the examiner is variable, and examination may not be routinely performed in some dialysis centers. For these reasons, other monitoring methods have focused on problems related to cannulation that can be quantified, such as difficult cannulation or prolonged time to achieve hemostasis after cannulation (>20 or 30 minutes after needle removal). In one study of AVGs, the positive predictive value for detecting a stenosis was 76% for prolonged bleeding, 58% for difficult cannulation, and 80%, overall, for physical examination.[56]

Monitoring can also be done by looking at dialysis adequacy, which is measured by urea reduction. Simply explained, AV access outflow stenosis reduces blood flow in the access so that dialyzed blood has time to mix with blood that has not yet been dialyzed. This "recirculation" of dialyzed blood reduces the efficiency of dialysis and can be measured by less urea reduction from the patient's circulating blood volume. Reduced urea reduction is calculated using blood samples from the patient, noting blood urea nitrogen (BUN) values from the arterial and venous cannulate and the systemic BUN level with the formula:

$$\text{Percentage recirculation} = \frac{\text{BUN}_{\text{systemic}} - \text{BUN}_{\text{arterial}}}{\text{BUN}_{\text{systemic}} - \text{BUN}_{\text{venous}}} \times 100\%$$

When the percentage recirculation is greater than 10% a stenosis should be suspected.[57] However, consistency of this method is poor for surveillance of access stenosis.[58]

Surveillance, using specialized tools or personnel, can be done by employing indirect or direct techniques. Indirect surveillance attempts to correlate some measure of AV access function (pressure or flow) with underlying stenosis. These techniques are usually done in the dialysis unit. Pressure measurements include static and dynamic methods. The static venous pressure ratio (SVPR) is calculated from pressure measurements obtained while the patient is not being dialyzed. Intra-access pressure is obtained through one of the cannulation needles and normalized to the systemic blood pressure. Calculation of the ratio of the two pressures yields the SVPR, which increases with progressive degrees of venous outflow stenosis.[59-61] Although a single ratio may suggest stenosis, it is analysis of the trend in a patient over time that is more reliable.[35]

Dynamic pressure measurements, which are not used as widely as static ones, call for measurement of intra-access pressure during the beginning of dialysis using a reduced dialytic blood flow rate (200 to 250 mL/minute). By comparing this pressure with baseline dynamic pressure measurements determined at an earlier time when the AV access was presumed to be patent, persistent changes of subsequent dynamic pressures on three successive sessions can predict stenosis.[61]

Whereas pressure measurements were widely used in the 1990s, current surveillance in the dialysis unit is often done with flow measurement. Using any of the techniques based on the Fick principle of dye dilution, saline is injected from the "upstream" cannulation needle ("arterial" cannula). With high flow, the effect of dilution within the access will resolve quickly, but with poor flow it will take longer to resolve. By measuring the rate of resolution and calculating the area under this curve, access blood flow can be determined. Initial flow measurements were done with a thermodilution technique,[62] but other dilution methods have also been described, such as ultrasound-detected flow velocity dilution.

Another method of flow determination, in-line measurement of flow with conductivity dialysance (also called ionic dialysance) provides flow measurements comparable to dilution techniques.[63,64] Therefore, accurate blood flow can be measured with either a Fick dilution method or an in-line technique. Either way, if parameters, such as AV access blood flow less than 600 mL/minute or a drop of blood flow greater than 25% over time are used, prediction of stensosis and thrombosis has been validated.[65,66]

Direct techniques of flow measurement are typically too cumbersome or expensive to perform in the dialysis center and are therefore not as widely used for surveillance. These techniques include duplex Doppler examination and, on occasion, magnetic resonance angiography (MRA). Nevertheless, both techniques are worth a brief review because they are in the realm of the radiologist.

Duplex ultrasound study has been validated for surveillance of AV access. Flow velocity measurements, luminal diameter reduction, and flow volume measurements are all found to be useful. Regarding flow velocity, peak systolic velocity (PSV) measurements are most often used for determination of significant stenosis. When the PSV at a stenosis is greater than or equal to two times the PSV immediately upstream, the positive predictive value for an angiographically demonstrated stenosis in a study of AVGs was 80%.[56] PSV greater than 4 meters/second is also often seen at angiographically proven stenoses that have a diameter reduction of greater than 50% of a normal reference segment. Direct visualization of a stenosis is also useful with significance usually attributed to luminal diameter narrowing of 50% or more. Finally, duplex ultrasound can be used reliably to measure AV access flow volume. Concordance with dilution methods has been established.[67] Duplex ultrasound findings correlate well with angiographically demonstrated stenosis.[68-70]

MRA has been used to detect AV access stenosis. Gadolinium contrast-enhanced MRA (CE-MRA) can accurately delineate stenoses.[71] Recent concern for nephrogenic systemic fibrosis associated with gadolinium in azotemic patients, however, will render CE-MRA obsolete for surveillance. It is possible to obtain accurate AV access MRA studies without gadolinium.[72] The reality, though, is that surveillance with MRA is expensive and often difficult to schedule. Without compelling reasons to perform these studies, surveillance of AV access with MR techniques is just not realistic.

Although there are many monitoring and surveillance techniques that can detect AV access stenosis, the ultimate question is whether any of this matters. Does detection of stenosis by any method lead to intervention that prolongs AV access patency? Casey and colleagues[73] recently published a meta-analysis of monitoring and surveillance of AV access. They searched various online databases and found only nine studies that met their criteria for analysis. Their conclusion was that there is only weak evidence yielding imprecise results that suggests surveillance prolongs AV access patency. Robbin et al[74] reviewed current concepts of AV access monitoring and surveillance. They also noted that although many techniques can detect stenosis, preemptive PTA has not reduced graft thrombosis and, therefore, the role of monitoring and surveillance is unclear. The goal, as they see it, is to detect those stenoses that will cause AV access thrombosis and then preemptively treat only those stenoses with a method that affords better patency.

Given concerns that not all stenoses lead to thrombosis, and that PTA of stenosis has not been shown to improve AV access patency, the mandate from CMS to perform routine monitoring and surveillance has been challenged. In a provocative paper entitled "Controversial Vascular Access Surveillance Mandate," Paulson and Work[75] review the shortcomings of surveillance and state that it does not prolong graft or fistula life, does not reduce graft thrombosis, and may lead to many unnecessary procedures. They propose using only physical examination (monitoring) and believe that surveillance needs further study before it is mandated. The final word on monitoring and surveillance has yet to be spoken.

CONCLUSION

ESRD has become a global problem of significance. In the United States there has been unremitting growth in the number of people with renal failure, and the cost for providing ESRD care represents a significant portion of the health care dollar. Kidney transplantation is the optimal solution, but most patients will not receive a kidney because there are not enough organs available. Most people wait for years before receiving a transplant during which time they usually rely on dialysis. Peritoneal dialysis, an effective and less expensive renal replacement solution than hemodialysis, is used by only 6% of ESRD patients in the United States—down from 15% in the mid-1980s. Hemodialysis is the most prevalent solution, but vascular access for hemodialysis remains a source of frustration, morbidity, mortality, and cost. A usable AVF is the best form of access from both clinical and cost perspectives, but as many as 60% of new AVFs will have early failure and up to half of these may need to be abandoned. An AVG has a much lower early failure rate than an AVF, but it requires more procedures to maintain overall patency and is more prone to infection. The per-person per-year costs for an AVG are greater than for a usable AVFs. However, an AVG remains a viable option for permanent hemodialysis access when an AVF cannot be created, or perhaps for some subsets of ESRD patients. Catheters are costly and morbid, and although their use has increased over the past decade, the current trend is to develop strategies that avoid catheter placement whenever possible. For established permanent AV access, there are many monitoring and surveillance methods, including physical examination, measurement of pressure or flow, and imaging techniques. They have all been shown effective for detecting stenosis, and CMS mandates routine monitoring and surveillance. At this time, however, there are no compelling data that detection of stenosis and subsequent interventions lead to better AV access patency.

REFERENCES

1. Grassmann A, Gioberge S, Moeller S, et al. End-stage renal disease—global demographics in 2005 and observed trends. *Artif Organs* 2006;30(12):895–897.
2. U.S. Renal Data System. *USRDS 2010 Annual Report: Atlas of Chronic Kidney Disease and End-Stage Renal Disease in the United States.* Bethesda, MD: National Institutes of Health, National Institute of Diabetes and Digestive and Kidney Diseases; 2010. Available at: http://www.usrds.org.
3. Haas G. Versuche der Blutauswaschung am Lebenden mit Hilfe der Dialyse. *Klin Wochenschr* 1925;4(1):13–14.
4. Konner K. History of vascular access for haemodialysis. *Nephrol Dial Transplant* 2005;20:2629–2635.
5. Combe C, Pisoni RL, Port FK, et al. Dialysis Outcomes and Practice Patterns Study: data on the use of central venous catheters in chronic hemodialysis. *Nephrologie* 2001;22(8):379–384.
6. Pisoni RL, Arrington CJ, Albert JM, et al. Facility hemodialysis vascular access use and mortality in countries participating in DOPPS: an instrumental variable analysis. *Am J Kidney Dis* 2009;53(3):475–491.
7. Dhingra RK, Young EW, Hulbert-Shearon TE, et al. Type of vascular access and mortality in US hemodialysis patients. *Kidney Int* 2011;60:1443–1451.
8. Xue JL, Dahl D, Ebben JP, et al. The association of initial hemodialysis access type with mortality outcomes in elderly Medicare ESRD patients. *Am J Kidney Dis* 2003;42:1013–1019.
9. Allon M, Daugirdas JT, Depner TA, et al. Effect of change in vascular access on patient mortality in hemodialysis patients. *Am J Kidney Dis* 2006;47:469–477.
10. Lee T, Barker J, Allon M. Tunneled catheters in hemodialysis patients: reasons and subsequent outcomes. *Am J Kidney Dis* 2005;46:501–508.
11. Rayner HC, Pisoni RL. The increasing use of hemodialysis catheters: evidence from the DOPPS on its significance and ways to reverse it. *Semin Dial* 2010;23(1):6–10.
12. Spergel LM. Has the fistula first breakthrough initiative caused an increase in catheter prevalence? *Semin Dial* 2008;21(6):550–552.
13. Brescia MJ, Cimino JE, Appel K, et al. Chronic hemodialysis using venipuncture and a surgically created arteriovenous fistula. *N Engl J Med* 1966;275:1089–1092.
14. Maya ID, O'Neal JC, Young CJ, et al. Outcomes of brachiocephalic fistulas, transposed brachiobasilic fistulas, and upper arm grafts. *Clin J Am Soc Nephrol* 2009;4:86–92.
15. Pisoni RL, Young EW, Dykstra DM, et al. Vascular access use in Europe and the United States: results from the DOPPS. *Kidney Int* 2002;61:305–316.
16. NKF K/DOQI clinical practice guidelines for vascular access. National Kidney Foundation-Dialysis Outcomes Quality Initiative. *Am J Kidney Dis* 1997;30:S150–S191.
17. Fistula First National Vascular Access Improvements Initiative. Available at: http://www.fistulafirst.org/. Accessed January 26, 2011.
18. Allon M, Robbin ML. Increasing arteriovenous fistulas in hemodialysis patients: problems and solutions. *Kidney Int* 2002;62:1109–1124.
19. Dember LM, Beck GJ, Allon M, et al. Effect of clopidogrel on early failure of arteriovenous fistulas for hemodialysis: a randomized controlled trial. *JAMA* 2008;299(18):2164–2171.
20. Patel ST, Hughes J, Mills JL Sr. Failure of arteriovenous fistula maturation: an unintended consequence of exceeding Dialysis Outcome Quality Initiative guidelines for hemodialysis access. *J Vasc Surg* 2003;38:439–445.
21. Biuckians A, Scott E, Meier GH, et al. The natural history of autologous fistulas as first-time dialysis access in the KDOQI era. *J Vasc Surg* 2008;47:415–421.
22. Ernandez T, Saudan P, Berney T, et al. Risk factors for early failure of native arteriovenous fistulas. *Nephron Clin Pract* 2005;101:c39–c44.
23. Huijbregts HJ, Bots ML, Moll FL, et al. Hospital specific aspects predominantly determine primary failure of hemodialysis arteriovenous fistulas. *J Vasc Surg* 2007;45:962–967.
24. Choi KL, Salman L, Krishnamurthy G, et al. Impact of surgeon selection on access placement and survival following preoperative mapping in the "Fistula First" era. *Semin Dial* 2008;21:341–345.
25. Fassiadis N, Morsy M, Siva M, et al. Does the surgeon's experience impact on radiocephalic fistula patency rates? *Semin Dial* 2007;20:455–457.
26. Hossny A. Brachiobasilic arteriovenous fistula: different surgical techniques and their effects on fistula patency and dialysis-related complications. *J Vasc Surg* 2003;37:821–826.
27. Baker LD, Johnson JM, Goldfarb D. Expanded polytetrafluoroethylene (PTFE) subcutaneous arteriovenous conduit; an improved vascular access for chronic hemodialysis. *Trans Am Soc Artif Intern Organs* 1976;22:382.
28. Dixon BS, Beck GJ, Vazquez MA, et al. Effect of dipyridamole plus aspirin on hemodialysis graft patency. *N Engl J Med* 2009;360:2191–2201.
29. Miller PE, Carlton D, Deierhoi MH, et al. Natural history of arteriovenous grafts in hemodialysis patients. *Am J Kidney Dis* 2000;36(1):68–74.
30. Beathard GA. Percutaneous transvenous angioplasty in the treatment of vascular access stenosis. *Kidney Int* 1992;42:1390–1397.
31. Kanterman RY, Vesely TM, Pilgram TK, et al. Dialysis access grafts: anatomic location of venous stenosis and results of angioplasty. *Radiology* 1995;195:135–139.
32. Turmel-Rodrigues L, Pengloan J, Baudin S, et al. Treatment of stenosis and thrombosis in haemodialysis fistulas and grafts by interventional radiology. *Nephrol Dial Transplant* 2000;15:2029–2036.
33. Lilly RZ, Carlton D, Barker J, et al. Predictors of arteriovenous graft patency after radiologic intervention in hemodialysis patients. *Am J Kidney Dis* 2001;37:945–953.
34. Vesely TM, Siegel JB. Use of the peripheral cutting balloon to treat hemodialysis-related stenoses. *J Vasc Interv Radiol* 2005;16(12):1593–1603.
35. National Kidney Foundation. K/DOQI clinical practice guidelines and clinical practice recommendations for vascular access 2006. *Am J Kidney Dis* 2006;48(suppl 1):S1–S322.
36. Haskal ZJ, Trerotola S, Dolmatch B, et al. Stent graft versus balloon angioplasty for failing dialysis-access grafts. *N Engl J Med* 2010;362:494–503.
37. Trerotola SO, Lund GB, Scheel PJ Jr, et al. Thrombosed dialysis access grafts: percutaneous mechanical declotting without urokinase. *Radiology* 1994;191:721–726.
38. Middlebrook MR, Amygdalos MA, Soulen MC, et al. Thrombosed hemodialysis grafts: percutaneous mechanical balloon declotting versus thrombolysis. *Radiology* 1995;196:73–77.
39. Valji K, Bookstein JJ, Roberts AC, et al. Pulse-spray pharmacomechanical thrombolysis of thrombosed hemodialysis access grafts: long-term experience and comparison of original and current techniques. *AJR Am J Roentgenol* 1995;164:1495–1500.

40. Uflacker R, Rajagopalan PR, Vujic I, et al. Treatment of thrombosed dialysis access grafts: randomized trial of surgical thrombectomy versus mechanical thrombectomy with the Amplatz device. *J Vasc Interv Radiol* 1996;7:185–192.

41. Trerotola SO, Vesely TM, Lund GB, et al. Treatment of thrombosed hemodialysis access grafts: Arrow-Trerotola percutaneous thrombolytic device versus pulse-spray thrombolysis. *Radiology* 1998;206:403–414.

42. Nassar GM, Ayus JC. Infections complications of the hemodialysis access. *Kidney Int* 2001;60:1–13.

43. Alpers FJ. Clinical considerations in hemodialysis access infection. *Adv Ren Replace Ther* 1996;3:208–217.

44. Minga TE, Flanagan KH, Allon M. Clinical consequences of infected arteriovenous grafts in hemodialysis patients. *Am J Kidney Dis* 2001;38(5):975–978.

45. Lok CE, Allon M, Moist L, et al. Risk equation determining unsuccessful cannulation events and failure to maturation in arteriovenous fistulas. *J Am Soc Nephrol* 2006;17:3204–3212.

46. Davidson I, Gallieni M, Saxena R, et al. A patient centered decision making dialysis access algorithm. *J Vasc Access* 2007;8:59–68.

47. Department of Health and Human Services. Medicare and Medicaid Programs; conditions for coverage for end-stage renal disease facilities; final rule: rules and regulations, part II. *Fed Regist* 2008;73:20370–20482.

48. Center for Medicaid and State Operations/Survey & Certification Group. *ESRD Interpretive Guidance Update, Ref: S&C-09-01.* Baltimore, MD: Department of Health & Human Services, Centers for Medicare & Medicaid Services; 2008.

49. Trerotola SO, Scheel PJ, Powe NR, et al. Screening for dialysis access graft malfunction: comparison of physical examination with US. *J Vasc Interv Radiol* 1996;7(1):15–20.

50. Asif A, Leon C, Orozco-Vargas LC, et al. Accuracy of physical examination in the detection of arteriovenous fistula stenosis. *Clin J Am Soc Nephrol* 2007;2(6):1191–1194.

51. Leon C, Orozco-Vargas LC, Krishnamurthy G, et al. Accuracy of physical examination in the detection of arteriovenous graft stenosis. *Semin Dial* 2008;21(1):85–88.

52. Beathard GA. An algorithm for the physical examination of early fistula failure. *Semin Dial* 2005;18(4):331–335.

53. Gelbfish GA. Clinical surveillance and monitoring of arteriovenous access for hemodialysis. *Tech Vasc Interv Radiol* 2008;11(3):156–166.

54. Allon M, Robbin ML. Hemodialysis vascular access monitoring: current concepts. *Hemodial Int* 2009;13:153–162.

55. Trerotola SO, Ponce P, Stavropoulos W, et al. Physical examination versus normalized pressure ratio for predicting outcomes of hemodialysis access interventions. *J Vasc Interv Radiol* 2003;14:1387–1393.

56. Robbin ML, Oser RF, Allon M, et al. Hemodialysis access graft stenosis: US detection. *Radiology* 1998;208:655–661.

57. Whittier WL. Surveillance of hemodialysis vascular access. *Semin Intervent Radiol* 2009;26(2):130–138.

58. Sherman RA. The measurement of dialysis access recirculation. *Am J Kidney Dis* 1993;22(4):616–621.

59. Besarab A, Sullivan KL, Ross RP, et al. Utility of intra-access pressure monitoring in detecting and correcting venous outlet stenoses prior to thrombosis. *Kidney Int* 1995;47(5):1364–1373.

60. Besarab A, Frinak S, Sherman RA, et al. Simplified measurement of intra-access pressure. *J Am Soc Nephrol* 1998;9:284–289.

61. Schwab SJ, Raymond JR, Saeed M, et al. Prevention of hemodialysis fistula thrombosis. Early detection of venous stenoses. *Kidney Int* 1989;36(4):1364–1373.

62. Krivitski NM. Theory and validation of access flow measurement by dilution technique during hemodialysis. *Kidney Int* 1995;48:244–250.

63. Lacson E Jr, Lazarus JM, Panlilio R, et al. Comparison of hemodialysis blood access flow rates using online measurement of conductivity dialysance and ultrasound dilution. *Am J Kidney Dis* 2008;51:99–106.

64. Whittier WL, Mansy HA, Rutz DR, et al. Comparison of hemodialysis access flow measurements using flow dilution and in-line dialysance. *ASAIO J* 2009;55:369–372.

65. Bosman PJ, Boereboom FTJ, Eikelboom BC, et al. Graft flow as a predictor of thrombosis in hemodialysis grafts. *Kidney Int* 1998;54:1726–1730.

66. Neyra NR, Ikizler TA, May RE, et al. Change in access blood flow over time predicts vascular access thrombosis. *Kidney Int* 1998;54:1714–1719.

67. Sands J, Glidden D, Miranda C. Hemodialysis access flow measurement. Comparison of ultrasound dilution and duplex ultrasonography. *ASAIO J* 1996;42(5):M899–M901.

68. Schwarz C, Mitterbauer C, Boczula M, et al. Flow monitoring: performance characteristics of ultrasound dilution versus color Doppler ultrasound compared with fistulography. *Am J Kidney Dis* 2003;42:539–545.

69. Gadallah MF, Paulson WD, Vickers B, et al. Accuracy of Doppler ultrasound in diagnosing anatomic stenosis of hemodialysis arteriovenous access as compared with fistulography. *Am J Kidney Dis* 1998;32:273–277.

70. Robbin ML, Oser RF, Lee JY, et al. Randomized comparison of ultrasound surveillance and clinical monitoring on arteriovenous graft outcomes. *Kidney Int* 2006;69:730–735.

71. Duijm LE, Liem YS, van der Rijt RH, et al. Inflow stenoses in dysfunctional hemodialysis access fistulae and grafts. *Am J Kidney Dis* 2006;48(1):98–105.

72. Laissy JP, Menegazzo D, Debray PM, et al. Failing arteriovenous hemodialysis fistulas: assessment with magnetic resonance angiography. *Invest Radiol* 1999;34:218–224.

73. Casey ET, Murad H, Rizvi AZ, et al. Surveillance of arteriovenous hemodialysis access: a systematic review and meta-analysis. *J Vasc Surg* 2008;48:48S–54S.

74. Robbin ML, Oser RF, Lee JY, et al. Randomized comparison of ultrasound surveillance and clinical monitoring on arteriovenous graft outcomes. *Kidney Int* 2006;69:730–735.

75. Paulson WD, Work J. Controversial vascular access surveillance mandate. *Semin Dial* 2010;23(1):92–94.

Interventional Management Strategies for the Failing or Failed Dialysis Access

MARK OTTO BAERLOCHER and ANNE C. ROBERTS

INTRODUCTION

Long-term hemodialysis access may be accomplished by creation of either an arteriovenous fistula (AVF; a direct, surgically created anastomosis between an artery and a vein), or an arteriovenous graft (AVG; an indirect conduit between an artery and a vein, usually made of synthetic material, such as polytetrafluoroethylene [PTFE]).

Current recommendations by the Dialysis Outcomes Quality Initiative (DOQI) practice guidelines[1] recommend the creation of an AVF over an AVG, which has led to the "Fistula First" campaign. As outlined in the DOQI practice guidelines, AVFs have several advantages over all other forms of vascular access, including a lower rate of thrombosis, lower rate of re-intervention, lower rate of infection, and longer access survival.[2–5] Due to these intrinsic advantages of AVFs, the cost of access creation and maintenance is lower,[2,6–8] the morbidity and hospitalization rates are lower, and the survival is greater.[9,10] The potential disadvantages of AVFs include failure of the draining vein to enlarge or to deliver blood flow at an adequate level, comparatively long maturation times prior to suitability for use (1 to 4 months), potentially greater difficulty in cannulating the vein when compared to AVGs, and potentially less favorable cosmesis.[1,11–13] The DOQI Work Group concluded that the potential advantages of AVFs outweighed their potential disadvantages.

There are various potential options for fistula location, including between the radial artery and the cephalic vein (generally a side-to-side anastomosis; also called a Brescia-Cimino fistula), brachial artery to cephalic vein, brachial artery to basilic vein, brachial artery to median antecubital vein, and femoral artery to saphenous vein.

The AVF types recommended by the DOQI guidelines are radiocephalic (wrist), followed by brachiocephalic (elbow).[1] There is substantial evidence that these AVFs have longer patency rates and lower complication rates including conduit stenosis, infection, and vascular steal phenomena compared to other access types, such as other types of AVFs, AVGs, or catheter-based dialysis.[1,3,11,14,15] Furthermore, the general principle of preserving more proximal vessels for future access placement applies (thus favoring a wrist AVF over an elbow AVF). If a wrist or elbow AVF is not a possibility, consideration of a transposed basilic vein fistula is recommended. The transposed brachiobasilic fistula involves dissecting free the basilic vein, tunneling the vein subcutaneously over the bicep muscle, and creating an end-to-side anastomosis between the vein and the brachial artery.[16]

The disadvantages of this approach are an increased likelihood of significant arm swelling and pain, a greater incidence of steal syndrome, and increased difficulty in creation, particularly in obese patients.[1] The failure rate of AVFs to mature and be suitable for dialysis is typically between 15% and 20%,[4,17,18] although more recent studies have reported fistula nonmaturation rates of 20% to 60%.[19] Failure of AVFs is more likely to occur in patients who are elderly, diabetic, smokers, anemic, and/or have high cholesterol.[17,20–22]

If creation of an AVF is not an option, an AVG is the next best form of long-term access and has several potential advantages. AVGs tend to be easier to cannulate (due to a larger surface area); have a shorter time for maturation; allow for multiple possible shapes, configurations, and insertion sites; and are relatively easy to construct surgically and repair either surgically or endovascularly.[1,23,24]

Traditionally, the preferred material for AVG construction has been PTFE due to longer patency, lower risk of disintegration from infection, and better availability.[1,25] Other materials, such as polyurethane, cryopreserved femoral vein, bovine mesenteric vein, and various hybrids, are currently being tested.[26] The site of AVG construction should generally be as distal as possible with the goal of preserving sites for future placement.[1,27]

The preferred sites for AVG construction are the antecubital loop graft and the upper arm curved graft (DOQI guidelines document). The arterial/inflow sites include the radial artery (wrist), brachial artery (antecubital fossa, distal arm, or just below the axilla), axillary artery, and femoral artery. The venous/outflow sites include the median antecubital vein, proximal and distal cephalic vein, basilic vein (elbow, or upper arm), axillary vein, jugular vein, and femoral vein.

Although AVGs may be used earlier than AVFs (within 14 days of placement),[1] AVFs tend to have better longevity with fewer interventions, if they become functional. AVFs have a reported primary patency rate at 1 year of 40%,[45] and a secondary patency rate between 60% and 90%.[1,28] AVGs are reported to have 1-year cumulative patency of 59% to 90%.[29]

PATIENT SELECTION

The primary involvement for the interventional radiologist is detection and/or treatment of access dysfunction, in particular access stenosis and/or thrombosis. Access dysfunction has been shown to have substantial negative consequences on patient morbidity and mortality,[30,31] quality of life,[31] and health care expenditures.[32] Progressive venous outflow stenosis is the primary cause of AVG thrombosis, and thrombosis that cannot be resolved is the primary cause of access loss.[33–36]

The DOQI Work Group thus recommends active, prospective surveillance of hemodialysis access for hemodynamically significant stenoses (at intervals of 1 month or less, depending on practicality, complexity, and cost) and, if present, correction of these stenoses. The underlying principle or assumption by the Work Group is that stenoses develop after variable amounts of time, and if detected and corrected early, underdialysis can be minimized and thrombosis prevented.[1] The DOQI Work Group strongly recommends formation of multidisciplinary hemodialysis teams to manage access care.[1,37] Patient education is a vital component of the surveillance strategy; specifically, the hemodialysis patient should be taught how to feel for a pulse and/or thrill, the indicators of infection, and ensuring hemodialysis access teams rotate the site of needle puncture and to proper access maintenance in terms of hygiene.[1]

There are various methods by which access surveillance and monitoring may be performed, including physical examination, sequential access flow, sequential dynamic pressures, sequential static pressures, and recirculation measurements.[1,38–40]

Physical examination of a hemodialysis access, whether AVG or AVF, should include each of three components: inspection, palpation, and auscultation.[1] Inspection can detect the presence of access aneurysms, can give a sense if there is an outflow stenosis (e.g., arm swelling is an indication of stenosis; also, the outflow vein should collapse with elevation of the arm), and may detect graft infection (erythema). On palpation, the outflow veins of both AVFs and AVGs should have a palpable thrill. Lack of a palpable thrill or a pulsatile outflow vein may be an indication that there is a problem with the access. A stenosis itself can often be palpated. An infected graft, aside from having an erythematous appearance, may feel abnormally warm to the touch. Auscultation may reveal stenoses depending on the presence and character of its associated bruit. Some stenoses may be asymptomatic but hemodynamically significant and detected only via routine surveillance. It is important to detect and treat these lesions early because lack of treatment may lead to progression to complete thrombosis.

Other indications of an access problem include prolonged bleeding/oozing following needle removal postdialysis, arm swelling/pain, and/or lack of either an outflow vein thrill or pulsatility[1,41,42] as well as more objective measurements of pressure and flow.

Normal flow in a graft should exceed 800 to 1,000 mL/minute.[1,43] The risk of graft thrombosis is increased when the flow is less than 800 mL/minute,[44–47] there is a decline in access flow with serial flow measurements,[45,47–52] and/or there is a decrease of 25% or more from a stable baseline that was greater than 1,000 mL/minute.[1,49,53]

Regardless of the specific surveillance technique(s) utilized, angiography is indicated when a possible stenosis is detected to definitively confirm its presence and to characterize the lesion. Should a stenosis be confirmed at the time of angiography, angioplasty is recommended if there is greater than 50% stenosis.[1]

When a graft develops a stenosis, there is a finite time available before which there is thrombosis; this time interval varies inversely with the access flow.[1] A graft with a flow of less than 450 mL/minute has fewer than 8 weeks before thrombosis occurs,[54] whereas one with a flow between 600 and 800 mL/minute has 3 months.[48]

Criteria for intervention in fistulas are not as well established because they maintain patency at lower flow rates than grafts. Some have suggested that flows above 400 to 650 mL/minute are sufficient.[1]

ENDOVASCULAR TREATMENT OPTIONS

The two predominant pathologies in either AVGs or AVFs are access stenosis and thrombosis. Stenosis precedes thrombosis and, if untreated or treated inadequately, thrombosis will eventually occur. If an intervention for a stenosis is performed, failure to increase the access flow by 20% or greater represents failure of the intervention.[1,53] Although there is suggestion that AVGs react differently than AVFs and as such the criteria for treatment success should also differ, there are sparse data available to make this distinction.[1]

Other potential complications that may occur with either AVGs or AVFs include venous hypertension and extremity edema, aneurysm and pseudoaneurysm formation, infection, and vascular steal syndrome.

Depending on the specific pathology and anatomic considerations, the core endovascular treatment options available to the interventional radiologist include regular balloon angioplasty, cutting balloon angioplasty, stent/stent-grafting, thrombolysis, and thrombectomy.

Prior to performing any attempted intervention, it is important to consent the patient not only for the planned intervention itself, but also for placement of a new tunneled hemodialysis catheter. If the intervention fails, or the graft is lost, the patient will still require hemodialysis. A tunneled central line should usually be placed in such circumstances during the same procedure once an intervention is deemed a failure. This allows the patient to undergo needed dialysis while awaiting placement of a new access.

ANATOMIC OR LESION CONSIDERATIONS

Stenosis

Once the decision has been made to perform angiography based on either physical examination and/or other objective measurements, venography should be performed from the inflow artery all the way to the central veins/superior vena cava (SVC). The arterial inflow may be studied by manually compressing the midportion of the graft/outflow vein during injection, inflation of a balloon with the catheter end hole directed toward the anastomosis, or by direct injection of the anastomosis.

For either an AVG or an AVF, the direction and location of the initial puncture should be made depending on the suspicion of lesion location. This could be based on the physical examination and/or previous interventions. For example, if there is suspicion for a central venous lesion, the initial puncture should be performed so that the catheter is directed centrally.

If there is not a clear lesion location suspected, one can use the statistics of the most common lesion locations. AVG stenoses are most commonly in the vein located within a few centimeters of the graft-venous anastomosis; therefore, a puncture of the proximal to mid graft directed toward the venous outflow would be appropriate. AVF stenoses are most commonly at the venous anastomosis; therefore, a puncture of the outflow vein directed retrograde toward the inflow would be appropriate.

Arteriovenous Grafts

Although venous anastomotic stenoses are the most common stenotic lesion in AVGs, the incidence of arterial inflow or arterial anastomotic lesions are present in 5% to 25% of cases.[1,39,55] Central vein stenosis and intragraft stenoses, although less common, are also possible problems.

In any event, AVG venography should be performed from the arterial inflow to the central veins/SVC at the beginning of the procedure to characterize the location, type, and number of lesions to plan any intervention. In many cases, particularly around the venous anastomosis, multiple oblique views may be necessary to delineate overlapping outflow veins. There is the potential for "pseudo-stenoses"; in particular, surgical draping that is tight around the arm may produce the appearance of a significant stenosis but resolves with loosening of the drape.

If present, a stenosis warrants intervention if it is at least 50% or greater, *and* there is an associated hemodynamic, functional, or clinical abnormality.[1,56,57] There is no convincing evidence that prophylactic correction of an *asymptomatic* stenosis greater than 50% prolongs graft patency or function, and it is therefore currently advised against.[1,33,58,59] The DOQI guidelines are less clear regarding reintervention. There are no guidelines (or clear data) on endovascular follow-up of an access with symptomatic stenosis, which is then treated. At our institution, we tend to perform repeat angiography and treatment of residual/recurrent stenoses at 4 to 8 weeks, particularly in patients with recurrent thromboses.

If deemed suitable for endovascular treatment, stenoses should be treated first with balloon angioplasty (FIGURE 89.1). The size of the balloon is chosen based on the size of the normal, patent vessel on either size of the lesion. Typically, balloon sizes will range from 5 to 8 mm. In the forearm and elbow, a typical initial balloon size is 6 mm. If there has been previous angioplasty performed at the same location, the previous balloon size is generally used initially for repeat angioplasty. Over time the vein may increase in size, requiring increasing balloon diameters. If there is an intragraft stenosis, the most common balloon size will be 6 mm, or alternately, 1 mm larger than the graft diameter. Central vein stenoses (typically in the subclavian or brachiocephalic veins, often caused by vessel injury from previous venous catheters) usually require balloons 10 to 12 mm or larger in diameter.

Regular pressure, high-pressure (i.e., with burst pressures of 20 to 30 mm Hg), and cutting balloons are available to the interventional radiologist. In some cases, the balloon may appear to inflate entirely, yet a postdilatation contrast study demonstrates a persistent significant stenosis. Such "elastic" lesions require further treatment. If initial dilatation did not result in pain, a larger balloon may be useful.

Lesions resistant to angioplasty may require high-pressure balloons and/or prolonged inflation times of up to 5 minutes (FIGURE 89.2A). Cutting angioplasty balloons are noncompliant balloons with three or four small atherotomes (depending on balloon size) along the balloon's longitudinal axis that are three to four times sharper than conventional surgical blades. When deflated, the vessel wall is protected from the atherotomes and, when inflated, the atherotomes expand radially, delivering longitudinal incisions in the vessel plaque with the theory that their hoop stress is relieved. The inflation pressures for cutting balloon are typically lower, in the range of 4 to 8 atm (FIGURE 89.2B). The theoretical advantage of cutting balloons is that they produce a more localized and controlled "fault line" of vessel wall injury with linear crack propagation than regular, high-pressure balloons.[60] Although there have been multiple papers written on cutting balloons,[61–68] there is no evidence that cutting balloons

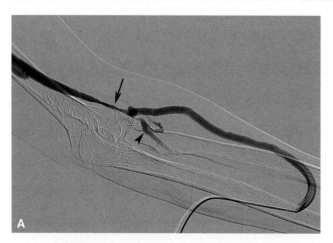
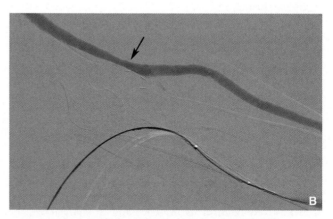

FIGURE 89.1 **(A)** Forearm loop graft with a tight stenosis at the venous anastomosis (*arrow*). This is a typical lesion seen with grafts. Note the flow into the venous collaterals (*arrowhead*) this is evidence of a hemodynamic significant obstruction to flow. **(B)** Post angioplasty with a good angiographic result. Note that the venous collaterals seen in 1a are not visualized. This suggests an improved hemodynamic result.

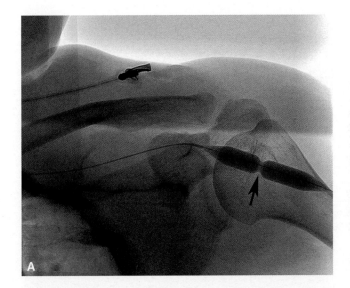

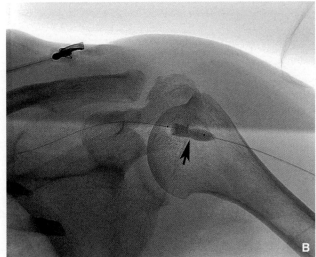

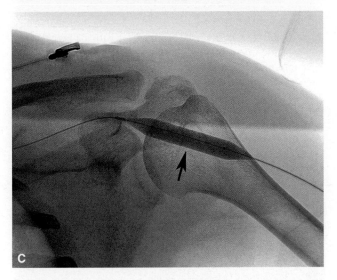

FIGURE 89.2 (A) There is a very tight stenosis in the cephalic vein. Despite 30 atmosphere high pressure balloon inflation a waist remains in the balloon (*arrow*). **(B)** Cutting balloon placed across the stenosis. The balloon is much shorter than the high-pressure balloon and is inflated to a much lower pressure (4-8 atmospheres). The atherotomes cannot be seen on fluoroscopy but are present in the center of the balloon (*arrow*). **(C)** Immediately following dilatation with the cutting balloon, the high-pressure balloon is replaced and now can be inflated completely without any waist (*arrow*).

are superior to standard balloons for simple stenoses.[69] They can, however, be useful in the treatment of venous stenoses that are resistant to regular or high-pressure balloon angioplasty (FIGURE 89.2C).

Uncovered stents are also an option in some scenarios, such as venous rupture, elastic recoil, and restenosis. Funaki et al.[70] treated 23 patients with venous rupture caused by balloon angioplasty with wallstent deployment, and reported a primary patency rate of the stents of 52% at 60 days, 26% at 180 days, and 11% at 360 days, with a secondary patency rate of 74%, 65%, and 56% at 60, 180, and 360 days, respectively. The disadvantage of an uncovered stent is its increased likelihood of intimal hyperplasia within the stent and at its proximal and distal ends. Stent should not be used in venous segments that may be used for future surgical revision, or across joints where bending may increase the strain on and likelihood of kinking/breaking of the stent.

According to the DOQI guidelines, uncovered stents should not be used primarily versus balloon angioplasty and are most appropriate in cases of angioplasty-induced venous rupture (FIGURE 89.3) or in patients with contraindications to surgical revision. Similarly, in the case of central venous stenoses in the subclavian or brachiocephalic veins, stents should generally be reserved for elastic lesions, rapidly recurring stenosis (within 3 months), or occluded vessels.[71] Stents used for the central veins should be oversized to avoid migration.[72,73]

Placement of a covered stent is a more recent innovation that has some data regarding its use.[74–80] Stent-graft placement has also successfully been used in central venous stenoses, (FIGURE 89.4)[76] and to treat pseudoaneuryms.[75] There has been debate recently regarding their primary use versus plain balloon angioplasty.[80] Generally, given their increased cost, stent-grafts should be used sparingly and not employed primarily prior to balloon angioplasty.

Following intervention performed for stenosis or thrombosis, repeat contrast injections should be performed to ensure patency and adequate flow. Anatomic success is considered achieved if the residual stenosis is less than 30%.[1,81]

In some patients, stenosis (and/or thrombosis) may recur in a short time frame, defined by the DOQI guidelines as a

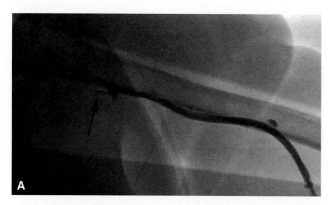
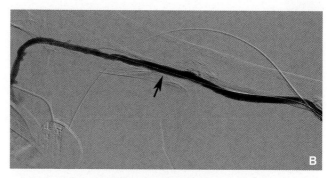

FIGURE 89.3 (A) There is a very tight stenosis in cephalic vein, which has ruptured following balloon angioplasty (*arrow*). **(B)** Rupture in cephalic vein treated with uncovered stent (*arrow*). Good flow through the vein, with no evidence of extravasation.

recurring lesion requiring two or more angioplasty procedures within a 3-month period. In such cases, it may be more cost-effective to pursue surgical revision.[1] These patients must be treated on a case-by-case basis. In some cases of early restenosis/rethrombosis the venous stenosis may have been underdilated.[82]

Arteriovenous Fistulas

AVFs have subtle differences in their evaluation. They may be difficult to access in some cases (FIGURE 89.5) and may require

direct puncture of the feeding artery (e.g., the brachial artery for a forearm fistula, accessed at the elbow with a 3 French dilator from the micropuncture set).[83,84] After sequential contrast injections of the entire fistula and central draining veins/SVC, a retrograde puncture of the draining vein within the arm may be performed for treatment of any apparent stenoses (FIGURE 89.6). If a retrograde access proves impossible, an antegrade approach via the artery may be performed with care.[83] Other techniques that may prove useful in obtaining fistula access include

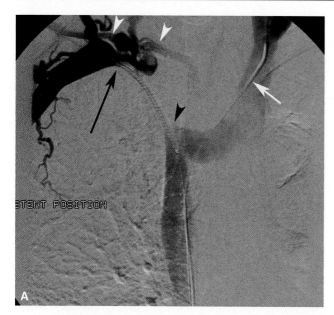
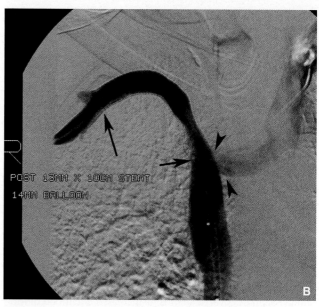

FIGURE 89.4 (A) Venogram demonstrates complete occlusion of right brachiocephalic vein (*black arrow*). There is no right internal jugular vein demonstrated, most likely indicating damage from previous dialysis catheter placement. Multiple collaterals are present (*white arrowheads*). A diagnostic angiographic catheter has been placed from a femoral approach to allow opacification of the left brachiocephalic vein (*white arrow*). This is to help with the precise positioning of the distal portion of the covered stent (*black arrowhead*) so that the stent graft does not cover the left brachiocephalic vein. **(B)** The stent graft has been positioned (arrows delineate the ends of the stent graft) and expanded with a 14 mm balloon. The collateral veins seen on the previous figure are no longer seen. There is still flow through the left brachiocephalic vein (*arrowheads*), the stent graft distal end is just above the brachiocephalic vein.

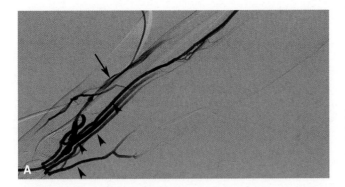

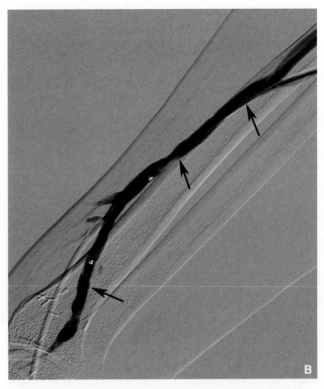

FIGURE 89.5 (A) Poorly maturing radiocephalic arteriovenous fistula, dialysis unit unable to access, and unable to use for dialysis. Using ultrasound guidance, the main outflow channel was identified, and accessed (*arrow*). Injection of contrast demonstrates the multiple outflow veins (*arrowheads*), which are filling because of stenoses within the main outflow vein. **(B)** Following 6 mm balloon angioplasty of the main outflow vein, the flow is now through the outflow vein (*arrows*) with no filling of the previously visualized collaterals.

ultrasound guidance and/or use of a tourniquet across the outflow vein(s).

Caution must be used when dilating any stenoses, frequently serial dilatations are required starting at a small balloon size (e.g., 3 or 4 mm) to avoid venous rupture. In some cases, the stenotic vein may be underdeveloped and require a staged procedure with initial angioplasty performed with a small balloon

and subsequent repeat angioplasty performed 1 to 3 weeks later with a larger balloon.

Results

The unassisted, primary patency rate of nonthrombosed AVGs at 6 months following technically successful balloon angioplasty of a stenosis is 40% to 50% according to the DOQI

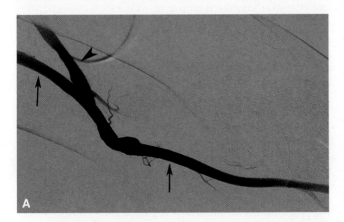

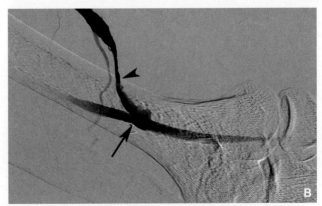

FIGURE 89.6 (A) Patient with poor flow in fistula during dialysis. The fistula is a brachiocephalic fistula, with access obtained within the fistula in the mid upper arm. Injection, performed with compression on the outflow vein, to opacify the arterial anastomosis, does not appear to demonstrate any abnormality. The brachial artery shown with arrows, the outflow cephalic vein show with arrowhead. **(B)** Same patient as in Figure 5A, now the arm has been placed in an oblique postion and repeat contrast injection demonstrates the relatively long area of stenosis in the vein (*arrowhead*) just distal to the anastomosis of the artery and vein (*arrow*). Stenosis of the draining vein is commonly just distal to the arterial anastomosis. This study demonstrates the importance of minimizing the overlap the artery and vein. The venous stenosis was treated with angioplasty with a good result.

guidelines, based on a number of reports.[1,24,85–88] By comparison, the target 1-year primary patency rate of surgically revised AVGs is 50%.[1] AVG survival has previously been shown to be inversely related to the degree of residual stenosis following angioplasty.[86]

According to the DOQI guidelines, the patency rate associated with primary stenting of AVG stenoses is not significantly different than that of primary PTA[1,89–91] and should therefore be reserved for angioplasty-induced AVG rupture, or those with angioplasty-resistant lesions with contraindications to surgical revision, due to the added cost.

However, a more recent study found the opposite, that primary treatment of stenotic, nonthrombosed AVGs with angioplasty plus stent-graft was superior to primary treatment with angioplasty alone. Haskal et al.[80] randomized 190 patients with AVGs and a venous anastomotic stenosis to undergo either angioplasty alone or angioplasty with placement of a stent-graft. The 6-month primary patency rate and incidence of freedom from subsequent interventions was 51% and 32%, respectively, in the stent-graft group, compared to 23% and 16% in the angioplasty-alone group ($p < .001$, $p = .03$). Still, at this point we advise that interventionists follow the DOQI guidelines' recommendations, reserving stents (either covered or uncovered) for select cases.

The patency rate for AVFs following treatment of stenosis is better than the corresponding data for AVGs. One-year primary and secondary patency rates have been reported as 39% and 79% for forearm AVFs and 57% in upper arm AVFs.[87] Glanz et al.[34] dilated 141 AVF stenoses and reported 1- and 2-year patency rates of 45% and 24%, respectively, whereas Clark et al.[92] reported primary, assisted primary, and secondary patency rates at 3 months of 84%, 88%, and 90%, respectively; 6-month rates of 55%, 80%, and 82%, respectively; and 1-year rates of 26%, 80%, and 82%, respectively.

Complications

Complications from treatment of AVG or AVF stenoses are relatively rare and include hematoma/bleeding, infection, and reaction to medication/contrast. A more serious complication is venous rupture, particularly in autologous fistulas. Initial treatment of a venous rupture is reinflation of the angioplasty balloon with a prolonged inflation time (5 to 10 minutes), which in many cases will successfully tamponade and seal the rupture. If repeat contrast injection demonstrates persistent extravasation, an uncovered or covered stent can be placed (FIGURE 89.3).[1,70,93,94] Uncovered stents are usually sufficient to treat smaller ruptures, whereas covered stents may be necessary for larger ruptures. If all of these options fail to control the rupture, as a last resort, occlusion of the graft/fistula using manual compression can shut down the access entirely. Vascular rupture should occur in less than 2% to 4% of cases, and rupture requiring blood transfusion or emergent surgery or resulting in limb threatening in less than 0.5% of cases.[71]

Thrombosis

Arteriovenous Grafts

The most common cause of AVG thrombosis is progressive stenosis.[48,58] Previous trials have shown that preemptively treating symptomatic stenoses reduces the rate of graft thrombosis and may increase the life span of the graft.[1,33,58]

Endovascular options for treatment of AVG thrombosis include pharmacologic thrombolysis, balloon angioplasty, and mechanical thrombolysis/thrombectomy, either on their own or often in combination. In general, thrombosis of either AVGs or AVFs should be treated as early as possible to avoid extension of the thrombus, which may increase the difficulty of achieving patency.

Pharmacologic thrombolysis may be used to declot most AVGs, unless there is a specific contraindication to the pharmacologic agent. If there is a contraindication to pharmacologic thrombolysis then mechanical thrombolysis can be used. Absolute contraindications to pharmacologic thrombolysis of a graft are similar to those for thrombolysis elsewhere in the body, including recent cerebrovascular accident/stroke/tumor/trauma (within 2 months), right-to-left cardiac shunt, or active hemorrhage (e.g., gastrointestinal bleed). Relative contraindications include recent major surgery or biopsy (within 2 weeks), serious trauma, severe uncontrolled hypertension, severe pulmonary hypertension, limited cardiopulmonary reserve, pregnancy, or recently postpartum.[95] An infected graft should not be declotted (either pharmacologically or mechanically) because this may lead to septic emboli.

There are several principles to be followed when declotting an AVG. First, there is usually an underlying stenosis in addition to the thrombus, which must be treated to ensure that the occlusion does not quickly recur. Second, substantial caution must be used at the arterial anastomosis to avoid sending arterial emboli distally to the wrist and hand. And, third, the interventionist must ensure that the venous outflow is patent prior to opening the arterial inflow.

Thrombolysis

There are several procedural variations possible when declotting a graft using thrombolytic agents, including the lyse-and-wait technique, lyse-and-go technique, and pulse-spray pharmacomechanical thrombolysis (PSPMT) (FIGURE 89.7).

In the lyse-and-wait technique, 2 mg of thrombolytic agent in 5 to 10 mL of normal saline is injected through an intravenous catheter into the venous limb of the graft over approximately 1 minute while the arterial and venous anastomoses are manually compressed.[96,97] This first part of the lyse-and-wait procedure is often performed in a holding room. After 30 minutes or longer, the patient is brought into the interventional suite, and venography is performed. Any significant venous anastomosis is then opened up with balloon angioplasty. Once the venous outflow is patent, attention is then turned to the arterial inflow, where there is often a thrombolytic-resistant arterial "plug" comprising densely packed platelets and fibrin.[98]

The arterial plug is treated with mechanical dislodgment and maceration using a compliant balloon (FIGURE 89.8). A guide wire is carefully passed from the venous side past the plug into the inflow artery. A compliant balloon, such as an 8.5-mm occlusion balloon (Cook Inc., Bloomington, IN) or over-the-wire Fogarty balloon (Baxter, Irvine, CA) is then placed beyond the plug, gently inflated so that it conforms to the native artery, and pulled back into the graft to drag the arterial plug with it. It may be necessary to repeat this process several times to dislodge the arterial plug. As mentioned previously, caution must be exerted during manipulation of

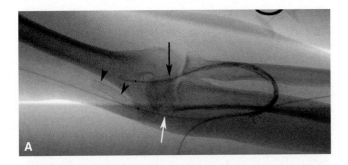

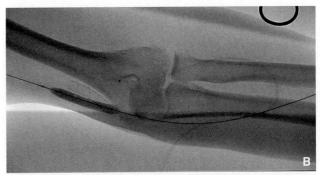

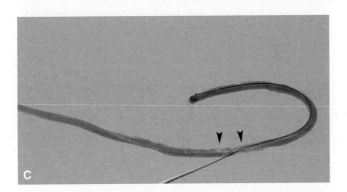

FIGURE 89.7 **(A)** Thrombosed forearm loop graft. Pulse spray catheters have been placed for PSPMT. One from the venous side of fistula with tip in arterial anastomosis (*black arrow*). One from level of loop extending to the venous outflow (*white arrow*), this was placed up the vein because of clot extending into the venous outflow. Note previously placed failed stent (*arrowheads*). The present graft was a replaced graft to another venous outflow because of the failed stent. **(B)** Following thrombolysis, the stenosis at the venous anastomosis is dilated with an appropriately sized balloon. **(C)** Following PSPMT and angioplasty of the venous stenosis there is now good flow in the graft. A small amount of residual clot (*arrowheads*) is present, but as long as there is good flow in the graft this clot will resolve.

the arterial plug when at the arterial inflow to avoid sending arterial emboli distally and to avoid damaging the native inflow artery. Should the plug become lodged within the graft, balloon angioplasty may be used at this point to macerate it because the risk of arterial emboli at this point no longer exists. Following the procedure, repeat angiography should be performed from the arterial inflow to the central draining veins/SVC. Repeat balloon angioplasty is used to macerate any remaining thrombus or treat any additional stenoses.

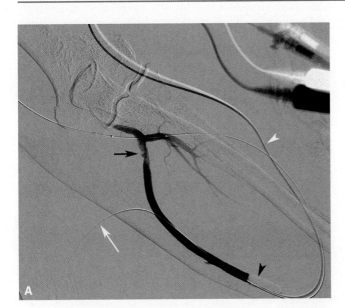

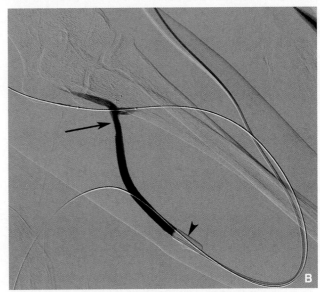

FIGURE 89.8 **(A)** Thrombolysis of the forearm loop graft using cross catheter technique access at the arterial side directed towards the venous outflow (*white arrow*), access at the venous side directed towards the arterial end (*white arrowhead*). An occlusion balloon is in place (*black arrowhead*) with the balloon inflated. This allows injection of contrast to fill the arterial end of the graft, and which shows adherent clot at the arterial anastomosis (*black arrow*). **(B)** Balloon catheter had been placed above the arterial anastomosis, into the arterial inflow, inflated and pulled back into the graft, dislodging the adherent arterial clot. Repeat injection with the balloon inflated (*black arrowhead*) now demonstrates that the arterial end of the graft is patent without adherent clot.

The lyse-and-go technique is very similar, except the initial injection of the thrombolytic agent is performed in the interventional suite rather than in a holding room. The advantage of the lyse-and-wait technique over the lyse-and-go technique of course is decreased time within the interventional room, allowing the interventionist to perform other procedures in the interim.

Another approach is the PSPMT (FIGURE 89.7). This technique utilizes crossed, specialized infusion catheters that have either multiple side slits or side holes along a portion of its length, usually between 4 and 30 cm. A tip-occluding wire (a wire with a small bulbous portion at its end) is used to block the distal end hole. Once the tip-occluding wire is in place, any thrombolytic agent injected into the catheter will be forced out of the multiple side slits/holes so that it is spread homogeneously along the entire length of the catheter through its side slits/holes, rather than solely from the end hole. The thrombolytic agent itself is injected through a hemostatic Touhy-Borst valve or Y-adapter.

In PSPMT, the graft is accessed toward its venous anastomosis, and a 5 French dilator placed over a guide wire past the venous anastomosis. Contrast is gently injected and the length of thrombosed graft/vein to the skin puncture site is measured. A pulse-spray catheter with this distance is then selected and placed into the graft. A second puncture, this time directed toward the arterial anastomosis, is then performed. Via this second puncture, a second pulse-spray catheter is placed over a wire so that its tip is just beyond the arterial anastomosis (i.e., with the two catheters overlapping). Again, caution must be exercised when manipulating wires and catheters at or near the arterial anastomosis to avoid causing distal arterial emboli.

At this point, with two crossing pulse-spray catheters in place, the end hole of each catheter is occluded using the special tip-occluding wire that is supplied with the pulse-spray catheter system. A hemostatic Y-adapter or Touhy-Borst valve is placed over each catheter. The thrombolytic solution (typically 2 to 4 mg of tPA in 10- to 20-mL normal saline) is divided equally into two reservoir syringes, and each syringe attached to one of Y-adapters. A 1-cc syringe is attached to the second port of each of the Y-adapters. Initially, 1 mL of the thrombolytic solution is injected through each catheter via the respective 1-cc syringe. At this point, aliquots of 0.2 to 0.3 mL of the thrombolytic solution are forcibly injected through each catheter via the syringe approximately every 15 to 30 seconds, until the entire dose has been administered. Solution remaining within the catheter is chased with an injection of saline, again in forceful 0.2- to 0.3-mL aliquots until an additional 1 mL of volume has been injected. If the length of occluded graft is greater than the length of the infusion catheters, they can be repositioned so that they cover the entire length after half of the dose has been administered.

At this point, the pulse-spray catheter pointing toward the arterial inflow is withdrawn so that its tip is just distal to the arterial anastomosis, and the tip-occluding wire is removed. A gentle injection of contrast is performed through this catheter in search of stenoses (typically venous stenoses). Stenoses are treated with balloon angioplasty. Following opening of the venous outflow, an arterial plug often remains, which is treated in a similar fashion to that described earlier.

An alternative to the use of specialized infusion catheters is placement of overlapping end-hole catheters (e.g., Kumpe catheters, Cook Inc., Bloomington, IN) with injection of thrombolytic solution through each catheter as they are pulled back, in essence lacing the thrombus with thrombolytic agent.

In addition to the thrombolytic (most commonly tPA, but alternatively streptokinase, urokinase, rPA, reteplase, TNK, tenecteplase), 3,000 to 5,000 units of heparin may be added to the thrombolytic solution. The potential concern is the increased risk of precipitation by their combination; however, most feel that the potential benefit outweighs this risk. Other pharmacologic adjuncts include the use of intravenous heparin (to minimize thrombus formation) and/or aspirin 325 mg orally (to minimize platelet aggregation).

Regardless of the treatment approach utilized, repeat contrast injections of the entire graft and outflow (from arterial inflow to central draining veins/SVC) are mandatory to confirm adequacy of treatment. If the patient is scheduled for same-day hemodialysis, short 6 or 7 French dialysis sheaths may be left in place.

Mechanical Thrombectomy

There are various types of mechanical thrombectomy devices currently available that may be used to mechanically remove thrombus.[99,100] The principle by which they work varies depending on the device but may incorporate a high-speed rotating component, ultrasound waves, a high-pressure saline/fluid jet, and/or a suction component.

The use of mechanical thrombectomy devices follows a similar principle to approaches discussed earlier involving thrombolytic therapy. The graft is accessed pointing toward the venous end, and contrast is injected via a catheter to measure the length of the clot. If a venous stenosis is visualized, some may choose to perform balloon angioplasty prior to use of a mechanical thrombectomy device, whereas others may choose to perform angioplasty after its use. The theoretical advantage of the former approach is the reduced risk of causing emboli to be sent distally through the inflow artery.[101] In either case, the catheter is exchanged for a sheath, through which the thrombectomy device is placed. Following use of the device and angioplasty of any venous stenoses, this process is repeated with a second puncture, performed toward the arterial end (FIGURE 89.9). Following subsequent removal of any arterial plug, repeat contrast injections are performed to confirm patency of the entire graft and venous outflow to the central draining veins/SVC.

Some interventionists may choose to use a single puncture technique, where the puncture is made at the apex of the loop graft. The thrombectomy device is then successfully directed toward each end of the graft (first toward the venous end, and then toward the arterial end). It may be technically difficult in some cases to redirect the catheter/sheath in the opposite direction using this technique.

Arteriovenous Fistulas

Thrombosed AVFs are often more complicated to treat given their more complicated anatomy. Use of ultrasound guidance and, potentially, arterial puncture may be helpful in gaining access. The occluded fistula may be treated with similar approaches as

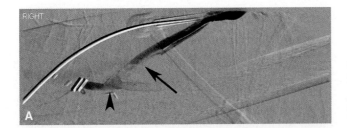

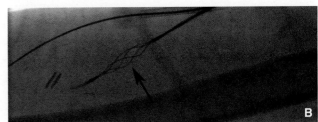

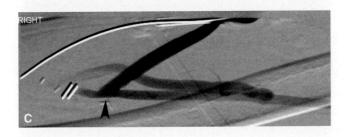

FIGURE 89.9 (A) Upper arm graft with thrombosis (arrow) in the graft just above the arterial anastomosis (*arrowhead*). **(B)** Mechanical thrombectomy using a Trerotola device (*arrow*) to remove the clot at the arterial end of the graft. **(C)** Following mechanical thrombectomy there has been removal of the clot at the arterial anastomosis (*arrowhead*).

with occluded grafts including thrombolysis techniques as well as mechanical thrombectomy devices (FIGURE 89.10).[102–104] In some cases, direct aspiration of the fistula thrombus may be useful, using 7 or 8 French aspiration catheters and a 20-mL syringe.[87] The fistula itself may be accessed in an antegrade or retrograde approach or, in some cases, via the brachial artery if necessary.[104]

Results

The outcomes of intervention in thrombosed AVGs with a stenosis have been shown to be poorer than those in nonthrombosed AVGs with a stenosis.[86] There are no clear data on the

benefit of one type of mechanical (percutaneous) thrombectomy device over another,[101,105] and the technical success and 1-, 3-, and 6-month primary patency rates of mechanical thrombolysis versus pharmacologic thrombolysis are comparable. The DOQI guidelines recommend a primary, unassisted, patency rate for percutaneous thrombectomy of 40%,[1] which is within the published range.[106–108]

There are no clear data comparing percutaneous versus surgical thrombectomy/revision; however, because the latter involves using additional vein segments, it is held to the higher standard of a 50% 6-month primary patency rate and a

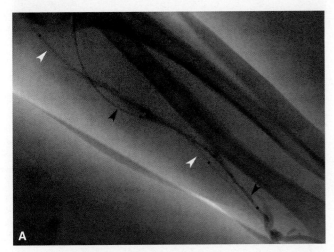

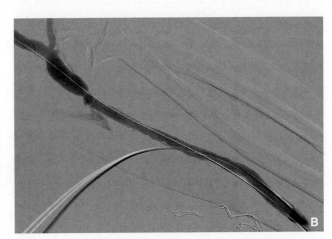

FIGURE 89.10 (A) This radiocephalic arteriovenous fistula has thrombosed. Access obtained using ultrasound to identify the thrombosed vein. Cross catheters placed for PSPMT. One catheter placed in the outflow vein from near the arterial anastomosis going towards the upper arm (*white arrowheads*). The other catheter placed from more distal in the arm going towards the arterial anastomosis (*black arrowheads*). **(B)** Fistula following thrombolysis and angioplasty of the stenosis at the arterial anastomosis. Now there is good flow through the fistula.

40% 1-year primary patency rate.[1] Where possible, percutaneous intervention is generally favored over surgical intervention with the goal of preserving as much vein length as possible for future use as becomes necessary.

AVFs have a substantially lower incidence of thrombosis compared to grafts, requiring fewer interventions and having longer access survival, with access events occurring 14% to 33% as compared to those of AVGs.[1,3,4,28] The DOQI guidelines set a target threshold of 50% unassisted AVF patency at 6 months following balloon angioplasty and 50% unassisted AVF patency at 1 year following surgery. Angioplasty of any underlying stenosis in addition to thrombectomy may result in greater patency rates—up to a primary, 1-year patency rate and a secondary, assisted patency rate of 50% and 80%, respectively.[87] Others have reported a primary, assisted patency rate of AVFs in the range of 60% to 80% at 6 months.[104]

Complications

Minor and major complications from treatment of AVG or AVF occlusions occur in up to 10% of cases[71] and include bleeding around the graft/fistula and/or from the puncture sites (particularly if a venous stenosis persists), arterial embolization, venous rupture from balloon angioplasty, reaction to medication/contrast, and pulmonary emboli. If bleeding from a puncture site is caused by a persistent venous anastomosis, control is usually achieved with immediate angioplasty of the stenosis. Pulmonary emboli are a possibility in any declotting procedure; however, only rarely are they symptomatic and very rarely are fatal.[109–111]

Arterial embolization should occur in less than 10% of cases[71] and typically requires mechanical removal. Mechanical removal may be achieved by carefully passing a guide wire and then an occlusion balloon past the embolus into the distal artery outflow, inflating the occlusion balloon, and carefully withdrawing the inflated occlusion balloon into the graft/venous flow to pull the embolus into a safer location. An alternate technique called the "backbleeding technique" involves inflating a balloon in the arterial inflow above the anastomosis and asking the patient to exercise his or her hand for 60 seconds.[112,113] The balloon is then deflated and repeat angiography performed with the hope that the arterial embolus will have been pushed via retrograde arterial flow back into the graft/venous outflow.

INFECTION

Arteriovenous Grafts

After cardiac causes, infection is the second leading cause of death in adult patients with chronic kidney disease stage 5 with AVGs having a greater incidence of infection than AVFs.[1,114] The frequency of dialysis sessions and low serum calcium are additional risk factors for access infection.[114] Subclinical access infection can result from retained graft material, particularly in abandoned/failed grafts. In such cases, indium-labeled white blood cell nuclear medicine scans or gallium scans may be necessary for diagnosis.[1] Management of access infection often requires more than antibiotic therapy; surgical removal of the infected graft material may be necessary.[1,115,116]

Arteriovenous Fistulas

Infections of AVFs are rare but can be fatal. When they do occur, they typically happen at the puncture/cannulation site.[1] AVF infections generally require both broad-spectrum antibiotic therapy and emergent surgical intervention with resection of the infected material (either artery or vein).[1] Antibiotic therapy should be broad-spectrum until infection sensitivities are determined and therapy is modified appropriately. Therapy should continue for 6 weeks. If it is necessary to resect an infected arterial segment, either an interposition vein graft may be used or a more proximal anastomosis created.[1]

VASCULAR STEAL

Both AVGs and AVFs cause a physiologic vascular steal phenomenon, where the blood flow from the inflow artery follows the path of least resistance and preferentially follows the venous outflow.[117] Most cases do not require any treatment or intervention other than regular surveillance for progression. In a minority of cases, insufficient arterial blood flow to the hand may occur. Patients who are elderly, hypertensive, diabetic, and/or have a history of peripheral arterial disease are at increased risk of symptomatic steal syndrome,[1] which can range from 1% to 4% for more severe symptoms (pain, fingertip necrosis) to 10% for milder symptoms (coldness, pain during dialysis) (FIGURE 89.11).[1,118,119] Although this

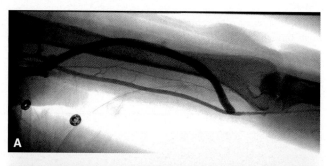
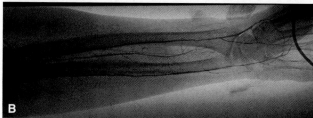

FIGURE 89.11 (A) Patient with cool, painful forearm and fingers following placement of an upper arm graft. Patient with pain with use of the arm, and some early ulceration of several finger tips. Angiogram performed which demonstrates rapid flow into the graft. Very little flow is seen distal to the graft. **(B)** Repeat angiogram performed with manual occlusion of the upper arm graft. Now there is more flow into the arm. The vessels in the arm are small and very diseased with multiple stenotic regions. The patient's symptoms are consistent with a vascular steal. The graft had to be removed because of the ischemic symptoms.

phenomenon usually occurs within days or weeks of the initial access placement surgery, it may in some cases occur months to years later.[1]

Clinical evaluation for ischemia is important in all hemodialysis patients because untreated ischemia can lead to gangrene and amputation.[1] Symptoms include coolness, pallor, pain during exercise and/or rest, skin changes (such as ulcers, necrosis, and gangrene), muscle weakness and/or wasting, and neurologic symptoms including tingling, and paresthesias.[120] If symptomatic vascular steal phenomenon is suspected, investigation and/or referral to a vascular surgeon is warranted. Vascular steal must be differentiated from other causes of hand pain, such as carpel tunnel syndrome and edema from venous hypertension.[1] Investigations may include digital blood pressure measurements, pulse oximetry, and duplex ultrasound.

Treatment options depend on the specific pathology. For example, an arterial stenosis proximal to the anastomosis may be appropriate for angioplasty.[121] In forearm AVGs, either coiling or ligation of the radial artery distal to the anastomosis may alleviate steal symptoms.[122,123] Potential surgical options include decreasing the diameter of the anastomosis or creating a new anastomosis distally.[1] In cases where limb viability is threatened, ligation of the outflow vein may be necessary.

ANEURYSM AND PSEUDOANEURYSM FORMATION

Aneurysms and pseudoaneurysms may form in either AVGs or AVFs from repeated puncture of a graft or vein.[124] These are often palpable as a pulsatile mass and/or visible to the eye. Untreated, these may involve the overlying tissues and lead to skin necrosis, graft infection, spontaneous bleeding or difficulty achieving hemostasis following needle withdrawal, hemorrhage, and even acute graft rupture.

The DOQI guidelines recommend repair of a severely degenerated graft or enlarging pseudoaneurysm. In the case of a pseudoaneurysm that is either enlarging and/or twice the size of the graft, surgical resection with graft interposition is recommended.[1,125] More recently, placement of a covered stent has been used to exclude the pseudoaneurysm.[126]

VENOUS HYPERTENSION

Many dialysis patients have undergone placement of central catheters, which puts them at risk for stenosis of the central veins, and these stenoses in combination with the high flow through the AVFs or AVGs may lead to symptoms of venous hypertension. Symptoms include swelling of the ipsilateral upper extremity, swelling of the breast, and, potentially, facial edema. The patient may have tenderness, pain, and associated erythema, which can mimic cellulitis.[127] Collateral veins will be evident in the ipsilateral extremity, the chest, and neck.[127] Aneurysmal dilatation of the AV access may also occur.[127]

Patients with a history of central venous catheters, pacemakers, or trauma to the extremity should be examined for evidence of collateral veins and arm edema. If there is a suspicion of central venous stenosis, then ultrasound, magnetic resonance imaging, and/or catheter venography can be performed for evaluation prior to access placement.[95,127] Patients who develop symptoms of venous hypertension while on dialysis should be examined with catheter venography with a plan for treatment if central stenosis or occlusion is verified (FIGURE 89.12).

Treatment options for central venous occlusions include balloon angioplasty, balloon angioplasty with placement of bare metal stents, and, more recently, placement of covered stents.[127] The DOQI guidelines recommend balloon angioplasty as the preferred treatment with stent placement reserved for acute elastic recoil or recurrent stenosis within 3 months.[1] The technical success rate for percutaneous transluminal angioplasty (PTA) is high (70% to 90%) but the primary patency rate for PTA rates are variable, ranging from 23% to 63% with a cumulative patency rate of 29% to 100%.[127] Angioplasty can be repeated multiple times and prolong the use of the access for potentially many years.[128] Bare metal stents have been used in central stenoses but are limited because of migration, shortening, or fracturing, and clearly incite intimal hyperplasia, leading to recurrent stenoses and repeat interventions to maintain patency.[127] Covered stents have been used in central stenoses/occlusion with reported primary patency, assisted primary patency, and secondary patency of 56%, 86%, and 100% at 12 months, respectively.[129] Although the patency rate may be improved, these stents will also require continued maintenance most likely from intimal hyperplasia developing at the ends of the stent.

THE FUTURE

Future changes in the maintenance of dialysis access will likely evolve in three primary areas—monitoring/surveillance, first-line therapy among existing treatments, and novel treatments.

In the future, the importance of well-organized and multidisciplinary access teams involved in all aspects of access maintenance, and in particular access surveillance, will increase, according to the recommendations of the DOQI guidelines and supported by clinical data.[37,130,131] More clinical data are necessary regarding the surveillance methods most predictive of impending access failure that are both practical and cost-effective. Trend analysis, whereby access measurements, such as flow and pressure, are plotted, and readily available during successive dialysis sessions, will likely play a more prominent role. The necessity, timing, and type of postintervention follow-up remains to be better elucidated.

Among the intervention options currently available, additional trials are necessary to further refine the best approach, including the construction of the access (e.g., the feeding artery, type and location of anastomosis) and the respective roles of cutting angioplasty balloons, stent-grafts, thrombolysis and thrombectomy devices, and concomitant medications, such as clopidogrel, aspirin, and Aggrenox.[132–135]

Finally, innovations will likely occur in all aspects of access care, including surveillance, surgical, and interventional. In particular, targeted delivery of various agents, such as medications, genes, cells, or virus particles, shows promise in the prevention

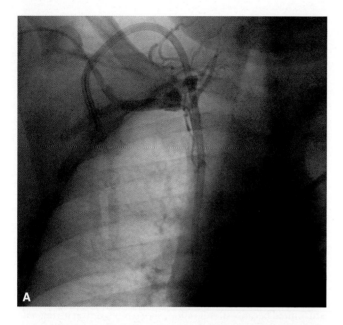

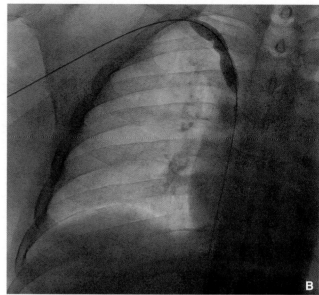

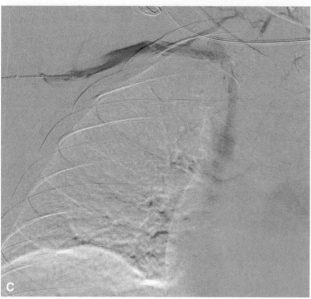

FIGURE 89.12 (A) Stenosis caused by dialysis catheter. Patient with a swollen right arm following placement of a right-sided fistula. There has been the development of collaterals around the region of the catheter. **(B)** Following removal of central venous catheter, the stenosis in the right brachiocephalic vein is dilated. **(C)** Following dilatation there is improvement in the flow through the vein. This is unlikely to be a long term solution, and this patient required repeated angioplasty to keep the vein open and to minimize swelling in the right arm. This is the type of situation where a stent graft might be a reasonable option.

of neointimal hyperplasia.[136] Given the ability of interventional radiologists to deliver these agents to an endovascular or perivascular target, we will likely continue to have a very important role in access management.

CONCLUSION

It is mandatory for any interventional radiologist working at a dialysis center to have expertise with all aspects of dialysis care, including familiarity with venous access, arteriovenous grafts, and AVF. Knowledge of dialysis care includes not only that of standard endovascular technique, but specifics unique to this subset of patients, such as when and how to intervene, how to treat complications that may arise, and when referral to surgery is necessary. It is strongly recommended that any interventional radiologist who is likely to be referred such patients become very

familiar with the DOQI guidelines as well as guidelines from the various interventional radiology societies, such as the Society of Interventional Radiology and Cardiovascular and Interventional Radiology Society of Europe.

Prompt and reliable service, proper follow-up, a solid background in the fundamentals of endovascular dialysis work, and a good relationship with the local dialysis unit and nephrologists can lead to a robust and very rewarding experience for those planning to offer this service.

REFERENCES

1. National Kidney Foundation KDOQI clinical practice guidelines and clinical practice recommendations for 2006 updates: hemodialysis adequacy, peritoneal dialysis adequacy and vascular access. *Am J Kidney Dis* 2006;48(suppl 1):S1–S322.

2. Mehta S. Statistical summary of clinical results of vascular access procedures for haemodialysis. In: Sommer BG, Henry ML, eds. *Vascular Access for Hemodialysis-II* S. Chicago, IL: Gore; 1991:145–157.

3. Pisoni RL, et al. Vascular access use in Europe and the United States: results from the DOPPS. *Kidney Int* 2002;61(1):305–316.

4. Perera GB, et al. Superiority of autogenous arteriovenous hemodialysis access: maintenance of function with fewer secondary interventions. *Ann Vasc Surg* 2004;18(1):66–73.

5. Huber TS, Buhler AG, Seeger JM. Evidence-based data for the hemodialysis access surgeon. *Semin Dial* 2004;17(3):217–223.

6. *The Cost Effectiveness of Alternative Types of Vascular Access and the Economic Cost of ESRD.* Bethesda, MD: National Institutes of Health, National Institute of Diabetes and Digestive and Kidney Diseases; 1995:139–157.

7. Eggers P, Milam R. Trends in vascular access procedures and expenditures in Medicare's ESRD program. In: Henry ML, ed. *Vascular Access for Hemodialysis-VII.* Chicago, IL: Gore; 2001:133–143.

8. Nassar GM, Ayus JC. Infectious complications of the hemodialysis access. *Kidney Int* 2001;60(1):1–13.

9. Dhingra RK, et al. Type of vascular access and mortality in U.S. hemodialysis patients. *Kidney Int* 2001;60(4):1443–1451.

10. Polkinghorne KR, et al. Vascular access and all-cause mortality: a propensity score analysis. *J Am Soc Nephrol* 2004;15(2):477–486.

11. Harland RC. Placement of permanent vascular access devices: surgical considerations. *Adv Ren Replace Ther* 1994;1(2):99–106.

12. Palder S, et al. Vascular access for hemodialysis. *Ann Surg* 1985;202:235–239.

13. Albers FJ. Causes of hemodialysis access failure. *Adv Ren Replace Ther* 1994;1(2):107–118.

14. Kherlakian GM, et al. Comparison of autogenous fistula versus expanded polytetrafluoroethylene graft fistula for angioaccess in hemodialysis. *Am J Surg* 1986;152(2):238–243.

15. Kinnaert P, et al. Nine years' experience with internal arteriovenous fistulas for haemodialysis: a study of some factors influencing the results. *Br J Surg* 1977;64(4):242–246.

16. Maya ID, et al. Outcomes of brachiocephalic fistulas, transposed brachiobasilic fistulas, and upper arm grafts. *Clin J Am Soc Nephrol* 2009;4(1):86–92.

17. Lok CE, et al. Reducing vascular access morbidity: a comparative trial of two vascular access monitoring strategies. *Nephrol Dial Transplant* 2003;18(6):1174–1180.

18. Bhalodia R, et al. Comparison of radiocephalic fistulas placed in the proximal forearm and in the wrist. *Semin Dial* 2011;24(3):355–357.

19. Allon M, Lok CE. Dialysis fistula or graft: the role for randomized clinical trials. *Clin J Am Soc Nephrol* 2010;5(12):2348–2354.

20. Gheith OA, Kamal MM. Risk factors of vascular access failure in patients on hemodialysis. *Iran J Kidney Dis* 2008;2(4):201–207.

21. Gagliardi GM, et al. Malnutrition, infection and arteriovenous fistula failure: is there a link? *J Vasc Access* 2011;12(1):57–62.

22. Pisoni R, Barker-Finkel J, Allo M. Statin therapy is not associated with improved vascular access outcomes. *Clin J Am Soc Nephrol* 2010;5(8):1447–1450.

23. Owens ML, et al. Vascular grafts for hemodialysis: evaluation of sites and materials. *Dial Transplant* 1979;8:521–530.

24. Kanterman RY, Vesely TM. Graft-to-vein fistulas associated with polytetrafluoroethylene dialysis grafts: diagnosis and clinical significance. *J Vasc Interv Radiol* 1995;6(2):267–271.

25. Butler HG III, Baker LD Jr, Johnson JM. Vascular access for chronic hemodialysis: polytetrafluoroethylene (PTFE) versus bovine heterograft. *Am J Surg* 1977;134(6):791–793.

26. Scott EC, Glickman MH. Conduits for hemodialysis access. *Semin Vasc Surg* 2007;20(3):158–163.

27. Raju S. PTFE grafts for hemodialysis access. Techniques for insertion and management of complications. *Ann Surg* 1987;206(5):666–673.

28. Huber TS, et al. Patency of autogenous and polytetrafluoroethylene upper extremity arteriovenous hemodialysis accesses: a systematic review. *J Vasc Surg* 2003;38(5):1005–1011.

29. Akoh JA. Prosthetic arteriovenous grafts for hemodialysis. *J Vasc Access* 2009;10(3):137–147.

30. Hakim RM, et al. Effects of dose of dialysis on morbidity and mortality. *Am J Kidney Dis* 1994;23(5):661–669.

31. Morbidity and mortality of dialysis. *NIH Consens Statement* 1993;11(2):1–33.

32. Rocco MV, Bleyer AJ, Burkart JM. Utilization of inpatient and outpatient resources for the management of hemodialysis access complications. *Am J Kidney Dis* 1996;28(2):250–256.

33. Besarab A, et al. Utility of intra-access pressure monitoring in detecting and correcting venous outlet stenoses prior to thrombosis. *Kidney Int* 1995;47(5):1364–1373.

34. Glanz S, et al. The role of percutaneous angioplasty in the management of chronic hemodialysis fistulas. *Ann Surg* 1987;206(6):777–781.

35. Rodkin R, et al. Streptokinase and transluminal angioplasty in the treatment of acutely thrombosed hemodialysis access fistulas. *Radiology* 1983;149:425–428.

36. Burger H, et al. Percutaneous transluminal angioplasty improves longevity in fistulae and shunts for hemodialysis. *Nephrol Dial Transplant* 1990;5:608–611.

37. Pflederer TA, et al. How to organize hemodialysis vascular access quality assurance efforts into a cohesive whole for better patient outcomes. *Contemp Dial Nephrol* 2000;21:18–21.

38. Roberts A, Valji K. Screening and assessment of dialysis graft function. *Tech Vasc Interv Radiol* 1999;2(4):186–188.

39. Sullivan KL, et al. Hemodynamics of failing dialysis grafts. *Radiology* 1993;186(3):867–872.

40. Basile C, et al. A comparison of methods for the measurement of hemodialysis access recirculation. *J Nephrol* 2003;16(6):908–913.

41. Beathard GA. Physical examination of AV grafts. *Semin Dial* 1996;5:74–76.

42. Trerotola SO, et al. Screening for dialysis access graft malfunction: comparison of physical examination with US. *J Vasc Interv Radiol* 1996;7(1):15–20.

43. Rittgers S, et al. Noninvasive blood flow measurement in expanded polytetrafluoroethylene grafts for hemodialysis access. *J Vasc Surg* 1986;3:635–642.

44. Asif A, et al. Inflow stenosis in arteriovenous fistulas and grafts: a multicenter, prospective study. *Kidney Int* 2005;67(5):1986–1992.

45. Bay WH, et al. Predicting hemodialysis access failure with color flow Doppler ultrasound. *Am J Nephrol* 1998;18(4):296–304.

46. Bosman PJ, et al. Graft flow as a predictor of thrombosis in hemodialysis grafts. *Kidney Int* 1998;54(5):1726–1730.

47. Lindsay RM, et al. Hemodialysis access blood flow rates can be measured by a differential conductivity technique and are predictive of access clotting. *Am J Kidney Dis* 1997;30(4):475–482.

48. May RE, et al. Predictive measures of vascular access thrombosis: a prospective study. *Kidney Int* 1997;52(6):1656–1662.

49. Neyra NR, et al. Change in access blood flow over time predicts vascular access thrombosis. *Kidney Int* 1998;54(5):1714–1719.

50. Rehman SU, et al. Intradialytic serial vascular access flow measurements. *Am J Kidney Dis* 1999;34(3):471–477.

51. Wang E, Schneditz D, Levin NW. Predictive value of access blood flow and stenosis in detection of graft failure. *Clin Nephrol* 2000;54(5):393–399.

52. Hoeben H, et al. Vascular access surveillance: evaluation of combining dynamic venous pressure and vascular access blood flow measurements. *Am J Nephrol* 2003;23(6):403–408.

53. Schwab SJ, et al. Hemodialysis arteriovenous access: detection of stenosis and response to treatment by vascular access blood flow. *Kidney Int* 2001;59(1):358–362.

54. Wang E, et al. Predictive value of access blood flow in detecting access thrombosis. *ASAIO J* 1998;44(5):M555–M558.

55. Kanterman RY, et al. Dialysis access grafts: anatomic location of venous stenosis and results of angioplasty. *Radiology* 1995;195:135–139.

56. May AG, et al. Critical arterial stenosis. *Surgery* 1963;54:250–259.

57. Berguer R, Hwang NH. Critical arterial stenosis: a theoretical and experimental solution. *Ann Surg* 1974;180(1):39–50.

58. Schwab SJ, et al. Prevention of hemodialysis fistula thrombosis. Early detection of venous stenoses. *Kidney Int* 1989;36(4):707–711.

59. Beathard GA. Thrombolysis versus surgery for the treatment of thrombosed dialysis access grafts. *J Am Soc Nephrol* 1995;6(6):1619–1624.

60. Tsetis D, Morgan R, Belli AM. Cutting balloons for the treatment of vascular stenoses. *Eur Radiol* 2006;16(8):1675–1683.

61. Vorwerk D. Cutting balloon angioplasty in dialysis fistulas: let us start to ask the right questions. *Cardiovasc Intervent Radiol* 2007;30(6):1171–1172.

62. Bittl JA, Feldman RL. Cutting balloon angioplasty for undilatable venous stenoses causing dialysis graft failure. *Catheter Cardiovasc Interv* 2003;58(4):524–526.

63. Sreenarasimhaiah VP, et al. Cutting balloon angioplasty for resistant venous anastomotic stenoses. *Semin Dial* 2004;17(6):523–527.

64. Song HH, et al. Cutting balloon angioplasty for resistant venous stenoses of Brescia-Cimino fistulas. *J Vasc Interv Radiol* 2004;15(12):1463–1467.

65. Wu CC, Wen SC. Cutting balloon angioplasty for resistant venous stenoses of dialysis access: immediate and patency results. *Catheter Cardiovasc Interv* 2008;71(2):250–254.

66. Murakami R, Tajima H, Kumita S. Cutting balloon-associated hemodialysis fistula rupture after failed standard balloon angioplasty. *Kidney Int* 2006;70(5):825.

67. Singer-Jordan J, Papura S. Cutting balloon angioplasty for primary treatment of hemodialysis fistula venous stenoses: preliminary results. *J Vasc Interv Radiol* 2005;16(1):25–29.

68. Funaki B. Cutting balloon angioplasty in arteriovenous fistulas. *J Vasc Interv Radiol* 2005;16(1):5–7

69. Vesely TM, Siegel JB. Use of the peripheral cutting balloon to treat hemodialysis-related stenoses. *J Vasc Interv Radiol* 2005;16(12):1593–1603.

70. Funaki B, et al. Wallstent deployment to salvage dialysis graft thrombolysis complicated by venous rupture: early and intermediate results. *AJR Am J Roentgenol* 1997;169(5):1435–1437.

71. Aruny JE, et al. Quality improvement guidelines for percutaneous management of the thrombosed or dysfunctional dialysis access. *J Vasc Interv Radiol* 2003;14(9, pt 2):S247–S253.

72. Verstandig AG, et al. Shortening and migration of Wallstents after stenting of central venous stenoses in hemodialysis patients. *Cardiovasc Intervent Radiol* 2003;26(1):58–64.

73. Sharma AK, Sinha S, Bakran A. Migration of intra-vascular metallic stent into pulmonary artery. *Nephrol Dial Transplant* 2002;17(3):511.

74. Vesely TM, Amin MZ, Pilgram T. Use of stents and stent grafts to salvage angioplasty failures in patients with hemodialysis grafts. *Semin Dial* 2008;21(1):100–104.

75. Keeling AN, et al. Successful endovascular treatment of a hemodialysis graft pseudoaneurysm by covered stent and direct percutaneous thrombin injection. *Semin Dial* 2008;21(6):553–556.

76. Kundu S, et al. Use of PTFE stent grafts for hemodialysis-related central venous occlusions: intermediate-term results. *Cardiovasc Intervent Radiol* 2011;34(5):949–957.

77. Salman L, Asif A. Stent graft for nephrologists: concerns and consensus. *Clin J Am Soc Nephrol* 2010;5(7):1347–1352.

78. Bent CL, et al. Effectiveness of stent-graft placement for salvage of dysfunctional arteriovenous hemodialysis fistulas. *J Vasc Interv Radiol* 2010;21(4):496–502.

79. Webb KM, et al. Outcome of the use of stent grafts to salvage failed arteriovenous accesses. *Ann Vasc Surg* 2010;24(1):34–38.

80. Haskal ZJ, et al. Stent graft versus balloon angioplasty for failing dialysis-access grafts. *N Engl J Med* 2010;362(6):494–503.

81. Gray RJ, et al. Reporting standards for percutaneous interventions in dialysis access. Technology Assessment Committee. *J Vasc Interv Radiol* 1999;10(10):1405–1415.

82. Murray SP, et al. Early rethrombosis of clotted hemodialysis grafts: graft salvage achieved with an aggressive approach. *AJR Am J Roentgenol* 2000;175(2):529–532.

83. Turmel-Rodrigues L, et al. Salvage of immature forearm fistulas for haemodialysis by interventional radiology. *Nephrol Dial Transplant* 2001;16(12):2365–2371.

84. Lui KW, et al. Ultrasound guided puncture of the brachial artery for haemodialysis fistula angiography. *Nephrol Dial Transplant* 2001;16(1):98–101.

85. Katz SG, Kohl RD. The percutaneous treatment of angioaccess graft complications. *Am J Surg* 1995;170(3):238–242.

86. Lilly RZ, et al. Predictors of arteriovenous graft patency after radiologic intervention in hemodialysis patients. *Am J Kidney Dis* 2001;37(5):945–953.

87. Turmel-Rodrigues L, et al. Treatment of stenosis and thrombosis in haemodialysis fistulas and grafts by interventional radiology. *Nephrol Dial Transplant* 2000;15(12):2029–2036.

88. Beathard GA. Percutaneous venous angioplasty in the treatment of stenotic lesions affecting dialysis fistulas. *Prog Cardiovasc Dis* 1992;34(4):263–278.

89. Patel RI, et al. Patency of Wallstents placed across the venous anastomosis of hemodialysis grafts after percutaneous recanalization. *Radiology* 1998;209(2):365–370.

90. Hoffer EK, et al. Prospective randomized trial of a metallic intravascular stent in hemodialysis graft maintenance. *J Vasc Interv Radiol* 1997;8(6):965–973.

91. Gray RJ, et al. Use of Wallstents for hemodialysis access-related venous stenoses and occlusions untreatable with balloon angioplasty. *Radiology* 1995;195(2):479–484.

92. Clark TW, et al. Outcome and prognostic factors of restenosis after percutaneous treatment of native hemodialysis fistulas. *J Vasc Interv Radiol* 2002;13(1):51–59.

93. Rajan DK, Clark TW. Patency of Wallstents placed at the venous anastomosis of dialysis grafts for salvage of angioplasty-induced rupture. *Cardiovasc Intervent Radiol* 2003;26(3):242–245.

94. Welber A, et al. Endovascular stent placement for angioplasty-induced venous rupture related to the treatment of hemodialysis grafts. *J Vasc Interv Radiol* 1999;10(5):547–551.

95. Ray E, Roberts AC. Hemodialysis access. In: Valji K, ed. *The Practice of Interventional Radiology*. Philadelphia, PA: Elsevier; 2012:581–602.

96. Cynamon J, et al. Hemodialysis graft declotting: description of the "lyse and wait" technique. *J Vasc Interv Radiol* 1997;8(5):825–829.

97. Cynamon J, Pierpont CE. Thrombolysis for the treatment of thrombosed hemodialysis access grafts. *Rev Cardiovasc Med* 2002;3(suppl 2):S84–S91.

98. Winkler TA, et al. Study of thrombus from thrombosed hemodialysis access grafts. *Radiology* 1995;197(2):461–465.

99. Vesely TM. Mechanical thrombectomy devices to treat thrombosed hemodialysis grafts. *Tech Vasc Interv Radiol* 2003;6(1):35–41.

100. Patel AA, Tuite CM, Trerotola SO. Mechanical thrombectomy of hemodialysis fistulae and grafts. *Cardiovasc Intervent Radiol* 2005;28(6):704–713.

101. Vesely TM. Techniques for using mechanical thrombectomy devices to treat thrombosed hemodialysis grafts. *Tech Vasc Interv Radiol* 1999;2(4):208–216.

102. Overbosch EH, et al. Occluded hemodialysis shunts: Dutch multicenter experience with the hydrolyser catheter. *Radiology* 1996;201(2):485–488.

103. Rocek M, et al. Mechanical thrombolysis of thrombosed hemodialysis native fistulas with use of the Arrow-Trerotola percutaneous thrombolytic device: our preliminary experience. *J Vasc Interv Radiol* 2000;11(9):1153–1158.

104. Rajan DK, et al. Procedural success and patency after percutaneous treatment of thrombosed autogenous arteriovenous dialysis fistulas. *J Vasc Interv Radiol* 2002;13(12):1211–1218.

105. Smits HF, et al. Percutaneous thrombolysis of thrombosed haemodialysis access grafts: comparison of three mechanical devices. *Nephrol Dial Transplant* 2002;17(3):467–473.

106. Falk A. Maintenance and salvage of arteriovenous fistulas. *J Vasc Interv Radiol* 2006;17(5):807–813.

107. Sofocleous CT, et al. Alteplase for hemodialysis access graft thrombolysis. *J Vasc Interv Radiol* 2002;13(8):775–784.

108. Beathard GA, Litchfield T. Effectiveness and safety of dialysis vascular access procedures performed by interventional nephrologists. *Kidney Int* 2004;66(4):1622–1632.

109. Soulen MC, et al. Mechanical declotting of thrombosed dialysis grafts: experience in 86 cases. *J Vasc Interv Radiol* 1997;8(4):563–567.

110. Petronis JD, et al. Ventilation-perfusion scintigraphic evaluation of pulmonary clot burden after percutaneous thrombolysis of clotted hemodialysis access grafts. *Am J Kidney Dis* 1999;34(2):207–211.

111. Kinney TB, et al. Pulmonary embolism from pulse-spray pharmacomechanical thrombolysis of clotted hemodialysis grafts: urokinase versus heparinized saline. *J Vasc Interv Radiol* 2000;11(9):1143–1152.

112. Tretotola S, et al. Backbleeding technique for treatment of arterial emboli resulting from dialysis graft thrombolysis. *J Vasc Interv Radiol* 1998;9:141–143.

113. Beathard GA. Management of complications of endovascular dialysis access procedures. *Semin Dial* 2003;16(4):309–313.

114. Gulati S, et al. Role of vascular access as a risk factor for infections in hemodialysis. *Ren Fail* 2003;25(6):967–973.

115. Deneuville M. Infection of PTFE grafts used to create arteriovenous fistulas for hemodialysis access. *Ann Vasc Surg* 2000;14(5):473–479.

116. Ryan SV, et al. Management of infected prosthetic dialysis arteriovenous grafts. *J Vasc Surg* 2004;39(1):73–78.

117. Sivanesan S, How TV, Bakran A. Characterizing flow distributions in AV fistulae for haemodialysis access. *Nephrol Dial Transplant* 1998;13(12):3108–3110.

118. Schanzer H, Eisenberg D. Management of steal syndrome resulting from dialysis access. *Semin Vasc Surg* 2004;17(1):45–49.

119. Tordoir JH, Dammers R, van der Sande FM. Upper extremity ischemia and hemodialysis vascular access. *Eur J Vasc Endovasc Surg* 2004;27(1):1–5.

120. Miles AM. Upper limb ischemia after vascular access surgery: differential diagnosis and management. *Semin Dial* 2000;13(5):312–315.

121. Guerra A, et al. Arterial percutaneous angioplasty in upper limbs with vascular access devices for haemodialysis. *Nephrol Dial Transplant* 2002;17(5):843–851.

122. Schanzer H, et al. Treatment of ischemia due to "steal" by arteriovenous fistula with distal artery ligation and revascularization. *J Vasc Surg* 1988;7(6):770–773.

123. Valji K, et al. Hand ischemia in patients with hemodialysis access grafts: angiographic diagnosis and treatment. *Radiology* 1995;196(3):697–701.

124. Charara J, et al. Morphologic assessment of ePTFE graft wall damage following hemodialysis needle punctures. *J Appl Biomater* 1990;1:279–287.

125. Ballard JL, Bunt TJ, Malone JM. Major complications of angioaccess surgery. *Am J Surg* 1992;164:229–232.

126. Hausegger KA, et al. Aneurysms of hemodialysis access grafts: treatment with covered stents: a report of three cases. *Cardiovasc Intervent Radiol* 1998;21(4):334–337.

127. Kundu S. Review of central venous disease in hemodialysis patients. *J Vasc Interv Radiol* 2010;21(7):963–968.

128. Ziegler TW, et al. Prolonging the life of difficult hemodialysis access using thrombolysis, angiography and angioplasty. *Adv Ren Replace Ther* 1995;2(1):52–59.

129. Anaya-Ayala JE, et al. Efficacy of covered stent placement for central venous occlusive disease in hemodialysis patients. *J Vasc Surg* 2011;54(3):754–759.

130. Allon M, et al. A multidisciplinary approach to hemodialysis access: prospective evaluation. *Kidney Int* 1998;53(2):473–479.

131. Cull DL, et al. The impact of a community-wide vascular access program on the management of graft thromboses in a dialysis population of 495 patients. *Am J Surg* 1999;178(2):113–116.

132. Dember LM, et al. Effect of clopidogrel on early failure of arteriovenous fistulas for hemodialysis: a randomized controlled trial. *JAMA* 2008;299(18):2164–2171.

133. Dixon BS, et al. Design of the Dialysis Access Consortium (DAC) Aggrenox Prevention of Access Stenosis Trial. *Clin Trials* 2005;2(5):400–412.

134. Dixon BS, et al. Use of aspirin associates with longer primary patency of hemodialysis grafts. *J Am Soc Nephrol* 2011;22(4):773–781.

135. Dixon BS, et al. Effect of dipyridamole plus aspirin on hemodialysis graft patency. *N Engl J Med* 2009;360(21):2191–2201.

136. Lee T, Roy-Chaudhury P. Advances and new frontiers in the pathophysiology of venous neointimal hyperplasia and dialysis access stenosis. *Adv Chronic Kidney Dis* 2009;16(5):329–338.

CHAPTER

90

Superior Vena Cava— Malignant Lesions

NARENDRA B. GUTTA and STEPHEN B. SOLOMON

OVERVIEW

Superior vena cava syndrome (SVCS) is a pattern of symptoms and signs resulting from obstruction of the superior vena cava (SVC) (FIGURE 90.1). Its total incidence is approximately 15,000 cases per year in the United States.[1]

APPLIED ANATOMY

The SVC carries blood from the head, arms, and upper trunk to the heart, which is about one-third of the total venous return to the heart (FIGURE 90.2). Obstruction of the SVC leads to flow of blood through multiple small collateral veins to the azygos vein or the inferior vena cava. These venous collaterals dilate over several weeks and the upper body venous pressure, which is markedly elevated initially at the time of obstruction, decreases over time.[2,3] The common collateral vessels include the azygos, intercostal, mediastinal, paravertebral, hemiazygos, thoraco-epigastric, internal mammary, thoracoacromioclavicular, and anterior chest wall veins[4] (FIGURES 90.3A and B). Four major venous collateral return patterns following SVC obstruction are described in the literature. Among these, symptoms tend to be more severe when obstruction is below the entry of the azygos vein[5] (FIGURES 90.4A and B).

ETIOLOGY

Malignant causes account for 70% to 90% of the SVCS cases. Non–small-cell and small-cell lung cancers account for about 50% and 25% of malignant SVCS cases, respectively. Hence lung cancer is the most common cause, accounting for almost 75% of malignant cases. Among non–small-cell lung cancers the most common histology found is adenocarcinoma. Of the remaining 25% of malignant SVCS cases, 10% are caused by lymphomas (non-Hodgkin being more common than Hodgkin), another 10% by metastases (most commonly from breast cancer), and the remaining less than 5% by germ cell tumors, thymoma, mesothelioma, and other rare malignancies. Of patients with small-cell lung cancer there is a higher likelihood to develop the syndrome (6% vs. 1%) compared to patients with non–small-cell lung cancer.[6–12]

The remaining 10% to 35% of cases of SVCS are due to benign causes, the most common of which is SVC thrombosis resulting from an intravascular device, which accounts for 70% of the benign cases. It should be noted that patients with known malignancy can also develop SVCS due to benign causes, such as central line or MediPort thrombosis.

CLINICAL PRESENTATION

Depending on the severity, the level of narrowing, and the acuteness of narrowing, the elevated upper body venous pressure determines the clinical presentation of SVCS.[1] Clinical presentation includes interstitial edema of the head, neck, upper trunk, and bilateral upper limbs with cyanosis, plethora, and distended subcutaneous vessels, which are visually very striking but generally of little consequence. Cough, hoarseness, dyspnea, stridor, and dysphagia as manifestations of laryngeal and/or pharyngeal edema are seen. Other findings also include those caused by cerebral edema, such as headache, confusion, and coma. Cerebral edema can also lead to cerebral ischemia, herniation, and possibly death due to raised intracranial pressure.[1] Only one death was directly attributed to SVCS in a large review of 1,989 cases, and it was a result of severe epistaxis.[13] SVC obstruction, which is apparent on computed tomography (CT) or magnetic resonance imaging (MRI) in the absence of symptoms is known as occult SVCS.[14]

DIAGNOSIS

Diagnosis is based on clinical features and imaging findings. During history and physical examination, emphasis should be given to the duration and severity of symptoms, history of any malignancy, previous interventions, any current or previous medications (especially antiplatelets and anticoagulants), any cardiopulmonary comorbidities, or presence of cerebral metastases. Based on clinical features of SVCS the differential diagnoses include cerebral metastasis or trachea-bronchial or cardiac compression.[15]

IMAGING

Imaging plays a very important role in the management of SVCS. Chest radiographs (posteroanterior [PA] and lateral views) are usually done during initial workup and also during the postprocedural follow-ups to look for possible stent migration (FIGURE 90.3D). The most useful imaging modality is contrast-enhanced CT scan of the chest. It helps to clearly identify the location and degree of narrowing, presence of intravascular thrombus, and the underlying etiology of SVCS (FIGURES 90.3A, 90.4A, and 90.5A). MRI of the chest is done sometimes, especially

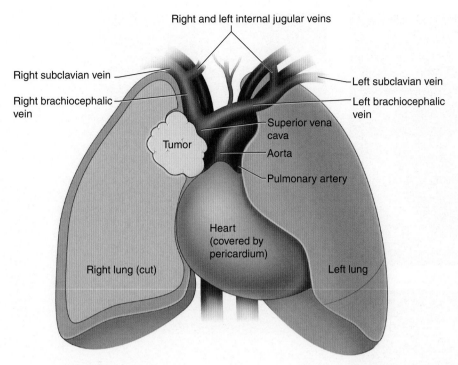

FIGURE 90.1 The vascular anatomy of the upper chest, including the heart, superior vena cava, inferior vena cava, and subclavian vessels. The tumor is shown compressing the superior vena cava.

for patients with contraindications to CT. Conventional venography is still considered the gold standard for technical assessment of the SVC. However, it is done primarily as part of the preintervention workup and when recurrence or deterioration of SVCS occurs on follow-up. Venography is useful to define the

SVC narrowing as well as the extent of any intravascular thrombus (FIGURES 90.3, 90.4, and 90.5). As part of any imaging study it is important to look for the location, extent of narrowing, along with the residual diameter of the SVC lumen, and also presence of any internal (bland or tumor) thrombus.

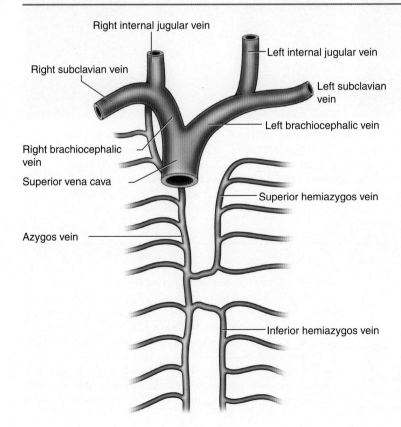

FIGURE 90.2 Anatomy of superior vena cava and its tributaries.

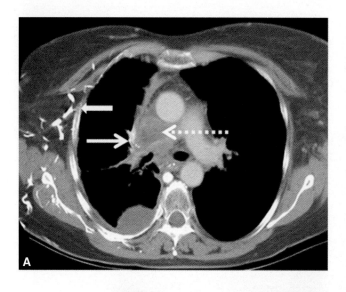
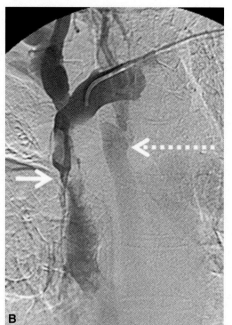
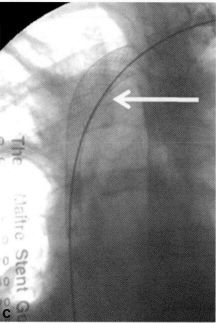
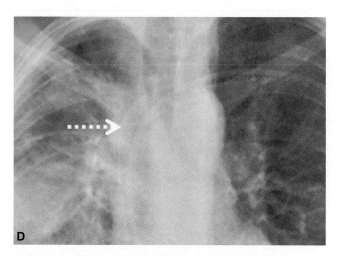

FIGURE 90.3 A. Contrast-enhanced axial CT scan of a 53-year-old woman with non–small-cell lung carcinoma (*dashed arrow*) shows severe stenosis of the superior vena cava (*arrow*) with chest wall collaterals (*block arrow*). This was initially treated with a 2-week course of radiotherapy but there was symptomatic recurrence. **B.** Superior venacavogram shows stenosis of the SVC (*arrow*) and network of collaterals that have developed via the azygos vein (*dashed arrow*). **C.** Superior vena cava successfully stented with a 16-mm diameter, 60-mm long wallstent (Boston Scientific, Inc., Newton, MA), extending from the SVC back into the left brachiocephalic vein (*arrow*). **D.** Postprocedure chest radiograph demonstrates the SVC stent (*dashed arrow*) to be unchanged in position.

▌MANAGEMENT

The management of malignant SVCS includes relief of the symptoms as well as treatment of the underlying cancer. It is dictated by the severity of the symptoms, its likelihood of response to a particular treatment option, and the underlying malignancy treatment itself.[15] In cases of acute life-threatening symptoms, such as significant cerebral edema causing confusion and obtundation, significant laryngeal edema causing stridor and potential airway compromise, significant hemodynamic compromise causing syncope without precipitating factors, hypotension, or renal insufficiency, treatment should be done on an emergency basis.[8,16] These patients should have stents placed expeditiously to reestablish venous flow. In most cases, SVCS symptoms are generally progressive over several weeks and get better over time as collaterals develop.[1]

The median life expectancy among SVCS patients is approximately 6 months, but estimates vary widely depending on the underlying malignancy.[7,8,17–19] Survival rate does

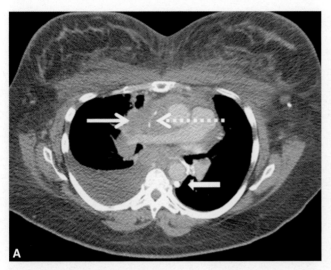
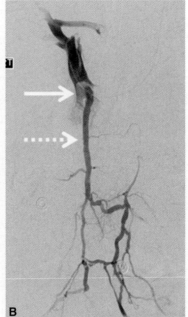
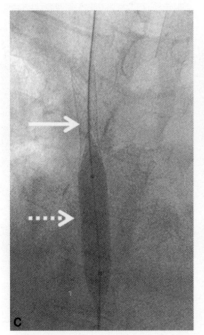
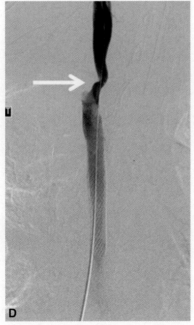
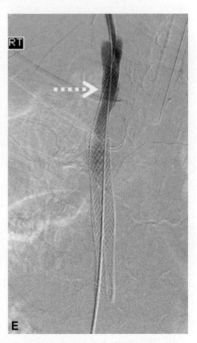

FIGURE 90.4 **A.** Contrast-enhanced axial CT scan of a 47-year-old woman with poorly differentiated non–small-cell lung cancer (*dashed arrow*) shows severe narrowing of the SVC (*arrow*) with collaterals (*block arrow*). **B.** The initial SVC-gram demonstrates complete obstruction of the SVC (*arrow*) with collateral flow through the azygos vein (*dashed arrow*). **C.** 14-mm diameter, 60-mm long wallstent (*arrow*) was deployed and then dilated with a 12-mm diameter balloon (*dashed arrow*). **D.** On repeat venography, a short segment residual narrowing (*arrow*) is seen at the top of the stent. **E.** Consequently, a second overlapping 14-mm diameter wallstent (*dashed arrow*) is deployed; the completion venography shows excellent flow through the SVC.

not appear to significantly differ from patients with the same tumor type and disease stage without obstruction of the SVC.[13,20–23]

To manage malignant SVCS it is necessary beforehand to have tissue diagnosis because treatments, such as radiation, chemotherapy, and/or steroids, may obscure histologic diagnosis at a later date. Radiation in particular can obscure a diagnosis in up to 42% of biopsy specimens obtained from the irradiated area after treatment.[24] Hence, initiation of such therapies before obtaining a diagnosis is unwarranted.

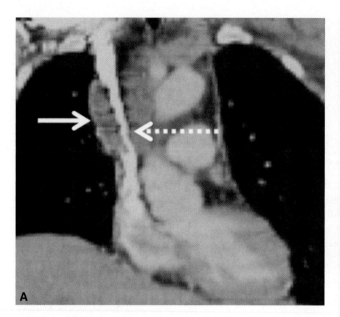
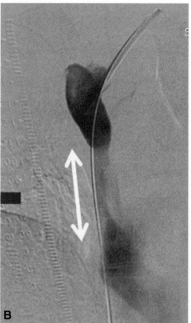
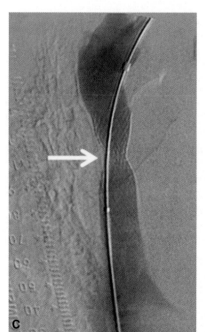
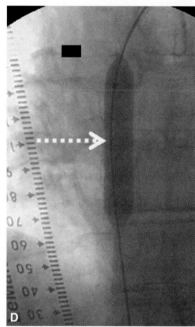
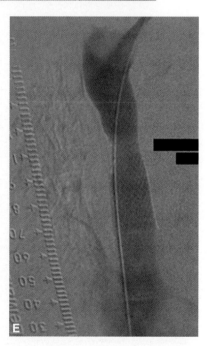

FIGURE 90.5 A. Contrast-enhanced CT scan (Coronal MPR) of a 43-year-old man with SVC obstruction due to poorly differentiated non–small-cell lung cancer (*arrow*) shows severe extrinsic narrowing of the SVC (*dashed arrow*). **B.** Superior venocavogram performed via an 8 French vascular sheath from a left jugular approach shows a focal area of narrowing (*double headed arrow*), which measured about 4 cm in length. This is consistent with the findings on the CT scan. **C.** The initial poststent (Smart stent, Cordis Medical, Johnson and Johnson, Warren, NJ) venogram demonstrates impingement of the stent focally (*arrow*), which was then (**D**) dilated with a 10-mm diameter balloon (*dashed arrow*). **E.** Postdilatation SVC-gram demonstrated improvement in the caliber of the vessel with good flow.

Medical Management

Elevating the patient's head helps to decrease the hydrostatic pressure and thereby the edema. It is usually of little benefit, however, if venous collaterals have not dilated enough. Oxygen supplementation is usually given to relieve shortness of breath.

Glucocorticoid therapy (dexamethasone, 4 mg every 6 hours) is commonly prescribed, although its effects have not been formally well studied, and there are only case reports to suggest the benefit. Because glucocorticoids significantly reduce tumor burdens of lymphoma and thymoma, they are more likely to reduce the obstruction in patients with these tumors than other tumor types.[20,25] Loop diuretics are occasionally used. However, in an observational study involving 107 patients with the SVCS due to various causes, the rate of clinical improvement (84% overall) was similar among patients receiving glucocorticoids, diuretics, or neither therapy.[8] Thus the use of loop diuretics is not suggested.

Surgery

Surgical bypass grafting (e.g., subcutaneous jugular–femoral graft) is infrequently used to treat the SVCS.[26] Polytetrafluoroethylene (PTFE) tube or autologous saphenous vein grafts are used for reconstruction. The more common surgical approach is sternotomy or thoracotomy with extensive resection and reconstruction of the SVC. The reported case series indicate an operative mortality rate of approximately 5% and patency rates of 80% to 90%.[22,27,28] Thymomas are relatively resistant to chemotherapy and radiotherapy compared to lymphomas and, therefore, surgery is more appropriate in cases of SVCS caused by thymoma.

Radiotherapy

Radiotherapy is commonly used to treat symptomatic malignant SVCS patients. Most tumor types causing the SVCS are sensitive to radiotherapy, but its use requires a prior tissue diagnosis. In a systematic review, complete symptomatic relief of SVCS was reported in 78% of patients with small-cell lung cancer and 63% of those with non–small-cell lung cancer at 2 weeks after radiotherapy.[6–8,10,13,20,29–33] Steroids are generally used in conjunction with radiotherapy because of concern about radiation-induced edema.

Systemic Chemotherapy

The general consensus for use of chemotherapy in patients with malignant SVCS is based on the tumor histology. Complete symptomatic relief of SVCS is seen with chemotherapy in approximately 80% of patients with non-Hodgkin lymphoma or small-cell lung cancer. Also, chemotherapy leads to rapid symptomatic relief of SVCS caused by germ cell tumors. But non–small-cell lung cancer shows poor response for chemotherapy with response seen in only 40% of cases.[8,21,25,30] In a review article that included 2 randomized and 44 observational studies, there was no clinically significant difference in the rate of relief from SVC obstruction whether chemotherapy, radiotherapy, or chemotherapy with radiotherapy was used in patients with either small- or non–small-cell lung cancers.[25]

Despite treatment with radiotherapy or chemotherapy, a significant proportion of patients (10% to 20%) fail to respond (primary failure) and symptoms persist. Reported recurrence or relapse rates (secondary failure) are between 20% and 50%.[10] Additionally, these therapies can take 2 to 4 weeks to show effectiveness with relatively high complication rates, particularly with high-dose radiotherapy. Because most patients with malignant SVCS have terminal illness, any increase in morbidity or decrease in quality of life due to delayed response to radiotherapy or chemotherapy is not clinically desirable. Therefore, SVC stenting may be a more favorable option not only for patients with acute SVCS but also for those with chronic SVCS.

▌ INTERVENTIONAL MANAGEMENT

Techniques

Catheter-directed thrombolysis—In cases of SVCS with bland thrombosis, thrombolytic therapy is useful. After thrombolysis or SVC stent placement, use of anticoagulants like warfarin, and antiplatelets like aspirin, in combination or alone, is controversial.[10,17,34]

Angioplasty—Angioplasty for the SVCS is generally performed in preparation for stent placement or in cases of incomplete expansion of the stent because of lack of durable benefit from angioplasty alone.[34,35]

Stenting—Since its first description by Charnsangavej et al.[36] in 1986, SVC stenting has become widely accepted in the management of SVCS and has recently been advocated as the first-line treatment option in patients with malignant obstruction.[37] Although the procedure is usually palliative, there is improvement in the quality of life of patients with malignant SVCS due to immediate resolution of symptoms.[38] Also, stenting allows the option for further management of the underlying malignancy with chemotherapy, radiotherapy, or combined-modality therapy.

▌ INDICATIONS

Primary Stenting

Primary stenting is recommended for SVCS patients with severe life-threatening symptoms, for those with poorly responding malignancies to conventional therapies (like mesothelioma), for those with contraindications to conventional therapies, for cases of thrombotic SVC obstruction, or for those planning to undergo cisplatin-based chemotherapy initiation for which hydration is required. In patients with severe life-threatening symptoms for which urgent intervention is required, primary stenting is advocated because stenting can be done even before a tissue diagnosis is available and it provides relief rapidly and safely.

Secondary Stenting

Secondary stenting is used for patients where primary conventional therapy failed (nonresponders) and also for those with recurrence (secondary failure) after initial response following conventional therapy or stenting itself.

▌ CONTRAINDICATIONS

Absolute contraindications—None.

Relative contraindications—Include brain metastasis, significant airway obstruction, or SVCS caused by thymoma. Brain metastasis is a relative contraindication because of the increased risk of cerebral hemorrhage when on anticoagulants after stenting. In patients with combined SVC and airway obstruction, resection of the tumor mass (complete or subtotal) or initial interventional management for airway obstruction (like stenting) followed by treatment of SVCS is recommended.[38–40] In SVCS cases caused by thymoma, stenting should be avoided if surgery is planned because it may complicate further resection.[11]

PREPROCEDURE TECHNICAL ISSUES

(a) **Choice of Stents.** Many endovascular stents with a variety of sizes and lengths are available to relieve the stenosis (FIGURES 90.3, 90.4, and 90.5). They may be classified into two categories: self-expanding stents and balloon-expanding stents.

The self-expanding stents, once released, continue to push radially outward against the stenosis until they reach their designed size. This may lead to perforation of the vessel wall, resulting in complications.[41–45] The self-expanding Z-stainless steel Gianturco (Cook Medical, Inc., Bloomington, IN) stents are generally rigid with a large diameter (up to 3 cm) and their placement through a tortuous vessel can be challenging. They are commonly used in large-diameter vessels. The open structure of the stent does not cause obstruction to the collateral side vessels bridged by the stent like the azygos vein, but it can potentially increase the stent occlusion rate due to tumor ingrowth and restenosis. Due to its short length, large diameter, and rigidity, multiple insertions of the Z-stent for long stenoses may represent a technical challenge, especially along tortuous venous anatomy. These stents also show high levels of fatigue and stent fractures with long-term use.[45] Use of these stents has been reduced recently because of the increasing availability of durable and more user-friendly self-expanding nitinol stents or wallstents (Boston Scientific, Inc., Newton, MA).

Unlike the Gianturco Z-stents, the nitinol self-expanding stents and wallstent stents (made of Elgiloy) are flexible, are easy to insert, and have a great efficacy in long stenoses. They have a smaller diameter (up to 1.6 cm) and are best suited for smaller vessels, such as brachiocephalic vein stenosis or along curvatures (FIGURES 90.3 and 90.4). Their meshlike structure prevents infiltration of the tumor through the stent. The main disadvantage of the wallstent is its weaker radial strength in larger diameters, its unpredictable length of foreshortening (usually 20% but can go up to 50%) when expanded, and its tendency to migrate postdeployment from the narrowest point to the normal portion of the vein if not correctly centered on the stenosis.[45–47] These issues rarely become clinically significant, however, because the length of the stents used is often two to three times longer than the actual length of obstruction. In a study published by Oudkerk et al.[48] higher early occlusion rates at 2 weeks were seen with the wallstent in comparison to the Gianturco Z-stent in their series of 30 patients with malignant SVC stenosis.

Almost all other self-expanding stents are also flexible, like the wallstent, because they are made of nitinol (nickel–titanium compound) mesh with super elasticity that allows the stent to expand to its designed size without any shortening of the length.[49]

Balloon-expanding stents are mounted on a balloon on the end of the delivery catheter. When the delivery catheter is positioned within the stenosis, the balloon is inflated, causing the stent to expand to a desired diameter; it is therefore less likely to cause perforation. Balloon-expanding stents have a high radial force when inflated.[50]

One advantage of balloon-expandable devices, relative to self-expanding stents, is precise stent positioning because they show lesser propensity to migrate once deployed across the lesion. Balloon-expandable stents also allow staged dilatation of the stenosis to a larger diameter. In general, the disadvantage of the balloon-expanded stents is their relative rigidity once released and expanded, which may lead to extrinsic deformation without elastic recovery, reocclusion, or stent fracture. A number of balloon-expandable stents, which are usually limited to diameters of 12 mm or less, have been used successfully to treat SVCS.[17,42]

Both self-expanding and balloon-expandable stents can be used in combination when there is residual stenosis after stent placement (FIGURE 90.4E). Overall there appears to be no significant difference in outcomes in the literature between the three general categories of stents detailed previously—the self-expanding stainless steel Gianturco Z-stent, balloon-expandable stents, and the self-expanding stents made of superelastic metals (e.g., nitinol, Elgiloy, etc.).[48,50,51] The specific type of stent selected for use is determined by the characteristics of the stenosis (diameter, length, and location) and the experience of the interventional radiologist.[45]

(b) **Unilateral Versus Bilateral Stenting.** In cases of obstruction of both brachiocephalic veins and the SVC, it is sufficient to relieve the obstruction in either the right or left brachiocephalic vein with collaterals, allowing drainage from both sides. Unilateral stent placement is preferred in SVCS because bilateral stent placement is technically more demanding, more expensive, more time consuming, and slightly more invasive. Also, comparative studies have shown increased incidence of occlusions and complications (including mutual obstruction of stents) following bilateral stenting.[10,37,52]

(c) **Covered Versus Bare Stents.** The choice of using covered or bare stents is based on the type of the tumor, type of obstruction (extrinsic compression vs. tumor invasion or internal thrombus), and the presence of significant collateral venous drainage, such as the azygos vein. Malignancies like lung cancer have a higher incidence of venous invasion with resultant tumor thrombus when compared with lymphoma or metastatic mediastinal nodal disease. Hence, in cases of SVCS with tumor or bland thrombus a wallgraft (Boston Scientific, Inc.) or a covered stent (e.g., Viabahn vascular prosthesis, W.C. Gore and Associates, Flagstaff, AZ), Fluency Plus stent-graft (C.R. Bard, Inc., Tempe, AZ), CAST or V12 covered stent (Atrium Medical, Hudson, NH), or others may be preferable. In cases of significant flow through the azygos vein, however, it is beneficial to use stents like the Gianturco stents, which have an open structure to bridge the azygos vein orifice.[45]

PROCEDURE

SVC stenting is a minimally invasive technique, usually done under local anesthesia with conscious sedation with standard monitoring (pulse, blood pressure, oxygen saturation, and electrocardiogram).

Preprocedural multiplanar CT or MRI helps to define the disease extent, the vessels involved, and presence of any thrombus[4,14] (FIGURES 90.3A, 90.4A, and 90.5A). Bilateral venography done in two different projections at the time of stenting helps to obtain information on disease extent, flow dynamics, collaterals, and presence of any thrombus and also to define the landing zones (FIGURES 90.3B, 90.4B, and 90.5B).

Access from the basilic, jugular, subclavian, or femoral veins is used, depending on disease extent. The most commonly used are internal jugular and femoral routes. However, the subclavian access route when compared with others is supposedly the more advantageous and simpler route despite a slight increased risk of pneumothorax.[10] In case of extensive SVC thrombus, thrombolysis or mechanical thrombectomy can be carried out to reduce the obstruction length and risk of emboli.[10,19,36,37,53,54]

Using a variety of hydrophilic guide wires and preshaped catheters (Multipurpose or Cobra, Cook) through a 7 to 9 French sheath, the stricture or obstruction can usually be crossed from either above (basilic, jugular, or subclavian veins) or below (via a femoral vein). A combined approach may sometimes be necessary to traverse tight lesions. After crossing the obstruction, a standard hydrophilic guide wire is exchanged for a 180- or 260-cm stiff guide wire. In case of strictures, predilatation to allow passage of the stent delivery system may be necessary. However, it is vital to confirm luminal reentry prior to balloon dilatation or stenting.[55] Short-acting opioids, such as fentanyl, should be given before ballooning or stenting tight strictures of the SVC because they can be painful. As far as sizing the balloons is concerned, many methods have been advocated by different authors, starting from routinely using 12-mm balloons[56] to oversizing by 1 mm[57] or slightly undersizing to the normal SVC diameter[58] or undersizing by 1 mm to the intended stent.[59] Therefore, balloon sizes used in the literature range from 12 to 20 mm[60] (FIGURES 90.4C and 90.5D).

Dilatation may also be required to help fully expand stents if they fail to do so sufficiently by 24 to 48 hours postprocedure (FIGURES 90.4C and 90.5D). Balloon dilatation should always be performed with caution, however, because this may result in catastrophic venous rupture.[59] Pressure measurements on both sides of the obstruction may be performed before and after stent implantation. Reduction in the pressure gradient to near zero with improved flow dynamics, underfilling of previously noted collaterals, and improved clinical symptoms are all signs of successful stent placement (FIGURES 90.4E and 90.5E).

CHANGES FOLLOWING STENT PLACEMENT

Sudden reversal of the abnormal caval pressure following successful stent placement results in improved right atrial pressure from restored venous return, leading to immediate increase in pulmonary capillary wedge pressure and cardiac output[45,61] (FIGURES 90.4E and 90.5E). This can lead to acute pulmonary edema, which can be fatal in patients with underlying coronary artery disease and heart failure.[43] Hence close hemodynamic monitoring during stenting is required to prevent or mitigate this type of complication.[61,62]

Endothelial intima usually covers stents and incorporates them into the physiologic vascular system within a few weeks' time following stent placement.[36] During this period the patient is at highest risk for thrombotic events. Anticoagulation is recommended following stent placement but optimal duration and methods of anticoagulation therapy remain controversial.[17,42,50,56] Following endovascular stent placements, clinical manifestations of SVCS usually resolve within 24 to 48 hours.

POSTPROCEDURE FOLLOW-UP

The need for long-term anticoagulants remains unclear. Most institutions recommend anticoagulation following stent placement but the type and duration of anticoagulation therapy varies

depending on the institution. There are no routine follow-up imaging protocols in the literature other than chest radiographs, which are done at 24 hours postprocedure to assess stent position/expansion (FIGURE 90.3D). This is also used as a baseline reference to check for future stent migration.[37,62,63] Most patients are usually assessed clinically along with chest radiograph and CT scan at each follow-up visit with repeat venography carried out only in cases of recurrence.

OUTCOMES

Overall both technical and clinical success rates are high for SVC stenting. In 80% to 95% of patients, SVC obstruction is relieved by stents with recurrence rates of 0% to 40% during the follow-up ranging from 3 days to 8 months. In a high proportion (78%) of these recurrent patients SVC patency is restored with reintervention.[10] Irrespective of the degree of obstruction prior to stenting patency rates are the same.[54]

To date, no randomized trials have been performed comparing stenting with either chemotherapy or radiotherapy. However, according to a Cochrane review, SVC stenting is the most rapid and effective treatment option for the relief of SVCS symptoms.[64] Also in many observational studies, endovascular stents have shown more rapid and sustained relief of symptoms when compared with conventional therapy.[10,19]

COMPLICATIONS AND THEIR MANAGEMENT

Overall SVC stenting complications rates compare very favorably with chemotherapy and radiotherapy.[25] For stent placement complication rates are in the range of 3% to 7% of which most are minor in nature.[10,17,18,34,35,44,57]

Minor complications include puncture site hematoma, chest pain, epistaxis, infection, and restenosis. Major complications include SVC rupture, pericardial tamponade, fatal pulmonary embolism, hemorrhage, right atrial stent migration causing cardiac arrhythmias, and death. According to a review article by Nguyen et al.,[45] 17 deaths (2%) were reported during or shortly after 884 malignant SVC stent placements from a total of 32 studies. Of the 17 deaths 7 (41%) were attributed to severe hemorrhage: 2 cerebral, 3 pulmonary, and 2 unspecified sites. Four deaths (23%) were attributed to cardiac events: two arrhythmias, one myocardial infarction, and one tamponade. Three deaths (17%) were attributed to respiratory failure. One death (6%) was due to documented pulmonary embolism, and in two cases (12%) cause of death was unknown. Fatal hemorrhages were mostly attributed to thrombolytic therapy administration, including streptokinase, urokinase, and tissue plasminogen activator, which were used to dissolve intracaval clot prior to stent insertion.[45]

As a major complication, stent migration into the right atrium can lead to cardiac arrhythmias. The predisposing factors for stent migration are poor patient selection, inaccurate vessel measurement, inadequate sizing of the stents, inaccurate positioning of the stents, and cardiac motion. These factors should be considered prior to stent deployment to minimize or prevent stent migration. It is also worth considering minimally shortening self-expanding nitinol stents (FIGURE 90.5) rather than wallstents, which can shorten unpredictably up to 50% at full expansion. Some authors recommend not to fully dilate the stent in the area of tightest obstruction and to leave both ends flared with a central waist to minimize stent migration. The main drawback of this technique is that it may increase the risk of perforation of the adjacent aorta and pericardium due to embedment of sharp stent filaments into the vessel wall at the flared ends.[60] In the event of stent migration, there are a number of endoluminal management options, which include retrieval either by snaring the stent directly or with balloon or guide wire assistance, or extending the stented segment with further stents.[65,66] It should, however, be borne in mind that most complications associated with SVC stenting have been minor and can be managed conservatively.

RECURRENCE

The reported symptomatic recurrence of the SVCS after chemotherapy or radiotherapy, or both, in patients with lung cancer (either small-cell or non–small-cell lung cancer) is nearly 20%.[30] In patients with primary conventional therapy failure, stents provided rapid symptomatic improvement as early as a few hours after the placement.[10] Stent effectiveness ranges from 81% to 100% and is unrelated to the type of stent used.[45] Relapse rates after primary stent placement range from 9% to 20% and nearly 78% of these relapses are successfully managed by repeat intravascular interventions.[10,17,35,44,62] In comparison, relapse rate after surgical reconstruction is nearly 10%.[27]

CONCLUSION

Malignant SVCS management is based on the severity of the symptoms, the underlying malignancy, and its anticipated response to treatment. Stenting is the treatment of choice for patients with acute life-threatening symptoms. It also is a very effective initial step for palliative treatment of chronic SVC syndrome because the clinical decision for subsequent elective chemotherapy or radiation therapy is not prejudiced. Also outcomes and complications compare very favorably with standard therapies (such as chemotherapy and radiotherapy); therefore, it has been advocated as the first-line treatment option.

REFERENCES

1. Wilson LD, Detterbeck FC, Yahalom J. Clinical practice. Superior vena cava syndrome with malignant causes. *N Engl J Med* 2007;356:1862–1869.
2. Kim HJ, Kim HS, Chung SH. CT diagnosis of superior vena cava syndrome: importance of collateral vessels. *AJR Am J Roentgenol* 1993;161:539–542.
3. Trigaux JP, van Beers B. Thoracic collateral venous channels: normal and pathologic CT findings. *J Comput Assist Tomogr* 1990;14:769–773.
4. Eren S, Karaman A, Okur A. The superior vena cava syndrome caused by malignant disease. Imaging with multi-detector row CT. *Eur J Radiol* 2006;59(1):93–103.
5. Stanford W, Jolles H, Ell S, et al. Superior vena cava obstruction: a venographic classification. *AJR Am J Roentgenol* 1987;148:259–262.
6. Armstrong BA, Perez CA, Simpson JR, et al. Role of irradiation in the management of superior vena cava syndrome. *Int J Radiat Oncol Biol Phys* 1987;13:531–539.
7. Yellin A, Rosen A, Reichert N, et al. Superior vena cava syndrome: the myth—the facts. *Am Rev Respir Dis* 1990;141:1114–1118.
8. Schraufnagel DE, Hill R, Leech JA, et al. Superior vena caval obstruction: is it a medical emergency? *Am J Med* 1981;70:1169–1174.
9. Rice TW, Rodriguez RM, Barnette R, et al. Prevalence and characteristics of pleural effusions in superior vena cava syndrome. *Respirology* 2006;11:299–305.
10. Nicholson AA, Ettles DF, Arnold A, et al. Treatment of malignant superior vena cava obstruction: metal stents or radiation therapy. *J Vasc Interv Radiol* 1997;8:781–788.
11. Detterbeck FC, Parsons AM. Thymic tumors. *Ann Thorac Surg* 2004;77:1860–1869.
12. Rice TW, Rodriguez RM, Light RW. The superior vena cava syndrome: clinical characteristics and evolving etiology. *Medicine (Baltimore)* 2006;85:37–42.
13. Ahmann FR. A reassessment of the clinical implications of the superior vena cava syndrome. *J Clin Oncol* 1984;2:961–969.
14. Bechtold RE, Wolfman NT, Karstaedt N, et al. Superior vena caval obstruction: detection using CT. *Radiology* 1985;157:485–487.
15. Yu JB, Wilson LD, Detterbeck FC. Superior vena cava syndrome—a proposed classification system and algorithm for management. *J Thorac Oncol* 2008;3(8):811–814.
16. Gauden SJ. Superior vena cava syndrome induced by bronchogenic carcinoma: is this an oncological emergency? *Australas Radiol* 1993;37(4):363–366.
17. Marcy PY, Magne N, Bentolila F, et al. Superior vena cava obstruction: is stenting necessary? *Support Care Cancer* 2001;9:103–107.
18. Greillier L, Barlesi F, Doddoli C, et al. Vascular stenting for palliation of superior vena cava obstruction in non-small-cell lung cancer patients: a future 'standard' procedure? *Respiration* 2004;71:178–183.
19. Tanigawa N, Sawada S, Mishima K, et al. Clinical outcome of stenting in superior vena cava syndrome associated with malignant tumors: comparison with conventional treatment. *Acta Radiol* 1998;39:669–674.
20. Ostler PJ, Clarke DP, Watkinson AF, et al. Superior vena cava obstruction: a modern management strategy. *Clin Oncol (R Coll Radiol)* 1997;9:83–89.
21. Sculier JP, Evans WK, Feld R, et al. Superior vena caval obstruction syndrome in small cell lung cancer. *Cancer* 1986;57:847–851.
22. Magnan PE, Thomas P, Guidicelli R, et al. Surgical reconstruction of the superior vena cava. *Cardiovasc Surg* 1994;2:598–604.
23. Maddox AM, Valdivieso M, Lukeman J, et al. Superior vena cava obstruction in small cell bronchogenic carcinoma: clinical parameters and survival. *Cancer* 1983;52:2165–2172.
24. Loeffler JS, Leopold KA, Recht A, et al. Emergency prebiopsy radiation for mediastinal masses: impact on subsequent pathologic diagnosis and outcome. *J Clin Oncol* 1986;4(5):716–721.
25. Rowell NP, Gleeson FV. Steroids, radiotherapy, chemotherapy and stents for superior vena caval obstruction in carcinoma of the bronchus: a systematic review. *Clin Oncol (R Coll Radiol)* 2002;14:338–351.
26. Dhaliwal RS, Das D, Luthra S, et al. Management of superior vena cava syndrome by internal jugular to femoral vein bypass. *Ann Thorac Surg* 2006;82:310–312.
27. Bacha EA, Chapelier AR, Macchiarini P, et al. Surgery for invasive mediastinal tumors. *Ann Thorac Surg* 1998;66:234–239.
28. Detterbeck FC, Jones DR, Kernstine KH, et al. Lung cancer: special treatment issues. *Chest* 2003;123(suppl 1):244S–258S.
29. Anderson PR, Coia LR. Fractionation and outcomes with palliative radiation therapy. *Semin Radiat Oncol* 2000;10:191–199.
30. Spiro SG, Shah S, Harper PG, et al. Treatment of obstruction of the superior vena cava by combination chemotherapy with and without irradiation in small-cell carcinoma of the bronchus. *Thorax* 1983;38:501–505.
31. Pereira JR, Martins SJ, Ikari FK, et al. Neoadjuvant chemotherapy vs radiotherapy alone for superior vena cava syndrome (SVCS) due to non-small cell lung cancer (NSCLC): preliminary results of randomized phase II trial [abstract]. *Eur J Cancer* 1999;35(suppl 4):260.
32. Wurschmidt F, Bunemann H, Heilmann HP. Small cell lung cancer with and without superior vena cava syndrome: a multivariate analysis of prognostic factors in 408 cases. *Int J Radiat Oncol Biol Phys* 1995;33:77–82.
33. Chan RH, Dar AR, Yu E, et al. Superior vena cava obstruction in small-cell lung cancer. *Int J Radiat Oncol Biol Phys* 1997;38:513–520.
34. Uberoi R. Cirse guidelines: quality assurance guidelines for superior vena cava stenting in malignant disease. *Cardiovasc Intervent Radiol* 2006;29:319–322.
35. Courtheoux P, Alkofer B, Al Refai M, et al. Stent placement in superior vena cava syndrome. *Ann Thorac Surg* 2003;75:158–161.
36. Charnsangavej C, Carrasco CH, Wallace S, et al. Stenosis of the vena cava: preliminary assessment of treatment with expandable metal stents. *Radiology* 1986;161:295–298.
37. Laniego C, Chacon JL, Julian A, et al. Stenting as first option for endovascular treatment of malignant superior vena cava syndrome. *AJR Am J Roentgenol* 2001;177:585–593.

38. Kim YI, Kim KS, Ko YC, et al. Endovascular stenting as a first choice for the palliation of superior vena cava syndrome. *J Korean Med Sci* 2004;19:519–522.

39. Takeda S, Miyoshi S, Omori K, et al. Surgical rescue for life-threatening hypoxemia caused by a mediastinal tumor. *Ann Thorac Surg* 1999;68:2324–2326.

40. Kvale PA, Simoff M, Prakash UBS. Lung cancer: palliative care. *Chest* 2003;123(suppl 1):284S–311S.

41. Thony F, Moro D, Witmeyer P, et al. Endovascular treatment of superior vena cava obstruction in patients with malignancies. *Eur Radiol* 1999;9:965–971.

42. Bierdrager E, Lampmann LEH, Lohle PNM, et al. Endovascular stenting in neoplastic superior vena cava syndrome prior to chemotherapy or radiotherapy. *Neth J Med* 2005;63:20–23.

43. Kee ST, Kinoshita L, Razavi MK, et al. Superior vena cava syndrome: treatment with catheter directed thrombolysis and endovascular stent placement. *Radiology* 1998;206:187–193.

44. Urruticoechea A, Mesia R, Dominguez J, et al. Treatment of malignant superior vena cava syndrome by endovascular stent insertion. Experience on 52 patients with lung cancer. *Lung Cancer* 2004;43:209–214.

45. Nguyen NP, Borok TL, Welsh J, et al. Safety and effectiveness of vascular endoprosthesis for malignant superior vena cava syndrome. *Thorax* 2009;64:174–178.

46. Dyet JF, Nicholson AA, Cook AM. The use of the Wallstent endovascular prosthesis in the treatment of malignant obstruction of the superior vena cava. *Clin Radiol* 1993;48:381–385.

47. Qanadli SD, El Hajjam M, Mignon F, et al. Subacute and chronic benign superior vena cava obstructions: endovascular treatment with self expanding metallic stents. *AJR Am J Roentgenol* 1999;173:159–164.

48. Oudkerk M, Kuijpers TJA, Schmitz PIM, et al. Self expanding metal stents for palliative treatment of superior vena caval syndrome. *Cardiovasc Intervent Radiol* 1996;19:146–151.

49. Chatziioannou A, Alexopoulos T, Mourikis D, et al. Stent therapy for malignant superior vena cava syndrome: should be first line therapy or simple adjunct to radiotherapy. *Eur J Radiol* 2003;47:247–250.

50. Elson JD, Becker GJ, Wholey MH, et al. Vena cava and central venous stenosis: management with Palmaz-balloon-expandable intraluminal stents. *J Vasc Interv Radiol* 1991;2:215–213.

51. Entwisle KG, Watkinson AF, Reidy J. Case report: migration and shortening of a self-expanding metallic stent complicating the treatment of malignant superior vena cava stenosis. *Clin Radiol* 1996;51:593–595.

52. Dinkel HP, Mettke B, Schmid F, et al. Endovascular treatment of malignant superior vena cava syndrome: is bilateral wallstent placement superior to unilateral placement? *J Endovasc Ther* 2003;10:788–797.

53. Miller JH, Mcbride K, Little F, et al. Malignant superior vena cava obstruction: stent placement via the subclavian route. *Cardiovasc Intervent Radiol* 2000;23:155–158.

54. Crowe MTI, Davies CH, Gaines PA. Percutaneous management of superior vena cava occlusions. *Cardiovasc Intervent Radiol* 1995;18:367–372.

55. Boardman P, Ettles DF. Cardiac tamponade: a rare complication of attempted stenting in malignant superior vena cava obstruction. *Clin Radiol* 2000;55:645–647.

56. Rosch J, Uchida BT, Hall LD, et al. Gianturco-Rosch expandable Z-stents in the treatment of superior vena cava syndrome. *Cardiovasc Intervent Radiol* 1992;15:319–327.

57. Smayra T, Otal P, Chabbert V, et al. Long term results of endovascular stent placement in the superior caval venous system. *Cardiovasc Intervent Radiol* 2001;24:388–394.

58. Brown KT, Getrajdamn GI. Balloon dilatation of the superior vena cava (SVC) resulting in SVC rupture and pericardial tamponade: a case report and brief review. *Cardiovasc Intervent Radiol* 2005;28:372–376.

59. Zollikofer CL, Antonucci F, Stuckmann G, et al. Use of the Wallstent in the venous system including haemodialysis-related stenosis. *Cardiovasc Intervent Radiol* 1992;15:334–341.

60. Ganesha A, Quen Hon L, Wrakaulle DR, et al. Superior vena caval stenting for SVC obstruction: current status. *Eur J Radiol* 2009;71(2):343–349.

61. Yamagami T, Nakamura T, Kato T, et al. Hemodynamic changes after self expandable metallic stent therapy for superior vena cava syndrome. *AJR Am J Roentgenol* 2002;178:635–639.

62. Kishi K, Sonomura T, Mitsuzane K, et al. Self-expandable metallic stent therapy for superior vena cava syndrome: clinical observations. *Radiology* 1993;189:531–535.

63. Hennequin LM, Fade O, Fays JG, et al. Superior vena cava stent placement: results with the Wallstent endoprosthesis. *Radiology* 1995;196:353–361.

64. Rowell NP, Gleeson FV. Steroids, radiotherapy, chemotherapy and stents for superior vena caval obstruction in carcinoma of the bronchus (Cochrane review). *Cochrane Database Syst Rev* 2001;(4):CD001316.

65. Brant J, Peebles C, Kalra P, et al. Haemopericardium after superior vena cava stenting for malignant SVC obstruction. The importance of contrast enhanced CT in the assessment of postprocedural collapse. *Cardiovasc Intervent Radiol* 2002;24:353–355.

66. Taylor JD, Lehmann ED, Belli AM, et al. Strategies for the management of SVC stent migration into the right atrium. *Cardiovasc Intervent Radiol* 2007;30(5):1003–1009.

Benign Disease of the Superior Vena Cava and Innominate Veins

ANDREW MISSELT and JAFAR GOLZARIAN

INTRODUCTION

Superior vena cava syndrome is the obstruction of the superior vena cava resulting in various clinical sequelae including head, neck, and upper extremity swelling and headaches, cyanosis, dyspnea, and hoarseness. The syndrome was first described by William Hunter, who in 1757 published an account of superior vena cava obstruction secondary to a syphilitic thoracic aortic aneurysm.

The superior vena cava and the innominate tributary veins are low-pressure vessels with relatively thin walls. Their anatomic proximity to adjacent structures, such as lymph nodes, lung, and large arteries, makes them susceptible to compression and stenosis.

Both benign and malignant processes can cause superior vena cava syndrome. Malignant causes of superior vena cava and innominate vein stenosis include bronchogenic carcinoma, lymphoma, and metastatic disease. Benign causes of superior vena cava and innominate vein stenosis include nonmalignant masses, such as cysts, goiter, teratoma, and thymoma; infectious and inflammatory processes, such as histoplasmosis, tuberculosis, and mediastinitis; vascular aneurysms; postsurgical anastomotic strictures; chronic or repeated central venous catheter use; and cardiac device leads from pacers and defibrillators.[1]

Including all causes, superior vena cava syndrome is estimated to affect approximately 15,000 people annually in the United States alone.[2]

The relative incidence of benign and malignant causes has changed over time. Benign causes of central venous stenosis predominated until they were supplanted by increasing rates of lung and mediastinal cancer in the mid- and late 1990s. At their peak, malignant causes accounted for 85% to 97% of all cases of superior vena cava syndrome.[2] Interestingly, increasing use of central venous catheters and implantable cardiac pacers and defibrillators has led to resurgence in the proportion of benign central venous stenosis relative to malignant etiology. In one series benign causes now account for up to 40% of cases of superior vena cava syndrome.[3]

Previously, mediastinal fibrosis accounted for most benign superior vena cava obstructions. However, recent studies have demonstrated that catheter and pacer wire-related stenoses now predominate the benign subset of superior vena cava obstruction (57% to 74%).[4–6]

CLASSIFICATION OF DISEASE

In 1987 William Stanford and colleagues[7] systematically reviewed the venograms of 67 patients with venous obstruction. Although their study cohort comprised patients with malignant superior vena cava obstruction, their analysis provides a useful venographic classification of superior vena cava obstruction that is broadly applicable. In the schema set forth by Stanford, superior vena cava obstruction can be stratified into four classes based on the pattern observed at venography (Table 91.1). The investigators found a correlation between advancing obstruction pattern and the presence of symptoms. Type I is described as up to a 90% stenosis of the superior vena cava with antegrade flow through the azygos vein. Type II is a greater than 90% stenosis or complete occlusion of the superior vena cava with antegrade flow in the azygos vein. Type III is a greater than 90% stenosis or complete occlusion of the superior vena cava with retrograde flow in the azygos vein. Type IV is occlusion of the superior vena cava in association with occlusion of one or more of the superior vena cava's tributary veins: the right innominate vein, the left innominate vein, and the azygos vein.

PATHOPHYSIOLOGY

Benign disease of the superior vena cava and the innominate tributary veins is caused by either extrinsic compression or intrinsic stenosis. Extrinsic compression is the result of mass effect from adjacent structures, such as arterial aneurysm or benign masses. Mediastinitis, either infectious or inflammatory, results in compressive forces as the surrounding fibrosis retracts and collapses the vein lumen. Intrinsic stenosis is the result of intimal trauma and pericatheter thrombus formation, which leads to smooth muscle ingrowth and the development

Table 91.1	
Stanford Venographic Classification of Superior Vena Cava Obstruction	
Type I	<90% of the SVC with patent azygos vein
Type II	90%–100% stenosis/occlusion of the SVC with patency of the azygos vein
Type III	90%–100% stenosis/occlusion of the SVC with reversal of flow in the azygos vein
Type IV	Occlusion of the SVC and occlusion of one or more SVC tributaries including the innominate veins and azygos vein

SVC, superior vena cava.

of cellular connective tissue.[8–10] This process results in stenosis.[8] Additionally, the process can be exacerbated by the strain of the high flow states caused by hemodialysis grafts or fistulas.[11,12]

Both extrinsic compression and intrinsic stenosis lead to venous compromise with impaired flow that can ultimately result in thrombosis of the vein itself. The process of thrombus formation further inflames and then scars the vein, resulting in worsening stenosis or occlusion.

The obstruction of the superior vena cava leads to impaired venous return from the head and upper extremities.[6] As the obstruction worsens, blood flow is diverted through collateral networks including the azygos, hemiazygos, intercostal, mediastinal, paravertebral, internal mammary, thoracoepigastric, thorococlavicular, and anterior chest wall veins.[13,14] Elevated pressure in the veins peripheral to the obstruction is the cause of the many observed clinical features of superior vena cava syndrome.[1] The more central the level of superior vena cava obstruction, the more severe the manifestation of the clinical syndrome.[15]

CLINICAL FEATURES

The clinical signs of superior vena cava syndrome include distention of the upper extremity veins, swelling of the face and upper extremities, and regionalized cyanosis. Clinical symptoms include headache, fatigue, dyspnea, cough, dysphagia, dizziness, impaired vision, nausea, syncope, and coma.[1,2]

In 1993, a rating system was devised to stratify the clinical signs and symptoms of superior vena cava syndrome (Table 91.2). In the Kishi scoring system grades were assigned to a series of clinical signs and symptoms. By summing the highest grade from each category a score was derived that was used to establish disease severity and evaluate treatment outcome.

TREATMENT OPTIONS

Traditional management of stenosis of the superior vena cava has differed based on the etiology. The primary treatment for malignant superior vena cava syndrome is either external radiation therapy or endovascular intervention with balloon angioplasty or stent placement.

Patients with benign causes of superior vena cava syndrome tend to be comparatively younger with longer life expectancies. For this reason, treatments need to be especially durable. Initial therapy for superior vena cava obstruction of benign etiology involves anticoagulation to prevent or limit thrombus formation. In some situations, sufficient collateral vessels may develop to alleviate the patient's symptoms.[1] Historically, surgery has been offered as the next treatment option for patients with intractable symptoms.[5,16–18]

More recently endovascular intervention has begun to rival surgical bypass for treatment of nonmalignant superior vena cava obstruction. Indeed some authors have concluded that endovascular intervention is now the first-line treatment for benign superior vena cava syndrome.[4]

Endovascular intervention may involve thrombolysis, balloon angioplasty, or stent placement. These interventions can be performed alone or in combination. Early use of thrombolysis for superior vena cava syndrome was focused on occlusions

Table 91.2	
Kishi Scoring System	
Neurologic symptoms	Grade
Stupor, coma, or blackout	4
Blurry vision, headache, dizziness, or amnesia	3
Changes in mentation	2
Uneasiness	1
Laryngopharyngeal or thoracic symptoms	Grade
Orthopnea or laryngeal edema	3
Stridor, hoarseness, dysphagia, glossal edema, or shortness of breath	2
Cough or pleural effusions	1
Nasal and facial signs or symptoms	Grade
Lip edema, nasal stiffness, epistaxis, or rhinorrhea	2
Facial swelling	1
Venous dilation	Grade
Neck vein or arm vein distension	1
Upper extremity swelling	1
Upper body plethora	1

induced by pacemaker wires.[19] Balloon angioplasty of the superior vena cava was first described by Rocchini et al.[20] in 1982. Shortly after this initial publication, several other authors published early accounts of balloon angioplasty of the superior vena cava.[19,21,22] Although balloon angioplasty marked a clear step forward in the realm of endovascular therapy, the procedure was limited by poor durability due to elastic recoil of the stenosis.[1] This observation led investigators to begin placing stents within the superior vena cava to provide a more durable result.[23–25]

TECHNICAL ASPECTS

Diagnosis of superior vena cava syndrome is made on clinical grounds. However, cross-sectional imaging is typically required for treatment planning (FIGURE 91.1). Ultrasound provides a useful overview of affected veins. Magnetic resonance (MR) or computed tomographic (CT) venography are the most useful tools for anatomic assessment of the obstruction and the existing collateral pathways and they play the primary role in preparation for intervention.[26] Thoughtful venography at the time of the intervention requires imaging in at least two projections to safely and accurately carry out the procedure.

By drawing on the clinical history, noninvasive imaging findings, and venographic appearance, the interventionist must determine if the vein is stenotic but patent or occluded. If the

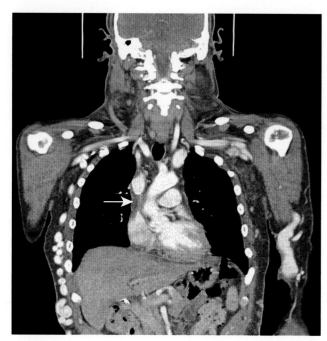

FIGURE 91.1 Coronal rendering of CT venogram demonstrates SVC occlusion (*arrow*) and extensive venous collaterals.

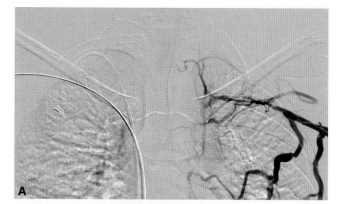

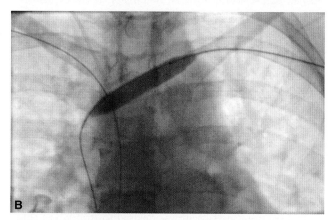

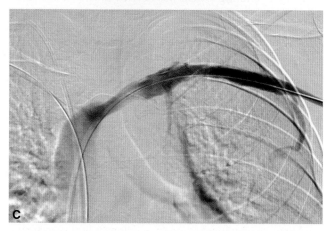

FIGURE 91.2 A. Frontal view of left arm venogram with occlusion of the left subclavian and innominate veins caused by prior central venous access. **B.** Balloon angioplasty of occluded segment. **C.** Postangioplasty venogram with restored patency of the previously occluded vein segment.

vein is occluded, it is necessary to recanalize the vein because guide wire access across the lesion is fundamental to further intervention.

If the vein is occluded with fresh thrombus, the guide wire typically passes without difficulty and the interventionist can proceed with thrombolysis. After excluding relevant contraindications to thrombolytic therapy (bleeding disorder, pregnancy, primary or metastatic disease of the brain or spinal cord, recent surgery, gastrointestinal bleeding, etc.), thrombolysis can proceed either via an infusion catheter or pulse-spray methodology. Catheter-directed thrombolysis has two main benefits. First, by lysing the acute thrombus there is less potential for it to embolize during subsequent balloon angioplasty and stent placement. Second, following a course of thrombolysis, the underlying stenosis or occlusion is often shorter than had been previously appreciated and may require fewer or shorter stents.[27]

If the occlusion is chronic, the obstructed vein is often little more than a scared remnant. In these situations, recanalization can be challenging. Recanalization techniques involve using various guide wires and support catheter to cross the occlusion, followed by balloon angioplasty to open the channel in preparation for balloon angioplasty and/or stent placement.[28] Occasionally it may be impossible to pass a wire through a particularly scarred segment of the occluded vein using conventional means. In these situations, sharp recanalization can be attempted using a Colapinto needle or other such device.[29]

Once the stenotic or occluded segment of the vein has been crossed, the interventionist can proceed with treatment using balloon angioplasty and/or stent placement. In central vein obstruction, balloon angioplasty should be performed primarily and the use of a stent(s) reserved for when there is a failure or complication of the percutaneous transluminal angioplasty

(PTA). The ideal technique of balloon angioplasty is to inflate a balloon (usually a noncompliant high resistant one) adapted to the size of the innominate vein or the superior vena cava for 3 to 5 minutes and repeated as many times as needed (FIGURE 91.2).

Both balloon-expandable and self-expandable stents have been used to treat superior vena cava stenosis[30,31] (FIGURE 91.3). The use of balloon-expandable stents in the central veins should

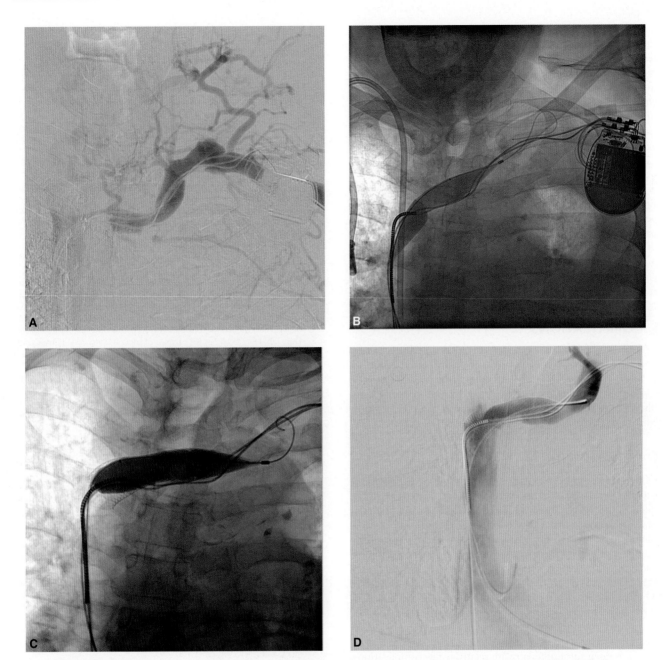

FIGURE 91.3 A. Left arm venogram demonstrates left innominate stenosis secondary to cardiac defibrillator leads. **B.** Balloon angioplasty of stenotic vein segment. **C.** Balloon angioplasty after stent placement (Wallstent, Boston Scientific, Inc., Newton, MA). **D.** Completion venogram following balloon angioplasty and stent placement documents restored patency of the vein segment.

be limited to straight segments within the thorax. Heparin anticoagulation during the procedure is favored by some, although its use is not universal.[32]

When placing a stent in the superior vena cava or innominate veins it is essential to maintain wire access across both the superior vena cava and inferior vena cava. By using this technique an inadvertently dislodged stent is constrained by the delivery wire and unable to travel into the heart.

When faced with a stenosis or obstruction that involves the superior vena cava as well as both innominate veins, recent publications have indicated that only the superior vena cava and

one innominate vein need to be revascularized to achieve clinical benefit. In comparative studies, unilateral innominate vein revascularization is favored because there is shorter procedure time, fewer complications, and less reocclusion.[32]

Pacer wires can cause innominate and superior vena cava stenosis. Removal of the pacer wire can be clinically undesirable or technically impossible. One frequently cited concern with the intervention in this setting is the possibility of a harmful interaction between the metallic stent and the pacer wire. This concern has led some interventionists to place temporary pacing wires during the stent implantation procedure to provide backup for pacemaker-dependent patients.[33] More recently, others have reported on stent placement over pacer wires without backup temporary pacers.[34,35] These authors note that pacemaker wires are not susceptible to damage or interference from an overlying implanted metallic stent for two reasons. First, pacemaker wires are well insulated by a coating of silicone rubber or polyurethane. Second, a pacemaker wire that has incited a venous stenosis is well embedded within the vessel wall and likely has no exposure to the lumen in which the stent is implanted.

OUTCOMES

Endovascular therapy provides a durable solution for superior vena cava syndrome of benign etiology. Whereas the reported primary patency rates of endovascular therapy are in the range of 57% to 79%, the primary assisted or secondary patency to 3 years is 96% to 100%.[31] These cumulative patency rates are comparable to open surgical repair, albeit with more frequent reintervention.

COMPLICATIONS

Complications from intervention on benign superior vena cava and innominate disease are rare with published incidence of between 3.2% and 7.8%.[32] Minor complications include access site hematoma, chest pain, epistaxis, and infection. Major complications include stent migration, pericardial tamponade, superior vena cava rupture, pulmonary embolism, and death.

CONCLUSION

Benign disease processes causing stenosis or occlusion of the superior vena cava and innominate veins are increasing in frequency, primarily caused by the increased use of implantable devices, such as catheters and pacer wires. Stenosis or occlusion of the superior vena cava and innominate veins can result in substantial morbidity. Whereas in the past, endovascular techniques had limited application in the treatment of superior vena cava of benign etiology, presently endovascular therapies are considered by many to be first-line treatments. Treatment option including thrombolysis, balloon angioplasty, and stent placement are often performed in conjunction with one and others. Endovascular treatment of superior vena cava syndrome results in similar outcomes as open surgical repair with relatively few complications.

REFERENCES

1. Yim CD, Sane SS, Bjarnason H. Superior vena cava stenting. *Radiol Clin North Am* 2000;38(2):409–424.
2. Schindler N, Vogelzang RL. Superior vena cava syndrome. Experience with endovascular stents and surgical therapy. *Surg Clin North Am* 1999;79(3):683–694, xi.
3. Rice T, Rodriguez RM, Light R. The superior vena cava syndrome: clinical characteristics and evolving etiology. *Medicine* 2006;85(1):37–42.
4. Rizvi AZ, Kalra M, Bjarnason H, et al. Benign superior vena cava syndrome: stenting is now the first line of treatment. *J Vasc Surg* 2008;47(2):372–380.
5. Kalra M, Gloviczki P, Andrews JC, et al. Open surgical and endovascular treatment of superior vena cava syndrome caused by nonmalignant disease. *J Vasc Surg* 2003;38(2):215–223.
6. Sheikh MA, Fernandez BB, Gray BH, et al. Endovascular stenting of nonmalignant superior vena cava syndrome. *Catheter Cardiovasc Interv* 2005;65(3):405–411.
7. Stanford W, Jolles H, Ell S, et al. Superior vena cava obstruction: a venographic classification. *AJR Am J Roentgenol* 1987;148(2):259–262.
8. Oguzkurt L, Tercan F, Torun D, et al. Impact of short-term hemodialysis catheters on the central veins: a catheter venographic study. *Eur J Radiol* 2004;52(3):293–299.
9. Hoshal VL Jr, Ause RG, Hoskins PA. Fibrin sleeve formation on indwelling subclavian central venous catheters. *AMA Arch Surg* 1971;102(4):353–358.
10. Forauer AR, Theoharis CGA, Dasika NL. Jugular vein catheter placement: histologic features and development of catheter-related (fibrin) sheaths in a swine model. *Radiology* 2006;240(2):427–434.
11. Morosetti M, Meloni C, Gandini R, et al. Late symptomatic venous stenosis in three hemodialysis patients without previous central venous catheters. *Artif Organs* 2000;24(12):929–931.
12. Kundu S. Review of central venous disease in hemodialysis patients. *J Vasc Interv Radiol* 2010;21(7):963–968.
13. Wan J, Bezjak A. Superior vena cava syndrome. *Hematol Oncol Clin North Am* 2010;24(3):501–513.
14. Eren S, Karaman A, Okur A. The superior vena cava syndrome caused by malignant disease. Imaging with multi-detector row CT. *Eur J Radiol* 2006;59(1):93–103.
15. Stanford W, Doty DB. The role of venography and surgery in the management of patients with superior vena cava obstruction. *Ann Thorac Surg* 1986;41(2):158–163.
16. Doty DB. Bypass of superior vena cava: six years' experience with spiral vein graft for obstruction of superior vena cava due to benign and malignant disease. *J Thorac Cardiovasc Surg* 1982;83(3):326–338.
17. Gloviczki P, Pairolero PC, Cherry KJ, et al. Reconstruction of the vena cava and of its primary tributaries: a preliminary report. *J Vasc Surg* 1990;11(3):373–381.
18. Doty DB, Doty JR, Jones KW. Bypass of superior vena cava. Fifteen years' experience with spiral vein graft for obstruction of superior vena cava caused by benign disease. *J Thorac Cardiovasc Surg* 1990;99(5):889–895.
19. Montgomery JH, D'Souza VJ, Dyer RB, et al. Nonsurgical treatment of the superior vena cava syndrome. *Am J Cardiol* 1985;56(12):829–830.
20. Rocchini AP, Cho KJ, Byrum C, et al. Transluminal angioplasty of superior vena cava obstruction in a 15-month-old child. *Chest* 1982;82(4):506–508.
21. Sherry CS, Diamond NG, Meyers TP, et al. Successful treatment of superior vena cava syndrome by venous angioplasty. *AJR Am J Roentgenol* 1986;147(4):834–835.
22. Capek P, Cope C. Percutaneous treatment of superior vena cava syndrome. *AJR Am J Roentgenol* 1989;152(1):183–184.
23. Elson JD, Becker GJ, Wholey MH, et al. Vena caval and central venous stenoses: management with Palmaz balloon-expandable intraluminal stents. *J Vasc Interv Radiol* 1991;2(2):215–223.
24. Gross CM, Krämer J, Waigand J, et al. Stent implantation in patients with superior vena cava syndrome. *AJR Am J Roentgenol* 1997;169(2):429–432.
25. Rosenblum J, Leef J, Messersmith R, et al. Intravascular stents in the management of acute superior vena cava obstruction of benign etiology. *JPEN J Parenter Enteral Nutr* 1994;18(4):362–366.
26. Kim H, Chung JW, Park JH, et al. Role of CT venography in the diagnosis and treatment of benign thoracic central venous obstruction. *Korean J Radiol* 2003;4(3):146–152. Available at: http://synapse.koreamed.org/DOIx.php?id=10.3348/Fkjr.2003.4.3.146.
27. Kee ST, Kinoshita L, Razavi MK, et al. Superior vena cava syndrome: treatment with catheter-directed thrombolysis and endovascular stent placement. *Radiology* 1998;206(1):187–193.
28. Ferral H, Bjarnason H, Wholey M, et al. Recanalization of occluded veins to provide access for central catheter placement. *J Vasc Interv Radiol* 1996;7(5):681–685.
29. Farrell T, Lang EV, Barnhart W. Sharp recanalization of central venous occlusions. *J Vasc Interv Radiol* 1999;10(2, pt 1):149–154.
30. Qanadli S, El Hajjam M, Mignon F, et al. Subacute and chronic benign superior vena cava obstructions: endovascular treatment with self-expanding metallic stents. *AJR Am J Roentgenol* 1999;173(1):159–164.
31. Kee ST, Kinoshita L, Razavi MK, et al. Superior vena cava syndrome: treatment with catheter-directed thrombolysis and endovascular stent placement. *Radiology* 1998;206(1):187–193.
32. Ganeshan A, Hon L, Warakaulle D, et al. Superior vena caval stenting for SVC obstruction: current status. *Eur J Radiol* 2009;71(2):343–349.
33. Slonim SM, Semba CP, Sze DY, et al. Placement of SVC stents over pacemaker wires for the treatment of SVC syndrome. *J Vasc Interv Radiol* 2000;11(2):215–219.
34. Teo N, Sabharwal T, Rowland E, et al. Treatment of superior vena cava obstruction secondary to pacemaker wires with balloon venoplasty and insertion of metallic stents. *Eur Heart J* 2002;23(18):1465–1470.
35. Lanciego C, Rodriguez M, Rodriguez A, et al. Permanent pacemaker-induced superior vena cava syndrome: successful treatment by endovascular stent. *Cardiovasc Intervent Radiol* 2003;26(6):576–579.

CHAPTER

92

Inferior Vena Cava Obstruction

KENNETH J. KOLBECK and JOHN A. KAUFMAN

INTRODUCTION

Obstruction of the inferior vena cava (IVC) can be caused by a wide variety of conditions including congenital absence, oncologic invasion, external compression from malignancy to obesity, thrombotic and embolic events, as well as iatrogenic adventures and misadventures.[1–17] Early case reports and reviews date back to the 1800s and provide a consistent description of the associated clinical findings.[18] Historically, most of these diagnoses were made at autopsy due to limited imaging and treatment options. As medical technology progressed, the etiology and diagnosis of IVC occlusion became relevant as treatment options emerged to assist in controlling symptoms.

The clinical signs and symptoms of an IVC occlusion are related to two major factors: the time frame in which the occlusion has developed and the level of occlusion. Acute occlusions have a high probability of producing bilateral lower extremity edema, abdominal and lower extremity discomfort or "heaviness," and, occasionally, ascites. With acute occlusions at or above the hepatic vein inflow, insufficient venous return to the heart can lead to fatal arrhythmias. Over time, collaterals develop gradually, reducing symptoms, frequently within 1 to 2 weeks.[19–22] The collateral pathways that develop highly depend on the level and extent of the caval occlusion with multiple combined drainage pathways available.[23,24]

IVC occlusions are frequently divided into three groups: peripheral/low/distal (below the renal veins), middle (between renal and hepatic veins), and central/upper/proximal (between hepatic veins and right atrium). Strictly peripheral occlusions frequently drain via gonadal venous collateral channels as the renal veins and suprarenal IVC remain patent. As the middle IVC segment becomes involved, intrahepatic collaterals to the portal vein and hepatic venous outflow become more prevalent. Occlusion of the IVC above the hepatic veins requires collateral pathways to develop with flow to the superior vena cava (frequently through paralumbar plexi as well as azygos, hemiazygos, and abdominal wall collateral veins). Not an exclusive process, any type of occlusion can result in a combination of these collateral draining pathways (FIGURE 92.1). If any of these collateral pathways are identified as prevalent on cross-sectional imaging, a hemodynamically significant occlusion of the IVC should be suspected. Similarly, the physical exam findings of bilateral lower extremity edema and dilated abdominal wall veins should suggest IV occlusion. Note that many of these collateral channels can develop with reversed flow in patients with cirrhosis or portal hypertension, so the differential diagnosis can be quite broad based on imaging findings alone.

The causes of IVC obstruction are frequently related to malignancy and other hypercoaguable states. However, less common causes include retroperitoneal fibrosis (idiopathic or radiation induced); congenital vessel absence; vascular webs (FIGURE 92.2); extension of deep venous thrombosis from femoral and/or iliac veins; functional IVC filter and massive trapped thromboembolism; femoral or direct IVC central venous catheters; peritoneal, retroperitoneal, or IVC surgery (including liver transplant); abdominal aortic aneurysms; pregnancy (compression via gravid uterus); compartment syndromes related to ascites; and even obesity.[1–17,25–30] The treatment of IVC occlusion also highly depends on the etiology. Symptomatic, acute thrombus within the IVC is commonly managed with thrombolytic techniques with or without filter placement as described previously (Chapters 87 to 91). Once the acute thrombus has been resolved, treating the underlying cause of the obstruction becomes an important consideration. For malignant direct vascular invasion or extrinsic compression from hepatic metastases, chemotherapy, radiation therapy, and surgical decompression can be considered; however, response times tend to be delayed. IVC stenting plays a key role in relieving symptoms in this group of patients.[31–43]

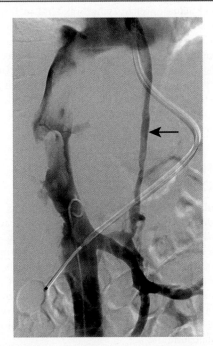

FIGURE 92.1 Inferior vena cavagram in a patient with an invasive right adrenal gland tumor with associated development of paralumbar venous collateral pathways (*arrow*).

1079

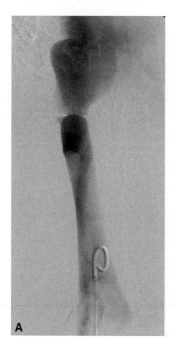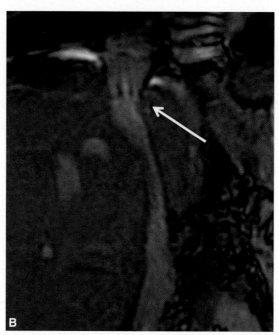

FIGURE 92.2 A. Inferior vena cavagram and (**B**) coronal T2 MR image of the same patient with an intrahepatic IVC web. No collateral drainage pathways have developed; however, the "jet" phenomenon on the MR image (*arrow*) suggests some level of hemodynamic compromise.

PATIENT SELECTION

Patients with significant symptoms, including lower extremity edema that alters daily activities, ascites that impacts mobility and breathing, or insufficient venous return to the heart, should be treated. As one would expect, patients with short segment stenosis and acute onset of symptoms tend to respond better than the converse. Long segment occlusions with multiple collateral channels are likely to have a lower technical success rate. Contraindications to treatment would include inability to obtain stable wire access across the lesion and inability to move obstruction lesion with angioplasty or stenting devices. The diameter of the normal IVC should be considered in the treatment planning, primarily ensuring that the selected stent is appropriately sized to prevent migration.

TREATMENT OPTIONS (ENDOVASCULAR AND OTHERS)

Endovascular treatment options of the symptoms related to IVC obstruction can generally be divided into two parts: breaking up flow-limiting thrombus followed by treating an underlying cause for the formation of the thrombus. Disrupting IVC thrombus as well as thrombi in collateral venous channels follows previously described thrombolysis techniques (Chapters 87 to 91). In short, a combination of both pharmacologic and mechanical thrombectomy agents can be used to disrupt the underlying thrombus and help establish inline venous return to the right atrium.

Identifying the etiology of the underlying venous obstruction (or cause of the thrombus formation) will lead to optimum

treatment options. Angioplasty, combined angioplasty and stenting, or primary stenting are endovascular treatment options for this lesion. For the most part, stenting either with or without present angioplasty is the most likely endovascular treatment option to have the most beneficial symptom control as well as long-term patency data.[44–46]

Collaboration with medical and surgical specialties may be of assistance and is recommended. Specifically, if symptoms trend toward significant improvement with anticoagulation alone, medical management may be appropriate. Alternatively, surgical interventions, such as venous bypass or tumor debulking, may also assist in symptom control without a need for interventional techniques. Without adequate comparative studies evaluating outcomes, the choice between medical management, endovascular techniques, and surgical debulking/bypass options is usually made on a case-by-case basis (primarily based on individual risk versus potential benefit).

ANATOMIC OR LESION CONSIDERATION

In patients with symptomatic IVC stenosis or occlusion, details of the length and location of the lesion will guide angioplasty and stenting options. In most cases, these symptoms are not emergent, allowing time for appropriate evaluation and planning. A computed tomography (CT) venogram, magnetic resonance (MR) venogram, or digital subtraction venography may be helpful in identifying the location of the lesion relative to key structures vital in stent placement decisions. In lesions near the right atrium at the hepatic venous confluence, the "landing zone" of the stents may be limited. Care must be taken in selecting and positioning a stent in these locations to minimize the risk of stent migration or malposition. For the most part, large-diameter, self-expanding stents are used in the IVC due to the dynamic nature of the cava diameter within the cardiac cycle and respiratory variation. Choosing a stent with enough radial force at the diameter and lengths needed (15- to 30-mm diameter, approximately 5- to 15-cm length) can be difficult. These diameters and lengths are rarely available "off the shelf" in most interventional radiology (IR) suites and frequently need to be ordered specifically for the patient (FIGURE 92.3). In some cases with a high-grade, focal lesion, a balloon-expandable stent may be appropriate (FIGURE 92.4).

Frequently, a diagnostic venogram prior to stent placement allows better evaluation of the length and location of the narrowing. These preliminary imaging studies allow more accurate measurements and assist in placement of the correct size/location of the stent (FIGURE 92.5). Another common step in evaluation of an IVC stenosis would include measuring a pressure gradient across the lesion. Although no clearly defined value for a hemodynamically significant gradient in the venous system has been established, commonly stented symptomatic lesions in our practice have minimum pressure gradients in the 5- to 7-mm Hg range (unpublished data).

TECHNICAL/DEVICE CONSIDERATIONS

The choice of stent used in the IVC is somewhat variable, primarily dominated by the diameters required (15 to 30 mm) to maintain adequate venous return to the heart. The IVC is a dynamic structure with both respiratory and cardiac variations. Historically, a self-expanding stent with a strong radial force that is tolerant of considerable respiratory and cardiac pressure and diameter fluctuations over the remaining lifetime of the patient is required. On some occasions, a balloon-expandable stent may be required to reinforce the self-expandable device. Although stenting across the renal vein or hepatic vein inflow is generally avoided, there are limited data to suggest that doing so would result in a suboptimal result.[47] The dominant concern of stent migration/malposition is the extension of the stent into the right atrium, resulting in potentially fatal arrhythmias.[48] Careful presenting image evaluation and cautious stent deployment limit the risks of these potentially fatal arrhythmias.

PLANNING THE INTERVENTIONAL RADIOLOGY PROCEDURE

Detailed analysis and review of any cross-sectional imaging with the assistance of multiplanar reformats will frequently help establish an appropriate range of stent diameters and lengths to have available at the time of the procedure. Stent diameters are frequently oversized by 15% to 40% depending on the extent of the stricture and adjacent vasculature. The "oversize" component helps reduce the risk of stent migration into the right atrium, which can result in a potentially fatal arrhythmia. The length of stent chosen should be sufficient to cross the lesion in its entirety with limited extension across major inflow veins (i.e., hepatic/renal if at all possible).

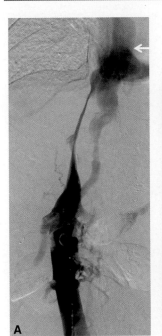
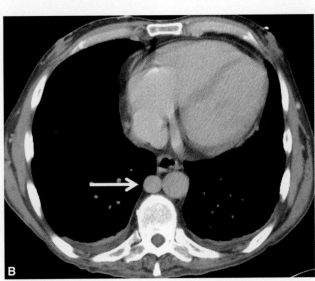
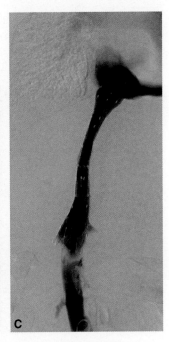

FIGURE 92.3 A. Inferior vena cavagram demonstrates extrinsic compression from multiple hepatic metastases. **B.** The stenosis created a hemodynamically significant narrowing in the intrahepatic IVC, resulting in dominant collateral outflow to the SVC via the azygos vein seen on both the venogram and accompanying CT (*arrow*). **C.** The placement of two overlapping self-expanding stents improved the flow through the IVC and eliminated flow through the dominant collateral channels.

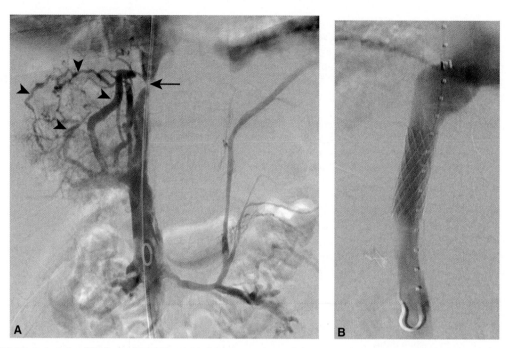

FIGURE 92.4 A. A focal high-grade intrahepatic IVC stenosis (*arrow*), likely from a congenital web, results in significant intrahepatic and paralumbar collateral vascularity (*arrowheads*). Both internal jugular vein and common femoral vein access were required for evaluation of the lesion in preparation for treatment. **B.** After angioplasty and placement of a balloon-expandable stent, no flow through the collateral channels was identified.

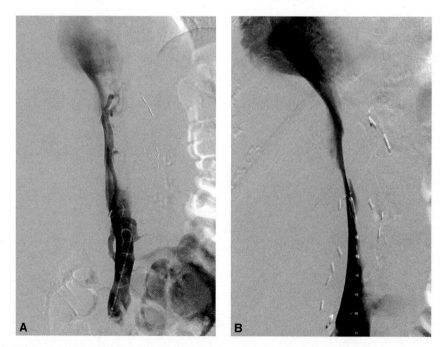

FIGURE 92.5 IVC narrowing caused by intrahepatic metastases (neuroendocrine tumor) with symptomatic venous out-flow obstruction (**A**). The initial inferior venacavagram demonstrates a long segment, intrahepatic stenosis with filling of right paralumbar collateral vessels. **B.** Oblique image helps define the length of compression and extent of luminal narrowing. **C.** Bilateral femoral access with measurement catheters assists in selecting the appropriate length and diameter of stent. **D.** Poststent cavagram demonstrates increased flow through the intrahepatic IVC and decreased flow through the collateral channels.

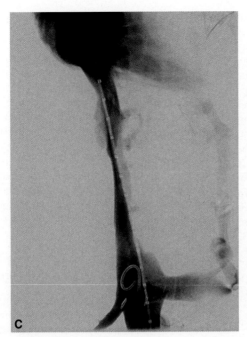
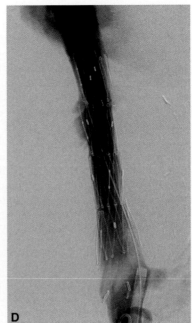

FIGURE 92.5 *(Continued)*

Understanding the relative position of fluoroscopic bony land-marks and the venous branch anatomy will assist choosing an appropriate stent length. Having a couple diameters and lengths to choose from at the time of the procedure is advisable because noninvasive imaging can occasionally misrepresent some key measurements.

Planning appropriate access (femoral vein or internal jugular vein, or both) is an important component to success and is frequently operator dependent. Factors include both the diameter of the anticipated devices as well as factors involved in deployment. Large-diameter sheaths (10 to 16 French) are occasionally required to deliver the appropriate stents and any potential required angioplasty devices. Given that the IVC-right atrial junction is frequently one endpoint of the stent, choosing an access site that allows the most accurate deployment at this location is advised. For example, devices deployed from one end to the other (i.e., in a "distal to proximal" fashion, such as "pin and pull" deployment) tend to have a slightly more accurate distal position relative to the proximal extent of the stent. A femoral approach with these devices may give the operator a slight advantage in the accurate delivery of the device at the cavoatrial junction.

SPECIFIC INTRAPROCEDURE TECHNIQUES

After establishing appropriate venous access (femoral or internal jugular, or both), repeat digital subtraction angiography of the IVC would be advised to confirm findings and measurements on the cross-sectional studies. Pressure measurements across the lesion may help establish an appropriate endpoint after stent placement because there are limited data defining a hemodynamically significant stenosis in the venous system.[49–51] As with any stenting procedure, obtaining and maintaining stable wire access across the lesion is vital. With external compression

lesions, a soft floppy tip wire is frequently all that is required to cross the lesion. With more chronic intravascular obstructions, a hydrophilic, steerable wire may be required. Exchange for a sturdy, "working wire" is recommended for the delivery of the large-diameter stents and angioplasty balloons. Advancing the dilator and sheath over the wire across the lesion (or "Dottering" the lesion) may help determine if present angioplasty may be required.

If the delivery sheath cannot be safely advanced across the lesion over the wire, angioplasty with an appropriate diameter balloon (8 to 14 mm) may be of assistance. External compression lesions (i.e., lymphadenopathy or hepatic metastases) tend to be displaced with inflation of the angioplasty balloon and return to the original position with balloon deflation (i.e., rebound/elastic lesions). More fibrotic lesions (i.e., retroperitoneal fibrosis or caval webs) are more likely to require higher radial force to disrupt the stenosis. Once a delivery sheath can be positioned safely across the narrowing, a controlled, steady, and accurate deployment of the stent can be attempted. Angiography during the initial stent positioning, just prior to deployment, either via the delivery sheath or an alternative access site is frequently useful in accurate deployment of the stent. After stent deployment, an additional venogram and pressure gradient measurements will likely assist in determining if additional steps are needed in controlling the patient's symptoms.

ENDPOINT ASSESSMENT

If the venous return to the right atrium has improved significantly after stenting (as determined by the rapid flow of contrast through the previously seen stricture, the lack of filling of previously noted collateral channels, and/or decreased pressure gradient), no further therapy may be required. If residual narrowing is identified, however, the decision about additional interventions becomes more complex. In many cases, moderate improvement in flow and small to moderate changes in the measured pressure gradient are enough to decrease clinical symptoms, so, frequently, a clinical trial is recommended prior to additional interventions. If symptoms improve in spite of a modest technical result, no further interventions would be advised. If symptoms persist after an appropriate clinical trial, however, further improvement in the venous return/opening any residual narrowing may be required. Reinforcing the stent with another self-expanding stent of the same or larger diameter will increase the radial force, hopefully increasing the diameter of the venous return channel. In more challenging situations, a balloon-mounted stent may be required to maximize the radial force and diameter of the IVC. In doing so, the dynamic motion of the IVC may be compromised.

PROCEDURAL COMPLICATIONS

In stenting the IVC, the most feared complication would likely be stent migration. In high-grade lesions in these large-diameter native vessels, the stent or balloon may migrate during deployment in a "watermelon seed" fashion (slipping above or below the "pinch point"). Properly centering the stent, with appropriate forward or back tension of the device, tends to reduce this problem. Similarly, choosing a longer stent, allowing more wall apposition above and below the narrowing, also tends to reduce migration during deployment. The risk of stent migration toward the heart, with the risk of lodging in the right atrium, ventricle, or pulmonary outflow tract and resulting in fatal arrhythmias, can be reduced with appropriate, stable wire access (well into the superior vena cava, or even "body floss" exiting from an internal jugular vein). Maintaining stable wire access and keeping the stent trapped on the wire may permit potential snare/reposition/recovery options. Surgical consultation is recommended because percutaneous attempts at repositioning can be high risk and frequently unsuccessful.

Alternative complications, such as caval injury and retroperitoneal bleeding or pulmonary emboli from underlying thrombus, should also be considered. Although frequently self-limited, severe bleeding from caval injury may require placement of a covered stent or even surgical bypass. If a covered stent is required (such as a thoracic aortic endograft), care must be taken to minimize the number of venous inflow covered.[52] Treatment of any complicating pulmonary emboli should be guided by the extent of symptoms.

OUTCOMES/PROGNOSIS

Although data are limited compared to that available for superior vena cava syndrome symptom relief, the outcome of returning patency to the IVC is also a relatively rapid process. Frequently within 24 to 48 hours, the dominant symptoms of caval occlusion, such as ascites and edema, tend to show improvement. The flow through the collateral drainage channels tends to be reduced quickly and these collaterals can thrombose as the IVC returns as the dominant venous return from the lower half of the body back to the right atrium.[36,53-55]

DISEASE SURVEILLANCE AND TREATMENT MONITORING ALGORITHMS

Once the IVC has been successfully opened (with or without a stent placed), recurrent clinical symptoms are frequently used for guidance of surveillance imaging and re-treatment. In some patients with a suitable body habitus, ultrasonography (US) can be used for evaluation of IVC patency. However, contrast-enhanced CT and MR also provide noninvasive means to monitor the lesion. Overall, the dominant prognostic factor relies on the underlying cause of the caval stenosis/obstruction. A benign etiology with complete resolution of the stenosis may not require significant follow-up imaging. Malignant lesions may require intermittent imaging depending on the growth of the lesion, response to treatment strategies, and recurrent symptoms.

EARLY AND LATE TREATMENT FAILURES AND OPTIONS FOR MANAGEMENT

Early and late treatment failures may be the result of a few different things. For example, stent collapse from external compression may require reinforcement with additional self-expanding or balloon-expanding stents. Tumor in growth may require placement of an endograft with fabric reducing the extent of the lumen narrowing via malignant invasion. Anticoagulation may be of assistance in hypercoaguable patients with incomplete expansion of the devices.[52]

PRACTICAL ADVANTAGES AND LIMITATIONS

The practical advantage of the percutaneous treatment of IVC stenosis/occlusion over surgical bypass techniques is related to the minimally invasive procedure, limited recovery time, and relatively rapid symptomatic improvement. When compared to surgical, radiation therapy, or chemotherapeutic options, the reestablishment of inline venous return to the right atrium from the lower half of the body can be done relatively quickly with minimal complications with IR techniques. The improved flow can rapidly reduce clinical symptoms, such as ascites, peripheral edema, and limb "heaviness." Unfortunately, most patients with a symptomatic stenotic/occluded IVC have a limited life span. Improving the quality of life in this group of patients with limited survival in a percutaneous, noninvasive technique is advantageous over more invasive surgical options. On rare occasions, the IVC stenosis/occlusion cannot be crossed with a wire catheter combination, limiting the universal application of this technique.

RELATIVE THERAPEUTIC EFFECTIVENESS COMPARED TO MEDICAL AND SURGICAL MANAGEMENT

The dominant drawback to a surgical approach in this disease would likely be related to the major abdominal/retroperitoneal operation required, prolonged recovery time, not to mention the potential thrombosis of the bypass graft as well as the native vessels involved. Similarly, relying exclusively on systemic chemotherapy or targeted radiation therapy to shrink the impact of an externally compressed lesion would likely be a time-intensive process. The percutaneous stenting of the symptomatic IVC occlusion can frequently produce clinical improvement within a relatively short time frame.

■ THE FUTURE

Given the relatively low incidence of the symptomatic IVC stenosis/occlusion problem, there is limited ongoing research dedicated specifically to this field. Future options include development of a stent that may be placed in benign temporary situations that may dissolve over time. Similarly, cytotoxic coated stents may assist in the treatment of malignancy-induced lesions. Stents in these lesions may end up being functioning as fiducial markers for radiation therapy or markers for endoluminal resection of these lesions. Finally, studies evaluating the long-term patency and the potential benefit and risks of anticoagulation in this group of patients would be worthwhile.

■ CONCLUSION

The percutaneous evaluation and management of IVC stenosis and/or occlusion is safe, results in a relatively quick therapeutic response, and can result in durable results. Stenting of the IVC is frequently required over angioplasty alone due to the resilient nature of most lesions (external compression via intrahepatic malignancy). The percutaneous approach demonstrates a satisfactory response with a shorter recovery time than most surgical or systemic chemotherapeutic options available in this patient population.

■ REFERENCES

1. Akerman S, Kaubisch A, Gucalp R, et al. Inferior vena cava syndrome from pancreatic adenocarcinoma: successful symptom palliation with endovascular stenting. *J Palliat Med* 2008;11:1066–1069.
2. Bass F, Redwine M, Kramer L, et al. Spectrum of congenital anomalies of the inferior vena cava: cross-sectional image findings. *Radiographics* 2000;20:639–652.
3. Brechtel K, Tepe G, Heller S, et al. Endovascular treatment of venous graft stenosis in the inferior vena cava and the left hepatic vein after complex liver tumor resection. *J Vasc Interv Radiol* 2009;20:264–269.
4. Chang T, Zaleski G, Lin B, et al. Treatment of inferior vena cava obstruction in hemodialysis patients using wallstents: early and intermediate results. *AJR Am J Roentgenol* 1998;171:125–128.
5. Debing E, Tielemans Y, Jolie E, et al. Congenital absence of inferior vena cava. *Eur J Vasc Surg* 1993;7:201–203.
6. Gasparis A, Kokkosis A, Labropoulos N, et al. Venous outflow obstruction with retroperitoneal Kaposi's sarcoma and treatment with inferior vena cava stenting. *Vasc Endovascular Surg* 2009;43:295–300.
7. Giannoukas A. Stent-grafts in the inferior vena cava. *J Endovasc Ther* 2011;18:255.
8. Hassan B, Tung K, Weeks R, et al. The management of inferior vena cava obstruction complicating metastatic germ cell tumors. *Cancer* 1999;85:912–918.
9. Kishi K, Sonomura T, Fujimoto H, et al. Physiologic effect of stent therapy for inferior vena cava obstruction due to malignant liver tumor. *Cardiovasc Intervent Radiol* 2006;29:75–83.
10. Meinhardt N, Pires Souto K, Knebel A, et al. Inferior vena cava syndrome and morbid obesity. *Obes Surg* 2008;18:1649–1652.
11. Melas N, Saratzis A, Saratzis N, et al. Inferior vena cava stent graft placement to treat endoleak associated with an aortocaval fistula. *J Endovasc Ther* 2011;18:250–254.
12. Park J, Chung J, Han J, et al. Interventional management of benign obstruction of the hepatic inferior vena cava. *J Vasc Interv Radiol* 1994;5:403–409.
13. Raju S, Hollis K, Neglen P. Obstructive lesions of the inferior vena cava: clinical features and endovenous treatment. *J Vasc Surg* 2006;44:820–827.
14. Rubinson R, Vasko J, Doppman J. Inferior vena caval obstruction from increased intra-abdominal pressure. *Arch Surg* 1967;94:766–770.
15. Sauter A, Triller J, Schmidt F, et al. Treatment of superior vena cava (SVC) syndrome and inferior vena cava (IVC) thrombosis in a patient with colorectal cancer: combination of SVC stenting and IVC filter placement to palliate symptoms and pave the way for port implantation. *Cardiovasc Intervent Radiol* 2008;31:S144–S148.
16. Stone D, Adelman M, Rosen R, et al. A unique approach in the management of vena caval thrombosis in a patient with Klippel-Trenaunay syndrome. *J Vasc Surg* 1997;26:155–159.
17. Wallace M. Transatrial stent placement for treatment of inferior vena cava obstruction secondary to extension of intracardiac tumor thrombus from hepatocellular carcinoma. *J Vasc Interv Radiol* 2003;14:1339–1343.
18. Osler W. Case of obliteration of vena cava inferior, with great stenosis of orifices of hepatic veins. *J Anat Physiol* 1879;13:291–304.
19. Hausler M, Hubner D, Delhass T, et al. Long term complications of inferior vena cava thrombosis. *Arch Dis Child* 2001;85:228–233.
20. Kim T, Chung J, Han J, et al. Hepatic changes in benign obstruction of the hepatic inferior vena cava: CT findings. *AJR Am J Roentgenol* 1999;173:1235–1242.
21. Pleasants J. Obstruction of the inferior vena cava with a report of eighteen cases. *Johns Hopkins Hosp Rep* 1911;16:363–548.
22. Razavi M, Hansch E, Kee S, et al. Chronically occluded inferior venae cavae: endovascular treatment. *Radiology* 2000;214:133–138.
23. Kapur S, Paik E, Rezaei A, et al. Where there is blood, there is a way: unusual collateral vessels in superior and inferior vena cava obstruction. *Radiographics* 2010;30:67–78.
24. Sonin A, Mazer M, Powers T. Obstruction of the inferior vena cava: a multiple-modality demonstration of causes, manifestations, and collateral pathways. *Radiographics* 1992;12:309–322.
25. Crochet D, Brunel P, Trogrlic S, et al. Long-term follow up of Vena Tech-LGM Filter: predictors and frequency of caval occlusion. *J Vasc Interv Radiol* 1999;10:137–142.
26. Hansen M, Miller G, Starks K. Pulse-spray thrombolysis of inferior vena cava thrombosis complicating filter placement. *Cardiovasc Intervent Radiol* 1994;17:38–40.
27. Doppman J, Rubinson R, Rockoff S, et al. Mechanism of obstruction of the infradiaphragmatic portion of the inferior vena cava in the presence of increased intra-abdominal pressure. *Invest Radiol* 1966;1:37–53.
28. Gaines P, Belli A, Anderson P, et al. Superior vena caval obstruction managed by the Gianturco Z stent. *Clin Radiol* 1994;49:202–208.
29. Hochrein J, Bashore T, O'Laughlin M, et al. Percutaneous stenting of superior vena cava syndrome: a case report and review of the literature. *Am J Med* 1998;104:78–84.
30. Kee S, Kinoshita L, Razavi M, et al. Superior vena cava syndrome: treatment with catheter-directed thrombolysis and endovascular stent placement. *Radiology* 1998;206:187–193.
31. Brountzos E, Binkert C, Panagiotou I, et al. Clinical outcome after intrahepatic venous stent placement for malignant inferior vena cava syndrome. *Cardiovasc Intervent Radiol* 2004;27:129–136.
32. Carrasco C, Charnsangavej C, Wright K, et al. Use of the Gianturco self-expanding stent in stenoses of the superior and inferior venae cavae. *J Vasc Interv Radiol* 1992;3:409–419.
33. Charnsangavej C, Carrasco C, Wallace S, et al. Stenosis of the vena cava: preliminary assessment of treatment with expandable metallic stents. *Radiology* 1986;161:295–298.
34. Elson J, Becker G, Wholey M, et al. Vena caval and central venous stenoses: management with Palmaz balloon-expandable intraluminal stents. *J Vasc Interv Radiol* 1991;2:215–223.
35. Fletcher W, Lakin P, Pommier R, et al. Results of treatment of inferior vena cava syndrome with expandable metallic stents. *Arch Surg* 1998;133:935–938.
36. Furui S, Sawada S, Irie T, et al. Hepatic inferior vena cava obstruction: treatment of two types with Gianturco expandable metallic stents. *Radiology* 1990;176:665–670.
37. Laing A, Thomson K, Vrazas J. Stenting in malignant and benign vena caval obstruction. *Australas Radiol* 1998;42:313–317.
38. Missal M, Robinson J, Tatum R. Inferior vena cava obstruction: clinical manifestations, diagnostic methods, and related problems. *Ann Intern Med* 1965;62:133–161.
39. Oudkerk M, Heystraten F, Stoter G. Stenting in malignant vena caval obstruction. *Cancer* 1993;71:142–146.
40. Sato M, Yamada R, Tsuji K, et al. Percutaneous transluminal angioplasty in segmental obstruction of the hepatic inferior vena cava: long term results. *Cardiovasc Intervent Radiol* 1990;13:189–192.

41. Tardy B, Mismetti P, Page Y, et al. Symptomatic inferior vena cava filter thrombosis: clinical study of 30 consecutive cases. *Eur Respir J* 1996;9:2012–2016.

42. Yamagami T, Nakamura T, Kato T, et al. Hemodynamic changes after self-expandable metallic stent therapy for vena cava syndrome. *AJR Am J Roentgenol* 2002;178:635–639.

43. Zamora C, Sugimoto K, Mori T, et al. Prophylactic stenting of the inferior vena cava before transcatheter embolization of renal cell carcinomas: an alternative to filter placement. *J Endovasc Ther* 2004;11:84–88.

44. Hartung O, Benmiloud F, Barthelemy P, et al. Late results of surgical venous thrombectomy with iliocaval stenting. *J Vasc Surg* 2008;47:381–387.

45. Nazarian G, Bjarnason H, Dietz C, et al. Iliofemoral venous stenoses: effectiveness of treatment with metallic endovascular stents. *Radiology* 1996;200:193–199.

46. Titus J, Moise M, Bena J, et al. Iliofemoral stenting for venous occlusive disease. *J Vasc Surg* 2011;53:706–712.

47. O'Sullivan G, Lohan D, Cronin C, et al. Stent implantation across the ostea of renal veins does not necessarily cause renal impairment when treating inferior vena cava occlusion. *J Vasc Interv Radiol* 2007;18:905–908.

48. Ploegmakers M, Rutten M. Fatal pericardial tamponade after superior vena cava stenting. *Cardiovasc Intervent Radiol* 2009;32:585–589.

49. Frazer J, Ing F. Stenting of stenotic or occluded iliofemoral veins, superior and inferior vena cavae in children with congenital heart disease: acute results and intermediate follow up. *Catheter Cardiovasc Interv* 2009;73:181–188.

50. Labropoulos N, Borge M, Pierce K, et al. Criteria for defining significant central vein stenosis with duplex ultrasound. *J Vasc Surg* 2007;46: 101–107.

51. Lee J, Ko G, Sung K, et al. Long-term efficacy of stent placement for treating inferior vena cava stenosis following liver transplantation. *Liver Transpl* 2010;16:513–519.

52. Makutani S, Kichikawa K, Uchida H, et al. Effect of antithrombotic agents on the patency of PTFE-covered stents in the inferior vena cava: an experimental study. *Cardiovasc Intervent Radiol* 1999;22:232–238.

53. Entwisle K, Watkinson A, Hibbert J, et al. The use of the wallstent endovascular prosthesis in the treatment of malignant inferior vena cava syndrome. *Clin Radiol* 1995;50:310–313.

54. Ishiguchi T, Fukatsu H, Itoh S, et al. Budd-Chiari syndrome with long segmental inferior vena cava obstruction: treatment with thrombolysis, angioplasty, and intravascular stents. *J Vasc Interv Radiol* 1992;3:421–425.

55. Zhang C, Fu L, Xu L, et al. Long-term effect of stent placement in 15 patients with Budd-Chiari syndrome. *World J Gastroenterol* 2003;9:2587–2591.

DANIEL Y. SZE

CHAPTER 93

Venous Compression Syndromes

INTRODUCTION

Blood flow within veins reflects not only cardiac output, but also respiratory, skeletal muscular, hydrostatic, and gravitational forces.[1,2] Normal veins are relatively inelastic but fully lined with an endothelial layer and can collapse and refill without formation of thrombus due to local production of thrombomodulin, heparan sulfate, tissue factor pathway inhibitor, tissue plasminogen activator, nitrous oxide, prostacyclin, interleukin-10, and other modulators.[3] Venous collapse is usually cyclical from respiratory phasicity and muscular contraction, but some veins are especially susceptible to extrinsic compression by rigid anatomic structures with potentially pathologic consequences. The most obvious consequence may be thrombosis, but even in the absence of frank thrombosis, symptoms of venous hypertension and congestion may occur. Predilection toward pathologic consequences is probably congenital but may be affected by habitus, habits, pregnancy and other mass effects, hormones, and drugs and may be exacerbated by specific repetitive musculoskeletal activities.

Veins are difficult to address by vascular surgical methods, such as bypass grafts.[4] The introduction of endovascular methods greatly increased treatment options, but structures extrinsic to the vein responsible for compression are not always reliably treated through the venous lumen. This chapter discusses three separate clinical entities of venous compression syndromes with starkly different demographics and treatment options.

ILIAC VEIN COMPRESSION SYNDROME (ALSO KNOWN AS MAY-THURNER SYNDROME, COCKETT SYNDROME)

Left-sided predominance for lower extremity deep venous thrombosis (DVT) was first described by German pathologist Rudolf Virchow in 1851,[5] who postulated that blood flow in the left iliac venous system was impeded by compression of the common iliac vein between the right common iliac artery and the lumbar vertebrae, resulting in left-sided thrombosis being approximately five times as common as right sided. Fifty years later, McMurrich[6] found common iliac venous adhesions in 35 of 107 cadavers, 32 of which occurred on the left side. He proposed that these adhesions were congenital, a conclusion contested by Ehrich and Krumbhaar in 1943,[7] who found obstructive lesions in 24% of 412 cadavers of different ages.

Only one-third of adhesions had developed in the first decade of life, so they concluded that these lesions were acquired.

These findings were confirmed by May and Thurner in 1957,[8] who found obstructive lesions in 22% of 430 cadavers. They subdivided anatomic lesions into three types of "spurs" or adhesions: (1) lateral, involving medial and/or lateral adhesions pinching off the lumen; (2) central, involving anteroposterior septae dividing the lumen into two or more channels; and (3) partial obliteration, involving a complex of synechiae with multiple irregular fenestrations. They reasoned that the constant pulsatility of the overlying right iliac artery caused mechanical trauma to the apposing left iliac anterior and posterior venous intima, resulting in proliferation and formation of spurs, which could then disturb blood flow and cause thrombosis.

The first report describing "iliac compression syndrome" in living patients was published by Cockett and Thomas in 1965,[9] who segregated 29 "major iliofemoral thrombosis" patients into acute and chronic. Of their patients, 55% were female, and a staggering 97% had left-side predominant symptoms. Mean and median ages were 23 and 20, respectively, and almost all patients had been temporarily confined to bed prior to thrombosis. Six patients were treated with surgical exploration, where it was found that obstruction was not relieved by lifting the artery off the vein because of the mature fibrous stricture caused by the vein being "so flattened at this point for so long that the inner walls have, as it were, stuck together."

A follow-up paper (where they modernized by replacing intraosseous phlebography with transfemoral venography?) further delineated anatomic and clinical patterns of presentation.[10] Specifically, four configurations of compression were identified: (1) usual right common iliac artery crossing over left common iliac vein, as found in 80% of patients; (2) complete overriding of the inferior vena caval bifurcation by the right common iliac artery; (3) compression of the (right) external iliac vein at the bifurcation of the right iliac artery; and (4) compression of either external iliac vein at the inguinal ligament. The mechanical impingement of the vein with associated fibrosis not only precipitated thrombosis in these patients, but also prevented adequate recanalization. Since then almost every conceivable anatomic variation of iliac vein compression syndrome (IVCS) has been reported of an iliac vein being compressed by a neighboring artery, including mirror image right common iliac vein compression by the left common iliac artery in a patient with left-sided inferior vena cava (IVC).[11] Other associated complications encountered have included rupture of the left iliac vein[12] or of a collateral pelvic varix.[13]

The eponym "May-Thurner syndrome" appeared in the literature in 1983 describing venography and surgical repair of three patients.[14] By then, numerous reports had been published describing surgical diversions expanding on Cockett's original reports, describing patency rates and clinical resolution in 40% to 88% of patients.[15]

Systemic thrombolysis was occasionally used to treat DVT starting in the 1960s[16] but had not become widely accepted even two decades later.[17–20] Local juxtathrombic infusion of thrombolytics[21] and the later development of intrathrombic infusion by multi-hole infusion catheter[22,23] allowed quicker and more effective local fibrinolysis while minimizing systemic exposure and complications. Balloon angioplasty techniques were easily transferred to application in iliac veins, first reported in 1991.[24] Numerous large series have since been published,[25–28] including a multicenter registry of patients treated for a variety of venous thrombotic conditions.[29] Based on the published record of safety, efficacy, and quality of life improvement,[30] endovascular treatment has become the standard of care where it is available, despite the paucity of rigorous level I data.[31] One small single-center randomized trial from Egypt was published in 2002 showing superior patency and decreased post-thrombotic reflux in patients treated by intrathrombic pulse-spray infusion of streptokinase,[32] and a larger randomized study in Norway[33] confirmed improved patency but did not find differences in reflux. There is currently a multicenter randomized prospective trial sponsored by the National Institutes of Health (NIH) that is underway in the United States (Acute venous Thrombosis: Thrombus Removal with Adjunctive Catheter-directed Thrombolysis, or ATTRACT),[34] Quality improvement and reporting guidelines have been established.[35,36]

Endovascular Treatment Options

Catheter-directed thrombolysis with intrathrombic infusion of a pharmacologic thrombolytic agent has become the standard of care for patients with DVT associated with IVCS (FIGURE 93.1). Agents currently available include recombinant tissue plasminogen activator or alteplase (r-tPA; Activase, Genentech, South San Francisco, CA), reteplase (rPA; Retavase, Centocor, Malvern, PA), tenecteplase (TNK, Genentech), and urokinase (Kinlytic, formerly known as Abbokinase, Microbix, Toronto, ON, Canada). More rapid resolution of thrombosis can usually be

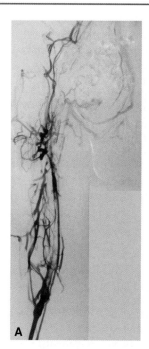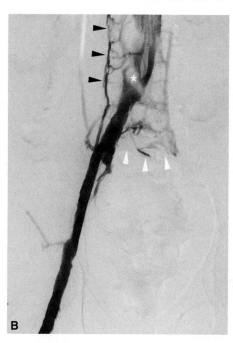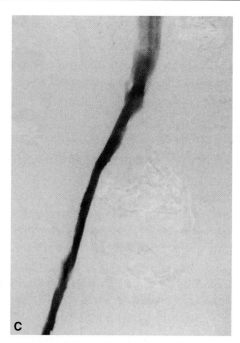

FIGURE 93.1 A. A 29-year-old female lawyer presented with subacute edema, pain, and discoloration of the left lower extremity and chest pain and shortness of breath after several long airplane flights. Initially, medical care was not sought, but ultrasound examination later diagnosed deep venous thrombosis, and this composite venogram of the left lower extremity and pelvis from popliteal vein access confirmed thrombosis of the superficial femoral, common femoral, external iliac, and common iliac veins. Collateral pathways were seen involving the deep femoral and pelvic wall veins, including veins crossing over into the patent right iliac system. **B.** After 20 hours of intrathrombus infusion of recombinant tPA, mechanical thrombolysis, and another 20 hours of infusion, repeat venography showed near complete resolution of the thrombosis in the femoral and iliac segments. A few ascending lumbar (*black arrowheads*) and presacral (*white arrowheads*) collateral veins were still seen, diverting blood flow around the May-Thurner lesion (*asterisk*) caused by the left common iliac vein being compressed between the right common iliac artery and the vertebral column. **C.** After placement of a 14-mm diameter, 60-mm long self-expanding stent and balloon venoplasty, rapid in-line flow across the lesion was achieved, and collateral veins were no longer filled.

accomplished by combining pharmacologic lysis with mechanical fragmentation and/or aspiration.[37-40] In a very small minority of patients with absolute contraindications to pharmacologic thrombolysis, purely mechanical thrombectomy and thrombolysis may be attempted. The array of currently available devices changes frequently but reflects a few proven mechanisms of action, including direct aspiration, Venturi effect aspiration, fragmentation by impeller or wire basket, enhanced distribution of pharmacologic agent, vessel wall scraping, or a combination thereof. Although full therapeutic anticoagulation was routinely performed during the entire thrombolytic infusion when urokinase was the standard, it appears that subtherapeutic heparin infusion through the sheath is sufficient and potentially safer when using tPA, rPA, or TNK.[41]

Removal of thrombus is not sufficient to address iliac compression syndrome because of the fixed obstructive lesion. Spurs and chronic thrombus may be remodeled by using balloon angioplasty, which may require large-diameter (12 to 18 mm) balloons. Balloon venoplasty alone is associated with a very high rate of recurrence due to persistent extrinsic compression, so stent placement is nearly always necessary to preserve patency (FIGURE 93.1).

Iliac compression syndrome is becoming increasingly recognized even without the occurrence of DVT in patients with left-sided symptoms of venous hypertension.[42] These patients also

benefit from balloon venoplasty and stent placement but may require simpler procedures using shorter stents (FIGURE 93.2).

Planning the Interventional Procedure

Ultrasound is usually performed to evaluate presence and extent of thrombosis, which can guide the decision on where to obtain venous access.[43] Frequently, cross-sectional imaging (computed tomography [CT] or magnetic resonance imaging [MRI]) is also performed to evaluate iliocaval thrombosis, site and degree of impingement, size and patency of collateral channels, thickness and inflammation of venous walls, anatomic variants, and presence of vascular malformations, malignancy, or mass lesions that may contribute to obstruction.[44,45] Associated venous pathologies, such as dilated gonadal veins, may also be detected. Because many of these patients are young and female, avoidance of ionizing radiation by using MRI instead of CT is probably most prudent.[46]

Cross-sectional imaging may also be confusing because impingement is found in a high proportion of the general population, most of whom are completely asymptomatic. Kibbe et al.[47] found that mean compression of the left common iliac vein in asymptomatic controls was 35%, and 24% had greater than 50% compression. Women demonstrated greater

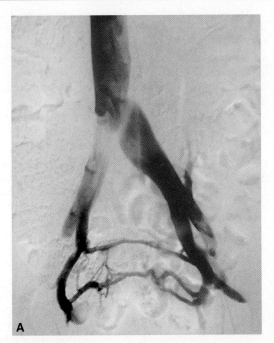
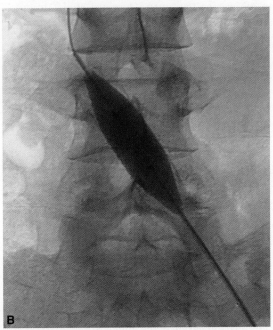

FIGURE 93.2 **A.** Left external iliac supine venogram from left femoral vein access in a 17-year-old woman who presented with chronic, lifestyle-limiting dependent edema and pain of the left lower extremity showed the stereotypical May-Thurner lesion of the left common iliac vein, retrograde flow in the left internal iliac vein, and presacral collateral veins draining into the right internal iliac vein. This patient had previously undergone technically successful but clinically ineffective stripping of the greater saphenous vein. There was no history and no evidence of deep venous thrombosis, so femoral access was chosen. **B.** Venoplasty with a 14-mm balloon was performed after deployment of a 14-mm diameter, 40-mm long self-expanding stent. **C.** Poststent venogram showed resolution of collateral flow and May-Thurner lesion. However, note the widened appearance of the common iliac vein, suggesting elastic recoil with flattening of the stent in the coronal plane. **D.** Curved planar reformat of a follow-up magnetic resonance venogram 9 years after treatment showed complete expansion of the stent and continued patency of all vessels, including the right iliac vein and inferior vena cava despite protrusion of the stent. The patient remained free of pain and edema but developed new small thigh varicosities. *(continued)*

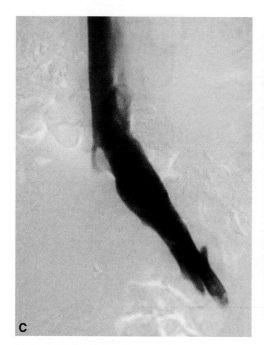
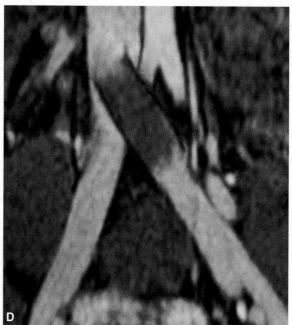

FIGURE 93.2 *(Continued)*

compression on average than men. Oguzkurt et al.[43] found greater compression in patients with left iliofemoral DVT than in asymptomatic controls, but the populations overlapped considerably. They advocated using 70% compression as a threshold for diagnosis. The degree of narrowing has been shown to be a powerful predictor of risk of DVT[48] but inversely related to risk of PE.[49]

Intravascular ultrasound has been promoted as a real-time adjunct to preoperative noninvasive imaging.[50,51] Although modification of the treatment scheme may result in up to half of patients, the relatively subtle contributions have not convincingly justified the added time and expense in most practices.

Technical and Anatomic Considerations

The diameter of an unobstructed common iliac vein in an adult ranges in diameter of approximately 12 to 18 mm. The cross-section of the impinged vein in an iliac compression syndrome patient is typically slit-like, measuring 1 or 2 mm in anteroposterior dimension but 20 or more mm in craniocaudal dimension. The appropriate diameter of stent to use may be estimated by measuring the contralateral common iliac vein, or by multiplying the craniocaudal dimension of the impinged vein by $2/\pi$.

The fibrosis in the region of venous impingement requires that the stent have a substantial radial hoop strength. Many practitioners wish to preserve the dynamic capacitative function of a vein by using self-expanding stents, whereas others find that the greater strength afforded by a balloon-expandable stent prevents recoil and recurrence of obstruction. Because most patients are female and young, the possibility of delayed stent collapse due to a gravid uterus must be considered. Stronger self-expanding stents are being developed, but until they are commercially available, increased hoop strength can be accomplished by using two superimposed stents.

The angle of confluence between the left and right common iliac veins is unfortunately rarely 90 degrees. Acute angulation between the two and the typical location of the impingement immediately adjacent to the confluence frequently requires that the cylindrical stent protrude from the left common iliac vein into the IVC, partially covering or "jailing" the right common iliac vein. Blood flow from the right lower extremity and pelvis must then partially flow through the interstices of the stent, theoretically causing turbulence and potential thrombus formation. This protrusion should be minimized, but if unavoidable, placement of a kissing stent in the right common iliac vein may be considered.

As is true of any thrombolysis, the maturity of the thrombus has great impact on the success of the procedure. Iliac compression syndrome patients all suffer from longstanding venous obstruction but may have any combination of acute and chronic thrombus. The more chronic thrombus, the less benefit is to be expected from lysis.[26] Additionally, the greater the extent of chronic thrombus, the greater the required length of stent placement (FIGURE 93.3). Stenting across potential hinge points, especially if using balloon-expandable stents, can be problematic. Additionally, placing stents over branches may cause stasis and thrombosis in those branches and can limit the ability of those branches to provide collateral drainage in case of stent occlusion. When stenosis and chronic thrombus extend peripherally from the site of vein impingement, flexible self-expanding stents should be used when crossing flex points, such as the psoas attachment and the inguinal ligament. Although crossing the hip joint and inguinal ligament was thought to be risky and prone to fracture and failure, this practice is now quite common and is associated with an acceptably low rate of complications.[41,52,53] Peripheral extension of stents into the thigh also shows promise but is still controversial.[54] Presence of chronic thrombosis lowers the likelihood of long-term patency after treatment.[55]

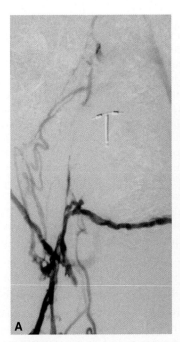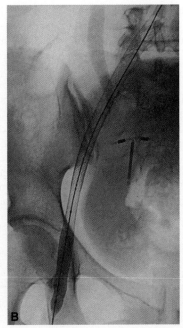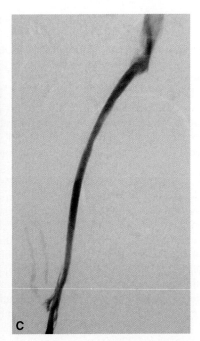

FIGURE 93.3 A. A 32-year-old woman, heterozygous for factor V Leiden, presented with persistent disabling edema and exercise intolerance after 10 months of anticoagulation treatment of an acute iliofemoral deep venous thrombosis suffered during pregnancy. Left lower extremity venogram from popliteal vein access in prone position showed poor recanalization of the femoral segment and no recanalization of the iliac segment. Circumflex iliac and anterior abdominal wall collateral vessels carried blood flow into the right iliac and left ascending lumbar systems. Note that the patient had an intrauterine contraceptive device placed to avoid the additional thrombotic risk of oral contraceptive use. **B.** The diseased segment was recanalized with catheters and hydrophilic guide wires, venoplastied seqeuentially to 10 mm and then 14 mm diameter, and stented with multiple overlapping self-expanding stents extending to the level of confluence of the superficial and deep femoral veins peripheral to the inguinal ligament. **C.** In-line flow was reestablished, but the superficial femoral vein peripheral to the stents still displayed linear filling defects indicative of chronic nonocclusive thrombus.

Specific Intraprocedural Techniques

Site of venous access can be chosen from a number of different options. Only a small minority of patients have valves in the iliac veins,[56] so anterograde and retrograde approaches are both feasible. In patients with no thrombosis, the access site that affords the most mechanical advantage is usually the left common femoral vein. Traversal of the site of impingement, introduction of large-diameter devices, and control of catheters and devices are all feasible and safe from this access. If thrombosis extends more peripherally, however, access to the popliteal vein or even a tibial vein may be preferable to allow lysis of the greatest length of vein. Introduction of large-diameter balloons, mechanical thrombolysis devices, and stents may be limited and may require a second site of access, such as the internal jugular vein or right common femoral vein.

Endpoint Assessment of the Procedure

Because most patients require stenting to relieve the impingement, the issue is not whether to stent, but rather how much is enough. Resolution of any pressure gradient greater than 2 mm Hg across the impingement is probably necessary for relief of symptoms, and in patients without thrombosis, a short (40 or 60 mm length) stent is usually sufficient. In patients with

thrombosis, stents may need to be extended into the external iliac and/or common femoral veins to reestablish inflow into the common iliac vein, using multiple overlapping long stents. It remains controversial how much residual thrombus necessitates additional stents. Saturation with a pharmacologic thrombolytic agent can result in continued and delayed lysis, and a certain degree of remodeling may occur even when the post-lysis venogram appears irregular. Rapid flow during venography is reassuring, but often the limb is so edematous that flow is sluggish despite wide patency of the veins.

In some practices, the use of cone beam c-arm CT has been implemented as part of the original procedure to obtain a three-dimensional depiction of stent configuration. Adequacy of coverage of the site of impingement, protrusion into the IVC, and recoil and collapse of the stent can all be examined.

Complications and How to Manage Them

Impingement of the left common iliac vein acts as a natural barrier against pulmonary embolus originating from that limb.[49] Treatment of the obstruction removes the barrier, theoretically increasing the risk for pulmonary embolus. Data from the Venous Registry suggested that clinically significant pulmonary embolus is rare during thrombolysis of DVTs with mortality in less than 1% of patients.[29] It has long been controversial whether the placement of an IVC filter is indicated as prophylaxis against these rare events. The commercial availability of retrievable IVC filters has changed the balance of risks because long-term adverse events associated with permanent caval filtration can now be avoided.

A dreaded intraprocedural complication is hyperacute thrombosis. The thrombophilia that led to DVT may remain uncorrected or uncorrectable, preexistent thrombus may act as a nidus of propagation, and vessel wall phlebitic inflammation and denudation of endothelium may all contribute to formation of new thrombus. Hyperacute thrombus is typically soft and amenable to both mechanical and pharmacologic lysis but must be considered a sign of failure of anticoagulation. Some patients may be resistant to heparin, and some may have antibodies (heparin-induced thrombocytopenia, or HIT). The addition or substitution of other anticoagulants, such as direct thrombin inhibitors (bivalirudin, argatroban), should be considered if efficacy of heparin alone is in question. Inhibition of platelet activation by administering glycoprotein 2b3a inhibitors, aspirin, and/or clopidogrel is controversial because anticoagulation is felt to be more effective in prevention of venous thrombosis.[57,58]

Some patients complain of pelvic or back pain after treatment, likely related to the stent pressing on the vertebral body of L4, L5, or S1. Rami of the lumbar and sacral plexuses may be pinched, which may contribute to the pain. A brief course of nonsteroidal or narcotic analgesics is usually sufficient because this discomfort typically resolves spontaneously within days.

Outcomes/Prognosis

Short-term procedural success approaches 100% in all reported series. Mid- and long-term clinical success is also encouragingly high but not perfect. One-year primary and secondary patencies have been reported as 80% to 90% and 90% to 100%, respectively, with similar 5-year patencies when available.[27,55,59–62] Corresponding with vessel patency, patient quality of life greatly improves after treatment.[30,63,64] However, some patients remain symptomatic, possibly from reflux and loss of valvular function,[30] although reflux may have only limited impact on the clinical success of iliac stenting.[65] Others may have a component of lymphedema, a diagnosis difficult to make until other potential causes have been eliminated.[66,67]

Disease Surveillance and Treatment Monitoring Algorithms

All patients should remain anticoagulated in the periprocedural period, usually with intravenous heparin or a subcutaneous surrogate (enoxaparin, fondaparinux), usually transitioning to oral vitamin K antagonist (warfarin) or a direct factor Xa inhibitor (rivaroxiban). The duration of anticoagulation varies with the patients' histories of thromboses and with identified genetic or malignant thrombophilias. Patients who never suffered thrombosis are generally discontinued from anticoagulation after about 3 months, at which time the stent should be covered by a layer of new endothelium and thus at low risk for platelet adhesion and thrombosis. Patients with paraneoplastic thrombotic syndrome (Trousseau syndrome) or genetic predispositions toward thrombosis (factor V Leiden mutation, prothrombin 20210A mutation, protein C or S deficiency, antithrombin III deficiency, homocysteinemia, etc.) generally require lifelong anticoagulation. Patients

with acquired and potentially correctable thrombophilia (pregnancy, paroxysmal nocturnal hemoglobinuria, anticardiolipin, lupus anticoagulant, and other antiphospholipid syndromes) may undergo intermediate term anticoagulation only while risk of rethrombosis is high.[68] The clinical significance of genetic mutations remains disputed, however, and greater emphasis should be placed on a patient's actual history of spontaneous thrombosis.[69]

Because a substantial proportion of patients may have components of venous reflux and/or lymphedema contributing to their symptoms, the use of compression stockings is recommended for those with persistent symptoms; 30 to 40 mm Hg pressure level is the most frequently prescribed and must be properly fitted or custom manufactured to provide optimal benefit.

Follow-up imaging is usually performed only if there are persistent or recurrent symptoms. Ultrasound, MRI, and CT are again the most frequently used modalities, similar to preprocedural imaging.

Early Failures and Options for Management

Early failures may be caused by propagation of residual thrombus, insufficient stent length, or collapse of stent. Diagnostic and therapeutic algorithms are essentially the same as for the original treatment. Of the cross-sectional imaging modalities, CT is usually the most useful to examine the stent and its relationship to vascular structures. Identification of a remediable technical issue, such as too short a stent or collapse of the stent, can be a welcome finding and reason for optimism. Repeat thrombolysis, venoplasty, and stent placement are generally successful.

Late Failures and Options for Management

Late failures may also reflect collapse or migration of the stent. Material fatigue in both self-expanding and balloon-expandable stents may result in progressive or sudden collapse with or without fracture of the material. Failure is often associated with a change in anatomy, such as compression from a gravid uterus, an arterial aneurysm, or a neoplasm. When reversible, the anatomic cause of failure should be addressed first, followed by re-treatment of the vein by lysis, venoplasty, and restenting. For instance, a pregnant patient may wait until after delivery to seek re-treatment to avoid radiation exposure to the fetus and to avoid high risk of early failure.[68] In some cases, such as invasive neoplasm, the addition of a stent-graft may provide more durable patency if ingrowth of tissue is the mechanism of failure.

The tight impingement of the iliac vein and the jagged design of most commercially available stents make stent migration a rare late complication. Migration peripherally may result in symptom recurrence, requiring re-treatment. Minor migration centrally may result in obstruction of the contralateral limb, which is usually asymptomatic. However, complete migration of the stent into the heart can be associated with life-threatening dysrhythmias as well as chest pain, cardiac valvular dysfunction, and perforation.[70] Stents are difficult to retrieve from the heart, and this complication may require open surgical retrieval.

Relative Therapeutic Effectiveness

The reported technical and clinical success rates exceed those of open surgical options, including for longer-term results. Surgical repairs are essentially only offered after recurrent failure of endovascular methods,[71] and endovascular repair has become the overwhelmingly dominant standard of care.

The Future

Thrombolysis of venous thrombosis and placement of stents to relieve iliac compression syndrome are performed off-label without the approval of the Food and Drug Administration (FDA). Currently, the economics of this field makes it unlikely to be profitable to obtain specific indications for devices and pharmaceuticals. However, when compelling level I evidence is generated, utilization may increase greatly.

Two areas of commercial research and development are geared toward treatment of this syndrome. First is the development of stents designed specifically for venous applications. Most companies are working toward providing greater hoop strength to resist the recoil caused by persistent compression by the overriding right iliac artery. Some are also exploring asymmetric stent designs to allow ostial stenting without protrusion into the vena cava and without jailing the contralateral right iliac vein. The second area of commercial research and development is in the area of long-term orally administered anticoagulants, including direct factor Xa inhibitors (rivaroxaban, apixaban) and direct thrombin inhibitors (dabigatran). These have the theoretical advantages over warfarin of being predictable in effect, greatly reducing the need for constant monitoring.

NUTCRACKER SYNDROME (ALSO KNOWN AS RENAL VEIN COMPRESSION SYNDROME)

The first anatomic description of the left renal vein being compressed between the aorta and the superior mesenteric artery (SMA) like a "nut caught in a nutcracker" was published by Grant in 1937.[72] El Sadr and Mina reported the first clinical case associated with left-sided varicocele in 1950.[73] In 1962, Vassilev[74] noted stagnation of contrast in the left renal vein in varicocele patients undergoing direct varicocele venography. Cope and Isard[75] found minor compression by aortic aneurysms or tortuosity or by retroperitoneal malignancy but did not find venographic or hemodynamic support for the existence of nutcracker phenomenon in over 500 patients studied. In retrospect, one of their published figures portrays an effaced renal vein and drainage via ovarian and lumbar vein collateral routes but is labeled "normal left renal vein." Chait et al.[76] and de Schepper[77] popularized the term *nutcracker* in 1971 to 1972. Chait et al. published arteriographic and venographic evidence of obstruction including dilatation of periureteric veins, delayed renal washout, and a 3-cm water gradient across the lesion in a varicocele patient. They also postulated that renal vein obstruction could be related to hematuria in patients with ureteric varicosities, varicoceles, or varices of the broad ligament.

Because effacement of the left renal vein with peripheral distention is found in 51% to 72% of the general population,[78,79] and most of those with this anatomy are asymptomatic, distinction has been raised between those with anatomic findings (nutcracker phenomenon) and those with symptoms (nutcracker syndrome).[80] Anatomically, patients may have a compressed left renal vein lying between the abdominal aorta and the SMA, the most common configuration called "anterior nutcracker." Compression of a retroaortic or circumaortic renal vein is called

"posterior nutcracker." Anterior nutcracker may also be associated with episodic obstruction of the third portion of the duodenum, which courses through the same space, a condition called "superior mesenteric artery syndrome" or Wilkie syndrome, but sometimes also confusingly called "nutcracker syndrome." Various anatomic anomalies have been described as causative factors, including ptotic left kidney, high insertion of left renal vein into the cava, and low or lateral origin of the SMA from the aorta or abnormal SMA branching.

The epidemiology of symptomatic patients with nutcracker syndrome is poorly understood. The published literature supports greater prevalence in women and people with tall, asthenic builds. Two distinct age groups have emerged as being the most commonly affected. Younger patients presenting in their second and third decades may enjoy spontaneous regression with conservative care, but a second peak of middle-aged multiparous women seem to suffer from more persistent symptoms.[81] The abundance of reports from Asia suggests a higher incidence there,[82] although no genetic or hereditary factors have been identified.

There are no accepted guidelines to define the pathologic nutcracker syndrome, but common symptoms associated with renal vein compression syndrome include hematuria, flank pain, varicocele or pelvic congestion syndrome, orthostatic proteinuria, and, possibly, orthostatic intolerance and chronic fatigue syndromes. Hematuria is the stereotypical presentation, where microhematuria is approximately four times as common as macrohematuria. Microhematuria is attributed to formation of valveless, thin-walled collateral channels that have been histologically shown to communicate with adjacent calyces. Macrohematuria is attributed to rupture of larger varices.[81]

Passage of clots causing renal and ureteral colic is one mechanism of associated pain. Flank pain may radiate to the posteromedial thigh and buttock and may be exacerbated by physical activity, by certain prolonged upright or supine positions, or by minor trauma, such as vibration within an automobile.[83] This pattern is more common in the younger patient with hematuria, whereas deep pelvic pain and other symptoms, such as dyspareunia, dysuria, dysmenorrhea, and perineal and buttock varices associated with pelvic congestion are more common in the older patient (FIGURE 93.4). Approximately 20% of patients with pelvic congestion were diagnosed with renal vein compression.[84] Similarly, 19% of male varicocele patients show left renal vein compression, and postsurgical recurrence is 100% in these patients[85] (FIGURE 93.5). Additionally, approximately two-thirds of male renal donors who underwent left renal vein ligation developed varicoceles.[86]

The third common clinical manifestation is orthostatic proteinuria. Diurnal variation in urinary protein excretion is normally approximately three- or fourfold greater during the daytime when subjects are upright. Pathologically elevated upright urinary protein excretion (>100 mg/m² body surface area, >25-fold greater than supine) is also very common, found in 20% of asymptomatic children 6 to 19 years old.[87] A high proportion of patients with orthostatic proteinuria demonstrate compression of the left renal vein (68%),[88] and in these patients, the left kidney is the source of proteinuria. Correction of compression successfully eliminates the proteinuria, but most of these young patients undergo spontaneous remission anyway. There are also data suggesting potential associations between renal vein obstruction with chronic fatigue syndromes and orthostatic intolerance syndromes.[83]

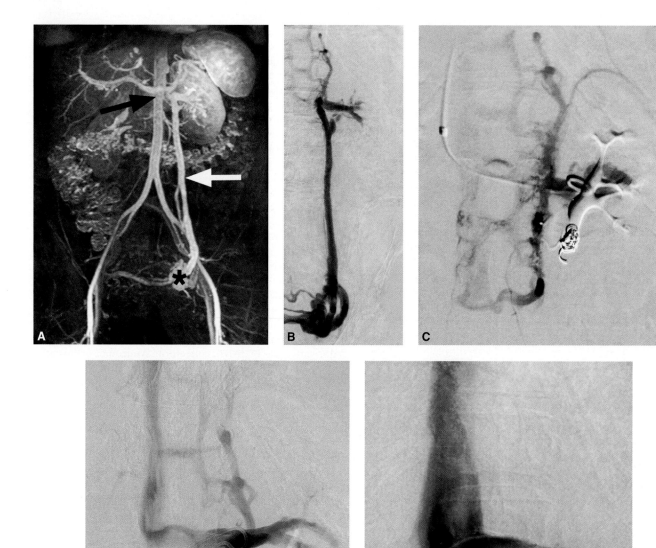

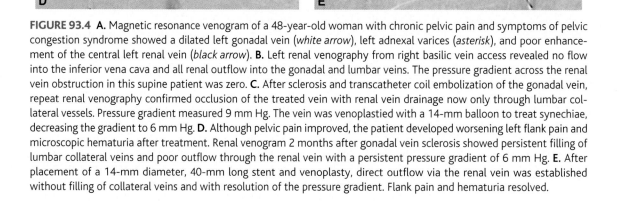

FIGURE 93.4 A. Magnetic resonance venogram of a 48-year-old woman with chronic pelvic pain and symptoms of pelvic congestion syndrome showed a dilated left gonadal vein (*white arrow*), left adnexal varices (*asterisk*), and poor enhancement of the central left renal vein (*black arrow*). **B.** Left renal venography from right basilic vein access revealed no flow into the inferior vena cava and all renal outflow into the gonadal and lumbar veins. The pressure gradient across the renal vein obstruction in this supine patient was zero. **C.** After sclerosis and transcatheter coil embolization of the gonadal vein, repeat renal venography confirmed occlusion of the treated vein with renal vein drainage now only through lumbar collateral vessels. Pressure gradient measured 9 mm Hg. The vein was venoplastied with a 14-mm balloon to treat synechiae, decreasing the gradient to 6 mm Hg. **D.** Although pelvic pain improved, the patient developed worsening left flank pain and microscopic hematuria after treatment. Renal venogram 2 months after gonadal vein sclerosis showed persistent filling of lumbar collateral veins and poor outflow through the renal vein with a persistent pressure gradient of 6 mm Hg. **E.** After placement of a 14-mm diameter, 40-mm long stent and venoplasty, direct outflow via the renal vein was established without filling of collateral veins and with resolution of the pressure gradient. Flank pain and hematuria resolved.

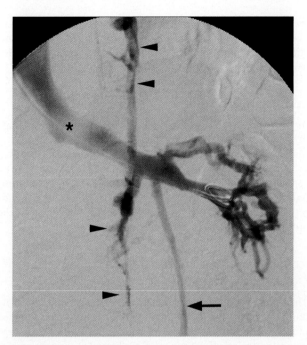

FIGURE 93.5 Left renal venography in a 22-year-old man with left-sided varicocele confirmed reflux down the gonadal vein (*arrow*) but also showed a nutcracker lesion (*asterisk*) with filling of lumbar collateral vessels (*arrowheads*). The pressure gradient was 3 mm Hg, which did not change after sclerosis of the varicocele, and the varicocele resolved without new symptoms of renal vein compression.

Endovascular Treatment Options

Therapies for renal vein compression syndrome range from observation to nephrectomy.[81] For patients severely symptomatic enough to consider open surgical reimplantation of the vein and/or SMA, balloon angioplasty and stent placement is an alternative option, first reported in 1996.[89] Because of the extrinsic mode of compression, balloon venoplasty alone would be expected to fail, and published reports have all advocated the use of stents. Fortunately, thrombosis of the renal vein is extremely uncommon so thrombolysis is rarely necessary. Dozens of reports of use of balloon-expandable, self-expanding, or self-expanding covered stents have been published, mostly single case reports.[90,91] Mean follow-up ranges up to 29 months, but existing data are inadequate to determine long-term efficacy and the comparative effectiveness of different stent types.

Anatomic or Lesion Considerations, Technical/Device Considerations, Treatment Selection Strategies, Planning the Interventional Procedure

Similar to iliac vein compression, the noncylindrical shape and angulated insertion of the left renal vein into the IVC in nutcracker syndrome requires careful planning prior to attempted endovascular treatment. Diameter of balloon and stent can be calculated according to the expected diameter of a cylinder based on the circumference of the compressed vein. Measurements should be based on cross-sectional imaging, such as CT or

MR, where three-dimensional multiplanar or volumetric reconstructions may allow more accurate measurements.

Intraprocedural Techniques, Endpoint Assessment

Venous access can be established either from the common femoral or internal jugular vein, depending on the angle between the left renal vein and IVC. Simultaneous pressure measurements in the IVC and the renal vein should be performed. Venography of the renal vein may benefit from the use of a multi-hole catheter, such as a pigtail catheter, to allow uniform filling of the vein and its outlets.

The renal vein may have synechiae similar to the spurs of IVCS, which can be disrupted by balloon venoplasty. However, the extrinsic compression also requires the placement of a stent if the impingement is to be relieved. Some authors have advocated the use of longer stents (60 or 80 mm length) to lessen the likelihood of migration,[90,91] even though the lesion may be adequately covered by a shorter stent.

Complications, Outcomes/Prognosis, Surveillance, Early and Late Failures

The published literature on outcomes is scant and there are no level I data. Single-center series show promising results with no significant in-stent restenoses or thromboses in short- and mid-term follow-up. Hematuria and pain may take up to 6 months to resolve, but some will show improvement or resolution within a week.[91] However, multiple accounts of stent migration, either peripherally or centrally, reveal the technical difficulty of placing and fixating a stent in a dynamic environment.[90,91]

PAGET-SCHROETTER SYNDROME (ALSO KNOWN AS AXILLOSUBCLAVIAN VEIN COMPRESSION SYNDROME, EFFORT VEIN THROMBOSIS, VENOUS THORACIC OUTLET [INLET] SYNDROME)

The pathologist Sir James Paget described spontaneous thrombosis of the subclavian vein as "gouty phlebitis" in 1875.[92] Austrian internist and laryngologist Leopold von Schroetter independently described spontaneous subclavian vein thrombosis and noted the musculoskeletal anatomy surrounding the vein and proposed a mechanical etiology in 1884.[93] The terms *Paget-Schroetter syndrome* and *effort vein thrombosis* were coined in the 1940s, and one of the first review articles was written by DeBakey et al. in 1942.[94]

Impingement of the subclavian vein is an unusual variation of thoracic outlet syndrome (sometimes corrected to "thoracic inlet syndrome"), which more commonly affects the brachial plexus and/or subclavian artery. Unlike cohesive neurovascular bundles elsewhere in the body, the subclavian vein courses through a different space than the artery and nerves, bounded by the first rib inferiorly, subclavius muscle and clavicle superiorly, costoclavicular ligament medially, and anterior scalene muscle posterolaterally. This space is restricted in the normal subject and the adjacent musculoskeletal structures do not move a great deal, but abduction and external rotation at the shoulder further narrow this space. Nearly all normal subjects significantly impinge the subclavian vein by this musculoskeletal motion, but only a small fraction become symptomatic.[95–98] The term *effort vein thrombosis* reflects the observation that most patients report an inciting musculoskeletal stress or effort that precipitated the onset of symptoms.

Paget-Schroetter syndrome is uncommon, affecting an estimated 5,000 patients per year in the United States.[99] Average age at presentation is in the early 30s, and men tend to present at a slightly earlier age than women. Approximately twice as many men as women are diagnosed, and probably related to hand dominance, more right-sided disease is reported than left. Although venous impingement and "pinch-off" syndrome may play a role in commonly seen iatrogenic subclavian vein thrombosis after venous catheterization, dialysis access creation, or pacemaker lead placement, this should be distinguished from primary axillosubclavian vein thrombosis or Paget-Schroetter syndrome.

Most of the literature promotes a combination of endovascular and open surgical treatment for Paget-Schroetter syndrome, exploiting endoluminal techniques for clearance of thrombus and extraluminal techniques for relief of musculoskeletal impingement. Large series document very high clinical success rates for early[100,101] as well as delayed[102,103] surgical decompression of the thoracic inlet. Techniques include transaxillary, supraclavicular, infraclavicular, paraclavicular, and laparoscopic methods of first rib resection; debulking of ligaments, muscles, fibrous bands, and osteophytes; and venolysis. However, there

are also data suggesting that surgical decompression is not necessary in up to half of these patients, who become asymptomatic after thrombolysis, anticoagulation, and a period of restraint from the inciting activity.[104–106]

Endovascular Treatment Options

As is true of other deep venous thromboses, mechanical, pharmacologic, or combination thrombolysis may be attempted after the diagnosis is made (FIGURE 93.6). Venous access to the brachial or basilic vein peripheral to the thrombosis allows diagnostic venography and use of thrombectomy devices and/or thrombolysis infusion catheters. Success of thrombolysis depends on chronicity of clot, but unlike May-Thurner syndrome, the options of balloon venoplasty and stenting are controversial.

Anatomic or Lesion Considerations, Technical/Device Considerations

The site of venous impingement in the thoracic inlet presents unique endovascular challenges. Patients may have hypertrophied muscles (subclavius, scalene), restrictive fibrous bands or ligaments (costoclavicular ligament, Roos bands[107]), supernumerary ribs, post-fracture calluses, or aberrant nerves (phrenic, brachial plexus) external to the vein contributing to impingement. None of these are amenable to decompression from within the vein

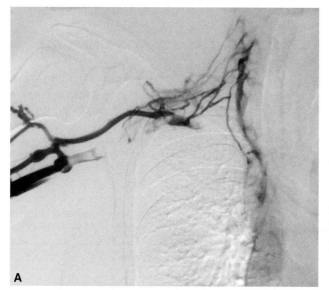
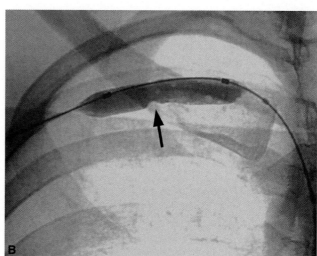

FIGURE 93.6 **A.** Right upper extremity venography via brachial access in a 19-year-old woman weight lifter who presented with pain and swelling after a workout revealed acute thrombosis of the subclavian and duplicated axillary veins with poorly formed collateral channels draining into the external jugular system. **B.** After 20 hours of intrathrombus thrombolytic infusion, much of the acute thrombosis had resolved and an incompletely inflated balloon was used to thrombectomize (Fogarty) the remaining adherent clot. Note the contour deformity on the inferior aspect of the balloon (*arrow*), caused by the fibrotic Paget-Schroetter lesion. These lesions typically do not respond well to balloon venoplasty and may, in fact, be further inflamed by aggressive dilatation. **C.** Venogram with the upper extremity in neutral position (parallel alongside the torso) after thrombolysis and thrombectomy confirmed the typical lesion of Paget-Schroetter syndrome. **D.** Evocative venogram in deep inspiration with the extremity abducted and externally rotated and head turned to the contralateral side (Wright's maneuver) showed complete occlusion of the subclavian vein at the thoracic inlet with poor filling of the collateral pathways. The patient has modified her exercise routine and remained asymptomatic despite deferring surgical decompression.

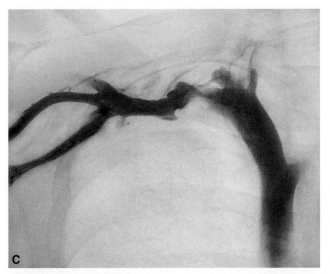
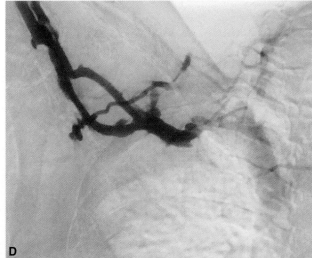

FIGURE 93.6 *(Continued)*

lumen. Additionally, chronic repetitive trauma and inflammation typically cause a focal venous wall thickening with synechiae or spurs even more robust than those found in May-Thurner syndrome. Impingement may also involve the site of confluence with the internal or external jugular veins and with supraclavicular collateral veins (FIGURES 93.7 and 93.8). Conservation of mass and the unyielding nature of the boundaries of the thoracic inlet render balloon venoplasty of limited use. In addition, the barotrauma

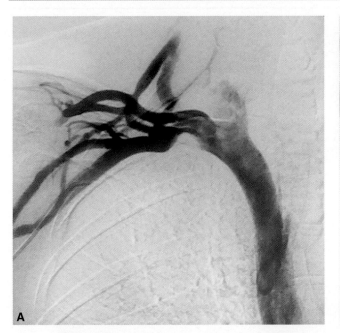
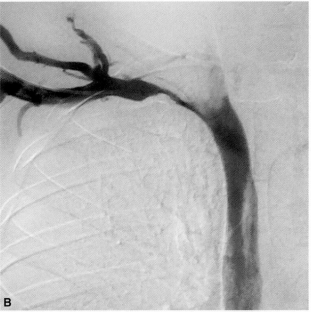

FIGURE 93.7 A. Right upper extremity venography in a 45-year-old woman weight lifter 3 months after successful thrombolysis of an acute deep venous thrombosis from Paget-Schroetter syndrome revealed persistent narrowing of the main subclavian vein and a well-developed collateral network posterior and superior to the clavicle. This patient initially deferred decompressive surgery, did not rethrombose on warfarin therapy, but remained symptomatic with athletic activity. **B.** Venography repeated with Wright's maneuver showed complete effacement of the collateral network and persistent high-grade stenosis of the subclavian vein. These collateral vessels, although effective at rest with the extremity in neutral position, did not facilitate the patient's return to athletic activities, and the patient elected to undergo decompressive surgery. **C.** In contrast, this 42-year-old man developed effective collateral channels that were not obstructed by evocative maneuvers and has remained asymptomatic without surgery. *(continued)*

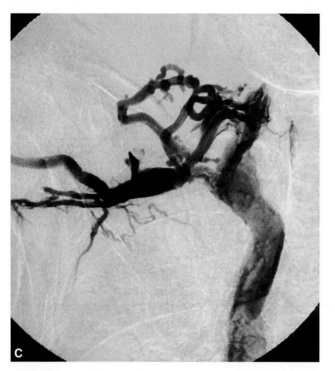

FIGURE 93.7 *(Continued)*

of venoplasty may actually accentuate the local inflammatory and thrombotic process. A certain degree of remodeling may be accomplished by placing a stent, but the musculoskeletal forces exerted on the vein far exceed a stent's ability to resist, and migration, fracture, and recurrent occlusion were so prevalent in early studies that placement of stents has become widely accepted as contraindicated in patients who have not undergone surgical decompression of the thoracic inlet[108] (FIGURE 93.9).

Planning the Interventional Procedure, Intraprocedural Techniques, Endpoint Assessment, Procedural Complications

Preoperative imaging may be as spartan as an ultrasound examination to confirm thrombosis. Although CT and MR may delineate the musculoskeletal structures impinging the vein, these have little impact on treatment planning. After attaining venous access peripheral to the thrombus, any pharmacologic and mechanical methods of thrombolysis may be employed, barring contraindications. Even in patients with documented pulmonary emboli, placement of superior vena cava filters is not routinely performed, in part because the volume of thrombus in the upper extremity veins is usually sublethal.

Perhaps the most difficult decision-making point of the procedure occurs after completion of thrombolysis, when

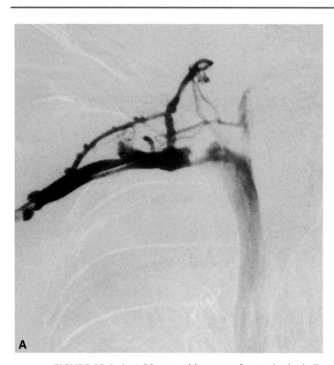

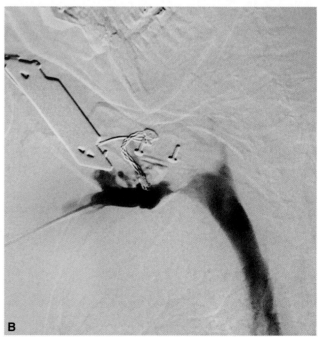

FIGURE 93.8 A. A 28-year-old woman, former basketball and volleyball player, presented with daily progressive discomfort and swelling 5 months after successful thrombolysis of effort vein thrombosis. She worked as a physician's assistant performing mostly telephone interviews and noted exacerbation of symptoms after prolonged telephone use. Right upper extremity venography showed a thoracic inlet lesion on the cranial aspect of the subclavian vein. **B.** Venography performed with the patient holding a telephone receiver between shrugged shoulder and ear showed compression and occlusion of the collateral channels and near-occlusion of the subclavian vein. She underwent decompressive surgery and purchased a headset.

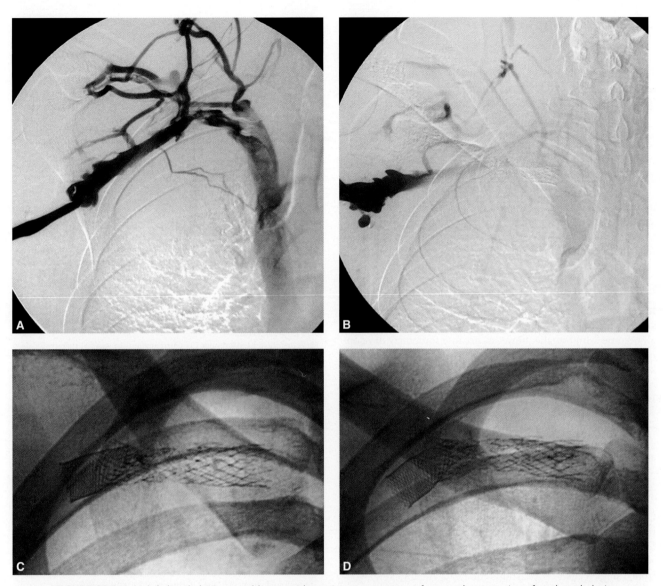

FIGURE 93.9 A. A left-handed 20-year-old man with persistent symptoms of venous hypertension after thrombolysis, venoplasty, and multiple stent procedures (in 1997) presented for surgical evaluation. Venography showed evidence of chronic nonocclusive thrombus in the subclavian vein and a well-developed system of collateral vessels while the extremity was in neutral position. **B.** With Wright's maneuver, the native vessel and nearly all of the collateral vessels were occluded. **C.** Radiograph of the stents while the arm was in neutral position revealed complete fracturing and disintegration of the nitinol stent (medial) and migration and compression of the woven steel stent (lateral). **D.** Radiograph with Wright's maneuver showed accentuation of deformation of both stents due to the overwhelming musculoskeletal forces exerted in the thoracic inlet. This patient underwent successful first rib resection and extensive venolysis without removal of stent fragments.

invariably a high-grade stenosis is found at the thoracic inlet. Flow may be sluggish and may be directed through collateral vessels, which may be poorly developed. Although most practitioners acknowledge the increased irritation and inflammation caused by balloon dilatation, a high proportion of patients are still treated thusly for fear of rethrombosis from persistent high-grade mechanical obstruction to flow.

The severity of external impingement may influence the surgical decisions on post-thrombolysis treatment. Several evocative maneuvers may be performed iteratively while performing venography. These include the Adson, Halsted, and Wright maneuvers, all of which replicate the various musculoskeletal positions and activities implicated in effort vein thrombosis.[109] Venography with evocative maneuvers may also delineate the existence and maturity of collateral channels and whether they are similarly affected by external impingement. Some of these maneuvers may also be performed during magnetic resonance venography for three-dimensional delineation of pathology.

Outcomes/Prognosis

Technical success of thrombolysis reflects chronicity of thrombus with nearly ensured success in patients with duration of symptoms of a week or less. Patients with chronic thrombosis may require more aggressive surgical techniques, such as jugular turndown or other reconstructions, to reestablish venous outflow.

Surveillance, Monitoring

Patients are usually placed on systemic anticoagulation for at least 3 months, and those with documented thrombophilia for longer periods up to lifetime. Surveillance is primarily expectant, and imaging is usually reserved for patients with residual or recurrent symptoms. Lifestyle modification is frequently necessary, such as discontinuation of anabolic steroids, overhead weightlifting, throwing, swimming, and other inciting physical activities.

Early and Late Failures

In patients who do not undergo immediate surgical decompression, up to 23% may demonstrate recurrent thrombosis.[105] Not all become symptomatic, however, because some may develop high-capacity collateral vessels. Even the development of collateral vessels may not ensure lack of symptoms because some of these vessels may also be impinged at the thoracic inlet. Failure and recurrence may be treated by repeat thrombolysis but usually invoke escalation of surgical therapy. Persistent symptomatic high-grade stenosis or rethrombosis after surgical decompression may be the only niche application of stenting, although durability of patency remains an issue.[110,111]

The Future

Controversy persists pertaining to patient selection and timing for surgical decompression. Authorities on treating Paget-Schroetter syndrome tend to be dogmatic in their treatment algorithms, supported by high rates of success in their noncontrolled single-center series. Thus, level I data are not likely to be generated comparing different algorithms.

▋ CONCLUSION

Extrinsic compression of veins by arterial, muscular, ligamentous, and skeletal structures more robust than veins is present in most normal subjects. Severe compression, insufficient collateralization, chronic repetitive trauma, and thrombosis may precipitate significant symptoms and disability. Intravascular thrombus may be amenable to mechanical and/or pharmacologic thrombolysis, and some impingements may be amenable to treatment by stenting.

▋ REFERENCES

1. Lowe GDO. Virchow's triad revisited: abnormal flow. *Pathophysiol Haemost Thromb* 2004;33:455–457.
2. Monos E, Berczi V, Nadasy G. Local control of veins: biomechanical, metabolic, and humoral aspects. *Physiol Rev* 1995;5:611–666.
3. Wakefield TW, Myers DD, Henke PK. Mechanisms of venous thrombosis and resolution. *Arterioscler Thromb Vasc Biol* 2008;8:387–391.
4. Alimi YS, Juhan C. New trends in the surgical and endovascular reconstructions of large veins for nonmalignant chronic venous occlusive disease. *Curr Opin Cardiol* 1998;13:375–383.
5. Virchow R. Uber die erweiterung kleinerer Gefasse. *Arch Path Anat* 1851;3:427.
6. McMurrich JP. The occurrence of congenital adhesions in the common iliac veins and their relation to the thrombosis of the femoral and iliac veins. *Am J Med Sci* 1908;135:342–346.
7. Ehrich WE, Krumbhaar EB. A frequent obstructive anomaly of the mouth of the left common iliac vein. *Am Heart J* 1943;26:737–750.
8. May R, Thurner J. The cause of the predominantly sinistral occurrence of thrombosis of the pelvic veins. *Angiology* 1957;8:419–427.
9. Cockett FB, Thomas ML. The iliac compression syndrome. *Br J Surg* 1965;52:816–821.
10. Cockett FB, Lea Thomas M, Negus D. Iliac vein compression—its relation to iliofemoral thrombosis and the post-thrombotic syndrome. *Br Med J* 1967;2:14–19.
11. Abboud G, Middulla M, Lions C, et al. "Right-sided" May-Thurner syndrome. *Cardiovasc Intervent Radiol* 2010;33:1056–1059.
12. Kim YH, Ko SM, Kim HT. Spontaneous rupture of the left common iliac vein associated with May-Thurner syndrome: successful management with surgery and placement of an endovascular stent. *Br J Radiol* 2007;80:e176–e179.
13. Dheer S, Joseph AE, Drooz A. Retroperitoneal hematoma caused by a ruptured pelvic varix in a patient with iliac vein compression syndrome. *J Vasc Interv Radiol* 2003;14:387–390.
14. Ferris EJ, Lim WN, Smith PL, et al. May-Thurner syndrome. *Radiology* 1983;147:29–31.
15. Greenfield LJ, Alexander EL. Current status of surgical therapy for deep vein thrombosis. *Am J Surg* 1985;150:64–70.
16. Hecker SP. Fibrinolytic therapy of thrombophlebitis. *Calif Med* 1964;101:23–29.
17. Rosch J, Dotter CT, Seaman AJ, et al. Healing of deep venous thrombosis: venographic findings in a randomized study comparing streptokinase and heparin. *AJR Am J Roentgenol* 1976;127:553–558.
18. Arnesen H, Hoiseth A, Ly B. Streptokinase or heparin in the treatment of deep vein thrombosis. *Acta Med Scand* 1982;211:65–68.
19. Graor R. Fibrinolytic therapy for deep vein thrombosis and pulmonary embolism. *Cardiovasc Interv Radiol* 1988;11:533–537.
20. Goldhaber SZ, Meyerovitz MF, Green D, et al. Randomized controlled trial of tissue plasminogen activator in proximal deep venous thrombosis. *Am J Med* 1990;88:235–240.
21. Harke H, Rahman S. A combined technique of local thrombolysis and regional neural blockade in severe venous occlusions. *Intensive Care Med* 1987;13:39–45.
22. Bookstein JJ, Saldinger E. Accelerated thrombolysis: in vitro evaluation of agents and methods of administration. *Invest Radiol* 1985;20:731–735.
23. Davis GB, Dowd CF, Bookstein JJ, et al. Thrombosed dialysis grafts: efficacy of intrathrombic deposition of concentrated urokinase, clot maceration, and angioplasty. *AJR Am J Roentgenol* 1987;149:177–181.
24. Okrent D, Messersmith R, Buckman J. Transcatheter fibrinolytic therapy and angioplasty for left iliofemoral venous thrombosis. *J Vasc Interv Radiol* 1991;2:195–200.
25. Semba CP, Dake MD. Iliofemoral deep venous thrombosis: aggressive therapy with catheter-directed thrombolysis. *Radiology* 1994;191:487–494.
26. Bjarnason H, Kruse JR, Asinger DA, et al. Iliofemoral deep vein thrombosis: safety and efficacy during 5 years of catheter-directed thrombolytic therapy. *J Vasc Interv Radiol* 1997;8:405–418.
27. O'Sullivan GJ, Semba CP, Bittner CA, et al. Endovascular management of iliac vein compression (May-Thurner) syndrome. *J Vasc Interv Radiol* 2000;11:823–836.
28. Patel NH, Stookey KR, Ketcham DB, et al. Endovascular management of acute extensive iliofemoral deep venous thrombosis caused by May-Thurner syndrome. *J Vasc Interv Radiol* 2000;11:1297–1302.
29. Mewissen MW, Seabrook GR, Meissner MH, et al. Catheter-directed thrombolysis for lower extremity deep venous thrombosis: report of a national multicenter registry. *Radiology* 1999;211:39–49.
30. Comerota AJ, Throm RC, Mathias SD, et al. Catheter-directed thrombolysis for iliofemoral deep venous thrombosis improves health-related quality of life. *J Vasc Surg* 2000;32:130–137.
31. Comerota AJ, Gravett MH. Iliofemoral venous thrombosis. *J Vasc Surg* 2007;46:1065–1076.
32. Elsharawy M, Elzayat E. Early results of thrombolysis vs anticoagulation in iliofemoral venous thrombosis. A randomized clinical trial. *Eur J Endovasc Surg* 2002;24:209–214.

33. Enden T, Klow NE, Sandvik L, et al. Catheter-directed thrombolysis vs. anticoagulant therapy alone in deep vein thrombosis: results of an open randomized, controlled trial reporting on short-term patency. *J Thromb Haemost* 2009;7:1268–1275.

34. Vedantham S. Catheter-directed thrombolysis for deep vein thrombosis. *Curr Opin Hematol* 2010;17:464–468.

35. Vedantham S, Thorpe PE, Cardella JF, et al., for the CIRSE and SIR Standards of Practice Committees. Quality improvement guidelines for the treatment of lower extremity deep vein thrombosis with use of endovascular thrombus removal. *J Vasc Interv Radiol* 2009;20:S227–S239.

36. Vedantham S, Grassi CJ, Ferral H, et al.; for the Technology Assessment Committee of the SIR. Reporting standards for endovascular treatment of lower extremity deep vein thrombosis. *J Vasc Interv Radiol* 2009; 20:S391–S408.

37. Kasirajan K, Milner R, Chaikof EL. Combination therapies for deep venous thrombosis. *Semin Vasc Surg* 2006;19:116–121.

38. Rao AS, Konig G, Leers SA, et al. Pharmacomechanical thrombectomy for iliofemoral deep vein thrombosis: an alternative in patients with contraindications to thrombolysis. *J Vasc Surg* 2009;50:1092–1098.

39. Lin PH, Zhou W, Dardik A, et al. Catheter-direct thrombolysis versus pharmacomechanical thrombectomy for treatment of symptomatic lower extremity deep venous thrombosis. *Am J Surg* 2006;192:782–788.

40. Cynamon J, Stein EG, Dym RJ, et al. A new method for aggressive management of deep vein thrombosis: retrospective study of the power pulse technique. *J Vasc Interv Radiol* 2006;17:1043–1049.

41. Semba CP, Razavi MK, Kee ST, et al. Thrombolysis for lower extremity deep venous thrombosis. *Tech Vasc Interv Radiol* 2004;7:68–78.

42. Raju S, Neglen P. High prevalence of nonthrombotic iliac vein lesions in chronic venous disease: a permissive role in pathogenicity. *J Vasc Surg* 2006;44:136–143.

43. Oguzkurt L, Ozkan U, Tercan F, et al. Ultrasonographic diagnosis of iliac vein compression (May-Thurner) syndrome. *Diagn Interv Radiol* 2007;13:152–155.

44. Baldt MM, Zontsich T, Stumpflen A, et al. Deep venous thrombosis of the lower extremity: efficacy of spiral CT venography compared with conventional venography in diagnosis. *Radiology* 1996;200:423–428.

45. Oguzkurt L, Ozkan U, Ulusan S, et al. Compression of the left common iliac vein in asymptomatic subjects and patients with left iliofemoral deep vein thrombosis. *J Vasc Interv Radiol* 2008;19:366–371.

46. Wolpert LM, Rahmani O, Stein B, et al. Magnetic resonance venography in the diagnosis and management of May-Thurner syndrome. *Vasc Endovasc Surg* 2002;36:51–57.

47. Kibbe MR, Ujiki M, Goodwin AL, et al. Iliac vein compression in an asymptomatic patient population. *J Vasc Surg* 2004;39:937–943.

48. Carr S, Chan K, Rosenberg J, et al. Correlation of the diameter of the left common iliac vein with the risk of lower-extremity deep venous thrombosis. *J Vasc Interv Radiol.* 2012;23:1467–1472.

49. Chan KT, Popat RA, Sze DY, et al. Common iliac vein stenosis and risk of symptomatic pulmonary embolism: an inverse correlation. *J Vasc Interv Radiol* 2011;22:133–141.

50. Ahmed HK, Hagspiel KD. Intravascular ultrasonographic findings in May-Thurner syndrome (iliac vein compression syndrome). *J Ultrasound Med* 2001;20:251–256.

51. Forauer AR, Gemmete JJ, Dasika NL, et al. Intravascular ultrasound in the diagnosis and treatment of iliac vein compression (May-Thurner) syndrome. *J Vasc Interv Radiol* 2002;13:523–527.

52. Andrews RT, Venbrux AC, Magee CA, et al. Placement of a flexible endovascular stent across the femoral joint: an in vivo study in the swine model. *J Vasc Interv Radiol* 1999;10:1219–1228.

53. Neglen P, Tackett TP Jr, Raju S. Venous stenting across the inguinal ligament. *J Vasc Surg* 2008;48:1255–1261.

54. Sharifi M, Javadpoor SA, Bay C, et al. Outcome of stenting in the lower-extremity venous circulation for the treatment of deep venous thrombosis. *Vasc Dis Management* 2010;7:E233–E239.

55. Lou WS, Gu JP, He X, et al. Endovascular treatment for iliac vein compression syndrome: a comparison between the presence and absence of secondary thrombosis. *Korean J Radiol* 2009;10:135–143.

56. LePage PA, Villavicencio JL, Gomez ER, et al. The valvular anatomy of the iliac venous system and its clinical implications. *J Vasc Surg* 1991;14:678–683.

57. Harvey RL, Lovell LL, Belanger N, et al. The effectiveness of anticoagulant and antiplatelet agents in preventing venous thromboembolism during stroke rehabilitation: a historical cohort study. *Arch Phys Med Rehabil* 2004;85:1070–1075.

58. Marsland D, Mears SC, Kates SL. Venous thromboembolic prophylaxis for hip fractures. *Osteoporos Int* 2010;21(suppl 4):S593–S604.

59. Jeon UB, Chung JW, Jae HJ, et al. May-Thurner syndrome complicated by acute iliofemoral vein thrombosis: helical CT venography for evaluation of long-term stent patency and changes in the iliac vein. *AJR Am J Roentgenol* 2010;195:751–757.

60. Kolbel T, Lindh M, Holst J, et al. Extensive acute deep vein thrombosis of the iliocaval segment: midterm results of thrombolysis and stent placement. *J Vasc Interv Radiol* 2007;18:243–250.

61. Lamont JP, Pearl GJ, Patetsios P, et al. Prospective evaluation of endoluminal venous stents in the treatment of the May-Thurner syndrome. *Ann Vasc Surg* 2002;16:61–64.

62. Oguzkurt L, Tercan F, Ozkan U, et al. Iliac vein compression syndrome: outcome of endovascular treatment with long-term follow-up. *Eur J Radiol* 2008;68:487–492.

63. Delis KT, Bjarnason H, Wennberg PW, et al. Successful iliac vein and inferior vena cava stenting ameliorates venous claudication and improves venous outflow, calf muscle pump function, and clinical status in postthrombotic syndrome. *Ann Surg* 2007;245:130–139.

64. Grewal NK, Martinez JT, Andrews L, et al. Quantity of clot lysed after catheter-directed thrombolysis for iliofemoral deep venous thrombosis correlates with postthrombotic morbidity. *J Vasc Surg* 2010;51:1209–1214.

65. Neglen P, Hollis KC, Olivier J, et al. Stenting of the venous outflow in chronic venous disease: long-term stent-related outcome, clinical, and hemodynamic result. *J Vasc Surg* 2007;46:979–990.

66. Raju S, Owen S Jr, Neglen P. Reversal of abnormal lymphoscintigraphy after placement of venous stents for correction of associated venous obstruction. *J Vasc Surg* 2001;34:779–784.

67. Szuba A, Razavi M, Rockson SG. Diagnosis and treatment of concomitant venous obstruction in patients with secondary lymphedema. *J Vasc Interv Radiol* 2002;13:799–803.

68. Hartung O, Barthelemy P, Arnoux D, et al. Management of pregnancy in women with previous left ilio-caval stenting. *J Vasc Surg* 2009;50:355–359.

69. Kyrle PA, Rosendaal FR, Eichinger S. Risk assessment for recurrent venous thrombosis. *Lancet* 2010;376:2032–2039.

70. Mullens W, de Keyser J, van Dorpe A, et al. Migration of two venous stents into the right ventricle in a patient with May-Thurner syndrome. *Int J Cardiol* 2006;110:114–115.

71. Garg N, Gloviczki P, Karimi KM, et al. Factors affecting outcome of open and hybrid reconstructions for nonmalignant obstruction of iliofemoral veins and inferior vena cava. *J Vasc Surg* 2011;53:383–393.

72. Grant JCB. *Method of Anatomy.* Baltimore, MD: Williams & Wilkins; 1937:158.

73. El Sadr AR, Mina E. Anatomical and surgical aspects in the operative management of varicocele. *Urol Cutaneous Rev* 1950;54:257–262.

74. Vassilev I. Radiographic study of the left spermatic vein in the course of idiopathic varicoceles [in French]. *Presse Med* 1962;70:704.

75. Cope C, Isard HJ. Left renal vein entrapment. A new diagnostic finding in retroperitoneal disease. *Radiology* 1969;92:867–872.

76. Chait A, Matasar KW, Fabian CE, et al. Vascular impressions on the ureters. *Am J Roentgenol Radium Ther Nucl Med* 1971;111:729–749.

77. de Schepper A. "Nutcracker" phenomenon of the renal vein and venous pathology of the left kidney [in Dutch]. *J Belge Radiol* 1972;55:507–511.

78. Buschi AJ, Harrison RB, Norman A, et al. Distended left renal vein: CT/sonographic normal variant. *AJR Am J Roentgenol* 1980;135:339–342.

79. Zerin JM, Hernandez RJ, Sedman AB, et al. "Dilatation" of the left renal vein on computed tomography in children: a normal variant. *Pediatr Radiol* 1991;21:267–269.

80. Shin JI, Lee JS. Nutcracker phenomenon or nutcracker syndrome? *Nephrol Dial Transplant* 2005;20:2015.

81. Menard MT. Nutcracker syndrome: when should it be treated and how? *Perspect Vasc Surg Endovasc Ther* 2009;21:117–124.

82. Ahmed K, Sampath R, Khan MS. Current trends in the diagnosis and management of renal nutcracker syndrome: a review. *Eur J Vasc Endovasc Surg* 2006;31:410–416.

83. Kurklinsky AK, Rooke TW. Nutcracker phenomenon and nutcracker syndrome. *Mayo Clin Proc* 2010;85:552–559.

84. Scultetus AH, Villavicencio JL, Gillespie DL. The nutcracker syndrome: its role in the pelvic venous disorders. *J Vasc Surg* 2001;34:812–819.

85. Pallwein L, Pinggera G, Schuster AH, et al. The influence of the left renal vein entrapment on outcome after surgical varicocele repair: a color Doppler sonographic demonstration. *J Ultrasound Med* 2004;23:595–601.

86. Das Adhikary S, Gopalakrishnan G. Varicocele: in search of a human model. *Urol Int* 2010;84:226–230.

87. Brandt JR, Jacobs A, Raissy HH, et al. Orthostatic proteinuria and the spectrum of diurnal variability of urinary protein excretion in healthy children. *Pediatr Nephrol* 2010;25:1131–1137.

88. Mazzoni MB, Kottanatu L, Simonetti GD, et al. Renal vein obstruction and orthostatic proteinuria: a review. *Nephrol Dial Transplant* 2011;26:562–565.

89. Neste MG, Narasimham DL, Belcher KK. Endovascular stent placement as a treatment for renal venous hypertension. *J Vasc Interv Radiol* 1996;7:859–861.

90. Hartung O, Grisoli D, Boufi M, et al. Endovascular stenting in the treatment of pelvic vein congestion caused by nutcracker syndrome: lessons learned from the first five cases. *J Vasc Surg* 2005;42:275–280.

91. Chen S, Zhang H, Shi H, et al. Endovascular stenting for treatment of nutcracker syndrome: report of 61 cases with long-term followup. *J Urol* 2011;186:570–575.

92. Paget J. *Clinical Lectures and Essays.* London, England: Longman, Green & Co; 1875.

93. von Schroetter L. Erkrankungen der Gefasse. In: *Nathnagel Handbuch der Pathologie und Therapie.* Vienna, Austria: Wein, Holder; 1884.

94. DeBakey M, Ochsner A, Smith MC. Primary thrombosis of the axillary vein. *New Orleans Med Surg J* 1942;95:62.

95. Adams JT, DeWeese JA. "Effort" thrombosis of the axillary and subclavian veins. *J Trauma* 1971;11:923–930.

96. Matsumura JS, Rilling WS, Pearce WH, et al. Helical computed tomography of the normal thoracic outlet. *J Vasc Surg* 1997;26:776–783.

97. Remy-Jardin M, Doyen J, Remy J, et al. Functional anatomy of the thoracic outlet: evaluation with spiral CT. *Radiology* 1997;205:843–851.

98. Panegyres PK, Moore N, Gibson R, et al. Thoracic outlet syndromes and magnetic resonance imaging. *Brain* 1993;116:823–841.

99. Illig KA, Doyle AJ. A comprehensive review of Paget-Schroetter syndrome. *J Vasc Surg* 2010;51:1538–1547.

100. Urschel HC Jr, Razzuk MA. Paget-Schroetter syndrome: what is the best management? *Ann Thorac Surg* 2000;69:1663–1668.

101. Molina JE, Hunter DW, Dietz CA. Paget-Schroetter syndrome treated with thrombolytics and immediate surgery. *J Vasc Surg* 2007;45:328–334.

102. Kunkel JM, Machleder H. Treatment of Paget-Schroetter syndrome: a staged, multidisciplinary approach. *Arch Surg* 1989;124:1153–1158.

103. Divi V, Proctor M, Axelrod D, et al. Thoracic outlet decompression for subclavian vein thrombosis: experience in 71 patients. *Arch Surg* 2005;140:54–57.

104. Lee WA, Hill BB, Harris EJ, et al. Surgical intervention is not required for all patients with subclavian vein thrombosis. *J Vasc Surg* 2000;32:57–67.

105. Lee JT, Karwowski JK, Harris EJ, et al. Long-term thrombotic recurrence after nonoperative management of Paget-Schroetter syndrome. *J Vasc Surg* 2006;43:1236–1243.

106. Johansen KH. Primary axillosubclavian venous thrombosis: observational care. In: Davies MG, ed. *Venous Thromboembolic Disease: Contemporary Endovascular Management.* Vol 2. Minneapolis, MN: Cardiotext; 2011:155–161.

107. Roos DB. Congenital anomalies associated with thoracic outlet syndrome: anatomy, symptoms, diagnosis, and treatment. *Am J Surg* 1976;132:771–778.

108. Urschel HC Jr, Patel AN. Paget-Schroetter syndrome therapy: failure of intravenous stents. *Ann Thorac Surg* 2003;75:1693–1696.

109. Sze DY, Shifrin RY, Semba CP. Current diagnostic and therapeutic strategies for effort vein thrombosis. *Tech Vasc Interv Radiol* 2000;3:12–20.

110. Kreienberg PB, Chang BB, Darling RC III, et al. Long-term results in patients treated with thrombolysis, thoracic inlet decompression, and subclavian vein stenting for Paget-Schroetter syndrome. *J Vasc Surg* 2001;33:S100–S105.

111. Molina JE. Reoperations after failed transaxillary first rib resection to treat Paget-Schroetter syndrome patients. *Ann Thorac Surg* 2011;91:1717–1721.

CHAPTER
94

Budd-Chiari Lesions

ROBERT K. KERLAN, JR. and JEANNE M. LABERGE

INTRODUCTION

The term *Budd-Chiari syndrome* (BCS) refers to the symptoms, signs, and pathologic findings caused by obstruction of hepatic venous outflow. The name of the syndrome is attributed to English internist George Budd who described the classic triad of abdominal pain, hepatomegaly, and ascites in 1845.[1] In 1899, Austrian pathologist Hans Chiari described the histopathologic features.[2]

BCS can be divided into two groups: primary and secondary. The primary form of this disorder is caused by acute or chronic thrombosis of hepatic venous structures or the inferior vena cava (IVC).[3] Primary BCS is quite rare in most of the world with an incidence estimated at 0.2 per million and a prevalence of 2 per million.[4,5] For yet unknown reasons, the disease is 10 times more common in Nepal and is the leading cause of hospitalization in patients with liver disease in that country.[6] Throughout Asia, stenosis of the suprahepatic IVC is the most common cause.

BCS is more common in women and young adults.[7,8] Primary BCS is usually associated or caused by a coagulation disorder. Table 94.1 lists the specific primary and secondary hypercoagulable disorders that are associated with hepatocaval thrombosis. The most common associated condition is myeloproliferative disease (MPD) being present in approximately 50% of cases. Other common disorders of coagulation that have been reported with BCS include factor V Leiden mutation, protein C deficiency, antithrombin III deficiency, antiphospholipid syndrome, and paroxysmal nocturnal hemoglobinuria (PNH). Secondary hypercoagulability can be seen in pregnancy, the immediate postpartum state, and a variety of other disorders. More than one cause is identified in 35% of patients. A hypercoagulability workup should be initiated in all patients who present with primary BCS.

Past literature made distinctions between patients who had acute clot within the hepatic venous system and IVC versus patients who presented with webs at the orifices of the major hepatic veins or cavo-atrial junction. It is likely that these morphologic manifestations reflect chronicity of thrombosis rather than a developmental abnormality.[9,10] Webs are a relatively common finding in chronically thrombosed recanalized veins throughout the body and their occurrence in the hepatocaval venous system almost certainly represents the sequelae of a previous thrombotic event. The occurrence of thrombus in that location should come as no surprise in hypercoagulable patients because the concentration of coagulation factors would be expected to be higher in the liver where most of the coagulation factors are produced.

A variant of primary BCS that occludes small hepatic venules has been observed in patients who are exposed to toxins or certain types of chemotherapy or who have undergone bone marrow transplantation. This was previously termed *hepatic veno-occlusive disease* (HVOOD) but is referred to as sinusoidal obstruction syndrome (SOS) in more recent literature.[11] This entity is distinct and requires biopsy for diagnosis, whereas other forms of Budd-Chiari can be diagnosed solely on the basis of imaging.

The secondary form of BCS is caused by external compression or obstruction by tumor thrombus of the hepatic venous

Table 94.1

Conditions Associated with Budd-Chiari Syndrome

Primary hypercoagulable conditions

Myeloproliferative disease

JAK2 V617F mutation

Paroxysmal nocturnal hemoglobinuria

Antiphospholipid syndrome

Factor V Leiden G1691A mutation

Factor II G20210A mutation

Inherited antithrombin deficiency

Inherited protein C deficiency

Inherited protein S deficiency

Hyperhomocysteinemia

Secondary hypercoagulable conditions

Oral contraceptives

Pregnancy

Behçet disease

Sarcoidosis

Connective tissue disease

Inflammatory bowel disease

Dehydration

structures by primary or metastatic tumor.[12,13] Benign causes of secondary BCS by cysts or surgical intervention following ortho-topic liver transplantation (OLT) are also well-described.[14,15]

Regardless of etiology, the pathophysiologic disturbance in BCS is elevation of hepatic sinusoidal pressure. This elevation in sinusoidal pressure leads to hepatomegaly, pain caused by cap-sular distension, ascites, portal hypertension, and deprivation of portal venular flow to the hepatic parenchyma. This deprivation of blood flow eventually leads to focal hepatocyte necrosis and hepatic fibrosis that further exacerbates the portal hypertension.

If the IVC is involved, or excessive hypertrophy of the cau-date lobe, there will be associated lower extremity swelling. The caudate lobe is commonly enlarged in BCS patients because this lobe has multiple veins draining directly into the IVC. Because of this spared venous drainage, the caudate has increased blood flow compared to other parts of the liver, resulting in hypertrophy.

The diagnosis of Budd-Chiari is usually established based on cross-sectional imaging. Ultrasound (US) with Doppler imaging, contrast-enhanced multiphasic abdominal computed tomography (CT), and magnetic resonance imaging (MRI) with vascular sequences can all readily establish the diagnosis.[16] The imaging characteristics of BCS differ in accordance to the acuity of the disease and the body's robustness of venovenous collateral formation.

All types of imaging will reveal hepatomegaly and ascites. Bizarre collateral veins either within the hepatic parenchyma or outside the liver are frequently observed. Moreover, if sig-nificant portal hypertension is present, the usual portosystemic venous collateral pathways will be visible.

The appearances of the hepatic veins are quite variable. Hepatic vein distension can be seen in veins containing throm-bus acutely or by an occlusive web chronically. However, when the hepatic venous thrombus is chronic, the hepatic veins may not be visible.

On US, an abnormal flow signal without phasicity may be observed within the hepatic vein. Absent flow signals will be encountered in patients with complete hepatic venous occlu-sion. Occasionally a filling defect within the vein will be encoun-tered, but often only a hyperechoic cord of the occluded vessel will be detected.

With multiphasic CT and MRI, the contrast enhancement of the peripheral hepatic parenchyma is usually patchy and enhancement of the enlarged caudate lobe is increased. An abnormal appearance or absence of the major hepatic veins is typical.

When the diagnosis is unclear on cross-sectional imaging, catheter venography can readily establish it. The venographic findings include a venous thrombus within hepatic veins, iso-lated webs at the cavo-atrial junction (FIGURE 94.1), focal webs or short segment occlusions at the origins of the hepatic veins, or the typical "spider web" collaterals of chronic occlusion (FIGURE 94.2).

PATIENT SELECTION AND ENDOVASCULAR TREATMENT OPTIONS

Selection of patients for specific therapeutic interventions depends on the clinical presentation. Four types of presentation have been described: fulminant, acute, subacute, and chronic. These classifications overlap but are generally based on the

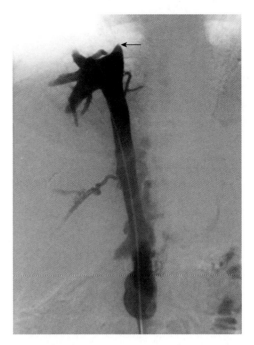

FIGURE 94.1 Inferior vena cavagram reveals a typical cavo-atrial web (*arrow*), causing hepatic venous outflow obstruction.

duration and severity of symptoms as well as the rate of disease progression.[17]

The fulminant form is characterized by jaundice, encepha-lopathy, and hepatic synthetic failure. The acute form is typi-fied by abdominal pain and ascites in an illness that has lasted days to weeks. Thrombus is usually present within the hepatic veins of these patients. Patients who have fulminant and acute

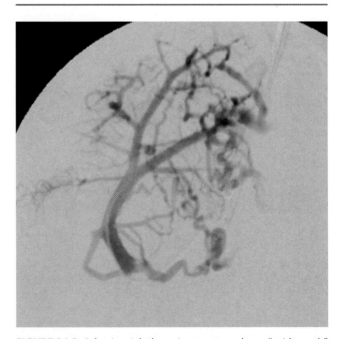

FIGURE 94.2 Selective right hepatic venogram shows "spider-web" collaterals typical of chronic Budd-Chiari.

BCS generally do not have well-formed portosystemic variceal communications.

Subacute and chronic forms are more often associated with obliteration of the hepatic veins or obstruction of the venous outflow by webs. The hepatic venous outflow obstruction may have been present for months to years. Extensive distortion of the liver with fibrosis and atrophy is often encountered in chronic patients. Portosystemic variceal communications are more commonly encountered in these patients.

The distinction of the various presentations may be blurred by an acute event, such as thrombosis of the last remaining patent hepatic vein or development of portal vein thrombosis. This may lead to a patient with chronic BCS present with an acute exacerbation of symptomatology, bringing them to medical attention.

Because the disease is secondary to venous obstruction rather than a primary hepatocellular injury, synthetic function is usually preserved and alterations in the liver function tests are relatively mild. The exception to this rule is patients with the fulminant variety who may develop extensive ischemic necrosis related to the venous obstruction.

Selection of patients for therapy depends on the presence of symptomatology. Some patients are asymptomatic and have Budd-Chiari discovered incidentally. However, in most patients, chronic obstruction of the venous outflow poses a threat of continued liver injury and the development of complications related to portal hypertension. These complications include life-threatening variceal bleeding and refractory ascites. Therefore, most patients with Budd-Chiari should be evaluated for interventions designed to relieve the venous obstruction. These interventions include anticoagulation, fibrinolytic therapy, correction of anatomic obstructions in the hepatic veins, portosystemic shunting, and OLT.

All patients with hypercoagulability should be treated with long-term anticoagulation, if they do not have an absolute contraindication. Oral anticoagulation with coumadin is typically used. Interestingly, patients with BCS are more prone to heparin-induced thrombocytopenia with unfractionated heparin, and low-molecular-weight heparin is recommended when immediate anticoagulation is required. Moreover, platelet counts should be carefully monitored (every other day at least) to detect this complication as early as possible.

Selective regional fibrinolytic therapy is appropriate for patients with acute thrombus occluding the major hepatic veins. Mechanical thrombectomy is more appropriate if the patient is actively bleeding or has had a recent significant hemorrhage.

Correction of the hepatic vein outflow stenosis should be performed in all patients with anatomically amenable short-segment lesions. This correction can be accomplished with endovascular techniques, as discussed later in this chapter. If hepatic vein patency can be reestablished, encephalopathy related to portosystemic shunting can be avoided.

When correction of the anatomic blockage in the hepatic vein is not feasible due to the underlying anatomy, portosystemic shunting should be performed. Because the hepatic synthetic function is generally intact, a portosystemic shunt can provide durable therapy in many patients and halt progressive liver damage. Whether the shunt is surgical or endovascular remains controversial. If a side-to side surgical shunt can be created to allow egress of blood hepatofugally through the portal vein, it is a reasonable and durable option in selected patients. Unfortunately, the presence of an IVC stenosis caused by caudate lobe hypertrophy may preclude creation of a shunt.

As an alternative, transjugular intrahepatic portosystemic shunts (TIPS) can be created. The downside of TIPS is recurrent shunt stenosis. There are currently no randomized prospective trials to provide scientific guidance for the selection of the appropriate shunt therapy.

OLT is reserved for patients with impaired synthetic function or lack of other therapeutic alternatives.

ANATOMIC OR LESION CONSIDERATIONS

The goal of all interventions in BCS is to relieve the vascular congestion of the hepatic sinusoids induced by hepatic venous outflow obstruction. The intervention should be directed to correct the underlying pathologic anatomy whenever possible, reserving TIPS for patients who are unsuitable for other forms of therapy.

Most patients with symptomatic BCS do not have acute thrombus within their hepatic venous system. However, when identified, the primary therapy should be removal of the thrombus. This can be accomplished with selective fibrinolytic therapy, pharmacomechanical thrombectomy, or a combination of both techniques. Once the thrombus has been removed, careful venography to assess for the presence of an underlying stenosis should be performed.

When a focal web is obstructing the hepatic vein orifices or suprahepatic IVC, balloon angioplasty is the indicated procedure. If there are residual areas of significant stenoses caused by elastic recoil, metallic stent placement is warranted. Due to the respiratory motion of the diaphragm, self-expanding stents rather than balloon-expandable stents should be placed. In so doing, both stent crushing and stent migration can be minimized.

When subacute or chronic BCS is present, the hepatic vein orifices are often completely obliterated. Despite the obliteration, some patients will harbor nearly intact hepatic veins proximal to the obstruction. In these patients, transhepatic hepatic venography (THHV) is useful for both depiction of the obstruction and to facilitate treatment of the stenosis.[18] This technique is described in detail later.

Unfortunately, many patients will have subtotal obliteration of the hepatic venous system. When effective drainage of the hepatic parenchyma cannot be achieved due to lack of hepatic venous side branches extending into the main hepatic trunk, TIPS is the only endovascular remedy.

TIPS in patients with BCS can be difficult because it may not be possible to catheterize the hepatic veins. When this situation is encountered, TIPS creation may require direct puncture of the IVC either in a conventional fashion or via an endovascular US-guided puncture of the extrahepatic portal vein through the caval wall (direct intrahepatic portosystemic shunt [DIPS]).[19]

TECHNICAL/DEVICE CONSIDERATIONS

Technical and device considerations depend on which intervention is being performed. However, most interventions require catheterization of the abnormal hepatic veins. This access is performed as follows.

The right internal jugular approach provides the most favorable angle for hepatic venous interventions and should be used when patent. If the vein is not patent, the left internal jugular should be used.

The internal jugular vein should be punctured with standard single-wall micropuncture technique using real-time US guidance to minimize vascular trauma and reduce incidence of access site bleeding in patients who are anticoagulated and may undergo fibrinolytic therapy. A 0.035-inch or 0.038-inch guide wire should be manipulated into the IVC to provide adequate purchase for sheath insertion.

After the wire has been manipulated into the IVC, a sheath should be selected of appropriate size and length to reach the hepatic veins. An angled 9 or 10 French 40-cm sheath (commonly used with TIPS creation) provides both support and steerability. Pressure measurements should be made in the infrahepatic IVC, suprahepatic IVC, and right atrium. An inferior vena cavagram is performed with the catheter tip positioned in the infrahepatic IVC to assess for the presence of caval compression and caval webs. The pressure measurements are important to confirm whether or not the patient would be a candidate for a surgical infrahepatic portosystemic shunt if endovascular interventions are unsuccessful.

Through the sheath, a 5 French selective catheter with an angled tip is inserted over a guide wire to engage the orifice of the hepatic vein. Gentle injections of contrast are made to confirm the diagnosis. Attempts should be made to catheterize the right, left, and middle hepatic veins. Although all hepatic veins should be addressed when feasible, opening a single, dominant hepatic vein is usually sufficient to relieve the patient's symptoms.

The interventions to be discussed may be performed in combination depending on the effectiveness of the procedure. For the sake of clarity, these procedures are divided into three groups: pharmacomechanical thrombolysis, hepatic vein reconstruction, and portosytemic shunt creation.

Pharmacomechanical Thrombolysis

As noted previously, removal of thrombus in patients with BCS is the least frequent intervention due to low incidence of this finding at presentation. However, in patients where the outflow obstruction is caused principally by acute thrombus, an attempt to remove the thrombus should be performed.

When fresh thrombus within the hepatic vein is encountered, pharmacomechanical thrombolysis should be attempted. No specific method has been demonstrated to be superior and, therefore, the combination of devices used is a matter of operator experience and preference. At our institution a 6 French rheolytic thrombectomy catheter (Angiojet DVX, Medrad, Warrendale, PA) is used. Initially, the clot is laced with a fibrinolytic agent. Many fibrinolytic agents are also available and the selection should be based on operator experience. At our institution, the thrombus would be laced with 10 mg of tissue plasminogen activator (Alteplase, Genentech, South San Francisco, CA). Subsequently, the rheolytic thrombectomy catheter is used to extract the thrombus. Using the rheolytic thrombectomy catheter in close proximity to the heart may lead to transient bradycardia; therefore careful monitoring of the patient is necessary during the procedure.

The thrombectomy catheter can be used in several veins during a single procedure but should not run longer than a total of 10 minutes due to the risk of hemoglobinuria and renal failure.

Following pharmacomechanical thrombolysis, the hepatic venogram(s) should be repeated to assess the therapeutic response. When significant thrombus persists, prolonged infusion of fibrinolytic agent into the residual clot should be performed through a multi–side-hole catheter designed for fibrinolytic infusion (multiple vendors). The venogram may then be repeated on the following day to assess the therpeutic response.

When the vein becomes cleared of the thrombotic occlusion and no obstructing lesion is present, the patient should be placed on aggressive anticoagulation to prevent reocclusion.

If an obstructing lesion is identified, the lesion should be treated as described next.

Hepatic Vein Reconstruction

When stenoses of hepatic veins or suprahepatic IVC are encountered, attempts at correction with endovascular therapy should be made. Stenoses at both the cavo-atrial junction as well as orifices of hepatic veins may respond durably to balloon angioplasty (FIGURE 94.3). Sometimes the stenoses are complex and extend several centimeters into the major hepatic veins. Some may be developmental or congenital, although it is likely that most represent a sequela of previous thrombosis as mentioned previously.

Technically, the procedure may be difficult because successful negotiation of a small, stenotic orifice with a catheter and guide wire requires a systematic search of the suprahepatic cava for successful engagement. However, the configuration of the hepatic sinus usually creates a shelf indicating the position of the major hepatic vein orifices.

As with thrombolytic therapy described earlier, it is useful to place a TIPS sheath to support the passage of guide wires and catheters into the stenotic hepatic veins. Following successful negotiation of the stenosis with a 5 French catheter into the hepatic vein, a stiff exchange guide wire is placed. Due to the large size of the veins, 0.035-inch catheter-balloon systems are preferred. Because the stenosis is often firm, a high-pressure balloon (multiple vendors) and mechanical inflator should be used for the dilatation. The balloon diameter should be as large as or slightly larger than the anticipated normal diameter of the vein. In most patients, this diameter ranges from 10 to 14 mm in size. If a focal resistant web is encountered, a 6-mm diameter cutting balloon (multiple vendors) may be useful to initiate the dilatation followed by a venoplasty with a conventional high-pressure balloon.

In some patients, the origin of the hepatic vein may be completely occluded. When this situation is encountered, THHV should be performed (FIGURE 94.4). This procedure is performed under conscious sedation from a right lateral approach. With either US or fluoroscopic guidance, a 21- or 22-gauge needle is advanced into the hepatic parenchyma. The needle is directed into the cephalic aspect of the liver where major hepatic venous trunks may be encountered. A contrast syringe is connected to the needle and the needle is slowly withdrawn under fluoroscopic observation. If a hepatic vein is opacified, images are made and analyzed. Often a trunk will be patent peripherally but completely occluded centrally. If the vein drains an

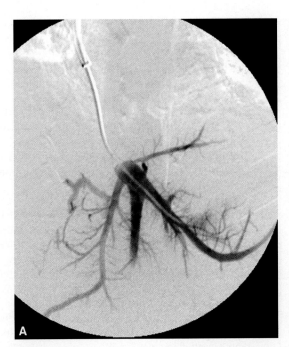 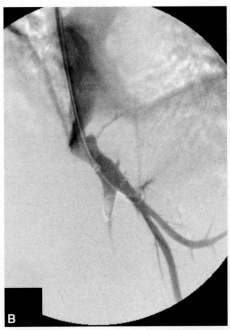

FIGURE 94.3 A 33-year-old woman with abdominal pain and ascites. **A.** Left hepatic venogram reveals focal high-grade stenosis at its junction with the IVC. The catheter occludes the lumen at the site of stenosis. **B.** Left hepatic venogram following inflation of a 10-mm diameter high-pressure angioplasty balloon across the stenosis. Minimal narrowing persists at the treated site.

adequate amount of liver, a 0.018-inch guide wire should be advanced through the needle and the vein catheterized. It is often possible to traverse highly stenotic or occluded segments

of hepatic veins from the antegrade approach when attempts at retrograde catheterization have failed. If a guide wire can be manipulated through the diseased segment of the hepatic vein

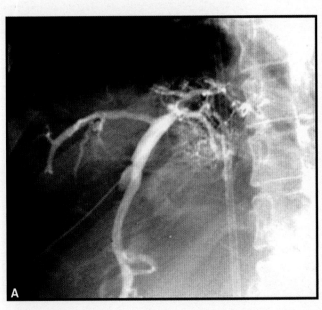 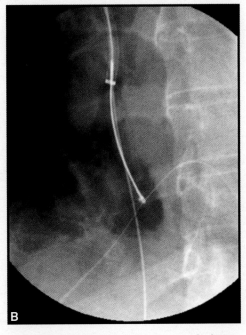

FIGURE 94.4 Transhepatic venography performed for hepatic vein reconstruction in a 38-year-old woman with chronic BCS. **A.** Right hepatic vein is opacified by contrast injected through a 22-gauge needle inserted from a right midlateral transhepatic puncture. **B.** A 0.014-inch guide wire is manipulated through the obstruction and captured by a snare in the IVC. The snare has been inserted from a right internal jugular approach. **C.** Angled 10 French sheath is advanced over the snared wire. Through this sheath hepatic vein reconstruction or TIPS can be performed. *(continued)*

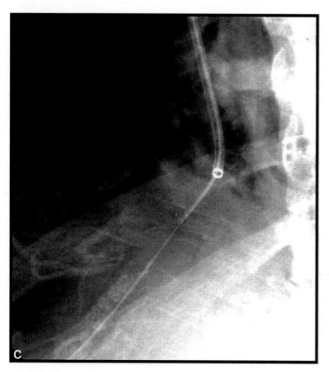

FIGURE 94.4 *(Continued)*

into the IVC, the wire can be snared and pulled through an internal jugular sheath. This wire can then be used to place an angioplasty balloon or stent, avoiding the necessity of creating a large tract through the hepatic parenchyma. Care must be exercised to avoid parenchymal damage from excessive tension on the wire traversing the liver substance.

Following the balloon dilatation, the hepatic venogram is repeated to assess the results. If there is less than a 30% residual stenosis, a durable result may be hoped for and the procedure terminated. If a persistent hemodynamically significant stenosis is present, a metallic stent should be placed (FIGURE 94.5).

Both balloon-expandable and self-expandable stents have been placed into the orifices of hepatic veins. However, due to the changing size of hepatic veins during the cardiac cycle and motion of the diaphragm during respiration, self-expanding stents are more appropriate. Either stainless steel or nitinol stents can be placed and sufficient length should be placed into the hepatic vein for stability. The stents should not extend into the atrium to avoid problems with arrhythmia and cardiac perforation. Metal stents can be placed across branching veins. In most cases a 12- or 14-mm diameter by 20- to 40-mm length stents are suitable.

Stent grafts should not be placed because these devices would occlude venous side branches.

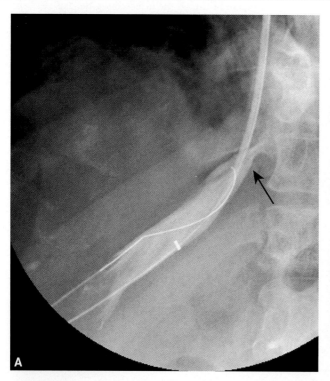
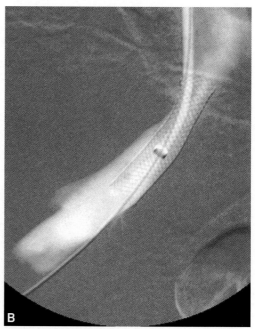

FIGURE 94.5 A 42-year-old woman with recurrent right hepatic vein stenosis following percutaneous transluminal angioplasty. **A.** Hepatic venogram shows highly stenotic hepatic vein orifice (*arrow*). **B.** A self-expanding metallic stent is placed, eradicating the recurrent stenosis.

Portosystemic Shunt Creation

When no suitable residual hepatic veins are available for reconstruction, a portosystemic shunt should be created. Although surgical options may be available, the prolonged durability afforded by TIPS using stent-grafts is an attractive option. Although the creation of TIPS is covered in Chapter 32, the hepatic morphology and absence of hepatic veins may make the procedure more difficult and modifications of the usual technique may be necessary.

The principal difficulty is in finding a suitable point to initiate the puncture from the systemic venous system into the portal system. There are three alternatives to initiate the puncture: residual hepatic vein, hepatic vein stump, or IVC.

The residual hepatic vein is used in many patients if sufficient purchase of the guide wire and sheath can be achieved. It is also possible to use the aforedescribed transhepatic hepatic vein catheterization technique to advance a guide wire into the IVC. This guide wire can be snared and pulled through a jugular access site, affording considerable support for the passage of a sheath designed for the puncture of the portal vein. Care must be taken not to lacerate the liver with the transhepatic wire, and it is generally wise to place a small catheter over this wire to reduce the likelihood of this complication.

When engagement of the hepatic vein is not possible, a transhepatic puncture can be made from the hepatic vein stump. The stump is consistently present at the level of the hepatic sinus and will support and direct the TIPS needle through the wall of the IVC into the hepatic parenchyma (FIGURE 94.6).

Direct puncture through the wall of the IVC can also be used to create TIPS in patients with BCS. The IVC immediately below the hepatic veins is surrounded by hepatic parenchyma and the risk of procedural bleeding is low.

Another alternative is direct intrahepatic portosystemic shunt (DIPS).[20] In this procedure intravascular US is used to directly guide a needle through the IVC wall and caudate lobe directly into the extrahepatic portal vein. A wire is advanced through the needle and a stent-graft is placed. In many patients with BCS the enlarged caudate lobe compresses the IVC at this level, making the technique unsuitable.

Alternatively, direct US-guided percutaneous puncture through a portal vein branch into a segment of patent IVC can also be performed.[21] The creation of a bridging wire from a portal vein branch to the IVC allows retrograde passage of suitable catheters and guide wires to place a decompressing stent.

Occasionally patients with BCS will present with occlusion of the portal vein in addition to hepatic vein outflow obstruction (FIGURE 94.7). This anatomy requires establishing a portosystemic shunt in conjunction with pharmacomechanical thrombolysis of the splanchnic venous system. To perform this procedure successfully, a US-guided transhepatic catheterization of the right portal vein may be necessary to serve as a target for portosystemic shunt creation. These procedures may be technically challenging.

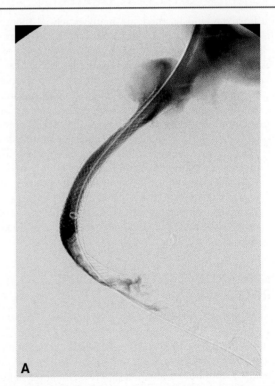

A

FIGURE 94.7 TIPS creation in a 46-year-old woman with BCS and portal and superior mesenteric vein thrombosis. **A.** Injection through TIPS shows thrombus throughout the main portal vein. **B.** Contrast injection into the SMV branch following pharmacomechanical and infusion thrombolysis confirms patency of SMV, portal vein, and TIPS. *(continued)*

FIGURE 94.6 Injection of contrast through Colapinto needle (Cook Inc., Bloomington, IN) positioned adjacent to the right hepatic vein stump immediately prior to transcaval portal venous puncture for TIPS creation.

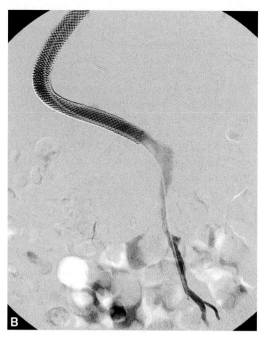

FIGURE 94.7 *(Continued)*

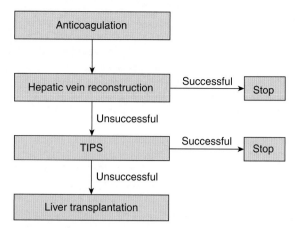

FIGURE 94.8 Flowchart for suggested management of complications related to portal hypertension secondary to hepatic vein outflow obstruction.

TREATMENT SELECTION STRATEGIES

As outlined previously, there are many potential therapeutic maneuvers for patients with BCS. The initial intervention should be anticoagulation to prevent progression of the occlusion. Whenever possible, addressing the primary issue of hepatic vein occlusion is preferable to the creation of a portosystemic shunt. If the occlusion is secondary to acute thrombus, the thrombus should be removed with pharmacomechanical thrombectomy. If the occlusion is secondary to obstructing webs, the webs should be dilated with a high-pressure balloon. If a residual stenosis is present following balloon dilatation, a self-expanding metallic stent should be placed. Only when no suitable residual hepatic can be identified for reconstruction should a portosystemic shunt be created. Percutaneous transhepatic venography can facilitate all of the procedures described earlier when necessary. This treatment strategy is outlined in FIGURE 94.8.

PLANNING THE INTERVENTIONAL PROCEDURE

Interventions for Budd-Chiari may be technically complex and require prolonged procedure times. Although conscious sedation may suffice in many patients, general anesthesia should be considered for complex cases.

Standard laboratory evaluation should be obtained to assess the coagulation profile, hematocrit level, and renal function. Correction of abnormal coagulation parameters and hydration for renal impairment should be implemented as appropriate.

Planning of the intervention must be made in conjunction with the available cross-sectional imaging. The appearance of the MRI or contrast-enhanced CT will suggest the most appropriate

intervention as well as the approach. In general, when the cavo-atrial junction is patent, an internal jugular approach is preferable to a femoral approach. This provides a more favorable angle for catheterization of obstructed hepatic veins and allows more effective transmission of both torque and force to the catheter and guide wire. Stenoses at the cavo-atrial junction may be better approached from the femoral approach. In some cases of cavo-atrial stenoses a combined internal jugular and femoral approach is useful. If it appears that a transhepatic approach is potentially necessary, the anterior and right lateral abdomen overlying the liver should also be prepped and draped.

Measurements of the diameter of the IVC and normal hepatic veins should be made on cross-sectional imaging. These measurements should be confirmed with a calibrating catheter during the procedure. Appropriate balloon and stent sizes should be available at the time of the intervention.

Prophylactic antibiotics should be administered when a transhepatic or portosystemic shunt procedure is being performed.

Because of the potential for complicating hemorrhage, it is wise to have a specimen in the blood bank for typing and crossmatching in patients undergoing pharmacomechanical fibrinolysis, percutaneous hepatic puncture, or portosystemic shunt creation.

PROCEDURAL COMPLICATIONS AND HOW TO MANAGE THEM SUCCESSFULLY

The most common significant complication following intervention for BCS is hemorrhage. The risk of hemorrhage is higher for BCS patients undergoing transhepatic or portosystemic shunt procedures compared to other patients with portal hypertension. This increased risk of bleeding is attributable to the numerous collateral veins carrying blood away from the liver in the presence of obstructed hepatic veins. Careful real-time US should be performed whenever transhepatic punctures are being performed to avoid the larger, visible collaterals. Moreover, preprocedural cross-sectional imaging should be carefully reviewed prior to the procedure to establish the safest route for a percutaneous puncture.

A higher risk of bleeding is also entailed due to the abnormal nature of the proximal hepatic veins. These hepatic veins are extrahepatic close to their junction with the IVC. Therefore, if a venous rupture occurs following percutaneous reconstruction, the bleeding can be impressive and occur either into the abdomen or pleural space. Prompt and robust resuscitative measures may be required to prevent life-threatening exsanguination. A stent-graft should be placed across the disrupted conduit when possible.

Lower rates of hemorrhage may be occult and obtaining serial hematocrit levels following the procedure is recommended.

The other complication that is of particular concern in BCS patients is observed in those who require stent placement. The proximal obstructing lesions require stent positioning across the hepatic-caval or cavo-atrial junction in many patients. Extending stents into the atrium itself should be avoided because perforations of the heart have been reported in patients with stents malpositioned too proximally.[22] Moreover, very proximal stent positioning may make subsequent OLT considerably more difficult and even require cardiopulmonary bypass in some patients.

The other unique feature of BCS interventions is the underlying hypercoagulability of most patients. Because of this hypercoagulability, consideration for intraprocedural anticoagulation should be given to avoid the formation of thrombus in the hepatic or portal system (during TIPS) while the procedure is being conducted. In most patients, postprocedural as well as long-term anticoagulation needs to be performed.

OUTCOMES/PROGNOSIS

The prognosis of patients with BCS depends on the severity of the disease at presentation. In a multicenter study of 237 patients,[23] BCS was classified into three groups (Rotterdam classification) based on encephalopathy, ascites, international normalized ratio (INR), and serum bilirubin. Five-year survival rates for classes 1, 2, and 3 were 89%, 74%, and 42%, respectively. The major therapeutic interventions in the study group were anticoagulation ($n = 171$) and principally open surgical portosystemic shunting ($n = 117$).

Using the aforedescribed interventional radiologic techniques in a cohort of 61 patients,[24] the 5-year survival rates for classes 1, 2, and 3 were 100%, 86%, and 77%, respectively. Therefore, the current data would suggest that minimally invasive interventions can provide acceptable outcomes and should be performed rather than open surgical interventions when possible.

The role of specific procedures was reviewed in a prospective cohort of 163 incident cases of BCS in a multicenter trial by the European Network for Vascular Disorders of the Liver.[25] Ten patients underwent thrombolysis of which four were successful in reestablishing patency. Thrombolytic therapy should be delivered directly into the thrombus via a catheter. Systemic thrombolytic therapy or therapy delivered regionally through the hepatic artery is usually unsuccessful.[26]

In the same multicenter trial, 14 patients had balloon angioplasty with durable patency established in 8 patients (57%). Better results were reported by Xue et al.[27] in 53 patients with hepatic outflow stenosis. Over 90% of patients benefited from hepatic vein or IVC interventions including balloon angioplasty and stent placement. In another group of 101 patients reported by Li et al.,[28] primary and secondary patencies at 2 years were 76% and 84%, respectively, following balloon dilatation of the hepatic veins and/or IVC. In this series, self-expandable stents were placed when residual stenosis was present following balloon dilatation. These results confirm previous studies that have documented the usefulness of hepatic vein and IVC interventions.[29,30] The American Association for the Study of Liver Diseases (AASLD) guidelines recommend percutaneous angioplasty/stenting for all symptomatic patients with stenoses amenable to treatment.[31]

Uniformly good results are reported using balloons and stents to treat hepatic vein or IVC stenosis secondary to liver transplantation. Lee et al.[32] reported clinical success in 12 of 14 patients following IVC stent placement with a median follow-up of 65.3 months. In the pediatric post-transplant population, Carnevale et al.[33] had a 100% clinical success treating 18 children with IVC or hepatic vein obstruction with stents and balloons with a 100% primary assisted patency rate at a mean follow-up of 42 months.

When reconstruction of the hepatic vein is not technically feasible, excellent results following TIPS in patients with BCS have been documented.[34–41] A series of 124 BCS patients undergoing successful TIPS was reported by Garcia-Pagán et al.[37] In this series, the 1- and 5-year transplant-free survival rate was 88% and 78%, respectively. The AASLD guidelines recommend TIPS for patients without ongoing improvement on anticoagulation, with or without hepatic vein recanalization. This recommendation was based on a compilation of retrospective surveys on 195 consecutive patients[24,42–51] with a technical success rate of 81%, 1-month mortality of 9%, and a subsequent transplantation rate of 9.2%. In a series of 35 patients by Rossle et al.,[52] the 1- and 5-year transplant-free survival were 93% and 74%, respectively. In a series of 20 patients by Zahn et al.[34] a 92% survival was report during a median follow-up of 4 years following TIPS.

Not only is the transplant-free survival rate acceptably high following TIPS, but symptomatic improvement of pain and ascites is observed in most patients who undergo the procedure. Moreover, it is an extremely effective technique in the prevention of bleeding from gastroesophageal varices.

TIPS may also be used to bridge patients to transplantation in BCS patients with altered hepatic synthetic function.[53] In some cases, liver function improves, making transplantation unnecessary.

As in other groups of patients undergoing TIPS, superior patency with diminished reintervention rates can be achieved by using stent-grafts rather than bare metal stents. In a comparative study of 16 patients, the primary patency at 2 years was 12% using bare metal stents and 56% using stent-grafts.[54] Despite the low primary patency rate, the assisted patency was high and the 3-year survival was 72%.

One situation where numbers are too small to provide reliable outcome data is BCS associated with portal vein and superior mesenteric vein (SMV) thrombosis. The risk of major bleeding in patients with transhepatic catheter-directed thrombolysis of the splanchnic veins has been reported to be as high as 50%.[55]

DISEASE SURVEILLANCE AND TREATMENT MONITORING ALGORITHMS

Whatever treatment is selected, close follow-up to assess for a therapeutic response is essential. Doppler US of the hepatic vasculature should be obtained the day following the procedure to serve as a baseline, and then periodically after that to assess hepatic vein or TIPS patency. A common algorithm is to obtain ultrasonographic examinations at 1 month, 3 months, 6 months, and 1 year following the intervention. US evaluation should be immediately obtained for any change in symptomatology. Moreover, the US examination can somewhat quantify the amount of ascites. If ascites completely resolves following the procedure and then reappears at a later time, catheter venography is indicated to reevaluate the hepatic venous or TIPS morphology.

EARLY FAILURES AND OPTIONS FOR MANAGEMENT

Doppler US 24 hours to 1 month following the procedure may indicate rethrombosis of the hepatic vein, recurrence of hepatic vein stenosis, or occlusion of the TIPS. Immediate reintervention is warranted to reestablish venous patency. The specific reintervention depends on the nature of the problem.

If a treated vein is thrombosed, catheter-directed fibrinolytic therapy is warranted to reopen the vessel. If hepatic vein stenosis recurs following balloon angioplasty, stent placement is indicated. If a TIPS becomes occluded it should be reopened with a combination of balloon dilatation and restenting.

LATE FAILURES AND OPTIONS FOR MANAGEMENT

Abdominal pain, recurrence of ascites, or variceal bleeding are highly suggestive of a failing intervention. Investigation with Doppler US and catheter venography are indicated to delineate the problem.

If the intervention has been balloon dilatation of the hepatic veins or IVC, recurrent stenoses are not unusual. If the durability of the initial intervention was significant, repeat high-pressure balloon angioplasty can be performed to correct the problem. If stenosis has recurred within a year, stent placement should be considered.

Unfortunately, the placement of a stent does not prevent recurrence of stenosis, and in-stent stenoses or stenoses at the margins of the stent are not infrequently observed. Dilatation with high-pressure balloons may correct the problem; however, stent extension may be necessary.

TIPS stenoses are commonly encountered with bare metal stents. As mentioned previously, using stent-grafts has improved the patency of TIPS considerably. In most cases of TIPS dysfunction, the stenosis develops at the hepatic venous end, requiring balloon angioplasty or stent extension to the margin of, or a short distance into, the IVC. Care should be taken not to extend the stent too far into the IVC because this may precipitate a caval stenosis and make liver transplantation more difficult. Stenosis of the portal venous end is unusual and can usually be corrected by stent extension.

TIPS thrombosis may also occur because many of these patients have an underlying hypercoagulable state. A TIPS thrombosis may be associated with portal vein thrombosis, requiring stent extension to the confluence of the superior mesenteric and splenic veins. Progressive splanchnic thrombosis can be difficult to treat; therefore, long-term anticoagulation is recommended in most patients with BCS.

PRACTICAL ADVANTAGES AND LIMITATIONS

The advantages of endovascular therapy for patients with BCS are readily apparent compared to open surgical procedures to correct hepatocaval stenoses or portosystemic shunts. The surgical procedures required carry with them a significant morbidity and, in some cases, require cardiopulmonary bypass to complete. Despite the risks of the open surgical procedure if exceptional durability was achieved, these procedures would be warranted in selected individuals. In general, the competitive endovascular procedures can be accomplished with less risk to the patient.

Endovascular techniques tend to be more effective in managing short stenoses in the hepatic veins adjacent to the IVC. The visualization of the venous morphology by venography is often superior to the visualization achieved with an open surgical exposure. Moreover, the procedures can be repeated and usually do not require general anesthesia. In selected patients, the endovascular procedures can be accomplished on an outpatient basis.

If portosystemic shunting is required in this patient population, the TIPS procedure can be superior to surgical shunts by providing a conduit to the suprahepatic cava. Although surgical portosystemic shunts have an established durability to the infrahepatic cava, compression of the intrahepatic IVC by an enlarged caudate lobe may necessitate the creation of a mesoatrial shunt. The patency of mesoatrial shunts is considerably lower than conventional infrahepatic portosystemic shunt procedures.[45]

With the exception of OLT in patients who cannot be managed with endovascular techniques or patients with severely altered synthetic function, endovascular therapy has replaced open surgical management of BCS in most centers.

RELATIVE THERAPEUTIC EFFECTIVENESS COMPARED TO MEDICAL AND SURGICAL MANAGEMENT

Medical management of patients with BCS is limited to long-term anticoagulation. However, anticoagulation alone is associated with steady improvement in 20% of patients without the necessity of any additional therapy.[56,57] In these asymptomatic patients, the progression of the thrombosis can be checked by the anticoagulant therapy and allow the development of decompressive collaterals. In some cases, spontaneous recanalization of obstructed veins may occur.

Historically, surgical intervention for cavo-atrial stenoses has been reasonably effective. In a series of 53 patients by Inafuku et al.,[58] 5- and 10-year patencies for this procedure has been reported to be 89.8% and 70.7%, respectively. However, this procedure is not commonly performed in most centers and has been replaced with endovascular interventions.

The current role of surgical shunting in BCS is less clear. Depending on the status of the intrahepatic IVC, several strategies have been used. These strategies include endovascular stenting of the IVC followed by the creation of an infrahepatic portosystemic shunt, creation of mesoatrial shunts, as well as creating shunts from the portal circulation that are sequentially anastomosed to the IVC and atrium. Despite these innovative techniques, the overall mortality has been excessive, averaging 25%.[59] Moreover, in series with medium- and long-term follow-up a shunt dysfunction rate of 30% has been noted.[60,61]

The results of surgical portosystemic shunting are not universally poor, however. A report of 45 patients by Tang et al.[62] showed surgical shunting to be a significant factor for survival by multivariate analysis.

Despite this, open surgical portosystemic shunting is not used as the primary strategy in most centers. TIPS has replaced this procedure for most patients but continues to suffer from the necessity of frequent surveillance and reinterventions.

THE FUTURE

As with many endovascular interventions, current therapy is limited by balloon and stent technology. Improvement in the durability of balloon dilatation may potentially be improved by drug-eluting balloons and stents that diminish the rate of restenosis. Biodegradable stents may also be developed that promote long-term patency. The advent of stent-grafts clearly improved the patency of TIPS; however, stent-grafts are not appropriate for hepatic vein recanalization due to the obstruction of side branches. Heparin-impregnated stent-grafts may offer an advantage in BCS patients who are usually hypercoagulable. The relative contributions of these potential technical advances will require rigorous investigation to ascertain their position in the management of this complex group of patients.

CONCLUSION

The management of patients with BCS is complex and requires the expertise of physicians from several specialties including medicine, surgery, and interventional radiology. Long-term anticoagulation must be performed to correct the underlying hypercoagulable disorder that incited the hepatic venous outflow obstruction. Surgical therapy for hepatocaval stenosis as well as open portosystemic shunting has been replaced in most centers by a variety of endovascular techniques. These techniques should be directed to reestablishing patency of the hepatic venous system when possible because this affords the most physiologic solution to the anatomic pathology. The reconstruction of hepatic vein obstruction requires expertise with both transluminal and transhepatic approaches. When reestablishment of hepatic venous outflow is not possible, the creation of a TIPS shunt can substantially prolong life. OLT should be reserved for patients who cannot be treated by other methods or who have severe hepatic synthetic dysfunction.

REFERENCES

1. Chung RT, Iafrate AJ, Amreon PC, et al. Case records of the Massachusetts General Hospital. Case 15-2006. A 46-year-old woman with sudden onset of abdominal distension. *N Engl J Med* 2006;354:2166–2175.
2. Horton JD, San Miguel FL, Ortiz JA. Budd-Chiari syndrome: illustrated review of current management. *Liver Int* 2008;28:455–466.
3. Valla D-C. Primary Budd-Chiari syndrome. *J Hepatol* 2009;50:195–203.
4. Okuda H, Yamagata H, Obata H, et al. Epidemiological and clinical features of the Budd-Chiari syndrome in Japan. *J Hepatol* 1995;22:1–9.
5. Valla D. Hepatic venous outflow tract obstruction etipathogenesis: Asia versus the West. *J Gastroenterol Hepatol* 2004;19:S204–S211.
6. Shrestha SM, Okuda K, Uchida T, et al. Endemicity and clinical picture of liver disease due to obstruction of the hepatic portion of the inferior vena cava in Nepal. *J Gastroenterol Hepatol* 1996;11:170–179.
7. Valla D, Benhamou JP. Obstruction of the hepatic veins and inferior vena cava. *Dig Dis* 1996;14:99–118.
8. Mori H, Hayashi K, Amamoto Y. Membranous obstruction of the inferior vena cava associated with intrahepatic portosystemic shunt. *Cardiovasc Intervent Radiol* 1986;9:209–213.
9. Okuda K. Obliterative hepatocavopathy-inferior vena cava thrombosis at its hepatic portion. *Hepatobiliary Pancreat Dis Int* 2002;1:499–509.
10. Kage M, Arakawa M, Kojiro M, et al. Histology of membranous obstruction of the inferior vena cava in the Budd-Chiari syndrome. *Gastroenterol* 1992;102:2081–2090.
11. Senzolo M, Riggio O, Primignani M. Vascular disorders of the liver: recommendations from the Italian Association for the Study of Liver (AISF) ad hoc committee. *Dig Liver Dis* 2011;43(7):503–514
12. Valla D-C. Hepatic vein thrombosis (Budd-Chiari syndrome). *Semin Liver Dis* 2002;22:5–14.
13. Okuda K. Inferior vena cava thrombosis at its hepatic portion (obliterative hepatocavopathy). *Semin Liver Dis* 2002;22:15–26.
14. Uddin W, Ramage JK, Portmann B, et al. Hepatic venous outflow obstruction in patients with polycystic liver disease: pathogenesis and treatment. *Gut* 1995;36:142–145.
15. Wang SL, Sze DY, Busque S, et al. Treatment of hepatic venous outflow obstruction after piggyback liver transplantation. *Radiology* 2005;236:352–359.
16. Brancatelli G, Vilgrain V, Federle MP, et al. Budd-Chiari syndrome: spectrum of imaging findings. *AJR Am J Roentgenol* 2007;188:168–176.
17. Cura M, Haskal Z, Lopera J. Diagnostic and interventional radiology for Budd-Chiari syndrome. *Radiographics* 2009;29:669–681.
18. Wilson MW, Ring EJ, LaBerge JM, et al. Percutaneous transhepatic hepatic venography in the delineation and treatment of Budd-Chiari syndrome. *J Vasc Interv Radiol* 1996;7:133–138.
19. Hoppe H, Wang SL, Petersen BD. Intravascular US-guided direct intrahepatic portocaval shunt with an expanded polytetrafluoroethylene-covered stent-graft. *Radiology* 2008;246:306–314.
20. Petersen BD, Clark TW. Direct intrahepatic portocaval shunt. *Tech Vasc Interv Radiol* 2008;11:230–234.
21. Boyvat F, Harman A, Ozyer U, et al. Percutaneous sonographic guidance for TIPS in Budd-Chiari syndrome: direct simultaneous puncture of the portal vein and inferior vena cava. *AJR Am J Roentgenol* 2008;191:560–564.
22. Martin M, Baumgartner I, Kolb M, et al. Fatal pericardial tamponade after Wallstent implantation for malignant superior vena cava syndrome. *J Endovasc Ther* 2002;9:680–684.
23. Darwish-Murad S, Valla D-C, de Groen PC, et al. Determinants of survival and the effect of portosystemic shunting in patients with Budd-Chiari syndrome. *Hepatology* 2004;39:500–508.
24. Eapen CE, Velissaris D, Heydtmann M, et al. Favourable medium term outcome following hepatic vein recanalisation and/or transjugular intrahepatic portosystemic shunt for Budd-Chiari syndrome. *Gut* 2006;55:878–884.
25. Darwish-Murad S, Plessier A, Hernandez-Guerra M, et al. Etiology, management, and outcome of the Budd-Chiari syndrome. *Ann Intern Med* 2009;151:167–175.
26. Sharma S, Texeira A, Texeira P, et al. Pharmacological thrombolysis in Budd Chiari syndrome: a single centre experience and review of the literature. *J Hepatol* 2004;40:172–180.
27. Xue H, Li Y-C, Shakya P, et al. The role of intravascular intervention in the management of Budd-Chiari syndrome. *Dig Dis Sci* 2010;55:2659–2663.
28. Li T, Zhai S, Pang Z, et al. Feasibility and midterm outcomes of percutaneous transhepatic balloon angioplasty for symptomatic Budd-Chiari syndrome secondary to hepatic venous obstruction. *J Vasc Surg* 2009;50:1079–1084.
29. Griffith JF, Mahmoud AE, Cooper S, et al. Radiological intervention in Budd-Chiari syndrome: techniques and outcomes in 18 patients. *Clin Radiol* 1996;51:775–784.
30. Martin LG, Henderson JM, Millikan WJ, et al. Angioplasty for long-term treatment of patients with Budd-Chiari syndrome. *AJR Am J Roentgenol* 1990;154:1007–1010.
31. DeLeve LD, Valla D-C, Garcia-Tsao G. Vascular disorders of the liver. *Hepatology* 2009;49:1729–1761.
32. Lee JM, Ko G-Y, Sung K-B, et al. Long-term efficacy of stent placement for treating inferior vena cava stenosis following liver transplantation. *Liver Transpl* 2010;16:513–516.
33. Carnevale FC, Machado AT, Moreira AM, et al. Midterm and long-term results of percutaneous endovascular treatment of venous outflow obstruction after pediatric liver transplantation. *J Vasc Interv Radiol* 2008;19:1439–1448.
34. Zahn A, Gotthardt D, Weiss KH, et al. Budd-Chiari syndrome: long term success via hepatic decompression using transjugular intrahepatic portosystemic shunt. *BMC Gastroenterol* 2010;10:25–30.

35. Boyer TD, Haskal ZJ; American Association for the Study of Liver Diseases. The role of transjugular intrahepatic portosystemic shunt (TIPS) in the management of portal hypertension: update 2009. *Hepatology* 2010;51:306–311.

36. Carnevale FC, Szejnfeld D, Moreira AM, et al. Long-term follow-up after successful transjugular intrahepatic portosystemic shunt placement in a pediatric patient with Budd-Chiari syndrome. *Cardiovasc Intervent Radiol* 2008;31:1244–1248.

37. Garcia-Pagán JC, Heydtmann M, Raffa S, et al. TIPS for Budd-Chiari syndrome: long-term results and prognostics factors in 124 patients. *Gastroenterology* 2008;135:808–815.

38. Darwish Murad S, Luong TK, Pattynama PM, et al. Long-term outcome of a covered vs. uncovered transjugular intrahepatic portosystemic shunt in Budd-Chiari syndrome. *Liver Int* 2008;28:249–256.

39. Corso R, Intotero M, Solcia M, et al. Treatment of Budd-Chiari syndrome with transjugular intrahepatic portosystemic shunt (TIPS). *Radiol Med* 2008;113:727–738.

40. Klein AS. Management of Budd-Chiari syndrome. *Liver Transpl* 2006;12:S23–S28.

41. Plessier A, Sibert A, Consigny Y, et al. Aiming at minimal invasiveness as a therapeutic strategy for Budd-Chiari syndrome. *Hepatology* 2006;44:1308–1316.

42. Ganger DR, Klapman JB, McDonald V, et al. Transjugular intrahepatic portosystemic shunt (TIPS) for Budd-Chiari syndrome or portal vein thrombosis: review of indications and problems. *Am J Gastroenterol* 1999;94:603–608.

43. Ryu RK, Durham JD, Krysl J, et al. Role of TIPS as a bridge to hepatic transplantation in Budd-Chiari syndrome. *J Vasc Interv Radiol* 1999;10:799–805.

44. Slakey DP, Klein AS, Venbrux AC, et al. Budd-Chiari syndrome: current management options. *Ann Surg* 2001;233:522–527.

45. Cejna M, Peck-Radosavljevic M, Schoder M, et al. Repeat interventions for maintenance of transjugular intrahepatic portosystemic shunt function in patients with Budd-Chiari syndrome. *J Vasc Interv Radiol* 2002;13:193–199.

46. Perello A, Garcia-Pagan JC, Gilabert R, et al. TIPS is a useful long-term derivative therapy for patients with Budd-Chiari syndrome uncontrolled by medical therapy. *Hepatology* 2002;35:132–139.

47. Blokzijl H, de Knegt RJ. Long-term effect of treatment of acute Budd-Chiari syndrome with a transjugular intrahepatic portosytemic shunt. *Hepatology* 2002;35:1551–1552.

48. Mancuso A, Fung K, Mela M, et al. TIPS for acute and chronic Budd-Chiari syndrome: a single-centre experience. *J Hepatol* 2003;38:751–754.

49. Kavanagh PM, Roberts J, Gibney R, et al. Acute Budd-Chiari syndrome with liver failure: the experience of a policy of initial interventional radiological treatment using transjugular intrahepatic portosystemic shunt. *J Gastroenterol Hepatol* 2004;19:1135–1139.

50. Molmenti EP, Segev DL, Arepally A, et al. The utility of TIPS in the management of Budd-Chiari syndrome. *Ann Surg* 2005;241:978–981.

51. Hernandez-Guerra M, Turnes J, Rubinstein P, et al. PTFE-covered stents improve TIPS patency in Budd-Chiari syndrome. *Hepatology* 2004;40:1197–1202.

52. Rossle M, Olschewski M, Siegerstetter V, et al. The Budd-Chiari syndrome, outcome after treatment with the transjugular intrahepatic portosystemic shunt. *Surgery* 2004;135:394–403.

53. Shrestha R, Durham JD, Wachs M, et al. Use of transjugular intrahepatic portosystemic shunt as a bridge to transplantation in fulminant hepatic failure due to Budd-Chiari syndrome. *Am J Gastroenterol* 1997;92:2304–2306.

54. Darwiah-Murad S, Lunog TK, Pattynama PMT, et al. Long-term outcome of a covered vs. unconvered transjugular intrahepatic portosystemic shunt in Budd-Chiari syndrome. *Liver Int* 2008;28:249–256.

55. Smalberg JH, Spaander MV, Jie KS, et al. Risks and benefits of transcatheter thrombolytic therapy in patients with splanchnic venous thrombosis. *Thromb Haemost* 2008;100:1084–1088.

56. Khuroo MS, Al-Suhabani H, Al-Sebayel M, et al. Budd-Chiari syndrome: long-term effect on outcome with transjugular intrahepatic portosystemic shunt. *J Gastroenterol Hepatol* 2005;20:1494–1502.

57. Min AD, Atillasoy EO, Schwartz ME, et al. Reassessing the role of medical therapy in the management of hepatic vein thrombosis. *Liver Transpl Surg* 1997;3:423–429.

58. Inafuku H, Morishima Y, Nagano T, et al. A three decade experience of radical open endvenectomy with pericardial patch graft for correction of Budd-Chiari syndrome. *J Vasc Surg* 2009;50:590–593.

59. Langlet P, Valla D. Is surgical portosystemic shunt the treatment of choice in Budd-Chiari syndrome? *Acta Gastroenterol Belg* 2002;65:155–160.

60. Bachet JB, Condat B, Hagege H, et al. Long-term portosystemic shunt patency as a determinant of outcome in Budd-Chiari syndrome. *J Hepatol* 2007;46:60–68.

61. Panis Y, Belghiti J, Valla D, et al. Portosystemic shunt in Budd-Chiari syndrome: long-term survival and factors affecting shunt patency in 25 patients in Western countries. *Surgery* 1994;115:276–281.

62. Tang TJ, Batts KP, de Groen PC, et al. The prognostic value of histology in the assessment of patients with Budd-Chiari syndrome. *J Hepatol* 2001;35:338–343.

CHAPTER

95

Pathophysiologic Basis and Hemodynamic Effects

BERTRAND JANNE D'OTHÉE and ZIV J. HASKAL

CHRONIC VENOUS INSUFFICIENCY: DEFINITION, ETIOPATHOGENY, AND EPIDEMIOLOGY

Chronic venous insufficiency (CVI), a condition characterized by insufficient venous return to the heart, is related primarily to retrograde blood flow in some of the veins of the lower extremities (venous reflux). CVI and reflux commonly result from valvular incompetence, with or without associated venous obstruction.[1] Recognized *causes* of venous insufficiency (FIGURE 95.1) include reflux related to valve incompetence, vein obstruction, and/or calf muscle pump failure (including muscle wasting, neuromuscular disease, and prolonged standing). At the early stage of disease, valvular incompetence results in venous reflux, whereas vein obstruction causes venous hypertension upstream. Later on, reflux and hypertension, the final endpoints of these etiopathogenic pathways, can cause and reinforce each other. Although overlapping terminology can be found in the literature, reflux is typically associated with CVI and venous hypertension with post-thrombotic syndrome (PTS).

Valvular incompetence causes venous reflux, the hallmark of CVI, which may affect any vein of the lower extremities. Valve incompetence may result from functional vein distension/deformation and/or from lesional valve damage. Vein/valve distension in the absence of lesion may result from exposure to progesterone (e.g., female gender, pregnancy), which relaxes the vein wall, or from an overflow of blood (e.g., coming from an arteriovenous shunt). Valve damage may originate from a superficial phlebitis, a deep venous thrombosis (DVT) with inflammation and distortion of the valvular architecture, or a leg injury.

Chronic *vein obstruction* causes venous hypertension, a characteristic feature of PTS. Chronic deep venous obstruction increases pressure in the deep and/or perforating veins (FIGURE 95.1), which eventually leads to flow reversal (reflux) in the perforators, eversion or incompetence of their valves, and hypertension in their superficial tributary veins. Hence the sequellae of an acute DVT can be related to valve incompetence/CVI—such as in case of partial or complete devalvulation after DVT—and/or to venous hypertension and PTS (as in case of permanent occlusion post-DVT). The natural history after acute lower extremity DVT shows that, at 1 year, thrombi fully resolve in 76% of the segments, 20% remain partially recanalized, and 5% are occluded. Venous occlusion is most prevalent in the femoral vein (21% at 1 year). On the contrary, calf veins show more rapid recanalization than proximal veins at any time point after acute DVT. Deep venous insufficiency is detected as early as 1 month after acute DVT, and the reflux is most predominant in popliteal veins (56%), followed by femoral veins (18%), with relative sparing of the calf veins.[2] In PTS, edema can be found in about two-thirds of patients, skin pigmentation in one-third, and venous ulcers in less than 5%.[3–7] Trophic skin changes occur within less than 5 years following the initial DVT episode.[3,5] The risk of such changes increases when the associated reflux is worse and when the initial DVT is more proximal and more extensive, involving multiple segments and vessels.[6–10]

Failure of the calf muscular pump is involved most commonly in patients with prolonged standing but may also occur in case of muscle wasting or neuromuscular disease.

Although both reflux and obstruction may increase pressure values in the venous lumen, very high-pressure values are typically associated with venous obstruction. However, reflux may also increase pressure quite significantly and cause by itself advanced venous disease, such as ulcers.

Several *predisposing factors* of varicose veins have been reported: in order of decreasing importance, they include age,

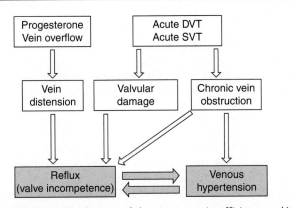

FIGURE 95.1 Etiopathogeny of chronic venous insufficiency and its relation to post-thrombotic syndrome.

female gender, genetics, occupation/prolonged standing position, prior pregnancy(ies), deficient calf muscular pump,[11] prior history of phlebitis or serious leg injury, and, possibly, other factors, such as obesity, heavy lifting and hematologic factors, which may play a role as well.[12,13] Females seem three to four times more likely to have varicose veins than men (range: 1 to 10 times); although they may be more likely to report them than men do, independent physical examinations demonstrate that this gender difference is real.[12] Varicose veins run in the family: 70% of patients with varicose veins have parents affected as well. Gravity and prolonged standing do increase the prevalence of superficial venous reflux.[14]

CVI remains a major health care problem today: Although its prevalence is difficult to precise, it is commonly estimated at approximately 40%,[12] including 25% of women and 15% of men. It affects between 15 and 25 millions of people in the United States,[15] of which 1.5 million seek treatment annually and, until the late 1990s, over 150,000 underwent surgical stripping any given year. It is estimated that, at age 50, at least 50% of people are affected and, at age 60, 72% of women and 40% of men are. Total health care expenditure associated with CVI is also major: 4.6 million workdays are missed annually in the United States due to venous disease, and the annual cost of managing CVI is estimated to 2% of the national health care budget in most European countries.[12,16–18]

HEMODYNAMICS OF CHRONIC VENOUS INSUFFICIENCY AND VENOUS REFLUX: BASIC PRINCIPLES

Two principles are crucial in summarizing the hemodynamics of CVI. The first one is that the large, bulging varicosities seen on inspection, the smaller reticular veins ("venulectasias"), and the telangiectasias ("spider veins") represent a *continuum*: they are all part of an interconnected venous network and are all caused by increased endovenous pressure, itself due to reflux (secondary to valvular incompetence or venous obstruction). Hence, no patient should ever be dismissed early because (s)he presents with "cosmetic" spider veins only: Such patients may in fact be at the early stage of disease, be symptomatic or not, and have significant reflux in their saphenous vein territories, which would benefit from treatment. Therefore, the remainder of this chapter includes all of these vein sizes under the denomination *varicose veins* unless specifically noted otherwise.

The second principle is best summarized by the "retrograde hydrostatic/valvular incompetence" hypothesis: This theory states that the development of CVI and chronic venous stasis changes are due to increased pressure inside the vein lumen (venous hypertension), which is itself caused by venous reflux originating from a more central vein in most cases. The absence of valves in the inferior vena cava, iliac, and common femoral veins,[19] the cyclic respiratory and cardiac variations in central venous pressure, and gravity cause the increased pressure upon the most cranial valves of the (superficial) femoral and greater saphenous veins (GSV). This increased pressure applies mainly on the proximal valve of the GSV because the superficial femoral vein is relatively

protected from overdistension thanks to the surrounding muscles and intracompartmental pressure. Therefore, the preferential pathway of reflux will be toward the GSV. If the most proximal, valveless segment of the GSV, near the saphenofemoral junction (SFJ), becomes too distended, the most proximal valve of the GSV may then become incompetent, which will in turn transmit the increased pressure to the next (more caudal) valve, and so on. The farther distally (caudally) the superficial venous reflux progresses, the longer the column of hydrostatic pressure and reflux becomes; as a result, the chances that a distal GSV valve near the calf keeps resisting this increased pressure and remains competent decrease accordingly, unless the reflux returns to the deep veins prior to reaching that valve.

This theory has been questioned using a variety of arguments from multiple different perspectives: functional, morphological, and biochemical studies[19] suggest that venous wall changes can occur anywhere along the venous tree regardless of the location and competence of the valves. However, such occurrences may be explained by failure to detect subclinical valvular incompetence or reflux. Although duplex ultrasonography (US) has dramatically helped our understanding of flow circuits in patients with CVI, it is by no means a perfectly sensitive technique, and its false negative results in detecting reflux might explain so-called failures of the retrograde reflux theory. All things considered, the retrograde hydrostatic/valvular incompetence theory remains perhaps the most widely accepted,[20] and the most appropriate one to explain symptoms evolution and resolution after treatment, and is the one followed in this chapter. Current therapeutic approaches, both endovenous thermal ablation (EVTA) techniques[11,21] and CHIVA surgery,[22–26] are based on this theory.

HEMODYNAMICS: IMPLICATIONS FOR PATIENT MANAGEMENT

As a result of the above, the key point in treating varicose veins and reflux is to start by identifying[20] and stopping the most central (proximal) source(s) of reflux first, before addressing the side branches (which can be treated either at the same treatment session or at a later stage). This principle is supported not only by our understanding of flow circuits and pathways of reflux gained from duplex US studies,[11] but also by the clinical successes observed after ligation of sources of reflux as applied in the CHIVA surgical approach ("Chirurgie hémodynamique de l'insuffisance veineuse en ambulatoire" or outpatient hemodynamic surgery of venous insufficiency).[27] Similar to the later development of EVTA, the CHIVA approach was a hemodynamic-based strategy[23,25,28]: instead of removing the refluxing veins (as stripping does), the CHIVA strategy aims at blocking the proximal sources of reflux in superficial veins and divert the flow toward the deep veins, thereby offering the theoretical potential advantage of allowing refluxing superficial veins to regain competence after eliminating the abnormal high-pressure constraint and potential functional valvular distension. By the time endovascular thermal ablation techniques started, few series detailing the clinical outcomes of CHIVA[23,28] had been published and provided low levels of scientific evidence and, subsequently, the CHIVA approach never developed into a mainstream strategy.

CLINICAL PRESENTATION

A simple clinical scoring system has been developed and validated that has fair sensitivity (75%) and high specificity (95%) for distinguishing CVI from leg symptoms of other causes. In this system, CVI is diagnosed when at least three of the following four criteria are met: sensation of heavy or swollen legs (82% sensitivity, 55% specificity); itching, impatient legs, or phlebalgia (55% sensitivity, 92% specificity); worsening in hot environments or improvement at cold temperatures (78% sensitivity, 71% specificity); and absence of worsening during walking (89% sensitivity, 62% specificity).[29] Clinical symptoms associated with CVI may vary with the venous system involved (superficial or deep, or both).[30] On the other hand, PTS with iliofemoral deep venous obstruction typically causes venous claudication, present in 44% of patients and significantly impairing quality of life.[31] Because CVI and PTS may coexist, both reflux and obstructive symptoms may be present in a given patient.

Objective signs and clinical stages of CVI are best described by the CEAP classification (Clinical, Etiology, Anatomy, Pathophysiology)[32] (Table 95.1). The severity CVI includes a continuum between the spider veins, varicosities, edema and skin trophic changes, and chronic venous ulcers. Most leg ulcers are venous in origin, and venous ulcers are predominantly caused by venous hypertension. One percent of adults experience leg ulceration at some point in their life,[33] and the prevalence of leg ulcers in patients with CVI is reported to be around 2%.[12] Up to 20% patients with venous ulcers show no clinically visible varicose veins.[20] Venous ulcers are a serious condition, however, with high risks of associated infection, delayed healing, and recurrence. The most severe forms of CVI may even lead to amputation.[16] Patient age and ulcer chronicity are independent risk factors for delayed ulcer healing.[34] The duration of ulcer

healing and the presence of untreated superficial venous reflux are independent risk factors for ulcer recurrence.[34]

Subjects in CEAP classes 2 and 3 are typically females (81%); reasons for this gender difference may include a higher prevalence of reflux and varicose veins due to pregnancies and a higher propensity to seek medical attention when cosmetic concerns arise. Males are slightly more prevalent (57%) in the more severe stages of CVI (CEAP classes 4 to 6), probably because they wait more to seek medical attention for this problem.[15]

A worsening CEAP class is associated with a higher prevalence of junctional reflux and larger saphenous trunks diameters (or cross-sectional areas, which are well correlated to diameters[15,35]) CEAP classes 2 and 3 show significantly larger saphenous trunk diameters than normal controls, except at the level of the malleoli, and classes 4 to 6 exhibit larger saphenous trunk diameters than classes 2 and 3 and a higher prevalence of SJF and saphenopopliteal junction (SPJ) involvement.[15] Deep venous reflux also increases as CEAP clinical changes become more severe, with significant axial reflux contributing to ulcer formation.[36] Advanced CVI is also associated with increased calf muscle deoxygenation,[37] as shown by near-infrared spectroscopy examinations during light-intensity exercise. However, noninvasive testing techniques (such as quantitative photoplethysmography, air plethysmography, and duplex US measurement of valve closure time) are unable to distinguish between limbs with nonulcerating skin changes (hyperpigmentation, brawny edema, and subcutaneous fibrosis) and ulcerated limbs.[38]

The CEAP classification is, however, a descriptive instrument that is relatively insensitive to changes over time,[39,40] and therefore the Venous Severity Scoring (VSS) system has been developed to address this drawback.[39,41] The three elements included in this system, namely, the Venous Disability Score (VDS), the Venous Segmental Disease Score (VSDS), and the Venous Clinical Severity Score (VCSS), can be used in an attempt to better assess the evolution of CVI severity over time and during follow-up in response to therapy.[41–45] Among these three, the VCSS is

---

Table 95.1

CEAP Classification

C component of CEAP classification	Description
C0	No visible or palpable signs of venous disease
C1	Spider veins ("telangiectasias") (<1 mm in diameter) Reticular veins ("venulectasias") (1 to <3 mm in diameter)
C2	Varicose veins (3 mm or larger in standing position)
C3	Venous edema; corona phlebectatica ("ankle flare")
C4	Skin changes ascribed to venous disease C4a: eczema ("stasis dermatitis") or brownish hyperpigmentation C4b: lipodermatosclerosis or atrophie blanche
C5	Healed ulcer (and skin changes as described above)
C6	Active ulcer (and skin changes as described above)

Eczema appears as an erythematous, blistering, weeping, or scaling eruption of the skin. Lipodermatosclerosis corresponds to a localized chronic induration of the skin; its acute form ("hypodermitis") presents with diffuse reddening and tenderness but, unlike cellulitis or erysipelas, there is no lymphadenitis and fever. Atrophie blanche (i.e., white atrophy) is a circumscribed, round area of atrophic white skin surrounded exclusive of healed ulcerations.

the most commonly used instrument and its validity and reliability has been studied for both varicose veins and deep venous obstruction, based on clinical and on duplex US findings.[43,45–52] It has even been suggested as a screening tool of CVI.[43] Other grading systems have been used as well, including—but not limited to—generic tools, such as the Short Form 36 (SF-36) and its variants, and disease-specific questionnaires, such as the Aberdeen Varicose Veins Questionnaire (AVVQ).[41,53]

CLINICAL—IMAGING/FUNCTIONAL CORRELATIONS

Anatomic Sources and Pathways of Reflux: Data from the Literature

Varicose veins are, in most cases, caused by superficial venous reflux due to valvular incompetence. In subjects with *primary chronic venous insufficiency* (i.e., in the absence of evident causes, such as prior DVT, superficial phlebitis, venous surgery, ablation, or sclerotherapy), the territory most commonly affected by superficial venous reflux by far is the GSV (60% to 86%),[15,19,54] followed by the small or short (or lesser) saphenous vein (SSV) (17%).[15,54] Nonsaphenous reflux is found in 8% to 9% of limbs.[15,55] Because the location of the visible varicosities is poorly correlated to the anatomic source(s) of reflux, additional imaging and functional evaluation is needed before treatment.

Similarly, in subjects with *chronic leg ulceration*, lesion location is a poor indicator of the source of reflux: medially located ulcers may be caused by GSV reflux (35%), reflux in medial perforating veins (15%), or even SSV reflux (6%). Similarly, ulcers located on the lateral side of the calf/ankle can be related to GSV incompetence (14%) or SSV incompetence (7% only).[20] In fact, the anatomic pattern in subjects with chronic leg ulcer is complex: there is a variety of systems (superficial, deep, and/or perforating veins) and levels (above-knee [AK] vs. [BK]) that can be involved. According to one series, combined reflux involving multiple systems is more common (64%) than not. Contrarily to prior beliefs, the advent of duplex US has shown that reflux affects the deep veins alone in only 6% of subjects with leg ulcers and the perforators alone in only 3%.[8] The most common patterns in venous ulcer patients are reflux involving all three systems (28%), isolated superficial venous reflux (23%), combined superficial and perforator reflux (21%), and combined superficial and deep reflux without perforator incompetence (12%). Combined deep and perforator reflux without superficial reflux has been described in 4% but likely reflects a failure of duplex US to detect the latter (i.e., a false negative result), and no reflux is found in the remaining 4% of subjects. So, overall, venous reflux in patients with leg ulcers is present in the superficial veins in 84% of cases, in the deep veins in 50%, and in perforating veins in 60%.

In terms of craniocaudal level involvement, superficial venous reflux is located in the GSV in 61% (AK 6%, BK 23%, both 32%), in the SSV in 9%, and in both in the remaining 30% (AK 3%, BK 9%, both 18%). Deep venous reflux may affect several segments at a time: common femoral vein in 46%, superficial femoral vein in 20%, popliteal vein in 66%, and calf veins in 29%. Isolated popliteal incompetence is present in only 25% of all subjects with deep venous reflux, and common and superficial incompetence in 20%. Perforator incompetence is rarely seen alone (3%): It is usually (97% of subjects) associated

with superficial or deep venous reflux. Most of the time (95%), associated incompetent veins are the BK GSV (70%), AK GSV (12%), or the SSV (13%). Of note, this series did not describe any venous obstruction findings, despite including 39% of patients with prior history of DVT and a few with iliac vein ligation or deep venous reconstructions (10/112 = 9%); therefore, the role of obstruction in this patient population remains unanswered.[8]

Reflux can also involve another superficial venous territory: the lateral subdermal venous system (LSVS) of Albanese.[56] This venous plexus is located on the lateral side of the lower thigh, knee, and upper calf. It appears typically as spider and reticular veins clinically, which are related to reflux through tiny perforators that are too small to see by US. Therefore, enlarged perforators are usually not detectable in such cases, even with modern US devices. Spider and reticular veins in this territory are usually treated by sclerotherapy because they are too small to accommodate the laser fiber or radiofrequency probe inside their lumen.

Incompetent perforating veins (or perforators) can be sources of significant reflux (i.e., retrograde flow from deep to superficial veins) with two main explanations advanced. One states that *high pressure* generated in the deep veins during muscular contractions (due to the lack of elasticity/extensibility of the perimuscular fascia and muscular compartments) exerts excessive pressure on the valves in the perforating veins, which then become incompetent and transmit their reflux to downstream superficial varicosities (causing the classical appearance of "blow-out" bulging varicosity at the exit outside of the fascia). The other hypothesis is that reflux in perforating veins may be caused by *volume overload* at reentry points of superficial venous reflux from incompetent superficial veins into the deep system.[57] These two explanations are not in contradiction and may in fact coexist in a given patient; they seem almost equally prevalent in the pathogenesis of new perforator incompetence (55% due to high pressure, 45% due to volume overload).[57] Although perforator incompetence/reflux is associated with subsequent worsening of the CEAP class after a median time of 31 months (range 14 to 52), this clinical worsening is attributable only partially to the perforator reflux because other veins also become incompetent during that time interval.[57]

Deep venous reflux may be found in 20% to 30% of patients with primary superficial venous incompetence. It is usually segmental, most commonly affecting the common femoral vein, and of short duration.[58] However, patients with femoral or popliteal reflux velocities greater than 10 cm/second have a high incidence of persistent symptoms after EVTA,[59] whereas patients with popliteal or femoral reflux velocities lower than 10 cm/second usually experience marked improvement in VCSS and venous filling index.

Pathways of Reflux: How Treatment Strategy Depends on the Diagnostic Findings

According to the valvular incompetence theory, in cases of pure reflux disease without associated obstruction, the endovenous pressure is higher at the ankle than in the thigh or groin when the entire GSV is incompetent. This explains why many patients report initial occurrence of varicose veins in the calf first, then followed years later by new onset of more cranial varicosities in the thigh. However, many other patients do not present this typical pattern because they develop different anatomic pathways of reflux, sometimes combined, and which can be quite complex.

Also, each of the venous territories discussed previously (GSV, SSV, LSVS, perforators, and deep veins) can be involved to various extents and at times combined. Therefore, the search for reflux has to investigate these pathways so that treatment strategy can then be adapted accordingly.

Common pathways/presentations and their therapeutic approach[60] are shown in FIGURES 95.2 and 95.3, respectively. In the simplest case where SFJ incompetence results in reflux following the entire GSV from groin to ankle (FIGURE 95.2A) (1% of limbs[15]), ablation could theoretically be performed along most of the GSV; however, treatment from the groin to near the knee is usually preferred (FIGURE 95.3A) due to the proximity of

superficial nerves and the GSV along the calf, which may result in post-treatment paresthesias. A more common pathway of reflux along the GSV involves only its thigh portion, in which case the reflux continues thereafter in side branch tributaries below or above the knee, that eventually enlarge to become bulging varicosities (FIGURE 95.2B). Such cases can be treated using a similar approach as above, from near the SFJ to near the knee (FIGURE 95.3B).

In a third type of presentation, SFJ incompetence may spare most of the GSV: the reflux then follows the anterior and/or the posterior thigh tributaries. In the former case, the first, most cranial segment of the anterior thigh tributary usually remains

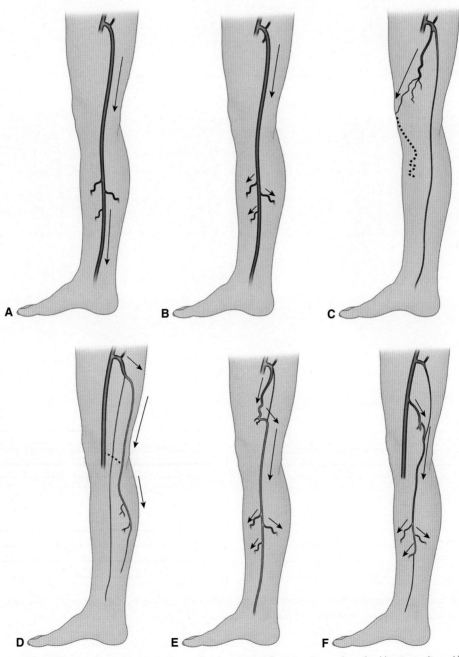

FIGURE 95.2 Common patterns of superficial venous reflux circuits, as described by Ganguli et al.[60]

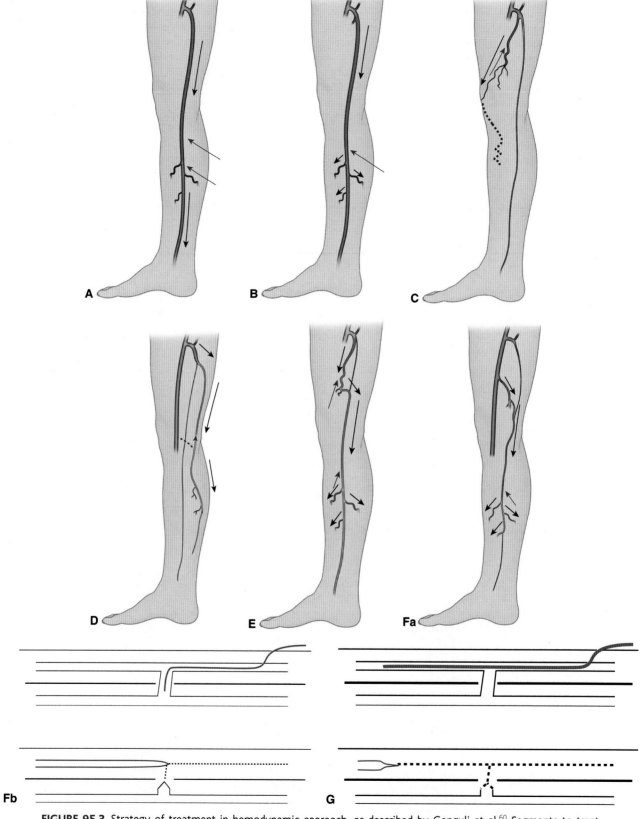

FIGURE 95.3 Strategy of treatment in hemodynamic approach, as described by Ganguli et al.[60] Segments to treat (by ablation or sclerotherapy) are represented in purple.

straight (FIGURE 95.2C) and deep enough to allow safe EVTA without risk of skin burns; more caudally, however, this vein becomes superficial and quite tortuous to eventually distend varicose tributaries in the distal thigh anterolaterally, around the knee, and/or in the anterolateral calf. At these levels, ultrasound-guided foam sclerotherapy can be used. Hence the single session of treatment will consist of an EVTA of the straight, cranial segment first, then followed by foam injection via the existing access just before sheath removal, with the foam being pushed down by external manual compression toward the knee (FIGURE 95.3C). This EVTA and sclerotherapy combination strategy makes sense even when the straight, cranial segment is too short (≤5 to 10 cm) to be successfully treated by ablation alone: ablation alone of such a short segment would invariably result in vein recanalization and recurrent reflux, and the additional distal sclerotherapy provides enough occlusion length to avoid that undesirable phenomenon.

In a fourth presentation type, where SFJ incompetence causes reflux in the posteromedial thigh tributary of the GSV, there is often communication between the GSV and SSV via a vein of Giacomini (FIGURE 95.2D). Hence, an incompetent vein of Giacomini can transmit reflux from the GSV to the SSV and, therefore, SSV reflux can exist as a result of saphenofemoral valvular incompetence even if the SPJ remains competent. This situation is probably not more common than in other superficial veins, but when reflux is found in the posteromedial thigh tributary of the GSV, the presence of an incompetent vein of Giacomini is common.[61] EVTA of the vein of Giacomini presents its own challenge in terms of patient positioning but can often be performed with the patient in semilateral decubitus with steep external rotation of the limb to treat (FIGURE 95.3D).

In a fifth type of presentation, the reflux may go through the SFJ and the anterior thigh tributary up to the proximal or mid-third of the thigh and then leave this vein via a tributary to join the GSV at mid-thigh and cause GSV reflux downstream (FIGURE 95.2E). In such case, duplex US can show the reflux from the mid-thigh downward but fails to demonstrate any GSV reflux at the proximal thigh level. This can be treated by ablations of two separate straight segments, each from its own access site, and likely subsequent thrombosis of the short, tortuous segment in between them (FIGURE 95.3E).

A sixth common pattern of superficial venous reflux involves perforator incompetence (FIGURE 95.2F), which commonly occurs at the mid-thigh or in the calf.[62,63] These perforating veins have various names depending on their anatomic level (Hunterian, Dodd, Boyd, and Cockett perforators) but their treatment strategy can be summarized along two approaches: (a) direct ablation of the superficial portion of the incompetent perforator and of part of its dependent superficial varicose tributary (FIGURE 95.3Fa-b), or (b) indirect approach ablating only the superficial varicose tributary but starting more cranially to prevent residual pressure in the blowout sac (FIGURE 95.3G). The direct and indirect approaches can also be applied to the EVTA of SPJ incompetence and reflux in the SSV,[64–70] which may help avoid heating in the popliteal fossa and its associated risks and discomfort.

Besides these, there are innumerable other variations or possible sources of reflux, including, but not limited to, posterolateral thigh perforator vein incompetence,[71] reflux involving one or both limbs of duplication of the GSV, which is present in 1% (true duplication within the saphenous canal) to 9% of

limbs (false duplication within the superficial fascia),[15] pelvic congestion syndrome transmitting its reflux to the GSV via the superficial inferior epigastric vein and/or perineal veins, and reflux developing from the thousands of tiny perforators and veins present in the normal venous anatomy (as demonstrated by autopsy studies).

When deciding the therapeutic strategy based on these findings, it is crucial to keep in mind that varicose veins in the legs can be caused by the presence of a more central venous obstruction, either in the femoral or popliteal veins or in the abdomen/pelvis (e.g., iliac or inferior vena cava compression or obstruction). In these cases, it is crucial to keep these leg varicosities open and to avoid treatments that close or remove them (such as EVTA, sclerotherapy, stripping, and phlebectomy) because these superficial leg varicosities are the only remaining collaterals that allow the leg to empty its venous blood to the heart. Should these collaterals become occluded, the risk of developing phlegmasia cerulea dolens would dramatically increase. In such cases, duplex US can suggest/detect proximal deep venous obstruction or compression by demonstrating disappearance of the phasic modulation of the spectral Doppler waveforms in the common femoral veins during the respiratory cycles. Duplex US is not the best technique to detect proximal deep venous obstruction or compression, however, and contrast venography or computed tomography (CT) or magnetic resonance (MR) venograms may be needed in doubtful cases. Any suspicion of proximal deep venous obstruction (i.e., popliteal, femoral, or above) should raise a flag: it is the most important contraindication to varicose veins ablation therapies. An isolated small thrombus in a calf vein is not as much of a concern: the risk becomes relevant only in case of obstruction/clots located at the popliteal level or more centrally.

■ REFERENCES

1. Lynch TG, Dalsing MC, Ouriel K, et al. Developments in diagnosis and classification of venous disorders: non-invasive diagnosis. *Cardiovasc Surg* 1999;7(2):160–178.
2. Yamaki T, Nozaki M. Patterns of venous insufficiency after an acute deep vein thrombosis. *J Am Coll Surg* 2005;201(2):231–238.
3. Franzeck UK, Schalch I, Jager KA, et al. Prospective 12-year follow-up study of clinical and hemodynamic sequelae after deep vein thrombosis in low-risk patients (Zurich study). *Circulation* 1996;93(1):74–79.
4. Heldal M, Seem E, Sandset PM, et al. Deep vein thrombosis: a 7-year follow-up study. *J Intern Med* 1993;234(1):71–75.
5. Prandoni P, Lensing AW, Cogo A, et al. The long-term clinical course of acute deep venous thrombosis. *Ann Intern Med* 1996;125(1):1–7.
6. Strandness DE Jr, Langlois Y, Cramer M, et al. Long-term sequelae of acute venous thrombosis. *JAMA* 1983;250(10):1289–1292.
7. Johnson BF, Manzo RA, Bergelin RO, et al. Relationship between changes in the deep venous system and the development of the postthrombotic syndrome after an acute episode of lower limb deep vein thrombosis: a one- to six-year follow-up. *J Vasc Surg* 1995;21(2):307–312; discussion 313.
8. Labropoulos N, Leon M, Geroulakos G, et al. Venous hemodynamic abnormalities in patients with leg ulceration. *Am J Surg* 1995;169(6):572–574.
9. McEnroe CS, O'Donnell TF Jr, Mackey WC. Correlation of clinical findings with venous hemodynamics in 386 patients with chronic venous insufficiency. *Am J Surg* 1988;156(2):148–152.
10. van Ramshorst B, van Bemmelen PS, Hoeneveld H, et al. The development of valvular incompetence after deep vein thrombosis: a follow-up study with duplex scanning. *J Vasc Surg* 1994;19(6):1059–1066.
11. Min RJ, Khilnani NM, Golia P. Duplex ultrasound evaluation of lower extremity venous insufficiency. *J Vasc Interv Radiol* 2003;14(10):1233–1241.
12. Lawrence PF, Gazak CE. Epidemiology of chronic venous insufficiency. In: Ballard JL, Bergan JJ, eds. *Chronic Venous Insufficiency: Diagnosis and Treatment.* London, England: Springer-Verlag; 2000:3–6.

13. Scott TE, LaMorte WW, Gorin DR, et al. Risk factors for chronic venous insufficiency: a dual case-control study. *J Vasc Surg* 1995;22(5):622–628.

14. Labropoulos N, Delis KT, Nicolaides AN. Venous reflux in symptom-free vascular surgeons. *J Vasc Surg* 1995;22(2):150–154.

15. Labropoulos N, Kokkosis AA, Spentzouris G, et al. The distribution and significance of varicosities in the saphenous trunks. *J Vasc Surg* 2010;51(1):96–103.

16. Tsai S, Dubovoy A, Wainess R, et al. Severe chronic venous insufficiency: magnitude of the problem and consequences. *Ann Vasc Surg* 2005;19(5):705–711.

17. Van den Oever R, Hepp B, Debbaut B, et al. Socio-economic impact of chronic venous insufficiency. An underestimated public health problem. *Int Angiol* 1998;17(3):161–167.

18. Ruckley CV. Socioeconomic impact of chronic venous insufficiency and leg ulcers. *Angiology* 1997;48(1):67–69.

19. Labropoulos N, Giannoukas AD, Delis K, et al. Where does venous reflux start? *J Vasc Surg* 1997;26(5):736–742.

20. Obermayer A, Garzon K. Identifying the source of superficial reflux in venous leg ulcers using duplex ultrasound. *J Vasc Surg* 2010;52(5):1255–1261.

21. Min RJ, Khilnani NM, Zimmet SE. Endovenous laser treatment of saphenous vein reflux: long-term results. *J Vasc Interv Radiol* 2003;14(8):991–996.

22. Cappelli M, Molino Lova R, Ermini S, et al. Comparison between the CHIVA cure and stripping in the treatment of varicose veins of the legs: follow-up of 3 years [in French]. *J Mal Vasc* 1996;21(1):40–46.

23. Escribano JM, Juan J, Bofill R, et al. Durability of reflux-elimination by a minimal invasive CHIVA procedure on patients with varicose veins. A 3-year prospective case study. *Eur J Vasc Endovasc Surg* 2003;25(2):159–163.

24. Zamboni P, Escribano JM. Regarding 'reflux elimination without any ablation or disconnection of the saphenous vein. A haemodynamic model for venous surgery' and 'durability of reflux-elimination by a minimal invasive CHIVA procedure on patients with varicose veins. A 3-year prospective case study'. *Eur J Vasc Endovasc Surg* 2004;28(5):567.

25. Criado E, Juan J, Fontcuberta J, et al. Haemodynamic surgery for varicose veins: rationale, and anatomic and haemodynamic basis [review article]. *Phlebology* 2003;18(4):158–166.

26. Criado E, Lujan S, Izquierdo L, et al. Conservative hemodynamic surgery for varicose veins. *Semin Vasc Surg* 2002;15(1):27–33.

27. Franceschi C. *Theory and Practice of the Conservative Haemodynamic Cure of Incompetent and Varicose Veins in Ambulatory Patients.* Precy-sous-Thil, France: Editions de l'Armancon; 1993.

28. Cappelli M, Lova RM, Ermini S, et al. Ambulatory conservative hemodynamic management of varicose veins: critical analysis of results at 3 years. *Ann Vasc Surg* 2000;14(4):376–384.

29. Carpentier PH, Poulain C, Fabry R, et al. Ascribing leg symptoms to chronic venous disorders: the construction of a diagnostic score. *J Vasc Surg* 2007;46(5):991–996.

30. Bradbury A, Evans CJ, Allan P, et al. The relationship between lower limb symptoms and superficial and deep venous reflux on duplex ultrasonography: The Edinburgh Vein Study. *J Vasc Surg* 2000;32(5):921–931.

31. Delis KT, Bountouroglou D, Mansfield AO. Venous claudication in iliofemoral thrombosis: long-term effects on venous hemodynamics, clinical status, and quality of life. *Ann Surg* 2004;239(1):118–126.

32. Allegra C, Antignani PL, Bergan JJ, et al. The "C" of CEAP: suggested definitions and refinements: an International Union of Phlebology conference of experts. *J Vasc Surg* 2003;37(1):129–131.

33. Baker SR, Stacey MC, Jopp-McKay AG, et al. Epidemiology of chronic venous ulcers. *Br J Surg* 1991;78(7):864–867.

34. Gohel MS, Taylor M, Earnshaw JJ, et al. Risk factors for delayed healing and recurrence of chronic venous leg ulcers—an analysis of 1324 legs. *Eur J Vasc Endovasc Surg* 2005;29(1):74–77.

35. Jeanneret C, Labs KH, Aschwanden M, et al. Venous cross-sectional area: measured or calculated? [in German]. *Ultraschall Med* 2000;21(1):16–19.

36. Welch HJ, Young CM, Semegran AB, et al. Duplex assessment of venous reflux and chronic venous insufficiency: the significance of deep venous reflux. *J Vasc Surg* 1996;24(5):755–762.

37. Yamaki T, Nozaki M, Sakurai H, et al. Advanced chronic venous insufficiency is associated with increased calf muscle deoxygenation. *Eur J Vasc Endovasc Surg* 2010;39(6):787–794.

38. Iafrati MD, Welch H, O'Donnell TF, et al. Correlation of venous noninvasive tests with the Society for Vascular Surgery/International Society for Cardiovascular Surgery clinical classification of chronic venous insufficiency. *J Vasc Surg* 1994;19(6):1001–1007.

39. Rutherford RB, Padberg FT Jr, Comerota AJ, et al. Venous severity scoring: an adjunct to venous outcome assessment. *J Vasc Surg* 2000;31(6):1307–1312.

40. Porter JM, Moneta GL. Reporting standards in venous disease: an update. International Consensus Committee on Chronic Venous Disease. *J Vasc Surg* 1995;21(4):635–645.

41. Vasquez MA, Munschauer CE. Venous Clinical Severity Score and quality-of-life assessment tools: application to vein practice. *Phlebology* 2008;23(6):259–275.

42. Kakkos SK, Rivera MA, Matsagas MI, et al. Validation of the new venous severity scoring system in varicose vein surgery. *J Vasc Surg* 2003;38(2):224–228.

43. Ricci MA, Emmerich J, Callas PW, et al. Evaluating chronic venous disease with a new venous severity scoring system. *J Vasc Surg* 2003;38(5):909–915.

44. Vasquez MA, Rabe E, McLafferty RB, et al. Revision of the venous clinical severity score: venous outcomes consensus statement: special communication of the American Venous Forum Ad Hoc Outcomes Working Group. *J Vasc Surg* 2010;52(5):1387–1396.

45. Meissner MH, Natiello C, Nicholls SC. Performance characteristics of the venous clinical severity score. *J Vasc Surg* 2002;36(5):889–895.

46. Kim YW, Lee BB, Cho JH, et al. Haemodynamic and clinical assessment of lateral marginal vein excision in patients with a predominantly venous malformation of the lower extremity. *Eur J Vasc Endovasc Surg* 2007;33(1):122–127.

47. Rasmussen LH, Bjoern L, Lawaetz M, et al. Randomized trial comparing endovenous laser ablation of the great saphenous vein with high ligation and stripping in patients with varicose veins: short-term results. *J Vasc Surg* 2007;46(2):308–315. Epub 2007 Jun 27.

48. Saarinen JP, Heikkinen MA, Rasku K, et al. Clinical and hemodynamical findings in legs with previous surgery of the great saphenous vein: role of the small saphenous vein. *J Cardiovasc Surg (Torino)* 2007;48(4):485–489.

49. Vasquez MA, Wang J, Mahathanaruk M, et al. The utility of the Venous Clinical Severity Score in 682 limbs treated by radiofrequency saphenous vein ablation. *J Vasc Surg* 2007;45(5):1008–1014; discussion 1015.

50. Krieger E, van Der Loo B, Amann-Vesti BR, et al. C-reactive protein and red cell aggregation correlate with late venous function after acute deep venous thrombosis. *J Vasc Surg* 2004;40(4):644–649.

51. Gillet JL, Perrin MR, Allaert FA. Clinical presentation and venous severity scoring of patients with extended deep axial venous reflux. *J Vasc Surg* 2006;44(3):588–594.

52. Gonzalez-Zeh R, Armisen R, Barahona S. Endovenous laser and echoguided foam ablation in great saphenous vein reflux: one year follow up results. *J Vasc Surg* 2008;17:17.

53. Mekako AI, Hatfield J, Bryce J, et al. A nonrandomised controlled trial of endovenous laser therapy and surgery in the treatment of varicose veins. *Ann Vasc Surg* 2006;20(4):451–457.

54. Engelhorn CA, Engelhorn AL, Cassou MF, et al. Patterns of saphenous reflux in women with primary varicose veins. *J Vasc Surg* 2005;41(4):645–651.

55. Garcia-Gimeno M, Rodriguez-Camarero S, Tagarro-Villalba S, et al. Duplex mapping of 2036 primary varicose veins. *J Vasc Surg* 2009;49(3):681–689.

56. Albanese AR, Albanese AM, Albanese EF. Lateral subdermic varicose vein system of the legs. Its surgical treatment by the chiseling tube method. *Vasc Surg* 1969;3(2):81–89.

57. Labropoulos N, Tassiopoulos AK, Bhatti AF, et al. Development of reflux in the perforator veins in limbs with primary venous disease. *J Vasc Surg* 2006;43(3):558–562.

58. Labropoulos N, Tassiopoulos AK, Kang SS, et al. Prevalence of deep venous reflux in patients with primary superficial vein incompetence. *J Vasc Surg* 2000;32(4):663–668.

59. Marston WA, Brabham VW, Mendes R, et al. The importance of deep venous reflux velocity as a determinant of outcome in patients with combined superficial and deep venous reflux treated with endovenous saphenous ablation. *J Vasc Surg* 2008;48(2):400–405; discussion 405–406.

60. Ganguli S, Tham JC, Janne d'Othee BM. Establishing an outpatient clinic for minimally invasive vein care. *AJR Am J Roentgenol* 2007;188(6):1506–1511.

61. Bush RG, Hammond K. Treatment of incompetent vein of Giacomini (thigh extension branch). *Ann Vasc Surg* 2007;21(2):245–248.

62. Corbett CR, McIrvine AJ, Aston NO, et al. The use of varicography to identify the sources of incompetence in recurrent varicose veins. *Ann R Coll Surg Engl* 1984;66(6):412–415.

63. Jiang P, van Rij AM, Christie R, et al. Recurrent varicose veins: patterns of reflux and clinical severity. *Cardiovasc Surg* 1999;7(3):332–339.

64. Janne d'Othee B, Walker TG, Kalva SP, et al. Endovenous laser ablation of the small saphenous vein sparing the saphenopopliteal junction. *Cardiovasc Intervent Radiol* 2010;33(4):766–771.

65. Yilmaz S, Ceken K, Alparslan A, et al. Endovenous laser ablation for saphenous vein insufficiency: immediate and short-term results of our first 60 procedures. *Diagn Interv Radiol* 2007;13(3):156–163.

66. Kontothanassis D, Di Mitri R, Ferrari Ruffino S, et al. Endovenous laser treatment of the small saphenous vein. *J Vasc Surg* 2009;49(4):973–979.e1.

67. Labropoulos N, Giannoukas AD, Delis K, et al. The impact of isolated lesser saphenous vein system incompetence on clinical signs and symptoms of chronic venous disease. *J Vasc Surg* 2000;32(5):954–960.

68. Nwaejike N, Srodon PD, Kyriakides C. Endovenous laser ablation for short saphenous vein incompetence. *Ann Vasc Surg* 2008;9:9.

69. Proebstle TM, Gul D, Kargl A, et al. Endovenous laser treatment of the lesser saphenous vein with a 940–nm diode laser: early results. *Dermatol Surg* 2003;29(4):357–361.

70. Theivacumar NS, Beale RJ, Mavor AI, et al. Initial experience in endovenous laser ablation (EVLA) of varicose veins due to small saphenous vein reflux. *Eur J Vasc Endovasc Surg* 2007;33(5):614–618.

71. Labropoulos N, Delis K, Mansour MA, et al. Prevalence and clinical significance of posterolateral thigh perforator vein incompetence. *J Vasc Surg* 1997;26(5):743–748.

CHAPTER 96

Chronic Venous Insufficiency and Varicose Veins: Imaging Evaluation and Indications for Intervention

BERTRAND JANNE D'OTHÉE and ZIV J. HASKAL

AVAILABLE IMAGING MODALITIES AND THEIR RELATIVE ROLES

Clinical examination alone is notoriously insufficient to evaluate patients with chronic venous insufficiency (CVI)[1] and, therefore, additional imaging/functional assessments are required. Until the advent of duplex ultrasonography (US) in the late 1980s, ascending phlebography (combined with varicography when necessary) and descending phlebography were the reference methods to assess varicose veins, sources of reflux, and presence of obstruction. All of them could be performed on the standing patient but required venipuncture and intravenous injection of iodinated contrast (with need to flush the vein with normal saline at the end of the examination to prevent phlebitis) and X-rays. For ascending phlebography, slow hand injection of iodinated contrast in a dorsal foot vein was performed,[2] first with tourniquets around the ankle and knee to opacify the deep veins alone, and then after release of the tourniquets to opacify both the superficial and deep veins. By comparison of venographic images obtained in similar projections with and without tourniquets, one could differentiate between superficial and deep veins and locate lesions and anomalies. Also, incompetent perforators and the dependent superficial veins they supplied could be readily identified at the initial, with-tourniquet phase when opacified because these veins were normally not seen at this early phase. When a clinically visible or palpable varicosity was not seen on ascending phlebography, a varicography[3-5] had to be performed, which consisted of direct puncture of the varix and iodinated contrast injection; the venograms hereby obtained demonstrated the communications between the varix and the major veins, hence allowing identification of the source(s) of reflux.

Similar to ascending phlebography, other imaging techniques, such as computed tomography (CT) and magnetic resonance imaging (MRI) with contrast injection in the foot have been used in the evaluation of varicose veins.[6,7] Potential advantages of these techniques include the rapidity of image acquisition with optimized protocols, the three-dimensional imaging capability (which might also be useful for planning of therapeutic interventions), and the incidental discovery of other diseases and allowing detection of perforating veins (PVs) as small as 1 mm, which remain difficult to detect with duplex US.[8] Probably the main indication for the use of these cross-sectional imaging techniques so far is the evaluation of abdominopelvic sources of reflux and demonstration of their communication with the leg varicosities, such as in pelvic congestion syndrome. Although such communications represent the only cause of reflux (i.e., in the absence of saphenous and perforator incompetence in the legs) in only 10% of leg varicosities, they may involve a variety of pathways including vulvoperineal varicosities (83%), round ligament varicosities (5%), persistent sciatic vein incompetence (5%), or others.[7] Additionally, MRI with phase contrast acquisition sequences may allow to measure velocity and blood flow, but the practicality, reliability/accuracy, and clinical significance of these measurements during compression maneuvers will have to be established. However, the role of CT and MRI has remained limited so far in routine clinical practice. Probably the main hindrance so far to their more widespread use is the difficulty to study the patient in orthostatism. This may be somewhat circumvented with use of the "semisupine position"[6] or completely avoided with orthostatic electron-beam CT, but the latter still carries the well-known drawbacks of ionizing radiation, potential for contrast reaction, and renal risks. Current MRI machines only allow small parts/organs to be positioned vertically; however, developing MRI machines that allow leg and abdominopelvic imaging would likely be extremely useful not only for evaluating complex cases of CVI in the legs, but also for the workup of patients with pelvic congestion syndrome (currently imaged with transvaginal duplex ultrasound during Valsalva maneuvers or by phlebography).

For all these reasons, duplex US has now become the reference method for the pretreatment evaluation of CVI.[9] Before the use of duplex US scanning became widespread, hand-held continuous wave Doppler examination had been suggested as an in-office screening tool because it misses great saphenous vein (GSV) or small saphenous vein (SSV) incompetence in no more than 11% of legs, and these false negatives represent cases with short-duration and low-velocity reflux of dubious clinical importance.[10-14] However, with growing use of duplex US and further studies showing less favorable results from hand-held devices,[15-17] there remains less incentive today in rich countries to forego duplex US and risk inappropriate, misguided treatment.

Data on the diagnostic accuracy of duplex US for the detection of venous reflux in the lower extremities are

Table 96.1

Diagnostic accuracy of duplex ultrasonography in the detection of venous reflux

#	Authors	Journal	Year	Number of patients	Number of limbs	SE (%)	SP (%)	Accuracy (%)	Gold standard
1	Szendro et al.[18]	J Vasc Surg	1986			84	88		Ambulatory venous pressure measurements
2	Rosfors et al.[30]	Angiology	1990	21	23			65	Descending phlebography
3	Gongolo et al.[19]	Radiol Med	1991	66		92	90		Descending phlebography
4	Masuda and Kistner[20]	Am J Surg	1992		25	90	84	88	Descending phlebography
5	Neglen and Raju[21]	J Vasc Surg	1992	32	56				Descending phlebography
6	Welch et al.[22]	J Vasc Surg	1992		28	90	94	93	Descending phlebography
7	Baker et al.[28]	Lancet	1993	52	98				Descending phlebography
8	Bohler et al.[23]	Thromb Haemost	1995	100	100			92	Ascending phlebography
9	Evers and Wuppermann[24]	Ultraschall Med	1995		120	93	95		Phlebography
10	Jing et al.[25]	Zhonghua Wai Ke Za Zhi	1995		40	92	100	94	
11	Magnusson et al.[29]	Eur J vasc Endovasc Surg	1995	44	56			74	Descending phlebography
12	Phillips et al[32]	Clin Radiol	1995	68	93	94			Ascending phlebography and varicography
13	Dixon[33]	Australas Radiol	1996			98	95		Clinical judgment of vascular surgeons
14	Depalma et al.[26]	J Vasc Surg	2000	30		95	100		Ascending and descending phlebography
15	Yamamoto et al.[27]	J Vasc Surg	2002	175	304	88	75		Surgical findings

SE, sensitivity; SP, specificity.

limited. Table 96.1 summarizes the findings of 15 studies[18–33] including a total of 943 limbs in 588 patients pooled over 16 years. Sensitivity values are in the 84% to 98% range, specificities in the 75% to 100% range, and accuracy values between 65% and 94%. Besides being less invasive, duplex US also offers the additional advantage over phlebography that it allows diagnosing isolated lower extremity valvular insufficiency (e.g., distal segmental reflux in the absence of more proximal incompetence).[30] Descending phlebography also underestimates reflux in the lower leg compared with duplex scanning.[28]

TECHNIQUE OF DUPLEX ULTRASONOGRAPHY FOR THE STUDY OF CHRONIC VENOUS INSUFFICIENCY

The duplex US examination is both (a) crucial clinically and (b) challenging technically. (a) Without a proper mapping of the flow circuit(s) and pathway(s) of reflux, treatment will be misguided and patients will experience symptom recurrence or worsening.[34] This examination is the very first step of the overall treatment plan and the most important one. (b) Additionally, it can be a very complex exam to perform, not only because of the difficulties of not moving the transducer while performing the compression maneuvers and of physiologic variations that may slightly influence flow measurements,[35] but also because of the frequent variability in the anatomy of leg veins. Not only are there a lot of anatomic variations between individuals, but also more than 90% of people have different venous anatomy between their right and left legs (Labropoulos)[37]. Superimposed onto these difficulties comes the investigational effort of finding out what is (are) the path(s) of reflux in a given patient. Due to this variability and complexity, there is no one best protocol for the examination: each study should be tailored to the individual patient and aimed at addressing the specific location of the symptoms and varicosities. A suggested protocol is shown in Table 96.2 for reference. The examination should answer the relevant questions (i.e., those that may change management) and the operator should at all times keep in mind what (s)he is searching for and why. For example, in a patient with obvious varicosities, simply answering that "there is no saphenous reflux" is not acceptable: in such case, another source of reflux (e.g., incompetent perforator) should be searched for and identified.

Morphology: Grayscale Ultrasonography and Its Limitations

The GSV[36] has a normal diameter of 4 mm or less. It is contained within the superficial fascia, which splits into a superficial and a deep layer as it surrounds the GSV. Therefore, the GSV may remain normal in size despite being incompetent and

Table 96.2

Suggested Protocol for Duplex Ultrasonography of Chronic Venous Insufficiency (Spider Veins, Varicose Veins, and Venous Stasis Ulcers)

1. **Deep veins study (part 1: patency):** patient supine
   Patent lumen: study patency from common femoral to popliteal vein by compressibility maneuvers under grayscale US

2. **Superficial veins study: patient standing;** for both greater (GSV) and small (SSV) saphenous veins, explore patency/anatomy and function

   Morphologic study (grayscale ultrasound)
   - Document vein patency (compressibility)
   - Measure maximal diameter on axial transverse images
   - Measure minimal depth: only needed if superficial vein lies <1 cm from the skin, between groin and upper calf (risk of skin burn during endovenous thermal ablation)
   - Document tortuosity or static valves that may hinder cranial passage of endovenous catheter
   - Search for any superficial side branch of the GSV (or SSV) starting within 10 cm of the saphenofemoral junction (or saphenopopliteal junction, respectively) and following a descending course; if present, study these branches the same way as the saphenous vein trunk (i.e., document patency, diameter, depth, tortuosity, and presence/absence of reflux)

   Incompetence study (duplex ultrasound)
   - Search for reflux in the saphenous veins and their relevant branches (e.g., cranial descending side branches, any enlarged perforator, or an enlarged SIEV); if reflux is detected, quantify it in terms of speed (more relevant than duration)
   - If no reflux found by compression maneuvers during spectral Doppler examination, try Valsalva maneuvers, or if vein of interest is large (10 mm diameter or more), try either maneuver during real-time grayscale US examination (with high gain setting)
   - If an enlarged pelviperineal varix (i.e., diameter >4–5 mm) is found, explore for reflux and document level of its connection to GSV territory relative to the saphenofemoral junction (e.g., superficial inferior epigastric vein)

3. **Perforating veins study:** patient standing; explore patency/anatomy and function
   - Document any enlarged perforator (i.e., >3–4 mm in diameter), whether connected to a truncal saphenous vein or to a nonsaphenous superficial varicosity: study patency, diameter, position relative to a fixed anatomic landmark (e.g., 20 cm above medial malleolus), and incompetence during compression maneuvers
   - If perforator is large and easily visible by grayscale US, use spectral Doppler to detect reflux by placing Doppler gate in this perforator; otherwise, examine a superficial vein segment in the more caudal, dependent varicosity (especially if "blow-out" appearance of superficial varicosity); if small perforator is difficult to see by grayscale US, may also image it by color Doppler imaging while performing distal compression maneuvers
   - Perforator study is particularly important in cases where symptoms/signs cannot be explained (e.g., absent saphenous reflux despite visible, symptomatic varicosities; or residual symptoms and reflux despite prior successful endovenous thermal ablation of incompetent saphenous vein)

4. **Deep veins study (part 2: incompetence):** patient standing
   Reflux: search for reflux in popliteal vein by using duplex US; if present, investigate farther proximally as well

carrying significant reflux to tributaries that become enlarged as soon as they exit the superficial fascia.[36] In fact, most GSVs and SSVs show mild focal dilatations rather than larger varicosities (which have <5% prevalence in each of CEAP [Clinical, Etiology, Anatomy, Pathophysiology] classes 2 to 6), and large varicosities are significantly more common in tributary and accessory veins than in the saphenous trunks.[37] Therefore, one should not assume that a normal-sized GSV is competent but should instead search for reflux at multiple levels before drawing such conclusion.

The SSV has a normal diameter of 3 mm or less.[36] Its cranial end is quite variable: it may connect directly with the popliteal vein in the popliteal fossa or more cranially with the superficial femoral vein in the thigh, and it can also end as a venous network rather than a single trunk.

Although the diameter of incompetent PVs is larger than that of competent PVs by both duplex US and intraoperative findings, diameter measurement alone cannot completely distinguish competent from incompetent PVs.[27]

Grayscale examination remains, however, a crucial element of the examination as the best criterion to rule out deep venous thrombosis (DVT) and obstruction is the absence of complete luminal compressibility.

General Principles of Spectral Doppler Examination Technique

To search for reflux, duplex US (which combines grayscale imaging and color and spectral Doppler techniques) is the functional and key component of the examination. The spectral Doppler signal sample must be obtained with the *imaging plane* aligned with the vessel longitudinal axis (not transverse), without compressing the vein with the transducer.

The *Doppler axis line* should be oriented obliquely relative to the skin surface, in the direction of the vessel, so that the angle between the vessel and the Doppler axis line is always acute.

The *gate* in which the Doppler signal is sampled is then properly positioned in the vessel and must be smaller than the vessel lumen: too small a gate will miss part of the Doppler signal, but too large a gate will include the vein walls and create corresponding artifacts.

The *Doppler angle* is then adjusted along the longitudinal axis of the vein to obtain an angle between 30 and 60 degrees; the Doppler axis line and the Doppler angle line should go in the same direction, which is the same direction as the vessel (i.e., the angle between both lines should be between 0 and <90 degrees).

The *Doppler gain* should be adjusted to have a tiny bit of grainy background noise superimposed onto the Doppler spectral waveform (too little noise will miss some of the Doppler signal and result in insufficient information contained in the waveform; too much noise will hide the waveform).

Color Doppler imaging is a useful adjunct but does not replace the spectral waveforms, which allow easier measurement of reflux duration. Also, color Doppler provides only an average estimate of velocity per pixel rather than the actual peak velocities. Lastly, spectral Doppler waveform analysis demonstrates longer reflux duration (mean ± SEM = 2.5 seconds ± 0.2) than that observed with color Doppler US (on average 0.7 second shorter, in the case of popliteal vein reflux, $p < .001$) in limbs with CVI.[38]

Functional Assessment with Duplex Ultrasonography: Criteria and Maneuvers to Detect Reflux

Unless an automatic inflation cuff is used, two operators are typically needed for the examination: one handling the ultrasound probe and ultrasound console, the other one performing the compression maneuvers. Presence of the interventionist who will performing the procedure is helpful to optimize the study performance and interpretation.

The duplex US evaluation of the patient with suspected or overt CVI can be described in two steps. First, the patient is examined supine to rule out the presence of deep venous obstruction. The common, superficial, and deep femoral veins and the popliteal vein are interrogated with grayscale US and compression maneuvers and color and spectral Doppler techniques.

Second, the patient is placed in orthostatism[2] with a safety belt around the abdomen and holding by hand a fixed point because of the non-negligible risk of patient fall during examinations on standing patients. The patient is instructed to relax and let drop the leg being studied and to bear his/her body weight on the contralateral leg.[36] This step is aimed at studying the superficial veins and detecting reflux in the superficial, deep, and perforating veins. The search for reflux should be performed with spectral Doppler waveform analysis rather than that with color Doppler US.[38] Normal valve closure time is equal or less than 0.5 second in the superficial veins and deep calf veins, 350 milliseconds in the PVs, and 1 second in the femoropopliteal veins.[39]

How to Study Superficial Veins' Function

In general, reflux lasting between 0.5 and 1 second (or perhaps 2 seconds) should be considered of borderline significance and might benefit from later clinical and duplex US follow-up rather than immediate intervention. Reflux that lasts for more than 1 second is considered hemodynamically significant[20,36] and deserves consideration for treatment. Reflux duration is a good parameter for identifying the presence of reflux, but not for quantifying it because descriptions of significant reflux as severe (>6 seconds), moderate (2 to 6 seconds), or mild (1 to 2 seconds) have limited clinical relevance. The saphenous vein diameter[40] (or cross-sectional area[41]), velocity,[42] and flow[40] (which, given the existence of the relation: flow = cross-sectional area × velocity, are all correlated among each other) are associated with the clinical severity on the CEAP classification, but neither of these variables is well correlated with duration of reflux. Hence, velocity and peak flow during reflux maneuvers are better parameters for evaluating reflux intensity than reflux duration because they are correlated with GSV dilatation/alterations and are associated with the disease's clinical severity.[40]

There are at least three techniques that can demonstrate reflux on duplex US, and their relative roles have yet to be fully investigated.[20,38,43] Each of them can yield positive results in the presence or absence of positivity of the other techniques. The most common—and probably the most sensitive—approach is peripheral compression maneuver (FIGURE 96.1A): the US transducer is positioned on the venous segment of interest, brief compression and release of the muscles located peripheral (i.e., distal) to that segment is applied, and the spectral Doppler waveform is analyzed. Normal tracings show no—or at most a very brief—protodiastolic flow reversal. Pathologic reflux is defined as above, whenever it lasts for more than 0.5 (or 1 to 2) second. Despite its apparent simplicity, the maneuver can be quite difficult to perform due to patient and/or transducer motion. Although automated cuff inflation systems and manual compression may be similarly useful in many patients, the evidence for this is limited[38,44] by small sample sizes and number of studies available and even contradicted by another study. The latter showed that the pneumatic cuff and the manual compression methods can induce equal peak velocities during the compression phase (median peak antegrade flow speed = 86 cm/second). The coefficient of variation for peak antegrade velocity in the superficial veins is significantly higher with the manual method (16.8%) than with the pneumatic cuff method (9.5%, $p < .001$). The values of sensitivity and specificity are 85% and 100%, respectively, for manual compression, and 78% and 100%, respectively, for the pneumatic cuff method.[45] Our preference is to use manual compression because it is deemed to allow faster compression and decompression, which may help avoid false negative results (missed reflux). Testing the competence of the saphenofemoral junction should be performed with the transducer on the groin while compression maneuvers are performed in the distal thigh or in the calf. Of note, reflux is more prominent and more easily detectable when the distance between the proximal transducer and the distal compression maneuver increases; that is, reflux in the GSV appears worse when compression is applied on the medial calf than on the medial thigh (because the former maneuver displaces a larger column of blood in the

vein than the latter). Methods that use thigh compression (as opposed to calf compression) or supine (vs. standing) position are less capable of discriminating normal limbs from limbs with CVI. Standing calf compression provides the greatest rates of sensitivity (91%), specificity (100%), and accuracy (95%).[38] Additionally, there is another advantage to leave more distance between the site of compression and the transducer: it avoids the transmission of the mechanical displacement of adjacent soft tissue (created during the compression maneuver) into the imaged area, and this transmission can cause low-frequency artifacts on the spectral Doppler waveforms.

A second technique to detect venous reflux consists of observing the spectral Doppler waveform in the venous segment of interest and asking the patient to perform deep inspiration and/or Valsalva maneuvers. In the author's experience, this appears much less sensitive overall than the manual compression technique but may in some cases show significant reflux despite negative manual compression maneuvers. The duration of reflux observed by this second technique is typically shorter than that from the manual compression technique (FIGURE 96.1B). The Valsalva maneuver can detect valvular incompetence only in the most central portions of the venous tree, such as the common femoral veins, but becomes less sensitive more distally toward the calf veins.[46]

The third technique (FIGURE 96.1C) uses real-time US only rather than spectral Doppler tracings. After increasing the overall grayscale gain, the operator observes the screen looking for

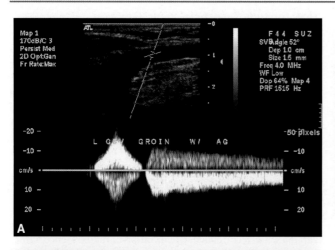
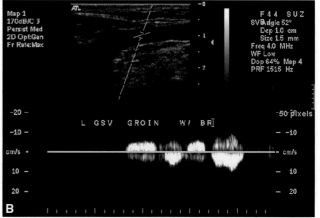
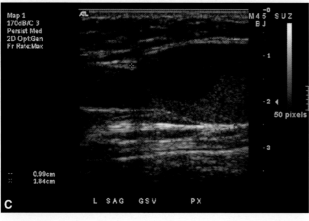

FIGURE 96.1 Diagnosis of venous reflux on duplex ultrasonography.

to-and-fro motion of the intraluminal echoes in the venous segment explored. This technique appears particularly useful to show reflux in markedly enlarged saphenous veins (>10 mm in diameter), especially when the first two methods are negative. In these patients with very large saphenous veins and varicose tributaries, the first two techniques may occasionally be falsely negative, which is inconsistent with the overall clinical picture and should not be confused with the absence of reflux. This technique could in theory be used with color Doppler as well, but this appears less useful than grayscale US.

How to Study Perforators' Function

The same principles apply to the evaluation of PVs. These veins are considered enlarged when their diameter is 3 to 4 mm or larger, but again, the absence of dilatation does not mean that the vein remains competent.

1. If the perforator is large and easily visible by grayscale US, one can use the spectral Doppler technique and place the Doppler gate in a straight segment of the perforator if available; otherwise, one can choose a spot in the dependent varicosity below. The maneuvers are otherwise similar as above: brief compression and rapid release distally to the transducer.
2. If the perforator is small, it may be difficult to see on grayscale images and then the best way to see and image them is to use color Doppler imaging while doing distal compression maneuvers.

How to Study Deep Veins' Function

Popliteal vein reflux lasting for more than 1 second after release of distal compression maneuver has been shown to be well correlated with the clinical severity of disease (Labropoulos)[39]. To search for popliteal vein reflux, brief manual compression and rapid release of pressure (total duration for both: <1 second) on the proximal or mid calf of the standing patient while the transducer is placed on the popliteal vein more proximally is performed. Popliteal reflux is usually more prominent (and easier to detect) when calf compression is applied in the anteroposterior direction rather than from side to side.

Special Cases: When Functional Assessment with Duplex Ultrasonography Is More Complex

The search for incompetent perforators in an initial simple study is arguably unnecessary if the examination has already answered all questions by demonstrating pathway(s) of reflux that explain all symptoms and visible varicosities. But there are specific situations in which the exploration of perforator competence is important.

1. Unexplained varicosities: If the patient has symptomatic and/or visible varicose veins in territories that do not appear directly connected to an incompetent GSV or SSV, one has to search for possible incompetent perforator(s) that may explain the patient's symptoms and/or visible varicosities. Of note, this indication is similar to the reason for which varicography used to be performed and when the standard method (ascending phlebography) did not demonstrate GSV or SSV reflux, direct puncture of these "unexplained varicosities" and varicography allowed to

visualize their connection with the normal venous network of the leg.
2. Change in caliber of a superficial vein at and below its connection with a perforator: If a large perforator is incidentally found to be connected to the GSV or SSV, it often represents only a side branch that drains the reflux from the incompetent GSV or SSV back into the deep venous system; in this case, the perforator drains antegradely from the superficial to the deep veins and is enlarged only because of overflow. Even if reflux is present in this perforator, this may be transient and caused by the overflow alone. This perforator is likely to recover normal caliber and function after successful closure of the superficial incompetent vein, and there is usually no need to test this perforator for reflux during the initial duplex US evaluation. Sometimes, however, an enlarged perforator may also represent an additional source of reflux into an already incompetent truncal vein (i.e., GSV or SSV). In such cases, the incompetent saphenous vein will typically enlarge further at and below the point where it connects to the incompetent perforator as a result of the additional source of reflux. In that case, one needs to test this perforator for reflux, obviously because it changes the treatment plan: this patient will require closure not only of the saphenous vein but also of the incompetent perforator.
3. After prior successful endovenous ablation of the GSV or SSV (and in the absence of detectable recanalization/reopening of the ablated vein), new or recurrent or persistent symptoms may occur and are typically caused by residual or new reflux coming from an incompetent perforator.

Is This Vein Suitable for Endovenous Thermal Ablation and/or Sclerotherapy?

Typical anatomic reasons why these therapies may be contraindicated include superficial location and excessive tortuosity of the incompetent vein to treat. If the GSV comes close to the skin (i.e., <1 cm depth), the risk of skin burn increases and endovenous thermal ablation (EVTA) may be contraindicated. However, this may be modulated during the tumescent anesthesia phase of the procedure by applying additional volume of tumescent fluid, which pushes the saphenous vein to be treated down deeper, further away from the skin. We have treated with endovenous laser ablation superficial venous segments that were immediately adjacent to the skin as long as they could be separated enough (i.e., at least 5 mm apart) from the skin during tumescent anesthesia. In these situations, the only real limitation is the rare cases where the vein is actually adherent to the skin and cannot be forced deeper by the tumescent anesthesia. In such cases, one can spare the superficial segment during ablation and decrease the number of joules given per centimeter near that segment.

The definition of excessive tortuosity of a saphenous vein segment to treat is highly variable and depends on the setting in which the procedure is performed. In a hospital setting with an angiographic room and contrast venographic capabilities, and more catheters and wires available, one can pass some difficult tortuosities that would be impossible to do in an office setting with limited catheters/wires choices available and no imaging other than US. Because of the reimbursement structure for EVTA in the United States, most of these procedures are performed in an office setting. Tortuosity, even minor, can then become a significant issue intraprocedurally. We do not use any specific rule other than having the interventional radiologist present during the initial duplex US evaluation and subjectively assess whether he or she feels the tortuosity can be passed with the materials available during the future procedure. If that fails, an alternative is to obtain a second venous access just cranial to the tortuous turn and perform ablations of two separate segments (as opposed to one continuous).

One should pay attention to any descending superficial venous side branches that connect to the proximal GSV in the groin or within 10 cm of the saphenofemoral junction: if such descending side branches are present, it is important to perform the same morphologic and functional study of these veins as that done for the GSV because these side branches may also carry reflux, or may become incompetent later, after successful closure of the incompetent GSV. Among these descending side branches, the two main ones are the anterior thigh tributary (ATT) and, slightly less commonly, the posteromedial thigh tributary (PMT). Both of these can vary in length, from a few centimeters only up to the entire length of the thigh. A superficial vein that is as small as 2 to 3 mm in diameter can be accessed percutaneously and treated in most cases by experienced operators; below that diameter, the vein is too small to accommodate 5 French micropuncture sheaths.

▌ INDICATIONS FOR INTERVENTION

Indications for treatment include *symptoms* from uncomplicated varicose veins and complications from varicose vein disease. Uncomplicated varicose veins are associated with a variety of symptoms: pain/aching, fatigue/heaviness, itching/burning sensation, leg cramps, calf/ankle swelling, restless legs,[47,48] and leg warmth. Clinical symptoms associated with CVI may vary with the venous system involved (superficial or deep, or both).[49]

Complications include blood stasis in the varicosities with subsequent superficial phlebitis and its complications, progression of disease, and—rarely—variceal bleeding. Variceal bleeding may lead to slow but continuous exsanguinations and eventually death by hemorrhagic shock; a classical presentation is that of an old patient waking up in the middle of the night to go to the bathroom, inadvertently hitting a leg varix, which starts bleeding and not noticing it, and going back to bed where the bleeding may continue for hours.

Although imperfect, there is some correlation between symptomatic severity and extent of venous reflux as seen by duplex US. The prevalence of primary venous reflux (i.e., in the absence of prior history of superficial or deep venous thrombosis, vein surgery, or sclerotherapy) is 14% in asymptomatic young individuals but raises to 77% in age-matched subjects with prominent but nonvaricose vein, and to 87% in age-matched subjects with clinically apparent varicose veins.[50] In subjects with clinically apparent varicose veins, reflux involving multiple segmental levels, reflux affecting both the greater and lesser saphenous veins, and deep venous reflux are more common (although deep venous reflux remains uncommon, affecting 20% of subjects at most).[50]

Data on the *natural history* of lower extremity varicosities[51] show that, at a median follow-up duration of 19 months, 73% of limbs remain stable, 11% develop worsening clinical stage, and a few percent more develop worsening reflux on duplex US without associated symptomatic progression. Similarly, a prospective longitudinal study with serial duplex US found, over a median observation time of 25 months (range: 9 to 52), no change in 67% of limbs, a change in the superficial veins in 15% of limbs, and a change in both superficial and perforating veins in 18% of limbs.[52] Although useful, these data do not provide long-term information. Secondary chronic venous disease (CVD) progresses faster than primary forms: progression of CVD is more rapid in post-thrombotic limbs when compared with those with primary CVD. The incidence of CVD in normal individuals is small and its progression is slow. Poor prognostic factors for progression to advanced CVD include the combination of reflux and obstruction, ipsilateral recurrent DVT, and multisegmental involvement.[53]

Therefore, the absence of symptomatic worsening does not mean that there is no indication to intervene or at least monitor. A typical example of this, encountered in multiple occasions by the authors, is the middle-aged to older woman who had very symptomatic varicose veins after pregnancies, did not undergo surgical stripping for the next two or three decades thereafter, and now presents with severe varicosities and reflux, sometimes even chronic venous stasis around the ankles, but no longer any complaint of pain because she has "learned to live with them." She now undergoes successful endovenous ablation with dramatic clinical and duplex US improvement, her quality of life improves spectacularly thereafter, and now states that she "did not remember how good life without these varices was" and "had forgotten that the symptoms were still present and bad." This relatively common real-life example might qualify as a particular type of recall bias or of reporting bias. It raises the key question of to what extent the presence and severity of symptoms matter in the decision-making process of intervening or not.

Accordingly, symptoms are not the only indication for treatment of CVI and the decision-making process is in fact much more complex. As seen previously, the absence of symptom complaints from patients does not mean that they are in fact symptomatic and will not benefit from intervention. Complications from varices are probably uncommon, but there are a lack of long-term data about the prevalence of superficial phlebitis or variceal bleeding in untreated patients. In daily clinical practice, patients' clinical presentations are frequently complex because at least three concerns may occur in various combinations that may warrant treatment: *symptoms, reflux, and concerns for future worsening and complications* from the varices. Additionally, a fourth concern is the *unesthetic appearance* of varices, which, although not in itself a medically warranted justification to undergo an invasive intervention, may influence in subtle, untold ways patients' decision to proceed with therapy. This is particularly relevant in the cases of leg varices, a medical condition that is immediately visible to the patient and to others, that usually does not require urgent treatment, that will remain stable for the next 2 years in at least two-thirds of cases, and for which the natural history remains partially unelucidated due to the lack of long-term data. There is a need (a) for acquisition of better long-term data on the natural history of untreated CVI and (b) for the development of decision support systems in this field.

FIGURE 96.2 presents a suggested *algorithm* taking into account these different clinical scenarios. The decision to treat patients who have symptoms suggestive of superficial CVI is usually straightforward, especially when the location of these symptoms matches the territory where reflux can be demonstrated: patients

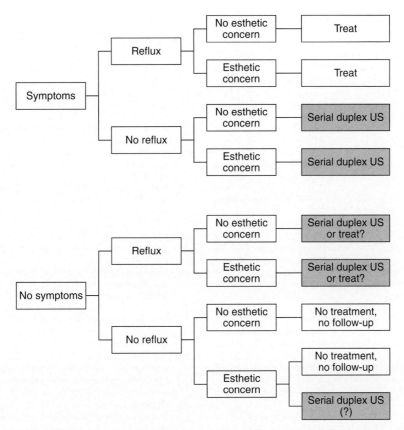

FIGURE 96.2 Suggested algorithm for the management of patients with CVI.

with both symptoms and reflux should be treated, regardless of whether they have an esthetic concern or not. At the other end of the spectrum, patients with no symptoms and no reflux lack a clear medical indication for intervention, regardless of whether they have esthetic concerns or not; typical examples are patients with spider veins alone. However, some symptomatic patients with only spider veins seen in inspection may in fact have significant reflux and deserve treatment, which will relieve symptoms. Hence symptomatic patients should at least undergo duplex US testing in search of reflux, even if they present with spider veins alone, and should not be dismissed as "cosmetic concern only."

When symptomatic varicose veins are present but no reflux can be demonstrated on duplex US, the first question is to rule out a false negative duplex US result. As pointed elsewhere, "Serial duplex US evaluation should probably be viewed as the preferred option for symptomatic patients with a negative initial examination and the presence of risk factors or physical findings suggesting a proximal deep venous obstruction/thrombosis."[54]

Asymptomatic patients with varicose veins and reflux could theoretically represent a false positive duplex US result. However, the repetition of reflux simulation maneuvers under duplex US often allows to confirm or infirm the finding. If reflux is confirmed, it is the authors' belief that these patients may benefit from treatment. The rationale for this is twofold: treatment (a) prevents future worsening of reflux and varices, and (b) may quite often result in spectacular symptomatic improvements in so-called asymptomatic patients, who had "learned to live with" these symptoms and had forgotten that life without them was

possible. But the alternative—watchful monitoring—is perfectly reasonable, too.

FIGURE 96.2 does not address all questions. For example, what is the best approach in a patient with isolated deep venous reflux? Or how to deal with a duplex US examination that shows distal superficial venous reflux but fails to demonstrate the proximal source convincingly: Is it just a false negative finding, and should it be treated? Many such questions are encountered in daily practice.

Lastly, the above considerations did not address in depth the question of *cosmesis*, which itself broadens the scope of the discussion. Traditional medical conception is that unesthetic appearance does not deserve treatment. Many private venous clinics, however, thrive on the performance of purely cosmetic interventions, including the endovenous ablation of large, nontortuous veins on the dorsum of the hands of older women. Whose decision is it: the patient's or the physician's? Current medical practice in the United States recognizes patients' right to decide on their health, but it is the authors' belief that physicians should at the same time strive to keep the system reasonable and avoid nonmedically necessary, purely cosmetic procedures.

▌ REFERENCES

1. Makris SA, Karkos CD, Awad S, et al. An "all-comers" venous duplex scan policy for patients with lower limb varicose veins attending a one-stop vascular clinic: is it justified? *Eur J Vasc Endovasc Surg* 2006;32:718–724.
2. Mahmutyazicioglu K, Gundogdu S, Ozdemir H, et al. Venous reflux: measurement variability due to positional differences [in Turkish]. *Tani Girisim Radyol* 2003;9:471–475.

3. Corbett CR, McIrvine AJ, Aston NO, et al. The use of varicography to identify the sources of incompetence in recurrent varicose veins. *Ann R Coll Surg Engl* 1984;66:412–415.

4. Savolainen H, Toivio I, Mokka R. Recurrent varicose veins—is there a role for varicography? *Ann Chir Gynaecol* 1988;77:70–73.

5. Keeling FP, Lea Thomas M. Varicography in the management of primary varicose veins. *Br J Radiol* 1987;60:235–240.

6. Koizumi J, Horie T, Muro I, et al. Magnetic resonance venography of the lower limb. *Int Angiol* 2007;26:171–182.

7. Jung SC, Lee W, Chung JW, et al. Unusual causes of varicose veins in the lower extremities: CT venographic and Doppler US findings. *Radiographics* 2009;29:525–536.

8. Min SK, Kim SY, Park YJ, et al. Role of three-dimensional computed tomography venography as a powerful navigator for varicose vein surgery. *J Vasc Surg* 2010;51:893–899.

9. Zygmunt J Jr. What is new in duplex scanning of the venous system? *Perspect Vasc Surg Endovasc Ther* 2009;21:94–104.

10. Campbell WB, Niblett PG, Ridler BM, et al. Hand-held Doppler as a screening test in primary varicose veins. *Br J Surg* 1997;84:1541–1543.

11. Darke SG, Vetrivel S, Foy DM, et al. A comparison of duplex scanning and continuous wave Doppler in the assessment of primary and uncomplicated varicose veins. *Eur J Vasc Endovasc Surg* 1997;14:457–461.

12. Kent PJ, Weston MJ. Duplex scanning may be used selectively in patients with primary varicose veins. *Ann R Coll Surg Engl* 1998;80:388–393.

13. Kim J, Richards S, Kent PJ. Clinical examination of varicose veins—a validation study. *Ann R Coll Surg Engl* 2000;82:171–175.

14. Campbell WB, Niblett PG, Peters AS, et al. The clinical effectiveness of hand held Doppler examination for diagnosis of reflux in patients with varicose veins. *Eur J Vasc Endovasc Surg* 2005;30:664–669.

15. Mercer KG, Scott DJ, Berridge DC. Preoperative duplex imaging is required before all operations for primary varicose veins. *Br J Surg* 1998;85:1495–1497.

16. Wills V, Moylan D, Chambers J. The use of routine duplex scanning in the assessment of varicose veins. *Aust N Z J Surg* 1998;68:41–44.

17. Daher A, Jones V, da Silva AF. The role of popliteal vein incompetence in the diagnosis of saphenous-popliteal reflux using continuous wave doppler. *Eur J Vasc Endovasc Surg* 2001;21:350–352.

18. Szendro G, Nicolaides AN, Zukowski AJ, et al. Duplex scanning in the assessment of deep venous incompetence. *J Vasc Surg* 1986;4:237–242.

19. Gongolo A, Giraldi E, Buttazzoni L, et al. Duplex study of primary venous insufficiency of the legs. First results and methodologic comparison [in Italian]. *Radiol Med* 1991;82:64–69.

20. Masuda EM, Kistner RL. Prospective comparison of duplex scanning and descending venography in the assessment of venous insufficiency. *Am J Surg* 1992;164:254–259.

21. Neglen P, Raju S. A comparison between descending phlebography and duplex Doppler investigation in the evaluation of reflux in chronic venous insufficiency: a challenge to phlebography as the "gold standard". *J Vasc Surg* 1992;16:687–693.

22. Welch HJ, Faliakou EC, McLaughlin RL, et al. Comparison of descending phlebography with quantitative photoplethysmography, air plethysmography, and duplex quantitative valve closure time in assessing deep venous reflux. *J Vasc Surg* 1992;16:913–919; discussion 919–920.

23. Bohler K, Baldt M, Schuller-Petrovic S, et al. Varicose vein stripping—a prospective study of the thrombotic risk and the diagnostic significance of preoperative color coded duplex sonography. *Thromb Haemost* 1995;73:597–600.

24. Evers EJ, Wuppermann T. Ultrasound diagnosis in post-thrombotic syndrome. Comparative study with color duplex, cw-Doppler and B-image ultrasound [in German]. *Ultraschall Med* 1995;16:259–263.

25. Jing Z, Lu P, Cao G. Comparative study of ultrasonic detection of popliteal vein reflux [in Chinese]. *Zhonghua Wai Ke Za Zhi* 1995;33:108–111.

26. Depalma RG, Kowallek DL, Barcia TC, et al. Target selection for surgical intervention in severe chronic venous insufficiency: comparison of duplex scanning and phlebography. *J Vasc Surg* 2000;32:913–920.

27. Yamamoto N, Unno N, Mitsuoka H, et al. Preoperative and intraoperative evaluation of diameter-reflux relationship of calf perforating veins in patients with primary varicose vein. *J Vasc Surg* 2002;36:1225–1230.

28. Baker SR, Burnand KG, Sommerville KM, et al. Comparison of venous reflux assessed by duplex scanning and descending phlebography in chronic venous disease. *Lancet* 1993;341:400–403.

29. Magnusson M, Kalebo P, Lukes P, et al. Colour Doppler ultrasound in diagnosing venous insufficiency. A comparison to descending phlebography. *Eur J Vasc Endovasc Surg* 1995;9:437–443.

30. Rosfors S, Bygdeman S, Nordstrom E. Assessment of deep venous incompetence: a prospective study comparing duplex scanning with descending phlebography. *Angiology* 1990;41:463–468.

31. Danielsson G, Eklof B, Grandinetti A, et al. Deep axial reflux, an important contributor to skin changes or ulcer in chronic venous disease. *J Vasc Surg* 2003;38:1336–1341.

32. Phillips GW, Paige J, Molan MP. A comparison of colour duplex ultrasound with venography and varicography in the assessment of varicose veins. *Clin Radiol* 1995;50:20–25.

33. Dixon PM. Duplex ultrasound in the pre-operative assessment of varicose veins. *Australas Radiol* 1996;40:416–421.

34. Stonebridge PA, Chalmers N, Beggs I, et al. Recurrent varicose veins: a varicographic analysis leading to a new practical classification. *Br J Surg* 1995;82:60–62.

35. Lurie F, Ogawa T, Kistner RL, et al. Changes in venous lumen size and shape do not affect the accuracy of volume flow measurements in healthy volunteers and patients with primary chronic venous insufficiency. *J Vasc Surg* 2002;35:522–526.

36. Min RJ, Khilnani NM, Golia P. Duplex ultrasound evaluation of lower extremity venous insufficiency. *J Vasc Interv Radiol* 2003;14:1233–1241.

37. Labropoulos N, Kokkosis AA, Spentzouris G, et al. The distribution and significance of varicosities in the saphenous trunks. *J Vasc Surg* 2010;51:96–103.

38. Araki CT, Back TL, Padberg FT Jr, et al. Refinements in the ultrasonic detection of popliteal vein reflux. *J Vasc Surg* 1993;18:742–748.

39. Labropoulos N, Tiongson J, Pryor L, et al. Definition of venous reflux in lower-extremity veins. *J Vasc Surg* 2003;38:793–798.

40. Morbio AP, Sobreira ML, Rollo HA. Correlation between the intensity of venous reflux in the saphenofemoral junction and morphological changes of the great saphenous vein by duplex scanning in patients with primary varicosis. *Int Angiol* 2010;29:323–330.

41. Jeanneret C, Labs KH, Aschwanden M, et al. Venous cross-sectional area: measured or calculated? [in German]. *Ultraschall Med* 2000;21:16–19.

42. Vasdekis SN, Clarke GH, Nicolaides AN. Quantification of venous reflux by means of duplex scanning. *J Vasc Surg* 1989;10:670–677.

43. Masuda EM, Kistner RL, Eklof B. Prospective study of duplex scanning for venous reflux: comparison of Valsalva and pneumatic cuff techniques in the reverse Trendelenburg and standing positions. *J Vasc Surg* 1994;20:711–720.

44. Markel A, Meissner MH, Manzo RA, et al. A comparison of the cuff deflation method with Valsalva's maneuver and limb compression in detecting venous valvular reflux. *Arch Surg* 1994;129:701–705.

45. Kakkos SK, Lin JC, Sparks J, et al. Prospective comparison of the pneumatic cuff and manual compression methods in diagnosing lower extremity venous reflux. *Vasc Endovascular Surg* 2009;43:480–484.

46. van Bemmelen PS, Beach K, Bedford G, et al. The mechanism of venous valve closure. Its relationship to the velocity of reverse flow. *Arch Surg* 1990;125:617–619.

47. Walters AS, LeBrocq C, Dhar A, et al. Validation of the International Restless Legs Syndrome Study Group rating scale for restless legs syndrome. *Sleep Med* 2003;4:121–132.

48. Zucconi M, Ferri R, Allen R, et al. The official World Association of Sleep Medicine (WASM) standards for recording and scoring periodic leg movements in sleep (PLMS) and wakefulness (PLMW) developed in collaboration with a task force from the International Restless Legs Syndrome Study Group (IRLSSG). *Sleep Med* 2006;7:175–183.

49. Bradbury A, Evans CJ, Allan P, et al. The relationship between lower limb symptoms and superficial and deep venous reflux on duplex ultrasonography: The Edinburgh Vein Study. *J Vasc Surg* 2000;32:921–931.

50. Labropoulos N, Giannoukas AD, Delis K, et al. Where does venous reflux start? *J Vasc Surg* 1997;26:736–742.

51. Labropoulos N, Leon L, Kwon S, et al. Study of the venous reflux progression. *J Vasc Surg* 2005;41:291–295.

52. Labropoulos N, Tassiopoulos AK, Bhatti AF, et al. Development of reflux in the perforator veins in limbs with primary venous disease. *J Vasc Surg* 2006;43:558–562.

53. Labropoulos N, Gasparis AP, Pefanis D, et al. Secondary chronic venous disease progresses faster than primary. *J Vasc Surg* 2009;49:704–710.

54. Lynch TG, Dalsing MC, Ouriel K, et al. Developments in diagnosis and classification of venous disorders: non-invasive diagnosis. *Cardiovasc Surg* 1999;7:160–178.

CHAPTER 97

Technical Strategies and Management of Varicose Veins

MICHAEL DARCY

INTRODUCTION

When managing symptomatic varicose veins, the approach can be dictated by the anatomy and the clinical condition of the patient. Although the focus is often on ablation of the major saphenous veins, nonsaphenous sources of reflux occur in 10% to 15% of cases.[1] Also, as the severity of the clinical class of venous insufficiency (CEAP class) increases, reflux via perforators is found with increasing frequency.[2] Thus with increasing severity of venous disease the approach to the patient may vary with increasing emphasis on managing perforators. Therapy needs to be targeted to the veins that are actually the source of the problem whether it is the great saphenous vein (GSV), small saphenous vein (SSV), perforators, or other accessory pathways. The strategy for managing the patient's unique pathology should be devised based on the comprehensive ultrasound exam as detailed in the Chapter 96.

The therapeutic approach will also be determined in large part by the size and morphology of the specific veins to be treated. There are multiple therapies that can be applied to venous reflux disease including surgical approaches, endovenous laser therapy (EVLT), radiofrequency ablation (RFA), sclerotherapy, and phlebectomy. Although there is considerable overlap in how these techniques are applied, the size and morphology of the pathologic veins usually dictates which technique is most appropriate. As technology advances the strategies also change. For example, in the past both EVLT and RFA required relatively long straight segments of vein to be able to introduce the devices. This pretty much limited their use to larger refluxing vessels such as GSV, SSV, or anterolateral trunk. Recently, smaller RFA and laser kits have been developed to allow introduction of these devices directly into perforators, thus allowing ablation techniques to move into the realm previously managed primarily by surgical ligation or phlebectomy. This chapter covers some of the technical strategies for managing different kinds of venous disease with a focus on the endovenous techniques.

TRUNCAL VEIN ABLATION

Technical/Device Considerations

Reflux down the larger truncal veins like GSV and SSV is most often managed by either surgery or ablation by EVLT or RFA. Because surgical stripping predated endovenous techniques, it is often the gold standard against which EVLT or RFA are compared. Some early reports indicated that surgery and endovenous techniques have similar efficacy. Rasmussen et al.[3] looked at outcomes 2 years after either surgical stripping or EVLT. According to the outcomes, 26% of the surgery

group and 37% of the EVLT patients developed recurrences, although in most of both groups the recurrence was from reflux from a source other than the GSV that was treated. Not only was the recurrence rate not significantly different, but there also was no difference in the clinical severity scores or quality of life scores.

Then some studies started to report improved efficacy for endovenous techniques. One such study was a meta-analysis that looked at 64 studies with a total of 12,320 treated limbs.[4] They found that the success rates for surgery, foam sclerotherapy, RFA, and EVLT were 78%, 77%, 84%, and 94%, respectively. When they compared individual modalities against each other, they found no significant difference between surgical therapy and RFA, but EVLT was statistically better than both surgery and RFA. As one might expect, studies comparing endovenous ablation to surgery often report fewer complications and less pain for those treated by ablation. In an earlier study, Rasmussen reported that although the efficacy was similar between surgery and EVLT, the surgical patients had more pain and more bruising than the EVLT patients.[5]

More recently, the improved efficacy of endovenous techniques over surgical stripping has again been questioned in several trials. Pronk et al.[6] randomized patients between surgery and EVLT with a 980-nm laser. They found no differences between the groups in the incidence of clinical varicosities at 1 year, the incidence of reflux, and the cosmetic results, but the surgical group actually had less pain and returned to full activity more quickly. Similarly another study with 2-year follow-up demonstrated no difference in clinical severity scores between the surgical and EVLT groups but both post-op bruising and long-term recanalization at 2 years were more common in the EVLT group.[7] These studies both questioned the superiority of EVLT versus surgery.

In more recent trials RFA has fared better. Two recent randomized trials found that surgery and RFA had comparable rates of GSV occlusion and recurrence rates, but in both studies the RFA patients had less pain and quicker return to normal activities.[8,9] Why are there discrepancies between the old and new studies? The most likely answer is evolution of the devices and techniques.

Both lasers and RFA devices have evolved in the last decade. Several lasers are available for EVLT including 810-, 940-, and 980-nm diode lasers as well as 1320-nm Neodynium YAG lasers. Recently 1,470-nm diode lasers have also become available. The lower wavelengths are absorbed more by hemoglobin; thus, the effect on the vein wall is more indirect with damage being primarily from the heated blood. At higher wavelengths, the laser energy is more specifically absorbed by the interstitial water of

1133

the vein walls. Therefore, the postulate is that higher wavelength lasers should be able to damage the vein wall more effectively and cause vein closure at lower total energy deposition because the energy is more specifically absorbed by the vein wall. Less heat used theoretically should lead to fewer side effects and complications.

Several studies have found that using higher wavelength lasers leads to less pain and ecchymosis.[10–12] For example, another study by Almeida et al.[13] found that 79% of their control group treated with a 980-nm laser had moderate to severe ecchymosis, but this occurred in only 10% of their patients treated with a 1,470-nm laser. Despite the lower complication rate the efficacy was still high in the 1,470-nm group with a 100% vein closure rate 1 month postprocedure.

Most of the studies comparing EVLT to surgery were done with older 980-nm lasers. So it is possible that the apparent changes in relative efficacy and complications between surgery and EVLT relate to improvement in surgical technique. Some of these studies need to be repeated with higher wavelength lasers to truly be able to assess the value of EVLT compared to surgery.

On the other hand, RFA technology has also evolved, and the recent studies[8,9] showing that RFA was better than surgery were done with the newer VNUS system (Covidien; Mansfield, MA). The older studies that showed that RFA was no better than surgery were primarily done using the older multipronged RFA device.

Similarly, the comparison between EVLT and RFA has also changed as technology has advanced. Originally, when compared to the multipronged RFA device, EVLT was shown to be superior even given the lower wavelength laser in use at that time.[4] Two recent studies compared the newer-generation VNUS RFA device to EVLT using 980-nm lasers.[14,15] In both studies, RFA was superior with the primary difference being less pain and bruising while still having similar efficacy to EVLT. Again these comparison studies do unfairly pit different generations of the technology against each other. The study that needs to be done now is to compare the VNUS system to newer-generation higher wavelength lasers.

Planning the Interventional Procedure

An important first step is picking the appropriate level to access the GSV. Whereas some practitioners access the GSV just above the knee, starting lower in the leg has benefits. Perforators below the knee can lead to persistent reflux into calf varicosities despite successful ablation of the GSV in the thigh. Theivacumar et al.[16] randomized 23 patients each to start access above the knee or in mid-calf. At 6 weeks after EVLT, 61% of patients in the above-knee group had residual varicosities requiring sclerotherapy as opposed to only 17% of patients with mid-calf access. Thus, a reasonable approach is to assess the vein with ultrasound and choose an access site that is peripheral enough to allow most of the vein to be treated but where the vein is still large enough to allow easy access. One disadvantage to mid-calf access is the greater potential for paresthesias because below the knee the saphenous nerve can run closer to the GSV; however, Theivacumar's study did not show any higher rates of paresthesias with below-knee access.

In patients with recurrent varicosities previously treated with surgery or sclerotherapy, the anatomy may be distorted. Thus, careful mapping of the veins is critical. As long as there is a long enough segment to introduce the laser fiber, EVLT can be used with a high degree of effectiveness. Nwaejike et al.[17] performed EVLT on 77 cases of recurrent varicosities, most of which had had prior ligation and stripping. Of the cases, 83% involved the GSV and 17% involved the SSV, and with 18-month median follow-up they had no clinical recurrences. To avoid other recurrences, access into collaterals or recanalized veins should be as low as is technically possible.

Specific Intraprocedural Techniques

Spasm can readily occur during attempted needle access. Prevention is better than having to treat spasm. The best way to prevent spasm is to take care to enter the vein in a single pass because making multiple needle passes around the vein increases the chances of spasm. Thus, accurate ultrasound identification and tracking of the needle tip is a critical skill. If spasm does occur, warm compresses, intravenous (IV) nitroglycerin infusion, or simply waiting may resolve the spasm. If not, puncturing the vein at a higher level may work. If the case is being done in an angiography suite, one can also inject contrast and use steerable wires and catheters to negotiate past the area of spasm (FIGURE 97.1). Although rarely needed, this can be extremely beneficial in some cases. Alternatively, in cases of severe spasm, the saphenous vein can be punctured near the saphenofemoral junction (SFJ) and the fiber can be fed retrograde down the saphenous vein (FIGURE 97.2). This is only feasible in nonobese patients and care must be taken to puncture close to the SFJ to avoid leaving a long segment of the upper vein untreated.

There may be difficulty advancing the wire up the GSV if there are large side branches. This is particularly true if there is reflux from a large perforator. This can be dealt with in several ways. A steerable guide wire or catheter can be used to steer up the GSV. This can usually be monitored by ultrasound but one can also use fluoroscopy with contrast injection to visualize the correct path (FIGURE 97.1). If the side branch is superficial enough, it can sometimes be manually compressed to help deflect the wire in the correct direction up the GSV.

When varicose veins recur after prior surgery or ablation, there is added complexity to the anatomy. There may be segment of vein occlusion that prevents treatment of the entire GSV at once. Additionally, when the GSV has recanalized, there are sometimes adhesions or synechiae that make it more challenging to advance a laser fiber or RFA probe up the length of the GSV. The use of directional wires and catheters can facilitate steering past these partial obstructions. Although ultrasound can be used to guide these manipulations, it is sometimes easier to do with fluoroscopic control (FIGURE 97.3). Despite the challenges inherent in some recanalized veins, ablative therapy can still generally be successfully performed. Anchala et al.[18] reported 100% technical success when using EVLT to treat recurrent reflux in patients who had previously undergone ligation and stripping.

Another study[19] looked at recurrent varicose veins arising from the previously treated GSVs and compared surgical approaches (ligation and phlebectomy) to EVLT. They had a

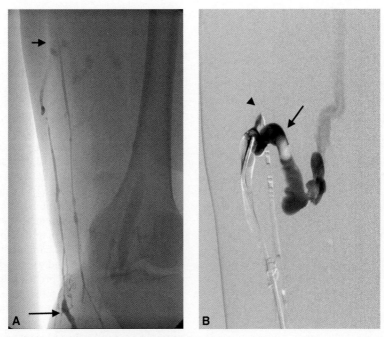

FIGURE 97.1 A. Contrast injection into the GSV in a patient in whom the wire could not be advanced above mid-thigh due to excessive spasm. The caliber of the unspasmed vein (*long arrow*) is seen below the knee. At the point where the wire would not advance up the GSV (*short arrow*) a large perforator vein is faintly seen medially. **B.** Venogram in the mid-thigh showing a large perforator (*arrow*) that the wire tended to enter. The GSV above the perforator tapers to severe spasm (*arrowhead*). After vasodilator injection, a steerable wire was able to be fluoroscopically directed up the GSV.

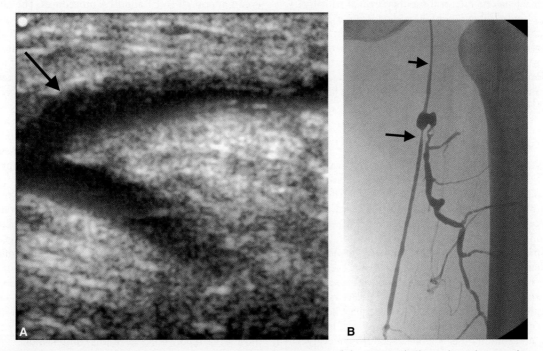

FIGURE 97.2 A. Patient with severe spasm preventing catheterization of the GSV in the lower leg. Ultrasound image shows the point (*arrow*) just peripheral to the saphenofemoral junction where the GSV was accessed in retrograde fashion. **B.** A venogram via the retrograde catheter (*short arrow*) in the upper GSV. Despite spasm (*long arrow*) of the GSV, the catheter was able to be manipulated down to the below-knee GSV, thus allowing a successful EVLT to be performed.

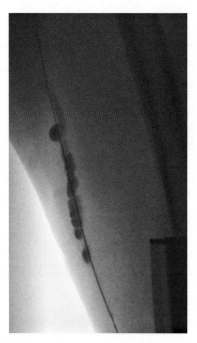

FIGURE 97.3 Patient with recurrent reflux down a recanalized GSV 1 year after successful EVLT. Despite the enlarged size of the GSV, postablation synechiae are seen as linear defects within the vein and these made it difficult to advance the wire without contrast and use of directional angiographic catheters and wires.

100% technical success rate in those they treated with EVLT, although they did exclude 37% of the patients from EVLT based on significant vessel tortuosity. The surgical treatment arm had higher post-op analgesia requirements (although the EVLT group reported more pain). The surgical arm also had more complications and a higher recurrence rate (29% vs. 19% for EVLT patients) during follow-up. Thus, ablation can be successfully applied to recurrent varicose veins.

Endpoint Assessment of the Procedure

Assessing the endpoint for EVLT or RFA is not really about completion of the ablation itself but what to do after the ablation. Typically, once the laser or RF probe is activated, the procedure continues until the device has been pulled back along the length of the vein. The progress can be monitored with ultrasound to confirm that the vein is occluded. However, this is not routinely done because there would be limited ability to advance the laser fiber or RFA probe back up the saphenous vein.

With EVLT there is no good way to monitor if a segment of vein has been adequately burned. Thus, with EVLT systems this is regulated by rate of pullback to achieve adequate heat deposition. The current recommendation is to pull the laser fiber back slowly and continuously at a rate of about 1 cm every 5 to 6 seconds. The VNUS RFA system uses a segmental pullback with a 7-cm segment of vein being treated at once for 20 seconds regulated by the RFA generator. This system does monitor the progress by means of a thermocouple on the RFA catheter. The ablation goal is to achieve a temperature of 120° while needing 20 W or less of power to maintain that temperature. If more

than 20 W of power is needed to maintain the temperature in the desired range, then the recommendation is to do a second 20-second ablation at that vein segment.

A question that is sometimes debated is whether or not one should proceed to treat the varicosities immediately after the ablation or wait and deal with any residual varicosities in a second procedure if needed. The proponents of the first approach argue that doing phlebectomy or sclerotherapy immediately after the ablation more completely manages the patient's problem quickly and efficiently. However, varicosities may shrink significantly as a result of the ablation of the major saphenous trunk alone. So others argue that adding phlebectomy or sclerotherapy immediately during the ablation procedure may subject patients to unnecessary procedures with their attendant discomfort, potential scarring, and risks. Carradice et al.[20] randomized patients to an initial procedure consisting of either ELVT or EVLT combined with phlebectomy. They found that the combined approach significantly decreased the need for subsequent procedures and led to better clinical severity scores at 6 weeks and 3 months, but by 1 year there was no difference between the groups. Alternatively Schanzer[21] looked retrospectively at how many patients ultimately required a second stage procedure after initial EVLT. He found that 58% of his patients required no further treatment after the EVLT. Thus, over half of the patients avoided an unnecessary secondary procedure.

Procedural Complications and How to Manage Them Successfully

Bruising and pain are probably the most common adverse events after both EVLT and RFA procedures. The rate at which they are reported varies widely from one series to another. For example, in papers dealing specifically with SSV, ablation bruising ranged from 27% to 100%.[22–24] The reported incidence also varies with the ablation device used. For example, the incidence has been shown in recent studies to be lower after newer VNUS RFA compared to EVLT.[13,14] Bruising is best managed by setting appropriate expectations prior to the procedure. By warning the patient that bruising is very common and will resolve spontaneously after several weeks, the patient's level of anxiety should be reduced. Postprocedural pain can almost always be managed with over-the-counter oral pain medications and only rarely are narcotics neccesary.

Phlebitis can develop in segments of the ablated vein in 1% to 4% of patients.[25–28] This is recognized as a warm, erythematous, and tender segment of vein. If the vein is superficial enough, there may be some erythema of the overlying skin. Typically, this can be managed conservatively with anti-inflammatory drugs and warm compresses. Needle aspiration of thrombus within the inflamed segment can be attempted and may lead to more rapid resolution of the symptoms.

Skin burn is a very uncommon complication of ablation. Although Chang and Chua[28] did report an incidence of 4.8%, most series report no cases of this complication.[26,29] Skin burn can occur by one of two mechanisms. Most often this probably results from inadequate tumescent anesthesia and the target vein being too close to the skin surface. However, Sichlau and Ryu[30] reported a case where ultrasonography showed that the burn was over a superficial tributary that arose from the GSV, but the burn was clearly medial to the ablated GSV. They postulated that the burn was caused by heated blood traveling from the GSV up the superficial tributary directly in the subcutaneous tissue beneath the site of the burn. Burns are generally very localized and conservative wound care is generally all that is needed.

Paresthesias can result from damage to an adjacent nerve traveling in close proximity to the vein being ablated. The nerves damaged are typically the saphenous nerve during GSV ablation and the sural nerve during ablation of the SSV. Incidence of paresthesias after GSV ablation is around 0% to 10%,[29,31,32] whereas the incidence after SSV ablation ranges widely from 1% to 40%.[22–26] This may take the form of numbness, tingling, or pain of various types and, although paresthesias are generally temporary, they can last for several months.

Deep venous thrombosis (DVT) is a complication that was expected to occur relatively often when ablation techniques were first developed, but in reality the rate in most large series is 0%.[26,29,33] One study specifically focused on rates of DVT after 2,470 cases of RFA and 350 of EVLT.[34] They found extremely low rates of DVT, 0.2% after RFA and 0.9% post-EVLT. Avoidance of this complication is critical and should be possible with careful attention to the position of the ablation device to ensure that it is not too close to the junction of the saphenous and deep veins. When true DVT is documented, standard anticoagulation should be considered.

For an overview comparing the complications of EVLT and surgery, one of the best sources is a systematic review done by Hoggan et al.[33] This was a review of 59 studies that included 6,702 legs treated by EVLA and 7,727 legs treated by surgery. The median rate of complications is shown in Table 97.1. These data indicate that pain and bruising were more common after EVLT but that the other complications were more common after surgery.

Outcomes/Prognosis

The acute outcomes after GSV ablation are quite good with veins being immediately occluded in 95% to 100% after initial treatment.[8,29,35] In most cases, the result is also durable with 1- and 2-year occlusion rates in the range of 99% and 93%, respectively,

Table 97.1
Median Complication Rates from Systematic Review

	EVLT (%)	Surgery (%)
Pulmonary embolism	0	0
DVT	0	0.3
Superficial thrombophlebitis	2.5	7.0
Paresthesias	3.4	8.8
Infection/cellulitis	0	1.5
Bruising	43.8	11.2
Edema	8.8	40.0
Pain/tightness	33.3	6.1

From Hoggan BL, Cameron AL, Maddern GJ. Systematic review of endovenous laser therapy versus surgery for the treatment of saphenous varicose veins. *Ann Vasc Surg* 2009;23:277–287.

being reported.[7,29,32,36] Another study showed that failure rates increased slightly from 7.7% to 13.1% when follow-up was carried out to 3 years.[37] Results for EVLT for SSV reflux are also quite good. Series that have reported specifically on SSV ablation have reported initial technical success of 99% to 100% with 94% to 97% persistent occlusion of the SSV at 1 year.[22–24,26]

In most series, endovenous techniques compare favorably to surgical stripping. For example, in a study with 2-year follow-up, Rasmussen et al.[3] discovered that 26% and 37% of patients in the EVLT and surgery groups, respectively, had developed recurrent varicose veins. This was not significant nor did the sources of reflux differ significantly between the groups.

In addition to occlusion of the target vein, relief of symptoms is another important parameter. In this regard, endovenous techniques fare well with symptom relief paralleling rates of vein occlusion. Endovascular therapy can also have significant effects on the major clinical sequela of venous reflux. It has been shown that lower extremity venous ulcers can heal as early as 1 week after EVLT of the GSV.[38] This same study reported cumulative healing of venous ulcers to be 82%, 93%, and 97% at 1, 6, and 12 months, respectively, post-EVLT.

Options for Failure Management

Regardless of whether failure occurs late or early, a careful ultrasound exam is necessary to determine the cause of failure. As already mentioned, the chance of recanalization of the ablated vein is relatively low. Thus, it is important that one also look for other sources of reflux including other truncal veins (such as the anterolateral trunk) or perforators below the prior level of ablation. Truncal vein reflux is typically treated with standard laser or RFA. However, if the previously treated vein is the source of reflux, a second attempt at ablation may be more technically challenging because the prior ablation attempt may have left webs or stenoses that may prevent easy passage of the guide wire.

Despite these challenges, recurrent varicosities can still be managed with a high degree of success using endovascular ablation. Nwaejike et al.[17] described 77 cases of recurrent varicose veins, most of which occurred after prior ligation and stripping. All were treated with EVLT with a distribution of 83% GSV and 17% SSV. With a median follow-up of 18 months, they had no clinical recurrences and no recanalizations. Another group compared EVLT to surgery as methods for dealing with recurrent varicosities of both the GSV[19] and the SSV.[39] In both of these studies EVLT was more successful than surgery in treating recurrent varicosities and did so with fewer complications.

■ PERFORATORS AND RESIDUAL VARICOSITIES

When patients have persistent varicose veins after an endovenous ablation of the main truncal veins, it is important to first determine if the veins simply failed to shrink as a result of long-term overdistension or if they are continuing to be pressurized by reflux from a perforator. Perforators can arise anywhere from mid-thigh down, although they are twice as common below the knee as above the knee.[40] Distinguishing if the varicosities are isolated or fed by a perforator is critical because local treatment alone may fail to prevent recurrences when a source of reflux is present. Managing perforator-related reflux is an area of vein treatment that is evolving since new devices have become available in recent years. Residual varicosities not associated with perforator reflux are usually tortuous channels not amenable to ablation techniques. Thus, direct treatment of these veins must be accomplished using phlebectomy or sclerotherapy techniques.

Planning the Interventional Procedure

Ablation can be used to deal with perforator reflux in two ways. If the perforator feeds a persistently patent truncal vein (for example, a below-knee saphenous segment) it may make sense to ablate the truncal vein across the connection point with the perforator. That way the truncal vein is also obliterated and eliminates the chance that another subtle unseen perforator might cause persistent flow into the truncal vein. Alternatively, if the perforator directly feeds superficial varicosities, then the perforator itself must be directly addressed. Specialized laser and RFA kits are available, which allow the thermal delivery device to be placed directly into the perforator, thus allowing the perforator to be obliterated right at its origin as it perforates up through the fascial layers (FIGURE 97.4). These kits have smaller, shorter laser or RFA sheaths and probes suitable for placement into the relatively shorter perforators.

Alternatively, perforators can be managed with phlebectomy. With this technique a small microincision is made over the perforator and a phlebectomy hook (FIGURE 97.5) is used to snag the vein and pull it up through the incision. Continued smooth traction is applied to the vein, pulling more and more of the vein out through the incision until finally the vein is avulsed. Although this can be done with tumescent anesthesia, special attention needs to be paid to deeper infiltration of anesthetic down around the vein as it passes through the fascia. Manual compression is then used to achieve hemostasis. This is typically

easily achieved because the process of avulsing the vein also usually causes some spasm of the remaining portions.

Managing isolated varicose veins (those not associated with refluxing perforators) involves either phlebectomy or sclerotherapy and often the choice is determined by the familiarity and comfort level of the practitioner with each technique. Size of the residual veins can sometimes be used as a guide to pick the most appropriate therapy. One algorithm that has been proposed is to sclerose reticular veins and varicose veins less than 4 mm with sodium tetradecyl sulfate and to treat varicose veins that are greater than 4 mm by phlebectomy.[41]

Endpoint Assessment of the Procedure

Similar to ablation of truncal veins, once the device has been pulled back along the length of a perforator, re-advancing back down into the vein is not likely to be possible. So generally the device is simply pulled back at the prescribed rate. Also, although ultrasound can be used to show that the vein is occluded, one probably could not distinguish a successful treatment of the vein versus spasm or complete compression related to good tumescent anesthesia. For isolated varicose veins the endpoint for phlebectomy and sclerotherapy differ slightly. In both cases, mapping the veins to be treated should be done prior to starting the procedure. For phlebectomy this is done with the patient standing and marking the skin with a marker. The endpoint is reached when all the veins in that distribution have been removed. Knowing if all the veins have been removed or not can be aided by using ultrasound or transillumination to look for residual vein fragments. Foam sclerotherapy is monitored by ultrasound and the procedure is stopped when all the planned target veins have been filled with foam sclerosant. Sometimes if

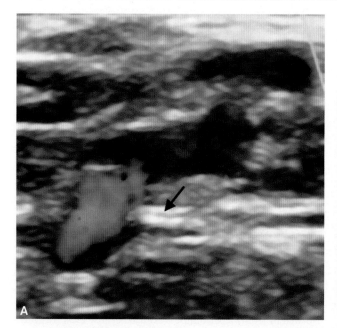 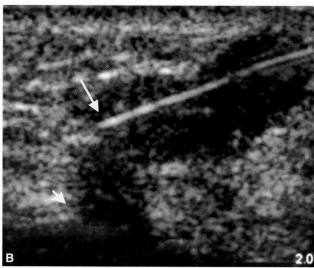

FIGURE 97.4 A. Ultrasound image documenting flow through a perforator in a patient who had persistent varicosities after GSV ablation. The arrow points to the fascial layer that the vein perforates through. **B.** After direct puncture into the most superficial part of the perforating vein, the laser fiber (*long arrow*) has been advanced close to the origin (*short arrow*) of the perforator.

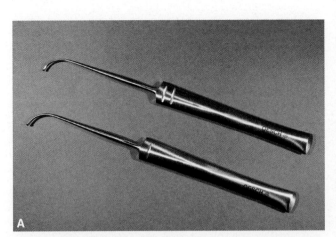
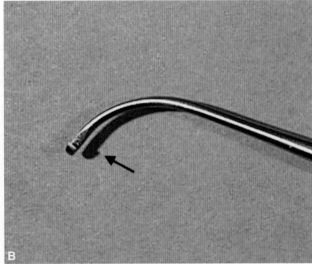

FIGURE 97.5 A. Typical vein hooks used for phlebectomy. **B.** Magnified view of the tip of the vein hook shows the barb that snags the vein. This is best appreciated in the shadow (*arrow*) of the hook.

a large number of veins need to be removed or sclerosed, some practitioners prefer to stage the procedure and quit after an arbitrary amount of time spent or after a certain number of incisions or punctures have been done.

Procedural Complications and How to Manage Them Successfully

Complications after phlebectomy are uncommon and usually mild. These were examined in detail in a review of 1,000 consecutive cases in which the total complication rate was 3.9%.[42] The complications encountered were blister formation (1.3%), localized superficial phlebitis (1.1%), telangiectasia (0.5%), pigmentation (0.4%), temporary dysesthesia (0.2%), skin necrosis (0.2%), and hematoma (0.1%). As infrequent as these are, complications tend to be less frequent after sclerotherapy. This was demonstrated in a randomized controlled trial in which blistering, bruising, and telangiectatic matting were seen more often after phlebectomy.[43]

Regarding sclerotherapy, a systematic review of 69 studies with over 9,000 patients revealed that serious events including pulmonary emboli occurred in less than 1% of cases.[44] Complications of particular interest and concern in this study were visual disturbances, which occurred in 1.4% of patients, and headache, which was seen in 4.2% of patients. Although this may seem unrelated, there is evidence that foam can travel centrally and even get into the arterial circulation. Ceulen et al.[45] demonstrated with echocardiography in 33 consecutive patients that microemboli got into the right heart in 100% of patients after a single 5-mL injection of 1% polidocanol foam despite using leg elevation and manual compression of the SFJ. In five of the patients, microemboli were also seen in the left atrium or left ventricle. It also appears that patients with GSV reflux have a higher incidence of right-to-left shunt. One study looked at 221 patients with symptomatic varicose veins and GSV incompetence.[46] Patients were tested for the presence of a right-to-left shunt using transcranial Doppler of the middle cerebral artery

after microbubble (created in agitated saline) injection. Right-to-left shunts were detected in 58.8%, which is significant compared to the 26% prevalence of patent foramen ovale reported in the general population. Thus, it should not be surprising that temporary visual disturbance was the most frequent (although still uncommon at a rate of 0.9%) complication seen in a larger French registry study of 1,605 sclerotherapy patients.[47] Fortunately, none of these progressed to a more serious neurologic complication and no treatment was necessary.

Outcomes/Prognosis

Success with phlebectomy for removing perforators is considered to be good but although phlebectomy has been utilized since the time of the Roman Empire, real data with objective evaluation of the perforators are lacking. Early studies on the endovascular ablation of perforators show that successful occlusion can be obtained in 98.5% of cases using a laser kit[48] and in 88% of cases using the RFA device.[49] Further studies are needed before one device can clearly be recommended over another.

Isolated varicosities can be treated effectively with both phlebectomy and sclerotherapy and, often, results depend on the individual practitioner's expertise with a given technique. With sclerotherapy, complete or partial obliteration of the varicose veins can be achieved in 93% to 99% of cases.[50,51] The success of phlebectomy is more operator dependent because removing long vein segments requires a fair amount of finesse with inexperienced operators often applying too much traction too rapidly, thus resulting is fragmentation of the vein into small pieces. With practice it is fairly easy to be able to extract long segments of vein (FIGURE 97.6). Good objective data on the technical success of phlebectomy are somewhat lacking. One randomized controlled trial did look at long-term recurrence rates for these techniques.[43] With 48 patients in each group, the rate of recurrent varicosities at 1 and 3 years was 3% after phlebectomy but for sclerotherapy recurrences at 1 and 3 years were 25% and 38%, respectively. The only downside to

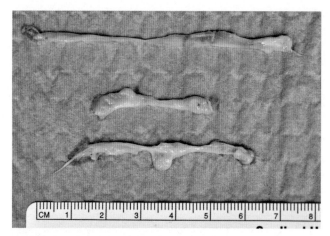

FIGURE 97.6 Multiple vein segments that were removed by phlebectomy. With gentle but firm traction the 7-cm segment had been removed through a single microincision.

phlebectomy was that there were more complications in the phlebectomy group including blistering, bruising, and telangiectatic matting.

Disease Surveillance and Treatment Monitoring Algorithms

Patients need to been seen early in follow-up to exclude complications of therapy, ensure adequate obliteration of the treated vein, and assess the need for additional treatment. This visit is typically within the first month after the treatment. If the treated veins are adequately obliterated, then further routine follow-up is probably not justified. Although patients can redevelop varicose veins, the indication to do further treatment would be based on the onset of new or recurrent symptoms. Thus, a pragmatic approach is to educate the patient about the possibility of varicose veins redeveloping (often arising from different sources), provide them with adequate contact information, and have them call as needed if new symptoms develop.

▌REFERENCES

1. Garcia-Gimeno M, Rodriguez-Camarero S, Tagarro-Villalba S, et al. Duplex mapping of 2036 primary varicose veins. *J Vasc Surg* 2009;49(3):681–689. Epub 2009 Mar 10.
2. Delis KT. Leg perforator vein incompetence: functional anatomy. Radiology. 2005;235(1):327–334. Epub 2005 Mar 8.
3. Rasmussen LH, Bjoern L, Lawaetz M, et al. Randomised clinical trial comparing endovenous laser ablation with stripping of the great saphenous vein: clinical outcome and recurrence after 2 years. *Eur J Vasc Endovasc Surg* 2010;39(5):630–635. Epub 2010 Jan 13.
4. van den Bos R, Arends L, Kockaert M, et al. Endovenous therapies of lower extremity varicosities: a meta-analysis. *J Vasc Surg* 2009;49(1):230–239.
5. Rasmussen LH, Bjoern L, Lawaetz M, et al. Randomized trial comparing endovenous laser ablation of the great saphenous vein with high ligation and stripping in patients with varicose veins: short-term results. *J Vasc Surg* 2007;46(2):308–315.
6. Pronk P, Gauw SA, Mooij MC, et al. Randomised controlled trial comparing sapheno-femoral ligation and stripping of the great saphenous vein with endovenous laser ablation (980 nm) using local tumescent anaesthesia: one year results. *Eur J Vasc Endovasc Surg* 2010;40(5):649–656. Epub 2010 Oct 5.
7. Christenson JT, Gueddi S, Gemayel G, et al. Prospective randomized trial comparing endovenous laser ablation and surgery for treatment of primary great saphenous varicose veins with a 2-year follow-up. *J Vasc Surg* 2010;52(5):1234–1241. Epub 2010 Aug 31.
8. Helmy ElKaffas K, ElKashef O, ElBaz W. Great saphenous vein radiofrequency ablation versus standard stripping in the management of primary varicose veins—a randomized clinical trial. *Angiology* 2011;62(1):49–54. Epub 2010 Aug 21.
9. Subramonia S, Lees T. Randomized clinical trial of radiofrequency ablation or conventional high ligation and stripping for great saphenous varicose veins. *Br J Surg* 2010;97(3):328–336. Epub 2009 Dec 26.
10. Kabnick LS. Outcome of different endovenous laser wavelengths for great saphenous vein ablation. *J Vasc Surg* 2006;43(1):88–93.
11. Proebstle TM, Moehler T, Gul D, et al. Endovenous treatment of the great saphenous vein using a 1,320 nm Nd:YAG laser causes fewer side effects than using a 940 nm diode laser. *Dermatol Surg* 2005;31(12):1678–1683; discussion 1683–1684. Epub 2005 Dec 13.
12. Doganci S, Demirkilic U. Comparison of 980 nm laser and bare-tip fibre with 1470 nm laser and radial fibre in the treatment of great saphenous vein varicosities: a prospective randomised clinical trial. *Eur J Vasc Endovasc Surg* 2010;40(2):254–259. Epub 2010 Jun 16.
13. Almeida J, Mackay E, Javier J, et al. Saphenous laser ablation at 1470 nm targets the vein wall, not blood. *Vasc Endovascular Surg* 2009;43(5):467–472.
14. Almeida JI, Kaufman J, Gockeritz O, et al. Radiofrequency endovenous ClosureFAST versus laser ablation for the treatment of great saphenous reflux: a multicenter, single-blinded, randomized study (RECOVERY study). *J Vasc Interv Radiol* 2009;20(6):752–759.
15. Shepherd AC, Gohel MS, Brown LC, et al. Randomized clinical trial of VNUS ClosureFAST radiofrequency ablation versus laser for varicose veins. *Br J Surg* 2010;97(6):810–818. Epub 2010 May 18.
16. Theivacumar NS, Dellagrammaticas D, Mavor AI, et al. Endovenous laser ablation: does standard above-knee great saphenous vein ablation provide optimum results in patients with both above- and below-knee reflux? A randomized controlled trial. *J Vasc Surg* 2008;48(1):173–178.
17. Nwaejike N, Srodon PD, Kyriakides C. Endovenous laser ablation for the treatment of recurrent varicose vein disease—a single centre experience. *Int J Surg* 2010;8(4):299–301.
18. Anchala PR, Wickman C, Chen R, et al. Endovenous laser ablation as a treatment for postsurgical recurrent saphenous insufficiency. *Cardiovasc Intervent Radiol* 2010;33(5):983–988. Epub 2009 Dec 26.
19. van Groenendael L, van der Vliet JA, Flinkenflogel L, et al. Treatment of recurrent varicose veins of the great saphenous vein by conventional surgery and endovenous laser ablation. *J Vasc Surg* 2009;50(5):1106–1113.
20. Carradice D, Mekako AI, Hatfield J, et al. Randomized clinical trial of concomitant or sequential phlebectomy after endovenous laser therapy for varicose veins. *Br J Surg* 2009;96(4):369–375.
21. Schanzer H. Endovenous ablation plus microphlebectomy/sclerotherapy for the treatment of varicose veins: single or two-stage procedure? *Vasc Endovascular Surg* 2010;44(7):545–549. Epub 2010 Aug 3.
22. Desmyttere J, Grard C, Stalnikiewicz G, et al. Endovenous laser ablation (980 nm) of the small saphenous vein in a series of 147 limbs with a 3-year follow-up. *Eur J Vasc Endovasc Surg* 2010;39(1):99–103. Epub 2009 Oct 20.
23. Park SJ, Yim SB, Cha DW, et al. Endovenous laser treatment of the small saphenous vein with a 980-nm diode laser: early results. *Dermatol Surg* 2008;34(4):517–524; discussion 24.
24. Park SW, Hwang JJ, Yun IJ, et al. Endovenous laser ablation of the incompetent small saphenous vein with a 980-nm diode laser: our experience with 3 years follow-up. *Eur J Vasc Endovasc Surg* 2008;36(6):738–742.
25. Huisman LC, Bruins RM, van den Berg M, et al. Endovenous laser ablation of the small saphenous vein: prospective analysis of 150 patients, a cohort study. *Eur J Vasc Endovasc Surg* 2009;38(2):199–202.
26. Janne d'Othee B, Walker TG, Kalva SP, et al. Endovenous laser ablation of the small saphenous vein sparing the saphenopopliteal junction. *Cardiovasc Intervent Radiol* 2010;33(4):766–771. Epub 2010 Jan 21.
27. Nwaejike N, Srodon PD, Kyriakides C. 5-years of endovenous laser ablation (EVLA) for the treatment of varicose veins—a prospective study. *Int J Surg* 2009;7(4):347–349.
28. Chang CJ, Chua JJ. Endovenous laser photocoagulation (EVLP) for varicose veins. *Lasers Surg Med* 2002;31(4):257–262.
29. Min RJ, Khilnani N, Zimmet SE. Endovenous laser treatment of saphenous vein reflux: long-term results. *J Vasc Interv Radiol* 2003;14(8):991–996.

30. Sichlau MJ, Ryu RK. Cutaneous thermal injury after endovenous laser ablation of the great saphenous vein. *J Vasc Interv Radiol* 2004;15(8):865–867. Epub 2004 Aug 7.

31. Pannier F, Rabe E. Mid-term results following endovenous laser ablation (EVLA) of saphenous veins with a 980 nm diode laser. *Int Angiol* 2008;27(6):475–481.

32. Rathod J, Taori K, Joshi M, et al. Outcomes using a 1470-nm laser for symptomatic varicose veins. *J Vasc Interv Radiol* 2010;21(12):1835–1840. Epub 2010 Nov 6.

33. Hoggan BL, Cameron AL, Maddern GJ. Systematic review of endovenous laser therapy versus surgery for the treatment of saphenous varicose veins. *Ann Vasc Surg* 2009;23:277–287.

34. Marsh P, Price BA, Holdstock J, et al. Deep vein thrombosis (DVT) after venous thermoablation techniques: rates of endovenous heat-induced thrombosis (EHIT) and classical DVT after radiofrequency and endovenous laser ablation in a single centre. *Eur J Vasc Endovasc Surg* 2010;40(4): 521–527. Epub 2010 Jul 27.

35. Schwarz T, von Hodenberg E, Furtwangler C, et al. Endovenous laser ablation of varicose veins with the 1470-nm diode laser. *J Vasc Surg* 2010;51(6):1474–1478. Epub 2010 Mar 30.

36. Min RJ, Khilnani NM. Endovenous laser treatment of saphenous vein reflux. *Tech Vasc Interv Radiol* 2003;6(3):125–131.

37. Spreafico G, Kabnick L, Berland TL, et al. Laser saphenous ablations in more than 1,000 limbs with long-term duplex examination follow-up. *Ann Vasc Surg* 2011;25(1):71–78. Epub 2010 Dec 22.

38. Teo TK, Tay KH, Lin SE, et al. Endovenous laser therapy in the treatment of lower-limb venous ulcers. *J Vasc Interv Radiol* 2010;21(5):657–662. Epub 2010 May 1.

39. van Groenendael L, Flinkenflogel L, van der Vliet JA, et al. Conventional surgery and endovenous laser ablation of recurrent varicose veins of the small saphenous vein: a retrospective clinical comparison and assessment of patient satisfaction. *Phlebology* 2010;25(3):151–157. Epub 2010 May 21.

40. Labropoulos N, Delis K, Nicolaides AN, et al. The role of the distribution and anatomic extent of reflux in the development of signs and symptoms in chronic venous insufficiency. *J Vasc Surg* 1996;23(3):504–510. Epub 1996 Mar 1.

41. Dietzek CL. Sclerotherapy: introduction to solutions and techniques. *Perspect Vasc Surg Endovasc Ther* 2007;19(3):317–324.

42. Olivencia JA. Complications of ambulatory phlebectomy. Review of 1000 consecutive cases. *Dermatol Surg* 1997;23(1):51–54. Epub 1997 Jan 1.

43. de Roos KP, Nieman FH, Neumann HA. Ambulatory phlebectomy versus compression sclerotherapy: results of a randomized controlled trial. *Dermatol Surg* 2003;29(3):221–226.

44. Jia X, Mowatt G, Burr JM, et al. Systematic review of foam sclerotherapy for varicose veins. *Br J Surg* 2007;94(8):925–936.

45. Ceulen RP, Sommer A, et al. (2008). Microembolism during foam sclerotherapy of varicose veins. *N Engl J Med* 358(14): 1525–1526.

46. Wright DD, Gibson KD, Barclay J, et al. High prevalence of right-to-left shunt in patients with symptomatic great saphenous incompetence and varicose veins. *J Vasc Surg* 2010;51(1):104–107. Epub 2009 Oct 20.

47. Guex JJ, Schliephake DE, Otto J, et al. The French polidocanol study on long-term side effects: a survey covering 3,357 patient years. *Dermatol Surg* 2010;36(suppl 2):993–1003. Epub 2010 Jul 16.

48. Proebstle TM, Herdemann S. Early results and feasibility of incompetent perforator vein ablation by endovenous laser treatment. *Dermatol Surg* 2007;33(2):162–168. Epub 2007 Feb 16.

49. Hingorani AP, Ascher E, Marks N, et al. Predictive factors of success following radio-frequency stylet (RFS) ablation of incompetent perforating veins (IPV). *J Vasc Surg* 2009;50(4):844–848. Epub 2009 Jul 7.

50. Nael R, Rathbun S. Effectiveness of foam sclerotherapy for the treatment of varicose veins. *Vasc Med* 2010;15(1):27–32. Epub 2009 Oct 3.

51. Thomasset SC, Butt Z, Liptrot S, et al. Ultrasound guided foam sclerotherapy: factors associated with outcomes and complications. *Eur J Vasc Endovasc Surg* 2010;40(3):389–392. Epub 2010 Jun 16.

SECTION XVI
Pharmacologic Therapies

Anticoagulation in Endovascular and Interventional Procedures

BRADLEY B. PUA and DAVID W. TROST

Physicians managing and treating patients for endovascular and interventional procedures will encounter anticoagulants and antiplatelets when performing the procedure and also in the management of these drugs prior to and after a procedure is performed. With the increasing number of foreign materials, such as stents, being implanted, the interaction between these materials and hemostasis becomes important. This interaction is highly complex and still not fully understood. Although this section gives an overview of the major topics that will arise, it is important to realize that many of the following statements should be viewed as guidelines and not hard and fast rules. The management of these hemostatic altering drugs, especially in the decision to hold them prior to certain procedures, is a topic that should be discussed with the prescribing physician to fully ascertain the risk-benefit profile.

This topic is addressed in four broad sections: Hemostasis and the Coagulation Cascade, Antiplatelet Agents, Anticoagulation Cascade Agents, and Fibrinolytics.

HEMOSTASIS AND THE COAGULATION CASCADE

Hemostasis refers to a process that encompasses the normal response to vascular injury. It includes the process of blood clotting, dissolution of clot, and subsequent vascular repair. Upon vascular injury, sympathetic factors cause vascular constriction that limits the amount of blood flow to the injured region. Endothelial damage results in release of factors that attract platelets and cause platelet activation and aggregation at the site of injury. These platelets adhere to exposed collagen of the injured endothelium, creating a temporary platelet plug. Platelet activation releases adenosine diphosphate (ADP) and thromboxane A_2 (TXA_2), among other factors, which influence the coagulation cascade as well as further activating additional platelets. To further stabilize this temporary platelet plug, a fibrin mesh is formed, of which thrombin and fibrinogen play a key role. The pathway that leads to the formation of the fibrin clot is termed the coagulation cascade (FIGURE 98.1); traditionally it is separated into the intrinsic and extrinsic pathways. The extrinsic pathway is activated as a result of tissue injury, whereas the intrinsic pathway is activated as a result of abnormalities in the vessel wall in the absence of external tissue injury. For example, the intrinsic pathway is activated by the vessel wall contacting negatively charged surfaces, such as circulating bacteria, or molecules associated with atherosclerosis, such as low-density lipoproteins (LDL), very-low-density lipoproteins (VLDL), and chylomicrons.

Platelet Adhesion and Activation

Platelet adhesion to collagen is mediated by von Willebrand factor (vWf). vWf is primarily produced and stored in platelets and acts as a glue to bind glycoprotein complexes on the platelet surface to collagen. vWf also binds factor VIII of the intrinsic pathway, stabilizing it in the circulation. The binding of platelet to collagen results in release in intracellular calcium, further stimulating aggregation.[1]

Concurrently, initial platelet activation is mediated by thrombin binding to the specific platelet cell surface receptors, resulting in a downstream transduction cascade, causing activation of phospholipase C-gamma (PLC-gamma) as well as release of intracellular calcium and activation of protein kinase C (PKC). This surge of intracellular calcium secondary to both collagen binding and platelet activation results in activation of phospholipase A_2 (PLA_2), which leads to a release of arachidonic acid and increased production and release of TXA_2. TXA_2 is a vasoconstrictor and further induces platelet aggregation.

PKC acts by activating various platelet proteins, one of which is ADP. ADP further stimulates platelet activation and exposure of certain receptors, such as the platelet glycoprotein complex, GPIIb-IIIa, which acts as a receptor for vWf and fibrinogen, resulting in platelet aggregation.

The Coagulation Cascade

The intrinsic pathway is initiated when proteins prekallikrein (PK), high-molecular-weight kininogen (HMWK), and factors XI and XII come in contact with a negatively charged surface. This is termed contact activation of the intrinsic pathway. This contact causes conversion of prekallikrein to kallikrein, which activates factor XII to factor XIIa. Factor XIIa converts factor XI to factor XIa in addition to converting more prekallikrein to kallikrein. In the presence of Ca^{2+}, factor XIa activates factor IX to factor IXa, which in turn activates factor X to factor Xa. Activation of factor Xa requires Ca^{2+}, factor VIIIa, and factor XIa. Factor Xa is where the intrinsic and extrinsic pathways converge.

The extrinsic pathway is initiated by release of tissue factor (TF), also known as factor III, in response to vascular injury. TF in addition to factor VIIa activates factor X to Xa in a similar fashion to activation via the intrinsic pathway. Activation of factor VII to VIIa is secondary to the actions of thrombin and/ or factor Xa. Multiple links between the extrinsic and intrinsic pathways exist; some examples include the ability of factor Xa to activate factor VII and the ability of the TF and factor VIIIa complex to activate factor IX.

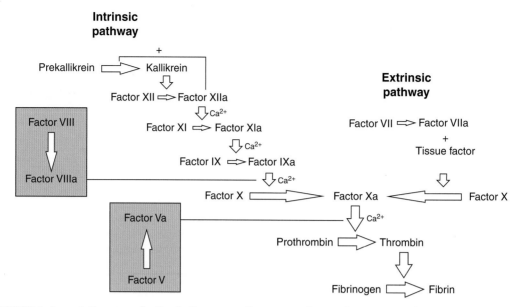

Intrinsic pathway

Extrinsic pathway

FIGURE 98.1 Coagulation cascade. Classically separated into two pathways, the intrinsic and extrinsic pathways leading to a common pathway of activation of factor X to factor Xa. Factor Xa activates prothrombin (factor II) to thrombin (factor IIa), which is responsible for converting fibrinogen to fibrin, finally leading to fibrin cross-linking and strengthening of the blood clot.

The common pathway begins upon activation of factor X to factor Xa. Factor Xa activates factor II (prothrombin) to factor IIa (thrombin) with cofactor factor Va. Thrombin is responsible for converting fibrinogen to fibrin monomers as well as factor XIII to factor XIIIa, which serves to cross-link fibrin monomers. Thrombin plays many roles in addition to activation of fibrin; one of these is its ability to activate thrombin-activatable fibrinolysis inhibitor (TAFI), which can reduce the rate of fibrinolysis secondary to inhibition of plasminogen activation.

Fibrinolysis

The fibrinolysis pathway marks the final portion of hemostasis in addition to providing a check for coagulation and clot formation (FIGURE 98.2). Fibrin degradation is controlled by a serine protease, plasmin, which is in normal circulation as a proenzyme, plasminogen. During clot formation, plasminogen normally binds to both fibrinogen and fibrin, thereby incorporating itself within the fibrin matrix. Two main endogenous enzymes exist that control this pathway, tissue plasminogen

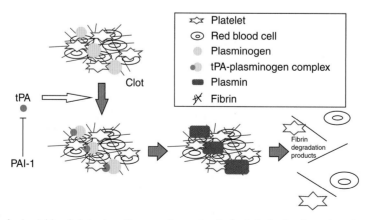

FIGURE 98.2 Fibrinolysis. A blood clot primarily comprises red cells (red clot), platelets, plasminogen, and fibrin cross-links. Upon activation by tPA, plasminogen that has been incorporated in the clot gets converted to plasmin, which acts to break down the fibrin cross-links, thereby weakening the clot, allowing for normal blood flow in the region to wash the fibrin degradation products away. Fibrinolysis is inhibited at the tPA level by plasminogen activator inhibitor–1 (PAI-1). High plasma levels of PAI-1 can lead to deposition of fibrin and formation of thrombus.

activator (tPA) and urokinase (UK). Activated tPA cleaves plasminogen to plasmin, which breaks the fibrin matrix, thereby facilitating clot dissolution. UK, less important in the vascular system, is found and produced as prourokinase in epithelial cells of excretory ducts (such as in the renal collecting system) and functions to break up clot in this region.

Blood Products

Multiple blood products, such as fresh-frozen plasma (FFP), cryoprecipitate, and platelets are available for use in maintaining or achieving hemostasis. As with any blood products, certain risks, such as the potential to contract viral diseases (HIV, hepatitis B and C), hemolysis caused by ABO-incompatibilities, acute lung injury, precipitation of graft versus host disease, must be weighed against the potential benefit of use.[2] In the setting of congenital factor deficiencies or complex cases of massive bleeding, it is often important to discuss obtaining hemostasis with an expert in the field. Under most normal circumstances, utilization of these products can follow the guidelines set forth in 1994 by the Development Task Force of the College of American Pathologists.[3] It must be noted that individual institutions may have local guidelines to be followed.

Fresh-frozen plasma is plasma separated from red blood cells and platelets of whole blood donations. FFP is frozen within 8 hours of collection and can be utilized up to 12 months after donation. It contains all blood coagulation factors and naturally occurring inhibitors. One bag yields approximately 200 to 250 mL volume. Most institutions dispense FFP by units (based on units of factors); actual minute volume discrepancies are secondary to additives, which vary of institution.

Common indications for use of FFP include: a history or clinical course suggestive of a coagulopathy caused by congenital or acquired deficiency of coagulation factors in the setting of active bleeding or prior to an operative or invasive procedure; massive blood transfusions where there is replacement of more than 1 circulating blood volume in a span of a few hours; an instance where reversal of warfarin effect is needed, either to stop bleeding or prior to an emergent surgery or procedure. If the indication is for use in documented coagulopathy with bleeding or prior to a procedure, coagulopathy must be proven with prothrombin time (PT) greater than 1.5 times the midpoint of normal range (usually >18 seconds); activated partial thromboplastin time (aPTT) greater than 1.5 times the top normal range (usually >55 to 60 seconds); or a coagulation factor assay of less than 25% activity.

The recommended dosage is usually two bags of FFP (400 to 460 mL). One unit (200 to 250 mL) may be adequate if PT is between 18 and 22 seconds or aPTT is between 55 and 70. Repeat PT and/or aPTT is obtained at the completion of transfusion and additional factors are given as necessary. The effect of FFP lasts approximately 5 to 6 hours owing to the short half-life of factor VII.

Platelets can be obtained from whole blood or plateletpheresis donations. The normal circulating platelet concentration is 150×10^9 to 400×10^9/L. The volume of plasma for 6 units of platelets is 250 to 350 mL. Platelets can be stored up to 5 days after collection.

It has been demonstrated that at platelet concentrations greater than 50×10^9/L, the bleeding risk for invasive procedures is minimal and with concentrations less than that associated with increased risk of bleeding.[4,5]

With each unit of infused platelets, platelet counts are expected to rise by 5 to 10×10^9/L. If there are no factors increasing platelet consumption, new platelets are not needed for 3 to 5 days, based on estimates of platelet survival. Any disorders that increase platelet consumption will increase this requirement. It is recommended that the platelet count be measured 10 minutes to 1 hour after transfusion. If the incremental increase in platelet counts does not achieve 7.5 to 10×10^9/L, these patients may have developed refractoriness to transfusion. These patients will require platelets from human leukocyte antigen (HLA)-matched and/or platelets cross-matched donors.

Cryoprecipitate is the cold precipitable protein fraction derived from FFP containing factor VIII:C, vWf, fibrinogen, and factor XIII. These factors are resuspended in 9 to 16 mL of plasma and are stored frozen, remaining effective for up to 1 year.

Indications for use of cryoprecipitate include hypofibrinogenemia, von Willebrand's disease (although factor VIII concentrate or desmopressin is preferred), and hemophilia A. Dosages are calculated based on factor deficit and need and is beyond the scope of this chapter.

Desmopressin (DDAVP) is a synthetic analog of antidiuretic hormone, which can be used in patients with uremia, liver disease, von Willebrand disease, and hemophilia to reverse antiplatelet effects. Although the exact mechanism is unclear, this drug increases plasma levels of factor VIII and vWf.[6] Typically, this drug is given at a 0.3-μg/kg dose diluted in 100 mL of normal saline and infused over 20 to 30 minutes. Discussion with a hematologist is recommended prior to usage of this drug.

Tests of the Coagulation Cascade

The aPTT, PT, international normalized ratio (INR), and thrombin time (TT) are in vitro tests that measure the time elapsed from activation of the coagulation cascade to generation of fibrin.

aPTT measures the time at which the intrinsic pathway is initiated (factor XII) to generation of fibrin. This test will be abnormal in deficiencies of or presence of inhibitors to factors XII, IX, XI, VIII, X, V, prothrombin, and fibrinogen. Common inherited disorders of this pathway include hemophilias A (factor VIII deficiency) and B (factor XI deficiency). Common acquired disorders of this pathway include vitamin K deficiency, hepatic dysfunction, and exogenous administration of anticoagulants.

PT measures the time at which the extrinsic pathway is initiated (factor VII) to generation of fibrin. An abnormal test suggests problems with factors VII, V, X, prothrombin, or fibrinogen. Rarely, an inherited factor VII disorder can be seen, which manifests with a prolonged PT and normal aPTT. Common acquired disorders of this pathway include liver disease, massive bleeding, and warfarin use.

INR was devised secondary to the variability of the measured PT by laboratory. Typically PT is measured by utilizing TF as a reagent. The time to blood clotting upon mixing prepared blood and TF is measured. Because manufactured TF is highly variable, each manufacturer assigns an International Sensitivity Index (ISI) for the TF it produces. This ISI and the measured individual PT is then used to calculate a standardized INR.

TT measures the time of conversion of fibrinogen to fibrin in the presence of thrombin. In this way, the test can delineate problems related to abnormalities in fibrinogen or an upstream inhibitor to thrombin activation. Dysfibrinogenemia is an inherited or acquired disease with abnormal fibrinogen and usually related to liver disease in its acquired form.

Anticoagulants

Anticoagulant medications are encountered at an increasing frequency secondary to advances in prevention and treatment of arterial and venous thromboembolism as well as atherosclerosis. Moreover newer agents are being developed with a focus on not only better efficacy and lower complication profile, but ease of administration and monitoring. The following is a collection of the most commonly used anticoagulants and antiplatelet agents with information on their associated pharmacokinetics, mechanism of action, and when available, recommendations on cessation of these drugs prior to an interventional procedure as well as suggestions for reinitiation of these drugs.

Although some clinical studies for cessation of various anticoagulants can be found in the surgical literature, these studies are rare because they relate to interventional procedures. Many of the following guidelines use data extrapolated from surgical data. It must be noted that clinical parameters and individual decision making play a large role. For example, performing a procedure in an area that is easily compressible (arterial puncture of the femoral artery) may be associated with lower risks than performing a procedure in an incompressible region (biopsy of an intraperitoneal organ). If surgical data are unavailable, guidelines can be extrapolated from pharmacokinetics and estimates on cessation of anticoagulants prior to a procedure can be made based on elimination half-life (assuming the drug is functionally eliminated within four to five half-lives).[7]

In 2009, the Society of Interventional Radiology (SIR) Standards of Practice Committee presented guidelines for periprocedural management of coagulation status in patients undergoing percutaneous interventional procedures.[8] When available, this committee utilized results from in-depth literature searches to create consensus for these guidelines. When such literature was not available, guidelines were based on consensus of practice patterns of 18 Certificate of Added Qualification (CAQ) certified interventional radiologists as compiled using a modified Delphi consensus method.[9] This committee separated recommendations based on perceived bleeding risks of the procedure, creating three categories: low-risk, moderate-risk, and high-risk procedures. The guidelines for discontinuing antiplatelet and anticoagulant agents prior to an interventional procedure are detailed in Tables 98.1 and 98.2, respectively. Table 98.3 provides dosing guidelines for administration of various thrombolytic drugs.

The pathophysiology and, therefore, treatment of arterial and venous thrombosis is different. Generally, arterial thrombosis is treated with drugs that target platelets, whereas venous thrombosis is treated with drugs that target proteins of the coagulation cascade.

▌ ANTIPLATELET AGENTS

The main utility of antiplatelet drugs is to limit the growth of the preexisting thrombus as well as prevent formation of arterial thrombus in patients with abnormal vessels walls, such as in patients with cardiovascular and peripheral vascular disease. Common classes of antiplatelet drugs include cyclooxygenase inhibitors (aspirin), ADP receptor inhibitors

(clopidogrel, ticlopidine), glycoprotein IIb/IIIa inhibitors (abciximab, tirofiban, eptifibatide), and adenosine reuptake inhibitors (dipyridamole).

In discussing this class of drugs, it is important to discuss the entity of late stent thrombosis. Drug-eluting stents have become popular over the last few years. These stents, impregnated with drugs, such as sirolimus, are designed to prevent smooth muscle cell proliferation and intimal hyperplasia, leading to stent reocclusion. Clinical trials have demonstrated the reduction in stent restenosis as compared with bare metal stents.[10] Interestingly, though, it is noted that after discontinuing antiplatelet drugs in patients with drug-eluting stents, there appeared to be a four- to fivefold rate of stent thrombosis as compared with bare-metal stents, an entity named late stent thrombosis.[11] There are many predictors of acute (<30 days) and late stent thrombosis (>30 days) that continue to be elucidated. This underscores the importance of discussing the risks and benefit of discontinuing antiplatelet drugs for interventional procedures in this subset of patients. When known, guidelines for discontinuing these drugs are listed in Table 98.1.

Aspirin (ASA), administered orally and absorbed in the upper gastrointestinal tract, is the most commonly used antiplatelet drug. ASA inhibits platelet cyclooxygenase-1 (COX-1), thereby interfering with the synthesis of TXA_2, a potent platelet activator. Among many other things, ASA is important in primary prevention of cardiovascular disease (myocardial infarction).[12] Benefits of ASA in patients with coronary artery disease (CAD) and carotid artery disease have been proven in large clinical trials.[13] However, its use in peripheral arterial disease (PAD) is still being questioned. Regardless, both the American College of Cardiology/American Heart Association Guidelines and Inter-Society Consensus for the Management of Peripheral Artery Disease (TASC II) support the use of ASA in patients with PAD.[14–16]

ASA's inhibition of platelet function has been measured within 60 minutes of administration.[17] Enteric-coated aspirin (ECASA) has documented delayed absorption and, therefore, onset of action.[18] Although the plasma half-life of ASA is only 20 minutes, its effects are long lasting secondary to its irreversible binding of COX-1, rendering its effects for the life of the platelet, about 10 days. It has been estimated that COX-1 activity recovers at a rate of 10% per day secondary to platelet turnover.[19] Although it will take 10 days for the total platelet population to be renewed, investigators have demonstrated that if as little as 20% of COX-1 activity is restored, hemostasis may be normal.[20,21]

Recent studies have demonstrated that low-dose ASA can be as efficacious in cardiovascular disease as high-dose ASA without the associated increased risk of gastrointestinal side effects.[22,23] In fact, a single dose of 100 mg of ASA can halt the production of TXA_2 in both normal individuals and those with atherosclerotic disease.[24] Additionally, low-dose ASA has shown preferential inhibition of platelet COX over endothelial COX.[25–27]

Interestingly, inhibition of the incorrect COX inhibitor was found to increase the risk of myocardial infarction and stroke. Two widely used anti-inflammatory drugs, rofecoxib and valdecoxib, were removed from the market for these reasons. These drugs targeted cyclooxygenase-2 (COX-2), which is important in COX-2 dependent synthesis of prostacyclin, a potent inhibitor of platelet activation.[28]

Although no recommendations exist in regard to discontinuing ASA prior to an interventional procedure, one survey has shown that most interventionists did not postpone procedures

Table 98.1		
Guidelines for Withholding Antiplatelet Agents Prior to an Interventional Procedure		
Antiplatelet	Mechanism	Delay prior to procedure
Aspirin	Inhibits COX-1, which interferes with synthesis of thromboxane A_2	**Studies** Renal biopsies: No difference in major bleeding complications between the group that discontinued ASA 5 d prior to the procedure and the group that remained on ASA Most interventional radiologists in a survey did not discontinue ASA prior to the procedure **SIR consensus panel** Low risk: do not withhold Moderate risk: do not withhold High risk: withhold 5 d
Ticlopidine	ADP receptor inhibitor	**Manufacturer**: Discontinue drug 10–14 d prior to procedure
Clopidogrel	ADP receptor inhibitor	**Study** Coronary artery bypass grafting: Patients who discontinued clopidogrel 5 d prior to the procedure did not suffer increased bleeding **SIR consensus panel** Low risk: do not withhold Moderate risk: withhold 5 d High risk: withhold 5 d
Abciximab	GPIIb/IIIa inhibitor	No official recommendations Based on clinical effects, discontinue at least 48 hr prior
Tirofiban	GPIIb/IIIa inhibitor	Platelet recovery after 3–8 hr
Eptifibatide	GPIIb/IIIa Inhibitor	Platelet recovery after 2–4 hr

Where available, studies determining the optimum time to discontinue antiplatelet drugs are listed with their recommendations. When these studies or manufacturer recommendations are not available, suggested guidelines are listed based on four to five half-life eliminations (*shaded*). Where available, SIR consensus panel recommendations are listed.[8]

in patients who had taken ASA.[29] In fact, one investigator found that concurrent ASA use did not increase the risk of development of groin hematomas after arterial puncture.[30] In areas that are not as easily compressible, such as the kidney, a different group retrospectively compared minor and major bleeding complications after native renal biopsies in patients continuing antiplatelet agents and those discontinuing them 5 days prior to the procedure.[31] They report no difference in major bleeding complications between both groups with a slight increase in minor complications (31% vs. 11.7%) in the group continuing antiplatelet; minor complication being defined as a hemoglobin drop of greater than or equal to 1 g/dL without the need for transfusion or intervention.

Adenosine diphosphate receptor inhibitors, as the name suggests, exert their effects by inhibiting binding of ADP to platelet receptors, hindering platelet activation. Additionally, these drugs can also inhibit ADP-induced binding of fibrinogen to platelets, thereby preventing aggregation. Prototypical examples in this class include ticlopidine and clopidogrel.

Ticlopidine (Ticlid, Hoffmann-LaRoche Inc., Nutley, NJ) has been used to decrease the risk of stroke and thrombosis after coronary artery stent placement. The use of this drug has fallen out of favor secondary to potential serious side effects including

aplastic anemia, neutropenia, and thrombotic thrombocytopenic purpura.[32] The manufacturer recommends discontinuing the medication 10 to 14 days prior to any elective procedure.

Clopidogrel (Plavix, Bristol-Myers Squibb/Sanofi Pharmaceuticals Partnership, New York, NY) is the most commonly used drug in its class of thienopyridine derivatives. Typical dosage of clopidogrel is 75 mg daily with some studies demonstrating that a higher loading dose of 300 mg may be needed to lead to a more rapid decrease in platelet function.[33] Plavix is predominately hepatically cleared, but its effects on platelet aggregation and bleeding times span up to 5 days owing to its irreversible binding of the ADP receptor.

Yusuf et al.[34] found that in 910 patients, those who discontinued clopidogrel 5 days or more prior to undergoing coronary artery bypass surgery did not suffer any increased bleeding problems postoperatively, while those that discontinued the drug less than 5 days prior to surgery had increased perioperative hemorrhage. If emergent reversal of clopidogrel is needed, there is some literature to suggest that a platelet transfusion may partially reverse the effects of clopidogrel, which, we surmise, may be secondary to overwhelming the amount of circulating drug.[35] There is no current literature evaluating the best time to restart clopidogrel after a procedure, although one group suggests restarting the day after completion of the procedure based on their experience with ASA.[36]

Clopidogrel has been found to be efficacious in many scenarios, ranging from therapy in acute coronary syndromes to PAD.[37–39] It has been shown that pretreatment with clopidogrel prior to coronary stenting improves stent patency.[40] Clopidogrel has also been used as an alternative to ASA in patients with PAD.[41] In fact the efficacy of clopidogrel vs. ASA was directly compared in the CAPRIE trial (Clopidogrel versus Aspirin in Patients at Risk of Ischaemic Events). This trial demonstrated a relative risk reduction in myocardial infarction, stroke, or cardiovascular death in the clopidogrel group with the subgroup with PAD receiving the greatest benefit.[42] Interestingly, although combination therapy of clopidogrel and ASA is used in patients undergoing infrainguinal angioplasty and/or stenting, the CHARISMA trial (Clopidogrel for High Atherothrombotic Risk and Ischemic Stabilization, Management and Avoidance) demonstrated no clear benefit in use of a combination of clopidogrel and ASA versus ASA alone in reducing myocardial infarction, stroke, or death from cardiovascular causes, even in the PAD subgroup.[43]

Glycoprotein IIb/IIIa (GPIIb/IIIa) Inhibitors

As stated previously, the final step of platelet aggregation is cross-linking of platelets with fibrinogen, via interaction of fibrinogen and platelet-cell surface receptors. The receptor comprises a dimer of glycoproteins IIb and IIIa, the target for this class of antiplatelet drugs. Mild or transient thrombocytopenia has been reported in this class of drugs with severe thrombocytopenia occurring rarely (0.3%).[44–46] This class is most commonly used in patients with acute coronary syndromes undergoing percutaneous coronary intervention (PCI).[47]

Abciximab (ReoPro, Centocor and Eli Lilly and Company, Malvern, PA, and Indianapolis, IN) is a chimeric mouse/human monoclonal antibody fragment that binds the GPIIb/IIIa complex. The drug is active within 2 hours of infusion and carries a short half-life of 30 minutes. The drug effect is prolonged though with its clinical effect being reduced at 48 hours; however, low-level receptor blockade can be seen up to 14 days after discontinuation.

Tirofiban (Aggrastat, Iroko Cardio, Philadelphia, PA) is a synthetic tyrosine derivative also given intravenously and can inhibit platelet function within 5 minutes. The drug is renally cleared and has a half-life of 90 to 180 minutes. The platelet inhibitory effects can last up to 3 to 8 hours.[48]

Eptifibatide (Integrillin, Millenium Pharmaceuticals, Inc., and Shering-Plough Corporation, Cambridge, MA, and Kenilworth, NJ) is newer, more specific, and is a competitive inhibitor of GPIIb/IIIa, resulting in a shorter time to clinical effect (2.5 hours). Platelets recover function within 2 to 4 hours after cessation of the drug.[49]

▌ANTICOAGULATION CASCADE AGENTS

Venous thromboembolism is the third leading cause of cardiovascular-associated death after myocardial infarction and stroke.[50] Thrombi that form in veins are generally rich with fibrin and red cells, named red clot. In discussing causes of venous thromboembolism, Virchow's triad of hypercoagulability, endothelial injury, and stasis come to mind. Interestingly,

the term *Virchow's triad* has an unclear history because Virchow may have never described the components of the triad.[51] Regardless of the details of the origin, the concept remains important in understanding venous thrombosis. Venous stasis refers to alterations in blood flow, whether it is the result of turbulence from cardiac sources or venous incompetence, such as the cause of varicose veins. Endothelial damage may be secondary to iatrogenic sources or from venous hypertension. Lastly, "hypercoagulability" refers to alterations in the composition of blood, whether it be secondary to increased number of cells, such as in cancer, hormonal factors in pregnancy, or factor deficiencies leading to a procoagulant state.

Two main classes of anticoagulants used for treatment and/or prevention of venous thrombosis include vitamin K antagonists, various forms of heparin (indirect thrombin inhibitor), and direct thrombin inhibitors. When known, guidelines for discontinuing this class of drug prior to an invasive procedure are listed in Table 98.2.

Vitamin K antagonists are used for long-term anticoagulation with **warfarin (coumadin)** being the most commonly prescribed. Warfarin inhibits vitamin K epoxide reductase, which is responsible for post-translational modification of multiple coagulation proteins (factor VII, IX, X, and prothrombin). The effective half-life of this drug is 20 to 60 minutes (mean 40) with its duration of clinical effect lasting 2 to 5 days.[52] The drug is orally administered and is nearly completely absorbed with peak blood levels at 4 hours. Warfarin efficacy is monitored by the INR and increases are seen only after the first 24 to 36 hours after the initial dose. The antithrombotic effect of warfarin does not peak until 5 days regardless of initial peaks in INR. This relates to the antithrombotic effect being associated with factor II (thrombin), whereas the INR is primarily the reflection of factor VII levels.[53] Additionally, it also lowers the levels of anticoagulant proteins C and S; hence, upon initiation of warfarin therapy, patients may be transiently hypercoagulable. Therefore, initiation of warfarin therapy is generally performed with concurrent use of another anticoagulant agent, such as heparin, until the INR reaches a satisfactory level for 2 days.

Clearance of warfarin involves the cytochrome p450 system in the liver. Therefore, hepatic insufficiency will increase the efficacy of warfarin, requiring lower dosages. Therapeutic warfarin levels can be markedly affected by diet/other medications and genetic makeup as well, requiring continued monitoring of the INR. This has implications for dosing because different individuals will respond differently to the same dosage. The genetic variation is owed to polymorphisms in the gene encoding for vitamin K, epoxide reductase, and in the cytochrome p450 gene, CYP2C9, that can account for up to 50% of variability in dosing.[54]

Common uses for warfarin include prevention of thrombosis and subsequent embolism formation in patients with atrial fibrillation, those with artificial heart valves, deep venous thrombosis (DVT), and/or pulmonary emboli.

The decision to withhold warfarin therapy prior to a procedure and the method by which this is accomplished is complicated and highly debated.[55] The decision should be individualized and based on the perceived risk and benefits of holding warfarin therapy and include a discussion with the patient as well as the physician who initiated the warfarin therapy. Complicating matters, discontinuing warfarin can result in a transient rebound hypercoagulable state, leading some physicians to

Table 98.2

Guidelines for Withholding Anticoagulant Agents Prior to an Interventional Procedure

Anticoagulent	Mechanism	Delay prior to procedure
Warfarin	Vitamin K antagonist	INR below 1.5 for major surgical procedures
Unfractionated heparin	Antithrombin inhibitor	Therapeutic infusion: Hold 4–6 hr prior Prophylactic subcutaneous injection: Hold 1 prior dose (8–12hr) ACT <200 prior to arterial sheath removal
Enoxaparin (LMWH)	Antifactor Xa > antifactor IIa inhibitor	Therapeutic subcutaneous—24 hr Prophylactic subcutaneous—12 hr **SIR consensus panel** Low risk: therapeutic—withhold 1 dose Moderate risk: therapeutic—withhold 1 dose High risk: withhold 24 hr or up to 2 doses
Fondaparinux	Antifactor Xa	Half-life is 17–21 hr; hold 4 d prior to procedure
Lepirudin	Direct thrombin (IIa) inhibitor	Half-life is 1.3 hr; hold 6.5 hr prior to procedure
Bivalirudin	Direct thrombin (IIa) inhibitor	**Manufacturer**: Normalization of coagulation times in 1 hr
Desirudin	Direct thrombin (IIa) inhibitor	Half-life is 2 hr; hold 10 hr prior to procedure
Argatroban	Direct thrombin (IIa) inhibitor	Discontinue 2–4 hr prior to procedure

Where available, studies determining the optimum time to discontinue anticoagulant drugs are listed with their recommendations. When these studies or manufacturer recommendations are not available, suggested guidelines are listed based on four to five half-life eliminations (*shaded*). Where available, SIR consensus panel recommendations are listed.[8]

suggest bridging therapy with another antithrombotic, typically one of the heparins.[56,57] The decision to use bridging therapy is highly complex and controversial and based on the patent's risk for thromboembolism and is beyond the scope of this chapter.[58] We must reiterate the importance of including the physician who prescribed warfarin in the discussions of discontinuing the drug. If the decision is to withhold warfarin therapy, the consensus seems to be that an INR of less than 1.5 is the goal prior to any major surgery, which we are extrapolating to include any interventional procedure.[59] It has been found that in most individuals with an INR of 2 to 3 (some therapeutic levels of INR are greater than this range), it requires 5 days for the levels to normalize to below an INR of 1.5.[60]

If normalization is decided upon and required for an emergent procedure, the effects of warfarin can commonly be reversed by FFP or oral vitamin K. As described in an earlier section, the suggested amount of FFP required is based on coagulation tests with 1 unit used if PT is between 18 and 22 seconds and to begin with 2 units of FFP if the PT is greater (most patients on therapeutic dosages of warfarin). Oral vitamin K is the preferred method of expedited reversal usually requiring dosages of 1 to 2 mg. The limitation of this method being that it may take up to 24 hours for there to be clinical effect.[61] If more rapid reversal is required, vitamin K can be given intravenously. This method is usually limited to patients who are supratherapeutic, requiring rapid reversal, because intravenous (IV) vitamin K has been rarely associated with anaphylaxis.[62] Dosages are based on INR: 0.5 to 1 mg IV if the INR is between 6 and 10 without bleeding; 3 to 5 mg IV if the INR is between 10 and 20 without bleeding; 10 mg IV if the INR is greater than 20 or with serious bleeding. If this method is used, PT/INR is checked every 4 to 6 hours.

In the postprocedure setting, warfarin is usually restarted immediately after the procedure. For patients with high risk of thromboembolism, heparin is usually given as a bridge regardless of whether a heparin bridge was used preprocedurally.[63]

Heparin, first used clinically in 1935, was the first antithrombotic agent available and currently the most common anticoagulant used.[64] Heparin binds to the protein antithrombin III and can inhibit the activity of factors IXa, Xa, Xia, and XIIa, plasmin, kallikrein, as well as thrombin. Unfractionated and fractionated forms of heparin exist, both with the similar targets in the coagulation pathway.

Unfractionated heparin (UFH) is isolated from porcine intestinal mucosa or bovine lung tissue. Because UFH binds to plasma proteins, platelets, and vascular endothelium, and bound heparin is inactive, bioavailability (<50 %) varies among individuals. UFH is effective within 3 minutes of IV injection and its effect is assessed by activated clotting time (ACT). For monitoring of long-term UFH therapy, aPTT is used.

Dosage of the drug depends on clinical indication. For prophylaxis of venous thromboembolism, 5,000 units of heparin is given subcutaneously either two or three times daily.[65] A recent meta-analysis suggests that twice a day (b.i.d.) dosing of subcutaneous heparin is associated with fewer major bleeding complications, but three times a day (t.i.d.) dosing offers better efficacy in preventing clinically relevant venous thromboembolic events.[66] There appears to be local treads in which dosing is preferred. Therapeutic doses of UFH require an initial large bolus of 80 units/kg followed by an infusion of 18 units/kg/hour with continued monitoring of aPTT (generally every 4 to 6 hours) with titration until therapeutic levels are achieved.[67]

Although utilization of heparin during routine diagnostic arterial or venous studies is rarely required, there is always a potential during an endovascular procedure for vessel damage inciting a thromboembolic event. The risks increase with the length of the procedure, its complexity, and decreasing vessel size. Anticoagulation is typically used when a vessel is temporarily occluded, whether it be during an open procedure with a vessel clamp/loop or with a balloon during an endovascular procedure. We must also be aware that indwelling guide wires, catheters, balloons, and sheaths are foreign materials that can serve as a nidus for thrombus formation. The more occlusive the device, the higher the risk of thrombosis.

Therapeutic doses of heparin are generally used in stenting or plasty procedures in both arteries and veins and on occasion during diagnostic exams when the catheter impedes flow through a tight stenosis. No firm recommendations are available for endovascular use of heparin. A group suggests that the dose be dependent on the vessel: brachiocephalic vessels (75 to 100 units/kg); aortoiliac (25 to 50 units/kg).[68] One study of coronary interventions used as little as 3,000 units without any increased risks of thromboembolism.[69] In adult patients, the authors use a dose of 3,000 to 5,000 units of IV bolus followed by 1,000 units every hour.[70] The intraprocedural effect of heparin is monitored by measuring the ACT with a target of 250 to 300 seconds. In the neurointerventional literature, one group suggests that the target ACT should be around twice the baseline.[71] In the pediatric population, patients undergoing angiography (diagnostic or therapeutic) who are less than 15 kg are routinely given 75 to 100 units/kg of IV heparin once arterial access is achieved to prevent thrombosis.[72] ACTs are measured at arterial puncture (baseline) and then 5 minutes after giving the bolus dose of heparin.

Heparinized flushes or infusion of subtherapeutic doses of heparin through the sideport of a vascular sheath have been used to prevent in-sheath clot formation at 150 units/hour during long arterial procedures. The utility of heparinized versus nonheparinized solutions to prevent vascular sheath clot formation is controversial. Indeed, one group looking specifically at risk of clot formation in femoral sheaths maintained overnight with and without a continuous heparinized drip (concentration of 2,000 units/L) through the sheath found no significant difference in number of clots, leading this group to suggest sheath exchange should repeat angiograms be necessary.[73]

The half-life of UFH is dose dependent and ranges from 30 to 90 minutes, at usual IV dosages. Heparin drips are generally discontinued 4 to 6 hours prior to any invasive procedure. Vascular sheath removal is performed with ACT below 200.[74]

Should rapid reversal of heparin effects be required, protamine can be used. **Protamine** is derived from salmon sperm and complexes with heparin in a 1:100 ratio (1 mg protamine:100 units heparin) and prevents binding of antithrombin (AT) to heparin. A suggested protocol for heparin reversal is 20 to 35 mg of protamine if ACT is greater than twice the baseline and 10 to 20 mg if less than twice the baseline.[75] Protamine is infused slowly to lower risk of anaphylaxis.

A risk unique to the use of heparin is **heparin-induced thrombocytopenia (HIT)**. It is a syndrome that occurs in 1% to 3% of patients receiving heparin (mostly unfractionated heparin). An IgG antibody develops against a complex of heparin and endogenous platelet-factor 4 and in the presence of exogenous

heparin, this antibody binds to platelets and leads to platelet cross-linking and subsequent thrombosis.[76] Treatment includes immediate cessation of all heparin, including in flushes.

Low-molecular-weight heparin (LMWH) is a newer form of heparin that is rapidly increasing in popularity. LMWHs are short segments of UFH created either synthetically or from depolymerization of standard UFH. LMWH offers more anti-Xa activity and less anti-IIa activity, leading to increased efficacy and lower bleeding risks.[77,78] Although LMWHs are associated with lower risks of HIT, once heparin-associated platelet antibodies are present due to prior exposure to UFH, up to 20% to 60% of patients will cross-react with LMWH, leading to the HIT syndrome.[79] Secondary to its size, LMWH has less affinity to bind to plasma proteins than unfractionated heparin, yielding up to 90% bioavailability after subcutaneous injection. This allows for a more reproducible response when dosing on a weight-adjusted basis without the need for monitoring.

The plasma half-life of LMWH is 90 to 180 minutes with a 4.4-hour subcutaneous half-life. Extrapolating from pharmacokinetics, one group found that at therapeutic doses of LMWH, a patient is no longer anticoagulated 21 hours after treatment is terminated. Generally, low (prophylactic) doses of LMWH should be withheld 12 hours prior to a procedure, whereas high (therapeutic) doses of LMWH should be withheld 24 hours prior to a procedure.[80] LMWH can be resumed anywhere from 2 to 8 hours after completing a procedure.

There is no current proven method to rapidly reverse or neutralize LMWH. Some animal studies have demonstrated that protamine can neutralize up to 60% of LMWH's antithrombin activity.[81] A group has suggested that if emergency reversal of LMWH is needed, the following protocol can be used: If LMWH was administered within 8 hours, protamine can be given at a dose of 1 mg per 100 antifactor Xa units LMWH (1 mg enoxaparin is equivalent to 100 antifactor Xa units); a second dose of 0.5 mg of protamine can be used per 100 antifactor Xa units if bleeding continues; smaller doses are used if the LMWH was injected more than 8 hours prior.[82]

A large number of LMWHs exist, varying in their methods of manufacture and size. Some of the more common include: tinzaparin, dalteparin, nadroparin, enoxaparin, and the synthetic fondaparinux, the latter two of which are described in more detail.

Enoxaparin (Lovenox, Sanofi-Aventis, Bridgewater, NJ) is used in both DVT prophylaxis and in treatment of venous thromboembolism. Low prophylactic dose is either 40 mg per day or 30 mg every 12 hours (q12). High (therapeutic) dose is 1 mg/kg every 12 hours. Enoxaparin is renally cleared and, therefore, a longer waiting period after discontinuing the drug prior to a procedure may be required. Some have demonstrated that the half-life of the anti-Xa activity of enoxaparin was prolonged as much as twofold in patients with renal failure.[83]

As with all LMWHs, aPTT is not useful in monitoring this drug. Although there is currently no standard in measuring the effects of enoxaparin, a group has suggested utilizing direct monitoring of antifactor Xa levels.[84] More recent literature suggest that there is a dose correlation of intravenous/intra-arterial enoxaparin with changes in ACT.[85] It must be stressed that enoxaparin is often given subcutaneously and thus will not affect ACT. It is in this capacity that utilizing antifactor Xa levels may have some utility.[86]

Fondaparinux (Arixtra, GlaxoSmithKline, Research Triangle Park, NC) is a synthetic version of heparin and specifically targets factor Xa. Currently, fondaparinux is the only indirect factor Xa inhibitor available in the United States and is increasingly used in patients with HIT.[87] Fondaparinux is also renally excreted and has a half-life of 17 to 21 hours. Therefore, assuming normal pharmacokinetics, this drug would need to be discontinued at least 4 days (five half-lives) prior to an invasive procedure. The manufacturer recommends that if fondaparinux were to be used in postoperative DVT prophylaxis, initial dose be postponed until 6 to 8 hours after the procedure.

Fondaparinux, in compariso to enoxaparin, has been found to be equally as efficacious with lower associated major bleeding complications in patients undergoing PCIs with acute coronary syndromes.[88] A recent randomized trial demonstrated nearly equivalent efficacy between fondaparinux and enoxaparin in treatment of acute symptomatic DVT.[89]

Prophylactic dosage is 2.5 mg daily subcutaneously, whereas therapeutic dosages of fondaparinux are weight based: 5mg (<50 kg), 7.5 mg (between 50 and 100 kg), or 10 mg (>100 kg).

Direct thrombin inhibitors, as the name suggests, work directly on inhibiting thrombin (factor IIa). These drugs are active against both soluble forms of thrombin as well as thrombin bound to thrombus, therefore, unlike heparin, has the theoretical potential to dissolve clot, not just prevent progression. Two forms exist, univalent and bivalent, which refer to whether or not the drug binds to an additional site other than the active site (bivalent). A host of direct thrombin inhibitors are undergoing clinical testing.[90] Common bivalent forms include lepirudin, bivalirudin, and desirudin. Common univalent forms include argatroban and dabigatran. Although the indications of direct thrombin inhibitors are increasing, this class of drug is currently mostly used in scenarios where heparin is indicated but cannot be utilized.

Lepirudin (Refludan, Berlex Laboratories, Montville, NJ) is a recombinant derivative of hirudin (the prototypic bivalent direct thrombin inhibitor), an anticoagulant found in saliva of medicinal leeches. Lepirudin binds at both the catalytic site of thrombin (preventing conversion of fibrinogen to fibrin) and at the fibrinogen binding site. This drug is renally excreted with a half-life of 1.3 hours.[91] Therefore, assuming normal renal function and five half-lives, 6.5 hours after discontinuing the drug would be a safe time to begin a procedure.

The normal dose (assuming normal renal function) is a bolus of 0.4 mg/kg followed by continuous infusion of 0.15 mg/kg/hour. The effective levels of lepirudin can be monitored by aPTT. The first aPTT is drawn 4 hours after initiation of infusion, and then checked 4 hours after every change in dose. Lepirudin has been proven to be a safe alternative in patients with HIT.[92]

Bivalirudin (Angiomax, The Medicines Company, Parsippany, NJ) is used primarily in patients with HIT undergoing PCI. It is also renally cleared with a half-life of 25 minutes. According to the manufacturer, aPTT, PT, TT, and ACT are abnormal with usage of this drug with normalization of coagulation times 1 hour after discontinuation.[93]

Desirudin (Iprivask, Canyon Pharmaceuticals, Hunt Valley, MD) is approved for use in the United States for preventing DVT in patients undergoing hip surgery. It has a half-life of about 2 hours and because it is also renally cleared, dosages are based on renal function.

Argatroban (GlaxoSmithKline Pharmaceuticals, Research Triangle Park, NC) derived from L-arginine, is a small (527 Da) synthetic direct thrombin inhibitor that binds reversibly to the active site of thrombin. Argatroban is most commonly used in patients with HIT and has been found to be associated with improved clinical outcomes without increased hemorrhagic complications in patients with HIT undergoing PCI.[94] For PCI, argatroban is approved for use in HIT at a dose of 25 g/kg/minute after a 350 g/kg initial bolus, titrated to ACT of 250 to 300 seconds.

Argatroban affects aPTT, PT, TT, and ACT. Coagulation times usually normalize 2 to 4 (half-life 40 to 50 minutes) hours after drug discontinuation. Argatroban is predominantly hepatically cleared with some renal excretion.[95]

Should argatroban be used in lieu of heparin as a bridge to oral anticoagulants, the manufacturer recommends concurrent administration of warfarin and argatroban for 4 to 5 days, at which point, if INR is above 4, argatroban should be discontinued and a repeat INR level checked in 4 to 6 hours.

Most direct thrombin inhibitors are administered subcutaneously, intramuscularly, or intravenously. Two new oral anticoagulants are being investigated, dabigatran and rivaroxaban. One of these, **dabigatran** (Pradaxa, Boehringer Ingelheim Pharmaceuticals, Ridgefield, CT) is a direct factor II inhibitor and inhibits free thrombin, fibrin-bound thrombin, and thrombin-induced platelet aggregation. The U.S. Food and Drug Administration recently announced approval of this drug to prevent stroke in patients with atrial fibrillation.[96]

FIBRINOLYTICS (THROMBOLYTICS)

The use of anticoagulation during endovascular procedures is generally to prevent thrombus formation. Occasionally, pathologic thrombosis has already occurred and the physician is faced with treating this state. Under normal circumstances, the body's own hemostatic functions release fibrinolytic enzymes to counter this thrombus. However, should the pathologic state overwhelm the normal process, thrombolytic agents can be administered. Intravascular administration of thrombolytic agents originated in the 1960s with treatment for pulmonary embolism. Thrombolytics are serine proteases that work by converting plasminogen to plasmin. Plasmin works on clot by breaking down both fibrinogen and fibrin (fibrinolysis).[97]

Systemic administration of thrombolytics has been shown to be superior to heparin administration alone in treatment of DVT.[98] Techniques for catheter-directed fibrinolysis/thrombolysis include mechanical or pharmacologic, or a combination of these. Dosages for pharmacologic thrombolysis are still controversial and current investigation is geared at discovering the lowest efficacious dose to lower bleeding risks (Table 98.3).

Common thrombolytics include first-generation thrombolytics: streptokinase and UK; second-generation thrombolytic: alteplase; and third-generation thrombolytics: reteplase and tenecteplase.

Table 98.3	
Dosing Guidelines for Administration of Thrombolytic Drugs	
Thrombolytic	Dose
Alteplase	**Consensus 2000:** A weight-adjusted dose of 0.001–0.02 mg/kg/hr or a non-weight-adjusted dose of 0.12–2 mg/hr[108] **Studies:** Low-dose regimen of 0.25–1 mg/hr for catheter-directed thrombolysis with doses not exceeding 40 mg[106,107]
Reteplase	**Consensus 2001:** A minimum dose of at least 0.25 unit/hr with a dose range of 0.25–1 unit/hr. Maximum dose amount 20 units with a maximum infusion time of 24 hr[112] **Study:** For lower-extremity arterial occlusions, doses of 0.5, 0.25, and 0.125 unit/hr are equally effective with more bleeding complications associated with the highest dose[113]
Tenecteplase	**Study:** The optimum dose for use in arterial and venous infusions has yet to be established; a low infusion dose of 0.125 mg/hr has similar success and complication rates as higher dosages[115]

Streptokinase, isolated from strains of beta hemolytic streptococci, was the first thrombolytic drug available for use. First isolated in 1933, it entered clinical use in the mid-1940s.[99] Streptokinase binds plasminogen to form a complex that facilitates further conversion of plasminogen to plasmin. Streptokinase has a short half-life of 16 minutes, which can be overwhelmed by administering a large initial bolus, raising the half-life to 83 minutes. The use of this drug has largely been abandoned secondary to its bacterial origins causing high levels of antistreptococcal antibodies resulting in allergic reactions.

Urokinase is a trypsin-like protease that directly cleaves plasminogen to plasmin.[100] UK is physiologic and normally produced in renal parenchymal cells; therefore, it is thought to be nonantigenic. Its thrombolytic potential is similar to that of streptokinase with a lower incidence of bleeding.[101] UK is extracted from human urine or cultures of neonatal kidney cells.

UK was approved in the United States in 1978 for treatment of pulmonary embolism and coronary artery occlusion. Due to its effectiveness, off-label usage of this drug for peripheral thrombolysis was common. Because this drug was obtained from fetal kidney cell cultures, some concerns for potential viral contamination of UK led the Food and Drug Administration (FDA) to ban its sale and distribution in January 1999.[102] This drug was reintroduced as Kinlytic (previously Abbokinase) and approved by the FDA in 2002 for treatment of massive pulmonary embolism. Likely due to prior concerns, the drug has changed manufacturers several times and is currently not available in the United States.[103] The 3-year hiatus when UK was not available opened the door for other thrombolytics, such as r-tPA to fill the void.

Alteplase (r-tPA, Activase, Genentech, San Francisco, CA), a serine protease produced by recombinant DNA technology, is currently the most widely used thrombolytic agent in the United States and has been used in situations, such as in acute stroke, acute pulmonary embolism, and acute myocardial infarction. It has also been FDA approved for restoration of central venous access device function (Cathflo, Activase). A common off-label use is catheter-directed venous and arterial thrombolysis. In a meta-analysis of prospective comparative trials comparing r-tPA to UK, r-tPA was found to be more effective in lysing acute peripheral arterial occlusions; however, it is associated with higher rates of total and minor bleeding.[104] A multicenter randomized trial has compared use of high-dose versus low-dose administration of tPA in patients with acute limb ischemia and found no differences in degree of limb salvage or complications.[105] This has led many to prefer the low-dose regimen of 0.25 to 1 mg/hour for catheter-directed thrombolysis in acute limb ischemia with doses not exceeding 40 mg.[106,107] In 2000, a consensus statement on guidelines for use of r-tPA suggested the following dosing regimen: a weight adjusted dose of 0.001 to 0.02 mg/kg/hour or a non-weight adjusted dose of 0.12 to 2 mg/hour.[108] Reports of concurrent utilization of therapeutic levels of heparin as well as tPA have demonstrated increased risks of major bleeding.[109] Therefore, it is advisable that only subtherapeutic heparin (300 to 500 units/hour) be administered concurrently through the sideport of the vascular sheath to prevent pericatheter thrombosis, keeping the aPTT below 60, although, as discussed in the **Heparin** section of this chapter, its efficacy for this purpose is questionable.

Reteplase (r-PA, Retavase; PDL BioPharma, Inc., Fremont, CA) is a deletion mutant of alteplase produced in *Escherichia coli*. Reteplase is currently approved for use in management of acute myocardial infarction for improvement of ventricular function following an acute event. The safety and efficacy of reteplase for treatment of acute arterial occlusion has been studied demonstrating high limb salvage rates with low risks of bleeding.[110] Utilization has also been studied in treatment of acute venous thrombosis in a retrospective study comparing UK, alteplase, and reteplase for catheter-directed treatment of DVT, which demonstrated no differences in success rates, infusion times, or complications between the three groups; however, it cited that both alteplase and reteplase were significantly less costly than UK.[111]

A consensus document published in 2001 suggested a minimum dose of at least 0.25 unit/hour with a dose range of 0.25 to 1 unit/hour. Maximum dose amount was 20 units with a maximum infusion time of 24 hours.[112] Another study evaluating differing doses of reteplase for lower-extremity arterial occlusions, doses of 0.5, 0.25, and 0.125 unit/hour were found to be equally effective with more bleeding complications associated with the highest dose.[113]

Tenecteplase (TNK-tissue plasminogen activator; Genentech, San Francisco, CA) is a fibrin specific recombinant plasminogen activator. It can selectively convert thrombus-bound plasminogen to plasmin. It is the only agent to have resistance against inactivation by plasminogen activator inhibitor-1. Although tenecteplase is approved for use only in treatment of acute coronary syndromes, studies for use in acute peripheral arterial and venous occlusions have been performed.[114] Although the optimum dose for use in arterial and venous infusions has yet to be established, a group has determined that a low infusion dose of 0.125 mg/hour appears to have similar success and complication rates as higher dosages.[115]

Third-generation thrombolytics, such as reteplase and tenecteplase, offer increased fibrin specificity over earlier generations and increased half-life over the second-generation drug alteplase. This increase in half-life allows for bolus dosing of third-generation drugs, which may be more pertinent in treatment of acute coronary syndromes than in peripheral thrombolysis. Because there have been reports linking decreased fibrinogen levels with fewer major bleeding complications, the increased fibrin specificity and decreased fibrinogenolysis of third-generation thrombolytics may be associated with fewer bleeding complications.[116]

▌ REFERENCES

1. Ruggeri ZM, Mendolicchio GL. Adhesion mechanisms in platelet function. *Circ Res* 2007;100:1673–1685.
2. Walker RH. Special report: transfusion risks. *Am J Clin Pathol* 1987;88:374–378.
3. Lundberg GD. Practice parameter for the use of fresh-frozen plasma, cryoprecipitate, and platelets. *JAMA* 1994;271:777–781.
4. NIH Consensus Conference. Platelet transfusion therapy. *JAMA* 1987;257:1777–1780.
5. Gaydos LA, Freireich EF, Mantel N. The quantitative relation between platelet count and hemorrhage in patients with acute leukemia. *N Engl J Med* 1962;266:905–909.
6. Mannucci PM, Ruggeri Z, Pareti F, et al. 1-deamino-8-arginine vasopressin: a new pharmacological approach to the management of haemophilia and von Willebrands disease. *Lancet* 1977;1:869–872.
7. Greenblatt DJ. Elimination half-life of drugs: value and limitations. *Ann Rev Med* 1985;36:421–427.
8. Malloy PC, Grassi CJ, Kundu S, et al. Consensus guidelines for periprocedural management of coagulation status and hemostasis risk in percutaneous image-guided interventions. *J Vasc Interv Radiol* 2009;20:S240–S249.
9. Fink A, Kosecoff J, Chassin M, et al. Consensus methods: characteristics and guidelines for use. *Am J Public Health* 1984;74:979–998.
10. Babapulle MN, Joseph L, Belisle P, et al. A hierarchical Bayesian meta-analysis of randomised clinical trials of drug-eluting stents. *Lancet* 2004;364:583–591.
11. Bavry AA, et al. Late thrombosis of drug-eluting stents: a meta-analysis of randomized clinical trials. *Am J Med* 2006;119:1056–1061.
12. Berger JS, et al. Aspirin for the primary prevention of cardiovascular events in women and men: a sex-specific meta-analysis of randomized controlled trials. *JAMA* 2006;295:306–313.
13. Antithrombotic Trialist Collaboration. Collaborative meta-analysis of randomized trials of platelet therapy for prevention of death, myocardial infarction, and stroke in high risk patients. *BMJ* 2002;324:71–86.
14. Berger JS, Krantz MJ, Kittelson JM, et al. Aspirin for the prevention of cardiovascular events in patients with peripheral artery disease: a meta-analysis of randomized trials. *JAMA* 2009;301:1909–1919.
15. Hirsch AT, Haskal ZJ, Hertzer NR, et al. ACC/AHA 2005 Practice guidelines for the management of patients with peripheral arterial disease. *Circulation* 2006;113:e463–e654.
16. Norgren L, Hiatt WR, Dormandy JA, et al. Inter-society consensus for the management of peripheral arterial disease (TASC II). *Eur J Vasc Endovasc Surg* 2007;33:S1–S75.
17. Jimenez AH, Stubbs ME, Tofler GH, et al. Rapidity and duration of platelet suppression by enteric-coated aspirin in healthy young men. *Am J Cardiol* 1992;69:258–262.
18. Latini R, Cerletti C, de Gaetano G, et al. Comparative bioavailability of aspirin from buffered, enteric-coated and plain preparations. *Int J Clin Pharmacol Ther Toxicol* 1986;24:313–318.
19. Burch JW, Stanford N, Majerus PW. Inhibition of platelet prostaglandin synthase by oral aspirin. *J Clin Invest* 1979;61:314–319.
20. Bradlow BA, Chetty N. Dosage frequency for suppression of platelet function by low dose aspirin therapy. *Thromb Res* 1982;27:99–110.
21. Patrono C, Ciabattoni G, Patrignani P, et al. Clinical pharmacology of platelet cyclooxygenase inhibition. *Circulation* 1985;72:177–184.
22. Patrono C, Collar B, Dalen J, et al. Platelet-active drugs: the relationships among dose, effectiveness, and side effects. *Chest* 1998;114:470S–488S.
23. Antiplatelet Trialists' Collaboration. Collaborative overview of randomised trials of antiplatelet therapy, I: prevention of death, myocardial infarction, and stroke by prolonged antiplatelet therapy in various categories of patients. *BMJ* 1994;308:81–106.
24. Patrignani P, Filabozzi P, Patrono C. Selective cumulative inhibition of platelet thromboxane production by low-dose aspirin in healthy subjects. *J Clin Invest* 1982;69:1366–1372.
25. FitzGerald GA, Oates JA, Hawiger J, et al. Endogenous biosynthesis of prostacyclin and thromboxane and platelet function during chronic administration of aspirin in man. *J Clin Invest* 1983;71:676–688.
26. Weksler BB, Pett SB, Alonso D, et al. Differential inhibition by aspirin of vascular and platelet prostaglandin synthesis in atherosclerotic patients. *N Engl J Med* 1983;308:800–805.
27. Clarke RJ, Mayo G, Price P, et al. Suppression of thromboxane A2 but not systemic prostacyclin by controlled-release aspirin. *N Engl J Med* 1991;325:1137–1141.
28. Grosser T, Fries S, FitzGerald GA. Biological basis for the cardiovascular consequences of COX-2 inhibition: therapeutic challenges and opportunities. *J Clin Invest* 2006;116:4–15.
29. Silverman SG, Coughlin BF, Seltzer SE, et al. Current use of screening laboratory tests before abdominal interventions: a survey of 603 radiologists. *Radiology* 1991;181:669–673.
30. Darcy MD, Kanterman RY, Kleinhoffer MA, et al. Evaluation of coagulation tests as predictors of angiographic bleeding complications. *Radiology* 1996;198:741–744.
31. Mackinnon B, Fraser E, Simpson K, et al. Is it necessary to stop antiplatelet agents before a native renal biopsy? *Nephrol Dial Transplant* 2008;23:3566–3570.
32. Gill S, Majumdar S, Brown NE, et al. Ticlopidine-associated pancytopenia: implications of an acetylsalicylic acid alternative. *Can J Cardiol* 1997;13:909–913.
33. Patrono C, Coller B, Fitzgerald GA, et al. Platelet-active drugs: the relationship among dose, effectiveness, and side effects: the Seventh ACCP Conference on Antithrombotic and Thrombolytic Therapy. *Chest* 2004;126:234S–264S.
34. Yusuf S, Zhai F, Mehta SR, et al. Effects of clopidogrel in addition to aspirin in patients with acute coronary syndromes without ST-segment elevation. *N Engl J Med* 2001;345:494–502.
35. Bhatt DL, Aranki S, Bryne J, et al. Issues in the management of antiplatelet therapy in patients undergoing surgical revascularization. A roundtable discussion. *J Invasive Cardiol* 2005;17:283.
36. Ho LM, Hodulik KL, Suhocki PV, et al. New classes of anticoagulation and antiplatelet agents: preprocedure management and safety guidelines for image-guided intervention. *J Comput Assist Tomogr* 2008;32:475–479.
37. Olin JW, Sealove BA. Peripheral artery disease: current insight into the disease and its diagnosis and management. *Mayo Clin Proc* 2010;85:678–692.
38. Yusuf S, Zhao F, Mehta SR, et al. Effects of clopidogrel in addition to aspirin in patients with acute coronary syndromes without ST-segment elevation. *N Engl J Med* 2001;345:494–502.
39. Sabatine MS, Cannon CP, Gibson CM, et al. Effect of clopidogrel pretreatment before percutaneous coronary intervention in patients with ST-elevation myocardial infarction treated with fibrinolytics. *JAMA* 2005;294:1224–1232.
40. Pekdemir H, Cin VG, Camsari A, et al. A comparison of 1-month and 6-month clopidogrel therapy on clinical and angiographic outcome after stent implantation. *Heart Vessels* 2003;18:123–129.
41. Hiatt WR, Krantz MJ. Masterclass series in peripheral arterial disease: antiplatelet therapy for peripheral arterial disease and claudication. *Vasc Med* 2006;11:55–60.

42. CAPRIE Steering Committee. A randomised, blinded, trial of clopidogrel versus aspirin in patients at risk for ischaemic events (CAPRIE). *Lancet* 1996;348:1329–1339.

43. Bhatt DL, Fiz KA, Hacke W, et al. Clopidogrel and aspirin versus aspirin alone for the prevention of atherothrombotic events. *N Engl J Med* 2006;354:1706–1717.

44. Bishara AI, Hagmeyer KO. Acute profound thrombocytopenia following abciximab therapy. *Ann Pharmacother* 2000;34:924–930.

45. Dasgupta H, Blankenship JC, Wood GC, et al. Thrombocytopenia complicating treatment with intravenous glycoprotein IIb/IIIa receptor inhibitors: a pooled analysis. *Am Heart J* 2000;140:206–211.

46. Rosove MH. Platelet glycoprotein IIb/IIIa inhibitors. *Best Pract Res Clin Haematol* 2004;17:65–76.

47. Kong DF, Califf RM, Miller DP, et al. Clinical outcomes of therapeutic agents that block the platelet glycoprotein IIb/IIIa integrin in ischemic heart disease. *Circulation* 1998;98:2829–2835.

48. Barrett JS, Murphy G, Peerlinck K, et al. Pharmacokinetics and pharmacodynamics of MK-383, a selective non-peptide platelet glycoprotein-IIb/IIIa receptor antagonist, in healthy men. *Clin Pharm Ther* 1994;56:377–388.

49. Phillips DR, Scarborough RM. Clinical pharmacology of eptifibatide. *Am J Cardiol* 1977;80:11B–20B.

50. Mackman N. Triggers, targets and treatments of thrombosis. *Nature* 2008;451:914–918.

51. Dickson BC. Venous thrombosis: on the history of Virchow's triad. *Univ Toronto Med J* 2004;81:166–171.

52. Majerus PW, Broze GJ, Miletich JP, et al. Anticoagulant, thrombolytic, and antiplatelet drugs. In: Hardman JG, Limbird LE, eds. *Goodman and Gilman's the Pharmacological Basis of Therapeutics.* 9th ed. New York, NY: McGraw-Hill; 1996:1347–1351.

53. Hirsh J, Dalen JE, Anderson DR, et al. Oral anticoagulants: mechanism of action, clinical effectiveness, and optimal therapeutic range. *Chest* 2001;119:8S–21S.

54. Krynetskly E. Building individualized medicine: prevention of adverse reactions to warfarin therapy. *J Pharmacol Exp Ther* 2007;322:427–434.

55. Jaffer AK, Brotman DJ, Chukwumerije N. When patients on warfarin need surgery. *Cleve Clin J Med* 2003;70:973–984.

56. Palareti G, Legnani C. Warfarin withdrawal. Pharmacokinetic-pharmacodynamic considerations. *Clin Pharmacokinet* 1996;30:300–313.

57. Douketis JD, Crowther MA, Cherian SS. Perioperative anticoagulation in patients with chronic atrial fibrillation who are undergoing elective surgery: results of a physician survey. *Can J Cardiol* 2000;16:326–330.

58. Spyropoulos AC. Bridging therapy and oral anticoagulation: current and future prospects. *Curr Opin Hematol* 2010;17:444–449.

59. Baker RI, Coughlin PB, Gallus AS, et al. Warfarin reversal: consensus guidelines, on behalf of the Australian Society of Thrombosis and Haemostasis. *Med J Aust* 2004;181:492–497.

60. White RH, McKittrick T, Hutchinson R, et al. Temporary discontinuation of warfarin therapy: changes in the international normalized ratio. *Ann Intern Med* 1995;122:40–42.

61. Hirsh J, Fuster V, Ansell J, et al. American Heart Association/American College of Cardiology Foundation guide to warfarin therapy. *Circulation* 2003;107:1692–1711.

62. Fiore LD, Scola MA, Cantillon CE, et al. Anaphylactoid reactions to vitamin K. *J Thromb Thrombolysis* 2001;11:175–183.

63. Kearon C, Hirsh J. Management of anticoagulation before and after elective surgery. *N Engl J Med* 1997;336:1506–1511.

64. Owen CA Jr. *A History of Blood Coagulation.* Rochester, MN: Mayo Foundation for Medical Education and Research; 2001.

65. Geerts WH, Pineo GF, Heit JA, et al. Prevention of venous thromboembolism: the Seventh ACCP Conference on Antithrombotic and Thrombolytic Therapy. *Chest* 2004;126:338S–400S.

66. King CS, Holley AB, Jackson JL, et al. Twice vs three times daily heparin dosing for thromboembolism prophylaxis in the general medical population. *Chest* 2007;131:507–516.

67. Raschke RA, Reilly BM, Guidry JR, et al. The weight-based heparin nomogram compared with a "standard care" nomogram: a randomized controlled trial. *Ann Intern Med* 1993;119:874–881.

68. Kandarpa K, Beacker GJ, Hunick MG, et al. Transcatheter interventions for the treatment of peripheral atherosclerotic lesions: part I. *J Vasc Interv Radiol* 2001;12:683–695.

69. Caussin C, Fsihi A, Ohanessian A, et al. Direct stenting with 3000 IU heparin. *Int J Cardiovasc Intervent* 2003;5:206–210.

70. Kaufman JA. Fundamentals of angiography. In: Kaufman JA, Lee MJ, eds. *2004 The Requisites: Vascular and Interventional Radiology.* Philadelphia, PA: Mosby; 2004:31–66.

71. Fujii Y, Takeuchi S, Koike T, et al. Heparin administration and monitoring for neuroangiography. *AJNR Am J Neuroradiol* 1994;15:51–54.

72. Marschalleck F. Pediatric arterial interventions. *Tech Vasc Interv Radiol* 2010;13:238–243.

73. Koenigsberg RA, Wysoki M, Weiss J, et al. Risk of clot formation in femoral arterial sheaths maintained overnight for neuroangiographic procedures. *AJNR Am J Neuroradiol* 1999;20:297–299.

74. Payne CS. A primer on patient management problems in interventional radiology. *AJR Am J Roentgenol* 1998;170:1169–1176.

75. Scott JA, Berenstein A, Blumenthal D. Use of the activated coagulation time as a measure of anticoagulation during interventional procedures. *Radiology* 1986;158:849–850.

76. Cines DB, Rauova L, Arepally G, et al. Heparin-induced thrombocytopenia: an autoimmune disorder regulated through dynamic autoantigen assembly/disassembly. *J Clin Apher* 2007;22:31–36.

77. Quinlan DJ, McQuillan A, Eikelboom JW. Low-molecular weight heparin compared with intravenous unfractionated heparin for the treatment of pulmonary embolism: a meta-analysis of randomized, controlled trials. *Ann Intern Med* 2004;140:175–183.

78. Kakkar W, Cohen AT, Edmonson RA, et al. Low molecular weight heparin versus standard heparin for prevention of venous thromboembolism after major abdominal surgery. *Lancet* 1993;341:259–265.

79. Mureebe L, Silver D. Heparin-induced thrombocytopenia: pathophysiology and management. *Vasc Endovascular Surg* 2002;36:163–170.

80. Tie ML, Koczwara B. Radiology interventions in patients receiving low molecular weight heparin: timing is critical. *Australas Radiol* 2001;45:313–317.

81. Massonnet-Castel S, Pelissier E, Bara L, et al. Partial reversal of low molecular weight heparin (PK 10169) anti-Xa activity by protamine sulfate: in vitro and in vivo study during cardiac surgery with extracorporeal circulation. *Haemostasis* 1986;16:139–146.

82. Hirsh J, Raschke R. Heparin and low-molecular-weight heparin: the Seventh ACCP conference on antithrombotic and thrombolytic therapy. *Chest* 2004;126:188S–203S.

83. Cadroy Y, Pourrat J, Baladre M, et al. Delayed elimination of enoxaparine in patients with chronic renal insufficiency. *Thromb Res* 1991;63:385–390.

84. Saw J, Kereiakes DJ, Mahaffey KW, et al. Evaluation of a novel point-of-care enoxaparin monitor with central laboratory anti-Xa levels. *Thromb Res* 2003;112:301–306.

85. Cavusoglu E, Lakhani M, Marmur JD. The activated clotting time (ACT) can be used to monitor enoxaparin and dalteparin after intravenous administration. *J Invasive Cardiol* 2005;17:416–421.

86. Laposata M, Green K, Elizabeth MVC, et al. College of American Pathologists Conference XXXI on Laboratory Monitoring of Anticoagulant Therapy: the clinical use and laboratory monitoring of low-molecular-weight heparin, danaparoid, hirudin and related compounds, and argatroban. *Arch Pathol Lab Med* 1998;122:799–807.

87. Nutescu EA, Shapiro NL, Chevalier A, et al. A pharmacologic overview of current and emerging anticoagulants. *Cleve Clin J Med* 2005;72:S2–S6.

88. Mehta SR, Granger CB, Eikelboom JW, et al. Efficacy and safety of fondaparinux versus enoxaparin in patients with acute coronary syndromes undergoing percutaneous coronary intervention: results from the OASIS-5 trial. *J Am Coll Cardiol* 2007;18:1742–1751.

89. Buller HR, Davidson BL, Decousus H, et al. Fondaparinux or enoxaparin for initial treatment of symptomatic deep venous thrombosis: a randomized trial. *Ann Intern Med* 2004;140:867–873.

90. Gomez-Outes A, Lecumberri R, Pozo C, et al. New anticoagulants: focus on venous thromboembolism. *Curr Vasc Pharmacol* 2009;7:309–329.

91. Refludan [package insert]. Montville, NJ: Berlex Laboratories; 2004.

92. Mudaliar JH, Liem TK, Nichols WK, et al. Lepirudin is a safe and effective anticoagulant for patients with heparin-associated antiplatelet antibodies. *J Vasc Surg* 2001;34:17–20.

93. Angiomax [package insert]. Parsippany, NJ: The Medicines Company; 2005.

94. Lewis BE, Matthai WH Jr, Cohen M, et al. Argatroban anticoagulation during percutaneous coronary intervention in patients with heparin-induced thrombocytopenia. *Catheter Cardiovasc Interv* 2002;57:177–184.

95. Argatroban [package insert]. Research Triangle Park, NC: GlaxoSmithKline Pharmaceuticals; 2009.

96. FDA approves Pradaxa to prevent stroke in people with atrial fibrillation. FDA Press Release. 2010-10-19.

97. Lord ST. Fibrinogen and fibrin: scoffold proteins in hemostasis. *Curr Opin Hematol* 2007;14:236–241.

98. Comerota AJ, Aldridge S. Thrombolytic therapy for acute deep vein thrombosis. *Semin Vasc Surg* 1992;5:76–81.

99. Mueller K. 1st experiences with highly purified streptokinae in thrombolysis in surgery [in German]. *Bruns Beitr Klin Chir* 1961;202:340–349.

100. Sobel GW, Mohler SR, Jones NW. Urokinase: an activator of plasma fibrinolysin extracted from urine. *Am J Physiol* 1952;171:768–769.

101. van Breda A, Katzen BT, Deutcsch AS. Urokinase versus streptokinase in local thrombolysis. *Radiology* 1987;165:109–111.

102. Valji K. Evolving strategies for thrombolytic therapy of peripheral vascular occulsion. *J Vasc Interv Radiol* 2000;11:411–420.

103. Urokinase executive summary. Mississauga, ON: Microbix Biosystems Inc.; November 2010.

104. Sander S, White CM, Coleman CI. Comparative safety and efficacy of urokinase and recombinant tissue plasminogen activator for peripheral arterial occlusion: a meta-analysis. *Pharmacotherapy* 2006;26:51–60.

105. Braithwaite BD, Buckenham TM, Galland RB, et al. Thrombolysis Study Group. Prospective randomized trial of high-dose bolus versus low-dose tissue plasminogen activator infusion in the management of acute limb ischaemia. *Br J Surg* 1997;84:646–650.

106. Knuttinen MG, Emmanuel N, Isa F, et al. Review of pharmacology and physiology in thrombolysis interventions. *Semin Intervent Radiol* 2010;27:374–383.

107. Rajan DK, Patel NH, Valji K, et al. Quality improvement guidelines for percutaneous management of acute limb ischemia. *J Vasc Interv Radiol* 2009;20:S208–S218.

108. Semba CP, Bakal CW, Calis KA, et al. Alteplase as an alternative to urokinase: Advisory Panel on Catheter-Directed Thrombolytic Therapy. *J Vasc Interv Radiol* 2000;11:279–287.

109. Swischuk JL, Smouse HB. Differentiating pharmacologic agents used in catheter-directed thrombolysis. *Semin Intervent Radiol* 2005;22: 121–129.

110. Hanover TM, Kalbaugh CA, Gray BH, et al. Safety and efficacy of reteplase for the treatment of acute arterial occlusion: complexity of underlying lesion predicts outcome. *Ann Vasc Surg* 2005;19:817–822.

111. Grunwald ME, Hofmann LV. Comparison of urokinase, alteplase, and reteplase for catheter directed thrombolysis of deep venous thrombosis. *J Vasc Interv Radiol* 2004;15:347–352.

112. Benenati J, Shlannsky-Goldberg R, Meglin A, et al. Thrombolytic and antiplatelet therapy in peripheral vascular disease with use of reteplase and/or abciximab. The SCVIR Consultants' Conference; May 22, 2000; Orlando, FL. Society for Cardiovascular and Interventional Radiology. *J Vasc Interv Radiol* 2001;12:795–805.

113. Castaneda F, Swischuk JL, Li R, et al. Declining dose study of reteplase treatment for lower extremity arterial occlusions. *J Vasc Interv Radiol* 2002;13:1093–1098.

114. Burkart DJ, Borsa JJ, Anthony JP, et al. Thrombolysis of acute peripheral arterial and venous occlusions with tenecteplase and eptifibatide: a pilot study. *J Vasc Interv Radiol* 2003;14:729–733.

115. Hull JE, Hull MK, Urso JA, et al. Tenecteplase in acute lower-leg ischemia: effiacy, dose, and adverse events. *J Vasc Interv Radiol* 2006;17: 629–636.

116. Hull JE, Hull MK, Uro JA. Reteplase with or without abciximab for peripheral arterial occlusions: efficacy and adverse events. *J Vasc Interv Radiol* 2004;15:557–564.

Principles of Thrombolytic Agents for Catheter-Directed Therapy

CHARLES P. SEMBA

First described in 1974 by Charles Dotter using low-dose streptokinase to treat arterial ischemia, catheter-directed thrombolysis remains a relevant and essential tool for the interventionist in the management of acute arterial and venous thrombus despite the advancements in endovascular thrombectomy and clot retrieval devices.[1] *Catheter-directed thrombolysis* refers to the technique of percutaneous intrathrombic insertion of an infusion catheter followed by administration of a thrombolytic agent (plasminogen activator) to enzymatically dissolute the fibrin strands and the obstructing thrombus. Catheter-directed intrathrombic infusions of plasminogen activators allow high concentrations of low-dose thrombolytic agent to be efficiently delivered directly into the targeted thrombus, thereby decreasing the time to lysis and reducing the risk of bleeding complications compared to high-dose nonselective systemic intravenous infusions. The technique allows for a minimally invasive and nonsurgical method to reduce the overall clot burden, restore blood flow, and assist in unmasking the underlying obstructing lesion, thus enabling adjunctive endovascular treatment or a reduced scope of surgical repair.

The objective of this chapter is to focus on the basic principles of the thrombolytic drugs and general approach toward catheter-directed thrombolysis; details of specific techniques are discussed in Section V (Arterial Occlusive Disease) and Section XV (Venous Disease and Endovascular Management).

▍ COAGULATION SYSTEM

The ability to produce clot is a complex orchestration of platelets, circulating proteins, and the damaged vascular wall (FIGURE 99.1). When the vascular wall is injured, initial formation of a hemostatic plug (*primary hemostasis)* involves platelet activation and adhesion.[2] Simultaneously, degranulation of adhered platelets and locally exposed proteins activate an enzymatic cascade (*secondary hemostasis)* to ultimately form cross-linked fibrin strands that serve as the structural scaffold to strengthen the aggregated platelet plug. The coagulation cascade generates fibrin through one of two pathways: *tissue factor (TF) pathway* (extrinsic) or *contact activation pathway* (intrinsic). Of the two pathways, TF pathway is the main generator of thrombin (factor IIa), as demonstrated by the observation that patients with deficiencies of factor XII (Hageman factor), high-molecular-weight kininogen (HMWK), or prekallikrein (PK) do not have bleeding disorders.[3]

The TF pathway provides an immediate response to injury by rapid generation of thrombin ("thrombin burst").[4,5] The pathway is initiated through the exposure of TF located on the surface of fibroblasts and smooth muscle cells that is expressed in the setting of vascular injury. TF combines with factor VII to form an activated complex (VIIa) that catalyzes the conversion

of factor X into its activated form (Xa) and, ultimately, the generation of thrombin (factor IIa). Thrombin serves a central homeostatic role of not only fibrin production but activates factors XIII (cross-linking the fibrin strands), V, VIII, and XI, further amplifying the cascade.

The contact activation pathway is initiated by the formation of an activated complex of HMWK, PK, and exposed collagen to activate factor XII.[3] Whereas the TF pathway activates immediately, the contact activation has a slower onset and is associated with coagulation involved in the setting of inflammation or hyperlipidemia.

The coagulation cascade is normally kept in balance by inhibitory pathways that help down-regulate the cascade, turn off platelet activation, and stimulate fibrinolysis. These processes include generation of *Protein C, antithrombin, tissue factor pathway inhibitor (TFPI), prostacyclin (PGI2),* and *plasmin.* Activated Protein C assists in degrading factors V and VIII. Antithrombin (antithrombin III, ATIII) is a protease inhibitor that breaks down thrombin and factors IXa, Xa, XIa, and XIIa. TFPI impedes with the interaction of TF and factors IXa and Xa. Prostacyclin is a potent platelet inhibitor produced by the vascular endothelium and prevents additional platelet degranulation.

▍ PLASMINOGEN-PLASMIN PATHWAY

Plasminogen is an inactive circulating plasma zymogen produced predominantly from the liver.[6] Conversion of plasminogen to plasmin by *tissue-type plasminogen activator* (tPA) is the sentinel event in the initiation of fibrinolysis (FIGURE 99.2). tPA is produced by vascular endothelial cells and has a high affinity for fibrin-bound plasminogen. Plasmin enzymatically cleaves fibrin into *fibrin degradation products* (FDP), thus breaking apart the structural integrity of the thrombus. Plasmin has naturally occurring inhibitors α₂-antiplasmin and α₂-macroglobulin, both produced by the liver. *Plasminogen activator inhibitor-1 (PAI-1)* is produced by endothelial cells and inhibits plasminogen activation.

▍ PLASMINOGEN ACTIVATORS

Five plasminogen activators (Table 99.1) are approved in the United States for the systemic intravenous treatment of acute myocardial infarction (AMI).[8,*] Although none of these agents are specifically approved for catheter-directed therapy, protocols have been developed empirically over the past four decades.

---

*Anistreplase (Eminase, formerly produced by Beecham) is a purified human plasminogen-streptokinase complex that has been acylated (anisoylated plasminogen streptokinase activator complex, APSAC) and was approved for AMI but is no longer manufactured or available.

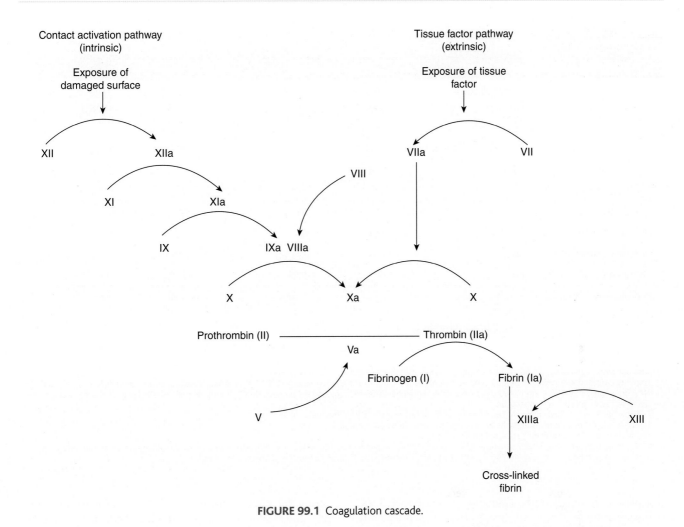

FIGURE 99.1 Coagulation cascade.

The development of plasminogen activators has mirrored technical improvements in biotechnology, protein engineering, and manufacturing techniques. Originally these proteins were only available from purified source tissue (e.g., human neonatal kidney cells or bacterial culture) but manufacturing processes have advanced and supplanted by recombinant DNA techniques that avoid the need to procure human donor tissue or expose the potential risks of passive viral contamination from source tissue. Additionally, pharmacologic features of the molecules have been modified to enhance fibrin specificity and simplifying the administration of these agents in the management of AMI.

First-generation plasminogen activators have been developed from human neonatal cell lines (urokinase, UK) or bacterial culture (streptokinase, SK) and were approved for systemic thrombolysis in the 1970s. Because of the risk of anaphylactic reaction and/or the need to procure human kidney cells, these agents are no longer manufactured or marketed in the United States. In the early 1980s, tissue plasminogen activator (alteplase, tPA) was introduced as a second-generation agent that uses recombinant DNA technology. Refinements in protein engineering in the 1990s allowed creation of novel plasminogen muteins (third-generation) using deletion mutations

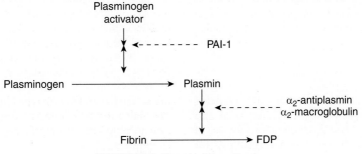

FIGURE 99.2 Plasminogen activation.

Table 99.1					
Comparison of Thrombolytic Agents					
	Streptokinase (SK)	Urokinase (UK)	Alteplase (tPA)	Reteplase (rPA)	Tenecteplase (TNK)
Trade name	Streptase[a]	Kinlytic[b]	Activase[c]	Retavase[d]	TNKase[c]
Source	β-hemolytic streptococci	HNK	cDNA	cDNA	cDNA
Plasma half-life (min)	~20–85	~16	~5	~15	~22
Fibrin selectivity	+	+	+++	++	++++
MW (kDa)	47	30	70	39	70
PAI-1 inhibition	Yes	Yes	Yes	Yes	No
Treatment time (AMI)	60 min	N/A	90 min	30 min	5 sec
Fibrinogen depletion[e]	N/A	N/A	31%	75%	4%–15%
Approved indication(s)	• AMI • PE • Peripheral thrombus	PE	• AMI • AIS • PE • Catheter occlusion[f]	AMI	AMI

[a]Formerly manufactured by CSL Behring—no longer manufactured or marketed in the United States.
[b]Formerly marketed as Abbokinase (Abbott Laboratories, Abbott Park, IL). Microbix Biosystems, Inc. (Toronto, Canada) acquired remaining product inventory and New Drug Application (NDA) from ImaRx Therapeutics in September 2008 and renamed the product Kinlytic. Currently not marketed in the United States.
[c]Genentech, Inc., South San Francisco, CA.
[d]EKR Therapeutics, Inc. (Bedminster, NJ) acquired rights for Retavase from PDL BioPharma in 2008.
[e]Fibrinogen depletion at 2 hours after therapeutic load for AMI compared to baseline.[7]
[f]Cathflo Activase (Genentech, Inc.) approved for catheter clearance.
AIS, acute ischemic stroke; AMI, acute myocardial infarction; cDNA, complementary (recombinant) DNA; HNK, human neonatal kidney cells; kDa, kiloDaltons; MW, molecular weight; N/A, not applicable; PAI-1, plasminogen activator inhibitor-1; PE, acute massive pulmonary embolism.

(reteplase, rPA) or substitution mutations (tenecteplase, TNK) to further improve fibrin specificity (FIGURE 99.3). Subsequently, systemic infusion times for AMI have decreased from 120 minutes (UK) to 30 minutes (rPA) to a single bolus delivered in 5 seconds (TNK).

From a historic perspective, UK was the dominant drug used for endovascular interventions in the United States prior to 1999 when the Food and Drug Administration (FDA) suspended sale and distribution of human-derived urokinase.[10] Forced to explore alternatives, interventionists developed techniques and protocols with second- and third-generation recombinant agents, particularly tPA and rPA; these agents have now essentially replaced first-generation agents.[11,12] SK and UK are still used in parts of Asia, Latin America, and Europe for catheter-directed thrombolysis.

The choice of the thrombolytic agent is a matter of regional practices and physician discretion. There are few well-controlled randomized comparative studies comparing superiority of one agent over another in treating peripheral limb ischemia or deep venous thrombosis (DVT) using catheter-directed techniques.[13]

Streptokinase

Streptokinase (SK) was the first commercially available thrombolytic agent approved in the United States for systemic treatment of AMI[14] and laid the foundations for use of plasminogen activators in catheter-based interventions for peripheral vascular thrombosis,[1] acute coronary thrombosis,[15] and treatment of organized pleural effusions, hemothorax, and infected fluid collections.[16] Previously manufactured under the trade name of Streptase, SK is no longer available in the United States.

SK is a 47 kDa bacterial protein expressed from Lancefield Group C β-hemolytic streptococci (Streptococcus equisimilis) and was first described by Tillett in 1933.[17] SK is an indirect plasminogen activator because it initially binds to plasminogen to form an intermediate SK-plasminogen complex that induces a conformational change in the bound plasminogen that exposes the catalytic site; the activated complex then cleaves other plasminogen molecules to plasmin. Because of its lack of affinity for fibrin, it cleaves both free circulating plasminogen and fibrin-bound plasminogen and can induce systemic fibrinolysis. It has been manufactured as a lyophilized powder in three vial configurations: 250,000, 750,000, or 1,500,000 units and has been approved for AMI, pulmonary embolism, systemic intravenous treatment of arterial and venous thrombosis, and dialysis cannula clearance.[18] The lyophilized powder requires reconstitution in 5 mL of sodium chloride 0.9% or dextrose 5% (Table 99.2). Its principal advantage is the significantly lower costs (per vial basis) compared to recombinant agents. Because SK is a nonhuman protein, it can be inactivated by circulating antibodies and invoke type I hypersensitivity (anaphylaxis). The half-life of SK ranges from approximately 20 minutes (due to action of any preexisting antibodies) to approximately 85 minutes.

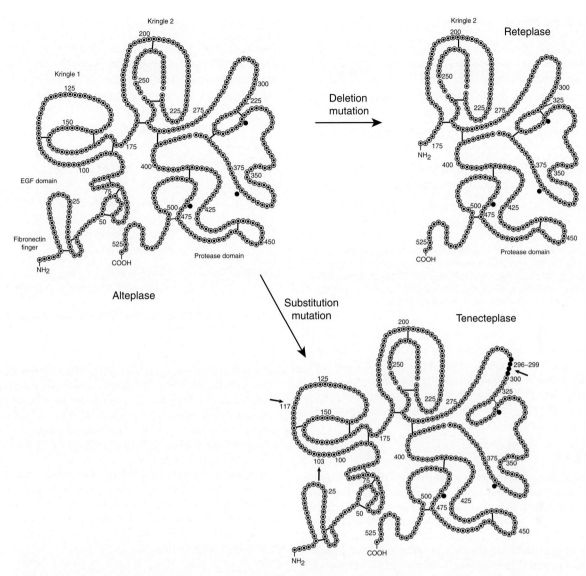

FIGURE 99.3 Recombinant DNA-derived plasminogen activators. Derivatives of alteplase can be produced using recombinant techniques involving deletion mutations (reteplase) or substitution mutations (tenecteplase) as described by Nordt and Bode.[9] For tenecteplase, three amino acid substitutions have occurred in kringle 1 and the protease domains (*arrows*).

Table 99.2

Preparation of Streptokinase for Catheter-Directed Thrombolysis

How supplied	• Sterile lyophilized powder in glass vials • 250,000-unit vial • 750,000-unit vial • 1,500,000-unit vial
Reconstitution	• 5 mL sodium chloride injection, USP, 0.9% per vial
Dilution	• Normal saline (0.9%) to 500 units/mL
Dosage	• Infusion 5,000–10,000 units/hr[19]

Urokinase

Urokinase (UK) is a double chain 30 kDa protein obtained from human neonatal kidney cells grown in culture. Similar to SK, UK activates both free circulating plasminogen and fibrin-bound plasminogen due to its low fibrin specificity. UK was the most commonly used agent for catheter-directed thrombolysis due to its broad range of therapeutic titration; however, the availability of UK was temporarily suspended by the FDA from 1999 to 2002 due to the theoretical potential for transmission of viral contaminants from human tissue culture and subsequently a revamped quality control process was required in its manufacturing.[20,21] No cases of transmission have ever been documented nor have any viral contaminants been isolated from the final purified protein. Production of UK in the United States was discontinued in 2004. Despite the lack of availability, the drug remains approved

Table 99.3	
Preparation of Urokinase for Catheter-Directed Thrombolysis	
How supplied	• Sterile lyophilized powder in glass vials • 250,000-unit vial
Reconstitution	• Sterile water for injection, USP to 50,000 units/mL
Dilution	• Normal saline (0.9%) to 1,000–2,000 units/mL
Dosage	• Bolus (if used) 60,000–250,000 units • 60,000–240,000 units/hr

Data from LeBlang SD, Becker GJ, Benenati JF, et al. Low-dose urokinase regimen for the treatment of lower extremity arterial and graft occlusions: experience in 132 cases. *J Vasc Interv Radiol* 1992;3:475–483; McNamara TO, Fischer JR. Thrombolysis of peripheral arterial and graft occlusions: improved results using high-dose urokinase. *AJR Am J Roentgenol* 1985;144:769–775.

Table 99.4	
Preparation of Alteplase for Catheter-Directed Thrombolysis	
How supplied	• Sterile lyophilized powder in glass vials • 2-mg vial • 50-mg vial • 100-mg vial
Reconstitution	• Sterile water for injection, USP to 1 mg/mL
Dilution	• Normal saline (NS) (0.9%) to 0.02 mg/mL (10 mg tPA in 490 mL NS) • If more volume required, maximum dilution is 0.01 mg/mL
Dosage	• Bolus (if used) 1–5 mg • Continuous infusion 0.5–1 mg/hr

Data from Semba CP, Sugimoto K, Razavi MK. Alteplase and tenecteplase: applications in the peripheral circulation. *Tech Vasc Intervent Radiol* 2001;4:99–106.

and registered in the United States for massive pulmonary embolism and in Canada for clot lysis and catheter clearance.[22] UK has been available as a lyophilized powder in 250,000-unit glass vials (Table 99.3). The principal drawback has been its current limited supply, significantly higher costs compared to the recombinant agents,[23] historically longer infusions times, and rare cases of anaphylactoid reactions.[24]

Alteplase

Tissue plasminogen activator is a naturally occurring glycosylated serine protease produced by human vascular endothelial cells and plays a role in the natural endogenous process of fibrinolysis. *Alteplase* is a 70 kDa human tPA produced using recombinant DNA technology and contains 527 amino acids. Alteplase consists of five functional domains: protease unit, two kringle domains, epidermal growth factor domain, and a fibronectin finger (FIGURE 99.3).[9] The protease domain is involved in cleaving plasminogen and is inhibited by PAI-1. Kringle 1 and epidermal growth factor are involved in hepatic clearance. Kringle 2 helps to stimulate the protease domain in the presence of fibrin and the fibronectin finger helps bind to fibrin.

Alteplase is a direct plasminogen activator but its affinity for fibrin-bound plasminogen is enhanced compared to first-generation agents and produces limited conversion of plasminogen to plasmin in absence of fibrin. Alteplase binds to fibrin within the thrombus and converts entrapped plasminogen to plasmin, which then initiates local fibrinolysis. Plasma clearance of alteplase is relatively rapid with a half-life of less than 5 minutes. Clearance is mediated by the liver.

Alteplase is produced using recombinant DNA technology.[25] Complementary DNA (cDNA) for natural human tPA is genetically inserted into a mammalian cell line (Chinese hamster ovarian cells). The fermentation process involves secretion of alteplase from the genetically modified cell lines into the tissue culture medium. The secreted protein is then separated, purified, and lyophilized into powder form.

Use of alteplase for catheter-directed thrombolysis was first described in 1986,[26] but its use was uncommon prior to 1999 in the United States until the unavailability of UK led to exploration of alternative plasminogen activators; however, tPA became

established as a suitable agent for catheter-directed thrombolysis in Europe in the late 1980s.[27,28] Initial empiric experiences in the United States used high doses and were accompanied by serious bleeding complications.[29] Protocols evolved to use significantly lower doses (Table 99.4) and the advent of a 2-mg vial obviated the need to freeze and store small quantities of alteplase aliquotted from 50- to 100-mg vials.

Alteplase is marketed under the trade name Activase (50 and 100 mg, Genentech, Inc., South San Francisco, CA) and is approved for the systemic treatment of acute ischemic stroke, AMI (90-minute infusion), and massive pulmonary embolism. A 2-mg vial of alteplase (Cathflo Activase, Genentech, Inc.) is approved for catheter clearance.

Reteplase

Reteplase is a 39 kDa nonglycosylated deletion mutation of tissue plasminogen (tPA) produced from cDNA genetically inserted into *Escherichia coli* and contains 355 of the 527 amino acids found in alteplase (FIGURE 99.3).[30] The protein is isolated as inactive inclusion bodies from *E. coli*, converted into its active three-dimensional form by an in vitro process, and purified by chromatographic separation. It has a plasma half-life of approximately 13 to 16 minutes and is cleared from the circulation primarily by the liver and kidneys.

Use of reteplase in catheter-directed treatment of arterial limb ischemia was initially reported in 2000 in a small dose-ranging study and has emerged as another thrombolytic alternative.[31] Reteplase is marketed under the trade name Retavase (EKR Therapeutics, Inc., Bedminster, NJ) and is supplied in 10-unit vials. It is approved for double bolus treatment of AMI (10 units + 10 units administered 30 minutes apart) (Table 99.5).

Tenecteplase

Tenecteplase (TNK) is a tissue plasminogen activator produced by recombinant DNA technology using an established mammalian cell line (Chinese hamster ovary cells).[32] TNK is a 527 amino acid glycoprotein developed by introducing the

Table 99.5
Preparation of Reteplase for Catheter-Directed Thrombolysis

How supplied	• 10-unit lyophilized powder in glass vials
Reconstitution	• Sterile water for injection, USP to 1 unit/mL
Dilution	• Normal saline (0.9%) to 0.01–0.05 mg/mL
Dosage	• Bolus (if used) 1–2 units • Continuous infusion 0.25–0.5 unit/hr

Data from Benenati J, Shlansky-Goldberg R, Meglin A, et al. Thrombolytic and antiplatelet therapy in peripheral vascular disease with use of reteplase and/or abciximab. *J Vasc Interv Radiol* 2001;12:795–805.

Table 99.6
Preparation of Tenecteplase for Catheter-Directed Thrombolysis

How supplied	• 50 mg sterile lyophilized powder in glass vials
Reconstitution	• Sterile water for injection, USP to 5 mg/mL
Dilution	• Normal saline to 0.01–0.05 mg/mL
Dosage	• Continuous infusion at 0.25–0.50 mg/hr

Data from Razavi MK, Wong H, Kee ST, et al. Initial clinical results of tenecteplase (TNK) in catheter-directed thrombolytic therapy. *J Endovasc Ther* 2002;9:593–598; Burkhart DJ, Borsa JJ, Anthony JP, et al. Thrombolysis of occluded peripheral arteries and veins with tenecteplase: a pilot study. *J Vasc Interv Radiol* 2002;13:1099–1102.

following modifications to the cDNA for natural human TPA: a substitution of threonine 103 with asparagine, and a substitution of asparagine 117 with glutamine, both within the kringle 1 domain, and a tetra-alanine substitution at amino acids 296 to 299 in the protease domain (FIGURE 99.3). TNK has higher fibrin specificity than tPA or rPA and is more resistant to inhibition by PAI-1.[33] In preclinical animal studies, TNK demonstrated significantly enhanced clot lysis ability and minimal plasminogen and fibrinogen depletion compared to known existing agents.[34] In human clinical trials for treatment of AMI, TNK demonstrated similar efficacy to alteplase, but major blood loss was reduced by 22%, need for blood transfusion was reduced by 23%, and minor bleeding decreased by 16%.[33] There was no significant difference in the rate of intracranial hemorrhage (0.9%).[33]

Use of TNK in catheter-directed treatment of arterial and venous thrombosis was initially reported in 2002 (Table 99.6).[35,36] TNK is marketed under the trade name TNKase (Genentech, Inc.) and supplied in 50-mg vials. Because only small quantities of TNK are required for peripheral thrombolysis, stability of 10-mg (2 mL) frozen/thawed aliquots has been reported.[37] TNK is approved for the treatment of AMI administered with a single 5-second intravenous bolus.

GENERAL CONSIDERATIONS FOR CATHETER-DIRECTED THROMBOLYSIS

Historically, the practice of catheter-directed thrombolysis has been highly variable.[38,39] In attempts to provide a framework of standardized techniques and definitions for interventionists, the Society of Interventional Radiology (SIR) and Cardiovascular-Interventional Radiology Society of Europe (CIRSE) have approved quality improvement guidelines for both arterial and venous thrombolysis.[40–42] The general principles are summarized next.

Indications—Arterial

Indications for catheter-directed thrombolysis include the management acute limb-threatening ischemia (category I or IIa) to eliminate the thrombus or embolus and restore reperfusion[43] (Table 99.7). Patients with category IIb limb ischemia may be candidates but risks and benefits need to be assessed on a case-by-case basis. Because the course of thrombolytic infusion may take several hours, patients with category III limb ischemia

Table 99.7
Clinical Categories of Acute Limb Ischemia

	Category	Description	Sensory loss	Muscle weakness	Arterial	Venous
			Clinical exam		Doppler signal	
I	Viable	Not immediately threatened	None	None	Audible	Audible
IIa	Threatened - marginal	Salvageable if promptly treated	Minimal (toe) or none	None	Often inaudible	Audible
IIb	Threatened - immediate	Salvageable with immediate revascularization	More than toes, associated with rest pain	Mild, moderate	Usually inaudible	Audible
III	Irreversible	Major tissue loss or permanent nerve damage	Profound, anesthetic	Profound, paralysis (rigor)	Inaudible	Inaudible

Table 99.8

Indications for Lower Extremity Venous Catheter-Directed Thrombolysis

Indication	Bleeding risk	Goals
Phlegmasia cerulean dolens	Low/moderate	Limb salvage survival
Acute iliofemoral DVT	Low	Prevent PTS
Acute femoropopliteal DVT	Low	Prevent PTS
Subacute/chronic iliofemoral DVT	Low	Alleviate/ prevent PTS

Acute DVT—venous thrombosis ≤14 days duration; *subacute DVT*—venous thrombosis 15 to 28 days duration; *chronic DVT*—venous thrombosis >28 days duration.
PTS, post-thrombotic syndrome.

should not be treated by catheter-directed infusion due to the high risk of irreversible tissue loss over time.

Indications—Venous

Catheter-directed treatment of acute DVT is a viable and accepted alternative to anticoagulation as a means to reduce the risk of post-thrombotic syndrome or limb salvage in the setting of massive venous thrombosis (Table 99.8).[41,44] Indications for treatment include *phlegmasia cerulea dolens* and acute/subacute iliofemoral DVT.

Contraindications

The most common complication of thrombolytic therapy is that bleeding and risks/benefits must be tailored to the individual patient. Contraindications can be classified as absolute and relative and are summarized in Table 99.9.[40,44]

Techniques

There is no single accepted protocol or method but catheter-directed techniques can be summarized in five general categories:

(1) continuous infusion, (2) bolus then infusion, (3) graduated infusions, (4) pharmacomechanical thrombolysis, and (5) combinations of more than one of these techniques.[38,39] *Continuous infusions* are the simplest (FIGURE 99.4). Once an infusion catheter is placed across the length of the thrombosed segment, a steady and constant infusion of thrombolytic agent is administered for several hours (typically overnight). *Bolus* (or *lacing*) involves delivery of a large concentration of thrombolytic drug directly into the clot through the intrathrombic catheter in attempts to immediately accelerate and initiate the fibrinolysis process; this is then followed by a lower continuous infusion. *Graduated infusions* is the process of using stepwise dosing regimen, typically a higher dose continually infused for a fixed period, then empirically lowered to a lower dose for the remainder of the infusion. *Pharmacomechanical thrombolysis* refers to either the use of high-velocity bursts of small volumes of the thrombolytic agent ("*pulse spray*") or use of a thrombolytic agent in conjunction with a mechanical device (balloon catheter or mechanical thrombectomy device) to macerate and physically fragment the clot and increase the surface area of clot exposed to the plasminogen activator.

Plasminogen Activator

There is no consensus on the optimal thrombolytic agent, and selection is based on physician preference and regional practice standards.[40,44]

Concomitant Anticoagulation

Use of intravenous unfractionated heparin during catheter-directed thrombolysis is highly variable. In treatment of arterial ischemia, doses have ranged from none to sub-therapeutic to full-therapeutic anticoagulation and no consensus position has been established.[40] For venous thrombolysis, published guidelines have recommended heparin use; however, the optimal regimen has not been established.[44]

Monitoring

Patients should be monitored closely during the infusion period for potential bleeding complications in an intensive care unit or step-down unit.[40,42] Serial monitoring of hematocrit, partial

Table 99.9

Contraindications for Thrombolytic Therapy

Absolute	Relative	
	Major	Minor
• Recent cerebrovascular event—including transient ischemic attacks within the last 2 mo	• Recent cardiopulmonary resuscitation (<10 d)	• Hepatic failure, particularly those with coagulopathy
• Active bleeding diathesis	• Recent major nonvascular surgery or trauma (<10 d)	• Bacterial endocarditis
• Recent gastrointestinal bleeding (<10 d)	• Uncontrolled hypertension: >180 mm Hg systolic or >110 mm Hg diastolic	• Pregnancy
• Neurosurgery (intracranial, spinal) within last 3 mo	• Puncture of a noncompressible vessel	• Diabetic hemorrhagic retinopathy
• Intracranial trauma within last 3 mo	• Intracranial tumor	
	• Recent eye surgery	

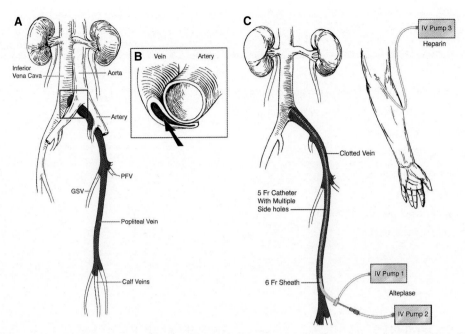

FIGURE 99.4 Typical setup for continuous infusion catheter-directed thrombolysis for acute left lower extremity ilio-femoral deep vein thrombosis (**A**) due to left common iliac vein entrapment by the right iliac artery (**B**, "May-Thurner syndrome").[45] Thrombolysis catheters are introduced into the iliofemoral thrombus via the popliteal vein and the thrombolytic agent introduced through the sheath and infusion catheter (**C**). Low-dose peripheral anticoagulation with heparin provided using upper extremity intravenous access. The goal of therapy is to lyse as much of the thrombus burden as possible, unmask the stenotic iliac vein, and angioplasty and stent the obstructed iliac segment to fully reconstruct the iliofemoral outflow. (Reprinted from Semba CP, Razavi MK, Kee ST, et al. Thrombolysis for lower extremity deep venous thrombosis. *Tech Vasc Interv Radiol* 2004;7:68–78, with permission from Elsevier.)

thromboplastin time PTT (if heparin is used), and platelets should be considered every 6 to 8 hours. Monitoring serial fibrinogen levels to assess for potential risk for bleeding complications from systemic fibrinolysis is controversial and no consensus has been established. Historically, maintenance of fibrinogen level greater than 100 mg/dL has been reported but there are no well-controlled studies to confirm that measuring serial fibrinogen levels are predictive of bleeding risk.[42]

Outcomes

There are few rigorously designed, prospective, multicenter studies evaluating comparative outcomes from arterial and venous thrombolysis and the body of literature represents mostly single center, nonrandomized observational studies. One of the complexities in analyzing clinical data across published studies is the varying techniques, definitions, patient selection, and outcome parameters used in reporting. Arterial limb salvage rates have ranged from 73% to 100%; the joint SIR/CIRSE statement suggests a threshold of 75% as a target clinical success rate in practice (as defined by returning the patient to his or her preocclusive clinical baseline after thrombus removal and use of adjunctive procedures).[40] Similarly, acute venous thrombolysis anatomic patency rates have ranged from 81% to 100% with immediate clinical improvements ranging from 76% to 100%; however, this must be considered in the light of variable reporting standards.[41]

Complications

Reporting standards recommend classification of thrombolytic complications into two categories, minor and major (Table 99.10).[43]

Bleeding is the most common complication. Although any bleeding complication is undesired, acceptable thresholds of major complications have been proposed for both arterial and venous thrombolysis[40,44] (Table 99.11).

Table 99.10
Classification of Complications by Outcomes

Minor	Major
• No therapy, no sequelae	• Requires therapy, minor hospitalization (<48 hr)
• Minor therapy or minor sequelae; includes overnight admission (<24 hr) for observation only	• Requires major therapy, unplanned increase in the level of care, or prolonged hospitalization (>48 hr)
	• Permanent adverse sequelae
	• Death

Table 99.11			
Major Complication Rates of Catheter-Directed Thrombolysis			
Complication		Reported range (%)	Suggested threshold (%)
Arterial	Major bleeding requiring transfusion and/or surgery	1–20	10
	Distal embolization not corrected with thrombolysis	1–5	5
	Compartment syndrome	1–10	4
	Intracranial hemorrhage	0–2.5	2
Venous	All major complications	0–24	18
	Major bleed	0–24	15
	Symptomatic pulmonary embolism	0–1	2
	Intracranial hemorrhage	0–1	1
	Death	0–1	1

FUTURE DEVELOPMENTS

Newer agents continue to be developed including direct fibrinolytic agents. *Desmoteplase* is a naturally occurring plasminogen activator isolated from the saliva of vampire bats (*Desmodes rotundus)* and is structurally similar to tPA. Its potential advantage is its very high fibrin specificity and long half-life (~2.8 hours) compared to tPA, making it an attractive single bolus systemic agent. Recombinantly derived, it is under investigation for the systemic treatment of acute ischemic stroke (H. Lundbeck A/S, Copenhagen, Denmark).[46] *Staphylokinase* (ThromboGenics, Inc., Leuven, Belgium), a recombinant protein that is normally produced by *Staphylococcus aureus*, was under investigation for the systemic treatment of AMI.[47] Similar to SK, staphylokinase does not directly activate plasminogen but forms an intermediate complex. *Recombinant urokinase* (r-UK; urokinase alpha, Abbott Laboratories) and *recombinant prourokinase* (r-proUK; Prolyse, Abbott Laboratories) were under investigation in peripheral limb ischemia, catheter clearance, and acute stroke but the development programs have been discontinued.[48–50]

Direct fibrinolytic agents are under development. *Ocriplasmin* is a 27 kDa recombinant derivative of human microplasmin (contains only the catalytic domain) that directly acts on fibrin instead of conversion of plasminogen to plasmin. Ocriplasmin (ThromboGenics, Inc.) is currently under development for intravitreal injection for treatment of ocular diseases[51] and acute ischemic stroke.[52] FDA approval for ophthalmic use was in 2012. *Recombinant plasmin* was under preclinical development for peripheral vascular occlusion[53] (Talecris Biotherapeutics, Research Triangle Park, NC) and thrombosed dialysis access[54] (BLX-155, Biolex Therapeutics, Pittsboro, NC). *Alfimeprase* (recombinant fibrolase) is a protease targeting fibrinogen. It is a recombinant enzyme that is normally produced from the venom of the southern copperhead snake (*Agkistrodon contortrix*). Alfimeprase was under investigation for peripheral arterial limb ischemia and catheter clearance but development was discontinued in 2007.[55]

REFERENCES

1. Dotter CT, Rösch J, Seaman AJ. Selective clot lysis using low-dose streptokinase. *Radiology* 1974;111:31–37.
2. Furie B, Fure BC. Mechanisms for thrombus formation. *N Engl J Med* 2008;359:938–949.
3. Gailani D, Renne T. Intrinsic pathway of coagulation and arterial thrombosis. *Arterioscler Thromb Vasc Biol* 2007;27:2507–2513.
4. Mackman N, Tilley RE, Key NS. Role of the extrinsic pathway of blood coagulation in hemostasis and thrombosis. *Arterioscler Thromb Vasc Biol* 2007;27:1687–1693.
5. Bode W. Structure and interaction modes of thrombin. *Blood Cells Mol Dis* 2006;36:122–130.
6. Castellino FJ, Ploplis VA. Human plasminogen: structure, activation, and function. In: Waisman DM, ed. *Plasminogen: Structure, Activation and Regulation.* New York, NY: Kluwer Academic/Plenum; 2003:3–9.
7. Moser M, Nordt T, Peter K, et al. Platelet function during and after thrombolytic therapy for acute myocardial infarction with reteplase, alteplase, and streptokinase. *Circulation* 1999;100:1858–1864.
8. Semba CP, Sugimoto K, Razavi MK. Alteplase and tenecteplase: applications in the peripheral circulation. *Tech Vasc Intervent Radiol* 2001;4:99–106.
9. Nordt TK, Bode C. Thrombolysis: newer thrombolytic agents and their role in clinical medicine. *Heart* 2003;89:1358–1362.
10. Dear Healthcare Provider Letter: Important Drug Warning: Safety information regarding the use of Abbokinase® (urokinase). U.S. Food and Drug Administration; January 25, 1999. Available at: http://www.fda.gov/Drugs/DevelopmentApprovalProcess/HowDrugsareDevelopedandApproved/ApprovalApplications/TherapeuticBiologicApplications/ucm113558.htm. Accessed January 8, 2011.
11. Semba CP, Bakal CW, Calis KA, et al. Alteplase as an alternative to urokinase. *J Vasc Interv Radiol* 2000;11:279–287.
12. Benenati J, Shlansky-Goldberg R, Meglin A, et al. Thrombolytic and antiplatelet therapy in peripheral vascular disease with use of reteplase and/or abciximab. *J Vasc Interv Radiol* 2001;12:795–805.
13. Robertson I, Kessel DO, Berridge DC. Fibrinolytic agents for peripheral arterial occlusion. *Cochrane Database Syst Rev* 2010;(3):CD001099.
14. Sikri N, Bardia A. A history of streptokinase use in acute myocardial infarction. *Tex Heart J* 2007;34:318–327.
15. Rentrop KP, Blanke H, Karsch KR, et al. Acute myocardial infarction: intracoronary application of nitroglycerin and streptokinase. *Clin Cardiol* 1979;2:354–363.
16. Tillett WS, Sherry S. The effect in patients of streptococcal fibrinolysin (streptokinase) and streptococcal deoxyribonuclease on fibrinous, purulent, and sanguinous pleural exudations. *J Clin Invest* 1949;28:173–190.
17. Tillett WS, Garner RL. The fibrinolytic activity of hemolytic streptococci. *J Exp Med* 1933;58:485–502.

18. Streptase® (Streptokinase Injection) [product monograph]. CSL Behring Canada, Inc.; March 2007. Available at: http://www.cslbehring.ca/docs/831/938/Streptase_app%2029mar07.pdf. Accessed January 8, 2011.
19. Berridge DC, Gregson RHS, Hopkinson BR, et al. Randomized trial of intra-arterial recombinant tissue plasminogen activator, intravenous recombinant tissue plasminogen activator, and intra-arterial streptokinase in peripheral arterial thrombolysis. *Br J Surg* 1991;78:988–995.
20. Hartnell GG, Gates J. The case of Abbokinase and the FDA: the events leading to the suspension of Abbokinase supplies in the United States. *J Vasc Interv Radiol* 2000;11:841–847.
21. Abbokinase® (urokinase) Dear Healthcare Professional Letter. U.S. Food and Drug Administration; October 10, 2002. Available at: http://www.fda.gov/Safety/MedWatch/SafetyInformation/SafetyAlertsforHumanMedicalProducts/ucm171213.htm. Accessed January 8, 2011.
22. Urokinase executive summary. November 2010. Microbix Biosystems, Inc. Available at: http://www.microbix.com/Public/Page/Files/1_UROKINASE%20BUSINESS%20OPPORTUNITY%20Web%20Edition%20Nov%202010.pdf. Accessed January 8, 2011.
23. Sugimoto K, Hofmann LV, Razavi MK, et al. The safety, efficacy, and pharmacoeconomics of low-dose alteplase compared with urokinase for catheter-directed thrombolysis of arterial and venous occlusions. *J Vasc Surg* 2003;37:512–517.
24. Perri JA, Stahfeld KR, Villella ER, et al. The management of anaphylactoid reactions to urokinase. *J Vasc Surg* 1994;20:846–847.
25. Activase® (alteplase) [package insert]. South San Francisco, CA: Genentech, Inc. April 2011.
26. Graor RA, Risius B, Young JR, et al. Peripheral artery and bypass graft thrombolysis with recombinant human tissue-type plasminogen activator. *J Vasc Surg* 1986;3:115–124.
27. Earnshaw JJ, Westby JC, Gregson RH, et al. Local thrombolytic therapy of acute peripheral arterial ischemia with tissue plasminogen activator: a dose-ranging study. *Br J Surg* 1988;75:1196–1200.
28. Berridge DC, Gregson RH, Hopkinson BR, et al. Intra-arterial thrombolysis using recombinant tissue plasminogen activator (rt-PA): the optimal agent, at the optimal dose? *Eur J Vasc Surg* 1989;3:327–332.
29. McNamara TO, Dong P, Chen J, et al. Bleeding complication associated with the use of rt-PA versus r-PA for peripheral arterial and venous thromboembolic occlusions. *Tech Vasc Interv Radiol* 2001;4:92–98.
30. Retavase® (reteplase) [package insert]. Bedminster, NJ: EKR Therapeutics, Inc. February 2009.
31. Davidian MM, Powell A, Benenati JF, et al. Initial results of reteplase in the treatment of acute lower extremity arterial occlusions. *J Vasc Interv Radiol* 2000;11:289–294.
32. TNKase® (tenecteplase) [package insert]. South San Francisco, CA: Genentech, Inc. May 2011.
33. ASSENT-2 Investigators. Single-bolus tenecteplase compared with front-loaded alteplase in acute myocardial infarction: the ASSENT-2 double-blind randomized trial. *Lancet* 1999;354:716–722.
34. Benedict CR, Refino CJ, Keyt BA, et al. New variant of human recombinant tissue plasminogen activator with enhanced efficacy and lower incidence of bleeding compared to recombinant TPA. *Circulation* 1995;92:3032–3040.
35. Razavi MK, Wong H, Kee ST, et al. Initial clinical results of tenecteplase (TNK) in catheter-directed thrombolytic therapy. *J Endovasc Ther* 2002;9:593–598.
36. Burkhart DJ, Borsa JJ, Anthony JP, et al. Thrombolysis of occluded peripheral arteries and veins with tenecteplase: a pilot study. *J Vasc Interv Radiol* 2002;13:1099–1102.
37. Semba CP, Weck S, Razavi MK, et al. Tenecteplase: stability and bioactivity of thawed or diluted solutions used in peripheral thrombolysis. *J Vasc Interv Radiol* 2003;14:475–479.
38. Razavi MK, Lee DS, Hofmann LV. Catheter-directed thrombolytic therapy for limb ischemia: current status and controversies. *J Vasc Interv Radiol* 2003;14:1491–1501.
39. Kessel DO, Berridge DC, Robertson I. Infusion techniques for peripheral arterial thrombolysis. *Cochrane Database Syst Rev* 2004;(1):CD000985.
40. Rajan DK, Patel NH, Valji K, et al. Quality improvement guidelines for percutaneous management of acute limb ischemia. *J Vasc Interv Radiol* 2005;16:585–595.
41. Vedantham S, Thorpe PE, Cardella JF, et al. Quality improvement guidelines for the treatment of lower extremity deep vein thrombosis with use of endovascular thrombus removal. *J Vasc Interv Radiol* 2006;17:435–448.
42. Working Party on Thrombolysis in the Management of Limb Ischemia. Thrombolysis in the management of lower limb peripheral arterial occlusion. A consensus document. *J Vasc Interv Radiol* 2003;7:S337–S349.
43. Patel N, Sacks D, Patel RI, et al. Society of Interventional Radiology (SIR) reporting standard for the treatment of acute limb ischemia with use of transluminal removal of arterial thrombus. *J Vasc Interv Radiol* 2003;14:S453–S465.
44. Vedantham S, Millward SF, Cardella JF, et al. Society of Interventional Radiology position statement: treatment of acute iliofemoral deep vein thrombosis with use of adjunctive catheter-directed intrathrombus thrombolysis. *J Vasc Interv Radiol* 2006;17:613–616.
45. Semba CP, Razavi MK, Kee ST, et al. Thrombolysis for lower extremity deep venous thrombosis. *Tech Vasc Interv Radiol* 2004;7:68–78.
46. Hacke W, Furlan AJ, Al-Rawi Y, et al. Intravenous desmoteplase in patients with acute ischemic stroke selected by MRI perfusion-diffusion weighted imaging or perfusion CT (DIAS-2): a prospective, randomized, double-blind, placebo-controlled study. *Lancet Neurol* 2009;8:141–150.
47. Moreadith RW, Collen D. Clinical development of PEGylated recombinant staphylokinase (PEG-Sak) for bolus thrombolytic treatment of patients with acute myocardial infarction. *Adv Drug Deliv Rev* 2003;55:1337–1345.
48. Ouriel K, Veith FJ, Sasahara AA. A comparison of recombinant urokinase with vascular surgery as initial treatment for acute arterial occlusion of the legs. Thrombolysis or Peripheral Arterial Surgery (TOPAS) Investigators. *N Engl J Med* 1998;338:1105–1111.
49. Deitcher SR, Fraschini G, Himmelfarb J, et al. Dose-ranging trial with a recombinant urokinase (urokinase alpha) for occluded central venous catheter in oncology patients. *J Vasc Interv Radiol* 2004;15:575–579.
50. Furlan A, Higashida R, Wechsler L, et al. Intra-arterial prourokinase for acute ischemic stroke. The PROACT II study: a randomized controlled trial. Prolyse in acute cerebral thromboembolism. *JAMA* 1999;282:2003–2011.
51. Stalmans P, Delaey C, de Smet MD, et al. Intravitreal injection of microplasmin for treatment of vitreomacular adhesion: results of a prospective, randomized, sham-controlled phase II trial (the MIV-IIT trial). *Retina* 2010;30:1122–1127.
52. Thijs VN, Peeters A, Vosko M, et al. Randomized, placebo-controlled, dose-ranging clinical trial of intravenous microplasmin in patients with acute ischemic stroke. *Stroke* 2009;40:3789–3795.
53. Comerota AJ. Development of catheter-directed intrathrombus thrombolysis with plasmin for the treatment of acute lower extremity arterial occlusion. *Thromb Res* 2008;122:S20–S26.
54. Biolex Therapeutics presents preclinical results for clot buster BLX-155. Available at: http://www.biolex.com/pdfs/Biolex%20ISTH%20Announcement%20July%202007.pdf. Accessed January 8, 2011.
55. Alfimeprase. *Drugs R D*. 2008;9:185–190.

Antirestenosis Agents and Attempts to Limit Intimal Hyperplasia

LINDSAY MACHAN

INTRODUCTION

Restenosis is the recurrence of a vascular narrowing after an initially successful treatment. It can occur after any surgical or endovascular intervention including balloon angioplasty, atherectomy, or stent insertion. Because it is the major factor limiting the longevity of endovascular procedures, it significantly impacts the choice between minimally invasive and open procedures for any individual patient. Restenosis after balloon angioplasty is caused by elastic recoil, constrictive remodelling, and neointimal hyperplasia. Because stents essentially prevent elastic recoil and vessel remodeling, neointimal hyperplasia is the largest component of in-stent restenosis (FIGURE 100.1).

Neointimal hyperplasia (also called intimal or myointimal hyperplasia) is an overexpression of the normal vascular healing process.[1] An endovascular intervention, such as stent implantation, causes disruption of the endothelium and results in a local change in vessel compliance (stiffness). These in turn immediately stimulate a healing response that is modulated by a complex interplay of events occurring in the lumen and the vessel wall.[2] On the luminal surface there is platelet activation and thrombus formation prior to endothelial re-coverage. Within the vessel wall there is acute inflammation, granulation tissue formation and the local release of chemotactic and growth factors, and oxygen-derived free radicals. In pathologic neointimal hyperplasia (as opposed to appropriately modulated intimal hyperplasia occurring after a normal vessel response to injury), there is excessive proliferation and migration of upregulated vascular smooth muscle cells, and oversecretion of an extracellular proteoglycan matrix. The ideal antirestenosis method should potently inhibit the overexpression of these processes yet still allow vascular healing (FIGURE 100.2).

It follows that certain methods of preventing restenosis (such as drug/device combinations) might be more effective in some body regions than others because the degree to which an intimal hyperplasia lesion is composed of vascular smooth muscle cells or proteinaceous matrix varies from vascular bed to vascular bed.[3] Other regional factors can cause profound differences in restenosis rates between different segments of the peripheral vasculature after endovascular intervention. These include repetitive deformation, burden of calcification, and vessel wall composition and thickness relative to luminal diameter. Regardless of vascular bed the three most significant determinants of restenosis rates are vessel diameter, length of lesion, and presence of diabetes.[4]

There are two common ways to describe restenosis: angiographic and clinical restenosis. In most clinical trials, angiographic restenosis is defined as a recurrent narrowing greater than 50% (the incidence of angiographic restenoses of 51% or greater may also be called the binary restenosis rate). If the narrowing occurs within the stent lumen, it is labeled in-stent restenosis (FIGURE 100.3A). If the narrowing is within the stent lumen or the 0.5 cm segment of artery immediately proximal or distal to the stent, it is called in-segment restenosis (FIGURE 100.3B).

Because patients with angiographic restenosis may be asymptomatic, many consider clinical restenosis the more relevant term. There are multiple ways to define clinical restenosis including recurrence of symptoms or a decline in noninvasive measurements. In the drug-eluting stent (DES) literature the most popular measures used are the incidences of target lesion revascularization (TLR rate), defined as the frequency of repeat procedure at the site of the initial intervention; and target vessel revascularization (TVR rate), the frequency of interventions performed anywhere along the entire length of the vessel into which the stent was inserted. Prevention of restenosis is more frequently attempted, and successfully performed, than treatment. Any tactic employed to prolong the efficacy of an intervention in

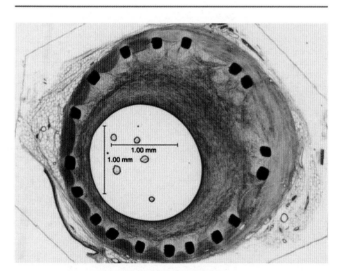

FIGURE 100.1 Stent-induced neointimal hyperplasia. Cross section of uncoated arterial stent (H and E stain). The lumen is narrowed by neointimal ingrowth. As the stent remains fully expanded, elastic recoil or constrictive remodeling are not components of in-stent restenosis.

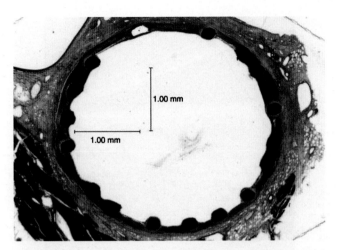

FIGURE 100.2 Ideal performance of a drug-eluting stent (H and E stain). Neointimal hyperplasia is prevented and there is endothelial coverage of the stent tynes.

essence impacts restenosis, thus systemic adjuvant medications, covered stent insertion, atherectomy, and resorbable stents are technically restenosis therapies. These are covered elsewhere in this text. In this chapter we focus on local pharmacologic treatments specifically targeted at the biologic cascade of restenosis.

DRUG-ELUTING STENTS

Introduction

A DES is a stent coated or embedded with single or multiple bioactive agents. Following implantation, the therapeutic material is released locally into the vessel wall adjacent to the stent as well as into the bloodstream. Multiple factors influence the amount of the active agent that ultimately enters the vessel wall and for how long it stays there.[5] These include physical characteristics of the drug, such as molecular size, solubility, and degree of protein binding; the rate of release of the drug from the stent surface; total dose of the drug applied to the stent; total surface area of contact between stent and vessel wall; characteristics of the vessel wall itself including composition (particularly the amount of fat and calcium) and mural thickness; and the rate of blood flow within the lumen (the zero sump effect). Publications will frequently compare DESs based on the dose of drug on the stent or whether the polymer is fast or slow release; however, the more critical issues are the concentration of the active agent achieved within the vessel wall and dwell time (the length of time the agent stays in the vessel wall). Both are profoundly affected by the aforementioned factors.

Since Food and Drug Administration (FDA) approval for coronary use in March 2003, DESs have made an impact on the practice of interventional cardiology similar in magnitude to the introduction of angioplasty in the 1980s. Improved clinical outcomes have resulted in a significant increase in both total number of endovascular coronary procedures and their complexity since that time.[6] Despite the broad acceptance by the cardiology community, experience in the peripheral arterial circulation has been much smaller; a small number of randomized multicenter studies and observational single center reports have been published. In the coronary circulation, surgical bypass to treat a blocked coronary artery involves the morbidity of a thoracotomy and a stay in the intensive care unit; therefore, an endovascular alternative does not have to be more durable to be an acceptable alternative. The consequences of open surgery in peripheral vascular disease are not as dire. Drug-eluting coronary stents profoundly decrease restenosis rates in comparison with bare metal stents, and reducing the restenosis rate improves patient clinical outcome.[7] In most peripheral vascular beds neither of these issues has definitively been proven. The clinical manifestations of coronary artery disease are sufficiently common that

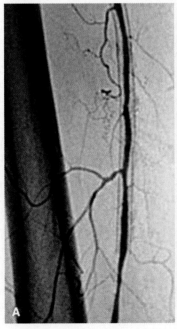

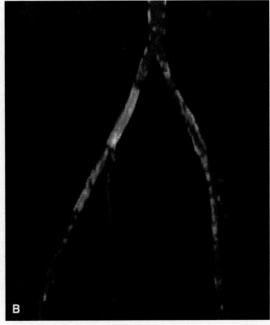

FIGURE 100.3 Types of angiographic restenosis. **A.** In-stent restenosis. SFA arteriogram 6 months postinsertion of a SMART stent demonstrating diffuse luminal narrowing due to neointimal hyperplasia. Note the separation of the outline of the stent from the narrowed arterial lumen. **B.** In-segment restenosis. Reconstructed MIP image from a CT angiogram demonstrating a tight eccentric stenosis immediately proximal to (within 0.5 cm of) the right common iliac artery stent.

MIP, maximum intensity projection; CT, computed tomography.

a company could justify the enormous expense of developing a coronary DES. In some peripheral vascular disease states the number of patients is so low that a product purpose-designed to treat that entity would not be commercially viable (e.g., mesenteric vascular ischemia).

DESs are complex devices made of three components: the stent, polymeric coating (or equivalent) connecting the drug to the stent and affecting its rate of release, and the drug itself. This chapter discusses only coated stents designed for the prevention of restenosis; however, stents that are resistant to thrombosis or designed as reservoirs for the release of agents, such as vasodilators, into the downstream vasculature have also been described.[8]

Stents

To date, most of the DESs used in the coronary circulation and all stents used in the periphery are conventional stents primarily designed to optimally traverse and treat stenoses with drug delivery a secondary consideration. It is ironic that stents have again become a means by which local tissue growth can be modified; Charles R. Stent, an English dentist who died in 1901, devised and lent his name to a curved mold used as a scaffold onto which oral skin grafts were applied to enhance their incorporation.[9] The active agent on DESs are typically applied as a thin layer on the surface of the stent opposing the vessel wall (abluminal surface). There are coronary stents purpose designed to enhance drug loading and delivery via laser cut reservoirs or slots that act as receptacles for drugs and polymer,[10] but no stents of this design have been employed in the peripheral circulation at this time.

Stent Coating

Identifying suitable carriers for stent-based drug delivery may be the most challenging aspect of DES development. The coating must be suitable for sterilization, be resistant to abrasion or flaking during stent implantation and expansion, and provide controllable drug release (both in concentration and time), all without thrombogenic or inflammatory effects on the vessel wall. The most commonly used vehicles are nonerodable polymer coatings, but others including phosphorylcholine, biodegradable or bioabsorbable polymers, and ceramic layers have been developed.[11] In some instnances drugs may be directly applied to the stent surface without a polymer (FIGURE 100.4), relying on the markedly lipophilic nature of the drug (e.g., paclitaxel) to create adequate concentration and dwell time in the surrounding vessel wall to achieve the desired inhibitory effect.[12]

Drugs

Several drugs have been evaluated as potential coatings for DESs.[13,14] They may be generally classified based on their mechanism of action as immunosuppressive, antiproliferative, anti-inflammatory, antithrombotic, modulators of extracellular matrix, or pro-healing (Table 100.1). Many of the agents listed are of research interest only. In practice this classification is somewhat arbitrary because a single agent may affect multiple steps in the restenotic process or have very different mechanisms of action depending on the tissue concentration. At this time, the three main groups of agents in clinical use for stent coating

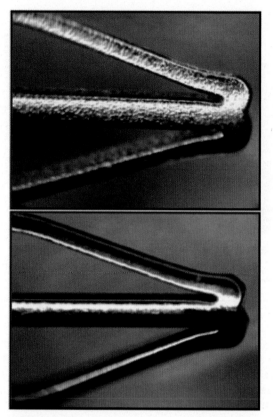

FIGURE 100.4 Coating of drug (paclitaxel) without polymer on the surface of a ZilverPTX stent (**top**). An uncoated stent is shown for comparison (**bottom**).

are sirolimus and analogues (the "limuses"), taxanes (paclitaxel), and prohealing.

Sirolimus and Analogues

Sirolimus-coated stents were the first commercially approved DESs for coronary artery disease. Sirolimus (Rapamycin, Wyeth, Ayerst, PA) is a macrolide antibiotic with potent immunosuppressive activity. It was originally isolated in the mid-1930s from *Streptomyces hygroscopicus* found in Easter Island soil samples (the island is called Rapanui by its natives; hence the name rapamycin). Rapamycin diffuses into smooth muscle cells and binds to an intracellular receptor, the FK506 binding protein. It inhibits cellular proliferation by blocking cell cycle progression from the G1 to S phase. After rapamycin was shown to profoundly inhibit intimal thickening in animal models of vascular injury, multiple trials confirmed the efficacy of rapamycin-coated coronary stents in humans using the Cypher stent (Cordis Corporation, Brunswick, NJ).[15,16] Human experience with rapamycin-eluting stents in the noncoronary circulation is discussed later in this chapter.

Stents coated with sirolimus analogues have largely supplanted sirolimus-coated stents in the coronary arteries.[17] Zotarolimus, also called ABT-578, is a sirolimus analog developed by Abbott Pharmaceuticals (Abbott Park, IL). It is mechanistically similar to sirolimus but has a shorter in vivo half-life. It is currently being developed by two companies for coronary use: the Zomaxx stent is produced by Abbott Vascular (Redwood City, CA) and the

Table 100.1

Drugs and Biologically Active Agents Used on Stents to Prevent Restenosis

Immunosuppressive drugs

Sirolimus (rapamycin)

Everolimus

ABT-578 (zotarolimus)

FK506 (tacrolimus)

Umirolimus (Biolimus A9)

Mycophenolic acid

Antiproliferative drugs

Paclitaxel

Angiopeptin

Tyrosine kinase inhibitor

Actinomycin D

C-myc antisense

Anti-inflammatory drugs

Corticosteroid

Tranilast

Antithrombosis agents

Heparin

Inhibitors of platelet aggregation

Extracellular matrix modulators

Batimastat

Prohealing agents

CD34 antibodies

Endothelial cells

Nitric oxide donors

Vascular endothelial growth factor

17-β-estradiol

Endeavor device by Medtronic (Minneapolis, MN). The immunosuppressant everolimus is a semisynthetic sirolimus analogue, also with a similar mechanism of action and a shorter half-life. Abbott Vascular coats its Xience coronary stent systems with this drug in both bioabsorbable polymer and durable polymer carriers. Umirolimus (Biolimus A9) is a highly lipophilic sirolimus derivative; thus, it is more rapidly absorbed into the vessel wall. Terumo (Tokyo, Japan) uses umirolimus on its Nobori coronary stent and Biosensors (Singapore) on the BioMatrix stent system.

Taxanes

The taxanes are a group of antimitotic agents with profound anti-inflammatory properties acting via a unique ability to interfere with microtubule function. Examples include paclitaxel, docetaxel, and 7-hexanoyltaxol (QP2). With rare exception, at present, paclitaxel is the only drug from the taxane family in use for the prevention of restenosis, being delivered via drug-eluting

stents, drug-eluting balloons, and nanoparticulate infusion.[18,19] Although it is the active ingredient in the broad-spectrum systemic chemotherapeutic agent Taxol (Bristol Myers Squibb, New York, NY), paclitaxel is intensely lipophilic, thus, ideal for local drug delivery. It is extracted from the bark and needles of the Pacific Yew tree. Additionally, synthetic and semisynthetic versions are now produced. Microtubules are intimately related to the functions of intracellular transport, signaling, protein secretion, and motility. Paclitaxel disrupts these cellular processes by forming stable dysfunctional microtubules.[20] The Taxus family of paclitaxel-eluting coronary stents are produced by Boston Scientific, Inc. (Natick, MA) using a polymer-based delivery system. The only commercially available self-expanding DES is the Zilver PTX, made by Cook Inc. (Bloomington, IN) with paclitaxel directly applied to the stent surface without polymer.

Prohealing Agents

Agents that accelerate endothelial coverage of a stent after implantation may reduce adverse effects, such as thrombosis.[21] It is also thought that functioning endothelium might maintain quiescence of the underlying media and adventitia, potentially reducing restenosis. The most common means of achieving this is coating the stent with CD34 antibody, which captures endothelial progenitor cells from the circulation, resulting in their deposit on the stent surface. OrbusNeich (Fort Lauderdale, FL) applies this technology to its Genous stent.

DRUG-ELUTING BALLOONS

The process of restenosis can be delayed when conventional angioplasty balloons are coated with the same agents used on DESs.[22,23] The drug most commonly used is paclitaxel, although limus-coated balloons have been described.[24] Because the balloon is in contact with the vessel wall and the active drug is lipophilic, therapeutic concentrations of drug can be achieved in the arterial wall from a single inflation. DESs contain low doses of drugs that are released slowly from a polymer stent coating. Sustained drug release may be necessary because drug distribution from a DES to the arterial wall is inhomogeneous or because the stent acts as a continual irritant. Approximately 85% of the stented vessel wall area is not covered by the stent struts, resulting in low tissue concentrations of the antiproliferative agent between struts (FIGURE 100.5A). To achieve antirestenotic efficacy in these areas, high drug concentrations on the stent struts are mandatory for stent-based local drug delivery with the consequence of delayed and incomplete endothelialisation of the stent struts. By contrast drug-eluting balloons are coated with free drug and usually an excipient (a polymer that helps in drug delivery). When the balloon is inflated most of the drug is released in 60 seconds or less. The therapeutic effects appear to be partly due to the fact that the drug is released precisely at the time of vessel wall injury and in part due to the dwell time of the active drug in the vessel wall. Angioplasty is considered to be a transient injury, thus a shorter duration of drug activity is needed. The duration of inhibition of cell proliferation far exceeds the time of balloon inflation, even though typically less than 10% of the drug on the surface of the balloon is actually delivered into the vessel wall.[25] Neointimal hyperplasia, one component of restenosis after balloon angioplasty, is diminished by paclitaxel (FIGURE 100.5B). In addition, it may surprise the reader to know that there is inhibition of elastic recoil and

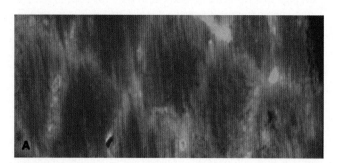
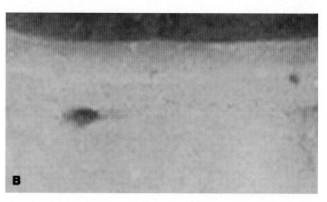

FIGURE 100.5 Drug distribution on arterial surface—fluorescent paclitaxel. **A.** Drug-eluting stent. A significant area of stented vessel wall is not covered by the stent, resulting in low tissue concentrations between tynes. **B.** Drug-eluting balloon. The balloon is uniformly coated with drug; therefore, drug is evenly distributed on the vessel surface.

negative remodeling, both also significant components of restenosis after angioplasty.[26]

In summary, the principal advantages of drug-eluting balloons are ease of use and the lack of a permanent prosthesis. Because there is no ongoing presence of stent, drug, or polymer, there is potentially less inflammation and more rapid endothelialization, which in turn should result in less late thrombosis and shorter and less intense antiplatelet therapy.

DRUG-ELUTING STENTS AND BALLOONS IN PERIPHERAL VASCULAR DISEASE

Superficial Femoral and Popliteal Arteries

Anatomic and Functional Considerations

As has been documented elsewhere in this text, in comparison with endovascular procedures in other peripheral arteries of similar size, interventional techniques for treating the superficial femoral–popliteal artery segment have poor long-term patency rates. The earliest efforts to improve this situation using DESs utilized drug and polymer combinations that worked effectively in the coronary circulation. In this region the diseased segments can be as long as 30 cm and the plaques are large and calcified, thus the burden of atherosclerotic disease is enormously greater and of different composition in the superficial femoral artery (SFA) compared with the coronary artery. Perhaps most significantly, the femoral artery differs from other arterial beds in that it is recurrently deformed in multiple directions with leg movement.[27] This deformation consists not just of flexion at the knee, but also compression within the adductor hiatus and rotation and longitudinal compression. The artery is fixed at the groin and knee and mobile between, so the elastic vessel of a young person accommodates to these forces well.[28] Atherosclerosis is characterized by circumferentially and longitudinally uneven loss of elastin and deposition of calcium within the vessel wall so that when an older, atherosclerotic patient bends his or her leg the effects of these forces are exaggerated, even to the point of abrupt kinking. These recurrent external deformations can not only in themselves serve as recurrent stimuli to the restenosis cascade,[29] they present continual stresses on an endoluminal stent (FIGURE 100.6), potentially resulting in stent fracture.[30] When designing a DES

for prevention of restenosis in the femoropopliteal segment, the burden of disease and recurrent mechanical distortions significantly impact stent design as well as choice of drug, dosage, and length of administration.

Experience with Drug-Eluting Stents

The first studies of DESs in the SFA were conducted using stents coated with drugs from the limus family. In the SIROCCO (Sirolimus-Coated Cordis Self-expandable Stent) I and II studies, a nitinol stent platform (SMART stent, Cordis Endovascular, Miami, FL) with a coating of sirolimus embedded in nonresorbable polymer was used.[31,32] The SIROCCO studies initially tantalized physicians with a significant improvement in the drug-eluting arm at 6 months; however, there was a progressive loss of drug effect and by 24 months there was no significant difference in patency rates between bare metal and sirolimus-eluting stents. The restenosis rates by duplex ultrasonography at 18 and 24 months were 18.4% and 22.9% for sirolimus-eluting

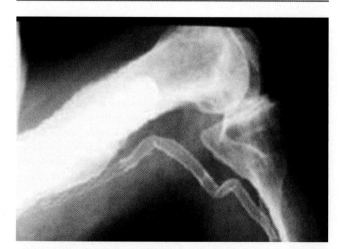

FIGURE 100.6 Lateral X-ray demonstrating distortion and kinking of a stent in the femoral–popliteal arterial segment with knee flexion.

(Image courtesy of R. Smouse, MD)

stents, and 12.8% and 21.1% for uncoated stents. In addition, the stent fracture rate was 11% at 6 months and 26% at 18 months.

STRIDES (Superficial Femoral Artery Treatment with Drug-Eluting Stents) was a single-arm study of 104 patients treated with a nitinol stent (Dynalink-E stent, Abbott Vascular, Inc., Santa Clara, CA) coated with everolimus and a nonresorbable polymer.[33] The results suggested improved patency over bare metal stents at 6 months; however, again, this improvement was not sustained. Duplex ultrasonography at 12 months demonstrated a patency rate of 68.5%, decreasing to 54.6% at 393 days. By comparison, the VIENNA Absolute trial recorded a 63% 12-month patency using an uncoated version of the same stent.[34] At the time of writing no other studies of stents coated with a drug from the limus family are being conducted in the SFA.

There have been two studies using paclitaxel-eluting stents in the femoropopliteal region, both using the Zilver PTX nitinol self-expanding stent coated with nonpolymeric paclitaxel[35,36] (FIGURE 100.7). The Zilver PTX study is the largest prospectively randomized trial of endovascular treatment ever performed in the SFA. It compared 236 patients treated with paclitaxel-coated stents with 238 treated by balloon angioplasty with provision for bailout stent placement. At 12 months primary patency in the primary DES group was 83.1% versus 32.8% for percutaneous transluminal angioplasty (PTA) and at 24 months 74.8% versus 26.5%. One hundred twenty patients had acute PTA failure and were randomly assigned to provisional paclitaxel-coated or uncoated stents. The provisional paclitaxel-coated stent group exhibited improved primary patency compared with the provisional uncoated stent group (89.9% vs. 73% at 12 months and 83.4% vs. 64.1% at 24 months). The higher patency rate in the drug-eluting arm appeared to convey a clinical benefit in the form of freedom from worsening symptoms of ischemia (90.5% vs. 72.3% at 12 months; 83.9% compared with 68.4%

at 24 months). This association of enhanced clinical efficacy with improved patency is not uniformly seen with DES trials in other vascular beds. The stent fracture rate for both coated and uncoated stents was 0.9% at 12 months.

The second study was a nonrandomized registry conducted outside the United States. Nine hundred femoropopliteal lesions in 787 patients were treated with Zilver PTX stents (FIGURE 100.8). The patients were a composite group including de novo and restenotic lesions, including in-stent restenosis. A 76% freedom from TLR rate was seen at 12 months in patients enrolled with in-stent restenosis. The overall 12-month Kaplan-Meier estimates included an 89% event-free survival rate, an 86.2% primary patency rate, and a 90.5% rate of freedom from TLR. No paclitaxel-related adverse events were reported. The 12-month stent fracture rate was 1.5%. Statistically significant improvement of ankle brachial index, Rutherford score, and walking distance/speed were seen at 12 months.

In summary, positive outcomes with DESs in the SFA have only been seen with polymer-free paclitaxel-coated stents to date. It is not clear how durable those results will be or how the data compare with other endovascular SFA treatments in previously untreated patients. The data are hopeful though, especially for certain patient subsets where no good endovascular solution exists, such as in-stent restenosis.

Experience with Drug-Eluting Balloons

The first significant human trial of drug-eluting balloons in peripheral vascular disease was the THUNDER (Local Taxane with Short Exposure for Reduction of Restenosis in Distal Arteries) trial.[37] It was a double-blind randomized study of 154 patients with stenotic or occluded superficial femoral or popliteal arteries using Paccocath paclitaxel-coated angioplasty balloons (Medrad, Warrendale, PA) compared with conventional balloon angioplasty alone or with an infusion of paclitaxel in iopromide. Paccocath balloons are standard angioplasty

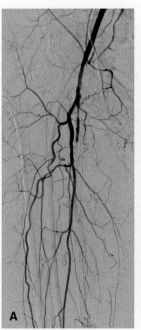 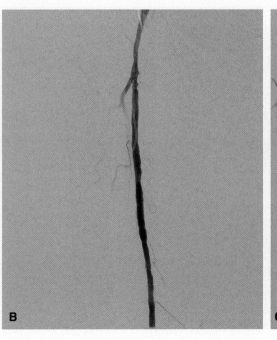 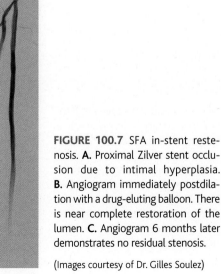

FIGURE 100.7 SFA in-stent restenosis. **A.** Proximal Zilver stent occlusion due to intimal hyperplasia. **B.** Angiogram immediately postdilation with a drug-eluting balloon. There is near complete restoration of the lumen. **C.** Angiogram 6 months later demonstrates no residual stenosis.

(Images courtesy of Dr. Gilles Soulez)

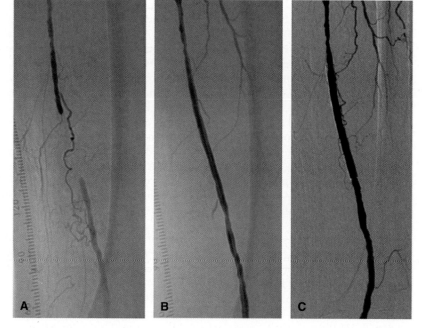

FIGURE 100.8 Treatment of SFA occlusion with a paclitaxel-eluting stent. **A.** Pretreatment angiogram demonstrating SFA occlusion in the adductor hiatus with above-knee reconstitution. **B.** Post-treatment angiogram after insertion of a Zilver PTX stent. **C.** Angiogram 12 months after stent insertion. There is minor intimal thickening at the proximal aspect of the stent; otherwise appearances are unchanged from time of insertion.

(Images courtesy of Dr. Michael Dake)

balloons coated with 3 μg/mm^2 of paclitaxel mixed with the iodinated contrast medium iopromide (FIGURE 100.9). The paclitaxel-coated balloon had significantly less restenosis at 6 months as well as a lower TLR rate and significantly less late lumen loss at 6, 12, and 24 months. A similar study also comparing Paccocath to balloon angioplasty for stenoses or occlusions in the femoropopliteal segment, the FEMPAC (Inhibition of Restenosis in Femoropopliteal Arteries: Paclitaxel-Coated Versus Uncoated Balloon) study, achieved similar results in 87 patients at 2-year follow-up.[38]

There are several other trials of drug-eluting balloons for which published data are not yet available.[39]

Tibial Arteries

Anatomic and Functional Considerations

Severe tibial atherosclerosis is typically associated with systemic diseases, such as diabetes or renal dysfunction, which will impact the outcome of any endovascular treatment. The distribution of drug in the arterial wall is likely to differ from the coronary circulation because flow rates are lower, and there is a higher frequency of severe calcification. The tibial arteries are not subject to the marked mechanical forces of the femoropopliteal segment but balloon-expandable stents can be crushed if the calf is subjected to compressive forces.

FIGURE 100.9 Treatment of focal popliteal artery stenosis using a drug-eluting balloon. **A.** Predilation angiogram demonstrating a focal popliteal artery stenosis. **B.** Post dilation there is residual irregularity at the angioplasty site. **C.** Angiogram 7 months postdilation. Appearance has improved due to positive remodeling.

(Images courtesy of Dr. Felipe Nasser)

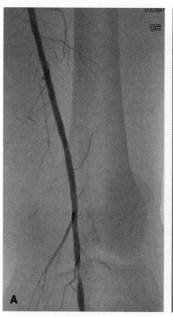
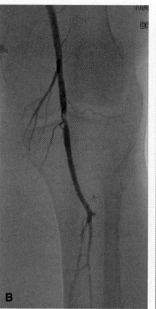
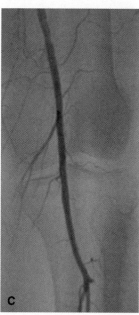

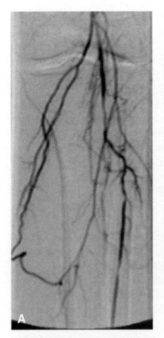
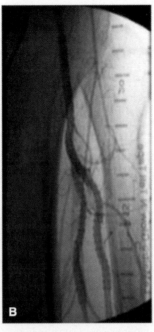

FIGURE 100.10 Tibial artery reconstruction with drug-eluting stents in a patient with chronic limb ischemia. **A.** Preprocedure angiogram demonstrates stenoses in proximal anterior tibial artery, minimal opacification of the tibial–peroneal trunk and peroneal artery and nonfilling of the posterior tibial artery. **B.** Patent tibial–peroneal trunk, anterior tibial artery and peroneal artery after insertion of multiple sirolimus-eluting Cypher stents.

(Images courtesy of Dr. Dimitris Siablis)

Although the tibial vessels are of similar size to coronary arteries, lesion lengths are much longer so a relatively small proportion of patients presenting with tibial artery blockage can be treated entirely with DESs designed for the coronary artery (FIGURE 100.10 and FIGURE 100.11). A common practice in these patients is angioplasty with long balloons and spot stenting for persistent stenosis. Adjunctive antiplatelet regimes are viewed as essential; however, consensus has not been reached on an optimal regime.

Experience with Drug-Eluting Stents

There are two randomized trials comparing drug-eluting to bare metal stents below the knee for which at least 1-year follow-up data are available. The Yukon-BTK study compared stents coated with polymer-free sirolimus to bare metal stents in 161 patients with intermittent claudication and critical limb ischemia (CLI).[40] In the DESTINY trial 140 patients with CLI were randomized to be treated with everolimus-eluting or bare metal stents.[41] A third randomized trial, ACHILLES, compared sirolimus-eluting stents with balloon angioplasty in 200 patients with severe claudication or CLI.[42] The results of these trials are summarized in Table 100.2.

The overall 1-year primary patency rate for tibial artery DESs pooled from the three randomized as well as published nonrandomized trials is 86% ± 5%, the mean TLR rate is 9.9% ± 5%, and the limb salvage rate is 96.6% ± 4%.[43] Although the data from these studies show significant improvements in patency and decreased incidence of reintervention in patients who receive DESs, a significant advantage in mortality or major or minor amputation rates have not been demonstrated in any study to date. It should be noted,

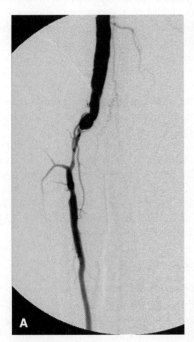
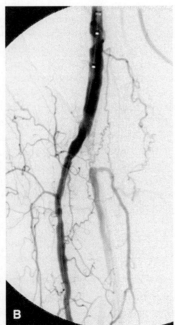
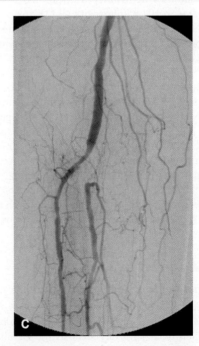

FIGURE 100.11 Drug-eluting stent for focal stenosis of the tibial artery. **A.** Preprocedure angiogram demonstrating a tight stenosis, narrowing the proximal 2 cm of the anterior tibial artery. **B.** Immediately post insertion of a paclitaxel-coated Taxus stent there is no residual stenosis. **C.** At 7 months, appearances are virtually unchanged.

Table 100.2

Twelve-Month Follow-Up of Randomized Trials of Drug-Eluting Stents in Tibial Arteries

Study	Destiny	Yukon-Btk	Achilles
DES	Everolimus	Non-polymeric sirolimus	Polymeric sirolimus
Control	BMS	BMS	Angioplasty
Patients	140	161	200
Primary patency (%)			
DES	85.2	80.6	80.6
Control	34.7	55.6	58.1
TLR			
DES	7.5	9.7	10.0
Control	34.7	17.5	16.5
Limb salvage			
DES	98.7	98.4	86.2
Control	97.1	96.8	80

however, that none of the studies were adequately powered to assess these endpoints.

Experience with Drug-Eluting Balloons

Initial experience with drug-eluting balloons below the knee has also been positive. In the first published report, tibial arteries were dilated with the In.Pact Amphirion paclitaxel-eluting balloon (Medtronic, Minneapolis, MN)[44]; 109 limbs were treated in 104 patients with CLI (82.6%) or severe claudication (17.4%). The mean lesion length treated was 17.6 cm. Angiography at 3 months demonstrated restenosis in 27.4%. Most restenotic lesions were focal; in only 9.5% was the entire treated segment renarrowed or occluded. Of 91 limbs remaining in the analysis at 1 year, clinical improvement was present in 83 (91.2%). Complete wound healing occurred in 74.2%. Major amputation occurred in four patients, resulting in a 95.6% limb salvage rate for patients with CLI. The DEBATE-BTK trial is a randomized study comparing the use of the In.Pact Amphirion balloon with uncoated balloons in 120 patients with chronic limb ischemia.[45] Preliminary 12-month data showed statistically significant differences in binary restenosis (29% of patients treated with a drug-eluting balloon vs. 72% treated with uncoated balloons) and reocclusion (14% vs. 50%).

Renal Arteries

Anatomic and Functional Considerations

The renal arteries have extremely high flow rates. Approximately 20% of the cardiac output flows through the paired arteries. Atherosclerotic renal artery stenosis most commonly occurs at the origin of the artery, including the portion that passes through the aortic wall; thus the plaque burden can be much larger than other arteries of similar size. The high intraluminal flow rates and large mural area could potentially affect drug

distribution delivered from a stent in comparison to other arteries with similar luminal diameter.

At this time consensus has not been reached on diagnosis or therapy of atherosclerotic renal artery stenosis. Notably lacking are prospective studies confirming clinical benefit of endovascular renal artery revascularization. The clinical aims of renal artery stenting are generally stated to be prevention of deterioration of renal function and resolution of or decrease in number of medications taken for hypertension.[46] Restenosis rates after renal artery stenting are typically reported as between 9% and 25% at follow-up times ranging from 5 to 12 months.[47]

Experience with Drug-Eluting Stents

The GREAT (Palmaz Genesis Peripheral Stainless Steel Balloon Expandable Stent in REnal Artery Treatment) trial prospectively randomized 52 patients to receive uncoated bare metal balloon-expandable Palmaz Genesis stents and 53 patients to be treated with sirolimus-coated Genesis stents (Cordis Endovascular, Miami, FL) as treatment for renal artery stenosis.[48,49] All stents were 5 or 6 mm in diameter. Ninety percent of the sirolimus was eluted within the first 30 days. The polymer and topcoat were the same as used for sirolimus-eluting coronary stents. When patients were reexamined 6 months post-treatment there was a reduction of restenosis (defined as ≥50% narrowing within the stent) from 14.3% for bare metal stents to 6.7% in the sirolimus-coated group, although it did not reach statistical significance, likely due to small sample size ($p = .30$). At 6 months and 1 year, TLR rates were 7.7% and 11.5% in the bare metal group and 1.9% at both time points in the drug-eluting group. However, 6.9% of the patients receiving a DES had worsening of their renal function compared with 4.6% in the bare metal group. This may have been compounded by the fact that pretreatment renal function was worse in the sirolimus patients than the bare metal group. In addition there was no significant difference between the two groups in improvement in blood pressure control or number of antihypertensive medications the patients had to take 6 months after stent insertion. At 2 years, the major adverse event rate was 23.7% for bare metal stent and 26.8% for the drug-eluting group.

The experience with DESs for treatment of renal artery in-stent restenosis has been disappointing. The largest reported series described the use of sirolimus-eluting stents in 22 renal arteries in 16 nonrandomized patients.[50] At a median follow-up of 12 months, restenosis was seen in 71.4% of patients.

Thus even though DESs resulted in a mild reduction in restenosis and reintervention rates, this difference did not result in improved clinical efficacy. There is no reduction, possibly a slight increase, in complication rates when using a DES. At the time of writing, no other clinical trials evaluating DESs in native renal arteries are under way, and there have been no reports on the use of drug-eluting balloons in the renal artery.

Dialysis Access

Anatomic and Functional Considerations

In both arteriovenous grafts and fistulas for dialysis access, the most common etiology of impaired function is venous neointimal hyperplasia. Although the basic histology is similar to neointimal hyperplasia seen after arterial interventions, there are several differences.[51,52] Clinically it is more aggressive. Veins have a poorly defined internal elastic lamina that could allow easier migration of smooth muscle and other cells after a vascular insult. There is lower nitric oxide and prostacyclin production than in arteries; thus veins have increased vasoconstrictor sensitivity. Other factors in dialysis patients are important: uremia results in endothelial dysfunction, which alters the vascular healing response, and repetitive punctures with large-bore dialysis needles is thought to contribute to venous hyperplasia because platelet thrombi that accumulate at the puncture site bathe downstream vessels in proinflammatory factors. Uptake and distribution after local delivery of an antirestenotic agent also will differ from an artery because the vein wall is thinner and of different composition.

Experience with Drug-Eluting Stents

A single randomized study assessing the efficacy of DESs in dialysis access has been performed. Tay et al.[53] compared the Zilver PTX paclitaxel coated stent to conventional balloon angioplasty in the treatment of venous anastomotic stenoses in 32 patients with failing arterio-venous dialysis grafts. In the PTA arm, either a normal balloon or high-pressure balloon was used. In the Zilver PTX arm, the stent was deployed across the stenosis following PTA (FIGURE 100.12) and postdilated if required. Mean duration of primary patency was 163.4 days for the Zilver PTX group and 103.9 days for PTA. Six-month primary patency was 46.2% versus 25.5%; 1 year secondary patency was 61.5% compared with 46.7%. None of the differences achieved statistical significance and the trial was halted prior to full enrollment.

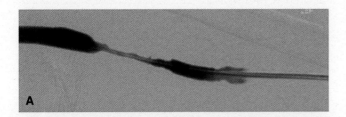

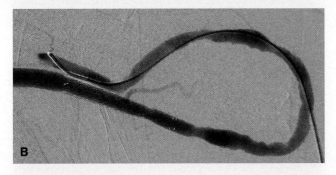

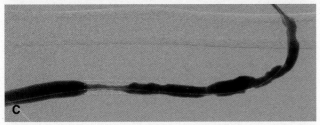

FIGURE 100.12 Drug-eluting stent in dialysis access. **A.** A tight stenosis is seen in the venous outflow of an A-V graft. **B.** Fistulogram at 6 months demonstrates the Zilver PTX stent placed across the stenosis is patent. **C.** At 9 months significant in-stent restenosis has developed.

Experience with Drug-Eluting Balloons

Angioplasty with paclitaxel-coated balloons has been compared with angioplasty with uncoated balloons in failing arteriovenous dialysis fistulas or prosthetic arteriovenous grafts.[54] Forty patients with significant venous outflow stenosis were prospectively randomized. At 6 months, cumulative target lesion primary patency was significantly higher after treatment with drug-eluting balloons (70% vs. 25% in the uncoated balloon group). Because high-pressure drug-eluting balloons are not available, many patients in the drug-eluting balloon group required additional treatment with a high-pressure balloon; therefore, further study is required to fully quantify the effectiveness of drug-eluting balloons in these patients.

THE FUTURE

In the near future efforts will primarily be dedicated to defining where drug-eluting balloons and stents are best suited to specific clinical scenarios in peripheral vascular disease. With better data and improved imaging, patient- and lesion-specific factors will be considered in addition to the gross anatomy. Anticoagulant and antiplatelet regimes have not yet been optimized for drug-coated devices in peripheral vascular disease and considerable work will be done in this area, both on a generic basis as well as creating an improved understanding of individual variations in response to these medications. Personalized medicine may find its way to the endovascular suite.

The intermediate future promises exciting advances in coatings that render devices nonreactive, improved bioabsorbable devices, nanoparticles both for device coating and for site-specific activity after systemic administration, refinement of gene therapy directed both at preventing restenosis and to promote neovascularity, drug delivery systems potentiated by outside energy including ultrasound and magnetism, and new therapeutic agents (including combination antithrombotic and antiproliferative coatings). Looming over all of these extraordinary technologies are the specters of increasingly stringent regulatory processes and cost constraints. It is ever more costly to fulfill the regulatory requirements for new devices and increasingly difficult to demonstrate the incremental improvements in outcomes over existing treatments to justify those costs. There is likely to be bittersweet solace in the not too distant future for frustrated interventionists; those bureaucrats whose jobs appear to be impedance of the adoption of new treatments for peripheral vascular disease may be rendered obsolete, as will the devices themselves—by a vaccine against atherosclerosis.[55]

SUMMARY

Both DESs and balloons demonstrate short-term efficacy in comparison with conventional angioplasty or bare metal stents in most peripheral applications, but comprehensive direct comparison between therapeutic modalities will be necessary to define specific roles for each technology. It is clear that there is no magic bullet, and that the remarkable success of drug-coated balloon-expandable stents in midsized coronary arteries cannot be repeated by merely applying the same drugs using the same dose and delivery methods in other vascular beds. Lessons have been learned. The SIROCCO trial taught us that profound inhibition of intimal hyperplasia can be achieved as in coronary arteries at 6 months, but a durable effect is quickly lost because of the very different milieu of the SFA. In the GREAT trial we saw that a reduction of restenosis does not necessarily confer a significant clinical benefit to the patient. Finally, perhaps most importantly, some technologies are now so expensive to develop and test that even if efficacy can be demonstrated, economics seems likely to prevent them from becoming clinical reality.

REFERENCES

1. Curcio A, Torella D, Indolfi C. Mechanisms of smooth muscle cell proliferation and endothelial regeneration after vascular injury and stenting: approach to therapy. *Circ J* 2011;75:1287–1296.
2. Marx SO, Totary-Jain H, Marks A. Vascular smooth muscle cell proliferation in restenosis. *Circ Cardiovasc Interv* 2011;4:104–111.
3. Neville RF, Sidawy AN. Myointimal hyperplasia: basic science and clinical considerations. *Semin Vasc Surg* 1998;11:142–148.
4. Serruys PW, Foley DP, Kirkeide RL, et al. Restenosis revisited: insights provided by quantitative coronary angiography. *Am Heart J* 1993;126:1243–1267.
5. Papafaklis MI, Chatzizisis YS, Naka KK, et al. Drug-eluting stent restenosis: effect of drug type, release kinetics, hemodynamics and coating strategy. *Pharmacol Ther* 2012;134:43–53.
6. Rao SV, Shaw RE, Bindis RG, et al. Patterns and outcomes of drug-eluting stent use in clinical practice. *Am Heart J* 2006;152:321–326.
7. Tung R, Kaul S, Diamond GA, et al. Narrative review: drug-eluting stents for the management of restenosis: a critical appraisal of the evidence. *Ann Intern Med* 2006;144:913–919.
8. Gertz ZM, Wilensky RL. Local drug delivery for treatment of coronary and peripheral artery disease. *Cardiovasc Ther* 2011;29:54–66.
9. Hedin M. The origin of the word Stent. *Acta Radiol* 1997;6:937–939.
10. Ramcharitar S, Vaina S, Serruys PW. The next generation of drug-eluting stents: what's on the horizon? *Am J Cardiovasc Drugs* 2007;7(2):81–93.
11. Ielasi A, Latib A, Colombo A. Current and future drug-eluting stent technology. *Expert Rev Cardiovasc Ther* 2011;9:485–503.
12. Dake MD, Van Alstine WG, Zhou Q, et al. Polymer-free paclitaxel-coated Zilver PTX Stents—evaluation of pharmacokinetics and comparative safety in porcine arteries. *J Vasc Interv Radiol* 2011;22:603–610.
13. Jukema JW, Ahmed TA, Verschuren JJ, et al. Restenosis after PCI: part 2, prevention and therapy. *Nat Rev Cardiol* 2011;11:79–90.
14. Sousa JE, Serruys PW, Costa MA. New frontiers in cardiology: drug-eluting stents: part I. *Circulation* 2003;107:2274–2279.
15. Marx SQ, Marks AR. Bench to bedside: the development of rapamycin and its application to stent restenosis. *Circulation* 2001;104:852–855.
16. Buch AN, Waksman R. Cypher versus Taxus: all smoke and no fire: lessons for future comparative drug-eluting stent trials in interventional cardiology. *Am J Cardiol* 2007;99:424–427.
17. Claessen BE, Henriques JP, Dangas GD. Clinical studies with sirolimus, zotarolimus, everolimus and biolimus A9 drug-eluting stent systems. *Curr Pharm Des* 2010;16:4012–4024.
18. Herdeg C, Oberhoff M, Baumbach A, et al. Local paclitaxel delivery for the prevention of restenosis: biological effects and efficacy in vivo. *J Am Coll Cardiol* 2000;35:1969–1976.
19. Serruys PW, Sianos G, Abizaid A, et al. The effect of variable dose and release kinetics on neointimal hyperplasia using a a novel paclitaxel-eluting stent platform: the Paclitaxel In-Stent Controlled Elution Study (PISCES). *J Am Coll Cardiol* 2005;46:253–260.
20. Chatterjee S, Pandey A. Drug eluting stents: friend or foe? A review of cellular mechanisms behind the effects of paclitaxel and sirolimus eluting stents. *Curr Drug Metab* 2008;9:554–566.
21. Klomp M, Beijk MA, Damman P, et al. Three-year clinical follow-up of an unselected patient population treated with the genous endothelial progenitor cell capturing stent. *J Interv Cardiol* 2011;24:442–449.
22. Barbash IM, Waksman R. Current status, challenges and future directions of drug-eluting balloons. *Future Cardiol* 2011;7:765–774.
23. Zeller T, Schmitmeier S, Tepe G, et al. Drug coated balloons in the lower limb. *J Cardiovasc Surg (Torino)* 2011;52:235–243.
24. Cremers JL, Toner L, Schwartz LB, et al. Inhibition of neointimal hyperplasia with a novel zotarolimus coated balloon catheter. *Clin Res Cardiol* 2012;101:469–476.
25. Speck U, Cremers B, Kelsch B. Do pharmacokinetics explain persistent restenosis inhibition by a single dose of paclitaxel? *Circ Cardiovasc Interv* 2012;5:392–400.
26. De Labriolle A, Pakala R, Bonello L, et al. Paclitaxel-eluting balloon: from bench to bed. *Catheter Cardiovasc Interv* 2009;73:643–652.
27. Choi G, Cheng CP, Wilson NM, et al. Methods for quantifying three-dimensional deformation of arteries due to pulsatile and nonpulsatile forces: implications for the design of stents and stent grafts. *Ann Biomed Eng* 2009;37:14–33.
28. Cheng CP, Wilson NM, Hallett RL, et al. In vivo MR angiographic quantification of axial and twisting deformations of the superficial femoral artery resulting from maximum hip and knee flexion. *J Vasc Interv Radiol* 2006;17:979–987.
29. Arena FJ. Arterial kink and damage in normal segments of the superficial femoral and popliteal arteries abutting nitinol stents—a common cause of late occlusion and restenosis? A single-center experience. *J Invasive Cardiol* 2005;17:482–486.
30. Scheinert D, Scheinert S, Sax J, et al. Prevalence and clinical impact of stent fractures after femoropopliteal stenting. *J Am Coll Cardiol* 2005;45:312–315.
31. Duda SH, Pusich B, Richter G, et al. Sirolimus-eluting stents for the treatment of obstructive superficial femoral artery disease: six-month results. *Circulation* 2002;106(12):1505–1509.
32. Duda SH, Bosiers M, Lammer J, et al. Sirolimus-eluting versus bare nitinol stent for obstructive superficial femoral artery disease: the SIROCCO II trial. *J Vasc Interv Radiol* 2005;16:331–338.
33. Lammer J, Bosiers M, Zeller T, et al. First clinical trial of nitinol self-expanding everolimus-eluting stent implantation for peripheral arterial occlusive disease. *J Vasc Surg* 2011;54:394–401.
34. Schillinger M, Sabeti S, Loewe C, et al. Balloon angioplasty versus implantation of nitinol stents in the superficial femoral artery. *N Engl J Med* 2006;354:1879–1888.
35. Dake MD, Scheinert D, Tepe G, et al. Nitinol stents with polymer-free paclitaxel coating for lesions in the superficial femoral and popliteal arteries above the knee: twelve-month safety and effectiveness results from the Zilver PTX single-arm clinical study. *J Endovasc Ther* 2011;18:613–623.
36. Dake MD, Ansel GM, Jaff MR, et al. Paclitaxel-eluting stents show superiority to balloon angioplasty and bare metal stents in femoropopliteal disease: twelve-month Zilver PTX randomized study results. *Circ Cardiovasc Interv* 2011;4:495–504.
37. Tepe G, Zeller T, Albrecht T, et al. Local delivery of paclitaxel to inhibit restenosis during angioplasty of the leg. *N Engl J Med* 2008;358:689–699.
38. Werk M, Langner S, Reinkensmeier B, et al. Inhibition of restenosis in femoropopliteal arteries: paclitaxel-coated versus uncoated balloon: femoral paclitaxel randomized pilot trial. *Circulation* 2008;118:1358–1365.
39. Chan YC, Cheng S. Drug-eluting stents and balloons in peripheral arterial disease: evidence so far. *Int J Clin Pract* 2011;65:664–668.
40. Rastan A, Tepe G, Krankenberg H, et al. Sirolimus-eluting stents versus bare-metal stents for treatment of focal lesions in infrapopliteal arteries: a double blind, multi-centre randomized clinical trial. *Eur Heart J* 2011;32:2274–2281.
41. Bosiers M, Deloose K, Callaert J, et al. Drug-eluting stents below the knee. *J Cardiovasc Surg (Torino)* 2011;52:231–234.
42. Schmidt A. The Achilles Study (DES for BTK). Presented at: LINC; Leipzig, Germany; 2012.
43. Rastan A, Noory E, Zeller T. Drug-eluting stents for treatment of focal infrapopliteal lesion. *Vasa* 2012;41:90–95.
44. Schmidt A, Piorkowski M, Werner M, et al. First experience with drug-eluting balloons in infrapopliteal arteries. *J Am Coll Cardiol* 2011;58:1105–1109.
45. Ferraresi R, Centola M, Biondi-Zoccai G. Advances in below-the-knee drug-eluting balloons. *J Cardiovasc Surg (Torino)* 2012;53:205–213.
46. Balk E, Raman G, Chung M, et al. Effectiveness of management strategies for renal artery stenosis: a systematic review. *Ann Intern Med* 2006;145:901–912.
47. Uder M, Humke U. Endovascular therapy of renal artery stenosis: where do we stand today? *Cardiovasc Intervent Radiol* 2005;28:139–147.
48. Sapoval M, Zahringer M, Pattynama P, et al. Low-profile stent system for treatment of atherosclerotic renal artery stenosis: the GREAT trial. *J Vasc Interv Radiol* 2005;16:1195–1202.
49. Zähringer M, Sapoval M, Pattynama PM, et al. Sirolimus-eluting versus bare-metal low-profile stent for renal artery treatment (GREAT Trial): angiographic follow-up after 6 months and clinical outcome up to 2 years. *J Endovasc Ther* 2007;14:460–468.
50. Kiernan TJ, Yan BP, Eisenberg JD, et al. Treatment of renal artery in-stent restenosis with sirolimus-eluting stents. *Vasc Med* 2010;15:3–7.
51. Lee T, Roy-Chaudhury P. Advances and new frontiers in the pathophysiology of venous neointimal hyperplasia and dialysis access stenosis. *Adv Chronic Kidney Dis* 2009;16:329–338.
52. Roy-Chaudhury P, Kelly BS, Melhem M. Vascular access in hemodialysis: issues, management, and emerging concepts. *Cardiol Clin* 2005;23:249–273.
53. Tay K, Irani F, Lo R, et al. Prospective randomised controlled trial comparing drug eluting stent (DES) versus percutaneous transluminal angioplasty (PTA) for the treatment of hemodialysis arterio-venous graft (AVG) stenoses: preliminary report. *J Vasc Interv Radiol* 2011;22:S6.
54. Katsanos K, Karnabatidis D, Kitrou P, et al. Paclitaxel-coated balloon angioplasty vs. plain balloon dilation for the treatment of failing dialysis access: 6-month interim results from a prospective randomized controlled trial. *J Endovasc Ther* 2012;19:263–272.
55. de Jager SC, Kuiper J. Vaccination strategies in atherosclerosis. *Thromb Haemost* 2011;106:796–803.

Note: Page numbers followed by *f* indicate figures; those followed by *t* indicate tables.

plaque modulation techniques, 546
  rotational aspiration atherectomy,
    546, 547*f*
intraprocedural techniques, 559–570
outcomes/prognosis, 571
patients with infrapopliteal disease,
    544–545, 545*f*
planning interventional procedure,
    558–559, 559*f*
relative therapeutic effectiveness
    compared to medical and surgical
    management, 572
surgical/endovascular
    revascularization, 545*f*
technical and device considerations
    access routes selection, 551, 551*f*
    aspiration devices, 555, 555*f*, 556*f*
    balloon catheters, 552–553
    crossing devices, 551–552
    debulking devices, 553
    drug-coated balloons, 553–555,
      554–555*f*
    guide wires, 551, 552*f*
    reentry devices, 552
    stents, 553, 553*f*, 554*f*
    support catheter, 551
below the knee (BTK) lesions and, 544
treatment selection strategies
    for complex lesions, 556, 557*f*
    for embolic lesions, 556, 558, 558*f*, 559*f*
    for focal lesion, 555–556, 557*f*
Critical limb-threatening ischemia, 575, 576
Critical temperature, 29
CRLM. *See* Colorectal liver metastases
Cross-sectional imaging
    for iliac vein compression syndrome, 1089
    ischemic anatomy, 761
Crosser device, 551, 552
    for chronic total occlusions, 551
CRP. *See* C-reactive protein
Crush-clamp/finger-fracture technique, 104
Cryoablation
    and cementoplasty, 216*f*
    for HCC, 64
    hydrodisplacement performed during, of
      paraspinal esophageal carcinoma
      metastasis, 213*f*
    of large painful HCC bone metastasis, 215*f*
    of lung cancer, 201–202
    outcomes/results, 216
    principles of, 181*f*
    for renal cell carcinoma, 179–180, 181*f*
    sterile glove for skin protection during, 213*f*
    therapy, 146
    in treatment of tumors, 213–214
Cryoplasty, 505, 535
Cryoprecipitate, 1145
Cryoprobes, 201
"Cryoshock," 64
Cryosurgery, immunologic implications
    of, 184
Cryotherapy, thermal ablations of liver
    metastases with, 117
Crystalloid
    infusion, 512
    isotonic, 505
CSS. *See* Churg-Strauss syndrome

CT. *See* Computed tomography
CT-US fusion, 41
CTA. *See* Computed tomography
    angiography
cTAG endoprosthesis, 666*t*, 670, 670*f*
CTCAE. *See* Common Terminology Criteria
    for Adverse Events
CTNNB1, 65
CTOs. *See* Chronic total occlusions
CTZ. *See* Chemoreceptor trigger zone
CUPI. *See* Chinese University Prognostic
    Index (CUPI) staging system
Curved planar reconstruction (CPR), 648
CUSA. *See* Cavitron ultrasound aspirator
Cushing syndrome, 190
Cut-down approach, of cephalic vein, 227
Cutaneous involvement, in Takayasu
    arteritis, 598
Cutaneous leukocytoclastic vasculitis, 603, 603*f*
Cutaneous polyarteritis nodosa (cPAN), 601
Cutting angioplasty balloons, 1050
Cutting balloon angioplasty (CBA), 505, 507
Cutting balloon catheter, 546, 552–553
Cutting Edge Trial, 1042–1043
Cutting/scoring balloon angioplasty, 535
CVA. *See* Cerebrovascular accidents
CVD. *See* Chronic venous disease
CVI. *See* Chronic venous insufficiency
CVX-300 Excimer laser, 583
Cyanoacrylate glue, 224, 698, 706
Cyanoacrylates, 717
Cyanosis, 907
Cyclists, 632
Cyclooxygenase-1 (COX-1), 1146
Cyclophosphamide
    for ANCA-associated vasculitis, 604
    for polyarteritis nodosa, 6020
    for Takayasu arteritis, 600
Cyclophosphamide, epirubicin, and
    vincristine (CEV), 196
CYP2C19, 437
CYP2C9, 1148
CYP3A4, 437
Cypher select stent, 548
Cypher stent, 1168
Cystathionine-beta-synthase (CBS), 632
Cystic adventitial disease, 405, 633, 633–634*f*
Cystic artery, 123
Cystic hygromas. *See* Lymphatic
    malformations
Cystic medial necrosis, 818
Cystostomy tube, 845
Cytarabine, 11
Cytochrome P450 3A4, 89
Cytochrome p450 gene, 1148
Cytokinesis, 7
Cytoplasmic ANCA (c-ANCA), 603
Cytoreductive nephrectomy, 178–179, 182
Cytotoxic agents
    alkylating agents, 8
    antimetabolites, 10–11
    antimicrotubule agents, 11–12
    other agents, 12
    platinum salts, 8, 10
    topoisomerase inhibitors, 11
Cytotoxic chemotherapy, in neuroendocrine
    tumors, 135

D
D-dimer test, 999
D2 blockers, 233*t*
D5W (5% dextrose in water), 37
Dabigatran, 1093, 1151
Dacarbazine, 135
Dacron, 537
    grafts, 727, 738, 910
Daflon, 288
Dalteparin, 1150
Dapsone, 600
Daunorubicin, 16
DaVinci robot, for partial nephrectomies, 179
DC Bead microspheres, 17, 159
DCE-MRA. *See* Dynamic contrastenhanced
    MRA
DCs. *See* Dendritic cells
DDAVP. *See* Desmopressin
DEB. *See* Drug-eluting beads
DEB-TACE. *See* Chemoembolization with
    drug-eluting beads
DeBakey and Stanford classifications, 748,
    750*f*, 762
DEBATE-BTK trial, 1174
DEBIRI. *See* Drug-eluting bead, irinotecan
Debulking devices, 553
    atherectomy and, 589
Deep venous insufficiency, 1115
Deep venous reflux, 1117, 1118
Deep venous thrombosis (DVT), 93, 981, 1115
    acute, 973*t*
        catheter-directed treatment of, 1162,
          1162*t*
        iliofemoral, 983, 984*t*, 1162
    chronic, 973*t*
    distal, 972, 972*t*
    endovascular treatment options, 983
        catheter-directed intrathrombus
          thrombolysis (CDT) infusions,
          983–985, 987
        endovascular thrombolysis
          procedures, 987
        percutaneous mechanical
          thrombectomy (PMT), 985
        pharmacomechanical catheter-
          directed thrombolysis (PCDT),
          985, 986*f*, 987
        therapeutic effectiveness, 987
    in endovenous laser therapy and
        radiofrequency ablation, 1137
    femoropopliteal, 983
    lower extremity
        classification based on, 972
        imaging evaluation, 972, 973*f*,
          973–974, 973*t*
        incidence of, 971–972
        indications for intervention, 978
        noninvasive diagnostic imaging
          techniques, 974–977
        post-thrombotic syndrome and,
          981–982
        prophylaxis and treatment, 227–228
        proximal, 972, 972*t*
        renal vein thrombosis and, 957
        systemic thrombolytic therapy, 982
        anatomic and clinical considerations,
          982–983